LATEST APPROVED METHODS OF TREATMENT
FOR THE PRACTICING PHYSICIAN

Edited by
# ROBERT E. RAKEL, M.D.

Chairman, Department of Family Medicine
Associate Dean for Academic and Clinical Affairs
Baylor College of Medicine, Houston, Texas

**W.B. SAUNDERS COMPANY**
**Harcourt Brace Jovanovich, Inc.**
Philadelphia
London   Toronto   Montreal   Sydney   Tokyo

Conn's **Current Therapy 1991**

**W. B. SAUNDERS COMPANY**
Harcourt Brace Jovanovich, Inc.

The Curtis Center
Independence Square West
Philadelphia, PA 19106

**Library of Congress Cataloging-in-Publication Data**

Current therapy; latest approved methods of treatment for the practicing physician. 1949–

v. 28 cm. annual.

Editors: 1949–      H. F. Conn and others.

  1. Therapeutics.      2. Therapeutics, Surgical.
  3. Medicine—Practice.      I. Conn, Howard Franklin,
  1908–1982 ed.

RM101.C87      616.058      49–8328 rev*

ISBN 0–7216–2583–5

*Editor:*  John Dyson
*Developmental Editor:*  David Kilmer
*Designer:*  Ellen Bodner
*Production Manager:*  Peter Faber
*Manuscript Editors:*  Tom Stringer, Sally Burke, and Terry Russell
*Illustration Coordinator:*  Peg Shaw
*Indexer:*  Dennis Dolan
*Cover Designer:*  Ellen Bodner

Conn's Current Therapy 1991                    ISBN 0–7216–2583–5

# Contributors

**GARRETT ADAMS, M.D., M.P.H.**

Associate Professor of Pediatrics, Chief, Division of Infectious Diseases, University of Louisville; Chief, Division of Infectious Diseases and Hospital Epidemiologist, Kosair Children's Hospital, Louisville, Kentucky
*Mumps*

**KEDAR KARIM ADOUR, M.D.**

Director of Research, Department of Otolaryngology-Head and Neck Surgery; Chairman, Cranial Nerve Research Clinic, Kaiser Permanente Medical Center, Oakland, California
*Acute Facial Paralysis*

**JOAQUIN S. ALDRETE, M.D.**

Professor of Surgery, Vice Chairman, Department of Surgery, University of Alabama at Birmingham; Attending Surgeon, University of Alabama Hospital and Veterans Administration Hospital, Birmingham, Alabama
*Acute Pancreatitis*

**RICHARD M. ALLMAN, M.D.**

Assistant Professor of Medicine, University of Alabama at Birmingham; University of Alabama Hospital and Birmingham Veterans Administration Medical Center, Birmingham, Alabama
*Pressure Ulcers*

**DAVID R. ANDERSON, M.D.**

Research Fellow of the Canadian Heart and Stroke Foundation, McMaster University, Hamilton, Ontario, Canada
*Pulmonary Embolism*

**JEFFREY L. ANDERSON, M.D.**

Professor of Medicine (Cardiology), University of Utah Medical School; Chief, Division of Cardiology, Latter Day Saints Hospital, Salt Lake City, Utah
*Premature Beats*

**KARL E. ANDERSON, M.D.**

Professor, University of Texas Medical Branch; Associate Member of Medical Staff, University of Texas Medical Branch, Galveston, Texas
*The Porphyrias*

**RODNEY U. ANDERSON, M.D.**

Professor of Surgery (Urology), Stanford University School of Medicine; Staff, Stanford University Hospital, Stanford, California; Staff, Santa Clara Valley Medical Center, San Jose, California
*Prostatitis*

**STEVEN W. ANDRESEN, D.O.**

The Cleveland Clinic Foundation, Cleveland, Ohio
*Disseminated Intravascular Coagulation; Thrombotic Thrombocytopenic Purpura*

**JACK ANSELL, M.D.**

Professor of Medicine and Pathology, University of Massachusetts Medical School; Attending Hematologist, University of Massachusetts Hospital, Worcester, Massachusetts
*Autoimmune Hemolytic Anemia*

**CAROLA A. S. ARNDT, M.D.**

Assistant Professor of Pediatrics, Mayo Medical School; Senior Associate Consultant, Pediatric Hematology and Oncology, Mayo Clinic and Foundation, Rochester, Minnesota
*Acute Leukemia in Childhood*

**ROBERT L. ATMAR, M.D.**

Fellow, Infectious Diseases, Department of Medicine, Baylor College of Medicine; Fellow, Infectious Diseases, Baylor College of Medicine Affiliated Hospitals, Houston, Texas
*Bacteremia*

**GEORGE F. ATWEH, M.D.**

Assistant Professor of Medicine, State University of New York Health Science Center at Brooklyn; Staff Physician, VA Medical Center, Brooklyn, New York
*Thalassemia*

**LAWRENCE D. BAILEY, JR., M.D.**

Fellow, University of Virginia, Charlottesville, Virginia
*Dysphagia and Esophageal Obstruction*

**WILLIAM F. BALISTRERI, M.D.**

Dorothy M. M. Kersten Professor of Pediatrics, University of Cincinnati Medical Center; Director, Division of Pediatric Gastroenterology and Nutrition and Division of Gastroenterology and Nutrition, Children's Hospital Medical Center, Cincinnati, Ohio
*Normal Infant Feeding*

**MARK BALLOW, M.D.**

Professor of Pediatrics, Department of Pediatrics, Division of Allergy and Clinical Immunology, State University of New York at Buffalo School of Medicine and Biomedical Sciences; Chief, Division of Allergy and Immunology, Children's Hospital, Buffalo, New York
*Anaphylaxis and Serum Sickness*

**SONIA BALSAN, M.D.**

Director of Research, Université René Descartes; Consultant, Hôpital des Enfants-Malades, Paris, France
*Rickets and Osteomalacia*

**DAVID H. BARCH, M.D.**

Assistant Professor of Medicine, University of Illinois at Chicago; Staff Physician, Westside VA Medical Center, Chicago, Illinois
*Constipation*

## RANDALL BARNES, M.D.

Assistant Professor, University of Chicago, Attending Physician, Chicago Lying-in Hospital, Chicago, Illinois
*Amenorrhea*

## MICHÉLE BARRY, M.D., D.T.M.

Associate Professor of Medicine, Yale University School of Medicine; Attending Physician, Yale–New Haven Hospital; Co-Director, Tropical Medicine and International Traveler's Clinic, New Haven, Connecticut
*Intestinal Parasites*

## CHARLES P. BARSANO, M.D., PH.D.

Associate Professor of Medicine, Division of Endocrinology, University of Health Sciences/The Chicago Medical School; Staff Physician, Medical Service, North Chicago VA Medical Center, North Chicago, Illinois
*Hypothyroidism*

## URIEL S. BARZEL, M.D.

Professor of Medicine, Albert Einstein College of Medicine; Attending Physician in Endocrinology and Metabolism, Montefiore Medical Center, Bronx, New York
*Osteoporosis*

## MARK L. BASSETT, M.D.

Visiting Fellow, Australian National University; Gastroenterologist, Royal Canberra Hospital, Canberra, Australia
*Hemochromatosis*

## CAROL A. BELL, M.D.

Clinical Professor of Pathology, University of Southern California; Clinical Professor of Pathology, University of California, Irvine; Director of Clinical Laboratories, Brotman Medical Center, Culver City, California
*Adverse Effects of Blood Transfusion*

## RICHARD G. BENNETT, M.D.

Clinical Professor of Medicine (Dermatology), University of Southern California School of Medicine, Los Angeles; Attending Physician, St. John's Hospital and Health Center, Santa Monica Hospital and Medical Center, Santa Monica; Los Angeles County–University of Southern California Medical Center, Los Angeles, California
*Nevi and Melanomas*

## MICHAEL L. BENNISH, M.D.

Assistant Professor, Departments of Pediatrics and Medicine, Tufts University School of Medicine; Assistant Pediatrician, Boston Floating Hospital for Children; Staff, New England Medical Center, Boston, Massachusetts; International Research Associate, International Centre for Diarrhoeal Disease Research, Bangladesh (ICDDR), Dhaka, Bangladesh
*Cholera*

## FRANK J. BIA, M.D., M.P.H.

Associate Professor of Medicine and Laboratory Medicine, Yale University School of Medicine; Attending Physician, Yale–New Haven Hospital; Co-Director, Tropical Medicine and International Traveler's Clinic, New Haven, Connecticut
*Intestinal Parasites*

## RICHARD P. BILLINGHAM, M.D.

Clinical Assistant Professor, University of Washington; Active Staff, Swedish Hospital and Northwest Hospital, Seattle, Washington
*Hemorrhoids, Anal Fissure, and Anorectal Abscess and Fistula*

## PHYLLIS R. BISHOP, M.D.

Resident, University of Mississippi Medical Center; Pediatric Resident, University of Mississippi Medical Center, Jackson, Mississippi
*Measles (Rubeola)*

## BRUCE R. BISTRIAN, M.D., PH.D.

Associate Professor of Medicine, Harvard Medical School; Chief, Section of Nutrition, New England Deaconess Hospital, Boston, Massachusetts
*Total Parenteral Nutrition in Adults*

## GEORGE L. BLACKBURN, M.D., PH.D.

Associate Professor of Surgery, Harvard Medical School; Surgeon, New England Deaconess Hospital; Consulting Surgeon, Cambridge Hospital, Falmouth Hospital, Children's Hospital, New England Baptist Hospital, and Faulkner Hospital, Boston, Massachusetts
*Obesity*

## JERRY G. BLAIVAS, M.D.

Professor and Vice-Chairman, Department of Urology, College of Physicians and Surgeons, Columbia University, New York, New York
*Benign Prostatic Hypertrophy*

## JANICE F. BLAZINA, M.D.

Assistant Professor, Department of Pathology, College of Medicine, The Ohio State University; Attending Staff, The Ohio State University Hospitals, Columbus, Ohio; Consulting Staff, Memorial Hospital of Union County, Marysville, Ohio
*Therapeutic Use of Blood Components*

## ERICH (E.) PETER BOSCH, M.D.

Professor, Department of Neurology, University of Iowa College of Medicine; Attending Neurologist, University of Iowa Hospitals and Clinics and Veterans Administration Medical Center, Iowa City, Iowa
*Peripheral Neuropathies*

## THOMAS BRANDT, M.D.

Professor of Neurology and Chairman, University of Munich; Director of Department of Neurology, Klinikum Grosshadern, University of Munich, Germany
*Episodic Vertigo*

## DAVID C. BREWSTER, M.D.

Associate Clinical Professor of Surgery, Harvard Medical School; Visiting Surgeon, Massachusetts General Hospital, Boston, Massachusetts
*Peripheral Arterial Disease*

## BRUCE BROECKER, M.D.

Clinical Associate Professor of Surgery, Emory University School of Medicine; Staff, Henrietta Egleston Hospital for Children and Scottish Rite Children's Hospital, Atlanta, Georgia
*Urinary Tract Infections in Female Children*

## KENNETH BROMBERG, M.D.

Assistant Professor of Pediatrics, SUNY Health Science Center at Brooklyn; Attending, Pediatrics and Infectious Diseases, Kings County Hospital, Brooklyn, New York
*Pertussis (Whooping Cough)*

## RICHARD B. BROWN, M.D.

Associate Professor of Medicine, Tufts University School of Medicine, Boston, Massachusetts; Chief, Infectious Disease

Division, Baystate Medical Center, Springfield, Massachusetts
*Streptococcal Pharyngitis*

## RONALD M. BUKOWSKI, M.D.

The Cleveland Clinic Foundation, Cleveland, Ohio
*Disseminated Intravascular Coagulation; Thrombotic Thrombocytopenic Purpura*

## JACK S. BURKS, M.D.

Executive Director, Rocky Mountain Multiple Sclerosis Center, Swedish Medical Center, Englewood, California
*Viral Meningoencephalitis*

## ROBERT A. BURNS, D.D.S., M.S.

Associate Professor, Departments of Dentistry and Pathology, Medical College of Ohio; Medical Staff, Medical College Hospital, Division of Dentistry; Chief, Section of Oral Pathology, Toledo, Ohio
*Diseases of the Mouth*

## WILLIAM W. BUSSE, M.D.

Professor of Medicine, University of Wisconsin Medical School; Staff, University of Wisconsin Hospital, Madison, Wisconsin
*Allergic Reactions to Insect Stings*

## JAMES H. BUTT, M.D.

Associate Professor of Medicine, University of Missouri–Columbia; GI Section Chief, Harry S Truman Memorial Veterans Hospital; Program Director, Division of Gastroenterology, University of Missouri–Columbia, Columbia, Missouri
*Ulcerative Colitis*

## RIAD CACHECHO, M.D.

Assistant Professor of Surgery, Boston University School of Medicine; Staff Surgeon, Associate Director, Surgical Intensive Care Unit at Boston University Hospital and Boston City Hospital, Boston, Massachusetts
*Thrombophlebitis in Obstetrics and Gynecology*

## BLAKE CADY, M.D.

Associate Professor of Surgery, Harvard Medical School; Chief of Surgical Oncology, New England Deaconess Hospital, Boston, Massachusetts
*Thyroid Cancer*

## JOANNA M. CAIN, M.D.

Associate Professor, University of Washington; Attending Physician, University of Washington Medical Center, Seattle, Washington
*Cancer of the Uterine Cervix*

## JEFFREY P. CALLEN, M.D.

Professor and Chief, Division of Dermatology, University of Louisville School of Medicine, Louisville, Kentucky
*Cutaneous Vasculitis*

## CAROL CAMFIELD, M.D.

Associate Professor of Pediatrics, Dalhousie Medical School, Dalhousie University; Izaak Walton Killam Hospital for Children, Halifax, Nova Scotia, Canada
*Epilepsy in Infants and Children*

## PETER CAMFIELD, M.D.

Professor of Pediatric Neurology, Dalhousie Medical School, Dalhousie University; Izaak Walton Killam Hospital for Children, Halifax, Nova Scotia, Canada
*Epilepsy in Infants and Children*

## CHARLES CAMISA, M.D.

Head, Section of Clinical Dermatology, Director, Dermatology Residency Program, Cleveland Clinic Foundation, Cleveland, Ohio
*Fungal Diseases of the Skin*

## J. ROBERT CANTEY, M.D.

Professor of Medicine, Acting Director, Division of Infectious Diseases, Medical University of South Carolina; Chief, Infectious Diseases, VA Medical Center; Consultant and Attending, Medical University Hospital and Charleston Memorial Hospital, Charleston, South Carolina
*Salmonellosis*

## THOMAS R. CARACCIO, Pharm.D., D.A.B.A.T.

Assistant Professor of Emergency Medicine at State University of New York at Stony Brook; Visiting Assistant Professor of Pharmacology and Toxicology at New York College of Osteopathic Medicine, Old Westbury, New York; Assistant Professor of Clinical Pharmacy, St. John's University College of Pharmacy, Jamaica, New York; Assistant Director, Long Island Regional Poison Control Center, Nassau County Medical Center, East Meadow, New York
*Acute Poisonings*

## SUSAN A. CARLIN, M.D.

Senior Instructor, Department of Pediatrics, Case Western Reserve University; Metro Health Medical Center (Primary Appointment); Rainbow Babies' and Children's Hospital, Cleveland, Ohio
*Otitis Media*

## ROBERT G. CARNEY, Jr., M.D.

Clinical Instructor, University of Illinois College of Medicine, Urbana–Champaign, Illinois
*Fixed Erythemas*

## VALERIAN A. CATANZARITE, M.D., Ph.D.

Formerly Assistant Professor of Obstetrics and Gynecology, Maternal-Fetal Medicine Division, Department of Obstetrics and Gynecology, University of Arkansas for Medical Sciences, Little Rock, Arkansas; Associate Director, Maternal-Fetal Medicine, Sharp Memorial Hospital, San Diego, California
*Antepartum Care*

## THOMAS R. CATE, M.D.

Professor of Medicine and Microbiology-Immunology, Baylor College of Medicine; Staff, Harris County Hospital District and The Methodist Hospital, Houston, Texas
*Management of HIV Infection*

## ROBERTO CEDILLO-RIVERA, M.D., Ms.C.

Assistant Professor in Pediatrics, Faculty of Medicine, Universidad Nacional Autonoma de Mexico; Associate Researcher, Clinical Research Unit of Infectious and Parasitic Diseases, Hospital de Pediatria, Centro Medico Nacional, Instituto Mexicano del Seguro Social, Mexico City, Mexico
*Typhoid Fever*

## RICHARD CHAMPLIN, M.D.

Professor of Medicine, University of Texas–M. D. Anderson Cancer Center; Staff, M. D. Anderson Cancer Center, Houston, Texas
*Aplastic Anemia*

**NICHOLAS P. CHRISTY, M.D.**

Writer in Residence and Senior Lecturer in Medicine, Columbia University College of Physicians and Surgeons; Attending Physician in Medicine, Presbyterian Hospital, New York, New York
*Hyperprolactinemia*

**GEORGE P. CHROUSOS, M.D.**

Chief, Pediatric Endocrinology Section, National Institute of Child Health and Human Development, Bethesda, Maryland
*Cushing's Syndrome*

**ALAN HOWARD COHEN, M.D.**

Associate Clinical Professor, Department of Medicine, University of California at San Diego; Staff Rheumatologist, Kaiser Permanante, San Diego; Attending Physician, VA Medical Center, La Jolla; Attending Physician, University Hospital, San Diego; Consultant, Balboa Naval Hospital, San Diego, California
*Polymyalgia Rheumatica and Giant Cell Arteritis*

**CAROL COLA, M.D.**

Assistant Professor of Medicine, University of Massachusetts Medical School; Staff Hematologist/Oncologist, University of Massachusetts Medical Center, Worcester, Massachusetts
*Autoimmune Hemolytic Anemia*

**REX B. CONN, M.D.**

Professor and Vice Chairman, Department of Pathology, Jefferson Medical College of Thomas Jefferson University; Active Staff, Thomas Jefferson University Hospital, Philadelphia, Pennsylvania
*Appendices and Index: Laboratory Values of Clinical Importance*

**KEVIN D. COOPER, M.D.**

Associate Professor and Director, Immunodermatology Unit, Department of Dermatology, University of Michigan Medical School; Staff, University of Michigan Hospitals and Ann Arbor Veterans Administration Hospital, Ann Arbor, Michigan
*Skin Diseases of Pregnancy*

**JAMES R. COUCH, M.D., Ph.D.**

Professor and Chairman, Division of Neurology, Department of Medicine, Southern Illinois University School of Medicine; Staff, Memorial Medical Center; Director of EEG Laboratory, Neurology, Neurorehabilitation, St. John Hospital, Springfield, Illinois; Consultant in Neurology, Marion Veterans Administration Hospital, Marion, Illinois
*Headache*

**JOHN H. CRANDON, M.D.**

Associate Professor of Surgery Emeritus, Tufts University Medical School, Boston, Massachusetts
*Scurvy and Vitamin C Deficiency*

**E. DAVID CRAWFORD, M.D.**

Chairman, Division of Urology, University of Colorado; Staff, University Hospital, Veterans Administration Medical Center, Denver, Colorado
*Malignant Tumors of the Genitourinary System*

**NANCY P. CUMMINGS, M.D.**

Assistant Clinical Professor, Stanford University; Staff, Stanford University Hospital, Menlo Park, California
*Asthma in Children*

**GREGORY D. CURFMAN, M.D.**

Assistant Professor of Medicine, Harvard Medical School; Assistant in Medicine, Massachusetts General Hospital, Boston, Massachusetts
*Acute Myocardial Infarction*

**JAMES J. CURRAN, M.D.**

Associate Professor of Clinical Medicine, University of Chicago Pritzker School of Medicine; Staff, University of Chicago Hospital, Chicago, Illinois; Consultant Rheumatologist, Oak Forest Hospital, Oak Forest, Illinois; Consultant Rheumatologist, St. Francis Hospital, Blue Island, Illinois; Consultant Rheumatologist, Illinois Valley Community Hospital, Peru, Illinois; Consultant Rheumatologist, South Chicago Community Hospital and Hyde Park Hospital, Chicago, Illinois
*Fibrositis, Bursitis, and Tendinitis*

**JAMIE DANANBERG, M.D.**

Lecturer in Internal Medicine, University of Michigan, Staff, University of Michigan Hospitals, VA Medical Center, Ann Arbor, Michigan
*Adrenocortical Insufficiency*

**GILBERT H. DANIELS, M.D.**

Associate Professor of Medicine, Harvard Medical School; Physician, Massachusetts General Hospital; Co-Director, Thyroid Clinic, Massachusetts General Hospital, Boston, Massachusetts
*Goiter*

**DAVID R. DANTZKER, M.D.**

Professor of Medicine, Albert Einstein College of Medicine, Bronx, New York; Chairman of Medicine, Long Island Jewish Medical Center, New Hyde Park, New York
*Chronic Obstructive Pulmonary Disease*

**SCOTT F. DAVIES, M.D.**

Associate Professor, University of Minnesota Medical School; Director, Pulmonary Medicine Division, Department of Internal Medicine, Hennepin County Medical Center, Minneapolis, Minnesota
*Histoplasmosis; Bacterial Pneumonia*

**CHARLES DAVIS, M.D.**

Staff, Infectious Disease Service, Brooke Army Medical Center and Wilford Hall Air Force Medical Center, Washington, D.C.
*Bacterial Meningitis*

**NATHAN C. DEAN, M.D.**

Clinical Assistant Professor of Medicine, University of Utah School of Medicine; Staff Department of Medicine, LDS Hospital, Salt Lake City, Utah
*Acute Respiratory Failure*

**G. WILLIAM DEC, M.D.**

Assistant Professor of Medicine, Harvard Medical School; Medical Director, Cardiac Transplantation Program, Massachusetts General Hospital; Director, Medical Intensive Care Unit, Massachusetts General Hospital; Assistant Physician (Medicine), Massachusetts General Hospital, Boston, Massachusetts
*Acute Myocardial Infarction*

**GAIL J. DEMMLER, M.D.**

Assistant Professor, Baylor College of Medicine; Staff, Texas Children's Hospital (Active), The Methodist Hospital (Courtesy), St. Luke's Episcopal Hospital (Provisional), Harris

County Hospital District (Consulting), Woman's Hospital of Texas (Consulting), Houston, Texas
*Rubella*

## RICHARD W. DEMMLER, M.D.

Assistant Professor of Family Medicine, Assistant Professor of Community Medicine, Baylor College of Medicine; Staff, St. Luke's Episcopal Hospital, Texas Children's Hospital, and The Methodist Hospital, Houston, Texas
*Urinary Incontinence*

## SUSAN E. DENSON, M.D.

Professor of Pediatrics and Acting Director, Division of Neonatal-Perinatal Medicine, University of Texas Medical School at Houston; Director, Newborn Services, Hermann Hospital; Attending Staff, Lyndon Baines Johnson General Hospital, Houston, Texas
*Resuscitation of the Newborn*

## RICHARD D. DeSHAZO, M.D.

Professor of Medicine and Pediatrics, and Chairman, Department of Internal Medicine, University of South Alabama College of Medicine, Staff, University of South Alabama Hospitals, Mobile, Alabama
*Anaphylaxis and Serum Sickness*

## JEAN DESLAURIERS, M.D.

Associate Professor of Surgery, Laval University; Head, Division of Thoracic Surgery, Centre de Pneumologie de Laval, Hôpital Laval, Sainte-Foy, Quebec, Canada
*Atelectasis*

## DOUGLAS S. DIEKEMA, M.D.

Fellow in Pediatric Emergency Medicine, University of Washington School of Medicine, and Children's Hospital and Medical Center, Seattle, Washington
*Disturbances due to Heat*

## ROBERT P. DILLARD, M.D.

Fellow in Pediatric Gastroenterology, Children's Hospital Medical Center, Cincinnati, Ohio; Associate Professor of Pediatrics, University of Kentucky Medical Center, Lexington, Kentucky
*Normal Infant Feeding*

## CHÉRIE M. DITRE, M.D.

Department of Dermatology, School of Medicine, University of Michigan Medical Center; University of Michigan Hospitals, Ann Arbor, Michigan
*Skin Diseases of Pregnancy*

## W. PAUL DMOWSKI, M.D., PH.D.

Professor, Rush Medical College of Rush University; Senior Attending Physician, Rush-Presbyterian-St. Luke's Medical Center; Attending Physician, Grant Hospital, Chicago, Illinois
*Endometriosis*

## NOUHA DOMLOGE-HULTSCH, M.D.

Research Associate, Department of Dermatology, Uniformed Services University of the Health Sciences, Bethesda, Maryland
*Bullous Diseases*

## WILLIAM DROEGEMUELLER, M.D.

Robert A. Ross Distinguished Professor and Chairman, Department of Obstetrics and Gynecology, University of North Carolina School of Medicine, Chapel Hill, North Carolina
*Pelvic Inflammatory Disease*

## JOHN D. EDWARDS, M.D.

Vascular Surgery Clinical and Research Fellow, Harvard Medical School and Massachusetts General Hospital, Boston, Massachusetts
*Peripheral Arterial Disease*

## MICHAEL H. ELLMAN, M.D.

Associate Professor of Clinical Medicine, University of Illinois; Director, Division of Rheumatology, Michael Reese Hospital and Medical Center, Chicago, Illinois
*Rheumatoid Arthritis*

## CRAIG A. ELMETS, M.D.

Associate Professor of Dermatology and General Medical Sciences (Oncology), Case Western Reserve University; Attending Physician, University Hospitals of Cleveland; Veterans Administration Medical Center; Cleveland, Ohio
*Sunburn and Photosensitivity*

## ROBERT J. ELSEN, M.D.

Clinical Fellow in Hyperalimentation, New England Deaconess Hospital, Boston, Massachusetts
*Total Parenteral Nutrition in Adults*

## ALLEN ERENBERG, M.D.

Professor, Department of Pediatrics, University of Kansas; Chairman, Department of Pediatrics, Kansas University Children's Center, University of Kansas Medical Center, Kansas City, Kansas
*Care of At-Risk Neonates*

## CALVIN B. ERNST, M.D.

Clinical Professor of Surgery, University of Michigan Medical School, Ann Arbor, Michigan; Head, Division of Vascular Surgery, Henry Ford Hospital, Detroit, Michigan
*Acquired Diseases of the Aorta*

## JOAN ESPLIN, M.D.

Fellow in Hematology and Oncology, University of Southern California School of Medicine; University of Southern California at Los Angeles Medical Center, Los Angeles, California
*Non-Hodgkin's Lymphomas*

## THOMAS G. EVANS, M.D.

Assistant Professor of Medicine, Division of Infectious Diseases, University of Utah School of Medicine, Salt Lake City, Utah
*Toxoplasmosis*

## GUODONG FANG, M.D.

Associate Professor of Medicine, Peking Union Medical College, Beijing, China
*Legionellosis (Legionnaires' Disease and Pontiac Fever)*

## SEBASTIAN FARO, M.D., PH.D.

Professor, Baylor College of Medicine; Vice-Chairman, Department of Obstetrics and Gynecology, and Director, Section of Infectious Diseases, Baylor College of Medicine; Staff, St. Luke's Episcopal Hospital, The Methodist Hospital, Ben Taub General Hospital, Houston, Texas
*Chlamydia Trachomatis Infection*

## GEOFFREY C. FARRELL, M.D.

Associate Professor of Medicine, University of Sidney; Head of Gastroenterology Unit, Westmead Hospital, Sydney, Australia
*Acute and Chronic Viral Hepatitis*

**SANDOR FELDMAN, M.D.**

Professor of Pediatrics, University of Mississippi Medical Center; Professor of Pediatrics, Chief, Pediatric Infectious Diseases, Children's Hospital Infection Control Officer, University of Mississippi Medical Center, Jackson, Mississippi
*Measles (Rubeola)*

**GARY G. FERGUSON, M.D.**

Professor of Neurosurgery, University of Western Ontario; Consultant Neurosurgeon, University Hospital, London, Ontario, Canada
*Trigeminal Neuralgia*

**KENNETH A. FOON, M.D.**

Professor of Medicine, State University of New York at Buffalo; Chief, Division of Clinical Immunology, Roswell Park Cancer Institute, Buffalo, New York
*The Chronic Leukemias*

**PIERRE FORGACS, M.D.**

Clinical Instructor, Harvard Medical School, Boston, Massachusetts; Staff, Section of Infectious Diseases, Lahey Clinic Medical Center, Burlington, Massachusetts
*Brucellosis*

**R. ARMOUR FORSE, M.D., Ph.D.**

Assistant Professor of Surgery, Harvard Medical School; Attending Surgeon, New England Deaconess Hospital, Boston, Massachusetts
*Obesity*

**JOSEPH F. FOWLER, Jr., M.D.**

Assistant Professor, Division of Dermatology, University of Louisville School of Medicine; Staff, Humana Hospital, University of Louisville; Chief of Dermatology, Veterans Administration Medical Center, Louisville, Kentucky
*Contact Dermatitis*

**GARY S. FRANCIS, M.D.**

Professor of Medicine, University of Minnesota; Director, Acute Cardiac Care, University of Minnesota Hospital, Minneapolis, Minnesota
*Congestive Heart Failure*

**HARRIS A. FRANKEL, M.D.**

Clinical Instructor, University of Nebraska Medical Center; Staff, Nebraska Methodist Hospital, Clarkson Memorial Hospital, and Immanuel Medical Center, Omaha, Nebraska
*Primary Intracerebral Hemorrhage*

**ANDREW J. FRIEDMAN, M.D.**

Assistant Professor, Harvard Medical School; Director, In Vitro Fertilization Program, Brigham and Women's Hospital, Boston, Massachusetts
*Leiomyomas of the Uterus*

**STEVEN M. FRUCHTMAN, M.D.**

Assistant Professor of Medicine, Mount Sinai School of Medicine; Director, Bone Marrow Transplantation and Executive Officer, Polycythemia Vera Study Group, The Mount Sinai Hospital, New York, New York
*Polycythemia Vera*

**WESLEY FURSTE, M.D.**

Clinical Professor of Surgery, Emeritus, Ohio State University; Senior Attending Staff, Department of Surgery, Riverside Methodist Hospitals, Columbus, Ohio
*Anaerobic and Necrotizing Infections, Including Gas Gangrene*

**JANICE LYNN GABRILOVE, M.D.**

Assistant Attending Physician, Memorial Sloan-Kettering Cancer Center; Assistant Member, Sloan-Kettering Institute; Assistant Professor of Medicine, Cornell University Medical College, New York, New York
*Neutropenia*

**ROBERT PETER GALE, M.D., Ph.D.**

Associate Professor of Medicine, UCLA School of Medicine; Staff, UCLA Medical Center, Los Angeles, California
*The Chronic Leukemias*

**GALE GARDNER, M.D.**

Clinical Professor, Department of Otolaryngology, University of Tennessee–Memphis; Staff, Baptist Memorial Hospital, Methodist Hospital, LeBonheur Children's Medical Center, VA Medical Center, Memphis, Tennessee
*Meniere's Disease*

**MARYA GENDZIELEWSKI, M.D.**

Clinical Assistant Professor of Medicine, SUNY Health Science Center of Syracuse; Assistant Attending Physician, University Hospital, Syracuse, New York
*Diabetes Insipidus*

**LAYNE O. GENTRY, M.D.**

Clinical Professor of Medicine, Microbiology and Immunology, Baylor College of Medicine; Chief of Infectious Disease Section, St. Luke's Episcopal Hospital, Houston, Texas
*Osteomyelitis*

**GERALD S. GILCHRIST, M.D.**

Helen C. Levitt Professor and Chairman, Department of Pediatrics, Mayo Medical School; Consultant in Pediatric Hematology and Oncology, Mayo Clinic and Foundation, Rochester, Minnesota
*Acute Leukemia in Childhood*

**ELI GLATSTEIN, M.D.**

Chief, Radiation Oncology Branch, National Cancer Institute; Professor of Radiology, Uniformed Services University of Health Sciences, Bethesda, Maryland
*Hodgkin's Disease: Radiation Therapy*

**W. PAUL GLEZEN, M.D.**

Professor and Head, Preventive Medicine Section, Departments of Microbiology and Immunology, and Pediatrics, Baylor College of Medicine; Associate Pediatrician, Harris County Hospital District, Houston; and Courtesy Staff, Infectious Diseases, Texas Children's Hospital, Houston, Texas
*Viral and Mycoplasmal Pneumonias*

**JEFFREY M. GOLDBERG, M.D.**

Assistant Professor, Division of Reproductive Endocrinology, Department of Obstetrics and Gynecology, Ohio State University Hospitals, Columbus, Ohio
*Dysfunctional Uterine Bleeding*

**MICHAEL P. GOLDEN, M.D.**

Associate Professor of Pediatrics, Indiana University Medical Center; Staff, James Whitcomb Riley Hospital for Children, Indianapolis, Indiana
*Diabetes Mellitus in Children and Adolescents*

**MICHAEL T. GOLDFARB, M.D.**

Lecturer, University of Michigan Medical School; Staff Attending Physician, University Hospital, Ann Arbor, Michigan
*Pruritus*

## FRANZ GOLDSTEIN, M.D.

Professor of Medicine, Jefferson Medical College of Thomas Jefferson University; Senior Staff, Lankenau Hospital, Philadelphia, Pennsylvania
*Diverticula of the Alimentary Tract*

## PHILLIP J. GOLDSTEIN, M.D.

Associate Professor of Obstetrics and Gynecology, Johns Hopkins University; Chief, Obstetrics and Gynecology, Sinai Hospital; Attending Physician, Johns Hopkins Hospital, Baltimore, Maryland
*Vaginal Bleeding in Late Pregnancy*

## MICHAEL S. GORDON, M.D.

Fellow, Medical Oncology/Hematology, Memorial Sloan-Kettering Cancer Center; Instructor, Cornell University Medical College, New York, New York
*Neutropenia*

## DAVID C. GORSULOWSKY, M.D.

Clinical Assistant Professor, University of California San Francisco; Staff Physician, University of California Hospitals and Veterans Administration Medical Center, San Francisco, California
*Papulosquamous Eruptions*

## CARMELO GRAFFAGNINO, M.D.

Resident in Neurology, Department of Clinical Neurological Sciences, The University of Western Ontario, University Hospital, London, Ontario, Canada
*Ischemic Cerebrovascular Disease*

## ROBERT A. GRAOR, M.D.

Staff, Department of Vascular Medicine and Department of Cardiology, The Cleveland Clinic Foundation, Cleveland, Ohio
*Deep Venous Thrombosis of the Lower Extremities*

## DEBORAH L. GRAY, R.N., M.S.N.

Adjunct Clinical Instructor, School of Nursing, Indiana University; Clinical Nurse Specialist, Section of Pediatric Diabetes, James Whitcomb Riley Hospital for Children, Indianapolis, Indiana
*Diabetes Mellitus in Children and Adolescents*

## RALPH G. GREENLEE, Jr., M.D.

Associate Professor, Department of Neurology, University of Texas Southwestern Medical Center; Staff Attending, Zale Lipshy University Hospital and Parkland Memorial Hospital, Dallas, Texas
*Primary Intracerebral Hemorrhage*

## JOSEPH GREENSHER, M.D.

Professor of Clinical Pediatrics, State University of New York at Stony Brook; Medical Director and Associate Chairman, Department of Pediatrics, Winthrop-University Hospital, Mineola; Associate Director, Poison Control Center, Nassau County Medical Center, East Meadow, New York
*Acute Poisonings*

## ROGER J. GREKIN, M.D.

Professor of Internal Medicine, University of Michigan; Chief, Endocrinology Section and Associate Chief of Staff for Research, VA Medical Center, Ann Arbor, Michigan
*Adrenocortical Insufficiency*

## GERALD C. GROGGEL, M.D.

Associate Professor of Medicine, College of Medicine, University of Vermont; Attending in Medicine, Medical Center Hospital of Vermont, Burlington, Vermont
*Glomerular Disorders*

## RONALD L. GROSS, M.D.

Assistant Professor of Ophthalmology, Glaucoma Service, Cullen Eye Institute, Baylor College of Medicine; Privileges at The Methodist Hospital, Ben Taub General Hospital, VA Medical Center, St. Luke's Episcopal Hospital, Texas Children's Hospital, Houston, Texas
*Glaucoma*

## JEFFREY P. GUMPRECHT, M.D.

Fellow in Infectious Disease, Albert Einstein College of Medicine, Bronx, New York
*Rat-Bite Fever*

## KLAUS E. GYR, M.D., M.P.H.

Head, Department of Internal Medicine, Kantonsspital Liestal, University of Basel, Basel, Switzerland
*Acute Infectious Diarrhea*

## VLADIMIR HACHINSKI, M.D., D.Sc.(Med)

Professor of Neurology, Richard and Beryl Ivey Professor and Chairman, Department of Clinical Neurological Sciences, The University of Western Ontario; Chief, Department of Neurological Sciences, University Hospital, London, Ontario, Canada
*Ischemic Cerebrovascular Disease*

## BÉLA B. HACKMAN, M.D.

Assistant Professor of Medicine (Cardiology), University of Tennessee; Attending Physician and Cardiologist, University of Tennessee Medical Center, William F. Bowld Hospital, Regional Medical Center at Memphis, Memphis, Tennessee
*Cardiac Arrest*

## YOON S. HAHN, M.D.

Professor of Neurological Surgery and Pediatrics, Chief of Pediatric Neurosurgery, Stritch School of Medicine, Loyola University of Chicago Medical Center, Maywood; Staff, Children's Memorial Hospital, Northwestern University, Chicago, Illinois
*Acute Head Injuries in Children*

## WILLIAM D. HAIRE, M.D.

Assistant Professor of Medicine, University of Nebraska College of Medicine; Active Staff, University of Nebraska Hospital, Omaha, Nebraska
*Vitamin K Deficiency*

## BRIAN C. HALPERN, M.D.

Director of Sports Medicine New Jersey, Marlboro; Clinical Instructor of Sports Medicine, University of Medicine and Dentistry of New Jersey Robert Wood Johnson Medical School, Piscataway, New Jersey
*Common Sports Injuries*

## C. R. HARMAN, M.D.

Assistant Professor, Department of Obstetrics, Gynecology and Reproductive Sciences, University of Manitoba; Director, Fetal Assessment Unit, Women's Hospital of Health Sciences Centre, Winnipeg, Manitoba, Canada
*Hemolytic Disease of the Fetus and Newborn*

## JOHN T. HARRINGTON, M.D.

Professor of Medicine, Tufts University School of Medicine, Boston, Massachusetts; Chief of Medicine, Newton-Wellesley Hospital, Newton, Massachusetts
*Acute Renal Failure*

## RICHARD L. HARRIS, M.D.

Associate Professor of Clinical Medicine, Department of Medicine, Baylor College of Medicine; Medical Epidemiologist, Chairman of Infection Control, The Methodist Hospital, Houston, Texas
*Bacteremia*

## STEPHEN L. HAUSER, M.D.

Associate Professor of Neurology, Harvard Medical School; Director, Neuroimmunology Unit, Massachusetts General Hospital, Boston, Massachusetts
*Multiple Sclerosis*

## MICHAEL G. HEGEWALD, M.D.

Cardiology Fellow, Oregon Health Sciences University; Cardiology Fellow, University Hospital and Veterans Administration Medical Center, Portland, Oregon
*Infective Endocarditis*

## R. PHILLIP HEINE, M.D.

Research Fellow, Division of Infectious Diseases, Department of Internal Medicine, University of North Carolina at Chapel Hill; Staff, University of North Carolina–North Carolina Memorial Hospital, Chapel Hill, North Carolina
*Pelvic Inflammatory Disease*

## JULIO HERNANDEZ, M.D.

Assistant Clinical Professor (ad honorem), University of Puerto Rico, San Juan, Puerto Rico; Consulting Staff, Chalmette General Hospital, Chalmette, Louisiana; Consulting Staff, Southern Medical Center and Montelepre Hospital, New Orleans, Louisiana; Consulting Staff, Metropolitan Hospital and University Hospital, San Juan, Puerto Rico
*Premalignant Lesions*

## CHRISTIAN HERRMANN, JR., M.D.

Professor Emeritus of Neurology, UCLA School of Medicine; Consultant in Neurology at UCLA Neuropsychiatric Institute and Hospitals and VA Medical Center, Los Angeles, California
*Myasthenia Gravis*

## LEONARD L. HESTON, M.D.

Professor of Psychiatry, University of Washington, Seattle, Washington
*Alzheimer's Disease*

## C. STRATTON HILL, JR., M.D.

Associate Professor of Medicine, Department of Neuro-Oncology, University of Texas M. D. Anderson Cancer Center; Director, Pain Service, M. D. Anderson Hospital, Houston, Texas
*Pain*

## JACK HIRSH, M.D.

Professor of Medicine, Department of Medicine, McMaster University; Director and Internist, Hamilton Civic Hospitals Research Centre, Henderson General Division, Hamilton, Ontario, Canada
*Pulmonary Embolism*

## IRA R. HOROWITZ, M.D.

Assistant Professor, Johns Hopkins University School of Medicine; Staff, Johns Hopkins Hospital, Francis Scott Key Medical Center, Sinai Hospital of Baltimore, Baltimore, Maryland
*Neoplasms of the Vulva*

## JOHN W. HOUSE, M.D.

President, House Ear Institute; Active Staff, The Hospital of the Good Samaritan; Provisional Staff, Huntington Memorial Hospital; Active Staff, St. Vincent Medical Center; Active Staff, Children's Hospital of Los Angeles; Attending Staff, Los Angeles County/USC Medical Center, Los Angeles, California
*Tinnitus*

## LAURENE L. HOWELL, M.D.

Assistant Professor, Department of Otolaryngology, Oregon Health Sciences University; Medical Staff, Oregon Health Sciences University; Consultant, Veterans Administration Hospital, Portland, Oregon
*Hoarseness and Laryngitis*

## MARK A. HUFTEL, M.D.

Postdoctoral Fellow, Allergy/Immunology, University of Wisconsin Medical School, Madison, Wisconsin
*Allergic Reactions to Insect Stings*

## FRANK L. IBER, M.D.

Professor of Medicine, Loyola University, Stritch College of Medicine; Chief of Gastroenterology, Hines VA Hospital; Co-Director, GI Fellow Training Program, Hines/Loyola Hospital, Chicago–Hines, Illinois
*Cirrhosis*

## DANIEL C. IHDE, M.D.

Professor of Medicine, Uniformed Services University of the Health Sciences; Deputy Chief, NCI-Navy Medical Oncology Branch, National Cancer Institute and National Naval Medical Center, Bethesda, Maryland
*Primary Lung Cancer*

## ABDOLLAH IRAVANI, M.D.

Professor of Pediatric Nephrology, University of Florida College of Medicine; Attending Physician, Shands Teaching Hospital; Director of Kidney Clinic and Blood Pressure Clinic, University of Florida Infirmary and Pediatric Renal Laboratory, University of Florida, Gainesville, Florida
*Bacterial Infections of the Urinary Tract in Women*

## ROBERT R. JACOBSON, M.D., PH.D.

Instructor in Medicine, LSU Medical School, New Orleans, Louisiana; Chief of the Clinical Branch, Gillis W. Long Hansen's Disease Center, Carville, Louisiana
*Leprosy (Hansen's Disease)*

## ANN JOHANSON, M.D.

Director, Clinical Affairs, Genentech Inc., South San Francisco, California; Clinical Professor/Pediatrics, University of Virginia, Charlottesville, Virginia
*Hypopituitarism*

## ROYCE H. JOHNSON, M.D.

Associate Professor of Medicine, University of California Los Angeles; Vice Chairman, Department of Medicine, Chief, Infectious Disease, Kern Medical Center; Active Staff, Kern Medical Center, Bakersfield, California
*Coccidioidomycosis*

## M. BASHAR KAHALEH, M.D.

Associate Professor of Medicine, The Medical University of South Carolina; Staff, Medical University of South Carolina Hospital, Charleston Memorial Hospital, and Charleston VA Hospital, Charleston, South Carolina
*Connective Tissue Disorders: Lupus Erythematosus, Dermatomyositis, and Scleroderma*

## THEMISTOCLES C. KAMILARIS, M.D., Ph.D.

Adjunct Scientist, Pediatric Endocrinology Section, National Institute of Child Health and Human Development, and Clinical Neuroendocrinology Branch, National Institute of Mental Health, Bethesda, Maryland
*Cushing's Syndrome*

## NERI M. KANDAWALLA, M.D.

Clinical Assistant Professor of Pathology, Ohio State University College of Medicine; Senior Active Staff, Riverside Methodist Hospital, Columbus, Ohio
*Anaerobic and Necrotizing Infections, Including Gas Gangrene*

## BEATRICE S. KANDERS, Ed.D., M.P.H.

Instructor in Surgery, Harvard Medical School; Scientific Director of Clinical Trials, New England Deaconess Hospital Nutrition Coordinating Center, Boston, Massachusetts
*Obesity*

## MATTHEW H. KANZLER, M.D.

Clinical Assistant Professor, Stanford University, Stanford, California
*Papulosquamous Eruptions*

## PAUL E. KAPLAN, M.D.

Bert C. Wiley Professor of Physical Medicine and Rehabilitation, Chairman, Department of Physical Medicine, College of Medicine, The Ohio State University; Medical Director, Clinical Division of Physical Medicine and Rehabilitation, The Ohio State University Hospitals, Columbus, Ohio
*Rehabilitation of the Stroke Patient*

## SAMUEL J. KEITH, M.D.

Clinical Associate Professor, Department of Psychiatry, Georgetown University School of Medicine, Washington, D.C.; Deputy Director, Division of Clinical Research, Associate Director for Schizophrenia Programs, National Institute of Mental Health, Rockville, Maryland
*Schizophrenia*

## ARTHUR L. KELLERMANN, M.D., M.P.H.

Assistant Professor of Medicine and Chief, Division of Emergency Medicine, University of Tennessee; Director, Emergency Department, Regional Medical Center at Memphis, Memphis, Tennessee
*Cardiac Arrest*

## MELANIE S. KENNEDY, M.D.

Associate Professor, Department of Pathology, College of Medicine, The Ohio State University, Attending Staff, The Ohio State University Hospitals, Columbus, Ohio; Consulting Staff, Memorial Hospital of Union County, Marysville, Ohio
*Therapeutic Use of Blood Components*

## WILLIAM R. KEYE, Jr., M.D.

Chief, Division of Reproductive Endocrinology and Infertility, Department of Obstetrics and Gynecology, William Beaumont Hospital, Royal Oak, Michigan
*Premenstrual Syndrome (PMS)*

## MOON H. KIM, M.D.

Professor of Obstetrics and Gynecology and Director of Reproductive Endocrinology, Ohio State University Hospitals, Columbus, Ohio
*Dysfunctional Uterine Bleeding*

## T. DOUGLAS KINSELLA, M.D.

Professor (Medicine), Assistant Dean (Research: Medical Bioethics), Faculty of Medicine, University of Calgary, Member, Attending Staff, Foothills Provincial Hospital, Calgary, Alberta, Canada
*Ankylosing Spondylitis*

## CRAIG S. KITCHENS, M.D.

Professor and Vice-Chairman, Department of Medicine, University of Florida College of Medicine; Chief, Medical Service, Veterans Administration Medical Center, Gainesville, Florida
*Hemophilia and von Willebrand's Disease*

## SAULO KLAHR, M.D.

Joseph Friedman Professor of Renal Disease, Director, Renal Division, Washington University School of Medicine; Physician, Barnes Hospital; Consultant in Nephrology, Jewish Hospital, St. Louis, Missouri
*Chronic Renal Failure*

## BRUCE KLEIN, M.D.

Assistant Professor of Pediatrics, University of Wisconsin Medical School; Staff, Department of Pediatrics, University of Wisconsin Hospital and Clinics, Madison, Wisconsin
*Blastomycosis*

## LAWRENCE S. KLEIN, M.D.

Assistant Professor of Medicine, Indiana University School of Medicine; Research Associate, Krannert Institute of Cardiology; Staff Physician, Indiana University Hospitals and Richard L. Roudebush VA Hospital, Indianapolis, Indiana
*Heart Block*

## MARK W. KLINE, M.D.

Assistant Professor of Pediatrics, Divisions of Infectious Diseases and Allergy/Immunology, Baylor College of Medicine; Attending Physician, Texas Children's Hospital, Houston, Texas
*Food-Borne Illness*

## MICHAEL O. KOCH, M.D.

Assistant Professor of Urology, Vanderbilt Medical School; Assistant Professor of Urology, Vanderbilt University Medical Center; Chief, Urology Service, Department of Veterans Affairs Medical Center, Nashville, Tennessee
*Genitourinary Trauma*

## JEROME B. KOPSTEIN, M.D.

Consultant in Dermatology, Windsor Western Hospital, Hotel Dieu Hospital, Grace Hospital, and Metropolitan Hospital, Windsor, Ontario, Canada
*Atopic Dermatitis*

## MABEL KOSHY, M.D.

Associate Professor in Clinical Medicine, University of Illinois at Chicago; Associate Professor in Clinical Medicine, Director, Sickle Cell Clinic, University of Illinois at Chicago, Chicago, Illinois
*Sickle Cell Disease*

## FREDERICK KOSTER, M.D.

Associate Professor, University of New Mexico School of Medicine; Staff Physician, Department of Medicine, University of New Mexico Hospital, Albuquerque, New Mexico
*Plague*

## MICHAEL S. KRAMER, M.D.

Professor of Pediatrics and of Epidemiology and Biostatistics, McGill University; Staff Pediatrician, Department of Pediatrics and Division of Adolescent and Youth Medicine, McGill University, Montreal, Quebec, Canada
*Fever*

## PETER J. KRAUSE, M.D.

Associate Professor of Pediatrics, The University of Connecticut School of Medicine; Chief, Pediatric Infectious Diseases, Hartford Hospital, Hartford, Connecticut
*Viral Respiratory Infections*

## JOHN N. KRIEGER, M.D.

Professor of Urology, University of Washington School of Medicine; Attending Surgeon, University of Washington Medical Center, Harborview Medical Center, and Children's Orthopedic Hospital; Consultant Surgeon, Seattle VA Medical Center, Seattle Washington
*Bacterial Infections of the Urinary Tract in Males*

## KAMALA KRISHNASWAMY, M.D.

Deputy Director, Food and Drug Toxicology Research Center, National Institute of Nutrition; Physician-in-Charge, Nutrition Unit, Osmania Medical College Hospital, Hyderabad, India
*Beriberi*

## ROGER KURLAN, M.D.

Associate Professor of Neurology, University of Rochester School of Medicine and Dentistry; Attending Neurologist, Strong Memorial Hospital, Rochester, New York
*Parkinson's Disease*

## NANCY JOSEPH LANCE, M.D.

Fellow, Combined Rheumatology Program of the University of Chicago and Michael Reese Hospital and Medical Center, Chicago, Illinois
*Rheumatoid Arthritis*

## GREGORY L. LANDRY, M.D.

Associate Professor of Pediatrics, University of Wisconsin Medical School; Head, Section of Sports Medicine, Head Medical Team Physician, University of Wisconsin–Madison Athletic Teams, Madison, Wisconsin
*Disturbances due to Heat*

## RENEE LANTNER, M.D.

Assistant Professor of Pediatrics and Medicine, Loyola University of Chicago Stritch School of Medicine; Staff, Loyola University Medical Center, Maywood, Illinois
*Anaphylaxis and Serum Sickness*

## FRANK L. LANZA, M.D.

Clinical Professor of Medicine, Section of Gastroenterology, Baylor College of Medicine; Attending Physician, Harris County Medical District, Ben Taub Hospital; Attending Physician, Memorial Southwest Hospital; Active Staff, Sharpstown General Hospital, Houston, Texas
*Tumors of the Stomach*

## RICHARD A. LARSON, M.D.

Associate Professor, Section of Hematology/Oncology, Department of Medicine, Pritzker School of Medicine, University of Chicago; Staff, University of Chicago Medical Center, Chicago, Illinois
*Acute Leukemia in Adults*

## LARRY A. LATSON, M.D.

Associate Professor of Pediatrics, University of Nebraska Medical Center; Director, Cardiac Catheterization Laboratory, Children's Memorial Hospital of Omaha; Associate Director of Heart Station, University of Nebraska Medical Center, Omaha, Nebraska
*Congenital Heart Disease*

## PAUL E. LAVOIE, M.D.

Associate Clinical Professor of Medicine, University of California, San Francisco; Teaching Attending, Department of Medicine, Pacific Presbyterian Medical Center; Active Staff, Pacific Presbyterian Medical Center; Consulting Staff, Children's Hospital and Medical Center, San Francisco, California
*Lyme Disease (Lyme Borreliosis)*

## J. DOUGLAS LEE, M.D.

Staff, Marshfield Clinic, Marshfield, Wisconsin; Associate Clinical Professor, Department of Medicine, University of Wisconsin, Madison, Wisconsin
*Relapsing Fever*

## ALEXANDRA M. LEVINE, M.D.

Professor of Medicine and Executive Associate Dean, University of Southern California School of Medicine; Head, Adult Hematologic Neoplasia Service, Los Angeles County–University of Southern California Medical Center and Kenneth Norris Jr. Cancer Hospital and Research Institute, Los Angeles, California
*Non-Hodgkin's Lymphomas*

## MACY I. LEVINE, M.D.

Clinical Professor of Medicine, University of Pittsburgh School of Medicine; Active Staff, Presbyterian-University Hospital; Active Staff, St. Margaret Memorial Hospital; Emeritus Staff, Montefiore Hospital, Pittsburgh, Pennsylvania
*Allergic Reactions to Drugs*

## JAMES H. LEWIS, M.D.

Associate Professor of Medicine, Division of Gastroenterology, Georgetown University School of Medicine; Attending Physician, Georgetown University Medical Center, Consulting Physician, National Institutes of Health, VA Medical Center, National Naval Medical Center, Washington, D.C.
*Peptic Ulcer*

## RICHARD P. LEWIS, M.D.

Professor of Medicine, Ohio State University College of Medicine; Attending Physician, Ohio State University Hospitals, Columbus, Ohio
*Mitral Valve Prolapse*

## CAROL B. LINDSLEY, M.D.

Professor of Pediatrics, University of Kansas School of Medicine; Director, Pediatric Rheumatology, University of Kansas Medical Center, Kansas City, Kansas
*Juvenile Rheumatoid Arthritis*

## LOUIS J. LING, M.D.

Medical Director, Hennepin Regional Poison Center, Hennepin County Medical Center, Minneapolis, Minnesota
*Narcotic Poisoning*

## BENJAMIN LIPTZIN, M.D.

Associate Professor of Psychiatry, Harvard Medical School; Assistant General Director, McLean Hospital, Boston, Massachusetts
*Delirium*

## ALAN S. LIVINGSTONE, M.D.

Professor of Surgery, Department of Surgery, University of Miami School of Medicine; Staff Surgeon, James M. Jackson Memorial Hospital, VA Medical Center, Miami, Florida
*Bleeding Esophageal Varices*

## SUSAN M. LOBEL, M.D.

Instructor in Obstetrics, Gynecology, and Reproductive Biology, Harvard Medical School; Fellow in Reproductive Endocrinology, Brigham and Women's Hospital, Boston, Massachusetts
*Leiomyomas of the Uterus*

## JACOB LOKE, M.D.

Associate Professor of Medicine, Department of Internal Medicine, Yale University School of Medicine; Attending Physician, Yale–New Haven Hospital, New Haven, Connecticut
*Primary Lung Abscess*

## MARIA V. LOPEZ-BRESNAHAN, M.D.

Clinical Fellow in Neurology, Department of Neurology, Harvard Medical School and Massachusetts General Hospital, Boston, Massachusetts
*Multiple Sclerosis*

## MARK C. MABERRY, M.D.

Assistant Professor, Department of Obstetrics and Gynecology, University of Texas Southwestern Medical Center; Attending Physician, Parkland Memorial Hospital, Dallas, Texas
*Vulvovaginitis*

## DAVID R. MacDONALD, M.D.

Assistant Professor of Neurology, Departments of Clinical Neurological Sciences and Oncology, University of Western Ontario; Attending Neurologist, London Regional Cancer Centre, Victoria Hospital; Consulting Neurologist, University Hospital, St. Joseph's Hospital, London, Ontario, Canada
*Brain Tumors*

## MALCOLM R. MACKENZIE, M.D.

Professor of Medicine, School of Medicine, University of California, Davis; Staff, University of California, Davis Medical Center, Sacramento, California
*Multiple Myeloma*

## JOHN H. MALFETANO, M.D.

Associate Professor, Department of Obstetrics and Gynecology, Albany Medical College; Director, Division of Gynecology-Oncology, Department of Obstetrics and Gynecology, Albany Medical College; Associate Attending, Department of Obstetrics and Gynecology, St. Peter's Hospital, Albany, New York
*Cancer of the Endometrium*

## WILLIAM MUIR MANGER, M.D., Ph.D.

Professor of Clinical Medicine, New York University Medical Center; Lecturer in Medicine, College of Physicians and Surgeons, Columbia Medical Center; Attending Physician, Bellevue Hospital, Assistant Attending Physician, Vanderbilt Clinic, Columbia-Presbyterian Medical Center, New York, New York
*Pheochromocytoma*

## PAUL MARCOUX, M.D.

Chief Resident in Medicine, University of Massachusetts Medical Center, Worcester, Massachusetts
*Platelet-Mediated Bleeding Disorders*

## JAY M. MARION, M.D.

Director, Cancer Center, Missouri Baptist Medical Center, St. Louis, Missouri; Staff, St. Luke's Hospital, Chesterfield, Missouri
*Hodgkin's Disease: Chemotherapy*

## BARRY J. MARSHALL, M.D.

Assistant Professor of Medicine, University of Virginia Health Sciences Center, Charlottesville, Virginia
*Gastritis*

## KAREN KELLEY MAVES, M.D.

Fellow, University of Iowa; Staff, University of Iowa Hospitals and Clinics, Iowa City, Iowa
*Asthma in the Adolescent and Adult*

## C. KENNETH McALLISTER, M.D.

Chief, Infectious Diseases, Brooke Army Medical Center; Clinical Professor of Medicine, University of Texas Health Science Center, San Antonio, Texas
*Gonorrhea*

## RICHARD W. McCALLUM, M.D.

Paul Janssen Professor of Medicine; Chief, Division of Gastroenterology, University of Virginia Health Sciences Center, Charlottesville, Virginia; Consultant, Veterans Administration, Salem, Virginia; Consultant, Roanoke Memorial Hospital, Roanoke, Virginia
*Dysphagia and Esophageal Obstruction*

## ALAN M. McGREGOR, M.D.

Professor and Head, Department of Medicine, King's College School of Medicine; Consultant Physician, King's College Hospital, London, England
*Thyroiditis*

## MARY ANN McRAE, M.D.

Assistant Professor, Department of Obstetrics and Gynecology, Southern Illinois University School of Medicine, Springfield, Illinois
*Ectopic Pregnancy*

## SHLOMO MELMED, M.D.

Professor of Medicine, UCLA School of Medicine; Director, Division of Endocrinology and Metabolism, Cedars-Sinai Medical Center, Los Angeles, California
*Acromegaly*

## MANI MENON, M.D.

Professor of Surgery and Physiology, Chairman, Division of Urological and Transplantation Surgery, University of Massachusetts Medical Center, Worcester, Massachusetts
*Renal Calculi*

## LEO C. MERCER, M.D.

Assistant Professor, Department of Surgery, Texas Tech University School of Medicine; Attending Staff, Surgical Service, Attending Staff, Emergency Medicine, Assistant Chief, Trauma Service, Assistant Medical Director, Intensive Care Unit, and Physician Advisor, Department of Utilization Management, R.E. Thomasen General Hospital, El Paso, Texas
*Cholecystitis and Cholelithiasis*

## DAVID E. MILLER, M.D., Ph.D.

Assistant Professor of Obstetrics and Gynecology, University of North Carolina at Chapel Hill School of Medicine, Chapel Hill; Active Staff, Wake Medical Center, Raleigh, North Carolina
*Postpartum Care*

## JOSEPH I. MILLER, Jr., M.D.

Associate Professor of Cardiothoracic Surgery, Emory University School of Medicine; Associate Professor, Emory University Hospital; Chief of Thoracic Surgery, Crawford Long Hospital; Chief of Thoracic Surgery, Emory University; Piedmont Hospital, Atlanta, Georgia
*Pleural Effusion and Empyema Thoracis*

## SUSAN M. MILLER, M.D., M.P.H.

Assistant Professor, Baylor College of Medicine, Departments of Family Medicine and Internal Medicine; Staff, St. Luke's Episcopal Hospital, Texas Children's Hospital, and Hermann Hospital, Houston, Texas
*Management of HIV Infection*

## EDITH P. MITCHELL, M.D.

Associate Professor of Medicine, University of Missouri–Columbia School of Medicine; Attending Physician, University of Missouri–Columbia Hospital and Clinics, Columbia, Missouri
*Nausea and Vomiting*

## DENNIS S. MIURA, M.D., Ph.D.

Assistant Professor of Medicine, Albert Einstein College of Medicine; Director, Clinical Arrhythmia and Electrophysiology Service, Jack D. Weiler Hospital of the Albert Einstein College of Medicine, New York, New York
*Tachycardias*

## HOWARD C. MOFENSON, M.D.

Professor of Clinical Pediatrics and Emergency Medicine, State University of New York at Stony Brook; Professor of Pharmacology and Toxicology, New York College of Osteopathy, Old Westbury; Professor of Clinical Pharmacy, St. John's University College of Pharmacy, Jamaica; Director, Long Island Regional Poison Control Center, Nassau County Medical Center; Staff, Winthrop University Hospital, Mineola, New York; Medical Director of Long Island Regional Poison Control Center, Nassau County Medical Center, East Meadow, New York
*Acute Poisonings*

## ARNOLD M. MOSES, M.D.

Professor of Medicine and Project Director, Clinical Research Center, State University of New York, Health Science Center; Attending Physician, University Hospital, Syracuse, New York
*Diabetes Insipidus*

## STEVEN R. MOSTOW, M.D.

Professor of Medicine, University of Colorado; Acting Chairman, Department of Medicine, Rose Medical Center, Denver, Colorado
*Epidemic Influenza*

## MAURY E. MULLIGAN, M.D.

Associate Clinical Professor of Medicine, University of California, Irvine; Staff Physician, Physician HIV Coordinator, VA Medical Center, Long Beach, California
*Brain Abscess*

## EDWARD S. MURPHY, M.D.

Associate Professor of Medicine, Oregon Health Sciences University; Director of CCU, University Hospital; Director, Catheterization Laboratory, Portland VA Hospital, Portland, Oregon
*Infective Endocarditis*

## RONALD S. MURRAY, M.D.

Director of Research, Rocky Mountain Multiple Sclerosis Center, Swedish Medical Center, Englewood, Colorado
*Viral Meningoencephalitis*

## WILLIAM L. NABORS, M.D.

Assistant Professor of Urology, Emory University, Atlanta, Georgia
*Malignant Tumors of the Genitourinary System*

## LILA E. NACHTIGALL, M.D.

Associate Professor of Obstetrics and Gynecology, New York University School of Medicine; Attending Staff, New York University Hospital, New York, New York
*Menopause*

## SALAH M. NASRALLAH, M.D.

Volunteer Associate Professor of Medicine, University of Maryland Hospital; Associate, Union Memorial Hospital; Associate, St. Joseph Hospital, Baltimore, Maryland
*Amebiasis*

## DAVID M. NATHAN, M.D.

Associate Professor of Medicine, Harvard Medical School; Director, Diabetes Clinic and Diabetes Research Center; Associate Physician, Massachusetts General Hospital, Boston, Massachusetts
*Diabetes Mellitus in Adults*

## RONALD NELSON, M.D.

Professor of Obstetrics and Gynecology, Loma Linda University, Loma Linda; Program Director, Obstetrics and Gynecology, White Memorial Medical Center, Los Angeles, California
*Dysmenorrhea*

## DAVID H. NEUSTADT, M.D.

Clinical Professor of Medicine, University of Louisville School of Medicine, Louisville, Kentucky
*Osteoarthritis*

## JEFFREY B. NEUSTADT, M.D.

Assistant Professor of Orthopaedic Surgery, Georgetown University School of Medicine, Washington, D.C.
*Osteoarthritis*

## VICTOR D. NEWCOMER, M.D.

Clinical Professor of Medicine and Dermatology, University of California at Los Angeles; Staff, University of California at Los Angeles Medical Center, VA Medical Center, Los Angeles; St. John's Hospital and Health Center, Santa Monica Hospital Medical Center, Santa Monica, California
*Pigmentary Disorders*

## STEPHEN R. NEWMARK, M.D.

Medical Director, Diabetes Center of Excellence, Humana Sunrise Hospital, Las Vegas, Nevada
*Pellagra*

## JOHN T. NICOLOFF, M.D.

Professor of Medicine, University of Southern California School of Medicine; Attending Staff, Los Angeles County–University of Southern California Medical Center, Los Angeles, California
*Hyperthyroidism*

## PETER T. NIEH, M.D.

Senior Staff Urologist, Lahey Clinic Medical Center, Burlington, Massachusetts
*Epididymitis*

## HOOSHANG M. NIKOO, M.D.

Active Staff, Nazareth Hospital, Philadelphia, Pennsylvania; Active Staff, Rolling Hill Hospital, Elkins Park, Pennsylvania
*Abortion*

## ROBERT C. NOBLE, M.D.

Professor of Medicine, University of Kentucky College of Medicine, Lexington, Kentucky
*Syphilis*

## PATRICK T. O'GARA, M.D.

Assistant Professor of Medicine, Harvard Medical School; Director, Coronary Care Unit, Massachusetts General Hospital, Boston, Massachusetts
*Acute Myocardial Infarction*

## JEFFREY P. OKESON, D.M.D.

Professor and Director of the Orofacial Pain Center, University of Kentucky College of Dentistry, Lexington, Kentucky
*Temporomandibular Disorders*

## STEVEN M. OPAL, M.D.

Assistant Professor of Medicine, Brown University Program in Medicine, Providence; Infectious Disease Consultant, Memorial Hospital, Pawtucket, Rhode Island
*Pyelonephritis*

## CHARLES N. OSTER, M.D.

Associate Professor, Department of Medicine, Uniformed Services University of the Health Sciences; Chief, Infectious Disease Service, Walter Reed Army Medical Center, Washington, D.C.
*Leishmaniasis*

## WILLIAM R. PANJE, M.D.

Professor, University of Chicago Pritzker School of Medicine; Staff, Mitchell Hospital, Wyler's Children's Hospital, Chicago, Illinois; Ingalls Memorial Hospital, Harvey, Illinois
*Sinusitis*

## DAVID M. PARENTI, M.D.

Associate Professor of Medicine, Division of Infectious Diseases, The George Washington University Medical Center, Washington, D.C.
*Tularemia*

## JAMES N. PARSONS, M.D.

Assistant Clinical Professor of Medicine, The Ohio State University; Attending Staff Physician, Mount Carmel Medical Center, Columbus, Ohio
*Anaerobic and Necrotizing Infections, Including Gas Gangrene*

## JOHN C. PARTIN, M.D.

Professor of Pediatrics, School of Medicine, and Director, Division of Pediatric Gastroenterology, State University of New York at Stony Brook, Stony Brook, New York
*Reye's Syndrome*

## ZBIGNIEW S. PAWLOWSKI, M.D.

Professor, Academy of Medicine; Chief, Clinic of Parasitic and Tropical Diseases, Poznań, Poland
*Trichinellosis*

## MARK A. PEPPERCORN, M.D.

Associate Professor of Medicine, Harvard Medical School; Physician, Beth Israel Hospital, Boston, Massachusetts
*Crohn's Disease*

## BRENT G. PETTY, M.D.

Associate Professor of Medicine, The Johns Hopkins University School of Medicine; Full-Time Active Staff, The Johns Hopkins Hospital, Baltimore, Maryland
*Viral Diseases of the Skin*

## JOSEPH G. PHANEUF, M.D.

Clinical Instructor, Department of Dermatology, The University of Texas Southwestern Medical Center at Dallas, Dallas; Medical Staff Member, Lewisville Memorial Hospital, Lewisville, Texas
*Spider Bites and Scorpion Stings*

## JAMES M. PIERCE, JR., M.D. (deceased)

Late Professor and Chairman, Department of Urology, Wayne State University School of Medicine; Staff, Harper-Grace Hospitals, Detroit Receiving Hospital, Rehabilitation Institute, Children's Hospital of Michigan, Detroit, Michigan
*Urethral Stricture in the Male*

## HAROLD PLOTNICK, M.D.

Clinical Professor of Dermatology, Wayne State University School of Medicine; Vice-Chief, Department of Dermatology, Harper Hospital and Detroit Receiving Hospital; Staff, Detroit Medical Center and Wayne State University Affiliated Hospitals, Detroit, Michigan
*Occupational Dermatitis*

## ROBERT POHL, M.D.

Associate Professor, Department of Psychiatry, Wayne State Univerity School of Medicine; Director, Outpatient Department, Lafayette Clinic, Detroit, Michigan
*Panic Disorder and Agoraphobia*

## SOLOMON POSEN, M.D.

Professor of Medicine, University of Sydney; Endocrinologist, Royal North Shore Hospital, Sydney, Australia
*Hyperparathyroidism and Hypoparathyroidism*

## WILLIAM A. PRIMACK, M.D.

Associate Professor of Pediatrics, Fallon Clinic, University of Massachusetts Medical School; Attending Pediatrician, St. Vincent Hospital; Associate Attending Pediatrician, University of Massachusetts Medical School; Courtesy Staff, Medical Center of Central Massachusetts, Worcester, Massachusetts
*Parenteral Fluid Therapy in Infants and Children*

## MARK PUCZYNSKI, M.D.

Associate Professor of Pediatrics, Medical College of Pennsylvania, Philadelphia; Chairman, Department of Pediatrics at Allegheny General Hospital, Pittsburgh, Pennsylvania
*Childhood Enuresis*

## G. FORREST QUIMBY, M.D.

Resident in Surgery, University of Massachusetts Medical Center, Worcester, Massachusetts
*Renal Calculi*

## B. ASHOK RAJ, M.D.

Associate Professor of Psychiatry, University of South Florida College of Medicine; Director, Senior Adult Unit, University of South Florida Psychiatry Centre, Tampa, Florida
*Anxiety Disorders*

## JAMES E. RASMUSSEN, M.D.

Professor of Dermatology and Pediatrics, University of Michigan; Clinic Chief, Outpatient Dermatology, and Chief, Pediatric Inpatient Department, The University of Michigan Medical Center, Ann Arbor, Michigan
*Bacterial Diseases of the Skin*

## ANDREW RAUBITSCHEK, M.D.

Senior Investigator, Radiation Oncology Branch, National Cancer Institute, National Institutes of Health, Bethesda, Maryland
*Hodgkin's Disease: Radiation Therapy*

## ALAN M. RAUCH, M.D.

Assistant Professor of Pediatrics, Division of Infectious Diseases, University of Texas Medical School; Staff, Hermann Hospital, M.D. Anderson Hospital and Tumor Institute, Houston, Texas
*Q Fever*

## JANET P. REALINI, M.D.

Associate Professor, Department of Family Practice, The University of Texas Health Science Center at San Antonio; Professional Staff, St. Luke's Lutheran Hospital; Courtesy Staff, Santa Rosa Medical Center Hospital, San Antonio, Texas
*Contraception*

## P. SUDHAKAR REDDY, M.D.

University of Pittsburgh School of Medicine, Director, Cardiac Catheterization Laboratory, Presbyterian-University Hospital, Pittsburgh, Pennsylvania
*Pericarditis*

## REES B. REES, M.D.

Clinical Professor Emeritus of Dermatology and Radiology, University of California School of Medicine; Honorary Staff Member, St. Luke's Hospital, San Francisco; Consultant, Santa Rosa Memorial Hospital, Santa Rosa, California
*Pruritis Ani and Vulvae*

## MICHAEL F. REIN, M.D.

Professor of Internal Medicine, Division of Infectious Diseases, University of Virginia; Attending Physician, University of Virginia Health Sciences Center, Charlottesville, Virginia
*Nongonococcal Urethritis*

## ARTHUR L. REINGOLD, M.D.

Professor of Epidemiology, School of Public Health, University of California Berkeley and School of Medicine, University of California San Francisco; Department of Medicine, University of California San Francisco, San Francisco, California
*Toxic Shock Syndrome*

## JAMES B. REULER, M.D.

Professor of Medicine, Oregon Health Sciences University; Chief, Section of General Medicine, VA Medical Center, Portland, Oregon
*Disturbances due to Cold*

## JAMES C. REYNOLDS, M.D.

Professor of Medicine, University of Pittsburgh; Professor of Medicine and Chief, Division of Gastroenterology, University of Pittsburgh Affiliated Hospital, Pittsburgh, Pennsylvania
*Irritable Bowel Syndrome*

## HARRIS D. RILEY, JR., M.D.

Distinguished Professor of Pediatrics, University of Oklahoma College of Medicine; Attending Physician, Oklahoma Children's Memorial Hospital, University of Oklahoma Health Sciences Center, Oklahoma City, Oklahoma
*Rocky Mountain Spotted Fever*

## INGRAM M. ROBERTS, M.D.

Associate Professor of Medicine, Division of Gastroenterology, Department of Medicine, George Washington University School of Medicine, Attending Physician in Internal Medicine and Gastroenterology, George Washington University Hospital, Washington, D.C.
*The Malabsorption Syndromes*

## CARLOS ROTMAN, M.D.

Assistant Professor of Obstetrics and Gynecology, Institute for the Study and Treatment of Endometriosis and Rush Medical College; Attending Physician, Rush-Presbyterian-St. Luke's Medical Center, Grant Hospital, Chicago, Illinois
*Endometriosis*

## ROSS RUDOLPH, M.D.

Head, Division of Plastic and Reconstructive Surgery, Scripps Clinic and Research Foundation, La Jolla, California; Associate Clinical Professor of Plastic Surgery, University of California, San Diego, San Diego, California
*Keloids*

## WILL G. RYAN, M.D.

Professor of Medicine, Rush Medical College; Senior Attending Physician, Rush-Presbyterian-St. Luke's Medical Center, Chicago, Illinois
*Paget's Disease of Bone*

## MARY ELLEN M. RYBAK, M.D.

Associate Professor of Medicine, University of Massachusetts Medical Center, Worcester, Massachusetts
*Platelet-Mediated Bleeding Disorders*

## ALFREDO A. SADUN, M.D., PH.D.

Professor of Ophthalmology and Neurological Surgery, University of Southern California; Estelle Doheny Eye Foundation; Kenneth Norris Jr. Cancer Hospital and Research Institute; Los Angeles County–University of Southern California Medical Center, Los Angeles, California
*Optic Neuritis*

## EDWARD C. SALTZSTEIN, M.D.

Professor and Associate Chairman, Surgery Department, Texas Tech University School of Medicine; Director of Surgical Services, R. E. Thomason General Hospital, El Paso, Texas
*Cholecystitis and Cholelithiasis*

## RAMON L. SANCHEZ, M.D.

Associate Professor, University of Texas Medical Branch at Galveston; Director of Surgical Pathology and Dermatopathology, University of Texas Medical Branch at Galveston, Galveston, Texas
*Cancer of the Skin*

## GEORGE A. SAROSI, M.D.

Chairman, Department of Internal Medicine, Maricopa Medical Center, Phoenix, Arizona
*Histoplasmosis*

## MICHAEL G. SARR, M.D.

Associate Professor of Surgery, Department of Surgery, Mayo Medical School; Consultant in General and Gastroenterologic Surgery, St. Mary's Hospital and Methodist Hospital; Consultant in Gastroenterology Research Unit, St. Mary's Hospital, Rochester, Minnesota
*Chronic Pancreatitis*

## THOMAS G. SAUL, M.D.

Associate Professor of Clinical Neurosurgery, Department of Neurosurgery, University of Cincinnati Medical Center; Director, Graduate Education Program in Neurological Surgery, Good Samaritan Hospital; Director, Neurosurgical Intensive Care Unit, Good Samaritan Hospital, Cincinnati, Ohio
*Acute Head Injuries in Adults*

## WILLIAM D. SAWYER, M.D.

China Medical Board of New York, Inc., New York; Adjunct Professor of Microbiology and Immunology and Professor of Medicine, New York Medical College, Valhalla, New York
*Typhus Fevers*

## JULIUS SCHACHTER, Ph.D.

Professor of Epidemiology, Department of Laboratory Medicine, University of California, San Francisco, San Francisco, California
*Psittacosis (Ornithosis)*

## ERNST J. SCHAEFER, M.D.

Professor of Medicine, Tufts University School of Medicine; Director, Lipid Clinic, New England Medical Center, Boston, Massachusetts
*Hyperlipoproteinemia*

## RICHARD K. SCHER, M.D.

Professor of Clinical Dermatology, Columbia University College of Physicians and Surgeons; Attending Dermatologist, Presbyterian Hospital, New York, New York
*Diseases of the Nails*

## ISAAC SCHIFF, M.D.

Joe Vincent Meigs Professor of Gynecology at Harvard Medical School; Chief of Vincent Memorial Gynecology Service at the Massachusetts General Hospital, Boston, Massachusetts
*Leiomyomas of the Uterus*

## MICHAEL J. SCHUMACHER, M.B.B.S.

Associate Professor, Department of Pediatrics, and Chief, Allergy-Immunology Section, University of Arizona Health Sciences Center, Tucson, Arizona
*Allergic Rhinitis due to Aeroallergens*

## DAVID A. SEARS, M.D.

Professor of Medicine, Baylor College of Medicine; Attending Physician and Chief of Medicine Service, Harris County Hospital District, Houston, Texas
*Iron Deficiency*

## DOUGLAS SEATON, M.D.

Consultant Physician, The Ipswich Hospital, Suffolk, England
*Silicosis*

## FRANCISCO SERAFIN, M.D.

Mexican Institute of Social Security; Associate Professor of Pediatrics and Associate Professor of Infectious Diseases and Clinical Microbiology, National Autonomous University of Mexico; Associate Director, Hospital de Pediatria, Mexico City, Mexico
*Tuberculosis and Other Mycobacterial Diseases*

## ALAN R. SHALITA, M.D., Sc.D.

Professor and Chairman, Department of Dermatology, State University of New York Health Science Center at Brooklyn; Chief of Dermatology, University Hospital of Brooklyn, Kings County Hospital Center, Brookdale Hospital Medical Center; Consultant Dermatologist, VA Medical Center; Interim Medical Director, Kings County Hospital Center, Brooklyn, New York
*Acne Vulgaris and Rosacea*

## JOHN D. SHANLEY, M.D.

Professor, University of Connecticut, Farmington; Staff, VA Medical Center, Newington, Connecticut
*Chickenpox (Varicella) and Zoster (Shingles)*

## ALAN B. SHAPIRO, M.D.

Clinical Instructor in Medicine, University of Illinois at Chicago; Gastroenterology Fellow, University of Illinois Hospital, Chicago, Illinois
*Constipation*

## DAVID V. SHEEHAN, M.D.

Professor of Psychiatry, University of South Florida College of Medicine; Director, Office of Research, University of South Florida Psychiatry Center, Tampa, Florida
*Anxiety Disorders*

## PHILIP D. SHENEFELT, M.D.

Assistant Professor, Section of Dermatology, Department of Internal Medicine, University of South Florida College of Medicine; Staff, Tampa General Hospital, James A. Haley Veterans Hospital, Tampa, Florida
*Parasitic Diseases of the Skin*

## ELIZABETH F. SHERERTZ, M.D.

Associate Professor of Dermatology, Bowman Gray School of Medicine of Wake Forest University, Winston-Salem, North Carolina
*Chancroid*

## BARRY SHERMAN, M.D.

Vice-President of Medical Affairs, Genentech Inc., South San Francisco, California; Clinical Professor of Medicine, Stanford University School of Medicine, Stanford, California
*Hypopituitarism*

## A. MAJID SHOJANIA, M.D.

Professor of Pediatrics and Associate Professor of Medicine and Pathology, Medical School of the University of Manitoba; Head of Department of Laboratory Medicine and Hematology Laboratory, Active Staff of Departments of Pediatrics and Medicine, St. Boniface General Hospital; Consulting Staff at Health Sciences Centre, Winnipeg, Manitoba, Canada
*Pernicious Anemia and Other Megaloblastic Anemias*

**IRA SHOULSON, M.D.**

Professor of Neurology, Pharmacology, and Medicine, University of Rochester School of Medicine and Dentistry; Attending Neurologist and Attending Physician, Strong Memorial Hospital, Rochester, New York
*Parkinson's Disease*

**STANFORD T. SHULMAN, M.D.**

Professor of Pediatrics, Northwestern University Medical School; Chief, Infectious Diseases, Children's Memorial Hospital, Chicago, Illinois
*Rheumatic Fever*

**RAYMOND G. SLAVIN, M.D.**

Professor of Internal Medicine and Microbiology; Director, Division of Allergy and Immunology and Allergy Research Laboratory, St. Louis University School of Medicine, St. Louis, Missouri
*Hypersensitivity Pneumonitis*

**CRAIG E. SMITH, M.D.**

Senior Fellow, Infectious Diseases Service, Brooke Army Medical Center, Fort Sam Houston, Texas
*Gonorrhea*

**LEE E. SMITH, M.D.**

Professor of Surgery, George Washington University Medical Center; Staff, George Washington University Hospital, Washington, D.C.
*Tumors of the Colon and Rectum*

**WILLIAM J. SNAPE, JR., M.D.**

Professor of Medicine and Director, Inflammatory Bowel Disease Center, University of California at Los Angeles School of Medicine, Los Angeles; Chief, Gastroenterology Section, Harbor-UCLA Medical Center, Torrance, California
*Gaseousness and Indigestion*

**CONSTANTIN R. SOLDATOS, M.D.**

Associate Professor of Psychiatry, University of Athens Medical School; Director, Sleep Disorders Unit, Eginition Hospital, Athens, Greece
*Insomnia*

**ROBERT STEFFEN, M.D.**

Senior Lecturer, University of Zurich; Head, Division of Epidemiology and Prevention of Communicable Diseases, Institute of Social and Preventive Medicine of the University, Zurich, Switzerland
*Acute Infectious Diarrhea*

**STEVEN N. STRUVE, M.D.**

Senior Fellow, University of Utah; Limited Term Instructor, University of Utah, Salt Lake City, Utah
*Acute Respiratory Failure*

**CIRO V. SUMAYA, M.D., M.P.H.T.M.**

Professor of Pediatrics and Pathology, Chief of Pediatric Infectious Diseases Division, Associate Dean for Continuing Medical Education, University of Texas Health Science Center; Staff Physician, Medical Center Hospital and Santa Rosa Medical Center, San Antonio, Texas
*Infectious Mononucleosis*

**ALVIN S. TEIRSTEIN, M.D.**

Professor of Medicine, Mount Sinai School of Medicine; Director, Division of Pulmonary and Critical Care Medicine, Mount Sinai Medical Center, New York, New York
*Sarcoidosis*

**UDHO THADANI, M.B.B.S.**

Professor of Medicine, Vice-Chief of Cardiology, University of Oklahoma Health Sciences Center; Staff Cardiologist, Oklahoma Memorial Hospital and VA Medical Center, Oklahoma City, Oklahoma
*Angina Pectoris*

**DAVID F. J. TOLLEFSON, M.D.**

Fellow, Vascular Surgery, Henry Ford Hospital, Detroit, Michigan
*Acquired Diseases of the Aorta*

**GARY D. TOLLEFSON, M.D., PH.D.**

Associate Professor, Department of Psychiatry, University of Minnesota–Minneapolis; Chairman, Department of Psychiatry, St. Paul–Ramsey Medical Center, St. Paul, Minnesota
*Affective Disorders*

**WILLIAM H. TOPPER, M.D.**

Associate Professor of Pediatrics, University of Kansas Medical Center School of Medicine; Faculty Physician, University of Kansas Medical Center, Kansas City, Kansas
*Care of At-Risk Neonates*

**BASIM M. UTHMAN, M.D.**

Instructor, Department of Neurology, University of Florida; Staff Neurologist, Neurology Service, Veterans Affairs Medical Center and University of Florida College of Medicine, Gainesville, Florida
*Epilepsy in Adolescents and Adults*

**FRANÇOIS VACHON, M.D.**

Professor, University of Paris; Head of the Department of Intensive Care for Infectious Diseases, Hôpital Bichat/Claude Bernard, Paris, France
*Tetanus*

**WILLIAM N. VALENTINE, M.D.**

Professor Emeritus, Department of Medicine Center for Health Sciences, University of California, Los Angeles, Los Angeles, California
*Nonimmune Hemolytic Anemia*

**J. CORWIN VANCE, M.D.**

Assistant Professor, University of Minnesota; Assistant Chief, Department of Dermatology, Hennepin County Medical Center, Minneapolis, Minnesota
*Verruca Vulgaris (Warts)*

**JOHN R. VAN GURP, M.D., PH.D.**

Chief Resident, Department of Dermatology, University of Michigan Medical Center, Ann Arbor, Michigan
*Pruritus*

**JON A. VAN HEERDEN, M.D.**

Fred C. Andersen Professor, Mayo Clinic and Mayo Foundation; Professor of Surgery, Mayo Medical School; Consultant in Surgery, Mayo Clinic and Mayo Foundation, Full Staff Privileges, St. Mary's Hospital and Rochester Methodist Hospital, Rochester, Minnesota
*Chronic Pancreatitis*

**LODEWYK H. S. VAN MIEROP, M.D.**

Graduate Research Professor and Chairman, University of Florida; Pediatric Cardiologist, Shands Teaching Hospital, Gainesville, Florida
*Snakebite*

## DONALD G. VIDT, M.D.

Chairman, Department of Hypertension and Nephrology, The Cleveland Clinic Foundation, Cleveland, Ohio
*Hypertension*

## MARSHA L. WAKEFIELD, M.D.

Assistant Professor of Anesthesiology, Medical College of Georgia; Staff, Medical College of Georgia Hospital and Veterans Administration Medical Center, Augusta, Georgia
*Obstetric Anesthesia*

## B. TIMOTHY WALSH, M.D.

Professor of Clinical Psychiatry, College of Physicians and Surgeons, Columbia University; Attending Psychiatrist, Columbia-Presbyterian Medical Center, and Research Psychiatrist, New York State Psychiatric Institute, New York, New York
*Bulimia Nervosa*

## PAUL F. WALTER, M.D.

Professor of Internal Medicine (Cardiology), Emory University School of Medicine; Staff, Emory University Hospital, Atlanta, Georgia
*Atrial Fibrillation*

## C. GILLON WARD, M.D.

Professor of Surgery, University of Miami School of Medicine; Medical Director, Burn Center, University of Miami–Jackson Memorial Medical Center, Miami, Florida
*Burns*

## ROBERT P. WARIN, M.D.

Emeritus Consultant Dermatologist, Department of Dermatology, Bristol Royal Infirmary, Bristol, England
*Urticaria*

## JAMES R. WARPINSKI, M.D.

Post-Doctoral Fellow, Allergy and Immunology, University of Wisconsin Medical School, Madison, Wisconsin
*Allergic Reactions to Insect Stings*

## DAVID A. WARRELL, D.M., D.Sc.

Professor of Tropical Medicine and Infectious Diseases, University of Oxford; Honorary Consultant Physician, Oxford Group of Hospitals, Oxford, England
*Malaria*

## JAY H. WARRICK, M.D.

Fellow in Rheumatology, Department of Medicine, Division of Rheumatology and Immunology, Medical University of South Carolina, Charleston, South Carolina
*Connective Tissue Disorders: Lupus Erythematosus, Dermatomyositis, and Scleroderma*

## SAMUEL R. WATKINS, JR., M.D.

Staff, Norton Children's Hospital, Baptist East Hospital, Humana Audubon Hospital, and Humana Hospital–Suburban, Louisville, Kentucky
*Genitourinary Trauma*

## JOHN M. WEILER, M.D.

Associate Professor, University of Iowa; Staff, VA Medical Center and University of Iowa Hospitals and Clinics, Iowa City, Iowa
*Asthma in the Adolescent and Adult*

## LOUIS WEINSTEIN, M.D., PH.D.

Lecturer in Medicine, Harvard Medical School; Professor of Medicine, Emeritus, Tufts University School of Medicine; Senior Consultant in Medicine, Brigham and Women's Hospital, Boston, Massachusetts
*Diphtheria*

## LOUIS M. WEISS, M.D., M.P.H.

Assistant Professor of Medicine, Division of Infectious Diseases and Assistant Professor of Pathology, Division of Parasitology and Tropical Medicine, Albert Einstein College of Medicine; Assistant Attending Physician, Jack D. Weiler Hospital of the Albert Einstein College of Medicine and Bronx Municipal Hospital Center, Bronx, New York
*Rat-Bite Fever*

## NANETTE K. WENGER, M.D.

Professor of Medicine (Cardiology), Emory University School of Medicine; Staff, Grady Memorial Hospital, Crawford W. Long Memorial Hospital, VA Medical Center, Atlanta, Georgia
*Rehabilitation After Myocardial Infarction*

## DAVID A. WHITING, M.D.

Clinical Professor of Dermatology and Pediatrics, The University of Texas Southwestern Medical Center at Dallas; Attending Dermatologist, Baylor University Medical Center, Children's Medical Center and Parkland Memorial Hospital; Medical Director, Baylor Hair Research and Treatment Center, Dallas, Texas
*Hair Disorders*

## D. L. WICKERHAM, M.D.

Research Associate Professor of Surgery, University of Pittsburgh, Pittsburgh, Pennsylania; Associate Director, National Surgical Adjuvant Breast and Bowel Project
*Diseases of the Breast*

## B. J. WILDER, M.D.

Professor of Neurology and Neuroscience, University of Florida College of Medicine; Chief, Neurology Service, Department of Veterans Affairs Medical Center, Gainesville, Florida
*Epilepsy in Adolescents and Adults*

## ROBERT F. WILLENBUCHER, M.D.

Fellow in Gastroenterology, Harbor-UCLA Medical Center, Torrance, California
*Gaseousness and Indigestion*

## NANCY ANDERSON WILMS, M.D.

Assistant Professor, Loma Linda University; Active Staff, Loma Linda University Medical Center, Jerry L. Pettis Memorial VA Hospital, Loma Linda Community Hospital, Loma Linda; San Bernardino County Medical Center, San Bernardino, California
*Granuloma Inguinale (Donovanosis); Lymphogranuloma Venereum*

## RICHARD E. WINN, M.D.

Chief, Pulmonary Medicine and Critical Care, Staff, Infectious Diseases, David Grant Medical Center, Fairfield, California
*Rabies*

## CHRISTOPHER M. WISE, M.D.

Associate Professor of Medicine (Rheumatology), Bowman Gray School for Medicine; Staff, North Carolina Baptist Hospitals, Inc., Winston-Salem, North Carolina
*Hyperuricemia and Gout*

## A. WODAK, M.D.

Lecturer, School of Medicine, University of New South Wales, Sydney; Director, Alcohol and Drug Service, St. Vincent's Hospital, Darlinghurst, New South Wales, Australia
*Alcoholism*

## NORMAN WOLMARK, M.D.

Mark M. Ravitch Professor of Surgery, University of Pittsburgh; Surgeon-in-Chief, Montefiore Hospital, Pittsburgh, Pennsylania
*Diseases of the Breast*

## KIM B. YANCEY, M.D.

Associate Professor of Dermatology, Uniformed Services University of the Health Sciences, Bethesda, Maryland
*Bullous Diseases*

## JESS R. YOUNG, M.D.

Chairman, Department of Vascular Medicine, Cleveland Clinic Foundation, Cleveland, Ohio
*Stasis Dermatitis and Stasis Ulcers*

## HERSCHEL S. ZACKHEIM, M.D.

Clinical Professor, University of California, San Francisco; Attending Staff, University of California, San Francisco; Sequoia Hospital District, Redwood City, California
*Cutaneous T Cell Lymphoma (Mycosis Fungoides and Sézary's Syndrome)*

## IRWIN ZIMENT, M.D.

Professor of Medicine, University of Los Angeles School of Medicine; Chief of Medicine, Olive View Medical Center, Sylmar, California
*Cough*

## DOUGLAS P. ZIPES, M.D.

Professor of Medicine, Indiana University School of Medicine; Attending Staff, Indiana University Hospital, Richard L. Roudebush VA Medical Center, Wishard Memorial Hospital, Indianapolis, Indiana
*Heart Block*

## FREDERICK P. ZUSPAN, M.D.

Professor, Department of Obstetrics and Gynecology, The Ohio State University College of Medicine; Staff, The Ohio State University Hospitals, Columbus, Ohio
*Hypertensive Disorders of Pregnancy*

# Preface

This 43rd edition of *Current Therapy* continues the tradition established by the late Howard Conn in 1949. Each year, a new edition is published offering fresh information from new authors who are recommended by authorities in that field. This year, more than 75% of the material is entirely new and the remainder is thoroughly revised and updated.

Premenstrual syndrome has been added as a new topic in view of the attention it has been receiving in the literature and in the public press.

Our goal is to provide the practicing physician with an up-to-date definitive reference for managing problems frequently encountered in practice. The authors are experts who recommend the drugs and therapeutic methods they have found most effective when a large number of possibilities exist. Often these recommendations are based on their extensive experience or recent research and may not yet be reported in the traditional literature.

The editorial staff at Saunders are experts in editing manuscripts so that the final product is concise and easy to read. The objective is to provide the busy physician with answers to specific questions that arise while caring for a patient.

In addition to the copy editors and John Dyson, Senior Medical Editor at W. B. Saunders, I want to thank Roxy Cuddy, my editorial assistant, and the pharmacologists in my department, Barry Carter and Lucinda Miller, who check the accuracy of every drug recommendation found in this text.

ROBERT E. RAKEL, M.D.

# Table of Contents

# SECTION 3. THE RESPIRATORY SYSTEM

# SECTION 4. THE CARDIOVASCULAR SYSTEM

# SECTION 5. THE BLOOD AND SPLEEN

# SECTION 6. THE DIGESTIVE SYSTEM

# SECTION 7. METABOLIC DISORDERS

# SECTION 8. THE ENDOCRINE SYSTEM

# SECTION 9. THE UROGENITAL TRACT

# SECTION 10. THE SEXUALLY TRANSMITTED DISEASES

# SECTION 11. DISEASES OF ALLERGY

# SECTION 12. DISEASES OF THE SKIN

# SECTION 13. THE NERVOUS SYSTEM

## SECTION 14. THE LOCOMOTOR SYSTEM

## SECTION 15. OBSTETRICS AND GYNECOLOGY

# SECTION 16. PSYCHIATRIC DISORDERS

# SECTION 17. PHYSICAL AND CHEMICAL INJURIES

# SECTION 18. APPENDIX AND INDEX

# Symptomatic Care Pending Diagnosis

## PAIN

method of
C. STRATTON HILL, JR., M.D.
*The University of Texas M.D. Anderson Cancer
    Center*
*Houston, Texas*

Pain is defined by the International Association for the Study of Pain as "an unpleasant sensory and emotional experience associated with actual or potential tissue damage or described in terms of such damage." Pain can also be defined in more clinical terms simply as acute or chronic. Acute pain, frequently associated with tissue damage, is seen primarily in trauma and acute disease processes. Chronic pain is also associated with ongoing painful medical conditions, such as rheumatoid arthritis, that have elements of tissue damage but can occur in settings where no cause for pain can be demonstrated, the so-called chronic pain syndrome.

Pain can also be classified by whether the nervous system is intact or damaged. Recognizing this classification is important because pain emanating from a damaged nerve or nervous system has distinct characteristics and responds differently to treatment than does pain emanating from a normal or intact nervous system. Pain distinguished by nerve damage is called *neuropathic,* or *deafferentation,* pain, the former term being preferred since it implies that the pain is due to functional abnormalities of the nervous system. Neuropathic pain may be perpetuated by sympathetic nervous system input, thereby requiring treatment directed toward eliminating or blocking input from this system, such as sympathic blockade or sympathectomy. Pain caused by tissue damage in the presence of a normal nervous system is called *nociceptive* pain.

### ACUTE PAIN

#### Etiology

An attempt to establish the etiology of any pain is essential because the fundamental goal in treating pain is to remove or correct its cause. Acute pain serves as a warning to the organism that there is a danger or threat to its integrity or existence. This is one of the fundamental differences between acute and chronic pain: acute pain serves a useful and meaningful purpose, whereas chronic pain does not. The etiology of acute pain is usually easy to establish. Causes of acute pain include mechanical injury, chemical irritation, burn, tissue stress such as ischemia, acute distention of hollow visceral organs or blood vessels, and spasm of smooth muscle. Fortunately, modern techniques make diagnosis of these conditions possible within a short time. Since most causes are correctable, pain relief is soon achieved.

Acute pain may occur during a chronic painful condition, such as cancer. Collapse of a vertebra due to metastatic disease, rupture of a viscus, or intestinal obstruction may cause increased intensity of pain in a cancer patient already suffering chronic pain. These acute pain episodes must be treated separately while maintaining treatment of the chronic pain. If the cause of the superimposed painful episode can be removed or otherwise treated, such treatment should be instituted. However, if treatment cannot dramatically relieve the pain, for example, radiation therapy for a collapsed vertebra, interim relief is required and will usually require the use of analgesic drugs. The choice of analgesic will depend on the intensity of the pain and whether it is nociceptive or neuropathic. Nociceptive pain usually responds to the commonly used non-narcotic and narcotic analgesics. Neuropathic pain, on the other hand, responds better to antidepressant and anticonvulsant drugs, usually is not dramatically relieved, and therefore becomes chronic; the dose required is not necessarily directly related to intensity of pain.

If a narcotic analgesic is being used to relieve the underlying chronic pain, it will be necessary to increase the dose. A dose higher than one that would control the acute pain in the absence of chronic pain is required. Physicians should not hesitate to provide these higher doses because narcotics have no "ceiling effect." However, if a non-narcotic is being used to relieve the underlying chronic pain, it will be necessary to switch to a stronger analgesic, usually a narcotic, because of the lack of response to the non-narcotic above a given dose level (ceiling effect) and the toxic effects of higher doses of non-narcotic analgesics. One should always keep in mind when using fixed combinations of a non-narcotic and narcotic (for example, Percocet, Percodan, Tylox) that with each increase in dose of the narcotic portion of the compound, there is a corresponding increase in the non-narcotic portion. Toxic doses of the non-narcotic are sometimes inadvertently reached.

## Treatment

### General

The ideal way to treat pain is to remove or otherwise correct the cause. Removal by surgical means, where appropriate, brings dramatic relief; other means may be less dramatic but equally effective. For example, treating muscle spasm with hot packs, ultrasound, and electrical stimulation requires days to weeks of therapy for relief. The emphasis in treating injuries or other self-limiting, pain-producing medical conditions should be on modalities that are more effective than drug therapy. Drug therapy should be considered merely an adjuvant to other modalities.

Physicians frequently voice their frustration with patients who begin a drug program for pain relief and who, when there is no relief after a period their physicians consider adequate, insist on continuing the initially prescribed drug program. Physicians become particularly concerned if the treatment regimen includes a narcotic for a benign condition such as low back pain, the etiology of which may be unclear because of a lack of objective, demonstrable physical or laboratory abnormalities. This frustration is easily avoided by making the proper diagnosis of the origin of the pain and applying the proper treatment modality. In addition, physicians should counsel their patients at the outset about the course of the pain and its outcome. The initial evaluation should include searching for clues that indicate a patient may have an interest in perpetuating his or her complaint for ulterior motives, such as monetary compensation for an accident or work-related injury.

### Nondrug Treatment

It is beyond the scope of this article to discuss the indications for treating acute pain with nondrug modalities, which are listed in Table 1, or the complications of such modalities. In fact, these modalities are not limited to treatment of acute pain but have application in the treatment of both acute and chronic pain and both benign

TABLE 1. **Nondrug Treatment Modalities for Acute Pain Control**

Physical therapy modalities for injured muscles, joints, etc.
Transcutaneous electrical nerve stimulation (TENS) and
   other electrostimulation techniques
Acupuncture
Cognitive and behavioral techniques
   Hypnosis and self-hypnosis
   Relaxation
   Guided imagery and distraction
   Biofeedback
   Behavior modification
Nerve blocks

and malignant conditions, once again emphasizing the need to assess the etiology of the pain and determine the appropriate treatment modality.

In general, nondrug procedures have specific indications; are provided by physiatrists, anesthesiologists, psychiatrists, psychologists, and physical therapists; and are frequently brought together in multidisciplinary pain clinics.

### Drug Treatment

Acetaminophen, nonsteroidal anti-inflammatory drugs (NSAIDs, including aspirin) and opiates (narcotics) are the principal drugs used to treat acute pain. Since acute pain is most frequently nociceptive, response to these drugs is usually gratifying and follows a predictable course. Choice of drug is determined by the severity of the pain, which is classified as mild, moderate, or severe.

Recommended doses for the NSAIDs depend on the specific drug prescribed. These drugs have a ceiling effect, and prescribing doses beyond that point will not provide additional relief. Narcotics, on the other hand, do not have such a ceiling, and recommended doses should be used merely as guidelines for attaining adequate pain relief. In fact, pain from severe conditions, such as acute renal colic and sickle cell crisis, may be so intense that the dose necessary to relieve it far exceeds the recommended dose. *Pain is a natural antagonist to the analgesic and respiratory depressant effects of narcotics; therefore, consideration of the dose size is of little practical importance in treating these very painful conditions. Pain relief, not dose size, is the end point.* However, one should use prudent increments when increasing the dose size, since a dose exceeding that required for pain relief can cause the potentially serious side effects characteristic of narcotics.

## CHRONIC PAIN

### Etiology

The two general categories for chronic pain are benign and malignant. Benign pain may be associated with chronic painful diseases in which nociception, or tissue damage, is apparent, such as rheumatoid or degenerative arthritis, osteoporosis, sickle cell disease, and diabetic neuropathy; or there may be no discernible disease process, such as in low back pain and the so-called chronic pain syndrome. Malignant pain is that associated with cancer. Pain in patients who have cancer may be caused by the tumor itself, tumor treatment, or unrelated benign painful conditions. Malignant pain due to the tumor frequently is associated with a nociceptive, or tissue damage, component, such as tumor invasion of nerves and soft tissue, bone destruction, etc. Pain secondary to cancer treatment is frequently neuropathic since treatment, such as surgery, radiation therapy, and chemotherapy, may damage nerves and nerve tissue. Treatment decisions will depend on distinguishing the type of pain the patient suffers; therefore, once again the importance of determining the etiology of the pain is demonstrated.

## Psychologic Aspect

A major difference between acute and chronic pain is the negative emotions elicited by the chronic pain experience. Among these are anxiety, depression, fear, frustration, anger, loneliness, abandonment, and isolation. In both benign and malignant chronic painful conditions, the psychologic aspect of this complex experience may be so dominant that adequate pain control will depend on treating the negative emotion(s), even though the nociceptive or neuropathic elements may be under adequate control. In addition, failure to recognize the role of negative emotions will frequently result in inappropriate pain treatment. For example, a physician might increase the dose of an analgesic rather than institute treatment for depression, which could be more appropriate. Patients frequently use the word pain to describe the complaint of disturbed emotional feelings. The practitioner should be alert to the patient's use of this word to express his or her poorly understood emotional feelings or as an expression of the more global, complex emotional condition known as suffering.

## Treatment

### Benign, Painful Medical Conditions

As with acute pain, treating the cause of pain in chronic, benign medical conditions, such as rheumatoid arthritis and vascular headaches, with drugs and other modalities known to be effective, or at least partially effective, is essential. The degree to which this treatment is suc-

cessful determines how much additional treatment specifically for pain will be required to achieve optimum pain relief.

When treatment of the underlying condition fails to relieve the pain, treatment of the pain itself is necessary. Nondrug treatment modalities, as listed in Table 1, may be effective. This approach should be the initial one. However, the initial effectiveness of some of these methods, for example, acupuncture and transcutaneous electrical nerve stimulation (TENS), is not sustained in a significant number of patients. Analgesic drugs must then be used. As with acute pain, the choice of drug depends on the intensity of the pain and whether the pain is nociceptive or neuropathic.

For nociceptive pain, non-narcotic analgesics such as aspirin, acetaminophen, and NSAIDs are used for mild to moderate pain. If the pain cannot be controlled with these drugs, narcotic analgesics should be used. For example, the pain of vascular and cluster headaches may be controlled most of the time by vasoconstrictors, beta-adrenergic blockers, calcium channel blockers, or other treatment. However, it is not uncommon for such patients to experience "breakthrough" headaches that respond only to narcotics. Relief of these headaches should be provided by a proper dose of narcotic, which usually exceeds "recommended" doses, and the patient should not be treated as if he or she were a drug-seeking street addict. There is a cultural and societal bias against the use of narcotics for chronic, benign painful conditions, even though they are the only means for providing adequate relief for the patient, but this is unjustified. Pain relief often means the difference between a patient's being a productive, independent member of society in contrast to an unproductive, dependent member. The chronic taking of narcotics is not synonymous with drug addiction. Drug dependency and drug addiction are separate entities.

Treatment of chronic, benign, painful conditions for which the etiology is unclear requires a special measured approach. The physician's initial assessment of the complaint will likely determine the success or failure of treatment. Perhaps the most important role the physician can play, and the one that is most likely to lead to successful treatment, is helping the patient understand the nature of his or her problem. If, on the other hand, the approach is one that indicates to the patient that the problem has a simple and rapid solution, treatment is likely to be fraught with stress and confrontation between physician and patient. It is beyond the scope of this article to discuss the various approaches one could use in addressing this problem, but in general, psychologic causes of pain should be a paramount focus of investigation. This is *not* to imply that the pain is imaginary. It is unlikely imaginary pain exists. The complaint should be considered legitimate and the patient respected. However, because of the frequency of psychologic causes for this condition and the higher risk of patients' becoming psychologically dependent on (addicted to) drugs, whether psychoactive or analgesic, drugs should be prescribed only if a clear indication for them exists. Nondrug treatments (Table 1) are applicable to treatment of this chronic condition.

### Malignant Painful Conditions

Unfortunately, primary treatment of a significant number of cancer patients fails, and an estimated 80 to 90% of these patients will experience pain as their disease progresses. Ultimately, nondrug treatment methods also fail, and strong narcotics must be used for pain relief. Ample data in the medical literature indicate inadequate treatment of these patients. For this reason, emphasis in this section will be on the drug treatment of malignant pain, although nondrug methods may initially be successful, should be used, and may indeed have continued usefulness as adjuvant treatment with strong narcotics.

**Pain due to Tumor.** In most instances, tumor-related pain is nociceptive, secondary to tumor invasion of or pressure on pain-sensitive structures. Non-narcotics and NSAIDs are useful for mild to moderate pain of this type. In addition, they are useful in combination with narcotics, and the combination seems to have a greater effectiveness than merely the sum of the analgesic strengths. NSAIDs in combination with narcotics are essential in the treatment of bone pain since narcotics alone fail to provide optimum relief for this type of pain.

Narcotics are classified as either pure agonists or agonist/antagonists. Drugs in the latter category have the capacity both to produce the characteristic agonist effects of narcotic drugs and to antagonize, i.e., reverse, them. Table 2 lists drugs in both categories. The pure agonists have almost 100% agonist activity, whereas the agonist/antagonists have predominantly agonist activity but also a significant amount of antagonist activity. The practical clinical significance of this difference in the two drug types is that because of the possibility of the antagonist action causing an abstinence (withdrawal) reaction, agonists/antagonists should not be given sequentially to a patient who has been receiving a pure agonist and may be physically dependent on it. Neither should doses of an agonist be used alternately with doses of an agonist/antagonist in a patient who is not physically dependent on a pure agonist

### TABLE 2. Commonly Used Narcotics

| Pure Agonist | Agonist/Antagonist |
|---|---|
| Morphine | Pentazocine (Talwin) |
| Hydromorphone (Dilaudid) | Butorphanol (Stadol) |
| Levorphanol | Nalbuphine (Nubain) |
| (Levo-Dromoran) | Buprenorphine (Buprenex) |
| Methadone (Dolophine) | |
| Meperidine (Demerol) | |
| Oxycodone (Roxicodone) | |
| Hydrocodone | |
| Codeine | |

because the patient will experience an unpleasant mental feeling, along with less effective pain control.

Chronic pain is best treated by the pure agonists. Studies done in hospices throughout the world, as well as in hospitals and home care settings, have shown that morphine is the drug of choice for treating chronic pain. Morphine is effective orally and, because of its availability in a variety of dosing forms, is acceptable to a majority of pain patients. As discussed earlier, recommended doses of narcotics should be used merely as guidelines for treating chronic pain since the dose required depends on the severity of pain. It is convenient to consider the management of chronic pain as one would consider the management of diabetes mellitus with insulin. There is no predetermined "recommended" or "standard" dose of insulin for the treatment of diabetes mellitus; an adequate dose of insulin is one that will control the diabetes. Likewise, there is no predetermined "recommended" or "standard" dose of morphine, and an adequate dose of morphine is one that will control the pain. To reiterate: *Pain is a natural antagonist to the analgesic and respiratory depressant effects of the opiates; therefore, one is unlikely to experience serious complications from narcotics in the face of unrelieved pain.*

**Pain due to Cancer Treatment.** Pain related to cancer treatment will primarily be due to nerve damage and therefore will be neuropathic. Table 3 outlines the clinical features of neuropathic pain. Significant features in the patient's history that distinguish neuropathic from nociceptive

### TABLE 3. Clinical Features of Neuropathic Pain

Pain onset is delayed after damage.
Pain persists in absence of ongoing obvious stimulus.
Pain sensation is frequently described as burning, electric shock–like, pressure, twisting or torque-like, paroxysmal, brief shooting or stabbing component, and other unfamiliar and strange sensations.
Pain is present in an area of numbness.
Stimulus that does not ordinarily cause pain, for example, touch, now causes pain in the affected area (allodynia).
Repetitive stimuli produce pronounced summation and after-reaction.

pain are the delay in onset after damage occurs and the pain's persistence in the absence of an obvious ongoing stimulus. In addition, the trauma necessary to cause damage to the nerve may seem insignificant, for example, cutting of a minor nerve during a surgical procedure, radiation to tissue, or neurotoxic chemotherapeutic drugs.

Treatment of this type of pain requires a different approach from that for nociceptive pain. Neuropathic pain responds better to drugs that are used primarily for the treatment of psychologic depression (antidepressants) and convulsive disorders (anticonvulsants). Antidepressants have been shown to possess analgesic properties, whereas anticonvulsants have not. Anticonvulsants are indicated for those patients who have an intermittently sharp, or lancinating, component to their pain. Treatment should start with an antidepressant, and if needed, an anticonvulsant can be added.

Treatment with these drugs requires the physician to explain to the patient the difference between the pain relief provided by these drugs and the relief provided by the usual analgesic drugs. Antidepressant and anticonvulsant drugs do not act as dramatically as non-narcotic and narcotic analgesic drugs do because of their different mechanism of action. The first-generation tricyclic compounds, for example, amitriptyline (Elavil), seem to be more effective than the second-, or greater, generation antidepressants, whose mechanism of action is more specific. In addition, the dose required for pain treatment is usually far less than that required for the antidepressant effect.

### Oral versus Parenteral or Novel Routes of Administration

Oral administration of narcotics is the preferred route for all indications for their use. Patients prefer this route because of ease and convenience. Only if this route is not available, for whatever reason, such as nausea or vomiting, should alternative routes be considered. Common parenteral routes of administration are intramuscular, intravenous, and subcutaneous. Novel routes, which are also parenteral, are epidural, intrathecal, and intraventricular. Rectal administration is essentially in the same category as oral administration, although less acceptable to patients.

Physicians often perceive that parenteral routes are preferable to the oral route because of a misunderstanding of biotransformation. Oral analgesics are biotransformed in the liver, after absorption, and portions of the dose are rendered void of their analgesic properties. The proportion

of the dose rendered ineffective varies with the drug prescribed. For example, for an oral dose of morphine to be equianalgesic to a parenteral dose, the oral dose must be larger than the parenteral dose by a factor of 3; i.e., 30 mg must be administered orally to achieve the equianalgesic effect of 10 mg administered parenterally. However, the "larger" oral dose is illusory, because biotransformation allows exactly the *same* amount of morphine, whether given as the "larger" oral dose or the "smaller" parenteral dose, to arrive at the binding sites of the central nervous system where pain control occurs. For this reason, physicians should acquaint themselves thoroughly with a limited number of narcotic analgesics in order to prescribe effectively for their patients.

# NAUSEA AND VOMITING

method of
EDITH P. MITCHELL, M.D.
*University of Missouri—Columbia*
*Columbia, Missouri*

Nausea and vomiting are controlled by a vomiting center in the medullary lateral reticular formation of the brain. The vomiting center lies close to the chemoreceptor trigger zone (CTZ) in the area postrema of the fourth ventricle and receives input from the cerebral cortex, primary sensory centers, cranial nerves, CTZ, and gastrointestinal tract. Emesis results when the vomiting center is stimulated from the CTZ or from afferent fibers in the cerebral cortex, gastrointestinal tract (particularly the duodenum), heart, and vestibular apparatus. Other processes known to stimulate the CTZ are various chemicals, drugs and toxic substances including apomorphine, cytotoxic agents, irradiation, uremia, and increased intracranial pressure. Impulses from the vomiting center are transmitted to the striated muscle of the thorax and abdomen and the smooth muscles of the gastrointestinal tract to initiate the vomiting reflex.

The mechanism by which the compounds interact with the CTZ or how impulses are initiated is not known. Several neurotransmitters appear to be involved, including dopamine, histamine, acetylcholine, serotonin, and endorphins.

## CAUSES OF NAUSEA AND VOMITING

Nausea and vomiting are common symptoms that may complicate diseases inside or outside the gastrointestinal tract and may be consequent to therapy. The objectives of management are to identify and treat the underlying causes. Some common causes of vomiting are given in Table 1. The recommended approach to management involves noting the onset, frequency, and severity of vomiting and the absence or presence of

TABLE 1. **Common Causes of Nausea and Vomiting**

Antineoplastic agents and irradiation
Gastrointestinal tract tumors, obstruction, and perforation
Disorders of gastrointestinal motility
Peptic ulcer disease and gastritis
Pancreatic tumors and pancreatitis
Cholelithiasis and cholecystitis
Chronic hepatic diseases
Infections
Intracranial processes—tumors, migraine, elevated intracranial pressure
Vestibular dysfunction
Motion sickness
Metabolic causes—ketoacidosis, uremia, hypercalcemia
Adrenal insufficiency
Medications—analgesics, digoxin, theophylline, anesthesia
Psychogenic causes

pain; and identifying predisposing factors such as previous abdominal surgery, chemotherapy, irradiation, infection, and congestive heart failure. Assessment of hydration and circulatory status is critical to management.

*Emesis Caused by Antineoplastic Agents*

Nausea and vomiting are the two most common and distressing complications of cancer chemotherapy and may result in medical complications such as esophageal tears, fractures, wound dehiscence, and anorexia; or metabolic complications such as volume depletion, electrolyte imbalance, weight loss, and metabolic alkalosis. Great variability is evident in the emetic properties of antineoplastic drugs, although specific agents such as cisplatin (Platinol), nitrogen mustard (Mustargen), dacarbazine (DTIC-Dome), and streptozocin (Zanosar) produce vomiting in virtually all patients. Table 2 outlines the emetic potential of commonly used antineoplastic agents.

The severity and duration of nausea and vomiting are affected by multiple variables, including dose and schedule of chemotherapy administration, and vary among patients, but may also be influenced by other factors. Table 3 outlines the factors influencing emesis caused by antineoplastic agents. Structural anatomic changes to the gastrointestinal tract from previous surgery, hepatic disease, or other concomitant medications may contribute to the nausea and vomiting experienced by patients. The psychologic state of the patient will greatly affect the amount of emesis experienced and the perception of its severity. Anticipatory

vomiting is a well-described entity reported in nearly 25% of patients and may be ameliorated by the prophylactic administration of antiemetics prior to giving chemotherapy.

## TREATMENT

### Antiemetic Agents

Management of nausea and vomiting associated with chemotherapy requires judicious use of various classes of antiemetics by the most effective and judicious route. Compounds that exert an effect on the CTZ, such as the phenothiazines, have shown the greatest potential as antiemetics. Antihistamines, which may be beneficial in motion sickness, have shown limited effectiveness in emesis associated with cancer chemotherapy. The commonly used antiemetics and their recommended doses are given in Table 4. The psychologic effect of treatment, however, is emphasized by the studies that have shown placebo treatment to be effective. Clinical management involves pharmacologic intervention, patient support, education, and behavioral or psychologic intervention.

**Phenothiazines.** The phenothiazine derivatives are the most commonly prescribed class of antiemetics and exhibit their major mode of action through disruption of dopaminergic transmission in the CTZ. They are well absorbed orally, parenterally, and rectally. Studies indicate that the halogenated derivatives with piperazine side chains—prochlorperazine (Compazine), thiethylperazine (Torecan), and perphenazine (Trilafon)—have greater activity than chlorpromazine (Thorazine). In a randomized double-blind study, the effectiveness of several antiemetic drugs was compared with placebo therapy in patients receiving 5-fluorouracil (Adrucil). Ten milligrams of thiopropazate* and 5 mg of prochlorperazine (phenothiazine derivatives) given orally three times daily demonstrated superior antiemetic effects compared with placebo. Major side effects of the phenothiazines include autonomic dysfunc-

*Not available in the United States.

TABLE 2. **Emetic Potential of Chemotherapeutic Drugs**

| High | Moderately High | Moderate | Low |
|---|---|---|---|
| Cisplatin | Semustine | 5-Fluorouracil | Busulfan |
| Dacarbazine | Carmustine | | Bleomycin |
| Mechlorethamine | Lomustine | Daunorubicin | 6-Thioguanine |
| Streptozocin | Cyclophosphamide | L-Asparaginase | |
| | Actinomycin D | Mitomycin C | Hydroxyurea |
| | Mithramycin | 5-Azacytidine | Etoposide |
| | Hexamethylmelamine | Melphalan | Vincristine |
| | Doxorubicin | Mitoxantrone | Vinblastine |
| | | Ifosfamide | Chlorambucil |

TABLE 3. **Factors Influencing Emesis Induced by Cancer Chemotherapy**

Structural and anatomic changes in the gastrointestinal tract
Concomitant use of other potentially emetic medications
Location of tumor
Psychologic state of patient
Emesis with previous chemotherapy
Chronic liver disease due to other causes
Antiemetic regimen
Prophylactic use of antiemetics
Alcohol use history

tion, hypotension, sedation, hepatotoxicity, and extrapyramidal effects. Extrapyramidal reactions can be treated with or prevented with diphenhydramine (Benadryl). Higher doses and intravenous administration, as in many investigational protocols, have allowed further improvement of the therapeutic efficacy, although these methods may be associated with increased adverse reactions.

**Substituted Benzamides.** Metoclopramide (Reglan) is the most frequently used drug of this class and is the only first line drug approved by the Food and Drug Administration for controlling chemotherapy-induced nausea and vomiting. Metoclopramide increases lower esophageal pressures and enhances gastric emptying, although other central effects contribute to its antiemetic activity. Intravenous administration and high oral dose have demonstrated efficacy. The adverse reactions observed in this class of compounds include mild sedation, akathisia, diarrhea, and acute dystonic reactions. With regimens containing lorazepam (Ativan) or diphenhydramine, akathisia and dystonic reaction are greatly reduced. The side effects may be relieved by orally or intravenously administered diphenhydramine. Concomitant administration of diphenhydramine, 25 to 50 mg, may prevent dystonic reactions.

**Butyrophenomes.** Haloperidol (Haldol) and droperidol (Inapsine) are the more commonly used drugs in the class and are structurally and pharmacologically similar to the phenothiazines. The major mechanism of action is dopaminergic interruption in the CTZ. The major side effect is sedation, and droperidol can only be given intravenously.

**Cannabinoids.** The cannabinoids dronabinol

TABLE 4. **Dosages and Schedules of Frequently Used Antiemetic Agents**

| | Trade Name | Common Dosage and Administration |
|---|---|---|
| *Phenothiazines* | | |
| Chlorpromazine | Thorazine | 10–25 mg PO q 4–6 hr; 10–25 mg IV q 3–4 hr; 50–100 mg rectally q 6–8 hr |
| Prochlorperazine | Compazine | 5–10 mg PO q 4–6 hr; 5–10 mg IM q 4–6 hr; 10–40 mg IV q 3 hr; 25 mg suppository q 4–6 hr |
| Thiethylperazine | Torecan | 10 mg PO, IM, or rectally q 6–8 hr |
| Perphenazine | Trilafon | 8–16 mg PO q d in divided doses |
| Promethazine | Phenergan | 25 mg PO, rectally, or IM q 4–6 hr |
| *Butyrophenones* | | |
| Haloperidol | Haldol | 1–3 mg q 2–6 hr IV |
| Droperidol | Inapsine | 1–2 mg PO or IM q 6–8 hr; 0.5–2.5 mg IV q 4 hr |
| *Substituted Benzamides* | | |
| Metoclopramide | Reglan | 1–3 mg/kg q 2 hr IV; 10 mg PO 30 min before meals |
| *Corticosteroids* | | |
| Dexamethasone | Decadron | 4–20 mg PO or IV q 4–6 hrs |
| Methylprednisolone | Solu-Medrol | 250–500 mg IV q 4–6 hrs |
| *Cannabinoids* | | |
| Dronabinol | Marinol | 5–10 mg/m$^2$ PO q 3–4 hr |
| Nabilone | Cesamet | 1–2 mg PO q 12 hr. |
| *Antihistamines* | | |
| Dimenhydrinate | Dramamine | 50 mg PO or IV q 4–6 hr |
| Meclizine | Antivert | 20–50 mg PO q 24 hr |
| Diphenhydramine | Benadryl | 25–50 mg PO or IV q 3–4 hrs |
| Hydroxyzine | Vistaril | 25–100 mg PO or IV q 6–8 hrs |
| *Anticholinergic* | | |
| Scopolamine | Transderm Scop | 1 patch behind ear q 3 days |
| *Miscellaneous* | | |
| Trimethobenzamide | Tigan | 100 mg PO or IM q 4–6 hr |
| Benzquinamide | Emete-Con | 50 mg IM q 3–4 hr; 25 mg IV (single dose, 1 mg/min) |
| Lorazepam | Ativan | 1–1.5 mg/m$^2$ IV q 4–6 hr |

(Marinol) and nabilone (Cesamet) have demonstrated efficacy in chemotherapy-induced nausea and vomiting and are specifically approved for this indication, but they are recommended for patients who fail to respond to standard antiemetic therapy. The mechanism of the antiemetic effect is not known. Adverse reactions include dizziness, somnolence, euphoria, ataxia, hypotension, and dysphoria and are more commonly seen in patients receiving high doses (above 15 mg per $m^2$) and in the elderly.

**Miscellaneous.** Lorazepam is the first benzodiazepine with well-documented antiemetic efficacy. Major adverse effects are sedation, prolonged amnesia, hypotension, and urinary incontinence. Antihistamines are effective in vestibular-mediated nausea and vomiting but have shown little effects on chemotherapy-induced emesis. However, their major role is in the prevention of extrapyramidal reactions. Scopolamine, an anticholinergic, has some usefulness. Barbiturates have no proven efficacy as single agents; however, their use in combination regimens has been advocated.

**Costicosteroids.** The glucocorticoids dexamethasone (Decadron) and methylprednisone (Medrol) have demonstrated antiemetic activity as single agents when compared with placebo. The mechanism of action remains unclear. Additional caution must be observed in patients with diabetes. Costicosteroids are extremely useful when combined with other agents.

### Combination Antiemetic Therapy

Combinations of antiemetic drugs provide superior management of symptoms than standard doses of single agents. The basic goal is to combine drugs with different mechanisms of activity and different side effects to allow enhanced tolerance. The most commonly used regimens combine the three drugs metoclopramide, dexamethasone, and lorazepam in varying doses. Other antiemetic combinations are given in Table 5.

### Delayed Emesis

Delayed emesis is defined as nausea and vomiting developing or persisting 24 hours or more following drug delivery. Nausea and vomiting can last 5 to 7 days and may cause profound symptoms. Continuation of oral antiemetic therapy for a period of days is an effective and safe method of controlling this problem. Two such regimens are given in Table 6.

### Anticipatory Emesis

Nearly 25% of patients exhibit this conditioned response, especially with poor control of emesis

TABLE 5. **Combination Antiemetic Regimens**

| | | |
|---|---|---|
| 1. | Metoclopramide | 2 mg/kg IV |
| | Dexamethasone | 20 mg IV |
| | Lorazepam | 1.5 mg/$m^2$ IV |
| 2. | Chlorpromazine | 25 mg IM |
| | Droperidol | 1 mg IV |
| | Methylprednisolone | 250 mg IV |
| 3. | Prochlorperazine | 10 mg IV |
| | Dexamethasone | 10 mg IV |

with prior chemotherapy. The prevalence of this syndrome may be reduced by the prophylactic administration of antiemetic therapy in patients receiving highly emetic chemotherapy.

### Nausea and Vomiting in Pregnancy

Morning or evening nausea and vomiting occur in 50 to 80% of women during the first trimester of pregnancy. Symptoms characteristically begin at the fourth to sixth week and end after the fourth or fifth month, but occasionally this problem may persist well into the second trimester of gestation. Although the nausea and vomiting may be quite distressing, this problem exerts no adverse effects on the pregnancy and does not presage other complications, though it is more common with multiple pregnancy and hydatidiform mole.

Hyperemesis gravidarum refers to persistent, protracted vomiting of pregnancy, causing nutritional deficiencies or acidosis or fluid and electrolyte disturbances.

The cause of nausea and vomiting during pregnancy is believed to be physiologically elevated estrogen levels. The incidence is not increased by parity, and patients do not have an increased incidence of toxemia of pregnancy or spontaneous abortion; the babies are usually not underweight or deformed.

For mild symptoms, reassurance and dietary advice are all that is required. Antiemetics are generally unnecessary. Pyridoxine (vitamin $B_6$), 50 to 100 mg per day orally, may be beneficial in some patients. The most commonly used drugs, if pharmacologic therapy is needed, are pheno-

TABLE 6. **Antiemetics for Delayed Emesis**

| Drug | Dosage and Schedule |
|---|---|
| 1. Metoclopramide | 0.5 mg/kg PO qid for 4 days |
| Dexamethasone | 8 mg PO bid for 2 days, followed by 4 mg bid for 2 days |
| 2. Prochlorperazine | 25 mg spansule PO q 6–8 hr for 4 days |
| Dexamethasone | 4 mg PO qid for 2 days, followed by 2 mg qid for 2 days, followed by 0.5 mg qid for 1 day |

thiazines and antihistamines. Prochlorperazine is effective in controlling nausea and vomiting associated with pregnancy. Metoclopramide may be helpful in the treatment of hyperemesis gravidarum. A sonogram should be taken because of the incidence of hydatidiform mole and multiple births. Studies have shown no association of either of these two drugs with teratogenic effects or congenital malformations. However, these drugs are not currently approved by the Food and Drug Administration, nor are there any drugs approved for this indication.

Management of nausea and vomiting of pregnancy should not involve drug therapy unless absolutely necessary. Initial treatment of patients with mild symptoms should include rest, frequent small meals, and reassurance. Hospitalization and intravenous fluids may be required for more severe symptoms. Although risks to the fetus appeared to be limited in previous clinical trials, drug therapy should only be instituted if protracted symptoms persist despite appropriate supportive measures.

### Postanesthesia Nausea and Vomiting

The incidence of nausea and vomiting during the perioperative and postoperative period is a major complication and occurs in nearly 80% of patients. The risks of nausea and vomiting include the surgical procedure and site, intraoperative complications, age, sex, duration of anesthesia, and type of preanesthetic and anesthetic. Postoperative complications are more likely to occur in patients who have pre-existing disease. Effective use of postoperative monitoring and avoidance of gastric inflation may help prevent this complication. Decreased morbidity is noted in patients who have adequate pain relief and who have no complications of hypertension, myocardial ischemia, dysrhythmias, hypotension, and hypercarbia. An increased incidence is noted in patients following gastrointestinal surgery, especially peptic ulcer disease.

General measures include treatment of underlying postoperative complications and judicious use of individualized drug therapy. Phenothiazines and antihistamines are useful antiemetics. Prochlorperazine, chlorpromazine, haloperidol, and benzamides are all effective but may cause prolonged somnolence, sedation, hypotension, and extrapyramidal reactions.

### Motion Sickness

The mechanism of motion sickness is not known. It develops when visual and vestibular inputs into the vestibulo-ocular reflex signal conflicting information about movement over an extended period of time. Symptoms related to autonomic dysfunction such as sweating, salivation, vomiting, and malaise develop. Motion sickness appears to depend on central cholinergic mechanisms and may be ameliorated or prevented by decreasing visceral sensations of motion as well as visual vineal stimulation. Reduction of anxiety with sedatives or psychotherapy offers benefit in some patients. Small meals of bland foods during the trip may reduce the tendency for nausea and vomiting. Anticholinergics and antihistamines are the most commonly used therapeutic agents and prophylactic administration is recommended in patients with severe symptoms. Scopolamine dimenhydrinate (Dramamine), cyclizine (Marezine), and meclizine (Antivert) are the most commonly used medications. The combination of promethazine (Phenergan), a phenothiazine, and ephedrine may provide relief in some patients. The symptoms of motion sickness vary in time and usually disappear immediately following cessation of motion.

# GASEOUSNESS AND INDIGESTION

method of
ROBERT F. WILLENBUCHER, M.D., and
WILLIAM J. SNAPE, Jr., M.D.
*Harbor-UCLA Medical Center*
*Torrance, California*

## GASEOUSNESS

Gaseousness, frequently associated with mild abdominal pain, represents a common primary care complaint. Increased stomach gas results in belching, whereas increased colonic gas results in flatus. Chronic eructation is secondary to air swallowing (aerophagy). Although aerophagy is associated with a variety of abdominal or thoracic disorders that cause discomfort, it is usually secondary to habit and does not contribute significantly to expelled flatus. There is convincing evidence that the majority of these patients with a chief complaint of "gas" do not have flatus production that is outside the range of normal (200 to 2000 ml per day). Because there are few readily available tests to confirm the production of excess flatus, the physician is usually forced to rely on historical information. Asking the patient to quantify the number of passages of flatus per day may be a crude indicator of intestinal gas production (average approximately 14 discrete passages per day). Hydrogen breath testing may be useful in these patients, since breath hydrogen appears to be correlated with colonic hydrogen production. However, hydrogen breath testing is also not widely available.

Colonic fermentation of sugars (especially lactose) and starches (oligo- and polysaccharides), which cannot be digested by the small bowel, is the major source of expelled flatus. Dietary sources of these substances include dairy products; a variety of fruits, vegetables, and legumes; and flours, including wheat, oat, corn, and potato flours. Only rice flour appears to be completely absorbed. Delayed colonic transit may contribute to gas production, as it allows for increased contact time of substrate with colonic flora.

Because most patients with complaints of abdominal pain, bloating, and gas will not actually have excess flatus, it is likely that the symptoms represent an underlying motility disorder—i.e. the irritable bowel syndrome (IBS). As with all patients with IBS, care should be taken to exclude organic disease of the colon. Patients with eructation, especially if recent in onset, should be carefully questioned for the presence of newly acquired abdominal or thoracic symptoms (cough, dyspnea, chest-abdominal discomfort). Any suggestion of organic disease should be fully investigated.

### Treatment

Patients with IBS respond best to treatment directed toward improving bowel function and alleviating symptoms. This is accomplished with judicious use of bulking agents, anticholinergics, bowel training, and reassurance. Treatment of eructation also requires reassurance and fostering patient awareness of air swallowing.

For patients with true excess intestinal gas production, dietary manipulations are most likely to be successful. Stepwise elimination of flatugenic foods such as milk and milk products, beans, onions, prunes, raisins, Brussels sprouts, and non-rice flours should be undertaken. If dietary manipulations are unsuccessful, pharmacotherapy can be considered (Table 1). Simethicone (Mylicon), activated charcoal, and enzyme preparations have been used in the past, but there is little evidence that they offer a significant advantage over placebo. Still, a trial of simethicone or activated charcoal may be justified. Prokinetic agents have also been advocated, but these agents were studied in heterogeneous patient groups in whom gastroesophageal reflux appeared to predominate. Because the currently available prokinetic agents have variable effects on colonic transit, it is unlikely that they would be uniformly effective. Cisapride,* a prokinetic agent with colonic effects currently under investigation in the United States, may prove to be useful in IBS patients with disordered transit as well as in selected patients with excess flatus.

### INDIGESTION

Indigestion is an imperfect term that describes symptoms from a heterogeneous group of disorders. This multiplicity of definitions may lead to much confusion for both the patient and the practitioner. For the sake of this discussion, indigestion will be synonymous with dyspepsia, which is defined as an upper abdominal pain or discomfort with or without relation to meals. A variety of disorders are associated with upper abdominal pain, including peptic ulcer disease, gastric cancer, gastroesophageal reflux, pancreatobiliary disease, and irritable bowel syndrome (IBS). Gastroesophageal reflux and pancreatobiliary disease usually can be differentiated from the others on the basis of historical risk factors and characteristic symptomatology. Abdominal pain and a disordered bowel habit suggest IBS. Of the remaining patients, in whom gastroesophageal reflux, pancreatobiliary disease, and IBS have been excluded, the majority will have nonulcer dyspepsia or essential dyspepsia in which no anatomic etiology can be identified. Excess gastric acid, environmental factors (e.g., smoking, analgesics), and psychosocial factors do not seem to play an etiologic role. The roles of disordered gastroduodenal motility and *Helicobacter*

---

*Investigational drug in the United States.

TABLE 1. **Treatment of Excessive Flatus**

| Medication | Dosage | Comments |
|---|---|---|
| *Bulking Agents* | | |
| Psyllium seed (Metamucil) | Individualized (1 tsp to 3 tbsp daily) | Increase dose gradually |
| *Anticholinergics* | | |
| Dicyclomine (Bentyl) | 10–20 mg PO qid | Appropriate when irritable bowel syndrome (IBS) is present |
| *Antiflatulents* | | |
| Simethicone (Mylicon-125) | 1 tab PO qid | After dietary manipulations have been attempted |
| Activated charcoal (Charcocaps) | 1 cap PO qid | |

TABLE 2. **Treatment of Indigestion**

| Medication | Dosage | Comments |
|---|---|---|
| *Antacids* | 30 ml 3–6 times daily | |
| *H₂ Blockers** | | |
| Cimetidine (Tagamet) | 300 mg PO qid | Patients over 40 or those not responding |
| Ranitidine (Zantac) | 150 mg PO bid | completely to empiric therapy should |
| Famotidine (Pepcid) | 20 mg PO bid | be investigated with upper endoscopy |
| *Anticholinergics* | | |
| Dichyclomine (Bentyl) | 10–20 mg PO qid | Appropriate when irritable bowel syndrome (IBS) is present |
| *Bismuth Preparations* | | |
| Bismuth subsalicylate (Pepto-Bismol) | 2 tabs PO qid | If *Helicobacter pylori* is demonstrated by endoscopic biopsies |
| *Prokinetic Agents* | | |
| Metoclopramide† (Reglan) | 10 mg PO 1/2 hr before meals and at bedtime | Only for patients with proven gastric stasis, as CNS side effects occur |

*This use of H₂ blockers is not listed in the manufacturer's official directive.
†This use of metaclopramide is not listed in the manufacturer's official directive.

*pylori* (formerly identified as *Campylobacter pylori*) remain controversial.

### Treatment

After the exclusion of the more readily identifiable disorders discussed earlier, patients less than 40 years of age with mild symptoms of recent onset can be treated empirically with antacids or H₂ blockers* (Table 2). Patients with severe or chronic symptoms, those with constitutional symptoms, and those who fail to respond to empiric therapy or who are more than 40 years old should have upper endoscopy to exclude the possibility of a gastric malignancy. Unless constitutional symptoms are present or pancreatobiliary disease is suspected, further tests, such as ultrasound or computed tomography, are usually of low yield. Treatment of essential dyspepsia is difficult. A trial of antacids or H₂ blockers may be successful, but these have no consistent advantage over placebo. If there is overlap with IBS, a trial of anticholinergics and treatment of constipation is reasonable after colonic pathology has been excluded. Patients who have normal upper endoscopic findings should have gastric (antral) biopsies at the time of the original examination to detect the presence of *Helicobacter pylori* and its related gastritis. *H. pylori* can be eradicated with bismuth preparations, although the addition of an antibiotic (e.g., amoxicillin) may be required. The symptomatic response to *H. pylori* eradication has been mixed. In patients with persistent symptoms, a radionuclide test of gastric emptying and, if abnormal, treatment with a prokinetic agent are warranted.

*This use of H₂ blockers is not listed in the manufacturer's official directive.

# ACUTE INFECTIOUS DIARRHEA

method of
ROBERT STEFFEN, M.D.
*University of Zurich*
*Zurich, Switzerland*

and

KLAUS E. GYR, M.D., M.P.H. & T.M.
*University of Basel*
*Basel, Switzerland*

Every day, in developing countries, 12,000 children die of acute, infectious diarrhea, 80% of whom are under 1 year of age. In many of these countries, diarrheal diseases are the leading cause of death and account for the greatest proportion of years of potential life lost. Even if the impact of acute diarrhea is less severe in our well-nourished population, dehydration and electrolyte imbalance are potentially fatal anywhere. Infants, the elderly, and malnourished persons are especially at risk of developing serious complications.

Definitions of acute diarrhea vary depending on the diet and the age of the patient. Usually acute diarrhea is defined as increased number of stools (greater than or equal to three or four per 24 hours, or less if accompanied by additional symptoms such as abdominal cramps, tenesmus, nausea, vomiting, fever, and blood with or without mucus in stools), increased water content of the stools (watery or pasty stools), and increased stool volume over a period not exceeding 2 weeks. Diarrheal episodes lasting longer are referred to as persistent diarrhea according to the World Health Organization (WHO). Grossly bloody stools and fever are indicative of invasive disease (dysentery) having damaged the intestinal mucosa, even if the stool volume is small.

No firm conclusions can be drawn from the symptoms or severity of the illness to the causative agent; for example, contrary to expectations *Shigella* may sometimes lead to mild watery diarrheas and some types of

*Escherichia coli* to severe bloody diarrheas. A careful history will indicate the severity and the chronology of the illness and will help distinguish infectious diarrhea from food poisoning (outbreak with short incubation time, symptoms usually less than 24 hours); osmotic diarrhea secondary to saline laxatives, some antacids, carbohydrate and other malabsorption syndromes, or alcohol; and the secretory diarrhea caused by irritative laxatives (such as castor oil and cascara). Ulcerative colitis, Crohn's disease, and occasionally malignant tumors may also begin as acute diarrhea. A broader differential diagnosis is needed in persistent diarrhea.

## LABORATORY WORK-UP

Acute infectious diarrhea in industrialized nations persisting after a few days of empiric treatment requires further assessment. Food handlers should always have their stools cultured. A positive test for fecal leukocytes (using a thin layer on a slide, with a drop of methylene blue added; five or more per high-power field is positive), grossly bloody stools, fever, rectal tenderness on examination, or severe diarrhea warrants a stool culture for invasive pathogens, such as *Helicobacter jejuni, Salmonella* spp., *Shigella* spp., *Yersinia enterocolitica, Vibrio parahaemolyticus, Aeromonas,* and *Plesiomonas.* If sheets of leukocytes are absent, one would concentrate on the investigation of enterotoxigenic organisms. Diarrhea following antibiotics may require stool cultures for *Clostridium difficile,* but for a proper diagnosis, direct evidence of *C. difficile* toxin either in the stool or from isolated organisms is required. Diarrhea persisting after travel to developing countries should primarily be assessed for various types of *E. coli, Salmonella, Shigella, Helicobacter, Aeromonas, Plesiomonas,* and parasites. Parasites can be evaluated in watery stools immediately after voiding or in samples preserved in polyvinylalcohol (PVA), merthiolate iodine formalin (MIF), or sodium acetate–acetic acid formalin (SAF) solutions. Serologic tests—e.g., for *Giardia*—cross-react widely with other protozoa. However, even with an elaborate and costly work-up, no more than two-thirds of the microbial agents will be detected. Apparently a large proportion of those that cannot be found by routine examination are of bacterial origin in adults; in children, viruses may play a greater role.

## CHARACTERISTICS OF THERAPEUTIC AGENTS

**Oral Rehydration.** Oral rehydration therapy (ORT) is the keystone of all national diarrheal disease control programs in developing countries because it is simple, highly effective, and inexpensive. A solution prepared from oral rehydration salts (ORS) is used both to treat clinically evident dehydration and to prevent dehydration. ORS contains, in grams per liter: NaCl, 3.5; trisodium citrate, 2.9 (or $NaHCO_3$, 2.5); KCl, 1.5; and glucose, 20. In the United States, Rehydralyte is a similar commercial preparation. ORT is effective because glucose-coupled sodium transport and absorption by the small intestine continue during the course of infection. Although ORT is highly effective for combating dehydration and its consequences, it does not diminish the amount or duration of diarrhea, which leads to a lack of confidence, particularly in mothers and in rushed travelers. Therefore, a new generation of ORS is currently being developed in which glucose has been replaced by polymers of glucose, individual amino acids, or cereals. Such cereal-based "improved ORS" requires cooking of, e.g., rice flour, and is not yet suitable for packaging in sachets.

The amount of ORT is 5% of body weight in mild, 6 to 9% in moderate, and 10% in severe dehydration, to be administered within 4 to 6 hours. ORT should be fed in small quantities at regular intervals. Plain water may also be given to minimize the monotony and the nausea or vomiting induced by ORS. After rehydration, the ongoing losses through stool or vomiting are corrected, using maintenance solutions with smaller amounts of sodium (40 to 50 mEq per liter)—e.g., Infalyte, Lytren, Pedialyte, and Resol. Cola drinks should be avoided because they contain caffeine, which may increase intestinal motility. ORT should be replaced by intravenous therapy only in rare cases of incessant vomiting with signs of dehydration either reappearing or worsening, or in unconsciousness.

**Antimotility Agents.** Opiates and their derivatives, such as codeine and paregoric, as well as loperamide (Imodium) and the less effective diphenoxylate (Lomotil) act primarily through their antimotility properties. None is recommended in infants and small children because the benefits are modest and they may cause serious adverse reactions. In dysenteric illness, such agents may prolong and worsen the symptoms; in severe diarrhea, they may cause fluid to pool within the bowel. On the other hand, loperamide given jointly with an antimicrobial agent brought faster relief than an antimicrobial agent alone in traveler's diarrhea.

**Antisecretory Drugs.** Chlorpromazine (Thorazine) and nicotinic acid (Nicobid), which inhibit adenyl cyclase; salicylic acid, indomethacin (Indocin), and somatostatin, which inhibit prostaglandin synthesis or induced secretion; and berberine have shown some benefit in experimental studies, but because of important side effects and/or limited efficacy, none can be recommended for routine treatment of acute diarrhea.

**Aciduric Bacteria.** Although normal aciduric bacteria in the human intestine inhibit the growth of certain bacterial pathogens, *Lactobacillus acidophilus, Bifidobacterium,* and *Streptococcus faecium* have hardly shown any beneficial effect in the treatment of acute diarrhea. The same applies for *Saccharomyces boulardii*.

**Adsorbents.** Charcoal, kaolin, and other adsorbents can bind and inactivate bacterial toxins, but results of clinical use have been disappointing. Moreover, some of these agents interfered with the beneficial effect of tetracycline (Sumycin). Studies to evaluate the antidiarrheal properties of cholestyramine (Questran) are under way.

**Antimicrobial Agents.** Antibiotics and other chemotherapeutic agents have been shown to reduce the severity and duration of dysenteric disease, as well as of cholera (tetracycline, in rare cases of resistance to trimethoprim-sulfamethoxazole, [Bacteria Septra], furazolidone [Furoxone], chloramphenicol [Chloromycetin], or erythromycin [ERYC, E-Mycin, E.E.S.]), of diarrhea due to *Helicobacter jejuni* (erythromycin to be started on the first day of illness), and of diarrhea caused by *Shigella* (depending on the resistance of isolates in the area—e.g., trimethoprim-sulfamethoxazole, ampicillin [Polycillin, Omnipen]). Antibiotics are not useful for treatment of nontyphoidal salmonellosis except when bacteremia develops.

No single antimicrobial agent has proved to be of value for the routine treatment of acute diarrhea; their use is often unnecessary and possibly disadvantageous because of adverse reactions, such as diarrhea or allergic rash. Bismuth subsalicylate (Pepto-Bismol), which may be considered a topical antimicrobial, results in only a modest improvement in acute diarrhea.

**Antiparasitic Agents.** Metronidazole (Flagyl) or the possibly even more effective ornidazole or tinidazole (not available in the U.S.) may be used. These agents, except for causing some nausea, are well tolerated. In amebiasis, such therapy may be combined with the use of diloxanide furoate. In giardiasis, quinacrine or furazolidone (Fluroxone [particularly in children]) may be used instead of nitroimidazoles.

## TREATMENT

The therapeutic regimen of acute diarrhea depends on its severity, the age of the patient, and his or her location (for dosages, see Table 1).

**Diarrhea in Native Populations in Developing Countries.** Oral or, if necessary, intravenous rehydration is the treatment of choice. Some practitioners tend to use also antibiotics and antidiarrheal agents, but these are necessary only in some patients with dysenteric symptoms and in cholera. Otherwise, they may even be harmful and are a burden on the meager budget of poor families.

**Diarrhea in Travelers Abroad.** One-third of the residents of industrialized countries who visit developing countries experience at least one episode of diarrhea. Travelers should have appropriate standby medication for self-therapy because they usually have a tight schedule and because they should preferably not consult doctors nor buy over-the-counter drugs in these countries. In all cases of traveler's diarrhea, the fastest cure is obtained by using loperamide (Imodium) and tri-

TABLE 1. **Dosage of Antidiarrheal Agents in Adults and Children**

| Drug | Adult Dosage | Pediatric Dosage |
|---|---|---|
| Oral rehydration-salts (ORS) | See text | See text |
| Loperamide (Imodium) 2-mg capsules 1-mg/5-ml liquid | 4 mg, then 2 mg after each loose stool to a maximum of 16 mg/day | 2–5 yr: 1 mg three times on day 1 |
| Bismuth subsalicylate (Pepto-Bismol) | 30 ml q 30 min for eight doses If needed, repeat on day 2 | 3–8 yr: 5 ml q 30 min for eight doses 6–9 yr: 10 ml q 30 min for eight doses 9–12 yr: 15 ml q 30 min for eight doses If needed, repeat on day 2 |
| Trimethoprim-sulfamethoxazole DS tablets 160/800 mg, or suspension 40/200 mg per 5 ml (Bactrim, Septra) | One DS tablet q 12 hr for 2–3 days | 0.5 ml/kg q 12 hr for 3 days: do not exceed adult dosage |
| Trimethoprim (Proteoprim, Trimpex) | 200 mg q 12 hr for 3–5 days | — |
| Norfloxacin (Noroxin) | 400 mg q 12 hr for 3–5 days | — |
| Ciprofloxacin (Cipro) | 500 mg q 12 hr for 3–5 days | — |
| Furazolidone (Furoxone), 100-mg tablets, 50-mg/15 ml liquid | 100 mg q 6 hr for 3–5 days | 8 mg/kg/day in three doses for *Giardia* for 7 days |
| Metronidazole (Flagyl) For *Giardia* For *Entamoeba histolytica* | 2 grams daily for 3 days 750 mg q 8 hr for 5 days | Use furazolidone 50 mg/kg/day in three doses for 10 days |
| Ornidazole, tinidazole (not available in U.S.) | Usually single dose | Usually single dose |

methoprim-sulfamethoxazole (Bactrim DS, Septra DS) usually for 1 to 3 days only. The mean duration of illness is reduced to 1 hour. For mild to moderate traveler's diarrhea without dysenteric symptoms, loperamide (Imodium) alone or bismuth subsalicylate (Pepto-Bismol) may be sufficient medication. Rehydration and electrolyte replacement can usually be achieved by fluid replacement (tea with sugar, orange juice) and by eating salted food. ORT is indicated for infants, children, and elderly patients. If traveler's diarrhea or other gastrointestinal symptoms persist after such empiric treatment over 1 to 2 weeks abroad or for a few days after returning home, a laboratory work-up is indicated. This may reveal *Entamoeba histolytica, Giardia lamblia,* or other pathogenic agents that require specific treatment usually beyond the possibilities of self-medication.

**Diarrhea in Patients in Industrialized Countries.** In infants, small children, and elderly patients, ORT as described earlier is the keystone to treatment. In older children and adults, it is usually sufficient to remind the patients of plentiful fluid intake.

Except for fecal leukocyte tests, all laboratory investigations require a few days, during which the adult patient may become impatient if specific treatment is withheld. In mild to moderate acute diarrhea without dysenteric symptoms, loperamide will usually bring fast relief; often, no further treatment is necessary. In severe or dysenteric diarrhea, trimethoprim-sulfamethoxazole (Bactrim DS, Septra DS), norfloxacin (Noroxin), ciprofloxacin (Cipro), or furazolidone (Furoxone) may be given if treatment is necessary before stool culture results are available. Thereafter, standard treatment for identified organisms is given, if the respective organism is to be treated by antimicrobial agents. Antibiotics are by no means not always indicated. However, they should be used more generously in infants under 2 months of age and in other patients with a high risk of bacteremia and complications thereof (e.g., patients with prosthetic valves).

## NUTRITIONAL ASPECTS OF ACUTE DIARRHEA AND PROPHYLAXIS

**Prophylaxis of Traveler's Diarrhea.** The risk of traveler's diarrhea can be reduced by selecting food and drink carefully. Generally safe foods include those served steaming hot, fruits that can be peeled by oneself, and bread; safe drinks include hot coffee or tea, carbonated beverages, bottled water, beer, and wine. Many travelers succumb to the temptation of room temperature buffets including cooked food that may have been recontaminated, salads, sauces, or desserts; they may also use ice cubes in their drinks. Raw or undercooked shellfish, seafood, and meat are especially dangerous, as they may transmit hepatitis A, flukes, tapeworms, trichinosis, etc.

Chemoprophylaxis of traveler's diarrhea is usually not encouraged because of the effective means for self-therapy. It is mainly prescribed for stays not exceeding 1 week abroad, particularly for travelers who are immunocompromised, who repeatedly suffered from severe diarrhea during previous travel, or in whom diarrhea might be dangerous. Bismuth subsalicylate (Pepto-Bismol) or trimethoprim-sulfamethoxazole (Bactrim DS, Septra DS) or doxycycline (*Vibramycin*) may be chosen, the latter two being more effective but also having a higher risk of adverse events.

**Food Consumption in Acute Diarrhea.** A reduction of food consumption is frequently observed as a result of anorexia. However, food should not be deliberately withheld during the diarrheal episode, because at least some macronutrients are still absorbed and because children who were fed showed better and more sustained weight gain than children who did not eat. After recovery, extra feeding should be encouraged.

# CONSTIPATION

method of
ALAN B. SHAPIRO, M.D., and
DAVID H. BARCH, M.D.
*University of Illinois at Chicago*
*Chicago, Illinois*

The first thing a physician must do when a patient complains of constipation is to clarify what the patient means by constipation. Constipation may refer to infrequent stools, passage of hard or small stools, straining with defecation, or inability to defecate at will. Stool frequency is the easiest factor to quantify, with approximately 95% of normal subjects having at least three stools per week. Any significant change in bowel habit, even within this "normal" range, should be evaluated to rule out an organic cause. Of particular importance is constipation of recent onset, since this is frequently due to significant underlying disease.

The assessment of constipation should focus on excluding anorectal and colonic pathology, as well as excluding metabolic, endocrine, and neurologic causes (Table 1). Particular attention should be addressed to the patient's medications (including over-the-counter medications and iron) because many drugs may cause constipation (Table 1). In addition, the patient should be questioned about chronic use of stimulant laxatives. Chronic use of these agents can produce severe structural abnormalities of the colon that may be identified

TABLE 1. **Causes of Constipation**

| **Metabolic-Endocrine** | **Neurogenic** | **Drugs** |
|---|---|---|
| Amyloidosis | Autonomic neuropathy | Analgesics |
| Diabetes | Cauda equina tumor | Antacids containing |
| Enteric glucagon excess | Cerebrovascular accident | calcium or aluminum |
| Hypercalcemia | Chagas' disease | Anticholinergics |
| Hypopituitarism | Hirschsprung's disease (aganglionosis) | Anticonvulsants |
| Hypothyroidism | Multiple sclerosis | Antidepressants |
| Pheochromocytoma | Neurofibromatosis | Antihypertensives |
| Porphyria | Parkinson's disease | Antiparkinsonian agents |
| Uremia | Spinal cord tumor or trauma | Barium sulfate |
| | Tabes dorsalis | Bismuth |
| **Colonic-Rectal** | | Diuretics |
| Anal fissure | | Heavy metal intoxication |
| Diverticular disease | | Iron sulfate |
| Irritable bowel syndrome | | Laxative abuse |
| Myotonic dystrophy | | Opiates |
| Obstruction | | Psychotherapeutic agents |
| Hernias | | |
| Rectal prolapse | | **Miscellaneous** |
| Strictures | | Dehydration |
| Tumors | | Immobility |
| Volvulus | | Menstruation |
| Scleroderma | | Pregnancy |

radiographically (cathartic colon). The initial evaluation should include a complete history and physical examination, diet history, stool testing for occult blood, complete blood count, serum electrolytes, and sigmoidoscopy. In addition, a barium enema should be obtained in those patients with recent onset of constipation, a change in stool caliber, a history of blood in the stool, occult blood–positive stool, weight loss, or any other features suggestive of serious colorectal pathology. Serum calcium determination, thyroid function tests, or additional studies should be obtained based on the patient's clinical picture.

## TREATMENT

After organic causes for the patient's constipation have been adequately excluded, a systematic approach to therapy should be initiated. All of the patient's medications (including nonprescription medications) should be reviewed, and those that may cause constipation should be discontinued or changed if possible. All stimulant laxatives should be discontinued. The patient should be encouraged to always respond to the urge to defecate and to set aside a routine time to attempt to move his or her bowels each day. This time should be scheduled after a meal, preferably after breakfast, to take advantage of the postprandial gastrocolic reflex. Regular exercise (walking or running) should be encouraged. A diet history is helpful to quantitate fiber intake, and the patient should be educated about the use of a diet with an adequate amount of natural fiber (greater than 30 grams per day). This may be accomplished through the use of bran cereals, whole wheat bread, fruits, and vegetables. In addition, the patient should be encouraged to increase fluid intake. These measures are often successful, and a 1-month trial of a high-fiber diet may be tried before instituting nondiet therapy. In our experience, patients are often unable to maintain a diet containing 30 grams of dietary fiber and we generally start with a fiber supplement.

The mainstays of therapy for chronic constipation are the bulk-forming agents. These include foods that are high in fiber as well as commercially available products that contain polysaccharides or cellulose derivatives. These agents (e.g. Metamucil, Citrocel, Fibermed) act by increasing water in the stool and by stimulating intestinal motility. These agents are available in a variety of forms that are all similar in efficacy, and they can be safely used for long-term therapy. It is important that these agents be taken with adequate amounts of fluid to prevent obstruction. They are contraindicated in patients with intestinal stricture (and relatively contraindicated in bedridden patients). Palatability is sometimes a problem, and patient compliance may be improved by mixing the powdered products with juices and other creative beverages. It may take several days before a beneficial effect is seen, and some patients may initially experience abdominal cramping, bloating, and flatulence. These symptoms generally subside during the first few weeks of therapy. The necessity of long-term, consistent compliance must be stressed to the patient on bulk-forming agents.

In patients with chronic constipation who are refractory to the preceding measures, there are a variety of other types of laxatives available, including emollient laxatives, lubricants, hyperosmotic agents, and saline laxatives. These agents are generally reserved for short-term use only and should be used with caution.

Emollient laxatives, such as docusate sodium (Colace) and docusate calcium (Surfak), are surfactants that primarily soften the stool by facilitating the mixture of water and fat in the fecal mass. Though not generally absorbed, they may enhance the absorption of other drugs. These agents are particularly useful for short-term therapy when straining at defecation is to be avoided, such as in acute perianal disease, after abdominal or rectal surgery, after myocardial infarction, or during pregnancy. Though occasionally useful, these agents are generally of little value in the treatment of chronic constipation.

The major lubricant laxative is mineral oil, which acts by coating the feces and allowing for easier passage of stool. It is primarily used to maintain soft stools for a short period of time and when straining at defecation is to be avoided. Though generally safe, chronic use may result in malabsorption of fat-soluble vitamins (A, D, E, and K). Aspiration of mineral oil may lead to lipoid pneumonia, and mineral oil should not be used in debilitated patients or before bedtime. Mineral oil should not be used with surfactants (Colace, Surfak), as this results in increased absorption and may lead to a foreign body reaction in systemic lymphoid tissue.

The hyperosmotic cathartics include lactulose and glycerin. Lactulose (Chronulac, Duphalac) is a nonabsorbable disaccharide that passes through the small bowel unchanged. In the colon, it is digested by bacteria to form short chain fatty acids. These acids are osmotically active, drawing water into the colon. In addition, these acids reduce colonic pH and stimulate colonic peristalsis. Although lactulose may cause cramping, flatulence, diarrhea, and electrolyte imbalances, this agent has been demonstrated to be safe and effective in the treatment of both chronic and acute constipation. The usual dosage is 15 to 45 ml per day, but occasionally higher doses are needed. We recommend lactulose in chronically constipated patients refractory to bulk forming agents alone, and it may be the treatment of choice in bedridden patients. The major drawback to lactulose therapy is its high cost. In patients who are lactose intolerant, administration of lactose (or milk) will relieve constipation through exactly the same mechanism as lactulose.

Glycerin is a hyperosmotic laxative given as a rectal suppository. It is ineffective if given orally. Glycerin suppositories usually induce defecation within 30 minutes. Glycerin is indicated for occasional use in acute constipation, but because it may cause rectal irritation, it should not be used on a regular basis.

Saline laxatives include magnesium hydroxide (milk of magnesia), magnesium citrate (citrate of magnesia), magnesium sulfate, and sodium phosphates (Phospho-Soda, Fleet Enema). The magnesium salts are given orally, and the sodium phosphates are used orally or rectally. The saline laxatives act primarily as osmotic agents. The onset of action is fast—within 3 hours when given orally and within 15 minutes when administered rectally. Adequate fluid must be taken with these products to prevent dehydration. These agents should not be used in patients with renal insufficiency, and patients who must restrict sodium intake should avoid the phosphate salts. These agents are best used for acute evacuation of the bowel in preparation for endoscopic or radiologic procedures and after GI studies to prevent barium impaction. Saline laxatives may be useful in the treatment of acute constipation, but these agents are not appropriate for long-term management of chronic constipation.

Stimulant laxatives consist of anthraquinones (cascara sagrada, senna, danthron, and casanthranol), diphenylmethanes (bisacodyl and phenolphthalein), and castor oil. The anthraquinones are hydrolyzed into active metabolites by colonic bacteria. Their effect is probably mediated by changes in fluid and electrolyte transport, and they act within 6 to 24 hours. With chronic use they may cause melanosis coli, a harmless dark pigmentation of the colonic mucosa. This pigmentation usually resolves after discontinuation of these agents. The use of danthron with docusate may cause hepatotoxicity similar in appearance to chronic active hepatitis. Bisacodyl (Dulcolax) may be given either orally or by rectal suppository. It acts by direct stimulation of the mucosal nerve plexus of the colon. When given orally, bisacodyl should not be chewed or taken with antacids or $H_2$ blockers, as this may lead to abdominal cramping or vomiting. Phenolphthalein (Ex-Lax, prunes) affects fluid and electrolyte transport in the colon and leads to the accumulation of intraluminal water. Phenolphthalein undergoes enterohepatic circulation; therefore, its duration of action may be up to 3 or 4 days. Although relatively safe, phenolphthalein may induce serious dermatologic reactions such as erythema multiforme, impair vitamin D and calcium absorption, or mimic Bartter's syndrome (hyperaldosteronism and hypokalemia). The chronic use of stimulant laxatives may result in severe cramping, fluid and electrolyte disturbances, malabsorption, and cathartic colon. Cathartic colon is diagnosed radiologically and usually affects the right colon and terminal ileum. Findings are similar to those seen in advanced ulcerative colitis, with shortening of the bowel associated with long, tapered areas of narrowing and absence of haustrations. These abnormalities may revert completely to normal after discontinuation of the laxative. Given the potential for adverse effects, we rarely recommend these agents, except for the use of bisacodyl as a preparation for diagnostic procedures. These agents are never indicated for regular daily use.

GoLytely and Colyte are oral electrolyte preparations containing sodium and potassium salts with polyethylene glycol 3350. These agents are indicated for bowel cleaning prior to colonoscopy, barium enema, and colorectal surgery, and are occasionally used for the acute management of constipation. These agents are not useful in the chronic management of constipation.

Cisapride is a new prokinetic agent that stimulates acetylcholine release at the myenteric plexus. It has been shown to decrease colonic transit time in patients with constipation due to neurologic disorders and in patients with severe idiopathic constipation secondary to colonic inertia. Experience with this agent is limited, and it is not yet available in the United States.

Surgical therapy for select patients with severe chronic idiopathic constipation due to colonic inertia has been reported by some centers; however, we feel that this is rarely indicated. Surgery is, of course, indicated for patients with Hirschsprung's disease or other anatomic abnormalities.

Fecal impaction is a separate clinical entity that deserves mention. Efforts to remove an impaction by administration of oral laxatives are not only ineffective but may also cause abdominal pain, vomiting, and other complications. Manual fragmentation and disimpaction are usually necessary as the initial measure. Once partial extraction of the fecal mass has been accomplished, enemas are used to clear the bowel. A mineral oil retention enema can provide additional lubrication, and this may be followed by standard sodium phosphate or tap water enemas as necessary. If these measures fail or if the impaction is more proximal, an orally administered osmotic agent such as lactulose or Colyte may be used in patients without evidence of obstruction. Soapsuds, hydrogen peroxide, and hot water enemas should never be used for the treatment of constipation or impaction, as these agents may precipitate acute colonic mucosal injury.

# FEVER

method of
MICHAEL S. KRAMER, M.D.
*McGill University Faculty of Medicine,*
*Montreal, Quebec, Canada*

Normally, the anterior hypothalamus regulates the set-point for core body temperature at $37 \pm 1°$ C and responds to an increase or decrease in environmental temperature by neural efferents that lead to heat loss or conservation, respectively. If the body is unable to compensate for a gain of heat, the core temperature rises above the set-point, a condition called *hyperthermia*. *Fever* is defined as an upward adjustment of the set-point. Unlike hyperthermia, therefore, fever does not represent a loss of temperature regulation, but rather an upward shift of the temperature regulated.

A considerable body of research has demonstrated that vertebrates and even many invertebrates are capable of developing a febrile response. Ectotherms, such as fishes, amphibians, and reptiles, lack the capacity to adjust body heat by intrinsic physiologic mechanisms. Instead, they rely on behavioral adaptation; they seek appropriate environmental temperatures and assume optimum heat-conserving positions. In humans, shivering, peripheral vasoconstriction, and increased metabolic rate result in an increase of the core temperature to between 38 and $41°$ C. In clinical fevers, the hypothalamus carefully modulates the rise in set-point so that temperatures rarely exceed $41°$ C, even in children.

Fever has been recognized as a cardinal sign of disease since the beginning of recorded history. Opinions have changed substantially, however, as to whether ill patients are better off with or without it. For Hippocrates and other ancients, fever was the body's defense mechanism for "cooking off" an excess of one of the four bodily humors: blood, phlegm, yellow bile, and black bile. In fact, the view that fever is beneficial persisted for over two millenia, as eloquently enunciated by the noted seventeenth-century English physician Thomas Sydenham: "Fever is Nature's engine which she brings into the field to remove her enemy." A change in this view occurred in the wake of experiments by the great nineteenth-century French physiologist Claude Bernard, who demonstrated that animals died when their body temperature was experimentally raised to 5 to $6°$ C above normal. Since that time, fever has become generally regarded as injurious to health.

Fever occurs as a result of the body's exposure to infecting microorganisms, immune complexes, or other sources of inflammation. The major pathophysiologic mechanism for its development involves the release of interleukin–1 (IL–1, formerly called endogenous pyrogen) from circulating monocytes and fixed tissue macrophages. IL–1 stimulates prostaglandin E production in the preoptic area of the anterior hypothalamus, which then brings about a rise in the temperature set-point by the physiologic and/or behavioral mechanisms mentioned earlier. IL–1 has a number of direct effects on the immune response, including release and production of neutrophils from the bone marrow, increased neutrophil oxidative activity, lactoferrin release, B cell proliferation and antibody production, and T cell activation. The lactoferrin release leads to a decrease in serum iron, which inhibits the growth of many microorganisms. But the fever induced by IL–1 has additional immunologic benefits above and beyond the direct effects of IL–1, including helper T cell proliferation, enhanced T cell cytotoxicity, B cell activity and antibody synthesis, and interferon production and function. Moreover, the growth of some organisms (including the polio virus, pneumococcus, gonococcus, and syphilis treponeme) are inhibited at febrile temperatures.

Fevers are not entirely without risks, however. Increased oxygen consumption and cardiac output could compromise the status of debilitated elderly persons or patients with severe pulmonary or cardiovascular disease. But in otherwise healthy children or adults, there is no evidence that fevers below 42° C are harmful. Children under the age of 5 years, and especially those under 3, are at risk for febrile convulsions, particularly at temperatures of 40° C or higher. Many such convulsions, however, occur early in the course of the febrile illness, while the temperature is rising and in many cases before the parents are even aware of the presence of the fever. Unfortunately, therefore, there is no convincing evidence that antipyretic treatment is effective in prophylaxis against febrile seizures. Febrile illnesses are often accompanied by other symptoms of the acute phase response, including headache, anorexia, malaise, fatigue, and myalgias. It is not clear, however, to what extent these symptoms are a consequence of fever per se, since many of them appear to be mediated by IL–1.

## TREATMENT

The first therapeutic decision concerning fever is whether or not to treat it. In patients with significant pulmonary or cardiovascular compromise or in severely debilitated elderly persons, lowering the hypothalamic set-point should be beneficial in reducing oxygen consumption and cardiac output. Even in the absence of strong evidence of prophylactic efficacy, it also seems reasonable to treat fevers in children under 5 years with a history of febrile convulsions or in patients of any age who experience convulsions without fever.

In otherwise healthy children and adults, the decision to administer antipyretic therapy should be based on balancing the likely risks and benefits of treatment. The risks of treatment remain largely theoretical and relate to the improved immune responses (vide supra) observed at febrile temperatures. Nonetheless, it is important to underline the fact that therapeutic blood levels of commonly used antipyretic medications do not reduce the production of IL–1. In fact, few adverse effects have been documented with therapeutic doses of antipyretic drugs in the intact human host, other than evidence of reduced lung mucociliary clearance and increased rhinovirus shedding in adults treated with aspirin, and a slight prolongation of time to scabbing in children with chickenpox who receive acetaminophen. The benefits of antipyresis also remain largely anecdotal. Many febrile adults and children appear less uncomfortable (less achy, more active, etc.) after antipyretic medication, although it is not clear whether such improvement is due to the antipyretic or analgesic properties of these agents.

Because many patients, and especially young children, often appear quite comfortable despite febrile temperatures, the best policy, given existing evidence, is to treat fevers when associated with significant discomfort. Although this is a natural policy to adopt for adults who elect to treat themselves, it is in marked contrast to the policy of many parents, who seem more focused on treating the thermometer rather than the child.

Once a decision has been made to treat a fever, the next decision involves the choice of therapy, which has traditionally comprised both pharmacologic and nonpharmacologic approaches. The major nonpharmacologic approach has been external cooling by removing clothing and/or bathing or sponging in cold or tepid water or application of isopropyl alcohol. Such measures are not very effective; moreover, they run counter to the physiologic mechanisms discussed earlier. Unless the hypothalamic set-point is lowered pharmacologically, the evaporation induced by application of water or alcohol to the skin will only lead to shivering (and therefore discomfort), as the body attempts to maintain the core temperature at the regulated set-point. The discomfort induced by cold water or alcohol bathing or sponging can be considerable. Isopropyl alcohol can also be absorbed through the skin, with appreciable blood levels and risk of systemic toxicity. Its use should therefore be discouraged.

The safe and effective mainstays of treatment are pharmacologic and include acetaminophen, aspirin, and other nonsteroidal anti-inflammatory drugs (NSAIDs). All appear to work by inhibiting production of prostaglandin E in the anterior hypothalamus in response to IL–1.

When antipyretic effect alone is desired, acetaminophen is usually the drug of choice. The dosage of acetaminophen is 10 to 20 mg per kg per dose, up to the maximum adult dose of 650 to 1000 mg administered every 4 hours. Table 1 indicates acetaminophen dosages by age and weight (in kg), based on the usually recommended dosage of 10 to 15 mg per kg per dose. A variety of dosage forms are available. The adult tablets contain either 325 mg (regular strength)

TABLE 1. **Recommended Dosages of Acetaminophen by Age and Weight***

| Age | Weight (kg) | Dose (mg q 4 hr) |
|---|---|---|
| <1 mo | 2.5–3.9 | 40 |
| 1–6 mo | 4.0–7.9 | 80 |
| 8–18 mo | 8.0–10.9 | 120 |
| 19 mo–3 yr | 11.0–14.9 | 160 |
| 4–5 yr | 15.0–20.9 | 240 |
| 6–7 yr | 21.0–27.9 | 320 |
| 8–9 yr | 28.0–35.9 | 400 |
| 10–11 yr | 36.0–44.9 | 480 |
| 12–13 yr | 45.0–59.9 | 650 |
| 14 yr–adult | ≥60 | 650–1000 |

*When age and weight categories do not coincide, base dosage on weight. Do not exceed 4 or 5 doses per day.

or 500 mg (extra strength). For young children, the forms include drops (80 mg per ml), syrup or elixir (80 mg per 5 ml), chewable tablets (80 mg each), and swallowable junior tablets (160 mg each). Acetaminophen is conjugated in the liver to form sulfate and glucuronide derivatives, with a small amount metabolized to toxic aryl intermediates by a cytochrome P–450–mediated pathway. This latter metabolite is quite hepatotoxic when present in quantities greater than the capacity of the liver to conjugate it with glutathione or other sulfhydryl donors. Adult dosage forms therefore represent a major hazard for accidental or intentional overdose.

Aspirin is a gastric irritant that increases the risk of gastric ulcer, hemorrhage, and perforation. Its inhibition of cyclo-oxygenase also interferes with platelet function and may increase the risk of bleeding; this is of particular importance in the postoperative patient. Aspirin is also associated with a risk of asthma exacerbation and even serious anaphylactic reactions, particularly in adults with a pre-existing history of asthma and nasal polyps. The adult form of aspirin is one of the most frequent causes of accidental poisonings in infants and toddlers and of suicide attempts in adolescents and adults. Overdose leads to a syndrome called salicylism, which is characterized by hyperventilation, depressed level of consciousness, and severe metabolic acidosis. Finally, there is unequivocal evidence linking the administration of aspirin to children with influenza, varicella, and other viral infections to the subsequent development of Reye's syndrome, a rare disease manifested by liver dysfunction and severe encephalopathy. As aspirin has become a progressively more rarely used antipyretic in children since the first reports of the aspirin–Reye's syndrome association in the early 1980s, so too has the incidence of, and mortality from, Reye's syndrome. In adults without a history of asthma or other allergic disease or peptic ulcer disease, and particularly those in need of aspirin's anti-inflammatory action (an action not shared by acetaminophen), the usual recommended dose is 650 mg (two 325-mg tablets) every 4 hours.

Other NSAIDs have also been used as antipyretic agents in children and adults, the most common being ibuprofen. Current evidence indicates that in doses of 5 to 10 mg per kg (up to a maximum adult dose of 400 mg), three or four times per day, ibuprofen is comparable in antipyretic efficacy with therapeutically equivalent doses of aspirin or acetaminophen. In acute overdoses, ibuprofen appears to be much safer than acetaminophen or aspirin. Like aspirin and other NSAIDs, ibuprofen can lead to gastric ulceration, perforation, and hemorrhage, particularly in the elderly, and, like aspirin, could exacerbate asthma or lead to anaphylactic reactions in asthmatics. Although there are no data linking ibuprofen to Reye's syndrome, the mechanism by which aspirin interacts with viruses to produce Reye's syndrome is not understood, and to the extent that such a mechanism may be shared by ibuprofen or other NSAIDs, one might suspect (at least on theoretical grounds) such a link with these medications. Because ibuprofen is also more expensive than aspirin or acetaminophen, and because it does not appear to carry any unique therapeutic benefits, it is difficult to recommend it as a drug of first choice, even in adults.

# COUGH

method of
IRWIN ZIMENT, M.D.
*Olive View Medical Center*
*Sylmar, California*

Numerous agents have been used in the treatment of cough, although only a select minority are available in the United States. Because acute coughs, particularly those accompanying viral respiratory illnesses, are usually self-limited to within 2 to 3 weeks, most cough medications appear to be useful even if they are only serving as placebos. Thus, the management of cough is frequently carried out with apparent success by simple agents of unproven value. More serious etiologies, such as lung cancer, may demand the use of highly effective narcotic antitussives. It is therefore reasonable to approach cough management with respect to the apparent severity of the cough, and to advance if necessary from simple measures to the prescription of potentially hazardous drugs. Special cases of cough will be discussed. Underlying all treatment approaches is the requirement to evaluate the cause of the cough and to treat this directly if possible. It is, of course, well known that smoking and its complications are major causes of cough.

## SIMPLE TREATMENT MEASURES

Airway irritation or inflammation may be palliated by inhaling warm moist air or steam with or without the addition of aromatic inhalants such as Friar's Balsam (compound tincture of benzoin).* Oral medications, including the popular over-the-counter cough candies and throat lozenges, may also help. Simple syrups may provide a soothing cover to irritated oropharyngeal receptor sites that initiate reflex coughing. Hot drinks of teas, soups, or other beverages with the addition of household adjuvants are extremely popular. Applying an embrocation or aromatic lubricant externally to the skin, neck, or lips is favored by many people, who have thus enabled proprietary products such as Vicks VapoRub and Tiger Balm* to achieve worldwide reputations that have not been supported by controlled studies.

Many proprietary cold remedies are also advertised to be effective for treating coughs. Alleviation of nasal inflammation and reduction of postnasal drip can undoubtedly result in an improvement in the cough that accompanies a common cold. Thus, topical or systemic vasoconstrictors, antihistamines, topical anticholinergic agents, and steroids can help alleviate the nasal symptoms and thereby may be of some value in the management of cough. However, the specific antitussive value of most of these drugs has not been demonstrated. Diphenhydramine (Benadryl, Benylin) and, to a lesser extent, tripelennamine have been reported to be more effective than other antihistamines, although the evidence for this is minimal. Antihistamines may be of further help in treating allergic coughs that are sometimes more of a problem than rhinitis in patients with allergy to pollen and other airborne antigens. An antihistamine with sedative properties is of added value at night.

In coughs caused by allergy or hypersensitivity or chemical irritation, steroid therapy could reduce the inflammatory response and thus benefit the cough. Viral infections that cause a hacking, nonproductive cough may also increase a latent tendency to bronchospasm, and in susceptible patients chronic asthma may follow. The inflammatory damage may render the airways very hyper-reactive, and this problem may persist. Early treatment with steroids may rapidly suppress the inflammation and can relieve the cough and prevent a subsequent liability to asthma. I have been impressed with the benefits of steroid administration for a few days if the patient does not present with any major contraindication to this therapy. A suggested regimen would be oral

---

*Not available in the United States.

prednisone or methylprednisolone, 40 mg on the first day, followed by 35 mg, 30 mg, 25 mg, 20 mg, and 10 mg on subsequent days, after which the drug can be stopped if the response has been favorable.

## DRUGS FOR SEVERE COUGH

A severe cough can be defined as one that is persistent and subjectively distressing to the patient or to those who have to live or work with the patient; it could also be one that threatens the patient's life or daily activities. An effective cough suppressant is also mandatory for patients undergoing eye surgery or those with fractured ribs.

For severe, nonproductive, distressing, or involuntary coughs that need to be suppressed, a narcotic medication is usually reliable (Table 1). In subjects with terminal diseases, such as cancer of the lung, morphine, hydromorphone (dihydromorphinone [Dilaudid]), or methadone (Dolophine) may be appropriate; but for individuals in whom the risk of narcotic addiction must be avoided, hydrocodone (dihydrocodeinone) (Hycodan) and codeine are safer although still somewhat addictive in susceptible patients. In other countries, heroin, dihydrocodeine, ethylmorphine, morpholinylethylmorphine, normethadone, and pholcodine are sometimes preferred. Analgesics such as hydrocodone, oxycodone (Percodan), and meperidine (Demerol) may be indicated to suppress pain as well as cough. In practice, morphine and hydrocodone are the most suitable agents for a severe distressing cough, but codeine, which is less effective, has the advantage of rarely leading to addiction. It may be necessary to use larger doses than are usually recommended to control persistent nonproductive coughs, and in the case of codeine as much as 40 to 60 mg every 4 to 6 hours may be prescribed in adults if side effects are not a problem.

As an alternative to narcotics, several nonnarcotic agents can be used. The most popular is dextromethorphan, which is usually given to adults in doses of 15 to 30 mg every 4 to 8 hours. This agent is generally well tolerated, and the dosage can be doubled to control a stubborn cough. An alternative drug is benzonatate (Tessalon); it is a local anesthetic that apparently acts on cough receptors in the lung. This agent can be particularly useful in coughs caused by interstitial lung diseases in which stretching of the damaged lung readily stimulates coughing. Benzonatate should be considered as the appropriate drug for any cough that is exacerbated by inhalation of a deep breath or by mild effort such as that of talking or moving. Lidocaine (Xylo-

TABLE 1. **Major Antitussive Products**

| Drug | Marketed Products | Adult Dosage Range (mg) ‡ | Relative Effects | |
|---|---|---|---|---|
| | | | Antitussive | Narcotic |
| Morphine | MSIR, Roxanol | 2–8 | + + + | + + + |
| Hydromorphone (dihydromorphinone) | Dilaudid | 0.5–2 | + + + | + + + |
| Methadone | Dolophine | 2.5–10 | + + | + + |
| Codeine | Bromarest-DC,* Dimetane-DC,* Medi-Tuss AC,* Medi-Tuss DAC,* Penntuss, Robitussin A-C,* Robitussin-DAC,* Ryna-C,* Ryna-CX,* Tussi-Organidin* | 5–20 | + + | + |
| Hydrocodone (dihydrocodeinone) | Hycodan,* Hycomine,* Tuss-end,* Tussionex* | 5–20 | + + | + |
| Pholcodine | Not available in United States | | + + | + |
| Noscapine (narcotine) | Conar,† Tusscapine† | 15–60 | + + | − |
| Dextromethorphan (dormethan) | Benylin DM,* Delsym, Hold, Robitussin-CF,* Robitussin-DM,* Tussi-Organidin DM* | 15–60 | + + | − |
| Benzonatate | Tessalon | 100–400 | + + | − |
| Caramiphen edisylate | Tuss-Ornade* | 10–30 | + | − |
| Carbetapentane (pentoxyverine) | Rynatuss,* Tussar* | 15–45 | + | − |
| Levopropoxyphene | Novrad† | 50–150 | + | − |

*Combination preparation.
†No longer marketed.
‡Single dose; may be repeated several times a day.

caine), in contrast, is not used in similar circumstances, although it is a valuable local anesthetic for preventing cough during bronchoscopy. The drug has also been given intravenously to suppress a severe cough. Cocaine and other topical anesthetics may be effective but are rarely suitable for use in clinical situations.

A surprising number of additional antitussive agents are known, most of which are not available in the United States. The drugs that have been marketed in the United States include caramiphen edisylate, carbetapentane (pentoxyverine), chlophedianol, levoproproxyphene, and noscapine; of these, only noscapine appeared to be as effective as dextromethorphan. For economic reasons, caramiphen, chlophedianol, levopropoxyphene, and noscapine have been withdrawn from the market in recent years. In other countries, the numerous available antitussives include alloclamide, aminothiazoline, benzobutamine, bibenzonium, brospasmin, butamyrate, clobutinol, cloperastine, codoxime, dibunate derivatives, dimemorfan, dimethoxanate, dropropizine, drotebanol, ethyl orthoformate, fedrilate, fominoben, glaucine, hydrocotarnine, isoaminile, levodropropizine, meprotixol, morclofone, oxeladin, oxolamine, picoperine, pipazetate, piperidione, prenoxdiazin, viminol, and zipeprol. There is no evidence to suggest that any of these agents offers any advantages over codeine, dextromethorphan, or benzonatate. Similarly, the many Oriental and Western folk medicine cough remedies have not been shown to be superior to established antitussives. Oriental medications that are readily available include Fritillary and Loquat Mixture, Ma-huang (ephedrine), Lo-han-kuo (mangasteen), and rhododendron extract. Popular Western folk medications include coltsfoot (which has the Linnaean name *Tussilago farfara*), horehound, eucalyptus, and extract of wild cherry.

## SPECIAL THERAPEUTIC CONCERNS

It is important to try and tailor therapy to the particular characteristics of a cough. The nonspecific measures just discussed may not be suitable in the following situations.

**Pulmonary Infection.** A new or persistent cough with or without sputum may result from bacterial infection, in which case the use of one or more specific antibiotics is required. Bronchitis may respond to almost any antibiotic and bronchodilator, whereas cystic fibrosis usually requires specific antistaphylococcal or antipseudomonal therapy. Bronchiectasis in exacerbation may present as a mixed infection, and broad-spectrum coverage is needed, as is the case with lung abscess or severe aspiration pneumonia in a compromised host. Legionnaires' disease and *Pneumocystis carinii* may present with a cough, and every effort must be made to diagnose and treat these conditions appropriately. Tuberculosis is becoming more common, and a persistent cough with an abnormal chest radiograph may be caused by typical or atypical mycobacterial infection, for which treatment with several drugs (e.g., isoniazid [Nydrazid], rifampin [Rifadin], and pyrazinamide) is required.

**Abnormal Sputum.** Persistent hyperviscous sputum in cystic fibrosis, the immotile cilia syndrome, or Young's syndrome may require postural drainage and chest percussion to alleviate the associated cough. Expectorants and other mucus-loosening drugs may help, with acetylcysteine (Mucomyst) being the best mucolytic agent and the saturated solution of potassium iodide (SSKI) or the organic iodide iodopropylidene glycerol (iodinated glycerol [Organidin]) being the most favored general mucokinetic agents. Occasionally, bronchoscopy and pulmonary lavage are required to remove inspissated secretions.

**Asthma.** Some patients with latent asthma present with a chronic cough. Routine examination and pulmonary function tests may not conclusively demonstrate bronchospasm, and an inhalation challenge test may be needed for diagnosis. However, in suspicious cases it may be reasonable to give an empiric trial of bronchodilator therapy with an adrenergic aerosol or oral theophylline. If there is evidence of bronchitis, a course of ipratropium (Atrovent) inhalation should be initiated.

**Allergy.** In some patients, airborne allergens cause an annoying cough rather than rhinitis or conjunctivitis. The diagnosis may be suggested by the presence of an atopic history or the finding of eosinophilia, increased serum IgE, a positive radioallergosorbent test (RAST), or a positive inhalation challenge test. The cough may respond best to a combination of codeine and chlorpheniramine in a slow-release preparation (Penntuss). In selected patients, a course of cromolyn (Intal) inhalation may be very effective, particularly in younger subjects with clear evidence of allergy or with coughing induced by cold air or exercise. Oral steroid therapy may be needed to control a cough that is exacerbated by breathing in aerosol particles, and once the condition is alleviated continuing treatment with an aerosol steroid can stabilize the condition. Aerosol steroids are particularly valuable in the patient with an allergic cough associated with both asthma and allergic rhinitis. In some patients, added benefit from the steroid aerosol may be noted if the steroid drug is breathed in through the mouth into the lungs and then exhaled through the nose.

**Nasal Disease.** A large proportion of persistent coughs result from nasal disorders, the most important being postnasal drip. The presence of allergic rhinitis, sinus infection, or nasal polyps may explain the cough, and treatment with vasoconstrictors, antihistamines, topical steroids, or intranasal cromolyn (Nasalcrom) should improve the nasal condition and alleviate the cough. In acute sinusitis, a course of antibiotic therapy is required.

**Heart Failure.** Heart failure can present as a cough, which may respond to diuretic and specific cardiac therapy. It is of interest that the angiotensin-converting enzyme inhibitors captopril (Capoten), enalapril (Vasotec), and lisinopril (Zestril, Prinivil), which may be useful in heart failure, can cause an annoying cough in a small minority of patients. It is thought that these inhibitors allow the accumulation of bradykinin by inhibiting its metabolism; this peptide is believed to induce the cough.

**Aspiration.** A proportion of cases of asthma, bronchitis, and chronic obstructive pulmonary disease are caused or exacerbated by aspiration, and in some patients a chronic cough may be the presenting symptom. If the history or evidence of a hiatus hernia, gastric reflux, or disordered swallowing suggests this possibility, radiologic studies may be justified to establish the diagnosis. Therapy may be limited to physical methods such as sleeping with the head raised, or avoiding large meals or bending down. Theophylline can induce relaxation of the gastroesophageal sphincter, and this may result in aspiration; if suspected as a cause, this drug should be removed from the patient's therapy. In selected cases, surgical procedures may be required to correct the cause of recurrent aspiration.

**Other Causes.** Psychologic causes or habit can account for some coughs, including hacking or throat clearing that may not be accompanied by sputum production. Many of these cases originate with a physical cause, but the cough may persist once the cause has been eliminated. Patient reassurance can usually be given without the need for an extensive work-up, but in more dubious cases it should be recognized that auditory, laryngeal, diaphragmatic, pericardial, chest wall, or gastric irritation can account for reflex coughing. In all cases, the physician should demonstrate that a thorough physical examination, chest radiographs, evaluation of sputum, and pulmonary function tests are normal before concluding that a persistent cough is of psychologic origin.

# HOARSENESS AND LARYNGITIS

method of
LAURENE L. HOWELL, M.D.
*Oregon Health Sciences University*
*Portland, Oregon*

Hoarseness is the most common symptom of any disorder of the larynx. The cause may be any number of diseases or pathologies in or around the larynx, or it may be faulty use or abuse of the vocal mechanism. The majority of voice problems of adults and children are due to misuse or abuse of normal vocal structures. Vocal abuse results from such behaviors as constant throat clearing, frequent cough, yelling, cheerleading, vocal strain in noisy environments, or conversing with hard-of-hearing co-workers or companions. Other contributing factors that can make the voice more vulnerable to misuse are dehydration, allergy symptoms, sinusitus with nasal obstruction or postnasal drainage, pharyngeal reflux, aging, and side effects of medication.

When the voice is altered due to misuse or abuse without laryngeal disease, it is termed a functional voice problem. Sometimes these are the most difficult to diagnose. In addition to attending to their general health, nutrition, and exercise, these patients need voice therapy by a speech pathologist in order to identify and eliminate the abusive habits.

If the voice problem is due to laryngeal disease or dysfunction (such as a vocal cord mass or paralysis), it is an organic voice disorder. These frequently require medical-surgical treatment, but some of these patients will also require voice therapy in order to maximize normal voice function.

The correct diagnosis requires a thorough history and laryngeal examination. Diagnosis of organic voice disorders requires either a direct or indirect examination of the larynx. Any patient with hoarseness persisting for more than two weeks needs a thorough visual inspection of the larynx.

## HOARSENESS IN CHILDREN

### Congenital Disorders

The differential diagnosis of hoarseness is quite different for neonates, children, and adults. The neonate with a hoarse cry or weak voice most likely has a congenital problem such as a laryngeal web, laryngeal cyst, hemangioma, or vocal cord paralysis. Partially obstructing laryngeal lesions usually cause laryngeal stridor. Stridor is a noise that occurs during inspiration, expiration, or both. When laryngeal stridor is present, an element of obstruction is present, and a prompt diagnosis must be made. This symptom cannot be ignored. The most common cause of stridor in the neonate is laryngomalacia. It is due to the flaccid nature of the supraglottic structures (generally the epiglottis and the aryepiglottic folds that extend from the epiglottis to the arytenoid laryngeal cartilages). Many children with laryngomalacia are asymptomatic except for the inspiratory stridor. Some infants will have increased symptoms when lying supine or when feeding or during upper respiratory infections.

**Treatment.** Symptoms are frequently improved with the infant in a prone position or with the neck flexed. The majority of infants improve with growth and maturity of the laryngeal structures, which usually occurs over 12 to 18 months. Close follow-up is required until this occurs.

Occasionally, a child will have severe laryngomalacia that requires surgical intervention. The epiglottis and aryepiglottic folds can be partially removed with the carbon dioxide laser. If the child exhibits obstructive apnea, right heart failure, or severe feeding problems, a tracheotomy may be necessary.

### Vocal Cord Paralysis

Vocal cord paralysis is the second most common congenital anomaly and may be unilateral or bilateral. Infants with bilateral paralysis generally have a normal cry but have significant airway compromise and stridor, especially when agitated.

**Treatment.** If respiratory distress is evident, the airway should be secured with intubation and subsequent tracheotomy. A direct laryngoscopy should be performed to observe for any evidence of vocal cord motion. The diagnostic work-up must include evaluation for a central cause such as hydrocephalus or Arnold-Chiari malformation. There are case reports of return of vocal cord function after placement of a ventricular shunt. If no cause is found, these children should be followed without additional surgical procedures for 2 or 3 years. If there is no return of function during this time, procedures to lateralize the cords to enlarge the airway can be considered. Any procedure used to enlarge the airway will sacrifice voice quality.

Unilateral vocal cord paralysis generally results in a poorer voice but a better airway. The degree of airway compromise may be well tolerated. In contrast to bilateral paralysis, unilateral paralysis may be due to a lesion along the peripheral nerve and requires investigation of the entire path of the recurrent laryngeal nerve. Radiologic evaluation of the chest should include a chest x-ray and barium swallow. If birth trauma is the cause of the paralysis, there is hope of return of function in a year or more. In idiopathic cases, no treatment is required unless airway obstruction or aspiration is a problem.

### Inflammatory Causes of Hoarseness and Stridor

Older children with new onset of stridor most likely have an infection. The most common infectious cause of stridor in children is laryngotracheobronchitis (LTB). The child presents with symptoms characteristic of upper respiratory infection and stridor progressive over 2 to 3 days. Affected children are usually less than 2 years of age, but ages can range from 6 months to 5 years.

The characteristic symptoms are a seal bark cough and biphasic stridor with chest retractions. The usual cause is parainfluenza virus.

**Treatment.** Moderate cases should be managed in an intensive care unit with aggressive medical therapy. Humidified air or oxygen should be supplied via a mist tent and nebulized treatments of racemic epinephrine (0.15 to 0.5 ml of 2.25% solution in 2 ml of normal saline) should be administered every 3 to 4 hours. Steroids are controversial, but dexamethasone sodium phosphate (Decadron) is frequently used in doses of 2 to 6 mg intravenously every 8 hours for 48 to 72 hours. Instrumentation of the airway should be avoided if possible, although deterioration of the airway does require intubation. A lateral neck x-ray will frequently show a characteristic steeple sign in the subglottic region.

LTB symptoms are caused by subglottic edema. Intubation in the narrowed airway raises the risk of subglottic stenosis, especially in young children with small airways.

**Epiglottitis.** Epiglottitis occurs less frequently than LTB but is more common in children ages 2 to 6 years. It is caused by a bacterial infection, usually *Haemophilus influenzae.* Symptoms escalate over 24 hours and include a sore throat, fever, lethargy, drooling, a muffled voice, and inspiratory stridor with chest retractions.

TREATMENT. If epiglottitis is suspected, the child should be managed expectantly for airway obstruction. The child should not be separated from the parents, and further diagnostic intervention should be delayed. Immediate plans must be made to secure an airway in the most controlled situation. If possible, the operating room and anesthesiologist should be alerted of the need for urgent intubation and possible tracheotomy. The child should be transported to the operating room accompanied by a parent. After an airway is secured, direct laryngoscopy confirms the diagnosis. Cultures should be taken from the epiglottis and blood.

Initial antibiotic therapy is directed at *Haemophilus influenzae* and modified after the culture results are available. This organism is frequently a β-lactamase producer and can be treated with a second- or third-generation cephalosporin. Appropriate choices include cefuroxime (Zinacef) administered at 50 to 100 mg per kg per day in divided doses every 8 hours or ceftazidime (Fortaz) administered at 100 to 200 mg per kg per day divided every 8 to 12 hours.

The child is observed for resolution of drooling, occurrence of an air leak around the endotracheal tube, and normalization of his white count and temperature, which usually occurs over 48 to 72 hours. It is usually safe to extubate the child at this point.

### Vocal Cord Nodules

Vocal cord nodules have also been referred to as screamer's nodules. They are the most common cause of hoarseness in school-age children. They are usually bilateral and are located at a characteristic area of the vocal cord: the junction of the anterior one-third and posterior two-thirds of the cords. This is actually the central vibratory portion of the cord because the cartilaginous attachment of the posterior cord extends submucosally for approximately one-third of the length of the cord.

**Treatment.** The nodules do not cause airway distress. They are caused by vocal abuse and generally resolve when the abusive behavior has been discontinued. Speech therapy and behavior modifications are appropriate interventions but are often unsuccessful until the child reaches a level of maturity that decreases yelling behavior.

Surgical intervention is inappropriate except for very large nodules or nodules that are persistent after the abusive behavior has been discontinued for an extended period of time.

### Laryngeal Papillomas

Squamous cell papilloma is the most common benign tumor of the larynx at any age, and there is a much higher incidence in children than in adults. The most common symptom is hoarseness, which is usually progressive. The onset of the disease generally occurs in younger children, with 60 to 70% presenting by age 6. The correct diagnosis is often delayed because the larynx is not examined.

These growths are wart-like in appearance and thought to be viral in origin, although this has not been proved. Papillomas in children tend to be multiple and have a high propensity for recurrence. Total airway obstruction can occur. The papillomas most commonly involve the vocal cords but can extend into the subglottis. Involvement of the trachea, bronchi, and lungs is infrequent unless a tracheotomy has been performed. The disease may subside spontaneously or may persist throughout most of the patient's life.

**Treatment.** Treatment with many topical and systemic agents has been tried in the past. Steroids, chemotherapeutic agents, podophyllin, vaccines, and estrogens have no value. The best currently available treatment is repeated excision with a $CO_2$ laser to minimize bleeding and damage to the surrounding normal mucosa. In spite of careful surgical intervention, many children do have persistent and permanent voice changes due to laryngeal scarring. Periodic biopsies should be taken at the time of excision because there is a low risk of malignant transformation. Radiation therapy was abandoned more than 20 years ago due to reported cases of malignant degeneration of papillomas after its use.

## HOARSENESS IN ADULTS

### Acute Laryngitis

Acute laryngitis is the most common cause of hoarseness in adults. It is the result of inflammation and swelling of the vocal cords and is most frequently caused by a virus. Other causes include bacterial infections, inhaled chemicals or caustic agents, inhaled smoke, or allergic reactions. Vocal cord abuse can cause inflammation and swelling, but it is usually less acute and more persistent.

**Treatment.** Treatment depends on the etiology. Acute laryngitis associated with a generalized, viral upper respiratory tract infection is treated symptomatically. Specifically, the voice should be rested as much as possible. Additional treatment includes increased inhaled humidification, forced hydration, and antitussive medications. If bacterial infection is confirmed or strongly suspected, especially if a persistent associated fever or cervical adenopathy exists, a broad-spectrum antibiotic, such as amoxicillin 500 mg three times daily for 10 days, should be used.

In noninfectious laryngitis, the irritating agent must be identified and eliminated. If hoarseness persists for more than two weeks, a complete view of the larynx must be obtained by either direct or indirect laryngoscopy.

### Chronic Laryngitis

This is caused by persistent inflammation and swelling of the vocal cords. The cords are usually thickened with mild erythema. It is rarely due to an infectious agent, although tuberculosis, blastomycosis, or other unusual granulomatous disease could be the cause.

The most likely etiology is one or more of a number of chronic irritants such as chronic cough, throat clearing, constant mouth breathing, postnasal drainage from chronic rhinitis, allergy or sinusitis, gastroesophageal reflux, or abuse of tobacco or alcohol. Occasionally, a patient will develop symptoms from occupational exposure to irritating chemicals.

Patients often try to overcome the abnormal or weak voice by using increasing muscle tension and effort with speaking. This leads to vocal strain and compounds the problem. It may also create severe tension and hyperfunction of the false vocal cords and larger muscles of the neck with resulting neck and throat pain. Some patients use a whispering voice with the erroneous idea that this rests the vocal cords.

Diagnosis is difficult and requires a careful history and diagnostic work-up. The work-up must be directed by additional history or physical findings that are suggestive of a specific cause. When appropriate, sinus radiographs, barium swallow, or allergy evaluation should be recommended.

**Treatment.** If no specific etiology can be identified, symptomatic treatment should be recommended and includes voice rest for several days, increased humidity and fluid intake, and avoidance of caffeine, alcohol, and dehydrating over-the-counter medications such as antihistamines. Smoking cessation is critical. Voice therapy by a speech pathologist is frequently a worthwhile therapeutic intervention. The speech pathologist will reinforce the symptomatic treatment recommendations and also help identify any abusive habits or poor compensatory habits that the patient has developed.

Chronic laryngitis can result in hyperkeratosis of the mucosal covering of the vocal cords. These changes appear as thickened or white patches. These areas may require biopsy if symptoms and appearance raise a concern for carcinoma. When vocal cords are biopsied, it is important to avoid the leading edge of the cord if possible and also to avoid removing any of the vocalis muscle.

Vocal cord stripping is recommended by some surgeons for chronic, diffuse inflammatory changes. Occasionally, the stripping does allow regrowth of more normal mucosa and improves the voice, but it does carry the risk of creating a depression of the cord or permanent scar between the vocalis muscle and overlying mucosa. Stripping of the mucosa anteriorly between the two cords frequently results in a permanent web formation.

### Polypoid Corditis

This is a severe form of chronic laryngitis that results in polypoid changes of the vocal cords. The patient has persistent and painless hoarseness. The cords do not appear red. The redundant tissue of the vocal cord edge may be so extensive that it has the appearance of a fluid-filled bag and moves above and below the glottis with respiration. These tissue changes have generally been so chronic that conservative treatment will not result in adequate shrinkage of the tissue.

**Treatment.** Most of the patients are smokers, but there also may be contributing factors such as those previously mentioned under the heading of chronic laryngitis. Cessation of smoking is mandatory. Preoperative voice therapy is often beneficial.

Surgical treatment is usually required and involves removal of the edematous mucosa with sparing of the anterior commissure mucosal bridge between the two cords. The condition will recur if the patient does not alter his or her habits.

### Vocal Cord Nodules

These discrete swellings are generally bilateral and occur at the free edge of the cords at the junction of the anterior one-third and posterior two-thirds of the cord. The site is the midpoint of the muscular vocal fold and undergoes maximal vibration with voicing.

The cause is vocal abuse or misuse. The vocal cords cannot adduct completely due to the protruding (kissing) nodules. This leads to breathiness, lower vocal pitch, vocal fatigue, and a sensation of something in the throat, which often precipitates habitual throat clearing.

**Treatment.** Treatment requires elimination of all vocal abusive habits (yelling, screaming, speaking in a noisy environment, hard glottal attacks when speaking or singing, throat clearing, and cough). Voice therapy is central to treatment. If the nodules do not completely disappear after this treatment, surgical removal can be considered. If the nodules are removed and the patient has not eliminated abusive habits, they will certainly recur.

### Vocal Cord Polyp

This lesion is most commonly unilateral and located at the same site on the vocal cord as nodules. The polyp appears soft and fluid filled and may be large enough to be displaced below and above the cord with respirations. The cause is usually a single abusive vocal event such as screaming at a sports competition. Once the polyp forms, vocal misuse may occur during attempts to compensate for the weighted vocal cord that is causing dysphonia.

**Treatment.** This lesion usually does not regress and requires surgical removal. Since it occurs on the leading edge of the cord, it is important to avoid surgical damage to the adjacent mucosa. Voice therapy should be considered prior to surgical removal in order to ensure there is no recurrence.

### Contact Ulcers/Granulomas

This lesion occurs over the vocal process, which is the mucosa-covered cartilaginous portion of the vocal cord. It is located at the posterior one-third of the glottis. Contact ulcers and granulomas arise over the cartilaginous area because of abrasion or excessive traumatic closure of the vocal processes during phonation. Low-pitched, emphatic vocalization will cause hyperactive contact of the processes and may be the cause. Contact ulcers can also occur from trauma caused by an endotracheal tube being passed over the vocal processes during intubation. Esophageal reflux is felt to be a contributing factor either by creating inflammation, which makes the area more vulnerable to injury, or by bathing the area with gastric acid after injury occurs. The usual symptoms include a relatively sudden onset of hoarseness and laryngeal pain occurring after prolonged vocalization. Pain may be referred to the ear as well. The ulcer base frequently attempts to heal and creates a bed of granulation tissue. With time granulation tissue enlarges into a discrete granuloma.

**Treatment.** Voice therapy is generally necessary to help the patient discontinue throat clearing and other vocal habits that originally precipitated the problem. Esophageal reflux should be carefully evaluated. If there is any element of reflux, it should be treated aggressively. When the patient has maximized medical and voice treatment, the granuloma can be removed surgically. Care is taken not to remove normal tissue around the vocal process.

With intubation granulomas, symptoms may include progression to partial airway obstruction or stridor. Large granulomas that are symptomatic may require somewhat urgent removal.

### Vocal Cord Bowing

Vocal cord bowing is a persistent gap between the vocal cords during adduction and can have several causes. The most common cause is atrophy of the vocalis muscle from aging, which is also called senile bowing. With loss of vocalis muscle mass, the cords are no longer able to completely adduct. The aging process results in redundant tissue with decreased elasticity that will allow the vocal cords to increase in length and flaccidity. Even with maximum muscle tension, it may not be possible to tense the cords across the laryngeal framework.

Bowing seen in younger adults may be due to hyperfunction of the laryngeal muscles which shorten the vocal framework. A third cause of bowing is from dysfunction of the cricothyroid muscle. This muscle is needed for maximal tension or stretch of the vocal cords. The cricothyroid is the only muscle innervated by the superior laryngeal nerve. An isolated superior laryngeal nerve paralysis will result in the inability to tense one cord even though it adducts and abducts normally.

**Treatment.** In cases of senile bowing, the patient's general health and stamina seem to play an important role. Regular exercise and improvement of respiratory function (i.e., abdominal breath support) may improve voicing. Voice therapy should be recommended to those patients who are distressed by their vocal quality. Some patients may show a dramatic improvement with instruction and practice maximizing their optimal vocal function.

A unilateral Gelfoam or Teflon injection into the lateral vocal cord may also improve the voice. Teflon should be used cautiously because it is permanent. If it is overinjected, the airway will be compromised. A thyroplasty procedure to medialize the vocal cord has also been described. This requires an incision in the neck and exposure of the lateral thyroid cartilage. An opening is made into the thyroid cartilage in order to allow dissection on its medial surface. Cartilage or Silastic is then placed adjacent to the vocal cord in order to displace it toward the midline. If the resulting medialization of the vocal cord allows better adduction, the voice will be improved.

## Vocal Cord Paralysis

The causes of vocal cord paralysis are varied. Paralysis may be a result of trauma, surgery (especially thyroid surgery), tumor, or neurologic disease. Approximately 30% of vocal cord paralysis is idiopathic. The vagus nerve has two branches to the larynx: the superior laryngeal nerve and the recurrent laryngeal nerve. The location of the paralyzed cord will depend on which branch of the nerve is affected. When the recurrent laryngeal nerve alone is involved, the cord will remain in the paramedian position which is approximately 1 or 2 mm from the midline. When both the superior laryngeal nerve and recurrent laryngeal nerve are involved, the cord sits in an intermediate or cadaveric position, which is more lateral. On examination, it is often difficult to make this distinction.

**Treatment.** If the recurrent laryngeal nerve alone is involved, the lesion must be in the neck or mediastinum, and a chest x-ray and barium swallow should be obtained. A CT scan of the neck should be considered. If both the recurrent laryngeal nerve and superior laryngeal nerve are affected, the base of the skull and parapharyngeal space are also suspect. About 60% of patients will have a cause identified. The idiopathic cases should be observed for a possible return of function.

With unilateral vocal cord paralysis, the patient may be able to compensate, using the unaffected cord to cross the midline with phonation and swallowing. The voice is usually slightly breathy and lower in pitch, and the singing voice loses its upper register. If the patient has a compromised voice or if aspiration is a problem, Gelfoam can be injected lateral to the vocalis muscle. This is a temporary treatment, and the Gelfoam will be absorbed in 2 to 4 months. If the patient has no return of function after 12 months and requires permanent treatment, a Teflon injection should be considered. This material is not reabsorbed. An alternative surgical treatment is a thyroplasty, which uses a small block of cartilage to medialize the cord. Voice therapy should be considered to educate the patient to avoid hyperfunction of the larynx and poor compensation.

Bilateral vocal cord paralysis generally causes significant airway obstruction and requires tracheotomy placement. Surgical intervention to improve the airway is possible. The goal of surgery is to eliminate the need for tracheotomy. Surgical intervention enlarges the airway through such procedures as external arytenoidectomy or endoscopic $CO_2$ laser arytenoidectomy. These procedures make the voice more breathy and increase the risk of aspiration.

An alternative treatment is a valve tracheotomy tube that allows inspiration of air through the tracheotomy tube and expiration through the vocal cords and mouth to permit voicing. The valve apparatus is removed at night to provide an unobstructed airway.

Many attempts have been made to reinnervate paralyzed vocal cords with neuromuscular grafts from various neck strap muscles. The nerve muscle pedicle grafts can be implanted into the posterior cricoarytenoid muscle, which is the only laryngeal abductor. Some surgeons have had encouraging results, although the success rate has been low in the majority of cases.

## Laryngeal Trauma

Intubation trauma to the vocal cords can cause abrasions and hoarseness. Such injuries are frequently self-limiting and heal spontaneously. As previously mentioned, vocal cord abrasion may result in ulceration and granuloma formation.

More severe damage to the arytenoid cartilage may actually dislocate it from its normal joint position on the cricoid cartilage. If this occurs, it is usually dislocated anteriorly and results in an immobile vocal cord. If this is not discovered and corrected within several days, the joint derangement will result in scarring and permanent fixation of the cord.

External trauma to the larynx most commonly occurs from motor vehicle accidents, although any blow to the neck can cause a laryngeal fracture and must be investigated to rule out laryngeal injury. Hoarseness may be delayed in onset. The patient may have mucosal tears with subsequent tissue emphysema from coughing and progressive airway obstruction. Severe injuries will require tracheotomy. Intubation should be avoided if possible since additional damage or total airway obstruction may result from attempts at intubation.

**Treatment.** Mild injuries can be treated conservatively with voice rest, humidification, avoidance of throat clearing and cough, short-term corticosteroid therapy and consideration of antacid or antireflux medications. The degree of injury can be determined only by visualization of the larynx. The flexible fiberoptic laryngoscope is an excellent adjunct for thorough examination of the larynx. If the patient has mucosal tears, evidence of hematoma, loss of the thyroid cartilage prominence, subcutaneous emphysema, or progressive hoarseness or stridor, tracheotomy will generally be required. If the airway is questionable, a tracheostomy should be performed.

When the patient is stable, a CT scan of the neck will better define the degree of injury. Severe injuries require open surgical repair. Best results from laryngeal repair are obtained if surgery is undertaken within the first 24 hours after injury. The surgical approach is generally through an anterior thyrotomy incision. Minimal débridement should be done, and primary repair of lacerations should be accomplished if possible. All fractures must be reduced. Internal fixation with a small-gauge wire may be required. An internal stent may be used as a lumen keeper. The stent is stabilized with sutures or wires that pass through the neck skin and tie over Silastic buttons on the surface. The stent is removed in a separate procedure in 2 to 6 weeks, depending on the degree of injury.

The final result will depend on the extent of the original injury, the return of vocal cord mobility, and the amount of scar formation.

### Laryngeal Carcinoma

The earliest symptom of carcinoma of the vocal cord is hoarseness. Very small lesions cause weighting and abnormal vibration of the affected cord. Early carcinomas do not cause pain, airway obstruction, or weight loss. Smokers are at the highest risk for throat cancer. All hoarse patients with a history of smoking need a careful laryn-

geal examination. If a cancer of the vocal cord is diagnosed at its earliest stage (normal vocal cord motion without spread above or below the cords), the likelihood of cure is 90 to 95%.

As the tumor enlarges, it infiltrates the underlying structures and causes vocal cord paralysis. The distance between the anterior commissure and the thyroid cartilage is very narrow. Spread to the thyroid cartilage is a Stage IV lesion, and this has the worst prognosis. Metastases to the neck occur very late with vocal cord cancer, owing to the sparse lymphatic channels that supply this area.

To diagnose laryngeal cancer, a biopsy is necessary. The most common cancer of the larynx is squamous cell carcinoma. Prior to biopsy, a routine evaluation of the general health of the patient as well as chest x-ray and laboratory data should be obtained. It is important to stage the tumor adequately, and this is done at the time of biopsy. Direct laryngoscopy and examination of the adjacent areas, such as the epiglottis, ventricles (space between the true and false vocal cords), and subglottis, are included.

**Treatment.** Stage I true vocal cord carcinoma has an excellent cure rate. Radiation therapy is frequently used to treat these small tumors because it maintains the voice in the majority of patients. Conservative surgery has also been used. Advanced laryngeal tumors require more extensive surgery, and some tumors may require combined surgical and radiation treatment. At present, no chemotherapy agent is known to cure laryngeal carcinoma. Tumors that require total removal of the larynx result in a permanent tracheal stoma. Voice rehabilitation includes many options today. Patients gain the use of some type of voice whether it be mechanical, esophageal speech or through a surgically placed tracheoesophageal shunt.

### Neurologic Disease

Voice disturbances can result from a variety of neuromuscular disorders. Essential tremor can affect the laryngeal muscles, causing a rhythmic, quivering voice. Palatal or laryngeal myoclonus produces a characteristic voice with hiccup speech. Amyotrophic lateral sclerosis is often manifested by dysarthria and progressive dysphagia with weakness of the vocal cord adductors and frequent aspiration.

Patients with paralysis agitans (Parkinson's syndrome) have difficulty initiating speech. Their voice is monotonal and low pitched and lacks volume or inflection. Disease progression causes deterioration of articulation with very poor intelligibility and frequent whispering. Involvement of the corticobulbar tracts results in a spastic bulbar (pseudobulbar or suprabulbar) palsy. The usual cause is vascular, but the disorder may also be caused by muscle system disease. Speech is slow and indistinct.

Paretic dysarthria results from weakness or paralysis of the articulatory muscles from involvement of cranial nerves either peripherally or at the motor nucleus of the medulla or lower pons. Fasciculations and atrophy of the tongue, pharynx, palate, or larynx may occur. Speech is very slurred and indistinct. Saliva may pool in the throat or the mouth, and this increases the risk of aspiration.

### Spastic Dysphonia

Spastic dysphonia is classically described as a strained, strangled voice with many breaks in phonation. There are two types described: adductor spastic dysphonia and abductor spastic dysphonia. The adductor variety is much more common.

**Treatment.** The most current information gives supporting evidence that this is a dystonia much like blepharospasm. The voice is frequently worse in stressful situations. Many treatments have been used including antianxiety medications and tranquilizers, biofeedback, psychotherapy, and voice therapy. In mild cases, voice therapy is frequently beneficial. The other treatments have been unrewarding.

Unilateral recurrent laryngeal nerve section has been recommended. The initial results with this surgical intervention are quite good, but long-term results are not as encouraging. The untreated vocal cord appears to become more hyperfunctional and allows the spastic voice quality to return.

A new treatment with potential benefit is currently being tested in several centers and will become available in the near future. The treatment is botulinum toxin (Botox) injected directly into the thyroarytenoid muscle. Botulinum toxin has been used in the treatment of blepharospasm for many years with good results. The toxin does not have a permanent effect and usually wears off in 3 to 4 months, allowing return of the characteristically strained voice. Repeated injections are required. Preliminary information indicates a very high success rate with few, if any, side effects. Even though this treatment is temporary, it may become the treatment of choice for this frustrating problem.

# INSOMNIA

method of
CONSTANTIN R. SOLDATOS, M.D.
*University of Athens*
*Athens, Greece*

The term "insomnia" applies to the condition of unsatisfactory quantity and/or quality of sleep. Insomniacs complain of difficulty in falling asleep, difficulty in staying asleep, awakening in early morning, or any combination of these symptoms. Not infrequently, however, patients suffer from poor quality of sleep, and the amount of their sleep may be judged subjectively and/or objectively to be within normal limits.

Insomnia is a prevalent condition both in the general population and in patient populations; surveys of the general public show a 20 to 30 per cent prevalence of insomnia, and physicians report that more than 20 per cent of their adult patients have had sleep problems. The prevalence of insomnia tends to be higher among women, older individuals, and psychologically disturbed and socioeconomically disadvantaged persons.

Chronic insomniacs report that at bedtime they feel tense, anxious, worried, or depressed and as if their thoughts were racing. They also report rumination about getting enough sleep, personal problems, health status, and death. Further, they often attempt to reduce tension by taking medication and drinking alcohol. In the morning, they typically feel physically and mentally tired, and during the day they report being depressed, worried, tense, irritable, and overly preoccupied.

## ETIOLOGIC CONSIDERATIONS

Insomnia is often a symptom of various psychiatric or medical conditions. It may also be a result of drug use. Amphetamines, energizing antidepressants, steroids, bronchodilators, and beta blockers are notorious for their sleep-disturbing effects. Rapidly eliminated benzodiazepine hypnotics such as triazolam often cause sleeplessness during the last few hours of nights during therapy (early morning insomnia) or intense sleep difficulty after their discontinuation (rebound insomnia). Substances other than drugs may lead to the development of insomnia: coffee and colas, as well as cigarette smoking, are associated with sleep disruption, particularly difficulty in falling asleep; use and abuse of alcohol are usually related to difficulty in staying asleep. Other common causes of insomnia include various environmental disturbances, stressful life events, and the process of aging. It should be emphasized that in most cases, multiple factors are involved in the etiology of insomnia.

Although insomnia is most often a secondary condition, when it is chronic and severe it becomes the focus of the patient's distress and is in fact perceived as a disorder itself. The most common cause of chronic insomnia is psychopathology. Extensive psychologic and psychiatric research has shown that chronic insomniacs tend to cope with stress and conflicts by internalizing their emotions, which leads to increased emotional arousal. This arousal causes physiologic activation, as indicated by the high levels of autonomic activity before sleep. In turn, this state of hyperarousal leads to difficulty in initiating sleep either at the beginning of the night or later on returning to sleep after a nocturnal awakening. Fear of sleeplessness further increases emotional arousal, thus perpetuating insomnia.

## DIAGNOSTIC ISSUES

An adequate assessment of insomnia can be accomplished in the physician's office. The cornerstone of this assessment is the sleep history, as outlined in Table 1. Through the sleep history, relevant clinical information that accurately describes the patient's sleep problem and its important correlates can be collected. In addition, a thorough medical work-up, a careful psychiatric assessment, and a complete drug history should be obtained.

For the diagnosis of chronic insomnia to be established, the following criteria are required: (1) the complaint of sleep disturbance is either difficulty in falling asleep or maintaining sleep or poor quality of sleep; (2) the complaint has occurred at least three times per week for at least 1 month; (3) the patient is preoccupied with sleeplessness and is excessively concerned about its consequences; and (4) the unsatisfactory quantity or quality of sleep either causes marked distress or interferes with social and occupational functioning.

## THERAPEUTIC PRINCIPLES

Insomniacs are so preoccupied with sleeplessness itself and invested in the secondary gain they receive that they are resistant to a systematic therapeutic approach. Thus, a major task of the physician is to overcome resistance and engage the patient in a comprehensive treatment plan. Such a plan should be multidimensional and should combine the following modalities: general measures for the improvement of sleep hygiene and the patient's lifestyle; psychotherapeutic techniques, selectively or in combination; and pharmacotherapy, only when indicated, as an adjunct.

### TABLE 1. **Steps in Taking the Sleep History***

Delineation of the specific sleep difficulty
Description of the condition's clinical course
Differentiation among various sleep disorders
Reassessment of previous diagnoses
Evaluation of sleep-wakefulness patterns on a 24-hr basis
Interview of bed partner
Evaluation for presence of other sleep disorders
Assessment of a family history of sleep disorders
Evaluation of the impact of the sleep disorder

*Reprinted from Kales A, Soldatos CR, and Kales JD: Taking a sleep history. Am Fam Physician 22:101–107, 1980, published by the American Academy of Family Physicians.

### General Measures and Psychotherapies

A number of general measures for improving the patient's sleep hygiene and overall lifestyle are relatively easy to implement (Table 2). These measures are often quite beneficial, especially when combined with other treatment modalities. The patient should be instructed to schedule times for hobbies and other interesting daytime activities. Particular emphasis should be given to increased exercise levels, although exercise close to bedtime should be avoided because of its arousing effect. Similarly, stressful situations and the use of coffee, colas, cigarette smoking, and other stimulating substances should be avoided close to bedtime.

It is important for the patient to observe a regular schedule for going to bed at night and arising in the morning; however, such a schedule must be reasonably flexible and take into account the fact that sleep cannot be forced on oneself. The patient can be taught that 7 to 8 hours of sleep per 24 hours is usually adequate and that any naps should be added up when the total duration of sleep is estimated. Special attention should be given to minimization of sleep-disrupting environmental stimuli, such as noise, light, and temperature extremes; uncomfortable beds should be corrected.

Any psychotherapeutic approach to treating insomnia should be tailored to meet the individual's needs. Most insomniacs require reassurance to alleviate their fear of sleeplessness; a full explanation should be offered of how anxiety becomes part of the vicious circle that exacerbates and perpetuates insomnia. Patients also need to be taught to reduce stress through effective management of emotions and appropriate expression of feelings. On an interpersonal level, they often need to become adequately assertive. From a technical standpoint, supportive, insight-oriented, and behavioral elements are usually combined for psychotherapy of insomnia. Although supportive psychotherapy can be performed successfully by almost any physician, appropriate referral is indicated for the application of highly specialized psychotherapeutic techniques.

### Pharmacotherapy

A hypnotic drug may be used only as an adjunct to the multidimensional treatment of insomnia.

### TABLE 2. **General Measures for Treating Insomnia**

Regular exercise, but not close to bedtime
Avoidance of stress and tension
Restricted use of sleep-disturbing substances
Flexible but not irregular, schedule for retiring and arising
Optimization of sleep duration
Improvement in sleep environment

Before prescribing a hypnotic, the physician must thoroughly assess the various factors involved in the etiology of the patient's insomnia and address them appropriately. A hypnotic can be quite beneficial in alleviating sleeplessness, thus providing the patient with a most needed sense of mastery. This beneficial effect, however, can be properly achieved only when certain principles are taken into account, as outlined in Table 3.

Because of their efficacy and safety, benzodiazepines have replaced other classes of hypnotics in the adjunctive treatment of insomnia. Benzodiazepines used as hypnotics in the U.S. market include flurazepam (Dalmane), temazepam (Restoril), and triazolam (Halcion). Because of their pharmacokinetics, these three drugs have different effects and side effects. Flurazepam and triazolam are absorbed rapidly and therefore are quite effective in inducing sleep; temazepam, a slowly absorbed formulation, has little efficacy for sleep induction. The long elimination half-life of flurazepam makes it possible for this drug to be effective during a 4-week period of nightly administration, whereas tolerance develops rather rapidly with triazolam and temazepam, both drugs having relatively shorter elimination half-lives.

Administration of slowly eliminated benzodiazepines, such as flurazepam, is often associated with higher degrees of daytime sedation. This side effect, however, is less of a problem with the 15-mg dose of flurazepam. Tolerance to daytime sedation develops much earlier than tolerance to the hypnotic effect of the drug. In contrast, rapidly eliminated benzodiazepines, such as triazolam, are practically devoid of this side effect, but they are more likely to cause rebound phenomena both during their administration (early morning insomnia, daytime anxiety) and after their withdrawal (rebound insomnia, rebound anxiety). Administration of triazolam has also been associated with episodes of amnesia, depersonalization, hallucinations, and other behavioral side effects.

Nonbenzodiazepine hypnotics are somewhat effective initially, but they lose most of their efficacy within about 2 weeks of nightly use. Thus, an escalation of their dosage often takes place, and a severe abstinence syndrome may occur with

TABLE 3. **Considerations During Use of Hypnotic Medication for Treatment of Insomnia**

Thorough evaluation of the patient should be done before treatment
Hypnotics should be used only as adjuncts
Limited amounts should be prescribed
Initial and continued efficacy should be considered
The patient has to be cognizant of side effects
Withdrawal problems need to be addressed
Drug interactions should be avoided

their abrupt withdrawal. Over-the-counter sedatives have been proved to be ineffective, and in high doses they may cause unwanted effects, such as confusional states, because of their atropine-like action. In the small subgroup of chronic insomniacs who are endogenously depressed, the use of tricyclic antidepressants is indicated. For psychiatric patients with the symptom of insomnia, neuroleptics with sedative effects should be prescribed.

### Treating the Elderly

Before any treatment, the elderly insomniac should be assessed for the presence of medical and psychiatric disorders. If conditions such as organic brain syndrome or depression are present, the treatment plan must be adjusted accordingly. For example, haloperidol (Haldol) should be prescribed to the organically impaired elderly insomniac with nocturnal agitation and confusion.

Monosymptomatic elderly insomniacs should be educated about the extent of age-related sleep changes. Special emphasis should be placed on the effects of daytime naps on nocturnal sleep. These naps should be generally discouraged. Instead, the elderly insomniac is advised to increase daytime activities and to try to be engaged in stimulating social contacts.

The use of hypnotic drugs should generally be avoided in the elderly because the age-related impairment of renal function may lead to retention of the drug, which is often associated with increased likelihood of daytime sedation, amnesia, and other side effects. If a hypnotic is needed, one that is lastingly effective may be preferable. All hypnotic drugs should be administered in about one-half the dosage intended for young adults.

# PRURITUS

method of
JOHN R. VAN GURP, M.D., PH.D., and
MICHAEL T. GOLDFARB, M.D.
*University of Michigan Medical Center*
*Ann Arbor, Michigan*

Itching is an unpleasant sensation that evokes the scratch response. It is thought that the sensation is initiated in the free nerve endings of the skin, then travels through unmyelinated C fibers to the dorsal horn of the spinal cord, ascending the contralateral spinothalamic tracts and eventuating in the cerebral cortex. Although gating of sensory afferent activity may influence the perception of itch, the scratch response is a spinal reflex.

Perhaps more accessible to therapeutic intervention are the known and postulated mediators and modulators of pruritus. Although histamine is the classic mediator, various other substances such as proteases, opioid and non-opioid peptides, prostaglandins, and serotonin may be active in the sensation of itch.

## DIAGNOSIS

The first step in the evaluation of the pruritic patient is to exclude a primary dermatologic disease or infestation (Table 1). Although specific diagnostic features such as morphology and distribution will usually lead to the correct diagnosis of a cutaneous eruption, distinguishing primary lesions from secondary excoriations, eczematization, and impetiginization may prove to be quite a challenging task. Careful examination may be required to discern the fine scale characteristic of asteatotic dermatitis. This condition tends to be more common in the elderly and worse during the winter months and is probably the most common cause of pruritus. When other family members are also affected, consideration should be given to a diagnosis of scabies or pediculosis. Cercarial dermatitis may be suggested by a history of swimming in a local lake, but other aspects of the history may be more consistent with aquagenic pruritus. Time and circumstances of onset as well as provocative and palliative factors elucidated in the history can often lead to the diagnosis or at least suggest an avenue of investigation. When indicated, adjunctive techniques such as skin scrapings are performed to confirm a diagnosis of scabies or dermatophytosis. A skin biopsy examination with special stains or direct immunofluorescence may be required to confirm a diagnosis of mastocytosis or one of the autoimmune bullous diseases.

After dermatologic disease has been excluded, the pruritic patient should then be evaluated for a potential underlying systemic condition (Table 2). Pruritus is a well known manifestation of chronic renal failure (especially those patients receiving hemodialysis), cholestatic liver disease, and myeloproliferative disorders such as Hodgkin's disease and polycythemia vera. Important but uncommon, patients with visceral malignancies have also been reported to present with pruritus and thus an appropriate work-up seems to be justified. The association of generalized pruritus and diabetes is suspect. Although anogenital pruritus is apparently more common in diabetics, candidiasis should be excluded. Pruritus is also reportedly more common in patients with hyper- and hypothyroidism. Drugs known to cause itching include opiates, amphetamines, quinidine, aspirin, vitamin B complex, and niacinamide, but a subclinical allergic reaction may occur with virtually any drug. Rare and unusual causes of pruritus include neurologic disease such as brain tumors, infarcts, and abscesses. Dumping syndrome, sicca syndrome, and even atypical angina have been associated with pruritus.

The findings of a careful history, physical examination, and review of systems will dictate the type and extent of laboratory work-up necessary for the diagnosis of pruritus of unknown origin. Initial laboratory screening often includes a complete blood count with differential, fasting blood glucose, thyroid and liver function tests, urea nitrogen, creatinine, and routine urinalysis. Serum iron studies; stool for ova, parasites, and occult blood; serum protein electrophoresis; chest x-ray; and CT scan of the abdomen and pelvis may be considered under appropriate circumstances.

## TREATMENT

Not uncommonly, the underlying cause of pruritus cannot be determined and therapy must be aimed at symptomatic treatment and avoidance of provocative factors. Teaching the patient to break the itch-scratch cycle and giving alternatives to scratching such as application of a cool,

TABLE 1. **Dermatologic Disorders Associated with Pruritus**

Asteatotic dermatitis
Nummular eczema
Atopic dermatitis
Lichen simplex chronicus
Prurigo nodularis
Contact dermatitis
Irritant dermatitis—e.g., fiberglass
Aquagenic dermatitis
Sunburn
Psoriasis
Pityriasis rosea
Mycosis fungoides, Sézary's syndrome
Urticaria
Dermatographism
Mastocytosis
Lichen planus
Polymorphous light eruption
Bullous pemphigoid
Dermatitis herpetiformis
Grover's disease
Herpes gestationis
Pruritic urticarial papules and plaques of pregnancy
Miliaria
Fox-Fordyce disease
Folliculitis
Scabies, pediculosis, and other arthropod infestations,
   bites, or stings
Cercarial dermatitis
Onchocerciasis
Dermatophytosis
Varicella

TABLE 2. **Systemic Conditions Associated with Pruritus**

Chronic renal failure
Cholestatic liver disease
Myeloproliferative disorders
Iron deficiency anemia
Thyroid disease
Diabetes
Pruritus gravidarum
Malignant neoplasms, carcinoid syndrome
Psychiatric illness
Parasitosis
Drug reaction

damp wash cloth and topical antipruritics can sometimes be helpful. Because dry skin can be a primary cause as well as exacerbate pruritus, patients should be instructed to avoid excessive bathing and to use a mild soap (Dove, Basis, Neutrogena, Purpose). Liberal use of emollients (Moisturel, Eucerin, Lubriderm) should be encouraged, especially immediately after bathing. Home humidifiers are helpful in dry climates. Loose fitting cotton clothes are preferable to wool and polyester garments. Fabric softeners and brighteners are also thought to sometimes cause or exacerbate pruritus. If possible, the patient should avoid warm environments, especially hot baths, as increased cutaneous blood flow will increase itching. Similarly, other vasodilators such as alcohol and spicy foods should be avoided. Stress and stimulants such as caffeine may also provoke itching.

### Topical Treatment

Preparations containing combinations of menthol (0.25 to 2%), phenol (0.5 to 1.5%), and camphor (1 to 3%) such as Sarna lotion may be applied several times daily for symptomatic relief of pruritus. Pramoxine-containing products (Pramegel, Prax) may also reduce itching; however, other topical anesthetics and topical antihistamines should be avoided because they can be potent sensitizers. Topical steroids should be reserved for specific steroid-responsive dermatoses.

### Systemic Treatment

Antihistamines with CNS sedative effects such as hydroxyzine (Atarax, Vistaril), 25 mg, diphenhydramine (Benadryl), 25 mg, cyproheptadine (Periactin), 4 mg, chlorpheniramine (Chlor-Trimeton), 4 mg, and trimeprazine (Temaril), 2.5 mg, given orally every 4 to 6 hours and/or prior to bedtime can be effective in alleviating pruritus. Dosages may be increased under proper supervision, and switching or combining agents is also occasionally helpful. Although nonsedating antihistamines such as terfenadine (Seldane) and astemizole (Hismanal) are useful where histamine plays a primary role, such as in urticaria, results are generally disappointing with most other pruritic disorders. Likewise, $H_2$ blockers are generally ineffective in the treatment of pruritus.

Psychotropic agents can also be useful under certain circumstances, especially when there is associated anxiety or depression. Doxepin (Sinequan), an antidepressant with antihistaminic properties, may be given in a dosage of 25 to 50 mg before bedtime. Pimozide (Orap) in a dosage of 4 mg twice daily is particularly useful for treatment of delusions of parasitosis. As with all medications, the physician and patient should be familiar with the potential side effects of these drugs.

Phototherapy with ultraviolet B (UVB) light can be especially effective in the treatment of renal and biliary pruritus as well as itching associated with other systemic and primary dermatologic disorders. Therapy can be initiated at 75% of the minimal erythemogenic dose at a frequency of three times per week.

Other treatment considerations include sequestrants such as cholestyramine (Questran), 5 mg twice daily, and dietary manipulation for treatment of both biliary (diet rich in polyunsaturated fatty acids) and renal (low-protein diet) pruritus.

# TINNITUS

method of
JOHN W. HOUSE, M.D.
*House Ear Clinic and House Ear Institute*
*Los Angeles, California*

As has been often stated, tinnitus is a symptom and not a disease. Therefore, when patients complain of noise in their ears or head, an evaluation is necessary to establish the etiology of their tinnitus. All patients complaining of tinnitus require an audiogram, including air conduction, bone conduction, and speech, to evaluate the nature of any hearing loss if in fact there is such a loss. Approximately 10 per cent of our patients who have a primary complaint of tinnitus have normal hearing. In addition to routine audiometric studies, a history is taken, and an otologic examination is performed by the otologist.

A unilateral sensorineural hearing loss, unilateral symptoms, or an asymmetric hearing loss may indicate serious pathology. In these cases a neuro-otologic evaluation is necessary. An auditory brain stem response (ABR) is performed as a screening test. If this result is positive, we proceed to magnetic resonance imaging (MRI) with gadolinium. When we are strongly suspicious of a retrocochlear lesion, we proceed directly to MRI without performing the ABR test. On the other hand, if the ABR result is negative, we rarely proceed to MRI.

In patients who describe the tinnitus as pulsatile, auscultation of the ear is performed by using Toynbee's tube. The neck and mastoid are auscultated by using a stethoscope. This objective type of tinnitus can be associated with arterial plaques, arteriovenous malformations, enlarged jugular bulb, or vascular tumors (e.g., glomus tympanicum or jugulare). In such cases, we obtain a high-resolution computed tomography scan with a bone program to look at the bony details of the jugular bulb, carotid artery, and middle-ear structures. If these studies are normal, we do not usually proceed to angiography. In rare cases we obtain vascular studies such as an arteriogram, jugular venogram, Doppler, or ultrasound studies.

## TREATMENT

Eighty-six per cent of patients with an ear disorder have associated tinnitus. Approximately 95 per cent of these patients are not particularly concerned about the tinnitus and are satisfied with an evaluation, an explanation, and any treatment of the underlying cause. A small number of patients are driven to distraction by the tinnitus and tend to focus on their complaints. Many of these patients complain of lack of sleep caused by the tinnitus. They also complain of difficulty in concentrating; in some cases they find everyday tasks difficult. We have evaluated the personality of these patients and have found that depression is a significant factor in their symptoms. We therefore recommend antidepressants as a first line treatment for these patients.

If the tinnitus is associated with a conductive hearing loss, correcting the hearing loss may be of benefit. Seventy-five per cent of patients with otosclerosis report resolution of the tinnitus after successful surgery. On the other hand, 5 per cent of patients report that the tinnitus is worse after surgery. Our experience with translabyrinthine removal of acoustic neuromas has shown that about one-half of the patients report improvement of the tinnitus, whereas the other half report that the tinnitus is worse. For this reason we do not recommend a cochlear nerve section for the treatment of tinnitus.

Because most tinnitus is associated with a sensorineural hearing loss, hearing aids can be helpful. We have found that most patients with a hearing loss and associated tinnitus report an improvement in the tinnitus while they wear hearing aids. The hearing aids act to improve the patients' performance and allow for environmental sounds to enter the ear, thus masking the tinnitus. We use tinnitus maskers on rare occasions. We have found that a small number of patients find the tinnitus masker to be helpful because they believe that it gives them some control of the tinnitus.

For many years we have been using biofeedback training as a treatment of tinnitus. Our experience has indicated that patients who are depressed or have anxiety attacks do well with biofeedback. Approximately 80 per cent of these patients report some relief or control of the tinnitus. Patients who are more severely disturbed tend to do poorly with biofeedback training. We believe that biofeedback training is successful in helping patients because the tinnitus is exacerbated by muscle tension around the neck and head and by constriction of the peripheral circulation. When patients learn to relax the muscles and to increase the peripheral circulation, the tinnitus tends to decrease. In addition the patients gain insight into the causes of the tinnitus and how it is exacerbated by tension and stress.

All patients complaining of tinnitus deserve an evaluation that should include at least routine audiometric studies. If any of these results are positive, further neuro-otologic or vascular studies are necessary. The general treatment is aimed at the underlying cause of the problem. A complete explanation of the situation is beneficial, and hearing aids, tinnitus maskers, biofeedback, and antidepressants may be helpful.

# Section 2

# The Infectious Diseases

## MANAGEMENT OF HIV INFECTION

method of
SUSAN M. MILLER, M.D., M.P.H., and
THOMAS R. CATE, M.D.

*Baylor College of Medicine*
*Houston, Texas*

Human immunodeficiency virus Type I (HIV) is the primary etiologic agent of the acquired immunodeficiency syndrome (AIDS). The Centers for Disease Control (CDC) estimates that 1 to 1.5 million U.S. citizens are infected with HIV and that more than 100,000 had developed AIDS by September 1989. HIV is a retrovirus that causes progressive impairment of the infected host's immune function. Death due to one or more of the opportunistic infections, cancers, or other conditions that define AIDS (Table 1) typically occurs within 10 years of the initiation of HIV infection. However, earlier stages of HIV infection are usually recognized and have been classified for reporting purposes (Table 2). Included are the initial infection that may be asymptomatic or manifested as an infectious mononucleosis-like illness with or without aseptic meningitis; a prolonged asymptomatic period during which hematologic or immunologic abnormalities may appear; persistent generalized lymphadenopathy; and finally, occurrence of constitutional disease, neurologic disease, and secondary infections, cancers, or other conditions that lead to debilitation and death. Occurrence or recurrence of the latter complications can be delayed by antiretroviral therapy, and many of the complications can be effectively treated or suppressed.

### BASELINE ASSESSMENT

The possibility of HIV infection should be considered in patients that fall into groups at risk for acquiring the virus through infected blood or secretions (Table 3). Transmission does not occur through casual contact or mosquitoes, but a low risk of transmission exists via blood or secretions on disrupted skin or through needle sticks; hence, universal blood and body fluid precautions should be followed. Sexually transmitted diseases and active tuberculosis in young adults are potential signals of HIV infection. The diagnosis should be considered in the differential for symptoms such as unexplained weight loss, prolonged fever or night sweats, fatigue, swollen lymph nodes, easy bruisability or petechiae, confusion, neuropathy, dyspnea, mouth sores, and prolonged diarrhea, as well as symptoms of the AIDS-defining complications.

## TABLE 1. Diseases Defining AIDS in an Adult with Proven HIV Infection*

**Viruses**
Herpes simplex virus—mucocutaneous >1 mo; bronchitis, pneumonitis, esophagitis
Cytomegalovirus—organs other than liver, spleen, lymph node
Papovavirus—progressive multifocal leukoencephalopathy

**Bacteria**
*Mycobacteria*—any with disease outside lungs, hilar and cervical nodes, or skin
*Salmonella*—recurrent, nontyphoidal septicemia

**Fungi**
*Candida*—disease of esophagus, trachea, bronchi, or lungs
Cryptococcosis—extrapulmonary
Histoplasmosis, coccidioidomycosis—outside lungs and hilar or cervical nodes

**Protozoa**
Pneumocystis carinii pneumonia
Toxoplasmosis of brain
Cryptosporidiosis, isosporiasis—diarrhea >1 mo

**Cancer**
Kaposi's sarcoma
Primary lymphoma of brain
Other non-Hodgkin's lymphoma—B cell or unknown immunologic phenotype, small noncleaved lymphoma or immunoblastic lymphoma

**Other**
Wasting syndrome—unexplained weight loss >10% and diarrhea or fever >1 mo
Dementia—cognitive and/or motor dysfunction interfering with work or daily living

*MMWR 1987; 36, August 14 Suppl. 35–155.

The primary means for diagnosis is testing serum for antibodies to HIV by an enzyme-linked immunosorbent assay (ELISA). Because of the health and societal implications of a positive test for HIV antibody, it is important to inform the patient about the purposes and meaning of the test; written consent for testing is required in some jurisdictions and should always be obtained when the test is being performed for case finding rather than for diagnosis of an illness or investigation of an exposure of others to the patient's blood or secretions. A positive result should be confirmed by an independent testing method (e.g., ELISA followed by a confirmatory Western blot). Testing for p24 antigen, one of the internal proteins of HIV, can be of use in following the effects of antiretroviral therapy and may rarely yield a diagnosis in the absence of a positive

TABLE 2. **Classification of HIV Infection***

I. Acute infection
II. Asymptomatic infection
III. Persistent generalized lymphadenopathy
IV. Other disease
    A. Constitutional disease
    B. Neurologic disease
    C. Secondary infections
    D. Secondary cancers
    E. Other conditions due to HIV or depressed immunity

*MMWR 1986; 35:334–339.

test for antibody. Attempts to diagnose HIV infection by culture or by a sensitive means for virus detection such as the polymerase chain reaction may be indicated in some circumstances. In any event, the patient should be told of the test results and counselled about safe sex and other methods for minimizing the risk of transmission of HIV.

In addition to HIV serology, studies on a patient known or suspected to be infected with HIV should include complete blood counts with differential, platelet count, quantitation of CD4 and CD8 T lymphocyte subsets, chemistry profile, a serologic test for syphilis, B-2 microglobulin or neopterin level, hepatitis B and toxoplasma serology, skin tests for tuberculosis and one or more control antigens, and a chest radiograph. A Pap smear needs to be performed in female patients. Vaccinations such as those against tetanus, pneumococci, and influenza should be reviewed and brought up to date as early in the course as possible. Hepatitis B vaccination is a consideration for those remaining free of infection with this virus, although actions to minimize the risk of HIV transmission should also minimize exposure to hepatitis. Attention should be paid to optimizing the nutritional value of the patient's diet.

When the patient's condition and support system permit, therapy is performed on an outpatient basis. Extensive use is made of visiting nurses and intravenous therapy within the clinic and at home. The following recommendations are those used for treatment of the retrovirus and the more common opportunistic infections in nonpregnant, HIV-infected adults.

## ANTIRETROVIRAL THERAPY

Treatment of HIV-infected patients with zidovudine (Retrovir, "AZT") will reduce replication of the virus, partially reverse immunosuppression, and delay the occurrence or recurrence of

TABLE 3. **Major Risk Behaviors and Groups for HIV**

Homosexual and bisexual activity
Intravenous drug abuse
Heterosexual partners of persons at risk, including prostitutes
Newborns of mothers at risk
Hemophiliacs treated prior to 1985
Transfusion recipients prior to mid-1985

complications; it is not curative. Recommendations about the stage of HIV infection at which zidovudine therapy should be initiated have recently been modified. Therapy should always be offered when the CD4 cell count is 200 per mm$^3$ or less or when the patient has developed a complication that defines AIDS, and is now recommended for patients with CD4 counts of 200 to 500 per mm$^3$ whether or not they have symptoms. Recent data suggest that treatment of the latter patients can delay the occurrence of complications, and furthermore, zidovudine is tolerated better by healthier patients. Zidovudine's role in pregnant and postexposure populations remains uncertain. Decreased susceptibility of HIV isolates to zidovudine has been noted following therapy, but the clinical significance of this finding is uncertain.

Recommendations for dosing of zidovudine have also changed. Initial recommendations were for two 100 mg capsules orally every 4 hours around the clock, but the high frequency of side effects with this dose and recognition that as few as five capsules per day were equally effective for slowing progression to AIDS among patients with CD4 counts of 200 to 500 per mm$^3$ have led to the frequent use of lower doses. The most recent recommendations are for 200 mg of zidovudine every 4 hours for 1 month, followed by 100 mg every 4 hours. We typically initiate therapy with 100 mg every 4 hours while awake (i.e., five capsules per day) or 200 mg every 8 hours, which seems to improve compliance; the dose may then be modified upward or downward according to the patient's tolerance and response to therapy. Attempts to achieve a dose of 200 mg every 4 hours may be warranted in patients with HIV disease of the central nervous system to facilitate delivery of the drug at the site of infection. Zidovudine therapy of HIV infection is continued indefinitely.

Patients initiating zidovudine therapy are generally followed at 2-week intervals for two visits to check for and attempt to alleviate side effects, and then on a monthly basis. Laboratory data obtained on these visits include a complete blood count, differential if the white blood cell count is 2000 per mm$^3$ or less, platelet count, creatinine, transaminases, lactic dehydrogenase, and creatinine phosphokinase. The most common side effects recognized by the patient are nausea, vomiting, headache, fatigue, insomnia, agitation, and pruritus. Seizures, myositis, hepatitis, and dystonic reactions have also been seen. However, the most common dose-limiting side effect is bone marrow suppression, particularly of the red cell series.

The anemia is frequently macrocytic. Vitamin B$_{12}$ deficiency has been detected in AIDS patients and should be checked for and corrected if present. The patient may also be receiving medications such as trimethoprim-sulfamethoxazole (TMP-SMZ) (Bactrim, Septra) or pyrimethamine (Daraprim) that can interfere with folate metabolism and, if so, should be supplemented with leucovorin (Wellcovorin). However, the anemia and macrocytosis are prominent side effects of zidovudine itself. Macrocytosis is not an indication for cessation of therapy.

Temporary cessation of zidovudine therapy, or at least dosage reduction, is advisable if chemotherapy for Kaposi's sarcoma is undertaken. Probenecid (Benemid) can elevate blood levels of zidovudine by interfering with its excretion and thus can potentiate its toxicity. The physician needs to be alert to the possibility of other drug interactions and modify therapy accordingly. If a patient receiving zidovudine has a persistent decline in hemoglobin, two alternatives are available: reduce zidovudine dosage and observe for marrow recovery, or maintain the current dosage and transfuse. We generally reduce zidovudine dosage and discontinue it altogether if transfusion requirements remain in the vicinity of 4 units every 1 to 3 months. The role of erythropoietin (r-HuEPO, EPREX) therapy in these situations is under investigation; preliminary data suggest a therapeutic effect if the serum erythropoietin level is less than 500 IU per liter.

Neutropenia is common in HIV-infected patients receiving zidovudine, and it may be necessary to reduce the dosage in order to maintain neutrophile counts above the danger level of 500 per mm³. Ganciclovir (Cytovene) used for treatment of cytomegalovirus infection commonly causes neutropenia, and it will likely be necessary to discontinue or severely reduce zidovudine dosing if ganciclovir therapy is required. Mild thrombocytopenia is a common finding as HIV infection progresses and may occasionally become severe; zidovudine therapy may improve this HIV-associated thrombocytopenia, but zidovudine can also rarely cause severe thrombocytopenia itself, thus necessitating dose reduction or discontinuation.

Two additional reverse transcriptase inhibitors are undergoing investigation: dideoxycytidine and dideoxyinosine. Both drugs show in vitro activity against HIV and, in early clinical studies, appear to cause less marrow suppression than zidovudine. The major toxicity of dideoxycytidine in relatively high doses is a stocking-glove peripheral neuropathy. Additional side effects include rash, mucositis, arthralgias, diarrhea, and marrow suppression. With lower doses of dideoxycytidine (0.75 mg orally every 8 hours) that still retain anti-HIV activity, the frequency of these side effects is reduced and they appear to be largely reversible. Studies are in progress to compare the efficacy of dideoxycytidine with that of zidovudine and to examine the effectiveness of alternating therapy with these two medications. Dideoxyinosine, another nucleoside analog, is available as a powder plus antacid to be dissolved in water and ingested every 12 hours on an empty stomach in a dose of about 4 mg per kg. Early side effects associated with its administration include neuropathy, pancreatitis, diarrhea, and encephalopathy. It is premature to state which of these nucleosides has the greatest antiviral activity. Future recommendations concerning their administration may be based on the toxicity profiles seen in individual patients. For example, one drug may be better tolerated than another by a given patient, even though both have similar antiviral profiles. Hence, drug substitution may, in the future, form the basis for managing complications of antiretroviral therapy.

## TREATMENT OF COMMON OPPORTUNISTIC INFECTIONS

### Protozoal Infections

*Pneumocystis carinii* **Pneumonia (PCP).** PCP is the most common major opportunistic infection complicating HIV disease. Prior to the use of primary PCP prophylaxis, it accounted for about 60% of initial AIDS diagnoses. Typical symptoms in patients with PCP include progressive shortness of breath, a nonproductive cough, fever, and weight loss. Physical findings in the chest can be minimal. Chest radiographs can be normal but commonly show bilateral interstitial infiltrates and occasional nodular lesions or a spontaneous pneumothorax. Arterial blood gases will typically reveal hypoxia and an increased A-a gradient. Although not routinely performed, gallium scanning will typically reveal increased uptake over the lungs in patients with PCP, even when the chest radiograph is relatively normal. The diagnosis may be established by microscopic detection of the organism in induced sputum or bronchoalveolar lavage fluid. Standard treatment regimens are oral/intravenous TMP-SMZ or intravenous pentamidine (see Table 4 for dosage).

The most common side effects of TMP-SMZ are nausea, vomiting, skin rash, bone marrow suppression, thrush, fever, and hepatotoxicity. Nausea or vomiting may be alleviated by shifting from oral administration to intravenous infusion, by decreasing the rate of drug infusion, or by modifying the dose based on pharmacokinetic monitoring. A mild rash may not require cessation of therapy if diphenhydramine (Benadryl) is given simultaneously. Co-administration of leucovorin may reduce bone marrow suppression.

TABLE 4. **Antimicrobials for Common Opportunistic Infections in HIV-Infected Adults**

| Disease | Medication | Daily Dose | Major Toxicities |
|---|---|---|---|
| *Pneumocystis carinii* pneumonia | Trimethoprim/sulfamethoxazole *or* | 15–20/75–100 mg/kg† | Drug fever, nausea, rash, marrow suppression |
| | Pentamidine isethionate | 3–4 mg/kg | Nephrotoxicity, nausea, hypotension, hypoglycemia, rash, marrow suppression, pancreatitis |
| *Toxoplasma* encephalitis | Pyrimethamine *plus* | 25 mg | Thrombocytopenia, neutropenia |
| | Sulfadiazine *plus* | 4–6 grams | Thrombocytopenia, neutropenia, rash, acute renal failure |
| | Leucovorin | 5–10 mg | |
| *Candida* (thrush) | Clotrimazole troche *or* | 30–50 mg | Mild transaminase increase, dental caries secondary to dextrose component |
| | Nystatin susp. *or* | 3 mU | Diarrhea, nausea, vomiting |
| | Ketoconazole | 200–400 mg | Nausea, hepatotoxicity, adrenal suppression, rash |
| Cryptococcal meningitis | Amphotericin *or* | 0.5–0.7 mg/kg | Fever, chills, renal failure, hypokalemia, marrow suppression, phlebitis |
| | Fluconazole | 200–400 mg | Nausea, vomiting, abdominal discomfort, rash, increased transaminase |
| Mycobacterial disease (see text) | Isoniazid | 300 mg | Hepatitis, neuropathy (reduced by pyridoxine), nausea, vomiting, allergy |
| | Rifampin | 600 mg | Nausea, allergy, hepatitis, thrombocytopenia |
| | Pyrazinamide | 25 mg/kg | Arthralgias, hyperuricemia, nausea, hepatitis |
| | Ethambutol | 15–25 mg/kg | Optic neuritis (acuity and color perception), hyperuricemia |
| | Streptomycin | 1 gram | Ototoxicity, nephrotoxicity |
| | Clofazimine | 100 mg | Darkened skin, abdominal pain |
| | Rifabutin* | 150–300 mg | Diarrhea, marrow suppression, hepatitis |
| | Amikacin | 500 mg | Nephrotoxicity, ototoxicity |
| | Ciprofloxacin | 1–1.5 gm | Nausea, vomiting, abdominal pain, headache, dizziness, photosensitivity |
| Neurosyphilis | Penicillin G | 18–24 mU | Allergic reaction |
| Herpes simplex | | | |
| Cutaneous | Acyclovir | 1 gram | Rash, nausea, diarrhea, vertigo |
| Disseminated | Acyclovir | 15 mg/kg | Nephrotoxicity, phlebitis, headache, encephalopathy, marrow suppression, rash, mild hepatotoxicity |
| Varicella-zoster | Acyclovir | 30 mg/kg | |
| Cytomegalovirus chorioretinitis | Ganciclovir | 2 wk: 10 mg/kg; then 5 mg/kg | Neutropenia, thrombocytopenia, rash, hypotension, nausea, vomiting, headache |

*Investigational drug.
†Milligrams per kilogram of body weight.

Nevertheless, about half of HIV-infected patients develop significant side effects or allergic reactions that prevent continued use of TMP-SMZ. An advantage of TMP-SMZ is its availability for oral administration. If the patient is allergic to sulfonamides and a nonparenteral therapeutic regimen is desired, less well proven considerations include dapsone 100 mg plus trimethoprim (Trimpex) 15–20 mg per kg orally each day or aerosolized pentamidine isethionate (NebuPent) given on a daily basis.

Intravenous pentamidine isethionate (Pentam) is the other standard treatment for PCP. Pain and sterile abscesses after intramuscular administration make the latter route undesirable. When given intravenously, pentamidine must be administered slowly over 60 minutes to diminish the risk of hypotension. Other adverse effects include bone marrow suppression, hypoglycemia, hypocalcemia, pancreatic islet cell necrosis, cardiac arrhythmias, nephrotoxicity, and hepatitis. Renal insufficiency requires dose adjustment. Pentamidine can be detected in tissue for several weeks after administration.

The duration of therapy for PCP is based on clinical response, severity of presenting symptoms, and complications of intervention but is typically 14 to 21 days. If the patient does not respond to therapy, we either change medications or repeat the bronchoscopy to rule out a second concurrent infectious process. High-dose corticosteroids may be used as an adjunct to antimicrobial therapy in an attempt to alleviate severe hypoxemia but are not recommended for uncomplicated PCP.

Chemoprophylaxis against PCP is recommended for HIV-infected persons with a prior history of this illness, a CD4 cell count of 200 per mm³ or less, or CD4 cells constituting less than 20% of total lymphocytes. Prophylactic regimens include aerosolized pentamidine in a dose of 300 mg once each month or 150 mg every other week, TMP-SMZ 160/800 mg once or twice daily 3 to 7 days a week, or dapsone 100 mg daily. No regimen is 100% successful. Aerosolized pentamidine may not be well tolerated in patients with reactive airway disease; moreover, breakthrough disease may occur in the lung apices, sometimes with a secondary pneumothorax, and extrapulmonary pneumocystosis is also seen. Allergic reactions, nausea, and vomiting are the usual limitations on chemoprophylaxis with TMP-SMZ or dapsone, but the latter regimens appear to be about equally as efficacious as aerosolized pentamidine and considerably less expensive.

**Toxoplasmosis of the Brain.** One of the most common opportunistic infections of the central nervous system in HIV-infected patients occurs with *Toxoplasma gondii*. It may present as meningoencephalitis, seizures, or focal neurologic deficits. Involvement of other organs has been reported but is not commonly recognized. Serology is unreliable for diagnosis, IgG antibodies may or may not be present in elevated titer, and IgM antibodies are not usually present. Contrast-enhanced computed tomography (CT) commonly reveals multiple ring-enhancing lesions in the brain parenchyma, although single and nonenhancing lesions may also be seen. Biopsy is required for definitive diagnosis, but we generally reserve this for patients who have failed an empiric course of therapy with sulfadiazine, pyrimethamine, and leucovorin. If the patient clinically responds to the therapy and shows improvement in follow-up CT scans, the diagnosis of toxoplasmosis of the brain is accepted.

Sulfadiazine can cause all of the numerous potential side effects of sulfonamides, and when given in the high dose used for treating toxoplasmosis of the brain, one must particularly avoid dehydration that might lead to crystalluria and acute renal failure. The major risk of pyrimethamine is marrow suppression, but this can be reduced by concomitant administration of leucovorin. A loading dose of 75 mg of pyrimethamine is given, followed by 25 mg daily. Lifelong suppressive therapy is generally required to avoid relapse. After 4 to 6 weeks, the sulfadiazine dose may be reduced to 1.0 gram per day for maintenance, continuing the daily pyrimethamine and leucovorin; it is possible that administration of these medications 3 days a week may be adequate for late secondary prophylaxis. For patients allergic to sulfonamides, it appears that clindamycin (Cleocin) may be substituted, using 900 mg

three times daily during the initial 4 to 6 weeks and 600 mg per day during maintenance; pyrimethamine and leucovorin should be given concomitantly.

**Cryptosporidium and Isospora belli.** These protozoa can cause chronic and sometimes severe diarrhea in immunosuppressed individuals. Diagnosis is by detection of the organisms in stool specimens. No curative therapy exists for cryptosporidiosis, and treatment is supportive with attention to nutrition, hydration, and electrolyte balance; polycarbophil (Mitrolan) or diphenoxylate-atropine (Lomotil) may provide some symptomatic relief. Treatment for *I. belli* consists of TMP-SMZ; pyrimethamine and metronidazole (Flagyl) have also been reported to be effective. Suppressive therapy may be required.

### Fungal Infections

**Candida.** Candidal infection of the oral or vaginal mucosa is extremely common in HIV-infected patients and typically responds to topical antifungal therapy. Spontaneous development of oral thrush in an HIV-infected individual may predict progression of disease in the next few weeks or months. The diagnosis of thrush can generally be made by its physical appearance and confirmed if necessary by examining scrapings in a wet-mount preparation. Topical therapy with nystatin oral suspension (Mycostatin) (swish and swallow 5 ml two to six times daily) or clotrimazole troches (Mycelex) (dissolve a 10 mg troche in the mouth two to six times daily) is generally effective. If left untreated, *Candida* esophagitis may result, causing pain on swallowing and interfering with nutrition. Esophagitis will usually respond to therapy with oral ketoconazole (Nizoral) or fluconazole, possibly combined with topical clotrimazole, but refractory disease may require intravenous therapy with amphotericin B. Since recurrences are common, suppressive therapy should be used.

**Cryptococcus.** Cryptococcal meningitis is a common life-threatening opportunistic infection in HIV disease. The most frequent clinical symptoms are headache and fever; findings such as photophobia or stiff neck and papilledema may not be present. A serum assay for cryptococcal antigen may yield the diagnosis, but this should be confirmed by a similar assay on cerebrospinal fluid in addition to microscopic examination (India ink) and cultures. Pulmonary and other sites may also be involved. Standard therapy consists of amphotericin B intravenously, with the initial objective being suppression of disease. Amphotericin is administered initially as a 1.0-mg test dose and then in escalating doses up to 0.5 to 0.7 mg per kg per day. Acute reactions may be minimized by slow infusion (2 or more hours) and by pretreatment with an antipyretic, diphenhydramine, meperidine (Demerol), and/or a low dose (25 mg) of intravenous hydrocortisone (Solu-Cortex). Attention must be paid to the renal, electrolyte, and hematologic toxicities of the medication, with appropriate corrective actions or dose reduction. After the acute disease is controlled, indefinite suppressive therapy must usually be maintained with 25 to 50 mg of amphotericin intravenously one to three times weekly. A tunnelled, long-lasting central line will greatly facilitate this therapy. The side effects of flucytosine, most notably bone marrow suppression, preclude the routine use of this oral medication in HIV-infected patients. However, oral fluconazole appears to be an effective and better tolerated alternative to amphotericin for the treatment of cryptococcal disease. We usually give a loading dose of 400 mg per day followed by 200 mg per day. Occasionally we give 400 mg per day, depending on a patient's response to therapy.

**Histoplasmosis and Coccidioidomycosis.** Disseminated histoplasmosis or coccidioidomycosis occurs with increased frequency in HIV-infected patients with the appropriate prior exposure and should be considered in any such patient with unexplained fever. Serology may suggest the diagnosis, but it is more commonly made by culture or demonstration of the organism in blood, bone marrow, bronchoalveolar lavage, or appropriate biopsy specimens. Treatment with amphotericin is required for suppression of the disease; full therapy with 2.0 to 2.5 grams of amphotericin has been recommended by some workers. In any case, indefinite suppressive therapy is required with amphotericin or ketoconazole (400 to 800 mg per day).

### Mycobacterial Infections

*Mycobacterium tuberculosis.* Coincident with the HIV epidemic has been a resurgence of tuberculosis, and occurrence of the latter disease is an indication for HIV serologic testing. In the baseline assessment of an HIV-infected patient, skin tests with 5 units of purified protein derivative (PPD) and at least one control antigen (e.g., *Candida*) should be performed. Only in the presence of a positive control would a negative PPD suggest no prior infection with *M. tuberculosis*. A reactive PPD in an HIV-infected patient (5 mm of induration versus 10 mm in other populations) requires an evaluation for active tuberculosis and, in the absence of the latter, isoniazid prophylaxis for a minimum of one year.

Pulmonary tuberculosis in an HIV-infected patient may present with hilar adenopathy and nonspecific infiltrates on chest radiographs rather than fibronodular disease extending toward the apex; apical cavitary disease is less likely. In patients with depressed CD4 counts, dissemination to the meninges and other organs is common. We treat *M. tuberculosis* infections with isoniazid, rifampin, and pyrazinamide; ethambutol and streptomycin are additional therapeutic considerations in patients with meningitis or disseminated disease. Pyridoxine, 50 mg per day, must be added for patients receiving isoniazid to reduce the risk of neuropathy. Drug susceptibility testing and follow-up cultures are essential. The duration of therapy has not been established; we have been treating tuberculosis in HIV-infected patients for at least one year after cultures were negative. Since many of the patients have underlying liver disease or receive other potentially hepatotoxic medications, it is important to be alert to hepatotoxic reactions with the antituberculous medications. Regular tests of visual acuity and red-green perception are also necessary for those receiving ethambutol.

*M. avium* **Complex (MAC).** MAC organisms are commonly found in dust and water, and infection with them is relatively common in HIV-infected patients. The presentation is typically not as pulmonary disease, but rather as a disseminated infection involving bone marrow, liver, spleen, lymph nodes, or the gastrointestinal tract. Cultures of bone marrow, blood, and stool are more critical for diagnosis than cultures of specimens from the respiratory tract. The clinical response of MAC infections to therapy is often disappointing. We typically employ three to four drugs including rifampin (Rifadin), ethambutol (Myambutol), clofazimine (Lamprene), or ciprofloxacin (Cipro). Rifabutin, a rifamycin derivative that has enhanced activity against MAC organisms, is under investigation. Intravenous amikacin (Amikin) has appeared useful as part of the initial management; parenteral therapy is continued for 6 to 8 weeks or until toxicity appears. Drug susceptibility testing on the original and follow-up isolates may help in adjusting therapy.

### Other Bacterial Infections

*Salmonella* **Bacteremia.** The immunologic defects that develop in HIV-infected individuals impair not only cellular immunity but also the ability to develop antibody responses to new antigens. Neutropenia may appear as a complication of the disease or of therapy. A variety of bacterial infections can and do occur in this setting. Although some may be chronic, such as sinusitis, acute infections are more likely to be complicated by bacteremia and secondary foci of infection (e.g., meningitis) than in otherwise normal individuals. Most of these infections respond well to conventional antimicrobial therapy, although relapses may occur if the infection is not completely eradicated. Recurrent, nontyphoidal salmonella bacteremia is notable as one of the AIDS-defining secondary infections. Therapy for the latter may be with such antimicrobials as ampicillin (Omnipen), ceftriaxone (Rocephin), or ciprofloxacin, and chronic suppressive therapy may be required.

**Neurosyphilis.** Many of the exposures that lead to acquisition of HIV also lead to exposure to syphilis. When these two infections exist concomitantly, the likelihood of progression to secondary and tertiary syphilis, notably neurosyphilis, increases. Furthermore, the latter may occur despite conventional benzathine penicillin G therapy for primary or secondary disease. An argument can be made for treating any stage of syphilis in an HIV-infected patient with antimicrobials adequate to eradicate organisms that may have reached the central nervous system, and we consider this a must when there is central nervous system disease of undocumented origin in a patient with positive serology for syphilis or an elevated titer without overt disease. Obtaining cerebrospinal fluid before therapy can be useful for determining the effect of treatment on any abnormalities, but the absence of abnormalities or a negative cerebrospinal fluid VDRL does not negate the indication for treatment. Therapy consists of 18 to 24 million units of aqueous crystalline penicillin G intravenously daily for 10 to 14 days, followed by weekly injections of 2.4 million units of benzathine penicillin G for 3 consecutive weeks. To facilitate outpatient therapy, we are exploring the efficacy of once daily intravenous ceftriaxone (1 or 2 grams) for 14 days in place of the intravenous penicillin. It is important to remain alert to the possible need for re-treatment.

### Viral Infections

**Herpes Simplex Virus (HSV).** Chronic, ulcerative, mucocutaneous infections with HSV are common in the perianal and oral areas in HIV-infected patients. Involvement of the esophagus may also occur and has to be differentiated from esophagitis of other etiologies. Cultures of swabs from the lesions will usually readily yield the virus. Oral therapy with 200 mg of acyclovir (Zovirax) five times daily is usually effective, but prolonged suppressive therapy with 200 mg three to four times daily is usually necessary to prevent recurrences. Rarely, treatment of acyclovir-resistant HSV virus may require intravenous vidarabine (Vira-A).

**Varicella-Zoster Virus (VZV).** Shingles due to VZV is also common in HIV-infected patients. We have seen therapeutic effects with early use of oral acyclovir in a large dose of 800 mg five times a day for 5 days, but intravenous therapy is indicated if there is evidence of dissemination or involvement of the ophthalmic branch of the trigeminal nerve.

**Cytomegalovirus (CMV).** CMV can be found almost universally in patients with AIDS, but presence of the virus per se does not warrant therapy. Diagnosis of invasive CMV disease in organs such as the lungs, stomach, colon, or liver requires histologic demonstration of the characteristic cytopathic changes in appropriate specimens. CMV adrenalitis may be suspected in a patient with hypoadrenalism, viremia, or viruria, and no other apparent cause of adrenal suppression. CMV chorioretinitis can be diagnosed by an experienced ophthalmologist on the basis of the characteristic hemorrhages, exudates, and vascular sheathing. Therapy with ganciclovir (Cytovene; DHPG) is indicated primarily in patients with sight-threatening chorioretinitis and can suppress the disease; the drug is less effective against other invasive CMV diseases.

Ganciclovir is administered intravenously. A 2-week induction period with twice daily administration of 5 mg per kg is followed by once daily maintenance therapy five to seven times per week. Prolonged or indefinite maintenance therapy is required to reduce the likelihood of relapses; even so, breakthroughs may occur. The major side effect of ganciclovir is bone marrow suppression, particularly neutropenia. Co-administration with zidovudine is associated with synergistic myelosuppression; hence, only reduced doses of zidovudine, if any, can usually be given to patients receiving ganciclovir, and such therapy should include close hematologic monitoring.

Foscarnet, an investigational drug, also exhibits anti-CMV virus activity. Early studies are encouraging, although the relapse rate and time to relapse are comparable to those with ganciclovir. Toxicities include renal dysfunction, anemia, penile ulceration, electrolyte abnormalities, and tremor, but apparently there is less marrow suppression than with ganciclovir.

### GENERAL COMMENTARY

The AIDS epidemic is placing considerable stress upon the medical care system in many communities, and it is incumbent upon all of us to use the available resources as effectively as possible. Many of the syndromes and secondary diseases that occur with HIV infection present in a chronic or subacute fashion. With specific treatment of obvious problems (e.g., thrush, fungal infections of the skin, mucocutaneous herpes) and therapy aimed at reducing symptoms (e.g., antipyretics, analgesics, skin emollients, nutritional supplements, antidiarrheal agents), most of these patients can be comfortably evaluated in the outpatient clinic. Thoughtful analysis is required of routine clinical and laboratory data; chest radiographs; arterial blood gases; skin tests (PPD and controls); CD4 and CD8 T lymphocyte subsets; serologies (e.g., tests for syphilis, cryptococcal antigen, and antibodies to *Toxoplasma,* coccidioidomycoses, and *Histoplasma*); results of microscopic examination of induced sputum, stool, and white blood cell buffy coat in selected circumstances; and bacterial, mycobacterial, and fungal cultures of sputum, stool, and blood. Special studies may be required such as a bronchial lavage for cytology and culture; contrast-enhanced CT scan of the head; lumbar puncture; biopsy and culture of bone marrow, a skin lesion, or lymph node; aspiration of fluid collections for analysis and culture; abdominal ultrasound; barium swallow or barium enema; or endoscopy. Each of the latter can also be done in the outpatient setting if back-up is available for emergencies. Observations of the effects of antiretroviral therapy by itself, a trial of oral TMP-SMZ aimed at PCP while awaiting bronchial lavage, or a trial of antituberculous therapy while awaiting cultures may be appropriate in selected circumstances. Thus, a major portion of the management of HIV-infected patients can be conducted in the outpatient clinic, even though most patients will, during the course of the disease, suffer one or more severe complications best managed in the hospital. Before hospitalization, if possible, an understanding should be reached with the patient and other responsible persons about the extent to which resuscitative measures will be employed if they should become indicated.

# AMEBIASIS

method of
SALAH M. NASRALLAH, M.D.
*Union Memorial Hospital*
*Baltimore, Maryland*

Amebiasis is primarily a colonic infection caused by the organism *Entamoeba histolytica.* The disease has worldwide distribution, but is most prevalent in underdeveloped and developing countries. It affects about 10% of the world's population. The reported prevalence rate in the United States varies between 2 and 5%. This rate is much higher among individuals in mental institutions, migrant workers, homosexual men, and patients with acquired immune deficiency syndrome (AIDS). Prevalence rates as high as 15 to 40% have been reported in homosexuals and AIDS patients. The disease is transmitted by ingestion of contaminated food or water. It may also be transmitted by intimate personal contact with infected individuals. The amebae invade the colonic epithelium, resulting in lysis of mucosal cells, with localized or diffuse mucosal damage

(intestinal amebiasis). Rarely, the organism may enter the mesenteric circulation and ascend into the portal venous system, causing infection in the liver or other organs (extraintestinal amebiasis). The organism possesses isoenzymes (zymodemes), which determine its pathogenicity. However, there is evidence that nonpathogenic *E. histolytica* isolates could become pathogenic in the presence of bacterial infections. This finding has given support to the recommendation of treating the asymptomatic carrier state.

The diagnosis of intestinal amebiasis is made by identifying *E. histolytica* in a freshly obtained stool specimen. Concentration techniques may be necessary to identify the cyst. Several substances may interfere with the recovery of the organism from the stools, such as the administration of bismuth, tetracycline, erythromycin, antacids, laxatives, soap, or hypertonic enemas. Thus, stool examination should be performed prior to the administration of any of these agents. Serologic tests in the form of indirect hemagglutination or gel diffusion are also helpful in diagnosing invasive or extraintestinal amebiasis. Results of these tests may be positive in more than 85% of patients.

## INTESTINAL AMEBIASIS

This condition has a wide spectrum of clinical manifestations, which range from the asymptomatic carrier state to fulminant disease. The infection may be mild, manifesting in the form of abdominal cramps and irregular bowel habits; or be more severe, with fever, bloody diarrhea, tenesmus, and lower abdominal pain. In severe untreated cases, progression to megacolon and perforation may also occur.

The acute illness, if not adequately treated, may become chronic, with recurrent episodes of diarrhea and abdominal pain. Rarely, amebiasis may involve the appendix and cecum, resulting in a mass lesion called ameboma.

### Treatment

There are two main classes of drugs that could be used in the treatment of amebiasis. The luminal amebicides act predominantly on organisms within the colonic lumen, and the tissue amebicides act mainly on the organisms that have invaded the tissues or are disseminated into the liver or other organisms. The choice of any of these drugs is dependent on the site of infection, but often treatment with both types of medications is necessary in the same patient. Pediatric dosages for all drugs are given in Table 1.

**Asymptomatic Carriers.** Controversy exists regarding the necessity of treating such individuals. However, the evidence that nonpathogenic *E. histolytica* could become pathogenic gives credence to treatment. The drug of choice would be

TABLE 1. **Pediatric Dosages of Amebicidal Drugs**

| Drug | Dose |
| --- | --- |
| *Tissue Amebicides* | |
| Metronidazole (Flagyl) | 30–50 mg/kg/day for 10 days* |
| Emetine | |
| Dehydroemetine‡ | 1 mg/kg/day (maximum 60 mg/day) IM for 5 days† |
| | 1–1.5 mg/kg/day (maximum 90 mg/day) IM for 5 days† |
| *Luminal Amebicides* | |
| Iodoquinol (Yodoxin) | 30–40 mg/kg/day for 20 days* |
| Diloxanide furoate (Furamide)‡ | 20 mg/kg/day for 10 days* |
| Paromomycin (Humatin) | 25–30 mg/kg/day for 7 days* |
| *Hepatic Amebicide* | |
| Chloroquine (Aralen) | 15 mg/kg/day (maximum 480 mg/day) for 14 days |

*Give in 3 divided daily doses.
†Give in 2 divided daily doses.
‡Available only from the Centers for Disease Control: telephone 404–639–3670 or 3356; nights and emergency (24 hr), 404–639–2888.

diloxanide furoate (Furamide),* in a dosage of 500 mg three times daily for 10 days. With such therapy, the cure rate is close to 80%. Its main side effects are increased flatulence and rash.

**Symptomatic Patients.** Invariably, patients with mild to moderately severe disease harbor the organism in the colonic lumen as well as the colonic wall. Thus, dual therapy with luminal and tissue amebicides is necessary. Metronidazole (Flagyl) is an effective tissue amebicide, which could be used orally or intravenously in a dosage of 750 mg three times daily for 10 days. Such treatment should be combined or followed with a luminal drug, such as diiodohydroxyquin (Iodoquinol) in a dosage of 650 mg three times daily for 20 days. This therapy is effective in about 70% of patients. Diloxanide furoate may be substituted for diiodohydroxyquin as a luminal amebicide. More recently, a nonabsorbable aminoglycoside, paromomycin (Humatin), has been used in a dosage of 25 to 30 mg per kg per day in three divided doses for a total of 7 days. Minor side effects, such as gastrointestinal discomfort with frequent loose stools, have been reported.

In the presence of fulminant disease or an ameboma that has not responded to intravenous metronidazole, dehydroemetine (Mebadin)* may be used in a dosage of 1 mg per kg per day for 5 days. Frequent monitoring with electrocardiography should be performed because the drug's main toxicity is cardiac, in the form of arrhythmias or ischemia.

There is controversy regarding treatment of

---

* Available from the Centers for Disease Control: Telephone 404–639–3670 or 3356; nights and emergency (24 hour), 404–639–2888.

homosexuals with asymptomatic infection. However, the potential change in the pathogenicity of the organism and the development of extraintestinal amebiasis without evidence of intestinal infection favor treatment of the asymptomatic patient.

## EXTRAINTESTINAL AMEBIASIS

The liver is a major site of extraintestinal amebic infection. Most frequently, the right lobe is involved, with a solitary abscess. This is well demonstrated by computed tomography scan and is confirmed by the indirect hemagglutination test. The condition is associated with right upper quadrant pain, fever, leukocytosis, prostration, and often intercostal tenderness. Rarely, the abscess may invade the diaphragm and rupture into the lung. Other reported extraintestinal sites of infection include the brain, the pericardium, the bladder, the kidney, and the pleura.

### Treatment

The treatment of choice in such individuals is the administration of metronidazole intravenously or orally in a dosage of 750 mg three times daily for 10 days. Dehydroemetine is also quite effective, but more toxic. Chloroquine (Aralen) phosphate is another drug that was used quite effectively in the past in a dosage of 1 gram (600 mg of base) daily for 2 days followed by 500 mg (300 mg of base) daily for 14 days. Because such therapy is aimed at the tissue phase of the infection, another luminal amebicide should be used to eradicate any organism present in the colon. Needle drainage is no longer necessary in the treatment of hepatic amebic abscess.

Surgical treatment of hepatic amebic abscess is not necessary, unless there is no therapeutic response to a tissue amebicide or the abscess has ruptured. A full course of metronidazole should be used before, during, and after surgery. A luminal agent should be given prior to discontinuing metronidazole.

# BACTEREMIA

method of
ROBERT L. ATMAR, M.D., and
RICHARD L. HARRIS, M.D.
*Baylor College of Medicine*
*Houston, Texas*

Bacteremia is a surprisingly common event and occurs in association with such activities as toothbrushing and during certain diagnostic and therapeutic procedures. It becomes important in patients when it causes clinically significant disease such as sepsis or prosthetic infection because of the considerable morbidity and mortality associated with these infections. The best approach to the management of bacteremia is prevention, but when this is not possible, prompt recognition of clinically significant bacteremia to allow appropriate diagnostic and therapeutic maneuvers is of the utmost importance.

Bacteremia is defined as bacteria in the blood stream. Sepsis is defined as the physiologic changes and the clinical consequences of microorganisms in the blood or tissues. There are numerous manifestations of sepsis (Table 1). It is not difficult to suspect sepsis in a febrile, hypotensive patient with rigors; however, signs of sepsis may be more subtle. Alteration of mental status may be the initial sign of sepsis in the elderly patient. Fever is usually present, but it may be absent in the elderly patient or in the patient with chronic liver or renal disease. Respiratory alkalosis, metabolic acidosis (lactic acidosis), or worsening renal function may be the first clue to sepsis in the intensive care unit. Septic shock is an advanced manifestation of sepsis in which there is circulatory failure resulting in inadequate tissue oxygenation and cell death. Because recognition of sepsis may be difficult, it is necessary for the clinician to maintain a high index of suspicion for its presence.

Once sepsis is suspected, a careful search for an underlying focus should be instituted. Identification of a focus of infection is helpful for selection of a therapeutic regimen before culture results become available. The most useful tool in identifying a source of infection is a careful history and physical examination. For example, a history of cough, sputum production, and pleuritic chest pain suggests a pulmonary focus, whereas recent passage of a kidney stone may suggest a urinary tract focus. The history and physical exam-

ination findings may also lead the physician to perform certain supplemental investigations (such as x-rays or sonograms), which will identify a focus of infection. It is important to obtain blood and other indicated cultures in all patients suspected of having sepsis so that antibiotic therapy may be adjusted for organism-specific treatment. Identification of a pathogen by blood culture may also suggest a focus in a patient who does not otherwise have a readily identifiable site of infection—for example, *Bacteroides fragilis* bacteremia suggesting an intra-abdominal focus.

## ADJUNCTIVE THERAPY

Because antibiotic therapy alone is frequently not sufficient for the treatment of sepsis, several other measures should be carried out while antibiotic therapy is being instituted. One of the most important additional steps in the treatment of bacteremia is the removal or drainage of septic foci. Potentially infected intravascular lines should be removed. Intra-abdominal abscesses, empyema, and most other abscesses require surgical drainage; infected or gangrenous tissue may need débridement; obstructions of the urinary and biliary tracts must be relieved; and infected prosthetic devices generally need to be removed.

Several of the manifestations of sepsis require additional therapy (Table 2). Hypoxemia is treated with supplemental oxygenation, whereas respiratory failure and adult respiratory distress syndrome require mechanical ventilation with or without positive end-expiratory pressure. Hemorrhagic disorders are treated with factor replacement and blood components (fresh-frozen plasma, packed red blood cells, and platelets) to control bleeding. Hyperglycemia is treated with insulin administration; hypoglycemia is treated by infusion of a 10% dextrose solution.

**Septic Shock.** Septic shock requires immediate recognition and therapeutic intervention. It is characterized by a range of hemodynamic findings, from a preshock state to a late shock state (Table 3). The preshock state is characterized by a decrease in the systemic vascular resistance and an increase in the cardiac output. The blood pressure is normal or slightly depressed. The acid-base status is usually a respiratory alkalosis caused by primary hyperventilation. As the preshock state advances to early shock and then late shock, the cardiac output declines and hypotension and metabolic acidosis develop. Persistence of hypotension and metabolic acidosis may result in multisystem organ failure and death.

Septic shock is characterized by hypotension. Septic patients are usually relatively volume depleted secondary to increased venous capacitance, increased vascular permeability, increased insen-

TABLE 1. **Manifestations of Sepsis***

| Common Manifestations | Less Common Manifestations or Those Seen Only in Severe Sepsis |
|---|---|
| Fever, rigors, myalgias | Hypothermia |
| Tachycardia | Shock (see Table 3) |
| Tachypnea (respiratory alkalosis) | Lactic acidosis |
| Hypoxemia | Adult respiratory distress syndrome |
| Proteinuria | Azotemia, oliguria |
| Leukocytosis (left shift, toxic granules, Döhle's bodies) | Leukopenia, leukemoid reaction |
| Eosinopenia | Thrombocytopenia |
| Hypoferremia | Disseminated intravascular coagulation |
| Irritability, lethargy | Anemia |
| Mild liver function abnormalities | Stupor, coma |
| Hyperglycemia in diabetics | Overt upper gastrointestinal tract bleeding |
| | Cutaneous lesions |
| | Hypoglycemia |

*From Harris RL, Musher DM, Bloom K, et al: Manifestations of sepsis. Arch Intern Med 1987, *147*:1895–1906. Copyright 1987, American Medical Association.

TABLE 2. **Manifestations of Sepsis That May Benefit from or Require Specific Therapy\*†**

| Manifestations | Therapy |
|---|---|
| Fever, rigors, myalgias | Antipyretics, cooling blanket |
| Hypotension | Volume replacement, dopamine (naloxone) |
| Hypoxemia | Supplemental oxygen administration |
| Respiratory failure, ARDS | Mechanical ventilation (PEEP) |
| Lactic acidosis | Bicarbonate administration |
| Azotemia, oliguria | Fluid and electrolyte management, reduction of renally cleared drugs |
| Thrombocytopenia | Platelet and/or RBC transfusions if active bleeding |
| DIC | Fresh-frozen plasma, platelet, and/or RBC transfusions if active bleeding (heparin) |
| Altered mentation | Monitoring or restraint of patient to prevent self-harm |
| GI tract bleeding | Nasogastric lavage or suction, RBC transfusions as needed (antacids, $H_2$ receptor antagonists) |
| Hyperglycemia | Insulin administration |
| Hypoglycemia | Constant 10% dextrose infusion |

\*From Harris RL, Musher DM, Bloom K, et al: Manifestations of sepsis. Arch Intern Med 1987, *147*:1895–1906. Copyright 1987, American Medical Association.

†Therapeutic maneuvers that may be effective are given in parentheses.

*Abbreviations:* ARDS = adult respiratory distress syndrome; PEEP = positive end-expiratory pressure; RBC = red blood cell; DIC = disseminated intravascular coagulation; GI = gastrointestinal; and $H_2$ = histamine$_2$.

sible fluid loss, or decreased fluid intake. A fluid challenge with either crystalloid or colloid is generally appropriate, and a pulmonary artery catheter may be useful in monitoring fluid therapy. The goal of fluid replacement is to restore adequate circulatory perfusion, which can be determined by organ function (mentation or urinary output) and which generally occurs at a systolic blood pressure of 90 to 100 mmHg. If a pulmonary artery catheter is used, a pulmonary capillary

TABLE 3. **Hemodynamics of Sepsis\***

| | Preshock | Early Shock | Late Shock |
|---|---|---|---|
| Blood pressure | → ↓ | ↓ | ↓ ↓ † |
| Systemic vascular resistance | ↓ | ↓ ↓ | → ↑ |
| Cardiac output | ↑ ↑ | ↑ | ↓ |
| Volume responsive | + + | + | − |
| Acid-base status | RA | RA, MA | MA |

\*From Harris RL, Musher DM, Bloom K, et al: Manifestations of sepsis. Arch Intern Med 1987, *147*:1895–1906. Copyright 1987, American Medical Association.

†Often pressor dependent.

*Abbreviations:* RA = respiratory alkalosis; MA = metabolic acidosis.

wedge pressure of 12 to 14 mmHg is recommended for guidance of fluid replacement therapy.

If volume replacement does not restore the perfusion pressure, vasopressor therapy should be initiated. Dopamine HCl as a constant infusion is the most commonly used pressor agent and should be titrated to maintain adequate perfusion. A low dose (1 to 2 µg per kg per minute) results in increased renal blood flow. At 5 to 10 µg per kg per minute, there is increased beta-adrenergic stimulation, which results in increased cardiac output while urinary sodium and volume excretion are maintained. At doses higher than 15 to 20 µg per kg per minute, alpha-adrenergic stimulation predominates and results in peripheral vasoconstriction and maintenance of blood pressure, usually at the expense of renal perfusion.

Steroids have been used for treatment of septic shock in the past, but there are now several well-designed, placebo-controlled trials showing that there is no long-term benefit from their use and that they may cause harm. In the absence of specific indications (e.g., Addison's disease), steroids should not be given.

Other therapies that must be considered investigational at this time include the use of the opioid antagonist naloxone in the treatment of septic shock and the use of monoclonal antibodies against gram-negative endotoxemia.

## SELECTION OF ANTIBIOTIC THERAPY

Selection of an appropriate antibiotic regimen requires knowledge of the organisms most likely to be responsible for the infection. Information that may be available to the clinician includes the following: (1) previous culture data, for example, a urine culture obtained several days earlier; (2) Gram's stain of specimens of body fluids; (3) expected flora (Table 4) of a site, such as enterococci and gram-negative bacilli in the urinary tract; and (4) hospital-specific resistance patterns in nosocomially acquired infections. At times, a clinical situation allows specific therapy from the outset—for example, penicillin in pneumococcal pneumonia or meningococcal meningitis—but more than one antibiotic is usually necessary to provide comprehensive antibacterial therapy until culture data become available.

When the physician selects the antibiotic regimen, the following should be considered.

(1) Initial treatment with two antibiotics is generally superior to treatment with one antibiotic because (a) the spectrum of antibacterial coverage is broadened with two antibiotics, (b) there may be synergy between the antibiotics for

TABLE 4. **Initial Antibiotic Selection Based on Likely Focus of Infection**

| Site or Type of Infection | Organisms | Antibiotics |
|---|---|---|
| Urinary tract | GNR | Aminoglycosides, ceftazidime |
| | GDS | Ampicillin, vancomycin |
| Pneumonia* | Pneumococcus, aspiration | Pencillin G |
|   Community-acquired | *Haemophilus influenzae* | Ampicillin |
| | *Legionella*, atypical pneumonias | Erythromycin |
|   Nosocomial | GNR† | Piperacillin, ceftazidime |
| | *Staphylococcus aureus* | Nafcillin, vancomycin |
| | *Legionella* | Erythromycin |
| Endocarditis, native valve | | |
|   Non-IVDA | Alpha streptococci, *S. aureus* | Penicillin, nafcillin |
|   IVDA | *S. aureus* | Nafcillin, vancomycin |
| | GNR† | Ticarcillin or ceftazidime and aminoglycosides |
| Meningitis | | |
|   Adult | Pneumococci, meningococci | Penicillin, chloramphenicol |
|   Postneurosurgery, immunosuppressed | *S. aureus, Staphylococcus epidermidis* | Nafcillin, vancomycin |
| | GNR† | Ceftazidime |
| Gastrointestinal and genital tracts | GNR | Ceftazidime, aminoglycoside |
| | GDS | Ampicillin, vancomycin |
| | Anaerobes | Clindamycin, piperacillin, metronidazole, chloramphenicol |
| Wound infection | *S. aureus* | Nafcillin, vancomycin |
| | GNR | Ceftazidime, aminoglycoside |
| Line sepsis | *S. aureus, S. epidermidis* | Vancomycin |
| | GNR | Ceftazidime, aminoglycoside |
| *Other Risk Factors* | | |
| Neutropenia | GNR | Ceftazidime or ticarcillin and aminoglycoside |
| | *S. aureus, S. epidermidis* | Vancomycin |
| Postsplenectomy | Pneumococcus, *H. influenzae*, meningococcus | Penicillin, ampicillin |
| Raw shellfish consumption | *Vibrio* | Tetracycline and aminoglycoside |
| | *Listeria* | Penicillin, ampicillin |
| | *Salmonella* | Chloramphenicol, ampicillin |
| Empiric | *S. aureus*, streptococci | Vancomycin |
| | GNR | Ceftazidime, aminoglycoside |

*Gram's stain of sputum may help direct initial therapy.
†Combination therapy with a penicillin or cephalosporin and an aminoglycoside should be given.
*Abbreviations:* GNR = gram-negative rod; GDS = group D streptococci; IVDA = intravenous drug abuse.

certain infections (e.g., enterococcal infections treated with ampicillin and an aminoglycoside), (c) development of resistance to the antibiotics may be prevented, and (d) the pharmacokinetics of the antibiotics may allow more continuous antibacterial coverage (i.e., when serum concentration of one antibiotic falls below the minimum inhibitory concentration of the bacteria being treated, the serum concentration of the other antibiotic may still be in the therapeutic range).

(2) Bactericidal agents (penicillins, cephalosporins, aminoglycosides) are preferred in the initial treatment of endocarditis, meningitis, and neutropenia. However, except for cefuroxime, first- and second-generation cephalosporins do not cross the blood-brain barrier and should not be used in the treatment of meningitis.

(3) Intravenous therapy should be instituted initially. This ensures that the antibiotics achieve adequate serum levels when dosed appropriately. Orally administered medications may not be absorbed because of an ileus, and medications given intramuscularly may have undependable absorption because of hypoperfusion during shock.

(4) Once culture data are available, the antibiotic regimen should be changed to the least toxic regimen that allows appropriate treatment.

(5) The appropriate length of therapy for most patients with bacteremia is not well defined but has generally been 10 to 14 days. Factors that may cause a change in the duration of treatment include the following: (a) organism, (b) host, (c) site of infection, and (d) clinical response of the patient. In some patients a switch from parenteral to oral therapy may be made to complete a course of treatment if a good clinical response has been achieved and an appropriate site is infected (e.g., in pyelonephritis).

Dosages of selected antibiotics are shown in Table 5.

**Empiric Therapy.** If a careful search for a site of

TABLE 5. **Dosage of Selected Antibiotics in Adult Patients with Normal Renal Function**

| Antibiotic | Dose | Usual Dosing Interval (hr) |
|---|---|---|
| β-Lactamase susceptible, nonantipseudomonal penicillins | | |
| Penicillin G | 1–2 million U | 4 |
| Ampicillin | 1–2 grams | 4–6 |
| β-Lactamase susceptible, antipseudomonal penicillins | | |
| Ticarcillin | 3 grams | 4 |
| Piperacillin | 3–4 grams | 4–6 |
| β-Lactamase resistant penicillins | | |
| Nafcillin | 1–2 grams | 4–6 |
| Methicillin | 1–2 grams | 4–6 |
| Penicillins with β-lactamase inhibitor | | |
| Ampicillin with sulbactam | 1.5–3 grams | 6 |
| Ticarcillin with clavulanate | 3.1 grams | 4 |
| First-generation cephalosporin | | |
| Cefazolin | 1–1.5 grams | 8 |
| Second-generation cephalosporin | | |
| Cefotetan | 1–2 grams | 12 |
| Third-generation cephalosporins | | |
| Ceftazidime | 1–2 grams | 8–12 |
| Cefotaxime | 1–2 grams | 4–8 |
| Carbapenem | | |
| Imipenem with cilastatin | 0.5–1 gram | 6–8 |
| Monobactam | | |
| Aztreonam | 1–2 grams | 6–8 |
| Aminoglycosides | | |
| Gentamicin | 1 mg/kg | 8 |
| Tobramycin | 1 mg/kg | 8 |
| Amikacin | 7.5 mg/kg | 12 |
| Others | | |
| Vancomycin | 15 mg/kg | 12 |
| Clindamycin | 300–600 mg | 8 |
| Erythromycin | 500–1000 mg | 6 |
| Doxycycline | 50–100 mg | 12 |
| Metronidazole | 7.5 mg/kg | 6 |
| Chloramphenicol | 25 mg/kg | 6 |
| Ciprofloxacin* | 250–750 mg | 12 |

*Not yet available in the intravenous form.

infection fails to reveal a likely source, the physician must make an empiric decision about the initial antibiotic regimen. Gram-negative bacilli and *Staphylococcus aureus* are the most common pathogens in this situation, and therapy should be directed to them. Ceftazidime or an aminoglycoside provides good coverage of gram-negative bacilli, and vancomycin is a good antistaphylococcal drug.

**Monitoring Therapy.** Once therapy is initiated, it is important to monitor the patient for adequacy of therapy and for signs and symptoms of antibiotic toxicity. If there is no clinical response after 1 to 3 days of antibiotic therapy, blood cultures should be repeated to evaluate the adequacy of therapy in eradicating the bacteremia; persistently positive blood cultures may be secondary to inadequate antibiotic therapy or to an undrained focus of infection.

All antibiotics have side effects for which patients should be monitored. Peak and trough levels of aminoglycosides and vancomycin should be checked and adjusted to the therapeutic range. Impaired hearing and tinnitus may occur during the administration of aminoglycosides and may be due to elevated serum levels. Rash is another common side effect of therapy with most antibiotics; it is usually mild and self-limited after treatment stops, but occasionally it can be severe. Diarrhea is another common, generally self-limited, side effect of virtually any oral or parenteral antibiotic; it resolves after discontinuation of the antibiotic. If the diarrhea persists, the patient should be evaluated for colitis caused by *Clostridium difficile*.

Laboratory tests may be useful in the monitoring of patients for antibiotic toxicity. Leukopenia may be seen during the administration of β-lactams or vancomycin; it usually resolves and is of little clinical significance if the antibiotic therapy is discontinued. Renal function may deteriorate during antibiotic therapy; aminoglycosides may cause renal tubular damage and β-lactams or sulfonamides may cause interstitial nephritis. Early recognition of toxicity and adjustment of antibiotic therapy may prevent more serious complications.

# BRUCELLOSIS

method of
PIERRE FORGACS, M.D.
*Lahey Clinic Medical Center*
*Burlington, Massachusetts*

Brucellosis has become a rare disease in the United States; about 100 to 200 new cases are seen each year, chiefly among farmers, veterinarians, employees of meat packing plants, and, rarely, laboratory workers. *Brucella abortus* usually is transmitted from animals to humans by cattle, *B. suis* by hogs, *B. melitensis* by goats, and, as recently discovered, *B. canis* by dogs. Ten per cent of infections occur in persons who drink raw milk or eat unpasteurized cheese, especially imported goat cheese. Human disease can be classified into two main categories: (1) acute—the duration of the disease is less than 3 months, systemic symptoms (chills, fever, and sweats) are present, involvement of specific organ systems may or may not occur, and blood cultures are positive or the serologic titer is high or rising; and (2) subacute or chronic—the duration of the disease is many months or years, symptoms are intermittent or continuous, and a specific organ, organ system, or tissue (skeletal system, genitourinary tract, spleen, lung, soft tissue, or heart valve) usually is involved.

Patients who have had symptoms of malaise, fatigue,

and depression for a long time and have a positive *Brucella* serologic test in low titer but no cultural recovery of *Brucella* organisms and no other objective evidence of illness probably do not have chronic brucellosis.

## TREATMENT

### In Vitro Sensitivity of *Brucella*

Many drugs are effective in vitro against most strains of *Brucella*. These include tetracyclines, aminoglycosides, rifampin (Rifadin), ampicillin, erythromycin, chloramphenicol, and trimethoprim-sulfamethoxazole (co-trimoxazole) (Bactrim). However, experience with ampicillin, first-generation cephalosporins, and chloramphenicol has been unfavorable, and these drugs are not used in the treatment of patients with brucellosis even when the organism is sensitive to them in vitro.

As in typhoid fever and tuberculosis, the bacteria in brucellosis are predominantly intracellular and the inflammatory response is usually granulomatous. This may explain some of the discrepancies between results achieved in vitro and in vivo. However, in vitro sensitivities should be performed because organisms resistant to a drug in vitro will probably be resistant in vivo.

### Choice of Drug Regimens

Five treatment regimens are available: (1) tetracycline and streptomycin (tetracycline, 500 mg orally every 6 hours for 3 to 6 weeks, and streptomycin, 500 mg intramuscularly every 12 hours for 2 to 4 weeks); (2) tetracycline alone (500 mg orally every 6 hours for 3 to 6 weeks); (3) sulfadiazine and streptomycin (sulfadiazine, 6 grams per day orally, and streptomycin intramuscularly, 500 mg every 12 hours); (4) trimethoprim-sulfamethoxazole (trimethoprim, 80 mg, and sulfamethoxazole, 400 mg), 6 tablets daily for 4 to 6 weeks (this use of trimethoprim-sulfamethoxazole is not listed in the manufacturer's official directive); and (5) rifampin, 600 mg per day alone or preferably in addition to doxycycline (Vibramycin), 100 mg orally every 12 hours for 4 weeks (this use of rifampin is not listed in the manufacturer's directive).

The first two regimens have been used most often and are effective; regimens 3 and 4 are alternative programs that are much less effective and should be used only when there is allergy to tetracycline, significant renal impairment, or pregnancy. In the United States, there is little experience with rifampin in patients with brucellosis.

Streptomycin or sulfa drugs should not be used alone in the treatment of patients with brucellosis because of frequent treatment failure and the occasional development of resistant organisms. The trimethoprim-sulfamethoxazole therapy is relatively new and is being evaluated; its effectiveness in chronic brucellosis is unknown, and relapses have been frequent (4 to 50%) when this regimen has been used in acute bacteremic brucellosis. Some strains of *Brucella,* especially *B. canis,* are resistant to streptomycin but are sensitive to other aminoglycosides in vitro; when this occurs, kanamycin or gentamicin should be substituted.

We prefer the combination of tetracycline and streptomycin in the therapy of all forms of brucellosis.

### Acute Brucellosis

The febrile patient should be in the hospital and under observation during therapy. Therapy with tetracycline alone is associated with a 30% incidence of relapse of acute infections of *B. abortus;* combination therapy reduces the relapse rate to less than 10%. Treatment of *B. melitensis* and *B. suis* infections with tetracycline alone is accompanied by relapse in two-thirds of the patients; adding streptomycin reduces the rate to about 14%. Combination treatment should be given for 3 weeks.

Occasionally patients are seen late during an attack of brucellosis with few symptoms but with positive blood cultures. They should be treated with tetracycline and streptomycin as outlined previously.

### Relapsing Brucellosis

In acute brucellosis, relapse after a course of therapy may occur because of persistence of organisms in their intracellular sites, in walled-off granulomas, or in suppurative foci. The diagnosis is often obvious—the patient becomes febrile and has fatigue, sweats, chills, arthralgias, backache, a rising *Brucella* titer, and positive blood cultures. If an organism can be cultured again, drug sensitivity testing should be performed even though relapse *does not* indicate that the organism has grown resistant to the previously administered antibiotic. Relapses should be re-treated with the original regimen for the same period or longer.

Response to appropriate therapy may be slow. Symptoms of malaise and fatigue may persist for months, splenomegaly may last for weeks to months, fever often occurs during the first week or two of therapy, and positive serology (in low titer) remains for years. These findings do not imply relapse. However, the patient should continue to improve at least gradually and should not have unexplained fever; the serology should neither persist at its peak nor increase 2 to 3 months after the completion of therapy.

Treated patients should have monthly examinations with blood cultures and serologic tests for 6 months. The patient with a positive blood culture at the completion of therapy, even when asymptomatic, should be re-treated. Re-treatment also should be considered for the patient who has unexplained fever and unchanged or increasing blood serologic titers even though the blood culture is negative.

The patient who has persistent malaise, fatigue, aches, and depression in the absence of other positive evidence of active disease should be re-evaluated frequently but not re-treated unless serologic titers increase or blood cultures become positive.

### Subacute or Chronic Localized Brucellosis

Chronic localized brucellosis is more difficult to treat, and tetracycline and streptomycin should be used for a longer period (at least 6 weeks and 4 weeks, respectively). Surgical drainage may be necessary for eradication of the foci of disease.

**Indications for Splenectomy in Brucellosis of the Spleen.** Splenectomy is rarely necessary in brucellosis but may be indicated for persistent moderate to severe hypersplenism or for drainage of a suppurative focus.

Splenic involvement is common in acute brucellosis, and occasionally hypersplenism ensues; however, this usually corrects itself with antibiotic therapy alone. In chronic brucellosis with hypersplenism, coexistent liver disease and portal hypertension should be ruled out before proceeding with splenectomy.

A more frequent indication for splenectomy is the coexistence of splenomegaly, splenic calcification, and recurrent fever of unknown cause. Laparotomy and splenectomy may be necessary for diagnosis and cure because in this situation appropriate antibiotic therapy often is insufficient to eradicate the infection. At the time of laparotomy, the surgeon should look for other suppurative foci, especially in the liver and retroperitoneum.

**Musculoskeletal Brucellosis.** *Brucella* spondylitis, or disk space infection, usually does not require surgical drainage for treatment, although *Brucella* arthritis may occasionally require synovectomy. Prepatellar bursitis responds to bursectomy and combined antibiotic therapy. *Brucella* osteomyelitis is a difficult therapeutic problem

requiring aggressive débridement and prolonged combined antibiotic therapy. Superinfection with *Staphylococcus aureus* may occur and should be treated appropriately.

**Brucella Endocarditis.** The mortality rate in brucellosis is low, but *Brucella* endocarditis accounts for more than 80% of the deaths that occur. *Brucella* organisms may invade normal, damaged, or prosthetic valves. The natural history of the illness is that of subacute endocarditis, usually of the aortic valve. In suspected cases, special culture media under cover of 10% carbon dioxide should be used and appropriate in vitro antibiotic sensitivity tests should be performed. Treatment with a combination of tetracycline for 2 to 3 months and streptomycin for 6 weeks has been effective in some patients. Valvular replacement should be contemplated in progressive aortic insufficiency or refractory heart failure and in infections of the prosthetic valve. A decline in *Brucella* antibody levels may be a useful prognostic sign.

Surgical drainage for chronic localized brucellosis should always be followed by combined antibiotic therapy.

### Herxheimer's Reactions

After the initiation of antibiotic therapy, increased fever and toxicity and sometimes hypotension may develop transiently in patients with brucellosis. When a severe reaction of this type occurs, corticosteroids (prednisone, 15 mg orally every 6 hours for 2 to 3 days, or equivalent doses of hydrocortisone sodium succinate [Solu-Cortef]) should be administered with the antibiotics. A Herxheimer reaction can be anticipated in the very ill patient with acute brucellosis, and initial doses of tetracycline and streptomycin should be reduced.

### Accidental Inoculation of Brucella Organisms

Veterinarians using live *Brucella* vaccines (strain 19) may accidentally inject themselves. Two types of disease may ensue. In the person who has had clinical or subclinical brucellosis (serologically positive), a marked local hypersensitivity reaction with pain, erythema, and occasionally gangrene develops within 48 hours. The treatment is tetracycline and 60 mg of prednisone orally each day in divided doses for 1 to 2 weeks. In the patient without previous clinical or subclinical illness, acute brucellosis develops 1 to 3 weeks later; tetracycline should be given for 3 weeks. When the patient has a past history of brucellosis and the injection site is in the distal part of an extremity where inflammation might compromise the circulation, corticosteroids together with antibiotic therapy should be started before the development of the local reaction.

### General Measures

The patient should be at rest for the first 2 to 3 weeks of treatment. This action by itself will result in symptomatic improvement. Any exposure to animals with brucellosis should be avoided during the initial convalescence because hypersensitivity-like reactions can occur. Prolonged asthenia and depression may accompany this infection.

### Vaccine Therapy and Desensitization

Blood transfusions, immune serum, *Brucella* vaccines, and *Brucella* phages are of no value and should not be used.

### Steroids

Steroids are used only rarely. Indications include severe Herxheimer reactions and some situations of accidental self-inoculation or (possibly) infection of the central nervous system.

# CHICKENPOX (VARICELLA) AND ZOSTER (SHINGLES)

method of
JOHN D. SHANLEY, M.D.
*University of Connecticut*
*Farmington, Connecticut*

Varicella, or chickenpox, is a common vesicular exanthem most often seen in childhood. It is one of the manifestations of primary infection by the human herpesvirus varicella zoster virus (VZV). Following acute infection, the virus persists in the host in an inactive or latent state. Zoster, or shingles, is a clinical illness characterized by local pain and a vesicular rash restricted to one or several dermatomes, which results from reactivation of latent infection.

## EPIDEMIOLOGY

Varicella is the result of primary infection with VZV. Transmission of varicella results from airborne transmission of respiratory droplet infection from patients with varicella or direct contact with the vesicular lesions of either varicella or zoster. The incubation period of varicella is 10 to 20 days, and transmission can occur 24 to 48 hours prior to the appearance of the rash. Healthy children need not be isolated from individuals with varicella. However, exposure of nonimmune adults, pregnant women, or individuals with impairment of cellular immunity should be avoided. In the USA, VZV is endemic, with infections occurring most commonly during childhood. Greater than 90% of individuals develop infection by age 15. Although most cases are clinically apparent, 50% of seropositive cases have no or an equivocal history of prior varicella. Varicella infections occur throughout the year but increase during the winter and spring. In tropical countries, varicella is much less common. Humans are the only reservoir of infection.

Zoster, or shingles, results from the reactivation of endogenous latent virus. There is no seasonal variation or epidemics. The risk of zoster progressively increases with age. Reactivation of infection is also more common in individuals with impairment of cellular immunity. However, zoster has poor predictive value for identifying individuals with underlying immune deficiency. The mechanism of reactivation is not known.

## DIAGNOSIS AND MANAGEMENT OF VARICELLA

The clinical presentation of varicella is generally sufficient to provide the diagnosis. Laboratory confirmation, while not often necessary, can be made by direct virus isolation or demonstration of viral antigens in vesicular lesions. Lesions generally appear on the head and neck, spreading to the trunk and extremities. The skin lesions evolve from papules to vesicles, to pustules, then scab and heal, generally without scarring. New crops of lesions continue to appear over 3 to 7 days, and lesions in all stages of evolution are present. Varicella in childhood is generally a benign illness, requiring only supportive care. Since pruritus is a major problem, nails should be trimmed to prevent excoriation. Baths in oatmeal or cornstarch or application of calamine lotion to lesions may provide relief. Skin lesions may be washed and blotted dry. Bathing may relieve discomfort from lesions in the perineum or vaginal area, but drying of the skin should be avoided. Because of the association of varicella with Reye's syndrome, use acetaminophen for antipyretic therapy, and avoid aspirin.

## DIAGNOSIS AND MANAGEMENT OF ZOSTER

Zoster, or shingles, can usually be diagnosed by the characteristic clinical syndrome of localized burning pain and a vesicular rash confined to a single dermatome. The illness is generally self-limited and will respond to the local supportive care described for varicella. Pain represents a major complication and will be discussed below. Antiviral therapy with oral acyclovir* 800 mg five times a day will hasten clinical resolution,

---

*This use of acyclovir is not listed in the manufacturer's official directive.

but its beneficial effects are offset by the expense of treatment.

## COMPLICATIONS OF VARICELLA

Although varicella is generally a benign illness, in certain circumstances it may produce serious, often life-threatening complications. Most often these complications occur in adults, neonates, and individuals with iatrogenic or disease-induced immune deficiency. Because of disruption of skin integrity, secondary bacterial infection of skin lesions leading to pyoderma or cellulitis is common, most often due to *Staphylococcus aureus* or group A beta-hemolytic streptococci. The development of spreading erythema, enlargement of lesions, or impetiginous changes suggests secondary bacterial infection. After culturing, antibacterial therapy directed toward staphylococci or streptococci should be instituted.

Roentgenographic evidence of pulmonary involvement occurs in approximately 15% of adults with varicella. Clinically apparent varicella pneumonia, while uncommon, can produce respiratory compromise and death. The development of cough, hemoptysis, tachypnea, or dyspnea in the face of varicella should raise concern for pulmonary involvement. Chest x-ray shows diffuse infiltrates with multiple nodular hilar and perihilar densities, a pattern distinct from secondary bacterial pneumonia. In the presence of clinically apparent lung involvement, intravenous antiviral therapy with acyclovir (Zovirax) (10 mg per kg every 8 hours for 7 days)* or vidarabine† (Vira A) (10 mg per kg per day given over 12 hours for 10 days) should be instituted promptly. Arterial $P_{O_2}$ should be monitored and respiratory support given as needed. The presence of secondary bacterial pneumonia should be ruled out.

There are a number of hemorrhagic complications of varicella thought to be the result of an immunopathologic process. Febrile purpuras are characterized by hemorrhage into the base of the skin lesions with associated thrombocytopenia. Postinfectious purpura with thrombocytopenia may develop after the resolution of acute varicella. Although platelet support and steroid therapy may be needed, both complications have good prognosis and respond to supportive care. Occasionally, purpura fulminans with generalized coagulopathy will develop, requiring intensive supportive care.

There are a number of neurologic complications of varicella, encephalitis and cerebellar ataxia

being the most common. Cerebellar ataxia is a self-limited process occurring in the late phases of varicella or within several weeks of resolution of the rash. Cerebellar ataxia will resolve without treatment. Encephalitis is characterized by changes in mental status or seizures that develop 5 to 7 days after the appearance of the rash. Symptoms progress to obtundation and coma. The pathogenesis is thought to be the result of demyelination rather than acute viral infection of the brain. The cerebrospinal fluid (CSF) profile typically shows a moderate increase in leukocytes, the majority being mononuclear cells, a normal glucose, and normal to slightly elevated protein. Care should include supportive measures including respiratory support, seizure control, and fluid restriction. Increased intracranial pressure can be managed by an initial dose of dexamethasone (Decadron) 10 mg IM or IV initially followed by 4 mg IM or IV every 6 hours. Mannitol 20% solution can be given at 1 to 1.5 grams per kg intravenously if the serum osmolality is less than 320 mOsm per liter. Antiviral treatment is generally not helpful unless visceral involvement is present. Examination of the CSF should be performed to rule out bacterial meningitis.

Other neurologic complications of varicella include transverse myelitis, radiculopathy, optic neuritis with blindness, and Guillain-Barré syndrome. Varicella precedes 20 to 30% of cases of Reye's syndrome, which should be considered in patients experiencing repeated vomiting.

Visceral involvement of varicella may involve the liver, leading to hepatitis. This is most common in immunocompromised patients. Parenteral antiviral therapy with acyclovir or vidarabine is indicated.

Ocular involvement with varicella may take the form of either keratoconjunctivitis or uveitis. Either topical or oral antiviral treatment may be helpful.

## COMPLICATIONS OF ZOSTER

As with primary infection, zoster is often complicated by secondary bacterial infection of the skin leading to pyoderma or cellulitis. Most often this is due to either *Staphylococcus aureus* or group A beta-hemolytic streptococci. If secondary infection develops, appropriate antibiotic therapy should be instituted.

Pain, either acute or postherpetic, is the main complication of zoster. Acute pain tends to resolve in conjunction with resolution of the rash and may be hastened by antiviral treatment. Postherpetic neuralgia, on the other hand, may develop into a long-standing and debilitating prob-

---

*Exceeds dosage recommended by the manufacturer.
†This use of vidarabine is not listed in the manufacturer's official directive.

lem. The occurrence of postherpetic neuralgia increases with age, especially over age 55. There are conflicting reports on the efficacy of antiviral treatment in postherpetic neuralgia. Interferon and vidarabine have both been shown to reduce the frequency and duration of postherpetic neuralgia. Studies of acyclovir have yielded mixed results. While accelerating the resolution of acute pain and rash, acyclovir does not appear to consistently prevent postherpetic neuralgia. The administration of steroids during the acute phase of zoster has been reported in two studies to reduce the frequency of postherpetic neuralgia. In a small, controlled study, triamcinolone, 16 mg administered three times a day for 7 days then 8 mg per day for a week, followed by 8 mg twice daily for a week, significantly reduced postherpetic pain. A large, controlled study of the efficacy of steroid treatment is in progress. At this writing, it is recommended that patients over the age of 55 who develop zoster be treated with a short, tapered course of corticosteroids. A variety of agents including tricyclic antidepressants, levodopa, anticonvulsants, and topical anesthetics have all been reported to improve postherpetic neuralgia but have not been rigorously studied.

Zoster is occasionally associated with neurologic complications. Encephalitis is most common and is generally self-limited. Zoster of the trigeminal nerve (herpes ophthalmicus) with contralateral hemiparesis is a serious complication, thought to be secondary to cerebral vasculitis. Zoster has also been associated with peripheral nerve palsy, Bell's palsy, and Ramsay Hunt syndrome.

## SPECIAL RISKS

Although varicella infection in childhood is generally well tolerated, there are a number of situations in which primary infection presents special risks. The literature suggests that adults are more likely to develop serious complications during primary varicella infection. The physician needs to be especially alert for signs of pulmonary involvement in these cases.

Although most women of childbearing age are VZV immune, pregnant women who develop varicella appear to be prone to complications, especially pneumonitis. Varicella infection during pregnancy may also lead to spontaneous abortion. Less than 5% of fetuses exposed in utero to maternal varicella develop congenital abnormalities, including microcephaly, cerebral atrophy, mental retardation, seizures, or cicatricial abnormalities of the limbs. If a pregnant woman with no history of varicella is exposed to VZV, her immune status should be rapidly assessed by antibody assay. In the varicella-nonimmune patient, passive immune treatment with varicella zoster immune globulin (VZIG) should be used to modify infection. VZIG is supplied by the American Red Cross, generally in vials containing 125 units in 1.25 ml. The recommended dose is 125 units per 10 kg given intramuscularly up to a maximum of 625 units. Currently, there is no evidence that this will protect the fetus.

Neonates are functionally immunocompromised, and exposure to varicella during the 5 days prior to or 2 to 3 days after birth may lead to life-threatening disseminated infection involving visceral organs. Passive antibody treatment with VZIG should be given as soon as possible after birth. Those who progress to varicella should be treated with parenteral acyclovir.

Varicella-nonimmune patients with abnormalities of host immunity, either iatrogenic or disease induced, are at increased risk of fatal complications during primary varicella infection. Generally, varicella follows a typical course, but it continues to progress with new lesion formation 5 to 6 days after the rash appears. This progression may be accompanied by visceral dissemination with pneumonitis, hepatitis, encephalitis, and disseminated intravascular coagulopathy, so-called malignant varicella. Immune deficiency may include diseases such as Wiskott-Aldrich syndrome, thymic dysplasia, or acquired immunodeficiency syndrome, or may result from malignancy or cytotoxic or corticosteroid treatment. In cases of known exposure of less than 96 hours duration, these VZV-nonimmune, immunocompromised individuals should receive varicella zoster immune globulin (VZIG), 125 mg per 10 kg. VZIG has been shown to moderate or prevent acute infection in immunocompromised patients but has no effect once clinical varicella occurs. In cases where clinical infection occurs, parenteral antiviral therapy with acyclovir (10 mg per kg every 8 hours for 10 days)* should be instituted as early as possible. Severe varicella will require intensive supportive measures.

Zoster, even in the severely immunocompromised patient, is generally a self-limited process. However, in individuals with immunodeficiencies, zoster may disseminate from the primary dermatome or develop into a protracted, nonresolving infection. In addition, zoster may delay chemotherapy for underlying malignancy. Parenteral antiviral therapy with acyclovir will shorten the course of infection.

### NOSOCOMIAL TRANSMISSION OF VARICELLA

It is important to emphasize that nosocomial transmission of varicella is a major problem,

---

*Exceeds dosage recommended by the manufacturer.

especially in pediatric services. Hospital-based epidemics are common and, because of the concentration of highly susceptible individuals, are of major concern. Individuals with varicella or zoster should not be hospitalized, if possible. If hospitalized, they should be placed in isolation in rooms with negative air pressure to the corridor. If exposure occurs, high-risk individuals should receive immune prophylaxis with VZIG. If possible, susceptibles should be discharged during the incubation period and those remaining placed in isolation. Nonimmune individuals can play a major role in transmission of infection and should avoid contact with patients with varicella or zoster.

# CHOLERA

method of
MICHAEL L. BENNISH, M.D.
*International Centre for Diarrhoeal Disease Research, Dhaka, Bangladesh; and New England Medical Center, Boston, Massachusetts*

## GENERAL BACKGROUND

Cholera is an acute watery diarrhea caused by infection of the small intestine with *Vibrio cholerae*, serogroup 01. Although sporadic cases of cholera have been reported in communities along the Gulf Coast of the United States as well as in other industrialized countries, the disease is most common in developing countries where fecal contamination of water supplies is widespread. During infection, *V. cholerae* organisms colonize the small intestine and produce a protein exotoxin that, by stimulating the production of cyclic AMP, causes an increase in intestinal chloride secretion and a decrease in sodium chloride absorption. Water accompanies this increased sodium chloride excretion, and when the volume of water exceeds the absorptive capacity of the colon, diarrhea results. The magnitude of the diarrhea varies, but children or adults with severe symptomatic *V. cholerae* infection may have stool volumes of 100 ml or more per kilogram body weight per day. This high rate of fluid loss results in the rapid and clinically very dramatic dehydration that is the primary complication of *V. cholerae* infection.

## CLINICAL FEATURES AND DIAGNOSIS

Cholera is characterized by a voluminous diarrhea in which the watery stool contains small flecks of mucus but little fecal matter. Cholera stool is not malodorous and is often described as "rice-water" in character—i.e., it resembles the water that rice has been washed in. Because the organism does not invade the epithelial lining of the intestine, there is little inflammatory response, and hence the stool contains few if any leukocytes and patients are afebrile. The stool is isotonic with plasma, with a sodium concentration that is slightly lower and with bicarbonate and potassium concentrations that are higher than those found in plasma (Table 1).

Vomiting is an almost invariable component of the disease, especially early in the illness, and contributes to the fluid and electrolyte abnormalities. Intestinal and extremity cramping is also an occasional feature.

If fluid replacement is not sufficient to keep pace with fluid loss, dehydration results. If untreated, the dehydration can be severe, leading to hypovolemic shock and death. The signs of dehydration are the same as those that occur with any diarrheal illness and include decreased skin turgor, sunken eyes, dry mucous membranes, and decreased urine output. The severity of dehydration is classified using standard criteria (Table 2). For practical purposes, mild dehydration is present when there is thirst in the absence of physical signs of dehydration; moderate dehydration is present if there are physical signs of dehydration without vascular collapse; and severe dehydration is present when there is vascular collapse. Because the sodium content of stools during cholera approximates that of serum, dehydration during cholera is usually isotonic in character. Subcutaneous turgor is the most consistent physical sign of dehydration during isotonic dehydration and is assessed by pinching the abdominal subcutaneous tissues between the thumb and forefinger. In patients without dehydration the subcutaneous tissue retracts immediately when the pinch is released; in patients with moderate or severe dehydration the subcutaneous tissues will remain erect (tented) following release of the pinch.

Definitive diagnosis of cholera depends on isolation of *V. cholerae* from the stool, and selective media are available for this purpose. For rapid diagnosis, dark-field examination of a fresh, unstained stool specimen is both a sensitive and a specific screening test. The presence of spiral-shaped organisms that have a characteristic "shooting star" pattern of motility and that are immobilized by the addition of specific antisera is diagnostic of cholera.

Whereas children may become dehydrated from diarrhea caused by a number of different enteric pathogens, severe dehydration in adults is uncommon in the absence of cholera. In any case, a bacteriologic diagnosis is not essential for the management of an individual with cholera, as therapy of any dehydrating diarrhea is guided by the extent of fluid loss rather than by the nature of the infecting organism.

## TREATMENT

### Fluid Therapy

The cornerstone of therapy of cholera is the replacement of the fluid and electrolyte losses that occur during the illness. If fluid replacement is instituted early, dehydration can be prevented; if treatment is delayed until dehydration is present, both the fluid deficit and the ongoing

TABLE 1. **Electrolyte Concentration in Cholera Stool and in Fluids Used for Rehydration and Replacement of Stool Losses**

| Solution | Electrolyte Concentration (mOsm/L) | | | | Osmolality |
|---|---|---|---|---|---|
| | $Na^+$ | $Cl^-$ | $K^+$ | $HCO_3$ | |
| Cholera stool | | | | | |
| Adults | 130 | 100 | 20 | 44 | 300* |
| Infants and children | 100 | 90 | 33 | 30 | 300* |
| WHO oral rehydration solution | 90 | 80 | 20 | 30† | 220‡ |
| Intravenous solutions | | | | | |
| Dhaka solution | 133 | 98 | 13 | 48 | 292 |
| Lactated Ringer's | 130 | 109 | 4 | 28§ | 271 |
| 5:4:1 solution | 129 | 97 | 11 | 44 | 281 |

*Osmolality includes unmeasured osmotically active molecules (primarily organic acids) in addition to electrolytes.
†As citrate.
‡From electrolytes only; also contains 111 mmol/L of glucose.
§As lactate.

fluid losses must be replaced. In either case, effective fluid replacement can be expected to reduce mortality to less than 1% of severely affected individuals, in comparison with 50% or more in the absence of effective treatment.

Treatment of secretory diarrheas including cholera was revolutionized by the finding that despite the poisoning of intestinal chloride absorption by cholera toxin (or the related heat-labile toxin of *Escherichia coli*), glucose-mediated sodium and water absorption in the small intestinal epithelium remains intact. This finding served as the basis for the development of oral solutions containing glucose, and sodium and bicarbonate in concentrations approximately equal to the concentrations found in the stool (see Table 1). With the assistance of UNICEF and the World Health Organization (WHO), oral electrolyte solutions are now available in powder form from pharmacies or community health workers in almost all developing countries where cholera is endemic. The contents of the packet are dissolved in a measured volume of water and the solution ingested at the onset of diarrhea. In the absence of such prepared packets, homemade solutions containing sucrose and salt (or with a cereal oligosaccharide, such as rice starch, in place of sucrose) may be used.

The most common reason for the failure of oral rehydration therapy is that insufficient amounts are ingested. Parents of affected children, and adult patients, must be instructed to ensure that a quantity of solution commensurate with the intestinal fluid loss is ingested. At our diarrhea treatment centre in Dhaka, Bangladesh, where over 5000 patients with cholera are treated yearly, a simple "cholera cot" is used for monitoring fluid losses and requirements. This plastic-lined jute cot contains a hole in the middle through which stool is collected into a calibrated bucket. Stool losses are measured every 2 to 4 hours by nurses or paramedical workers, who then ensure that fluid replacement proportional to stool losses is given.

Patients with a very rapid rate of intestinal fluid loss (greater than 200 to 250 ml per kilogram per day), and those with persistent and severe vomiting, will require intravenous fluid therapy in addition to oral solution. Different intravenous fluids have been used for the treat-

TABLE 2. **Classification of Dehydration and Fluid Deficit Based on Clinical Signs and Symptoms**

| Sign or Symptom | Degree of Dehydration | | |
|---|---|---|---|
| | *Mild or None* | *Moderate* | *Severe* |
| Mentation | Alert | Restless or lethargic | Infants or young children may be comatose; older children and adults are apprehensive |
| Thirst | Present | Present | Present |
| Radial pulse | Normal | Rapid | Rapid and feeble or impalpable |
| Respiratory pattern | Normal | Tachypneic | Tachypneic, labored |
| Blood pressure | Normal | Normal | Hypotensive |
| Mucous membranes | Moist | Dry | Dry |
| Elasticity of subcutaneous tissues | Pinch retracts immediately | Pinch retracts slowly | Pinch retracts slowly |
| Eyes | Normal | Sunken | Sunken |
| Urine flow | Normal | Scant and dark | Scant or absent |
| Approximate fluid deficit | ≤50 ml/kg | 51–90 ml/kg | >90 ml/kg |

TABLE 3. **Effects of Four-Hour Rapid Rehydration***

| | Time | | |
| --- | --- | --- | --- |
| Serum Concentration of: | Admission | 4 hr After Admission | 24 hr After Admission |
| Sodium (mmol/L) | 132 | 135 | 134 |
| Potassium (mmol/L) | 4.4 | 3.8 | 3.7 |
| Total $CO_2$ (mmol/L) | 13.4 | 19.4 | 21.9 |
| Creatinine (mg/dl) | 1.6 | 1.2 | 0.9 |
| Protein (g/L) | 102 | 72 | 73 |

*Mean serum protein, electrolyte, and creatinine concentrations in 32 children with cholera and moderate or severe dehydration rehydrated over 4 hours with Dhaka solution.

ment of patients with cholera (see Table 1). In general, they all contain relatively high concentrations of sodium and bicarbonate. There are not decided differences in the efficacy of these solutions, and the choice of intravenous solution depends on availability. If intravascular volume is maintained and urine output sustained, the kidneys should be able to moderate electrolyte imbalances.

Patients with dehydration require replacement of their fluid deficit in addition to the replacement of ongoing losses. In patients with severe dehydration, or with moderate dehydration and either vomiting or a high rate of fluid loss, fluid replacement is best given intravenously. If facilities for intravenous fluid administration are not available, oral rehydration solution may be given by a stomach tube. The volume of fluid replacement is guided by the degree of dehydration (see Table 2). Patients at the Treatment Centre of the International Centre for Diarrhoeal Disease Research in Dhaka have their fluid deficit completely corrected within 4 hours of admission, with half of the fluid replacement occurring within the first hour of admission. This rapid rehydration is safe and is more practicable than the slower rehydration regimens recommended for use in developed countries. Total serum protein and specific gravity, both of which can be easily estimated with an inexpensive refractom-

eter, are good guides to the adequacy of replacement therapy. Patients who are dehydrated will have an increased serum protein concentration and an increased serum specific gravity because of the loss of intravascular water and electrolytes. Severely dehydrated patients will inevitably have a serum specific gravity greater than 1.030, which will fall to 1.020 to 1.025 with adequate rehydration. The pattern of changes in serum electrolytes, creatinine, and protein during the 4-hour rapid rehydration of moderately or severely dehydrated children with cholera is shown in Table 3.

### Antimicrobial Therapy

Although appropriate fluid replacement alone ensures survival during cholera, antimicrobial therapy facilitates management by reducing both the volume and the duration of diarrhea. Although sporadic resistance to tetracycline has been reported, most V. cholerae organisms remain susceptible, and tetracycline remains the drug of choice for treating V. cholerae infections. Short courses of tetracycline, as used in the treatment of cholera, have not been associated with discoloration of permanent teeth in children. If preferred, furazolidone is a suitable alternative for children less than 8 years old. Treatment options and drug dosages are shown in Table 4.

### Complications Other Than Dehydration

Metabolic abnormalities are the major complications in addition to dehydration occurring during cholera. Severe hypoglycemia due to deficient gluconeogenesis can result in seizures and other neurologic abnormalities. Hypoglycemia is most often seen in malnourished children who have not eaten for 10 hours or more and have thus depleted their glycogen stores. Feeding during diarrhea could presumably prevent the hypoglycemia by obviating the need for gluconeogenesis. Treatment of established hypoglycemia requires the administration of dextrose intravenously. This can be achieved by giving bolus intravenous

TABLE 4. **Antimicrobial Therapy of Cholera**

| | Adults | Children <12 yr of Age |
| --- | --- | --- |
| Treatment of choice | Tetracycline, 500 mg q 6 hr for 3 days | Tetracycline, 50 mg/kg/day divided into four doses for 3 days |
| Alternative treatment regimens | Furazolidone (Furoxone), 100 mg q 6 hr for 3 days or Doxycycline (Vibramycin), 300 mg as a single dose | Furazolidone (Furoxone), 5 mg/kg/day divided into four doses for 3 days |

glucose or preferably by routinely including dextrose in all intravenous fluids used in the treatment of patients with cholera.

Hypokalemia as a result of stool loss of potassium is also most common in malnourished children. The hypokalemia may be masked on admission by the concomitant acidosis. With correction of the acidosis, potassium moves from the extracellular to the intracellular space and the hypokalemia becomes apparent. Because of the almost invariable fall in serum potassium during therapy (see Table 3), we administer potassium containing fluids from the beginning of therapy, rather than waiting until urination occurs. In severely dehydrated patients, urination may not occur until 4 or more hours after the initiation of fluid therapy.

Acidosis is a result of both bicarbonate loss in the stool and increased lactate production due to anaerobic glycolysis. Restoration of intravascular volume will diminish lactate production, and the bicarbonate contained in the intravenous solution will replenish plasma bicarbonate concentrations. Too vigorous bicarbonate therapy, however, can result in tetany as a result of a decrease in the proportion of ionized to bound calcium. Halting the bicarbonate infusion will result in the resolution of the tetany.

## PREVENTION

Compared with other enteric pathogens, the number of V. cholerae organisms required to establish infection is quite high. Diminished gastric acidity predisposes the patient to infection. Because of the high infectious dose, persons from developed countries traveling to or living in cholera endemic areas are at minimal risk of acquiring the disease. Immunization with current cholera vaccines (which are at any rate of limited efficacy) are not recommended for such persons. For persons living in endemic areas, access to potable water is likely to have the greatest impact in reducing disease transmission. In the absence of potable water, boiling of drinking water or the addition of alum potash should also be effective in preventing disease. The latter is available in many villages in developing countries.

# DIPHTHERIA

method of
LOUIS WEINSTEIN, M.D., PH.D.
*Harvard Medical School*
*Boston, Massachusetts*

## CLINICAL FEATURES

*Corynebacterium diphtheriae* is acquired by contact with patients with active disease or with asymptomatic carriers of the organism. Although most strains of the organism produce the toxin responsible for most of the clinical features of diphtheria, nontoxigenic organisms may rarely be involved. The incubation period of the disease is, on average, 2 to 4 days; it may be as short as 1 or as long as 7 days.

The diagnosis of diphtheria is established by two methods: (1) methylene-blue stains of the exudate; with experience, the organism can be identified by this technique in 75 to 85% of cases; and (2) culture of the membrane on Loeffler's medium is uniformly positive after 8 to 12 hours of incubation at 37° C in most patients who have not been treated with an antimicrobial agent prior to this study. If, however, an antibiotic has been administered, for even 1 day before the culture is obtained, 5 or more days may be required before it becomes positive. In some cases, the organism cannot be recovered.

Although the pharynx is the most common site of the diphtheritic membrane, it must be emphasized that the lesion may extend to other areas in the respiratory tract or, in some instances, be present as isolated disease in the nose (unilateral serosanguineous discharge), larynx, skin (round, deep, punched-out ulcer covered by a gray, yellow, or brown membrane), uterine cervix, vagina, vulva, urinary bladder, urethra (after prostatectomy), penis (after circumcision), tongue, buccal mucosa, gums, or esophagus.

The earliest faucial diphtheritic membrane consists of small, separated collections of soft exudate and resembles the follicular pharyngitis or tonsillitis produced by streptococci or some viruses. It is easily removed and is not followed by bleeding. Unless the possibility of diphtheria is considered, patients may be mistakenly treated with penicillin or erythromycin. If this is continued for 1 to 2 or more days, recovery of the organism is, in most instances, impossible.

As the disease progresses, the follicular areas coalesce to form a thin white to light yellow membrane that covers the tonsils, pharynx, or both, and is easily removed. Finally, the membrane becomes thicker, is yellow, white, gray, or black (hemorrhagic) in color and is tightly attached to the underlying mucosa and surrounded by a narrow zone of inflammation. Removal of the membrane causes bleeding. Mild, moderate, or severe pharyngeal discomfort is present. Fever is usually low grade (100 to 101° F). The white blood count usually does not exceed 15,000 per mm³, with a mild shift to the left; it may be as high as 25,000 per mm³ when the disease is severe.

Two mechanisms, toxin-induced and obstructive phenomena, are involved in the pathoanatomy and pathophysiology of diphtheria. Most of the clinical manifestations of the disease are related to the activity of the toxin. The diphtheritic membrane is, in essence, the factory in which the toxin is manufactured. Both obstructive and toxin-induced phenomena are present when the larynx alone is involved or when the faucial membrane descends into the larynx, from which it may spread into the bronchial tree and pulmonary alveoli. Involvement of the larynx may lead to total obstruction that, unless treated appropriately, may be fatal. Both diffuse obstruction and increased activity of toxin are problems when the lung is involved. The risk of a fatal outcome is increased when the pulmonary membrane begins to break up as the disease improves. This may lead to sudden death as large pieces of the membrane are coughed up and trapped between the vocal cords; this results in sudden, complete obstruction of the airway. Another problem is created by the very large surface area presented by the bronchial tree and alveoli over which very high concentrations of toxin are absorbed.

## TREATMENT

### General Management

All patients with diphtheria must be hospitalized because, although not very ill initially, they may rapidly progress to cardiovascular or neurologic dysfunction. Strict isolation practices are mandatory. When possible, patients should be housed in single rooms. This may not be possible in the face of a large outbreak of the disease when cases must be admitted to wards. This may present a problem for the following reasons. Because it is now standard practice to treat for 10 days with an antibiotic active against *C. diphtheriae,* most patients are free of the organism in 3 to 4 days and therapy is stopped. Once this occurs, patients are susceptible to acquiring the organism when fresh cases of diphtheria are admitted to the ward in which they reside.

The duration of bed rest is short in patients with a relatively benign course. Those in whom cardiac or neurologic complications appear require longer periods of rest in bed or in a chair.

Isolation is continued until two cultures (48 hours apart) of the pharynx or nose taken 48 to 72 hours after antimicrobial therapy is discontinued are negative. Because these patients may acquire the organism as fresh cases are admitted to the ward, it is best to move them to a "clean" area.

### Antitoxin

Treatment with antitoxin is the prime approach to the management of diphtheria. The fatality rate in patients who have not been treated with antitoxin has been reported to be as high as 35%; it may be 90% in those in whom the larynx is involved. The time in the course of the disease when treatment is carried out is important in determining the outcome. The fatality rate in persons receiving antitoxin on the first day of the disease is about 20%. In contrast, delay in treatment for 5 days is associated with death in about 65% of cases.

Because diphtheritic antitoxin is produced in horses, it is mandatory that all patients be tested for sensitivity to horse serum prior to treatment. This is carried out by injecting 0.1 ml of the ⅟₁₀₀₀ dilution of the antitoxin intradermally. A positive reaction is characterized by the development of urticaria surrounded by erythema within 20 minutes. Pseudopodial extensions from the site of the reaction indicate high-grade hypersensitivity.

The ophthalmic reaction is a more sensitive indication of sensitivity. It is of less value in children in whom a positive response may be obscured by reddening of the conjunctiva that may develop when they cry. This test involves the placement of one drop of ⅟₁₀ dilution of 0.1 ml of the antitoxin in the conjunctival sac of one eye. A positive response is indicated by the development of itching, watering, and diffuse redness. The installation of 0.1 ml of physiologic saline in the other eye serves as a control.

Antitoxin is administered 20 minutes after sensitivity to horse serum has been eliminated. It is important to point out that some adults with negative histories of reactions to horse serum, but with histories of allergy to a variety of other substances, should first be given 0.1 to 0.5 ml of antitoxin intramuscularly. If no reaction develops, antitoxin is administered in four to six equal doses over 30 to 60 minutes. Depending upon the severity, the dosage range may be 20,000 to 120,000 units or 40 to 240 ml. Nonsensitive children may be given the full dose of antitoxin in a single injection.

Although the intravenous administration of antitoxin has been considered unnecessary, it is clear that maximal levels are not produced when it is given by the intramuscular route alone. It has been my practice to administer half of the required quantity intramuscularly and the remainder intravenously. This is indicated most often in patients with severe or complicated diphtheria. The intravenous route *should never be used first* because it is associated with a greater risk of very severe hypersensitivity reactions. The initial intramuscular dose may desensitize some individuals who might react to antitoxin when it is given intravenously. If local or systemic reactions have not developed within 30 to 60 minutes after the intramuscular injection, intravenous administration is associated with little or no risk. The optimal site for the injection of antitoxin is low in the thigh because, should a reaction develop, the absorption of antitoxin may be interrupted by applying a tourniquet above the point of inoculation. *Patients who develop reactions in the skin and eye must never be treated intravenously.* However, if the disease is severe and therapy critical, desensitization should be attempted. This involves the administration of no more than 0.1 ml of ⅟₁₀₀,₀₀₀ dilution of antitoxin subcutaneously and is followed by doubling the first dose every 30 minutes. In the absence of a reaction, repeated doses are given until the required total quantity is administered.

The use of antitoxin may need to be abandoned in those who develop severe reactions during treatment. However, this may not be necessary in all cases because patients can be desensitized. This is usually attempted only when reactions in the skin are doubtful and involves an initial injection of no more than 0.1 ml of a 1/100,000 dilution of antitoxin. These patients may tolerate increasingly larger doses more rapidly. Reactions occurring prior to or during treatment should be treated with 0.01 ml per kg or 0.03 per square meter of a 1/100 dilution of epinephrine. The total dose should not exceed 0.5 ml.

The clinical manifestations of a reaction to antitoxin include lumbar or abdominal pain, urticaria, wheezing, dyspnea, cyanosis, or shock. Artificial respiration or treatment for shock may be required.

It is important to be aware that only that portion of toxin still free in solution in tissue fluid, lymph, and blood can be neutralized. Once fixed to cells, it is not neutralized by antitoxin. It has been suggested that the older the patient and the longer the duration of the disease, the larger the dose of antitoxin required. This is, in my opinion, questionable. Little benefit can be expected from the administration of even very large doses of antitoxin to those who come to medical attention late in the disease.

Although the use of specific quantities of antitoxin, as described below, has been recommended, it is clear that these are entirely empiric and probably excessive. This is based, for the most part, on the thesis that the more severe the diphtheria, the larger the dose required. Several carefully controlled studies have indicated that this does not hold. My experience with over 300 cases of diphtheria has made it clear that the time in the course of the disease when it is administered is more important than the size of the dose. Treatment after the disease has been present for more than 48 hours was found to be associated with a higher incidence of complications such as laryngeal obstruction, myocarditis, and neurologic dysfunction.

Antitoxin must be given as early in the course of diphtheria as possible. Delay in treatment increases the risk of complications and death. It has been suggested that larger quantities of antiserum are necessary when therapy is given late. However, since, as pointed out above, toxin is fixed instantaneously to the tissues and then cannot be neutralized by even the most massive doses of antitoxin, the beneficial effect of increasing the amount of antiserum is very questionable. The diphtheritic membrane frequently increases in size for 24 hours after the treatment; this does not indicate too small a dose or the need for additional serotherapy.

Physicians with little or moderate experience with this disease should employ the following recommended schedules on adults: (1) diphtheria with the faucial membrane limited to a small area on one tonsil or the nares—5,000 to 10,000 units of antitoxin; (2) disease involving both tonsils or one tonsil and its adjacent pillars—20,000 to 40,000 units; (3) nasopharyngeal, uvular, or laryngeal involvement—40,000 to 60,000 units; (4) extensive membrane, extreme toxicity, hemorrhages in mucous membranes and skin, swelling of neck (malignant diphtheria)—60,000 to 100,000 units.

The following schedule is recommended for children: (1) involvement of anterior nose and tonsils—10,000 to 20,000 units; (2) pharyngeal, uvular, or laryngeal disease—20,000 to 40,000 units; (3) nasopharyngeal infection—40,000 to 75,000 units.*

All instances of nasal diphtheria do not, in my opinion, require the use of antitoxin. It may not be necessary to treat the disease if it involves *only the anterior area of the nose.* My experience with a number of children with this problem has indicated that this type of diphtheria may be very chronic (months) and produce no clinical manifestations. Examination frequently disclosed the presence of a small foreign body in the anterior nose. When this was removed, the small membrane covering the mucosa disappeared in less than a week. Diphtheria involving the posterior nasal area presents a much more serious problem because the disease may spread to the larynx. Administration of antitoxin is critical in this situation.

Diphtheritic laryngitis is probably the most life-threatening form of the disease for two reasons: (1) the area covered by the membrane is fairly large and offers a large surface for the absorption of toxin; (2) there is a very high risk of total occlusion of the airway. This situation must be monitored constantly. Examination of the larynx by laryngoscopy is desirable. It may be necessary, in some cases, to remove part or all of the laryngotracheal membrane. However, it must never be torn away from the underlying tissues. Although intubation was the management of choice (O'Dwyer's tube) in the past, it is best to perform a tracheostomy. Relief of the obstructed airway should never be delayed until cyanosis develops; attempts at intubation, at this point, may produce cardiac arrest. Progressive restlessness accompanied by the use of the acces-

---

*Dosage is lower than that recommended by the manufacturer.

sory muscles of respiration is a strong signal for intubation or tracheostomy and the administration of oxygen. As a rule, the tracheal tube may be removed safely after about 5 to 6 days.

## Antimicrobial Therapy

All patients with diphtheria should be treated with an antimicrobial agent. However, it must be emphasized that this plays absolutely no role in altering the course of the disease. Its primary purpose is eradication of the organism and prevention of its spreading to other individuals. While penicillin G was almost universally effective some years ago, an increasing number of strains of *C. diphtheriae* have become resistant to this drug. At present, erythromycin appears to be the most effective agent. It is my practice to administer 250 to 500 mg of this drug orally, in four equally divided doses for 7 to 10 days. This therapy is also effective in eradicating the organism from the pharynx of healthy carriers.

## Complications

The potentially serious and, at times, life-threatening complications of diphtheria include laryngeal obstruction, bronchopulmonary invasion, myocarditis, dysfunction of the peripheral and central nervous systems, and shock.

A very important problem is presented by patients in whom diphtheria is restricted to the larynx. Because a membrane is not present in the pharynx, a mistaken diagnosis of simple croup may be entertained and treatment with inhaled warm steam instituted. If this fails after a few hours, laryngoscopy must be carried out. This will disclose the characteristic membrane when *C. diphtheriae* is involved. Because of the very high risk of total obstruction and death, every effort must be made to remove the laryngeal membrane with minimal injury to the underlying mucosa. If this fails, tracheostomy must be carried out.

Myocarditis has been said to complicate the course of diphtheria in about 10% of patients. However, my experience with more than 300 patients with this disease, all of whom had electrocardiography every other day, disclosed cardiac involvement in about two-thirds of the cases. The ECG abnormalities ranged from mild to very severe. Although infection by the *mitis* strain of *C. diphtheriae* was present in some who had only mild to moderate myocarditis, it was striking that 10% of those who developed the most severe electrocardiographic abnormalities and who had the highest fatality rate (90%) were infected by this strain. The ECG findings in this group included incomplete or complete bundle branch block, atrial or ventricular fibrillation, extrasystoles, tachycardia, alteration in the cardiac sounds, and cardiac failure; the right side was the first to fail. In contrast to the very high fatality rate in those with severe diphtheritic myocarditis, only 5% of those with mild to moderate cardiac involvement died. A few of the patients who succumbed to the disease after several weeks were found at autopsy to have a varying degree of myocardial fibrosis. It has been reported that some patients who survived an episode of diphtheria early in life and died many years later were found, at autopsy, to have myocardial abnormalities unrelated to atherosclerosis or hypertension.

While it was accepted, for many years, that the administration of digitalis to patients who developed cardiac failure following diphtheritic myocarditis was of either little or no value, it was, in fact, dangerous. These studies were carried out primarily in children. There is some suspicion that excessive doses of the drug had been administered. More recent experience suggests that digitalis has a salutary effect when given in appropriate dosage and when blood levels are monitored and maintained at safe levels. Restriction of salt and water is helpful. Treatment with quinidine is indicated for the management of arrhythmias; procainamide (Pronestyl) and other agents may be of value in controlling ventricular arrhythmias. More recently available drugs—angiotensin-converting enzyme inhibitors (ACE) such as enalapril (Vasotec)—may be of value in this type of cardiac disease.

Peripheral neuritis may appear at any time after the onset of diphtheria. In some cases, paralysis of the soft palate and posterior pharyngeal wall may appear early in the course of the disease. Neurologic dysfunction develops most often in the second to sixth week of the disease and involves the cranial nerves, most commonly N III, VI, VII, IX, and X. However, other cranial nerves may be involved and lead to paralysis of the extremities, diaphragm, or intercostal muscles. Sensory loss is quite uncommon and, when it occurs, is usually minor. The Guillain-Barré syndrome is rare and usually develops 2 to 3 months after the onset of diphtheria. The clinical manifestations include symmetrical decrease of sensation in a glove-and-stocking distribution and albumino-cytologic dissociation in the spinal fluid. Most patients with this disorder experience full return of neurologic function, without treatment, within a year. Rarely, however, this syndrome may become life-threatening because of progressive respiratory dysfunction and other types of paralysis. Hemodialysis may have a salutary effect when this occurs. Peripheral vascular collapse (shock) may develop suddenly in some patients with severe diphtheria. Although the usual methodology for control of this syndrome is employed, many patients die, despite intensive therapy.

## PREVENTION

Susceptibility to diphtheria is determined by the results of the Schick test. This involves the intradermal injection of 0.1 ml (1/50 MLD) of purified toxin. The injection of the same quantity of toxoid serves as a control. The results of the tests are read 72 to 96 hours later. A reaction positive to toxin but negative to toxoid indicates lack of immunity. A negative reaction to both effects immunity to the disease. A positive reaction to both the toxin and toxoid demonstrates high grade immunity. When the reaction to both toxin and toxoid is positive, but the one to toxin persists after the reaction to toxoid disappears, immunity is lacking.

Although most children and young adults have been fully immunized against diphtheria and have received adequate "booster" doses to maintain their immunity, the results of a recent study carried out in my laboratory that involved Schick testing of a large number of patients ranging in age from 16 to 90 years indicated that the incidence of positive reactions was very low in the young, but uncomfortably high (60%) in the elderly. This reflects the failure to monitor immunity to diphtheria in all age groups routinely and to administer a "booster" dose when it is found to be inadequate to protect against the disease.

Until relatively recently it has been impossible to give diphtheria toxoid to adults because of the high frequency of severe constitutional reactions. The present availability of highly purified preparations of the toxoid has minimized the risk of untoward sequelae and has made immunization of individuals in all age groups practical. A small number of immunized persons, even those with negative Schick reactions, may still develop diphtheria.

Many cases of active diphtheria are contracted from asymptomatic carriers. Until the development of effective antimicrobial therapy, it was very difficult or impossible to eliminate the carrier state. This can now be readily accomplished by treatment with penicillin or erythromycin.

Diphtheria is a preventable disease. Active immunization should be initiated shortly after birth and involves the administration of a combination of diphtheria, pertussis, and tetanus (DPT) vaccines. The initial dose is given when babies are 2 months of age and is followed by additional doses at 4, 6, and 18 months of age. A "booster" dose is administered at the time of entry to kindergarten. Children 7 or more years of age and adults who have not been immunized earlier should receive two doses of a combination of tetanus and diphtheria toxoids 4 weeks apart and a "booster" injection one year later. A "booster" dose should be administered every 10 years following completion of primary immunization. Immunization for diphtheria does not always produce complete protection. Fully immunized persons may become carriers of *C. diphtheriae* or develop mild disease after contact with a patient with diphtheria. Fully immunized pregnant women who have had "booster" doses of the vaccine may confer protection against the disease on their embryos.

Unimmunized individuals who come in contact with an active case of diphtheria should be given 5000 units of antitoxin; protection lasts for about 2 weeks. They should then be actively immunized.

# FOOD-BORNE ILLNESS

method of
MARK W. KLINE, M.D.
*Baylor College of Medicine*
*Houston, Texas*

Food-borne illness should be suspected when two or more persons experience similar gastrointestinal or neurologic symptoms within 72 hours of ingestion of food from the same source. A variety of bacterial, chemical, parasitic, and viral agents have been etiologically linked to food-borne illness. Most forms of food-borne illness are self-limited and require only supportive or symptomatic therapy. However, epidemiologic characteristics, clinical symptoms, and certain diagnostic studies can be helpful in elucidating the specific cause in given cases and in determining the potential need for more specific therapy.

### EPIDEMIOLOGY AND CLINICAL MANIFESTATIONS

The etiologic agents of confirmed food-borne disease outbreaks reported to the Centers for Disease Control between 1972 and 1986 are shown in Table 1. A total of 2745 outbreaks of known cause were confirmed during that time.

In general, food-borne illness with an incubation period of less than 1 hour has a chemical cause (e.g., scombroid, mushroom poisoning, or heavy metal poisoning). An incubation period of 1 to 7 hours is consistent with disease caused by preformed bacterial toxins (e.g., that produced by *Staphylococcus aureus* or *Bacillus cereus*). Ciguatera is a chemical intoxication with a similar incubation period. Disease with an incubation period of 8 to 14 hours implies toxin production in

TABLE 1. **Etiologic Agents of Confirmed Food-Borne Disease Outbreaks Reported to the Centers for Disease Control, 1972–1986***

| Agent | Percentage of Outbreaks |
|---|---|
| *Bacterial* | |
| Salmonella | 27.4 |
| S. aureus | 14.4 |
| C. botulinum | 8.0 |
| C. perfringens | 6.8 |
| Shigella | 3.6 |
| B. cereus | 1.9 |
| Campylobacter | 1.8 |
| Other | 2.6 |
| *Chemical* | |
| Ciguatera | 7.5 |
| Scombroid | 6.6 |
| Mushrooms | 2.3 |
| Heavy metals | 1.9 |
| Other | 5.5 |
| *Parasitic* | 5.4 |
| *Viral* | 4.1 |

*Adapted from Hughes JM, and Tauxe RV: Food-borne disease. *In* Mandell GL, Douglas RG, Jr, and Bennett JE (eds.): Principles and Practice of Infectious Diseases. Churchill Livingstone, New York, 1990, p. 893.

vivo. Etiologic agents include *Clostridium perfringens* and *B. cereus*. Most other etiologic agents of food-borne illness are associated with disease incubation periods of longer than 14 hours. These agents include *Salmonella, Clostridium botulinum, Shigella, Campylobacter,* and parasites and viruses.

*Salmonella, Shigella,* and *Campylobacter* typically produce abdominal cramps and diarrhea. Fever is common, but vomiting occurs in only a minority of individuals. Most food-borne illness outbreaks caused by these organisms occur during the summer months. Implicated foods often include poultry and dairy products. *S. aureus* and "short-incubation" *B. cereus* infection produce vomiting predominantly, although diarrhea may also occur. Fever is distinctly uncommon. Another form of *B. cereus* infection, occurring after an incubation period of 8 to 14 hours, is characterized by abdominal cramps and diarrhea without vomiting. Food-borne illness caused by *S. aureus* occurs most commonly during the summer months; *B. cereus* infection occurs year-round. *S. aureus* is frequently acquired from contaminated ham, poultry, or eggs; *B. cereus* is transmitted from rice, meats, or vegetables. *C. perfringens* produces abdominal cramps and diarrhea, usually without either fever or vomiting. Implicated foods often include beef, poultry, and gravies. *C. botulinum* is associated with vomiting, diarrhea, and descending weakness or paralysis. Constipation may occur late in the course of illness. Outbreaks of botulism are often associated with ingestion of home-canned vegetables, fruits, and fish.

Ciguatera is characterized by diarrhea, vomiting, paresthesias, hypotension, and muscle weakness. Disease generally follows consumption of reef fishes (e.g., barracuda, grouper, snapper, and jacks). Scombroid poisoning is characterized by symptoms resembling those of a histamine reaction, including flushing of the skin, itching, diarrhea and vomiting, headache, and heart palpitations. Most cases follow consumption of dark-fleshed, saltwater fish (e.g., tuna, mackerel, bonito, skipjack, and mahi-mahi). Outbreaks of ciguatera and scombroid have predominantly affected coastal areas.

Mushroom poisoning produces diverse clinical manifestations, including psychotic reactions, signs of parasympathetic hyperactivity, disulfiram-like reactions, and vomiting and diarrhea. Heavy metal poisoning produces vomiting and abdominal cramps. Outbreaks are often associated with ingestion of acidic or carbonated beverages that have been in prolonged contact with corroded metallic surfaces.

## LABORATORY DIAGNOSIS

*Salmonella, Shigella,* and *Campylobacter* infections can be diagnosed by appropriate cultures of stool. Botulism is confirmed by isolation of *C. botulinum* from stool or by demonstration of botulinal toxin in serum or stool. Confirmation of food-borne illness caused by other bacterial organisms can be difficult and may require specialized cultures, typing of organisms, or assays for toxin production. Diagnostic confirmation of chemical agents of food-borne illness generally requires specialized studies of clinical specimens or foods. In part, because of the limitations of available diagnostic studies, about half of reported outbreaks of food-borne illness defy etiologic diagnosis.

## TREATMENT

Most food-borne illness is self-limited, and affected individuals require only supportive or symptomatic treatment. Dehydration is common when vomiting and diarrhea occur concomitantly, especially in infants or elderly individuals. Mild or moderate degrees of dehydration (5% or less) can often be corrected with a commercial oral rehydration solution (e.g., Pedialyte). Current recommendations are that such solutions contain approximately 90 mEq of sodium and 20 mEq of potassium per liter and 2% glucose. Severe vomiting, refusal to drink, or severe dehydration (10%) mandate intravenous rehydration. Patients with hypotension or signs of poor perfusion should receive an initial fluid bolus of normal saline intravenously, 10 to 20 ml per kg of body weight. Intravenous fluid therapy can then be initiated with 5% dextrose in one-half normal saline with 20 to 30 mEq of KCl per liter or a similar fluid. This solution can be amended, depending on initial serum electrolyte determinations. If the serum bicarbonate concentration is less than 10 to 12 mEq per liter, NaHCO$_3$ in a concentration of 20 to 30 mEq per liter should be added to the solution. The rate of intravenous fluid administration ordinarily should be calculated to provide for maintenance fluid requirements, replacement of ongoing fluid losses, and correction of the fluid deficit during 18 to 24 hours. Hypernatremia (serum sodium concentration >150 mEq per liter) mandates replacement of the fluid deficit over a more prolonged period, usually 48 hours or longer. Ideally, the serum sodium concentration should not fall at a rate faster than 0.5 mEq per liter per hour. More rapid falls in serum sodium concentration may result in cerebral edema and seizures.

Promethazine HCl (Phenergan) can be given orally or rectally (25 mg by either route) for symptomatic therapy of persistent vomiting. Symptomatic therapy for diarrhea usually is not warranted and is best avoided if there are signs of bowel inflammation (fever, blood in the stool, or fecal leukocytes). Loperamide (Imodium), given orally in an initial dose of 4 mg, followed by 2 mg after each loose stool, can be effective in symptomatic treatment of severe noninflammatory diarrhea. The total daily dose should not exceed 16 mg. All agents used for symptomatic therapy of vomiting or diarrhea are best avoided in children.

Antibiotic therapy is sometimes useful for persons with food-borne illness caused by *Salmonella typhi*, *Shigella*, or *Campylobacter*. Antibiotics should be avoided in patients with uncomplicated gastrointestinal infections caused by nontyphoid salmonellae.

Patients with food-borne botulism, ciguatera, mushroom poisoning, or heavy metal poisoning may benefit from induced emesis (syrup of ipecac: younger than 1 year, 5 to 10 ml; 1 to 12 years, 15 ml; adult, 15 to 30 ml) or gastric lavage and administration of a cathartic agent (MgSO$_4$, 30 to 45 grams* orally). Antitoxin should be administered as soon as possible to persons with symptoms of food-borne botulism. Antitoxin generally is available through local or state health departments. Patients with ciguatera may benefit from analgesics and antihistamines. Atropine, 0.4 mg, given intramuscularly, is useful in treating symptomatic bradycardia and hypotension. Patients with mushroom poisoning and parasympathetic hyperactivity may also benefit from atropine administration. Scombroid poisoning is best managed with oral or intravenous antihistamine therapy.

---

*Exceeds dosage recommended by the manufacturer.

# ANAEROBIC AND NECROTIZING INFECTIONS, INCLUDING GAS GANGRENE

method of
WESLEY FURSTE, M.D.,
NERI M. KANDAWALLA, M.D., and
JAMES N. PARSONS, M.D.
*Ohio State University*
*Columbus, Ohio*

## PROPHYLAXIS

Prophylaxis of anaerobic and necrotizing infections (Tables 1 and 2) requires optimal, meticulous surgical technique and the indicated use of antibiotics. Table 1 consists of diagnoses that have been reported in the literature or that have been used in clinical practice. Closely related diagnoses are grouped together. Table 1 is more for retrospective than prospective use, inasmuch as the most important considerations in these infections are (1) determination, by surgical exploration, of the extent of necrotic tissue, (2) removal of this tissue, (3) production of an aerobic environment, and (4) supportive and adjunctive therapy.

**Surgical Wound Care.** The most effective prevention of the precipitating anaerobic conditions continues to be early and adequate wound care. Such surgical care includes wide incision, thorough débridement of all devitalized and potentially devitalized tissues, removal of contaminating dirt and all foreign bodies, and effective drainage. Adequate débridement is especially important in irregular deep wounds in which there are loculations and recesses that favor growth of anaerobic bacteria. Dead and devitalized tissues and foreign bodies must be removed at the time of the initial operation. In war wounds and in wounds for which treatment has been inordinately delayed, thorough débridement should be coupled with delayed surgical closure of the wound. The wound should be left open from 4 to 7 days after the débridement, and then delayed surgical closure should be accomplished if the wound has remained clean and shows no evidence of infection.

These surgical principles should be observed when elective surgery is performed for lesions of any of the body cavities or of the extremities.

**Antibiotics.** Antibiotic therapy is of prophylactic value when combined with proper surgical procedures. Experimental and clinical experience affirms this principle but indicates that antibiotic therapy alone cannot be relied on to prevent the occurrence of clostridial myositis. Penicillin G,

TABLE 1. **Diagnoses of Anaerobic and Necrotizing Infections, Including Gas Gangrene**

A. Deep infections with muscle involvement and with or without abscess
  1. Gas gangrene
    a. Gas gangrene resulting from soft tissue trauma; clostridial myositis; clostridial myonecrosis
    b. Abdominal wall gas gangrene; postoperative clostridial sepsis of the abdominal wall; clostridial myonecrosis of the abdominal wall
    c. Metastatic gas gangrene; gas gangrene without a visible wound; nontraumatic gas gangrene
    d. Uterine clostridial infections
    e. Gas gangrene of the heart
    f. Gas gangrene of the brain
  2. Streptococcal myositis; anaerobic streptococcal myonecrosis; anaerobic streptococcal myositis
  3. Infected vascular gas gangrene; nonclostridial gas gangrene; nonclostridial myositis
  4. Synergistic necrotizing sepsis; synergistic necrotizing cellulitis*
B. Superficial infections with or without abscess
  1. Hemolytic streptococcal gangrene
  2. Acute, infectious, staphylococcal gangrene
  3. Anaerobic cellulitis; crepitant phlegmon; clostridial cellulitis
  4. Necrotizing fasciitis*; synergistic gangrene; nonclostridial anaerobic cellulitis; anaerobic cutaneous gangrene; Fournier's gangrene†
  5. Panophthalmitis
C. Sample clostridial contamination of wounds
D. Infiltration of injection or aspiration of gas into wounds
  1. Wounds with gas not produced by bacteria
  2. Injection of gas into wounds
    a. Therapy ($H_2O_2$)
    b. Pranksters' jokes
    c. Malingerers
    d. Psychiatric problems
  3. Aspiration and dissemination of air into wounds by muscular activity
E. Gas in tissues after industrial accidents
  1. Magnesiogenous pneumagranuloma
F. Gas in tissues after injections of chemicals
  1. Injection of drugs
  2. Accidental injection of a foreign agent
    a. Benzene

*These are similar infections but are in different locations.
†If there is extension to the tissues of the abdominal wall below the deep fascia, such as the anterior sheath of the rectus muscle, Fournier's gangrene is a synergistic necrotizing sepsis rather than just a necrotizing fasciitis.

clindamycin, metronidazole, chloramphenicol, and the cephalosporins are effective against most strains of *Clostridium perfringens* (Table 3).

Penicillin G administered intravenously in doses of 1 to 2 million units every 4 hours is the antibiotic of choice, to be used in conjunction with adequate surgical intervention for the prevention of gas gangrene. Massive doses of penicillin can prolong the period during which surgical intervention short of amputation can be effective.

**Antitoxins.** Gas gangrene antitoxins have no place in the prophylaxis of gas gangrene.

There may be multiple species of clostridia involved, each requiring a specific antitoxin for

TABLE 2. **Microorganisms Reported to Produce Gas in Human Tissues**

| Gram's Stain Result | Aerobes | Anaerobes |
| --- | --- | --- |
| Gram-positive | | Cocci<br>  *Peptostreptococcus* (anaerobic *Streptococcus*) (usually with group A *Streptococcus* [*Streptococcus pyogenes,* beta-hemolytic *Streptococcus*] or *Staphylococcus aureus*)<br>Bacilli<br>  *Clostridium perfringens* and other clostridia |
| Gram-negative | Bacilli<br>  *Escherichia coli*<br>  *Klebsiella pneumoniae*<br>  *Enterobacter* species<br>  *Proteus* species<br>    (all usually in mixed infections) | Bacilli<br>  *Bacteroides fragilis* (usually with other anaerobic gram-negative bacilli) |

TABLE 3. **Antibiotic Treatment of Anaerobic and Necrotizing Infections Based on Gram's Stain Results, Cultures, and Sensitivity Tests**

| Gram's Stain Result | Presumptive Microorganism | Antibiotics |
|---|---|---|
| Gram-positive cocci | Anaerobic *Streptococcus* | Penicillin G<br>Clindamycin<br>Metronidazole<br>Chloramphenicol<br>Cephalosporins |
| Gram-positive bacilli | *Clostridium* species | Penicillin G<br>Clindamycin<br>Metronidazole<br>Chloramphenicol<br>Cephalosporins |
| Gram-negative bacilli | *Bacteroides* species | Clindamycin<br>Metronidazole<br>Cefoxitin<br>Chloramphenicol<br>Ticarcillin<br>Mezlocillin |
| | Coliforms | Gentamicin<br>Tobramycin<br>Amikacin<br>Cephalosporins<br>Ampicillin<br>Ticarcillin<br>Mezlocillin<br>Chloramphenicol |

neutralization of its exotoxin. Moreover, the antitoxin cannot be distributed to neutralize the exotoxin being produced in the nonviable, avascular tissue involved. In addition, there are often significant reactions to the large amounts of antitoxin that have been recommended. Large series of cases have not unequivocally proved the desirability of prophylactic gas gangrene antitoxin.

Even more important than such considerations, however, are studies of the hemolytic action of *C. perfringens* alpha-toxin. It has been shown that the amount of hemolysis has a high correlation with the phospholipase C activity of the toxin. In addition, the influence of such factors as enzyme concentratiion and concentration of red blood cells has been studied. The problem with the previous data was that the analyses were performed on only a qualitative basis. Ikezawa, however, used enzyme kinetics to study the mechanism of hemolysis by *C. perfringens* alpha-toxin. His work was of special interest with regard to the role of antitoxin.

As a summary of Ikezawa's work, it may be stated that (1) when antitoxin is added before the enzyme metal substrate (EMS)* complex is formed, the result is complete inhibition of lysis, (2) only partial inhibition is observed when antitoxin is added after the EMS complex is formed,

and (3) the calcium ion is essential for the hemolytic reaction.

**Hyperbaric Oxygen Therapy.** Hyperbaric oxygen therapy remains experimental and unproved as a prophylactic therapeutic measure in gas gangrene. Experimental evidence indicates that it has little value without adequate surgical débridement.

### THERAPY

For proper treatment, there must be an accurate diagnosis with respect to which tissues are involved and the types of bacteria and their drug sensitivities. Deep and spreading infections may require mutilating operations; superficial and localized infections may require only multiple incisions; and pure gas infiltrations and contaminations may require only diagnostic incisions. The extent and depth of a gas-forming infection are easily and—relatively safely—determined by longitudinal incisions of the skin, superficial fascia, and deep fascia.

An immediate Gram's stain provides a rapid determination of the type of bacteria, and subsequent culture and sensitivity tests can yield a more definitive bacterial identification for decisions about subsequent antibiotic therapy.

The major goals of treatment in a soft tissue infection include (1) complete removal of necrotic tissue, (2) limitation of the spread of infection, (3) control of bacteremia, (4) correction of deficits

---

*Enzyme (phospholipase C) metal (calcium ion) substrate (red blood cells).

of fluid and electrolytes, and (5) prevention of organ failure (e.g., renal and cardiac).

**Radical Surgical Wound Care.** Treatment should be initiated as soon as a clinical diagnosis is established. Optimally, treatment consists of multiple incisions for decompression and drainage of the fascial compartments, excision of the involved muscles, or open amputation when necessary, followed by immobilization of the affected part. *Early and meticulous operation is the primary and most effective means of treating clostridial myositis.* If the diagnosis is made early, while the gangrene is relatively localized, radical decompression of the involved fascial compartments by extensive longitudinal incisions and excision of infected muscle usually arrests the progress of infection and eliminates the need for amputation. If the diagnosis is delayed and made when the process is extensive and has caused irreversible gangrenous changes, open amputation of the guillotine type becomes necessary.

Gas gangrene of the abdominal wall or perineum presents special problems, but the same surgical principles apply. *Multiple incisions, fasciotomy,* and *extirpation of* as much *involved tissue* as is technically feasible should be undertaken.

Marlex, Mersilene, and Prolene mesh may be used for temporary and permanent containment of abdominal viscera after extensive clostridial myonecrosis of the abdominal wall. Débridement is carried out through parallel incisions with maximum preservation of skin and subcutaneous tissues. Mesh is used temporarily until the infection is completely controlled. The mesh is then removed, and the skin and subcutaneous tissues are reapproximated. Such a procedure gives excellent wound coverage and markedly shortens the hospital stay.

On occasion, a postabortal infection may be caused by *C. perfringens.* Women infected with this organism may be critically ill with bacteremia, shock, and renal failure. Parenteral antibiotic therapy and heroic measures, such as peritoneal dialysis or hemodialysis, may be necessary. Hysterectomy is also often indicated.

In contrast to deep and anaerobic infections, treatment of superficial infections may require only débridement of the wound. Devitalized tissues must be excised. When the infection extends along fascial planes beyond the traumatized area of the wound, long incisions must be made to open these areas and to excise the necrotic fascia. After débridement, the wounds should be copiously irrigated with antibiotic isotonic solutions, such as 0.1 per cent cefazolin in normal saline solution, before a dressing is loosely applied. Such wounds are obviously not closed primarily.

**Antibiotics.** These drugs add much to the successful care of patients with gas-forming infections. The selection of optimal antibiotic therapy depends on identification of the pathogens involved.

Major considerations in anaerobic bacteriology include proper specimen collection, immediate transport to the laboratory, and prompt inoculation and placement of the specimen under aerobic and anaerobic conditions. Special collection and transport methods to ensure the survival of even the most fastidious anaerobic organisms should be instituted, such as the following:

1. The syringe technique can be effective in the case of abscess. The skin is decontaminated, and pus is removed with a needle and syringe. All air is eliminated, the needle is inserted into a cork or rubber stopper, and the specimen is carried promptly to the laboratory, where it must be processed immediately.

2. Specimens can be collected in rubber-stoppered tubes that have been gassed with $CO_2$ or $N_2$.

3. Transport systems containing reducing agents that help to maintain a low oxidation-reduction potential are commercially available.

It is important to remember in the interpretation of the smear and the culture that the presence of gram-positive rods or other organisms in either smear or culture does *not necessarily* indicate that *infection* is present. Colonization of uninfected wounds by microorganisms is not uncommon. The clinical picture should be considered before the institution of unwarranted antimicrobial therapy. Although an infection occasionally develops in these contaminated lesions, in most cases thorough cleaning and débridement will suffice.

Antimicrobial drugs are useful in the management of patients with soft tissue infections. These drugs limit the spread of infection within the tissues and are critical in the treatment of bacteremia. Note, however, that antibiotics used without adequate surgical measures often cannot control these infections, and their use must be coupled with the other modalities outlined.

Major considerations in the selection of antimicrobial agents include a knowledge of the bacterial pathogens involved and their antibiotic susceptibilities, the patient's sensitivity to antibiotics (e.g., penicillin allergy), and factors such as hepatic or renal insufficiency, which may affect drug metabolism and excretion.

The initial choice of an antibiotic should be based on the findings of the gram-stained smear of wound exudate, with therapy later modified as indicated by the results of the culture and sensitivity tests. Because these infections are often mixed and contain both aerobic and anaerobic organisms, more than one antibiotic is frequently necessary. Antibiotics are given intravenously and in high doses.

Table 3 gives the antibiotics commonly used in the management of necrotizing soft tissue infections but does not include all available antibiotics. By using Gram's stain as a guide, patients with a large number of gram-positive bacilli or gram-positive cocci in chains can be treated with penicillin G, 3 to 4 million units intravenously every 4 hours. *C. perfringens* is often isolated from these lesions. Patients who are allergic to penicillin may be given intravenous therapy with clindamycin, 600 mg every 6 hours, chloramphenicol, 12.5 mg per kg every 6 hours, or metronidazole, 500 mg every 6 hours.

For patients from whom a gram-stained smear of exudate shows pleomorphic gram-negative bacilli or pale gram-negative rods with tapered ends, clindamycin, chloramphenicol, or metronidazole may be selected. *Bacteroides* species and fusobacteria are often cultured in these cases.

When multiple morphologic forms are seen by Gram's stain—as in many cases—a combination of penicillin and chloramphenicol or a combination of clindamycin and an aminoglycoside is often effective.

Aminoglycosides that are used include gentamicin, tobramycin, and amikacin. The intravenous dose of gentamicin and tobramycin is 1.5 to 1.7 mg per kg every 8 hours, and that for amikacin is 7.5 mg per kg every 12 hours. Aminoglycoside serum levels should be monitored to ensure adequate therapy and reduce toxicity, particularly in patients with impaired or changing renal function.

If gentamicin-resistant strains of *Pseudomonas* are present, tobramycin, 1.5 to 1.7 mg per kg every 8 hours intravenously, or amikacin, 7.5 mg per kg every 12 hours intravenously, may be used.

These recommendations are guidelines. Other agents with broad activity against aerobic and anaerobic bacteria are also available. These agents include broad-spectrum penicillins and first-, second-, and third-generation cephalosporins. Because of some gaps in coverage, these drugs should be reserved for use against isolates with known antibiotic susceptibility. In addition, the aminoglycosides and metronidazole have no activity against anaerobic or aerobic bacteria, respectively, and must be used together with another agent in mixed aerobic-anaerobic infections.

Because the degree of activity of antibiotics is not always predictable, it is important to collect specimens for culture before starting antibiotic therapy. Such information may be used later to choose the most appropriate antibiotic. The selection and dose of an antibiotic depend on the clinical setting, the isolated pathogen or pathogens, and specific host features that may modify response and toxicity. Final therapy will be determined largely by these factors and especially by the culture and sensitivity results.

**Antitoxin.** Antitoxin therapy is not recommended, for the reasons already given in the section on prophylaxis.

**Hyperbaric Oxygen.** The administration of hyperbaric oxygen is controversial. Good results have been reported in certain medical centers. The following factors, however, must be considered: (1) oxygen penetrates poorly into necrotic tissue; (2) there are certain associated hazards, such as oxygen toxicity with disorientation and convulsions; (3) seriously ill patients are difficult to manage in a hyperbaric oxygen chamber; and (4) the apparatus is frequently not available. When this treatment is used, 100 per cent oxygen at 3 atmospheres pressure for 1 to 2 hours at 8-hour intervals is recommended. One salient advantage of hyperbaric oxygen is that the involved tissues quickly become demarcated, so that the extent of resection is readily apparent. Hyperbaric oxygen treatment may be worthwhile for a patient with gas gangrene before radical excisional surgery, *provided the apparatus is reasonably convenient and provided there is no delay in the indicated and necessary surgical intervention.*

**Tetanus Prophylaxis.** For all wounds, the best possible tetanus prophylaxis—including, when indicated, the administration of adsorbed tetanus toxoid and/or tetanus immune globulin—is to be effected. *Although gas gangrene is a complication primarily of severe wounds, tetanus may occur after wounds of any size and even in individuals in whom no wound can be demonstrated.*

**Special Considerations for HIV Infections.** Since the immune processes of the body are greatly altered by human immunodeficiency virus (HIV) infection, these individuals may not respond to tetanus toxoid with an adequate anamnestic response. They should receive, in addition to tetanus toxoid, tetanus immune globulin.

**Adequate Supportive Therapy.** The general supportive measures of value in the management of gas gangrene include maintenance of satisfactory hematocrit levels, monitoring of the fluid and electrolyte balance, adequate immobilization of the infected and injured parts, respiratory and ventilatory therapy, and relief of pain. Blood or blood product transfusions may be necessary to correct the profound anemia with which this condition is frequently associated; such transfusions are one of the mainstays of postoperative management. Plasma is usually reserved for the correction of coagulation factor deficiencies seen with disseminated intravascular coagulation. Platelet transfusions may also be necessary.

**Exchange Transfusions.** Exchange transfusion is another technique advocated for cases with hemolysis caused by the toxemia. This approach has been used in uterine and abdominal wall gas gangrene. It is a measure of desperation that has not been proved to be effective in controlled trials.

**Control of Renal Failure.** Hemodialysis or peritoneal dialysis may be needed to control renal insufficiency related to septic shock or rhabdomyolysis, the latter being characterized by elevation of serum creatine kinase levels.

**Secondary Operative Procedures.** Secondary operative procedures to facilitate healing of the wound and normal function of the extremity should be performed as indicated. These procedures should obviously be postponed until after the infection has been brought completely under control.

# EPIDEMIC INFLUENZA

method of
STEVEN R. MOSTOW, M.D.
*Rose Medical Center*
*Denver, Colorado*

Outbreaks of influenza are an annual phenomenon, and epidemics of influenza causing excess mortality have occurred in nearly each of the past 20 years. There are three immunologic types of influenza virus (A, B, and C), but large epidemics of disease associated with death are caused primarily by type A. The most recent outbreaks have been caused by A/Shanghai ($H_3$ $N_2$), A/Taiwan ($H_1$ $N_1$), and B/Yamagata. Why these viruses are constantly changing, how much change is necessary (antigenic drift) to cause outbreaks, what forces are operative when major changes (antigenic shift) in the hemagglutinin and neuraminidase occur and lead to pandemics, and what happens to the virus between outbreaks are all questions that remain unanswered.

## DIAGNOSIS

The diagnosis of influenza is a clinical one. Although influenza virus is characterized as a respiratory virus, the illness usually includes severe systemic symptoms. A nonproductive cough is frequent, and half the patients have a mild to moderate sore throat, fever, substernal chest pain, profound myalgias, headache, and insomnia; these chief complaints force the patient to seek medical advice. The virus can be cultivated in tissue cultures in some but not all diagnostic virus laboratories. It takes about 5 days to identify the virus. New rapid diagnostic tests, though not available currently, should be available for office use by 1992. Serologic tests are available, but results take too long to be clinically useful. Thus, the basic therapy is based on a clinical diagnosis and is specifically directed against the virus and also against the symptoms.

## TREATMENT

### Uncomplicated Cases

1. Amantadine HCl (Symmetrel) or rimantadine HCl should be considered for most patients with severe systemic symptoms due to influenza.
   a. The usual dosage of amantadine hydrochloride is 100 mg (one capsule or two teaspoons of the liquid) twice a day. In persons over 65 years of age, the daily dosage is 100 mg. For patients with significant renal impairment, dosage adjustments are well outlined in the *Physician's Desk Reference* (*PDR*). Rimantadine doses are exactly half that of amantadine (rimantadine should receive FDA approval in 1990).
2. Analgesics are administered for fever, sore throat, myalgia, and headache. For adults, the dose of aspirin (acetylsalicylic acid) is 0.6 grams (10 grains) every 4 hours, but 0.9 gram (15 grains) may be necessary to control severe myalgia or very high temperature (>40° C; 104° F). The patient should be warned that the aspirin may cause drenching sweats. In the adult, if aspirin is contraindicated, 650 mg of acetaminophen (Tylenol) may be given every 4 hours. For children (up to 12 years old), aspirin is contraindicated because of the association of influenza, aspirin, and Reye's syndrome. Thus for children (6 to 12 years old), the use of acetaminophen is recommended in a dosage of 325 mg every 4 to 6 hours.
3. Cough suppressants such as codeine phosphate or various elixirs containing codeine are useful, if necessary, to permit the patient some uninterrupted sleep. If insomnia is a troublesome problem, promethazine hydrochloride (Phenergan) with codeine may be a helpful combination, since one of the beneficial side effects of this mild antihistamine is drowsiness.
4. Humidification of room air may help to relieve the dry, hacking cough associated with the disease. A cold water vaporizer is preferred, as steam vaporizers introduce the risk of scalding burns and should not be used for young children or demented adults.
5. Bed rest should be encouraged, especially while the patient is febrile. When possible, early ambulation is recommended.
6. Diet should be very light. Soups and liquids should be emphasized to maintain adequate

hydration until the patient can tolerate more substantial meals.

7. Reassurance should be given that although the patient may not feel up to par for 2 or 3 weeks, he or she will eventually get better. A gradual rather than an abrupt return to full pre-illness physical activity is recommended.

8. Smoking, both active and passive, should be forbidden for the duration of the illness. An explanation that smoking further paralyzes the already damaged (by virus) ciliated lining of the airways is usually sufficient.

9. Antibiotics should not be used prophylactically, especially because their use may selectively encourage superinfection by drug-resistant bacteria. There are no data to support the claim that prophylactic antibiotics prevent the more serious complications of influenza such as bronchitis and pneumonia.

### Complicated Cases

Most complications occur in the elderly, especially in those with significant chronic illness such as heart and pulmonary disease. Any patient with influenza, a fever, and an underlying disease needs to be examined periodically for the onset of lower respiratory tract complications.

#### Lower Respiratory Tract Complications

**Bronchitis.** A negative chest film in the presence of rales and purulent sputum, with or without fever, usually signifies the onset of bronchitis, which generally requires treatment. Prior to therapy, sputum smear and culture should be carried out, especially since staphylococcal infection must be recognized as early as possible. Ordinary bronchitis in adults is best treated with an oral dose of 200 mg per day of doxycycline (Vibramycin) or a double-strength trimethoprim-sulfamethoxazole (Septra, Bactrim) tablet twice a day for 5 to 7 days. If the smear or culture reveals only pneumococci, penicillin alone is adequate. In children, ampicillin is often recommended in a dosage of 50 to 100 mg per kg per day. Tetracyclines should be avoided in young children because of discoloration of developing teeth.

**Bronchiolitis.** Hyperinflated lungs, wheezing, and hypoxia in the absence of pneumonia signify the onset of bronchiolitis, which can be of primarily influenzal cause. This disease can be devastating, usually because of gas exchange problems. Therefore, determination of arterial blood gas levels and judicious use of oxygen based on arterial gas results are important. Treatment with amantadine (4.4 to 8.8 mg per kg per day)

should be considered in these cases due to influenza A.

The role of antibiotics is less clear. If the sputum is not purulent, antibiotics need not be given, as this primarily is a viral disease. If the sputum is purulent, however, antibiotics should be given as outlined above.

**Pneumonia.** The incidence of staphylococcal pneumonia is significantly higher following influenza epidemics, and the patient with staphylococcal pneumonia is at the risk of death. Therefore, it is recommended that all patients with suspected or confirmed pneumonia during an influenza epidemic be hospitalized. Patients with active influenza virus infection should probably be separated from other uninfected patients with other diseases, although patients with influenza can be boarded together. Because it is so vitally important to rule out staphylococcal pneumonia, the following procedures should be carried out immediately after the admission of a patient with clinical evidence of pneumonia:

1. Baseline chest x-ray. Cavitary disease suggests staphylococcal infection.
2. Sputum smear to rule out staphylococcal infection (large, round, gram-positive cocci in clusters).
3. Pretreatment sputum and two blood cultures.
4. Antibiotic treatment based on results of Gram's stain:
   a. If the sputum smear reveals many polymorphonuclear leukocytes (PMNs) and staphylococci, therapy should be started immediately with a penicillinase-resistant antibiotic (cefazolin [Ancef, Kefzol], 3 grams per day; oxacillin [Bactocill, Prostaphlin] or nafcillin [Nafcil, Unipen], 6 to 9 grams per day; or vancomycin [Vancocin], 2 grams per day). These antibiotics should be emergently administered intravenously because of this life-threatening situation.
   b. If PMNs and pneumococci (gram-positive diplococci) predominate, low doses of intravenous penicillin (6 million units per day) should be given on a 4-hour basis.
   c. If there are many PMNs and *Haemophilus influenzae* (gram-negative pleomorphic rods) or a mixed flora predominates, cefuroxime (Kefurox, Zinacef) (4.5 grams per day) or other β-lactamase–resistant antibiotics should be given intravenously.
   As the patient improves, especially after he or she becomes afebrile, other routes of administration, including oral, should be considered.
5. Arterial blood gas measurements should be determined if the patient is in severe respiratory distress or if the patient has a history of severe chronic obstructive lung disease.

### Upper Respiratory Tract Complications

There is usually an increased incidence of otitis media and sinusitis following influenza. Therapy involves drainage (medically with decongestants or surgically if indicated) and antibiotics. In children under 4 years of age, antibiotics resistant to β-lactamase are indicated because of the high incidence of *Haemophilus influenzae* as the causative agent. Be sure to confirm whether or not *H. influenzae* produces β-lactamase.

### Cardiovascular Complications

Myocarditis is a rare complication of influenza and usually presents with the sudden onset of congestive heart failure or an arrhythmia or both. Judicious use of digitalis, diuretics, rest, and salt restriction forms the keystone of therapy, but these patients should also be treated with amantadine as outlined above.

**Congestive Heart Failure.** Any patient with preexisting heart disease is prone to develop congestive heart failure secondary to the increased metabolic demands associated with fever. Therefore, control of temperature as outlined above is important in patients with severe heart disease.

### Neurologic Complications

Reye's syndrome (children) and encephalitis (adults) are uncommon complications of influenza. Consultation with a neurologist or neurosurgeon should allow a rational plan of monitoring and supportive measures to be formulated. Steroids should be avoided on theoretical grounds in any acute viral infection of the brain, but there is no evidence to contraindicate using such preparations in a patient who is rapidly deteriorating because of progressing cerebral edema.

## PREVENTION OF DISEASE

### Vaccine Approach

Although influenza vaccines have been in existence for 40 years, effectiveness varies considerably. Well-controlled studies revealed that the vaccine is about 70% effective in completely preventing any disease due to influenza virus. However, in those not completely protected, vaccine is also very effective in modifying disease. For instance, 80 to 90% of recipients who develop mild disease do not develop fever or require a stay in bed. All vaccines are prepared in a purified form that obviates side effects. However, a vaccine is not effective unless it is made from current influenza viruses. Thus physicians should confirm that the vaccine is up to date, with regard to both the shelf life and the antigenic composition.

Vaccine is available in two forms. The whole-virus vaccine is more immunogenic but causes more adverse reactions. The split-virus vaccine is less immunogenic but causes fewer adverse reactions. Only split-virus vaccine should be used for children, even though a second dose may be necessary to provide immunity. Neither the whole nor the split vaccine should be administered to persons with a history of severe reaction to influenza vaccine in the past.

Influenza vaccine is recommended yearly in the fall for all of those at risk of death from influenza—these include persons of any age with chronic or debilitating illness and all those over 65 years of age. Vaccine is also recommended for persons whose community functions are essential. Health care personnel should also receive vaccine in order to decrease the chances of spreading the virus to patients and to keep health care facilities operational during an epidemic.

### Chemoprophylaxis and Chemotherapy

Amantadine prophylaxis (100 mg once daily), will reduce the incidence of epidemic influenza by about 70%. It has been shown to be more effective in the presence of serum antibody if the antibody is relevant for the influenza strain causing disease. The drug is active at several points in the virus reproductive cycle, but its most important action is to prevent viral uncoating, thus blocking the exposure of the viral genome to the nucleus of the infected cell. Neither amantadine nor rimantadine is effective against influenza B infections or outbreaks.

Amantadine treatment has also been shown effective in reducing the total duration of fever in cases of influenza A. In other words, its net therapeutic effect is much like that of aspirin, but its routine use to reduce fever alone is not encouraged. Amantadine has been shown to decrease the peripheral airway resistance caused by influenza A virus. In patients with severe hypoxia secondary to influenza A infection, amantadine should always be considered. Amantadine will also reduce the potential spread of the virus when taken therapeutically (100 mg twice a day).

The side effects (drowsiness, inability to concentrate, feeling of detachment, depression, and dizziness) are not often seen at normal doses but occur more frequently in elderly persons. Amantadine should be used with extreme caution in patients with compromised renal function, since it is not easily dialyzed.

The prophylactic administration of amantadine should be reserved for those chronically ill patients, both vaccinated and unvaccinated, who are at risk of death from influenza. It is especially important for those who are more likely to be exposed, such as senile patients with cardiac or respiratory disease living in homes where there are school children or adults with widespread outside contacts. It should be remembered that to be maximally effective the drug should be given prior to and for the duration of the exposure to the influenza A virus.

# LEISHMANIASIS

method of
CHARLES N. OSTER, M.D.
*Walter Reed Army Medical Center*
*Washington, D.C.*

Leishmaniasis is a group of diseases caused by infection with one of the protozoan parasites of the genus *Leishmania*. Human diseases that result from these infections can be grouped into three syndromes: (1) cutaneous leishmaniasis, caused by *L. major, L. tropica,* and *L. aethiopica* in the Old World and *L. mexicana* and *L. braziliensis* in the New World, characterized by papular, nodular, or ulcerative skin lesions; (2) mucocutaneous leishmaniasis (espundia), caused by *L. braziliensis,* characterized by skin lesions that are followed in months or years by ulcerative, destructive lesions of the oral, nasal, and pharyngeal mucosa; and (3) visceral leishmaniasis (kala-azar), caused by *L. donovani,* characterized by widespread infection of the reticuloendothelial system with fever, hepatosplenomegaly, anemia, and leukopenia. Although these diseases are not commonly seen in the United States, physicians must be alert to the possibility of leishmaniasis in people who have lived or traveled in areas of the world where these diseases are endemic. When leishmaniasis is suspected, the diagnosis should be established by demonstrating amastigotes in tissue obtained by aspiration or biopsy or by culturing promastigotes in vitro after inoculating tissue.

## TREATMENT

The drug of choice for all forms of leishmaniasis is one of the pentavalent antimonial compounds. Sodium stibogluconate (Pentostam)* is used in the United States, Asia, most of Europe, and the English-speaking countries of Africa, whereas meglumine antimoniate (Glucantime)† is used in Central and South America and the French-speaking parts of Europe and Africa. In the United States, sodium stibogluconate is available from the Centers for Disease Control (telephone 404–639–3670; nights and emergency [24 hour] 404–639–2888).

---

*Investigational drug in the United States.
†Not available in the United States.

Sodium stibogluconate is provided as a solution containing 100 mg of antimony per ml. It can be given either intramuscularly or intravenously, although the latter route is preferred because the intramuscular injections are painful. When given intravenously, the dose should be diluted 1:10 in 5% dextrose in water and given over 10 to 15 minutes through a peripheral vein. If the undiluted drug is injected intravenously, thrombophlebitis commonly results. Sodium stibogluconate is rapidly excreted by the kidneys, with clearance equivalent to the clearance of creatinine, and little drug accumulates in tissue, even with prolonged courses. Therefore, this drug should be used with caution in patients with decreased creatinine clearance, although there are no guidelines for its use in these patients.

**Old World Cutaneous Leishmaniasis.** Although ulcers caused by *L. tropica* and *L. major* are usually self-healing in 6 months to a year, sodium stibogluconate accelerates healing and should be offered to all patients. Alternatively, patients with mild disease can be managed without antimony treatment. The most effective dosage of sodium stibogluconate has not been determined, but 10 mg per kg of body weight per day for 10 to 20 days is probably adequate. Response to treatment is indicated by reduction in the erythema and induration of the ulcer margin in the first few weeks after therapy and then by gradual but progressive healing of the lesion. There is no adequate test for cure, so patients should be seen periodically for 1 year after treatment. A recurrence of the lesion should be retreated with sodium stibogluconate in the same dosage used initially.

Alternative drugs for the treatment of leishmaniasis, such as amphotericin B (Fungizone) or pentamidine isethionate (Pentam), are too toxic to be used for Old World cutaneous lesions. Local heat therapy (raising the temperature at the site of the lesion to 40° to 41° C for 2 to 3 hours a day for 2 weeks) may be helpful in some patients, although *L. tropica* and *L. major* are less responsive to heat than are *Leishmania* causing New World cutaneous leishmaniasis.

Cutaneous leishmaniasis acquired in Ethiopia or Kenya may be due to *L. aethiopica*. This organism is less susceptible to pentavalent antimonials and generally does not respond to sodium stibogluconate in a dosage of 10 mg per kg per day. Higher dosages, up to 20 mg per kg twice daily for 30 days, may be needed for cure. Alternatively, local heat treatment (raising the skin temperature to 40° to 41° C 12 hours a day for several weeks) has been used successfully in a few patients.

Diffuse cutaneous leishmaniasis of the Old World is caused by *L. aethiopica* and can be treated according to the earlier recommendations for simple cutaneous disease caused by this organism, although the response is generally poor. Pentamidine,* 4 mg per kg given once weekly for several months, may control the disease; however, pentamidine can cause serious toxicity, even when used in this low dosage.

**New World Cutaneous Leishmaniasis.** Only *L. mexicana* has been found to cause cutaneous leishmaniasis in southern Texas and in Mexico. In the rest of Central and South America, cutaneous leishmaniasis may be due to *L. mexicana* or *L. braziliensis*. Because disease caused by these two species cannot be reliably differentiated clinically, and because it is possible for espundia to develop after cutaneous infections with *L. braziliensis,* every patient with American cutaneous leishmaniasis should be treated, no matter how mild the disease. Sodium stibogluconate should be given at a dosage of 20 mg per kg per day, as a single intravenous infusion, for 20 consecutive days. Patients with New World cutaneous leishmaniasis should be followed for 1 year after treatment. Relapses can be treated with repeated courses of sodium stibogluconate in the same dosage.

A controlled clinical trial that compared sodium stibogluconate, 20 mg per kg intramuscularly per day for 20 days, with oral ketoconazole (Nizoral), 600 mg per day for 28 days, and placebo demonstrated equal efficacy of the ketoconazole and the sodium stibogluconate, both of which were better than placebo. This study limited the maximal daily dose of sodium stibogluconate to 850 mg (average dosage of 13 mg per kg per day), so it is uncertain whether ketoconazole is as effective as sodium stibogluconate given at a dosage of 20 mg per kg per day. However, this study did demonstrate the efficacy of ketoconazole as an alternative therapy for American cutaneous leishmaniasis.

**Mucocutaneous Leishmaniasis.** Espundia usually responds to pentavalent antimonials, but relapse after treatment is common. The dosage of sodium stibogluconate is the same as suggested earlier for New World cutaneous leishmaniasis, but patients should probably receive at least 4 weeks of therapy. Relapses can be treated with repeated courses of sodium stibogluconate. Those patients who fail to respond to pentavalent antimonials should be treated with amphotericin B,† administered by slow intravenous infusion in gradually increasing doses, to a maximum of 1 mg per kg per day; thereafter, the drug can be administered every other day until a total of 1.5 to 2 grams

*This use of pentamidine is not listed in the manufacturer's official directive.

†The manufacturer recommends a 1-mg test dose.

has been administered. Pentamidine isethionate, 4 mg per kg given intravenously or intramuscularly three times per week for several months, may also be an effective alternative, although there has been little experience with this regimen.

Diffuse cutaneous leishmaniasis of the New World can be treated in the same way as that of the Old World (see earlier). Diffuse cutaneous leishmaniasis of the New World also responds poorly to treatment.

**Visceral Leishmaniasis.** Patients with kala-azar acquired in India respond well to sodium stibogluconate, 10 mg per kg per day for 20 days. All other patients with visceral leishmaniasis should be treated with sodium stibogluconate, 20 mg per kg per day, as a single daily intravenous infusion, for 30 days. Signs of response to treatment include return of the temperature to normal, usually within 72 hours of starting therapy; improvement of the anemia and leukopenia over several weeks; and regression of the hepatosplenomegaly slowly, over weeks to months. Patients who do not respond to the initial course of treatment or who relapse after this treatment should be treated with sodium stibogluconate, 20 mg per kg per day, for 60 days. Patients who fail to respond to this regimen can be treated with pentamidine or amphotericin B, in the same dosage as for mucocutaneous leishmaniasis (see earlier). Patients should be followed for at least 1 year after treatment to detect possible relapses.

### Toxicity of Sodium Stibogluconate

Side effects of sodium stibogluconate, when used in a dosage of 10 to 20 mg per kg per day, are usually mild and well tolerated. Patients may complain of myalgia and arthralgia, which respond to nonsteroidal anti-inflammatory agents. Less frequently, patients note anorexia, nausea, vomiting, headache, lethargy, and pruritus. Thrombophlebitis is common when the undiluted drug is given intravenously; this can be prevented by diluting the drug (1:10) in 5% dextrose in water. Liver enzyme elevations, up to five times normal, are frequently seen and are not a reason to stop the drug; these abnormal values return to normal when treatment is stopped. Electrocardiograms taken during treatment often show nonspecific ST and T wave changes or T wave inversion; again, these abnormalities are not cause to interrupt therapy, and they quickly revert to normal when therapy is completed. With high dosages of sodium stibogluconate (>30 mg per kg per day), the corrected QT interval may become prolonged. This finding may be a harbinger of sudden death due to an arrhythmia; therefore, electrocardiograms should be performed daily when high dosages of sodium stibogluconate are given. If the corrected QT interval is prolonged to greater than 0.50 second, therapy should be withheld until the QT interval returns to normal. Thereafter, sodium stibogluconate should be reintroduced at a lower dosage.

# LEPROSY
## (Hansen's Disease)

method of
ROBERT R. JACOBSON, M.D., PH.D.
*Gillis W. Long Hansen's Disease Center*
*Carville, Louisiana*

Leprosy is a chronic infectious disease caused by *Mycobacterium leprae*. Because of the mobility of modern peoples, it is seen at least occasionally in nearly every country, but is common only in a number of Third World countries in tropical or semitropical areas. The World Health Organization (WHO) estimates that there are about 11 million cases worldwide. The United States now has over 6000 cases, and the number of new cases detected annually in the United States is currently about 200. These are found mostly among aliens, particularly those from Southeast Asia, Mexico, and the Philippines. Cases among native-born Americans currently constitute about 15% of the total.

Leprosy is best viewed as a spectrum of diseases, and the problems encountered in treatment vary considerably from one end of the spectrum to the other. Although most people (>95%) are not susceptible, those who are initially develop indeterminate leprosy. This may be self-healing, but is always treated if it is diagnosed. When self-healing or treatment does not intervene, the disease eventually progresses to one of the advanced forms. Those with the most intact immune response, relatively speaking, keep the infection localized, manifesting tuberculoid leprosy, which is referred to as polar tuberculoid disease, or TT in the Ridley-Jopling classification. On the other hand, those with a poor immune response to the infection allow it to become generalized, exhibiting polar lepromatous (LL) disease. Between the two extremes is a broad borderline (dimorphous) region where the disease may be classified borderline tuberculoid (BT), midborderline (BB), or borderline lepromatous (BL).

Classification is based on findings of physical examination, skin biopsy, and skin scrapings. Bacteria in biopsy sections and skin scrapings are evaluated to determine the morphologic index (MI), and their numbers are quantified using the bacterial index (BI). The MI is the percentage that appear fully intact and presumably viable and is usually 5% or less in patients with newly diagnosed disease. The BI is a semilogarithmic scale ranging from 0, which indicates none found in 100 oil immersion fields, to 6+ (>1000 per oil immersion field). Indeterminate, TT, and most BT cases have a BI of 0 on skin scrapings at diagnosis,

and only rare bacilli are detected on biopsy specimens. The BI on biopsy specimens and skin scrapings in BB, BL, and LL cases usually ranges from 2 to 3+, 3 to 5+, and 4 to 6+, respectively. The WHO classifies those with a BI of 0 on skin scrapings at all sites at the time of diagnosis (indeterminate, TT, and most BT) as paucibacillary and those with a BI of 1+ or above at any site as multibacillary.

## TREATMENT

### AntiLeprosy Drugs

At present, five drugs are widely used to treat leprosy: dapsone, clofazimine (Lamprene), rifampin (Rifadin),* and ethionamide (Trecator-SC)† and prothionamide.‡ Dapsone and clofazimine are weakly bactericidal against *M. leprae*, rifampin has potent bactericidal activity, and ethionamide and prothionamide are intermediate in activity. Other drugs with some activity against *M. leprae*, such as certain aminoglycosides, thiacetazone,‡ and acedapsone (DADDS [Hansolar])‡ are seldom used owing to cost, delivery (intramuscular rather than oral administration), or toxicity problems, or because they have only bacteriostatic activity against *M. leprae*. Technically, only dapsone and clofazimine are approved by the U.S. Food and Drug Administration for the treatment of leprosy. However, rifampin is regularly used, both in the United States and throughout the world, for this purpose and ethionamide and prothionamide to a lesser extent, because there is no question as to the effectiveness of any of these drugs against *M. leprae*. Because *M. leprae* cannot be grown in artificial media, drug sensitivity testing is usually done utilizing the mouse footpad technique. Sensitivity to dapsone, rifampin, clofazimine, and ethionamide is routinely tested at the Gillis W. Long Hansen's Disease Center (GWLHDC).

**Dapsone.** Dapsone is available as 25- and 100-mg tablets, and the usual dosage is 100 mg daily for adults and 0.9 to 1.4 mg per kg for children. Because of its safety, low cost, and effectiveness, it is included in all treatment regimens, unless the patient is infected with fully dapsone-resistant bacilli or has had a serious adverse reaction to dapsone. Its most common side effect is anemia, but, except for occasional patients with glucose-6-phosphate dehydrogenase (G6PD) deficiency, it is rarely severe enough to require discontinuation of the drug. Gastrointestinal complaints also

---

*This use of rifampin is not listed in the manufacturer's official directive.

† This use of ethionamide is not listed in the manufacturer's official directive.

‡Not available in the United States.

rarely necessitate its discontinuance with the dosages used to treat leprosy. The most serious complications of dapsone therapy are agranulocytosis and the "dapsone syndrome" (infectious mononucleosis–like syndrome). Fortunately, both are relatively rare. Other reported side effects are uncommon and include various rashes, peripheral neuropathies, hepatitis, cholestatic jaundice, hypoalbuminemia, the nephrotic syndrome, psychoses, and fever. Methemoglobinemia occurs, but is rarely a problem in patients receiving the standard antileprosy dosage of dapsone. It may be severe, however, if an overdose is taken and may require the use of supportive measures and methylene blue.

DADDS is the diacetyl derivative of dapsone. Although not obtainable in the United States, it is used in some countries as a long-acting parenteral preparation. It yields low blood levels of dapsone, which might encourage the development of dapsone-resistant *M. leprae,* making its use under any circumstances of uncertain efficacy.

**Rifampin.** Rifampin is available as 150- and 300-mg capsules, and the usual adult dosage is 600 mg daily, although it has been given intermittently at intervals of up to 1 month in dosages ranging from 600 to 1500 mg. Strains of *M. leprae* resistant to it can appear in as few as 3 to 4 years if it is given as monotherapy. It should therefore be used only in combination drug regimens. Its major side effect has been hepatotoxicity, but this has usually not been a major problem, except in patients receiving it in combination with ethionamide, which is also hepatotoxic. In general, it is discontinued only if the alanine aminotransferase (ALT) level rises to 2½ times the upper limit of normal. Thrombocytopenia is occasionally observed in patients taking the drug, but the platelet count rarely drops below 100,000 per mm³, which would require discontinuation of rifampin therapy. The drug may also produce a reddish-orange to reddish-brown discoloration of urine, feces, saliva, sputum, sweat, and tears. Other reported side effects include an influenza-like syndrome, fatigue, drowsiness, headaches, dizziness, pruritus, various rashes, eosinophilia, and rarely kidney damage. The drug also affects the metabolism of other medications. Those treating patients with leprosy should be aware that it decreases plasma levels of corticosteroids and reduces the effectiveness of oral contraceptives. Thus, higher dosages of corticosteroids may be necessary for the management of leprous reactions and alternate methods of contraception may be required.

**Clofazimine.** Clofazimine is available as 50- and 100-mg capsules. It is extremely useful in the management of leprosy. It not only treats the disease, but in higher dosages also suppresses reactive episodes. The usual adult dosage for treatment is 50 to 100 mg daily, but dosages as high as 300 mg daily* may be used to suppress reactive episodes. Although clofazimine-resistant *M. leprae* are rarely reported with monotherapy, it should be given only in combination with other antileprosy drugs.

The most obvious side effect is pigmentation of the skin. The severity of this is proportional to the dosage being given and the extent of infiltration of the skin by the disease process. The color can range from a reddish hue to a purplish-black. It tends to be blotchy, being most pronounced in areas where skin lesions are present. The pigmentation occurs in essentially all patients with active disease, and its absence may indicate that the patient is not taking the drug. As the disease process clears from the skin, the coloration slowly diminishes and nearly disappears in patients with inactive disease. Discontinuation of the drug also leads to clearance of most of the pigmentation within 6 to 12 months, although traces of it may remain for several years.

The most serious toxic effect is on the gastrointestinal tract. Patients receiving 50 to 100 mg daily may have mild crampy or burning midabdominal to epigastric pain, which is sometimes associated with mild nausea and/or diarrhea. Patients receiving greater than 100 mg daily for control of reactions, however, may develop severe crampy abdominal pain, diarrhea, nausea, vomiting, and weight loss, which with continued treatment may progress to symptoms suggesting a partial or complete bowel obstruction. This usually clears rapidly if the drug is temporarily discontinued.

Other side effects include an anticholinergic activity, resulting in diminished sweating and tearing, and phototoxicity reactions, which are uncommon.

**Ethionamide (Trecator-SC).** Ethionamide is available only as 250-mg tablets, and the usual adult dosage is 250 to 500 mg daily. Resistance to the drug develops rapidly if it is given as monotherapy, and it should therefore be used only as part of a combination drug regimen. Its most common side effects are various gastrointestinal complaints, such as a metallic taste in the mouth, nausea, vomiting, abdominal pain, diarrhea, anorexia, and hepatotoxicity. These usually clear rapidly if the drug is discontinued. Giving ethionamide and rifampin together increases the chance of hepatotoxicity considerably, and patients taking this combination must be followed closely for evidence of such toxicity, particularly during the first year of therapy. The drug is normally dis-

---

*Exceeds dosage recommended by the manufacturer.

continued if the ALT level rises to 2½ times the upper limit of normal. Other side effects include postural hypotension, mental depression, drowsiness, peripheral neuropathies, and asthenia.

### Treatment Regimens

**Patients with Newly Diagnosed Leprosy.** Patients with newly diagnosed disease in the United States are generally infected with fully sulfone-sensitive *M. leprae* (no growth in mice treated with 0.0001% dietary dapsone). Bacilli from occasional patients show varying degrees of primary resistance to dapsone in mouse footpad testing. Clinically, however, those treated with dapsone monotherapy in the past have shown a normal initial response to standard dosages, unless their bacilli were fully dapsone resistant—i.e., there was growth in mice treated with 0.01% dietary dapsone. Such resistance is rare in new cases. Thus, dapsone probably remains useful in essentially all newly diagnosed disease. Standard therapy for paucibacillary adult patients seen at the GWLHDC is 100 mg of dapsone plus 600 mg of rifampin daily for 6 months, followed by dapsone monotherapy for 3 years in indeterminate and TT cases and for 5 years in BT patients. Multibacillary patients receive dapsone plus rifampin for 3 years, followed by dapsone monotherapy for 10 years after inactivity (no bacilli found on skin scrapings or biopsy specimens) in BB patients, and indefinitely in BL and LL cases as a prophylactic measure to prevent reactivation. Because the BI generally falls at the rate of 0.5 to 1 per year, it usually requires 2 to 6 years for BB patients, and 5 to 10 years for BL and LL patients, to reach an inactive status.

Adding a third drug to this regimen, giving either clofazimine or ethionamide daily, may further increase its effectiveness. It would also avoid the small chance that the patients are infected with fully dapsone-resistant *M. leprae,* so that in effect they would be receiving only monotherapy with rifampin. Unfortunately, it is often difficult to convince new patients to take clofazimine because of the disfiguring effect of the pigmentation. Giving ethionamide in combination with rifampin considerably increases the danger of serious hepatotoxicity. Mouse footpad studies on bacilli from all new cases, as done at the GWLHDC, avoid the danger that primary dapsone resistance will be missed, but this test is expensive and not available to most of those treating this disease. Fortunately, this danger has so far proved more theoretical than real.

**Patients Infected with Dapsone-Resistant *M. leprae.*** This usually refers to secondary dapsone-resistant infections—i.e., those that resulted from prolonged intake of dapsone or other sulfones as monotherapy irregularly or in low dosages, resulting in relapse with fully dapsone-resistant *M. leprae* 5 to 20 years or longer after the start of therapy. Rarely, as noted earlier, patients with newly diagnosed disease may also be infected with fully dapsone-resistant bacilli.

The treatment of choice for adults is 50 to 100 mg of clofazimine daily, given for the same time intervals as dapsone for newly diagnosed disease, plus 600 mg of rifampin daily for the first 6 months in paucibacillary cases and for the first 3 years in multibacillary cases. If the patients do not accept the pigmentation produced by clofazimine, 600 mg of rifampin with 250 mg of ethionamide daily may be substituted for the clofazimine-rifampin combination. Both the rifampin and the ethionamide are then continued for the same interval as the dapsone in individuals with newly diagnosed leprosy.

**World Health Organization Treatment Regimens.** Leprosy control is a major problem in many Third World countries. Patient compliance is frequently poor, case-finding and follow-up efforts are inadequate, and budgets are unrealistically small. Personnel may be poorly trained and motivated and too few in number. Furthermore, the incidence of primary and secondary resistance is often high and is steadily rising, creating the possibility that dapsone, which is inexpensive and has proved to be safe and effective for long-term administration, could be lost as a first-line antileprosy drug. This would have serious adverse effects on most control programs.

In 1981, the WHO organized a study group to make recommendations for the "chemotherapy of leprosy for control programs" (WHO Technical Report Series No. 675–1982). They proposed two regimens. Adult patients with paucibacillary disease would be given 100 mg of dapsone daily, unsupervised, and 600 mg of rifampin, once monthly, supervised, both for a total of 6 months. Therapy is then discontinued. Multibacillary cases should receive 100 mg of dapsone daily, plus 50 mg of clofazimine daily, unsupervised, plus 600 mg of rifampin with 300 mg of clofazimine once monthly, supervised. Therapy is continued for at least 2 years, and preferably to a BI of 0, and then discontinued. The once-monthly rifampin and the relatively short period of treatment are controversial. A single dose of 600 mg of rifampin has been shown to have a marked bactericidal effect against *M. leprae* in humans, but whether giving it monthly is as efficacious as daily administration remains uncertain. There is also evidence that shorter periods of treatment may be possible if two or more bactericidal drugs are given to patients with leprosy, but the study in question did not involve the use of rifampin given only monthly. On the other hand, the WHO regimens have certain advantages. Cost is relatively low; compliance should improve; and, if relapse does occur after therapy is discontinued, it should be with *M. leprae* having the same drug sensitivity pattern as those that originally infected the patient. Trials to date with these regimens have found an extremely low relapse rate, even when the multibacillary regimen is given for only 2 years, but long-term follow-up on larger numbers of patients is needed.

**Follow-up of Patients on Treatment.** Patients are followed at varying intervals, depending on the severity of their disease, complications, the drugs they are receiving, etc. For example, patients receiving only dapsone with no complications may need to be seen only every 3 months, whereas those with severe reactions may require weekly or more frequent follow-up. It is generally useful to see the patient relatively frequently at first because complications are most likely to occur during the first 1 to 2 years. Later, as the danger of reaction diminishes and the patient has gained an understanding of his or her disease, the follow-up visits can be less frequent. Isolation of patients is not necessary because therapy rapidly renders them noninfectious, thus providing "chemical isolation," and close contacts have already generally received maximal exposure prior to the time the diagnosis was established. Pregnancy has little effect on the disease process, except for increasing the likelihood of reaction.

Clinically, there is a gradual clearance of skin lesions. Within 3 to 4 months of the start of appropriate therapy, the MI should fall to 0, but, as noted earlier, the BI on skin scrapings or biopsy specimens falls slowly. Routine follow-up laboratory studies would include a complete blood count, urinalysis, creatinine determination, and liver function tests. Drug toxicity, however, is uncommon after the first year of treatment, and serious toxicity may manifest itself clinically before it is detected in the laboratory. If possible, skin scrapings should be done from several of the most active sites at 6-month intervals. Routine follow-up biopsies are not done unless skin scrapings are unavailable.

## REACTIONS

About half the patients with leprosy have reactive episodes of varying degrees of severity during the course of their disease. Some have them before treatment is started, but most occur during therapy, particularly during the first year. Reaction should not be regarded as a side effect of any drug; rather, it is apparently due to destruction of bacilli by whatever cause and the immune response to bacterial antigens released. Chemotherapy should be continued in spite of reactive episodes, and the episodes themselves should be suppressed as needed by other therapy.

Reactions can be broadly divided into two main categories: erythema nodosum leprosum (ENL, or type 2 reactions), occurring almost exclusively in BL and LL patients, and reversal (type 1) reactions, occurring throughout the leprosy spectrum, except for the lepromatous (LL) pole. A third type of reaction known as the Lucio phenomenon may only be an extreme variation of ENL, and it occurs in patients with diffuse lepromatous leprosy who are from Mexico and some other areas. It is occasionally seen in the United States and is managed with corticosteroids. A fourth type, known as downgrading reactions, is also uncommon. It represents inflammation associated with progression of the disease process in untreated patients and is usually managed just by initiation of antileprosy therapy.

### Erythema Nodosum Leprosum

ENL usually manifests with fever and painful erythematous nodules, but peripheral neuritis, orchitis, lymphadenitis, iridocyclitis, nephritis, periostitis, and arthralgias may also occur. Mild episodes may require no therapy, or symptomatic measures, such as aspirin administration, may suffice. Several drugs are useful for the management of severe episodes.

Corticosteroids are effective in all patients and should always be used if an acute neuritis is present to prevent permanent nerve injury. Usually, 60 mg of prednisone daily is sufficient. When the initial episode has been completely controlled for several days, an attempt may be made to taper the drug dosage, over a period of 2 to 4 weeks. The reaction often recurs, however, and the dosage has to be increased again. If, as often happens, the process becomes chronic and recurs whenever attempts to reduce or discontinue the prednisone are made, prolonged therapy may be needed. In these patients, I try to taper the prednisone to alternate-day therapy. When an alternate-day schedule is reached, the dosage is reduced still more slowly until either the drug is eliminated or the lowest possible maintenance level is reached. However, because steroid-associated side effects are often a problem, other forms of therapy should be considered in chronic cases.

Thalidomide, which is investigational in the United States, is effective in most patients. The initial regimen is 100 mg four times daily, and the reaction is usually controlled within 48 to 72 hours. The dosage is then tapered over 2 weeks to a maintenance level, usually 100 mg daily. Regular attempts are made to discontinue it, but patients may need to continue taking thalidomide for months to years before it can be discontinued without recurrence of the reaction. Side effects are few, drowsiness being the most common. It cannot, of course, be given to fertile females because of its well-known teratogenicity. Information regarding procurement of the drug may be obtained from the GWLHDC in Carville, LA.

Clofazimine is also effective for the control of ENL. A dosage of 100 mg two or three times daily* usually is necessary, and the reaction should come under control during a period ranging from a few weeks to a few months, depending on its severity. Normally, reaction control is maintained with prednisone in these patients, and the dosage of prednisone is gradually diminished as the clofazimine begins to act. Because gastrointestinal symptoms may develop with high dosages, the dosage should be reduced to 100 mg daily within a year if possible. Pigmentation from the clofazimine is usually quite marked in these patients, and they should be fully cognizant of this before therapy is started.

### Reversal Reactions

Clinically, these usually are evidenced by fever and edema and erythema of pre-existing lesions, which may progress to ulceration. Neuritis and adenopathy may also occur. If there is danger of a motor or sensory deficit or ulceration, high dosages of corticosteroids must always be used—e.g., 60 to 120 mg of prednisone daily. The reaction usually is controlled within 24 to 48 hours, and only a short course of therapy may be necessary if the patient has minimally active disease and no neuritis. Those with neuritis may require prolonged treatment (3 to 6 months), however, if neural damage is to be reversed. Patients with prolonged reaction may sometimes be managed with alternate-day steroids as noted for ENL, and some investigators have found clofazimine to be useful in these patients.

### Other Complications

Neuritis may occur independently of any reactive episode. Immediate treatment with high dosages of corticosteroids is necessary to avoid permanent injury and recover lost function insofar as possible.

Iridocyclitis is a medical emergency and is probably best managed by an ophthalmologist.

Atropine drops and corticosteroid drops must be started at once if permanent damage is to be avoided. Tear substitutes are used in patients with lagophthalmos and/or decreased lacrimation.

Orchitis may occur with or independently of a reactive episode. It usually responds quickly to corticosteroids, but sterility may result.

Injuries are common in all patients with leprosy who have significant degrees of sensory and/or motor loss. The patient must be taught how to avoid them by frequent inspections of involved skin and the use of protective measures, such as wearing gloves or special footwear. When an injury does occur in an insensitive area, it must be protected from further damage during healing.

### CONTROL MEASURES

These include appropriate patient education and management, evaluation of contacts, and prophylaxis. Patient education is vital if treatment is to be successful. Prolonged compliance with any regimen is unlikely unless the patient fully understands the necessity for it. The family's cooperation is also important.

Evaluation of contacts in countries of low endemicity, such as the United States, is limited to the household. They should be checked for evidence of the disease at 6- to 12-month intervals for at least 5 years and know to seek immediate attention if suspicious changes occur at any time.

Possible prophylactic measures include bacille Calmette-Gúerin (BCG) and dapsone therapy. The usefulness of BCG remains uncertain, but it probably does not protect against development of the more severe types of the disease. Three years of dapsone prophylaxis has been recommended by the Centers for Disease Control for household contacts younger than age 25 years of multibacillary patients. Compliance is often a serious problem, and it is uncertain whether such prophylaxis prevents or only delays the onset of the disease in those contacts destined to undergo development of multibacillary disease. The WHO does not recommend dapsone prophylaxis.

### FUTURE PROSPECTS

Considerable research is under way, sponsored by such agencies as the National Institutes of Health and the GWLHDC in the United States and internationally by WHO's Therapy of Leprosy (THELEP) and Immunology of Leprosy (IMMLEP) Scientific Working Groups. Emphasis has been placed on new drug development and improved utilization of existing drugs, cultivation of *M. leprae* in artificial media, antileprosy vac-

---

*Exceeds dosage recommended by the manufacturer.

cine development, serodiagnostic tests for the early detection and follow-up of this disease, and the clarification of the immunopathology involved. Considerable progress has already been made. For example, preliminary trials with antileprosy vaccines are under way. New bactericidal drugs, such as ofloxacin,* also show considerable promise and may allow further shortening of leprosy chemotherapy.

# MALARIA

method of
DAVID A. WARRELL, D.M., D.Sc.
*University of Oxford*
*Oxford, England*

Humans are the natural vertebrate hosts of four species of *Plasmodium*—*P. falciparum, P. vivax, P. malariae,* and *P. ovale*—and, on rare occasions, can be infected with the primate malarias—*P. brasilianum, P. inui, P. knowlesi, P. simium, P. shortti,* and *P. cynomolgi.* In all cases, infection results from inoculation into the blood stream of sporozoites by female *Anopheles* mosquitoes. Sporozoites disappear into hepatocytes and develop into schizonts. After 6 to 16 days, merozoites are released into the blood and invade erythrocytes. In the liver, the development of some sporozoites of *P. vivax* and *P. ovale* becomes arrested, and they remain dormant as hypnozoites, which are capable of causing relapses months or years later. *P. falciparum* and *P. malariae* have no persisting hepatic phase, but may survive in the blood in small numbers to give rise to recrudescent infections. Inside erythrocytes, the parasites develop from rings through trophozoites to pigmented multinucleated schizonts. These schizonts rupture, releasing merozoites, which can infect new erythrocytes, but cannot reinvade the liver. In the case of *P. falciparum* alone, erythrocytes containing mature trophozoites and schizonts stick to the walls of small blood vessels and become sequestered in various organs and tissues, notably the brain. Some of the merozoites that invade erythrocytes become male (micro) or female (macro) gametocytes. When these gametocytes are taken up by mosquitoes, they complete a sexual cycle, resulting in sporozoites, which are injected with the mosquito's saliva during a blood meal. The prepatent period (the interval between the infecting mosquito bite and the appearance of parasitemia) is usually 9 to 10 days for *P. falciparum,* 8 to 13 days for *P. vivax,* 9 to 14 days for *P. ovale,* and 15 to 16 days for *P. malariae.* Incubation periods (intervals between the bite and the first symptom) are a few days longer. Almost all antimalarial drugs are blood schizonticides, acting on the asexual erythrocytic forms of the parasites. Drugs such as primaquine, proguanil,† tetracycline, and possibly pyrimethamine are primary tissue

schizonticides, acting on the pre-erythrocytic or exoerythrocytic forms in the liver. Primaquine and other 8-aminoquinolines are hypnozoiticides, needed to prevent relapses after *P. vivax* and *P. ovale* infections. Quinine, mefloquine,* and 4- and 8-aminoquinolines are gametocyticides for *P. vivax, P. ovale,* and *P. malariae,* and primaquine also kills the gametocytes of *P. falciparum.*

## EPIDEMIOLOGY

Currently, the endemic area for malaria spreads throughout most tropical regions from Central and South America, Haiti, and the Dominican Republic in the Caribbean, to Africa, the Middle East, the Indian subcontinent, and Southeast Asia, including parts of China and the western Pacific. *P. falciparum* is replaced by *P. ovale* in West Africa and is absent from the eastern Mediterranean. *P. vivax* has been the dominant species in most parts of the Indian subcontinent, but there is a resurgence of *P. falciparum.* In parts of Africa, Papua New Guinea, and elsewhere, species of *Anopheles* mosquito are such efficient vectors that infants and children are frequently infected and gradually acquire immunity. In these endemic regions, severe disease occurs only in infants and young children. However, immunity lapses in people who move outside the endemic area for several years. Thus, people from the Indian subcontinent who emigrate to Europe or North America may become vulnerable to infection by the time they return home on holiday. Outside the endemic area, autochthonous malaria may occur sporadically—e.g., in the region of international airports. Infection may also be acquired by blood transfusion, transplacentally, by contaminated needles (e.g., among intravenous drug abusers), and via marrow and tissue transplants.

## CLINICAL FEATURES

**Falciparum Malaria.** The prepatent period is usually 9 to 10 (shortest, 5) days and the incubation period 7 to 14 (mean, 12) days. Almost 90% of patients with imported falciparum malaria evidence symptoms within 1 month of leaving the endemic area, and two-thirds of those with vivax or ovale malarias experience symptoms within 6 months, but, unusually, this may be delayed for a year or more. The diagnostic tertian fever (fever occurring every third day) is rarely seen, and even the dramatic malaria chill is uncommon. There is nothing specific about the clinical picture of malaria. Fever usually starts abruptly and continues irregularly or with daily spikes, and there are headache, backache, myalgias, postural syncope, prostration, and vomiting. Gastrointestinal symptoms, including abdominal pain and diarrhea (which may be profuse and watery), are relatively common. Useful physical signs include anemia; jaundice; tenderness and enlargement of liver and spleen and the absence of lymphadenopathy; rash; and localizing signs. Severe, life-threatening falciparum malaria is characterized by impaired consciousness (cerebral malaria), severe

---

*Investigational drug in the United States.
†Not available in the United States.

---

*Not available in the United States.

anemia, spontaneous bleeding, jaundice, hypoglycemia, shock (algid malaria), renal failure, lactic acidosis, pulmonary edema, and secondary bacterial infections (Table 1). In cases of strictly defined cerebral malaria (unrousable coma with asexual parasitemia and exclusion of other causes of encephalopathy), the mortality is 15 to 20%.

**Vivax, Ovale, and Malariae Malarias.** Fever and chills are as severe as in falciparum malaria and, in untreated cases, tertian periodicity may be seen with vivax and ovale malarias and quartan (every fourth day) fever in *P. malariae* infection. Unless the persisting hepatic cycle of vivax and ovale malarias is eliminated with primaquine, relapses may occur every 2 to 3 months for up to 8 years or even longer. *P. malariae* infection may recrudesce after more than 50 years. Vivax malaria is life-threatening only in debilitated patients or as a result of rupture of the acutely enlarged spleen. Malariae malaria is an important cause of nephrotic syndrome in parts of Africa and has caused a few deaths in immunocompromised patients infected by blood transfusion.

## DIAGNOSIS

Malaria must be excluded in any febrile patient who has traveled to an endemic area, has received a blood transfusion, or has been exposed to other rare routes of infection. The differential diagnosis includes other infections that cause chills and rigors (lobar pneumonia, ascending cholangitis, pyelonephritis, and viral hepatitis), jaundice (viral hepatitis, leptospirosis, yellow fever, and relapsing fevers), hyperpyrexia (heat stroke), gastrointestinal symptoms (traveler's diarrhea and typhoid), and encephalitides (viral, bacterial, fungal, and protozoal encephalitides). Laboratory diagnosis depends on finding asexual parasites in thick or thin blood films. Gametocytes indicate recovery from infection and are useful for distinguishing falciparum from vivax malaria. Ideally, the film should be made at the bedside and stained immediately with a Romanovsky's stain such as Wright's, Field's, Leishman's, or Giemsa's stain. A simple technique employs Field's stain for both thick and thin films. The thin film is first fixed in anhydrous methanol, and the thick film is dried rapidly using a small hair dryer. Thrombocytopenia is common in falciparum and vivax malarias. The total leukocyte count may be normal or low, but, in severe falciparum malaria, there is a neutrophil leukocytosis. Biochemical abnormalities include hyponatremia: bilirubinemia (usually indirect, resulting from hemolysis, but sometimes direct, caused by hepatocellular damage or even cholestasis); moderately increased serum aminotransferase levels; and reduced antithrombin III levels. Hypoglycemia is common in severe infections. Levels of C-reactive protein, complement components, fibrinogen, and other acute phase proteins are increased, and high levels of cachectin (tumor necrosis factor) have been recorded in severe disease.

## TREATMENT

### Principles of Antimalarial Chemotherapy

In severe falciparum malaria (see Table 1), effective plasma concentrations of an appropriate

### TABLE 1. Clinical Features of Severe or Complicated Malaria

| Principal Manifestations | Other Features |
| --- | --- |
| Cerebral malaria (unrousable coma) | Impaired consciousness, but rousable |
| Severe normocytic anemia | Hyperparasitemia |
| Renal failure | Jaundice |
| Pulmonary edema | Hyperpyrexia |
| Hypoglycemia | Prostration |
| Circulatory collapse | Inability to swallow tablets |
| Spontaneous systemic bleeding and disseminated intravascular coagulation | |
| Generalized convulsion | |
| Acidemia | |
| Macroscopic hemoglobinuria | |

schizonticidal drug, preferably greater than the measured in vitro or in vivo minimal inhibitory concentration when this is known, should be achieved as quickly and safely as possible and sustained for long enough to ensure rapid clearance of asexual parasitemia. In these circumstances, the use of single-dose regimens to ensure compliance, the prevention of late recrudescences (R1 resistance), and the destruction of gametocytes are of minor importance. Unpleasant side effects, such as cinchonism (with quinine and quinidine) or pruritus (with chloroquine), may be acceptable in the treatment of a life-threatening infection and should not limit dosage.

In patients with severe falciparum malaria, it is important to start chemotherapy as soon as the infection is proved or suspected (Tables 2 through 4). In severely ill patients with negative blood smear findings, therapeutic trial is indicated if the patient has been exposed to infection. Treatment should be initiated via the parenteral route, preferably by intravenous infusion over periods of 2 hours or more. The course of treatment should be completed by the oral route as soon as the patient is able to swallow tablets. The dosage should be calculated according to body

### TABLE 2. Chemotherapy of Malaria

| | Country Where Infected | |
| --- | --- | --- |
| **Species** | *Chloroquine-Sensitive Area* | *Elsewhere or Unknown* |
| *P. falciparum* (or unknown) | Chloroquine or quinine | Quinine *or* quinidine ± tetracycline (Pyrimethamine-sulfonamide) (Mefloquine†) (Halofantrine†) |
| | **All Areas** | |
| *P. vivax* *P. ovale* *P. malariae* | Chloroquine* | |

*Followed by primaquine for *P. vivax* and *P. ovale*.
†Not available in the United States.

TABLE 3. **Chemotherapy of Malaria: Patients Who Can Swallow Tablets***

| Chloroquine | 10 mg/kg of base followed by 5 mg/kg 6, 24, and 48 hr later (normal adult dosage, 3 tablets followed by 1 tablet 6, 24, and 48 hr later) (total dose 25 mg/kg of base) |
|---|---|
| Quinine or quinidine | 8.4 mg/kg of base tid for 7 days with tetracycline,† 250 mg 4 times per day for 7 days |
| Pyrimethamine-sulfon-amide (e.g., Fansidar) | Pyrimethamine, 1.5 mg/kg, and sulfadoxine, 30 mg/kg, as a single dose (normal total adult dose 3 tablets) |
| Mefloquine‡ | 15 mg/kg of *base* (maximal dose 1 gram) divided into 2 equal doses given 6 hr apart (normal total adult dose 4 tablets) |
| Halofantrine‡ | 8 mg/kg of base q 6 hr for 3 doses (normal total adult dose 6 tablets) |
| Primaquine | 15 mg of *base* per day on days 4–17§ *or* 45 mg once per wk for 8 wk |

*Chloroquine syrup and halofantrine suspension are available for young children.

†Except in children less than 8 yr old and pregnant women.

‡Not available in the United States.

§Double dose or duration for Chesson-type strains of *P. vivax* in Solomon Islands, the Philippines, Thailand, Indonesia, etc.

weight. The response to treatment is monitored by examining the patient, recording the temperature, and repeating the blood film studies at least every 6 hours.

**Chemotherapy of Severe Falciparum Malaria.** Quinine is the drug of choice (Table 4), unless it is certain that the infection was acquired in an area where there is no high-grade resistance to chloroquine. In the United States, quinine dihydrochloride is available only from the Centers for Disease Control (telephone 404–639–3670; nights and emergency [24 hour] 404–639–2888); however, quinidine gluconate injection may be available for cardiac use and can be used to initiate treatment. Unless the patient has been given quinine, quinidine, or mefloquine* within the previous 12 to 24 hours, a loading dose should be given to ensure that therapeutic plasma concentrations are achieved quickly. The dosage of quinine or quinidine should be halved if the plasma concentration exceeds 15 mg per liter at any stage or if parenteral treatment has to be continued for more than 72 hours.

In the remaining parts of the endemic area where *P. falciparum* is still sensitive to chloroquine, this is the treatment of choice, as chloroquine (Aralen) is less toxic than quinine and may be more rapidly effective. However, physicians may prefer to use quinine in all cases of severe falciparum malaria because of the risk of chloroquine resistance, even when the infection has been acquired in a predominantly chloroquine-sensitive area of the world. If it is not possible to give quinine or chloroquine by intravenous infusion, quinine dihydrochloride (30 mg per ml concentration) can be given by intramuscular injection or chloroquine can be administered by a subcutaneous or intramuscular injection. In areas of quinine resistance, tetracycline should be given (but not in children younger than 8 years old nor in pregnant women).

**Chemotherapy of Uncomplicated Falciparum Malaria.** The treatment of choice for chloroquine-resistant falciparum malaria or malaria of unknown origin is mefloquine (marketed as Lariam in France, Switzerland, Britain, and Germany). Alternatively, quinine sulfate can be given for 5 to 10 days, alone or in combination with tetra-

*Not available in the United States.

TABLE 4. **Chemotherapy of Severe Malaria: Parenteral Regimens**

| Quinine | IV infusion | 5.6 mg/kg of *base* in 30 min (loading)* using constant rate infusion pump |
|---|---|---|
| | *then* | 8.4 mg/kg of *base* in 4 hr q 8 hr until patient can swallow,† then quinine tablets to complete 7 days' treatment |
| | *or* | IV infusion 16.7 mg/kg of *base* in 4 hr (loading)* |
| | *then* | 8.4 mg/kg of *base* in 4 hr q 8 hr until patient can swallow, then quinine tablets to complete 7 days' treatment |
| | *or* | IM (anterior thigh), same dosage regimen |
| Quinidine | IV infusion | 10 mg/kg of *gluconate base* in 1–2 hr (loading)* |
| | *then* | 0.02 mg/kg/min by infusion pump for 72 hr or until patient can swallow, then quinine tablets to complete 7 days' treatment |
| Chloroquine | IV infusion | 10 mg/kg of *base* in 8 hr |
| | *then* | 15 mg/kg of *base* in 24 hr‡ |
| | *or* | 5 mg/kg in 4–6 hr every 12 hr ⎱ to total dose of |
| | IM/SC | 2.5 mg/kg q 4 hr ⎰ 25 mg/kg of *base* |

*Loading dose should not be used if patient received quinine, quinidine, or mefloquine within preceding 12–24 hr.

†Parenteral quinine is not commercially available in the United States. However, quinine dihydrochloride is investigational and can be obtained from the Centers for Disease Control, telephone 404–639–3670 nights and emergency (24 hr) 404–639–2888.

‡Exceeds dosage recommended by the manufacturer.

cycline, pyrimethamine-sulfadoxine (Fansidar), or clindamycin (Cleocin)—depending on the sensitivity of local strains. Halofantrine* (Halfan) may soon be marketed in Europe and North America.

**Chemotherapy of Vivax, Ovale, and Malariae Malarias.** Chloroquine is effective in all parts of the world. There has been a single report of chloroquine-resistant vivax malaria from Papua New Guinea. Persistent hepatic cycles in vivax and ovale malarias acquired by mosquito bite are eliminated using primaquine. The Chesson-type strain of *P. vivax* in Thailand, Indonesia, Papua New Guinea, and the Solomon Islands is relatively resistant to primaquine and requires double the normal dosage. In patients with mild glucose-6-phosphate dehydrogenase (G6PD) deficiency, primaquine-induced hemolysis can be reduced by giving 45 mg as a single dose each week for 8 weeks (children, 0.75 mg per kg per week for 8 weeks). Severe infections should be treated with parenteral chloroquine or quinine. Mixed infections (with *P. falciparum*) are common, but may be difficult to diagnose.

## Toxic Effects of Antimalarial Drugs

Quinine at plasma concentrations greater than 5 mg per liter produces cinchonism—giddiness, tinnitus, high-tone deafness, tremors, blurred vision, nausea, vomiting, and dysphoria—and levels greater than 20 mg per liter may cause blindness, deafness, hypotension, electrocardiographic abnormalities, and central nervous system depression. Hypoglycemia caused by hyperinsulinemia is the most common important side effect of quinine.

Quinidine has similar side effects to quinine, but is relatively more cardiotoxic.

Mefloquine commonly causes abdominal symptoms (nausea, vomiting, abdominal pain, and diarrhea) and rarely may produce cardiac arrhythmias, postural hypotension, and an acute transient encephalopathy.

Chloroquine at plasma concentrations greater than 250 ng per ml causes dizziness, diplopia, difficulty in visual accommodation, dysphagia, nausea, and vomiting. High plasma concentrations following parenteral administration may cause vasodilation, hypotension, cardiotoxicity, and death. Large overdoses can be treated with diazepam and epinephrine. Hypokalemia is an additional problem in these cases. Pruritus is a common side effect in black-skinned patients. A cumulative dose of more than about 100 grams can cause irreversible neuroretinitis.

---

*Not available in the United States.

TABLE 5. **Principles of Management of Severe Falciparum Malaria**

Early antimalarial chemotherapy using optimal dosages of an appropriate agent administered by controlled rate IV infusion

Prevention, or early detection and treatment, of complications (e.g., convulsions, hypoglycemia, and hyperpyrexia)

Correction of fluid, electrolyte, and acid-base imbalance

Proper nursing care (e.g., of unconscious patients)

Avoidance of harmful ancillary treatments (e.g., corticosteroids)

---

Primaquine may cause hemolysis in patients with severe deficiencies of erythrocyte enzymes, such as G6PD and NADH-methemoglobin reductase.

Pyrimethamine-sulfonamide combinations (e.g., Fansidar), given prophylactically, are associated with a risk of mortality between 1:11,000 and 1:25,000, Stevens-Johnson syndrome, and toxic epidermal necrolysis.

Dapsone-pyrimethamine combination (Maloprim)* used prophylactically in double the recommended dosage, and rarely in the recommended dosage (1 tablet per week), has caused agranulocytosis, which is usually reversible. Hemolysis and methemoglobinemia (producing ashy cyanosis of nail beds, etc.) are not uncommon in patients congenitally deficient in erythrocyte NADH-methemoglobin reductase. A few cases of nodular eosinophilic interstitial pneumonia have been described.

Proguanil* is the least toxic of all antimalarial drugs, but may cause mouth ulcers, gastrointestinal symptoms, and hair loss in a few recipients.

### General Management (Table 5)

Febrile patients should be nursed in bed because of the tendency to postural hypotension. A high temperature contributes to symptoms and causes febrile convulsions in children and fetal distress in pregnant women. Hyperpyrexia may cause irreversible neurologic damage. Patients should be cooled by sponging with tepid water and fanning, the use of hypothermia mattresses, and the administration of antipyretics, such as acetaminophen (15 mg per kg by mouth, via nasogastric tube, or rectally). Patients with severe malaria should be treated in an intensive care unit and, especially if they are unconscious, given the benefit of expert nursing care. Convulsions can be controlled with diazepam and prevented by a single intramuscular injection of phenobarbital (10 mg per kg†) on admission to the hospital.

---

*Not available in the United States.
†Exceeds dosage recommended by the manufacturer.

A number of unproven and potentially harmful ancillary treatments have been suggested for cerebral malaria. Dexamethasone (Decadron) in dosages of 2 and 11 mg per kg over 48 hours was found, in two double-blind, placebo-controlled trials, to increase morbidity and to not reduce mortality. Other treatments for which there is no convincing evidence include osmotic or diuretic agents, such as mannitol; plasma expanders, such as dextrans; epinephrine; heparin; prostacyclin; and cyclosporine (Sandimmune).

## Management of Complications

*Fluid and electrolyte imbalances* should be corrected. Patients may show clinical evidence of hypovolemia associated with hyponatremia, hypoalbuminemia, and oliguria. Failure to restore an adequate circulating volume may lead to the development of hypotension, shock, lactic acidosis, and renal failure, but it is easy to precipitate pulmonary edema in these patients by excessively vigorous fluid replacement. Fluid requirements should be carefully calculated, taking into account the volume of blood transfused and the fluid used as the vehicle for infusion of antimalarial drugs. Jugular venous pressure, central venous pressure, or pulmonary artery wedge pressure should be monitored and not allowed to rise above +5 cm $H_2O$. Cautious rehydration increases urinary flow in the majority of patients who are admitted to the hospital with oliguria and raised serum creatinine levels. If urinary output remains low, increasing intravenous dosages of furosemide (Lasix), up to a total dose of 1 gram, and dopamine infusion can be tried, but are rarely effective. Indications for dialysis include hyperkalemia, fluid overload, metabolic acidosis, and clinical manifestations of uremia. Hemodialysis or hemofiltration is preferable, but peritoneal dialysis can be effective; it may need to be continued for long periods. The initial dosage of antimalarial drugs need not be reduced in patients who are in renal failure.

*Anemia* is an inevitable consequence of hemolysis of infected erythrocytes and of other disturbances—e.g., hemolysis or splenic removal of unparasitized erythrocytes and dyserythropoiesis. If the hematocrit falls below 20%, fresh compatible whole blood should be transfused while the patient is carefully monitored for signs of fluid overload.

*Hypoglycemia* is increasingly reported as a complication of falciparum malaria in patients with severe disease, pregnant women, and young children. In pregnant women, hypoglycemia may be asymptomatic, but most patients have convulsions, impairment of consciousness, extensor posturing, or the more familiar cardiovascular and neurologic symptoms of this disturbance. Quinine and quinidine cause hypoglycemia by stimulating insulin release, but, especially in patients with hyperparasitemia and in pregnant women and young children, hypoglycemia may develop before antimalarial chemotherapy and without hyperinsulinemia. Patients with severe malaria should be screened repeatedly for hypoglycemia and, if there is any doubt, given a therapeutic trial of intravenous 50% dextrose in water. In children, a continuous infusion of 5% dextrose in water (80 ml per kg per 24 hours) may prevent quinine-induced hypoglycemia, but, in adults, hypoglycemia may arise during infusion of 5 or 10% dextrose in water. Quinine- or quinidine-induced hyperinsulinemia can be prevented and reversed by the somatostatin analogue SMS201–995, given as a single subcutaneous dose of 50 µg, followed by glucagon, 1 mg.

*Metabolic (lactic) acidosis* results from impaired tissue perfusion, hypovolemia, reduced hepatic clearance of lactate, and, in patients with a large parasite burden, lactate generated by parasite metabolism. Treatment should be aimed at improving perfusion and oxygenation by correcting hypovolemia, clearing the airway, increasing inspired oxygen concentration, and treating septicemia, a frequently associated complication. In cases of severe acidosis (pH less than 7.2), treatment with sodium bicarbonate, tromethamine (tris [hydroxymethyl] aminomethan), or dichloroacetate (which stimulates pyruvate dehydrogenase) may be considered.

*Hypotension and shock* (algid malaria) may result from pulmonary edema, massive gastrointestinal hemorrhage, splenic rupture, or uncorrected dehydration. However, many of the patients with this clinical presentation are found to have gram-negative septicemia. Appropriate antimicrobial cover should be given and the hemodynamic problems corrected with plasma expanders and selective vasoconstrictors, such as dopamine.

*Hyperparasitemia,* usually defined as infection of more than 10% of circulating erythrocytes, carries a mortality exceeding 60%. In some 60 reported cases, exchange transfusion using cell separators, hemofiltration, or manual methods appeared to reduce the parasitemia more rapidly than would have been expected using optimal chemotherapy alone, and there was striking clinical improvement in some cases. Other merits of the method are the isovolumetric correction of anemia; restoration of clotting factors, platelets, and albumin; and the removal of putative circulating toxins, mediators, and metabolites. However, the risks of transmitting infection and precipitating hemodynamic changes must be balanced against these potential benefits. Total exchange requires approximately 10 liters of blood in an adult patient.

*Pulmonary edema* is a particularly dangerous complication of severe falciparum malaria. It may be precipitated by excessive parenteral fluid therapy, but may also develop in association with normal or low pulmonary arterial wedge pressures. The latter condition resembles adult respiratory distress syndrome. The probable cause is a primary increase in pulmonary capillary permeability associated with reduced plasma oncotic pressure. Pulmonary capillary hydrostatic pressure may be reduced by tipping the patient's head up and giving potent vasodilators, such as isosorbide dinitrate (Isordil), sodium nitroprusside (Nipride), or nitroglycerin. Administration of oxygen and mechanical ventilation with positive end-expiratory pressure may be beneficial.

*Disseminated intravascular coagulation* is frequently described in cases of imported severe falciparum malaria in nonimmune subjects. Vitamin K, fresh whole blood plasma, or concentrates of platelets and clotting factors should be given, but heparin has proved dangerous.

*Hemoglobinuria* may be precipitated by oxidant antimalarial drugs in patients with G6PD deficiency and other erythrocyte enzyme deficiencies. Some patients with severe infections also have massive intravascular hemolysis, which has been attributed to quinine. This blackwater fever carries a high mortality. Treatment with mannitol and bicarbonate may protect the kidneys from damaging effects of hemoglobin and other products of hemolysis.

*Splenic rupture* is the only potentially fatal complication that is more common in vivax malaria than in falciparum malaria. It should be excluded in patients who develop abdominal pain or shock. Ultrasound is useful for detecting free blood in the peritoneum and a tear in the splenic capsule.

### Malaria in Pregnancy

In nonimmune and semi-immune women, malaria appears to be particularly dangerous during pregnancy, causing maternal death, abortion, stillbirth, premature delivery, and low birthweight. Normal therapeutic doses of quinine and chloroquine can be used with confidence, even in the third trimester. There is no evidence that these drugs stimulate the uterus or harm the fetus. However, hypoglycemia is a frequent problem and can be induced by quinine treatment. Fetal distress results from placental pathologic changes, maternal high fever, and hypoglycemia. Inducing labor, performing cesarean section, or speeding up the second stage of labor with forceps or vacuum extractor should be considered in patients with severe falciparum malaria. A sudden increase in peripheral vascular resistance after separation of the placenta may precipitate acute pulmonary edema, and so fluid balance is particularly critical in women who go into labor.

### Malaria in Children

Children develop severe manifestations of falciparum malaria more rapidly than adults, but also respond more rapidly to treatment. The clinical picture is different from that in adults. Cough, vomiting, diarrhea, and convulsions are more common than in adults, whereas jaundice, pulmonary edema, and renal failure are relatively rare. Hypoglycemia is common and is usually associated with an appropriately low plasma insulin concentration. It is particularly important to detect and correct hypoglycemia as early as possible to prevent permanent neurologic sequelae. The principles of management are the same as for adults. Febrile convulsions and convulsions associated with cerebral malaria are common and probably warrant the prophylactic use of anticonvulsants in all young children requiring hospital admission for the treatment of malaria. The unpleasantly bitter flavor of chloroquine and quinine can be disguised by grinding up the tablets with something sweet or using pediatric syrups or suspensions. The risk of the child's vomiting back the tablets can be reduced by enforcing a period of quiet bed rest and by lowering the fever. Chloroquine, quinine, and mefloquine seem to be well absorbed when given as suspensions by nasogastric tube, but antimalarial drugs have proved less bioavailable when given by suppository.

## PROPHYLAXIS

### Prevention of Malaria in Travelers

The geographic extent and seasonality of malaria transmission can be discovered from sources such as "Vaccination Certificate Requirements and Health Advice for International Travellers" published by the World Health Organization in Geneva. Brief stopovers in a malaria endemic area may expose the traveler to malaria, even if the ultimate destination is malaria free. Most capital cities in Southeast Asia and Latin America are free of malaria.

Almost 2000 cases of imported malaria are reported in Britain each year, with 2 to 12 deaths; the figures from the United States are similar. It is important to remember that none of the currently recommended chemoprophylactic drugs is totally effective, and all have some adverse effects. A risk/benefit analysis is appropriate before prescribing chemoprophylaxis. Even those who have taken chemoprophylaxis should consult a physician and mention the risk of malaria if any febrile illness develops after their return from a malaria endemic area. Standard advice to all travelers is

1. Prevent mosquito bites by excluding these insects (especially during the usual biting hours from dusk to dawn) by using pyrethrum-impregnated nets or insect-proofed rooms, protective clothing, and knock-down insecticides.

2. Repel mosquitoes with deet (N,N-diethyl-m-toluamide)–containing ointments or by burning mosquito coils. Bites can be avoided by staying in insect-proofed rooms after dark. An alternative to chemoprophylaxis is presumptive treatment. The traveler carries a therapeutic course of a drug such as mefloquine, halofantrine, pyrimethamine-sulfonamide (Fansidar), quinine, or chloroquine, which is taken immediately when feverish symptoms develop.

### Chemoprophylaxis

The standard chemoprophylaxis regimen recommended in North America is once-weekly chloroquine: for adults 300 mg of base (two tablets) and for children 5 mg of base per kg per week. In Europe, the usual advice is to combine daily proguanil* (adults, 200 mg or two tablets; children, 3 mg per kg) with weekly chloroquine. These drugs are safe even in pregnancy and relatively free of side effects (but see earlier). However, people who have prolonged (longer than 3 months) or unusually heavy exposure (for example, those working outside after dark, those on military expeditions, and field workers) or who are particularly vulnerable to severe infection (e.g., infants, pregnant women, and splenectomized and immunosuppressed patients) are not adequately protected by these regimens in the zone of chloroquine-resistant P. falciparum. There is currently no satisfactory chemoprophylaxis for this group, but once-weekly pyrimethamine-dapsone (Maloprim)* (adults, one tablet) and chloroquine (adults, two tablets) is favored in Europe and Australia. The Centers for Disease Control no longer recommends pyrimethamine-sulfonamide (Fansidar) for prophylaxis because of the high risk of fatal skin complications (see earlier). In the future, mefloquine or halofantrine may be available for prophylaxis, but it would clearly be undesirable to jeopardize the long-term therapeutic value of these compounds by using

*Not available in the United States.

them for large-scale prophylaxis. There have been some encouraging early results of studies using proguanil-sulfonamide and proguanil-dapsone combinations. Doxycycline may be effective, but carries risks of photosensitization and disturbance of intestinal bacterial flora. Chloroquine should be started 2 weeks before travel, and all prophylactic drugs should be continued for at least 4 weeks after returning from the endemic area because most have their principal action on the erythrocytic forms, which may not emerge until 2 to 4 weeks after the infecting mosquito bite. Chloroquine is effective in preventing the erythrocytic cycle of P. vivax, P. ovale, and P. malariae, but does not prevent the establishment of a persistent hepatic infection by P. vivax and P. ovale. After prolonged exposure in a vivax-infested area, a course of primaquine should be given for this purpose.

# BACTERIAL MENINGITIS*

method of
CHARLES DAVIS, M.D.
Walter Reed Army Medical Center
Washington, D.C.

Bacterial meningitis is a rapidly fatal but treatable medical emergency. If untreated, this condition is associated with a mortality of greater than 90%. However, with prompt, aggressive treatment, the survival may exceed 90%, depending on the infecting pathogen. To obtain such a favorable response, the diagnosis must be made without delay and one must administer early, aggressive therapy, which is bactericidal, is given in high dosage, and penetrates inflamed meninges. Anticipation and proper management of complications may be lifesaving.

### THERAPY

Early and aggressive treatment of bacterial meningitis is crucial. In the acutely ill patient, death may ensue within a few hours. A delay of 30 to 60 minutes, while evaluating the cerebrospinal fluid (CSF) may worsen the prognosis in the acutely and seriously ill patient. Initial therapy is often empiric. The antimicrobial agent chosen must be highly active against the infecting pathogen, penetrate the CSF in the presence of inflamed meninges, and be bactericidal. A lumbar puncture and blood cultures should be performed prior to therapy and without undue

*The views of the author do not purport to reflect the position of the Department of the Army or the Department of Defense.

## TABLE 1. Most Likely Infecting Pathogens on the Basis of Clinical Setting*

| | Neonates | Children | Adults | Presumed Immunocompromised | Closed Head Trauma | Penetrating Head Trauma, Postneurosurgery | CSF Shunt | Meningomyelocele |
|---|---|---|---|---|---|---|---|---|
| **Gram Positives** | | | | | | | | |
| S. pneumoniae | X | X | X | X | X | | | |
| Streptococcus spp. (Groups A, B, C, D, and G) | X | | | X | X | X | X | X |
| S. aureus | | | | X | X | X | X | X |
| S. epidermidis | | | | | | X | X | |
| L. monocytogenes | X | | X | X | | | | |
| **Gram Negatives** | | | | | | | | |
| H. influenzae | X | X | | | X | | | |
| N. meningitidis | | X | X | | | | | |
| Gram-negative bacilli | X | | | X | | X | X | X |
| **Empiric Therapy**† | 1 | 2 | 3 | 4 | 5 | 6 | 7 | 8 |

*Therapy is given intravenously unless stated otherwise.

†1 = ampicillin plus cefotaxime or gentamicin; 2 = ampicillin plus cefotaxime or chloramphenicol; 3 = penicillin G or ampicillin; 4 = ampicillin plus ceftazidime; 5 = penicillin G; 6 = nafcillin plus ceftazidime plus an aminoglycoside (intravenously and intrathecally); 7 = vancomycin plus ceftazidime; 8 = nafcillin plus ceftazidime.

delay, unless there is evidence of increased intracranial pressure or a space-occupying lesion. In this case, therapy should be instituted and the lumbar puncture delayed until these processes have been ruled out by either computed tomography (CT) or magnetic resonance imaging. In the absence of identification of a specific pathogen or positive Gram's stain or antigen detection assay result, selection of empiric antimicrobial therapy is based on consideration of the patient's age, the clinical setting, the presence of underlying disease, and the immune status of the

## TABLE 2. Antimicrobials for Common Pathogens of Bacterial Meningitis

| Organism | Drug of Choice | Alternative Drug | Duration of Therapy |
|---|---|---|---|
| **Gram Positives** | | | |
| S. pneumoniae | Penicillin G | Chloramphenicol or third-generation cephalosporin* or cefuroxime or vancomycin | 10–14 days |
| Streptococcus spp. (Groups A, B, C, G) | Penicillin G | Same as above | 10–14 days |
| Streptococcus, Group D | ampicillin plus an aminoglycoside | Vancomycin plus an aminoglycoside | |
| S. aureus | | | 3–6 wk |
|   Penicillin sensitive | Penicillin G | Vancomycin | |
|   Penicillin resistant | Nafcillin or oxacillin | Vancomycin | |
|   Methicillin resistant | Vancomycin | — | |
| Staphylococcus, coagulase negative | | | 3–6 wk |
|   Penicillin resistant | Nafcillin or oxacillin | Vancomycin | |
|   Methicillin resistant | Vancomycin | — | |
| L. monocytogenes | Ampicillin | Trimethoprim-sulfamethoxazole | 3–6 wk |
| **Gram Negatives** | | | |
| H. influenzae | | | 10–14 days |
|   Beta-lactamase negative | Ampicillin | Chloramphenicol or third-generation cephalosporin* or cefuroxime | |
|   Beta-lactamase positive | Chloramphenicol | Third-generation cephalosporin* or cefuroxime | |
| N. meningitidis | Penicillin G | Chloramphenicol or third-generation cephalosporin* or cefuroxime | 7–10 days |
| Enterobacteriaceae | Cefotaxime | Third-generation cephalosporin* or cefuroxime | 10–14 days after CSF cultures are negative |
| P. aeruginosa, Acinetobacter, Serratia | Piperacillin plus tobramycin (IV and IT) | Ceftazidime or imipenem plus tobramycin (IV and IT) | 10–14 days after CSF cultures are negative |

*Cefotaxime, ceftazidime, ceftizoxime, or ceftriaxone.

*Abbreviations:* IV = intravenously; IT = intrathecally; CSF = cerebrospinal fluid.

TABLE 3. **Dosage Recommendations for Treatment of Bacterial Meningitis\***
**(Assumes Normal Renal and/or Hepatic Functions)**

| Antimicrobial | Neonates | | Children (<12 yr) | Adults |
|---|---|---|---|---|
| | <1 wk | >1 wk | | |
| Amikacin† | 15 mg/kg/day (2) | 15 mg/kg/day (2) | 15 mg/kg/day (3) | 15 mg/kg/day (3) |
| Ampicillin | 100 mg/kg/day (2) | 100 mg/kg/day (3) | 200 mg/kg/day (6) | 200 mg/kg/day (6), maximum 2 grams q 3 hr |
| Cefotaxime | 100 mg/kg/day (2) | 150 mg/kg/day (3) | 200 mg/kg/day (3) | 200 mg/kg/day (3), maximum 2 grams q 4 hr |
| Ceftazidime | 100 mg/kg/day‖ (2) | 150 mg/kg/day (3) | 150 mg/kg/day (3) | 150 mg/kg/day (3), maximum 2 grams q 8 hr |
| Ceftizoxime | 100 mg/kg/day (2) | 150 mg/kg/day (3) | 200 mg/kg/day (3) | 200 mg/kg/day (3), maximum 3–4 grams q 8 hr |
| Ceftriaxone | 200 mg/kg/day‖ (2) | 200 mg/kg/day‖ (2) | 100 mg/kg/day (2) | 100 mg/kg/day (2), maximum 2 grams q 12 hr |
| Cefuroxime | 100 mg/kg/day (3) | 100 mg/kg/day (3) | 100 mg/kg/day (3) | 240 mg/kg/day (3), maximum 3 grams q 8 hr |
| Chloramphenicol† | 25 mg/kg/day (4) | 50 mg/kg/day (4)‡ | 50 mg/kg/day (4) | 100 mg/kg/day (4), maximum 1–1.5 grams q 6 hr |
| Gentamicin† | 5 mg/kg/day (2) | 5 mg/kg/day (2) | 5 mg/kg/day (3) | 7.5 mg/kg/day (3) |
| Imipenem | — | — | — | 80 mg/kg/day‖ (4), maximum 1 gram q 6 hr |
| Nafcillin | 200 mg/kg/day (6) | 200 mg/kg/day (6) | 200 mg/kg/day (6) | 200 mg/kg/day (6), maximum 2 grams q 6 hr |
| Oxacillin | 50 mg/kg/day (2) | 75 mg/kg/day (3) | 200 mg/kg/day (6) | 200 mg/kg/day (6), maximum 2 grams q 4 hr |
| Penicillin G | 150,000 U/kg/day (3) | 250,000 U/kg/day (4) | 300,000 U/kg/day (6) | 300,000 U/kg/day maximum 4 mU q 4 hr |
| Piperacillin | — | — | — | 300 mg/kg/day (6), maximum 3 grams q 4 hr |
| Tobramycin† | 4 mg/kg/day (2) | 4 mg/kg/day (2) | 5 mg/kg/day (3) | 7.5 mg/kg/day (3) |
| Trimethoprim-sulfamethoxazole | — | — | 10 mg/kg/day of trimethoprim (4)§ | 10 mg/kg/day of trimethoprim (4) |
| Vancomycin† | 30 mg/kg/day‖ (2) | 30 mg/kg/day‖ (2) | 60 mg/kg/day‖ (4) | 40 mg/kg/day (4), maximum 500 mg q 6 hr |

\*Number of divided doses per day in parentheses.
†Blood levels need to be monitored.
‡Older than 2 wk of age.
§Indicated only for children older than 2 mo of age.
‖Exceeds dosage recommended by the manufacturer.

patient (Table 1). Specific therapy should be directed against the causative organism when identification and susceptibilities are available (Tables 2 through 4).

### Antibiotic Dosing and Modifications

The most effective and least toxic bactericidal antimicrobial should be used. Its selection is

TABLE 4. **Antimicrobials That Can Be Given Intrathecally or Intraventricularly\***

| Antimicrobial | Total Daily Child's Dose | Total Daily Adult Dose | Dosing Interval |
|---|---|---|---|
| Amikacin (Amikin) | 5.0 mg | 20 mg | 24 hr |
| Gentamicin (Garamycin) | 2.5 mg | 8 mg | 24 hr |
| Tobramycin (Nebcin) | 2.5 mg | 8 mg | 24 hr |
| Vancomycin (Vancocin) | — | 20 mg | 24 hr |

\**Note:* These preparations should be preservative free.

based on susceptibilities. The antimicrobial agent must be bactericidal (because of impaired opsonic activity and inefficient phagocytosis within the CSF), be capable of crossing the blood-brain barrier, and be given in high dosage to achieve a CSF level of at least 10-fold higher than the minimal bactericidal concentration for the microorganism. Suggested dosing regimens are shown in Tables 3 and 4.

Beta-lactam antimicrobials are the mainstays of therapy. Penicillin G is the drug of choice for *Streptococcus pneumoniae*. In the event of penicillin resistance, either chloramphenicol, a third-generation cephalosporin, or vancomycin may be selected. When *Haemophilus influenzae* is suspected, chloramphenicol, a third-generation cephalosporin (cefotaxime [Claforan], ceftazidime [Fortaz], ceftizoxime [Cefizox], or ceftriaxone [Rocephin], or cefuroxime [Zinacef] should be included in the empiric therapy until susceptibility data are available. Enteric gram-negative bacilli can often be treated with a high-dose intravenous third-generation cephalosporin; however, *Pseu-*

TABLE 5. **Conditions Associated with Recurrent Bacterial Meningitis**

**Anatomic Defects**
  Congenital
    Cranial or lumbosacral midline dermal sinuses
    Dermoid cysts
    Myelomeningocele
    Basiethmoid or cribriform plate defects
  Trauma
    Fracture of paranasal sinuses, cribriform plate, petrous bone
  Surgical CSF fistulas
**Immune System Defects**
  Splenectomy
  Hypogammaglobulinemia
  Leukemia and lymphoma
  Hemoglobinopathies
  Defects in complement components (alone or in combination)
**Parameningeal Focus of Infection**
**Resistant Organism**
**Idiopathic**

domonas aeruginosa requires the addition of an intrathecal aminoglycoside to a synergistic intravenous regimen.

The duration of treatment depends on the bacteria responsible for the meningitis. Seven to 10 days of therapy are usually sufficient for meningococcal meningitis and 10 to 14 days for *S. pneumoniae* and *H. influenzae* meningitis. *Staphylococcus, Listeria,* and gram-negative bacilli meningitis in neonates require longer lengths of therapy. Intravenous therapy should be given throughout the treatment course in an effort to maintain an adequate CSF concentration of antimicrobial in the face of decreasing inflammation.

Infected intraventricular or intravascular foreign bodies must be removed, in most cases, before the infection can be eradicated. If the removal of a CSF shunt is impossible or inadvisable, intraventricular (or intrashunt) antimicrobials should be added.

A subsequent lumbar puncture is not necessary for most cases of bacterial meningitis, particularly if the patient is showing a good clinical response. The lumbar puncture should be repeated, however, if the initial diagnosis is unclear, if the clinical response to therapy seems inadequate, or there is the suggestion of a possible relapse of infection. The CSF should be re-evaluated when the meningitis is caused by a gram-negative bacilli or *Listeria,* which entails ensurance of CSF sterilization after 24 to 48 hours of therapy to assess the need for additional therapeutic modalities.

## Adjunctive and Supportive Therapy

The pathophysiology of brain injury and neuronal death in bacterial meningitis involves a combination of altered cerebral metabolism, cerebral edema, increased intracranial pressure, decreased cerebral blood flow, altered cerebrospinal fluid dynamics, and leukocyte-mediated injury to neuronal tissue.

Tissue damage may also occur after the initiation of appropriate antimicrobial therapy. Therapy usually involves a β-lactam antimicrobial, resulting in rapid bacterial lysis and death. Enhanced inflammation contributes to the inherent morbidity and mortality of disease.

There should be frequent physical examinations to assess for evidence of cerebral edema, which necessitates the usage of osmotic agents and controlled ventilation. Fluid volume should be restored and restricted to approximately two-thirds of the daily requirements, with careful monitoring of daily input and output, body weights, and electrolyte levels in an effort to prevent syndrome of inappropriate antidiuretic hormone. The patient should receive nothing by mouth for the first 48 hours to prevent aspirations. The administration of vasopressors and ventilatory support may be required. Seizures may occur because of cerebral cortical irritation or ischemia, especially within the first 48 hours, requiring anticonvulsants. A cranial CT scan should be performed in individuals with recurrent or persistent seizures, evidence of increased intracranial pressure, persistently bulging fontanelles, or prolonged fever. Recent studies suggest that, although controversial, dexamethasone

TABLE 6. **Postexposure Prophylaxis for Bacterial Meningitis of Close Contacts and Index Cases***

|  | Children | | Adults |
|---|---|---|---|
|  | <1 mo | 1 mo–12 yr |  |
| *N. meningitidis* |  |  |  |
|   Rifampin | 5 mg/kg q 12 hr for 4 doses | 10 mg/kg q 12 hr for 4 doses | 600 mg q 12 hr for 4 doses |
|   Sulfadiazine† | 500 mg once/day for 2 days | 500 mg q 12 hr for 4 doses | 1 gram q 12 hr for 4 doses |
| *H. influenzae* |  |  |  |
|   Rifampin | 10 mg/kg once/day for 4 days | 20 mg/kg once/day for 4 days (maximum 600 mg/day) | 600 mg once/day for 4 days |

*Note: The meningococcal vaccine and the *H. influenzae* Type b vaccines should not be used in place of chemoprophylaxis.
†Sulfadiazine should only be used if the organism is known to be susceptible to sulfa.

(Decadron) decreases cytokine and prostaglandin production, as well as inflammation, reducing morbidity, mortality, and sequelae. I would suggest the addition of dexamethasone in children and in severely ill adults with altered mental status and evidence of increased intracranial pressure.

One should carefully evaluate for a predisposing source. X-ray films of the paranasal sinuses and mastoids and CT scans are obtained when there are focal neurologic deficits, which may require surgical drainage.

## RECURRENT MENINGITIS

The incidence of recurrent meningitis is not known. However, this condition is most often associated with congenital, traumatic, and surgical CSF fistulas and immunodeficiency (Table 5). A congenital communication to the middle ear is the most frequently recognized defect. Deafness, CSF otorrhea, and bulging of the tympanic membrane with an air-fluid level may be clues to the diagnosis. Congenital basiethmoid or cribriform plate defects and dermal sinus tracts should also be considered in the setting of recurrent meningitis. Radioisotope studies, polytomography, and CT are often helpful diagnostic studies. Cases of immunodeficiencies have included deficiencies of single components of complement (C2, C5, C6, C7, C8), as well as combinations (C3, C4, C9, factor B, and properdin), IgG2 deficiency, and lymphoma with asplenia. There should also be a thorough search for a parameningeal focus of infection that may require surgical drainage.

Recurrent meningitis has been largely due to *S. pneumoniae*, followed by *H. influenzae* and *Neisseria meningitidis*. Congenital, traumatic, and surgical fistulas should be repaired surgically after the infection has been treated medically. There are no controlled studies demonstrating the efficacy of immunoglobulin preparations, vaccine immunizations, or prophylactic antibiotics. However, in cases resulting from immunodeficiency and non–surgically correctable defects, polyvalent pneumococcal and meningococcal vaccines should be offered, as well as low-dose penicillin prophylaxis.

## PREVENTION OF MENINGITIS

Patients with undiagnosed cases of meningitis should be placed in respiratory isolation until a firm diagnosis has been established or until meningococcal or *H. influenzae* meningitis has been treated for at least 24 hours. Secondary cases of meningococcal and *H. influenzae* meningitis may result from close exposure to an index case.

Postexposure chemoprophylaxis is recommended for close contacts of an index case of meningococcal meningitis (Table 6). Close contact is defined as household members, nursery school and day care attendees, roommates, boyfriend or girlfriend, nursing home residents, members of closed populations such as military recruits living in the same barracks, and medical personnel who have mouth-to-mouth contact or direct contact with respiratory aerosols of the index case. Secondary cases may occur within 1 week (usually within 30 days) of the index case. Thus, close contacts of index cases should be identified and prophylaxis instituted without delay, with the intent of eradicating the nasopharyngeal and oropharyngeal carriage of the organism. Rifampin is the prophylactic agent of choice, unless the organism is known to be susceptible to sulfa. The quadrivalent meningococcal vaccine may not be adequate for prophylaxis against secondary cases, as it does not provide protective antibody soon enough. To eliminate the nasopharyngeal or oropharyngeal carriage of the organism in the index case, rifampin, as recommended for prophylaxis, should be administered at the end of therapy.

Rifampin is also the prophylactic agent of choice to prevent secondary cases of meningitis as a result of *H. influenzae* exposure and should be administered to all household contacts and siblings younger than 4 years old (Table 6). The index case should also receive this prophylactic regimen prior to the completion of therapy.

Although colonization has been documented with other microorganisms associated with meningitis, the risk for infection and transmission has not been established.

# INFECTIOUS MONONUCLEOSIS

method of
CIRO V. SUMAYA, M.D., M.P.H.T.M.
*University of Texas Health Science Center*
*San Antonio, Texas*

Infectious mononucleosis (IM) is the prototype primary symptomatic infection produced by the Epstein-Barr virus (EBV). Most infections by this virus in early childhood are usually asymptomatic, whereas primary infections not occurring until adulthood are more likely to be manifested as IM. IM is diagnosed by a triad of characteristic clinical, hematologic, and serologic findings. The typical clinical manifestations include fever, malaise, cervical lymphadenitis, tonsillopharyngitis, and splenic and/or liver enlargement. Children, particularly the very young, may present with some other findings, including failure to thrive or increased rates of skin rashes, abdominal pain, and associated upper respiratory tract infections. Minimal hematologic features include a relative lymphocytosis and the presence of atypical lymphocytes equal to or greater than 10% of the leukocytes. The serologic findings include a positive typical heterophil antibody test (rapid slide test), although this antibody response often is undetectable in children less than 4 years of age. A heterophil antibody also may not be detectable (1) early in the disease course; (2) at any time during the course of about 5 to 10% of otherwise classic episodes of IM in adults; (3) and in IM or IM-like episodes due to other etiologic agents such as cytomegalovirus, *Toxoplasma gondii*, and possibly others. In these cases, the determination of EBV-specific antibody titers may be required to make a satisfactory diagnosis. EBV-specific serologic testing also may be useful to identify EBV infections that instead of producing an IM picture are associated with isolated manifestations such as those affecting the neurologic system (meningoencephalitis, Bell's palsy), hematologic system (thrombocytopenia, aplastic anemia), or liver (hepatitis). It is believed that EBV enters the human body through exchange of saliva that harbors the virus. After IM or other forms of primary EBV infection, clinical or subclinical, a lifelong infection of the body's B lymphocytes by the virus regularly ensues. The latent state in peripheral blood B lymphocytes appears to persist because of the continual production of virus in oropharyngeal epithelium. The high rate (75% or more) of secretion of EBV in oropharyngeal salival secretions in children and adults with acute IM declines only minimally over the following months. Actually, at any time approximately 6 to 16% of seropositive adults and a lower number of seropositive children in the general population have detectable EBV in oropharyngeal salivary secretions. The role that this high, prolonged, and presumably intermittent incidence of virus excretion plays in transmission of infections is unclear, but current data indicate that the transmission rate even among susceptibles—i.e., nonimmunes—is relatively low. IM also occurs uncommonly among intimate contacts of an index case, except possibly in young family member contacts. And even in the latter setting, the development of subsequent IM episodes in family members may be months to years later, suggesting a familial susceptibility to this disease but not necessarily a relation to viral transmission from the index case. The transmission of EBV via blood products occurs but at a much lower rate than that attributed to cytomegalovirus. Several months should elapse before an individual with IM donates blood. Isolation of the patient with acute IM is not required.

## COMPLICATIONS

Acute IM is self-limiting in almost all cases, with patients recovering in 2 to 4 weeks. Complications, however, may develop early or late in the disease course. Fortunately, these complications are usually short in duration and seldom produce permanent sequelae.

**Respiratory.** Upper airway obstruction from tonsillar enlargement and generalized airway inflammation may be a life-threatening complication. An interstitial pneumonitis occurs in a small percentage of cases and more so in young children.

**Neurologic.** Encephalitis, aseptic meningitis, Guillain-Barré syndrome, Bell's palsy, optic neuritis, transverse myelitis, and psychosis have been reported. Sometimes these neurologic manifestations may occur very early in the course and be so prominent that they obscure the diagnosis of IM.

**Splenic Rupture.** Splenic rupture should be considered whenever abdominal pain accompanies IM. It is a rare complication (0.2% of adult patients) but may be life-threatening. Splenic rupture is most commonly noted in the second or third week of illness and may occur without any apparent trauma.

**Hematologic.** Thrombocytopenia, granulocytopenia, and, less frequently, autoimmune hemolytic anemia may accompany IM. The thrombocytopenia may be profound and lead to hemorrhaging. Despite the common occurrence of granulocytopenia, including values for segmented band forms of neutrophils of less than 500 per mm³, significant bacterial superinfections are uncommon.

**Hepatic.** Liver transaminase levels are commonly elevated, although not reaching the values usually seen with hepatitis A and B infections. Jaundice is an uncommon manifestation, occurring in less than 5% of cases.

**Chronic EBV Disease.** On rare occasions, patients may suffer a severe, persistent, and apparently EBV-induced disease that may consist of pancytopenia, significant lymphadenopathy, pneumonitis, immunoglobulin disturbances, fever, hepatitis, and widespread lymphoproliferative lesions. Antibodies to EBV antigens of the replicative cycle (viral capsid and early) are extremely elevated, whereas the response to EBV nuclear antigen is low or absent. The course may eventuate in death. This clinical entity is distinct from the currently popularized illness characterized predominantly by a prolonged fatigue syndrome associated with multiple symptoms (subjective fever, sore throat, painful lymph nodes, neuropsychological abnormalities) but few if any objective physical findings. It is now theorized that the mildly unusual EBV serum antibody profile, as well as increased serum antibody responses to other viruses, found in patients with chronic fatigue syndrome is an epiphenomenon reflecting the underlying general immunologic aberration that exists. It is important to search for identifiable and treatable diseases that may appear as chronic fatigue syndrome.

**Lymphoproliferative Complications in the Immunocompromised Host.** Although IM and other EBV infections in immunocompromised patients in general run a course similar to that in immunocompetent individuals, there is some greater risk for the development of significant lymphoproliferative lesions. An X-linked lymphoproliferative syndrome characterized by a combined variable immunodeficiency and vulnerability to severe EBV infections has been described in young males. In these patients, the primary EBV infection may produce fatal IM, acquired agammaglobulinemia, aplastic anemia, or malignant B cell lymphomas. Patients with other immunodeficiencies as recent recipients of transplants or those with acquired immunodeficiency such as AIDS may develop EBV-associated lymphoproliferative disorders including fatal B cell lymphomas.

## TREATMENT

Symptomatic or supportive measures are the cornerstone of management of uncomplicated IM. Reduction of activity and bed rest usually are dictated by the tolerance of the patient. Contact sports should be avoided during the acute phase and probably throughout the time the spleen is palpable—i.e., clinically enlarged. Corticosteroids are not recommended for routine IM because there is no clear evidence that any benefit is gained. It is probably appropriate to administer corticosteroids to very ill patients or to those with significant manifestations such as severe thrombocytopenia, airway obstruction, and neurologic or other systemic complications. In these cases, corticosteroids in doses equivalent to 60 to 80 mg of prednisone per day can be given intravenously or orally with tapering to complete the therapy over 5 to 14 days. It is important to realize, though, that there is no clear evidence that corticosteroids are beneficial in the management of these complications. Moreover, careful consideration should be given to the potential side effects of corticosteroid administration, including bacterial superinfection. Acyclovir (Zovirax) produces no apparent modification of the clinical course of uncomplicated IM, although it does reduce viral shedding from salival secretions. The intravenous administration of this drug (1500 mg per M² per day divided in three daily doses) to patients with severe, life-threatening forms of IM or other forms of EBV infections has yielded equivocal results. This therapy is given for a variable duration (5 to 14 days), taking into account the presence of a therapeutic response. Interestingly, the use of acyclovir therapy has been associated at times with a regression and apparent resolution of EBV-related lymphoproliferative lesions and possibly even lymphomas in renal transplant recipients. Recent reports of the clinical efficacy of therapeutic agents as metronidazole (Flagyl), tinidazole,* and cimetidine (Tagamet) for IM require greater scrutiny and evaluation before their general use can be advocated.

The insertion of an artificial airway appears to be replacing emergency tonsillectomy as the treatment necessary for complete airway obstruction produced by profound upper respiratory tract inflammation. There is evidence, albeit mainly anecdotal, that the use of corticosteroids for imminent airway obstruction from progressively increasing tonsillar and oropharyngeal inflamma-

* Not available in the United States.

tion may eliminate or reduce the subsequent need for these emergency invasive procedures. Nonoperative management of splenic rupture in IM patients has been reported. Patients with streptococcus group A–positive throat cultures should be treated with penicillin or erythromycin (for penicillin-allergic patients).

There is limited interest for the development of a vaccine against EBV.

# MUMPS

method of
GARRETT ADAMS, M.D., M.P.H.
*University of Louisville School of Medicine*
*Louisville, Kentucky*

Classic mumps is acute parotitis due to infection with mumps virus, a paramyxovirus. Transmission of virus by respiratory secretions to susceptible individuals results in late winter and spring outbreaks. Communicability occurs from 1 or 2 days (up to 7) before parotid swelling to 5 days (up to 9) after its onset. Patients should be isolated for the usual period of communicability. The incubation period is usually 16 to 18 days (range, 12 to 25 days) from exposure. During epidemics, infection in symptomatic patients is easily recognized by swelling of one or more salivary glands accompanied by glandular pain when salivation is stimulated; however, 25 to 50% of infected patients are asymptomatic. Elevated serum amylase values may be seen. Laboratory confirmation may be made by recovery of virus from saliva, urine, or CSF, and demonstration of a fourfold increase in antibody levels between acute and convalescent serum samples. Because infection confers permanent immunity, recurrent parotitis probably does not represent recurrent mumps infection. Parainfluenza virus and other agents also cause parotitis.

## TREATMENT

There is no specific treatment for mumps infection. Adequate fluids and nutrition should be provided. Mumps hyperimmune serum is not recommended and is no longer available.

## COMPLICATIONS

Mumps infection involves many organs of the body, including the meninges. Viral meningitis may occur before, during, after, or in the absence of glandular swelling. Without appropriate viral diagnostic studies, these infections might not be recognized to be caused by mumps virus. Aseptic meningitis in the late winter and early spring is most likely due to mumps. Most cases of mumps meningitis are manifested by headache for a day or two and respond to rest and supportive care. Mumps encephalitis is more severe and has a worse prognosis; however, the treatment remains supportive. Transverse myelitis has also been reported. Transient acute sensorineural hearing loss, especially of higher tone frequency, has been reported in 4% of adults with mumps.

Orchitis occurs in up to 38% of postpubertal males. In the case of unilateral orchitis, sterility is not a concern but it can occur rarely following bilateral orchitis. Analgesics and physical support of the testes are recommended. Application of ice may also be helpful. The value of steroid use is unknown. Rarely, nerve blocks for pain relief and incision of the tunica albuginea to relieve swelling have been used. Oophoritis and mastitis are reported in postpubertal females. Myocarditis, pancreatitis, diabetes mellitus, nephritis, arthritis, and thyroiditis are other rare complications of mumps infection.

## PREVENTION

Prevention is available by immunization with an attenuated live viral vaccine usually combined with measles and rubella (MMR) and administered at 15 months of age. The vaccine strain used in the United States, the Jeryl Lynn strain, has an excellent safety record, unlike the Urabe strain of mumps virus used in Canada and Europe (not in the U.S.), which has been associated with cases of postvaccinal mumps meningitis. However, vaccine efficacy studies in the U.S. have demonstrated failure rates of 9 to 25%. Nevertheless, widespread use of mumps vaccine in the United States has reduced mumps incidence by 98%. There has recently been a relative resurgence of mumps, particularly in adolescents and young adults who represent a cohort of individuals not vaccinated in infancy. These new cases are due, not to vaccine failure, but to failure to vaccinate. Mumps vaccine should be given to all persons (pregnancy excluded) without documentation of (1) physician-diagnosed mumps, (2) immunization with live mumps vaccine after 12 months of age, or (3) laboratory evidence of immunity. Because serologic testing is inconvenient and there is no harm in giving vaccine to an immune individual, if previous immunization or infection is in doubt, as a practical policy immunization is usually given without prior antibody testing. For example, a father whose child has mumps but who is unsure of his immune status could be given mumps vaccine without testing. He should understand that the immunization would probably not provide immunity soon enough to prevent infection from the current exposure, but it would prevent future infection.

There is evidence that use of mumps vaccine during outbreaks may contribute to outbreak control. Mumps immunity in the future will be further bolstered by the new recommendation for a measles vaccine booster to be given as MMR around 12 years of age.

Note that infection with human immunodeficiency virus (HIV) is not a contraindication for MMR vaccine. HIV-infected patients may have severe measles if they become infected without the benefit of immunization.

# PLAGUE

method of
FREDERICK KOSTER, M.D.
*University of New Mexico School of Medicine
Albuquerque, New Mexico*

Plague is the clinical infection with the encapsulated gram-negative bacterium *Yersinia pestis*, acquired incidentally by humans during the natural flea-animal-flea-humans transmission cycle. Plague is a worldwide disease but uncommon in the United States. In the fourteenth century, a quarter of the population of Europe died during epidemics of the "Black Death" in both urban and rural areas where rats provided an abundant animal reservoir for the infected fleas. The disease is now transmitted in rural areas by fleas infecting wild rodents and other animals such as rabbits and prairie dogs. In the United States most of the cases occur in New Mexico, with sporadic cases in California, Colorado, Arizona, Utah, and Oregon. When the disease occurs in endemic locations, it is frequently recognized and treated promptly and appropriately, but when patients acquire the disease in the western United States and travel to other areas before the manifestations have appeared, physicians may not recognize the possibility of plague, resulting in inappropriate or tardy treatment. The majority of cases are acquired by people whose occupation brings them in contact with infected animals or through hunting and recreational activities. Areas with abandoned autos, old tires, and wood piles provide shelter for rodents, which bring infected fleas closer to rural homes. When domestic pets living in rural or semirural areas come into contact with dead or ill flea-infected animals infected with plague, the fleas may be brought home and subsequently infect humans. It remains possible that urban epidemics could still appear since urban rat populations have occasionally been found to be infected with the organism. At present, males and females are about equally infected, and about 60% of cases occur in individuals who are less than 20 years of age.

### CLINICAL MANIFESTATIONS

The primary challenge in making the diagnosis is to first consider the possibility of plague in the differential diagnosis. A history of possible exposure in endemic areas is usually present. Usually the exposure occurs 2 to 7 days before the patient seeks medical attention. Plague presents in three ways: bubonic, septicemic, and primary pneumonic plague. In addition to fever, 85 to 90% of the infected people have a bubo, a painful lymphadenopathy, often with surrounding edema and erythema. Inguinal-femoral nodes are most commonly involved, but axillary, cervical, epitrochlear, and other nodes can be infected depending on the site of the flea bite. Single node involvement is most common, but multiple nodes may be found, and this indicates a poorer prognosis. A history of a flea bite, or the evidence of the flea bite, is usually absent. About 10 to 15% of patients have septicemic plague, in which no lymphadenopathy is detected on initial examination but blood cultures are positive. These patients present only with systemic symptoms, including fever, malaise, nausea, vomiting, diarrhea, or shock. Cough, pulmonary infiltrates, or mediastinal lymphadenopathy occurs in approximately 10% of patients, and this is usually considered to be pneumonia secondary to plague elsewhere in the body. In 1% of cases, plague can be acquired from aerosol spread of the organism and be a primary infection in the lung. Primary pneumonic plague usually has an extremely rapid course with death in 2 to 3 days.

The characteristic bubo is usually obvious, but at times there may be no bubo or it may simply be missed on physical examination when a high level of suspicion is not maintained. An initial rapid diagnosis may be made by aspirating the bubo under strict precautions with personnel wearing masks and avoiding aerosolization of the aspirate. Bacteriologic stains using the Gram or preferably the Wayson method may show organisms with characteristic bipolar staining resembling a safety pin. However, a fluorescent antibody stain is more satisfactory and can usually be performed on an emergent basis through state public health laboratories. Aspirated material should be cultured, and at least two blood cultures should be obtained. The laboratory should be informed that plague is suspected so that lab personnel may protect themselves and perform the appropriate stains. Blood cultures are positive in about 80% of cases and may become positive after only 2 to 3 days of incubation. The level of bacteremia may be so high that organisms can be seen microscopically in a Giemsa stain of the blood smear. Diseases that similarly present with buboes and systemic signs of toxicity include streptococcal or staphylococcal lymphadenitis, tularemia, incarcerated inguinal hernia, acute appendicitis, cat-scratch fever, and sepsis of unknown origin. Some of these potential diagnoses could lead to therapy that is inappropriate for plague. Serologic diagnostic techniques are readily available and accurate, but the tests do not become positive until the second week of illness and thus are not useful as a guide for initial therapy.

## TREATMENT

Untreated bubonic plague has a mortality rate of approximately 50%. Moreover, bubonic plague may progress rapidly over 1 to 2 days to septicemic plague with secondary pneumonia and a higher mortality rate. Thus, treatment must begin as soon as possible, usually before a definite diagnosis has been made. First, the patient should be strictly isolated by mask, gown, and glove barriers worn by health care personnel. Isolation should be maintained for 48 hours in the absence of signs of pulmonary involvement and for 96 hours in the presence of pneumonic disease. All cases of plague must be reported immediately to the state public health authorities so that contact tracing may be done (see below).

Streptomycin remains the drug of choice for treatment of all types of plague because of extensive successful experience. Although no in vivo studies exist to confirm equal efficacy of gentamicin, in vitro studies and some clinical experience suggest that gentamicin is probably equally effective and could be used for presumptive treatment of bacterial sepsis if plague is in the differential diagnosis. In addition, if the patient is in shock and the absorption of intramuscular drug is in doubt, the use of intravenous gentamicin (Garamycin) is preferable. The dose of streptomycin is 30 mg per kg per day given intramuscularly in two divided doses for 10 days. Toxicity from streptomycin in the treatment of plague is rarely seen, but in pregnant women and in the elderly with pre-existing auditory or vestibular disease, it may be desirable to avoid streptomycin. In milder cases of bubonic plague, streptomycin treatment can be shortened to 3 to 5 days if the fever and all systemic signs have disappeared. A 10-day course of antibiotic treatment can be completed using oral tetracycline, 15 mg per kg per day in four divided doses, except in children in whom tetracycline will stain developing teeth. When meningitis is suspected or proved or when abscesses or unusual locations are involved, chloramphenicol should be given because it crosses the blood-brain barrier and penetrates into all tissue sites and abscesses. Trimethoprim-sulfamethoxazole (Bactrim) may also be effective. Antibiotic treatment is continued for a minimum of 10 days, and longer in occasional cases, because small numbers of organisms may persist in large buboes. Relapse of plague meningitis has been reported. Superinfection of buboes with other organisms can occur and may require reaspiration for diagnostic purposes and subsequent change of antibiotics to treat the responsible organisms. Occasionally, large abscessed buboes need to be incised and drained if severe local pain persists. Antibiotic sensitivity tests should not be used as a guide for antibiotic treatment. While Y. pestis is often reported as being sensitive to ampicillin, penicillins and cephalosporins are ineffective in vivo.

## PREVENTION

The best way to prevent plague is to avoid situations where it may be acquired. Exposure may be subtle and difficult to avoid, however, since even a stroll through a prairie dog colony may result in infection. Persons in endemic areas should avoid wild rodents and carnivores, especially carcasses during summer. Children should be taught not to handle such carcasses. Persons whose houses are in rural or semirural locations in endemic areas should take measures to remove potential rodent food and habitats from around their houses. Appropriate measures should be taken to control fleas on household pets. A vaccine is available and has been shown to reduce the frequency and severity of plague and may be indicated for individuals whose occupation places them at high risk for the disease.

People who have been exposed to a patient with proven plague are at increased risk by two mechanisms. Household contacts may have about a 5% chance of developing plague, which is probably flea-borne. Aerosolized organisms during diagnostic studies are a risk to health care and laboratory workers. Household contacts and people who have been in a waiting room with a patient who has a cough and pulmonary infiltrates due to plague are also exposed to aerosolized organisms. A common practice is to treat such high-risk contacts with tetracycline (15 mg per kg per day) or a sulfonamide (40 mg per kg per day) for 5 to 7 days.

# PSITTACOSIS
(Ornithosis)

method of
JULIUS SCHACHTER, Ph.D.
*University of California, San Francisco*
*San Francisco, California*

Psittacosis is a chlamydial infection contracted by humans through exposure to infected avian species. The term psittacosis is also applied to chlamydial infection of psittacine species (parrots and related birds), whereas the term ornithosis is used for chlamydial infection of other avian species (such as turkeys, pigeons, etc.). The causative agent, *Chlamydia psittaci,* is an obligate intracellular bacterium. Infected birds shed the organism in their feces, and human infection usually results from aerosolization of the fecal material. The incubation period for humans is generally 1 to 2 weeks. Onset may be either acute or insidious. There are two forms of human psittacosis. In one, pneumonitis or atypical pneumonia is the predominant finding. The second form is associated with a toxic or almost septic condition in which neither pneumonic findings nor symptoms are prominent. Fever and chills are almost always present. Severe headache is very common, as is a nonproductive cough. Splenomegaly is a frequent finding. Often there are radiologic findings of considerable pneumonitis in the total absence of any signs of respiratory distress. Marked leukopenia is found in approximately 25% of cases. Prior to the introduction of antibiotics, case fatality rates often exceeded 20%. Seroepidemiologic studies have found that subclinical infections are common.

## DIAGNOSIS

The organisms to be considered in the differential diagnosis would be other causes of atypical pneumonia. The major pathogens include *Mycoplasma pneumoniae, Coxiella burnetii,* and influenza virus. Typhoid should be considered in the differential diagnosis of the toxic form. The physician's index of suspicion is often crucial in determining a diagnosis, and patients with atypical pneumonia should be questioned concerning avian contact.

Although chlamydial infection in birds can be severe and fatal, it is well known that asymptomatic shedders can be a source of human disease. Most cases of human psittacosis have been due to exposure to pet birds, but the disease is recognized to be an occupational hazard in the poultry industry. In the United States, turkeys are an important reservoir, and they have been a common source of outbreaks as a result of processing infected flocks. In Europe the duck appears to be the major reservoir.

A newly described chlamydial species, *C. pneumoniae* (formerly called TWAR agents), is also recognized to be a cause of pneumonitis. This organism has no known animal reservoir and appears to depend on person-to-person transmission. Seroprevalence rates indicate infection is very common, starting early in childhood and reaching levels as high as 45% of the adult population. Infection with either species can result in induction of high complement-fixing (CF) antibodies to the chlamydial genus-specific CF antigen. More specific tests are required to distinguish among these infections.

Diagnosis of psittacosis is usually made by serology. A fourfold rise in antibody titer by CF or microimmunofluorescence test (this test is an indirect fluorescent antibody test using chlamydial elementary bodies as antigen) is considered diagnostic. A CF titer of 1:32 or greater in a patient with symptoms consistent with psittacosis is considered suggestive. Antibodies to *C. psittaci* are usually elevated within 2 weeks of infection; those with *C. pneumoniae* may take 4 weeks. Isolation of *C. psittaci* requires the use of living cells (cell culture or embryonated hens' eggs or mice). This procedure is not recommended, as *C. psittaci* has been a common cause of laboratory infections.

## TREATMENT

Tetracyclines are considered the drugs of choice for chlamydial infection. For psittacosis the usual recommendation is 2 grams a day for at least 2 weeks. Erythromycin should be used for treatment of pregnant women or children less than 9 years of age. Response to therapy is often rapid, but it can be slow. Treatment should be continued for at least 1 week—perhaps 14 days after disappearance of fever. Early cessation of therapy often results in relapse. Rifampin* is the most active antibiotic in vitro, but there is relatively little experience with its use in clinical settings.

There is no indication for isolation of patients with *C. psittaci* infection. Although person-to-person transmission has been reported, it is uncommon. Psittacosis is reportable.

## PREVENTION

Infected avian sources should be identified. If a single bird is involved, medicated feed can be given to it. If the bird is recently acquired from a pet shop, the pet shop should be quarantined. All birds on the premises should be appropriately treated. If exposure has been through poultry, it may be necessary to investigate the relevant farm and initiate mass therapy of birds. Other humans who may have had similar exposure to the infected premises should be closely monitored.

Because virtually all species of birds harbor *C. psittaci* there is no practical approach to control infections from sources other than pet birds. Feral birds can always introduce infections into poultry. Chlortetracycline-impregnated seeds or mashes are used to treat exotic pet birds being imported into the United States. These birds undergo a quarantine that is specifically directed against velogenic Newcastle disease virus and are coincidentally treated prophylactically for chlamydial infection. Thus there is no routine monitoring for either effective tetracycline blood levels or chlamydial infection. There are continued sources of human exposure. Typically 100 to 200 human cases are reported to the Centers for Disease Control each year.

# Q FEVER

method of
ALAN M. RAUCH, M.D.
*University of Texas Medical School*
*Houston, Texas*

Q fever is a zoonosis caused by the rickettsial organism *Coxiella burnetii*. *C. burnetii* is highly infectious, with a single inhaled organism able to cause clinical

infection. Infectious organisms are found in urine, feces, milk, and in greatest numbers in the products of conception (placenta, amniotic fluid, and fetal membranes) of infected animals. Q fever infection of humans usually occurs in individuals exposed to cattle, sheep, or goats; but other animal reservoirs, including cats and rodents, have been reported. The incubation period for Q fever ranges from 4 to 39 days.

Human Q fever infection is often mistaken for a viral illness and may be asymptomatic. Definitive diagnosis is made on the basis of serologic testing. Symptomatic Q fever generally presents as a febrile illness characterized by severe headache, with pneumonia or hepatitis as the predominant disease process. The disease is usually self-limited. However, chronic Q fever endocarditis, a potentially fatal condition, sometimes occurs in patients who have pre-existing valvular heart disease or prosthetic valves.

## TREATMENT

Owing to the severity of the headache typically associated with Q fever, analgesics are often required. Optimal antibiotic treatment for acute Q fever is not well defined, though numerous studies show that early treatment with appropriate antimicrobials reduces the severity and duration of illness. The most widely accepted therapy is with drugs of the tetracycline group, most often with doxycycline (Vibramycin), 100 mg every 12 hours, or tetracycline (Sumycin), 500 mg every 6 hours. Alternatively, patients have been successfully treated with standard doses of chloramphenicol (our preference in pediatric patients). Combination therapy with rifampin (Rifadin), 300 mg every 12 hours, and erythromycin is a reasonable approach in patients who have atypical pneumonia in whom Q fever is a diagnostic consideration. Trimethoprim-sulfamethoxazole (Bactrim, Septra), one double-strength tablet every 12 hours, may be considered in patients who are intolerant of the preceding therapies.

Diagnosis of chronic Q fever culture–negative endocarditis is based upon Phase I *C. burnetii* titers that are severalfold higher than Phase II titers, the inverse of what is seen in acute Q fever infection. Appropriate treatment for Q fever endocarditis remains controversial. Surgical resection of infected valvular lesions may be required. Long-term antibiotic therapy, often for periods of 2 years or longer, is required when medical management of this condition is successful. Various single and combination therapies have been used successfully in the medical management of Q fever endocarditis. The tetracycline family of drugs remains the mainstay of therapy; however, many drug regimens have been used in successful management of this condition, including trimethoprim-sulfamethoxazole in combina-

---

*This use of rifampin is not listed in the manufacturer's official directive.

tion with tetracycline, doxycycline, or rifampin in the dosages used for acute Q fever. Management of patients undergoing therapy for Q fever endocarditis requires regular monitoring of Phase I and Phase II titers, with declines in Phase I titers parallelling therapeutic efficacy.

## PREVENTION

Livestock used in research settings should be serologically screened for *C. burnetii* prior to being incorporated into research facilities. Animal research facilities should be isolated so that there is no exposure of patients to potentially infected animals. In addition, exposure of nonessential personnel to animal research facilities that use livestock should be restricted. People who have pre-existing anatomic cardiac lesions should be cautioned about the risk of of chronic Q fever following exposure to potentially infected livestock. Similarly, pregnant women should be cautioned, owing to the theoretical risk to the unborn fetus.

### Vaccination

A Phase I vaccine has been used successfully in Australia to protect individuals having occupational exposure to livestock. Currently a purified preparation of *C. burnetii* is being tested by U.S. Army researchers for potential use in vaccination and skin testing. Vaccination should be considered in individuals who are at high risk of infection, specifically persons who have occupational exposure to livestock and livestock products.

# RABIES*

method of
RICHARD E. WINN, M.D.
*David Grant Medical Center*
*Fairfield, California*

"Mad dog!" cried the panic-stricken townsperson, and the men ran for their guns as the women scurried to clear the streets of children. Although immortalized in books and movies of the Old West and into the twentieth century, this scenario was described as long ago as 2500 B.C. and continues today as a grisly part of life in many parts of the world. In the Middle East, where wolves contribute to human cases; in Mexico, where dogs most frequently cause disease; and in Asia, rabies

*The views expressed herein are those of the author and should not be construed as representing the views of the U.S. Army, the U.S. Air Force, or the Department of Defense.

is an accepted risk of daily living. As many as 20,000 deaths per year have been reported from India alone. In Latin and South America, deaths range from 600 to 1000 per year with the highest incidence in Ecuador. Underestimates of the true number of cases of rabies are commonplace, owing to inadequacies in case reporting in underdeveloped countries. Despite the extremely high death rate when clinical rabies occurs and the lack of specific treatment regimens, the real tragedy of human rabies is that it occurs at all, since effective prevention is available through passive and active immunization. In fact, not a single death from rabies has been documented when appropriately administered rabies immune globulin and rabies vaccine have been given.

## PATHOPHYSIOLOGY

Rabies in both animals and man is caused by a rhabdovirus. The virus is bullet-shaped when examined by electron microscopy. Propagation and transmission of the virus in nature are facilitated by the unique pairing of salivary excretion with neuroexcitatory biting behavior in the affected host.

After exposure to the virus, usually through a bite injury, a latent interval ensues (hours to weeks) wherein the microorganism persists in the muscle cell or soft tissue or replicates locally. Following this latent period, the rabies virus invades the peripheral nerves and ascends to the central nervous system. Once in the central nervous system, spread of the virus throughout the brain is rapid and thorough. Afterward, progression of virus occurs centrifugally, and the highest concentrations of virus are in areas that are richly innervated such as the cornea, skin of the head and neck, and the buccal cavity, among others. High viral concentrations occur in the saliva by way of efferent secretory nerves in acinar salivary cells and are usually maximal at the time of host behaviors that ensure transmission to another host.

Host viral transport is virtually solely accomplished through nervous tissue; no substantial viremia has been detected.

Structurally, the glycoprotein of the rabies virus appears to be the major determinant of neuroinvasiveness. Viral transport appears to be critically dependent on an intact neuronal microtubulin network; disruptions produced experimentally interdict viral progression.

Both gross and histologic central nervous system abnormalities are remarkable for their relative infrequency. Inflammatory reaction is notably minimal in areas where Negri bodies (intracytoplasmic inclusions of rabies ribonucleoprotein), the pathognomonic histologic finding of rabies, are found. Most recently, spongiform encephalopathy has been observed in experimentally induced rabies lesions.

During the period of viral latency, clinical rabies may be prevented through the use of immunization; however, once the virus gains access to the peripheral nerves, death is a virtual certainty. The usual cause of death is respiratory failure or hemodynamic collapse.

## EPIDEMIOLOGY

Rabies is prevalent in most of the world, but there are several island countries, particularly in the Pacific, as well as parts of Europe, the Americas, and Asia, where rabies has been prevented or has been eradicated through assiduous quarantine practices and animal control programs. In India, Iran, and many Third World countries, rabies remains in epidemic proportions in animal populations with spillover to the local populace directly or through intermediate domestic animal vectors.

In the United States, until the mid-twentieth century, most cases of human rabies were attributed to domestic dog exposures. In 1960 wild animal rabies exposures surpassed domestic animal exposures as causes of human disease. Owing to an intense education program and mandatory domestic animal vaccination program, rabies from domestic animals has been practically eliminated. Since 1980 the number of human cases reported to the Centers for Disease Control has averaged one per year.

Worldwide there are numerous different wild animal hosts for rabies (donkeys, camels, wolves, vampire bats). In the United States, skunks, raccoons, bats, and foxes account for greater than 90% of cases. Since 1980, cats, cattle, and dogs have been responsible for most domestic animal rabies cases. Since the 1970s there has been a dramatic increase in the prevalence of wild animal rabies in the U.S. primarily due to four separate epizootics, two involving skunks and two involving raccoons. Rabies is now rampant in skunks in the North Central and South Central states while raccoon rabies affects West Virginia and Virginia. A further raccoon epizootic began in the southeastern U.S. and has spread to the Middle and South Atlantic states. This second raccoon epizootic appears to have been spread by importation of infected raccoons from the southeast. Control of the feral rabies problem is aggravated by several factors including prolonged incubation times in wild animals and unpredictable response to vaccines and impracticality of their administration in wild animal populations. Recent investigations into field trials of oral rabies vaccines appear promising as initial approaches to the problem. The use of anticoagulants has had some impact on vampire bat populations in Central and South America.

## CLINICAL HUMAN RABIES

Although documented transmission of rabies has occurred through mucosal exposure (licks, conjunctiva), inhalation (laboratory, bat cave aerosols), and tissue transplantation (corneal transplant), the most frequent exposure is from a biting injury. The incubation period after exposure is variable and depends on several factors:

1. The site of the bite, with proximity to the head shortening the time period.

2. Severity of the bite (correlates with the viral inoculum).

3. Viral strain (virulence).

4. Host age/immunologic status, with children being at risk for a shortened interval.

5. Previous vaccination status.

There are limited data suggesting that incomplete immunization may accelerate the incubation period. In general, the usual range for the incubation period is 18 to 78 days (99% within 1 year). If the bite is on the head, the incubation period is usually less than 50 days and can be as short as 2 1/2 weeks. The incubation times of bites on the extremities range from 6 weeks to 78 days.

Clinical rabies most commonly is divisible into three phases: the prodrome, the acute neurologic period (furious or agitated type), and the paralytic phase (dumb rabies).

The prodrome may be preceded or accompanied by paresthesias or pain at the inoculation site. Itching was an early symptom in many cases observed in Thailand. Excoriation of skin may result from frenetic scratching attempts. Retro-ocular pain occurred in the majority of patients with rabies secondary to corneal transplant. Nonspecific prodromal symptoms consist of fatigue, sore throat, anorexia, headache, fever, cough, and gastrointestinal discomfort with nausea, vomiting, or diarrhea. They usually last from 2 to 10 days.

During the acute neurologic period, the "classic" manifestations of rabies are observed, including hydrophobia, aerophobia, choking behavior, and drooling, owing to difficulty swallowing (laryngeal and diaphragmatic spasm). Patients may experience marked anxiety, terror, or excitement early in the course, progressing to frank disorientation, meningeal irritation, hypertension, and seizures. Hyperesthesia is common; priapism and recurrent ejaculation have been described as initial signs. Paroxysms of hydrophobia or aerophobia may be precipitated by the mere sight of water or hearing a fan. Muscle fasciculations, hyperventilation, diplopia, and photophobia may also be witnessed.

The paralytic phase may follow the acute neurologic period, although it may occur as the initial phase following the prodrome in 70% of cases. Paralysis may be ascending, symmetric, or asymmetric usually leading to a decline in mental status to coma.

Initial enthusiasm for intensive care support of rabies has been tempered by a dismal outcome. Although patients may be managed through a wide array of complications such as adult respiratory distress syndrome (ARDS), hypothermia, myocarditis, and diabetes insipidus, disease progression has been relentless, and despite prolongation of life (up to 133 days), death has been universal owing to cardiac arrest or arrhythmia. Heavy sedation is often required to relieve pain and anxiety. The mean interval from onset of clinical rabies to death is 10 days.

Only three individuals have recovered from carefully documented rabies infections. All three received either pre- or postexposure prophylaxis before the onset of clinical disease. Interferon and ribavirin have prolonged life, but no cures have been effected.

## LABORATORY DIAGNOSIS

Laboratory abnormalities of routine chemistries, blood counts, cerebrospinal fluid, and arterial blood gases are nonspecific and variable.

Diagnosis depends on direct analysis of brain tissue in animals. Negri bodies are present in 80% of nerve tissues examined. Culture of saliva or brain homogenates can be performed in weanling mice. Negri bodies are usually seen in necropsy specimens of mouse brain.

Antemortem human diagnosis may be made using serum-neutralizing antibodies (SNA). These antibodies usually develop 7 to 10 days after clinical infection. Measurements of SNA can be performed by using indirect fluorescence, by rabies fluorescent focus inhibition testing (RFFIT), immunoadherence hemagglutination (IAHA), or dot immunobinding. The "gold standard" appears to be the RFFIT, which is used in most state reference laboratories. The IAHA test gives similar results to the RFFIT but can be performed rapidly (24 hours), is inexpensive relative to RFFIT, and may be performed on less-sophisticated equipment. Dot immunobinding uses inactivated antigen and also yields results comparable to the RFFIT. In the presence of encephalopathy, the presence of measured cerebrospinal fluid (CSF) rabies antibody is highly suggestive of infection.

Rabies antigen testing can also be performed by fluorescent staining of tissue obtained from buccal mucosa, corneal touch impressions, or the skin. Saliva may also be examined. Corneal impressions may be positive for antigen before the development of SNA. Skin biopsies are usually taken from the hair-covered areas of the neck or scalp where hair follicles are richly innervated. These areas also may be positive before SNA appear. It is emphasized that these areas will be free of antigen during the incubation period.

## TREATMENT

There is no specific therapy for clinical rabies. Interferon and antiviral drugs have been tried without success. Corticosteroids have been unsuccessful and may compromise development of neutralizing antibodies.

Postexposure prophylaxis using both rabies immune globulin and vaccine is efficacious at preventing clinical disease when used appropriately in the incubation period. All deaths following postexposure prophylaxis have occurred after variances in suggested administration of immunoglobulin or vaccine. One case has been reported in which vaccine was given in the buttock rather than the deltoid muscle and rabies later developed. This situation may be analogous to the inefficacy of hepatitis B vaccine when administered intragluteally.

The current recommendation after exposure is to (1) wash the wound thoroughly; (2) administer rabies immune globulin (RIG), 20 IU per kg (50% infiltrated around the wound, 50% in buttock); and (3) give five intramuscular injections of human diploid cell vaccine (HDCV) in the deltoid muscle (1.0 ml) on days 0, 3, 7, 14, and 28. An alternative immunization schedule is to give two doses of HDCV on day 0 with RIG and additional single doses on days 7 and 21. An earlier seroconversion (day 14) may be seen with this method. Antibody production should be examined after the last dose of vaccine and at 2 to 3 weeks. SNA levels ≥1:5 by RFFIT confer protection. If RIG is unavailable in 24 hours, equine rabies antiserum may be used. Adverse effects are seen in 46% of recipients and include serum sickness. If available, interferon may be used for wound infiltration and intramuscular administration and at the wound site and works like RIG. If HDCV is unavailable, duck embryo vaccine or (least preferred) Semple-type vaccines can be used (Fig. 1).

Health care time and costs of the evaluation and prophylaxis of rabies in the U.S. and elsewhere are considerable. Knowledge of the circumstances of exposure, type of animal incriminated, region of the country where the exposure occurred, quarantine of domestic animals, or brain tissue analysis of wild animals can greatly reduce the incidence of overprophylaxis of rabies (Fig. 2).

## INFECTION CONTROL

Despite the lack of any recognized cases of human-to-human transmission of rabies, other

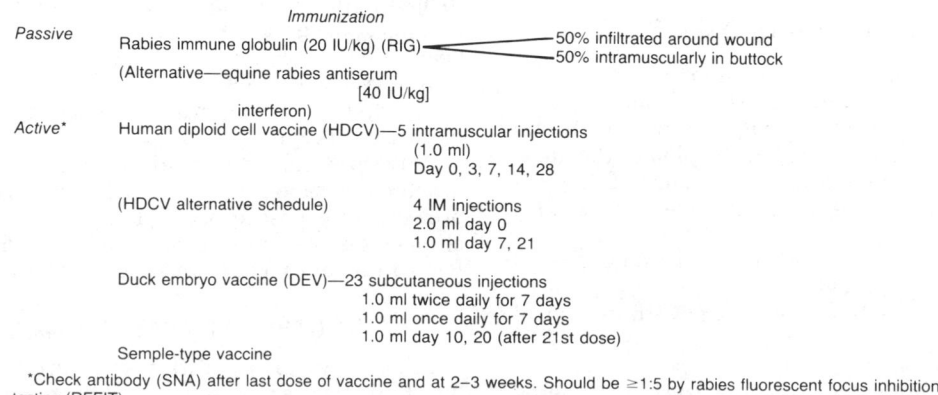

**Figure 1.** Recommendation for post-exposure prophylaxis.

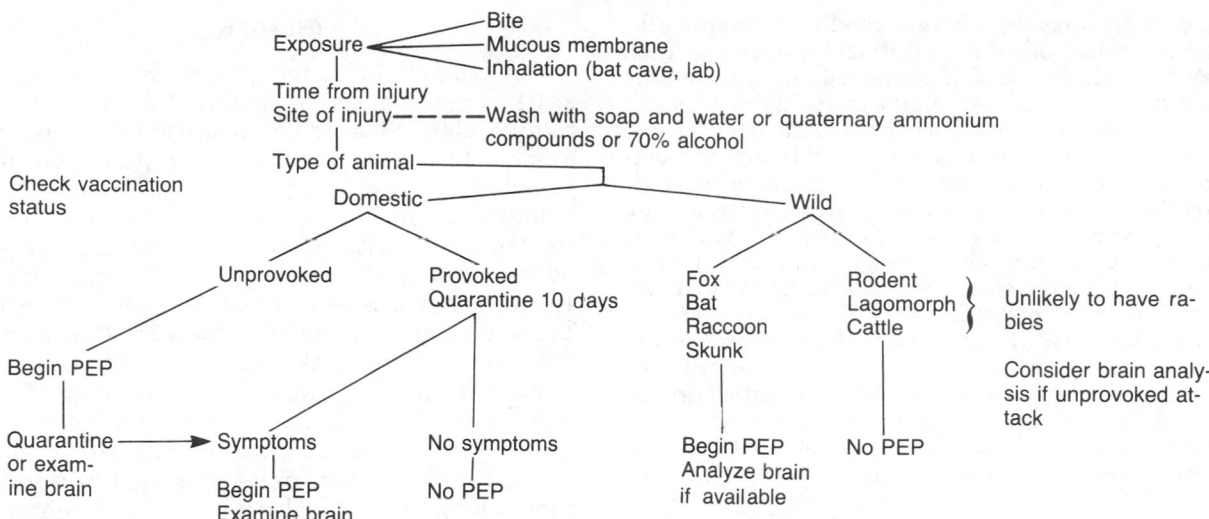

**Figure 2.** Suggested approach to possible rabies exposure. PEP = post-exposure prophylaxis.

than tissue (cornea) transplants, the potential exists for this possibility owing to salivary excretion of the virus and exposure to wounds or mucous membranes. Other culture-positive body fluids have included tracheal secretions, sputum, CSF, and tears. Several tissue and organ specimens have been positive. Unspun urine, blood, serum, and feces have never been positive.

To prevent exposure, rabies should be considered in the differential diagnosis in any patient with encephalitis or encephalopathy. Barrier precautions using gowns, gloves, masks, and goggles should be worn when patient contact is anticipated. Contact isolation procedures should be followed. Any exposure to potentially infectious fluids should immediately be cleaned with soap and water. If a reasonable suspicion exists as to the potential for a valid rabies exposure, postexposure prophylaxis should be undertaken.

# RAT-BITE FEVER

method of
LOUIS M. WEISS, M.D., M.P.H., and
JEFFREY P. GUMPRECHT, M.D.
*Albert Einstein College of Medicine*
*Bronx, New York*

Rat-bite fever is a single designation for two similar systemic febrile illnesses caused by different bacterial species transmitted by the bite of rodents. Depending upon the etiologic agent producing the disease, rash, arthritis, adenitis, or a local lesion at the site of the bite is common. Illness due to rat bite has been known in India for over 2000 years, and the characteristic syndrome of rat-bite fever was reported in the United States in 1839. In Japan, rat-bite fever or sodoku (*so;* rat; *doku;* poison) was also well known. In 1926, it was

recognized that one of the forms of rat-bite fever could be transmitted in an epidemic way through food (Haverhill fever or erythema arthriticum epidemicum). These diseases are worldwide in distribution and most commonly affect individuals exposed to rodents, especially rats. The responsible pathogens are *Spirillum minus* (sodoku) and *Streptobacillus moniliformis* (Haverhill fever). Both are part of the normal oropharyngeal flora of various rodents, especially rats, which may excrete the organism in urine. *S. moniliformis* is found in 50 to 100% and *S. minus* in 25% of wild or laboratory rats. Infection is acquired through contact, usually bites or scratches, with rodents or occasionally from contact with carnivores, such as cats, that feed on rodents. *Streptobacillus moniliformis* has also been associated with food- or water-borne spread, presumably owing to contamination with rodent excreta.

## BACTERIOLOGY

*Streptobacillus moniliformis* is a microaerophilic, pleomorphic, nonmotile, gram-negative rod that forms branching filaments and bead-like chains. It requires 10% $CO_2$ and serum or Panmede supplementation of media for optimal growth. The organism can be recovered from routine blood culture media; however, sodium polyanethol sulfonate (Liquoid) at concentrations of 0.0125% inhibits growth. A lysis centrifugation system may improve the yield from blood culture if this organism is suspected. L-Forms have been described in culture. *Spirillum minus* is a gram-negative spiral rod demonstrating darting motility on dark-field microscopy that does not grow on any media. *Spirillum minus* has traditionally been considered a spirochete, but recently it has been suggested that this organism belongs to the *Campylobacter* genus. Animal inoculation is required for isolation and definitive diagnosis. The organism can be identified in blood or material obtained from skin lesions or lymph nodes by dark-field examination or Giemsa's stain.

## CLINICAL MANIFESTATIONS

Following inoculation of the pathogen from the rodent bite, two similar but distinct diseases may develop. Both illnesses are associated with fever, chills, headache, and other constitutional symptoms. Both may be relapsing, and if untreated the disease may recur for several months. A 10% mortality rate, mostly from endocarditis, has been attributed to untreated disease. A rapidly fatal case of disseminated *S. moniliformis* infection was reported in an infant who received several rat bites. In food- or water-borne disease due to *Streptobacillus moniliformis,* pharyngitis is common. Complications of both pathogens, though rare, include amnionitis, anemia, fever of unknown origin, chronic arthritis, myocarditis, endocarditis, meningitis, hepatitis, and localized abscesses. *Streptobacillus moniliformis* infection is associated with arthritis and *Spirillum minus* infection with regional adenopathy and an ulcer or eschar at the site of the rodent bite. The distinguishing features between the illnesses are summarized in Table 1.

## DIAGNOSIS

The diagnosis of rat-bite fever should be considered in individuals with fever, a history of animal exposure, and leukocytosis. Supporting evidence would include arthritis, a false-positive test for syphilis, and a rash. Several case reports exist of laboratory workers developing the illness following rodent bites. Streptobacillary disease accounts for most of the cases in the United States, whereas *S. minus* infection has been reported mainly from Asia. Confirmation of the diagnosis requires either isolation of the organism for *Streptobacillus moniliformis* or, in the case of *S. minus* infection, direct visualization of characteristic spirochetes in blood, exudate, or lymph node tissue by Giemsa's or Wright's stain or dark-field microscopy. Gas-liquid chromatographic analysis of fatty acids has also been used for rapid diagnosis of *S. moniliformis* infection. In *S. moniliformis* infection, serum agglutinins appear with 10 days of illness. A titer greater than 1:80 or a fourfold rise in titer is considered diagnostic. No specific serologic test exists for *S. minus.*

## TABLE 1. Distinguishing Features of Rat-Bite Fever Syndromes

|  | *Streptobacillus moniliformis* | *Spirillum minus* |
| --- | --- | --- |
| Incubation period | <10 days | ≥7 days |
| Reaction at site of inoculation | Rare | Ulceration or eschar at onset of fever at site of inoculation of organism |
| Lymphadenopathy | Rare | Frequent in nodes adjacent to the area of ulceration |
| Rash | Morbilliform and petechial | Maculopapular with red/brown coloration |
| Joint involvement | Arthralgia and arthritis common | Rarely arthralgia |
| False-positive test for syphilis | <25% | ≥50% |

## THERAPY

The drug of choice for rat-bite fever caused by either organism is penicillin. Patients should receive 400,000 to 600,000 units intravenously every 4 to 6 hours or 600,000 units of procaine penicillin intramuscularly every 12 hours. Individuals who do not require hospitalization can be treated orally with penicillin V, 500 mg every 6 hours. Response to therapy is often dramatic. A 10- to 14-day course of therapy is recommended. Treatment of *S. minus* infection is often associated with a Jarisch-Herxheimer reaction. In patients allergic to penicillin, tetracycline (500 mg every 6 hours) or doxycycline (100 mg every 12 hours) can be used. In cases of endocarditis therapy, 12 to 24 million units of penicillin per day should be given for at least 4 weeks. Streptomycin, 15 mg per kg per day in two divided doses, may be added to enhance activity against L-forms, which are penicillin resistant. Ciprofloxacin (Cipro), cefuroxime (Zinacef), and cefotaxime (Claforan) have in vitro activity against *S. moniliformis.*

Prevention of rat-bite fever involves careful pest control and the wearing of gloves when handling rodents. All rodent bites should be thoroughly cleaned with an antiseptic solution. No studies exist to demonstrate a value of the prophylactic administration of antibiotics after a rat bite. However, the prophylaxis of individuals with known valvular heart disease seems justifiable given the ability of these organisms to cause endocarditis. Penicillin V, 500 mg every 6 hours; or tetracycline, 500 mg every 6 hours, for 3 days would be reasonable prophylaxis.

# RELAPSING FEVER

method of
J. DOUGLAS LEE, M.D.
*Marshfield Clinic*
*Marshfield, Wisconsin*

Relapsing fever is an acute febrile illness caused by the genus *Borrelia* that occurs in a worldwide distribution in epidemic (louse-borne) and endemic (tickborne) forms. The major differences between the forms are outlined in Table 1.

## CLINICAL MANIFESTATIONS

This is a bacteremic disease causing mild to life-threatening illness. The relapsing nature of the illness is due to sequential alterations in the antigenic makeup of the organism, which allow cyclic re-emergence of the spirochete into the blood stream of the host causing fever. Febrile episodes last 3 to 5 days with

TABLE 1. **Features of Relapsing Fever**

|  | Endemic | Epidemic |
|---|---|---|
| Organism | *Borrelia* spp. | *Borrelia recurrentis* |
| Vector | Tick | Human body louse |
| Reservoir | Rodents/ticks | Humans |
| Distribution | Worldwide | Third World |
| Severity | Less severe | More severe |
| Jarisch-Herx-heimer re-action | 20–30% | 80 + % |

afebrile intervals of about 8 days. The bacteremia may affect multiple systems, and in the extreme case, encephalopathy, myocarditis, renal failure, liver failure, hypotension, disseminated intravascular coagulation (DIC), hemorrhage, or death may occur. Typically, the acute onset of fever, headache, and myalgia without a source for the fever in an individual with tick or louse exposure is suggestive. The occurrence of the remittent fever is highly suggestive, and examination of peripheral blood by dark-field, Wright's, or Giemsa's stain during a febrile episode is diagnostic when extracellular spiral organisms are seen.

## TREATMENT

Treatment includes general support, antibiotics, and management of Jarisch-Herxheimer reaction. Where health care resources are limited, outpatient therapy of mild to moderately ill patients may be appropriate.

Very ill patients should be hospitalized, with intravenous dextrose in normal saline or half-normal saline given rapidly in an amount dictated by the initial state of hydration and cardiac compensation. Persistently hypotensive individuals may also benefit from the administration of oncotic agents, such as albumin in a dose of 0.5 to 1.5 grams of protein per kg, to allow intravascular volume expansion.

Fever can be managed with tepid water baths or alcohol sponging. Pain may be controlled with meperidine (Demerol), 25 to 100 mg intramuscularly or 10 to 25 mg intravenously. Codeine or other nonantipyretic analgesics may also be used.

### Antibiotic Therapy

The recommendations for antibiotic treatment of relapsing fever are different for endemic and epidemic disease. Epidemic disease can be treated with a single dose of any of the drugs listed in Table 2 to achieve a very low relapse rate. Erythromycin and tetracycline are generally considered drugs of choice.

For tick-borne disease, there are no large series to determine the minimal effect of therapy. Table 3 outlines therapy and duration of therapy for tick-borne fever as seen in the United States.

TABLE 2. **Louse-Borne Relapsing Fever: Antibiotics**

| Drug | Dose | Route | Number of Doses |
|---|---|---|---|
| PAM*† | 1,200,000 U | IM | 1 |
| Tetracycline | 500 mg | PO | 1 |
| Tetracycline | 250 mg | IV | 1 |
| Doxycycline | 100 mg | IV/PO | 1 |
| Erythromycin | 500 mg | IV/PO | 1 |
| Chloramphenicol | 500 mg | IV/PO | 1 |

*Penicillin aluminum monostearate.
†Not available in the United States.

### Jarisch-Herxheimer Reaction

Most patients with epidemic relapsing fever and a small percentage of patients with endemic relapsing fever experience a rise in temperature and a fall in blood pressure, white count, and peripheral vascular resistance within 2 hours of the initial dose of antibiotics. This may result in significant prolonged hypotension, and this is not modified by the use of steroids, antipyretics, or narcotics. Intensification of the initial support measures, particularly optimizing intravascular volume, is important at this stage. There is evidence that meptazinol,* an opiate antagonist, suppresses certain features of this reaction, but its effect on mortality is not clear and its use should not be routine, particularly in mildly ill patients (100 mg by slow intravenous infusion with antibiotic injection, 30 minutes later, at the onset of chills, and again if blood pressure falls significantly).

### PREVENTION

Relapsing fever is prevented by avoiding vector exposure. Patients with louse-borne relapsing fever should be deloused by applying 1% lindane (Kwell) for 10 minutes to the skin surface, with particular attention to hair-bearing areas, or by using 0.5% malathion lotion (Prioderm) or pyrethrin liquid with piperonyl butoxide (RiD). Lindane use should be repeated in one week to assure cure in the hair-bearing areas. Removal of lin-

*Not available in the United States.

TABLE 3. **Tick-Borne Relapsing Fever: Antibiotics***

| Drug | Dose | Frequency | Route |
|---|---|---|---|
| Penicillin | 500 mg | qid | IV/PO |
| Ampicillin | 500 mg | qid | IV/PO |
| Doxycycline | 100 mg | bid | IV/PO |
| Tetracycline | 500 mg | qid | IV/PO |
| Erythromycin | 500 mg | qid | IV/PO |
| Chloramphenicol | 500 mg | qid | IV/PO |

*All 5- to 10-day courses orally if patients are able.

dane from the skin after 10 minutes is important in children and infants as the drug is absorbed and is potentially toxic. Other agents, such as pyrethrins, piperonyl butoxide (Rid), malathion (Prioderm lotion or 1% powder), or 10% DDT powder, may be used. The use of insecticides in lice-infested dwellings should be considered. Household contacts should also be deloused. Personal clothing and bedclothes should be hot laundered and ironed to avoid reinfection or dusted with 1% malathion or 10% DDT powder. Tick-borne relapsing fever is avoided by the use of pyrethrins on clothing or deet insect repellents.

The use of doxycycline (Vibramycin), 100 mg a day, is recommended for short-term visitors in areas endemic for louse-borne relapsing fever. This will also cure typhus.

# RHEUMATIC FEVER

method of
STANFORD T. SHULMAN, M.D.
*The Children's Memorial Hospital*
*Chicago, Illinois*

The treatment of rheumatic fever is divided into therapy of the *acute attack,* including antibiotics, anti-inflammatory agents, bed rest, anti-chorea medications, and cardiac drugs; and *chronic therapy* following the acute attack (Table 1).

## ACUTE RHEUMATIC FEVER (ARF)

Patients with suspected or confirmed ARF should be hospitalized to obtain a full medical evaluation, to observe their progress before and after the onset of therapy, and to impress upon them and their families the long-term consequences of rheumatic heart disease and the likelihood for recurrence. A 10-day course of an antistreptococcal antibiotic (oral penicillin or erythromycin, or intramuscular benzathine penicillin) should be administered even to those patients whose throats no longer can be shown to harbor group A streptococci.

Anti-inflammatory agents (salicylates and glucocorticosteroids like prednisone) are highly effective in suppressing the inflammatory activity of ARF. In fact, the very dramatic clinical response of arthritis to aspirin may be useful in establishing the diagnosis of ARF. The available controlled studies that compare the effect of salicylates and prednisone in ARF, assessing the ultimate incidence of residual cardiac disease up to 15 years later, provide no consistent evidence that steroids prevent cardiac damage. Steroids do, however, promptly suppress acute inflammation, particularly cardiac inflammation, and on rare occasions can be lifesaving. In patients who are only mildly to moderately ill and in whom the diagnosis of ARF is not completely clear, it is frequently wise to withhold anti-inflammatory agents to observe the progression of disease—i.e., to witness the migratory nature of the arthritis of ARF to confirm the diagnosis.

Salicylates should be utilized for anti-inflammatory therapy of ARF patients with no evidence of cardiac disease or those with mild carditis (i.e., unassociated with cardiomegaly or congestive failure). Aspirin should be given at 50 to 100 mg per kg per day (the higher per kg dose for smaller children) in four divided doses, and prompt amelioration of arthritis and other inflammatory parameters should be noted. The full salicylate dose should be maintained for 2 weeks and half that dose for another 2 to 3 weeks.

Prednisone should be reserved for ARF patients who demonstrate significant cardiac involvement, with cardiomegaly and/or congestive failure and/or pericarditis. Prednisone is usually administered at 2 mg per kg per day for 2 to 4 weeks and is then gradually tapered over several weeks. During the steroid taper, salicylates are added at about 50 to 70 mg per kg per day to

TABLE 1. **Treatment of Rheumatic Fever**

**Acute Rheumatic Fever**
*Antistreptococcal antibiotics*
　1.2 million U benzathine penicillin IM
　　　　*or*
　Oral penicillin or erythromycin for 10 days

*Anti-inflammatory agents*
　*Aspirin:* 50–100 mg/kg/day in four divided doses for patients without cardiac involvement or with mild carditis
　　　　*or*
　*Corticosteroids:* prednisone 2 mg/kg/day in four doses for 2–4 weeks in patients with moderate or severe carditis, then taper with addition of salicylates

*Cardiac drugs (if needed)*
　Diuretic therapy as indicated
　Cautious digitalization as indicated

*Choreic drugs (if needed)*
　Phenobarbital or tranquilizers as indicated (see text)

**Chronic Rheumatic Disease**
*Rheumatic prophylaxis (for all patients)*
　1.2 million U benzathine penicillin IM monthly (0.6 million U if <60 lb)
　　　　*or*
　Sulfadiazine PO 500 mg bid (500 mg once daily if <30 kg)
　　　　*or*
　Penicillin V PO 250 mg bid

*SBE prophylaxis (for patients with cardiac disease)*
　As recommended by the American Heart Association

prevent a clinical rebound of inflammatory activity.

Congestive cardiac failure is usually controlled by bed rest and steroids. Occasionally diuretic therapy is necessary, and rarely careful digitalization is required.

Treatment of chorea, a self-limited feature, generally requires more than anti-inflammatory therapy. Most patients benefit significantly from quiet, nonstressful surroundings and administration of phenobarbital or diazepam (Valium) or other tranquilizer. The latter medications must be given on a trial-and-error basis, since patients vary considerably in their responsiveness to treatment and a single drug is not beneficial in all cases.

## CHRONIC RHEUMATIC DISEASE

Individuals who have had an attack of ARF with or without cardiac disease or who are found to have chronic rheumatic heart disease (RHD) are at risk for recurrent attacks of ARF following streptococcal pharyngitis. Thus, they should receive *continuous* antistreptococcal prophylaxis to prevent recurrences of ARF. Three standard regimens are considered satisfactory for this purpose, in order of preference: (1) monthly intramuscular injection of 1.2 million units of benzathine penicillin (0.6 million units for those less than 60 pounds); (2) 500-mg tablets of sulfadiazine twice daily; and (3) 250 mg tablets of penicillin V twice daily.

The advantage of parenteral penicillin is that one does not depend upon daily patient compliance; however, the injections may be painful. Strict compliance with this regimen has been shown to result in healing of valvular heart disease (as reflected by disappearance of murmurs) in the majority of patients, in addition to prevention of recurrent attacks of ARF. The advantage of sulfadiazine over oral penicillin relates primarily to the induction of penicillin-resistant oral flora by the latter, which theoretically could predispose a patient to an episode of bacterial endocarditis due to a penicillin-resistant organism. Erythromycin has been suggested for the rare patient who is intolerant of both penicillin and sulfadiazine. A subject of considerable controversy is the optimum duration of rheumatic fever prophylaxis. Most investigators, including the American Heart Association, recommend lifelong prophylaxis for patients with RHD because the risk of recurrent ARF persists long beyond childhood, albeit in a diminished way. In patients without residual cardiac involvement, prophylaxis can probably be safely discontinued at age 21 if at least 5 years has elapsed from the last attack of ARF.

In addition to rheumatic fever prophylaxis, patients with RHD require subacute bacterial endocarditis (SBE) prophylaxis on an episodic basis related to dental or surgical procedures, or gastrointestinal or genitourinary tract instrumentation, as recommended by the American Heart Association.

# LYME DISEASE
## (Lyme Borreliosis)

method of
PAUL E. LAVOIE, M.D.
*Pacific Presbyterian Medical Center*
*San Francisco, California*

Lyme borreliosis is a recently described spirochetal infection caused by *Borrelia burgdorferi*. It is already recognized as the most common tick-borne infection in the United States. It is transmitted primarily by hard-shelled vegetation inhabiting ticks of the *Ixodes ricinus* complex. These include *Ixodes dammini* in northeastern United States, *Ixodes scapularis* in southeastern United States, and *Ixodes pacificus* in far western United States. This disease has been reported from 43 states, most European countries, Russia, China, northern and South Africa, and Australia. The nymphal stage occurs in spring and summer and accounts for most human attacks. The attachment is recognized in only 25 to 30% of patients, most likely because of the vector's tiny size.

### CLINICAL DESCRIPTION

Although the infection often presents in a characteristic manner, many atypical presentations have been described in recent years, often leading to diagnostic confusion. It is a multisystem disorder affecting skin, joints, nervous system, and heart most commonly, but involvement of other systems has also been described. The key to diagnosis is the pathognomonic rash, erythema chronicum migrans. Unfortunately, it is often not present. The disease is described in stages, but considerable overlap between stages has been seen. Its pathogenesis appears to be predominantly immunologic.

*Stage I: Early Manifestations*

A few days to a month following a tick bite, the central erythematous papule becomes macular and expands gradually, at times to greater than 60 cm. Erythema chronicum migrans is typically flat, annular, with diffuse erythema early. Pain and pruritus are variable but usually not prominent. Central cyanosis leading to vesiculation may occur early. Late central clearing is common, leading to a ring pattern. Slow resolution typically occurs, but similar migrating annuli may occur elsewhere. The rash often does not occur and is especially infrequent in children. Constitutional symptoms, including fever, fatigue, malaise, myalgias, arthralgias, transient and migratory synovitis, tendinitis, bursitis, axial stiffness, pharyngitis, headaches, and lymphadenopathy, are common. Nonproductive cough, hepatosplenomegaly, hepatitis, orchitis, periorbital edema, conjunctivitis, iritis, and panophthalmitis are less common. Symptoms often wax and wane within an individual. They may remit within weeks, even without treatment, or persist for extended periods.

*Stage II: Cardiac and Early Neurologic Manifestations*

Onset is typically weeks to months following infection. This stage often appears prior to resolution of Stage I. Cardiac affliction affects about 10% of untreated subjects and often presents as syncope due to high-grade atrioventricular (AV) conduction disorders. Most commonly first-degree AV block is seen. It often resolves spontaneously or with therapy but may persist. Cardiomegaly, left ventricular dysfunction, pancarditis, and cardiac death have all been reported.

In untreated patients 20% develop neurologic injury. Cranial palsies, especially facial nerve, often symmetrical, are the most common presentations. Cranial nerves II, III, V, VI, VIII, IX, and XII have also been involved. The triad of cranial neuritis, meningitis, and radiculoneuritis (Garin-Bujadoux-Bannwarth syndrome) is commonly seen in Europe. Encephalitis, myelitis, ataxia, chorea, and mononeuritis multiplex may occur.

Borrelia lymphocytoma, a nodular cutaneous lesion often of the ear lobe, is recognized in Europe.

*Stage III: Chronic Arthritis and Neurologic Manifestations*

Typically, months to years following infection, inflammatory arthritis appears in 60% of untreated patients. It becomes chronic in 10%. The knees are most commonly affected, but any synovial joint may be affected. Symmetrical polyarthritis may be seen. The radiologic and pathologic findings are indistinguishable from rheumatoid arthritis. Panniculitis, myositis, and dermatomyositis have been described. Ulnar fibrous nodules clinically resembling rheumatoid nodules may be seen.

Acrodermatitis chronica atrophicans is often seen in Europe and has been seen in the United States. The inflammatory phase may resemble lymphedema or venous stasis while the atrophic stage can be confused with other cutaneous sclerosing disorders. Peripheral neuropathies with both axonal and myelin sheath injuries are often associated. Multifocal encephalitis, central nervous system (CNS) demyelination leading to multiple sclerosis presentations, psychoses, and dementia have been recognized.

## PREGNANCY

Transplacental infection was recognized in 5 of 19 pregnancies reported in one study. Injuries there included fetal wastage, syndactyly, cortical blindness, prematurity, and neonatal rash. The organism has been cultured from fetal organs and from two neonatal deaths, one resulting from aortic thrombosis.

## LABORATORY FINDINGS

Serology remains the mainstay of laboratory diagnosis. Unfortunately, the sensitivity of available tests is exceedingly low in early disease and is too often inadequate in late disease. Of the 19 mothers in the above quoted study on transplacental infection, 80% were falsely seronegative. Threshold for serodiagnosis has been set at three standard deviations (S.D.) above the control mean in some laboratories rather than the customary 2 S.D. This was done to reduce cross-reactivity with other spirochetal infections, but unfortunately, cross-reactivities with treponemal and other borrelia infections occur at and above that higher threshold. T cell stimulation studies support the concept of seronegative disease. T cell assays are not available commercially. Intradermal testing of delayed hypersensitivity may follow this in vitro assay. An antibody capture assay reporting only a 7% false negativity in late disease has recently been described. A urine antigen capture assay is under study. Direct culture of the organism is too often unsuccessful to be useful as a clinical assay. Elevation of serum IgM and transaminases as well as microhematuria is seen at times, especially in early disease. CSF assays often reveal only a mild pleocytosis and elevation of total protein. Lack of evidence for CNS in situ formation of borrelia antibodies should not exclude the diagnosis of neuroborreliosis. Conversely, malignant-appearing cells may be seen in the CSF leading to a misdiagnosis of CNS lymphoma. It is generally agreed that the diagnosis of Lyme borreliosis should be based on clinical factors and not excluded because of negative serology.

## TREATMENT

### General Considerations

Prevention remains the most important approach. Thorough covering by light-colored clothing whose openings are tightly closed offers the first line of defense. Careful tick checks should be done at the end of an outdoor day and more often if possible. Hairy and crural regions are special targets of the ticks. Gentle traction on the tick near its attachment is the best removal method.

Standard treatment for early disease (Stage I) has typically consisted of common oral antibiotics administered over a 2-week period. Penicillin V 500 mg, tetracycline 250 to 500 mg, or erythromycin 250 mg, all given four times a day, has been the usually recommended regimen. Recently, the adequacy of these as well as standard regimens for later stages has been questioned. This has been stimulated by numerous reports of treatment failure or late relapses following all available forms of oral and parenteral treatment. According to a sizable European dermatologic study, 27% of early and 47% of late disease patients later developed extracutaneous signs and symptoms following standard treatment. The causes of these difficulties are likely manifold. Surely the very slow reproduction rate of this microbe in vitro (12 to 20 hours) and its suspected much slower reproduction rate when the microbe has become established in host parenchyma are probable contributors. Evidence for long asymptomatic intervals of many years is accumulating. This latency is reminiscent of lues.

*B. burgdorferi* is sensitive to common spirochetal antibiotics including the penicillins, tetracyclines, some cephalosporins, erythromycin, and chloramphenicol (Chloromycetin). Erythromycin's benefit in vivo is far less than its in vitro sensitivity would indicate. Rifampicin, sulfonamides, aminoglycosides, and quinolones appear to have no role in this infection.

## Stage IA: Hematogenous

This is the earliest and usually asymptomatic stage when parenchymal infection has not yet occurred. It accompanies the tick bite and likely lasts for only a few days during which a low-grade spirochetemia exists. Treatment with the above noted standard oral agents may be adequate. The use of doxycycline at 2.5 to 3 mg per kg per day or amoxicillin at 25 to 30 mg per kg per day in divided doses for 2 weeks is preferred. Tetracycline should not be used in children under age 8 years. Erythromycin at 30 mg per kg per day in divided doses for 20 days may be used in penicillin-allergic children, although its efficacy is likely less than the agents it replaces.

## Stage IB: Parenchymous

Experience with hamsters indicates that parenchyma is invaded within 7 days of experimental infection. Too often patients are seen initially weeks following spirochetal inoculation; therefore, the likelihood of parenchymous infection becomes high. Once systemic symptoms and signs are present, parenchymous infection likely exists. Antibiotics that cross the blood-brain barrier are then required. Doxycycline (Vibramycin) at 2.5 to 3 mg per kg per day or minocycline (Minocin) at 2 to 2.5 mg per kg per day or amoxicillin (Amoxil, Polymox) 1500 mg with probenecid (Benemid) 500 mg (in adults) three times a day appears to adequately penetrate CNS tissues and offer acceptable antibiotic effect. Children under age 8 should receive amoxicillin 60 mg per kg

per day in divided doses. Those who are penicillin allergic may receive erythromycin at 30 mg per kg per day in divided doses, but its weaker effectiveness should be kept in mind. Studies of various oral third-generation cephalosporins and a new erythromycin class drug are in progress. These should be considered in this penicillin-allergic age group when they become available.

Persistent symptoms including fatigue, headaches, myalgias, and arthralgias have been noted in about half of all patients with this disease. These symptoms have been considered immunologically based by many. Molecular mimicry, where natural host proteins mimic spirochetal antigens, has been offered as one such mechanism promoting ongoing immune response. Longer antibiotic therapy has been beneficial to a number of these patients in uncontrolled observations suggesting that persistence of the infection in parenchymous sites may be the cause of these ongoing symptoms. Borreliae have been shown in deep tissues following 2 months of accepted oral antibiotic treatment. Such findings strongly support suspicion that parenchymal infection is probably not eradicable with short-term treatment. Treatment well beyond clearance of the last symptoms seems appropriate until controlled studies define optimal type and duration of therapy to achieve bacteriologic cure. To date there is no evidence of the spirochete's developing resistance to established antibiotics.

## Stage II: Cardiac and Neurologic Treatment

This stage clearly implies parenchymous infection. It is also the stage of potentially dramatic and organ-threatening presentations. When cardiac signs are limited to mild PR interval prolongation, then the oral antibiotics and dosing mentioned for Stage IB parenchymous disease above should be applied. Duration of treatment should be at least 4 months, pending results of controlled studies. Nonsteroidal anti-inflammatory drugs (NSAID) such as high-dose aspirin (3 to 4 grams daily in adults) or equivalent should also be applied in the early weeks. Temporary restriction of physical activity may be appropriate.

In addition to minor conduction defects, this infection is known to cause major conduction defects (PR interval $\geq 0.3$ seconds), which often present as syncope or as inflammation of any or all three layers of the heart (endocardium, myocardium, pericardium). Death may ensue. Hospitalization is often indicated, and temporary pacemaker placement may be required. In this setting of acute threat to vital organs, intravenous antibiotics appear to have their greatest applicability. High-dose penicillin, 20 million units per day in divided doses, has been favored until recently. Ceftriaxone (Rocephin) 2 grams intravenously per day for 14 days now seems more appropriate based upon its superior tissue penetration and spirochetal sensitivity. It is also more easily administered in the home setting, allowing shorter hospital stays. Continued oral antibiotic treatment as previously described for Stage IB parenchymal infection should follow for at least 4 months or until resolution of symptoms, whichever is longer. NSAID treatment may be beneficial, but a rapidly tapering course of corticosteroids over 1 week is preferred for these life-threatening presentations. Prednisone starting at 1 mg per kg the first day is suggested.

Acute CNS presentations (meningitis, encephalitis, myelitis) typically require hospitalization. Intravenous ceftriaxone at 2 grams daily for 14 days has become favored for reasons mentioned above. In addition, its penetration of the blood-brain barrier is far superior to that of penicillin. Treatment with oral antibiotics as described for Stage IB parenchymal infection should follow for at least 4 months or until resolution of symptoms, whichever is longer. Less dramatic CNS presentations, e.g., headaches and memory difficulties, also are usually adequately treated by this oral regimen.

Peripheral nervous system afflictions should be treated according to the method suggested for Stage IB parenchymal infection. Duration should also be at least 4 months or until resolution of symptoms, whichever is longer. A rapidly tapering course of corticosteroids over 1 week, e.g., prednisone starting at 1 mg per kg the first day, may be additionally beneficial to patients presenting with recent onset (less than 2 weeks) cranial neuropathy, e.g., facial palsy or sudden deafness.

## Stage III: Chronic Arthritis and Neurologic Disorders

A general consensus is arising among clinicians most familiar with this disorder that late disease is the most difficult to treat and refractoriness to various treatment modalities is often seen. Intravenous ceftriaxone 2 grams per day for 14 days has recently been favored in publications for this stage. Unfortunately, its long-term efficacy in practice falls below what has been published. It is conceivable that late disease represents the greatest adaptation of the microbe to its host environment. In turn, its reproduction rate may be far slower than its in vitro rate, leading to greater need for prolonged therapy as well as optimal antibiotic tissue penetration. Treatment of the kind outlined in Stage IB parenchymal disease is at times more efficacious

than a short course of intravenous ceftriaxone. Unfortunately, symptomatic flares as a result of treatment are often seen. This likely represents tissue deposition of immune complexes formed as a result of antibiotic-induced release of antigen from its parenchymous sites. Interruption of treatment typically aborts the flares. A treatment approach that allows for ongoing clearance of immune complexes via scheduled interruption of treatment seems to be most efficacious when flares recur as a function of prolonged oral therapy. Using amoxicillin 1500 mg and probenecid 500 mg twice a day or even daily seems to offer the greatest comfort, especially in the case of chronic arthritis. Doxycycline or minocycline can similarly be interrupted by giving doses as described in Stage IB parenchymal disease on an every-other-day schedule. Treatment should be continued beyond clearance of symptoms or at least 4 months, whichever is longer.

In a 1981 report, hydroxychloroquine (Plaquenil) was shown be beneficial for chronic Lyme arthritis. It appears to improve the efficacy of prolonged oral antibiotic treatment in cases where antibiotics alone are insufficient. Standard dosing at 6 mg per kg per day is recommended along with the usual ophthalmologic precautions.

### Pregnancy

Maternal treatment to prevent transplacental infection is not established. A standard, short course of oral penicillin given to the mother soon after appearance of erythema migrans did not prevent fetal infection and neonatal death in the only reported case of this circumstance. Two weeks of ceftriaxone 2 grams intravenously per day in early pregnancy and amoxicillin 1 gram three times a day for 6 weeks in late pregnancy have been protective to offspring in recent uncontrolled observations on eastern Long Island, N.Y. Six weeks of amoxicillin 500 mg four times a day given at various gestational times has resulted in no apparent fetal injuries in 12 pregnancies in Wisconsin.

The likelihood of placental infection is highest early in the disease when hematogenous spread is active. Very low-grade spirochetemia likely occurs in later stages and may continue for indefinite periods. Protection against this phenomenon should require lower serum antibiotic levels than those required for CNS penetration. Amoxicillin 500 mg orally four times a day should be adequate. Continuation throughout gestation would seem to offer the greatest protection, pending results of studies defining optimum treatment.

Maternal immunologic reaction to treatment of

the Jarisch-Herxheimer type could be acutely injurious to the fetus and could lead to fetal wastage, but this has not been reported.

## ASYMPTOMATIC TICK BITE

As we learn more about the potential severity of late disease and the difficulties with effecting adequate treatment, consideration for treatment at the earliest time becomes rational. In the first days following a bite by an infected tick, potential for eradicating the infection is highest because the infection is presumed to be only hematogenous. In regions of high endemic tick infection, early treatment of asymptomatic tick bites by the method previously described for Stage IA hematogenous seems prudent. Serologic reactivity will likely not occur, but late disease should be prevented. In regions of low endemic infection, such prophylactic treatment offers no benefit statistically.

# ROCKY MOUNTAIN SPOTTED FEVER

method of
HARRIS D. RILEY, Jr., M.D.
*University of Oklahoma Health Sciences Center*
*Oklahoma City, Oklahoma*

Rocky Mountain spotted fever (RMSF), an acute infectious disease, is the most prevalent and severe of the rickettsioses. The etiologic agent is *Rickettsia rickettsii,* an obligate intracellular parasite of several species of ticks and rodents and possibly of mammals. It is transmitted to man by the bite of the adult tick. A variety of ixodid (hard-shelled) ticks serve as both reservoir and vector for the disease. The western wood tick, *Dermacentor andersoni,* and the eastern dog tick, *D. variabilis,* are the principal vectors. RMSF of the United States is identical to Sao Paulo fever, Colombian spotted fever, fiebre maculosa, fiebre petequial, and the fiebre manchada of Mexico.

Despite its name, the disease is more common in the southern, southwestern, and eastern United States. Since 1960 the number of reported cases in the United States has increased steadily, and the increase has been particularly striking since 1970. The true incidence is likely higher than the reported incidence. Persons of all ages are susceptible to the disease, but most of the cases occur in children. There is a striking seasonal distribution, with most cases occurring during the spring and summer. This parallels both the activity of ticks and the behavior of individuals that brings them in contact with the ticks.

The incubation period in man is 2 to 12 days, with a mean of 7 days. Since about one-fourth of patients have no history of a tick bite or of the presence of ticks on the body, the absence of such a history should not prevent the physician from suspecting the disease.

The severity of the disease ranges from cases that are clinically quite mild to fulminant forms. In untreated patients the mortality rate ranges from 10 to 40%. Appropriate treatment has reduced this to between 5 and 10%. Prognosis is influenced by age and other factors, but the most important influence in successful treatment of the infection is early diagnosis and institution of therapy.

## CLINICAL ASPECTS

The most prominent clinical features of RMSF are headache, fever, rash, and edema. However, many patients have nonspecific features such as nausea, vomiting, abdominal pain, diarrhea, arthralgia, myalgia, and neurologic manifestations. The onset of symptoms may be either abrupt or gradual. The neurologic manifestations, particularly when alterations in mental status and vomiting are present, may suggest a diagnosis of meningoencephalitis.

The rash of RMSF is the earliest dependable and most important diagnostic sign. It typically begins on the ankles and wrists and spreads centrally. In the early stages it is maculopapular but in many cases (more than half) assumes a petechial character. Some patients do not have a typical rash, and in others, the rash may not appear until later in the disease. Variability in the nature of the rash is common, and failure to recognize this may result in a delay in diagnosis, which can be catastrophic. When looked for, many patients show generalized nonpitting edema. Conjunctivitis, splenomegaly, and a variety of neurologic manifestations may occur.

RMSF may be confused clinically with other infectious diseases, including meningococcal infections, enteroviral infections, atypical measles, infectious mononucleosis, and others. The rash of drug eruptions may be confusing. A newly recognized rickettsial disease, ehrlichiosis, may clinically resemble RMSF. It is caused by *Ehrlichia canis,* an intraleukocytic parasite that infects a variety of wild and domestic animals, including dogs. The clinical findings are similar to those of RMSF, except that rash is usually absent.

RMSF cannot be clearly identified in the early stages on the basis of routine laboratory procedures. Urinalysis is usually normal, but specimens may contain traces of albumin and, sometimes, casts. Leukopenia, present in the first week, evolves into moderate leukocytosis in the second. There may be mild to moderate normochromic normocytic anemia, thrombocytopenia, and multiple coagulation disturbances, including hypofibrinogenemia and evidence of disseminated intravascular coagulation.

Serial determinations of serum proteins usually show a progressive decrease, particularly of the albumin fraction. Serum electrolyte measurements frequently demonstrate hyponatremia and hypochloremia. These abnormalities may be associated with increased aldosterone excretion.

Mild CSF mononuclear pleocytosis with slight elevation of the protein content is common. The leukocyte count almost never exceeds 300 per mm³. The glucose concentration is normal.

Liver function abnormalities include decreased

serum protein and usually transient elevations of enzymes and bilirubin. Blood urea nitrogen (BUN) may be increased.

## TREATMENT

Early diagnosis and prompt initiation of effective treatment are vitally important in achieving successful results in the management of rickettsial diseases. Therapy may be considered in two general categories: specific antirickettsial measures and supportive care.

### Specific Antirickettsial Therapy

Both tetracycline and chloramphenicol are effective in the treatment of Rocky Mountain spotted fever. However, each drug must be administered early in the course of the disease; the drugs are rickettsiostatic, not rickettsiocidal. In patients seen late in the course of the disease or in fulminating disease, irreversible pathologic changes may have taken place that decrease the effectiveness of antimicrobial agents. If antimicrobial treatment is initiated in the first 3 or 4 days of illness, the likelihood of a satisfactory result is much greater. Although the drugs are equally effective, tetracycline is generally preferred because of the frequent hematologic complications of Rocky Mountain spotted fever and the known dose-related bone marrow depression that accompanies the use of chloramphenicol. The recommended dosage of the tetracyclines (or chloramphenicol) for children is 50 to 100 mg per kg per day orally in four divided doses. The maximum daily dose is 2 grams for children and 4 grams for adults. If indicated by the patient's condition, the intravenous route may be used. By this route, 30 to 40 mg per kg every 24 hours of either drug should be administered in three equal doses. Antibiotic therapy should be continued until the patient is afebrile for 48 hours; this is usually 5 to 9 days after initiation of treatment. Sulfonamides should not be used in the treatment of rickettsial infections because the severity of illness has been observed to increase with their use.

Although the response to treatment is usually apparent within the first day or so, fever usually persists for several days following the initiation of antibiotic therapy. If antimicrobial therapy is discontinued too soon, a relapse may occur. Isolation of the patient is not required.

Because of its likelihood to stain developing teeth, tetracycline should not be used to treat pregnant or lactating women or children less than 8 years of age. Complicating hepatic necrosis has been associated occasionally with the intravenous use of tetracycline; oral therapy should be instituted as soon as it is possible for the patient to tolerate this route.

Hematocrit, white blood cell, and differential counts should be determined at least twice weekly during therapy with chloramphenicol to monitor for hematologic complications.

A not infrequent differential diagnostic dilemma is that of the patient with fever and petechial rash—features common to both RMSF and meningococcemia. At the time the patient is first seen, it may be impossible to distinguish with certainty between these two life-threatening infections, both of which require immediate therapy. In such instances, in addition to the antirickettsial therapy outlined, penicillin G in large doses (250,000 units per kg per day in children), administered intravenously, may be employed to combat the possible meningococcal infection. Sulfonamides should not be used. They are no longer considered appropriate therapy for meningococcal disease and, as mentioned, make rickettsial infections worse.

Both tetracycline and chloramphenicol have been associated with serious side effects, particularly in children, and this aspect must be weighed before the decision is made to initiate treatment based on questionable clinical suspicion alone. On the other hand, the potentially fatal outcome of Rocky Mountain spotted fever must be considered as well.

### Supportive Care

In addition to specific antimicrobial therapy, it is of utmost importance to provide adequate supportive therapy. The pathologic hallmark of Rocky Mountain spotted fever is a vasculitis. This results in certain important pathophysiologic changes, particularly in patients who are severely ill. These include hypoproteinemia, circulatory collapse, hypotension, oliguria, acidemia, edema, and depression of serum sodium and chlorides. The maintenance of an adequate blood volume and handling of circulatory collapse are of prime importance. Fluid and electrolyte therapy must be carefully monitored. Because of the vascular leak and secondary hypoproteinemia, these patients frequently require large amounts of replacement fluid. Albumin or plasma may be used in addition to electrolyte solutions. If anemia is severe, blood transfusions may be necessary. Measurement of pulmonary artery and wedge pressures can provide a guide to volume replacement in patients with evidence of circulatory collapse. Injudicious use of intravenous fluids may lead to increased tissue edema and cardiopulmonary failure.

Thrombocytopenia and coagulopathies occur

frequently in RMSF. The platelet level should be monitored serially and frequently, as more than half of the patients will exhibit some degree of thrombocytopenia. Rapidly progressing disease with an extensive hemorrhagic rash may have associated disseminated intravascular coagulation (DIC), which is manifested by thrombocytopenia, prolonged prothrombin and partial thromboplastin times, hypofibrinogenemia, and an increase in serum fibrin split products. The most important aspect of its management is proper treatment for the underlying disease. The next aim of therapy, especially in the patient who is bleeding, is replacement of the coagulation factors, platelets, or both, to hemostatic levels. In some patients, however, the treatment of the underlying disease may be inadequate or too slow, or replacement therapy may not be effective. Management must then be aimed at medically interrupting the DIC with anticoagulation; heparin is usually employed for this purpose, but its use is controversial. It should be remembered that in most cases, once the underlying disease is properly identified and treated, therapy of the DIC is generally supportive, and anticoagulant therapy is rarely indicated except in special situations.

Supplemental therapy with corticosteroids has been reported to be of value in patients first treated late in the course of the disease; the value, if any, of corticosteroids appears to be related to their antitoxemic effect. Insufficient information is available to warrant use of these agents in most cases.

Renal insufficiency occasionally occurs and should be handled in standard fashion. Necrosis of the tips of the fingers or toes, nose, ear, scrotum, and other sites may result from the severe vasculitis. After the acute illness has subsided, such patients may require surgical correction.

### PREVENTION

The most effective individual prophylaxis against spotted fever is prevention of the attachment of a tick to the skin or removal of it as quickly as possible if it becomes attached. Personal prophylactic measures should include (1) application of repellents such as diethyltoluamide (deet) or dimethylphthalate to clothing and exposed parts of the body; (2) in heavily infested areas, the wearing of clothing that interferes with attachment of ticks, i.e., boots and a one-piece outer garment, preferably impregnated with repellent; and (3) daily inspection of the entire body, including the hairy parts, to detect and remove attached ticks. While it may be feasible for most persons to avoid tick-infested areas in

certain localities in the Rocky Mountain states, it is more difficult to avoid contact with ticks in the East or South, where dog ticks are the vectors. Since victims are seldom aware of crawling ticks or even of the process of attachment, frequent inspection of the scalp, skin, and clothing is necessary in tick-infested areas. Patient education is thus crucial.

In spite of all precautions, some ticks will reach the body. They seldom attach immediately on skin contact and rarely transfer infection until they have fed for several hours. In endemic tick-infested areas, careful search must be made, systematic removal practiced, and children examined at least twice daily.

Attached ticks must be removed with forceps or gauze-protected fingers. In removing ticks, care should be taken to avoid crushing the arthropod, since this may result in contamination of the bite wound or aerosol transmission. Touching the tick with gasoline or whiskey sometimes encourages detachment, but gentle traction with small forceps applied close to the mouth parts, which are readily removed, is usually necessary. The site of the bite should be cleansed thoroughly with soap and water. Precaution is indicated in removing engorged ticks from animals by hand, since infection through minor abrasions on the hands is possible.

At present there is no commercially available vaccine. Investigation of a more antigenic antigen replicated in chick-embryo cells continues and is encouraging. The administration of prophylactic antibiotics after tick exposure is not effective in preventing the disease.

# RUBELLA

method of
GAIL J. DEMMLER, M.D.
*Baylor College of Medicine*
*Houston, Texas*

### CLINICAL MANIFESTATIONS

Rubella is a mild illness characterized by a 2- to 3-week incubation period; a prodrome of malaise, low-grade fever, and mild upper respiratory symptoms; followed by a 2- to 3-day period of erythematous, maculopapular rash and mild postauricular and suboccipital lymphadenopathy. Polyarthralgia and polyarthritis also can occur, especially in adults. Extremely rare, yet serious, complications include encephalitis, myocarditis, and thrombocytopenia. Asymptomatic infection with rubella also can occur.

Congenital rubella syndrome can occur after a woman experiences a primary infection with rubella virus during the first or early second trimester of pregnancy. In contrast to the mild, self-limited illness of postnatal rubella, congenital rubella syndrome is a devastating disease. The classic manifestations of congenital rubella include intrauterine growth retardation, hepatosplenomegaly, thrombocytopenia, petechiae and purpuric skin lesions, microcephaly, cataracts, glaucoma, "salt and pepper" chorioretinitis, patent ductus arteriosus or pulmonary artery stenosis, sensorineural deafness, and meningoencephalitis. Late onset illnesses that result from congenital infection with rubella virus include diabetes mellitus and progressive hearing loss.

## DIAGNOSIS

Postnatal rubella can be diagnosed serologically. A seroconversion, a fourfold or greater rise in rubella-specific IgG antibody titer, or the presence of rubella-specific IgM antibody is diagnostic of a recent primary infection with rubella virus. The hemagglutination-inhibition (HAI) test was used for many years to determine the presence of rubella antibody. However, more sensitive tests, especially enzyme-linked immunosorbent assay (ELISA) and latex agglutination (LA), are now widely available. In addition, many clinical laboratories can determine the presence of rubella-specific IgM antibody.

Congenital rubella can be diagnosed serologically by the presence of rubella-specific IgM antibody in cord blood. In addition, the persistence of rubella-specific IgM antibody beyond the time of expected decline of passively acquired maternal antibody can help establish if a congenital infection with rubella virus has occurred. Rubella virus also can be isolated in tissue culture from a throat swab, nasal wash, buffy coat, urine, or cerebrospinal fluid specimen. Virus can be isolated from the throat of persons experiencing postnatal rubella as early as 7 days before onset of rash and for up to 7 days after the rash. Viral cultures for rubella in congenitally infected infants may be positive for up to 1 year after birth.

## TREATMENT

There is no specific antiviral therapy available for rubella. If postnatal rubella is complicated by arthritis, aspirin may be used (60 mg per kg per day for children, and 2 grams per day for adolescents and adults divided in four equal doses). Supportive therapy is indicated for complications such as severe thrombocytopenia and encephalitis.

Congenital rubella also is treated supportively. Expert cardiologic consultation may be required to diagnose and treat cardiac anomalies. Thrombocytopenia, especially if severe or symptomatic, may require platelet transfusions. Cataracts in babies usually require early surgery and optical correction with contact lenses, so that early expert ophthalmologic consultation is important. In addition, auditory assessment should be performed and hearing aids, if indicated, should be

fitted as soon as possible. Later in infancy, special education and physical therapy may be necessary.

## Isolation

Children with postnatal rubella should be excluded from school or day care for 7 days after onset of the rash. Infants with congenital rubella are contagious for 6 months and, ideally, should not be in a group care setting until they are a year old, since some children shed small quantities of virus for up to a year. Contact isolation is required for hospitalized patients with postnatal or congenital rubella. Pregnant women who are not rubella immune should not care for rubella-infected patients or children.

## Care of Exposed Pregnant Women

If a pregnant woman is exposed to rubella and she does not know her rubella immune status, a blood specimen should be obtained immediately and tested for rubella-specific IgG antibody. If antibody is present in this first specimen, the exposed person is immune and not at risk. Similarly, if a woman is known to be rubella immune from a previous test, she is not at risk. If rubella IgG antibody is not present at the time of exposure, however, a second blood specimen should be obtained 2 to 3 weeks post-exposure. If the repeat test is negative for rubella IgG antibody, a third test should be obtained 6 weeks post-exposure before it is safe to say infection did not occur. Of course, a positive rubella IgG antibody test in the second or third specimen indicates infection did occur around the time of exposure. Ideally, all blood specimens should be tested simultaneously in the same laboratory. A rubella IgM antibody test, if available, also can be performed on the specimens.

The gestational age at which maternal infection occurred is crucial in determining the risk to the fetus. Fetal infection and adverse outcome are most likely to occur when rubella is acquired during the first 12 weeks of pregnancy, though babies with symptomatic congenital rubella have been born to women infected with rubella as late as the twenty-fourth week of gestation. Women who experience a primary rubella infection during the first trimester and early second trimester of pregnancy should be carefully counseled by their physician. A thorough understanding of the pathogenesis of congenital rubella, as well as a deep compassion for the persons involved, is necessary if termination of the pregnancy is considered. If termination is not an option, administration of immune globulin (0.55 ml per kg intramuscularly) is recommended in the hope it may modify infection in the fetus to some degree. Rubella vaccine given immediately after exposure does not prevent illness and is not recommended in pregnant women.

## IMMUNIZATION

The live rubella virus vaccine with strain RA27/3 induces lifelong rubella antibody in greater than 98% of recipients. It is administered as a single 0.5-ml dose subcutaneously, either alone or, more commonly, in combination with mumps and measles vaccine (MMR). The vaccine may be given simultaneously with other immunizations such as diphtheria, tetanus, and pertussis (DTP) vaccine and oral poliovirus vaccine (OPV).

Rubella vaccine is effective if administered to children who are 12 months of age or older. Commonly, it is administered at 15 months of age as MMR. During measles epidemics, the vaccine can be administered to infants as young as 6 months of age. All human immunodeficiency virus (HIV)–infected children, regardless of symptoms, should receive rubella vaccine. Postpubertal females who are not known to be immune should be immunized. Prenatal screening for rubella immunity should be routine and vaccine should be administered immediately post partum in those women found to be susceptible. Breast-feeding is not contraindicated after rubella vaccination. Adults, both male and female, who work in educational institutions, day care centers, or health care facilities should be immune to rubella. The rubella vaccine is generally well tolerated but can cause rash, low-grade fever, and mild lymphadenopathy in children 5 to 12 days post-vaccination. Transient arthralgias and arthritis can occur in adults, especially females, 7 to 21 days post-vaccination.

Contraindications to rubella vaccine include pregnancy because of the theoretical risk to the fetus. Women of childbearing age should wait at least 3 months after vaccination before becoming pregnant. However, if a woman who is pregnant inadvertently receives the vaccine, she can be reassured that congenital rubella syndrome from rubella vaccine has never been reported, and termination of pregnancy after receipt of vaccine during pregnancy is not recommended. Patients who are immunocompromised (those with leukemia, lymphoma, generalized malignancy, etc.) or who are receiving large doses of corticosteroids, alkylating agents, antimetabolites, or radiation should not receive the live rubella vaccine. Three months after cessation of any immunosuppression, it is generally permissible to administer rubella vaccine, though the interval may vary depending on the type and intensity of immunosuppression. The vaccine should not be administered within 3 months of the administration of immune globulin because immune globulin may neutralize vaccine virus and prevent successful vaccination. However, vaccine may be given post partum at the same time as anti-Rho(D) Ig or after blood product transfusion. Minor illnesses, such as upper respiratory illness, are not contraindications to rubella vaccine.

# MEASLES
## (Rubeola)

method of
PHYLLIS R. BISHOP, M.D., and
SANDOR FELDMAN, M.D.
*University of Mississippi Medical Center*
*Jackson, Mississippi*

Measles and smallpox simultaneously appeared in France, during the Saracen invasion of the ninth century. Measles was first declared a unique clinical entity in 1675 with its separation from smallpox. It was known as *morbilli,* Italian for "a little plague," until the mid 1700s when Sauvages first called it rubeola.

During the prevaccine era there were more than 500,000 U.S. cases of measles annually with a mortality rate of 1–2 in 1000. Since the introduction of the first measles vaccine in 1963, the number of measles cases has declined 98 to 99%. In underdeveloped countries, mortality from measles complications still approaches 10%.

### ETIOLOGY, TRANSMISSION, PATHOLOGY, AND EPIDEMIOLOGY

Measles is caused by a single-stranded ribonucleic acid (RNA) virus in the Paramyxoviridae family. The virus is readily transmitted by respiratory droplets from an infected source and may remain infective up to several hours in the environment. Infectious virions invade the respiratory epithelium where local replication occurs, followed by a primary viremia. In the reticuloendothelial system, the virus replicates rapidly, resulting in a secondary viremia. The widely disseminated infection causes acute inflammatory changes in the conjunctiva, oral mucosa, and respiratory tract epithelial cells. There is generalized lymphoid hyperplasia and perivascular cuffing of small vessels, rarely complicated by hemorrhage. Central nervous system (CNS) involvement is not uncommon, and brain edema and demyelinization may occur acutely.

Measles has a worldwide distribution and is one of the most communicable of all infectious diseases. In temperate climates it has a winter-spring pattern of occurrence, with epidemics and endemics every 2 or 5 years.

## CLINICAL COURSE

The prodromal phase of measles begins 10 to 11 days after exposure and corresponds to the onset of the secondary viremia. Its duration is 3 to 4 days, and symptoms include fever greater than 101° F and at least one of the following: cough, coryza, or conjunctivitis (Fig. 1). On the third day of the prodrome, pathognomonic Koplik spots (which represent inflammation of submucous glands) appear on the oral mucosa. They are pale, raised papules on dull red bases that which are most consistently found on the buccal surface opposite the molars.

The eruptive phase begins late on the third or fourth day with a rise in temperature, frequently to 104° to 105° F. The distinctive maculopapular rash begins on the face and spreads to the trunk and limbs within 3 days. The lesions are irregular in shape and size, often coalescing into patches with sharp margins. They are a deep rose color ("red measles"), more purple than red, and minute hemorrhages may occur. Desquamation is minimal and may include the palms and the soles. The peripheral white blood cell (WBC) count is decreased and there is a relative lymphocytosis. By the seventh day of the illness, the temperature returns to the normal range and the rash begins to fade ("7-day measles").

## COMPLICATIONS

### Respiratory Tract

Respiratory tract complications include otitis media, cervical adenitis, laryngitis, laryngotracheitis, and bronchopneumonia. Bronchopneumonia occurs in 10% of patients and is the most common serious complication of measles. It is usually due to a secondary bacterial infection and is the leading cause of measles-related deaths. Giant cell pneumonia (Hecht's pneu-

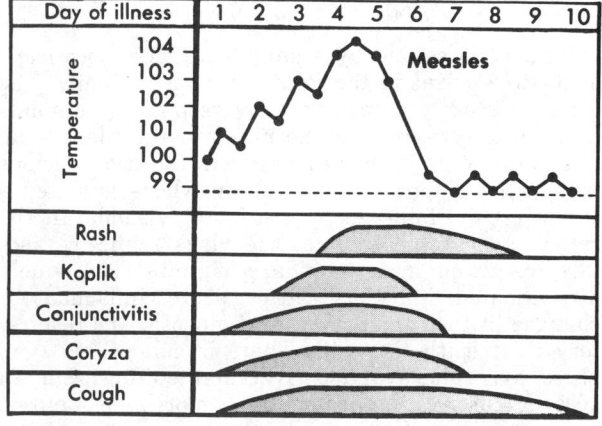

**Figure 1.** Schematic diagram of clinical course of a typical case of measles. Rash appears 3 to 4 days after onset of fever, conjunctivitis, coryza, and cough. Koplik spots usually develop 2 days before rash. (From Krugman S, et al: Infectious Diseases of Children, ed 8, St. Louis, 1985, The CV Mosby Co. Used by permission.)

monia), owing to viral invasion of the lung, may occur in the immunocompromised patient.

### Gastrointestinal

Diarrhea, minimal in developed countries, is responsible for significant morbidity and mortality in Third World countries. Gastrointestinal hemorrhages are very rare.

### Central Nervous System

Acute encephalitis occurs in 1 in 1000 cases. Mortality is 15%, and permanent neurologic sequelae are found in 25% of the survivors. Encephalitis usually appears within the first 6 days of rash but may occur later. Its onset is heralded by a resurgence of fever, headache, change in consciousness, and occasionally seizures. Studies have shown that up to 50% of measles patients show EEG abnormalities, suggesting asymptomatic CNS involvement. In acute measles encephalitis virus may be isolated from the cerebrospinal fluid (CSF) and brain.

Subacute sclerosing panencephalitis (SSPE) is a slowly progressive demyelinating and degenerative cerebral disease with onset years after measles infection. It occurs in 1 in 100,000 cases of natural measles versus 1 in 2 to 3 million recipients of the measles vaccine. Initial symptoms are subtle intellectual decline, myoclonus, or ataxia. Less commonly, dysarthria and seizures may be presenting features. Progression is variable over months to years but is ultimately fatal. Typical EEG findings are bursts of high voltage slow waves with myoclonus. Diagnosis is based on clinical findings and high levels of measles antibody in the CSF and serum.

Immunosuppressive measles encephalitis, or "delayed acute" encephalitis, is an opportunistic infection of measles in the immunocompromised host. Incubation period is 5 weeks to 6 months with CNS invasion by neurovirulent variants of the measles virus. Symptoms include progressive neurologic deterioration, convulsions, twitching, coma, and death. Computed tomography (CT) of the brain shows atrophy. Antibody to measles virus has been inconsistently found in the CSF of these patients.

## TREATMENT AND NATURAL IMMUNITY

There is no specific antiviral chemotherapy for the treatment of measles, although ribavirin (Virazole) in two uncontrolled studies has been associated with amelioration of symptoms and decreased duration. Immune serum globulin (0.5 ml per kg, to a maximum of 15 ml) is recommended postexposure in the immunocompromised host. Isolation of the infected individual should be from onset of prodrome to 4 to 5 days posteruption of rash. Natural infection confers lifelong immunity.

## Atypical Measles

Atypical measles has been reported in individuals receiving the killed measles vaccine in whom there was subsequent exposure to the wild virus. Its pathogenesis is thought to be hypersensitivity to measles virus in a partially immune host. The prodrome lasts 1 to 2 days and is characterized by high fever, headache, abdominal pain, and myalgia. Koplik's spots are not found. In contrast to prototypical measles, the rash begins peripherally and may be hemorrhagic, urticarial, maculopapular, or vesicular. Severe lobar pneumonia is a prominent finding. The measles virus is transmissible from the onset of the prodrome to 4 to 5 days after rash eruption. Management is symptomatic.

## CURRENT VACCINATION RECOMMENDATIONS

Revaccination is recommended for all adults born after 1956 without a previous history of two doses of live measles vaccine on or after their first birthday, physician-diagnosed measles, or laboratory evidence of immunity. Furthermore, it is strongly recommended that medical facilities adhere strictly to this policy for their employees. Since 1986, there has been a recrudescence of measles. The incidence increased 300% in the first half of 1989 as compared with a similar period in 1988. The American Academy of Pediatrics (AAP) and the Immunization Practices Advisory Committee (ACIP) of the Centers for Disease Control (CDC) advise a two-dose schedule for the measles vaccine. The committees agree on administration of the initial measles-mumps-rubella (MMR) vaccine at 15 months. Controversy arises in the scheduling of the second dose. ACIP recommends that the second MMR be given on entry into kindergarten or first grade. This would coincide with the standard requirement for the booster DPT and polio, eliminating the need for an additional provider visit and having the children "captive." However, the AAP advises that the second dose be administered on entry into middle or junior high school, since the risk of measles substantially increases after age 12 for individuals receiving the 15-month MMR. The reader is advised to contact local health department officials for further recommendations on the timing of the second dose.

In high-risk situations such as inner city areas and in countries where more than five cases of measles in preschoolers have occurred in the last 5 years, the age for initial MMR should be lowered to 12 months. During extensive local outbreaks, the monovalent measles vaccine may be administered as early as 6 months. Vaccine before age one does not preclude the need for two subsequent doses of MMR.

For international travel, ACIP recommends that adults should have two prior doses of measles vaccine or physician-documented infection or positive measles serology or they should receive a dose of measles vaccine before departure. Children 12 to 14 months should receive one dose of MMR prior to traveling, and infants 6 to 11 months receive one dose of monovalent measles vaccine before traveling.

Human immunodeficiency virus (HIV) antibody–positive children who are asymptomatic should receive the MMR at 15 months of age. Infants symptomatic of HIV infection should be considered for immunization, since they are at risk for severe infection.

A recent report suggests that during immunosuppressive therapy for leukemia, some previously vaccinated patients have become seronegative. It is suggested that previously vaccinated cancer patients and other immunosuppressed patients successfully completing therapy be evaluated for antibody status to measles (mumps and rubella) or be revaccinated. Initial or repeat vaccination may be administered 3 or more months after termination of immunosuppressive therapy.

The measles vaccine is contraindicated in pregnancy or in those who plan to conceive within 3 months of vaccination. The vaccine is also contraindicated in the patient receiving immunosuppressive therapy and in those with previous anaphylactic reaction to neomycin.

# TETANUS

method of
FRANÇOIS VACHON, M.D.
*Hôpital Bichat/Claude Bernard*
*University of Paris*
*Paris, France*

Tetanus (lockjaw) is a severe disease that is caused when the anaerobic telluric toxin-producing *Clostridium tetani* is introduced into the body at the site of a wound. It is characterized first by trismus, then by a generalized permanent contracture of voluntary muscles, with tonic spasms. There is a high risk of respiratory arrest at any time. Until modern treatment, the mortality was high, but now intensive care obtains good results.

## TREATMENT

### Serotherapy

The toxin can be neutralized by intramuscular or intravenous injections of antitoxin if it is not already fixed onto the nervous tissues. Studies in intensive care units have not shown any obviously significant advantages of high doses of antitoxin, because of the side effects of heterologous antitoxin and the cost of homologous serum. Many investigators still recommend the use of small doses of antitoxin serum (500 to 1000 IU of homologous serum or 1500 to 10,000 IU of heterologous serum). However, the death rate has been found to increase in the absence of early serotherapy, particularly in countries with few intensive care facilities or none at all.

Serotherapy is thought to be of more benefit when administered by the intrathecal route. Animal experiments suggest that the antitoxin is able to combine with the fixed toxin in the intraneuronal areas when antitoxin is given intrathecally. Several studies have substantiated the beneficial effects of intrathecal antitoxin administration, especially where intensive care facilities are not available. Various studies may have yielded different results because of differences in the experimental protocols: dosage, type of antitoxin, and site of injection (lumbar or suboccipital) are only some of the variables that can affect outcome. The precise protocol for correct intrathecal administration (route of injection, dosage, type of antitoxin) is still to be determined, and no specific antitoxin for this technique is yet commercially available. The present antitoxin preparations are stabilized with phenol byproducts and cannot be safely injected into the cerebrospinal fluid.

### Surgical Wound Care

Wounds are often not explored because they seem too minor or because they have already healed (even though they may contain foreign material detected on x-ray films) or because they are apparently too trivial to have attracted attention (e.g., ingrowing toenail). A lot of these wounds should, however, be opened and excised if they harbor the possibility of proliferating tetanus bacilli. Ignoring them facilitates progression and exacerbation of the disease, with the possibility of relapse after the acute phase is over because of the persisting release of free toxin from the wound if the patient has not been vaccinated or treated at the time with serotherapy.

A large dirty wound that does not heal easily must be washed, excised, and fully opened.

Chronic wounds (e.g., varicose ulcers) are treated in a classic manner. Particular situations may warrant more specific treatment, such as curettage or hysterectomy in tetanus following abortion, limb amputation in the case of major

and irreversible injuries of the limb, or excision of ulcerated tumors.

In addition, penicillin G, 3 to 6 million U per day, is given. Larger dosages are used in the case of extensive necrotic or dirty wounds. Any patient with penicillin intolerance should be treated with erythromycin or other appropriate antibiotics.

### Intensive Care of Generalized Tetanus

**Respiratory Assistance.** From the onset of generalized tetanus, the primary risk is that of asphyxia. Treatment includes tracheostomy (or tracheal intubation) as the only technique that can prevent glottic spasm. While ensuring a patent airway, it allows aspiration of saliva from the trachea and is easily completed by artificial ventilation as required.

Tracheostomy should be performed as soon as the spasms start to spread and should not be delayed until respiration is impaired. This course is recommended, particularly if the circulation period has been short. Some authors recommend prolonged intubation, but most investigators consider that tracheostomy is safer for a disease whose course is expected to last 2 to 3 weeks or longer.

**Control of Spasms.** The administration of muscle relaxants is the second course of treatment allowing the control of tetanic spasms and preventing the blocking of respiratory muscles. Many drugs have been used. In my experience, the following preparations merit attention:

Diazepam (Valium) has a remarkable muscle-relaxant action and has transformed the treatment of tetanus since 1965. Its hemodynamic side effects are usually negligible, even when high dosages are used. An injection of 10 mg or more intravenously can depress respiration, and respiratory assistance is usually necessary when the total daily dose equals 120 mg.*

The serum concentration of diazepam reached after oral administration can vary some 20-fold in different patients. Absorption is poor following intramuscular injection, and this mode of administration is not suitable for prolonged treatment. When the treatment is stopped, a secondary release from the tissues, especially from the body fat, ensures a sufficient concentration of the drug for about a week. Therefore, it is better to use large dosages at the start of treatment and to reduce the dosage quickly afterwards. Smaller dosages should be given in the case of hepatic insufficiency.

Clorazepate (Tranxene), which belongs to the same group of drugs, can be used as an alternative.

---

\* Exceeds dosage recommended by the manufacturer.

Dantrolene (Dantrium) has also been proposed for use in the treatment of tetanic spasm. Its antispasmodic action is adequate, but it seems to have more side effects than diazepam.

Carbamates are used in some countries (particularly meprobamate [Equanil]), but are of relatively little value.

Barbiturates are used only in conjunction with diazepam, during severe tetanus, or when curarization is necessary. Rapid-acting barbiturates allow control of acute episodes, but can cause hemodynamic disorders. In the dosages that are needed to treat tetanus, all barbiturates depress respiration; consequently, artificial ventilation is often required. The dosage must be modified in the presence of renal or hepatic failure.

Central analgesics have marked effects on spasms. From the hemodynamic point of view, phenoperidine* and fentanyl (Sublimaze) are the best tolerated at present. When they are injected intermittently, their action is short (30 minutes), and after a few days their effect is less pronounced.

Nondepolarizing neuromuscular blocking agents are used if necessary for treatment of tetanus. Pancuronium bromide (Pavulon) is particularly valuable because of its minimal cardiovascular effects and the lack of histamine release. It is excreted via the kidneys and does not accumulate; plasma concentrations rapidly fall below the activity threshold when administration is stopped, even after a 1- to 3-week course.

### Where and How to Treat

The main problem in the treatment of tetanus is the control of spasms. The dosage of drugs required to achieve this depresses ventilatory function, and the complications of the disease itself combine with this effect to make respiratory assistance necessary. Therefore, effective management is only possible in a special unit with the facilities for providing all areas of treatment. Many of the problems that arise are side effects of the treatment, especially in elderly patients.

Pharmacologic agents designed to restore cholinesterase levels to normal have been tried in tetanus, but have not met with success.

Tracheostomy is carried out under local anesthesia after premedication, including atropine, 0.25 mg, and meperidine (Demerol), 1 mg per kg. Intravenous diazepam, 5 to 10 mg per hour, is started immediately, and the dosage is increased as required up to a maximum of about 7 to 10 mg per kg per day. During 2 to 5 days, administration via the enteral route, via a nasogastric tube, is gradually substituted for the parenteral route. The total daily dose is distributed evenly every 2 to 3 hours and adjusted daily for optimal control of the spasms. The average daily dose for an adult is 250 mg.

Artificial ventilation is initiated according to the effects of diazepam on the level of consciousness and the respiratory status.

Treatment is eventually progressively reduced, depending on the patient's condition. The average duration of treatment is 2 to 3 weeks. In elderly and obese patients, the drugs must be withdrawn sooner.

Actual recovery does not really begin until 5 to 15 days after diazepam has been discontinued; the tracheostomy tube is not removed until the patient is able to swallow normally.

The need for additional treatment is conceded when prolonged spasms persist, despite a rapid increase of the dosage of diazepam to the maximum compatible with safety, and also when injections of diazepam, 10 mg intravenously, provide only short periods of sedation (less than 5 minutes) or no sedation at all. Additional drugs are then prescribed, such as rapid-acting barbiturates (thiopental sodium [Pentothal], 2 to 4 grams per day in adults) for 2 or 3 days and central analgesics, particularly phenoperidine* intravenously, as required.

**Curarization.** If treatment fails to improve the patient's condition, intermittent injections of a nondepolarizing muscle relaxant may prove useful and are usually the prelude to continuous curarization.

Whether to paralyze the patient is a difficult decision because of the hazard that can be associated with prolonged curarization. It is not an acceptable treatment for milder cases of tetanus, and most workers believe that it must be reserved for the severe forms that cannot be controlled by sedation. The circulating blood volume must be adequate, and sedation is continued. Curare may be administered intravenously or via a subcutaneous needle continuously by means of an infusion pump. Pancuronium bromide (Pavulon) has been the preferred preparation for curarization; dosages vary in adults and are determined individually for each patient at about 0.25 mg per kg per day. Serum concentrations, however, are variable (between 0.27 and 0.48 microgram per ml).

As for patients dependent on artificial ventilation, curarized patients require constant surveillance. Adequate sedation must be provided. The balloon of the tracheostomy cannula must remain inflated continuouously, and tracheal aspirations must be frequent and brief to avoid hypoxia.

---

* Not available in the United States.

* Not available in the United States.

When the clinical course allows, curare is withdrawn and replaced by diazepam for a few days. The average duration of treatment is 15 to 20 days.

Cardiac activity must be monitored for at least 10 days after the administration of curare has been stopped.

**Other Aspects of Therapy.** The patient should be placed in a private, quiet room, and efforts should be made to reduce all external stimuli as much as possible.

Careful attention to fluid and electrolyte balance is required. A high water and sodium intake is necessary, usually between 3000 and 4000 ml per day, because of increased sweating. Nasogastric feeding can usually be started after 3 to 4 days. A high caloric and protein intake is essential, at least 3000 calories and 120 grams of protein per day. Defecation must be controlled. In curarized patients, paralytic ileus may prevent enteral feeding, and intravenous feeding should then be substituted.

Catheterization of the bladder is usually needed to prevent urinary retention.

The importance of nursing care and physiotherapy has been stressed. Insertion of a padded tongue depressor can protect the tongue from being bitten during tonic contractions. Particular attention must be given to incomplete closure of the eyelids during curarization.

Pulmonary embolism used to be a frequent cause of death during tetanus, but preventive treatment with subcutaneously administered heparin has markedly reduced its incidence.

Hyperbaric oxygen therapy has been proposed by some authors, but does not seem to be widely used.

Circulatory disorders are not rare during tetanus, and they vary in nature and severity. In the early stages of the disease, they are generally related to hypovolemia and often become manifest as hypotension after the administration of sedatives.

Disorders specific to tetanus are more severe; they are probably not frequent, but their incidence is difficult to evaluate. In the past decade, several studies have been devoted to the pathogenesis and treatment of these autonomic dysfunctions. Signs of sympathetic hyperactivity appear a few days after the onset of the disease and consist of large and rapid variations in heart rate, arterial pressure, and (if they are measured) cardiac output and systemic vascular resistance. There appears to be a parallel increase in both alpha- and beta-adrenergic activities of either peripheral or central origin. Many types of drugs have been tried in such situations with varying and sometimes contradictory results:

Beta-adrenergic blockers, such as propanolol (Inderal) or pindolol (Visken), do not control the disorders fully. Labetalol (Trandate, Normodyne) has been found to be effective.

Although they control hypertension, alpha blockers, such as phenoxybenzamine (Dibenzyline) and phentolamine (Regitine) have been abandoned in tetanus treatment because of the severe secondary hypotension that is likely to appear.

Central nervous system depressants, particularly chlorpromazine (Thorazine), which also has an alpha-adrenergic blocker action, can control the disorder with few side effects.

Recovery occurs slowly, and rehabilitation with active and passive re-education of the muscles must be started early to avoid stiffness of the joints and muscles. This type of disability is marked in 10 to 15%; 3% of people affected by tetanus develop ossification adjacent to the joints, especially the elbow.

### Neonatal Tetanus

The treatment of neonatal tetanus is not different from that of the adult form, except that, if barbiturates are used, they must be prescribed at low dosages because of a possible deleterious effect on cerebral development. Only the techniques, particularly those for ventilation and feeding, are different, requiring specially trained medical staff for the management of the acute phase, which often lasts 4 to 6 weeks. In centers frequently treating neonatal tetanus, mortality should not be higher than 20%. Although neonatal tetanus has almost disappeared in Western countries, it remains a serious problem in countries with few or no technical resources.

The main features of treatment of the neonate with tetanus are: early control of spasms with diazepam, 0.3 to 1 mg per kg intravenously; passage of a nasojejunal tube to allow administration of water, electrolytes, food, and drugs; and injections of antitoxin (10,000 IU intramuscularly or 500 to 1000 IU intrathecally). Nonetheless, this treatment does not prevent a high mortality, between 70 and 90%. In nondeveloped countries, this is the form of treatment that is most frequently adopted.

Sedative drugs are administered, but the dosages are reduced to avoid undue respiratory depression.

This treatment protocol can be improved at little cost by providing facilities for isolating the patient (which can be difficult in some societies) and for performing tracheostomy as required. Even though artificial ventilation may not be available, tracheostomy prevents the occurrence of severe apnea due to glottic spasms and ensures a patent airway. A nasogastric tube can also then be inserted for parenteral feeding. These measures would entail the setting up of special care units, with the expectation that the mortality in this age group would fall to about 25%; the cost could be relatively low.

# TOXOPLASMOSIS

method of
THOMAS G. EVANS, M.D.
*University of Utah*
*Salt Lake City, Utah*

Toxoplasmosis, or infection by the parasitic protozoan *Toxoplasma gondii,* is a common and frequently missed diagnosis in the United States and throughout the world. Many hosts, including humans, ingest viable tissue cysts or sporulated oocysts, which develop into invasive trophozoites (tachyzoites). This invasive form of the organism then spreads hematogenously and disseminates to all tissues. After the tachyzoites have spread throughout the body, immune system control results in the formation of tissue cysts in most immunocompetent hosts. These cysts can survive for the life of the individual and later lead to further invasive trophozoites. Disease can therefore be characterized either as an acute infection or as a reactivation of latent infection.

Only in the cat gut does the organism undergo a definitive sexual stage, which results in the oocyst. Humans can thus become infected by contact with cat feces in food or the environment, by ingestion of tissue cysts in a variety of uncooked meat, through transplacental infection of the fetus, through white blood cell transfusions, or by organ transplantation of infected tissues. Depending on the environment and eating habits, 3 to 70% of individuals in the United States are infected with *T. gondii.* In many European countries, such as Holland and France, this percentage is much higher. Because the overwhelming majority of these infected individuals have asymptomatic disease, which requires no treatment, the decision to treat is based on a number of other factors; the most important of these are the immune status of the patient, the relationship of infection to pregnancy, the location of the infection, and the severity of the initial response.

## TREATMENT

The treatment of the various syndromes of toxoplasmosis is not based on large studies, but rather on a wealth of clinical experience. Table 1 summarizes the syndromes that do and do not require treatment and lists acceptable therapies.

### Acute Infection

In immunologically normal adults and children, symptomatic infection with *T. gondii* usually results in a mononucleosislike syndrome, characterized by lymphadenopathy. This is a self-resolving illness, which rarely requires treatment. Indications for treatment include severe myocarditis, hepatitis, encephalitis, and, rarely, episodes of pneumonitis. Many experts would also include primary laboratory infection as a reason to treat, as these infections may be more severe than naturally acquired infections. Treatment of choice is pyrimethamine (Daraprim), 25 mg per day; leucovorin (folinic acid), 10 mg per day; and sulfadiazine, 75 mg per kg per day with a maximum of 6 grams per day. These drugs act synergistically against the trophozoites, but do not eliminate the tissue cysts that have developed. Treatment is continued for 4 to 6 weeks.

Primary infection during pregnancy represents a serious risk to the fetus. Although the likelihood of infection of the fetus increases from approximately 20% during the first trimester to 60% during the third, infection is more severe when it is acquired earlier in pregnancy. French investigators have shown that treatment of the maternal infection given as soon as infection is diagnosed or suspected reduces congenital transmission. Therapy consists of spiramycin (Rovamycine), 3 grams per day in divided doses for the entirety of the pregnancy. The fetus can then be monitored by amniocentesis and ultrasonography to attempt to document infection before delivery. If abnormalities are discovered during the second or third trimester, pyrimethamine and sulfadiazine should be added to the spiramycin therapy. An alternative regimen for the infected fetus used in these studies was to alternate spiramycin, 3 grams per day for 3 weeks, with 3 weeks of daily pyrimethamine (50 mg) and sulfadiazine (3 grams per day), along with leucovorin.

In the congenitally infected infant, treatment is always indicated to attempt to prevent the serious sequelae that can occur at birth or later in life. If the mother is known to have acquired the infection during pregnancy, treatment should be started immediately. In the asymptomatic or symptomatic infant, pyrimethamine, 1 mg per kg every other day (maximum 25 mg), plus leucovorin, 5 mg every other day, and sulfadiazine, 75 to 100 mg per kg per day given in two divided doses, should be administered during the first 21 days. In the symptomatic infant, the initial two dosages of pyrimethamine are often given as 2 mg per kg. In the asymptomatic infant, spiramycin should be begun after the 3-week initial therapy above and continued until a definitive diagnosis of congenital toxoplasmosis is either confirmed or eliminated.

In the symptomatic infant or confirmed asymptomatic case, treatment should continue for a minimum of 6 months; most authorities prefer a

TABLE 1. **Treatment Regimens for Toxoplasmosis**

| Syndrome | Treatment | Duration of Treatment |
|---|---|---|
| *Acute Infection* | | |
| Adult, asymptomatic | None | |
| Adult, severe (hepatitis, pneumonitis) | Pyrimethamine,* 25 mg/day, plus sulfadiazine, 75 mg/kg/day in 4 divided doses (maximum 6 grams) plus leucovorin, 10 mg/day | 4–6 wk |
| Pregnant female† | Spiramycin, 3 grams/day in 3–4 divided doses | Throughout pregnancy |
| With evidence of fetal infection | Same as severe disease in adult | 2nd and 3rd trimester |
| Congenital infection, suspected | Pyrimethamine,* 1 mg/day qid (maximum 25 mg), plus sulfadiazine, 75–100 mg/kg/day in 2 divided doses, plus leucovorin, 5 mg qid | 21 days or until definitive testing results |
| Congenital infection, proven‡ | As above and then alternate 21-day cycles with 45–60 days of spiramycin, 100 mg/kg/day in 2 divided doses (maximum 3 grams) | 12 mo |
| *Reactivation* | | |
| Ocular‡ | Same as severe disease in adult; as an *alternative*, substitute clindamycin, 300–600 mg q 6 hr, for sulfadiazine | 1 mo |
| Encephalitis | | |
| AIDS, acute‡ | Pyrimethamine,* 50–100 mg/day, plus sulfadiazine, 6–8 grams/day in 3–4 divided doses; as an *alternative*, substitute clindamycin, 2400–4800 mg/day in 3–4 divided doses, for sulfadiazine | 4–6 wk or until resolution of symptoms |
| AIDS, maintenance | Pyrimethamine, 25–50 mg/day, plus sulfadiazine, 2 grams/day in 4 divided doses, plus leucovorin, 10–20 mg/day; as an *alternative* substitute clindamycin, 300–600 mg q 6 hr, for sulfadiazine | Indefinite |
| Immunodeficient patients‡ | Similar to AIDS, acute (usually slightly lower doses) | 4–6 wk after resolution of symptoms |

*Pyrimethamine is often given as a loading dose during the first 2 to 3 days of treatment at 200 mg/day in 2 divided doses in the adult and at 2 mg/kg in the infant.

†Pyrimethamine should not be used during the first trimester.

‡Many experts would add prednisone, 1 mg/kg/day, then tapering, for treatment of these conditions.

12-month regimen, although there are few data to substantiate either regimen. Treatment can be administered by continuing the above dosages of pyrimethamine, folinic acid, and sulfadiazine, or by alternating this regimen with 4- to 6-week cycles of spiramycin, 100 mg per kg per day.

## Reactivation

Ocular toxoplasmosis is usually due to reactivation of infection in adults. The disease in the eye results in chorioretinitis and requires ophthalmologic monitoring. Treatment is usually the same as that of severe primary infection in the adult (see earlier). When the macula or optic nerve is involved, or widespread lesions appear, corticosteroids may be added at relatively high dosages (1 mg per kg of prednisone per day) to decrease inflammation. Many ophthalmologists also substitute clindamycin (Cleocin), 1200 to 2400 mg per day in three or four divided doses), for sulfadiazine, because clindamycin is concentrated by the choroid.

Infection due to reactivation in the immunosuppressed patient has given birth to a renewed interest in therapy for toxoplasmosis. Nearly 10% of patients with the acquired immune deficiency syndrome (AIDS) develop toxoplasmosis, almost always as a severe encephalitis. Others at risk include transplant recipients, individuals with lymphoma, and patients with immunologic diseases, such as systemic lupus erythematosus, that require immunosuppressive therapy. In the AIDS patient, the onset of neurologic symptoms accompanied by multiple ring-enhancing lesions demands the immediate initiation of therapy for toxoplasmosis with pyrimethamine, 50 to 100 mg per day, plus leucovorin, 10 mg per day, and sulfadiazine, 6 to 8 grams per day in divided doses. Often, a 100- to 200- mg loading dose of pyrimethamine is used. In the sulfa-intolerant patient, clindamycin, 1800 to 3600 mg per day, should be substituted. The leucovorin dose can be increased if there is severe hematologic toxicity from the pyrimethamine.

If there is no improvement in the patient or the lesions during the ensuing 10 to 14 days, diagnosis of the lesion with brain biopsy should be pursued. Corticosteroids should be added for most patients who have significant edema associated with their infection. High-dose therapy should continue for 3 to 4 weeks or until no further improvement can be noted.

Primary treatment failure results in 10 to 20% of patients, but this does not necessarily indicate drug resistance. However, alternatives include switching from sulfadiazine to clindamycin and increasing all drug dosages to a maximal range, including up to 4800 mg per day of clindamycin. In event of failure at these high dosages, trimetrexate can be considered, but little clinical evidence is available for its effectiveness in humans. Spiramycin is not effective in primary or suppressive therapy of toxoplasmosis encephalitis. In addition, there is in vitro evidence that zidovudine may antagonize therapy for toxoplasmosis. Referral to national trials of investigational agents should be considered for treatment failures.

Because these regimens do not eliminate the tissue cysts and do not alleviate the underlying immune defect in AIDS, toxoplasmosis in AIDS patients should be treated for life. A variety of suppressive regimens have been suggested, but, in general, the patient should be continued on the same therapy as the primary treatment at lower dosages. Thus, 25 to 50 mg per day of pyrimethamine plus 10 mg of leucovorin is combined with either sulfadiazine, 2 to 4 grams per day, or clindamycin, 900 to 1800 mg per day, in three or four divided doses.

### Drugs

Pyrimethamine (Daraprim) is a lipid-soluble inhibitor of *T. gondii* dihydrofolate reductase. It penetrates most tissues well, including the cerebrospinal fluid. It is more active than trimethoprim, another member of the same class of compounds, against *T. gondii,* but may be less active in vitro than trimetrexate. The usual dosage is 25 mg per day, but in severe encephalitis associated with AIDS, some investigators have raised the dosage to as high as 75 to 100 mg per day. One to 2 mg per kg is a standard pediatric dosage.

Toxicities associated with the compound include bone marrow suppression, resulting in leukopenia, thrombocytopenia, and anemia. This side effect can be reduced with the use of folinic acid (leucovorin), at usual dosages of 10 mg per day. Folic acid interferes with the antiparasitic effect of the drug and should not be used. Complete blood counts should be monitored at least every 2 weeks in patients taking pyrimethamine. Other side effects include mild gastrointestinal upset, with diarrhea, nausea, and vomiting, as well as occasional headache. The compound is teratogenic during the first trimester and should not be used during early pregnancy.

Many sulfa drugs are effective against *T. gondii;* however, sulfadiazine and trisulfapyrimidines are the most active. Sulfisoxazole and sulfamethoxazole are less active and should be avoided. Toxicities include crystalluria; hypersensitivity reactions, including severe rash and high fever; the Stevens-Johnson syndrome; and leukopenia. Gastrointestinal side effects, such as nausea, vomiting, and diarrhea, can occur. Patients should be well hydrated with oral or intravenous fluids to avoid the renal effects. More than half of the individuals with AIDS who are treated with sulfonamides experience rash, fever, or neutropenia. Alternatives consist of lowering the dosage by 25 to 50%, with further monitoring, or discontinuing the drug. Typical dosages of sulfadiazine are 6 to 8 grams per day in divided doses.

Spiramycin (Rovamycine) is a macrolide antibiotic that has been widely used outside of the United States (especially in France) and is not yet available commercially in the United States. It is readily obtainable by request to the U.S. Food and Drug Administration (FDA). Spiramycin is typically administered at dosages of 3 to 4 grams per day in divided doses to the adult and as 100 mg per kg to children. Potential toxicities include gastrointestinal pain and upset. Rash is rarely seen.

Clindamycin (Cleocin) is now frequently used in the treatment of toxoplasmosis in AIDS patients who cannot tolerate sulfonamides or as primary therapy in ocular toxoplasmosis. Side effects include the possibility of *Clostridium difficile*–associated diarrhea or pseudomembranous colitis, rash, fever, granulocytopenia, and gastrointestinal upset. Dosages recommended vary, are based mostly on small or anecdotal series, and range from 900 to 2400 mg per day in divided doses. Because clindamycin has low concentrations in the brain, some investigators have used dosages as high as 3600 mg per day in severe cases or treatment failures of AIDS-related toxoplasmosis encephalitis.

The failure of many regimens in AIDS patients has resulted in a flurry of study of new drugs. Potential agents include the dihydrofolate reductase inhibitor trimetrexate, which is available from the FDA as an Investigational New Drug for failed therapy of pneumocystis pneumonia. The in vitro activity is superior to that of pyrimethamine, but large-scale clinical data on this compound are still lacking. The macrolide antibiotics roxithromycin or azithromycin, which are related to spiramycin, also have in vitro activity with little clinical data. Interferon-gamma has significant in vitro activity and is effective in animal models of toxoplasmosis. Clinical studies of this immune modulator in AIDS encephalitis have begun, but results are not yet available.

# TRICHINELLOSIS

method of
ZBIGNIEW S. PAWLOWSKI, M.D.
*Academy of Medicine*
*Poznań, Poland*

Trichinellosis, or trichinosis, is caused by an intestinal nematode *(Trichinella spiralis),* which produces larvae that invade muscle tissue. The infection is contracted chiefly by ingesting raw infected pork. Other meats, such as horse, wild boar, bear, or walrus, may occasionally be the source of trichinellosis. Many cases of *T. spiralis* infection remain asymptomatic or abortive, with only eosinophilia and a few transient symptoms. Others have a mild or moderate clinical expression. Some have a severe course, with a fully developed trichinellosis syndrome owing to allergic vasculitis and myositis; life-threatening neurologic or cardiovascular complications may occur.

## TREATMENT

The efficacy of treatment of human trichinellosis depends on the intensity of infection, the strain of infecting *T. spiralis,* the duration of infection (early infection, acute disease, late phase of disease), and the character and intensity of the host response.

### Intestinal Infection

The production of newborn *T. spiralis* larvae that migrate to various tissues of the human host is stopped by ridding the small intestine of adult worms. Therefore, treatment against intestinal *Trichinella* is obligatory in any case of infection: proved or only suspected, symptomatic or asymptomatic, severe or mild, and early or late (up to 6 weeks after ingestion of infected meat). Currently, the following drugs are in use: pyrantel (Antiminth, Combantrin),* 10 mg per kg per day for 5 days, mebendazole (Vermox),† 200 mg per day for 5 days, or albendazole (Zentel),‡ 400 mg per day for 3 days. In case of pregnancy and for children younger than 2 years of age, the risk of treatment (pyrantel is safer than the others) should be weighed against the potential danger of disease.

Mebendazole or albendazole (see the dosages earlier) may prevent symptomatic trichinellosis when given in the first few days after ingestion of infected meat. Piperazine and thiabendazole are no longer used in human trichinellosis.

### Acute Severe Trichinellosis

In acute trichinellosis, symptoms common to some other infections are found, such as fever, myalgia, and general weakness, in addition to characteristic allergic signs—i.e., periorbital edema, conjunctival hemorrhages, and high eosinophilia. Corticosteroids are the drug of choice in acute trichinellosis because of their anti-inflammatory and antiallergic action. The usual dosage is 40 to 60 mg of prednisone per day, until the fever and allergic signs disappear. Severe cases may require higher dosages of lifesaving corticosteroids. Bed rest is always necessary, and any cardiac, circulatory, neurologic, or pulmonary complications may need additional, intensive, specific treatment.

Mebendazole (Vermox), 5 mg per kg per day (maximum 400 mg),§ or albendazole (Zentel), 400 mg (or even up to 800 mg) per day for 5 days, should be used in severe trichinellosis, especially that caused by sylvatic or polar strains, which may respond poorly to corticosteroids alone. However, to prevent a systemic hypersensitivity response caused by antigenic substances liberated from destroyed *T. spiralis* muscle larvae, corticosteroids should be given with these drugs.

### Moderate or Mild Trichinellosis

Corticosteroids prolong the intestinal infection and increase the number of larvae parasitizing

---

*This use of pyrantel is not listed in the manufacturer's official directive.
†This use of mebendazole is not listed in the manufacturer's official directive.
‡Not available in the United States.
§Exceeds dosage recommended by the manufacturer.

the muscle tissue by depressing the host inflammatory and immune responses to *T. spiralis*. The use of corticosteroids is therefore justified only in patients with fever, allergic symptoms, high leukocytosis, and eosinophilia. In moderate trichinellosis, the dosage of corticosteroids is 20 to 40 mg of prednisolone per day. In mild infections, corticosteroid therapy is not necessary, as antipyretic and analgesic treatment alone give a satisfactory result.

### Late Phase of Trichinellosis

After the third week of the disease, metabolic and circulatory disorders dominate the clinical picture of severe trichinellosis. Profound hypoalbuminemia may require replacement human serum therapy. Some cardiac symptoms caused by hypokalemia are controlled by restoration of the correct electrolyte balance.

Trichinellosis is a self-limited disease in both the intestinal and the muscular phases, and complete recovery usually occurs within a few months. In sporadic cases, myalgia and weakness have been shown to persist for several years. In those cases, evidence of an active process by muscle biopsy examination may justify the use of larvicidal drugs, such as mebendazole or albendazole, under a cover of corticosteroids. However, symptomatic treatment and proper mental and physical rehabilitation should be tried first, as they are usually effective. Many people live quite well despite having some *T. spiralis* larvae encapsulated in their muscle.

# TULAREMIA

method of
DAVID M. PARENTI, M.D.
*The George Washington University Medical
   Center
Washington, D.C.*

Tularemia is an infectious illness caused by *Francisella tularensis*, a gram-negative aerobic coccobacillus. Tularemia is distributed throughout the northern hemispheres between 30 and 71 degrees latitude, particularly in rural areas where animal reservoirs have their habitats. The organism can infect wild and domestic mammals and arthropods such as ticks, deerflies, and mosquitoes.

In the United States, most cases have been reported from Arkansas, Oklahoma, Missouri, Tennessee, and Texas. Transmission of *F. tularensis* is most often associated with contact with infected tissues or body fluids of rabbits or hares and the bites of infected ticks. Transmission can also occur following contact with water contaminated by sick or dying animals, or through ingestion or inhalation of contaminated material. The illness occurs most frequently in hunters, trappers, or farmers, with peaks of transmission in the summer (tick-associated) and winter (hunting-related) months. The disease is generally sporadic; however, small outbreaks have been reported.

Tularemia may present clinically in three or more forms, somewhat dependent on the route of inoculation. All forms have the associated systemic symptoms of fever, chills, malaise, and fatigue. The most common presentations are ulceroglandular (75 to 85%), typhoidal (5 to 15%), and oculoglandular (1 to 2%). *F. tularensis* penetrates mucous membranes of both intact and traumatized skin. Following an incubation of 3 to 5 days, a papule develops at the site of inoculation. Rapid ulceration of the lesion occurs followed by fever and lymphadenopathy. Primary lesions develop on the hand in rabbit-associated cases and on the trunk or lower extremity in tick-associated cases. Similarly, adenopathy is noted in either the axilla (rabbit-associated) or the groin (tick-associated).

Oculoglandular fever develops when the conjunctiva is the initial site of infection. Purulent conjunctivitis develops in association with lymphadenopathy in the head and neck region, especially in the preauricular area. Periorbital swelling, chemosis, and nodular or ulcerated lesions of the conjunctiva may also be evident. Disseminated infection involving the lung, pericardium, and meninges has also been noted.

Diagnosis is made by recovery of the organism from blood or infected lymph node. The organism does not grow well on standard media, and isolation requires use of sulfhydryl-rich media such as glucose cysteine blood agar, thioglycolate broth, or charcoal yeast extraction medium. Cultures and clinical material may be hazardous to laboratory personnel if aerosolized; therefore, the laboratory should be alerted to the potential presence of *F. tularensis* and isolation should be attempted with caution. Improved recovery from blood has been noted with radiometric culturing systems, although blind subculturing may be necessary. Serologic diagnosis is made by tube agglutination, microagglutination, or enzyme-linked immunosorbent assay (ELISA). Titers are positive in 50 to 70% of patients by the third week of the illness. Newer diagnostic methods include immunofluorescence and in situ hybridization of infected tissues.

## TREATMENT

*F. tularensis* is sensitive to a variety of antibiotics in vitro, including the aminoglycosides, chloramphenicol, tetracycline, erythromycin, and the third-generation cephalosporins. The majority of clinical experience has been with streptomycin at 15 to 20 mg per kg per day intramuscularly in divided doses, and this remains the drug of choice for all forms of tularemia. Patients should be treated for a total duration of 7 to 14 days. Gentamicin, at 3 to 5 mg per kg per day intravenously or intramuscularly in divided doses, is probably an equivalent alternative.

Chloramphenicol and tetracycline have also

been used successfully in the treatment of tularemia. Clinical relapse may be as high as 30% with short-course therapy; therefore, treatment should be continued for at least 14 days. Both should be given as an initial loading dose of 30 mg per kg followed by 30 mg per kg per day in divided doses. There is little clinical experience with other antimicrobial agents.

Resolution of fever is usually evident within 48 hours, but resolution of lymphadenopathy or hepatitis can take days to weeks. Suppurative buboes may require aspiration or incision and drainage. Mortality rates of 2 to 3% have been reported since the advent of antimicrobial therapy. Poor outcome is related to underlying disease, pulmonary involvement, and delays in antimicrobial therapy.

## PREVENTION

Tularemia is best prevented by avoiding contact with infected animals. Rubber gloves and protective clothing should be worn while dressing rabbits or hares. Protection against tick exposure by clothing that fits tightly around the wrists or ankles is helpful; the use of tick repellents is also of value. A live attenuated vaccine has been developed that is partially protective in humans. Immunization of those at very high risk such as laboratory workers or animal handlers may be indicated. Inquiries concerning the vaccine should be directed to the Drug Service, Centers for Disease Control, Atlanta, Georgia.

# SALMONELLOSIS

method of
J. ROBERT CANTEY, M.D.
*Veterans Affairs Medical Center*
*Charleston, South Carolina*

Salmonellae are gram-negative rods of the family Enterobacteriaceae. They are highly similar biochemically, although *S. typhi* and *choleraesuis,* both single serotypes, can be differentiated biochemically from each other and from *S. enteriditis,* the latter actually consisting of a group of more than 2000 strains. Salmonellae can be differentiated by serotyping. The older or Kauffmann-White schema, based on somatic antigens, divided *Salmonella* into five groups (A to E), whereas the schema used most often at present is based on determination of major and minor somatic antigens and on two phases of flagellar antigens. Most clinical laboratories report only the biochemical groups and depend on reference laboratories for serotyping.

Salmonellae cause disease largely as a result of their ability to invade the intestinal mucosa. Although salmonellosis was previously thought to be a small intestinal disease, recent evidence suggests that colon involvement is more common than had been thought. The number of bacteria necessary to cause diarrheal disease in volunteer studies has ranged from $10^6$ to $10^9$, but evidence from outbreaks and person-to-person spread suggests a much lower inoculum, perhaps less than 100 organisms.

Salmonellae are a major cause of sporadic and food-borne diarrhea throughout the world. They infect many animal species, and, in contrast to other species of enteric pathogens, a single strain can infect many different host species, facilitating spread of the organism. More than 35,000 bacteriologically confirmed cases are reported annually in the United States. The majority of cases are sporadic, with 25% of cases occurring under the age of 5 and half of those occurring under the age of 1 year. The impoverished children of the inner city are most at risk. Salmonellae are often causes of traveler's diarrhea, reflecting a major role in morbidity and mortality in the young and elderly populations of developing parts of the world.

Food-borne outbreaks are common, and eggs and poultry are well known vehicles. Milk-borne outbreaks, associated with faulty pasteurization of raw milk, have recently been in the news. It is rare to trace food-borne outbreaks to an animal source; rather, a very small inoculum of bacteria is thought to proliferate during food preparation and storage. Nosocomial outbreaks continue to be reported and they may be persistent, lasting for months, readily spreading from person to person among patients as well as health care personnel.

Salmonellae are sensitive to a variety of antibiotics in vitro, but it cannot safely be assumed that infected patients will respond, based on in vitro sensitivity. For example, salmonellae are sensitive to cefamandole in vitro but the drug is not reliably effective in patients. Ampicillin, amoxicillin, chloramphenicol, and trimethoprim-sulfamethoxazole (Bactrim, Septra) are known to be effective in vivo. Ciprofloxacin (Cipro) is reported to be effective in *Salmonella* gastrointestinal infections. Experience with the newer cephalosporins is inadequate to recommend their use except in specific focal infections.

Resistance to antibiotics among salmonellae has been on the increase, particularly among animals fed antibiotic containing growth supplements. Ampicillin resistance is found in 25 to 45% of United States *Salmonella* isolates. Trimethoprim-sulfamethoxazole resistance has been reported from Asia and western Europe. Chloramphenicol resistance is rare but has been reported in Spain, North Africa, and, less frequently, South America and Asia.

## ENTEROCOLITIS

*Salmonella* enterocolitis is a self-limited illness, with an incubation period of 6 to 48 hours, that begins with fever, malaise, nausea, and vomiting. Abdominal pain and tenderness, which may be periumbilical or lower abdominal in location, and diarrhea, which is usually loose and moderate in volume, follow. Rarely, stools may be large in volume (cholera-like) or there may be tenesmus and dysentery-like stools. Grossly bloody stools have been reported as well. The duration of the enterocolitis is 3 to 5 days, although diarrhea may continue for a week. The disease is more severe among the young, the old, and immunosuppressed patients.

Stool examination reveals a moderate number of polymorphonuclear leukocytes and, occasionally, red blood cells. Stool cultures are diagnostic and may remain positive for several weeks. Occasionally, they may remain positive for 6 months, but chronic carriage greater than a year is rare in non-typhoidal *Salmonella* infections. Blood cultures are positive in 5% of patients.

The major cause of morbidity in diarrheal disease is dehydration. In adults rehydration is best managed by the oral route, unless the patient has developed orthostatic hypotension. Water in the volume prescribed by the thirst mechanism is usually sufficient, except in the elderly, whose thirst mechanism may be defective. Caffeine or lactose containing liquids should be avoided. Infants and young children may best be rehydrated using oral rehydration solutions conforming to World Health Organization standards.

Antimotility agents, such as loperamide (Imodium) or diphenoxylate with atropine (Lomotil), are not recommended in diarrheas that are due to invasive organisms, particularly if fever or bloody or mucoid stools are present. Anti-nausea medications, such as prochlorperazine (Compazine), 5 to 10 mg three or four times daily orally; 25 mg twice daily via rectal suppository; or by intramuscular injection, 5 to 10 mg every 4 hours as needed (not to exceed a total daily dose of 40 mg), may be useful. Promethazine hydrochloride (Phenergan) is an alternate therapy, given orally, by suppository, or intramuscularly 25 mg every 4 to 6 hours. Dosages should be adjusted for children.

Antibiotic therapy does not shorten the duration of diarrhea and may prolong fecal carriage of the organism. However, in infants less than 3 months of age, in patients with complicating underlying illness or immunosuppression, or in otherwise normal patients with a prolonged or relapsing course, treatment with 160 mg trimethoprim and 800 mg sulfamethoxazole (two single-strength or one double-strength tablet) twice each day in adults, or 4 mg per kg of trimethoprim in children, also twice each day, should be considered. If the organism is known to be sensitive, ampicillin, 2 to 4 grams per day in four doses in adults, or 50 to 100 mg per kg per day in four doses in children, can be used. The oral quinolones are also effective, and ciprofloxacin in a dosage of 250 mg twice each day may be used in

adults, but this is contraindicated in children. The duration of therapy is 5 days.

## BACTEREMIA AND FOCAL INFECTIONS

Bacteremia is associated with more severe constitutional symptoms, is not necessarily associated with intestinal disease, and generally has a low mortality. It occurs in 5 to 10% of cases of uncomplicated acute enterocolitis. It is more common and likely to be prolonged or recurrent in immunosuppressed patients, particularly AIDS patients.

Extraintestinal focal infections ordinarily follow bacteremia. Meningitis is most common in infants, and osteomyelitis is a complication in sickle cell disease. Joint infections are occasionally seen. Endovascular infections, which are difficult to eradicate and occur in the older patient, may involve heart valves and other vascular prostheses, atherosclerotic plaques, and aneurysms. Focal infections may also present in a manner similar to that of other Enterobacteriaceae infections.

Antibiotic therapy is advisable in bacteremias and focal infections. Depending on antibiotic sensitivity, ampicillin, 100 to 200 mg per kg per day (maximum of 12 grams), divided into six doses; or trimethoprim-sulfamethoxazole, 10 mg per kg per day of trimethoprim (maximum of 320 mg) in three to four divided doses parenterally or two to three times each day orally, may be used. A higher dose of trimethoprim-sulfamethoxazole may be advisable in some situations but requires monitoring the white blood cell count for evidence of bone marrow toxicity. Chloramphenicol, 50 mg per kg per day (maximum of 3 grams) in four divided doses orally or parenterally, is usually efficacious but is known to fail in some focal infections, including meningitis and arthritis. Cefotaxime (Claforan), 6 grams per day in three divided doses, and ceftriaxone (Rocephin), 2 grams per day in two divided doses, have been found to be effective in meningitis, septicemia, and focal infections. Ciprofloxacin in a dose of 500 to 750 mg twice each day may also be useful, particularly in osteomyelitis. Typical courses of therapy are 14 days for bacteremia, 2 to 3 weeks for meningitis, and 6 weeks or longer for osteomyelitis and endovascular infection. AIDS patients may require chronic therapy to prevent relapses. Surgical drainage and débridement may be advisable for certain localized infections. Infected aneurysms are very difficult to treat without reconstructive surgery.

## ENTERIC FEVER

*Salmonella* enteric fever, rare in the developed world, is characterized by sustained high fever, malaise, headache, a dry cough, and abdominal pain. Diarrhea may occur, especially initially, but constipation is more common in the latter stages of the disease. The average duration of untreated disease is 4 weeks. Physical findings include bradycardia; hepatomegaly; splenomegaly; abdominal tenderness and distention; diminished bowel sounds; segmental ileus, evident as palpable loops of bowel or by roentgenography; and, in a minority of patients, rose spots on the abdomen. Laboratory findings include leukopenia and abnormal liver function tests. Diagnosis is by positive blood cultures. Stool cultures are often positive, particularly in the later (intestinal) stages of the disease. Among non-typhoidal salmonellae, *S. paratyphi A, S. schottmuelleri,* and *S. choleraesuis* are most commonly associated with enteric fever. Serology is of little diagnostic value. Convalescence is prolonged, even with adequate therapy. Relapse may occur, in spite of adequate antibiotics. Complications can be life threatening and include intestinal perforation and intestinal hemorrhage.

Careful attention must be paid to fluid and electrolyte balance. Salicylates should not be used because they may produce a profound hypothermia. High-dose corticosteroids (dexamethasone, 3 mg per kg initially, followed by eight doses of 1 mg per kg every 6 hours) may be beneficial,* but only for patients with stupor, delirium, obtundation, or coma. Depending on antibiotic sensitivity, ampicillin, 100 to 200 mg per kg per day (maximum of 12 grams), divided into six doses; trimethoprim-sulfamethoxazole, 10 mg per kg per day of trimethoprim (maximum of 320 mg [some investigators have recommended a maximum of 640 mg]) in three to four divided doses parenterally or two to three times each day orally; or chloramphenicol, 50 mg per kg per day (maximum of 3 grams) in four divided doses orally or parenterally, have been proved efficacious. A loading dose of 15 to 20 mg per kg of chloramphenicol is given in enteric fever. Oral amoxicillin, 100 mg per kg per day in three divided doses, has proved to be an effective alternative to chloramphenicol if the infecting organism is sensitive to ampicillin. The dose is usually decreased by one-third for chloramphenicol or one-half for ampicillin when the fever breaks, usually at 48 to 72 hours. Therapy should be continued for 14 days. The cephalosporins and quinolones cannot be recommended for the treatment of enteric fever at this time.

## ASYMPTOMATIC CARRIER STATE

A small portion of patients may excrete non-typhoidal salmonellae in the stool for 6 months,

---

*Exceeds dosage recommended by the manufacturer.

but chronic carriage for a period greater than 1 year is very rare. The gallbladder is important in *S. typhi* chronic carriage, but its role in the carriage of non-typhoidal salmonellae is uncertain. Carriage can be a major problem, particularly in institutionalized patients, in food handlers, or in persons involved in child care. For that reason, it may occasionally be advisable to attempt termination of the carrier state by the use of long-term, high-dose oral antibiotics. Appropriate therapy includes 160 mg trimethoprim and 800 mg sulfamethoxazole (two single-strength or one double-strength tablet) twice each day in adults, or 4 mg per kg trimethoprim in children, also twice each day; or amoxicillin 500 mg four times each day in adults or 250 mg four times each day in children. Therapy is continued for 4 to 6 weeks. Ciprofloxacin, in doses ranging from 500 mg twice each day for 4 weeks to 750 mg twice each day for 3 weeks (in adults only), appears to be more effective than the latter two drugs, although it is comparatively expensive. Follow-up cultures for a prolonged period of time are necessary to ensure permanent elimination of the organism.

# TYPHOID FEVER

method of
ROBERTO CEDILLO-RIVERA, M.D., Ms.C.
*Instituto Mexicano del Seguro Social*
*Mexico City, Mexico*

Typhoid fever is an acute, systemic infection caused by *Salmonella typhi*, found exclusively in humans. It is found worldwide and mainly affects developing countries. The infection is acquired through ingestion of water or food contaminated by feces of patients or carriers. Bacteria penetrate the intestinal mucosa, are disseminated in the blood stream, and primarily infect the reticuloendothelial system. The disease is characterized by fever, malaise, headache, diffuse abdominal pain, and leukopenia. The diagnosis is confirmed by isolation of *S. typhi* from blood or bone marrow. Serologic tests may be of use for diagnosis when they are performed after 1 week of evolution of the illness. Early recognition and prompt antibiotic therapy are necessary to prevent complications and death. Lethality of untreated or inadequately treated disease is up to 15% as a result of complications such as septic shock, hemorrhage, and intestinal perforation.

## THERAPY

### Antimicrobial Agents

Since the introduction of chloramphenicol in 1948, mortality from typhoid fever has decreased from 10 to 15% to 1 to 3% and the duration of illness from 5 weeks to 1 week; however, the appearance of bacterial strains that are resistant to chloramphenicol has obliged physicians to search for alternative drugs.

**Chloramphenicol.** Most strains that cause endemic typhoid fever are sensitive to chloramphenicol, and the therapeutic results with this drug are superior to those obtained with other antibiotics; hence, chloramphenicol is the drug of choice. The recommended dosage in adults is 3 grams per day, and that in children is 100 mg per kg per day, divided into four doses. Treatment must be maintained for 10 to 12 days, and a reduction of fever generally occurs within 3 to 5 days; lower doses of chloramphenicol delay fever control until the seventh day. The total dose regimen should not exceed 30 grams. The route of choice is oral; when this route is not possible, the intravenous route is used until the switch to oral medication can be made. Chloramphenicol should not be given intramuscularly because this route is painful and low and variable drug serum levels are achieved.

Chloramphenicol does not change the rate of occurrence of carriers, and it is ineffective for the treatment of these patients. Relapses occur in 5% of patients, and case fatality rates range from 1 to 3%. The major side effect of chloramphenicol is its hematologic toxicity and that it generally corresponds to reversible hematopoietic depression, which is dose related. Irreversible aplastic anemia occurs in approximately 1 in 40,000 to 50,000 recipients and is not dose related.

Since 1972, chloramphenicol-resistant strains of *S. typhi* have been reported during epidemics in Mexico, Southeast Asia, and India. In this situation, alternative drugs should be used.

**Furazolidone.** As a result of experience in India and Mexico, we consider furazolidone (Furoxone) as the drug of second choice. We recommend a high dosage: 800 mg per day in adults and 10 to 15 mg per kg per day in children, divided into four doses, for 10 to 12 days.* Control of fever is obtained after 5 to 7 days of treatment. One disadvantage of the use of this drug is that it can be administered only by the oral route, but it has the advantage of being less expensive than other drugs. Side effects are gastrointestinal discomfort and headache. *S. typhi* is sensitive to furazolidone in vitro.

**Amoxicillin.** Amoxicillin (Amoxil) is a congener of ampicillin but with superior intestinal absorption and thus higher serum levels than the latter. The recommended dosage in adults is 3 grams

per day divided into three doses and in children is 100 mg per kg per day. Treatment should be continued for 14 days. The clinical response to this drug is slower than that with chloramphenicol; fever disappears after 7 days of treatment. Certain chloramphenicol-resistant strains of *S. typhi* that have appeared since 1972 may also carry plasmid-mediated resistance to ampicillin and amoxicillin. The resistance of endemic strains of these antibiotics is higher than that for chloramphenicol and furazolidone. Rashes and gastrointestinal upsets occur with amoxicillin use, as with ampicillin.

**Trimethoprim-Sulfamethoxazole.** Trimethoprim-sulfamethoxazole (Bactrim) is less effective than those drugs mentioned earlier, and therapeutic failures have been reported in 8 to 10% of infections with sensitive strains of bacteria. As with amoxicillin and ampicillin, the resistance of endemic strains to this drug combination is higher than that for chloramphenicol and furazolidone. However, it is considered to be an acceptable choice for treatment of cases resistant to the above-mentioned drugs. The recommended dosage is 160 mg of trimethoprim and 800 mg of sulfamethoxazole orally every 12 hours in adults and 8 mg of trimethoprim and 40 mg of sulfamethoxazole per kg per day in children, divided into two doses, for 12 to 14 days. Fever disappears after 5 to 7 days of treatment. The most frequent side effects are nausea, vomiting, and rash.

**Cephalosporins and Quinolones.** Third-generation cephalosporins, such as cefotaxime (Claforan), ceftriaxone (Rocephin), and cefoperazone (Cefobid), and new quinolones, such as norfloxacin (Noroxin) and ciprofloxacin (Cipro), have good activity in vitro against *S. typhi*. The clinical studies performed thus far indicate that these new classes of antimicrobial agents offer significant potential improvement for the treatment of typhoid fever; however, they must now be considered as alternative treatments for resistant strains of *S. typhi*.

### Supportive Measures

In addition to antimicrobial therapy, the following measures must be taken: bed rest during the febrile period; normal low-residue diet, even enriched in calories; and physical measures to control fever (the use of antipyretics should be avoided because they may cause hypothermia and hypotension). Intravenous fluids must be given as necessary to those patients who are unable to maintain hydration orally. Corticosteroids have been used in some patients with severe toxicity, but in our experience this measure is not useful

---

*These doses exceed the manufacturer's recommended dosages.

and increases the risk of gastrointestinal bleeding, intestinal perforation, and superinfections.

## Management of Complications

**Intestinal Complications.** Hemorrhage occurs in 10% of patients. It appears more frequently during the second week of the illness, and its major clinical sign is melena; hypovolemic shock related to acute anemia can develop. Treatment involves blood transfusions and management of the shock.

Intestinal perforation occurs in 3 to 5% of patients and is more common during the second and third weeks of the disease. It is manifested by severe abdominal pain with signs of peritoneal irritation, perforation of hollow viscera, and septic shock. Treatment is based on (1) correction of shock; (2) administration of additional antimicrobial agents to treat peritoneal infection caused by aerobic and anaerobic bacteria by using amikacin together with metronidazole or cefoxitin; and (3) surgical correction, which may vary from the single closure of the perforation with drainage to intestinal resection with ileostomy.

**Septic Extraintestinal Complications.** Hepatitis, myocarditis, pneumonia, osteoarthritis, meningitis, typhoidic status, parotitis, and nephritis usually respond to basic antimicrobial treatment but in some cases may require drainage or surgery.

**Septic Shock and Intravascular Coagulation.** Special measures in addition to antimicrobial treatment are required for these complications (see specific articles).

**Relapses.** Relapses occur despite adequate antimicrobial therapy in about 5% of patients. Symptoms are usually less severe than those of the initial episode and occur 10 to 20 days after the cure. Treatment is the same as that given initially unless chloramphenicol was used at the maximal dose, in which case an alternative drug is preferred.

**Carrier State.** Approximately 10% of patients continue to eliminate the bacillus for weeks or months. This is a self-limited condition and these *convalescent carriers* do not need treatment. It is only necessary to insist on strict hygienic measures and to prevent these persons from working as food handlers. If after a year *S. typhi* organisms are still being eliminated in the stool, these subjects are considered to be *chronic carriers* (about 1%). Women and older adults are at increased risk of becoming typhoid carriers. The gallbladder is the common site of infection. Many of these patients have gallstones and gallbladder dysfunction, which make management difficult. Treatment involves a medical or combined medical-surgical approach: cholecystectomy accompanied by 4 weeks of amoxicillin, 2 grams three times a day, can cure the carrier state in about 90% of cases. If only medical treatment is indicated, there have been therapeutic successes with 4 to 6 weeks of amoxicillin, 6 grams per day. Early reports indicate that third-generation cephalosporins and new quinolones, cited earlier, are also useful in the treatment of chronic carriers.

## Prevention

The rational prevention of typhoid fever is based on hygienic education, environmental sanitation, and improvement of the quality of life. However, during epidemics and in subjects who travel from nonendemic areas to epidemic areas, vaccination is in order. One of the most effective vaccines available is prepared by acetone extraction, which preserves the Vi antigen and confers protection for up to 3 years in 90% of the subjects immunized. The vaccine is administered parenterally in two doses of 0.5 ml at 1-month intervals. Side effects are fever, malaise, and adverse local reactions.

A new live oral vaccine has been developed by using a mutant strain of *S. typhi* (Ty21a). It has been tested in a field trial in Egypt with good results (95% of protection for at least 3 years); however, in Chile the vaccine provided protection in only 67% of those immunized. The advantage of this vaccine is the lack of notable adverse reactions, and it will probably be a good alternative for prevention of typhoid fever.

# TYPHUS FEVERS

method of
WILLIAM D. SAWYER, M.D.
*China Medical Board of New York, Inc.*
*New York, New York*

Two species of *Rickettsia* are responsible for the diseases of the typhus fever group. These are *Rickettsia prowazekii,* the cause of epidemic (louse-borne) typhus and recrudescent typhus (Brill-Zinsser disease), and *Rickettsia typhi,* the cause of murine (endemic) typhus. The three diseases present similarly but differ in severity and in epidemiology.

Certain other rickettsial diseases are sometimes known as a form of typhus. Scrub typhus, caused by *Rickettsia tsutsugamushi,* differs clinically and epidemiologically from the typhus fevers. The spotted fever group of diseases, sometimes called tick typhus, results from infection by different rickettsial species in different parts of the world. The most severe form, Rocky Mountain spotted fever, which is caused by *Rickettsia rickettsii,* is found in the United States.

Although they are not called typhus and are quite

different clinically, two other rickettsial infections are considered here because they respond to the same therapy: Q fever, caused by *Coxiella burnetii,* and rickettsial pox, caused by *Rickettsia akari.*

The *Rickettsia* species are widely distributed in nature, are transmitted primarily by arthropod vectors, and have various mammalian reservoirs. Except for epidemic typhus and Brill-Zinsser disease, human infection is incidental to the perpetuation of the organisms in nature. The global distribution of the rickettsial diseases depends on the ecology of the arthropod vectors and the mammalian reservoirs. Epidemic typhus, for example, is transmitted primarily from human to human by lice. Conditions such as war and disaster promote such transmission and can lead to major outbreaks of disease.

The common rickettsial diseases in the United States are Rocky Mountain spotted fever, endemic typhus, and Q fever. Epidemic typhus, Brill-Zinsser disease, and rickettsial pox occur only rarely. Rocky Mountain spotted fever, transmitted by ticks, occurs throughout the country, but most often in the south Atlantic and Gulf states. The reservoir is ticks and a variety of wild mammals. The peak period of the disease is in the spring and summer when ticks are most active. The incidence is highest in rural and suburban areas where humans are exposed to ticks. Endemic typhus is an infection of rats and other rodents that is transmitted to humans by fleas. Rickettsialpox is an infection of the house mouse and other rodents that is transmitted to humans by mites. Cases of both diseases occur when there is interaction of the requisite species. Q fever is an infection of small mammals, cattle, sheep, and goats that is transmitted both by ticks and by inhalation of dried infected material from mammals with the disease.

In humans the rickettsiae may multiply locally at the site of inoculation and, in some instances, produce a local lesion. The organisms spread throughout the body and multiply within and injure the endothelial cells of the small blood vessels. The injury and inflammation lead to leakage and extravasation of blood elements into the tissues and also lead to thrombosis with resultant damage to tissues. The specific manifestations of each disease relate to the location of the dominant organ involved and the consequences of the angiitis.

The key features of the diseases are an acute, febrile illness that develops after an incubation period of a few days to 3 weeks, a rash (except for Q fever), and the consequences of the angiitis such as decreased effective circulating blood volume, azotemia, electrolyte imbalance, delirium, stupor, coma, myocarditis, hepatitis, a consumptive coagulopathy, and shock. The clinical manifestations and epidemiologic setting are the basis of initial diagnosis. Specific serologic tests provide confirmation. The nonspecific Weil-Felix reaction may help during the second week of illness. Rocky Mountain spotted fever is the most severe rickettsial disease. It may be fulminant and fatal before the results of serologic tests can be obtained. Antirickettsial therapy must not be delayed in cases of clinically suspected Rocky Mountain spotted fever until a diagnosis is made.

## THERAPY

Prompt antirickettsial therapy is the principal concern in the treatment of rickettsial diseases. Patients who are cooperative and mildly ill can be treated as outpatients. Those who may be unreliable or who are moderately or severely ill should be hospitalized to ensure proper antimicrobial treatment and to attend to complications that tend to occur in the second week of untreated disease.

Supportive care is vital for the severely ill patient and must be directed to the complications, for example, azotemia, hypovolemia, and hypoproteinemia. Corticosteroids in large doses for up to 3 days may be tried in severely toxic patients.

General therapeutic measures include provision of a nutritious diet, protection of the agitated patient from injury, and skin and mouth care. The severe headache that is common in these diseases is most often intractable and not eased by the usual drugs.

### Specific Therapy

Both tetracycline (or an equivalent congener) and chloramphenicol are highly effective in the treatment of the typhus group of infections and the other rickettsial diseases. Other common antibiotics are ineffective. Chloramphenicol is preferred in cases in which typhoid fever is included among the possible causes of illness and in children younger than the age of 8 years. Clinical response begins quickly. Fever remits and dramatic overall improvement typically occurs in the first 2 days of antimicrobial therapy. In Rocky Mountain spotted fever, the vascular lesions may be so extensive that permanent tissue damage occurs despite effective antibiotic treatment.

Patients who can tolerate oral medication should receive one of the following drugs:
1. Tetracycline
   a. Initial dose: 25 mg per kg
   b. Daily dose: 25 mg per kg per day in four equal doses every 6 hours
2. Chloramphenicol
   a. Initial dose: 50 mg per kg
   b. Daily dose: 50 mg per kg per day in four equal doses every 6 hours

Intravenous preparations should be administered to patients who are unable to tolerate oral treatment. Warnings on package inserts should be observed. Oral therapy should replace intravenous administration as soon as possible. Adults and children should receive one of the following drugs:
1. Tetracycline
   a. Initial dose: 15 mg per kg infused in 30 to 45 minutes

b. Daily dose: 25 mg per kg per day infused in equal doses every 6 hours
2. Chloramphenicol sodium succinate
   a. Initial dose: 20 mg per kg infused in 30 to 45 minutes
   b. Daily dose: 50 mg per kg per day infused in equal doses every 6 hours

Treatment should continue until the patient is improved and has been afebrile for 24 to 48 hours. Treatment with these drugs stops the proliferation of organisms and hence treats the disease. The antibiotics do not, however, eradicate the organisms. Eradication depends on the host's immune response, which is relatively slow to develop. A relapse may follow cessation of therapy, especially if the treatment was instituted early in the course of the disease and was short. Such a relapse responds quickly to a new course of the same antibiotic.

Doxycycline is a long-acting derivative of tetracycline. A single oral dose is effective in the treatment of typhus and is both convenient and safe. This is probably the treatment of choice for the typhus fever group, especially in situations such as refugee camps or disasters when medical service is limited. A single dose of doxycycline is not, however, reliable therapy for Rocky Mountain spotted fever. For this disease, doxycycline should be continued until the patient has improved and been afebrile for 24 to 48 hours. Doxycycline should be given as follows:

1. Doxycycline
   a. Single dose: 100 or 200 mg

### PREVENTION

Prevention of rickettsial disease relies primarily on reducing human contact with the arthropod vectors, for example, delousing and using insect repellents, and on reducing the number of reservoir hosts and vectors. A commercial vaccine for epidemic typhus is available. It consists of killed rickettsiae prepared as a formalin-treated suspension of infected yolk sac. The vaccine prevents or ameliorates the disease.

Local health authorities should be informed of the occurrence of a case of rickettsial disease.

# PERTUSSIS
## (Whooping Cough)

method of
KENNETH BROMBERG, M.D.
*SUNY Health Science Center at Brooklyn*
*Brooklyn, New York*

Some patients infected with *Bordetella pertussis* have an upper respiratory tract infection followed by the gradual onset of sudden prolonged coughing spells. These spells end with vomiting and a whoop caused by the patient's inspiratory effort against a narrowed glottis. Many patients do not exhibit these typical symptoms. The term "pertussis," which means intensive cough, is preferred to the term "whooping cough" because, although all symptomatic patients cough, they do not all whoop.

Pertussis has an incubation period of 1 to 3 weeks. In classic pertussis, the first clinical symptoms are those of an upper respiratory tract infection and the disease is indistinguishable from that of any other upper respiratory tract infection. During a 1- to 2-week period, the frequency and intensity of the cough increases, while the upper respiratory tract symptoms are still present. This is the catarrhal stage. The second, or paroxysmal, stage begins as cough becomes the predominant feature. The paroxysmal stage lasts from 2 to 4 weeks. Episodes of coughing begin suddenly, especially at night, and continue for much longer than seems possible. As the patient coughs for up to 30 seconds, signs of hypoxia develop, with central and peripheral cyanosis. This expiratory effort leads to distended neck veins, bulging eyes, and occasionally periorbital and subconjunctival hemorrhages. The increase in pressure can lead to intracerebral hemorrhages; an intra-abdominal defect, such as an inguinal hernia, may become manifest. When vomiting occurs, it can lead to significant malnutrition and metabolic alkalosis. The whoop is heard during inspiration at the end of a coughing attack. The patient enters the convalescent stage as the cough gradually subsides. Exacerbations and remissions of these clinical symptoms may go on for several months. Infections with viral organisms may trigger a recurrence of the paroxysmal stage, but these exacerbations resolve quickly.

Many patients, especially those who have received partial or complete immunization against *B. pertussis,* adults, and infants less than 6 months of age, may exhibit less typical symptoms. Immunized children may have upper respiratory tract symptoms. Adults may have a chronic cough. Infants may primarily manifest apnea and cyanosis. However, all of these patients exhibit the common symptom of cough. Cough severe enough to cause vomiting is a helpful clinical indicator of infection with *B. pertussis.*

In the United States, most deaths from pertussis are seen in children younger than 1 year of age. Pertussis may pose a problem for immunocompromised patients; *B. pertussis* has caused serious disease in older patients with human immunodeficiency virus (HIV) disease and is a major killer of malnourished children in underdeveloped countries.

Laboratory diagnosis is appropriate in both typical and atypical cases. Samples for diagnosis should be obtained using Dacron-covered wire swabs that are inserted into the nasopharynx. These swabs are then used to inoculate culture plates and to make slides for direct antigen detection. If a laboratory is experienced in isolating *B. pertussis,* the sensitivity of culture increases. The major problem with culture is the overgrowth of *B. pertussis* by other organisms because *B. pertussis* may take 7 days to grow. An experienced observer can detect the colonies of *B. pertussis* before they are obscured by overgrowth. *B. pertussis* is best isolated using a commercially available charcoal agar with supplemental antibiotics (Oxoid CM119). Detection of the organism by immunofluorescent staining (direct antigen detection) is a rapid and potentially sensitive technique. The major limitation is the quality of available reagents. When monoclonal antibodies against the organism are available, fluorescence may become widely available. Serologic study is of use in retrospective diagnosis. Bacterial agglutination is easy to perform, but lacks sensitivity. Serologic tests that may detect current infection are under development.

The white blood cell count is of value in the diagnosis of pertussis when an absolute lymphocytosis is present. Its absence does not eliminate the possibility of infection. Lymphocytosis is less common in infants and adults. The most difficult aspect of diagnosis is considering the possibility of pertussis. When pertussis is considered in the differential diagnosis of respiratory illness, diagnosis becomes less difficult.

*B. parapertussis* may cause a similar but milder illness. *B. parapertussis* grows in 3 days on media used for the isolation of *B. pertussis*. *B. parapertussis* is isolated infrequently from patients with pertussis. Although adenovirus can be isolated from patients with pertussis, the virus is unlikely to be responsible for the clinical findings, and its detection is more likely representative of reactivation of latent adenovirus infection.

## TREATMENT

**General Measures.** Supportive care is the major mode of therapy. Although antimicrobial therapy may alter the course of disease if given early in infection, diagnosis usually occurs too late for any effect to be seen. Antimicrobial therapy eliminates carriage of the organism and thus prevents infection in contacts. Physical isolation is of value until the patient has received antimicrobial therapy for a long enough period to be noninfectious.

All patients younger than 1 year of age and any patient showing signs of cyanosis must be hospitalized. The mainstay of therapy is supplemental oxygen administration and gentle suctioning of the voluminous secretions until the patient is no longer cyanotic. However, it is important that young patients be observed for apnea. Patients must be isolated in such a way as to be readily observed. A patient placed in a mist tent for the administration of supplemental oxygen may develop airway obstruction from increased mucus production. Suctioning might be needed on an emergency basis and would be delayed if the patient were placed in a back room for isolation or was invisible inside an oxygen tent. The need for isolation and oxygen administration must be balanced with the need for careful observation. Suctioning cannot be done frequently because any stimulus may trigger an attack of coughing and cyanosis. Noxious stimuli, such as inhaled irritants, should be avoided. Cough suppressants are contraindicated, as the patient's mucociliary clearance is already compromised by pertussis and bacterial superinfection is a major risk in these patients. Adults may be given codeine for cough in the convalescent stage, but the coughing is hard to suppress.

Maintenance of adequate nutrition is important. Attacks of vomiting may make this difficult. Frequent feeding, continuous nasogastric feeding, or even intravenous hyperalimentation may be necessary.

**Specific Therapy.** Most patients become culture negative after several weeks so that any drug associated with significant risk is not justified. Orally administered erythromycin is the drug of choice for the elimination of nasopharyngeal carriage because it is effective and carries little risk. Therapy for 10 days has been associated with relapse, so a course of 14 days has been recommended. Although any form of erythromycin (base, ethylsuccinate [EES], proprinate, stearate, or estolate) is well absorbed on an empty stomach, only the estolate and EES ethylsuccinate forms are well absorbed with food. Although cholestatic jaundice has been associated with the estolate form in adults, this is uncommon in children. Thus, estolate in a dosage of 40 to 50 mg per kg per day divided every 6 hours (maximum dose 2 grams per day) is the treatment of choice for the elimination of carriage in children. Any other erythromycin preparation may be used in adults (2 grams per day divided every 6 hours). Some authorities recommend trimethoprim-sulfamethoxazole or amoxicillin for the elimination of carriage. These drugs are less well studied than erythromycin. Physical isolation of the patient should be maintained for the first 5 days of therapy.

Pertussis immune globulin has not been shown to be of value. However, because some aspects of pertussis are mediated by toxins, high-titered intravenous gamma globulin preparations may someday be shown to be of value in preventing disease.

Antimicrobials given early in the course of

TABLE 1. **Pertussis Vaccination in Disease Contacts**

| Vaccine Status (Full Doses of DTP) | Interval Since Vaccination | Action |
|---|---|---|
| 0 | | Immunize |
| 1 or 2 | <2 mo | None |
| 1 or 2 | >2 mo | Immunize |
| 3 | <6 mo | None |
| 3 | >6 mo | Immunize |
| 4 | <3 yr | None |
| 4 | >3 yr | Immunize |

disease may result in a less severe course and if given prophylactically may abort infection. However, there have been failures of prophylaxis. These failures may have been due to the dosage or duration of therapy.

Beta-adrenergic agents, such as albuterol or steroids, may be of value in severely affected infants, but they have not proved effective.

## COMPLICATIONS

**Respiratory Tract.** Bacterial pneumonia is the most common complication of pertussis. Atelectasis is seen in patients with pertussis and may be difficult to distinguish from early pneumonia. In the nonintubated patient, the causes of pneumonia are similar to those in patients without pertussis (*Streptococcus pneumoniae, Haemophilus influenzae* Type b, and occasionally *Staphylococcus aureus*). A cephalosporin, such as cefuroxime or ceftriaxone, would be appropriate initial therapy. In the patient with pertussis who requires mechanical ventilation because of respiratory failure or intractable cyanosis, pneumonia would necessitate broad-spectrum antimicrobial therapy. Otitis media is frequently seen with pertussis and can be treated with a fixed combination of erythromycin and sulfisoxazole if the otitis did not develop while the patient was taking erythromycin. Otherwise, amoxicillin or trimethoprim-sulfamethoxazole is appropriate.

**Central Nervous System.** Seizures, if prolonged, should be treated with anticonvulsants. Maintenance of oxygenation is critical and may necessitate mechanical ventilation.

## MANAGEMENT OF CONTACTS

Contacts younger than the age of 7 years should be given a dose of diphtheria-tetanus-pertussis (DTP) vaccine (Table 1). Erythromycin should be given to all contacts to eliminate secondary spread and to abort infection. This second goal may not be attainable. The primary means of treating pertussis is prevention. Whole-cell vaccine is effective. Pertussis vaccine associated with death and severe neurologic damage may not be related on a cause-and-effect basis. A recent study of an acellular vaccine showed it to be less effective than whole-cell vaccine; however, the development of acellular pertussis vaccines that are as effective as whole-cell vaccine should eliminate many of the current objections to vaccination. Acellular vaccines have fewer local side effects but will not decrease the infrequent occurrence of neurologic abnormalities, since the neurologic abnormalities are not caused by the vaccine.

# The Respiratory System

## ACUTE RESPIRATORY FAILURE

method of
STEVEN N. STRUVE, M.D., and
NATHAN C. DEAN, M.D.
*University of Utah School of Medicine*
*Salt Lake City, Utah*

Our tissues require oxygen to utilize nutrient substrate efficiently. Oxidative metabolism in turn produces $CO_2$ that must be eliminated from the body. The respiratory system, the cardiovascular system, and the hematologic system are integrally involved in performing the task of oxygen uptake and $CO_2$ excretion. The lungs allow the diffusion of oxygen from the alveoli to the pulmonary capillaries, where oxygen binds with hemoglobin. The heart pumps oxygen-rich blood to the tissues, where it moves down a concentration gradient into cells and ultimately mitochondria. Carbon dioxide diffuses from the cells back into the venous blood stream and is transported to the lungs for elimination. The coordinated efforts of the heart, lung, and blood are responsible for realizing the goal of adequate tissue oxygenation. A defect in any one of these systems (e.g., low cardiac output, a severe anemia) might prevent the attainment of this goal.

## CLASSIFICATION

The lungs must achieve both oxygenation of the blood and elimination of carbon dioxide. Thus, lung failure can involve failure to remove $CO_2$ (ventilatory failure) or failure to oxygenate (oxygenation failure). Acute ventilatory failure is diagnosed when the arterial $PCO_2$ is greater than 45 in conjunction with acidemia. Oxygenation failure generally is diagnosed when the $PO_2$ is less than 60. However, blood gases must be interpreted in light of the clinical situation. For example, ventilatory failure is present when the $PCO_2$ rises from 30 torr to 40 torr in a patient with status asthmaticus. Moreover, a $PO_2$ of 55 is appropriate for a man at the summit of Pike's Peak.

### Ventilatory Failure

The level of carbon dioxide in the blood is directly related to how much is being produced and is inversely related to how much is being eliminated ($PCO_2 = CO_2$ production–alveolar ventilation).

By far, the most common cause of ventilatory failure is impaired $CO_2$ elimination. Impaired $CO_2$ elimination is categorized into four general areas:

1. Impaired central nervous system (e.g., drugs, cerebral vascular accidents)
2. Impaired efferent-afferent neural control (amyotrophic lateral sclerosis, cervical spine trauma)
3. Impaired bellows (muscle weakness, as in severe hypophosphatemia, or chest wall deformities such as kyphoscoliosis)
4. Impaired airways and/or pulmonary parenchyma (emphysema, upper airway obstruction)

Increased $CO_2$ production is a very uncommon cause of an elevated $PCO_2$. $PCO_2$ will not rise because of increased $CO_2$ production if everything else is normal. However, if $CO_2$ elimination is marginal, an increase in $CO_2$ production can have a profound effect on arterial $PCO_2$. Some causes of increased $CO_2$ production include agitation, thyrotoxicosis, fever, and overfeeding.

### Hypoxemic Respiratory Failure

There are five general causes of hypoxemia:
1. Alveolar hypoventilation
2. Impaired diffusion
3. Breathing a gas mixture with a decreased oxygen concentration
4. Ventilation-perfusion mismatching
5. Right-to-left shunting of blood

Alveolar hypoventilation causes hypoxemia because of Boyle's law. Boyle's law indicates that the sum of partial pressures of all gases within a particular volume must equal the total pressure within that volume. In the alveolus, the pressure is near atmospheric and the gases involved include oxygen, $H_2O$ vapor, $CO_2$, and nitrogen. If we assume nitrogen to be constant, the amount of oxygen within the alveolus is defined by the alveolar-air equation that relates alveolar oxygen tension ($PA_{O_2}$) to the concentration of inspired oxygen ($FI_{O_2}$) and the partial pressure of $CO_2$ ($PCO_2$):

$$PA_{O_2} = FI_{O_2} \times (P_B - PH_2O) - Pa_{CO_2}/RQ$$

$P_B$ is the barometric pressure, $PH_2O$ is the water vapor pressure at body temperature (47 mmHg at 37° C), and RQ is the respiratory quotient (generally estimated to be 0.8). As $PCO_2$ increases, the alveolar oxygen concentration ($PA_{O_2}$) decreases if all other variables remain unchanged. Therefore, if hypoventilation causes an increase of $PCO_2$ by 4 mmHg, there will be a decrease of alveolar oxygen tension ($PA_{O_2}$) by about 5 mmHg.

Impaired diffusion is a rare cause of hypoxemia. It may be a factor in patients with severe interstitial lung disease during heavy exercise.

Breathing a gas mixture with a low concentration

of oxygen can cause hypoxemia. The most common cause of a reduced $F_{I_{O_2}}$ is altitude.

Efficient gas exchange depends on the ability to match alveolar air (ventilation) adequately with blood volume (perfusion). If a portion of the lung is well perfused but not well ventilated, there is a ventilation-perfusion mismatch. The ratio of ventilation to perfusion ($\dot{V}/\dot{Q}$) is low. A low $\dot{V}/\dot{Q}$ ratio is the most common cause of hypoxemia.

The fifth general cause of hypoxemia is a "shunt." A shunt occurs when venous blood bypasses ventilated portions of the lungs and is dumped unoxygenated into the arterial circulation. There are two types of shunts: anatomic and physiologic. Anatomic shunts are those in which venous blood bypasses the gas exchanging portion of the lungs altogether. Examples include a small amount of bronchial artery blood and a small amount of left coronary blood. Physiologic shunts are those that occur within the lung where portions of the lung are perfused but not ventilated. A physiologic shunt is an extreme case of $\dot{V}/\dot{Q}$ mismatching in which ventilation is zero. Physiologic shunting occurs when alveoli become filled with blood, pus, or serum, such as in alveolar hemorrhage, severe pneumonia, or pulmonary edema.

Clinically, a shunt can be distinguished from a $\dot{V}/\dot{Q}$ mismatch by the response to oxygen. If hypoxia is caused predominantly by a shunt, increasing the inspired oxygen will result in only a small increase in $P_{O_2}$. However, increased levels of inspired oxygen when the predominant lesion is $\dot{V}/\dot{Q}$ mismatch will correct hypoxemia.

A measure of the lung's efficiency to exchange gas is called the alveolar to arterial oxygen difference ($P[A-a]_{O_2}$). $P(A-a)_{O_2}$ is calculated by subtracting the directly measured arterial $P_{O_2}$ from the alveolar oxygen concentration derived from the alveolar-air equation. $P(A-a)_{O_2}$ can be determined only if the $F_{I_{O_2}}$ is accurately known (patient breathing room air or intubated). Furthermore, the normal value increases as $F_{I_{O_2}}$ increases. Therefore, $P(A-a)_{O_2}$ is easiest to interpret and follow if the patient is not breathing supplemental oxygen. The normal $P(A-a)_{O_2}$ results from the presence of anatomic shunts and small amounts of normal $\dot{V}/\dot{Q}$ mismatching. The normal value with the patient breathing room air increases with age (less than 10 in young adults and less than 30 in an 80-year-old). In $\dot{V}/\dot{Q}$ mismatching, physiologic shunts, and oxygen diffusion problems, the efficiency of gas exchange is impaired and the $P(A-a)_{O_2}$ difference widens. In contrast, alveolar hypoventilation and breathing a low $F_{I_{O_2}}$ do not impair the efficiency of the lung and the $P(A-a)_{O_2}$ is normal. Thus, calculation of $P(A-a)_{O_2}$ and observing the response to increasing levels of inspired oxygen will help decipher the general cause of hypoxemia.

## TREATMENT

The treatment of respiratory failure differs with the etiology, the classification (oxygenation failure versus ventilatory failure), the presence or absence of spontaneous respirations, and the ability to protect and maintain a clear airway. Furthermore, manipulations of the cardiovascular and hematologic systems may become paramount in achieving delivery of sufficient oxygen to the tissues and elimination of $CO_2$. The initial evaluation of respiratory failure includes a quick assessment of the patency of the airway and the presence and quality of spontaneous respirations. Is there stridor? Is the gag reflex absent? Is the chest moving appropriately with inspiratory efforts? If a problem is detected, immediate measures include clearing the airway, maintaining a patent airway (head tilt, oropharyngeal airway, or endotracheal tube), and providing adequate oxygen and ventilation.

### Oxygen Therapy

The method of providing adequate oxygenation differs depending on the degree of hypoxia, whether or not the mechanism involves $\dot{V}/\dot{Q}$ mismatching or shunting, and the presence or absence of hypercapnia. Most patients with mild to moderate hypoxemia ($P_{O_2}$ greater than 50), owing predominantly to $\dot{V}/\dot{Q}$ mismatch, can be adequately supplemented with low-flow oxygen.

The most common and best tolerated technique for providing low-flow supplemental oxygen is the nasal cannula. This augments $F_{I_{O_2}}$ by 3 to 4% per liter per minute of $O_2$ flow.

Excess oxygen therapy can be harmful to patients who demonstrate hypoxemia due to $\dot{V}/\dot{Q}$ mismatch but who also have hypercapnia (chronic obstructive pulmonary disease [COPD]). Sufficient supplemental oxygen must be given to provide adequate oxygenation to the tissues. However, $\dot{V}/\dot{Q}$ mismatching may worsen when these patients are given oxygen, thereby increasing wasted ventilation and making it more difficult for the lungs to eliminate $CO_2$. Excessive supplemental oxygen may worsen $CO_2$ retention, leading to acidosis, $CO_2$ narcosis, and eventually apnea and death. Therefore, small increments in $F_{I_{O_2}}$ should be employed until the $P_{O_2}$ is about 60. Blood gases and mental status should be monitored frequently, as ventilatory support may become necessary.

Hypoxic patients whose mechanism is predominantly shunting often have a high minute ventilation and may require a higher concentration of oxygen at a faster flow rate. Furthermore, because high oxygen concentrations for long periods of time can damage the lung, it is useful to know the $F_{I_{O_2}}$. Most high-flow oxygen devices generally work by entraining room air, thereby diluting the original concentration of oxygen (Venturi's principle). For 100% oxygen, no room air is entrained and the flow to the patient is lower. If 40% oxygen is desired, a substantial amount of room air is entrained and the flow of gas to the patient is much greater.

Extremely tachypneic patients can have inspired flow rates in excess of 100 liters per minute. Thus, it is important to assess whether or not the patient's inspiratory demands are being met by the high-flow system. If the system is a nebulizer, water vapor particles are delivered with the gas. The disappearance of the stream of water vapor from the mask's exhalation ports during inspiration is reflective of room air being entrained (overbreathing). Overbreathing with non-nebulizer masks can be assessed by placing a flimsy piece of tissue paper next to the mask exhalation port. Movement of the tissue paper toward the port during inspiration is indicative of overbreathing. If overbreathing is present, the patient must be given higher flow rates of oxygen to maintain the desired $FI_{O_2}$.

Very high $FI_{O_2}$ can be delivered with a non-rebreather mask. A reservoir bag larger than the patient's tidal volume fills with 100% oxygen. If the mask is tight fitting, very little room air will be entrained and an $FI_{O_2}$ approaching 1.0 can be delivered. However, difficulty in attaining a proper mask fit and valve resistance problems often limit the delivered oxygen fraction to much less than 1.0.

## Mechanical Ventilation

Intubation and mechanical ventilation are often initiated for clinical reasons rather than for specific blood gas or respiratory mechanical criteria. The patient's inability to protect his or her airway is a clear indication for intubation, as is apnea. Hemodynamic instability with impending cardiovascular collapse is a nonpulmonary indication for beginning mechanical ventilation. Other indications for mechanical ventilation include refractory hypoxemia, progressive acidosis, or hypercapnia. Commonly used specific criteria for mechanical ventilation include a vital capacity less than 1 liter, a sustained respiratory rate greater than 35, a maximal inspiratory pressure less than 20 cm $H_2O$, a $Pa_{O_2}$ less than 50 on supplemental oxygen, or an acute increase in $PCO_2$ to greater than 55. These specific criteria must be tempered by clinical judgment.

There exist many different types of ventilators and modes of ventilation. General types include volume cycled, time cycled, and pressure cycled. The goal of mechanical ventilation is to deliver a minute ventilation (respiratory rate times tidal volume) with an enriched oxygen concentration sufficient for adequate tissue oxygenation.

The usual tidal volume delivered by a ventilator is in the range of 10 to 15 ml per kg, compared with a normal spontaneous tidal volume of 5 ml per kg. These high tidal volumes are thought to prevent atelectasis; however, they may also cause high airway pressures that enhance the risk of barotrauma.

A sufficient rate is that which maximizes patient comfort while attaining a minute ventilation that normalizes acid-base status. If one is using a volume ventilator, this is most easily accomplished by the assist-control mode (volume control, depending on the ventilator being used). An estimated rate is set and if the patient desires more, additional patient-initiated breaths are delivered with a full preset tidal volume.

Advantages to the assist-control mode of volume ventilators include minimal work of breathing for the patient. This allows the diaphragm and respiratory muscles to rest. This technique should be used for patients with respiratory muscle fatigue, hemodynamic instability, interstitial lung disease acidosis, or any condition in which the work of breathing needs to be minimized.

A difficult problem arises when patients have too fast a respiratory rate. This can result from setting too small a tidal volume or having a patient with a high ventilatory drive. A tendency to hyperventilate is common in patients with diffuse lung disease, liver disease, toxic sensorium from drugs, or sepsis. Rapid respiratory rates may not allow adequate time for exhalation. If the lung does not deflate adequately, high intrathoracic pressure (auto-PEEP*) develops and may result in reduced cardiac output or barotrauma. The requirement for adequate exhalation time is magnified in patients with COPD, in whom reduced lung elastic recoil and high airway resistance limit air flow.

Furthermore, hyperventilation can lead to respiratory alkalosis, causing CNS irritation, seizures, vasodilatation, cardiac irritability, and arrhythmias. If the patient's pH is 7.55 or greater, corrective steps need to be taken. The patient can be sedated to blunt his or her ventilatory drive, or the mode of ventilation can be changed to intermittent mandatory ventilation (IMV) or continuous positive airway pressure. Adjusting inspiratory flow rates and/or tidal volume to match the patient's demand also can be helpful.

IMV incorporates a preset tidal volume and a backup respiratory rate similar to assist-control. However, when the patient desires to breathe faster than the mandatory backup rate, he or she draws a spontaneous tidal volume. The size and frequency of the spontaneous tidal volume are determined by the patient. This technique is used

---

*PEEP = positive end-expiratory pressure.

for patients with an inappropriately high minute ventilation, or as a weaning tool by gradually reducing the backup rate.

Some patients with high ventilatory drives do not require mechanical ventilation yet still require airway protection and help with oxygenation. A reasonable alternative for these patients is continuous positive airway pressure (CPAP). In CPAP, the patient breathes spontaneously and a preset pressure is maintained throughout the respiratory cycle. Maintaining this pressure often allows a reduction in $F_{I_{O_2}}$ while maintaining an acceptable $P_{O_2}$. CPAP can be instituted by an option on most volume ventilators or by way of a retardant valve at the exhalation end of a "T tube" connected to a high-flow gas source. One disadvantage of CPAP through mechanical ventilators is that the work of breathing may be increased because of the resistance in initiating gas flow. The level of CPAP chosen should be as low as possible to obtain an acceptable $P_{O_2}$ (greater than 60 mmHg) with a relatively safe $F_{I_{O_2}}$ (less than 0.6). Other disadvantages of CPAP include the lack of backup mandatory ventilation. Thus, careful monitoring with transcutaneous $O_2$ saturation monitors and in-line pressure monitors with alarms is paramount. Furthermore, respiratory rates, level of agitation, and blood gases must be followed to prevent unrecognized hypercapnia.

Another mode of ventilation is "pressure support." This mode relies on patient effort to determine tidal volume and frequency. The mode differs from CPAP in that inspiratory efforts trigger ventilator air flow until the preset airway pressure is attained. Air flow continues as long as the patient is making a sufficient inspiratory effort to keep airway pressure below the preset limit. Some patients find pressure support more comfortable, possibly because of high initial inspiratory flow or possibly because they have more control. The advantages to pressure support ventilation may include overcoming the circuit resistance associated with spontaneous breathing through a ventilator. By decreasing the level of "pressure support" over time, this mode of ventilation can be an effective weaning technique.

There are many new modes of ventilation currently being touted as beneficial, including pressure-controlled inverse ratio ventilation, pressure release ventilation, and jet ventilation. These are all unproven methods, are potentially dangerous, and should be employed only by experienced clinicians in research protocols.

A major complication of high $F_{I_{O_2}}$ is the toxicity of oxygen on the lung. Prolonged use of an $F_{I_{O_2}}$ of 1.0 can cause lung damage indistinguishable from that of the adult respiratory distress syndrome (ARDS). Lower oxygen concentrations are safer but still dangerous. Therefore, the $F_{I_{O_2}}$ should be as low as possible to maintain good arterial oxygenation (i.e., arterial oxygen saturation greater than or equal to 90%). When a hypoxemic patient is placed on a ventilator, it is best to start with an $F_{I_{O_2}}$ of 1.0 to effect immediate and adequate oxygenation. Then, one should decrease the $F_{I_{O_2}}$ to the lowest level able to maintain oxygen saturation greater than or equal to 90%.

If the $F_{I_{O_2}}$ cannot be safely reduced below 0.6, other measures need consideration to decrease the chances of oxygen toxicity. Positive end-expiratory pressure (PEEP) is often used in this circumstance. PEEP increases the resting volume of the lung (functional residual capacity [FRC]), recruits alveoli that may have been collapsed, and decreases shunting. PEEP levels greater than 5 cm $H_2O$ should be restricted to those patients with a diffuse bilateral pulmonary lesion, such as pulmonary edema, ARDS, and diffuse interstitial pneumonia. Its effects may be counterproductive in patients with localized pathology such as lobar pneumonia. PEEP can increase chances of barotrauma or cardiovascular collapse. It can even worsen hypoxemia if used inappropriately. PEEP can decrease venous return to the right atrium and increase pulmonary vascular resistance. These cardiovascular effects of PEEP are more pronounced in hypovolemic patients: PEEP levels of less than 15 in euvolemic patients generally are tolerated well from a cardiovascular standpoint. Relative contraindications to the use of PEEP include pre-existing barotrauma, hypotension, cardiogenic shock, and hypovolemia. If hemodynamic problems arise with the use of PEEP, invasive monitoring should be considered.

Complications of mechanical ventilation include barotrauma and cardiovascular instability. Both of these complications can be minimized by keeping intrathoracic pressures (peak airway pressure, mean airway pressure, PEEP) as low as possible while maintaining an adequate $P_{O_2}$ (60 mmHg). Peak pressures in excess of 50 cm $H_2O$ are a matter of concern. Sometimes decreasing the tidal volume or adjusting the inspiratory flow rates will correct this problem. Other measures include aggressive treatment of bronchospasm, suctioning, and, if necessary, sedation. Barotrauma will occasionally occur even with optimal ventilator management. Early recognition of the occurrence of pneumothorax is vital to avoiding disaster. A rapid increase in peak pressure or a rapid decline in oxygen saturation or blood pressure can be clues. Often pneumothoraces occur but do not cause catastrophic collapse and are discovered only on a chest radiograph. Patients on mechanical ventilators often have a myriad of invasive tubes and lines (e.g., nasogastric tube, endotracheal tube, subclavian or jugular line). Monitoring line and tube position and discovering occult barotrauma mandate a chest radiograph daily on most ventilated patients.

### Weaning from Mechanical Ventilation

Before a patient is weaned from mechanical ventilation, it is important to review why the patient was intubated. Obviously, the condition that originally led to intubation must have improved. Patients should also be awake, cooperative, and able to mobilize secretions. Moreover, the $F_{I_{O_2}}$ should be less than 0.5., PEEP should be 5 cm of water or less, and the patient should be able to breathe spontaneously through the endotracheal tube without assistance for at least 30 minutes. Spontaneous respiratory mechanics are additional useful predictors of a successful extubation. These include a maximal inspiratory pressure greater than 20 cm $H_2O$, a vital capacity greater than 10 ml per kg, a tidal volume greater than 5 ml per kg, and a resting minute ventilation less than 10 liters per minute.

There are many methods of weaning from mechanical ventilation. No method has proved superior, and the key factor in successful weaning is improvement in the patient's condition. The three most common include IMV, pressure support, and "T piece" trials with or without CPAP. IMV weaning allows the patient to assume the work of breathing gradually. This is performed by gradually reducing the mandatory respiratory rate and allowing the patient to take more spontaneous breaths. Eventually the mandatory rate will be low enough that the patient is essentially breathing without assistance.

Pressure support weaning incorporates a gradual decrease of inspiratory pressure assistance. The patient gradually assumes more of the work of maintaining a tidal volume. Again, eventually the patient is receiving minimal ventilatory assistance and can be extubated.

The T tube technique utilizes a high-flow gas device that connects to a T tube. The patient is disconnected from the ventilator and connected to the T tube for increasing lengths of time. When the patient is able to sustain ventilation for an extended period, weaning is accomplished.

Being weaned from a ventilator can be very stressful and dangerous for patients. Not all attempts are successful, and well-defined end points need to be specified. Accepted criteria for failure include acute hypoxia ($Pa_{O_2}$ less than or equal to 55), acute hypercapnia, sustained respiratory rates greater than 35, hypotension, severe hypertension, arrhythmia, or agitation. A patient who fails a weaning attempt should be placed back on the pre-attempt ventilator settings and allowed to rest.

Manipulation of clinical variables before a weaning trial contributes to success, and review of these variables after a failure is paramount. The variables include minimizing sedation over the preceding 24 hours; ensuring normal electrolytes, including phosphate, calcium, and magnesium; and avoiding malnutrition. Calming the patient by discussing what to expect is also important.

The recognition of respiratory failure by the patient and the physician can be one of the most frightening experiences either individual will encounter. The successful treatment and returned health of the patient can also be one of the most rewarding.

# ATELECTASIS

method of
JEAN DESLAURIERS, M.D.
*Unité de Recherche, Centre de Pneumologie*
*Hôpital Laval*
*Sainte-Foy, Québec, Canada*

Atelectasis is usually an acquired disorder that is characterized by the collapse of a lung, a lobe, a segment, or an acinar unit from any cause. The loss of volume reflects the resorption of air from distal lung units, a situation that occurs when normal communication between air passages (central or peripheral) and alveoli is interrupted (resorption atelectasis).

The clinical relevance of atelectasis is threefold: (1) It may be the only indication of an occult thoracic pathology such as an endobronchial obstructing neoplasm. (2) It can predispose the lung to bacterial pneumonia not only because retained mucus is an ideal medium for bacterial growth but also because decreased blood flow impairs local defense mechanisms. Indeed, it has been shown that atelectasis affects the antibacterial function of alveolar macrophages and decreases mucociliary clearance. (3) Perfusion of underventilated areas of the lung may result in significant shunting of blood, with resultant hypoxemia.

Proper management of atelectasis depends on a clear understanding of its mechanisms and on the presence and the severity of secondary complications.

## TREATMENT

### Segmental or Lobar Atelectasis in Nonoperative Patients

Segmental or lobar atelectasis in nonoperative patients is mainly due to airway obstruction by a neoplasm, a foreign body, or an inflammation. The diagnosis can sometimes be suspected from a review of previous chest radiographs, but bronchoscopic examination is mandatory to determine the cause, the site, and the degree of obstruction. Biopsies of intraluminal masses can readily be performed. If the obstruction is in the distal bronchial tree and cannot be seen by the endoscopist, or if it is extrinsic, bronchial brushings or transbronchial biopsies can be obtained for histopathologic examination.

In all of these situations, management should be that of the primary lesion.

## Atelectasis in the Postoperative or Critically Ill Patient

Atelectasis in postoperative or critically ill patients is mainly the cumulative result of decreased tidal volume, absence of sigh mechanism, and ineffective cough. It can present as "plate" atelectasis in lung bases or as lobar atelectasis when secretions are retained and mucous plugging occurs. Atelectasis is a common problem after thoracic or upper abdominal operations and often causes significant venoarterial shunting.

The incidence of postoperative atelectasis can be decreased substantially by proper prophylactic measures. In all patients, medical operability must be carefully assessed with reference to age, weight loss, coexisting diseases, and cardiopulmonary function. Patients should be prepared preoperatively by physiotherapy training, and the nature of the surgery and its possible complications should be properly explained. Bronchodilators or antibiotics should be given preoperatively when indicated. The surgery itself should be performed rapidly and with minimal tissue trauma. The anesthetist must be familiar with modern techniques of intubation, one-lung anesthesia, and perioperative monitoring. The anesthetist must make sure that residual anesthetic effects are minimized. Postoperatively, active chest physiotherapy must be started early, and modern analgesia methods should be routinely used. Most important, imminent atelectasis must be recognized and treated vigorously.

Once atelectasis has developed, active respiratory therapy is the mainstay of treatment. This therapy includes chest physiotherapy with deep breathing and cough exercises, frequent changing of body positions, early ambulation, and postural drainage with percussion maneuvers. To facilitate vigorous coughing and deep breathing, control of pain must be optimal. The use of intercostal block therapy, cryotherapy, or spinal narcotics (epidural analgesia) is preferred to systemic analgesia. When these conservative measures fail to initiate proper cough and/or to reverse atelectasis, therapeutic bronchoscopy is indicated.

In most circumstances, bedside flexible bronchoscopy under local anesthesia suffices. Large mucous plugs are first aspirated from major bronchi. The bronchoscope is then advanced into lobar or segmental bronchi where any inspissated mucus is carefully suctioned. Individual segments of the lung are then lavaged with a sterile saline solution. In some cases, selective lobar re-expansion can be achieved with a balloon-cuffed bronchoscope. Unstable or hypoxic patients may require endotracheal intubation to enable a safe bronchoscopy through the endotracheal tube.

Because the primary objective in preventing atelectasis is to maintain the best possible tidal volumes and functional residual capacities, any maneuver that emphasizes inflation is likely to be useful. Acceptable techniques include incentive spirometry and continuous positive airway pressure (CPAP). The current belief is that intermittent positive pressure breathing is of little use and that medications such as albuterol (Ventolin), which may be useful in relieving bronchospasm and/or potentiating clearing of secretions, are best given by nebulization.

Incentive spirometer devices are designed to ensure a large inspired volume. They stress a sustained inspiratory effort and are recommended by most investigators. CPAP techniques are similarly effective, but their use requires trained personnel and more cooperative patients.

## Compression Atelectasis

Compression or passive atelectasis is defined as a reduction in lung volume secondary to a contiguous pulmonary abnormality or to a space-occupying lesion within the chest wall or pleural space. Primary therapy should be aimed at removing the underlying cause.

Accumulation of fluid or gas in the pleural space can readily be treated by needle aspiration or tube thoracostomy. When the disease process is more chronic, the lung may have to be surgically decorticated. In most of these cases, proper anatomic expansion of the lung can be achieved, although pulmonary function does not always return to normal.

## Decreased Ventilation

Several disorders can be associated with alveolar hypoventilation and secondary atelectasis. In these cases, atelectasis is secondary to the loss of surface tension within the alveoli, or decreased distending pressure and alveolar size, or the failure to generate an adequate negative inspiratory pleural pressure. The physiologic consequences depend on the amount of lung involved.

Decreased ventilation results from either a decreased central drive or faulty chest wall or lung mechanics. Although central origins include various rare brain disorders, decreased ventilation is more commonly associated with improper use of narcotic analgesia. In patients with trauma or in postoperative patients, for example, intercostal block therapy (bupivacaine [Marcaine] every 8 to 12 hours) can be effective while avoiding the central depression that is associated with intramuscular administration of analgesics. As noted earlier, spinal analgesia, particularly with morphine, can also be useful.

Decreased ventilation may also occur in patients in whom there is interference with chest wall mechanics or respiratory muscle function. One example of this problem is seen in patients with flail chests, when pain and instability of the chest wall can lead to hypoventilation, atelectasis, and ultimately respiratory failure. Prevention of atelectasis in these patients may be achieved through adequate pain control, aggressive respiratory therapy, and, on occasion, open stabilization of the chest wall. In the post-thoracotomy patient, the function of intercostal and diaphragmatic muscles can be severely perturbed. Because both of these muscles are important for normal respiration, this malfunction can lead to significant hypoventilation and atelectasis. Therapy should be primarily aimed at preventing surgical damage to the phrenic nerve, relieving pain, and/or encouraging deep breathing exercises.

# CHRONIC OBSTRUCTIVE PULMONARY DISEASE

method of
DAVID R. DANTZKER, M.D.
*Long Island Jewish Medical Center*
*Albert Einstein College of Medicine*
*New Hyde Park, New York*

Chronic obstructive pulmonary disease (COPD) is a condition characterized by reduced expiratory flow rates that are relatively stable over periods of several months' observation. Three pathologic entities are included under the general umbrella of COPD. The most important is emphysema: an anatomic alteration of the lung characterized by an abnormal enlargement of airspaces distal to terminal bronchioles accompanied by destruction of the alveolar walls. The degree of emphysema correlates best with the presence of severe airway obstruction and is usually present in at least moderate amounts in patients with any degree of functional impairment. The etiology of the emphysema is thought to be an imbalance in the protease and anti-protease levels in the lung leading to lung destruction. The most graphic example of this can be seen in patients with a deficiency of alpha₁-antitrypsin (AAT). Subjects who possess the ZZ variant of AAT have very low levels of AAT and are at high risk for the development of emphysema. Cigarette smoking is thought to act as the major risk factor for the development of emphysema through its ability to increase the protease levels in the lung while at the same time decreasing the anti-protease activity.

The earliest manifestation of COPD is thought to occur in the small airways, which may show inflammation or fibrosis of the terminal or respiratory bronchioles with narrowing and goblet cell metaplasia. Smoking has also been incriminated in the development of these lesions. Although small airway lesions undoubtedly contribute to the airflow obstruction in some patients with COPD, the correlation with the degree of impairment is not as close as with emphysema.

Chronic bronchitis is a disease of the large airways manifested by excessive mucus production and chronic cough. Although bronchitis is present in the majority of patients with functionally significant COPD, it is also common in many cigarette smokers who demonstrate no reduction of expiratory airflow. It is now generally felt that cough and sputum production do not have a significant independent effect on the development of airflow obstruction and that the reduced expiratory flow seen in the setting of chronic bronchitis is due mostly to the concomitant presence of emphysema, small airway disease, and bronchospasm.

The basis for the bronchospasm in COPD is unknown, but increased bronchial reactivity is commonly found. The degree of reversible bronchial tone in these patients is small when compared with that seen in asthma. However, even small changes in airway diameter may cause significant alterations in the work of breathing when the airway has already been narrowed by structural changes.

The important physiologic consequences of COPD are the increased work of breathing and the abnormal pulmonary gas exchange. The increased work of breathing contributes to the sense of dyspnea and places significant limits on exercise tolerance. The abnormal pulmonary gas exchange leads to hypoxemia and, with increasing severity, to hypercapnia and respiratory failure.

## TREATMENT

The treatment of COPD is primarily directed at the relief of symptoms. There is very little that can be done to correct the basic underlying pathophysiology, with the exception, perhaps, of smoking cessation and AAT replacement.

### Bronchodilators

Clinically useful drugs that relax bronchial smooth muscle fall under three categories: beta-adrenergic agonists, cholinergic antagonists, and methylxanthines. These drugs form the cornerstone of the treatment of COPD.

The airways are richly invested with beta$_2$-adrenergic receptors that when stimulated lead to bronchodilatation. Beta-adrenergic agonists are potent bronchodilators and generally the first choice for the immediate treatment of bronchospasm in patients with COPD. Even in patients who do not demonstrate immediate reversibility of airflow limitation following the acute administration of these agents, long-term results are often favorable. Beta$_2$-specific agents have less toxicity than that attributed to nonspecific adrenergic agonists like epinephrine and isoproterenol but, more importantly, have an increased duration of action (Table 1). Whenever possible, these agents should be given by aerosolization through the use of a metered dose inhaler (MDI), which can be coupled to a spacer or collapsible bag (InsperEase) in patients unable to coordinate the technique easily. In patients who cannot master the MDI it may be necessary to utilize a simple powered nebulizer. Oral administration is usually not advisable because the dose required is much higher than that needed for aerosolization and the side effects are also increased. These include muscle twitching, insomnia, and tachycardias. In addition, it is much more difficult to titrate the correct oral dose, owing to variability of absorption and metabolism.

There are many different beta$_2$ agonists on the market, but the differences among them are too small to recommend any in particular. The most important thing is to be certain to use them in sufficient amounts. Most therapeutic failures are due to underdosing or to patients not receiving the drug at all because of poor MDI technique. Watching the patient use an MDI until it is apparent that he or she correctly coordinates breathing with activation is key to the successful use of any MDI-based therapeutic regimen. Initially, the patient can be started on a regular dose of 2 or 3 actuations three or four times per day with additional doses as required up to 16 to 24 actuations per day. The use of the MDI prior to tasks requiring increased exertion is often useful. Little clinically significant tolerance develops with prolonged use.

Stimulation of the cholinergic nerves to the airways results in increased smooth muscle tone, and it is not surprising that anticholinergic drugs should be effective bronchodilators. These agents were, in fact, the first bronchodilators and have been used in one form or another for hundreds of years. The introduction of ipratropium bromide (Atrovent) provided an anticholinergic agent that, unlike atropine, was poorly absorbed from the airways and thus had a much lower risk of extrapulmonary side effects such as tachycardia, dry mouth, blurred vision, urinary obstruction, and constipation. The usual recommended dosage is 40 µg (2 actuations of the MDI at 4- to 6-hour intervals. In patients with severe disease, higher doses may be required. Increasing the dose of ipratropium also tends to increase the duration of action. There is no clinical evidence of tachyphylaxis. Anticholinergic agents are very efficacious in treating COPD, and many investigators have found them to be equally effective or in some cases more effective bronchodilators than beta$_2$-adrenergic agonists. The combination of an anticholinergic and beta$_2$-adrenergic inhaler has in some, but not all, studies been shown to be additive and should be tried when single-agent therapy is ineffective.

The mechanism by which the methylxanthine bronchodilators (theophylline, aminophylline) produce bronchodilation remains an enigma. Present theories favor a role as an adenosine receptor blocker. Methylxanthines are about 50% as potent as beta-adrenergic agents in their bronchodilating ability. Their role in the treatment of COPD is now controversial because many studies have shown no appreciable improvement in flow rates when they are added to adequate doses of beta-adrenergic agents, either in stable patients or in those with an acute exacerbation. However, other studies have noted symptomatic improvement and even an improvement of exercise tolerance in patients with stable COPD following the initiation of theophylline therapy. This improvement has been ascribed to other, putative non-bronchodilator effects of these drugs such as their positive inotropic potential or their purported ability to improve respiratory muscle function. In patients who fail to respond adequately to a combination of beta agonists and anticholinergics, a trial of theophylline is reasonable. The usual adult dosage is 10 to 12 mg per kg per day but may vary widely depending on the presence of factors that alter the metabolism of theophylline (Table 2). This dosage may be effectively given using sustained-release preparations in a twice-a-day regimen. Effectiveness is related to the blood level, which is usually kept in the range of 8 to 16 µg per ml. Above these levels, there is rarely a significantly increased efficacy and gastrointestinal, cardiac, and neurologic toxicity becomes unacceptable. Some patients fail to tolerate even these low therapeutic levels. Methylxan-

TABLE 1. **Beta-Adrenergic Bronchodilators**

| Drug | Role of Administration | Duration of Action (hr) |
|---|---|---|
| Epinephrine | Subcutaneous | 1–2 |
| Isoproterenol | Aerosolized | 1–2 |
| Beta$_2$-specific agonist | Aerosolized | 4–6 |

TABLE 2. **Factors Affecting the Clearance of Methylxanthine Drugs**

**Increase Clearance**
Cigarette smoking
Charcoal-broiled meat
Rifampin
Phenobarbital
Childhood

**Decrease Clearance**
Erythromycin
Cimetidine
Allopurinol
Ciprofloxacin
Propranolol
Oral contraceptives
Viral infection and vaccination
Heart failure
Liver disease

thines should be tried particularly in patients who complain of regular nocturnal symptoms, since these agents have a sufficiently long enough duration of action to be present in therapeutic amounts in the early morning when symptoms are often at their worst. Because of the high incidence of side effects, methylxanthines should be continued on a chronic basis only if there is clear objective evidence of improved function or at least symptomatic improvement following their initiation.

### Corticosteroids

Intravenous corticosteroids should be used in all patients admitted to the hospital with an exacerbation of COPD as long as no contraindication exists, since they speed the rate of recovery. Doses of methylprednisolone (Solu-Medrol) higher than 40 mg four times a day have no demonstrable increase in efficacy, and the dose should be tapered as clinical improvement is noted. The usefulness of long-term corticosteroid administration in relatively stable COPD is not as clear, although studies suggest that a small subset of these patients will benefit from chronic steroid therapy. Because of the serious side effects of prolonged steroid administration, especially in a population of older individuals, objective demonstration of an increase in expiratory flow rate after a short course (2 weeks) of moderate doses of prednisone (Deltasone) (30 to 40 mg per day) should be sought before committing the patient to chronic therapy. If there is improvement, the smallest dose consistent with continued success should be used. Although there have been some suggestions that every-other-day usage or substitution with inhaled corticosteroids can reduce the side effects, there are no studies that have yet demonstrated their efficacy in COPD.

### Antibiotics

There is scant evidence that infection is a common cause of COPD exacerbations, although colonization of the airways with potentially pathogenic organisms is common. A single recent study, however, suggested that antibiotics increased the rate of recovery of patients with COPD if a worsening of symptoms was accompanied by an increase or change in the character of the sputum. In patients who meet these criteria or those with clear-cut systemic signs of infection, it is appropriate to begin antibiotics. Sputum smears and cultures are not particularly useful in this patient population and it is more reasonable to treat empirically for the most common pathogens: *Streptococcus pneumoniae* and *Haemophilus influenzae*. Adequate treatment would include ampicillin (Omnipen), amoxicillin (Larotid), or erythromycin (E-Mycin) (all 2 grams per day); or trimethoprim-sulfamethoxazole (Bactrim, Septra) (one double-strength tablet twice a day). Prophylactic therapy with antibiotics is not useful.

### Vaccines

Vaccines against specific strains of influenza have been shown to be very effective in preventing the development of clinical illness and should be given to all patients with symptomatic COPD. In the case of an influenza A outbreak, unvaccinated patients can obtain protection from amantadine (Symmetrel) therapy (100 mg twice a day, reduced to 100 mg every day in elderly patients). Pneumococcal vaccine has been shown to be immunogenic in healthy subjects, but its ability to prevent pneumonia in debilitated patients with COPD is less certain. Nevertheless, it is worthwhile giving because the complication rate is very low. Only a single dose of the vaccine is recommended.

### Expectorants and Mucolytic Agents

The presence of excessive and difficult to clear mucus is one of the most vexing problems in the treatment of COPD. Although many purported expectorants and mucolytics are available, none have been demonstrated to be efficacious in well-controlled clinical trials, although iodinated glycerol (Organidin) was recently shown to result in subjective improvement. Dehydration probably increases the viscidness of sputum, but overhydration or bland saline nebulization has no beneficial effects and vigorous intravenous hydration of patients with COPD risks the development of congestive heart failure. The appropriate use of beta-adrenergic agents and corticosteroids is associated with improved clearance of sputum.

### Alpha₁-antitrypsin (AAT) Replacement (Prolastin)

AAT replacement has been demonstrated to significantly increase AAT levels in the serum and lungs of patients with AAT deficiency. Patients whose AAT level is less than 11 $\mu$M, which includes those who are zz, null null, or z null AAT phenotypes, are at high risk for the development of emphysema and should be considered for AAT replacement. Treatment should be reserved for patients who, in addition, have abnormal lung function as defined by spirometry, since anywhere from 5 to 50% of patients at risk do not develop clinically significant emphysema. AAT replacement is very expensive (about $25,000 per year), requires weekly intravenous administration, and has not yet been shown to protect the lung against the development of emphysema. AAT replacement clearly has no role in patients with emphysema who do not have severe reductions in AAT levels.

### Oxygen

Hypoxemia is an invariable consequence of COPD. As a result, $O_2$ transport to the tissues may be compromised and pulmonary hypertension may develop, leading to cor pulmonale. Both factors have been associated with a decreased survival. In patients admitted to the hospital with an acute exacerbation of COPD, supplemental $O_2$ is almost always necessary to increase the $PaO_2$ to clinically acceptable levels ($PaO_2$ greater than 60 torr). For stable patients with chronic hypoxemia who meet the criteria set up by the Nocturnal Oxygen Therapy (NOT) Trial (Table 3), continuous low-flow $O_2$ (1 to 4 liters per minute) is associated with a significantly greater survival. Some patients with COPD demonstrate significant $O_2$ desaturation only when asleep or during exercise. Because experimental studies have demonstrated the development of pulmonary hypertension with as little as 6 hours per day of hypoxemia, nocturnal $O_2$ therapy should be considered for patients in whom prolonged nocturnal desaturation can be demonstrated, particularly if other physiologic consequences are already evident such as cor pulmonale or polycythemia. In these patients, a formal sleep study should be performed to rule out the presence of coexistent obstructive sleep apnea prior to prescribing $O_2$ because it may worsen the apneic episodes. $O_2$ therapy for patients who only desaturate during exercise should be reserved for patients in whom an objective improvement in exercise tolerance with $O_2$ can be demonstrated. In all cases, the goal should be to maintain an arterial $O_2$ saturation of greater than 90%.

An increase in the arterial $PcO_2$ is common during supplemental $O_2$ therapy in markedly hypoxemic patients who are hypercapnic to begin with. The mechanism of the increasing hypercapnia is complex but can only be ascribed in part to depression of ventilatory drive. The increase in the $PaCO_2$ cannot be predicted in any individual patient, nor can the absolute level of $PaCO_2$ that will result in $CO_2$ narcosis be predicted. Therefore, no fixed level of $PaCO_2$ can be defined as being too high and $CO_2$ narcosis should be defined on the basis of clinical examination. Usually this complication can be avoided by careful attention to the level of inspired $O_2$, increasing the $O_2$ concentration carefully and using only enough to reach the clinical goal of 90% saturation. It is important, however, to remember that it is hypoxia and not hypercapnia that kills patients and if adequate oxygenation cannot be achieved without risking $CO_2$ narcosis, mechanical ventilation is required.

### Vasodilators

Many drugs have been shown to dilate pulmonary arteries whose tone is abnormally increased. The most clinically important ones include the calcium channel blockers, hydralazine (Apresoline), and prostacyclin.* In patients with COPD, these drugs can reduce pulmonary vascular resistance both at rest and during exercise while at the same time increasing cardiac output. However, it is unclear whether the modest pulmonary hypertension associated with COPD is an independent risk factor or that it leads to functional limitation. In addition, there are a number of potential problems associated with the use of vasodilators, including worsening hypoxemia and systemic hypotension with decreased organ perfusion. Thus, unless long-term clinical trials can show improved survival, the routine use of vasodilators in patients with cor pulmonale is not advisable.

### Digitalis

Digitalis has not been shown to improve cardiac function in patients with isolated right ven-

TABLE 3. **Criteria for Continuous Oxygen Therapy**

Arterial $PO_2$ <55 torr
*or*
Arterial $PO_2$ <59 torr
*and*
Right heart failure or erythrocytosis

*Not available in the United States.

tricular failure associated with cor pulmonale. In addition, there is an increased risk of digitalis-induced arrhythmias in this patient group.

### Diuretics

Edema is a common finding in patients with cor pulmonale, and when it becomes excessive the cautious use of diuretics is indicated. Excessive diuresis must be avoided, however, since an increased right-sided filling pressure is often advantageous in the setting of pulmonary hypertension.

### Nutrition

Reduced body weight and poor nutritional status have been correlated with increased mortality and reduced pulmonary function in patients with COPD. Whether or not nutritional status is the independent variable or body weight is falling because of increasing demands or there is some other factor contributing to both the worsening lung function as well as the nutritional impairment is unclear at this time. Although it seems logical to provide supplemental nutritional support to severely debilitated patients with COPD, there is no evidence that increasing the weight of the typical patient with emphysema is of any use and may be detrimental if it increases metabolic $O_2$ requirements.

### Physical Therapy and Rehabilitation

Chest physiotherapy (percussion and postural drainage) is employed on the assumption that it improves the mobilization and clearance of secretions. Although this has not been proved, it is appropriate to attempt this modality in hospitalized patients with excessive secretions who have inadequate cough, which is the most efficient method of clearing the airways, or who develop areas of atelectasis that do not rapidly clear. Fiberoptic bronchoscopy is not any more effective than chest physiotherapy as a means of sputum removal.

Exercise rehabilitation programs improve exercise tolerance and efficiency but do not increase the maximum level of exercise achievable, improve pulmonary function, or alter morbidity or mortality. In highly motivated patients, exercise rehabilitation programs can improve the quality of life.

### Hospitalization

The patient with COPD should be hospitalized when acute exacerbations significantly compromise pulmonary gas exchange or cardiac function, or when the tenuous state of the patient makes outpatient treatment of related or unrelated medical or surgical problems risky.

Some hospitalized patients with exacerbations of COPD may progress to the point at which mechanical ventilation is required to maintain acceptable oxygenation and acid-base status. The decision to intubate the patient should be made by the physician in conjunction with the patient and family and should be based on the patient's overall physical status including the presence or absence of other complicating diseases. For patients whose only medical problem is COPD, it is usually impossible to predict the likelihood of reversibility confidently, and thus intubation and mechanical ventilation are generally advisable unless the patient declines or the prognosis of other underlying conditions precludes the likelihood of recovery.

### Smoking Cessation

Perhaps the most important factor in the management of patients with COPD is smoking cessation. Smokers who develop COPD have an accelerated rate of decline in lung function when compared with nonsmokers ($FEV_1$ decreases 80 ml per year versus 30 ml per year). Following cessation of smoking, the rate drops to that in the nonsmoker.

A smoking cessation program should address all of the forces responsible for the smoking behavior: biologic, behavioral, and psychologic. This may take many forms, including counseling, individual and group behavior modification programs, and adverse conditioning. Pharmacologic intervention using nicotine polacrilex (Nicorette) may be useful to minimize the effects of nicotine withdrawal. Under the best of circumstances, a 20 to 30% success rate can be expected.

# PRIMARY LUNG CANCER

method of
DANIEL C. IHDE, M.D.
*National Cancer Institute*
*Bethesda, Maryland*

Lung cancer has long been the most common cause of death from malignant neoplasms in American men, and has recently become so in American women. In the United States, approximately 95% of these cancers in men and 80% in women are caused by cigarette abuse and thus are potentially preventable. Fortunately, there is now evidence that the decline in cigarette smoking that began in the 1960s has led to falling lung cancer mortality in individuals under the age of 50. However, because of the large numbers of current smokers and the delay between smoking cessation and reduced lung cancer rates, it is expected to be at least another decade before overall lung cancer mortality begins to diminish.

Although there are four major pathologic cell types of bronchogenic carcinoma, there are only two relevant categories for therapeutic planning. Squamous (epidermoid) carcinoma, adenocarcinoma, and large cell carcinoma, termed *non–small cell lung cancer* (NSCLC), comprise three-fourths of all cases; whereas most remaining patients have small cell (formerly called oat cell) lung cancer (SCLC). In contrast to patients with SCLC, those with NSCLC sometimes follow a more indolent clinical course, more often have no clinically detectable distant metastases at diagnosis, can more often undergo potentially curative surgical resection, and less frequently respond to radiotherapy or cytotoxic chemotherapy.

## CLINICAL PRESENTATION AND DIAGNOSIS

Presenting symptoms and signs of lung cancer are extremely varied and arise from a myriad of sources (Table 1). Although any of these findings can occur in any cell type of lung cancer, patients with small cell and adenocarcinoma more often present with distant metastases, squamous and small cell carcinomas more frequently produce symptoms caused by central endobronchial tumor or enlarged regional lymph nodes, and adenocarcinoma more commonly originates in peripheral lung fields and induces a pleural effusion. SCLC

TABLE 1. **Clinical Presentations of Lung Cancer**

**Symptoms and Signs of Primary Tumor**
Cough; hemoptysis; dyspnea, atelectasis, wheezing, or pneumonitis from endobronchial obstruction; pain from peribronchial nerve or chest wall involvement; dyspnea from pleural effusion; superior sulcus (Pancoast's) syndrome with brachial plexus invasion

**Symptoms and Signs of Regional Lymph Node and Soft Tissue Metastases**
Superior vena cava syndrome; hoarseness from recurrent laryngeal nerve paralysis; dysphagia from esophageal compression; diaphragmatic paralysis from phrenic nerve involvement; pericardial tamponade

**Symptoms and Signs of Distant Metastases**
Bone pain or fracture; neurologic dysfunction from brain metastases or spinal cord compression; abdominal pain or jaundice from liver metastases; peripheral lymph node enlargement; subcutaneous nodules

**Paraneoplastic Syndromes**
Hypercalcemia; hypertrophic pulmonary osteoarthropathy; migratory thrombophlebitis/Trousseau's syndrome; syndrome of inappropriate secretion of antidiuretic hormone; ectopic Cushing's syndrome; Eaton-Lambert (myasthenia-like) syndrome; sensory neuropathy, cerebellar or retinal degeneration, limbic encephalitis

**Distant Metastases from Carcinoma of Unknown Primary Site**

**Incidental Finding on Routine Chest X-Ray**

less often presents with chest wall involvement, as a superior sulcus (Pancoast's) tumor or a carcinoma of unknown primary site, or with hypercalcemia or pulmonary osteoarthropathy.

Once lung cancer is suspected, pathologic confirmation of the diagnosis is usually obtained from endobronchial tumors by sputum cytology or bronchoscopy, from peripheral or large mediastinal lesions by percutaneous needle aspirate or transbronchial biopsy, from less accessible enlarged mediastinal lymph nodes by mediastinoscopy or mediastinotomy, from malignant pleural effusions by thoracentesis or pleural biopsy, or from a metastatic site such as supraclavicular node or liver. Thoracotomy may occasionally be required for diagnosis.

## PRETREATMENT EVALUATION

Most lung cancer patients who are cured undergo surgical removal of the primary tumor. Therefore, the physician's initial evaluation should center on determining if thoracotomy with intent to perform a potentially curative surgical resection is possible. If not, the remaining critical question is whether SCLC or NSCLC is present, since cytotoxic chemotherapy administered with expectation of substantial survival prolongation will be given to all patients with SCLC. Review of diagnostic pathologic material by an experienced pathologist is mandatory because SCLC can sometimes be mistaken for poorly differentiated squamous or adenocarcinoma, and crushed material obtained by needle aspiration or small bronchoscopic biopsy can sometimes be confused with SCLC.

**Non–Small Cell Lung Cancer.** Staging, or determining the degree of tumor dissemination, is used to select the most appropriate therapy for NSCLC. Patients are first evaluated to assess whether they are operative candidates. Either unfavorable tumor extent or inability to tolerate thoracotomy or pulmonary resection for medical reasons can render a patient inoperable. Thoracotomy is performed in operable cases. At thoracotomy, if the tumor can be completely excised with pathologically negative margins, it is resected.

The staging process consists of a combination of clinical (physical examination and imaging studies) and limited operative (bronchoscopy, mediastinoscopy, mediastinotomy, thoracentesis, or pleural biopsy) procedures. Many surgeons omit pathologic evaluation of the mediastinum if thoracic CT scan does not reveal involvement or if a decision on resectability of enlarged mediastinal metastases can be made only at thoracotomy. Only staging tests that unequivocally establish that the tumor is inoperable should prevent thoracotomy. Imaging studies of distant metastatic sites are often omitted unless symptoms, physical findings, or abnormal blood test results suggest involvement.

The new international TNM (tumor, nodes, metastases) staging system for lung cancer is presented in Table 2. Stage I and II and some Stage IIIa lesions are potentially surgically resectable. Some Stage IIIb patients have clearly unresectable tumors that can potentially be encompassed within a radiation portal, whereas Stage IV patients with distant metastases are currently incurable. Approximately one-third of pa-

TABLE 2. **International TNM Staging System for Lung Cancer***

**Tumor (T)**

TX  Occult carcinoma (malignant cells in sputum or bronchial washings but tumor not visualized by imaging studies or bronchoscopy)

T1  Tumor 3 cm or less in greatest diameter, surrounded by lung or visceral pleura, but not proximal to a lobar bronchus on bronchoscopy

T2  Tumor $\geq$3 cm in diameter, or with involvement of main bronchus at least 2 cm distal to carina, or with visceral pleural invasion, or with associated atelectasis or obstructive pneumonitis extending to the hilar region but not involving the entire lung

T3  Tumor invading chest wall, diaphragm, mediastinal pleura, or parietal pericardium; or tumor in main bronchus within 2 cm of but not invading carina; or atelectasis or obstructive pneumonitis of entire lung

T4  Tumor invading mediastinum, heart, great vessels, trachea, esophagus, vertebral body, or carina; or ipsilateral malignant pleural effusion

**Nodes (N)**

N0  No regional lymph node metastases

N1  Metastases to ipsilateral peribronchial or hilar nodes

N2  Metastases to ipsilateral mediastinal or subcarinal nodes

N3  Metastases to contralateral mediastinal or hilar, or to any scalene or supraclavicular nodes

**Distant Metastases (M)**

M0  No distant metastases

M1  Distant metastases

**Stage Groupings**

| Occult | TX | N0 | M0 |
|---|---|---|---|
| Stage I | T1–2 | N0 | M0 |
| Stage II | T1–2 | N1 | M0 |
| Stabe IIIa | T3 | N0–1 | M0 |
| | T1–3 | N2 | M0 |
| Stage IIIb | T4 | N0–2 | M0 |
| | T1–4 | N3 | M0 |
| Stage IV | Any T | Any N | M1 |

*Modified from American Joint Committee on Cancer: Manual for Staging of Cancer, 3rd ed. Philadelphia, JB Lippincott, 1988, pp. 115–121.

tients with NSCLC have Stage I or II disease at diagnosis, one-third have Stage IIIa or IIIb, and the final third have Stage IV.

The most important prognostic factors are TNM stage and ambulatory or performance status. The predictive accuracy of TNM stage is greater if based upon pathologic evaluation of thoracotomy specimens rather than upon preoperative staging procedures alone.

**Small Cell Lung Cancer.** Because chemotherapy is always given, staging procedures do not identify SCLC patients who can be treated with surgery or irradiation alone. However, staging will detect tumor lesions that can be used to assess response, establish prognosis, and, when chest irradiation is given only to patients with apparently localized disease, aid in treatment selection. The common sites of distant metastases—liver, brain, and bone—should be evaluated with imaging studies and bone marrow examination if signs, symptoms, or blood tests are suspicious for involvement. Before chest irradiation is administered, absence of tumor in all these sites should be documented. Evaluation of ambulatory status and general medical condition is extremely important, since bedridden patients tolerate aggressive chemotherapy only with greatly increased morbidity.

The most commonly used staging system is divided into limited (confined to the hemithorax of origin and regional nodes and encompassable within a tolerable radiotherapy portal) and extensive (tumor beyond these bounds) stages. At diagnosis, approximately one-third of patients have limited and two-thirds, extensive disease. Stage and performance status are the major prognostic factors.

## THERAPY

### Non–Small Cell Lung Cancer

**Occult Lung Cancer.** Treatment of occult lung cancer requires tumor localization. Endoscopic examination of the upper aerodigestive tract is needed to exclude a primary cancer in the oral cavity, pharynx, or esophagus. Repetitive fiberoptic bronchoscopy will usually identify the primary tumor. Once lung cancer is diagnosed, treatment is dependent upon the stage of the tumor.

**Surgical Resection.** Surgical resection is the treatment of choice for NSCLC confined within the pleural reflection (Stages I and II). Preoperative assessment of the extent of lung resection that the patient can tolerate is important in choosing the appropriate surgical procedure. Lobectomy, pneumonectomy, segmentectomy or wedge resection, and sleeve resection of central tumors may each be indicated in specific situations. An optimal procedure removes the entire tumor with adequate margins and allows the greatest possible conservation of normal lung tissue. Operative mortality with modern surgical techniques is 3% for lobectomy and 5 to 8% for pneumonectomy; it increases with age.

Certain patients with Stage IIIa cancer may benefit from complete resection of their tumor. Such patients have low-volume ipsilateral or subcarinal mediastinal node metastases with less advanced primary tumors or locally extensive primary tumors with minimal or no lymph node involvement. In these selected cases, 5-year survival as high as 25 to 30% has been reported. Low-dose preoperative irradiation is often given to superior sulcus tumors to facilitate potentially curative surgical resection.

**Chest Irradiation.** Chest irradiation is given with curative intent to three groups of NSCLC patients, including those with unresectable locoregionally advanced tumor (Stages IIIa and selected IIIb), patients with clinically staged Stage I or II cancer who are inoperable for medical reasons, and as a postoperative adjuvant in patients who have undergone potentially curative surgical resection.

Radiotherapy induces objective tumor regression at least half the time. Five-year survival of 4 to 8% is consistently reported among patients completing radiotherapy administered with curative intent. Such treatment is not initiated in patients with poor performance status, bulky tumors and poor pulmonary function, or pleural effusion, and is not completed when distant metastases, progressive intrathoracic tumor, or clinical deterioration develops. A dose of 55 to 60 Gy (5500 to 6000 rad) is administered with daily fractionation using megavoltage equipment. Careful treatment planning to define a target volume with the minimum feasible dose to adjacent critical structures (normal lung, heart, spinal cord) is required. Better outcome occurs in patients who are fully ambulatory with lesser tumor volume or who have superior sulcus tumors. In the 40 to 60 Gy range, increasing tumor dose is associated with a higher objective response rate and decreased frequency of local tumor recurrence, but not with better survival, presumably because of frequent occult distant metastases.

Medically inoperable patients with Stage I or II cancer and sufficient pulmonary reserve are given chest irradiation with curative intent. Five-year survival of 15 to 20% is reported.

The role of postoperative irradiation in patients who have received potentially curative surgical resection is controversial. The frequency of tumor recurrence in the ipsilateral lung and mediastinum is reduced with properly administered radiotherapy. However, the only randomized study in carefully staged Stage II and IIIa patients failed to demonstrate improved survival.

The major acute toxicity of chest irradiation in lung cancer is esophagitis. A common delayed side effect is radiation fibrosis on chest radiograph, but this is usually asymptomatic. Radiation pneumonitis, which is occasionally fatal, occurs more often with increasing doses of irradiation and volume of irradiated lung. Consequences are worse in patients with impaired pulmonary function.

**Chemotherapy.** Cytotoxic chemotherapy does not have an established role in patients with NSCLC. Single-agent chemotherapy is associated with objective response rates of 15 to 20% at best. Some recent combination regimens, most of which contain cisplatin (Platinol) and a vinca alkaloid or etoposide (VePesid), produce objective response rates of 20 to 40% in fully ambulatory patients. Patients who are less than fully ambulatory, however, have inferior response rates and survival and more frequently experience toxicity. Median survival in most large studies of cisplatin-based drug combinations in fully ambulatory patients who are incurable by surgery or irradia-

tion is 5 to 9 months, not strikingly different from data reported in similar patients with distant metastases receiving supportive care alone. Whether currently utilized chemotherapy programs improve survival in patients with distant metastatic disease remains unsettled. Results of the few randomized studies with contemporary regimens are conflicting.

Cisplatin-based chemotherapy programs have only recently been studied in the adjuvant setting. Two randomized studies in patients with completely or marginally resected Stage II and IIIa NSCLC have demonstrated improved disease-free survival with combination chemotherapy compared with immunotherapy and no treatment, respectively, but survival was only marginally prolonged. Survival benefit has been shown for another combination program when added to potentially curative chest irradiation in a single randomized trial in fully ambulatory patients.

Further clinical investigation to clarify the role of chemotherapy is needed. At present, no chemotherapy program is sufficiently effective to be considered standard treatment for any stage of NSCLC. Outside a clinical trial setting, a patient with distant metastatic disease or one who is not a candidate for potentially curative surgery or irradiation may be offered a published combination chemotherapy regimen provided that the patient (1) is fully ambulatory; (2) has evaluable tumor lesions, so that therapy can be stopped if tumor regression does not occur; and (3) understands the limitations of current treatment but still desires it.

**End Results.** Anticipated median and 5-year survival (which is tantamount to cure of the original tumor in most cases) rates by stage with current therapy are summarized in Table 3.

## Small Cell Lung Cancer

**Chemotherapy.** After cyclophosphamide (Cytoxan), was demonstrated in 1969 to double median survival in extensive stage patients, chemotherapy became the cornerstone of management for

TABLE 3. **Estimated Survival by Stage with Current Optimal Therapy in Non–Small Cell Lung Cancer***

| Clinical Stage | Median Survival (months) | 5-Year Survival (%) |
|---|---|---|
| I | 48 | 45 |
| II | 20 | 25 |
| IIIa | 12 | 15 |
| IIIb | 8 | <5 |
| IV | 4 | <1 |

*Modified from Mountain CF: A new international staging system for lung cancer. Chest 89(Suppl): 225S–233S, 1986.

SCLC. The high objective response rates and substantially prolonged survival achieved with present chemotherapy programs, with or without chest irradiation, represent a striking contrast to the at best quite modest benefits of chemotherapy in NSCLC.

Many single chemotherapeutic agents produce objective response rates of 30 to 50% or more in previously untreated patients, and combination chemotherapy is even more effective. Complete response rates of 40 to 60% and 80 to 95% complete plus partial responses are routinely observed in limited stage tumors. Equivalent figures in extensive disease are 15 to 30% and 65 to 85%, respectively. Unfortunately, the majority of even complete responders will suffer relapse, although SCLC can now be permanently eradicated in about 5% of all patients.

Drugs with well-documented activity include cyclophosphamide, etoposide (VP–16), doxorubicin (Adriamycin), vincristine, methotrexate (Mexate), lomustine (CCNU), cisplatin, and carboplatin (Paraplatin). Multiple published combination regimens containing two to four drugs yield approximately equivalent results. Moderately intensive drug doses that induce leukopenia of 1000 to 2500 cells per $\mu$l are optimal, maximum response to treatment virtually always occurs by 12 to 18 weeks, and continuation of chemotherapy beyond that point is of little or no benefit. Although administering two combination regimens in an alternating fashion is a common practice, survival is not consistently improved by this strategy in randomized clinical trials.

The most common acute toxicities produced by virtually all chemotherapy programs utilized in SCLC are neutropenia-associated fever and infection and thrombocytopenic bleeding. Nausea, vomiting, and alopecia are also frequent. Side effects of specific drugs, such as congestive heart failure with doxorubicin and peripheral neuropathy with cisplatin and vincristine, are also observed. Treatment-related mortality rates of 1 to 4% in limited and 3 to 7% in extensive disease can be anticipated; patients with poor ambulatory status are more vulnerable. Completely bedridden patients, because of their greatly increased risk of treatment-related morbidity and mortality, should be given less aggressive therapy, possibly with a single drug.

**Chest Irradiation.** SCLC is highly responsive to thoracic radiotherapy, with objective regression rates of approximately 90%. Most authorities agree that adding chest radiotherapy to chemotherapy does not affect survival in extensive disease. In limited stage patients, however, randomized trials comparing chemotherapy and chest irradiation with chemotherapy alone have repeatedly documented reduced failure rates at the primary tumor site, at the expense of greater pulmonary, hematologic, and esophageal toxicities. Mature results of several of these trials demonstrate modest but significant survival advantage for combining the two forms of treatment, particularly for programs designed in a fashion in which chemotherapy doses are not delayed for the delivery of irradiation. Increased survival with combined modality treatment is most evident beyond 1 to 2 years. However, 2-year survival with added chest radiotherapy in the most promising of these randomized trials is only 20 to 30%, emphasizing that the major factor needed to improve survival for most patients is better systemic therapy.

**Surgical Resection.** Although surgical resection of SCLC was generally abandoned in the 1970s, the fact that the rare patients with pathologically staged Stage I and II tumors experience actuarial 5-year survival of at least 20 to 40% following surgical resection has recently been recognized. Whether this better survival is due to the surgical procedure or to the less aggressive biology of resectable tumors is not certain. If a patient without a preoperative pathologic diagnosis has resectable SCLC at thoracotomy, the tumor should be resected. In patients with a known

TABLE 4. **Survival Benefits of Chemotherapy in Small Cell Lung Cancer***

| Therapy | Median Survival (mo) | | 2-Year Survival (%)† | |
|---|---|---|---|---|
| | *Limited Stage* | *Extensive Stage* | *Limited Stage* | *Extensive Stage* |
| None | 3 | 1.5 | 0 | 0 |
| Surgical resection | 5‡ | — | 4‡ | — |
| Chest irradiation | 8‡ | — | 10‡ | — |
| | 4–8§ | — | 4–7§ | — |
| Cyclophosphamide | 6 | 3 | 0 | 0 |
| Combination chemotherapy ± chest irradiation | 12–16 | 7–11 | 10–25 | 0–4 |

*From Ihde DC: Chemotherapy of lung cancer. *In* Brain MC, and Carbone PP (eds): Current Therapy in Hematology/Oncology—3. Toronto, BC Decker, 1988, pp. 213–217.

†Disease-free survival.

‡Operable patients only.

§All limited stage patients.

diagnosis of SCLC, thoracotomy should be performed only after complete staging including negative mediastinoscopy. In either case, postoperative combination chemotherapy is required.

**Prophylactic Cranial Irradiation.** The brain is a frequent site of relapse after chemotherapy for SCLC. Randomized trials of elective or "prophylactic" cranial irradiation have documented reduced occurrence of brain metastases without evidence of increased survival. Its value would be accepted without question except for the occasional profound and frequent subtle neuropsychologic impairment of long-term survivors who received prophylactic brain radiotherapy. If prophylactic cranial irradiation is utilized, it should be given in low doses per fraction, preferably only to patients completely responding to therapy.

**End Results.** The major impact of chemotherapy on survival, compared with survival in the prechemotherapy era with supportive care alone, surgical resection, or chest irradiation, is illustrated in Table 4. Current treatment produces a four-to-fivefold increase in median survival in both limited and extensive disease. Only a minority of patients, however, mostly those with limited disease, live more than 2 years, although approximately two-thirds of 2-year disease-free survivors will not develop recurrent SCLC. An increased death rate from second smoking-related neoplasms and other diseases is still present.

### Palliative Therapy

The majority of lung cancer patients except those with surgically resected Stage I NSCLC either develop recurrence after initially successful treatment or never have their tumors controlled at all. Thus, palliation of symptoms will at some point be the physician's major goal in over 85% of patients.

Chemotherapy of the previously untreated SCLC patient temporarily palliates most cancer-related symptoms except those from brain or spinal epidural metastases. Superior vena cava syndrome is usually successfully managed with chemotherapy alone. In contrast, palliation is infrequently achieved with chemotherapy in patients with progressive tumor.

Radiotherapy plays the major palliative role in relapsing SCLC and in most symptomatic surgically unresectable NSCLC patients. Chest irradiation in lower than curative doses provides palliation for many symptoms due to locoregional lung cancer, especially pain; superior vena cava obstruction; and dyspnea, hemoptysis, and pneumonitis due to bronchial obstruction. Atelectasis and vocal cord paralysis are less often improved. Irradiation also frequently relieves pain or neurologic symptoms from bone, brain, or spinal epidural metastases.

Malignant pleural effusions are often difficult to treat, but long-term control can sometimes be obtained with early tube thoracostomy and instillation of sclerosing agents. Endoscopic laser or photodynamic therapy sometimes palliates symptoms of endobronchial tumor obstruction in previously irradiated patients.

# COCCIDIOIDOMYCOSIS

method of
ROYCE H. JOHNSON, M.D.
*Kern Medical Center*
*Bakersfield, California*

Coccidioidomycosis was originally described in 1892 and is caused by *Coccidioides immitis*, a dimorphic fungus. It exists in the soil in the mycelial phase. As mycelia mature they produce arthroconidia, which easily fracture off and become airborne. These may infect a new soil site, and, if inhaled by a susceptible host, produce primary pulmonary infection. In tissue the arthroconidia transform to spherules that reproduce by endosporulation. The fungus may be recovered on simple bacteriologic or mycologic media and will grow in the mycelial phase. (It is very dangerous to work with these cultures unless special precautions are taken.)

This fungus has a specific geographic distribution in South, Central, and North America. Most cases seen in the United States are related to exposure in the southwest. Occasionally fomite acquisition occurs. There is no interhuman or animal transmission of disease.

The predominant pathologic finding is granulomatous inflammation. Spherules with endosporulation are diagnostic, although not always easily found.

Of those infected, 60% have no or trivial symptoms. The remainder develop pulmonary or systemic symptoms within 1 to 3 weeks of exposure. Cough, productive or nonproductive, or chest pain may predominate. Alternatively, fever with night sweats and a flulike syndrome may be more significant than the respiratory symptoms. Erythema nodosum or, less commonly, erythema multiforme may be presenting complaints. In mild disease the chest radiograph shows little or no change. In more severe involvement, focal infiltrates, often with significant perihilar and even paratracheal adenopathy, are demonstrated. Diminishing acute infiltration with persistent or increasing hilar adenopathy defines progressive primary coccidioidomycosis. The disease may also present as an exudative pleural effusion with or without infiltrate.

Chronic pulmonary involvement also occurs. The most benign form is fibrosis. Pulmonary nodules may occur. These are important because of the confusion with carcinoma. Pulmonary cavities are frequently seen and these may be asymptomatic, although they

TABLE 1. **Systemic Chemotherapy of Coccidioidomycosis**

| Drug | Indications | Dosage | | | |
|------|-------------|--------|--|--|--|
| | | *Route* | *Initial* | *Optimal* | **Total** |
| Amphotericin B (Fungizone) | Severe or potentially severe disease | IV | 1–5 mg | 1 mg/kg, not >50 mg | 1–3 gm, occasionally more |
| Ketoconazole (Nizoral) | Mild to moderate stable disease | PO | 400 mg | 400 mg | 3 months to years |

often cause significant hemoptysis and occasionally become superinfected or rupture and produce pneumothorax.

Less than 1% of all cases of coccidioidomycosis will disseminate. Extrapulmonary foci include almost any body site. Infections of skin, bones, joints, and soft tissue predominate.

Meningitis is the most serious manifestation of coccidioidomycosis. Untreated, death is uniform, usually within 1 year. Presentation and cerebrospinal fluid analysis are compatible with a chronic meningitis. Headache is the most common presenting symptom. Alteration in consciousness, psychologic disturbance, fever, stiff neck, and focal neurologic deficits are also common. Cerebrospinal fluid analysis reveals a predominant monocytic pleocytosis (occasionally, neutrophils predominate in very early disease). Significant eosinophilia is also occasionally seen. Hypoglycorrhachia and an increased protein level complete the typical analysis. The cerebrospinal fluid coccidioidal antibody titer is usually positive. The serum IgG and IgM antibody analysis is positive in disseminated disease, except in severely immunocompromised patients.

## THERAPY

Treatment of coccidioidomycosis is currently less than optimal. What is needed is an antifungal drug that penetrates all body compartments, is available for oral and parenteral administration, and is nontoxic. Unfortunately we have only amphotericin B (Fungizone) and the imidazoles, currently ketoconazole (Nizoral), available for clinical use (see Table 1).

It is clear that many cases of primary coccidioidomycosis, even primary cutaneous disease and disseminated disease of limited extent, may recover spontaneously. The indications for therapy in pulmonary disease are twofold. The actual extent and severity of the pulmonary infection itself is the first indication. An extensive pneumonia with prostration or duration of pneumonic symptoms for greater than 6 weeks is a general indication for therapy. Second, the risk of extrapulmonary dissemination is an additional indication for therapy of pulmonary disease. The risk factors for metapulmonary dissemination are indicated in Table 2. Disseminated coccidioidomycosis virtually mandates systemic chemotherapy.

While no trials of imidazole therapy for primary pulmonary disease have been done, many clinicians use ketoconazole for primary disease of moderate extent or in individuals with significant risk of dissemination. Amphotericin B is reserved for more severe clinical presentation and individuals considered to be at high risk for dissemination or those in whom imidazole therapy has failed.

Even in disseminated disease, an indolent skin lesion or an isolated joint might be managed by initial ketoconazole therapy. More extensive and severe disease should be treated with amphotericin B. Treatment failure by either drug often suggests a trial of the other.

Persistence of a pulmonary cavity over an extended period (6 to 24 months), large size, or the presence of hemoptysis calls for surgical therapy with or without concomitant medical therapy.

Amphotericin B given by local injections or irrigation, particularly in a joint space or at surgical sites of osteomyelitis, may prove beneficial either as primary therapy or as an adjunct to systemic and surgical therapy. Intra-articular injections of amphotericin B prepared in sterile water of appropriate volume can be injected. The dose is escalated from 5 to 15 mg, depending on patient tolerance, and continued three times a week for 2 to 4 weeks. Subsequently the frequency of injections is gradually decreased and total treatment continued for approximately 6 months.

Surgical removal of involucrum and sequestrum is important in the treatment of osteomyelitis. Adjunctive in-and-out irrigation tubes may be placed at surgery and the site irrigated continuously with 50 to 100 mg of amphotericin in 1 liter of sterile water every 24 hours. This can be continued for 7 to 14 days, tube patency permitting.

Coccidioidal meningitis is the most difficult

TABLE 2. **Risk Factors for Dissemination of Coccidioidomycosis**

| | |
|--|--|
| Age | Very young or very old |
| Sex | Male > female |
| Race | Noncaucasian |
| Skin Test | Negative > positive |
| Serum Complement Fixation Titer | >1:64 = increased risk |
| Pregnancy | Increased risk third trimester and post partum |

therapeutic problem. Intrathecal administration of amphotericin B is the treatment of choice. The drug can be administered by lumbar or cisternal puncture and ventricular or cisternal Ommaya reservoirs. Each route of administration has advantages and disadvantages. Usually therapy is initiated with alternating lumbar and cisternal punctures at doses of 0.1 mg of amphotericin B 4 ml D5W. Glucocorticoids, such as methylprednisolone (Solu-Medrol), in doses of 5 to 10 mg is often administered as a preinjection or concomitantly with the amphotericin B. The subsequent amphotericin dose is increased by 0.1 mg after each cycle of lumbar and cisternal injections, as tolerated by the patient. Complications of therapy and individual patient problems may necessitate the use of cisternal or ventricular Ommaya reservoirs as either primary or secondary therapy.

In the treatment of coccidioidomycosis, ketoconazole is usually given in doses of 400 mg (two 200 mg tablets). Higher doses have been used, especially in attempts to treat central nervous system infections where doses of 800 to 2000 mg* have been used. Efficacy is not yet proved, but such doses may be of benefit in individual cases. The whole daily dose is taken at one time in order to decrease the suppressive effects of the drug on steroidogenesis, particularly androgenic steroids. The drug is best absorbed in an acid milieu, and antacid therapy or $H_2$ blockers prevent absorption. An acidic drink may promote absorption. Gastrointestinal intolerance, gynecomastia, and drug-induced hepatitis (rarely fatal) are the major side effects.

Amphotericin is initiated with a test dose and slowly escalated. This is done because of rare problems with hypotension, hypertension, and possible cardiac toxicity. An initial test dose of 1 mg has often been used; however, it has been our practice to initiate 5-mg doses and increase the dose at 8- to 12-hour intervals in 10-mg increments until a dose of 1 mg per kg, or 50 mg, is reached, whichever is least. The drug is then administered at that level on a daily basis until clinical stability is attained. Subsequently ambulatory therapy three times a week may be undertaken until the total course of therapy is completed. Home amphotericin therapy has been administered in selective cases.

For relatively mild diseases, such as a skin lesion, a total dose of 1 gram of amphotericin B may suffice. For more severe lesions of soft tissue 2 grams may be needed. Three grams is most often used for significant osteomyelitis and other severe disseminated disease. Repeated courses of up to 9 grams total are rarely needed.

The immediate signs of amphotericin B toxicity are fever, chills, nausea, vomiting, and headache. Acetaminophen (Tylenol) 650 mg and diphenhydramine (Benadryl) 50 mg are routinely used as premedication. Prochlorperazine (Compazine) 10 mg or metoclopramide (Reglan) 50 mg is added as needed for gastrointestinal symptoms. Severe chills are specifically treated by parenteral meperidine (Demerol) in small doses of 25 to 50 mg administered as premedication or during acute episodes.

The major problem with amphotericin therapy is nephrotoxicity. Creatinine monitoring is crucial. A creatinine level greater than three would indicate a need to discontinue the drug until the level has decreased to below three. Monitoring the blood urea nitrogen is not helpful. The other major toxicity of the drug is bone marrow suppression, particularly anemia. Evaluation of electrolytes, particularly $K^+$ and $Mg^{++}$, and correction of abnormalities are necessary.

Both fluconazole and intraconazole are experimental imidazoles currently under trial that may soon be available for use and may augment or supplant ketoconazole and perhaps some of the indications for amphotericin B. It is hoped that newer antifungal agents will become available to make the treatment of coccidioidomycosis less arduous and more efficacious.

# HISTOPLASMOSIS

method of
SCOTT F. DAVIES, M.D.
*Hennepin County Medical Center*
*Minneapolis, Minnesota*

and

GEORGE A. SAROSI, M.D.
*Maricopa Medical Center*
*Phoenix, Arizona*

Histoplasmosis, the disease caused by the thermal dimorphic fungus *Histoplasma capsulatum*, is endemic throughout the world but is most common by far in the central and south central United States. The organism grows as a mold (with hyphae) in nature. Soil enriched by bird or bat droppings or by decaying vegetation best supports growth of the fungus. Disturbance of contaminated soil creates an infective aerosol. An alveolitis develops when the spores are inhaled. Once in the lung, the organism converts to the yeast phase of growth, multiplying by binary fission. The primary host defense is the monocyte-macrophage system. Any illness that interferes with this system predisposes to dissemination of the yeast from the lung and decreases tissue response in the lung and at distant sites.

Several classification schema exist. For purposes of this discussion, a simplified system will be used, divid-

---

*Exceeds dosage recommended by the manufacturer.

ing the illness into acute pulmonary histoplasmosis, chronic cavitary pulmonary histoplasmosis, and progressive disseminated histoplasmosis.

## TREATMENT

### Acute Pulmonary Histoplasmosis

After inhaling the spores, the vast majority of infected individuals clear the infection without much problem. Treatment is not required since recovery is the rule. Occasionally, especially with heavy exposure in a closed space, an overwhelming primary infection may occur with severe diffuse infiltration of both lungs. These patients are severely ill; unless diagnosed and treated rapidly they may die from progressive respiratory failure. This form of acute pulmonary histoplasmosis must be treated quickly with amphotericin B (AMB). The exact dose required for cure is unclear. We believe a total dose of 500 to 1000 mg, depending on patient response, is usually adequate. Forty to 50 mg per day are given for 10 to 20 days until the patient is well. Extending treatment to a total dose of 2 to 2½ grams (as used for other severe forms of histoplasmosis) is seldom needed. Ketoconazole (Nizoral) an orally administered imidazole, is not recommended for the treatment of severe acute pulmonary histoplasmosis. It is less potent than AMB, and the response to therapy is slower—not what is needed when gas exchange is severely impaired and life is threatened.

### Chronic Cavitary Pulmonary Histoplasmosis

This form of histoplasmosis occurs almost exclusively in middle-aged or older cigarette smokers. The lungs of such patients may have abnormal air spaces from centrilobular emphysema, most common in the upper lobes. Spores inhaled into these spaces are harder to clear. The majority of infected patients still recover spontaneously, but do so slower than normal, with symptoms lasting many weeks or a few months. Occasionally a progressive disease develops which slowly advances and destroys adjacent lung tissue. The radiographic appearance is similar to reinfection tuberculosis with fibrosis and cavitation. Patients have low-grade fever, night sweats, cough, anorexia, and weight-loss, also similar to symptoms of tuberculosis. The disease is slowly progressive and rarely disseminates. If untreated, chronic respiratory failure may develop from the combination of the underlying disease and new lung destruction by histoplasmosis.

Since many patients with chronic cavitary pulmonary histoplasmosis recover spontaneously, we observe most patients for 6 weeks. If there is no improvement in symptoms or chest roentgenogram, or if the patient is worse, treatment is started. Ketoconazole, 400 mg once daily, is the initial therapy. The patient is seen monthly for clinical evaluation and a chest roentgenogram. If there is no improvement, the daily dosage may be increased monthly in 200-mg increments up to 800 mg. Higher doses increase toxicity without improving chances of recovery. In practice most patients respond well to the 400-mg dose, and higher doses are rarely used. Therapy is continued for 6 to 12 months.

Occasionally a patient will fail to respond to ketoconazole, even at the higher doses, or, after initial improvement, will relapse when therapy is stopped. These patients should be treated with AMB to a total dose of 35 mg per kg. After an initial 10-mg dose (see below), a daily dose of 40 to 50 mg, depending on body weight, is given for the first 5 days (or longer if necessary). If the patient is stable, the final dose is continued three times weekly until the desired total dose is reached, usually 12 to 18 weeks.

For chronic cavitary pulmonary histoplasmosis, amphotericin B is usually reserved for ketoconazole treatment failures. However, patients with disease that is life-threatening at onset or rapidly progressive during the initial observation period should be treated with amphotericin B from the start, because of greater potency and faster response.

### Progressive Disseminated Histoplasmosis

During usual episodes of primary pulmonary histoplasmosis, the yeast spreads to the draining lymph nodes and then through the blood to the entire body. The yeast spores are removed from the circulation by the cells of the reticuloendothelial system. With onset of effective delayed hypersensitivity, granulomas develop in draining lymph nodes and in the liver, spleen, and bone marrow, checking the infection. Old calcified granulomas in the lung, hilar and mediastinal nodes, and in the liver and spleen are radiographic markers of remote histoplasmosis with uneventful healing.

In some patients delayed hypersensitivity is not adequate owing to age, current illness, or current therapy. Infants and the very old may have poor cell-mediated immunity, and progressive dissemination of histoplasmosis may occur. Hodgkin's disease is an example of an illness with deficient cell-mediated immunity, even without therapy. More commonly, therapy with glucocorticoids and with cytotoxic agents used for a variety of malignant and nonmalignant conditions is the major insult to this arm of the immune system. With advanced disease, malnutrition and debility further depress host resistance. When the immune response is deficient, a primary pulmonary infection may spread unchecked. The result is progressive disseminated histoplasmosis, which is highly lethal and requires immediate therapy. Another mechanism for progressive disseminated histoplasmosis is reactivation of old, inactive infection in immunosuppressed patients.

The epidemic of acquired immune deficiency syndrome (AIDS) has brought a new level of T cell immunosuppression, more profound than that seen before and affecting a large number of patients. As the T-helper count decreases, cases of progressive disseminated histoplasmosis increase. Histoplasmosis can be the first opportunistic infection in patients with the human immunodeficiency virus (HIV), and thus the AIDS defining illness. T cell immunosuppression insufficient to predispose to *Pneumocystis carinii* pneumonia can still predispose to progressive disseminated histoplasmosis (very similar to tuberculosis). In highly endemic areas, 5% or more of HIV-infected patients develop progressive disseminated histoplasmosis. Many of these cases represent rapid progression of a primary infection, acquired while immunosuppressed. However, cases are also being seen in San Francisco and New York City, which are nonendemic areas for histoplasmosis. Many of these patients have remote but not recent exposure to highly endemic areas, providing indirect evidence for reactivation of dormant disease as the mechanism of infection.

The treatment for progressive disseminated histoplasmosis is AMB. The dose is rapidly increased to 50 mg. It is given daily until the disease stabilizes and then three times weekly to the desired total dose. When the patient is stable enough for three times weekly dosing, outpatient therapy is usually possible. With lesser degrees of immunosuppression, a total of 40 mg per kg is usually curative. Treatment is successful in patients with solid organ transplants and patients receiving glucocorticoid therapy for collagen diseases and other nonmalignant disorders. Prior to AIDS, Hodgkin's disease was the one setting in which cure was difficult and relapses common. With AIDS it is doubtful any patient can be cured, and new strategies for continuous suppression have had to be developed.

Amphotericin B is the treatment of choice for progressive disseminated histoplasmosis complicating HIV infection. We treat such patients three times weekly (each dose 40 to 50 mg) for the first 2 grams. Then we continue treatment with 50 mg each week, continued indefinitely to prevent relapse.

Although ketoconazole has been used with some success in patients with progressive disseminated histoplasmosis, it must be tried only in patients with mild illness without a recognizable immune defect. It has not been useful in patients with AIDS, either for primary treatment or for preventing relapses.

### Amphotericin B

Introduced in 1957, this agent has been the mainstay of therapy for histoplasmosis and other fungal infections. It is highly effective, and newer therapies must be compared with amphotericin B as the current "gold standard." The downside of AMB is substantial toxicity and the need for intravenous therapy. Dose-related renal toxicity is most common. During therapy the serum creatinine should be checked weekly. On a three times weekly schedule, renal toxicity is less, which is the reason we switch to this dosing regimen once the patient is stable and nontoxic. We still follow the creatinine closely and reduce the dose of AMB if serum creatinine increases beyond 2.5 mg per dl. AMB also causes substantial renal tubular injury with much potassium wasting. Serum potassium should be monitored weekly, and sufficient oral potassium supplementation must be given to prevent severe hypokalemia.

Amphotericin B is reconstituted with 5% dextrose in water. We mix each dose in 250 ml and give it over 2 hours, rather than a more customary longer infusion time. Shorter infusion makes outpatient administration easier and, though not proven, seems to reduce infusion reactions which include chills, fever, nausea, vomiting, and headache. We premedicate our patients with 650 mg of aspirin and 50 mg of diphenhydramine (Benadryl) 30 minutes before the infusion. However, narcotics are most effective for blocking infusion reactions. If aspirin and diphenhydramine do not work, we use 25 to 50 mg of intravenous meperidine (Demerol) before the infusion. Oral codeine (30 to 60 mg) may suffice for some patients. As the treatment course progresses, the reactions may become less severe and the narcotic no longer necessary.

Rarely, hypotension due to peripheral vascular collapse has been reported, often with the initial dose of amphotericin B. For this reason some authorities recommend an initial test dose of 1 mg. However, severe hypotension may occur even with the test dose, perhaps as often. Therefore, we begin with a 10-mg dose. If tolerated, the additional 30 to 40 mg designated for that day can be given immediately afterwards. There is no evidence that gradual stepping up of the dose reduces the severity of infusion reactions. If there is a problem with the first 10-mg dose, then intravenous narcotics are used before the subsequent doses. As soon as is practical (guided by the clinical situation), we switch to three times weekly dosing and continue as an outpatient.

### Ketoconazole (Nizoral)

This oral agent is preferred therapy for immunocompetent patients with non–life-threatening forms of histoplasmosis. It is well tolerated, especially in doses of 400 mg per day. Above this dose nausea and vomiting are more common. The drug is fungistatic rather than fungicidal, and long periods of treatment (at least 6 months) are necessary. It requires gastric acidity for absorption. Thus, $H_2$ blockers and antacids should not be used simultaneously, even if the patient has gastrointestinal side effects.

Ketoconazole suppresses testosterone production. Gynecomastia and impotence are problems in males, especially at high doses. Adrenal hypofunction, also due to blocking of steroid synthesis, occurs rarely. Hepatotoxicity is an important, though uncommon, problem. Hepatic failure may occur in very severe cases.

### Itraconazole

This is a new triazole compound not released yet for clinical use. Investigational use in small numbers of patients with histoplasmosis suggests that it is as effective as, and perhaps more effective than, ketoconazole. It has fewer side effects than ketoconazole. No definite statement can be made about usefulness in histoplasmosis at this time. It is unlikely to be as effective as amphotericin B for severe infections. It may be useful in treating milder illness. It probably will be tried in direct comparison with weekly amphotericin B for long-term suppression of histoplasmosis in AIDS.

# BLASTOMYCOSIS

method of
BRUCE KLEIN, M.D.
*University of Wisconsin*
*Madison, Wisconsin*

Blastomycosis, one of the important endemic systemic mycoses of North America, derives from infection with the thermal dimorphic fungus *Blastomyces dermatitidis*. The organism is believed to be a soil saprophyte which dwells primarily in the southeastern, south central, and upper midwestern regions of the United States. Primary infection in humans follows inhalation of conidia (asexual spores) into the lungs. At body temperature, the conidia convert to yeast forms which can be distinguished from other yeasts by their size, refractile cell wall, and broad-based buds. The acute primary pulmonary infection may be asymptomatic or may produce an influenza or atypical pneumonia syndrome. Although acute blastomycotic pneumonia may resolve spontaneously, progressive forms of disease involving the lungs, the extrapulmonary organs (usually the skin, bones, joints, or prostate gland), or both develop in some patients. Reactivation of a latent focal infection probably occurs less often than progression of primary infection. Primary cutaneous infection occurs infrequently through direct inoculation from a needle puncture, dog bite, or scalpel wound. Opportunistic infection among immunocompromised patients is uncommon. Although the majority of patients in case series of blastomycosis are 20 to 50 years of age, up to 10% are under 20.

The diagnosis of blastomycosis is confirmed by culture of the organism from body fluids such as sputum, pus, or urine, or from biopsied tissue. Cytologic and histopathologic studies with special stains should always be performed on fluid and tissue specimens; the characteristic morphology of the yeast form of *B. dermatitidis* usually allows a presumptive diagnosis well before the results from culture are available.

### TREATMENT

Before chemotherapy for blastomycosis was available, patients often had a progressive downhill course, and the mortality rate approached 80%. With the advent of effective antifungal therapy in the 1950s, the mortality rate declined to 10%, and it became accepted that all patients should be treated. This approach came under question after the description of self-limited pulmonary blastomycosis in 1974. To date, at least 76 patients with spontaneously resolving disease have been described. While some experts now advocate that selected patients do not require antifungal therapy, others disagree, countering that such patients are at risk to exacerbate and develop miliary disease or endobronchial spread, both associated with high mortality, or to develop reactivation of a latent focal infection at a later date. I believe that the majority of patients with blastomycosis require specific antifungal therapy. The decision whether or not to treat and, if so, with which drug should be based on the acuity, severity, and extent of disease upon presentation (Table 1).

Asymptomatic patients, patients who are already improving when the diagnosis is established, and those who present acutely (generally within 3 to 4 weeks of illness onset) with mild symptoms unassociated with respiratory distress

TABLE 1. **Management of Blastomycosis**

| Disease Form | Severity | Treatment |
| --- | --- | --- |
| Acute pulmonary | Asymptomatic, resolving, or mild | Observe |
| | Mild to moderately severe | Ketoconazole |
| | Life-threatening | Amphotericin B |
| Subacute or chronic pulmonary or extrapulmonary | Mild to moderately severe | Ketoconazole |
| | Life-threatening | Amphotericin B |
| Central nervous system (usually meningeal) | — | Amphotericin B |

or hypoxemia could be observed carefully and antifungal therapy withheld. To date, such patients have been identified mainly during epidemics of blastomycosis. These patients, however, represent the minority of blastomycosis patients because epidemic disease is far less common than sporadically occurring disease. Observation should include biweekly clinical and roentgenographic evaluation until spontaneous resolution takes place. Progression of pulmonary infection or evidence of extrapulmonary spread should signal the need for treatment.

In the more common subacute or chronically progressive forms of pulmonary blastomycosis and the nonmeningeal extrapulmonary forms which are mild to moderately severe, ketoconazole therapy is indicated. When pulmonary or extrapulmonary involvement is extensive, particularly if respiratory embarrassment or meningeal spread is documented, amphotericin B is the drug of choice. Serial chest roentgenograms, sputum cultures, or other studies according to infected sites should be performed to assess the therapeutic response. Clinical improvement generally occurs by the second week of therapy, but complete healing may not occur until after 2 or more months of therapy.

Accidental lacerations, bite wounds, or needle punctures with *B. dermatitidis* should be treated by careful, vigorous cleansing with tincture of iodine, an iodophor, or chlorhexidine. Systemic antifungal therapy is not indicated for primary cutaneous blastomycosis in the normal host. The lesion should be observed carefully to document resolution.

### Amphotericin B

Amphotericin B, a polyene macrolide antibiotic, is produced by *Streptomyces nodosus*. Polyene refers to the conjugated double bonds that comprise a portion of the closed macrocyclic ring of carbon atoms in the structure of the drug. The lipophilic polyene structure is probably the major site responsible for the mechanism of action of amphotericin B. Combination of the polyene with cytoplasmic membrane sterols, particularly er-

gosterol, in fungi leads the membrane to become porous.

Amphotericin B is considered the "gold standard" of antifungal therapy. Since its introduction in 1956, the drug has remained the most effective antifungal agent available for treatment of blastomycosis. Rates of clinical responses to this drug have ranged from 66 to 93% and have been greatest in adults who have received a total of at least 1.5 to 2 grams, or 25 to 35 mg per kg of body weight.

Amphotericin B may be administered in a variety of schedules. If a 1-mg test dose infused intravenously over 30 to 60 minutes is tolerated, an initial therapeutic dose of 0.25 mg per kg is administered over a 2- to 4-hour period on the first day. The dose should be increased in increments of 0.25 mg per kg each day to the desired maintenance dose. In acutely ill patients, 0.3 to 0.6 mg per kg (maximum, 50 mg) is administered daily until clinical improvement is noted. For patients less seriously ill or those who have improved after initial daily therapy (usually by 1 to 2 weeks after treatment is begun), 0.6 to 1.0 mg per kg (maximum, 50 mg) can be given three times weekly rather than daily. The latter schedule usually permits treatment to be administered on an outpatient basis. A total dose of at least 25 to 35 mg per kg should be achieved. Relapse may occur in 10 to 20% of patients within 5 years of completion of treatment (usually within 1 year); in these instances patients should be retreated with amphotericin B.

Unfortunately, amphotericin B produces frequent side effects and considerable toxicity including fever, shaking chills, shock, adult respiratory distress syndrome, anemia, and especially azotemia. Most patients treated with amphotericin B in daily doses in excess of 0.3 mg per kg, or who have received a total dose of at least 3 mg per kg, will show evidence of incomplete renal tubular acidosis with hypokalemia. Amphotericin B toxicity can be ameliorated appreciably by pretreatment regimens that include premedication with acetaminophen (10 mg per kg orally; maximum, 1000 mg) and diphenhydramine hydrochloride (1.25 mg per kg orally; maximum 100 mg) 30 minutes prior to beginning the infusion;

and if rigors persist, by giving an intravenous bolus of meperidine (1.1 mg per kg; maximum, 50 mg) immediately prior to beginning the infusion. If severe febrile reactions continue despite these regimens, patients should receive an intravenous bolus of hydrocortisone (0.5 to 0.7 mg per kg; maximum, 50 mg) immediately prior to beginning the infusion. The nephrotoxic effects of amphotericin B can be reduced by preventing the insidious dehydration that typically occurs during therapy, by salt and volume loading to maintain urine output (greater than 30 ml per kg daily), and by aggressively replacing lost bicarbonate and potassium when the metabolic effects of renal tubular acidosis are apparent in the serum electrolytes ([$K^+$] less than 4.0 mEq per liter; [$CO_2$] less than 20 mEq per liter). The electrolytes and serum creatinine should be monitored closely, especially early in therapy when the daily dosage is being incremented rapidly, and when other nephrotoxic drugs are being given concomitantly. Temporary interruption or decrease of dosage may be indicated if serum creatinine increases to more than three times normal, or more than 3.0 mg per dl in adolescents.

Despite the proliferation of methods for measurement of amphotericin B in biologic fluids, routine determination of serum, urine, or cerebrospinal fluid concentrations of the drug has no definite clinical value.

## Azole Antifungal Agents

Orally administered, less toxic, and equally effective antifungal agents have long been sought as alternatives to amphotericin B. Since the early 1970s, azole drugs have been extensively evaluated for the treatment of systemic mycoses. The basic structural unit of the antifungal azoles is a five-membered azole ring attached by a carbon nitrogen bond to other aromatic rings. Imidazoles contain two nitrogen atoms in the azole ring; triazoles contain a third nitrogen atom in the ring. The primary mechanism of action of antifungal azoles involves inhibition of ergosterol biosynthesis due to suppression of cytochrome $P^{450}$ activity, which is necessary for the demethylation of 14-alphamethylsterols to ergosterol, the principal sterol in the fungal cell membrane.

**Ketoconazole.** Ketoconazole, an oral imidazole antifungal drug with broad spectrum in-vitro and in-vivo activity against various superficial and deep fungal pathogens, represents a considerable advance in the treatment of blastomycosis. A recent multicenter, prospective, randomized trial of ketoconazole has shown that the drug is a safe, well-tolerated, and effective alternative to amphotericin B for treatment of mild to moderately severe nonmeningeal forms of the disease. In that study, a cure rate of 89% was recorded among patients treated for at least 6 months; the rates were 100% in those who received a high dose (800 mg per day) and 79% in those who received the low dose (400 mg per day).

Treatment is initiated with a dose of 400 mg per dl (6 mg per kg daily in preadolescent children over 2 years of age). The lower initial dose is preferred because of the greater likelihood that higher doses will cause more toxic or adverse effects. The drug is administered once daily, preferably each morning with or just after a meal, since absorption from the gastrointestinal tract is enhanced in the presence of gastric acid. In patients who tolerate the initial dose and have no evidence of clinical progression of disease, the dosage of 400 mg per dl should be maintained for a minimum of 6 months. Therapy must be continued until cultures are persistently negative and radiographic resolution, or at least stabilization, is evident. In patients whose disease is progressive or who develop a new focus of infection during the initial month of therapy on 400 mg per dl, the dosage can be advanced by increments of 200 mg per dl (3 mg per kg daily in preadolescent children over 2 years of age) every 4 to 6 weeks to a maximum of 800 mg per dl (12 mg per kg daily in preadolescent children over 2 years of age). For patients who cannot tolerate ketoconazole or whose disease progresses significantly despite treatment, ketoconazole should be discontinued and amphotericin B begun.

Because *B. dermatitidis* is uniformly susceptible to ketoconazole, routine susceptibility testing of a patient's isolate is not recommended. In patients whose disease progresses, the serum ketoconazole concentration should be determined, and the physician should carefully review concomitant drugs to look for possible causes of decreased absorption of ketoconazole (antacids, anticholinergics, and $H_2$ blockers) or an adverse drug-drug interaction (rifampin and isoniazid).

Although ketoconazole is generally well tolerated in the dosage range of 400 mg per dl or less, higher dosages, particularly the high-dose regimen of 800 mg per dl, may be associated with more adverse or toxic effects, especially gastrointestinal and endocrinologic. Anorexia, nausea, and vomiting, the most common adverse effects, may be ameliorated by evening or split-dose administration of the drug. The increased frequency of gynecomastia, impotence, menstrual irregularities, and rarely weakness due to adrenal insufficiency, in adults who have received high-dose ketoconazole derives from the drug's ability to block adrenal and gonadal steroid synthesis. These endocrine-mediated effects are reversible when the drug is withdrawn. Hepatotoxicity, primarily hepatocellular and idiosyncratic, has been associated with use of ketoconazole, including rare fatalities. Hepatic injury is usually reversible upon discontinuation of the drug. Liver function tests should be monitored before starting treatment and at frequent intervals during treatment. Although transient minor elevations of liver enzymes may occur during therapy, the drug should be stopped if abnormalities greater than three times normal persist, if the abnormalities worsen, or if they become accompanied by symptoms of possible liver injury.

**Itraconazole.** Recent studies suggest that new investigational antifungal oral azole drugs, including the triazole itraconazole, will offer important additions to the current armamentarium. Although this compound has not yet been approved by the Food and Drug Administration, it has been extensively studied in in-vitro and in-vivo animal model systems and, to a lesser degree, in humans. As with ketoconazole, itraconazole is active in vitro against a broad range of fungal organisms, including *B. dermatitidis*. Preliminary reports of itraconazole therapy for nonmeningeal, non–life-threatening forms of blastomycosis in humans indicate that it may offer effective therapy with the distinct advantage of minimal toxicity. In an ongoing drug trial sponsored by the National Institutes of Health, response rates of over 90% have been accomplished with dosages of 200 mg to 400 mg daily among 44 patients thus far enrolled. The majority of these patients have had no drug toxicity. Precise recommendations on the role and usage of itraconazole in the treatment of blastomycosis await the completion of this and other studies.

### Other Treatment Modalities

2-Hydroxystilbamidine isethionate is a comparably effective alternative to amphotericin B only for treatment of noncavitary pulmonary disease or cutaneous disease. Unacceptably high relapse rates have been noted in the treatment of patients with more extensive disease. The dose is 3 to 5 mg per kg administered by slow intravenous infusion daily to achieve a total dose of at least 8 grams. The availability of ketoconazole, a less toxic, equally effective alternative to amphotericin B, which can be administered orally for treatment of non–life-threatening forms of blastomycosis, would seem to abrogate almost any indication for 2-hydroxystilbamidine.

Surgery plays little role in the treatment of blastomycosis, except possibly to drain large abscesses or accumulations of empyema fluid, to repair a bronchopleural fistula, and to débride devitalized bone in some cases of osteomyelitis.

# PLEURAL EFFUSION AND EMPYEMA THORACIS

method of
JOSEPH I. MILLER, Jr., M.D.
*Emory University School of Medicine*
*Atlanta, Georgia*

The basic management of pleural effusion and empyema thoracis is outlined in Figure 1.

A thoracentesis should be performed when any fluid is present in the chest. If the fluid is clear or watery and the cultures and Gram's stain are negative, management is frequently by a simple thoracentesis. Characteristics of a transudative effusion are as follows: (1) the fluid is clear, (2) the pH is less than 7.35, and (3) the protein is less than 3.5 grams per ml. This is most frequently seen in sympathetic effusions, secondary to diseases of the abdomen, in congestive heart failure, or as a consequence of trauma. If the pleural effusion has a negative culture and Gram's stain but has a pH greater than 7.35 and a protein greater than 3.5 grams per ml, it is referred to as an exudative pleural effusion. If there is a clear, watery effusion, a pH greater than 7.2, and a glucose concentration greater than 60 mg per ml, and the effusion reoccurs, repeat thoracentesis can be performed. However, if the pH is less than 7.0, with the glucose level less than 40 and a lactate dehydrogenase (LD) concentration greater than 1000 IU per ml, a chest tube should be inserted. If the pleural fluid culture is positive or has a positive Gram's stain, a chest tube should be inserted. Other factors indicative or suggestive of a parapneumonic effusion of bacterial origin are a pH less than 7.0, a glucose concentration less than 40, or an LD greater than 1000.

The term *empyema* refers to a collection of pus in a natural body cavity. A pleural empyema is accumulation of pus within the pleural space and is referred to as empyema thoracis. Empyema in the pleural space must be considered a surgical disease. The success in management is proportional to the promptness of the treatment, and prevention and treatment have the same goal. The pleural empyema may be unilateral or bilateral, may be localized or diffused, and may be acute or chronic. The distinction between acute and chronic empyema is a matter of time and is largely arbitrary. In general, chronicity may be determined by the nature of the causative organism but usually implies failure of diagnosis and management in the acute stage.

The infected fluid may be thick or watery, odorless or putrid, clear or cloudy, unilateral or

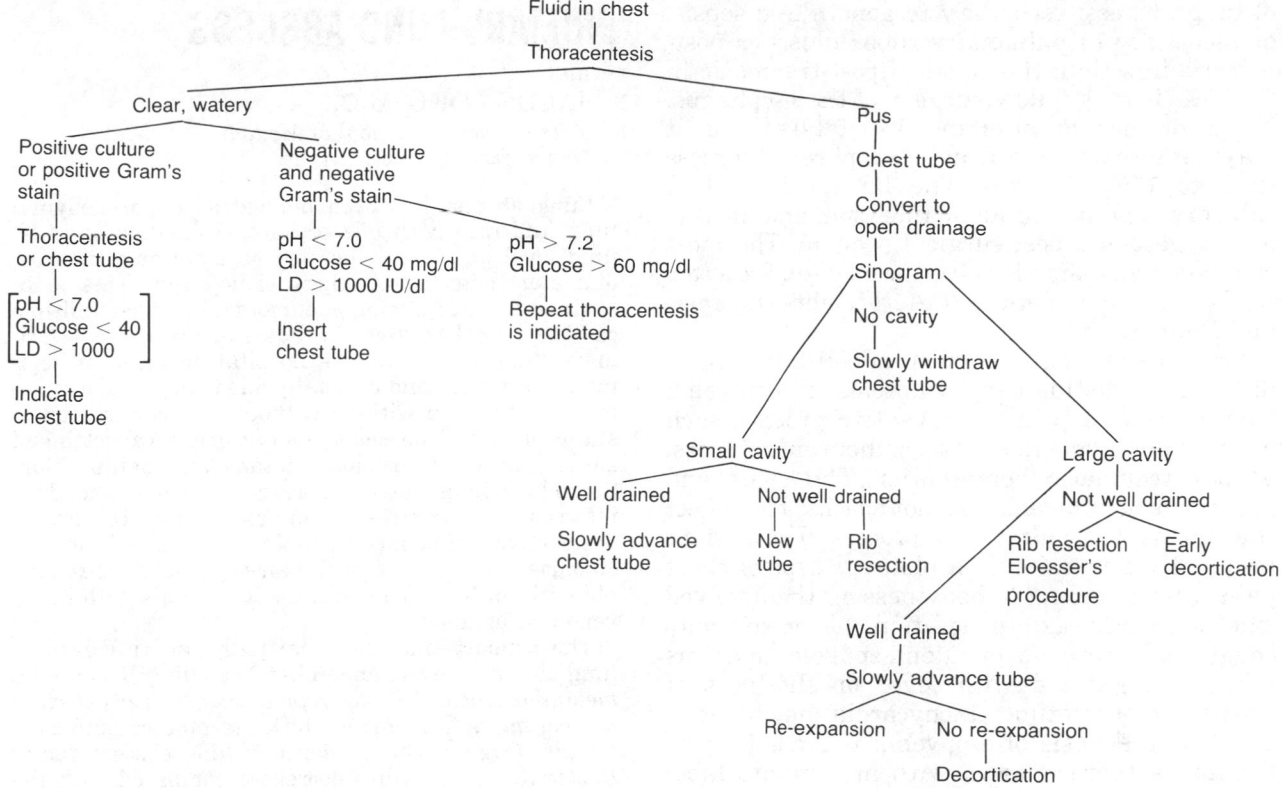

**Figure 1.** Management of empyema thoracis and pleural effusion.

bilateral, localized or loculated, or diffuse and involving the entire pleural space.

Laboratory values are useful in defining an empyema when the fluid is yellow or clear. Empyema thoracis, with clear empyema fluid, has been defined as a pleural fluid with positive bacterial cultures or a white cell count greater than 15,000 cells per mm³ and a protein level greater than 3 grams per ml. When the pleural fluid pH is less than 7, the pleural glucose level is greater than 40 mg per ml, and the pleural LD is greater than 1000, combined with a positive Gram's stain of the pleural fluid, the fluid is also defined as an empyema.

The distinction between acute and chronic empyema is generally made between 4 and 6 weeks. Some individuals consider an empyema chronic if it fails to respond to treatment within a reasonable period of time; others define chronicity in terms of pathologic changes in the surrounding tissue of the pleural space—i.e., when the walls become thick and fibrous. The time when a pleural symphysis can be postulated is reached when the sediment in the pleural fluid reaches 75 to 85% of the total.

The etiology of empyema most frequently follows a pyogenic pneumonia in approximately 50% of cases. Other causes are secondary to rupture

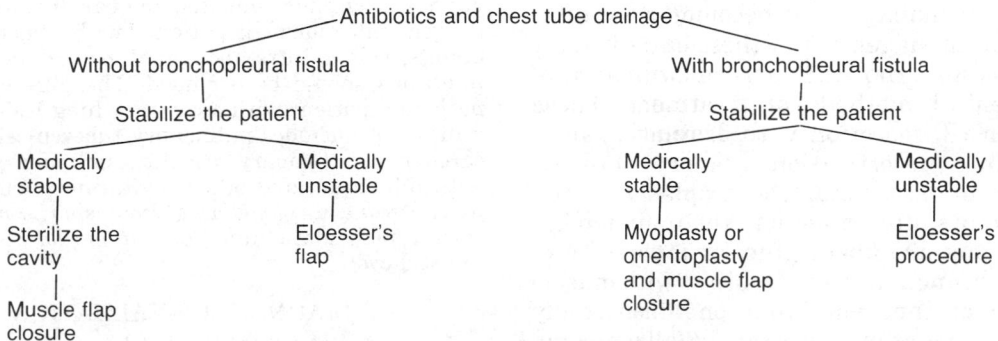

**Figure 2.** Management of post-resectional empyema.

of lung abscess, secondary to generalized sepsis, or secondary to pulmonary tuberculosis or post-mycotic infection; the cause is post-traumatic in 3 to 5%. It may follow surgery of the esophagus, lungs, or mediastinum in 25% of cases, and it may be an extension from a subphrenic abscess in 8 to 11% of cases. The largest individual category is parapneumonic infection, and the second largest is a post-surgical sequela. The most common organisms involved are *Staphylococcus, Klebsiella, Escherichia coli, Aerobacter aerogenes,* and *Proteus.*

From a symptomatology standpoint, it may be difficult to distinguish symptoms of empyema from those of a primary causative process, such as pneumonia, mediastinitis, subphrenic abscess, or post-traumatic hemothorax. The signs and symptoms of empyema are not specific but reflect the underlying pulmonary process. The patient frequently complains of a pleuritic type of chest pain, with a feeling of heaviness on the involved side of the thorax. In addition, he or she may cough and bring up purulent sputum, and this may be associated with fever or shortness of breath, and sometimes tachycardia may be present. The diagnosis of empyema is made by performing a thoracentesis, with appropriate laboratory or bacteriologic confirmation. Once the definitive diagnosis is made, closed chest tube thoracostomy should be performed immediately. This is outlined in Figure 1. Subsequent management of the chest tube with the presence of pus in the pleural space is as outlined in Figure 1. The chest tube is converted to open drainage at an appropriate time, generally between 10 and 12 days. A sinogram is performed, and subsequent management depends on the size of the cavitiy, whether it is large or small, and whether or not it is well drained.

The surgical management of empyema is most frequently accomplished by closed chest tube thoracostomy. The majority of cases can be easily treated with this procedure. When the empyema is secondary to a complication from surgery of the lung, esophagus, or other mediastinal structures, surgical management becomes more difficult. Surgical management of these cases is most often referred to a thoracic surgeon, with a number of potential methods of treatment. These include open rib resection with drainage, Eloesser's procedure, decortication in appropriate circumstances, or occasional thoracoplasty. When empyema occurs after resection, the main modalities of therapy are fibrin glue, or myoplasty of the primary bronchial leak combined with muscle flap closure of the remaining pneumonectomy space. Management of post-resectional empyema is outlined in Figure 2.

# PRIMARY LUNG ABSCESS
method of
JACOB LOKE, M.D.
*Yale University School of Medicine*
*New Haven, Connecticut*

Lung abscess has been defined as a parenchymal lung infiltrate with one or several cavities and air-fluid level (arbitrarily defined as 2 cm or greater in diameter) detected on chest radiograph. This is in contrast to a necrotizing pneumonia, in which multiple cavities less than 2 cm in diameter are present. Primary lung abscess can be hospital acquired or community acquired and is usually due to aspiration pneumonia associated with or without changes in mental status or loss of consciousness in the clinical setting of surgery, previous antibiotic therapy, and malnutrition. Secondary lung abscess may result from secondary infections of lung cysts, bullous cavities in chronic obstructive pulmonary disease, obstructive lung carcinomas, foreign body in the airways, septic thrombophlebitis, or bacteremic disease in patients with intravenous drug abuse.

The primary microbacterial pathogens involved in lung abscess are the anaerobes, including *Bacteroides melaninogenicus, Peptostreptococcus, Fusobacterium nucleatum,* and microaerophilic streptococci and *Bacteroides fragilis.* The incidence of lung abscess due to *Bacteroides fragilis* has decreased compared with the other anaerobes cited, but this anaerobe is clinically important because it is usually resistant to penicillin and the major source of it is from an intra-abdominal process. In addition to the anaerobes that are present as indigenous normal flora of the oral pharynx, other bacterial organisms present include *Actinomyces, Branhamella, Haemophilus, Mycoplasma, Staphylococcus,* and *Streptococcus* species. In hospital-acquired lung abscess, the aerobes or facultative organisms have to be considered and include *Staphylococcus aureus, Klebsiella,* Enterobacteriaceae, and *Pseudomonas.*

The clinical presentation of a patient with lung abscess usually is subacute or chronic, although an acute course can be seen with high fever, chills, sweats, cough and foul smelling sputum, hemoptysis, and pleuritic chest pain. Predisposing conditions such as chronic alcoholism, esophageal dysfunction, seizure disorder, drug abuse, or changes in mental status that lead to aspiration pneumonia should be sought. Also, the patient should be evaluated for periodontal disease; gingivitis; chronic sinusitis; and ear, tonsillar, or pharyngeal infections. In patients with abdominal complaints, pelvic, intra-abdominal, or subdiaphragmatic infections should be excluded. The differential diagnosis in a patient with a cavitary lung lesion on chest radiograph includes pulmonary tuberculosis, cavitary carcinoma, pulmonary vasculitis, pulmonary embolism with infarction, and other cavitating pneumonia due to *Nocardia, Legionella, Mycoplasma, Pneumocystis carinii,* melioidosis, fungi or *Entamoeba histolytica,* or hydatid cyst.

## DIAGNOSTIC EVALUATION

Sputum culture is not helpful for anaerobic pulmonary infection because the normal flora of the mouth and upper airways has a large number of anaerobes, but sputum examination is of value to exclude other bacterial organisms such as mycobacterial disease, gram-positive and gram-negative organisms, or fungal disease. Sputum for cytologic examination should be sent for those patients who are heavy cigarette smokers with or without evidence of pulmonary lung infection but who have a cavitary lesion on chest radiograph. Diagnostic techniques of percutaneous transtracheal aspiration, fiberoptic bronchoscopy with double sheath–protected catheter device, and percutaneous transthoracic needle aspiration lung biopsy have been used to obtain anaerobic culture specimens in order to avoid the contamination by the anaerobes present in the upper airways. The preceding techniques are seldom used in the majority of the medical centers, so that most of the time when the sputum examination is non-diagnostic, broad-spectrum antibiotics are initially given if the patient is very ill, and antibiotic therapy is narrowed depending on the clinical response of the patient and the chest radiographic improvement. Fiberoptic bronchoscopy is usually performed to exclude foreign body, endobronchial abnormalities or stenosis, or a lung carcinoma. When pleural fluid is present it should be tapped and sent for aerobic and anaerobic culture and examined for white blood cell and differential count, Gram's stain, pH, protein, and lactate dehydrogenase. In cases in which a peripheral lung abscess is suspected, computed tomography of the chest is useful to determine whether the cavitary lung lesion is a peripheral lung abscess or a loculated empyema.

## THERAPY

Medical therapy with prolonged antibiotic administration is the mainstay of therapy for lung abscess. Initially, antibiotics are given intravenously for 7 to 10 days and subsequently orally for a total course of antibiotic treatment of 4 to 6 weeks. Because anaerobes are usually involved, aqueous penicillin G, 1 to 2 million units intravenously every 4 hours, is given, followed by oral penicillin VK, 500 mg four times daily. In acutely ill patients, metronidazole (Flagyl) (15 mg per kg intravenously over 1 hour as the loading dose followed by a maintenance dose of 7.5 mg per kg intravenously over 1 hour every 6 hours) is given also for a β-lactamase producing pathogen. Clindamycin (Cleocin) may be preferred, since the relapse and failure rate is less than that with penicillin therapy. Clindamycin is given intravenously—600 mg every 8 hours and then orally 300 mg four times a day. Seriously ill patients who have been on previous antibiotic therapy in the hospital or patients with underlying diseases such as diabetes, alcoholism, malnutrition, drug abuse, or immunosuppression, should receive broader antibiotic coverage. Initially this may include oxacillin or a cephalosporin such as cefoperazone (Cefobid) and an aminoglycoside. Patients should respond symptomatically within 7 to 10 days. When empyema is present, the pleural fluid should be drained. Failure of therapy requires a change of antibiotics that may include imipenem-cilastatin (Primaxin). In patients with progressive lung infiltrate, persistent fever, and empyema, thoracotomy with rib resection and open drainage may be required. Rarely pulmonary resection is needed. In elderly debilitated patients who cannot tolerate pulmonary resection, external drainage of the abscess may be indicated. Complications of lung abscess include intrabronchial hemorrhage; spillage of abscess to other parts of the lung; bronchopleural fistula; pneumothorax; and vascular thrombosis with sloughing of lung tissue and pulmonary gangrene, residual lung cavities, and bronchiectasis.

# OTITIS MEDIA

method of
SUSAN A. CARLIN, M.D.
*Case Western Reserve University*
*Cleveland, Ohio*

Otitis media is the most common bacterial illness of infants and young children. About two-thirds of infants experience one or more episodes of otitis media by the age of 2 years. Management of otitis media in children can be divided into three categories: management of the acute episode, management of recurrences, and management of chronic otitis media with effusion.

## MANAGEMENT

### Acute Otitis Media

Symptoms and signs of acute otitis media typically include ear pain, fever, and irritability accompanied by a viral upper respiratory infection. Spontaneous perforation of the tympanic membrane may occur with subsequent otorrhea and improvement in pain. Young infants in particular may be asymptomatic.

Careful examination of the tympanic membrane by pneumatic otoscopy after removal of cerumen is necessary to diagnose otitis media. A bright light source and the largest size speculum that will occlude the ear canal painlessly and still allow visualization of the tympanic membrane are the keys to successful pneumatic otoscopy. Presence of decreased mobility or a visible air-fluid level is the most reliable sign of middle ear effusion. The tympanic membrane may appear opaque, yellow, red, or gray in color and may bulge laterally as effusion accumulates.

Middle ear fluid cultures should be obtained by

tympanocentesis prior to starting antibiotics in the following high-risk patients: neonates, the immunocompromised, patients who are critically ill, and those who present with a complication of otitis media such as mastoiditis. Initial antimicrobial therapy should provide coverage against the most common bacterial pathogens in acute otitis media, which are *Streptococcus pneumoniae* (30%), *Haemophilus influenzae* (20%), and *Moraxella* (formerly *Branhamella catarrhalis*) (10 to 15%). Ten to thirty percent of *H. influenzae* and 75% of *M. catarrhalis* produce the β-lactamase enzyme. *Streptococcus pyogenes, Staphylococcus aureus,* and anaerobes are detected in less than 10% of cases. In neonates less than 6 weeks of age, perinatally acquired organisms such as *Escherichia coli, Klebsiella, S. aureus,* and group B streptococci should be considered in addition to the usual upper respiratory pathogens. Cultures of the nasopharynx do not correlate with cultures of middle ear fluid in children with acute otitis media.

Amoxicillin (40 mg per kg per day in three divided doses) continues to be the initial drug of choice in treating otitis media. Advantages of amoxicillin include its acceptability to patients, the rarity of serious toxicity, and cost. Increasing resistance to amoxicillin due to bacterial production of the β-lactamase enzyme is the major disadvantage of this drug.

Amoxicillin–clavulanic acid (Augmentin) (40 mg per kg per day in three divided doses) provides activity against β-lactamase producing *H. influenzae* and *M. catarrhalis* in addition to the coverage provided by amoxicillin. Clavulanic acid binds itself irreversibly to the β-lactamase enzyme of bacteria, protecting amoxicillin from enzymatic degradation. Gastrointestinal upset and diarrhea present more of a problem than with amoxicillin alone, but adjusting the dosage slightly downward can sometimes alleviate this problem. It is significantly more expensive than amoxicillin.

Trimethoprim-sulfamethoxazole (Bactrim) (8 mg per kg per day trimethoprim in two divided doses) has the advantage of activity against pneumococci and β-lactamase producing organisms but does not adequately cover group A streptococci or *S. aureus*. Hematologic abnormalities, photosensitivity, and hypersensitivity reactions due to sulfonamides are occasional side effects that require prompt discontinuation of therapy.

Erythromycin-sulfisoxazole (Pediazole) (50 mg per kg per day erythromycin in four divided doses) provides adequate coverage of all the expected organisms, including ampicillin-resistant *H. influenzae, M. catarrhalis,* group A streptococci, and *S. aureus*. Erythromycin may produce gastrointestinal upset, which may necessitate discontinuation of the drug, in addition to the previously mentioned concerns regarding sulfonamide drugs. High cost and four times per day dosing are additional disadvantages.

Cefaclor (Ceclor) (40 mg per kg in three divided doses) is effective in vitro against the common otitis media pathogens, including β-lactamase producing organisms, but many clinical failures have been reported at the recommended 40 mg per kg per day dosage. Cefaclor is expensive, and a risk exists of a serum sickness–type reaction with fever, arthritis, and arthralgias. This risk increases in children who are given multiple courses of the drug. Clinical experience is still limited with other new cephalosporins, cefuroxime (Ceftin) and cefixime (Suprax); both provide broad-spectrum coverage against common otitis media pathogens.

The usual length of antibiotic treatment is 10 days. Most children with acute bacterial otitis media are significantly improved in 48 to 72 hours after treatment is initiated. If ear pain, fever, and irritability persist after this time, consideration should be given to tympanocentesis and/or a change in antibiotic therapy to include coverage against β-lactamase producing bacteria. Knowledge of the resistance pattern of bacteria found in a particular community is important. Acetaminophen (10 to 15 mg per kg as needed every 4 to 6 hours) for pain and fever and local heat may provide symptomatic relief for earache.

Patients should be re-examined with pneumatic otoscopy 1 month after their episode of acute otitis media and monthly thereafter until resolution of the middle ear effusion is observed. Tympanometry may also be useful in following the course of persistent effusion. Approximately 40% of children under age 2 have persistent middle ear effusion 1 month after diagnosis of acute otitis media, 20% after 2 months, and 10% after 3 months. Asymptomatic children with persistent middle ear effusion do not require repeated courses of antibiotics during this time, but parents should be instructed to bring the child in promptly if symptoms of otitis media recur. If the middle ear effusion resolves within a 3-month period, no further follow-up is required.

Antihistamines, decongestants, and corticosteroids have not been proved beneficial and are not recommended for treatment of either acute otitis media or persistent middle ear effusion. Parents should be advised to avoid bottle propping and exposing infants to cigarette smoke, both of which are known to increase the risk of otitis media. Breastfeeding has been found to have a protective effect against otitis media and should be encouraged.

## Recurrent Otitis Media

Those children who develop frequent recurrences of otitis media can present a frustrating management problem to both parents and the physician. Recurrent ear disease may cause significant morbidity from discomfort and pain, intermittent hearing loss, and concerns about speech acquisition.

If the recurrences are infrequent and middle ear effusion clears promptly, it is appropriate to treat each episode individually. The bacteriology of otitis media in cases of recurrent infection is similar to that of acute otitis media even when the recurrence occurs within 1 month after initial treatment. In the case of closely spaced recurrences, if amoxicillin was used as initial drug, an antibiotic with coverage against β-lactamase producing pathogens should be instituted.

For children with closely spaced episodes of otitis media (more than three episodes in 6 months or more than 2 episodes if the child is less than 6 months old), daily antibiotic prophylaxis has been shown to be helpful in reducing the frequency of attacks. Either amoxicillin, 20 mg per kg in a single daily dose, or sulfisoxazole (Gantrisin), 50 to 75 mg per kg per day in two divided doses, can be used, particularly during the respiratory virus season (November to May). These children should be examined periodically while on prophylaxis to detect onset of any new middle ear effusion.

If multiple episodes of acute otitis media occur despite daily antibiotic prophylaxis, referral to an otolaryngologist is warranted for tympanostomy tubes. In addition, consultation should be considered for patients with persistent signs and symptoms of eustachian tube dysfunction, such as pain, hearing loss, atelectasis, or vertigo.

## Chronic Otitis Media With Effusion

Further treatment is indicated for the minority of children who have persistent middle ear effusion for 3 months. Because bacterial pathogens have been isolated in approximately one-third of middle ear aspirates in patients with chronic middle ear effusions, these children should receive a 10-day course of antimicrobial therapy prior to referral to an otolaryngologist. Because the bacteria and the resistance pattern isolated from chronic middle ear effusions are similar to those found in acute otitis media, re-treatment with amoxicillin provides adequate coverage in most circumstances. If ampicillin-resistant bacteria are prevalent in a particular community, one might choose a beta-lactamase–resistant antibiotic. If this treatment does not prove to be successful, placement of tympanostomy tubes is indicated. Recent evidence suggests that adenoidectomy plus bilateral myringotomy may be sufficient treatment in older children (4 to 8 years) with persistent middle ear effusion, thereby avoiding the possible complications of tympanostomy tubes.

# BACTERIAL PNEUMONIA

method of
SCOTT F. DAVIES, M.D.
*University of Minnesota Medical School*
*Hennepin County Medical Center*
*Minneapolis, Minnesota*

The treatment of bacterial pneumonia is usually empiric. More than half the time the specific etiology of the infection is never known. A large number of potential pathogens exist and an extensive diagnostic work-up would cost several thousand dollars and still leave many pneumonias undiagnosed.

Pneumonia is also a serious infection with a mortality which is at least 10% overall and several times that high in elderly patients with underlying cardiac and pulmonary diseases. The uncertainty of treating a severe infection without an etiologic diagnosis can be uncomfortable.

A host of powerful antibiotics exist, all active against many (but not all) pathogens causing pneumonia. There is probably not a "right" antibiotic for any specific patient; rather there is a choice of effective drugs that, alone or in combination, will treat the organisms that are the usual causes of pneumonia in similar patients. Treatment can be narrowed in the event a specific pathogen is identified, but identification occurs less than half the time.

Treatment of pneumonia is not as clear cut as, for example, treatment of urinary tract infections, where a specific pathogen is isolated from the urine (cheaply and noninvasively) and antibiotic sensitivities for the specific isolate are available the next day. In treating pneumonia the clinician has to consider the clinical features of the illness and especially the nature of the host. He or she must decide on the extent of the diagnostic work-up. Giving strong weight to the epidemiology of pneumonia (different types of patients get different types of pneumonias), empiric therapy must be started with appropriate antibiotics. Finally, if the patient does not get better with the initial treatment, the clinician must have a rational plan for performing more diagnostic tests or adding more treatment. The remainder of this article will review the epidemiology of bacterial pneumonia, suggest an initial diagnostic work-up, offer a number of appropriate antibiotic choices, and finally, give the author's approach when empiric therapy fails.

## EPIDEMIOLOGY

Aspiration of oropharyngeal flora is the cause of most bacterial pneumonias. The factors that determine whether an individual gets pneumonia are the virulence of the organisms, the quantity of material aspirated, and the integrity of the local and systemic host defenses. The oropharyngeal flora is very different in different hosts. Similarly, certain hosts are more likely to aspirate large amounts of secretions, and certain hosts are less able to defend themselves against an inoculum of bacteria.

In general, patients with pneumonia can be divided into three groups, each with a different spectrum of likely pathogens.

A normal host is colonized by anaerobic and microaerophilic bacteria of low virulence, including peptococci, peptostreptococci, microaerophilic streptococci, *Fusobacterium,* and *Bacteroides* species. Very few organisms are aspirated, and host defenses eliminate them in most cases. Bacterial pneumonia is distinctly unusual. However, perhaps 10% of normal hosts are colonized by *Streptococcus pneumoniae,* especially in the winter months. This organism has a greater chance, when aspirated, of causing pneumonia. Thus, 85% of the uncommon bacterial pneumonias seen in normal hosts are pneumococcal pneumonias. In rare circumstances, particularly with a larger inoculum, the mixed flora of the mouth can cause a mixed anaerobic pneumonia. Other causes of bacterial pneumonia are distinctly unusual.

Intermediate hosts include alcoholics, smokers with chronic bronchitis, diabetics, intravenous drug users, and, most important, all persons greater than 65 years of age. Such patients are often colonized by *Streptococcus pneumoniae* but also by common gram-negative bacteria including *Haemophilus influenzae,* and *Klebsiella pneumoniae* and by other organisms including *Branhamella catarrhalis* and *Staphylococcus aureus.* Many intermediate patients have reasons to aspirate more organisms (including poor oral hygiene and episodic changes in level of consciousness) and have a variety of local or systemic host defects. Bacterial pneumonia is at least several times more common than in normal hosts. Pneumococcal pneumonia is still the most common bacterial pneumonia but accounts for only 40% of cases. All the other organisms mentioned above also contribute. For patients infected with the human immunodeficiency virus (HIV positive), the dominant pulmonary pathogen is *Pneumocystis carinii.* And yet, approximately 10% of all pulmonary infections in HIV-positive patients are bacterial pneumonias, and the range of pathogens is the same as for other intermediate hosts.

Certain hospitalized patients are a third group of hosts who have different types of bacterial pneumonias. The important risk factors are patient related and not environmental. At risk are patients with indwelling lines and tubes, incapable of performing activities of daily living without help. Many are incontinent, many are hyperglycemic, some are acidotic, and many have moderate to severe dysfunction of one or more organs including brain, lungs, heart, liver, and kidneys. Such patients are often colonized by gram-negative organisms potentially resistant to multiple antibiotics. *Pseudomonas aeruginosa* is the most important, but *Serratia* sp. and *Enterobacter* sp. are also important. Many hospitalized patients aspirate, and most have one or more local or systemic immune defects. In this group

bacterial pneumonia is fairly common, and pneumococcal infections are only about 5% of the total. All the organisms that cause pneumonia in intermediate hosts (especially *Klebsiella pneumoniae*) are seen in hospitalized patients. Many other infections, however, are caused by bad gram-negative rods with more potential for antibiotic resistance.

Several important types of bacterial pneumonia are acquired by inhalation of organisms rather than by aspiration. Pneumonia caused by *Legionella* sp. mimics other bacterial pneumonia but does not respond to the usual therapy. Infections tend to be more severe in intermediate hosts, probably because of host defense abnormalities, and so the diagnosis is made more commonly in this group. However, normal hosts may also have severe infections, and outbreaks of nosocomial infections have occurred in specific hospitals, probably owing to contaminated water or air-conditioning systems. Mycoplasmal pneumonia, also acquired by inhalation, is a common cause of so-called atypical pneumonia (see below) in normal hosts. The illness is most common in children and young adults but may occur in any age group and may cause severe illness.

## DIAGNOSTIC WORK-UP

Bacterial pneumonia is almost surely present if the patient has these four findings: (1) new or increasing infiltrate on chest roentgenogram; (2) purulent sputum; (3) white blood count that is high, low, or left shifted with immature forms; and (4) fever greater than 100° F. Absence of one or more findings does not disprove the diagnosis but raises the odds of a nonbacterial or even noninfectious pulmonary illness. The initial work-up should include a careful history and physical examination, a chest roentgenogram, a complete blood count with differential counting of the white blood cells, and a Gram's stain and culture of expectorated or induced sputum. If the patient is sick enough to be hospitalized (lobar or greater pneumonia; toxicity; markedly abnormal vital signs; dyspnea; significant underlying disease, especially alcoholism with current binge) then blood cultures should also be done. If the chest roentgenogram shows more than a small amount of pleural fluid, it should be sampled by thoracentesis to rule out empyema and to obtain cultures. Positive cultures of blood or pleural fluid prove a specific pathogen. A positive sputum Gram's stain showing predominant gram-positive diplococci, including intracellular organisms, strongly suggests pneumococcal pneumonia, and a Gram's stain showing predominant gram-negative rods points away from pneumococcal pneumonia and toward a gram-negative pneumonia. Sputum cultures are helpful only if a pathogen is isolated which fits the clinical picture and the Gram's stain. The sensitivity of the isolate to various antibiotics can be determined. However, finding an organism on a Gram's stain of sputum or isolating an organism from a sputum culture never proves a specific etiology. If the patient is severely ill, the whole range of potential pathogens should be treated, based on epidemiology. One should never bet the life of an alcoholic with lobar pneumonia on a

Gram's stain showing gram-positive cocci, because he or she might just have klebsiella pneumonia. Remember that infected pulmonary secretions contain $10^5$ organisms per ml, while oral secretions, particularly with poor dentition, may contain more than $10^{10}$ organisms per ml. Each bacterium coughed from the lung may pass by 100,000 or more oropharyngeal bacteria before ending up in the specimen cup. Screening the sputum to make sure there are more than 25 neutrophils and less than 10 epithelial cells per high-power field helps somewhat to exclude gross contamination by oral secretions. However, this certainly does not make sputum cultures highly specific for the exact pulmonary pathogen causing the pneumonia.

A more extensive work-up is not necessary except in unusual circumstances. If the patient is critically ill and requires immediate intubation, fiberoptic bronchoscopy with bronchoalveolar lavage of a radiographically involved segment of the lung can be done. Quantitative cultures of lavage fluid have high specificity if they show $10^5$ colonies of a single pathogen; such cultures are also very sensitive for the presence of bacterial infection if obtained before antibiotic therapy. The high cost of the procedure itself and the battery of tests that it generates preclude its use in every pneumonia. Similarly, cultures for unusual bacterial and nonbacterial agents of pneumonia and serodiagnostic tests for these agents are not routinely done initially unless there are clinical clues that suggest an unusual pneumonia or if the clinical course is progressive without a specific diagnosis (see below). The initial treatment is empiric. Unless the blood cultures are positive (perhaps 10 to 20% of hospitalized patients), the exact etiology is never known.

Atypical pneumonia is a term used when the sputum is not grossly purulent and the infiltrates are patchy and bilateral, or even diffuse. Many patients have a longer prodrome with myalgias and other systemic features including arthralgias and headache. Viral pneumonia, mycoplasma pneumonia, and primary fungal pneumonias are all possible, as is pneumocystis pneumonia in appropriate patients. Diagnostic tests depend on the circumstances. An influenza culture is appropriate in winter months, especially if there is an outbreak of influenza in the community. Serum IgM for *Mycoplasma* is appropriate for a college student whose roommate had a similar illness 2 weeks ago. Serologic testing for histoplasmosis is appropriate in an endemic area, especially if the infiltrate is nodular. Diagnostic tests for pneumocystis pneumonia are appropriate if the patient is HIV positive or belongs to a high-risk group. Induced sputum should be examined first. If the sputum is negative, fiberoptic bronchoscopy with bronchoalveolar lavage should be done.

Lobar pneumonia, grossly purulent or even bloody sputum, pleuritic chest pain or pleural fluid, and marked left shift of the white blood count all argue strongly for usual bacterial pathogens and against the organisms causing atypical pneumonia.

## TREATMENT

### Appropriate Antibiotic Therapy

Table 1 lists several appropriate choices for each of the three groups of patients. Table 2 gives

### TABLE 1. Choice of Antibiotic Therapy for Bacterial Pneumonia

**Normal Host**
Penicillin G
Erythromycin
Second- or third-generation cephalosporin

**Intermediate Host**
Second-generation cephalosporin
   Cefuroxime (Zinacef)
   Cefotetan (Cefotan)
   Cefamandole (Mandol)
Third-generation cephalosporin
   Cefotaxime (Claforan)
   Ceftriaxone (Rocephin)
   Ceftizoxime (Cefizox)
Ticarcillin-clavulanate (Timentin)
Ampicillin-sulbactam (Unasyn)
Imipenem-cilastatin (Primaxin)
Ciprofloxacin (Cipro) plus penicillin G
Trimethoprim-sulfamethoxazole (Bactrim)

Clindamycin is never used alone as empiric therapy but may be added for putrid sputum or if anaerobes are isolated from blood or pleural fluid.

**Hospitalized Patient**
Ceftazidime
Ticarcillin-clavulanate
Imipenem-cilastatin
Mezlocillin (Mezlin) (or piperacillin [Pipracil] or ticarcillin [Ticar] or ticarcillin-clavulanate) plus amikacin (or gentamicin or tobramycin or netilmicin or aztreonam)*
Ceftazidime plus amikacin (or gentamicin or tobramycin or netilmicin or aztreonam)*
Vancomycin plus ceftazidime (or imipenem-cilastatin or ticarcillin [Nebcin, Netromycin, Azactam] clavulavate)—some add amikacin (or gentamicin or tobramycin or netilmicin or aztreonam)†

Add vancomycin or nafcillin or oxacillin to regimens without vancomycin when gram-positive cocci in clusters are seen on Gram's stain of the sputum.
*Preferred when *Pseudomonas* is documented from sputum or blood cultures.
†Preferred with neutropenia ($<500/mm^3$).

usual adult dosing (with normal renal function) for the antibiotics mentioned. If a specific pathogen is isolated from blood or pleural fluid, more selective treatment can be given, directed at the pathogen independent of the host. Otherwise, empiric therapy is given based on patient factors. General concepts regarding therapy will be briefly outlined.

Penicillin is the treatment of choice for bacterial pneumonia in normal hosts. Because a higher percentage of patients with pneumonia respond to a cell-wall–active antibiotic than to erythromycin, the latter agent should not be used routinely for bacterial pneumonia but should be reserved for penicillin-allergic patients or those with clinical features suggesting mycoplasma infection. In particular, patients with grossly purulent sputum or pleuritic pain should get a cell-wall–active agent. Therapy should be broader than penicillin alone if the patient is critically

TABLE 2. **Common Dosing of Antibiotics Used for Bacterial Pneumonia (Adults with Normal Renal Function)*** 

| | |
|---|---|
| Penicillin G | 1.2 million U bid IM (benzathine penicillin G) or 2 million U IV q 4–6 hr |
| Erythromycin | .5–1.0 grams q 6 hr |
| Cefuroxime | .75–1.5 grams q 8 hr |
| Cefotetan | 1–3 grams q 12 hr |
| Cefamandole | .5–2.0 grams q 4–6 hr |
| Cefotaxime | 1–2 grams q 6–8 hr |
| Ceftriaxone | 1–2 grams q 12–24 hr |
| Ceftizoxime | 1–4 grams q 8–12 hr |
| Ticarcillin-clavulanate | 3.1 grams q 4–8 hr |
| Ampicillin-sulbactam | 1.5–3 grams q 6 hr |
| Imipenem-cilastatin | .5–1 gram q 6 hr |
| Ciprofloxacin | .5–.75 grams q 12 hr PO |
| Trimethoprim-sulfamethoxazole | 2.5–5 mg/kg q 6 hr (higher dose only for *Pneumocystis* pneumonia) |
| Clindamycin | .6–.9 grams q 6–8 hr |
| Ceftazidime | 1–2 grams q 8–12 hr |
| Mezlocillin | 3 grams q 4 hr |
| Piperacillin | 3 grams q 4 hr |
| Ticarcillin | 3 grams q 4 hr |
| Amikacin | 15 mg/kg/day (q 8–12 hr dosing; check levels) |
| Gentamicin | 3–5 mg/kg/day (q 8 hr dosing; check levels) |
| Tobramycin | 3–5 mg/kg/day (q 6 hr dosing; check levels) |
| Netilmicin | 4–6.5 mg/kg/day (q 8 hr dosing; check levels) |
| Aztreonam | 1–2 grams q 6–8 hr |
| Vancomycin | 1 gram q 12 hr |
| Nafcillin | 1–2 grams q 4 hr |
| Oxacillin | 1–2 grams q 4 hr |

*Assume intravenous administration except when other route indicated.

ill, especially if the sputum Gram's stain is not highly convincing for pneumococci. Treatment such as that for intermediate patients (see Table 1) is appropriate for such patients. If the respiratory illness is biphasic, the bacterial pneumonia may be complicating influenza. Such patients should also be treated as intermediate patients, but special consideration should also be given to *Staphylococcus aureus*. If the Gram's stain shows gram-positive cocci in clusters, a highly potent antistaphylococcal agent (vancomycin, nafcillin, or oxacillin) should be added.

Intermediate hosts should never be treated with penicillin alone. Therapy must cover *H. influenzae* and *K. pneumoniae* but need not cover *P. aeruginosa* or other highly antibiotic-resistant gram-negative pathogens. Some authorities recommend concurrent initial therapy with erythromycin to cover *Legionella* infections. In practice this is seldom done, except in areas with a high incidence of *Legionella* infection. Rather, further diagnostic tests are done if the initial therapy fails, and erythromycin is added at that time (see below). Patients with poor dentition and risk

factors for gross aspiration are at risk for anaerobic infections. Where this is a major concern agents such as ticarcillin/clavulanate (Timetin)or imipemen/cilastatin (Primaxin), can be used rather than a second- or third-generation cephalosporin (although the cephalosporins in general have some activity against anaerobes and clinical failure with these agents is uncommon). Clindamycin (Cleocin) is highly effective against anaerobes but has no gram-negative activity and cannot be used alone for intermediate patients. Clindamycin is the best treatment for anaerobic lung abscess but is not generally necessary for bacterial pneumonia. It can be used when the sputum is putrid or if anaerobes are recovered from pleural fluid or uncommonly from blood. Metronidazole (Flagyl) is not very effective for pleuropulmonary anaerobic infections and should not be used as a substitute for clindamycin. Ciprofloxacin (Cipro) is a newer antibiotic, a quinolone, which is well absorbed orally and very effective against the gram-negative organisms commonly seen in intermediate hosts. However, the pneumococcus is still the single most common bacterial pathogen in this group, and ciprofloxacin is at best a second-rate antipneumococcal agent. For this reason it should not be used alone for empiric therapy but can be used in combination with penicillin.

There is some controversy about the treatment of the third group of patients, hospitalized patients or those with similar severe illnesses being nursed in a nursing home or at home. Some new antibiotics, including ceftazadime (Fortaz), ticarcillin-clavulanate, and imipenem-cilastatin have a very wide spectrum of activity against gram-negative bacteria including significant anti-*Pseudomonas* activity. These are appropriate for pneumonia in hospitalized patients if no pathogen or a pathogen other than pseudomonas has been identified. However, current evidence suggests that combination therapy, including an aminoglycoside, should be used if *Pseudomonas* is recovered from blood or even as the sole pathogen from sputum samples showing many gram-negative rods on the Gram's stain. It should also be mentioned that profoundly neutropenic patients, usually after cancer chemotherapy, are a special category of hospitalized patients who require even broader empiric therapy including vancomycin for coagulase-negative and coagulase-positive staphylococci. Therapy is initiated for fever, even without infiltrates. If the patient remains febrile for 5 days, empiric antifungal therapy with amphotericin B (Fungizone) is added to the empiric antibacterial regimen.

Duration of therapy is variable. For proven pneumococcal pneumonia, penicillin can be stopped once the patient has been afebrile for 3 days. For serious gram-negative pneumonias, intravenous therapy should be continued for at least 2 weeks. For patients with moderate illness and no definite etiology, intravenous therapy is continued until the patient has been afebrile for 24–48 hours. Then a switch is made to an appropriate oral agent and it is continued for 7 to 10 days. Penicillin VK is appropriate for normal hosts. Amoxicillin-clavulnate (Augmentin), trimethoprim-sulphamethoxazole (Bactrim), oral cephalosporins (cefuroxime [Ceftin] or cefaclor [Ceclor]), and ciprofloxacin are all reasonable choices for intermediate hosts. Oral cephalosporins and ciprofloxacin are reasonable for hospitalized patients, although many of these patients are more seriously ill and require long courses of intravenous therapy.

### Failure of Empiric Therapy

Patients with overwhelming pneumonia may die in the first few days despite appropriate therapy. If the blood cultures are positive and the antibiotic therapy is correct, life support and drainage of localized pus (empyema, purulent pericarditis) are all that can be done. However, if the blood cultures are negative and the illness is progressing despite empiric antibiotics, there is always the possibility that the infection might be due to an organism not covered by the empiric therapy. After 48 to 72 hours with no improvement or clear progression, further diagnostic tests should be done. Sputum smears and cultures for *Legionella* and tuberculosis should be sent. These are the two most common causes of bacterial pneumonia (or mycobacterial pneumonia in the case of tuberculosis) not covered by usual empiric therapy. Fiberoptic bronchoscopy, including bronchoalveolar lavage and if possible transbronchial biopsy, is the best diagnostic test and should be done once smears for tuberculosis are negative. Cultures for routine bacteria are not very helpful after several days of antibiotics, but those organisms are already being treated. Smears and cultures for *Legionella,* tuberculosis, fungi, pneumocystis, and viruses should be done, as appropriate. Diagnostic tests for rare illnesses like tularemia, melioidosis, psittacosis, and Q fever can be considered in specific instances. At this point it is reasonable to add erythromycin (1 gram four times daily intravenously) to cover *Legionella* infection.

If a specific diagnosis is not made from these tests and the illness progresses despite the initial therapy (a broad-spectrum, cell-wall antibiotic) and erythromycin, selected patients will require open lung biopsy as a final attempt to make a specific diagnosis. In other cases the severity of underlying illnesses or the rapid progression of the acute pneumonia (with hypotension and multiorgan failure) precludes open biopsy. Even when open lung biopsy is performed, a new, treatable pathogen often is not found. Many times the antibiotics are indeed appropriate, and the problem is the nature of the host or the severity of the infection.

# VIRAL RESPIRATORY INFECTIONS

method of
PETER J. KRAUSE, M.D.
*University of Connecticut School of Medicine*
*Hartford, Connecticut*

Viral respiratory infections are the most common type of acute illnesses seen by physicians in the United States. All age groups are affected. Transmission occurs within families, at work, and in school. The most important viral respiratory pathogens in adults in the United States are influenza viruses and in children the respiratory syncytial virus. Other important causes of viral respiratory illness include rhinovirus, adenovirus, parainfluenza viruses, coronavirus, herpes simplex virus, enteroviruses, and Epstein-Barr virus. Syndromes caused by these viruses include rhinitis, parotitis, stomatitis, pharyngitis, laryngitis, bronchitis, bronchiolitis, pneumonia, the common cold, influenza-like illness, and mononucleosis-like illness. Specific diagnosis can be made by rapid viral antigen tests, culture, and serology. In most cases of mild upper respiratory illness, specific laboratory identification is unnecessary and treatment is symptomatic. Only a limited number of antiviral agents for some viral pathogens are currently available; however, new antiviral compounds are being developed.

## RHINORRHEA AND NASAL CONGESTION

Symptomatic relief of nasal congestion can be achieved by the use of sympathomimetic amines, antihistamines, or mechanical suctioning to relieve nasal obstruction. Sympathomimetic amines can be administered as nasal drops or spray two to three times per day for no more than 3 days (0.1 per cent xylometazoline [Otrivin] or 0.05 per cent oxymetazoline [Afrin]) or can be given orally. Half-strength formulations are available for children. Antihistamines are probably beneficial for patients with viral rhinorrhea only if there is an accompanying allergic rhinitis. Combination oral sympathomimetic amines and antihistamines are available. Use of saline nose drops and gentle suctioning with a bulb aspirator is recommended in infants because of concern about untoward reactions to drugs. Humidification of room air may be helpful, as it tends to loosen tenacious nasal mucus. Sympathomimetic amines can cause rebound congestion with chronic use, transient increase in blood pressure, and nervousness. They are contraindicated in patients taking monamine oxidase (MAO) inhibitors or tricyclic antidepressants. Antihistamines can cause drowsiness.

## PHARYNGITIS

Pharyngitis due to viral pathogens may be difficult to distinguish from group A streptococcal pharyngitis, and the latter should be ruled out with a throat culture. Symptomatic treatment of viral pharyngitis may be obtained with throat lozenges or salt water gargle. Aspirin or acetaminophen (Tylenol) may be used, but aspirin should be avoided in children 16 years and younger with chickenpox or influenza because of the association with Reye's syndrome. In severe cases of pharyngitis, 2% viscous xylocaine (Lidocaine) can be topically applied or used as a gargle. Excessive use should be avoided because of the possibility of paralysis of the epiglottis with subsequent aspiration. In young children, severe pharyngitis may cause dehydration because of refusal to take liquids.

## CROUP

Croup is a term used to describe several respiratory illnesses characterized by constriction of the upper airway and varying degrees of inspiratory stridor, cough, and hoarseness. Epiglottitis is a life threatening condition caused by *Haemophilus influenzae*, type b, which must be distinguished from viral croup and managed in a different manner. Treatment of most mild forms of viral croup such as spasmodic croup consists simply of administration of moist air. The treatment of more severe viral croup (laryngotracheobronchitis) depends on the severity of illness. Therapeutic choices include cool water vapor, which can be delivered by bathroom shower, nebulizer, or mist tent; racemic epinephrine; corticosteroids; supplemental oxygen; or assisted ventilation. Racemic epinephrine (Vaponephrin) should be reserved for patients admitted to the hospital in whom transient improvement in air flow may prevent the need for intubation. It is administered by mask or in some cases by IPPB* nebulization as a 2.25% solution (0.25 to 0.5 ml) added to 3 ml of water or normal saline. It is generally given every 3 to 4 hours but may be repeated more frequently if serious side effects such as marked tachycardia do not occur. The use of

---

*Intermittent positive-pressure breathing.

corticosteroids for croup is controversial despite numerous studies. Recent studies indicate that dexamethasone (Decadron) is useful in severely ill patients when given once at 0.3 to 0.5 mg/kg and repeated in 2 hours.

## BRONCHITIS AND BRONCHIOLITIS

Treatment of acute bronchitis is primarily directed at control of *cough*. Moderate to severe cough can be treated with dextromethorphan given orally every 6 to 8 hours, 15 to 30 mg in adults and 0.25 mg per kg in children. If this does not work, preparations containing codeine (10 to 20 mg in adults and 0.2 to 0.25 mg per kg body weight in children) given every 4 hours can be used. Expectorants are generally not helpful. Bronchiolitis is an acute viral lower respiratory tract illness characterized by cough, coryza, fever, expiratory wheezing, hyperaeration, tachypnea, and respiratory distress that occurs in the first 2 years of life. Supplemental oxygen is the primary therapy. Mist therapy, bronchodilators, and steroids have not been shown to be helpful.

## RIBAVIRIN

Ribavirin (Virazole) is a synthetic nucleoside that has been shown to be of benefit to children with respiratory syncytial virus lower respiratory tract disease and adults with influenza. It should be reserved for patients with severe disease or those with underlying pulmonary, cardiac, or immunologic impairment who have moderate to severe disease. Ribavirin is administered by aerosol via face mask, mist tent, or ventilator. It is administered for 12 to 18 hours per day for 3 to 7 days. Special care must be taken with the use of ribavirin for patients on ventilators to prevent precipitation of the drug within the ventilator, and constant monitoring of such patients is mandatory. Pregnant health care workers should avoid caring for patients on ribavirin because of the remote possibility that the drug is a human teratogen.

## AMANTADINE

Amantadine hydrochloride (Symmetrel) specifically inhibits the replication of influenza A (but not influenza B) virus and is used for prophylaxis and therapy of influenza A virus infections. Amantadine efficacy in prevention of influenza A has ranged from 50 to over 90%, rates comparable with those of influenza A vaccine. It has also been shown to reduce the duration of fever and other systemic signs with a more rapid return to normal daily activities when given within 24 to

48 hours after onset of illness. The usual dosage in adults and children over 9 years of age is 100 mg given orally twice per day. Prophylaxis is continued throughout the period of risk (4 to 8 weeks), while treatment is for 3 to 7 days. The dose for children under 9 years of age is 2.2 to 4.4 mg per kg body weight every 12 hours with a maximum single dose of 75 mg. Side effects are uncommon but include minor gastrointestinal and central nervous system complaints. These are more common in the elderly and in patients with impaired renal function.

# VIRAL AND MYCOPLASMAL PNEUMONIAS

method of
W. PAUL GLEZEN, M.D.
*Baylor College of Medicine*
*Houston, Texas*

## VIRAL PNEUMONIA

Respiratory virus infection can be implicated in the etiology of a large proportion of pneumonia episodes in adults as well as children. Although the death rate attributed to pneumonia has been declining in recent years, the frequency of occurrence has remained high and essentially unchanged. The overall rate has ranged from 1.0 to 1.6 per 100 persons per year, with the higher rates occurring during years when influenza virus epidemics were more intense. These rates can be translated to totals of 2.5 to 3.3 million episodes per year in the United States. The seasonal occurrence of these pneumonia episodes implicates etiologic roles for certain respiratory viruses; 85 per cent of pediatric pneumonia cases have occurred during the relatively discrete outbreaks caused by influenza, parainfluenza, and respiratory syncytial (RS) viruses, whereas 40 per cent of adult pneumonia cases occurred during annual influenza virus epidemics. Knowledge of the seasonal pattern of occurrence of these viruses, their major clinical manifestations, and the usual age distribution for these manifestations aids etiologic assessment of patients with pneumonia. Outbreaks of parainfluenza virus Types 1 and 2 have occurred in the autumn (usually odd-numbered years only) and were accompanied by epidemics of croup in children between 6 and 24 months of age. RS virus epidemics have occurred in winter and were most evident by the common manifestation of bronchiolitis in infants. Influenza epidemics can be charted by frequent bulletins published by public health officials. Influenza epidemics are usually heralded by the increased frequency of febrile respiratory illnesses in school-age children and young adults and come in midwinter after the peak of RS virus activity. Parainfluenza virus Type 3 activity has been greatest in the spring, after activity of the other major viruses has declined.

RS virus is the most common cause of pneumonia in infancy. The illness usually commences with rhinorrhea, low-grade fever, and cough for 2 or 3 days followed by a progressive increase in respiratory rate and development of subcostal and intercostal retractions. The chest roentgenogram reveals scattered peribronchial and perihilar infiltrates, involving multiple lobes. Air trapping may be present. Diffuse interstitial infiltrates may be present, but scattered linear shadows resulting from subsegmental areas of atelectasis are probably more common. Atelectasis of the right upper lobe or middle lobe is not uncommon. Influenza and parainfluenza viruses may give a similar picture but are less likely to produce air trapping than RS virus. Most of these illnesses are self-limited and resolve within 3 weeks. Some adenoviruses (Types 1, 2, 5, and 6) may give a similar clinical picture, but Types 3, 7, and 21 may produce a destructive process that results in obliterative bronchiolitis with permanent damage to the lungs. Measles virus pneumonia in infancy may produce a similar process. Pneumonitis caused by *Chlamydia trachomatis* should be differentiated from viral pneumonias in infants. *C. trachomatis* pneumonitis has an afebrile and indolent course with progressive cough and respiratory distress during 2 to 3 weeks. Infants with this infection usually present between 6 to 12 weeks of age and often have a history of conjunctivitis during the first 2 weeks of life. Influenza viruses are the most common cause of viral pneumonia in adults in civilian populations, but adenovirus Types 4 and 7 have been predominant types in military recruits. Onset usually occurs with fever (temperature up to 39° C) with chills and muscle aches, dry hacking cough, pharyngitis, and conjunctival irritation. Influenza commonly involves the trachea and major bronchi and is accompanied by pneumonitis in about 5 per cent of persons. Influenza pneumonitis may progress rapidly with paroxysmal cough, breathlessness, and thin, bloody sputum. Secondary bacterial invasion is common. The major bacterial pathogens involved are pneumococci, staphylococci, and *Haemophilus influenzae*. Pneumonitis may also be present in approximately 15 per cent of adults with varicella.

## Treatment

Ribavirin (Virazole) is a broad-spectrum antiviral drug that is licensed for treatment of RS virus pneumonia and bronchiolitis. The drug is administered by small particle aerosol, which limits its use to hospitalized patients. Use is further limited by cost, so that treatment is recommended particularly for persons who are likely to develop life-threatening infections. Because ribavirin may be teratogenic and dispersed throughout the room, health care workers who are pregnant should not prepare or administer it and should avoid rooms where it is being given. Antigen detection by enzyme-linked immunosorbent assay allows rapid identification of infected patients. The patients who are recommended for treatment include infants with congenital heart disease, bronchopulmonary dysplasia, or other chronic lung conditions; infants less than 8 weeks of age; and immunocompromised patients of any age, particularly patients undergoing bone marrow transplantation or patients with acquired immunodeficiency syndrome. Any child presenting with $Pa_{O_2}$ levels less than 65 mmHg or with increasing $Pa_{CO_2}$ levels should be considered for therapy. The drug can be administered successfully through a ventilator, but its use must be monitored closely by trained respiratory therapists. Ribavirin also has been demonstrated to be effective against influenza viruses A and B and parainfluenza viruses. Ribavirin aerosol should be considered for treatment of hospitalized patients with life-threatening infections with these viruses.

Amantadine (Symmetrel), another licensed antiviral drug, is effective against influenza A viruses. The drug is administered orally and can be prescribed for hospitalized patients or ambulatory patients. To have a therapeutic effect, the drug should be started as early as possible in the course of the illness. The dose for children is 5 mg per kg body weight per day administered in two divided doses for 5 days. The total dose should not exceed 150 mg per day for children younger than 10 years of age. For persons aged 10 years or older, the daily dose is 100 mg twice daily. Adults may be given 200 mg as a loading dose to initiate therapy, followed by 100 mg twice daily for 5 days. The dose in elderly patients (older than 65 years) should be 100 mg once daily. Amantadine is not effective for influenza B virus or other respiratory viruses. Amantadine is well tolerated when administered in these dosages, but an occasional patient (about 1 in 20) may complain of nervousness, insomnia, anorexia, or nausea. These symptoms disappear when the drug is stopped. Rimantadine, an analogue of amantadine, should be licensed soon; because of its slower absorption, rimantadine therapy is generally free of the side effects attributed to amantadine. Rimantadine is equally effective for treatment of influenza A virus infections.

Hospitalization is recommended for all infants younger than 4 months of age with lower respiratory tract disease. Only about 10 per cent of patients above that age with viral pneumonia require hospitalization, but bed rest and careful follow-up are recommended until improvement is clinically obvious. Telephone contact, at least, is important during the first few days to watch for signs of bacterial superinfection, which would be indicated by persistence or exacerbation of fever, increased respiratory rate, decreasing appetite, and general deterioration. If any suspicious signs or symptoms occur, the patient should be seen and re-evaluated.

For children we have found certain clinical features to help in differentiating viral infection from bacterial infection. A scoring system has been developed that can assist the physician to decide about initiating antibiotic therapy. The chest x-ray film is scored for features that are characteristic of bacterial or viral pneumonia. Positive scores are applied for features of bacterial infections and negative scores for features of viral infections. The outline for the scoring system is shown in Table 1.

The scores for the chest film are summed and additional positive scores of +1 are added for total white blood cell count of 20,000 per $mm^3$ or more, absolute polymorphonuclear neutrophil (PMN) count of 10,000 per $mm^3$ or more, immature PMN count of 500 per $mm^3$ or more, and temperature of 103° F or higher. For hospitalized

TABLE 1. **Scoring System for Pediatric Chest X-Ray Films***

| Characteristic | Score |
|---|---|
| 1. Infiltrate | |
|   a. Well-defined lobar, lobular, segmented (rounded) | +2 |
|   b. Poorly defined, patchy, lobular, alveolar | +1 |
|   c. Interstitial, peribronchial | −1 |
| 2. Location | |
|   a. Single lobe | +1 |
|   b. Multiple lobes in one or both lungs but as in 1a | +1 |
|   c. Multiple sites, perihilar as in 1c | −1 |
| 3. Fluid in pleural space | |
|   a. Minimal blunting of costophrenic angle | +1 |
|   b. Obvious fluid | +2 |
| 4. Abscess, pneumatocele, or bullae | |
|   a. Equivocal | +1 |
|   b. Definite | +2 |
| 5. Atelectasis | |
|   a. Subsegmental (usually multiple sites) | −1 |
|   b. Lobar involving right, middle, or upper lobe | −1 |
|   c. Lobar involving other lobes | 0 |

*Developed with Dr. Tuenchit Khamapirad.

children 6 months of age or older, another +1 is added. A score of 0 or less usually indicates a viral infection, whereas a score of 1 or more usually indicates a bacterial infection. Viral pneumonias for the common etiologies have yielded average scores ranging from −1.5 to −3.0. In contrast, pneumococcal pneumonias averaged +4.4 and staphylococcal pneumonias averaged +6.3. Pneumonia caused by *H. influenzae* Type b had scores that averaged only +1.5 and may be the most difficult to distinguish from viral infections. Low total white blood cell counts (<5000) were encountered with both influenza virus infections and staphylococcal pneumonias in infants. Because bacterial superinfection may occur during the course of a viral infection, reassessment may be necessary at intervals if the patient's condition is not improving.

When clinical assessment can be combined with methods for rapid detection of viral and bacterial polysaccharide antigens in respiratory secretions, the diagnosis may be clear-cut and treatment can be rationally applied. The presence of a predominant bacterial pathogen in the upper respiratory tree (nasopharynx or trachea) does not establish the diagnosis of bacterial pneumonia; however, if clinical features of bacterial infection are present, specific therapy can be directed to the predominant bacteria.

Fluid intake should be encouraged to maintain adequate hydration. Cough depressants are not recommended for children younger than 2 years of age, but an antitussive such as dextromethorphan may be used in older children and adults who are afebrile and have a persistent, nonproductive cough. Aspirin is not recommended for children, but an antipyretic such as acetaminophen may be used for temperatures of 102° F or higher. Antipyretics should not be used routinely at any age because regular use may mask the early signs of bacterial superinfection.

For patients who require hospitalization because of respiratory distress or systemic toxicity, baseline arterial blood gas values should be obtained to assess the need for oxygen therapy. Supplemental humidified oxygen should be administered to maintain the arterial $P_{O_2}$ value between 80 and 100 mmHg. If the $P_{CO_2}$ value climbs to 40 or 45 mmHg, tracheal intubation and ventilatory assistance may be necessary. Bronchodilators should be administered to infants with caution; these medications should be stopped if clear evidence of benefit is lacking. Chest physical therapy is recommended only for patients with lobar atelectasis.

## MYCOPLASMAL PNEUMONIA

*Mycoplasma pneumoniae* is probably the most common cause of pneumonia in school-age children and young adults who are free of chronic underlying conditions. It is rarely seen in infants but is occasionally present in preschool children and older adults. The agent has been responsible for indolent, smoldering epidemics that often begin in summer and peak in autumn. Cases may occur at any time of the year but are unusual from midwinter through spring.

The average incubation period, which usually includes prodromal symptoms, is 18 days. Onset of symptoms is gradual and starts with a scratchy sore throat and intermittent low-grade fever for a few days before a dry cough begins. Cough, malaise, and low-grade fever gradually become more persistent and severe during several more days. On examination of the chest, rales are usually present in both lower lobes, and the chest roentgenogram often shows bilateral patchy infiltrates, usually involving the lower lobes. Cold agglutinin titers of 1:32 or higher support the diagnosis of *M. pneumoniae* infection.

### Treatment

Most patients do not require hospitalization for treatment of mycoplasmal pneumonia. Both erythromycin and tetracycline are effective antibiotics. Erythromycin is preferred for children under 10 years of age because of the problem of tetracycline-caused staining of teeth in younger children. Either antibiotic can be used for older children and adults. Usually 7 days of therapy is adequate. Rest at home with plenty of fluids is usually adequate supportive care. Antitussives may be required in some cases, with attention to cautions mentioned earlier. Children with sickle cell disease when they are infected with *M. pneumoniae* may present with a clinical picture similar to that of an acute bacterial pneumonia, and this possibility should be kept in mind when patients with hemoglobinopathies develop pneumonia.

*M. pneumoniae* infection may be accompanied by nonpneumonic complications such as erythema multiforme, Stevens-Johnson syndrome, central nervous system disorders, and hematologic problems such as hemolysis and thrombocytopenia.

# LEGIONELLOSIS
## (Legionnaires' Disease and Pontiac Fever)
method of
GUODONG FANG, M.D.
*Peking Union Medical College*
*Beijing, China*

Legionellosis refers to the clinical syndromes produced by members of the Legionellaceae family. Eighteen species have been implicated in human disease, including *Legionella pneumophila*, *L. micdadei* (also called the Pittsburgh pneumonia agent), *L. bozemanii*, *L. dumoffii*, *L. longbeachae*, *L. jordanis*, *L. gormanii*, *L. feeleii*, *L. hackeliae*, *L. maceachernii*, *L. wadsworthii*, *L. birminghamensis*, *L. cincinnatiensis*, *L. oakridgensis*, *L. anisa*, *L. cherrii*, *L. sainthelensis*, and *L. tucsonensis*. These bacteria are ubiquitous in natural water and can be isolated from potable water systems and cooling towers. The source for most sporadic cases is unknown, whereas the epidemic breakouts have been readily linked to environmental water sources contaminated by *Legionella* species. The postulated modes of transmission include inhalation of aerosols, aspiration, and direct inoculation, but the precise mode of transmission for many patients remains uncertain.

## CLINICAL MANIFESTATIONS

Two forms of infection have been documented. The non-pneumonic type, Pontiac fever, is a flu-like syndrome, including fever, chills, headache, malaise, and myalgias, but without pneumonia. The symptoms resolve within several days without specific antibiotic therapy. Diagnosis is demonstrated by antibody seroconversion to the responsible *Legionella* species.

The second type, pneumonia, is the major and most common form of *Legionella* infection. Extrapulmonary infection, including endocarditis, pericarditis, and pyelonephritis, has been reported. Wound infections have been caused by contaminated water infecting wounds. Most *Legionella* pneumonias are caused by *L. pneumophila*, so-called legionnaires' disease. The incubation period is estimated to be 2 to 10 days after exposure.

The clinical symptoms and signs of *Legionella* pneumonia are generally nonspecific when compared with pneumonia of other etiologies, although gastrointestinal symptoms, especially diarrhea, are prominent. Hyponatremia occurs frequently and may be a helpful clue for diagnosis. The Gram's stain of sputum typically reveals many neutrophils but few, if any, bacteria.

Definitive diagnosis depends on specialized laboratory tests. The most reliable method is culture of respiratory tract secretions on selective media (buffered charcoal yeast extract agar with antimicrobial agents that inhibit competing bacteria and fungi). The optimal specimens are from transtracheal aspirates, but specimens can also be obtained via bronchoscopy.

Direct fluorescent antibody staining is a rapid method with visualization of the organisms in respiratory secretions, pleural fluid, and lung tissue. Serologic testing for antibody is more widely available, but fourfold seroconversion may require 4 to 8 weeks, making this test less useful to the clinician. Detection of *Legionella* antigen in urine, a sensitive and specific test, is commercially available for *L. pneumophila*, serogroup 1. DNA probe appears to be a potentially useful adjunct to culture.

## TREATMENT

*Legionella* is an intracellular parasite, and drugs that penetrate into cells, including eryth-romycin, rifampin, the tetracyclines, and the quinolones, have activity against *Legionella* in vitro and in vivo.

Erythromycin, 1 gram intravenously every 6 hours, is recommended as initial therapy for legionnaires' disease (Table 1). Our experience with a few patients who seemed to be initially stable but who deteriorated abruptly has led to the routine use of an intravenous regimen at the outset. Once a clinical response has been demonstrated (usually within 5 days), oral therapy may be substituted in a dose of 500 mg every 6 hours. The dosage of erythromycin should be decreased in patients with hepatic or renal failure to prevent ototoxicity. Relapse has been reported in immunocompromised patients; therefore, 3 weeks of therapy has been recommended for such patients. The side effects caused by erythromycin include nausea, vomiting, and hepatotoxicity. Ototoxicity occurs with the 4-grams-per-day dosing and is reversible when the drug is discontinued.

For patients who are immunocompromised, are critically ill, or show multilobar infiltrates on chest x-ray, I recommend the combination of intravenous erythromycin, 1 gram every 6 hours, and rifampin (Rifadin), 600 mg every 12 hours, as initial therapy.

The side effects of rifampin are mainly liver function abnormalities, especially hyperbilirubinemia. Rash, fever, leukopenia, hemolysis, and anemia are rarely seen if the duration of therapy is less than 2 weeks. Rifampin should never be used as sole therapy because of the possibility of emergence of resistant organisms.

The tetracyclines, including doxycycline (Vibramycin) and minocycline (Minocin), trimethoprim-sulfamethoxazole (Bactrim, Septra), ciprofloxacin (Cipro), and imipenem (Primaxin) have been effective in anecdotal cases.

TABLE 1. **Antibiotic Therapy
for Legionnaires' Disease**

| Antibiotic Therapy of Choice | Route | Dose |
|---|---|---|
| Erythromycin | IV | 1 gram q 6 hr |
| | PO | 500 mg q 6 hr |
| *Alternative Agents* | | |
| Rifampin* (Rifadin) | PO | 600 mg q 12 hr |
| | IV | 600 mg q 12 hr |
| Tetracycline (Sumycin, Achromycin-V) | PO | 0.5–1.0 gram q 6 hr |
| Trimethoprim-sulfamethoxazole (Bactrim, Septra) | IV | 160/800 mg q 8 hr |
| | PO | 160/800 mg q 12 hr |
| Doxycycline (Vibramycin) | PO | 100 mg q 12 hr |
| Minocycline (Minocin) | PO | 100 mg q 12 hr |
| Ciprofloxacin (Cipro) | PO | 750 mg q 12 hr |
| Imipenem (Primaxin) | IV | 500 mg q 6 hr |

*Must be used in combination with another agent.

## PROGNOSIS

The mortality of patients receiving erythromycin for treatment of community-acquired *Legionella* is low (about 10%), and is related to the severity of underlying illness and the timing of initiation of antibiotic therapy. Mortality in immunocompromised patients with nosocomial infection is substantially higher and may approach 40%.

The radiographic extent of pneumonia may worsen even in the face of appropriate antibiotic therapy, but this is not predictive of clinical failure. Small to moderate pleural effusions occur in one-third of patients and usually resolve spontaneously. Cavitation can be seen in patients receiving corticosteroids or immunosuppressive medications; these cavities usually resolve over time with appropriate antibiotic therapy.

## PREVENTION

*Legionella* colonization of a hospital water system may be linked to occurrence of nosocomial *Legionella* infection. I recommend routine environmental culturing for *Legionella* in hospitals with large numbers of transplant recipients. Several methods have been successfully used to decontaminate potable water systems, including temperature elevation of water to 60 to 70° C followed by flushing of distal sites (faucets, showerheads) with hot water, hyperchlorination, and ultraviolet light treatment.

Low-dose erythromycin or trimethoprim-sulfamethoxazole has been successfully used for prophylaxis for transplant patients in hospitals with endemic nosocomial legionnaires' disease, although such prophylaxis is not routinely recommended.

# PULMONARY EMBOLISM

method of
JACK HIRSH, M.D., and
DAVID R. ANDERSON, M.D.
*McMaster University*
*Hamilton, Ontario, Canada*

Pulmonary embolism is responsible for approximately 250,000 deaths per year in the USA. Most of these deaths occur in hospitalized patients, in whom pulmonary embolism is the most common preventable cause of death. The vast majority of pulmonary emboli arise from venous thrombi in the deep veins of the leg. Less frequently, clinically important pulmonary emboli arise from axillary or subclavian vein thrombosis, from an inferior vena caval thrombosis, or from a mural thrombus in the right side of the heart. Patients with a potential risk for developing venous thromboembolism can be classified as being at low, moderate, or high risk based on fairly well-defined and easily recognized clinical criteria. The risk of venous thromboembolism increases with age and is much more common in sick hospitalized patients than in otherwise healthy patients. The risk is also increased by prolonged immobilization, inflammation, malignant disease, lower limb or pelvic trauma or surgery, other major surgery, cardiac failure, or paralysis due to stroke or paraplegia.

## DIAGNOSIS

The clinical diagnosis of pulmonary embolism is non-specific. Consequently, more than half of all patients with clinically suspected pulmonary embolism do not have pulmonary embolism when pulmonary angiography is performed.

The chest radiograph is not specific for pulmonary embolism and may show no abnormality. It is very useful, however, since it may reveal other causes for the patient's condition (e.g., pneumothorax, acute pulmonary edema) and is required for the interpretation of the lung scan findings.

The ECG is frequently normal or non-specific, and the findings of right axis shift and $S_1$, $Q_3$, and $T_3$ pattern are uncommon and also non-specific.

Perfusion lung scanning is extremely useful because when it is normal it excludes a diagnosis of pulmonary embolism, and when there is a large perfusion defect (segmental or greater) with normal ventilation, the result can be used to diagnose pulmonary embolism. Other lung scan findings cannot be used to either rule out or rule in pulmonary embolism, and in these patients pulmonary angiography is often required to make a correct management decision. Objective tests for venous thrombosis are also useful because 70% of pulmonary emboli are associated with venographically detected deep vein thrombosis of the legs. However, because approximately 30% of patients with proven pulmonary embolism do not have detectable venous thrombosis, a diagnosis of pulmonary embolism cannot be ruled out on the basis of negative test results for venous thrombosis. An approach to the diagnosis of pulmonary embolism is summarized in Figure 1.

## PROPHYLAXIS

In the absence of prophylaxis, the frequency of postoperative fatal pulmonary embolism ranges from 0.1 to 0.8% in moderate-risk patients undergoing elective general surgery to 0.5 to 2.0% in patients undergoing elective hip surgery and 3 to 6% in patients undergoing emergency hip surgery for fractured hip. Prophylaxis against clinically important venous thromboembolism is available for most high-risk groups and is both effective and cost effective (Table 1).

Prophylaxis is directed at either suppressing activation of blood coagulation or increasing venous flow in leg veins. These objectives can be

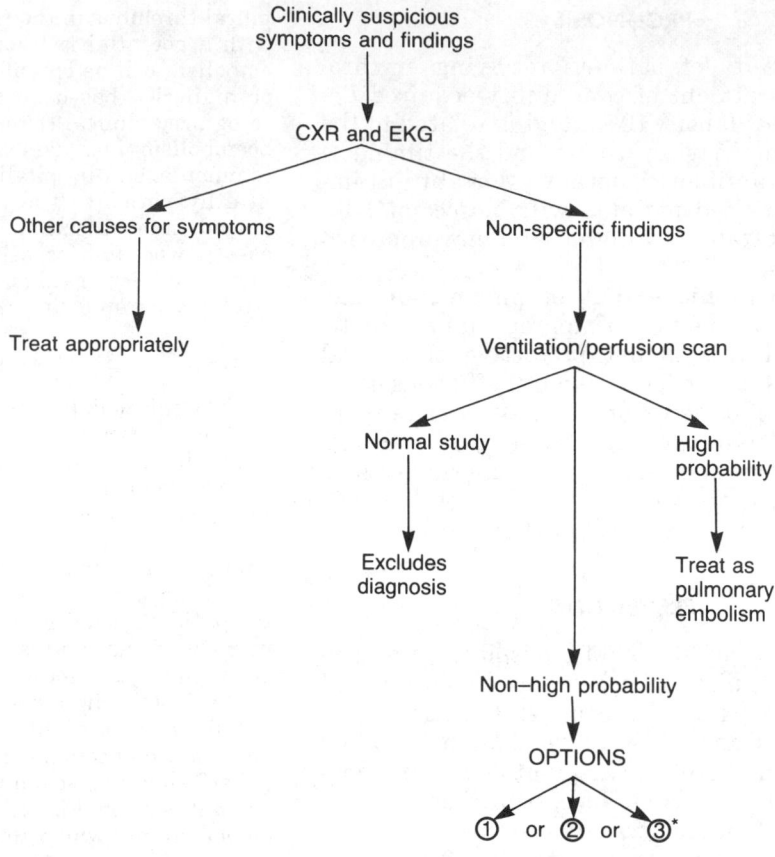

SEVERAL OPTIONS:
1. Pulmonary angiography.
2. Venogram—30% will have negative venogram.
3. Serial impedance plethysmograph over 10–14 days. If positive, venography; if negative, withhold anticoagulants.*

*This approach is experimental and is not recommended for patients with underlying cardiopulmonary disease or with a high clinical probability of pulmonary embolism.

**Figure 1.** Diagnosis of pulmonary embolism.

achieved by using one of the following prophylactic approaches: low-dose subcutaneous heparin, intermittent pneumatic compression of the legs, graduated compression stockings, intravenous dextran, oral anticoagulants, adjusted dose subcutaneous heparin, and low-molecular-weight heparins. The use of these prophylactic approaches in moderate-risk patients results in a 60 to 70% reduction of clinically important thromboembolic events. However, not all of these prophylactic approaches are equally effective in the very-high-risk patient. Oral anticoagulants, adjusted dose heparin, and low-molecular-weight heparins all appear to be highly effective in very-high-risk groups, and adjusted dose heparin and low-molecular-weight heparins reduce the risk of clinically important venous thromboembolism by approximately 70% in high-risk patients who undergo major orthopedic procedures.

## TREATMENT

The objectives of treating patients with pulmonary embolism are to prevent death from either the initial or recurrent pulmonary embolism, to prevent recurrent pulmonary embolism from the associated venous thrombosis, to reduce morbidity from the acute event, and to prevent thromboembolic hypertension.

### Preventing Death from Pulmonary Embolism

Untreated, patients with pulmonary embolism have a mortality rate of greater than 25%, which can be reduced markedly by appropriate treatment. The therapeutic approaches available for patients with pulmonary embolism are anticoagulants, thrombolytic agents, vena caval interruption, and pulmonary embolectomy. Anticoag-

TABLE 1. **Risk Categories for Venous Thromboembolism**

| Risk Category | Risk of Venous Thromboembolism (%) | | | Effective Prophylaxis |
| --- | --- | --- | --- | --- |
| | *Calf Vein Thrombosis* | *Proximal Vein Thrombosis* | *Fatal Pulmonary Embolism* | |
| *High Risk* | 40–80 | 10–20 | 1–5 | 1. Adjusted dose subcutaneous heparin |
| 1. General surgery in patients >40 yr with recent history of deep venous thrombosis or pulmonary embolism | | | | *or* |
| 2. Extensive pelvic or abdominal surgery for malignant disease | | | | 2. Low-molecular-weight heparin† |
| 3. Major orthopedic surgery of lower limbs | | | | *or* |
| | | | | 3. Sodium warfarin (Coumadin) adjusted to keep International Normalized Ratio at 2.0–3.0, starting treatment on the first postoperative day |
| *Moderate Risk* * | 10–40 | 2–10 | 0.1–0.7 | 1. Subcutaneous heparin 5000 U bid |
| 1. General surgery in patients >40 yr lasting 30 min or more | | | | *and/or* |
| 2. Immobilization with major medical illness, including stroke, cardiac disease, chronic respiratory disease, bowel disease, and malignancy | | | | 2. Compression leg stockings |

*Risk is increased by advancing age, malignancy, prolonged immobility, varicose veins, and cardiac failure.
†Approved for use in a number of European countries but not approved in Canada or the USA.

ulants prevent the growth of the associated venous thrombosis and by so doing prevent recurrent pulmonary embolism. In addition, anticoagulants prevent thrombotic extension of the existing pulmonary embolism. Anticoagulants are highly effective in preventing death and recurrent embolism in patients with pulmonary embolism. Most patients who present with pulmonary embolism are clinically stable. The mortality rate in patients with pulmonary embolism who are treated with heparin in adequate doses and who are hemodynamically stable at the time of presentation is less than 5%. However, the mortality rate is approximately 20% in patients who have persistent hypotension due to major pulmonary embolism.

Vena caval interruption prevents recurrent pulmonary embolism by intercepting emboli that arise in the deep veins of the legs or pelvis. Vena caval interruption, usually with a Greenfield filter, is considered when anticoagulant therapy is contraindicated because of the risk of serious hemorrhage. Vena caval interruption is also indicated in the small percentage of patients who experience recurrent pulmonary embolism despite an adequate anticoagulant dose and response.

Thrombolytic therapy accelerates the dissolution of pulmonary emboli and so has the potential to prevent death in the hemodynamically com-

promised patient who would otherwise have not survived the many hours or days required for spontaneous thrombolysis. Thrombolytic therapy with streptokinase, urokinase, or tissue plasminogen activator is more effective than heparin alone in correcting the angiographic and perfusion scan defects produced by pulmonary emboli and may be more effective than heparin in preventing death in patients with shock due to massive pulmonary embolism. Thrombolytic therapy is recommended in hemodynamically compromised patients with massive pulmonary embolism and in patients with submassive embolism with underlying cardiac or pulmonary disease in whom even a small or moderate embolus may be life-threatening.

Surgical removal of the embolus by pulmonary embolectomy has the potential to rapidly restore the obstructed pulmonary circulation, but this procedure requires open heart surgery and may be difficult to organize on an urgent basis. Because the surgery is major and the patient unstable, the procedure itself carries considerable risk. For these reasons, urgent pulmonary embolectomy is usually restricted to patients with a saddle embolism lodged in the main pulmonary artery or in patients with massive embolism whose blood pressure cannot be maintained despite thrombolytic therapy and vasopressor agents.

Pulmonary thromboendarterectomy relieves chronic thromboembolic obstruction in patients with thromboembolic pulmonary hypertension who have proximal pulmonary arterial obstruction. In recent years, this procedure has been found to be effective in selected patients with chronic thromboembolic pulmonary hypertension.

### Anticoagulant Therapy

Anticoagulant therapy with heparin followed by sodium warfarin (Coumadin) is the mainstay of treatment for most patients with venous thromboembolism. Most information on the effectiveness of heparin has come from clinical trials in patients with venous thrombosis. However, the results of these studies are directly applicable to most patients with pulmonary embolism.

Heparin can be given by continuous intravenous infusion, by intermittent intravenous injection, or by subcutaneous injection. Heparin is equally safe and effective when administered by continuous infusion or by high-dose subcutaneous injection. In one study in which thrombosis recurrence was more common in the group treated with subcutaneous heparin, the initial dose of subcutaneous heparin was subtherapeutic in the majority of patients randomized to this group. When heparin is administered by the intravenous route, less bleeding occurs with continuous intravenous infusion than with intermittent intravenous injection. The incidence of clinically important recurrence is less than 5% and that of clinically important bleeding is between 5% and 10% when heparin is administered by either continuous intravenous infusion or subcutaneous injection.

Heparin has a half-life that varies considerably among individuals. After a single intravenous injection, there is an initial rapid disappearance as a result of a saturable clearance mechanism followed by a more gradual linear clearance with a mean heparin half-life of approximately 60 minutes. Intravenous heparin has an immediate anticoagulant effect, and when administered as a single bolus this effect lasts for 3 to 5 hours, depending on the dose. High-dose subcutaneous heparin injections produce a measurable heparin effect in 1 to 2 hours, and peak heparin levels are usually obtained at approximately 3 hours; the effect of subcutaneous heparin injections may last for 12 hours or more, depending on the dose.

The anticoagulant response to heparin varies considerably from patient to patient. Therefore, in order to achieve an adequate effect the amount of heparin administered must be monitored by an appropriate laboratory test.

Tests used to monitor heparin therapy include global tests of blood coagulation such as the activated clotting time and the activated partial thromboplastin time (APTT), and heparin assays that measure the interaction of heparin with either thrombin or activated Factor X. The responsiveness of APTT reagents to heparin varies from reagent to reagent. Therefore, for individual batches of APTT reagents, the responsiveness should be established by adding heparin to normal pooled plasma and determining the range of APTT ratios that correspond to a heparin level of 0.2 to 0.4 U per ml (using a protamine titration thrombin clotting time assay) or to a heparin level of 0.3 to 0.7 U per ml using a chromogenic anti–Factor Xa assay. For many of the reagents in present use, the therapeutic range for the APTT is a ratio of 1 1/2 to twice the mean laboratory control value. The mean dose of heparin administered by intravenous infusion that is required to produce a heparin effect in the therapeutic range is approximately 30,000 U per 24 hours. The mean heparin dose is about 10% higher if heparin is administered by high-dose subcutaneous injection. Approximately 70% of patients achieve therapeutic heparin levels with heparin doses of between 25,000 and 35,000 U per 24 hours. There is good evidence that the risk of recurrent thromboembolism is influenced by the patient's anticoagulant response and that clinically important recurrence is less than 5% if the APTT is maintained in the therapeutic range.

Patients treated with heparin by continuous intravenous infusion are given a bolus of 5000 to 10,000 U followed by continuous infusion of 30,000 U per 24 hours. The APTT should be performed approximately 6 hours after the bolus injection, at which time the heparin response reflects the effect of the continuous intravenous infusion. The test used to monitor heparin therapy should then be repeated once more in the first 24 hours and then twice daily until an appropriate heparin dose is determined. Thereafter, the test used to monitor heparin therapy can be performed once daily.

If heparin is given by subcutaneous injection, it should be given twice daily and the dose adjusted according to the result of the monitoring test, which is performed 6 hours after each injection. The heparin dose should be adjusted to produce a heparin response in the middle of a therapeutic range 6 hours after each injection. Monitoring should be performed twice daily until the appropriate dose is determined and then once daily.

It has been common practice to administer heparin for a period of 7 to 10 days, to start oral anticoagulants after 4 to 5 days, and to overlap heparin with oral anticoagulants for 4 to 5 days.

This approach has recently been challenged by a study in patients with venous thrombosis and submassive pulmonary embolism that demonstrated that 9 days of heparin with a 4-day warfarin overlap was not superior to 4 days of heparin with 4 days of overlapping warfarin. The rationale for a period of overlap between heparin treatment and oral anticoagulants is based on experimental studies demonstrating a delay before the antithrombotic effects of oral anticoagulants are expressed, and on the short circulating half-life of protein C, a natural vitamin K–dependent anticoagulant. This rapid reduction in protein C levels results in the potential for the early anticoagulant effect of warfarin to be counteracted by the prothrombotic effect of low levels of protein C. Thus, by overlapping heparin and warfarin for 4 days, the early prothrombotic state is neutralized by the anticoagulant effect of heparin.

Patients with proximal vein thrombosis and with pulmonary embolism require continuing anticoagulant therapy after hospital discharge to prevent recurrent episodes. There is good evidence that 3 months of treatment with either oral anticoagulants or adjusted dose subcutaneous heparin is effective in preventing recurrent thromboembolism in patients with proximal vein thrombosis, and because the majority of patients with pulmonary embolism have proximal vein thrombosis, it would seem reasonable to treat these patients for at least 3 months. The use of oral anticoagulants is more convenient and less expensive than subcutaneous heparin. If oral anticoagulants are used, the dose should be adjusted to maintain the prothrombin time (PT) ratio at 1.3 to 1.5 using a North American thromboplastin (International Normalized Ratio [INR] of 2.0 to 3.0).

An alternative approach to oral anticoagulants is the use of adjusted dose subcutaneous heparin on an outpatient basis. With this regimen, heparin is given twice daily with subcutaneous injection and the dose adjusted to maintain the APTT 6 hours at the lower therapeutic range (APTT 1 1/2 times control, heparin level 0.2 U per ml). The heparin regimen is particularly convenient if there is difficulty in laboratory monitoring because of geographic inaccessibility, since the dose can be adjusted in hospital and the patient sent home without further monitoring. The use of subcutaneous heparin is also the treatment of choice for patients who require out-of-hospital anticoagulant therapy and who are pregnant.

### Thrombolytic Therapy

Thrombolytic therapy with streptokinase, urokinase, and tissue plasminogen activator has been shown to be effective in producing early lysis of acute pulmonary embolism. None of the studies using thrombolytic therapy have been large enough to have the power to demonstrate clinically important differences in mortality when a thrombolytic agent is compared with heparin. Thrombolytic therapy should not be used in all patients with acute pulmonary embolism, since most will recover uneventfully if treated with anticoagulants. However, based on available evidence, it would be reasonable to use thrombolytic therapy in patients who have no contraindications, if they have massive embolism or submassive embolism with evidence of circulatory collapse, syncope, or acute cor pulmonale. The dosage regimens used for the three thrombolytic agents are shown in Table 2.

Thrombolytic therapy with streptokinase and urokinase is administered for 12 to 24 hours, whereas thrombolytic therapy with tissue plasminogen activator is administered for 2 hours. Thrombolytic therapy should be followed by heparin and oral anticoagulants.

Bleeding occurs more frequently with thrombolytic therapy than with heparin. The risk of hemorrhage increases with the duration of thrombolytic infusion and usually occurs at a site of previous surgery or trauma. Intracranial hemorrhage occurs in approximately 1% of patients treated with thrombolytic therapy, about twice as frequently as with heparin treatment. Costs associated with thrombolytic therapy are greater than with heparin, but cost would not be an important consideration if thrombolytic therapy reduces mortality from pulmonary embolism.

### Treatment of Other Complications of Pulmonary Embolism

**Pain.** Pleuritic chest pain may be severe in some patients with pulmonary embolism. Pain should be controlled with regular analgesia. Pain control improves patient comfort and improves oxygenation by facilitating deep breathing and thus reducing the risk of atelectasis. Acetaminophen with codeine given every 4 hours usually provides adequate pain relief. The dose of the medication can gradually be tapered after 48 to 72 hours as the discomfort begins to subside.

**Hypoxemia.** Hypoxemia occurs commonly in patients with large pulmonary emboli. Hypoxic patients frequently have "air hunger" and may become confused and agitated. Hypoxia also leads to an increase in pulmonary hypertension and may lead to arrhythmias, especially in patients with underlying cardiopulmonary disease. For these reasons, continuous oxygen therapy is recommended in all hypoxic patients with acute

TABLE 2. **Recommended Doses for Thrombolytic Therapy***

1. *Streptokinase:* The standard regimen for streptokinase therapy is 250,000 U as a loading dose over 20–30 min followed by a continuous infusion of 100,000 U/hr for 24 hr.

2. *Urokinase:* Different dosing schedules of urokinase have been used. One approach is to give 4400 U/kg/hr as a bolus followed by a continuous infusion of 4400 U/kg/hr for 12 hr.

3. *Tissue plasminogen activator (tPA):* Experience with this agent in the treatment of pulmonary embolism is limited. Optimal dosage regimens are under investigation. One effective approach is 100 mg of tPA as a continuous infusion over 2 hr.

*Heparin should be started without a bolus after the partial thromboplastin time (PTT) falls below twice the control value.

pulmonary emboli. Oxygen can be administered intranasally or by a face mask; the latter method is more effective but less comfortable for the patient. Oxygen saturation should be measured regularly by ear or finger oximetry in hypoxic patients. Oxygen administration should be adjusted to ensure an arterial oxygen saturation of at least 90%.

**Hypotension.** Hypotension may occur with massive pulmonary embolism or in patients with submassive pulmonary emboli who have serious underlying cardiorespiratory disease. The mortality rate of this subgroup of patients is high with anticoagulant therapy, and thrombolytic therapy should be strongly considered. Intravenous fluid should be used liberally initially, and the patient nursed in the Trendelenburg position. If a fluid challenge does not improve the blood pressure, vasopressor agents are indicated. Emergency embolectomy should be considered only in patients who fail to respond to aggressive medical management including thrombolytic therapy.

### Prevention of Late Effects of Pulmonary Embolism

It is unknown whether thrombolytic therapy for acute pulmonary emboli prevents the development of thromboembolic pulmonary hypertension. In the randomized trials comparing heparin with either streptokinase or urokinase in patients with acute pulmonary embolism, follow-up serial lung scanning performed at 2 weeks, 3 months, and 1 year after treatment demonstrated no apparent difference in the rate of lysis between heparin and thrombolytic agents after the first week of treatment. A subsequent study in a subgroup of these patients reported that pulmonary capillary blood volume and pulmonary diffusion lung capacity were significantly better at 2 weeks and at 1 year in patients treated with thrombolytic therapy than in those treated with heparin. However, the clinical significance of these pulmonary function findings is unknown.

Most patients who survive the initial episode of acute pulmonary embolism make a full recovery. However, a small proportion develop thromboembolic pulmonary hypertension. Thromboembolic pulmonary hypertension may be more common in patients with underlying chronic heart or lung disease or in patients who sustain recurrent pulmonary embolism, but in most instances pulmonary hypertension is insidious in onset and there are no obvious predisposing factors. When a diagnosis of thromboembolic pulmonary hypertension is made, the patients should be treated with long-term anticoagulant therapy. Most patients show a steady deterioration and will die unless the obstruction is relieved.

There has been a renewed interest in performing pulmonary thromboendarterectomy in patients with chronic thromboembolic pulmonary hypertension. The selection of appropriate patients has been improved by the preoperative use of pulmonary artery angioscopy, and postoperative complications due to reperfusion non-cardiac pulmonary edema have been markedly reduced by the use of high-dose preoperative corticosteroids. The results of pulmonary thromboendarterectomy in a fairly large series of patients with thromboembolic pulmonary hypertension have been encouraging, although it should be stressed that potential candidates should be carefully screened to ensure that they have an operative lesion (e.g., that the obstruction is proximal), and even with improved perioperative care the mortality rate from the procedure is still high.

### Practical Recommendations

The majority of patients with pulmonary embolism should be treated with high-dose heparin followed by oral anticoagulant therapy for 3 months. High-dose heparin should be given by continuous intravenous infusion. Therapy should be initiated with a bolus injection of 5000 to 10,000 U of heparin. The initial dose of continuous intravenous heparin should be 30,000 U per 24 hours. Heparin should be administered for 5 to 10 days and oral anticoagulants commenced after 96 hours of commencing heparin.

The dose of heparin should be adjusted to maintain the APTT at 1.5 to 2.0 times control. The dose of warfarin should be adjusted to maintain the PT at an INR of 2.0 to 3.0 (equivalent to a

PT of 1.3 to 1.5 using a typical North American thromboplastin).

Indefinite anticoagulant therapy should be considered for patients with continuing risk factors or those with recurrent venous thromboembolism.

Thrombolytic therapy is indicated in patients with clinically major embolism in whom there are no contraindications. Inferior vena caval interruption should be reserved for patients in whom anticoagulants are contraindicated or who suffer recurrent pulmonary embolism despite adequate anticoagulant therapy.

# SARCOIDOSIS

method of
ALVIN S. TEIRSTEIN, M.D.
*The Mount Sinai Medical Center*
*New York, New York*

Sarcoidosis is a multi-system granulomatous disease. The diagnosis rests on demonstration of non-caseating epithelioid granulomas with no identifiable cell or inciting agent, in a patient with a compatible clinical picture. In institutions where interest in the disease is great, diagnostic specific Kveim-Siltzbach skin test material is produced. Because sarcoidosis can affect any tissue, the clinical presentations and indications for therapy vary greatly. The most commonly affected organs that require treatment are the lungs, eyes, skin, liver, spleen, heart, neuromuscular systems, bones, joints, and lymph nodes; also seen is the syndrome of hypercalcemia with its attendant renal complications.

## TREATMENT

It must be emphasized that most patients with sarcoidosis will not require treatment. Of the more than 9000 patients in the sarcoidosis registry at the Mount Sinai Medical Center, New York, only 25% have been treated. The cornerstone for treatment of any affected organ is an oral adrenocorticosteroid, usually prednisone. The regimen we employ is as follows:

Prednisone, 30 mg daily for first month
Prednisone, 20 mg daily for second month
Prednisone, 35 mg every other day for third month
Decrements of 5 mg every other day each month thereafter

Most patients will require treatment for 9 to 18 months.

Many patients receiving prednisone will experience disease rebound, usually when the dose is less than 20 mg every other day, or up to 6 months after completion of treatment. Rarely, sarcoidosis may exacerbate after years of quiescence. Exacerbations are much more common after cessation of prednisone than after spontaneous disease remissions.

Chloroquine, 250 mg twice daily, or hydroxychloroquine (Plaquenil), 200 mg twice daily, has been effective in treating cutaneous sarcoidosis and hypercalcemia. With these medications, surveillance every 6 months for retinal toxicity is necessary, but the complications are far less severe than those of prednisone. There have been sporadic reports of the efficacy of methotrexate, 5 to 10 mg a week, or chlorambucil (Leukeran), 8 mg daily, in patients who have failed steroid therapy. When one prescribes these cytotoxic medications, complete blood counts must be monitored.

Many other therapies have also been recommended. However, it must be emphasized that it is very difficult to evaluate the results of treatment objectively in a disease that spontaneously clears in the majority of patients.

### Indications

**Pulmonary Sarcoidosis.** Sarcoidosis usually presents with a typical chest x-ray pattern: Stage I—hilar and right paratracheal lymph node enlargement and clear lung fields; Stage II—Stage I plus symmetrical pulmonary infiltrations; and Stage III—pulmonary infiltrations alone. The x-ray of patients with chronic pulmonary infiltrations may exhibit signs of fibrosis. These are frequently classified as Stage II and IIIb or Stage IV. The treatment of pulmonary sarcoidosis remains controversial. Should physicians treat symptoms, radiographic abnormalities, or pulmonary dysfunction? The single best guide is function studies, but persisting pulmonary infiltrations must also be considered. Our scheme for therapy of pulmonary sarcoidosis is outlined in Table 1.

TABLE 1. **Scheme for Therapy of Pulmonary Sarcoidosis**

| Duration | Chest X-Ray Stage | Pulmonary Function Test | Treatment |
|---|---|---|---|
| >6 mo | I | VC and/or $FEV_1$ > 70% | None |
| <6 mo | II, III | VC and/or $FEV_1$ > 70% | None |
| >6 mo | II, III | VC and/or $FEV_1$ > 70% | Prednisone |
| <6 mo | II, III | VC and/or $FEV_1$ < 70% | Prednisone |

*Abbreviations:* VC = vital capacity; $FEV_1$ = forced expiratory volume in 1 second.

Briefly, prednisone therapy is indicated for pulmonary sarcoidosis if the vital capacity (VC) and/or the forced expiratory volume in 1 second (FEV$_1$) is less than 70% of predicted and/or if radiographic stage II or III chest x-ray pattern persists for more than 6 months. Prednisone is rarely, if ever, indicated for radiographic stage I disease alone. Fortunately, most studies confirm that symptoms parallel pulmonary function. Symptoms without significant pulmonary dysfunction are rarely indications for treatment.

**Ocular Sarcoidosis.** All patients with sarcoidosis should have yearly slit lamp examinations. Blindness due to sarcoidosis occurred prior to institution of steroid treatment. Today, almost all patients with uveitis can be successfully controlled with steroid eye drops.

**Cutaneous Sarcoidosis.** Erythema nodosum is a non-specific vasculitis involving the skin in a variety of conditions such as streptococcal infections and drug reactions as well as sarcoidosis. This non-granulomatous skin lesion and its frequently accompanying ankle arthritis are almost always controlled with non-steroidal anti-inflammatory agents such as aspirin, ibuprofen, and indomethacin.

Granulomatous involvement of the skin is a major manifestation of chronic sarcoidosis and predictably will require prolonged treatment. For this reason, chloroquine is the first drug of choice. Relapses are very common. Some patients, particularly those with disfiguring facial lesions such as lupus pernio, will require prednisone, orally or by direct injection into the skin lesion.

**Hypercalcemia and Hypercalciuria.** Hypercalcemia can cause nausea, vomiting, muscle weakness, renal calcinosis, renal calculi, and renal failure. Low calcium diet and chloroquine have been successful in restoring normal calcium levels. If the patient is acutely ill, prednisone will effect a rapid reduction in serum calcium with clearing of symptoms and improvement in renal function.

**Cardiac Sarcoidosis.** Cardiac sarcoidosis occurs with two major clinical presentations: (1) tachy-bradyarrhythmias and (2) cardiomyopathy.

Tachybradyarrhythmias are common in sarcoidosis. Most are benign and asymptomatic. Occasionally patients will experience severe palpitations due to tachyarrhythmia and syncope due to heart block. These patients respond poorly to steroid treatment and are best treated with antiarrhythmic agents (quinidine, verapamil, and procainamide) for tachycardia and permanent pacemaker for heart block. Cardiomyopathy due to granulomatous involvement of the heart muscle leads to decreased ventricular function, reduced ejection fraction, and chronic congestive heart failure. Prednisone plus inotropic agents is

indicated. Unfortunately, the response to treatment is poor and many of these patients will die. They may be candidates for heart or heart-lung transplantation.

**Neuromuscular Sarcoidosis.** Neuromuscular sarcoidosis presents with a variety of syndromes, with facial palsy the most common. Involvement of other cranial nerves, hypothalamic-induced diabetes insipidus, seizures, and skeletal muscle myopathy occur. Prednisone, occasionally in doses as high as 60 mg per day for prolonged periods, is the best treatment.

**Hepatosplenic Sarcoidosis.** Every patient with sarcoidosis has granulomatous invasion of the liver and spleen. This is usually manifested as enlargement of these organs with elevation of alkaline phosphatase (sometimes to quite high levels), minimal elevations in aspartate aminotransferase (AST) and alanine aminotransferase (ALT), WBC 3000 to 4000 per ml, mild anemia, and thrombocytopenia. On occasion, a patient with hepatic sarcoidosis will experience high fevers and progress to liver failure. Prednisone is the drug of choice for severe hypersplenism and hepatic failure or fever. Elevated enzymes and alkaline phosphatase, in themselves, are not indications for prednisone therapy. Very rarely, portal hypertension with bleeding esophageal varices occurs, requiring surgical intervention. Hypersplenism may be so severe and unresponsive to prednisone that splenectomy is required.

**Lacrimal Gland, Parotid Gland, and Lymph Node Enlargement.** Occasionally, the salivary glands and lymph nodes become so enlarged that they are cosmetically unacceptable to the patient. For these less than absolute indications for treatment, a trial of chloroquine for at least 6 weeks should be attempted before employing prednisone therapy.

### Laboratory Tests as Diagnostic Aids and Guides to Therapy

During the past decade, serum angiotensin converting enzyme (SACE) levels, bronchoalveolar lavage (BAL) cell count differentials, and $^{67}$gallium citrate ($^{67}$Ga) radionuclide scans have

TABLE 2. **Clinical Applications of SACE, BAL, and $^{67}$Ga Scan**

|  | SACE | BAL | $^{67}$Ga |
|---|---|---|---|
| Diagnostic | No | No | May locate biopsy site |
| Therapeutic guide | No | No | May indicate persisting activity |

*Abbreviations:* SACE = serum angiotensin converting enzyme; BAL = bronchoalveolar lavage; $^{67}$Ga = $^{67}$gallium citrate.

been touted as important diagnostic aids and therapeutic guides in sarcoidosis.

**SACE.** SACE is elevated in 50 to 70% of all patients with sarcoidosis. SACE is also elevated in a variety of other, non-sarcoidal diseases. Thus, SACE is not a diagnostic test. Most, but not all, patients with active sarcoidosis will exhibit an elevated SACE. Many of these patients will be asymptomatic with normal organ function. An elevated SACE, by itself, is not an indication for treatment of sarcoidosis.

**BAL.** BAL cell count differentials reveal an elevated percentage of $CD_4$ (helper) T lymphocytes in most but not all patients with active sarcoidosis. BAL lymphocytosis may be found in other non-sarcoidal diseases. Thus, BAL is not diagnostic for sarcoidosis. Some authorities suggest repeating BAL to monitor the results of therapy. However, the eventual patient outcome is not related to BAL results. BAL is expensive and uncomfortable. Therefore, BAL is not a practical therapeutic guide for sarcoidosis.

**$^{67}$Ga.** The radioisotope $^{67}$gallium is picked up by active granulomas, such as those in sarcoidosis. In the rare patient in whom the $^{67}$Ga scan demonstrates simultaneous activity in the lacrimal and parotid glands and hilar and right paratracheal lymph nodes, the scan is diagnostic for sarcoidosis. For the majority of patients, there is no indication for routine use of the $^{67}$Ga scan. $^{67}$Ga scanning is most valuable in evaluating patients with chronic pulmonary sarcoidosis whose chest x-ray suggests severe fibrosis. A positive $^{67}$Ga scan may indicate the presence of active granulomas, which may respond to prednisone therapy. Occasionally, the $^{67}$Ga scan may locate an active site in the lungs or elsewhere, which may be biopsied for diagnosis.

The clinical applications of SACE, BAL, and $^{67}$Ga scan are summarized in Table 2.

# SILICOSIS

method of
DOUGLAS SEATON, M.D.
*The Ipswich Hospital*
*Suffolk, England*

Silica, or silicon dioxide, is the most abundant mineral constituent of the earth's crust. As such, it exists in different physical forms, the most common being quartz. Silicosis is a mineral dust disease, or pneumoconiosis, that is caused by inhalation of particles of silica of respirable size. Casual contact with silica dust is insufficient to cause the disease, which requires continued exposure that may arise in the occupations indicated in Table 1. Miners, tunnelers, and quarry

**TABLE 1. Some Occupations and Industries Associated with a Risk of Silicosis**

| | |
|---|---|
| Mining | Manufacture of |
| Tunneling | Silica flour |
| Quarrying | Pottery and ceramics |
| Stone masonry | Glass and enamel |
| Foundry working | Silica-based abrasives |
| Sandblasting | Refractory bricks |

workers whose excavations involve the removal of quartz-bearing rock such as sandstone, granite, and slate are at risk, as are workers who cut, crush, finish, or clean such stone. The mouldings used for castings in foundries are made from bonded sand, and the heat of the molten metal that is poured into them produces a fused silica compound that is polished off the casting, a task known as fettling. Fettlers and other foundry workers may also be exposed to silica dust when replacing the silica brick linings of furnaces and kilns. These so-called refractory bricks are produced from sandstone, and persons involved in their manufacture may also develop silicosis. The ceramic industry has traditionally used quantities of silica-containing substances such as crushed flint for the manufacture of china and earthenware pottery, although modern substitutes are now being found. Sandblasting involves the production of a high-speed jet of finely ground sand used for cleaning stone and polishing metal. Safe substitutes such as carborundum are available, and the practice of sandblasting has long been illegal in the European Community but may still be practiced in parts of the United States. Finely ground silica, known as silica flour, may be encountered in the manufacture and use of a wide range of substances including polishes, scouring powders, and toothpaste; it is also used as a filler in rubber and plastics. The glass and enamel industries make use of sand and quartz in polishing or as a component.

## CATEGORIZATION AND CLINICAL COURSE

The usual form of silicosis occurs after years of exposure to siliceous dust in an occupational setting and is termed "chronic." The condition is frequently unaccompanied by symptoms or signs and may declare itself only as a chance finding on a routine chest radiograph. At an early stage, various numbers of small nodular opacities are seen in the upper and middle zones of the lungs. This radiographic appearance is similar to that found in simple coal workers' pneumoconiosis (CWP), although the opacities in silicosis tend to get larger as time passes even though exposure may have ceased. The opacities, as well as tending to be larger (3 to 10 mm in diameter), are more dense than those in CWP, and calcification of small nodules may be seen. "Simple" chronic silicosis may progress, so that numbers of small opacities aggregate to form larger, more conglomerate shadows. When such opacities exceed a diameter of 1 cm on the radiograph, the condition is referred to as "complicated" chronic silicosis, and progressive massive fibrosis (PMF) is said to be occurring. Such larger opacities, which sometimes cavitate, are associated with fibrosis and distortion of surrounding lung with compensatory emphysema and bullae formation. Pleural thickening is sometimes found, as is so-called eggshell calcification of the hilar lymph nodes, a radiographic sign that is almost pathognomonic of silicosis, although it also rarely occurs in sarcoidosis.

Although there is little functional abnormality in simple chronic silicosis, except perhaps when the small opacities are profuse, silicotic PMF is associated with a mixed restrictive and obstructive impairment of ventilatory capacity and a reduction of diffusing capacity ($DL_{CO}$). These measurable impairments of lung function are matched by exertional dyspnea, which is often accompanied by cough and production of sputum. Further disease progression may result in respiratory failure with pulmonary hypertension and right-sided heart failure, although such advanced disease is now rare except in settings where dust control legislation does not exist or has been blatantly ignored. Chronic silicosis has a protracted time course lasting many years, but a heavier occupational exposure over a few years may produce a similar but more rapid clinical and radiographic progression that is termed "accelerated silicosis." Heavy occupational exposure to silica dust for a few weeks or months may produce an even more aggressive form of disease called "acute silicosis." In acute silicosis the history is one of accelerating breathlessness and cough, usually culminating in respiratory failure within months. Rather than showing the nodular pattern of chronic silicosis, the chest radiograph shows more diffuse shadowing, often in the middle or lower zones, that may be confused with pulmonary edema or bronchopneumonia if the patient's occupation is overlooked.

The course of silicosis may be complicated by tuberculosis, several epidemiologic surveys having established that this infection is more common in patients with silicosis than in matched control populations. This situation probably exists because the main defense against *Mycobacterium tuberculosis* in the lungs is provided by macrophages, for which silica particles are highly toxic. It follows that this complication is likely to be particularly evident in populations in which tuberculosis is endemic, probably as a result of reactivation of old primary infection. A high index of suspicion is advised in advanced silicosis, in which the cavitation of PMF may be tuberculous rather than ischemic and in which soft-looking infiltrates may be part of a tuberculous process, which requires repeated and regular examination and culture of sputum for diagnosis. Opportunistic mycobacterial infections may also occur in endemic areas, *Mycobacterium avium–intracellulare* and *Mycobacterium kansasii* being important pathogens for patients with silicosis in the southeastern United States. Other complications include pneumothorax, which may occur in any disease associated with fibrosis and bullae formation, and scleroderma, which has been reported to occur with increased frequency in silicosis.

## PATHOLOGY

The physicochemical processes by which silica exerts its toxic effects in lung tissue are poorly understood.

Crystals of quartz are known to be cytotoxic for lung macrophages that ingest them and cause cellular disruption with release of proteases and other inflammatory and fibrogenic factors. The resultant inflammation causes a characteristic histopathologic response, the hallmark of which is the silicotic nodule, an "onion skin" arrangement of hyalinized collagen, reticulin, and fibroblasts that arises close to respiratory bronchioles and pulmonary arterioles. Both the bronchioles and arterioles may be involved and destroyed as the fibrosis progresses. Particles of silica may be demonstrated in the periphery of these nodules by using polarized light and x-ray defraction techniques, but, in an apparent paradox, the amount of silica demonstrated bears no clear relationship to the extent of the fibrotic reaction found. PMF results in large areas of diffuse and coalescent fibrosis surrounded by silicotic nodules. These lesions may cavitate as a result of avascular necrosis. Although the pathology of accelerated silicosis is primarily similar to that of chronic silicosis, the pathology of acute silicosis is quite different, silicotic nodules being either absent or few in number, the alveolar walls containing a mixed inflammatory cell infiltrate, and the alveolar spaces being filled with thick eosinophilic material that gives a positive periodic acid-Schiff stain reaction. A positive reaction is also found in pulmonary alveolar proteinosis, from which acute silicosis may be histologically distinguished by the presence of interstitial pneumonitis. Macroscopically, the lungs in chronic silicosis are pigmented, with areas of pleural fibrosis and adhesions. The hilar nodes are often enlarged and the cut surface of the lung contains hard, fibrotic nodules. PMF is characterized by coalescence of these lesions, and cavitation may be present.

## PREVENTION

Avoidance of exposure to respirable silica dust prevents silicosis, and national and international health agencies are concerned first with making employers and workers aware of the hazards and, when a suitable alternative substance cannot be found, with promoting acceptance of an acceptable and enforceable dust standard. The standard of 100 μg per m$^3$ of respirable quartz, although not ideal, is likely to prevent most severe disease. Dust is removed from the environment by enclosure of processes, by good ventilation, and by use of water suppression where appropriate. When this standard cannot be achieved despite these measures, appropriate breathing equipment (including a suit, headgear, and an isolated supply of clean respirable air) should be provided for the worker. In addition to dust control measures, workers in at risk occupations should be protected by evaluation of chest radiographs, taken at not more than intervals of 4 years, so that early radiographic change can be detected and appropriate measures taken to prevent further exposure. Early radiographic changes that have taken many years of exposure to become manifest are not likely to result in much further deterioration, whereas similar changes that have arisen as a result of relatively short but heavier exposure are likely to continue apace with serious consequences for the patient. Acute silicosis is usually fatal within a matter of a few months.

## MANAGEMENT

No treatment influences the progress of silicosis once it has developed, and the usual symptomatic measures include antibiotics for the control of acute respiratory infection, bronchodilators if airflow is limited, oxygen when hypoxemia supervenes, and diuretics in right-sided heart failure. Various other, more specific attempts at treatment have been tried with negative or inconclusive results. These include the inhalation of aluminum powder and the use of D-penicillamine or corticosteroids. A negatively charged polymer, polyvinyl pyridine-$N$-oxide, when inhaled or injected, may prevent silicic acid from bonding with surface components of lung macrophages and has been shown to protect experimental animals from the effects of silica. It has, however, also been found to be carcinogenic in animals. Whole-lung bronchial lavage has been attempted in acute silicosis but is not known to alter the dismal prognosis of this disease, in which the only present hope of prolonging life may be lung transplantation.

Pulmonary tuberculosis complicating silicosis should be treated according to standard therapeutic guidelines. The earliest effective drug regimens appeared to control tuberculosis about as well in patients with silicosis as in those without the disease. Although controlled trials of modern short-course antituberculous drugs are not available for silicosis, these drugs have nevertheless been shown to be effective in tuberculous patients with CWP and are probably also effective in silicosis. Careful follow-up is mandatory in these patients, as in all patients with tuberculosis. After a 2-month induction course with three or four drugs (rifampicin, isoniazid, ethambutol, pyrazinamide), the physician should be prepared to continue the maintenance drugs (usually rifampicin and isoniazid) for longer than the usual 6- or 9-month course, according to the extent of the disease, its apparent response to treatment, and the compliance of the patient.

# HYPERSENSITIVITY PNEUMONITIS

method of
RAYMOND G. SLAVIN, M.D.
*St. Louis University School of Medicine*
*St. Louis, Missouri*

Hypersensitivity pneumonitis is a disease process caused by sensitivity to an inhaled organic dust. In the acute form, associated with intermittent intense exposure to the organic dust, the individual responds 4 to 6 hours later with low-grade fever, chills, chest pain, cough, and dyspnea. In the chronic form, associated with prolonged, low-grade exposure, the clinical presentation is more insidious, with progressively increasing cough, dyspnea, malaise, weakness, and weight loss.

The antigens responsible for hypersensitivity pneumonitis can be grouped into the following categories with an example of each: thermophilic actinomycetes (*Micropolyspora faeni*), fungi (*Cryptostroma corticale*), amebae (*Naegleria gruberi*), animal proteins (bird excreta), and chemicals (toluene diisocyanate).

The diagnosis of hypersensitivity pneumonitis should be suspected in any patient presenting with interstitial pneumonitis or pulmonary fibrosis. Pulmonary function testing reveals a largely restrictive component including decreases in pulmonary compliance and in carbon monoxide diffusing capacity. A careful history eliciting the onset of symptoms following exposure with remission on avoidance together with positive serum precipitins to the appropriate antigen is presumptive evidence of hypersensitivity pneumonitis.

## THERAPEUTIC APPROACH

### Avoidance

Clearly the most important aspect in the management of hypersensitivity pneumonitis is recognition and avoidance of the causative antigen. A number of interventions will decrease the formation of antigens in conducive environments. For example, the growth of thermophilic *Actinomyces* spores in compost can be suppressed by treatment with a 1% solution of propionic acid. Water that remains for long periods of time in older air conditioners or humidification units may become a fertile source for the growth of thermophilic organisms. Therefore, the water needs to be changed and the units cleaned on a regular basis.

In occupational situations in which organic dust generation is inevitable, efforts should be made to reduce the workers' exposure through mechanical handling of dusty material, improved ventilation, and electrostatic air purifiers. The use of personal dust respirators or masks is limited because of inconvenience. The best device available has a maximal filtering capacity of 99% for fine particles. The remaining 1% can produce new attacks in highly sensitive individuals. If the disease is not yet manifest, a filter with 95% filtering capacity such as a 3M disposable mask model 8710 is adequate.

When these environmental control measures cannot be carried out or are inadequate, the patient should be removed from that work area.

### Therapy (Table 1)

In most cases of hypersensitivity pneumonitis, no treatment is necessary other than avoidance

TABLE 1. **Treatment of Hypersensitivity Pneumonitis**

*Acute form*
Remove patient from exposure; may entail hospitalization
Oxygen
Prednisone 40–60 mg/day with slow tapering
Supportive measures—rest, antitussives, antipyretics

*Repeated acute or subacute form*
Decrease exposure as much as possible
Long-term corticosteroid therapy emphasizing alternate-day therapy

*Chronic form*
Trial with corticosteroids but continue only if radiographic findings and physiologic testing indicate a response

of the causative antigen. Corticosteroid therapy, however, can greatly accelerate clinical improvement and should be instituted in very ill patients with gross radiographic or physiologic abnormalities such as hypoxemia. Oral therapy with prednisone in an initial daily dosage of 40 to 60 mg is usually adequate and should be continued until there is significant clinical, radiographic, and pulmonary function test evidence of improvement. The prednisone dosage then may be tapered slowly over a period of 4 to 6 weeks until resolution of clinical and radiologic signs is complete. In cases of severe hypoxemia, oxygen should be administered in amounts sufficient to keep the $P_{O_2}$ level between 60 and 100 mmHg. Other supportive measures include rest, antitussives, and antipyretics.

On occasion, despite the physician's best efforts, the patient may elect to return to the same work place or occupation. In these instances, long-term continuous corticosteroid therapy may have to be administered with an emphasis on alternate-day therapy.

The chronic form of hypersensitivity pneumonitis occurs either following repeated acute episodes or as a result of long-term, low-grade exposure. A therapeutic trial of steroids can be given but should be continued only if radiographic findings and physiologic testing indicate a beneficial response.

# SINUSITIS

method of
WILLIAM R. PANJE, M.D.
*University of Chicago Medical Center
Chicago, Illinois*

Sinusitis is defined as an inflammation of the paranasal sinuses. Environmental agents such as cigarette smoke, industrial pollutants, motor vehicle emissions, viruses, bacteria, and immune deficiency diseases can produce sinusitis. Sinusitis can be acute, subacute, or chronic, depending on length of inflammation/infection. Acute sinusitis is treated medically while chronic sinusitis is a surgical condition. Subacute sinusitis may require prolonged medical therapy. If it is recalcitrant to therapy, subsequent surgical therapy may be necessary.

## ACUTE SINUSITIS

Acute sinusitis usually follows or in some cases is coexistent with an upper respiratory infection (Table 1). Facial pain, especially over the cheeks and between the eyes, as well as dental discomfort suggests infection of the paranasal sinuses. Nasal purulence, congestion, fever, and accentuation of facial pain with straining are all clinical indicators of acute sinusitis.

Reliable culture data are difficult to obtain in evaluating both normal sinuses and the etiologic organism of sinusitis. Only direct sinus aspiration provides reliable data. Quantitative culture techniques can help distinguish true pathogens from resident flora or contaminants. Nasal cultures are highly unreliable as to the etiologic agent.

Nevertheless several studies of adult community-acquired maxillary sinusitis revealed *Streptococcus pneumoniae* and unencapsulated *Haemophilus influenzae* represented over 50% of the isolates. Anaerobic bacteria, including *Bacteroides* species, are found in up to 10% of cases when appropriate anaerobic culture techniques are used. *Staphylococcus aureus* was found in earlier studies in up to 8% of cultures, but using more recent, stricter culture techniques, this organism has not been as prevalent, suggesting contamination may have misled earlier estimations. Of note, *Branhamella catarrhalis* is much more common in children as a cause of acute sinusitis, accounting for nearly 20% of cases. Again, *S. pneumoniae* and *H. influenzae* predominate in children.

Anaerobic organisms play a much larger role in chronic sinusitis in both adults and children. Frederick found anaerobes in 52% of 83 surgical specimens from patients with chronic sinusitis, including 31%, in

TABLE 1. **Microbial Causes of Acute Sinusitis**

| Microorganisms | % of Cases |
|---|---|
| Bacteria | |
|   *S. pneumoniae* | 20–35 |
|   *H. influenzae* | 6–26 |
|   *S. pneumoniae* and *H. influenzae* | 1–9 |
|   Anaerobic bacteria (*Bacteroides*, anaerobic gram-positive cocci, *Fusobacterium* sp., etc.) | 0–10 |
|   *S. aureus* | 0–8* |
|   *S. pyogenes* | 1–3 |
|   *B. catarrhalis* | 2† |
|   Gram-negative bacilli | 0–25‡ |
| Viruses | |
|   Rhinovirus | 15 |
|   Influenza | 5 |
|   Parainfluenza | 3 |

*Seen less frequently in more recent studies.
†Up to 20% in children.
‡Up to 75% in nosocomial sinusitis.

whom anaerobes were the only organism isolated. Anaerobes are the most common pathogens of sinusitis from a dental source, often with a mixture of *Bacteroides* and anaerobic, gram-positive streptococci.

Gram-negative bacteria predominate in nosocomial sinusitis. In Caplan and Hoyt's study of 34 cases of nosocomial sinusitis in a trauma unit, *Pseudomonas aeruginosa* was most commonly isolated (12), followed by *Klebsiella pneumoniae* (7), *Enterobacter* species (7), *Proteus mirabilis* (5), and *Escherichia coli* (3).

Fungi can infect the sinuses rarely; *Aspergillus, Mucor, Candida, Penicillium, Pseudallescheria boydii,* and others are involved. *Aspergillus* infection can be noninvasive, causing mycetoma or allergic aspergillosis, or invasive. There is usually recalcitrant nasal obstruction and rhinorrhea unresponsive to typical therapy. The infection may mimic a malignancy of the paranasal sinuses. Allergic aspergillosis of the sinuses has been recently described and is similar to allergic bronchopulmonary aspergillosis.

*Candida albicans* can cause noninvasive sinusitis in patients receiving prior antibiotic therapy or with diabetes mellitus. It has not been identified as a common pathogen in immunocompromised patients or patients with nosocomial sinusitis.

Unusual organisms causing sinusitis have been reported in patients with acquired immune deficiency syndrome (AIDS). In a recent study of 12 AIDS patients with sinusitis, *Pseudallescheria boydii* was isolated as often as the two most common bacterial isolates, *H. influenzae* and *S. pneumoniae*.

Viruses can be isolated in up to 15% of aspirates from patients with signs and symptoms of acute sinusitis. They may be isolated in pure culture or together with a significant colony count of one of the common bacterial sinus pathogens. Rhinovirus is most commonly isolated; other viruses include parainfluenza adenovirus and influenza.

## TREATMENT

Antibiotic therapy of acute sinusitis (Table 2) should be directed against the most common pathogens: *S. pneumoniae, H. influenzae,* and *Branhamella catarrhalis*. Empiric therapy is appropriate, except in complicated or refractory cases.

Oral cephalosporins, with the *exception* of ce-

TABLE 2. **Antimicrobial Therapy of Acute Sinusitis**

| Antibiotic | Recommended Oral Dose in Adults |
|---|---|
| Ampicillin | 500 mg q 6 h |
| Amoxicillin | 500 mg q 8 h |
| Amoxicillin-Clavulanate | |
| (Augmentin) | 500 mg q 8 h |
| Cefaclor (Ceclor) | 500 mg q 6 h |
| Cefuroxime (Axetil) | 250 mg q 12 h |
| Trimethoprim-sulfamethoxazole | |
| (160/800 mg) | |
| (Bactrim, Septra) | 1 tablet q 12 h |

faclor and cefuroxime axetil, penicillin V, and erythromycin should not be used against many of the common pathogens because of inadequate sinus fluid levels.

Antibiotic treatment of acute sinusitis should be done for at least 14 days. Additional treatment of acute sinusitis should include rest, humidity, hydration, decongestants, and expectorants. Antihistamines should be avoided.

### Subacute Sinusitis

Subacute sinusitis is a sinus infection that lasts longer than 2 weeks but less than 4 weeks. Subacute sinusitis is usually caused by inadequate treatment of acute sinusitis, i.e., antibiotic inappropriate to infective organism, antibiotic not prescribed or taken for sufficient duration of time, or coexisting illness, e.g., mononucleosis.

Chronic sinusitis is relatively asymptomatic in well-developed countries rich in food, proper hygiene, and availability of antibiotics. The patient typically complains of one or all of the following: persistent nasal congestion, postnasal drip, purulent nasal drainage, halitosis, anosmia, and occasionally sinus headache. Usually the headache associated with chronic sinusitis is a pressure-like feeling over the central face and behind the eyes, often relieved with antibiotics but not nasal decongestants. When headache occurs with chronic sinusitis, the physician must be concerned with accentuation of the sinus infection which, if not treated, will lead to a complication.

Complications of sinusitis include orbital cellulitis, subperiosteal abscess, cavernous sinus thrombosis, osteomyelitis of the skull, meningitis, or brain abscess. The orbital complications are the most common, especially in children. Periorbital cellulitis and abscess may follow an upper respiratory infection with purulent rhinorrhea and ethmoid sinusitis. Life-threatening complications of sinusitis, including cavernous sinus thrombosis, osteomyelitis of the skull, meningitis, or brain abscess, usually follow inappropriate medical treatment or not executing proper surgical drainage of the sinuses.

Acute sinusitis should be treated medically. Chronic sinusitis is a surgical disease. Failure to provide adequate sinus drainage, if not responsive to the "big 3"—antibiotics, decongestants, bedrest, will lead to sinus complications. All types of complications arising from sinusitis are a surgical emergency. Persistent facial pain (longer than 24 hours) following the diagnosis of acute sinusitis and administration of antibiotics indicates the need for surgical consultation.

Immunocompromised patients present a particularly labile situation regarding the management of their sinusitis. We have found from our own work that this special class of patients should have aggressive medical and surgical intervention directed toward antibiotic, fungal, and drainage therapy. In patients so managed, we had no deaths. Patients having clinical and radiologic evidence of sinusitis before chemotherapy had a very high incidence of subsequent septicemia and death.

# STREPTOCOCCAL PHARYNGITIS

method of
RICHARD B. BROWN, M.D.
*Baystate Medical Center*
*Springfield, Massachusetts*

Streptococcal pharyngitis caused by *Streptococcus pyogenes* (the group A, beta-hemolytic streptococcus) represents one of the most common bacterial infections and most often is noted in children and young adults. However, it is uncommon in individuals under the age of 3. It must be distinguished from other important causes of infections of the throat and tonsils. Table 1 depicts other etiologies for pharyngitis with which the clinician must be familiar. Groups C and G streptococci may also cause pharyngitis indistinguishable from that caused by *S. pyogenes*. However, they are unlikely to cause nonsuppurative complications. Prompt documentation and treatment of infection caused by *S. pyogenes* is important to limit duration of clinical illness; prevent rheumatic fever; limit the likelihood of spread; and decrease local suppurative complications.

Although streptococcal pharyngitis is typically a self-limited illness with resolution within 1 week, treatment administered within 24 to 48 hours may result in still more rapid improvement of clinical status. As recently as 1985, rheumatic fever was thought to have virtually disappeared from the United States, although it was still recognized as a major cause of cardiovascular disease in underdeveloped countries. Since then, several large outbreaks of rheumatic fever have occurred in middle class and military settings, demonstrating that the disease remains with us. Therapy of streptococcal pharyngitis during the first 7 to 9 days of clinical illness can greatly reduce the likelihood of this nonsuppurative complication. Spread of streptococcal pharyngitis is person to person via droplets of nasal secretions or saliva and is most prominent in close quarters. Risks include proximity to infected persons and clinical activity and treatment status of the patient. Potential for spread is higher in patients with clinical illness than in convalescents or carriers, as organism burden is substantially greater and these organisms may be more virulent. Suppurative complications following streptococcal pharyngitis are uncommon but potentially life-threatening. They include peritonsillar cellulitis or abscess, retropharyngeal abscess, and metastatic spread of infection via either the carotid artery or jugular vein. Bacterial supraglottitis may be caused by *S. pyogenes* and may closely mimic streptococcal pharyngitis.

## CLINICAL PRESENTATION

Classical presentation is that of an acute febrile constitutional illness associated with throat pain. Temperature is often greater than 102° F. Physical findings include red throat and enlarged tonsils associated with varying amounts of yellow-white exudate that may be easily removed with a swab without resultant bleeding. In patients with large tonsils, especially if asymmetric, physical examination should include careful palpation of the tonsillar area to rule out the presence of peritonsillar abscess. Anterior cervical lymph nodes are typically enlarged and tender, especially those at the angle of the mandible. Unfortunately, 25 to 50% of patients may present with more subtle findings of low-grade fever, less severe throat pain, and nonexudative disease. Symptoms and signs negating the diagnosis of streptococcal pharyngitis include hoarseness, diarrhea, rhinitis, conjunctivitis, and posterior cervical adenopathy.

Scarlet fever represents disease caused by a strain of *S. pyogenes* that produces erythrogenic toxin and is now seen in only a small percentage of patients. Intense erythema is typically noted early in the disease, may begin on the trunk and work centrifugally, blanches on pressure, and is classically described as sandpaper on an erythematous base. Pastia's lines (petechiae caused by enhanced capillary fragility) may be noted in skin folds such as the antecubital fossa. Diseases to be ruled out include Kawasaki's disease and toxic shock syndrome, but in the setting of exudative pharyngitis, it is highly suspicious of streptococcal pharyngitis.

Laboratory data, if obtained, demonstrate an elevated leukocyte count with a predominance of polymorphonuclear leukocytes and band forms. Acute phase reactants are usually elevated but are of no diagnostic significance.

## DIAGNOSIS

Diagnosis cannot be reliably made on clinical grounds. Twenty to 50% of patients will be misidentified solely on interpretation of history and physical examination. This may result either in treatment for nonstreptococcal illness or withholding of therapy for streptococcal disease. A throat culture positive for *S. pyogenes* has been the "gold standard" for diagnosis but suffers from several problems, including time delays, potential for sampling errors, and cost. Recently,

TABLE 1. **Differential Diagnosis of Streptococcal Pharyngitis**

| Common | Uncommon |
| --- | --- |
| Epstein-Barr virus | *Corynebacterium hemolyticum* |
| *Neisseria gonorrhoeae* | *Yersinia enterocolitica* |
| Adenovirus | *Corynebacterium diphtheriae* |
| *Mycoplasma hominis* | *Haemophilus influenzae* |
| Vincent's angina | *Francisella tularensis* |
| | Supraglottitis |

a variety of antigen detection "rapid methods" have become commercially available, and these offer high specificity and reasonable sensitivity, with results available in minutes. The clinician must be aware of the brand of test employed, as sensitivity and specificity criteria may vary among manufacturers. Thus a positive rapid test is usually predictive of *S. pyogenes* pharyngitis while a negative test does not rule it out. Gram's stain of pharyngeal exudate provides another rapid method that may also be valuable in denoting the presence of polymorphonuclear leukocytes and organisms consistent with streptococci. However, training in interpretation is necessary in order for this to prove clinically valuable. A reasonable approach is to obtain swabs for rapid methods (Gram's stain or antigen detection). If either is positive in the appropriate clinical setting, therapy can be initiated. If negative, throat culture should be obtained and therapy may be withheld pending results. The presence of scarlet fever, however, should prompt initiation of treatment.

Conclusive proof of infection (rather than colonization) with *S. pyogenes* is available only by demonstrating a serologic response to the organism. Although methods to do this are available (antistreptolysin-O, streptozyme, etc.), they are rarely useful in the management of acute pharyngitis. Such tests should be reserved for the patient with possible rheumatic fever or poststreptococcal glomerulonephritis, where documentation of recent infection with this organism is needed. Rarely the tests may also be indicated for patients with unusual epidemiologic considerations. It should also be noted that prompt treatment of *S. pyogenes* pharyngitis may obliterate the serologic response.

## TREATMENT

Therapy is directed toward eradication of the offending pathogen, maintenance of hydration, and relief of pain. Table 2 depicts antibiotic treatment regimens. In all instances, therapy must be continued for 10 days, as likelihood of eradication of the organism increases until this time. Intramuscular benzathine penicillin G provides acceptable levels of antibiotic over the entire time period and, thus, ensures compliance.

TABLE 2. **Treatment Regimens for Streptococcal Pharyngitis**

| Agent | Dose |
|---|---|
| Benzathine penicillin G | 600,000 U IM for children weighing <60 lb.*; 1,200,000 U IM for persons weighing >60 lb |
| Penicillin VK | 250 mg PO bid or tid for children under age 12; 500 mg PO bid or tid for older children or adults |
| Erythromycin | 20–40 mg/kg daily in 2–4 divided doses; maximum dose of 1 gram daily |
| Cephalexin | 250–500 mg bid or tid |

*Preparation containing 900,000 U benzathine penicillin G plus 300,000 U procaine penicillin G may be substituted in children.

However, it may be more sensitizing than oral regimens and is associated with pain at the injection site. Penicillin VK is typically employed for oral therapy and can be safely used at a twice daily dosing regimen in compliant populations. If questions of compliance arise, thrice daily dosing is acceptable. Either a first-generation cephalosporin or erythromycin may be employed as alternative therapy for patients intolerant of penicillin. The former should not be used in patients with significant penicillin allergies. Neither ampicillin nor amoxicillin offers advantages over any of these agents. Antibiotics not to consider for treatment include trimethoprim-sulfamethoxazole, tetracyclines, and sulfas, as all have been associated with treatment failures.

### Suppurative Complications

With prompt medical care and initiation of antimicrobial therapy, local complications are now unusual. They should be suspected in patients with persistent complaints following several days of appropriate treatment, those who present with significant painful swallowing, and those in whom physical examination reveals fluctuance around the tonsil(s) or tonsillar asymmetry. Incision and drainage of tonsillar or peritonsillar abscess should be performed if fluctuance is demonstrated, and a parenteral antibiotic is indicated. Epiglottitis (an illness easily confused with pharyngitis) can be diagnosed by lateral neck films. If demonstrated, the patient should be hospitalized for intravenous antibiotics directed toward *S. pyogenes, S. pneumoniae,* and *Haemophilus influenzae* (which may be ampicillin-resistant) and for careful management of the airway.

### SPECIAL CONSIDERATIONS

Most patients should not receive follow-up throat cultures after successful treatment of streptococcal pharyngitis. Cultures may remain positive in approximately 10% of persons, yet have no clinical or epidemiologic significance. Such persons typically carry small burdens of organisms and are unlikely to either transmit the disease to others or become ill. Persons with a history of rheumatic fever are an exception to this rule.

Occasionally, patients will clinically relapse following treatment. In this situation, repeat assessment is indicated to rule out suppurative complications and to document the etiology of the process. Alternative causes of pharyngitis should be explored, and special cultures for *Neisseria gonorrhoeae* and *H. influenzae* may be indicated.

If *S. pyogenes* is again demonstrated, therapy should be reinitiated. If the patient has enlarged tonsils, therapy with higher doses of antibiotic is needed, as organisms may be sequestered deep in tonsillar crypts. Alternatively, a β-lactamase–producing organism such as *Staphylococcus aureus* may be simultaneously present and be capable of inactivating penicillin. An agent such as cephalexin 500 mg four times daily takes both of these issues into consideration. If sequestered organisms are a consideration, therapy may be extended to 2 to 3 weeks.

Culturing of household contacts for *S. pyogenes* is infrequently indicated. It should only be performed when persons are symptomatic or at high risk for rheumatic fever.

## PREVENTION

Routine measures to prevent streptococcal pharyngitis are not indicated. However, patients at risk for rheumatic fever or poststreptococcal glomerulonephritis are candidates for long-term prophylaxis aimed at preventing streptococcal infection. The most reasonable strategy is to administer intramuscular benzathine penicillin G 1,200,000 units monthly. For persons in endemic areas for rheumatic fever, a treatment regimen of every 3 weeks may be indicated. Alternative oral regimens include penicillin VK 25 to 250 mg or sulfadiazine 500 to 1000 mg twice daily.

# TUBERCULOSIS AND OTHER MYCOBACTERIAL DISEASES

method of
FRANCISCO SERAFIN, M.D.
*Mexican Institute of Social Security*
*Mexico City, Mexico*

The mycobacterial category includes acid-resistant organisms, so named because of their characteristic of resisting the action of fast acids and alcohol after carbolfuchsin staining. Four groups are known within this category: (1) tuberculous bacillus, which includes human, bovine, murine, avian, and cold-blood types; (2) tuberculoid bacillus, which comprises the also called atypical mycobacteria, classified at present in the four Runyon groups; (3) acid-resistant saprophitic bacilli; and (4) leprosy and Johne's bacillus.

In more than 95% of cases, the disease is produced by human *Mycobacterium tuberculosis*. The remaining cases are divided between bovine *M. tuberculosis* and atypical mycobacteria.

Tuberculosis has a worldwide distribution, and in developing countries, it constitutes a major health

TABLE 1. **Toxicity of Major Antituberculous Drugs**

| Drug | Toxicity |
| --- | --- |
| Isoniazid (INH) | Hepatitis, peripheral neuritis, rash, fever |
| Ethambutol (Myambutol) | Optic neuritis |
| Streptomycin | Deafness, renal failure |
| Rifampin (Rifadin) | Hepatitis, fever, thrombocytopenia |
| Pyrazinamide | Hyperuricemia, hepatitis, arthralgia |
| Thiacetazone* | GI distress, bone marrow depression, hemolytic anemia, rash, hepatitis |

*Not available in the United States.

problem, although developed countries also register some cases. According to World Health Organization estimates, 3 million people die yearly and 10 to 20 million have the disease.

The classification of tuberculosis and of diseases caused by tuberculoid bacilli is no longer as complex as it was some years ago, and it takes into account whether there is infection or disease, or if neither is present; its location (lungs, pleura, bones or joints, etc.); the bacteriologic state (positive, negative, or pending); the state of chemotherapy; and radiographic image (cavitation or not, nonprogressive or progressive).

## DIAGNOSIS

A definite diagnosis can be made only when the tuberculous bacillus is isolated from the biologic material collected from the patient, such as tracheal smear, gastric, pleural, peritoneal, or cerebrospinal fluids, urine, bone marrow, or tissue samples obtained through biopsy. When there is no isolation of the bacillus, a presumptive diagnosis can be arrived at using other elements: history of contact with tuberculous patient; suggestive clinical framework; positive tuberculin skin test (induration of 10 mm or larger); compatible radiographic image; and therapeutic test.

## TREATMENT

Drugs for treating tuberculosis are divided into two groups, according to their effectiveness. Major drugs are isoniazid (INH), ethambutol, streptomycin, rifampin, and pyrazinamide. Other drugs are cycloserine, viomycin, kanamycin, capreomycin, ethionamide, and thiazetazone.* These last are used when resistance of the organisms is such that the patient cannot be treated with an adequate combination of major drugs. All antituberculous drugs have toxic effects which partly depend on the susceptibility of each individual and on the dosage administered. Table 1 summarizes the main toxic effects of most commonly used antituberculous drugs.

---

*Not available in the United States.

TABLE 2. **Daily Treatment**

| Regimen A | Regimen B* | Regimen C |
|---|---|---|
| Isoniazid (INH) 20 mg/kg/day up to 300 mg per day, one intake | INH 20 mg/kg/day up to 300 mg per day, one intake | *Intensive 8-Week Phase* Streptomycin 20 mg/kg/day up to 1 gram per day IM |
| Rifampin 20 mg/kg/day up to 600 mg per day, one intake | Thiacetazone† 150 mg per day | INH 20 mg/kg/day up to 300 mg per day, one intake |
| For 12 months | For 12 to 18 months | Ethambutol 20 mg/kg/day up to 1200 mg per day, one intake |
| | | *Support Phase* (12-month completion) |
| | | INH 20 mg/kg/day up to 300 mg per day, one intake |
| | | Ethambutol 20 mg/kg/day up to 1200 mg per day, one intake |

*Probably the lowest cost-effective regimen.
†Not available in the United States.

For the treatment of active cases, use of one or more major drugs is recommended with the purpose of reducing resistant stocks and increasing the antibacterial effect.

There are several primary treatment regimens:

**Daily Treatment.** A daily dose of two or three major drugs is administered over 12 months. Table 2 depicts three regimens.

**Intermittent Treatment.** This consists of an intensive phase of 1 to 3 months of daily treatment, combining two or three major drugs, followed by a fully supervised, twice weekly administration

of two of the drugs for 9 months to 1 year. Two regimens are described in Table 3.

**Short-Course Treatments.** These extend for less than 12 months. The shortest last 6 months, and there are also 8- and 9- month treatments. The regimen that offers the best results is one combining INH and rifampin in one daily administration over 9 months. This regimen has produced 2.5% of relapses in a period of 7 to 30 months.

The benefits of short course treatment are better acceptance by the patient and consequent higher degree of cooperation, reduced chronic toxicity, and lower cost. Table 4 proposes several short regimens, 6, 8, and 9 months in duration, which have a potential index of success of over 95%, according to the experience of the Pan American Health Organization.

There are no reasons for prolonging treatment

TABLE 3. **Intermittent Treatment**

**Regimen One**

| | |
|---|---|
| | *Intensive phase* (1 month) |
| Isoniazid (INH) | 20 mg/kg/day up to 300 mg/day, one daily intake |
| Rifampin | 20 mg/day up to 600 mg/day, one daily intake |
| | *Support phase* (8 months) |
| INH | 40 mg/kg/day up to 900 mg/day, twice weekly |
| Rifampin | 20 mg/kg/day up to 600 mg/day, twice weekly |

**Regimen Two**

| | |
|---|---|
| Streptomycin | 20 mg/kg/day up to 1 gram daily IM, one application |
| INH | 20 mg/kg/day up to 300 mg/day, one daily intake |
| Ethambutol | 20 mg/kg/day up to 1200 mg/day, one daily intake |
| | *Support phase* (8-month completion) |
| INH | 40 mg/kg/day up to 900 mg, one twice-weekly intake |
| Streptomycin | 20 mg/kg/day up to 1 gram twice weekly IM |
| INH | 40 mg/kg/day up to 900 mg, one twice-weekly intake |
| Ethambutol | 40 mg/kg/day up to 1200 mg, one twice-weekly intake |

TABLE 4. **Short-Course Treatment**

| 6-mo Regimens | 8-mo Regimens | 9-mo Regimens |
|---|---|---|
| 1. IR daily for 6 mo | *1. SRIZ daily for 2 mo TI daily for 6 mo | 1. SRIZ daily for 2 mo RI daily for 7 mo |
| 2. SRIZ daily for 2 mo RI daily for 4 mo | 2. RIZ daily for 2 mo IZ twice weekly for 6 mo | 2. ERI daily for 2 mo RI daily for 7 mo |

S = streptomycin 20 mg/kg/day, up to 1 gram/day, IM.
R = rifampin 20 mg/kg/day, up to 600 mg/day, one oral intake.
I = isoniazid 20 mg/kg/day, up to 300 mg/day, one oral intake (40 mg/kg/day, up to 900 mg/day twice weekly).
Z = pyrazinamide 30 mg/kg/day, up to 2 grams/day, one oral intake.
T = thiacetazone 150 mg/day; not available in the United States.
E = ethambutol 20 mg/kg/day, up to 1200 mg/day, one oral intake.
*Probably the most effective low-cost regimen for developing countries.

TABLE 5. **Nontuberculous Mycobacteria Frequently Related to Human Disease**

| Species | Affected Tissue | Recommended Drugs |
|---|---|---|
| *M. marinum* | Skin | INH-rifampin and ethambutol |
| *M. ulcerans* | Skin | Rifampin–ethambutol–trimethoprim-sulfamethoxazole |
| *M. avium-intracellulare* | Lungs—disseminated infection | INH-rifampin, ethambutol, streptomycin, pyrazinamide, ethionamide |
| *M. kansasii* | Lungs—disseminated infection | INH-rifampin, ethambutol, streptomycin |
| *M. fortuitum* | Skin, lungs, prosthetic devices | Amikacin, cefoxitin, rifampin, sulfonamide erythromycin, doxycycline |
| *M. chelonei* | Skin, lungs, prosthetic devices | Cefoxitin, amikacin, rifampin, erythromycin, sulfonamides |

in disseminated or extrapulmonary forms of tuberculosis. In tuberculosis of the central nervous system, chosen drugs are INH and rifampin, given their better diffusion. In special cases, such as meningeal tuberculosis, endobronchial cases with obstructive mediastinal adenitis, and constrictive pericarditis, antituberculous drugs can be used together with prednisone, 1 to 2 mg per kg per day. However, there are no control studies demonstrating the effectiveness of glucocorticoids in these clinical forms.

## RE-TREATMENT AND DRUG RESISTANCE

The need for re-treatment may arise from inadequate use or premature interruption of drug administration, resulting in a relapse. Re-treatment must be given with different drugs from those previously used. It is necessary to effect sensitivity tests in order to select medications to which the germ is susceptible. When INH resistance is suspected, although not yet confirmed, a good regimen to begin with consists of streptomycin, pyrazinamide, and rifampin and INH. If resistance to streptomycin is suspected, capreomycin can be substituted. Both cases call for daily doses over 6 to 8 weeks until sensitivity is determined, and the choice of treatment is made accordingly.

## CHEMOPROPHYLAXIS

It has been demonstrated that isoniazid administration in doses of 10 mg per kg per day in children and up to 300 mg per day in adults can reduce the possibilities of developing the disease in individuals exposed to risk. The treatment must be carried out over a year, and it is indicated in the following cases:

1. Intrahousehold contacts and persons who have a close relationship with an individual with recently diagnosed tuberculous disease and a positive sputum.

2. Tuberculin-positive persons in whom radiographic studies suggest nonprogressive tuberculous disease, those with negative bacteriology, or those who underwent inadequate treatment.

3. Persons who have become tuberculin-positive during the last year.

4. Tuberculin-positive persons under special clinical circumstances frequently related to tuberculosis: prolonged treatment with corticosteroids, immunosuppressive therapy, leukemia, Hodgkin's disease, diabetes mellitus, silicosis, gastrectomy, and measles or vaccination against it.

## INFECTIONS DUE TO NONTUBERCULOUS MYCOBACTERIA

The importance of these mycobacteria as causes of infection has gradually increased. They are considered opportunistic germs, and consequently immunocompromised individuals are particularly susceptible to them. They affect the lungs or other tissue according to the mycobacteria, and some, such as *M. avium-intracellulare, M. kansasii, M. fortuitum,* and *M. chelonei,* can cause generalized infection. *M. kansasii* is frequently observed in patients with AIDS.

Diagnosis requires a high degree of suspicion and the isolation of the germ from sputum or, whenever possible, from biopsy. In the latter case, it is possible to determine with certainty the linkage between the isolated mycobacteria and the disease, whereas if isolated from sputum, it is necessary to confirm correspondence by repeating isolation in several samples.

In the treatment of nontuberculous mycobacterial infections, both antituberculous drugs and other antimicrobial agents are used; sensitivity tests are of great help for treatment choice. Table 5 mentions organs commonly affected by each nontuberculous mycobacteria and useful drugs. Dosages are as indicated in the preceding tables. Regimens with three to five drugs are recommended, in accordance with sensitivity tests, for periods from 12 to 18 months.

Children in particular develop mycobacterial lymphadenopathy. Low maxillary and cervical chains are highly affected. *M. scrofulaceum* and *M. avium-intracellulare* are the most frequent pathogens, although there are also cases caused by *M. fortuitum* and *M. chelonei.* Treatment for these cases is surgical excision and antituberculous drugs.

# The Cardiovascular System

## ACQUIRED DISEASES OF THE AORTA

method of
DAVID F. J. TOLLEFSON, M.D.
*Henry Ford Hospital*
*Detroit, Michigan*

and

CALVIN B. ERNST, M.D.
*University of Michigan Medical School and*
*Henry Ford Hospital*
*Detroit, Michigan*

Aneurysmal and occlusive disease are the two major categories that comprise acquired diseases of the aorta. The pathophysiologic mechanisms of these diseases have changed over the years, and currently, aneurysmal disease is usually secondary to atherosclerosis and mural degenerative disease. Aneurysms resulting from inflammation, infection, trauma, and pseudoaneurysmal formation following previous aortic operations occur much less frequently. Obliterative disease results primarily from atherosclerosis, but inflammatory disease, such as Takayasu's arteritis, may also affect major visceral aortic branches.

### PERIOPERATIVE ASSESSMENT

Acquired diseases of the aorta, when due to atherosclerosis, are only part of a generalized process that affects other vessels, especially the coronary arteries. Successful management of aortic occlusive or aneurysmal disease not only requires appropriately timed and performed operative procedures but also comprehensive assessment of the risks to the patient of such intervention. History and physical examination do not always detect occult cardiac disease. Preoperative coronary arteriography of vascular surgical patients has documented severe correctable coronary artery disease in 14% of individuals with a negative cardiac history and normal electrocardiogram (ECG). Stress electrocardiography and stress thallium testing, while useful in detecting occult cardiac disease, cannot always be used in elderly patients who cannot adequately exercise or who, because of medication like beta-adrenergic–blocking drugs, cannot achieve a stressed heart rate. Dipyridamole (Persantine) thallium studies have shown promise in identifying individuals with occult coronary artery disease. Patients identified to be at risk as a result of abnormal stress testing require cardiac catheterization to identify correctable lesions.

Pulmonary function is often compromised in this patient population, owing to a history of heavy smoking. Cessation of smoking, antibiotic treatment of pulmonary infection, and the judicious use of bronchodilators guided by preoperative pulmonary function studies can minimize postoperative pulmonary morbidity and mortality. Renal function, occasionally mildly compromised following aortography, should be allowed to return to normal before operative intervention.

Aortic reconstructive operations are facilitated by use of arterial pressure monitoring lines, Swan-Ganz catheter monitoring of cardiac performance, and double-lumen endotracheal tubes when the operative approach requires entrance into the left chest. Two-dimensional transesophageal echocardiography provides assessment of segmental wall motion abnormalities indicative of early myocardial ischemia. This new modality detects such ischemic events before either ST-segment ECG changes or abnormal pulmonary arterial pressures develop.

### MANAGEMENT

#### Abdominal Aortic Aneurysms

The incidence of infrarenal abdominal aortic aneurysms in an unselected population approximates 3%. Although distal embolization and acute thrombosis are inherent risks, aneurysmal rupture is the chief cause of death. Untreated, patients with abdominal aortic aneurysms have a 5-year survival of 29%, with 63% of deaths due to rupture. Mortality of acute rupture remains nearly 50%, contrasted with an operative mortality of 3% for elective aortic reconstruction. Risk of rupture relates primarily to aneurysm size, with those measuring greater than 5 cm at greatest risk.

Although many abdominal aortic aneurysms are first discovered by routine physical examination or abdominal x-ray, ultrasonography and computerized tomography (CT) are the best tests to evaluate and document the size of the aneurysm. Aortography inherently underestimates the size of aortic aneurysms. It is mainly used to identify concomitant disease of the visceral vessels and the extent of lower extremity arterial compromise. A lateral aortogram is essential to adequately study the splanchnic circulation.

An abdominal aortic aneurysm can be repaired through either transabdominal or retroperitoneal approaches. The latter method is especially useful in elderly, high-risk patients, those with compromised pulmonary function, or patients with a hostile abdomen secondary to previous operations. For aortic replacement, a knitted Dacron graft is used in the elective setting, whereas a woven Dacron graft is used for ruptured aneurysms. Recently, expanded polytetrafluoroethylene grafts have gained popularity.

Depending on the status of the iliac arteries, a bifurcated graft anastomosed to either the iliac or femoral arteries is used. For disease confined to the aorta, a tube graft between the infrarenal and distal aorta is employed. The old aneurysmal wall is wrapped around the graft to isolate it from the gut and prevent development of an aortoenteric fistula. Other complications of operation include distal embolization, which occurs in less than 1% of patients, and ischemic colitis, which may develop in 6% of patients. Ischemic colitis can be prevented by restoring arterial blood flow to at least one hypogastric artery or the inferior mesenteric artery (IMA).

Inflammatory aneurysms, which comprise 5% of infrarenal abdominal aortic aneurysms, are characterized by a dense, invasive fibrosis throughout the retroperitoneum, commonly involving the duodenum, ureters, and inferior vena cava. These aneurysms are technically challenging to repair, and therefore, it is helpful to identify such lesions preoperatively. Diagnosis is suspected in individuals complaining of weight loss, those with elevated erythrocyte sedimentation rates, and those with CT documentation of a thickened aneurysm wall with medial deviation of the ureters. Following aneurysm repair, the inflammatory process may regress.

### Descending Thoracic Aortic Aneurysms

Owing chiefly to atherosclerosis and medial degeneration, descending thoracic aortic aneurysms also result from trauma, infection, and aortitis. Thoracic and abdominal aortic aneurysms, either metachronous or synchronous, occur in 25% of patients. Atherosclerotic aneurysms should be repaired if symptomatic or if the aneurysm diameter measures greater than two times that of the native aorta. Aortic repair, using a

woven Dacron tube graft, is accomplished through a left posterior lateral thoracotomy. The major complication is paraplegia, which occurs in about 3 to 5% of patients.

### Ascending Aortic Aneurysms

While atherosclerosis may be superimposed, ascending aortic aneurysms usually result from medial degeneration or dissection in over 95% of patients. Associated aortic valvular disease is common, especially aortic insufficiency. Aortography is diagnostic. Treatment requires replacement of the involved segment with a woven Dacron graft using cardiopulmonary bypass. If aortic valvular disease is also present, the aortic valve is replaced with a composite valve graft.

### Transverse Aortic Arch Aneurysms

Owing to either atheroclerosis or medial degeneration, transverse aortic arch aneurysms can involve all or part of the ascending and transverse aorta. Complications are serious as a result of either compression of the upper mediastinal structures or rupture. Computed tomography and aortography are key to diagnosis and proper evaluation. Treatment requires graft replacement of the involved aorta. Cardiopulmonary bypass with cardioplegia and profound hypothermia, to protect the brain and myocardium, are required during aneurysm repair.

Takayasu's aortitis, initially thought to be limited to the Orient, has now been identified worldwide. It is due to an inflammatory process of unknown etiology, resulting in an obliterative process involving the aortic arch and its branches. Treatment in the early stages of the disease is nonsurgical, using steroids to relieve systemic symptoms and appropriate therapy for hypertension and heart failure. Surgical intervention is used in the late fibrotic stage of the disease for symptoms such as transient ischemic attacks, exercise ischemia of the arm, and renovascular hypertension. Graft interposition and bypass techniques are preferred to repair aortic arch branches.

### Thoracoabdominal Aneurysms

Thoracoabdominal aortic aneurysms, due to either atherosclerosis or medial degeneration, present a formidable therapeutic challenge because of the extent of disease which involves most of the aorta. Untreated, 5-year survival is 19%, with more than half of patients dying from rupture of the aneurysm. Aortography and CT evaluation of the entire aorta are essential for proper planning of an operation. Operative intervention is recommended if the aneurysm diameter measures greater than twice the size of the normal aorta and the patient's overall condition is satisfactory to tolerate operation.

Treatment requires graft replacement of the involved thoracoabdominal aorta. Arterial flow to the viscera and kidneys must be re-established. A left thoracoabdominal approach is used with general anesthesia via a double-lumen endotracheal tube to allow selective collapse of the left lung during aneurysm repair.

Operative mortality of approximately 9% with 5-year survival of 60% has been reported. Complications include postoperative bleeding, respiratory and renal failure, and spinal cord ischemia resulting in paraplegia or paraparesis. Postoperative paraplegia has defied attempts at prevention. Paraplegia is unpredictable, and its incidence is related to the size of the aneurysm. Postoperative coagulation problems are common. Prompt replacement of coagulation factors, prevention of hypothermia, and avoidance of heparin sodium intraoperatively can help to ameliorate the coagulopathy.

### Aortic Dissection

Owing primarily to medial degeneration, aortic dissection is classified based on the presence or absence of involvement of the ascending aorta. Type I dissection involves the entire aorta; Type II is confined to the ascending aorta; and in Type III, the dissection usually originates in the descending aorta at or just distal to the left subclavian artery and can extend to the aortic bifurcation. Hypertension is frequent, especially in the elderly. Patients with Marfan's syndrome are particularly vulnerable to aortic dissection. Following a primary intimal tear, the dissection can proceed proximally or distally, creating a false lumen that can rupture with fatal hemorrhage. Rupture also occurs into the pericardial sac, causing cardiac tamponade, acute aortic valvular insufficiency, or occlusion of the coronary artery ostia with resultant myocardial infarction. Aortic dissections can cause stroke, renal failure, mesenteric insufficiency, or lower extremity ischemia.

Diagnosis traditionally has been by aortography, although dynamic CT imaging has recently become popular. Treatment is initially nonoperative. Nitroprusside (Nipride) and propranolol (Inderal) are used to decrease the blood pressure and force of cardiac contraction. Dissections involving the ascending and transverse aortic arch are treated surgically with graft replacement using cardiopulmonary bypass. Aortic valve re-

placement may be required, as is coronary artery saphenous vein bypass grafting, depending on the extent of proximal dissection.

Dissection of the descending thoracic aorta is treated medically unless rupture is impending, the dissection is continuing as evidenced by progressive pain, or obstruction of a major aortic branch develops. Dissections treated medically are monitored with serial CT examinations. Operative intervention is recommended if there is progressive dilation to twice normal size.

### Traumatic Thoracic Aortic Aneurysms

Traumatic thoracic aortic aneurysms are pseudoaneurysms that develop just distal to the left subclavian artery following a sudden deceleration injury, usually resulting from a motor vehicle accident. Patients with a history of sudden deceleration and a chest x-ray suggesting widening of the superior mediastinum, a shift of the trachea to the right, a downward shift of the left mainstem bronchus, or right shift of a previously placed nasogastric tube should undergo aortography to confirm the diagnosis. The role of CT scanning has not yet been determined. Emergency operation is essential, since the risk of rupture is extreme in the early stages. At times, primary aortic repair is possible, but often correction of the defect requires graft interposition. Traumatic aneurysms discovered late may progressively expand, causing symptoms due to compression of adjacent structures. Repair is similar to that for descending thoracic aneurysms.

### Abdominal Aortic Occlusive Disease

Progressive obliteration of the abdominal aorta and its branches, producing variable symptoms depending on the degree and extent of disease, is almost always due to atherosclerosis. Isolated involvement of the aortoiliac segment is infrequent and characteristically occurs in young individuals, with an equal representation in both sexes. Symptoms, seldom limb-threatening, consist of intermittent claudication involving buttock, thigh, and hip. When associated with male impotence, such aortoiliac disease is termed Leriche's syndrome. The majority of symptomatic individuals also have generalized arteriosclerosis affecting coronary, carotid, and femoropopliteal arteries. These individuals, often having diabetes and hypertension, are frequently elderly and can present with advanced, limb-threatening ischemia. Diminished or absent pulses and a history of progressive intermittent claudication suggest the diagnosis of aortoiliac occlusive disease.

Noninvasive vascular laboratory tests confirm

the diagnosis, and arteriography defines the extent of disease. Noninvasive testing is particularly helpful in distinguishing between vasculogenic claudication and neurogenic claudication. Neurogenic claudication is often secondary to low back disorders or spinal stenosis and mimics vasculogenic claudication. At rest, ankle-arm indices may be similar and normal in both conditions. However, ankle pressure measurements taken after treadmill exercise will be significantly decreased in patients with vasculogenic claudication and remain normal in those with neurogenic claudication.

Untreated, patients with stable intermittent claudication seldom require amputation. Such events occur with a frequency of 1% per year of survival. Five-year survival of untreated patients approximates 75%, most succumbing to myocardial infarction. Consequently, a conservative stance should be adopted when managing patients with aortoiliac occlusive disease.

Drug therapy has been uniformly ineffective in managing aortoiliac occlusive disease.

Endovascular procedures, such as balloon angioplasty and catheter atherectomy, are still in the evolutionary stages and should be used only for the same indications as surgical intervention. Laser technology is of unproven efficacy and remains an experimental procedure.

Indications for aortoiliac reconstruction include limb-threatening ischemia or activity-limiting intermittent claudication. Trivial intermittent claudication does not require aortic reconstruction. While aortoiliac endarterectomy was popular in the past, aortofemoral bypass grafting has become the preferred procedure. Although graft patency is 85 to 90% at 5 years and 70 to 75% at 10 years, long-term patient survival is compromised as a result of associated atherosclerosis, especially involving the coronary arteries.

# ANGINA PECTORIS

method of
UDHO THADANI, M.B.B.S.
*University of Oklahoma Health Sciences Center*
*Oklahoma City, Oklahoma*

The term "angina pectoris," signifying a painful manifestation of ischemic heart disease, was first used in 1772 by Heberden. The discomfort of angina pectoris is characterized by its substernal or retrosternal location; many patients do not complain of actual pain but describe a feeling of discomfort, tightness, or suffocation. Pain often radiates to the neck, jaw, or left arm.

The term "chronic stable angina" implies that symptoms are stable for at least 3 months. Pain or a feeling of discomfort, tightness, or suffocation is precipitated by exercise or emotion and is relieved by rest and/or sublingual nitroglycerin; occasional episodes of rest angina may occur but are relieved after sublingual nitroglycerin. Symptoms such as faintness, fatigue, or dyspnea on exercise are considered angina equivalents but are non-specific. Their recognition is nevertheless important, especially in the elderly, in whom the symptoms of angina equivalent may be the only manifestation of ischemic heart disease. The combination of exercise-induced and occasional rest angina has been termed "mixed angina."

The term "unstable angina" was introduced by Fowler in 1971. Some investigators use the term "acute coronary insufficiency." In recent years the term "unstable angina" has been used to describe four different clinical conditions:

1. Angina at rest with pain lasting for 5 to 30 minutes, which may not be relieved by sublingual nitroglycerin; this form has been called "preinfarction angina" or "intermittent coronary syndrome."
2. Angina of recent onset precipitated by minimal exertion.
3. Angina on effort with a recent change in severity in patients with a previous history of stable angina.
4. Angina occurring within 4 weeks of acute myocardial infarction (post-infarct angina).

"Variant angina," also known as "Prinzmetal's angina," is associated with electrocardiographic ST segment elevation and is due to coronary artery spasm. Affected patients experience pain at rest and invariably have normal exercise tolerance.

The basic underlying pathophysiologic mechanism that produces anginal pain is myocardial ischemia due to an imbalance between myocardial oxygen requirement and myocardial oxygen supply. Other manifestations of myocardial ischemia—i.e., electrocardiographic ST segment changes, metabolic abnormalities, and functional impairment of the left ventricle—may occur with or without associated anginal pain. In the absence of anginal pain, these manifestations are believed to indicate silent myocardial ischemia. How the anginal pain is produced is not known, but it may be related to stretching of the ischemic myocardium or stimulation of the nerve endings due to accumulation of metabolites or a change in the pH.

The pathophysiologic mechanisms that bring about an imbalance between myocardial oxygen requirement and myocardial oxygen supply are different in various anginal syndromes and have an impact on management.

## CHRONIC STABLE ANGINA

### Pathophysiology

The underlying cause of chronic stable angina is usually atherosclerotic coronary artery disease. Recent evidence suggests that atherosclerotic coronary arteries are not able to dilate normally either during exercise or when provoked pharmacologically. Further, the atherosclerosis process is often eccentric, and a normal portion of the coronary artery can undergo dynamic changes in tone, which if augmented can produce critical stenosis. In patients with stable angina pectoris, the resting coronary blood flow is often adequate to meet myocardial oxygen demand. However, during exercise, an increase in heart rate, blood pressure, and contractility increases myocardial oxygen demand, which cannot be met by an equal increase in coronary blood flow, and this produces an imbalance between myocardial oxygen requirement and oxygen supply and leads to myocardial ischemia. Because of the fixed nature of the obstructive lesions in the coronary arteries, the symptoms can be produced by exercise at identical workloads and rate pressure products. As the disease becomes more severe, effort tolerance decreases progressively. In some patients, an increase in coronary tone may bring about a reduction in blood flow and aggravate ischemia. Some patients with classic exertional angina have a variable angina threshold. This is probably due to superimposed coronary artery spasm, resulting in decreased coronary blood flow.

Some patients with classic exertional angina do not have underlying coronary artery disease. In these patients, maximum coronary flow reserve is impaired because of abnormally high tone in the coronary arteries or precapillary sphincters. Some of these patients also have small vessel disease. An increase in myocardial oxygen demand during stress cannot be matched by an increase in supply. In some patients with hypertension, aortic stenosis, or hypertrophic cardiomyopathy, the preceding mechanism has been shown to account for myocardial ischemia and angina pectoris in the presence of normal coronary arteries.

One of the manifestations of myocardial ischemia is chest pain, but prior to the onset of chest pain there is evidence of contractile failure of the myocardium resulting in increased left ventricular end-diastolic pressure and an increase in resistance to blood flow in the subendocardial tissue. The subendocardial ischemia produces ST segment depression, and when the area of ischemia is large, one may observe changes in systolic and diastolic left ventricular function. Depending upon the extent of ischemia, global ejection fraction may or may not decrease but regional function invariably shows some abnormality.

## Management

The overall prognosis of patients with chronic stable angina pectoris is relatively good, with an annual mortality rate of 1.6 to 3.3%. The Canadian classification of exertional angina (Table 1)

TABLE 1. **Grading of Angina of Effort by the Canadian Cardiovascular Society***

I. "Ordinary physical activity does not cause . . . angina," such as walking and climbing stairs. Angina with strenuous or rapid or prolonged exertion at work or recreation.

II. "Slight limitation of ordinary activity." Angina only with walking or climbing stairs rapidly, walking uphill, walking or stair climbing after meals, or in cold, or in wind, or under emotional stress, or only during the few hours after awakening. Walking more than two blocks on the level and climbing more than one flight of ordinary stairs at a normal pace and in normal conditions do not cause angina.

III. "Marked limitation of ordinary physical activity." Walking one to two blocks on the level and climbing one flight of stairs in normal conditions and at normal pace cause angina.

IV. "Inability to carry on any physical activity without discomfort—anginal syndrome may be present at rest."

*Adapted from Campeau L: Circulation *54:* 522, 1976. By permission of the American Heart Association, Inc.

is a useful practical guide for outlining management. In addition to the clinical history, high-risk groups can usually be identified by exercise testing. Using a Bruce protocol for the treadmill exercise, patients who cannot exercise more than 6 minutes due to chest pain and those with ST segment depression during Stage I or II have a 60 to 70% chance of three-vessel coronary artery disease; some of them also have associated left main disease. A decrease in systolic blood pressure rather than an expected rise during exercise and a maximal heart rate of less than 120 beats per minute at the termination of exercise in the absence of beta-blocker therapy often indicate severe underlying coronary artery disease. Patients who cannot exercise 6 minutes or who have an abnormal response to exercise should have left ventricular function determined non-invasively by radionuclide techniques. In patients whose electrocardiogram is abnormal at rest, radionuclide ventriculography and/or exercise thallium perfusion studies provide important information of prognostic value. Patients with poor left ventricular function and a limited exercise response should undergo coronary angiography to determine if they are in a high-risk subgroup with left main or three-vessel disease.

Major risk factors for coronary artery disease are hypertension, smoking, and hyperlipidemia. In addition to this, diabetes mellitus and a family history of coronary artery disease are also associated with increased risk of coronary artery disease. Therefore, the patient should be screened for hypertension and hyperlipidemia and treated appropriately with dietary modification and pharmacologic therapy if necessary. Smoking increases the risk of myocardial infarction in both males and females. It is, therefore, absolutely essential to tell patients to stop smoking. Diabetic patients should get special counseling and management to adequately control their blood glucose levels. Conditions exacerbating angina should be sought in all patients. Treatment of anemia, thyrotoxicosis, hypertension, and arrhythmias may achieve a relief of angina pectoris.

The treatment strategy is to lower myocardial oxygen demand with drugs or increase coronary blood flow to the ischemic region with coronary artery bypass surgery or balloon angioplasty.

In patients with stable angina pectoris who do not have left main disease or triple vessel disease with poor left ventricular function (ejection fraction less than 50%), the prognosis is excellent and there is no difference between medical and surgical treatment as far as long-term mortality is concerned. Therefore, proper patient counseling is essential. The patient should be told that the disease has a relatively benign prognosis and can be managed medically. Therapeutic options like coronary bypass surgery and coronary angioplasty should also be discussed, and the patient should be told about the benefits and risks of these procedures compared with medical therapy.

### Pharmacologic Treatment

Three classes of drugs are available to treat stable exercise-induced angina pectoris: nitrates, beta blockers, and calcium channel entry blockers.

**Nitrates.** Nitrates are effective antianginal and anti-ischemic agents. Nitroglycerin and other organic nitrates are potent smooth muscle relaxants primarily affecting the vascular smooth muscle. Nitrates produce venous pooling in the systemic and pulmonary beds. Nitrate-induced venodilation reduces end-diastolic and systolic ventricular dimensions and wall stress. In addition, nitrates reduce afterload and lower arterial pressure. The reduced pre-load and afterload decrease myocardial oxygen requirements at any level of stress and are the primary mechanisms by which nitrates alleviate myocardial ischemia

in patients with stable angina pectoris. There is also conclusive evidence that nitrates increase blood flow to ischemic areas by increasing the collateral flow and dilating the eccentrically stenotic coronary arteries. A reduction in end-diastolic left ventricular pressure also facilitates subendocardial perfusion.

In patients with variable angina threshold, which is best explained on the basis of dynamic changes in vascular tone, nitrates prevent the dynamic increase in vascular tone and thus halt a reduction in coronary blood flow.

In patients with classic symptoms of angina pectoris despite normal coronary arteries, nitrates are as effective as calcium channel blockers in reducing coronary vascular tone and improving myocardial blood flow during pacing-induced stress.

SHORT ACTING NITRATES (Table 2). Sublingual nitroglycerin is highly effective when taken prophylactically; it improves exercise tolerance. In patients who experience angina only during exercise, discontinuation of effort will invariably relieve angina. However, when angina is not relieved, sublingual nitroglycerin tablets (0.3 to 0.6 mg) or sublingual nitroglycerin spray delivering 0.4 mg of nitroglycerin per puff is highly effective in relieving angina within a few minutes. There is no evidence that sublingual nitroglycerin taken intermittently leads to development of tolerance, but its effects are very short lasting and it is not possible to provide continuous antianginal prophylaxis with this preparation.

LONG-TERM PROPHYLAXIS OF ANGINA WITH NITRATES (Table 2). Various nitrate preparations are available and are widely used for this purpose. There is evidence, however, that it is not possible to provide continuous antianginal and anti-ischemic prophylaxis throughout the dosing intervals with any of the nitrate preparations. The efficacy of nitroglycerin patches is rapidly lost within 24 hours of application, with complete loss of efficacy in 3 to 7 days. Even during intermittent four-times-daily therapy with isosorbide dinitrate in doses ranging from 15 to 120

TABLE 2. **Nitrates for Stable Angina Pectoris**

|  | Preparation | Onset of Action | Usual Dose |
|---|---|---|---|
| For the relief of anginal attack | Sublingual nitroglycerin | 1–3 min | 0.3–0.6 mg* ×3 |
|  | Translingual (Nitrolingual) spray | 1–3 min | 0.4 mg* |
| For long-term antianginal prophylaxis | Isosorbide dinitrate (Isordil) | 30–45 min | 15–30 mg bid or tid† |
|  | Oral nitroglycerin (Nitro-Bid) | 30–45 min | 6.5–18 mg bid or tid† |
|  | Nitroglycerin patch (Transderm-Nitro) | >60 min | 15–60 mg NTG/24 hr (apply for only 12 hr)‡ |

*May be repeated q 5 min for up to three times.
†Last dose should be taken at 5 or 6 p.m.; qid therapy produces tolerance.
‡Patches should be applied in the morning and removed 12 hr later. Continuous therapy with patches is ineffective.

mg four times a day, attenuation of circulatory and antianginal effects is seen within a week of therapy. This attenuation is characterized by reduced peak and duration of effects following long-term therapy as compared with the first dose effects. Recent studies have shown that this tolerance toward the morning dose can in part be overcome by the intermittent use of long-acting oral nitrates or nitroglycerin patches. It is recommended that one use isosorbide dinitrate, 20 to 40 mg twice or three times a day, with the last dose administered at 2:00 p.m. or 5:00 p.m. However, even with these dosing regimens, it is not known if the last dose given at 2:00 p.m. or 5:00 p.m. is effective. An alternative is to apply the nitroglycerin patch first thing in the morning and remove the patch before retiring to bed. Nitroglycerin patches releasing more than 15 mg of nitroglycerin per 24 hours have been shown to exert antianginal effects for 8- to 12-hour periods when used intermittently, but there are no data to support the application of patches beyond 12 hours.

Buccal nitroglycerin, 2.5 to 6.5 mg prescribed three times a day with the last dose administered at 5:00 p.m., has been shown to be effective and does not produce tolerance toward the morning dose of the medication. This preparation of nitrates is widely used in Europe but has not gained wide acceptance in the USA. Patients should be advised not to use this medication at night, for fear of inhalation.

In most patients with stable angina who have pain only during daily activities, intermittent nitrate therapy may suffice. However, patients are unprotected in the early hours of the morning when the incidence of myocardial infarction, sudden death, and myocardial ischemia is high. Therefore, another class of antianginal agent— i.e., a beta blocker—should be used in addition to nitrates, for the treatment of angina pectoris.

About 10% of patients do not respond to nitrates, and another 10% experience intolerable headaches, which may necessitate discontinuation of nitrate therapy. Some patients are very sensitive to nitrates and may experience syncope due to a marked fall in blood pressure induced by nitrates. Patients should be warned against this and asked to lie down and raise their legs if they experience fainting while taking nitrates. All patients should, however, be advised to carry sublingual nitroglycerin tablets or nitroglycerin spray with them for emergency use.

**Beta Adrenergic Blockers.** These agents work by a competitive inhibition of the beta adrenergic receptors. There are two kinds of beta receptors: $beta_1$ and $beta_2$. Blockade of $beta_1$ receptors, located primarily in the cardiac tissue, leads to reduction in heart rate and cardiac contractility, especially during exercise. In addition, there is a fall in free fatty acids due to prevention of lipolysis. Blockade of $beta_2$ receptors, located in the bronchial and vascular smooth muscle, produces bronchoconstriction and vasoconstriction.

Beta blockers are very effective in the management of patients with stable angina pectoris. These agents improve exercise tolerance and reduce myocardial ischemia. This effect is achieved primarily by $beta_1$ adrenoceptor blockade, which produces a reduction in myocardial oxygen demand due to a reduction of heart rate and contractility. In addition, beta blockade attenuates a rise in systolic blood pressure during exercise. This beneficial effect of $beta_1$ blockade is in part offset by dilation of the left ventricle, which increases myocardial oxygen demand. This is especially important in patients who have enlarged hearts prior to initiation of therapy.

There are numerous beta blockers available (Table 3). All have in common the property of blocking $beta_1$ receptors. In addition, some of the beta blockers also block $beta_2$ receptors and are known as non-cardioselective beta blockers; beta blockers that block only $beta_1$ receptors are known as cardioselective agents. Some of the newer agents also have the ability to block the $alpha_1$ receptors or dilate the blood vessels directly, and these agents, together with agents that also possess partial agonist activity (intrinsic sympathomimetic activity), are known as vasodilator beta blockers. The ancillary property (quinidine-like effect, also referred to as local

TABLE 3. **Beta Adrenoceptor Antagonists for Stable Angina**

| Drug | Cardioselectivity | ISA | Lipid Solubility | Usual Dose |
|---|---|---|---|---|
| Acebutolol* (Sectral) | + | + | Low | 200–400 mg tid |
| Atenolol (Tenormin) | + | 0 | Low | 50–200 mg once daily |
| Metoprolol (Lopressor) | + | 0 | Low | 50–200 mg bid |
| Nadolol (Corgard) | – | 0 | Moderate | 40–240 mg once daily |
| Pindolol* (Visken) | – | + + + | Moderate | 10–30 mg bid |
| Propranolol (Inderal) | – | 0 | High | 80–320 mg divided in two, three, or four daily doses |
| Inderal-LA | – | 0 | High | 80–320 mg once daily |
| Timolol (Blocadren) | – | 0 | Moderate | 10–30 mg bid |

*These agents have been approved for use only in hypertension by the FDA; are also effective in angina.

anesthetic or membrane stabilizing effect) is not related to beta blockade and has no clinical bearing on the effectiveness of beta blockers. Beta blockers are either lipid- or water-soluble, which determines the duration of their effects and has a bearing on the potential adverse effects.

All beta blockers, irrespective of other properties like cardioselectivity, intrinsic sympathomimetic activity, or membrane stabilizing property, are equally effective in patients with stable angina pectoris who do not have concomitant disease. These agents also reduce the episodes of silent myocardial ischemia. Cardioselective agents such as atenolol (Tenormin) and metoprolol (Lopressor) are preferable in patients with angina pectoris who have associated peripheral vascular disease, diabetes, or a history of asthma. However, caution should be used in patients with asthma or obstructive airway disease; even cardioselective agents may aggravate bronchial constriction.

Some patients cannot tolerate beta blockade, owing to effects such as fatigue, extreme bradycardia, dyspnea, or cold extremities. In these patients, an alternative class of antianginal drugs should be used. Beta blockers with low lipid solubility have a lower incidence of central nervous system side effects than lipid-soluble agents. Beta blockers should be used with caution in patients with severely impaired left ventricular function because they may precipitate heart failure.

**Calcium Channel Entry Blockers.** Calcium channel blockers work primarily by reducing afterload and contractility, but may also dilate stenotic coronary arteries and improve blood flow. Unlike beta blockers, which have similar mechanisms of action, the three calcium channel blockers have different pharmacologic effects and different contraindications to therapy (Table 4). Nifedipine (Procardia) and nicardipine (Cardene) are dihydropyridine derivatives and cause the least depression of cardiac function but may produce

troublesome palpitations and edema in some patients due to vasodilation. On the other hand, verapamil (Isoptin) may cause constipation; this could be an important problem in elderly patients. Diltiazem (Cardizem) is often well tolerated, but may produce a slowing of the heart rate in some patients. Calcium channel blockers should be used with caution in patients with impaired left ventricular function; even nifedipine may cause worsening of heart failure.

All three agents are very effective in the management of patients with stable angina pectoris, and many of the studies have shown that these are as effective as beta blocking agents. Patients who cannot tolerate beta blockers are excellent candidates for treatment with calcium channel blockers. Patients with angina who have associated obstructive airway disease or peripheral vascular disease or hypertension are excellent candidates for therapy with these agents.

**Combination Therapy.** Before combining different agents, one should attempt to optimize treatment with a given single agent. When taking appropriate doses, many of the patients respond to monotherapy. However, when monotherapy fails and the patient is still experiencing angina, it is often advisable to add another therapeutic agent of a different class. Therefore, treatment of angina must be individualized, but some guidelines may be useful. Nitrates should be used in conjunction with beta blockers. Nitrates are very effective during the daytime, but because they do not provide continuous prophylaxis, concomitant therapy with a beta blocker with a long half-life or a long acting beta blocker provides additional protection during the hours when nitrates are not exerting any effects. Further, the two agents complement each other. Nitrates reduce or prevent cardiac dilation induced by beta blockade, whereas beta blockers prevent nitrate-induced reflex tachycardia.

There are few data regarding the usefulness of combinations of nitrates and calcium channel

TABLE 4. **Calcium Channel Blockers for Stable Angina Pectoris**

| | Bioavailability (%) | Effect on AV Nodal Delay | Usual Dose | Contraindications |
|---|---|---|---|---|
| Nifedipine (Procardia) | 45–70 | 0 | 10–40 mg tid or qid | Aortic stenosis, pre-existing tachycardia |
| Procardia XL | 45–70 | 0 | 30–120 mg once daily | Aortic stenosis, pre-existing tachycardia |
| Nicardipine (Cardene) | 35 | 0 | 20–40 mg tid | Aortic stenosis, pre-existing tachycardia |
| Diltiazem (Cardizem) | 40–67 | + + | 60–120 mg qid | Sick sinus syndrome, pre-existing AV block, digoxin toxicity, moderately severe myocardial depression |
| Verapamil (Calan/Isoptin) | 20–35 | + + | 90–120 mg tid | Same as for diltiazem |

blockers in the management of patients with stable angina pectoris. Because both nitrates and nifedipine or nicardipine may increase heart rate and reduce blood pressure, it is advisable to use a combination of nitrates plus verapamil or diltiazem, although the superiority of this combination over monotherapy with calcium blockers alone is not established.

A combination of beta blocker and calcium channel blocker is often used. There are some studies to show that combination therapy is more effective than monotherapy. It is safe to combine a beta blocker with nifedipine, but caution should be exercised in combining a beta blocker with verapamil because extreme bradycardia or even heart block may develop in some patients. Combination of a beta blocker with verapamil may precipitate heart failure. Combination of a beta blocker and diltiazem is usually well tolerated, but some patients may develop heart block.

The role of triple therapy in stable angina pectoris is questionable. Triple therapy in some patients may be less effective than double therapy.

**General Recommendations for Drug Therapy.** In patients who have minimal symptoms, intermittent use of sublingual nitrates may suffice. In patients who are moderately symptomatic, it is worthwhile to try beta blockers or calcium channel blockers or long acting nitrates. If the symptoms do not improve, a different agent should be tried. If some improvement occurs with one agent but the patient is still symptomatic, a combination of a beta blocker and nitrate preparation or calcium channel blocker should be considered. Efficacy of treatment should be assessed by serial exercise testing but may not be feasible, and relief of symptoms during daily activities may become a guide to therapy.

### Coronary Artery Bypass Surgery

Because of the relatively good prognosis in patients with stable angina pectoris, surgical therapy is recommended as initial therapy only in high-risk patients—i.e., those with left main disease or three-vessel disease and impaired left ventricular function. In the presence of good left ventricular function, the survival of patients treated with medical therapy or surgery is similar whether they have one-, two-, or three-vessel disease. Surgery may enhance the quality of life, but one should recognize that the immediate mortality of surgery is 1 to 4% and the incidence of myocardial infarction is 5 to 9%. Therefore, in patients with good left ventricular function, surgery is recommended only if symptoms persist despite medical therapy or if they are severe enough to interfere with the patient's lifestyle.

Even when medical therapy fails in patients with one- and two-vessel disease, an alternative to surgery is balloon angioplasty.

### Percutaneous Transluminal Coronary Angioplasty

Coronary balloon angioplasty is a safe alternative to bypass surgery and is often successful in patients with one-, two-, and even three-vessel disease. The procedure is, however, invasive and is associated with a 1 to 3% complication rate and therefore should be reserved for patients in whom symptoms persist despite medical therapy or in those who manifest myocardial ischemia during Stage I or II of the treadmill exercise test utilizing the Bruce protocol despite medical therapy. Patients who do not like to take medications are also good candidates for balloon angioplasty. Whether balloon angioplasty prolongs survival in patients with one-, two-, or three-vessel disease in the presence of normal ventricular function is not known. Restenosis of a dilated artery within the first 6 months remains a problem in some 20% of the patients, but a repeat procedure is often successful. Dilation of a stenotic artery often improves exercise tolerance and is a good alternative to surgery in symptomatic patients with one- or two-vessel disease at the present time. When patients are considered for balloon angioplasty, it is recommended that a cardiac open heart surgery team be on standby for emergency coronary bypass surgery in case complications occur. Following angioplasty, patients should be routinely followed because recurrence of symptoms within 6 months often indicates restenosis. Routine exercise testing or thallium exercise perfusion studies are often useful when done sequentially following angioplasty. Progression of disease is often indicated by recurrence of symptoms beyond a 6-month period.

## UNSTABLE ANGINA

### Pathophysiology

Unstable angina, until recently, was considered to result from progression of an atherosclerotic plaque, and superimposed coronary artery spasm at the site of the lesion was thought to precipitate ischemic episodes. Recent evidence has clearly shown that the culprit lesion in unstable angina is a fissuring of an atherosclerotic plaque, which predisposes the patient to platelet deposition and thrombus formation. In some patients, plaque progression may be contributory, and there is also evidence that in some patients with unstable angina, chest pain or myocardial ischemia is produced due to an increased myocardial oxygen demand rather than a reduction in blood flow. In patients with stable angina who start experiencing angina at lower levels of exertion, the mechanism responsible may be plaque progression. However, in patients with angina at rest and those experiencing frequent episodes of angina (crescendo angina), the underlying mechanism is invariably a complicated plaque with plaque rupture and deposition of platelets and/or thrombus formation. Even in patients in whom there is a progression of a plaque, platelets might deposit at the stenotic site and further reduce luminal diameter and blood flow.

During an episode of chest pain in patients with unstable angina, there is often electrocardiographic evidence of ST segment depression or ST-T wave changes. However, some patients experience classic chest pain without any ST-T changes. The usual duration of chest pain in unstable angina is 15 to 30 minutes, and up to three sublingual nitroglycerin tablets (0.4 to 0.6 mg per tablet) may be required for relief of pain.

### Management

Patients with unstable angina should be hospitalized. Any precipitating circumstance—e.g., loss of blood due to gastrointestinal hemorrhage or marked increase in blood pressure, thyrotoxicosis, or hypotension—that may produce unstable angina needs appropriate treatment.

Until recently, unstable angina was considered to be a medical emergency and many affected patients were taken immediately to the cardiac catheterization laboratory for coronary angiography and subsequent coronary bypass surgery. Recent identification of pathophysiologic mechanisms and the results showing that surgical therapy does not reduce mortality and may even increase the incidence of myocardial infarction have changed this approach.

#### Pharmacologic Treatment in the Initial Phase

Aspirin is a highly effective therapy that according to Veterans Administration and Canadian studies reduces the development of acute myocardial infarction as well as mortality by approximately 50% as compared with placebo. A recent study from Canada has shown that therapy with aspirin or intravenous heparin is equally effective and the combination of the two agents is more effective than therapy with either agent alone, but the incidence of bleeding complications increases during combination therapy. The present recommendation, therefore, is to use aspirin provided that there are no contraindications. A dose of 80 to 320 mg given once a day is sufficient to prevent platelet aggregation and is usually effective in the management of patients with unstable angina pectoris. An alternative is

to use intravenous heparin for 48 to 72 hours aiming to maintain the partial thromboplastin time at one and a half to twice normal. There is some concern of rebound increase in angina when heparin is suddenly stopped. Therefore, one should institute aspirin therapy prior to discontinuing heparin. Aspirin should be continued indefinitely.

Although both aspirin and heparin are effective in reducing the incidence of myocardial infarction and mortality in patients with unstable angina pectoris, these agents do not relieve chest pain or myocardial ischemia immediately. Intravenous nitroglycerin relieves ischemic and anginal episodes rapidly and plays an important role in the initial management of patients with unstable angina. How nitroglycerin works in patients with unstable angina is not entirely clear, but it probably works predominantly by venodilator effects with resultant decrease in ventricular volumes and end-diastolic pressures. In addition, nitrates, by dilating coronary arteries, may increase blood flow. There is also evidence that nitrates inhibit platelet aggregation in vitro and reduce platelet deposition and vasoconstriction at the site of endothelial injury, and this effect of nitrates may improve blood flow to the ischemic regions.

It is recommended that intravenous nitroglycerin be used, provided that the systolic blood pressure prior to institution of therapy is 100 mmHg or higher. Intravenous nitroglycerin (5 to 10 µg per minute) should be started if there are no contraindications to nitrate therapy. The dose can be titrated upward every 5 to 10 minutes with the aim of relieving angina or until a fall in systolic blood pressure to 90 mmHg has occurred. On the other hand, in patients who are asymptomatic at the time of hospitalization, it is recommended that intravenous nitroglycerin be titrated with the aim of reducing mean arterial pressure by 10 to 15 mmHg. If anginal pain recurs, the dose can be titrated upward as often as necessary (up to 1000 µg per minute or higher) and if adverse effects develop, discontinuation of therapy is warranted. Intravenous nitroglycerin should be used for a period of 24 to 72 hours, and it is recommended that one gradually taper off nitroglycerin and institute therapy with oral nitrates. In the acute phase of unstable angina, there is no role for intermittent nitrate therapy. Nitroglycerin ointment, 1 inch to 1 1/2 inch applied every 6 hours, has also been used with effectiveness; similarly, isosorbide dinitrate, 60 mg four times a day in combination with nitroglycerin ointment, has been shown to be beneficial. It is, however, preferable to use intravenous nitroglycerin because it can be easily titrated upward to achieve therapeutic effects and in case an adverse reaction occurs, it can be rapidly titrated downward or discontinued.

Headaches that may be experienced by patients during intravenous nitroglycerin therapy often are not a major problem, but in some patients headaches are severe and unresponsive to analgesics, which necessitates discontinuation of therapy. In some patients, excessive hypotension may be a problem, especially in patients with unstable angina following an inferior myocardial infarction with right ventricular involvement. Even when one uses very high doses of intravenous nitroglycerin, methemoglobinemia is not usually a problem unless the patient has severe concomitant obstructive airway disease.

In patients who do not respond to intravenous nitroglycerin, it is recommended that concomitant therapy with a beta blocker be instituted. A combination of beta blocker and nitrates has been shown to be superior to oral nitrate therapy alone. However, vasodilatory beta blockers may aggravate myocardial ischemia and should be avoided.

An alternate to intravenous nitroglycerin is monotherapy with intravenous atenolol 5 mg, followed by 5 mg 10 minutes later and then oral therapy with 100 mg daily. Used in this manner, atenolol reduces mortality and the incidence of myocardial infarction in patients with unstable angina.

Use of calcium channel blockers as initial therapy of unstable angina is not recommended. However, in patients who are symptomatic despite therapy with nitrates and beta blockers, the addition of nifedipine is worth a trial. However, caution should be exercised because the adverse effects of combination therapy may increase during concomitant therapy. The role of thrombolytic agents, streptokinase, and tissue plasminogen activator (tPA) in unstable angina is not well defined, and these agents are not recommended for routine use at the present time.

### Pharmacologic Treatment in the Late Phase

Once the patient with unstable angina has been stabilized for at least 24 hours or longer, intravenous therapy with nitroglycerin should be gradually tapered and oral nitrate therapy (isosorbide dinitrate, 30 mg, two to three times a day) started, with the first dose of oral therapy prescribed 1 to 2 hours prior to discontinuation of the intravenous infusion for fear of a rebound increase in angina. Because intermittent nitrate therapy does not provide 24-hour antianginal prophylaxis, it is recommended that concomitant therapy with a long-acting beta blocking agent or a calcium channel blocker like diltiazem or verapamil be used in order to provide 24-hour

antianginal and anti-ischemic effects. Therapy with aspirin, 80 to 325 mg once daily, should be continued indefinitely.

Subsequently, patients can be stratified into a low- or high-risk group by performing an exercise test. Gated blood pool studies to evaluate left ventricular function or thallium perfusion study to assess the myocardium at risk are also useful in identifying a high-risk group. High-risk patients should undergo coronary angiography, and patients with left main disease and those with triple vessel disease and decreased left ventricular function should be considered for coronary bypass surgery.

### Non-Pharmacologic Treatment

Patients who remain symptomatic despite high-dose intravenous nitroglycerin, beta blockers, aspirin, and heparin therapy need urgent coronary angiography with or without preceding insertion of an intra-aortic balloon pump. Urgent balloon angioplasty or coronary bypass surgery is often necessary in this subgroup of patients, but 10 to 13% of these patients have normal coronary arteries and in this group of patients, medical therapy is indicated. The incidence of myocardial infarction following bypass surgery and angioplasty is 5 to 8% and it is recommended that antiplatelet therapy with aspirin be continued even after these procedures.

## VARIANT (PRINZMETAL'S) ANGINA

In this syndrome, angina occurs primarily as a result of coronary artery spasm either at the site of an atherosclerotic lesion, which is the case in the majority of patients, or in one or more branches of normal coronary arteries. In addition to coronary artery spasm, many affected patients give a history of migraine or Raynaud's phenomenon. The pain usually occurs at rest, and exercise tolerance is invariably normal. During an episode of pain, if an electrocardiogram is taken, it usually shows ST segment elevation; under these circumstances, no further diagnostic procedures are indicated. These patients are prone to ventricular arrhythmias and conduction disturbances. Sudden death or syncope may occur. In patients who give a history suggestive of variant angina but in whom it is not possible to obtain an electrocardiogram during an episode of chest pain, a 24-hour Holter monitor may show episodes of ST segment elevation. An alternative is to give intracoronary or intravenous ergonovine to reproduce chest pain, electrocardiographic ST segment elevation, or focal coronary artery spasm during coronary angiography.

### Management

Both nitrates and calcium channel blockers are very effective. Because of the development of tolerance to nitrates during sustained therapy, it is recommended that calcium channel blockers be used, as tolerance development does not seem to be a problem. Non-selective beta blockers are usually contraindicated because these agents may aggravate coronary artery spasm. Coronary artery bypass surgery or balloon angioplasty is not recommended unless the patient has a severe proximal lesion of a dominant coronary artery. However, because of the underlying pathophysiologic mechanism, these patients may continue to experience symptoms despite surgery or balloon angioplasty, and long-term therapy with calcium channel blockers is recommended.

# CARDIAC ARREST

method of
BÉLA B. HACKMAN, M.D. and
ARTHUR L. KELLERMANN, M.D., M.P.H.
*The University of Tennessee*
*Memphis, Tennessee*

Despite a progressive decline in cardiovascular mortality over the past 20 years, heart disease remains the leading cause of death in industrialized countries. Of the 700,000 deaths attributable to heart disease in the United States each year, almost half occur suddenly, within an hour of the onset of symptoms. Although a majority of cardiac arrest victims have had prior evidence of heart disease, sudden cardiac death is the first sign of trouble in 20 to 25%.

## ETIOLOGY AND RISK FACTORS

About four out of every five cardiac arrests occur in the context of chronic coronary heart disease; a variety of other conditions account for the remainder (Table 1). In patients with coronary disease, underlying myocardial fibrosis due to prior infarction is present in

TABLE 1. **Common Causes of Cardiac Arrest**

| |
|---|
| Coronary heart disease |
| Valvular heart disease |
| Hypertrophic cardiomyopathy |
| Dilated cardiomyopathy |
| Cardiac conduction abnormalities |
|    Prolonged QT syndromes |
|    Pre-excitation syndromes |
|    Heart block |
| Drug effects |
|    Intoxication |
|    Proarrhythmia |
|    Metabolic (i.e., hypokalemia) |
| Pulmonary embolism |
| Cerebrovascular occlusion and hemorrhage |

over 50%. Although most arrests are thought to be precipitated by acute myocardial ischemia, only one-fourth of patients develop evidence of an acute myocardial infarction.

Because sudden cardiac death is so commonly associated with atherosclerotic coronary artery disease, the risk factors for cardiac arrest generally parallel those for atherosclerosis. Certain factors, such as cigarette smoking, hypercholesterolemia, and hypertension, are amenable to intervention. Others, including male sex, family history, advanced age, and co-morbid conditions, are not. When complex ventricular ectopy and poor left ventricular function accompany structural heart disease of any etiology, the risk for sudden death is particularly high.

## MECHANISMS AND RATES OF SURVIVAL

Because the onset of cardiac arrest is sudden and unpredictable, most arrests occur outside of the hospital, usually in the home of the victim. In 50 to 70% of cases, paramedics arriving shortly after collapse find the victim in ventricular tachycardia (VT) or ventricular fibrillation (VF). Brady-asystolic rhythms and electromechanical dissociation (EMD) are encountered less frequently and are generally associated with prolonged arrest, extensive cardiac disease, or severe disease of other organ systems. Under ideal circumstances, 50 to 60% of victims found in VF or tachycardia can be resuscitated and roughly half of these survive to hospital discharge. In contrast, the prognosis for patients found in other rhythms is much worse. Regardless of circumstances, fewer than 5% survive to be discharged from the hospital.

Hospitalized patients who suffer cardiac arrest are more frequently found in bradyarrhythmias and EMD. In contrast to victims of out-of-hospital cardiac arrest, in-hospital victims tend to be older and have a higher prevalence of severe cardiac disease, renal failure, pneumonia, sepsis, diabetes, and cancer. Not surprisingly, rates of survival are poor in these patients. As in out-of-hospital arrest, the ventricular tachyarrhythmias appear to be the only rhythms significantly associated with survival.

### RESUSCITATION AND PREDICTORS OF SURVIVAL

The predictors of survival following cardiac arrest have been well established. Some, such as whether or not the arrest was witnessed, are a matter of chance. Others reflect the patient's individual characteristics, among them age and general medical condition. These "fate" factors cannot be altered to improve survival. In contrast, other determinants, sometimes termed "program" factors, can be favorably influenced by the configuration and efficiency of the emergency medical service (EMS) system. These include prompt recognition of cardiac arrest; rapid activation of the EMS system; the availability of bystander CPR; and a short time interval from collapse to provision of basic and advanced cardiac life support, especially defibrillation.

## Early Recognition and Activation of the EMS

The effectiveness of any EMS system depends on prompt recognition of cardiac arrest and rapid activation of the emergency response team. When cardiac arrest is witnessed and help is summoned quickly, survival is five times greater than if the arrest is unwitnessed or unrecognized. In the community, public education programs to increase public awareness of cardiac arrest may reduce delays in calling for help. Widespread adoption of a "universal" emergency telephone number (i.e., "9-1-1") facilitates public access to emergency services dramatically. In the hospital setting, all personnel, including maintenance and housekeeping staff, must be trained to recognize cardiac arrest and to summon help immediately. As in the community, an established emergency phone number is crucial to ensure rapid activation of the hospital emergency response team.

## Basic Life Support (BLS)—Cardiopulmonary Resuscitation (CPR)

Early initiation of CPR significantly improves a victim's chances of survival after cardiac arrest (for the technique of CPR, see Figure 1). In cases of out-of-hospital cardiac arrest, survival of victims receiving CPR within 4 minutes is almost twice that when CPR is delayed beyond 4 minutes. Ideally, the bystander who witnesses the arrest or first discovers the victim should begin CPR. Bystander-initiated CPR, by markedly reducing the time from collapse to CPR, nearly doubles a victim's chances of being discharged from the hospital. Mass community training programs have raised the rates of bystander CPR in

- *Establish unresponsiveness*
- *Call for assistance*
- *Position the airway:*
  Tilt the head back by lifting the chin forward or pulling up on the angles of the jaw.
- *Establish apnea:*
  Listen at the mouth and nares for air movement, watch the chest for rise and fall.
- *Ventilate:*
  Form tight seal with mask or mouth, pinch nose if mouth to mouth; blow hard enough to make the chest rise, deliver 2 ventilations immediately.
- *Establish pulselessness:*
  Palpate the carotid artery for pulsations.
- *Begin chest compressions:*
  Place heel of hands in mid sternum 1–2 inches cephalad to the xiphoid process, lock elbows, and compress about 1.5–2 inches at a rate of 80/min.
- *Alternate ventilations and compressions:*
  *For one* man CPR, deliver 2 ventilations for each 15 chest compressions; for *two* man CPR, deliver 1 ventilation for each 5 chest compressions.

**Figure 1.** Technique of cardiopulmonary resuscitation (CPR).

some communities, but such programs require a pool of dedicated instructors, a motivated populace, and a major commitment of health care resources.

Given the fact that the majority of cardiac arrests occur in the home, a member of the victim's family is most likely to witness cardiac arrest. Therefore, families of persons at high risk for cardiac arrest should receive training in CPR. Currently, practicing physicians infrequently recommend such training.

Recently, two independent groups have shown that emergency CPR instructions can be provided over the telephone to callers reporting cardiac arrest. Comparable levels of performance with that achieved by conventionally trained individuals can be obtained. Telephone CPR instruction by EMS dispatchers may be a highly focused and cost-effective way to increase rates of bystander CPR.

## Advanced Cardiac Life Support—Defibrillation

The most crucial determinant of outcome following cardiac arrest is the interval of time from collapse to the provision of definitive care, principally defibrillation. If victims of out-of-hospital ventricular fibrillation receive definitive care within 6 minutes, they are three times more likely to survive than if care is delayed. Until recently, only paramedic units have had the training and authority necessary to provide prehospital defibrillation. In the mid-1980s, efforts to reduce the delay between collapse and delivery of the first defibrillatory shock concentrated on training first-responding basic emergency medical technicians (EMTs) to operate standard manual defibrillators. Although this program was promising, the costs of training and skills maintenance were found to be high.

Fortunately, computer driven defibrillators (automatic external defibrillators, or AEDs) are now available that automatically interpret the patient's rhythm and advise the rescuer if a shock is indicated. These devices have been shown to significantly reduce training and retraining costs. In rural and suburban settings where prehospital defibrillation has not been previously available, EMT defibrillation programs using manual or automatic defibrillators have been shown to improve survival in out-of-hospital cardiac arrest. Uncontrolled studies suggest that similar benefits may be achieved even in urban areas with existing paramedic services. A controlled trial is in progress.

Within the hospital setting, designated personnel capable of rapid response and trained in advanced cardiac life support (ACLS) must be

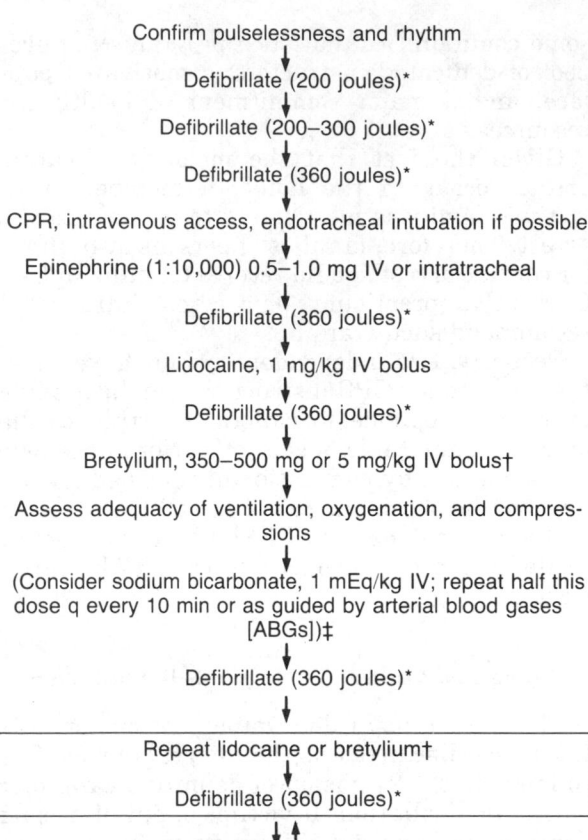

\*Assess pulse and rhythm after each shock.

†Repeat bretylium at 700 to 1000 mg or 10 mg/kg IV bolus; lidocaine at 0.5 mg/kg q 8 min to a total dose of 3 mg/kg may be substituted for bretylium.

‡Sodium bicarbonate is of questionable value during cardiac arrest.

**Figure 2.** Algorithm for ventricular fibrillation and ventricular tachycardia. Pulseless ventricular tachycardia is treated identically to ventricular fibrillations.

available at all times. Figures 2 through 5 summarize the current consensus approach to the treatment of four major dysrhythmias associated with cardiac arrest.

### Termination of Resuscitation

In general, if an organized rhythm and pulse have not returned after 15 to 20 minutes of determined CPR and advanced cardiac life support, success with further treatment is extremely unlikely. The outcome for patients experiencing out-of-hospital cardiac arrest who have failed prehospital resuscitation is uniformly dismal; multiple studies have confirmed that fewer than 2% survive to hospital discharge despite continued attempts at resuscitation in the emergency department. Those who do survive are almost invariably left with severe neurologic impairment. Therefore, in patients rushed to the emer-

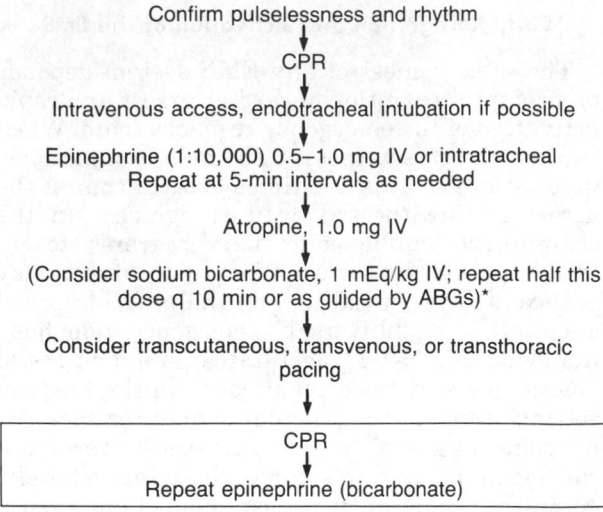

If patient is hypothermic, core temperature should be normalized. Fine ventricular fibrillation may appear to be asystole, and an attempt at defibrillation may therefore be considered.

\*Note: Sodium bicarbonate is of questionable value during cardiac arrest.

**Figure 3.** Algorithm for asystole.

gency department after failed field resuscitation, continued efforts should be brief and limited to confirming that prehospital measures were adequate. Exceptions to this rule are patients who are unsuccessfully intubated, those who respond transiently in the field, and those who are profoundly hypothermic. In these cases, survival is possible even following prolonged arrest and resuscitation. Even so, most authorities now agree that lack of response to 30 minutes of adequate treatment virtually precludes survival in all but the most severely hypothermic patients.

Similar guidelines may be applied to hospitalized patients suffering cardiac arrest. Because

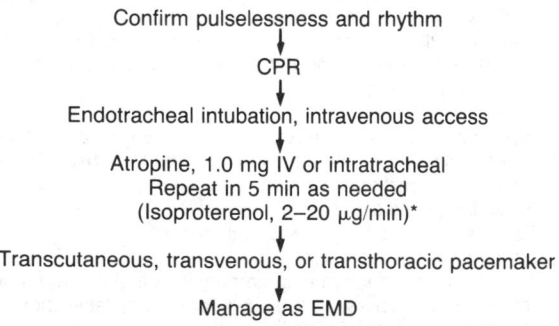

\*Use only if transcutaneous pacing is not immediately available while preparations are being made for transvenous or transthoracic pacing.

**Figure 4.** Algorithm for bradycardia–heart block. This algorithm is intended to be used for bradycardia or heart block only in the context of *full arrest*.

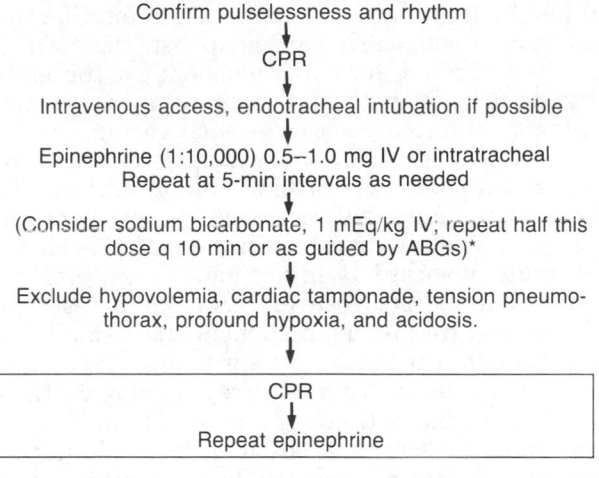

Confirm pulselessness and rhythm
↓
CPR
↓
Intravenous access, endotracheal intubation if possible
↓
Epinephrine (1:10,000) 0.5–1.0 mg IV or intratracheal
Repeat at 5-min intervals as needed
↓
(Consider sodium bicarbonate, 1 mEq/kg IV; repeat half this
dose q 10 min or as guided by ABGs)*
↓
Exclude hypovolemia, cardiac tamponade, tension pneumo-
thorax, profound hypoxia, and acidosis.
↓
CPR
↓
Repeat epinephrine

*Sodium bicarbonate is of questionable value during cardiac arrest.

**Figure 5.** Algorithm for electromechanical dissociation.

severe non-cardiac disease is frequently present in hospitalized patients and usually determines long-term outcome, the decision to attempt resuscitation in a chronically ill individual should be made in advance and explicitly communicated to personnel responsible for the patient's care. Chart documentation and specific orders regarding resuscitation clarify this decision and minimize confusion regarding the patient's or family's wishes.

## POSTRESUSCITATION MANAGEMENT

The potential for long-term survival following cardiac arrest is determined by the "fate" and "program" factors outlined earlier. Maximizing this potential, however, requires meticulous care in the early hours and days following successful resuscitation. Following an initial phase of stabilization and recovery, those who survive must be carefully evaluated to reduce their chances of recurrence.

### Postresuscitation Complications

**Recurrent Arrhythmia.** Most cases of cardiac arrest are precipitated by VT-VF, and virtually all survivors are initially found in these rhythms. Because the risk of recurrence is highest during the first 24 hours after arrest, it is prudent to continue the antiarrhythmic drug successfully used during the resuscitation for at least this interval of time. If no drugs were used (e.g., a patient who responded to the initial series of shocks), lidocaine is the drug of first choice. Should lidocaine fail to suppress complex ventricular ectopy, procainamide (Pronestyl) and bretylium (Bretylol) should be tried in succession. In

unusual cases, single drugs do not provide adequate suppression and combination therapy (i.e., procainamide and lidocaine) may be required. Antiarrhythmic therapy is continued for 24 to 48 hours after clinical stability has been achieved. (See Table 2 for antiarrhythmic drug dosing.)

**Coma.** Anoxic brain damage is the most frequent cause of death after successful resuscitation from cardiac arrest. Prognosis is closely related to the duration of coma; early awakening is associated with improved survival and better neurologic outcomes. Although most patients who regain consciousness do so by 72 hours (greater than 90%), late awakenings can occur. Because the duration of coma and extent of neurologic damage are directly related to the length of time from collapse to the re-establishment of effective cardiac function, rapid provision of basic and advanced life support is essential to reduce the frequency and severity of neurologic sequelae. Interventions designed to lessen anoxic brain damage after resuscitation, such as induced hypothermia and the administration of high doses of barbiturates, calcium channel blockers, or free radical scavengers, remain investigational. Current therapy for anoxic encephalopathy is largely supportive.

**Shock.** Cardiovascular collapse is second only to anoxic encephalopathy as a cause of death following cardiac arrest. In some instances, it is secondary to extensive myocardial infarction; more frequently, it is due to diffuse myocardial and vascular dysfunction caused by prolonged hypoxia and acidosis. Initial management should focus on correction of hypoxia, acid-base, and electrolyte abnormalities. Volume infusion and therapy with inotropic or pressor agents are often needed and, optimally, should be guided by measurements of cardiac output, ventricular filling pressure, and systemic vascular resistance using a pulmonary artery catheter. First, hypovolemia should be excluded by infusion of normal saline to achieve a left ventricular filling pressure (pulmonary capillary wedge pressure) of 15 to 16

TABLE 2. **Antiarrhythmic Drug Dosage**

| Compound | Usual Intravenous Loading Dose | Usual Maintenance Infusion Rate |
|---|---|---|
| Lidocaine (Xylocaine) | 1.5 mg/kg followed in 10 min by 0.5 mg/kg | 2–4 mg/min |
| Procainamide (Pronestyl) | 50 mg every 5 min to a total of 1 gram* | 1–4 mg/min |
| Bretylium (Bretylol) | 5–10 mg/kg over 8–10 min | 2 mg/min |

*Or until the arrhythmia is suppressed, hypotension occurs, or the baseline QRS widens by ≥50%.

mmHg. If volume expansion alone fails to improve the shock state or if filling pressures are normal to high from the outset, further therapy is guided by blood pressure and systemic vascular resistance measurements. In general, low cardiac output syndromes with normal to high blood pressure and systemic resistance respond well to inotropic agents with vasodilator properties (e.g., dobutamine [Dobutrex] or amrinone [Inocor]). When elevated filling pressures and pulmonary congestion are encountered, reduction of central blood volume with diuretics or additional vasodilation with nitroprusside (Nipride) may be required. If low output is accompanied by low blood pressure and resistance, an agent with both pressor and inotropic effects such as dopamine is preferred. The addition of a "pure" pressor agent, such as norepinephrine, may be needed to support blood pressure in some patients. Refractory shock should prompt a search for treatable complications of resuscitation such as pneumothorax, pericardial tamponade, or intra-abdominal injuries.

### Identification of High-Risk Patients

**Evaluation of Survivors.** The optimal evaluation and long-term treatment of patients who survive cardiac arrest are still in evolution. However, high-risk patients have been identified who may benefit from intensive evaluation and pharmacologic or nonpharmacologic treatment. Other groups of patients appear to be at a relatively low risk for recurrence and have little to gain from aggressive antiarrhythmic therapy.

**Risk Group Stratification.** Because survivors who have sustained an acute Q-wave myocardial infarction have a much lower risk of recurrence than those whose arrest occurred in the absence of an acute infarction, serial cardiac enzyme values and electrocardiograms must be obtained in all patients. Triggering factors such as drug toxicity (cocaine, phenothiazines, tricyclic antidepressants, digitalis, antiarrhythmics) and profound electrolyte imbalance (hypokalemia, hypomagnesemia) must be routinely sought. After stabilization, most patients should undergo cardiac catheterization with coronary angiography and echocardiography to characterize underlying structural heart disease.

On the basis of this evaluation, most patients will fall into one of four groups:

1. *Patients with cardiac arrest within 24 hours of an acute myocardial infarction.* Roughly one-fourth of patients with underlying coronary artery disease who experience cardiac arrest will evolve evidence of an acute Q wave myocardial infarction. If the cardiac arrest occurred within 24 hours of infarction, prognosis appears to be no different from patients sustaining infarction not associated with early cardiac arrest. Risk stratification and long-term management are therefore the same as for patients with similar myocardial infarctions uncomplicated by early cardiac arrest.

2. *Patients with coronary disease and cardiac arrest without acute myocardial infarction.* The bulk of patients with coronary disease who experience cardiac arrest do not develop evidence of acute myocardial infarction. These patients have a high incidence of recurrent arrest and deserve aggressive management. It is this large subgroup of cardiac arrest survivors who appear to benefit most from electrophysiologic (EP)–guided antiarrhythmic drug selection, antiarrhythmic surgery, and possibly the implantation of an automatic implantable cardioverter-defibrillator (AICD). Cardiac catheterization and a functional assessment using exercise or dipyridamole thallium scanning should be performed prior to electrophysiologic studies. Optimal antiischemic medical therapy and revascularization, if indicated, can then be accomplished to ensure a stable myocardial substrate during electrophysiologic testing.

3. *Patients with a reversible precipitating cause of cardiac arrest.* This group includes patients who have experienced cardiac arrest clearly caused by drug intoxication or proarrhythmic effects (cocaine, digitalis, antiarrhythmics, phenothiazines, or tricyclic antidepressants) or profound electrolyte abnormalities (hypokalemia, hypomagnesemia). After reversal of the underlying cause of arrest, these patients may undergo noninvasive screening for cardiac disease with echocardiography, exercise thallium testing, and 48-hour ambulatory ECG monitoring. If no significant spontaneous or exercise-induced arrhythmia is found, electrophysiologic testing and long-term antiarrhythmic therapy are usually not indicated.

4. *Patients with noncoronary heart disease or no identifiable heart disease.* The proper approach to patients with noncoronary heart disease or no identifiable heart disease is less clear. The risk of recurrence is often high in this heterogeneous group, and therapy to prevent recurrence is desirable. In general, empiric antiarrhythmic drug therapy has not proved to be of value for prevention of recurrence in these patients. Therapy guided by electrophysiologic testing is essential in the management of some patients (e.g., patients with pre-excitation syndromes) but is of uncertain utility in others (e.g., dilated cardiomyopathy). In still others (e.g., those with hypertrophic cardiomyopathy or the idiopathic long QT syndromes), electrophysiologic testing has been proved to be of no value. The assistance of an experienced electrophysiologist is essential to se-

lect an appropriate management strategy for patients with these complex problems.

## PREVENTION OF CARDIAC ARREST

### Prevention of Coronary Heart Disease

Because coronary heart disease is responsible for the vast majority of cardiac arrests, it stands to reason (although the hypothesis is unproved) that preventing coronary disease will reduce the incidence of sudden cardiac arrest. Cessation of smoking is arguably the single most effective way to reduce the risk of coronary disease. Reduction of dietary calories and saturated fat and regular aerobic exercise will reduce serum cholesterol and improve the ratio of atherogenic low density to protective high density lipoproteins. For patients with severely elevated cholesterol, modern drug therapy is spectacularly effective in reducing serum cholesterol levels and, to a lesser extent, coronary risk. Finally, although antihypertensive therapy with older drugs has not significantly reduced the incidence of coronary disease, newer drugs (especially the angiotensin converting enzyme [ACE] inhibitors and calcium channel agents) that produce less metabolic perturbation may be effective in reducing coronary risk in hypertensive patients.

### Primary Prevention of Cardiac Arrest in Patients with Structural Heart Disease

Although patients with established structural heart disease (particularly coronary heart disease with prior infarction) accompanied by left ventricular dysfunction and spontaneous ventricular ectopy are at high risk for sudden cardiac death, prophylactic treatment with antiarrhythmic drugs has not been shown to be effective. Indeed, several studies, including the ongoing CAST (Cardiac Arrhythmia Suppression Trial), have shown that many available antiarrhythmic drugs can actually *increase* mortality when used to treat patients with asymptomatic ventricular arrhythmia. Therefore, antiarrhythmic therapy for ventricular arrhythmias should be limited to patients who have sustained ventricular tachycardia or highly symptomatic nonsustained ventricular ectopy (e.g., with near-syncope, syncope, or sudden cardiac death).

### Prevention of Drug-Induced Cardiac Arrest

Although only a small fraction of cardiac arrests are induced by proarrhythmic and toxic drug effects or by electrolyte abnormalities, many of these arrests are preventable. Hypomagnesemia and hypokalemia are commonly caused by excessive diuretic therapy and should be assiduously avoided in all patients taking diuretics, most importantly those with structural heart disease and those taking digitalis glycosides. In such patients, it is prudent to keep serum potassium levels in the upper range of normal. Digitalis toxicity is a common clinical problem in patients with heart disease and can be avoided by close attention to drug interactions, renal function, and potassium balance, all of which may require changes in digitalis dosage or potassium replacement. Type I-A antiarrhythmics (e.g., quinidine), and drugs with similar electrophysiologic properties, such as the phenothiazines and tricyclic antidepressants, typically prolong the QT interval in patients who experience drug-induced arrest. Thus the electrocardiogram must be closely monitored for excessive QT prolongation in all patients taking these compounds. Other antiarrhythmic drugs (especially flecainide [Tambocor] and encainide [Enkaid]) do not appear to produce warning signs before their proarrhythmic effects become manifest. Because proarrhythmia is often unpredictable and frequently occurs early in the course of treatment, antiarrhythmic therapy is most safely initiated in the hospital under monitored conditions.

# ATRIAL FIBRILLATION

method of
PAUL F. WALTER, M.D.
*Emory University School of Medicine*
*Atlanta, Georgia*

Atrial fibrillation is a relatively common arrhythmia and is more common than the other atrial tachyarrhythmias. It may occur in sustained or paroxysmal form. Atrial fibrillation occurs in patients with mitral valve disease, coronary artery disease, systemic arterial hypertension, dilated cardiomyopathy, and constrictive pericarditis. It is a common arrhythmia following heart surgery. Atrial fibrillation is uncommon in patients with congenital heart disease, except for adults with atrial septal defect. It appears in association with diseases that are not primarily cardiac problems, such as hyperthyroidism, chronic obstructive lung disease, and pulmonary embolus. In susceptible persons with otherwise apparently normal hearts, the arrhythmia is occasionally precipitated by an alcohol spree. Heart failure from any cause may initiate atrial fibrillation; on the other hand, the onset of rapid atrial fibrillation may precipitate heart failure in the diseased but otherwise compensated heart. It is occasionally detected in apparently healthy persons, when it is called "lone fibrillation."

Atrial fibrillation may be asymptomatic, but most patients complain of palpitations, fatigue, or dyspnea.

It exacts two hemodynamic penalties. The loss of a synchronized atrial contraction decreases ventricular filling, and the rapid, irregular ventricular response abbreviates diastolic filling time and increases left atrial pressure. A decrease in cardiac output and congestive heart failure may result. Atrial fibrillation also predisposes to systemic emboli.

## TREATMENT

Since atrial fibrillation is associated with so many diverse cardiac and noncardiac disorders and the hemodynamic changes are so variable, intelligent management is impossible without thorough assessment of all the patient's medical problems. Hemodynamic consequences of atrial fibrillation range from the extremes of pulmonary edema in a patient with tight mitral stenosis to minor palpitations in a person with no other cardiac or pulmonary disease. The patient's hemodynamic status must be appraised and a search made for factors that may contribute to the development of atrial fibrillation. Occasionally, eliminating sympathomimetic amines and correcting metabolic acidosis, hypoxemia, respiratory alkalosis or acidosis, or electrolyte abnormalities may restore sinus rhythm. When myocardial ischemia, congestive heart failure, pericarditis, pneumonia, and pulmonary embolus coexist, their concomitant treatment may speed the resolution of atrial fibrillation. Atrial fibrillation may be the major clinical finding suggesting the possibility of hyperthyroidism, especially in elderly people.

### Medical Emergencies Produced by Atrial Fibrillation

In some patients with severe mitral stenosis, coronary atherosclerotic heart disease, hypertrophic cardiomyopathy, or the Wolff-Parkinson-White syndrome, the abrupt onset of atrial fibrillation with a rapid ventricular response may produce hemodynamic changes that threaten life and require immediate, synchronous, direct current cardioversion. In patients with tight mitral stenosis, the rapid, irregular ventricular response decreases diastolic filling time and results in an abrupt increase in left atrial pressure with resultant pulmonary edema. Myocardial ischemia and a marked decrease in cardiac output may occur with the appearance of atrial fibrillation in patients with severe coronary artery disease. The rapid ventricular rate and loss of atrial contribution to ventricular filling may cause angina, hypotension, and pulmonary congestion when the left ventricle is stiff and noncompliant, as occurs with hypertrophic cardiomyopathy.

Atrial fibrillation is a threat to patients with the Wolff-Parkinson-White syndrome when the refractory period of the accessory pathway is so short that the pathway can conduct 250 or more impulses per minute to the ventricle. In this situation, the electrocardiogram shows an irregular ventricular response as rapid as 300 beats a minute and wide, bizarre QRS complexes. Immediate, synchronous cardioversion is imperative in these patients because the development of ventricular fibrillation is a definite risk. Digitalis and verapamil (Isoptin) are contraindicated because they may facilitate accessory pathway conduction, accelerate the ventricular rate, and increase the risk of ventricular fibrillation.

### Control of the Rapid Ventricular Response

For most patients with atrial fibrillation, emergency cardioversion is not needed, and medical treatment is sufficient. The initial medical treatment is designed to slow atrioventricular (AV) conduction and thereby decrease the ventricular rate. Factors facilitating rapid AV node conduction such as fever, drugs, or hypokalemia should be corrected. Slowing of AV node conduction may be achieved with digitalis glycosides. Digoxin 0.50 mg should be administered intravenously over 5 minutes. This initial dose may be followed by the administration of digoxin, 0.25 mg every 2 to 3 hours until a total dose of 1.5 mg has been given or the ventricular rate is less than 100 beats a minute. It is preferable to obtain an electrocardiographic rhythm strip prior to giving supplemental doses of digoxin in order to detect signs of digitalis intoxication, such as ectopic ventricular depolarizations or AV junctional rhythm. The serum potassium and magnesium must be determined and any deficit corrected. If the ventricular response remains too rapid following 1.5 mg of digoxin, additional doses of 0.125 mg may be given every 2 to 3 hours until the ventricular rate is controlled or the total digoxin dose is 2 mg.

The patient's physiologic state must be considered when determining the appropriate ventricular rate. Generally, ventricular rates ranging from 60 to 90 beats per minute at rest and 90 to 115 beats per minute during moderate exercise are ideal. Digoxin may not produce such a controlled ventricular response in patients with fever, anemia, hyperthyroidism or increased sympathetic activity. Ordinarily, the resting heart rate would exceed 90 beats per minute if these patients were in sinus rhythm. Aggressive digoxin therapy in such circumstances may precipitate digitalis intoxication before the ventricular response has slowed satisfactorily. It is no longer necessary to give extraordinarily large doses of digoxin—greater than 2 mg—in the first 24 hours for the treatment of acute atrial fibrillation since beta-adrenergic blocking drugs or calcium-entry blocking drugs may be given concurrently to help slow the ventricular rate.

Beta-adrenergic blocking drugs such as propranolol (Inderal) or metoprolol (Lopressor) are given when a rapid ventricular rate persists despite digoxin therapy. However, patients with hyperthyroidism, hypertrophic cardiomyopathy, or mitral valve prolapse should receive beta-blocking drugs at the outset. One mg of propranolol is given intravenously every 5 minutes until the ventricular rate is controlled or a total dose of 0.10 mg per kg has been administered. The blood pressure, ventricular rate, and respiratory status are monitored before each dose. Beta-blocking drugs are contraindicated in patients with reactive airway disease or severe left ventricular dysfunction. Patients with chronic bronchitis without hyper-reactive airways usually tolerate metoprolol without increased bronchospasm. All beta-blocking drugs may aggravate heart failure when increased sympathetic activity is needed to support a failing circulation. However, when heart failure is directly related to atrial fibrillation, the beneficial effect of slowing the ventricular response may exceed the drug's negative inotropic action.

Verapamil (Calan, Isoptin), a calcium-entry blocker, exerts a depressant effect on AV nodal conduction and may be used when beta blockers are contraindicated. Unlike beta blockers, verapamil does not cause bronchial constriction and is particularly useful in patients with reactive airway disease. Rapid control of the ventricular rate can be achieved with intravenous verapamil, but its effect on AV node conduction is brief, so that after 30 minutes the ventricular response gradually accelerates. The usual intravenous dose is 2.5 to 10 mg. Careful blood pressure monitoring is mandatory since arterial hypotension is a common complication. Verapamil rarely restores sinus rhythm. The drug's negative inotropic action precludes its use in the presence of advanced heart failure. Verapamil should not be given in combination with beta blockers since the depressant effects on AV nodal conduction and the negative inotropic actions are probably additive.

Chronic control of the ventricular response generally can be accomplished with digoxin, given alone or in combination with a beta-blocking drug or a calcium-entry blocker. The requisite daily dose of digoxin varies from 0.25 to 0.5 mg per day. Propranolol, 20 to 80 mg given orally four times a day, or metoprolol, 25 to 100 mg given orally every 12 hours, is used in conjunction with digoxin for patients with hyperthyroidism, hypertrophic cardiomyopathy, angina pectoris, or poorly controlled ventricular rates. Verapamil, 80 to 120 mg orally every 6 to 8 hours, or diltiazem (Cardizem), 60 mg orally every 8 hours, may be useful when beta-blocking drugs are contraindicated or poorly tolerated.

### Conversion to Normal Sinus Rhythm

A return to normal sinus rhythm is ideal for all patients with atrial fibrillation, but restoration of sinus rhythm cannot be achieved nor can sinus rhythm be maintained in some patients. The hemodynamic benefits of sinus rhythm are greatest in patients with organic heart disease, especially those with mitral stenosis or a noncompliant left ventricle. However, nearly all people with or without associated heart disease note an improved exercise tolerance when their cardiac rhythm is sinus rather than atrial fibrillation. Reducing the risk of arterial embolization is another bonus proffered by sinus rhythm.

Atrial fibrillation precipitated by an acute reversible problem such as myocardial infarction, respiratory failure, cardiothoracic surgery, pericarditis, or an alcohol binge usually converts to sinus rhythm upon resolution of the initiating problem and medical management of the atrial fibrillation. The ventricular rate should be controlled with digoxin, beta-blocking drugs, or calcium-entry blockers as outlined previously. In some instances, treatment with digoxin may be all that is necessary to restore sinus rhythm. The mechanisms by which digoxin converts atrial fibrillation to sinus rhythm are not completely understood. Digoxin slows AV conduction by vagal and direct membrane effects, but it has no demonstrable antifibrillatory action on atrial myocardium. The conversion to sinus rhythm may result from slowing of the ventricular response and an attendant increase in cardiac output and coronary blood flow and a reduction in atrial stretch. If atrial fibrillation persists after the acute medical problem has been resolved, cardioversion may be attempted.

Every patient with persistent atrial fibrillation requires individual assessment to determine whether cardioversion is worthwhile. The enthusiasm for electroversion has waned with the realization that most patients with chronic heart disease relapse within a few months following successful cardioversion. Elective cardioversion is suggested when atrial fibrillation is of recent onset and minimal heart disease is present. Cardioversion is recommended when atrial fibrillation produces or seriously aggravates heart failure or angina pectoris. When atrial fibrillation persists after control of hyperthyroidism and for

6 weeks following successful mitral valve surgery, cardioversion may be attempted.

Cardioversion is usually avoided in certain patient groups, including:

1. Patients over 65 to 70 years of age.

2. Patients in whom atrial fibrillation has been present for 1 year or more, unless successful cardiac surgery has been performed.

3. Patients having considerable cardiac enlargement, especially when the left atrium is greatly enlarged, because sinus rhythm is rarely sustained after cardioversion.

4. Patients in whom previous cardioversion has been followed by a return to atrial fibrillation, despite adequate prophylactic doses of a Class IA antiarrhythmic drug (quinidine, procainamide [Procan], disopyramide [Norpace]).

5. Patients having a ventricular rate less than 80 beats a minute in the absence of digoxin or any drug that slows AV nodal conduction.

6. Patients with the tachycardia-bradycardia syndrome unless a pacemaker is in place, because prolonged asystole may follow the cardioversion.

Atrial fibrillation of recent onset may be converted by medical therapy in approximately 75% of patients. After the ventricular rate is controlled, quinidine, 800 to 1200 mg per day, disopyramide, 400 to 600 mg per day, or procainamide, 3 to 4 gm per day, is begun. Continuous electrocardiographic monitoring is essential. The electrocardiographic appearance of marked QTU interval prolongation of QRS complex widening precludes further administration of Class IA antiarrhythmic drugs. If this medical regimen does not restore sinus rhythm after 4 days, it should be abandoned and plans made for electrical cardioversion.

Anticoagulation with warfarin (Coumadin) should be started 3 weeks before elective cardioversion. Warfarin should be continued for at least 2 weeks afterward to prevent late embolic complications resulting from delayed resumption of atrial systole and relapse of some patients into atrial fibrillation. To prevent hemorrhagic complications, the prothrombin time should be maintained at 1.5 times control using the rabbit brain thromboplastin standard. For atrial fibrillation of several days duration, the usual clinical practice is not to use anticoagulant drugs. Reversion of atrial fibrillation with drug therapy is not entirely analogous to cardioversion. Cardioversion involves some physical trauma from the electrical shock, which may result in disruption of a thrombus. Although there are no controlled trials that examine the issue of anticoagulation for drug reversion of atrial fibrillation, it seems prudent to follow the recommendations for anticoagulation as outlined for electrical cardioversion.

The patient is prepared for electrical cardioversion by pretreatment with quinidine 1.2 grams or disopyramide 300 mg daily, 24 to 48 hours before the procedure. Such pretreatment may reduce relapse into atrial fibrillation immediately following cardioversion. The serum potassium and magnesium levels should be checked and any deficit corrected. Digoxin is withheld on the day of the procedure. Cardioversion should follow an overnight fast. The room should be equipped for cardiac monitoring and cardiopulmonary resuscitation. A 12-lead electrocardiogram and rhythm strip are recorded. The cardioversion should be postponed if a digitalis toxic arrhythmia is found. Continuous electrocardiographic monitoring is essential during cardioversion and for a minimum of 6 hours afterward. Sedation is accomplished by administering diazepam (Valium) or midazolam (Versed) intravenously in incremental doses every 1 to 2 minutes until the patient is not fully arousable. Alternatively, a short-acting anesthetic methohexital (Brevital) may be administered by an anesthesiologist.

Synchronization of the defibrillator should be tested before administering the first shock. Once synchronization with the QRS complex is ensured, the paddles may be applied. A posterior paddle positioned medial to the left scapula and an anterior paddle located on the left of the sternum may be employed. A liberal amount of electrocardiogram paste or specifically prepared cardioversion pads should be used to reduce electrical resistance and to prevent skin burns.

For most adults, an initial energy setting of 100 watt-seconds is satisfactory, but a higher level may be chosen for patients with lung disease or obesity because electrical conductance is decreased. If the initial shock is not successful, the operator should proceed in 50 watt-second increments to a maximum of 300 watt-seconds. Lidocaine, 100 mg intravenously, is given if ventricular extrasystoles follow a shock. There is rarely an indication for exceeding energies of 300 watt-seconds, since the incidence of complications is higher when 400 watt-seconds is used. Complications of cardioversion include hypotension, electrocardiographic evidence of myocardial damage, cardiac arrhythmias, and pulmonary edema. The genesis of the last complication is incompletely understood, but it may be a manifestation of electrical damage to the myocardium.

### Prevention of Atrial Fibrillation

Patients in whom atrial fibrillation complicates an acute reversible illness may be maintained on digoxin for 4 to 6 weeks and then have the drug discontinued. In patients with ischemic heart disease, a maintenance antiarrhythmic program may need to be continued indefinitely. Digoxin alone is usually insufficient prophylactic therapy for patients with chronic heart disease, and a Class IA antiarrhythmic agent—quinidine, disopyramide, or procainamide—should be given concurrently. Disopyramide may be preferred in patients with hypertrophic cardiomyopathy. It is prudent to decrease the dose of digoxin when quinidine and digoxin are given together, since quinidine predictably increases the serum digoxin level. If digoxin and a Class IA antiarrhythmic drug fail to prevent recurrences, a beta-blocking drug may be added. Class IC (flecainide [Tambocor], encainide [Enkaid]) and Class III (amiodarone [Cordarone]) antiarrhythmic drugs may be effective, but they are not approved for this indication in the United States at the time of this writing.

Recurrent episodes of atrial fibrillation pose a serious problem for some patients with the Wolff-Parkinson-White syndrome when accessory pathway conduction allows for a ventricular response greater than 250 beats a minute. A combination of a Class IA antiarrhythmic drug and a beta-blocking drug may prevent further episodes. However, drug therapy should be guided by electrophysiology testing. If a successful medical regimen cannot be found, surgical ablation of the accessory pathway is mandatory.

### Atrial Fibrillation with a Slow Ventricular Response

Untreated atrial fibrillation accompanied by a ventricular response of less than 90 beats a minute suggests abnormal AV nodal conduction. Disease of the atria and sinus node frequently accompanies the slow AV conduction. Treatment is not necessary if a patient is asymptomatic. Symptoms of episodic dizziness or syncope, worsening angina pectoris, or congestive heart failure require further investigation. A 24-hour ambulatory electrocardiogram may reveal periods of extreme ventricular slowing that correlate with episodes of dizziness or syncope. The detection of symptoms occurring at a time of marked ventricular slowing requires the insertion of a permanent, demand ventricular pacemaker. Cardioversion is inadvisable when the untreated ventricular rate is slow because sinus node and escape pacemaker function is frequently abnormal and severe bradycardia may follow the termination of atrial fibrillation.

### Systemic Thromboembolism

Paroxysmal or sustained atrial fibrillation is associated with an increased incidence of systemic arterial emboli. The issue of anticoagulation in atrial fibrillation hinges on the balance between efficacy and risk. Sodium warfarin (Coumadin) is used in patients with chronic atrial fibrillation or recurrent atrial fibrillation, when it is associated with mitral valve disease, dilated cardiomyopathy, hypertrophic cardiomyopathy, recent myocardial infarction, enlarged left atrium, prosthetic valves, or a history of systemic embolus.

# PREMATURE BEATS

method of
JEFFREY L. ANDERSON, M.D.
*Latter Day Saints Hospital*
*Salt Lake City, Utah*

Premature or ectopic beats may arise singly or in repetitive sequences from the atria, ventricles, or (rarely) from the conduction system itself and may be caused by the mechanisms of (1) abnormal automaticity; (2) re-entry; or (3) triggered activity. Therapy is often required when they cause debilitating symptoms or initiate tachyarrhythmias that are symptomatic, such as atrial fibrillation (AF) or ventricular tachycardia (VT). Therapy is required only occasionally when beats are asymptomatic. Premature beats may arise in association with a host of pathologic processes, including fibrosis, ischemia, hemodynamic stress, electrolyte imbalance, and neurogenic factors. Occasionally, no associated structural heart disease is clinically apparent.

## ATRIAL PREMATURE COMPLEXES

Atrial premature complexes (APCs) are common, even in otherwise normal individuals, increase with age, and are usually asymptomatic or cause only minor symptoms. APCs are frequent in organic heart disease, particularly with increased atrial pressures, atrial enlargement, or intra-atrial conduction abnormalities. They may also occur in apparently normal hearts and may be increased by sympathetic nervous system activity, caffeine, or alcohol. By themselves, APCs rarely justify treatment with antiarrhythmic drugs and are usually asymptomatic or mildly symptomatic. Therapy may be justified when they trigger symptomatic sustained arrhythmias such as paroxysmal supraventricular tachycardia or atrial fibrillation or flutter.

## VENTRICULAR PREMATURE COMPLEXES

Ventricular premature complexes (VPCs) may be classified as acute and chronic arrhythmias. Chronic arrhythmias may be divided into benign, prognostically important, and malignant, based on the presence and degree of underlying heart disease, hemodynamic consequences, and estimated associated risk of sudden cardiac death (Table 1). Drug treatment is not indi-

TABLE 1. **Categories of Ventricular Premature Complexes (VPCs)**

| Characteristic | Acute | Chronic | | |
| | | *Benign* | *Prognostically Important* | *Malignant* |
|---|---|---|---|---|
| Presentation | In-hospital monitoring | Palpitations or no symptoms | Palpitations, dyspnea, or no symptoms | Presyncope, syncope, cardiac arrest |
| Organic heart disease | Usually present | Absent or minimal | Present | Present, usually advanced |
| Treatment objective | Suppress if arrhythmia hemodynamically or prognostically significant | Reassure Avoid therapy, unless symptoms severe | Treat underlying disease (e.g., with beta blockers) Relieve symptoms ?Prevent sudden cardiac death (antiarrhythmic therapy not shown to be of benefit; may be harmful) | Prevent recurrent ventricular tachycardia and fibrillation or sudden cardiac death |

cated for benign arrhythmias unless severely symptomatic, but aggressive treatment (usually in consultation with an arrhythmia specialist) is indicated when VPCs are associated with malignant arrhythmias. Whether prognostically important arrhythmias should be treated, especially when asymptomatic, has been controversial. The Cardiac Arrhythmia Suppression Trial (CAST) recently addressed this question. Although arrhythmias were effectively suppressed by encainide (Enkaid) and flecainide (Tambocor), total mortality was *increased* (risk ratio 2.5) by active therapy; specifically, sudden death mortality was increased (risk ratio 3.6). The third treatment in CAST, moricizine, is ongoing. However, an overview of all earlier drug trials with Class I antiarrhythmic agents for postinfarction VPCs suggests an adverse or at best a neutral rather than a beneficial trend. Thus, at present, asymptomatic, but prognostically important, VPCs should not be treated with Class I antiarrhythmic agents.

## DIAGNOSIS AND MONITORING THERAPY

The history and physical examination usually must be supplemented with electrocardiographic studies for arrhythmia diagnosis and evaluation. The standard electrocardiogram (ECG), even with a rhythm strip, is diagnostic only when very frequent premature beats or ongoing tachyarrhythmia is present. Ambulatory electrocardiographic monitoring (for 24 to 48 hours) allows identification and quantification of frequently occurring arrhythmias and association with symptoms. When symptoms ascribed to arrhythmias are infrequent, an event recorder (such as a transtelephonic monitor with a memory loop) may be useful. The patient carries this portable device with him or her over a prolonged period (1 month or more), activating it when symptoms suggesting arrhythmias occur. Exercise testing is useful when symptoms occur with exertion; the possibility of exercise aggravation of arrhythmia during treatment and latent ischemia can also

be assessed. Electrophysiologic study is an invasive procedure, useful for diagnosis and therapeutic monitoring of sustained, re-entrant ventricular tachycardia or fibrillation (VT/VF) and selected supraventricular tachyarrhythmias. Because of the adverse potential, including arrhythmia aggravation, of Class I antiarrhythmic agents, therapeutic effects should be confirmed by appropriate noninvasive or invasive monitoring.

## ANTIARRHYTHMIC DRUG CLASSIFICATION

Antiarrhythmic drug action has been separated into four classes by Vaughan Williams (Table 2).

TABLE 2. **Classification of Antiarrhythmic Drug Action**

**Class Action**

I Sodium-channel blockade (slows conduction)
  A. Moderate action
    Prototype: quinidine (Quinaglute, Quinidex)
    Others: procainamide (Pronestyl, Procan-SR), disopyramide (Norpace), moricizine*
  B. Mild action
    Prototype: lidocaine (Xylocaine)
    Others: tocainide (Tonocard), mexiletine (Mexitil)
  C. Strong action
    Prototype: flecainide (Tambocor)
    Others: encainide (Enkaid), propafenone (Rythmol)

II Blockade of beta-adrenergic receptors
    Prototype: propranolol (Inderal)
    Others: acebutolol (Sectral), esmolol (Brevibloc)†

III Prolongation of repolarization (potassium-channel blockade)
    Prototypes: bretylium (Bretylol) (IV), amiodarone (Cordarone) (PO)
    Others: sotalol*

IV Calcium-entry channel blockade
    Prototype: verapamil (Calan, Isoptin)†
    Others: diltiazem‡ (Cardizem)

*Investigational, under FDA review
†For supraventricular arrhythmias only
‡This use of diltiazem is not listed in the manufacturer's official directive.

Membrane sodium-channel blockade is a Class I action; blockade of beta-adrenergic receptors comprises a Class II action; Class III effect involves prolongation of the action potential, believed to be caused by blockade of membrane potassium currents; and blockade of calcium-entry channels is a Class IV action. Three subdivisions of Class I have been proposed, based on the intensity and duration of sodium-channel blockade. Agents with moderate action are grouped in Subclass IA and include the traditional antiarrhythmic agents quinidine, procainamide (Pronestyl), and disopyramide (Norpace). Agents with mild (transient) action are grouped in Subclass IB and include the lidocaine (Xylocaine) family, including tocainide (Tonocard) and mexiletine (Mexitil). The most intense sodium-channel blockade is provided by agents in the new Subclass IC, such as flecainide (Tambocor), encainide (Enkaid), and propafenone (Rythmol).

## RELATIVE EFFECTIVENESS OF ANTIARRHYTHMIC DRUGS

The effectiveness of an antiarrhythmic drug varies in individual patients, and the selection of an effective drug is mostly empiric. Table 3 summarizes the relative efficacy from studies that used ambulatory (Holter) monitoring and treadmill testing of patients who required therapy for symptoms associated with benign or prognostically important VPCs. Suppression of more than 75% of VPCs was defined as effective. Drugs with Class IA action show a moderate rate of response; Class IB drugs a somewhat lower rate; and Class IC the highest rate. Beta blockers show a relatively low response rate, and amiodarone a high rate (but its use is restricted because of toxicity). Calcium blockers are rarely effective for VPCs. Electrophysiologic testing was used to assess relative efficacy among those with malignant arrhythmias (VT or VF). In patients with malignant ventricular arrhythmias monitored by electrophysiologic study, all drugs show a lower response rate for VT/VF, in the range of 25 plus or minus 10%.

Less quantitative information is available for response rates of APCs and related supraventricular arrhythmias, but relative effects can be assessed. Class IA and Class IC agents are generally effective, but IB agents are generally ineffective or rarely used. A beta blocker, a calcium-channel blocker, or digoxin may be initially tried because of their ease of administration and relative safety. However, they are less effective in suppressing APCs and AF than in suppressing sinus and AV nodal re-entrant tachycardias or controlling rate during AF.

## ADVERSE REACTION POTENTIAL OF ANTIARRHYTHMIC DRUGS

Consideration of adverse potential of antiarrhythmic therapy is as important in therapeutic decision making as considerations of efficacy (Table 4).

### Noncardiac Adverse Effects

Noncardiac toxicity causing subjective adverse effects may preclude therapy in one-fourth to one-third of patients given Class IA drugs, but for different, drug specific reasons (Table 4). Up to 40% of patients are intolerant of tocainide and mexiletine because of neurologic (tremor, ataxia) and gastrointestinal (nausea, anorexia) reactions. Flecainide and encainide have the lowest incidences of intolerable adverse effects requiring discontinuation (about 5 to 10%); most commonly, blurred vision, lightheadedness, or headaches are noted. Beta blockers may cause a fatigue syndrome of variable severity. The adverse effects of amiodarone are in part dose and time related and may be a manifestation of organ toxicity.

Serious organ toxicity is of greater concern with certain antiarrhythmic drugs. Among Class I agents, organ toxicity is of greatest concern with quinidine, procainamide, and tocainide. Amiodarone has the greatest potential for organ toxicity over the long term, including potentially fatal pulmonary fibrosis, which restricts its use to patients with refractory, malignant arrhythmia, as guided by an arrhythmia specialist.

### Cardiac Adverse Effects

Cardiac adverse reactions may take the form of proarrhythmia, negative inotropic effects, and conduction system depression. All drugs have the potential to worsen previous arrhythmia or induce new arrhythmia. Quinidine has a particular propensity to cause torsades de pointes, or polymorphic VT associated with a long QT interval, even in patients without a prior history of malignant arrhythmia. The risk is present but somewhat less with procainamide and disopyramide. Class IC drugs have the greatest potential for arrhythmogenic activity in those with malignant arrhythmias, and an increase in sudden death postinfarction has recently been demonstrated for use of these agents for treatment of asymptomatic arrhythmias after myocardial infarction.

Many arrhythmia patients have impaired left ventricular function that may be aggravated by antiarrhythmic therapy. Disopyramide, followed by flecainide, beta blockers, and verapamil, shows the greatest negative inotropic potential.

Depression of function of the sinus and AV

TABLE 3. **Relative Effectiveness of Antiarrhythmic Drugs**

| Class | Drug | Ventricular | | Supraventricular‡ |
|---|---|---|---|---|
| | | Benign or Prognostically Important* | Malignant† | |
| IA | Quinidine | + + + | + + | + + + |
| | Procainamide (Pronestyl) | + + + | + + | + + |
| | Disopyramide (Norpace) | + + + | + + | + +/+ + + |
| | Moricizine | + + + | +/+ + | ? |
| IB | Lidocaine (Xylocaine) (IV) | + + | + | + |
| | Tocainide (Tonocard) | + + | + | + |
| | Mexiletine (Mexitil) | + + | + | + |
| IC | Flecainide (Tambocor) | + + + + | + + | + + +/+ + + + |
| | Encainide (Enkaid) | + + + + | + + | + + +/+ + + + |
| | Propafenone (Rythmol) | + + + | + + | + + + |
| II | Propranolol (Inderal) | + + | + | + + |
| | Acebutolol (Sectral) | + + | + | + + |
| III | Bretylium (Bretylol) (IV) | + | + + | + +? |
| | Amiodarone (Cordarone) | + + +/+ + + +§ | + +/+ + + | + + +/+ + + + |
| | Sotalol | + + + | + + + | + +/+ + + |
| IV | Verapamil (Calan, Isoptin) | + | 0/+ | + + |

*Evaluated by ambulatory electrocardiographic (Holter) monitoring or treadmill exercise testing. Scale of patient response (based on suppression of >75% of ventricular premature complexes): +, <50%; + +, 51–60%; + + +, 61–70%; + + + +, 71–85%. For supraventricular arrhythmias, scale is relative and qualitative.

†Induced by programmed electrical stimulation. Scale of patient response: +, ≤15%; + +, 16–30%; + + +, 31–40%; + + + +, >40%.

‡Includes atrial premature complexes, paroxysmal atrial fibrillation and flutter (for conversion and prophylaxis), paroxysmal supraventricular tachycardias, and supraventricular arrhythmias associated with Wolff-Parkinson-White syndrome.

§Although effective, amiodarone is not indicated for benign or potentially malignant arrhythmias because of toxicity.

nodes and the His-Purkinje system may be of concern in certain patients, particularly those with pre-existing disease. This is of greatest concern with Class IC agents, which may also raise the energy threshold for pacemaker capture in those requiring pacing.

Drug interaction is another important consideration in selecting and monitoring therapy. Quinidine interacts significantly with digoxin, reducing clearance and increasing digoxin blood levels. Amiodarone interacts with many other cardiovascular agents, including anticoagulants (such as warfarin), digoxin, and other antiar-

rhythmic drugs, potentiating the effects of these drugs. Dosage reduction (by up to one-third to one-half) of these various drugs is often indicated.

## GUIDELINES FOR ANTIARRHYTHMIC DRUG SELECTION

A review of benefit and risk allows formulation of tentative algorithms for use of drugs for therapy (Table 5).

**Benign Arrhythmia.** For *asymptomatic* and mildly symptomatic *benign arrhythmia*, treatment is not advised, but reassurance and lifestyle

TABLE 4. **Selected Safety Comparisons of the Oral Antiarrhythmic Agents**

| Class | Drug | Adverse Potential | | | |
|---|---|---|---|---|---|
| | | Noncardiac Side Effects | Organ Toxic Potential | Proarrhythmic Risk | Negative Inotropy |
| IA | Quinidine | + + + | + + | + +/+ + + | 0/+ |
| | Procainamide | + + | + + | + + | + |
| | Disopyramide | + + | + | + + | + + + |
| IB | Tocainide | + + + + | + + | +/+ + | + |
| | Mexiletine | + + + + | + | +/+ + | + |
| IC | Flecainide | + | 0/+ | + + + | + + |
| | Encainide | + | 0/+ | + + + | +/+ + |
| II | Beta blockers | +/+ + | 0/+ | + | + + |
| III | Amiodarone | + + | + + + + | + | + |
| IV | Verapamil | + | 0/+ | + | + + |

0 to + + + + = negligible to greatest relative adverse effect risk.

### TABLE 5. Proposed Treatment Algorithms or Chronic Ventricular Premature Complexes (VPCs)

**Asymptomatic, Benign VPCs**
1. Reassure patient; general measures
2. No antiarrhythmic drug

**Asymptomatic, Prognostically Important VPCs**
1. Beta blocker
2. Avoid Class IC agents, ? also avoid other Class I agents
3. None, or refer to a study center (CAST, VA studies)
4. Select high-risk patients for individualized therapy—electrophysiologic study

**Malignant Ventricular Arrhythmias**
1. Class IA (procainamide, quinidine)
2. Class IB (mexiletine)
3. IA plus IB
4. Class IC (selected patients)
5. Amiodarone

**Symptomatic, Benign or Prognostically Important Ventricular Arrhythmias**
1. Beta blocker
2. Class IA (procainamide, quinidine)
3. Class IB (mexiletine) alone or with IA
4. Class IC (avoid for MI, ? other CAD patients)

changes may be indicated (such as reduction in emotional or physical stress and use of caffeine, tobacco, and alcohol).

**Acute Ventricular Arrhythmias.** Acute ventricular arrhythmias, occurring during intercurrent illness such as myocardial infarction and the postoperative period, are often treated for 1 or 2 days with intravenous therapy. Lidocaine is usually the drug of first choice, although beta blockers may be used when ischemia or sympathetic nervous drive is important. Procainamide is used as the drug of second choice. Bretylium is reserved for treatment of refractory, recurrent VT and associated rhythms.

**Postinfarction (Prognostically Important) Ventricular Premature Complexes.** An implication of the recent CAST study is that asymptomatic, prognostically important, VPCs should *not* be treated with flecainide and encainide, and therapy is also *not* currently indicated with other Class I agents, in the absence of additional indications. Only the beta-blocking agents can be recommended for prophylaxis, based on mortality data from postinfarction studies. Additional therapy should be directed at reduction in ischemia and other risk factors. Only when VPCs are significantly symptomatic or unusually complex should additional therapy be considered.

**Malignant Ventricular Arrhythmias.** Because of their proarrhythmic potential, Class IC agents are generally reserved for second line therapy of VT or VF. Class IA, Class IB, and combined Class IA and IB therapy form the first approach to drug treatment. Therapy may be monitored noninvasively, or preferably, invasively. Amiodarone is moderately effective but is reserved for second or third line therapy because of its potential for organ toxicity. Sotalol, an investigational beta blocker with Class III activity that may be approved for use in the near future, is often effective, even in patients with VT or VF in the setting of ischemic heart disease, and may become an agent of first choice. If an effective antiarrhythmic regimen is not found, implantation of an automatic defibrillator or arrhythmia surgery should be considered.

**Symptomatic Non–Life-Threatening Arrhythmias.** Given concerns about the safety of antiarrhythmic drugs, a conservative approach to symptomatic but benign arrhythmias is appropriate. Only when symptoms are well documented and debilitating should specific therapy be given. Often, an initial trial with a beta blocker is appropriate before considering a Class I agent. In young patients, disopyramide is a useful Class IA agent with low organ toxicity. Class IC therapy, no longer officially indicated in patients with non–life-threatening arrhythmias, may be effective and well tolerated but poses concern about uncertain proarrhythmic potential.

**Supraventricular Arrhythmias.** For arrhythmias involving the sinus or AV nodes, digitalis, beta blockers, and calcium-channel blockers may be useful. For refractory arrhythmias involving the AV node or re-entry in the atrium or through an atrioventricular bypass tract (such as Wolff-Parkinson-White syndrome), Class I therapy is often required, in addition, for prevention and treatment. Class IA agents have been traditionally used; Class IB agents are usually ineffective. Class IC agents are active against these arrhythmias. Recently, flecainide received a favorable review by the advisory committee to the Food and Drug Administration for use in paroxysmal supraventricular tachycardia and paroxysmal atrial fibrillation in patients with serious symptoms and without structural heart disease. Amiodarone, effective for these arrhythmias, may be appropriate for selected patients with severely symptomatic/potentially life-threatening supraventricular arrhythmias (such as some of those associated with Wolff-Parkinson-White syndrome), although it is not officially approved for these uses in the United States.

# HEART BLOCK
method of
LAWRENCE S. KLEIN, M.D., and
DOUGLAS P. ZIPES, M.D.
*Krannert Institute of Cardiology*
*Indianapolis, Indiana*

Heart block refers to an abnormality of cardiac impulse conduction. This may be a normal, physiologic phenomenon, such as from enhanced vagal tone, or it may be pathologic. Management depends on the degree of block, the site of block, the severity of symptoms, and the clinical setting. For example, recurrent episodes of Wenckebach block (Type I second-degree atrioventricular [AV] block) may be asymptomatic in an athlete and require no therapy, while transient complete AV block accompanying acute anterior myocardial infarction may require permanent pacing, regardless of the presence of symptoms.

Over 100,000 new pacemakers are implanted in the United States each year. Although in recent years the sick sinus syndrome has formed a larger segment of the pacemaker population, implantation for AV block continues to be one of the major indications for permanent cardiac pacing. Thus, an understanding of the mechanisms, presentation, and therapy of sinus nodal dysfunction and the different types of AV block is important for the practicing physician. AV block may be classified into three types: first degree, second degree, and third-degree (complete) heart block. Some experts add a fourth category, high degree. Simply described, first degree AV block means all P waves conduct, but with delay; second degree, intermittent block of one P wave; high degree, intermittent block of more than one consecutive P wave; and third-degree, no P waves conduct.

## TREATMENT

### Sinus Nodal Dysfunction

Sinus nodal dysfunction refers to a heterogeneous group of disorders often referred to as the "sick sinus syndrome." The syndrome includes (1) persistent sinus bradycardia not due to reversible factors; (2) sinus arrest or exit block (sudden, unexpected failure of atrial activity); (3) combinations of sinoatrial and AV conduction abnormalities; or (4) tachycardia-bradycardia syndrome (alternation of atrial tachycardia, atrial flutter, or atrial fibrillation with marked sinus bradycardia or sinus arrest).

The etiology of sinus nodal dysfunction may be either intrinsic (structural abnormality of the sinus node or perinodal tissues) or autonomic. Reversible causes of sinus nodal dysfunction include excessive vagal tone, hyperkalemia, hypercapnea, hypothermia, increased intracranial pressure, and sepsis. Pharmacologic agents that can depress sinus nodal function include beta blockers, calcium channel blockers, sympatholytic agents such as methyldopa or clonidine, Type I and Type III antiarrhythmic agents such as procainamide (Procan), flecainide (Tambocor) or amiodarone (Cordarone), cimetidine (Tagamet), lithium, amitriptyline (Elavil), and phenothiazines such as chlorpromazine (Thorazine). Patients with the sick sinus syndrome are often sensitive to the effects of digitalis.

Symptoms of sinus nodal dysfunction are inter-mittent and unpredictable. Sinus bradycardia and prolonged sinus pauses can be normal in healthy young adults, especially at night. It is crucial to correlate the electrocardiographic (ECG) abnormality suggesting sinus nodal dysfunction and the patient's symptoms.

Treatment of sinus nodal dysfunction includes withdrawal of drugs that may exacerbate the problem. If these agents cannot be safely withdrawn, permanent pacing may be necessary. Although vagolytic or adrenergic therapy (atropine or isoproterenol) may temporarily increase the sinus rate, chronic drug therapy is usually associated with intolerable side effects. Therefore, the treatment of choice for most patients is permanent cardiac pacing, once the relationship between symptoms and bradyarrhythmia has been established. Aminophylline may benefit some young patients with vagally mediated sinus nodal dysfunction. Prognosis of patients with sinus nodal dysfunction, especially older patients, is related more to the underlying heart disease than to the sinus nodal dysfunction itself. Implantation of a permanent pacemaker certainly will relieve symptoms in properly selected patients, although pacemakers have not been demonstrated to improve survival in all studies. Atrial pacing is usually not sufficient because of the commonly associated AV conduction abnormality that, if not apparent at the time of diagnosis, may subsequently develop as the conduction disease progresses.

### First-Degree Atrioventricular Block

First-degree AV block results in prolongation of the PR interval to greater than 0.20 seconds on the surface ECG. The site of conduction delay may be in the AV node, the bundle of His, the bundle branch-Purkinje system, or a combination of these sites. Conduction delay in the AV node is the most common cause of first-degree AV block. If the QRS complex is normal, then the site of conduction delay is proximal to the bundle branch system, but it may be within the His bundle in as many as 13% of patients. The remaining patients have delay in the AV node. In patients with bundle branch block and first-degree AV block, the site of conduction delay is in the Purkinje system in 10 to 30% of the patients.

The most common causes of first-degree AV block include enhanced vagal tone, intrinsic (structural) AV nodal disease, acute inferior wall myocardial infarction, myocarditis, and a number of pharmacologic agents (digitalis, beta blockers, and calcium-channel blockers). First-degree AV block caused by AV nodal delay does not require any specific therapy, nor is it a contraindication to the administration of digitalis, beta blockers, calcium channel blockers, or Class I antiarrhythmic agents, although these patients may have some risk of developing higher grades of AV block when these agents are given. In patients with first-degree AV block caused by delay of conduction in the His-Purkinje system, no specific therapy is required. However, these patients should be followed, and if higher grades of AV block do occur, a permanent pacemaker may be necessary.

### Second-Degree Atrioventricular Block

Second-degree AV block may be classified as Type I (Wenckebach block) or Type II.

**Type I Second-Degree Atrioventricular Block.** Type I second-degree AV block is characterized by a progressive prolongation of the PR interval until a P wave fails to conduct to the ventricle. Typically, while there is progressive prolongation of the PR interval, the absolute increment in the PR interval decreases, so that the RR intervals progressively shorten. This form of AV block may result from conduction delay and block within the AV node, the bundle of His, or the bundle branch-Purkinje system.

**Type I Second-Degree Atrioventricular Block within the Atrioventricular Node.** Type I second-degree AV block occurs in the AV node in the majority of patients with Type I AV block. Also known as Wenckebach block, Type I AV block is characterized by progressive shortening of the RR intervals, a phenomenon that occurs more commonly if the degree of block is 4:3 or less. If the conduction ratio is 5:4 or greater, progressive RR shortening is less easily detected. Type I AV block may resemble Type II block when there are long Wenckebach cycles during which the last several beats of the cycle show relatively constant PR intervals. Type I AV nodal block does not carry the risk of paroxysmal AV block that is associated with Type II second-degree AV block.

Type I second-degree AV block within the AV node is found in a number of clinical situations, including acute inferior wall myocardial infarction, during sleep (especially in young patients or athletes), digitalis toxicity, and after the administration of beta blockers or calcium-channel blockers. It is also a normal phenomenon during atrial pacing at rapid rates or during rapid atrial tachycardias. When it occurs in the setting of acute myocardial infarction, Type I second-degree AV block within the AV node is usually a transient phenomenon and often subsides within 48 hours of the event. Usually, small doses of atropine restore 1:1 AV conduction or convert the rhythm to longer Wenckebach conduction ratios.

Often, no therapy at all is indicated. A temporary pacemaker is recommended for (1) a ventricular rate of less than 40 beats per minute despite atropine, (2) congestive heart failure or ventricular arrhythmias related to the bradycardia, or (3) progression to higher grade AV block. If Type I second-degree AV block is due to drug toxicity, withholding the drug and administration of atropine may be all that is necessary.

**Type I Second-Degree Atrioventricular Block within the His-Purkinje System.** This form of conduction delay and block occurs infrequently, almost always in the setting of bifascicular conduction system disease. The precise identification of the site of block (within the His bundle or His-Purkinje system) requires His bundle recording studies, details of which are beyond the scope of this article. Since Type I second-degree AV block within the His-Purkinje system ultimately progresses to higher grades of block or to complete heart block (see below), it has the clinical implications of Type II second-degree AV block. The implantation of a permanent pacemaker is justified in these patients.

**Type II Second-Degree Atrioventricular Block (Mobitz II).** Type II second-degree AV block is characterized by a sudden and unexpected nonconducted P wave without antecedent increase in conduction time on the surface electrocardiogram. Therefore, unlike Type I second-degree AV block, the PR intervals of the conducted beats prior to the blocked P wave remain constant, and virtually always, some form of bundle branch block is present. Type II AV block is less common than Type I AV block, but the former indicates more significant conduction system disease because the site of block is almost always distal to the AV node and usually below the bundle of His. Therefore, slower, less reliable escape rhythms control ventricular discharge, and the risk of progression to complete heart block is high. Because Type II second-degree AV block usually progresses to complete heart block, a permanent pacemaker is recommended in these patients, even if they are asymptomatic. The purpose of prophylactic pacing is to prevent the patient from having symptomatic events (for example, syncope).

### High-Degree Atrioventricular Block

High-degree AV block is manifested as 3:1 (or greater) AV conduction ratios. The site of AV block may be in the AV node, bundle of His, or the bundle branch–Purkinje system. The site of block can be precisely localized by His bundle recordings during AV block. However, clinical and ECG criteria can lead to a correct diagnosis in most instances. Features suggesting high-degree AV block caused by AV nodal block include (1) normal QRS complexes; (2) Wenckebach's AV block prior to the development of high-degree AV block; (3) block due to inferior wall myocardial infarction, digitalis intoxication, or drug therapy with beta blockers or calcium-channel blockers; and (4) reversion to 1:1 conduction after atropine administration. Clinical and ECG features suggesting AV block in the His-Purkinje system include (1) bundle branch block during conduction of QRS complexes; (2) no history of digitalis, beta blockers, or calcium-channel blockers; or (3) either no change or an increase in the ratio of AV block with acceleration of the sinus rate or after administration of atropine.

Patients with high-degree AV block in the His-Purkinje system should have a permanent pacemaker implanted, regardless of the presence of symptoms. If high-grade AV block is due to block in the AV node, then a pacemaker may not be indicated if the patient is asymptomatic, the block is drug-related, or the ventricular response increases after administration of atropine, isoproterenol, or exercise. However, a pacemaker is indicated if the patient is symptomatic, has congestive heart failure due to AV block, or a ventricular rate of less than 40 beats per minute without an increase in the ventricular response after exercise or the administration of atropine, regardless of the site of block.

### Complete Heart Block

Total absence of AV conduction occurs if heart block is complete. The ventricular rate is controlled by pacemakers located in the lower AV junction, the His bundle, the bundle branch–Purkinje system, or the ventricle at rates ranging from 20 to 60 beats per minute. Complete heart block may be due to block within the AV node, His bundle, or bundle branch–Purkinje system. Block below the His bundle occurs in over 60% of patients with complete AV block (acquired complete heart block), with the His bundle being the site of block in approximately 15%. Block within the AV node forms the remainder of this group (most of whom have congenital complete heart block). If the QRS escape complex is normal, block is probably within the AV node. However, in patients with block within the His bundle, the QRS complex is usually normal also, unless concomitant bundle branch block is present. When complete heart block is due to block within the AV node, the ventricles are driven by a junctional pacemaker and the heart rate is usually 40 to 60 beats per minute. These pacemakers are usually stable and increase their

discharge rate during exercise. If complete heart block is due to block within or below the His bundle, the ventricles are driven by pacemakers in the His-Purkinje system. These pacemakers are frequently unstable and have intrinsic rates less than 40 beats per minute.

A permanent pacemaker is indicated for all patients who are symptomatic and for all patients who have block within or below the bundle of His. A pacemaker may not be required in asymptomatic patients who have a normal QRS escape mechanism due to AV nodal block and in whom the junctional pacemaker is found to accelerate following exercise.

### Bifascicular and Trifascicular Blocks

Electrocardiographically, the intraventricular conduction system is composed of three fascicles: the right bundle branch, the left anterior fascicle, and the left posterior fascicle of the left bundle branch. Right bundle branch block combined with left anterior hemiblock is the most common form of bifascicular block and is seen in approximately 1% of hospitalized patients. Progression to complete AV block in these patients is estimated to be less than 5% per year. The combination of right bundle branch block and left posterior hemiblock is less common but more likely to progress to complete heart block, presumably because of the amount of myocardium that must be involved to impair conduction in these two fascicles.

The incidence of progression to complete heart block in patients with left bundle branch block is less than that in patients with right bundle branch block combined with either left anterior hemiblock or left posterior hemiblock. Progression to complete AV block is more likely to occur if left axis deviation and left bundle branch block are present. Thus, patients with bifascicular block do not progress to complete heart block frequently enough to warrant prophylactic permanent cardiac pacing in the asymptomatic patient.

**Temporary Pacing in Patients with Acute Myocardial Infarction.** Bifascicular blocks occur in approximately 10 to 15% of patients with acute myocardial infarction. These patients usually have extensive (and usually anterior) myocardial infarctions. The most commonly encountered bifascicular block includes right bundle branch block combined with left anterior hemiblock. The combination of right bundle branch block and left posterior hemiblock is quite uncommon. The reported risk of progression to complete AV block in patients with an acute myocardial infarction and bifascicular block varies from 10 to 50%. More important, one-third of acute MI patients who develop complete AV block do so without recorded progression through first- or second-degree AV block. Thus, in patients with acute myocardial infarction, temporary pacing is recommended for those who develop the new onset of alternating bundle branch block, right bundle branch block, and either left anterior or left posterior fascicular block (i.e., bifascicular block), or left bundle branch block with PR prolongation. Temporary pacing is not recommended in patients with new onset of left anterior hemiblock or patients with pre-existing left bundle branch block or right bundle branch block (with or without axis deviation) because the risk of progression to complete heart block is low. The indications for pacing are not as clear for patients with new right bundle branch block with normal axis or new left bundle branch block with a normal PR interval. We generally do not use temporary transvenous pacing in these patients, especially with the advent of transthoracic pacemakers that deliver high-energy, long-duration pulses for external pacing through special large skin patches. Thus, one can be more conservative than in the past with these patients since they can be paced quickly through the skin should complete AV block occur.

A temporary pacemaker is not recommended in patients who develop PR prolongation, second-degree Type I (Wenckebach) AV block, or AV dissociation without complete AV block in association with an acute myocardial infarction. However, temporary pacing is recommended for all patients who develop new second-degree Type II AV block or complete AV block in this setting.

Implantation of a permanent pacemaker in patients who suffer an acute myocardial infarction and develop bifascicular block or transient second-degree or third-degree AV block is usually recommended. However, it has not been clearly determined that the incidence of subsequent sudden death is lower in those patients in whom a permanent pacemaker is implanted. The need for prophylactic permanent pacing in patients with persistent bifascicular block (without documented AV block) after myocardial infarction is controversial. Permanent prophylactic pacing for bifascicular block in these patients is not routinely recommended.

# TACHYCARDIAS

method of
DENNIS S. MIURA, M.D., PH.D.
*Albert Einstein College of Medicine*
*New York City, New York*

The understanding of clinical tachyarrhythmias is based on cellular electrophysiologic techniques that have been developed over the past 30 years. A tachycardia is present when the heart rate exceeds 100 beats per minute. Basic electrophysiologic mechanisms of tachycardias are generally caused by an abnormality of impulse initiation (automaticity), abnormal impulse conduction, or a combination of both. Abnormal impulse initiation refers to an acceleration of an ectopic focus during electrical diastole. Normal automatic mechanisms occur in the sinoatrial node; abnormal automatic mechanisms may result from ischemia, myocardial infarction, or diseased myocardium of any cause. Other types of abnormal automatic mechanisms include triggered rhythms, which refer to a spontaneous repetitive activity arising from early or late after-depolarizations in an ectopic focus. Abnormal impulse conduction, on the other hand, may occur as a result of conduction block or re-entry. Combinations of these abnormalities of impulse generation and conduction have been noted as well.

The treatment of patients with a symptomatic tachycardia requires the following:

1. Interpretation of available clinical information, including medications.

2. A careful evaluation of the electrocardiogram (ECG) with a determination of the dominant rhythm disorder.

3. Determination of the origin of the P wave, its configuration, regularity, morphology, and relationship to the QRS complex.

4. Determination of the origin of the QRS complex when the atrial or ventricular rhythm disorders are independent.

5. Determination of the need for and goals of therapy.

A general inspection of the ECG is necessary to determine the rate, frequency, regularity, and atrioventricular (AV) relationships. The next step is to determine the presence or absence of P wave. If a true P wave is definitely present, one should determine the relationship between the P wave and the QRS complex. When the P wave is present, one should determine whether the P wave is of sinus or ectopic origin.

Diagnosis and treatments of the specific types of tachycardia can be subdivided into the treatment of supraventricular tachycardias vs. that of ventricular tachycardias. The distinction between the supraventricular and ventricular tachycardias can be difficult, especially if the QRS complex is wide. The relationship of the P wave to the wide complex tachycardias can be paramount to the diagnosis and treatment of these types of arrhythmias. If the diagnosis is not apparent on the surface ECG, invasive electrophysiologic techniques may be used to determine the mechanisms of the tachycardia.

## TREATMENT

### Sinus Tachycardia

Sinus tachycardia is defined as a sinus rate greater than 100 beats per minute and is usually the result of a physiologic response to stress such as exercise, fever, anemia, and elevated circulating levels of catecholamines. This tachycardia is

TABLE 1. **Paroxysmal Supraventricular Tachycardia (PSVT)**

| Mechanism | Rate (Beats/Min) | Mode of Initiation | | Response to Vagal Maneuver | Agents That May Slow or Terminate Tachycardia |
|---|---|---|---|---|---|
| | | APB | VPB | | |
| Re-entrant | | | | | |
| AV nodal re-entry | 150–180 | + | + | Slows, may terminate | Digitalis, propranolol, verapamil, procainamide |
| Concealed bypass tract (CBT) | 150–200+ | + | + | Variable | Propranolol, verapamil |
| Sinus node re-entry | 130 | + | + | Carotid sinus pressure slows, may terminate | Propranolol, verapamil |
| Intra-atrial re-entry | | + | − | AV block without terminating | |
| Automatic atrial tachycardia | <175 | − | − | AV block without terminating | |

usually benign, and a thorough search for the precipitating physiologic event should be done.

## Multifocal Atrial Tachycardia

If the atrial rate is greater than 100 beats per minute with at least three distinct, differing P wave morphologies, and irregular variations are seen in the PP interval, the diagnosis of multifocal atrial tachycardia (MAT) may be made. This tachycardia is often seen in the elderly or in severely ill patients with respiratory and metabolic abnormalities. Treatment should be directed at correction of the underlying acid-base disturbance or metabolic problems underlying the patient's clinical state. Digitalis toxicity can be associated with this rhythm disorder. Atrial tachycardia with block whose rates are 130 to 250 beats per minute is in the differential diagnosis from MAT. A constant P wave morphology differing from the P wave in normal sinus rhythm makes this diagnosis.

## Atrial Flutter—Atrial Fibrillation

Both of these types of atrial rhythm disorders are due to rapid rates in the atrium. Atrial flutter generally has a regular rate of 300 beats per minute and on the surface the ECG has a sawtooth appearance. The atrial P wave rate can vary, however, from 250 to 400 beats per minute. The ventricular response is somewhat slower ow-ing to AV block. The QRS complex can vary with the P wave in a 2:1 to 3:1 relationship, depending on the patient's age and medications. The treatment of atrial flutter is directed at increasing the level of AV block so that the ventricular response rate is no greater than 100 beats per minute. The primary treatment is to prevent paroxysmal atrial flutter by Class I membrane active antiarrhythmic agents. Conversion to sinus rhythm can be done by antiarrhythmic agents or electrical cardioversion.

Atrial fibrillation, on the other hand, has a faster atrial rate (greater than 350 per minute) which appears to be chaotic on the ECG baseline. Paroxysmal atrial fibrillation has a rapid ventricular response, since the AV node can conduct up to the patient's physiologic rates. Therapy is directed at converting this rhythm to sinus rhythm immediately by antiarrhythmic agents or electrical cardioversion. Chronic atrial fibrillation due to atrial enlargement or valvular disease tends to be resistant to conversion to sinus rhythm. If the patient is converted to sinus rhythm by electrical means, antiarrhythmic medications such as quinidine (Quinaglute), procainamide (Procan) and disopyramide (Norpace) may be initiated to maintain sinus rhythm. If the atrial fibrillation has been prolonged in time and if the atria are enlarged, this approach tends to be ineffective. The therapy then is to decrease the ventricular response rates by increasing the level of AV block. This is done with digoxin as

TABLE 2. **Agents Useful in Treating Supraventricular Tachycardia**

| | Intermittent Intravenous Dosing | | | |
|---|---|---|---|---|
| | Initial Dose (mg) | Maximum Dose (mg) | Unit Dose (mg) | Dosing Interval (min) |
| Digoxin | 0.50 | 2.0 | 0.25 | 120–240 |
| Procainamide | 1000 | 1000 | 100 | 5 |
| Propranolol | — | 10 mg | 1 | 5 |
| Quinidine | 600 | 200–300 | 100 | 20 |
| Verapamil | 5.0 | 15 | 5.0 | 5 |
| Adenosine | 6 | 12 | 6 | 1–2 |

TABLE 3. **Effect of Carotid Sinus Pressure (CSP) on Tachyarrhythmias**

| Arrhythmia | Possible Responses to CSP | | | | |
| --- | --- | --- | --- | --- | --- |
| | No Effect | Gradual Slowing of Rate | Abrupt Conversion to Sinus Rhythm | AV Block and Decreased Ventricular Rate Response | Other Responses |
| Sinus tachycardia | | + | | | |
| PSVT-AV nodal re-entry | + | | + | | |
| PSVT–concealed bypass tract | + | | + | | Slight slowing |
| Automatic atrial tachycardia | + | | | + | |
| Atrial flutter | + | | | + | Atrial fibrillation |
| Atrial fibrillation | + | | | + | |
| Ventricular tachycardia | + | | | | AV dissociation |

the drug of choice. If digoxin therapy is insufficient to control ventricular response rates, a small amount of verapamil (Isoptin) or propranolol (Inderal) may be added to the medical regimen. Note that in patients with chronic atrial fibrillation with mitral valve disease, the risk of a thrombotic event is increased and anticoagulation therapy should also be considered.

### Paroxysmal Supraventricular Tachycardia

When atrial rate suddenly changes to 150 to 250 beats per minute, the diagnosis of paroxysmal supraventricular tachycardia (PSVT) should be considered. Two basic mechanisms have been postulated for PSVT. These are the re-entry mechanisms and enhanced automaticity. Table 1 shows a summary of paroxysmal supraventricular tachycardia caused by re-entry and by abnormal impulse initiation. Therapy is usually directed at agents that may slow or terminate the tachycardia. These are generally agents that affect the AV node and the response of the ventricle to the rapid rates in the atrium. Nonpharmacologic mechanisms to terminate paroxysmal supraventricular tachycardias can also be used. These include (1) the Valsalva maneuver, (2) squatting with the Valsalva maneuver, (3) the gag reflex, and (4) the diving reflex (face in cold water).

These are vagal maneuvers that increase the block at the level of the AV node, which may terminate many supraventricular tachycardias. If the supraventricular tachycardia persists, intravenous antiarrhythmic drugs may be used in an attempt to convert the patient to sinus rhythm. Table 2 lists various medications currently available. A new agent, adenosine (Adenocard), with an extremely short half-life has recently been approved and can be given in an attempt to terminate the tachycardia within 30 seconds. The next choice would be intravenous verapamil (Isoptin). If the person is hemodynam-

ically compromised or has angina symptoms, electrical cardioversion should be used in place of the pharmacologic maneuvers.

Chronic therapy should be directed at the underlying problems that may be associated with patients with PSVT. Avoidance of the trigger mechanisms may limit the frequency of recurrence. These may include excessive use of caffeine, nicotine, or beta stimulants used in the treatment of pulmonary diseases. Chronic antiarrhythmic prophylaxis should be used in patients with frequent or hemodynamically compromising PSVT episodes.

### Supraventricular Tachyarrhythmias Associated with Pre-excitation Syndromes

Pre-excitation syndromes are based on proposed and theorized anatomic AV connections between the atria and ventricles. These were presented as four basic anatomic groups: accessory AV pathways, nodoventricular pathways, fasciculoventricular pathways, and AV nodal bypass tracts of three types: (1) atrio-His tract, (2) intranodal tract, and (3) posterior intranodal tract. The site and conduction properties of bypass tracts and their antegrade and retrograde refractoriness will determine a tract's ability to sustain the various types of arrhythmias. Two types of circus movement tachycardias (CMT) are initiated by a premature atrial beat. The first type is an orthodromic CMT, which requires normal conduction of the atrial impulse to proceed down the AV conduction system with a retrograde conduction through the bypass tract, completing a re-entry pathway. A reversed (antidromic) CMT is primarily a result of conduction being initiated antegrade down the accessory pathway and retrograde through the AV nodal system. This type of tachycardia is a wide complex re-entry tachycardia. Most patients with pre-excitation syndrome present with a history of nonsustained PSVT. Therapy is therefore directed at minimizing the occurrence of the atrial premature beats, narrowing the intervals in which the premature beat can initiate the tachycardia, and prolonging the refractoriness in the circuit so that the re-entry impulse may block in either the AV node or the accessory pathway. Membrane-active agents that slow conduction velocity appear to have the most effect on these types of arrhythmias.

If a patient has a supraventricular tachycardia, such as atrial fibrillation, with an accessory pathway with a short refractory period, this condition could be life-threatening. The ventricular responses to the supraventricular tachycardia could be 1:1 owing to rapid conduction down the accessory pathway, and patients may be severely hemodynamically compromised. These patients should be treated with surgical interruption of the abnormal pathway. If the tachycardia and ventricular responses are sufficiently slow and hemodynamically stable, alternative modes of therapy other than antiarrhythmic drugs may be considered. These include antitachycardia pacing and catheter ablation of the accessory pathway or AV node.

### Narrow Complex Tachycardia

When the patient presents with a tachycardia of QRS duration less than 120 milliseconds, the differential diagnosis for the tachycardia increases owing to the number of sites or re-entry pathways with which the tachycardia could have originated. Table 3 and Figure 1 outline the methods by which the tachycardia can be analyzed. The branching diagram shows that atrioventricular block produced by carotid sinus pressure (CSP) should be the initial step to make the diagnosis.

CSP should almost always be used to aid in the diagnosis of supraventricular tachyarrhythmias. If no significant bruits are present over the carotid arteries, the patient should be placed in a prone position, and continuous ECG recording should be done. Continuous external pressure is applied in a circular motion to massage the right and left carotid sinuses sequentially for 3 to 5 seconds. This maneuver activates a baroreceptor reflex that results in a vagal discharge with effects on various tachyarrhythmias as summarized in Table 3. Look for a QRS alternation, i.e., differences in amplitude to the QRS from beat to beat. Location of the P wave relative to the QRS

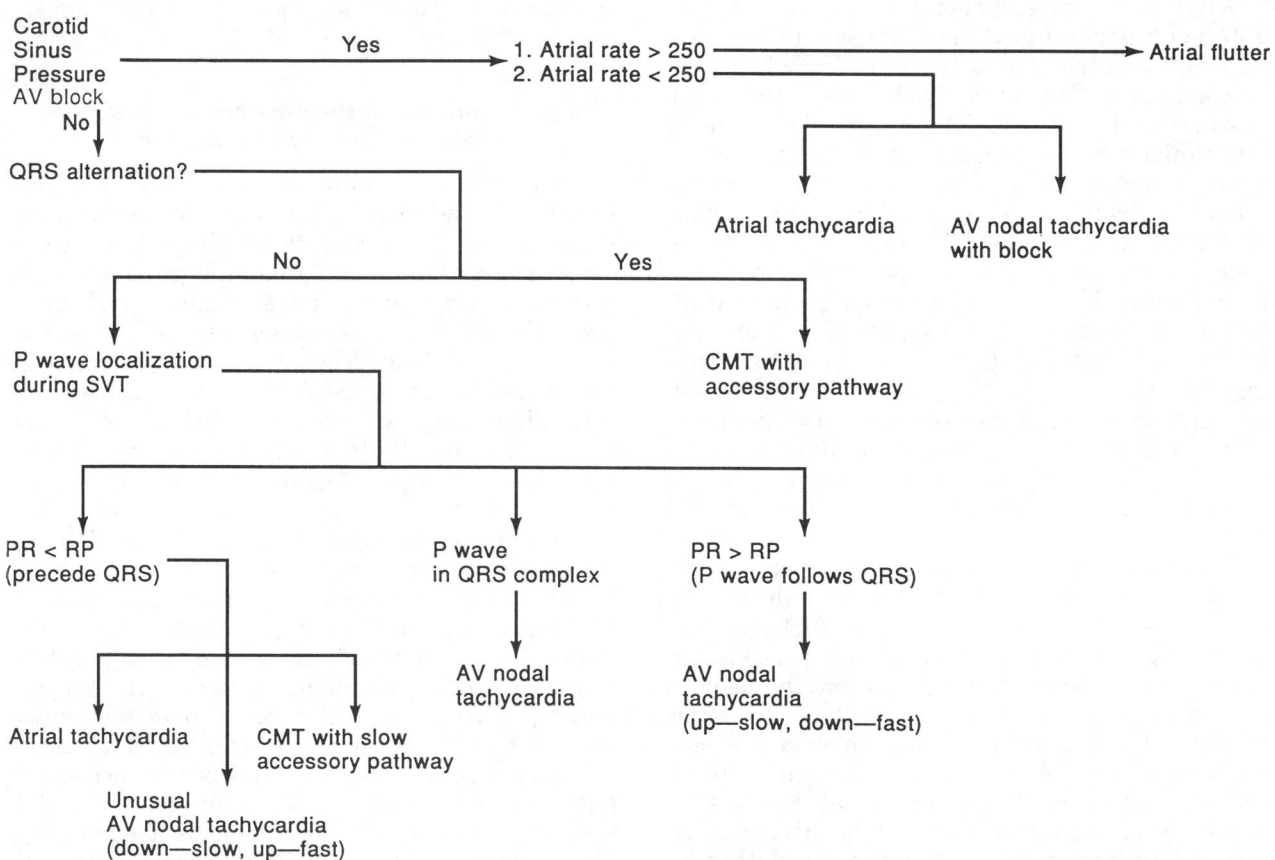

**Figure 1.** Algorithm for analyzing narrow complex tachycardia (QRS < 0.12 sec).

TABLE 4. **Steps in the Diagnosis of a Wide Complex Tachycardia (QRS >0.12 sec)**

| | |
|---|---|
| AV dissociation | Present—VT |
| QRS width? | >0.14 sec—VT<br>   Rule out a. SVT with pre-existing BBB<br>           b. SVT with antegrade conduction over AP |
| Left axis deviation (Left of −30°)? | Present, Favors VT<br>   Rule out a. SVT with pre-existing BBB<br>           b. SVT with antegrade conduction over Kent (septal<br>             or right-sided) or Mahaim bundle |
| QRS configuration?<br>   RBBB-shaped<br>   LBBB-shaped | $V_1$: Mono or biphasic QRS suggests VT<br>$V_6$: R/S <1 suggests VT<br>$V_1$: $R_{Tachy} < R_{SR}$ suggests SVT<br>    $R_{Tachy} > R_{SR}$ suggests VT<br>$V_{1,2}$: $R_{Tachy}$ >30 msec suggests VT<br>$V_{1,2}$: Notching downslope S wave suggests VT<br>$V_{1,2}$: Beginning QRS to nadir S >70 msec suggests VT<br>$V_6$: qR suggests VT |

complex is essential to determine the site of origin of the ectopic focus. What is the P wave axis? Treatment of the narrow complex tachycardia depends on the type of arrhythmia with which the tachycardia was initiated.

### Wide Complex Tachycardia

When a patient presents with a wide complex tachycardia, the schema outlined in Table 4

should be used to quickly determine whether the tachycardia is supraventricular or ventricular in origin. The differential diagnosis includes ventricular tachycardia, supraventricular tachycardia with aberrant conduction, and supraventricular tachycardia with an accessory pathway. Unfortunately, the baseline ECG should also be available, since the patient may have a myocardial infarction, evidence of an accessory pathway, or an abnormal QRS duration prior to presenta-

TABLE 5. **Selected Pharmacokinetic and Clinical Data for Antiarrhythmic Agents by Classification**

| Drug | Usual Oral Dose (mg) | Route | Half-Life | Elimination Mechanism | Adverse Reactions |
|---|---|---|---|---|---|
| **IA** Quinidine<br>Quinidine gluconate<br>(Quinaglute) | 200–600 q 6 h<br>324–972 q 6 h | PO, IV | 4–6 hr | Liver | Diarrhea, nausea, thrombocytopenia, cinchonism, hypotension, dermatitis |
| Procainamide sustained release (Procan SR) | 250–1000 q 3–4 hr<br>500–2000 q 6 hr | PO, IV | 3.5 hr | Liver, kidney | Nausea, agranulocytosis, rash, fever, ANA positive, SLE syndrome |
| Disopyramide sustained release (Norpace CR) | 100–300 q 6 hr<br>200–400 q 12 hr | PO | 4–10 hr | Liver, kidney | Urinary retention, constipation, heart failure |
| **IB** Lidocaine | — | IV | 1.5 hr | Liver | Dizziness, confusion, tremor, convulsions |
| Phenytoin (Dilantin) | 300–400 q 12–24 hr | PO, IV | 24 hr | Liver | Hypotension, ataxia, nystagmus, gingival hyperplasia |
| Mexiletine (Mexitil) | 200–400 q 8 hr | PO | 12–16 hr | Liver, kidney | Dizziness, confusion, tremor, nystagmus, ataxia, nausea |
| Tocainide (Tonocard) | 150–600 q 8 hr | PO | 11 hr | Liver, kidney | Dizziness, confusion, tremor, rash, lupus syndrome, nausea |
| **IC** Flecainide (Tambocor) | 100–200 q 12 hr | PO | 14–20 hr | Liver, kidney | Nausea, heart failure, blurred vision |
| Encainide (Enkaid) | 25–50 q 8 hr | PO | 2.4–4 hr | Liver, kidney | Nausea, tremor, blurred vision, dizziness, heart failure |
| Propafenone (Rythmol) | 150–300 q 8 hr | PO | 5–8 hr | Liver | Depressed cardiac output, neurologic symptoms |
| **II** Propranolol (Inderal) | 10–80 q 6 hr | PO, IV | IV 3.3 hr<br>PO 4.6 hr | Liver | Fatigue, depression, nausea, depressed cardiac output |
| **III** Bretylium (Bretylol) | — | IV | 8 hr | Kidney | Hypotension, parotid gland swelling, nausea |
| Amiodarone (Cordarone) | 200–400 q day | PO | 30–45 days | ? | Skin discoloration, cornea deposits, thyroid function abnormalities, pulmonary fibrosis |
| **IV** Verapamil (Isoptin) | 40–120 q 6–8 hr | PO, IV | 3.7 hr | Liver | Bradycardia, asystole, constipation, lethargy, headache, depressed cardiac output |

tion with a wide complex tachycardia. The first step is to assume that the tachycardia is ventricular in origin, since it occurs statistically more frequently. A differential diagnosis in tachycardias with a QRS duration greater than 120 milliseconds is shown in Table 4. If the patient is hemodynamically stable, there is time to make the diagnosis of tachycardia. If the patient is hemodynamically unstable, electrical cardioversion should be done immediately.

### Ventricular Tachycardia

Ventricular tachycardia (VT) is considered to be any wide complex tachycardia that occurs below the levels of the AV node. Wide complex tachycardia that is determined to be ventricular in origin in a hemodynamically unstable patient should always be treated with immediate electrical cardioversion. Most patients who present with ventricular tachycardia have ischemic heart disease or left ventricular dysfunction. If the rhythm disorder is hemodynamically unstable, the rhythm may degenerate to ventricular fibrillation and may be fatal. Recurrent VT, untreated, has an annual recurrence rate of 40 to 50% in many studies. Prophylaxis of patients who have recurrent ventricular tachycardia is an attempt to prevent the sudden cardiac death syndrome. Prophylactic antiarrhythmic drug therapies as outlined in Table 5 may be effective when combined with electrophysiologic evaluation of the tachyarrhythmia to test drug efficacy. It should be emphasized that empiric antiarrhythmic drug therapy in patients with recurrent VT has been found to exacerbate arrhythmias in 5 to 15% of patients. Encainide, flecainide, and amiodarone should be used *only* in severe, life-threatening arrhythmias. When recurrent episodes of monomorphic, nonsustained ventricular tachycardia occur frequently and predictably, treatment with conventional antiarrhythmic drugs can be initiated and their efficacy assessed by Holter recordings. If the ventricular tachycardia does not occur spontaneously with sufficient frequency to guide this type of therapy, electrophysiologic methods to induce the VT are available.

### Ventricular Fibrillation

Ventricular fibrillation is an irregular rhythm that is ventricular in origin. This is a medical emergency, since no cardiac output can be maintained during this condition. Electrical defibrillation is the current treatment method of choice. An electrical device that senses hemodynamically unstable ventricular tachycardia or ventricular fibrillation can be implanted in these patients.

These devices can deliver up to 30 joules through pads that are placed around the heart to electrically defibrillate the rhythm disorder. This device can be used for a variety of ventricular tachyarrhythmias or in patients in whom VT drug resistance is found.

# CONGENITAL HEART DISEASE

method of
LARRY A. LATSON, M.D.
*University of Nebraska Medical Center*
*Omaha, Nebraska*

Approximately eight of every 1000 children born has some type of congenital heart defect identified in childhood. Thus, in the United States, there are approximately 30,000 infants born each year with a clinically detectable congenital cardiac defect. Only about 20% of these patients will require surgery or specific cardiac medications during childhood, but all affected children need to be identified and properly diagnosed so that they can be followed closely for the development of any complications from their defects and so that they are adequately counselled for bacterial endocarditis prophylaxis. In addition to the patients easily identified in childhood, it is estimated that an additional 1% of the population may have a minor congenital defect such as a bicuspid aortic valve that is relatively silent in childhood but can lead to significant consequences in young adult life. The most common congenital heart defects can be classified into three groups according to their major hemodynamic consequence: a left-to-right shunt, obstruction to flow, or cyanosis.

### OVERVIEW OF CONGENITAL HEART DEFECTS

*Left-to-Right Shunts*

By far, the largest group of patients with a congenital heart defect includes those who have one of the three common lesions leading to a left-to-right shunt: ventricular septal defect (VSD), patent ductus arteriosus (PDA), and atrial septal defect (ASD). VSD is the most common isolated congenital heart defect, accounting for approximately 30% of all patients with congenital heart disease. PDA and ASD each account for approximately 7 to 10% of patients with congenital heart disease. The most significant effects of a left-to-right shunt lesion are an increase in pulmonary blood flow and excessive volume work for the left ventricle (VSD and PDA) or right ventricle (ASD). The left-to-right shunt through a VSD or PDA occurs under high pressure and is much more likely to be significant in young patients. Patients with an ASD most commonly do not manifest the signs of a large left-to-right shunt until they are over 1 to 2 years of age.

The primary symptoms of patients with a large left-to-right shunt are caused by the increased work of breathing and increased calorie needs of the patient.

Thus the typical infant with a large left-to-right shunt is tachypneic at rest, may have difficulties feeding because of the tachypnea, and may gain weight poorly because of the increased need for calories. The primary goals of medical treatment in these patients are to reduce the work of breathing by reducing pulmonary edema (primarily with diuretics) and, if necessary, increasing the caloric intake.

*Obstructive Lesions*

This is the second most common group of congenital cardiac defects and includes primarily aortic stenosis, pulmonary stenosis, and coarctation of the aorta (each approximately 5% of congenital heart defects). These lesions tend to present as either asymptomatic murmurs or as true emergencies in the early neonatal period if the obstruction is critical. Critical aortic stenosis and coarctation, with or without hypoplasia of the left ventricle, are the most common causes of cardiovascular collapse in the first 1 to 2 weeks of life. Even infants with critical lesions often are asymptomatic in the first few days of life when the PDA is widely patent and pulmonary resistance is high. The PDA then serves as a pathway for perfusion to the systemic circulation. Closure of the PDA in these patients, however, is accompanied by very poor peripheral perfusion and cardiovascular collapse. A hallmark of these lesions is the disparity between the weak pulses (either all over or in the legs) and the increased precordial activity of the heart on palpitation. Patients with critical pulmonary stenosis may have cardiovascular collapse but tend to present with much more cyanosis than those with left-sided obstructive lesions.

Patients with less than critical obstructive lesions are often asymptomatic, even if the degree of obstruction is graded as severe. Treatment of mild obstructive lesions in childhood is expectant until (or unless) the pressure gradient across the lesion becomes significant. Once the degree of obstruction has become more severe, intervention in the catheterization laboratory or operating room is generally indicated.

*Cyanotic Lesions*

These are the least common, but often most dramatic, group of congenital heart defects and include predominantly transposition of the great vessels, tetralogy of Fallot, and hypoplastic right heart lesions (tricuspid atresia and pulmonary atresia with intact ventricular septum). These lesions each account for 2 to 5% of patients with congenital heart disease. Because of the cyanosis, these lesions are generally detected in infancy. The most characteristic finding in these patients is that they are cyanotic but usually quite comfortable at rest. This is in contrast to infants with cyanosis secondary to respiratory disease who usually have retractions or grunting and who appear to be in distress. It is imperative that patients with suspected cyanotic heart disease be sent for early diagnosis and treatment because these lesions are quickly fatal without treatment but have a very good prognosis with appropriate therapy.

## TREATMENT

### Neonate with Suspected Congenital Heart Disease

**The Asymptomatic Neonate with a Heart Murmur.** Most heart murmurs in neonates are secondary to relatively minor abnormalities, many of which will resolve spontaneously (such as a PDA in the process of closing, transient tricuspid insufficiency, physiologic pulmonary branch stenosis, or very small VSD). The decision of when to refer a patient with a heart murmur for further evaluation is often difficult. Any patient with possible *symptoms* of heart failure, significant cardiomegaly, or definite cyanosis should be referred immediately. If the significance of clinical signs on physical exam alone is uncertain, then supporting information can readily be obtained from a chest x-ray and pulse oximeter. The electrocardiogram is useful if it is abnormal, but it may be normal even with very severe cardiac malformations.

Echocardiography is the procedure of choice for noninvasive diagnosis of congenital heart defects. Most of the congenital heart defects requiring early intervention will result in at least some abnormalities that can be detected by echocardiographers with only limited experience in pediatric echocardiography. However, echocardiographers who do not have special training and a great deal of experience in pediatric echocardiography may miss the exact diagnosis, and if there are any questions, the patient should be referred for more definitive evaluation at a specific pediatric cardiology center. Echocardiography is expensive and is not needed in most cases if the patient is truly asymptomatic.

The parents of any child with a heart murmur should be informed about the murmur and some discussion of possible symptoms should be undertaken. It may be advisable to see patients with a murmur earlier or more often than the routine patient until the diagnosis is clear. Development of any significant symptoms should prompt referral for further evaluation from a pediatric cardiology center.

**The Cyanotic Neonate.** Persistent cyanosis in a neonate demands early and aggressive evaluation and treatment. The most common etiologies of cyanosis include respiratory system abnormalities (most commonly lower airway disease, such as hyaline membrane disease or pneumonia), central nervous system depression resulting in hypoventilation, or intracardiac right-to-left shunting secondary to congenital heart disease or persistent pulmonary hypertension of the newborn.

Lower airway disease generally causes significant distress and affected infants appear uncom-

TABLE 1. **Differentiation of Causes of Cyanosis in the Neonate**

| | Appearance | ABGs in Room Air | | $Pa_{O_2}$ on 100% $FI_{O_2}$ |
| --- | --- | --- | --- | --- |
| | | $Pa_{O_2}$ | $Pa_{CO_2}$ | |
| Lung disease | Retractions, distress | ↓ | N to ↑ | >120 mmHg |
| CNS depression | Poorly responsive | ↓ | ↑ | >150 mmHg |
| Intracardiac R–L shunt | Comfortable | ↓ | N to ↓ | <100 mmHg |

*Abbreviations:* ABGs = arterial blood gases; R–L = right to left; N = normal.

fortable and show signs of increased work of breathing. Those with central nervous system depression or intracardiac right-to-left shunts often have normal lung function and mechanics and, at least initially, may appear comfortable but cyanotic. Arterial blood gases in room air (or relatively low oxygen concentrations) and with the patient on 100% oxygen may be very helpful in distinguishing the major causes of cyanosis (Table 1). Hypoxemia from lower respiratory disease, hypoventilation, and ventilation/perfusion abnormalities will be at least partially overcome by administration of 100% oxygen and the $Pa_{O_2}$ will rise to well over 100 mmHg at least transiently. Patients with a significant intracardiac right-to-left shunt however will have very little response to 100% oxygen and only rarely will the systemic $Pa_{O_2}$ rise to above 100 mmHg in such patients.

It must be remembered that many patients with cyanotic congenital heart disease will have little or no cardiac murmur (especially those with transposition of the great vessels). A chest x-ray and electrocardiogram are useful if they show definite abnormalities, but they may initially appear normal even in the presence of severe cyanotic heart defects. Any infant who does not show an increase in the $Pa_{O_2}$ to above 100 mmHg in the first hours of aggressive medical treatment must be suspected of having an intracardiac right-to-left shunt. Occasionally patients with persistent pulmonary hypertension of the newborn or severe pneumonias or pulmonary hypoplasia may have a large intracardiac right-to-left shunt through the normal foramen ovale or PDA. Right-to-left shunting through the PDA can be detected by finding a lower $Pa_{O_2}$ in the descending aorta (umbilical artery catheter) than in the right radial artery. Intracardiac right-to-left shunts (either through the normal foramen ovale or through a congenital defect) will result in uniformly low $Pa_{O_2}$ readings.

If the facilities to thoroughly evaluate the neonate with possible cyanotic heart disease are not immediately available, then early consultation with a pediatric cardiology center is essential. If a significant congenital heart defect cannot be ruled out after telephone consultation, then transport to a pediatric cardiology center should be undertaken. If cyanotic congenital heart disease is a strong possibility, infusion of prostaglandin E$_1$ (PGE$_1$) will usually be recommended prior to transport. PGE$_1$ will result in dilation of the PDA in nearly all neonates less than several days of age and also reduces pulmonary vascular resistance. Although these effects may not be particularly helpful in infants who do not have congenital heart defects, PGE$_1$ very definitely is lifesaving in those who have ductus dependent circulations. Therefore, when the diagnosis is uncertain, the benefits outweigh the risks. Facilities must be available to mechanically ventilate the neonate when PGE$_1$ is first instituted since it may cause apnea in a significant percentage (Table 2).

**The Neonate with Possible Heart Failure.** Congestive heart failure secondary to obstructive heart defects (critical aortic stenosis/atresia or coarctation) most often develops over the first few days to weeks of life, rather than presenting in the first hours after delivery. While the PDA is widely patent and pulmonary resistance is relatively high, perfusion to the body can be maintained adequately by ejection of right ventricular blood through the PDA to the descending aorta

TABLE 2. **Intravenous Drip Drugs for Critically Ill Neonates with Heart Defects**

| Drug | Dose | Major Beneficial Effect | Major Detrimental Effect |
| --- | --- | --- | --- |
| PGE$_1$ (Prostin VR) | .05–.1 µg/kg/min | Dilates ductus Reduces pulmonary resistance | Apnea, hyperthermia, flushing |
| Dopamine (Dopastat) | 2–5 µg/kg/min | Dilates renal arteries (dopaminergic effect) | |
| | 5–20 µg/kg/min | Raises systemic BP (alpha effect) | Tachycardia, reduces peripheral perfusion |
| Isoproterenol (Isuprel) | 0.05–0.5 µg/kg/min | Increases contractility Reduces pulmonary resistance Improves peripheral perfusion | Tachycardia (may be severe) Hypotension if hypovolemic |
| Dobutamine (Dobutrex) | 2–20 µg/kg/min | Increases contractility and cardiac output | Tachycardia |

(as in fetal life). Closure of the PDA, however, is disastrous because perfusion to the body is abruptly diminished and, at the same time, severe pulmonary hypertension or pulmonary edema develops. The clinical hallmarks of the common congenital heart defects leading to early severe heart failure are signs of decreased perfusion, with or without a significant decrease in absolute blood pressure, and a noticeable discrepancy between the readily palpable hyperactivity of the heart and diminished pulses in some or all of the extremities. A chest x-ray in these patients will always show cardiomegaly and usually will show signs of pulmonary congestion or edema.

Early diagnosis is again essential because surgical treatment is available for many of the lesions that cause severe cardiovascular collapse. Early consultation with a pediatric cardiology center should be undertaken. $PGE_1$ [prostaglandin $E_1$ (Prostin VR)] may often be recommended in these patients since many of the defects causing this clinical picture can be improved if the ductus is widely patent. Patients who are severely ill will require mechanical ventilation to reduce their energy requirements and to improve pulmonary edema. Intravenous diuretics may help relieve symptoms in patients who are less ill. Intravenous catecholamine drips (especially dopamine [Intropin] and dobutamine [Dobutrex]) may be necessary to reverse severe cardiovascular collapse until improved systemic perfusion can be achieved by $PGE_1$ or surgery (see Table 2).

### Infant (1 Month to 1 Year) with Known or Suspected Congenital Heart Disease

**The Infant with Congestive Heart Failure.** The congenital cardiac lesions causing chronic congestive heart failure in older infants are predominantly the left-to-right shunt lesions. In most cases, the degree of left-to-right shunting is at least partially dependent on the pulmonary artery resistance. Thus, it is very common for there to be little in the way of symptoms (and often no murmur) in newborns with lesions such as large VSDs, because the pulmonary resistance is high and reactive in the early neonatal period. The symptoms of congestive heart failure typically develop over the first several weeks of life as pulmonary resistance drops and may not peak until 5 to 6 months of life. The primary symptoms of heart failure in this age group are tachypnea at rest, increased diaphoresis, and failure to thrive.

Many of the lesions causing large left-to-right shunts can be repaired if necessary in early infancy. However, some lesions, especially VSDs,

may spontaneously decrease in size or even close completely in the first several years of life. Therefore, these lesions are often treated medically for a fairly long period of time in order to allow any spontaneous improvement. Lesions that have little chance of improving spontaneously (such as atrioventricular canal or very large VSDs) will generally require surgical intervention prior to 1 year of age. The exact timing for surgery in an individual patient may depend on multiple factors, including degree of failure to thrive, degree of pulmonary hypertension, and the experience of a particular center with a particular lesion.

The cornerstones to treatment of the infant with chronic congestive heart failure are diuretic therapy and caloric supplementation (Table 3). Powerful diuretics, such as furosemide (Lasix), are usually required. Diuresis helps to reduce pulmonary edema, which reduces the work of breathing and hopefully allows the patient to feed better. If large doses of furosemide (Lasix) are required, the addition of either spironolactone (Aldactone) or oral potassium supplements may be needed to maintain normal body potassium. Most centers continue to treat patients with chronic left-to-right shunts with digoxin (Lanoxin). Although this drug has some mild beneficial clinical effect, the inotropic state of these infants is usually normal and the effects on symptoms are usually minimal. Because side effects of high doses of digoxin can be very serious, we generally treat our patients with low to moderate doses and are quick to discontinue digoxin if there are any questions about significant side effects.

Since patients with a large left-to-right shunt

TABLE 3. **Recommended Treatment of Chronic Congestive Heart Failure in Children**

*Diuresis*
Furosemide (Lasix)—0.5–2 mg/kg/dose 1–3 times daily
If using over 2 mg/kg/day, addition of spironolactone (Aldactone) 2–6 mg/kg/day* in one or two doses may be needed (crushed tablets recommended over suspension since drug not highly soluble)

*Caloric Supplementation*
Glucose polymer (Polycose powder)—7.6 kcal/tsp—maximum 3 tsp/4 oz of formula
MCT Oil (coconut oil)—7.6 kcal/ml—maximum 3 ml/4 oz of formula
Gradually increase additives by adding approximately ⅓ of maximum amount of one of the other additives to formula and watch for diarrhea (more common with Polycose) or vomiting (more common with MCT Oil) for 24–48 hours before advancing again

*Digoxin (Lanoxin)*
Maintenance dose is 8–10 μg(0.008–0.01 mg)/kg/day PO in two divided doses in term neonates and older children
Loading doses and IV administration are not recommended unless rapid effects are required (as in treatment of supraventricular tachycardia)

*Exceeds dosage recommended by the manufacturer.

have a greatly increased energy requirement, they commonly require 130 to 150 kcal per kg per day in order to grow normally. At the same time, their fluids need to be restricted to prevent the development of worsening pulmonary edema. Therefore, formulas with a high caloric density are usually given to these infants. We find that standard formulas supplemented with glucose polymer (Polycose) or coconut oil (MCT Oil) are generally well tolerated. In patients who are able to consume an adequate volume of formula by mouth, we gradually increase the additives in the formula to give them 1 kcal per ml. Patients with more severe heart failure may not be able to ingest this much formula without tiring excessively. In these infants, we supply the formula via a nasogastric tube. In many patients, continuous nasogastric drip of formula is better tolerated by both the parents and the patient than is long-term intermittent gavage.

Infants with large left-to-right shunts are highly susceptible to lower respiratory tract infections, and these must be treated aggressively. Infections with respiratory syncytial virus may be particularly devastating.

**The Infant with Cyanosis.** Any older infant with cyanosis should undergo complete evaluation as early as is feasible, even though the child may be otherwise doing well. Treatment on an urgent basis may not be necessary in patients who are not noted to be cyanotic until several months of age, but early diagnosis is essential so that parents and all physicians involved with the treatment of the child have an understanding of the likely progression of the symptoms and a tentative treatment plan can be formulated.

Cyanosis, per se, often causes very little symptomatic impairment in small infants. Patients with lesions such as transposition of the great vessels or tetralogy of Fallot generally require fewer medications than patients with large left-to-right shunts and often grow better. Progression of these lesions can be estimated by changes in the resting oxygen saturation (by pulse oximetry) and by the hemoglobin. Resting arterial oxygen saturations (not $Pa_{O_2}$) of over 75% are generally well tolerated, but resting saturations under 65% leave very little reserve and may be associated with problems. Increased hemoglobin is a normal response to hypoxemia, and hemoglobin concentrations of less than 20 grams% per dl are well tolerated, but higher levels may result in hyperviscosity. Patients with cyanotic heart lesions should be given adequate iron in the diet to maintain normal red cell indices.

Patients who have a large interventricular communication and pulmonary blood supplied only through a stenotic valve (such as unshunted tetralogy of Fallot or some patients with tricuspid atresia) may be prone to hypercyanotic spells ("tet spells"). These spells are characterized by a relatively abrupt increase in cyanosis associated with some apparent discomfort, as though the patient is short of breath. The patients typically become hyperpneic and agitated but may become unresponsive if severe cyanosis persists, so early treatment of hypercyanotic spells is essential. The mechanism of a spell is a relative decrease in the proportion of blood going to the lungs as compared with the systemic circulation. Therefore, treatment efforts must primarily be aimed at increasing the amount of blood entering the lungs. This can best be done by calming the patient as much as possible (to reduce the need for systemic cardiac output) and raising the systemic blood pressure by gently drawing the knees against the chest. Administration of oxygen to patients having a spell has some slight value if they do not object to having the oxygen blown in their face, but it is detrimental if it causes them to struggle. If necessary, a rapid infusion of fluid to increase intravascular volume can be given after an intravenous line is started. In very refractory cases, infusion of phenylephrine (Neo-Synephrine) to raise blood pressure or propranolol (Inderal) to reduce muscular subpulmonary obstruction may be necessary. Patients who have a significant hypercyanotic spell are generally candidates for either palliative or corrective surgery in the near future.

### The Infant with an Asymptomatic Murmur

Most of the transitory, functional murmurs of neonates (such as closing PDAs, transient tricuspid insufficiency, or physiologic pulmonary branch stenosis) will have disappeared by 1 month of age. On the other hand, the murmurs of small left-to-right shunts (such as VSD) may be first noted or be louder at 1 month. Murmurs noted at this age should be very carefully evaluated clinically. The most common *pathologic* murmur in infants in this age group is a small VSD. This murmur is relatively soft and well localized to a small area along the lower left sternal border. Murmurs that are unusually loud, that are well heard in the back, or that radiate to the upper right sternal border and into the neck should be evaluated more extensively. Remember that patients with moderate or even severe aortic or pulmonic stenosis can be entirely asymptomatic, but they need to be identified for possible early treatment because of a risk of sudden death.

Infants with asymptomatic murmurs generally require little in the way of special treatment. However, functional murmurs must be separated from those caused by structural heart disease

TABLE 4. **Bacterial Endocarditis Prophylaxis (American Heart Association, 1984)**

| Procedure | Patients with Congenital Heart Disease or Acquired Valvular Disease (Type A) | Patients with Artificial Valve Replacements or Who Are High Risk (Type B) |
|---|---|---|
| *All Dental Procedures (Including Professional Cleaning) and Upper Respiratory Tract Surgical Procedures* | | |
| Oral treatment | Penicillin V: Over 60 lb—2.0 grams PO 1 hr before procedure, then 1.0 gram PO 6 hr after procedure (one dose only) Under 60 lb—1.0 gram PO 1 hr before procedure, then 500 mg PO 6 hr after procedure (one dose only) | |
| Parenteral treatment | Aqueous penicillin 50,000 U/kg (2 million U max.) IV or IM 30 min.–1 hr before procedure, then one dose 6 hr after procedure; may use aqueous penicillin G, 25,000 U/kg, 1 million U max. for this dosage or penicillin V as in oral treatment. | Ampicillin 50 mg/kg (2.0 grams max.) and gentamicin 2.0 mg/kg (80 mg max.) IM or IV 30 min.–1 hr before procedure, then penicillin 1.0 gram, PO 6 hr after procedure. Alternatively, parenteral B regimen should be repeated 8 hr after procedure (one dose only) |
| Penicillin Allergic Patients | Erythromycin 20 mg/kg (1 gram max.) PO 1 hr before procedure, then 10 mg/kg (500 mg max.) PO 6 hr after procedure (one dose only) | Vancomycin 20 mg/kg (1.0 gram max) IV slowly 1 hr before procedure. No repeat dose is necessary. |
| *Genitourinary/Gastrointestinal* | Ampicillin 50 mg/kg (2.0 grams max.) IM or IV and gentamicin 2.0 mg/kg (80 mg max.) IM or IV 30 min. before procedure, then repeat 8 hr after procedure (one dose only) | Ampicillin 50 mg/kg (2.0 grams max.) IM or IV and gentamicin 2.0 mg/kg (80 mg max.) IM or IV 30 min before procedure, then repeat 8 hr after procedure (one dose only) |
| Penicillin Allergic Patients | Gentamicin 2.0 mg/kg (80 mg max.) IM or IV and vancomycin 20 mg/kg (1.0 gram max.) IV slowly 1 hr before procedure, then repeat 8–12 hr after procedure (one dose only) | Gentamicin 2.0 mg/kg (80 mg max.) IM or IV and vancomycin 20 mg/kg (1.0 gram max.) IV slowly 1 hr before procedure, then repeat 8–12 hr after procedure (one dose only) |

Reprinted from Revised American Heart Association recommendations for SBE prophylaxis, *Nebraska Medical Journal,* November 1985.

because of the need for prophylaxis for bacterial endocarditis and possible continued follow-up of patients with cardiac defects.

### The Older Infant and Child with Congenital Heart Disease (Over 1 Year)

Murmurs present in early infancy and continuing past 1 year of age merit careful clinical evaluation and possible referral for pediatric cardiology evaluation. Most small ventricular septal defects that will close spontaneously do so within the first 1 to 2 years of life. Many functional murmurs will first appear at 1 to 5 years of age, but these generally are murmurs that were not audible in early infancy. Distinguishing functional murmurs from pathologic murmurs can be very difficult. In general, functional murmurs are poorly localized, do not radiate along the paths of blood vessels, are harmonic in quality rather than harsh, and decrease significantly or disappear when the patient is sitting or standing. If there is any question about whether a murmur

is caused by a heart defect, evaluation by a qualified specialist is highly recommended. It is essential that patients with functional murmurs not be restricted from any activities and that they be reassured that their hearts are entirely normal. Conversely, it is essential that patients with true congenital defects have these identified clearly so that any necessary treatment and follow-up can be planned.

The vast majority of patients with congenital heart defects do not require any exercise limitations. However, patients with lesions known to be progressive (such as congenital aortic stenosis) may require intermittent stress testing to be certain that their lesions are not progressing to the point of needing intervention. Contact sports may be discouraged in some postoperative patients, particularly if they have artificial valves. Good dental care and bacterial endocarditis prophylaxis is recommended for all patients with any type of congenital heart defect (Table 4). Because the severity of many congenital defects can change with age (either for better or for worse), nearly all patients with congenital heart defects will require intermittent evaluations by a qualified pediatric or adult cardiologist for life (or until the defect spontaneously closes). In asymptomatic patients, these evaluations may only need to be done every 1 to 3 years, but they are essential so that patients can be checked for slow progression or late sequelae of their lesions. Although there may be little that can be done to prevent the progression of many congenital heart defects (such as premature deterioration of abnormal valves), the adverse effects can be detected early and treated in a timely manner before the patient becomes acutely ill.

# MITRAL VALVE PROLAPSE

method of
RICHARD P. LEWIS, M.D.
*The Ohio State University*
*Columbus, Ohio*

Mitral valve prolapse (MVP) is one of the most common cardiovascular disorders. It affects approximately 5% of the adult population. Despite this high prevalence, MVP has been clearly recognized for only 25 years. Recognition was dependent on modern cardiac imaging techniques, most notably echocardiography.

The entity we now call MVP has been described clinically for at least 150 years, mostly by physicians working for the military. It has been variously called "soldier's heart," "effort syndrome," "DaCosta's syndrome," and "neurocirculatory asthenia." It represented the single greatest cause of disability among military draftees during World War I. Although it was considered a "functional" cardiovascular disorder, some clinicians (Osler, Albutt, P.D. White) recognized that such patients could develop severe mitral regurgitation later in life. Osler also noted that in the civilian population, the condition was most commonly seen in young women. The descriptions of the syndrome by these earlier physicians (including the presence of clicks and murmurs) are remarkably similar to those of the MVP syndrome as we know it today, leaving little doubt that MVP is not a new disease.

## PATHOLOGY

Patients with MVP have some symptoms that are directly related to the diseased mitral valve, and others are best characterized as due to autonomic dysfunction. What is still unclear is why the association exists between these two phenomena.

The primary abnormality in the mitral valve is dissolution of both collagen and elastin. The cause is unknown. The degenerative process affects a variable amount of the valve leaflets ranging from one scallop to the entire valve. The chordae tendineae are variably involved in the same manner, and mitral annulus dilatation also frequently occurs. Similar changes are often present in the tricuspid valve but rarely in the semilunar valves. As a result of collagen degeneration (which increases with age), "myxomatous" deposition and scarring occur, which produces a thickened valve leaflet. The valve leaflets also become stretched and in certain areas may be quite thin. These enlarged and thickened valves are termed "floppy" valves. The floppy valve is not necessarily incompetent. When mitral regurgitation occurs, it is usually a result of associated mitral annulus dilatation and chordae tendineae elongation or rupture. MVP is now the major cause of isolated mitral valve surgery in the Western world.

MVP is an autosomal dominant characteristic. Although it may be associated with most of the identifiable dyscollagenoses, such patients account for less than 1% of all MVP cases. Nonetheless, a collagen defect (or defects) is suspected as the cause of "primary" MVP. Half of such patients have a tall, slender habitus with arm span greater than height, hyperdistensible joints, chest deformities (scoliosis, pectus excavatum, straight back), hypomastia in women, and mild aortic root dilatation. Echographic MVP can occur as a secondary phenomenon in hypertrophic cardiomyopathy, atrial septal defect, and anorexia nervosa due to a small left ventricular cavity.

Complications related to the mitral valve include progressive mitral regurgitation, bacterial endocarditis, and cerebral emboli. In addition, arrhythmias can be produced or aggravated by the abnormal mitral valve. Therapy of these complications will be discussed later.

## THE MITRAL VALVE PROLAPSE SYNDROME (MVPS)

MVPS consists of symptoms not directly related to the mitral valve in patients who have MVP. These symptoms include palpitations, chest pain, dyspnea, fatigue, light-headedness, syncope, and anxiety. In addition, migraine headaches, functional gastrointestinal syndromes, Graves' disease, and sleep disorders are associated with MVPS.

Most of these symptoms appear to have a neurohumoral basis. Symptomatic patients with MVP have increased daytime adrenergic tone and increased adrenergic sensitivity, and at times, they may also exhibit increased parasympathetic tone. Plasma volume may be lower than normal, related to either a blunted renin-angiotensin system or excessive elaboration of atrial natriuretic hormone. Understanding of the neurohumoral basis for symptoms in the MVPS is critical to appropriate therapy.

Echo Doppler studies show that in many symptomatic patients with MVP there is minimal abnormality of the mitral valve (i.e., no thickening or redundancy and absent or minimal mitral regurgitation). Such patients undoubtedly have involvement of only a small portion of one leaflet, usually the posterior leaflet. The majority of these patients are females. Symptoms are most severe between ages 20 and 50, coinciding with menses. In males, symptoms are often precipitated by prolonged physical or emotional stress (such as being drafted into the military).

Not all recent investigators accept the concept of MVPS. Such has been the case since DaCosta's description in 1871. However, as was noted by Albutt in 1918, the "group of symptoms is too uniform to be fictitious or fantastic." Recent documentation of neurohumoral abnormalities by numerous investigators provides convincing evidence that MVPS is not a primary psychiatric disorder.

## DIAGNOSIS

The history and physical examination still remain the foundation for the diagnosis of MVP. The clinical history of patients with MVPS is remarkably similar as most describe all the typical symptoms to a greater or lesser degree. In the presence of a click or typical mid- or late systolic murmur and the typical body habitus, the diagnosis is virtually assured. Occasionally, postural maneuvers are required to elicit the click and murmur, and it is now recognized that on a given day neither a click nor murmur may be present, and repeated examinations may be required.

Echocardiography is an extremely useful adjunct and should be performed in all patients suspected of having MVP. The criteria for diagnosis are now better defined. Generally, the combination of M-mode, two-dimensional echocardiography, and Doppler studies (including color flow) is required for proper echographic assessment of MVP. The diagnosis of MVP should be made on the basis of echocardiography alone only when classic findings are present.

In addition to aiding in the diagnosis of MVP, the echo is the most useful technique for stratifying high- and low-risk patients. Numerous studies have documented that patients with thickened, redundant valves, particularly if associated with some degree of mitral regurgitation, are the ones most likely to develop progressive mitral regurgitation, bacterial endocarditis, and probably sudden death. Although the exact prevalence of this more severe form of MVP is not clear, it probably represents no more than half of the total MVP population.

## LONG-TERM PROGNOSIS

MVP patients seen at referral medical centers are not representative of the entire population of MVP patients since referral patients have more symptoms. It is estimated that referral patients represent approximately half of the total MVP population.

Although the long-term prognosis for most patients with MVP is excellent, there is nonetheless a significant (but still unknown) percentage of patients who develop complications. For example, a recent study of 300 MVP patients followed at a large referral center showed only 51% were free of symptoms or evidence of progressive mitral regurgitation during a follow-up period averaging 6 years. The age of this cohort was somewhat older (42 years) than that for some series, which may contribute to the relatively high incidence of complications. In this population, over the 6-year follow-up period, 6% showed an increasing murmur intensity, 9% had supraventricular tachycardia, 18% developed ventricular tachycardia, 6% developed sub-

acute bacterial endocarditis, 9.5% required mitral valve replacement, and 3.5% had a cerebrovascular accident. Sudden death occurred in 1%. Although these percentages clearly overstate the prevalence in the entire MVP population, the incidence of complications of MVP is significantly higher than was originally suspected on the basis of short-term follow-up of relatively young individuals. In view of this, the importance of defining high- and low-risk groups of patients with MVP is clear.

## THERAPY

The therapeutic approach to a patient with MVP depends on the nature of the symptoms and the initial risk stratification. Thus, a young women with minimal MVP on physical examination and echocardiography and symptoms of the MVPS should be approached differently from a middle-aged male with a systolic murmur and a thickened, redundant mitral valve.

### MVP Syndrome

Explanation of the physiologic basis for the symptoms, reassurance of the benignity of the disorder, and lifestyle modifications can be remarkably effective in most of these patients. Prior to establishment of the diagnosis, these patients are often anxious and hypochondriacal. However, it is our opinion that most of these patients are not truly psychoneurotic. Their anxiety is targeted to concern over specific symptoms ("why is my body doing this to me?"), rather than a diffuse anxiety state. MVPS patients are often unusually aware of bodily functions and tolerate symptoms poorly, especially when they do not understand the basis for them. Most patients respond favorably to being given a diagnosis instead of being told their symptoms are in their head. Occasionally, however, explanation and reassurance are not adequate, and laboratory testing to establish the benign nature of the process may be required.

MVPS patients are sensitive to drugs or agents that affect the central nervous system. These include caffeine, alcohol, tobacco, antihistamines, tranquilizers, antidepressants, and many cardiac medications. Removal of the offending agent may result in significant improvement.

Regular daily exercise may improve the sense of well-being and minimize the dysautonomic symptoms. Light exercise usually suffices but must be *faithfully* performed. In more severe cases, referral to a cardiac rehabilitation program may be useful.

A major characteristic of the MVPS is the intermittency of symptoms and aggravation or precipitation of symptoms by emotional or physical stress. The military experience illustrates this for males. In females, symptoms are often most prominent in the premenstrual period. Therapy, therefore, need not always be continuous but can often be used intermittently (e.g., beta-blocking agents).

Chest pain is generally the most worrisome symptom for patients with MVPS. The pain is usually atypical for ischemia and clearly of chest wall origin, perhaps related to the narrow anteroposterior chest diameter associated with excessive adrenergic activity which produces a forceful cardiac impulse. Unfortunately, false-positive electrocardiographic changes frequently occur with exercise testing in females, and this may lead to a diagnosis of ischemic heart disease. Our experience has been that radionuclide exercise testing is more specific, but often a satisfactory level of exercise is not achieved to rule out ischemia. Thus, coronary arteriography is not infrequently required to finally convince the patient (and the doctor) that the pain is not ischemic. Beta-blocking agents and anti-inflammatory agents may be useful in refractory cases of chest pain not relieved by the finding of a normal coronary arteriogram.

There are some patients with MVP who have typical angina pectoris in spite of normal coronary arteries. These patients may truly have ischemia related to abnormal coronary vascular regulation. Nitrates, beta blockers, or calcium-channel blockers will usually improve symptoms in this small subset.

Exercise intolerance and exertional dyspnea are usually due to several factors. Many patients with MVP are asthenic and lack adequate musculature to perform vigorous activity. They often have avoided strenuous activity all their lives. However, diminished plasma volume can produce inadequate venous return and a low cardiac output with upright exercise, and this is an important factor in many patients. Adequate salt intake and avoidance of diuretics as well as regular daily exercise frequently improve exercise capacity.

Fatigue is usually intermittent and may be profound. It responds readily to rest. It often follows excessive physical or intellectual activity and most likely has a metabolic basis which has not yet been defined. Many patients with MVPS appear as if they "do not have a rheostat" and vary from feeling "great" to being so fatigued they cannot function. Fatigue in these patients is often misdiagnosed as depression, and treatment with antidepressants will not improve the symptom (it often makes it worse). Reassurance and lifestyle modification to minimize stress and excessive activity are the most effective approaches to this symptom. Fatigue may also be aggravated or precipitated by beta-blocker therapy, calcium-channel–blocking agent therapy, or Class I antiarrhythmic therapy.

Postural hypotension is common and may produce light-headedness or even syncope. Approximately one-third of symptomatic patients with MVPS have a low resting arterial blood pressure. When they assume the upright position, there is marked sinus tachycardia. Hypovolemia and increased adrenergic responsiveness play a major role in this symptom complex. Adequate salt intake and avoidance of diuretics is critical, but occasionally fludrocortisone acetate (Florinef) (0.1 mg twice daily) must be added. In some instances, postural symptoms are associated with marked sinus bradycardia, rarely requiring pacemaker therapy.

Syncope is a complex symptom that has multiple causes in patients with MVP. It is frequently recurrent. These patients are predisposed to develop vasodepressor syncope, which is the most common cause. Avoidance of precipitating factors is the major goal of therapy. Cardiac arrhythmias also may produce syncope, and when arrhythmic syncope is suspected on the basis of monitoring, an invasive electrophysiologic study (EPS) should be considered. This is particularly true if syncope is recurrent or is associated with bodily injury. The results of the EPS help guide therapy (see later).

Palpitation is probably the most common symptom of MVPS. Almost unique to MVPS, palpitations may occur with sinus rhythm, probably reflecting increased adrenergic responsiveness. This symptom responds to beta-blocker therapy. Arrhythmias are extremely common in MVP and have a complex etiology relating to both anatomic and metabolic factors. For reasons that are unclear, there is an increased incidence of dual atrioventricular (AV) node pathways, anomalous atrioventricular pathways, and sinus or AV node dysfunction in MVP. The floppy mitral valve may also play a direct role in arrhythmogenesis by mechanical stimulation of the atrium or ventricle. Upon this anatomic substrate is superimposed episodic excessive vagal or adrenergic tone, hypokalemia (probably from $beta_2$ adrenergic stimulation), and hypersensitivity to cardiac stimulants.

Ambulatory monitoring reveals that most patients with palpitations have frequent premature atrial or premature ventricular contractions or both. Typically, there is excessive sinus tachycardia during the day and excessive sinus bradycardia at night. PVCs may be induced or aggravated during exercise. Thus, an exercise test should be performed in most patients with MVP who have palpitations and PVCs.

When there is a history of sustained rapid heart

action or syncope, an EPS should be strongly considered. Atrial tachycardia, atrial flutter and fibrillation, and ventricular tachycardia are often induced, and abnormalities in sinus or AV node function can also be elicited. The EPS should include tilt, autonomic interventions, and frequently, the administration of caffeine or alcohol. The tilt study has proved extremely useful in eliciting the tendency to develop a vasodepressor response. Paroxysmal asystole (probably secondary to excessive vagal tone) almost exclusively occurs in patients with MVPS and may be elicited by tilt. These patients may require a pacemaker.

Tachyarrhythmias are often unusually responsive to beta-adrenergic–blocking agents, and these are the preferred initial therapy. In addition, interdiction of stimulants such as caffeine, alcohol, and nicotine is important as well as therapy of hypopotassemia and hypomagnesemia. When SVT is due to atrial flutter or fibrillation, digitalis should be used in conjunction with a beta blocker. Class I agents should be avoided if possible. However, Class I agents or verapamil (Isoptin) may be required for paroxysmal atrial tachycardia. Those with Wolff-Parkinson-White syndrome with antegrade conduction require Class I agents (or surgery). When short runs of ventricular tachycardia are present, Class I agents should be used with caution as there is no convincing evidence that this arrhythmia carries a dire prognosis in MVP.

Sudden death is common enough that MVP is a recognized cause of sudden death by forensic pathologists. It is nonetheless a rare event. The usual mechanism is thought to be ventricular fibrillation. It may occur in the absence of significant mitral regurgitation. As yet, there is no clearly defined high-risk subset of patients for sudden arrhythmic death. However, patients with syncope or presyncope and ventricular ectopy should undergo EPS. If sustained ventricular tachycardia or ventricular fibrillation is inducible (or has been documented as occurring spontaneously), amiodarone should be considered if beta-blocking agents fail. Implantation of an automatic defibrillation device should also be considered.

Neuropsychiatric symptoms were discussed earlier. Anxiety is best treated by treating the symptoms. Panic disorder and agoraphobia are common in MVPS. Panic attacks may respond to beta-blocker therapy used on an as needed basis. Psychiatric consultation may be required in more difficult cases.

## THERAPY OF ANATOMIC COMPLICATIONS OF MVP

Cerebral vascular accidents occur with increased frequency in younger patients with MVP.

Most cerebral ischemic attacks under age 40 are in patients with MVP. These are generally considered to be platelet emboli originating from the abnormal mitral valve. Fortunately, the emboli usually produce minimal residual problems. However, massive strokes sometimes occur and most likely represent embolized red thrombi (which develop at the junction of the left atrium and mitral valve). Although it is not clear whether patients with thickened, redundant valves are more likely to develop cerebral emboli, it is our current approach to recommend low-dose aspirin in patients with thickened mitral valves and, of course, in all patients who have had antecedent cerebrovascular ischemia events.

A high-risk subset for cerebral ischemia are patients with mitral valve prolapse who also have migraine. Recently, increased platelet aggregability during migraine attacks has been documented and is thought to be related to increased adrenergic tone. Migraine occasionally results in permanent central nervous system injury, possibly due to in situ platelet thrombi. In such patients, cigarette smoking and birth control pills should be interdicted. Furthermore, beta-blocker therapy may also help reduce increased platelet aggregability.

If atrial fibrillation develops either intermittently or permanently, warfarin (Coumadin) should be added.

Bacterial endocarditis is an established complication of MVP but occurs mostly in patients with thickened valves. It requires standard therapy with intravenous antibiotics. It is uniquely responsive to medical therapy and often does not produce surgical degrees of mitral regurgitation at the time, although it is clearly a factor in progressive mitral regurgitation.

Standard endocarditis prophylaxis as well as specific therapy of periapical disease is indicated in all patients with thickened valves or documented mitral regurgitation. In those patients in whom only a click is present, the risk of endocarditis is low, but it must be remembered that the mitral regurgitation may progress with age, so careful follow-up is required if prophylaxis is not recommended. The recent simplified recommendations for SBE prophylaxis for dental work make compliance much more likely (penicillin V 2 grams orally 1 hour before and 1 gram orally 6 hours after).

Progressive mitral regurgitation is the most common serious complication of MVP. It usually occurs in later life (mean age 60) and is more common in males. Patients with thickened and redundant valves are the most likely subset to develop this complication, which may occur in up to 10% of such individuals. It is not known if this process can be delayed. It is logical, for instance, that therapy for hypertension should be beneficial, but this is unproved. The higher incidence in males suggests that excessive physical activity may increase the likelihood of degenerative changes in the floppy mitral valve.

Progressive mitral regurgitation usually also requires mitral annulus dilatation and stretching or rupture of the chordae tendineae. It can occur over a period of months to years or suddenly if several chordae rupture simultaneously. Therefore, the patient may present with either the acute or chronic mitral valve regurgitation syndrome. Standard medical therapy of congestive heart failure (digitalis, diuretics, converting enzyme inhibitors) should be given, but mitral valve surgery is the definitive therapy unless severe left ventricular dysfunction is present.

Recent surgical experience with ring annuloplasty combined with valve repair has been extremely favorable compared with mitral valve replacement. Operative mortality is lower, and postoperative left ventricular function is better. Long-term results so far have been remarkably good. Because of this new surgical approach, surgery is being considered earlier, before left ventricular dysfunction develops. Mitral valve replacement may nonetheless be necessary in some patients with more advanced disease.

Atrial fibrillation may develop as a complication of progressive mitral valve regurgitation, but it is hoped that permanent atrial fibrillation related to left atrial dilatation can be avoided with early surgical intervention.

Athletes with MVP may present a difficult problem. Patients with evidence of significant mitral regurgitation, life-threatening ventricular arrhythmias, or poorly controlled rapid supraventricular arrhythmias should probably avoid competitive sports. Mild aortic root dilatation is occasionally present, and the risk of this finding is still unclear. It is not as great as for those patients with Marfan's syndrome, but it is currently our policy to recommend that patients with clear-cut dilatation of the aortic root not participate in competitive athletics. Patients with milder degrees of MVP can usually compete in sports.

Pregnancy is generally very well tolerated in patients with MVP. This is most likely because the increased blood volume and decreased systemic vascular resistance minimize mitral regurgitation. Arrhythmias usually are not exacerbated. However, at the time of delivery, SBE prophylaxis should be administered. Sympathomimetic agents should be used with caution in patients with premature labor in view of potential adrenergic hypersensitivity.

# CONGESTIVE HEART FAILURE

method of
GARY S. FRANCIS, M.D.
*University of Minnesota*
*Minneapolis, Minnesota*

Even the definition of congestive heart failure provokes considerable controversy. It is above all a clinical syndrome that can complicate virtually any form of heart disease, and it has at least two components: cardiac dysfunction and reduced exercise tolerance. The most common causes of congestive heart failure in the United States are as follows:

1. Coronary artery disease with destruction of contractile muscle tissue
2. Systemic hypertension
3. Chronic alcoholism
4. Diabetes mellitus
5. Idiopathic dilated cardiomyopathy
6. Valvular heart disease

Of course, these etiologic factors may coexist with each other, particularly coronary artery disease, hypertension, and diabetes mellitus. In the United States, an estimated 400,000 individuals develop heart failure annually; it is thus the most common inpatient diagnosis of patients older than age 65 years. The therapy is closely related to the etiology. For example, patients with acute aortic insufficiency and infective endocarditis are managed by urgent valve replacement, whereas patients with idiopathic cardiomyopathy are treated with diuretics and vasodilators. This discussion will focus on patients with congestive heart failure caused by a large, dilated heart. Treatment of both acute and chronic heart failure will be considered.

## ACUTE CONGESTIVE HEART FAILURE (PULMONARY EDEMA)

Patients with acute pulmonary edema are usually unable to give a detailed history because of breathlessness. They commonly come to the emergency room in acute respiratory distress, diaphoretic, somewhat cyanotic, and unable to lie down or give more than two or three words of history at a time. The differential diagnosis includes acute exacerbation of chronic obstructive lung disease and acute asthma. Arterial blood gas analyses, a portable chest x-ray film, and an echocardiogram (when the patient is stable) are extremely useful to confirm the diagnosis of heart failure.

Low-flow oxygen via Venturi's mask (40 to 60%) should be initiated and adequate oxygenation ensured by obtaining arterial blood gas measurements. If adequate oxygenation cannot be accomplished with a mask or if severe carbon dioxide retention occurs, the patient may have to be intubated and mechanically ventilated.

Morphine sulfate should be given in dosages of 2 to 5 mg intravenously every 15 minutes to alleviate anxiety and to further reduce venous pressure. Because of possible respiratory depression and hypotension, morphine should be used with great care. The total dose should not exceed 15 mg. If respiratory depression occurs, naloxone, 0.4 mg, should be given intravenously every 2 to 5 minutes as necessary.

Furosemide (Lasix), 40 mg intravenously, should be administered. If the blood urea nitrogen level is raised, large intravenous doses of furosemide (>100 mg) may be necessary. Oral furosemide is poorly absorbed in acute heart failure. Sublingual nitroglycerin (Nitrostat) is also useful in the early stages of pulmonary edema. If the systolic blood pressure is 90 mmHg or higher, nitroprusside (Nipride) should be started at 10 to 15 μg per minute. Fifty milligrams of nitroprusside should be mixed in 250 ml of 5% dextrose in water to a concentration of 200 μg per ml. The dose should be rapidly increased as needed to control breathlessness, not to allow the systolic blood pressure to go below 90 mmHg. Nitroprusside in excess of 300 μg per minute is rarely necessary. The infusion should be maintained for 24 to 48 hours, with close attention paid to blood pressure, arterial blood gas levels, urinary output, electrolyte values, and renal function. Nitroprusside has a balanced effect on arterial resistance and venous capacitance. It reduces the systolic wall tension on the heart and lowers pulmonary capillary wedge pressure. Nitroprusside is particularly valuable because of its immediate onset of action and extremely short half-life. Toxicity is rare.

Acute pulmonary edema occasionally occurs in the setting of rapid atrial fibrillation or atrial flutter. Rather than trying to slow the atrial arrhythmia with intravenous digoxin, electrical cardioversion is preferred. Immediate restoration of normal sinus rhythm, rather than gradual slowing of the ventricular response, is desirable in acute pulmonary edema.

Patients who present with hypotension and acute pulmonary edema have a grave prognosis. Restoration of blood pressure becomes an immediate goal. Dopamine (Intropin), 500 mg in 500 ml of 5% dextrose in water (1000 μg per ml), should be administered at 5 to 20 μg per kg per minute to restore blood pressure to a systolic level of 90 to 100 mmHg. Dopamine in dosages of less than 2 μg per kg per minute may cause additional arterial dilation and lowered blood pressure, so large doses are necessary to promote a "pressor" effect. Dopamine enhances myocardial contractility directly and produces peripheral vasoconstriction related to alpha-adrenergic receptor activation in peripheral arteries. When hypotension and acute pulmonary edema coexist, insertion of a Swan-Ganz pulmonary artery catheter and an arterial catheter is strongly encouraged. Cuff blood pressure measurements are notoriously inaccurate in patients with severe hypotension. When blood pressure is restored (systolic blood pressure >100 mmHg), nitroprusside can be added to dopamine, 15 to 300 μg per minute, to augment cardiac output and further reduce pulmonary capillary wedge pressure. The combination of dopamine and nitroprusside can usually maintain circulatory homeostasis after blood pressure is stable. Dopamine use is limited by tachycardia and arrhythmias.

Dobutamine (Dobutrex), 500 mg in 500 ml of 5% dextrose in water (1000 μg per ml), markedly improves cardiac output but has little or no peripheral vasoconstrictor activity. It usually does not restore blood pressure in patients with severe hypotension. However, dobutamine is appropriate therapy for severe heart failure if blood pressure is adequate (systolic blood pressure >90 mmHg). The usual dosage of dobutamine is 3 to 20 μg per kg per minute; as with dopamine, its use is limited by tachycardia and arrhythmias. Dobutamine is sometimes added to nitroprusside to augment cardiac output.

The therapy for acute pulmonary edema, perhaps more than any condition, must be tailored to the individual patient's needs. Table 1 offers useful therapies, but success is predicated on a firm understanding of the pathophysiology of acute heart failure and of the pharmacology of the various agents.

## CHRONIC HEART FAILURE

As in acute heart failure, a thorough search for etiologic factors should be performed. Almost always, an electrocardiogram, a chest x-ray film, and an echocardiogram are required, in addition to a careful history and physical examination. Cardiac catheterization is frequently necessary. I generally also perform an exercise test to assess the degree of disability.

Nearly all patients should follow a regimen that includes a low-sodium diet (2 grams), a diuretic (furosemide, 20 to 40 mg per day), and a vasodilator (Table 2). There is now firm evidence that vasodilator therapy improves survival, even in patients with Class II and III heart failure. The role of digitalis is less clear, and I reserve it for patients with an obviously dilated heart, an $S_3$ gallop, and resting tachycardia. I prefer to begin therapy with furosemide and a vasodilator regimen, and I add digitalis later if the patient does not improve. Because furosemide tends to

TABLE 1. **Treatment of Acute Pulmonary Edema**

| Generic Name | Trade Name | Route of Administration | Average Dosage | Limiting Factors | Comments |
|---|---|---|---|---|---|
| Furosemide | Lasix | IV | 40–100 mg | | Correct hypokalemia |
| Oxygen | | Venturi's mask | 50–60% | $CO_2$ narcosis | Monitor blood gas levels |
| Morphine sulfate | | IV | 2–5 mg q 10–15 min | Respiratory depression | May reverse respiratory depression with naloxone, 0.4 mg q 2–5 min |
| Nitroprusside | Nipride | IV | 15–300 µg/min | Hypotension | May be combined with dopamine if BP is stable |
| Dopamine | Intropin | IV | 3–20 µg/kg/min | Tachycardia, arrhythmias | Use only for hypotension or combine with nitroprusside if BP is stable |
| Dobutamine | Dobutrex | IV | 3–20 µg/kg/min | Tachycardia, arrhythmias | Not useful for hypotension |
| Nitroglycerin | Nitrostat | SL | 1/150 grain | Hypotension | May repeat q 5–10 min if BP is stable |
| Heparin | | SC | 5000 q 8 hr | Bleeding, thrombocytopenia | |

*Abbreviations:* SL = sublingual; BP = blood pressure.

promote hypokalemia, supplemental potassium (20 to 40 mEq per day) is usually necessary.

One vasodilator regimen that has been shown to improve survival is hydralazine (Apresoline), 300 mg per day in divided doses, with isosorbide dinitrate (Sorbitrate or Isordil), 40 to 60 mg three times per day. Experience indicates that patients with large, dilated hearts respond best to vasodilator therapy. If peripheral edema or pulmonary congestion recurs, metolazone (Zaroxolyn), 2.5 to 10 mg, should be added to furosemide on a temporary basis, usually for 1 or 2 days. Patients should be instructed to weigh themselves daily and to use metolazone or an extra dose of furosemide on those days that they note a gain in weight (2 to 3 pounds) or feel edematous or congested.

Converting enzyme inhibitors may also be used as first-line vasodilator therapy, and they have been shown to prolong survival. Captopril (Capoten) should be started at 6.25 mg every 8 hours and should be titrated to 25 to 50 mg three times

per day. The blood urea nitrogen level may rise, which usually responds to a reduction in diuretic dose. Captopril should be avoided in patients who have recently undergone vigorous diuresis or who are severely hyponatremic (serum sodium level <130 mEq per liter) because precipitous hypotension may ensue. Asymptomatic hypotension that is induced by converting enzyme inhibitors need not be treated, but symptomatic hypotension usually responds to leg raising or careful rehydration. Converting enzyme inhibitors should probably not be used in patients with systolic blood pressures less than 80 mmHg, although this decision must be individualized. Enalapril (Vasotec) can be used instead of captopril if desired; captopril and enalapril appear to be equally effective. The usual starting dosage of enalapril is 2.5 or 5 mg twice daily, and the dosage should be increased to 10 mg twice daily over several weeks as maintenance therapy. Potassium and diuretic therapy can frequently be reduced when using converting enzyme inhibitor therapy. Potassium-

TABLE 2. **Treatment of Chronic Congestive Heart Failure**

| Generic Name | Trade Name | Starting Dosage | Maintenance Dosage | Limiting Factors | Comments |
|---|---|---|---|---|---|
| Furosemide | Lasix | 40 mg/day | 40–100 mg/day | Hypokalemia | |
| Metolazone | Zaroxolyn | 2.5 mg | | Dehydration, hypokalemia | Should be used as intermittent supplement |
| Captopril | Capoten | 6.25 mg tid | 6.25–50 mg tid | Hypotension, cough, rash, hyperkalemia | Renal function and $K^+$ level should be monitored |
| Enalapril | Vasotec | 2.5 mg bid | 2.5–10 mg bid | Hypotension, cough, rash, hyperkalemia | Renal function and $K^+$ level should be monitored |
| Hydralazine | Apresoline | 25–75 mg qid | 300 mg/day | Lupus, hypotension, nausea, vomiting, edema | Dosage is highly variable |
| Isosorbide dinitrate | Isordil, Sorbitrate | 10–20 mg tid | 10–60 mg tid | Headache, hypotension | Headaches usually respond to acetaminophen (Tylenol) |
| Digoxin | Lanoxin | | 0.125–0.375 mg/day | Toxicity | |

sparing agents should be avoided in patients taking angiotensin-converting enzyme inhibitors because of potentially dangerous hyperkalemia, except under unusual circumstances. The most frequent complications of the use of converting enzyme inhibitors are hypotension, nonproductive cough, rash, and renal insufficiency. Renal function and serum electrolyte levels should be monitored 1 week and sometimes sooner after initiating converting enzyme inhibitor therapy for heart failure. If the blood urea nitrogen or serum creatinine levels rise after starting this therapy, a reduced diuretic dose frequently improves these abnormalities without the need for reducing the dose of converting enzyme inhibitor. Clinical improvement sometimes requires 3 to 4 weeks of therapy. These agents have had a positive influence on the treatment of congestive heart failure, are generally well tolerated, and are effective in all degrees of severity of heart failure.

Digitalis (digoxin) is still widely used to treat heart failure. The usual dosage is 0.25 mg daily but will vary according to renal function. Loading doses are rarely necessary for chronic heart failure. Unlike the situation with vasodilator therapy, it is not known if digoxin improves survival in patients with heart failure. Except for patients with rapid atrial fibrillation, long-term clinical benefit from digoxin therapy has remained controversial. Monitoring serum digoxin levels is not routinely necessary unless toxicity or a subtherapeutic response is suspected. I use digoxin in patients with large, dilated hearts and an $S_3$ gallop.

Ventricular arrhythmias are common in patients with heart failure. To date there are no controlled data to indicate that treatment of these arrhythmias prolongs survival. Symptomatic ventricular arrhythmias should be treated, but this has proved to be a difficult task, may require the use of multiple antiarrhythmic drugs, and should be based on electrophysiologic studies. This problem is an important one that will require a large, randomized controlled trial to solve.

# INFECTIVE ENDOCARDITIS

method of
MICHAEL G. HEGEWALD, M.D., and
EDWARD S. MURPHY, M.D.
Oregon Health Sciences University
Portland, Oregon

Infective endocarditis is a microbial infection implanted on the endothelial surface of the heart. Endocarditis develops with endothelial injury and the formation of a platelet fibrin clot that becomes infected when transient bacteremia occurs with an adherent microorganism. Endothelial trauma typically occurs from areas of turbulent blood flow, usually from valvular regurgitation or stenosis and congenital heart lesions. Intravenous drug abusers without any underlying valvular heart disease may traumatize the endothelial surface of their valves with the foreign particles they inject. Transient bacteremia is common with dental and medical procedures.

The overall survival rate with infective endocarditis is about 75%. The most frequent cause of death is congestive heart failure. Mortality is higher in patients with advanced age and other underlying diseases. Endocarditis is uniformly fatal if left untreated, and survival depends in large measure on the promptness of initiation of therapy, the nature of the infecting organism, and the patient population involved. A successful outcome depends on accurate identification and treatment of the infecting organism and management of complications.

The underlying lesions predisposed to endocarditis are changing, with mitral valve prolapse and degenerative or calcific valvular lesions becoming more common than rheumatic heart disease. With the increasing number of elderly people, degenerative, calcific valvular lesions (not always previously clinically recognized) are increasing in frequency and account for up to 25% of endocarditis cases. Up to one-third of patients with endocarditis have no known underlying cardiac disease.

## DIAGNOSIS

*History*

The history can identify factors that predispose to endocarditis as well as the associated symptoms of endocarditis. The classical presentation of fever, chills, weight loss, and peripheral emboli in patients with pre-existing valvular disease is uncommon. In many cases the presentation will be subtle, and one should be suspicious of endocarditis in patients with congestive heart failure and emboli, combined congestive heart failure and renal failure with active urinary sediment, or a prosthetic valve with emboli or progressive congestive heart failure. In patients with prior antibiotic therapy or advanced age, fever may be present in only 70% of cases. In less than 50% of cases the clinician can identify an antecedent bacteremic event that correlates with the infecting organism. See Table 1 for the clinical manifestations of endocarditis.

TABLE 1. **Clinical Manifestations of Endocarditis**

| | Intravenous Drug Abuse (%) | Culture Negative (%) | Native Valve (%) | Infants and Children (%) | Age > 60 (%) | Early Prosthetic Valve (%) | Late Prosthetic Valve (%) | Gram Negative (%) |
|---|---|---|---|---|---|---|---|---|
| Fever | 98 | 90 | 95 | 92 | 70 | 94 | 98 | 100 |
| New or changing murmur | 75 | 100 | 90 | 60 | 67 | 65 | 50 | 83 |
| Sepsis or shock | — | <5 | 40 | — | 27 | 33 | <5 | — |
| CNS manifestations | 8 | — | 20 | 21 | 35 | 30 | 30 | 35 |
| Peripheral emboli | 20 | 33 | 20 | 30 | — | 10 | 20 | 50 |
| Splenomegaly | — | 30 | 40 | 65 | 12 | 25 | 20 | 30 |
| Leukocytosis | — | — | 50 | — | 62 | 50 | 40 | — |

## Physical Examination

The initial examination should focus on finding the portal of entry of infection, extent of cardiac involvement, hemodynamic status, and complications of the disease. It is important to perform serial examinations daily, or more frequently, in critically ill patients, to monitor for changing heart murmur, a pericardial rub, and the onset of congestive heart failure. Clinically the hemodynamic status of the patient should be monitored closely because the progression of heart failure can be frighteningly rapid. Patients with aortic insufficiency and worsening congestive heart failure or hemodynamic deterioration will require urgent cardiac valve replacement. Signs of peripheral embolization should be searched for, including splinter hemorrhages, Osler's nodes, Janeway's lesions on the hands, and Roth's spots in the fundi. An oral exam should be performed looking for petechiae and poor dentition. If patients have poor dentition, dental roentgenograms should be performed and an oral surgeon should be consulted. The skin also should be examined, looking for evidence of abscesses or infected IV sites.

## Laboratory Studies

Initially an ECG should be performed daily and then repeated at weekly intervals to monitor for conduction abnormalities. Atrioventricular (AV) block will occur in approximately 14% of patients with endocarditis and is more common with aortic than with mitral valve involvement. Conduction disturbances are important because they may indicate extension of an infection to perivalvular structures, including AV node and interventricular septum.

When available, echocardiography should be used to determine the site of valvular involvement, examine other valves for vegetation, characterize the underlying cardiac disease, demonstrate extravalvular extension of infection (perivalvular abscess), evaluate left ventricular function, and assess the hemodynamic consequences of the valvular lesion. The ability of echocardiography to detect vegetations in clinically proven endocarditis is approximately 50%. Small vegetations cannot be detected. It is unclear if the size of the vegetation independently predicts the need for future cardiac surgery or future embolic events, but the presence of a vegetation is associated with worsened prognosis. Destructive lesions of the valve, including flail mitral or tricuspid leaflets, torn aortic leaflets, and subannular aneurysms of the aortic root, can also be diagnosed. Doppler studies can identify and quantitate the severity of mitral and aortic insufficiency. The presence of aortic insufficiency detected by Doppler is a serious finding and requires careful monitoring of hemodynamic status; if deterioration occurs, urgent surgery is required.

A urinalysis should be done to look for proteinuria, hematuria, or red blood cell casts. These findings may be secondary to embolic renal infarcts or acute glomerulonephritis from immune complex deposition. Evidence of a urinary tract infection may identify the portal entry of infection.

## GENERAL PRINCIPLES OF MANAGEMENT

General principles in the management of patients with endocarditis include: (1) establishing a microbiologic diagnosis before initiating treatment; (2) instituting parenteral therapy with bactericidal antibiotics; (3) monitoring the effects of therapy with microbiologic studies, including minimum bactericidal concentration (MBC) and bactericidal titer; (4) searching for the portal of entry of infection; (5) determining hemodynamic status and evaluating for complications; (6) teaching appropriate prophylaxis.

The most important principle in managing patients with endocarditis is to establish a microbiologic diagnosis. Most patients with endocarditis have been chronically ill for some time, and unless they appear septic or acutely ill, it is important to identify the infecting organism before starting treatment. If patients have not received antibiotic therapy during the previous 2 weeks, three sets of blood cultures over a 24-hour period should be adequate. These should identify the organism in greater than 95% of patients. If patients have received prior treatment with antibiotics or have prior negative cultures, blood should be cultured with special techniques to inactivate antibiotics (antimicrobial removal devices). If patients are toxic or severely ill and empiric therapy needs to be started immediately, three sets of blood cultures taken at 10-minute intervals should be obtained before starting treatment. The bacteremia of endocarditis is usually continuous, and blood cultures do not need to be taken over prolonged periods of time or to correlate with fever spikes. However, the number of organisms shed is low, and fewer than 100 colonies may be cultured per milliliter of blood. Since a larger sample of blood increases the chance of culturing an organism, at least 30 ml of blood should be obtained with each venipuncture. Blood cultures should be repeated 3 or 4 days after initiation of treatment to determine efficacy of treatment. Persistent positive blood cultures indicate possible myocardial or peripheral abscess formation, resistant organisms, inadequate therapy, or erroneous microbiology laboratory data.

Follow-up blood cultures should be obtained after therapy since fastidious organisms may have relapses 2 months after therapy is completed.

### Microbiology Laboratory

The microbiology laboratory should be alerted if the patient has suspected endocarditis. Most organisms causing endocarditis can usually be cultured after less than 1 week of incubation. However, more fastidious organisms, including *Haemophilus, Eikenella,* cardiobacterium, actinobacillus, nutritional variant streptococci, and fungi, may require up to 4 weeks to grow. For this reason, we recommend incubating cultures for up to 4 weeks.

Once the causative organism has been identified, further microbiologic studies are needed to guide therapy. The minimum inhibitory concentration (MIC) and MBC should be determined. The MIC is the lowest concentration of antibiotics that inhibits the growth of bacteria, and the MBC is the lowest concentration of antibiotics that kills greater than or equal to 99.9% of the organisms in a test tube. Serum antibiotic levels should be drawn to determine the peak concentration of antibiotic, and these levels should exceed the MBC in order for therapy to be effective. In order to define which antibiotic regimen the organism is most susceptible to, the MBC should be determined with different antibiotics and combinations of antibiotics. This is particularly important with resistant organisms as combination therapy may be necessary. Serum concentrations of antibiotics should be periodically measured to see if therapeutic levels are continually maintained or to see if toxic levels occur. Although debated, the serum bactericidal titer should also be obtained to establish the effectiveness of antibiotic administration. A serum sample should be taken at the time of peak serum antibiotic concentration, usually 1 hour after intravenous administration. The serum is then diluted until the highest dilution of serum that kills greater than or equal to 99.9% of the organisms is found. A serum bactericidal titer of at least 1:8 is preferred.

### TREATMENT

The most common organisms causing endocarditis are staphylococci and streptococci, which account for 75% of cases. *Streptococcus viridans* is the most common streptococcal agent. Enterococci and *Streptococcus bovis* also occur and will probably increase in frequency with an older patient population becoming infected. Both gram-negative and fungal endocarditis are also increasing in frequency and are most often seen in addict-associated infective endocarditis or nosocomial-acquired infections usually secondary to infected intravascular devices. *Candida albicans* is usually seen only in patients with indwelling catheters or prosthetic valves.

If patients have an acute form of endocarditis and appear toxic, empiric therapy should be started immediately after blood cultures have been obtained. Empiric antibiotic therapy should include the combination of penicillin G, nafcillin (Nafcil), and gentamicin. This regimen should be effective for treating the most common organisms: staphylococci, streptococci, and enterococci. In patients who are penicillin-allergic, vancomycin (Vancocin) and gentamicin should be substituted. Patients with prosthetic valvular endocarditis should initially be treated with vancomycin and gentamicin to cover *Staphylococcus epidermidis* and corynebacterium, in addition to the other organisms involved in native valve endocarditis. Patients who are intravenous drug abusers may have unusual organisms, but the initial empiric therapy is unchanged. After the infecting organism has been identified, antibiotic therapy should be adjusted according to susceptibility data. See Table 2 for antibiotic treatment dosage and duration of treatment.

All organisms require at least 4 weeks of empiric therapy, except nonenterococcal streptococcal endocarditis which can be treated in 2 weeks. In order to discharge patients earlier, in special circumstances antibiotics may be administered intravenously at home or on an outpatient basis. The optimal duration of treatment is under active clinical investigation.

### MANAGEMENT OF COMPLICATIONS

Complications of infective endocarditis often predominate the clinical picture. Complications can be caused by heart failure secondary to valvular insufficiency, tissue invasion with myocar-

TABLE 2. **Antibiotic Treatment of Infective Endocarditis**

| Infecting Organism | Regimen of Choice* | Duration (wk) | Alternate Regimen | Duration (wks) |
|---|---|---|---|---|
| *Streptococci* | | | | |
| *Penicillin-Sensitive†* | | | | |
| α-Streptococci *(S. viridans)* | 1. Penicillin G | 4 | 1. Vancomycin | 4 |
| Nonenterococcal group D streptococci | 2. Penicillin G or procaine penicillin and streptomycin | 4 2 | 2. Cefazolin or cephalothin§ | 4 |
| β-Streptococci (groups A, B, C, E, F, H, etc.) | 3. Penicillin G or procaine penicillin and streptomycin‡ | 2 2 | | |
| *S. pneumoniae* | | | | |
| *Relatively Penicillin-Resistant†* | | | | |
| α-Streptococci in setting of rheumatic fever prophylaxis (e.g., *S. mitis, S. sanguis*) | 1. Penicillin G | 4 | 1. Vancomycin | 4 |
| | 2. Penicillin G or procaine penicillin and streptomycin | 4 2 | 2. Cefazolin or cephalothin | 4 |
| *S. bovis* | | | | |
| Nutritionally deficient variant, *S. viridans* | | | | |
| *Penicillin-Resistant†* | | | | |
| Enterococci *(S. faecalis)*‖ | 1. Penicillin G or ampicillin and streptomycin or gentamicin | 6 6 | 1. Vancomycin¶ and streptomycin or gentamicin | 6 6 |
| *Staphylococci* | | | | |
| *Penicillin-Sensitive* | | | | |
| *S. aureus* | 1. Pencillin G | 4–6 | 1. Vancomycin | 4–6 |
| *S. epidermidis (albus)* | | | 2. Cephalothin or cefazolin | 4–6 |
| *Penicillin-Resistant* | | | | |
| Methicillin-sensitive** | | | | |
| *S. aureus* | 1. Nafcillin | 4–6 | | |
| *S. epidermidis* | 2. Oxacillin | 4–6 | | |
| Methicillin-resistant | | | | |
| *S. aureus* | 1. Vancomycin | 4–6 | | |
| *S. epidermidis* | 1. Vancomycin and rifampin and gentamicin | 6 | | |
| *Gram-Negative Bacilli* | | | | |
| *Haemophilus parainfluenzae* | 1. Ampicillin and gentamicin or tobramycin ± chloramphenicol | 4–6 4–6 | | |
| Other *Haemophilus* sp. | 1. Penicillin†† and streptomycin | 3–4 3–4 | Penicillin-allergic patients may require desensitization, followed by a course of penicillin or ampicillin | 3–4 |
| | 2. Ampicillin | | | |
| *Pseudomonas aeruginosa* | 1. Piperacillin‡‡ and tobramycin or gentamicin or amikacin | 6 6 | Third-generation cephalosporin (e.g., ceftazidime), based on results of organism sensitivity testing | 6 |
| *Serratia marcescens* | Piperacillin‡‡ or cefoxitin or trimethoprim-sulfamethoxazole and tobramycin or gentamicin | 6 6 | Third-generation cephalosporin, based on results of organism sensitivity testing | 6 |
| Other gram-negative bacilli | Therapy depends on antimicrobial sensitivity testing—combination antimicrobial therapy often required | 4–6 | | |
| *Miscellaneous Causes* | | | | |
| *Neisseria* sp. | Aqueous penicillin G | 4–6 | 1. Penicillin-allergic patients will require desensitization followed by course of penicillin | |
| | | | 2. Cefoxitin | |
| | | 4–6 | 3. Third generation cephalosporin | |
| *Corynebacterium* sp. | 1. Aqueous penicillin G and gentamicin | 4–6 4–6 | Vancomycin | |
| | 2. Vancomycin for gentamicin-tolerant *Corynebacterium* | 4–6 | | |

TABLE 2. **Antibiotic Treatment of Infective Endocarditis** *Continued*

| Infecting Organism | Regimen of Choice* | Duration (wk) | Alternate Regimen | Duration (wks) |
|---|---|---|---|---|
| Diphtheroids | 1. Vancomycin | | | |
| Anaerobes | | | | |
| *Bacteroides fragilis* | 1. High-dose penicillin if penicillin-sensitive | 4–6 | | |
| | 2. Metronidazole | 4–6 | | |
| Other | High-dose penicillin | | | |
| *Candida* sp.§§ | Amphotericin B and 5-fluorocytosine and surgery | for 6 wk after surgery | | |
| *Aspergillus* sp.§§ | Amphotericin B and 5-fluorocytosine or rifampin and surgery | for 6 wk after surgery | | |

*Dosages given assume the patient has normal hepatic or renal function; appropriate dosage adjustments must be made where there is significant functional impairment:

| | | | |
|---|---|---|---|
| Amikacin | 5 mg/kg IV q 8 hr | Metronidazole | 750 mg q 8 hr, PO or IV |
| Amphotericin B | 1.5–3 grams IV total dose (0.75–1.25 mg/kg/day) | Nafcillin | 8–12 grams/day IV |
| | | Oxacillin | 8–12 grams/day IV |
| Ampicillin | 12–18 grams/day IV | Piperacillin | 300 mg/kg/day IV, divided q 4–6 hr |
| Aqueous penicillin G | 10–20 million U/day IV continuously, or in frequent, divided doses | Procaine penicillin | 1–2 million U IM q 6 hr |
| | | Rifampin | 300 mg PO q 8 hr |
| Cefoxitin | 1–2 grams IV q 6 hr | Streptomycin | 10 mg/kg (not to exceed 500 mg) IM q 12 hr |
| Carbenicillin | 30–40 grams/day IV | | |
| Cefazolin | 2 grams IV q 6–8 hr | Tobramycin | 1 mg/kg IM or IV q 8 hr |
| Cephalothin | 2 grams IV q 4–6 hr | Trimethoprim-sulfamethoxazole | 10–20 mg/kg trimethoprim (with appropriate sulfamethoxazole equivalent) |
| Chloramphenicol | 3–6 grams/day IV | | |
| 5-Fluorocytosine | 150 mg/kg/day PO in divided doses | | |
| Gentamicin | 1 mg/kg IM or IV q 8 hr | Vancomycin | 10 mg/kg (not to exceed 500 mg) IV q 6 hr |

†Penicillin-sensitive organisms are those inhibited by penicillin G concentration in broth (MIC) of ≤0.1 μg/ml. Relatively resistant organisms, MIC of >0.1 to 1.0 μg/ml. Resistant organisms, MIC >1.0 μg/ml.

‡The 2-week regimen is not recommended for patients with complicated cases with shock, extracardiac foci of infection, prosthetic valve endocarditis, or infection with nutritionally deficient variants of *S. viridans*.

§For minor penicillin allergy (e.g., rash). There is not enough experience with the 2-week therapy with cephalosporins.

‖Although therapy for 6 weeks is commonly recommended for enterococcal endocarditis, 4 weeks may be used in mitigating circumstances, such as unacceptable drug toxicity, and if the course is otherwise uncomplicated.

¶Cephalosporins should not be used for enterococcal endocarditis.

**Because of the risk of methicillin-associated nephritis, its use is not recommended.

††β-Lactamase production may require use of second- and third-generation cephalosporins.

‡‡Other ureidopenicillins (ticarcillin, mezlocillin, carbenicillin) may be substituted. May require concomitant colistin or polymixin B.

§§Surgery should be considered early.

Modified from Cheitlin, M. D., and Morelli, R. L.: Conn's Current Therapy 1986. Philadelphia, W. B. Saunders Co., 1986.

dial abscess formation and rupture, embolic phenomenon, and resistant or metastatic infection. Management of these complications often requires surgical intervention, and a cardiac surgeon should be consulted. The timing of surgery is a difficult decision. It may be critical to the patient's survival. Operating too early may unnecessarily subject the patient to the risks of the surgery and the chronic risk of having a prosthetic valve in place. Procrastination may increase the risk of complications and worsen chances of survival. It is difficult to anticipate complications, and the decision of when to operate needs to be individualized for each patient and clinical situation. If criteria for surgery are present, there is little to be gained by delaying and prompt surgery is recommended. The absolute and relative indications for surgery are shown in Table 3.

### Congestive Heart Failure

Heart failure caused by valvular insufficiency is the most serious complication of endocarditis and is the leading cause of death among patients with endocarditis. Patients with endocarditis and congestive heart failure have decreased mortality when treated with surgical versus only medical treatment. Patients with congestive heart failure secondary to aortic insufficiency have a worse prognosis than heart failure secondary to mitral regurgitation. If surgery is delayed, patients with

TABLE 3. **Indications for Surgery in Infective Endocarditis**

**Generally Accepted Indications**

Congestive heart failure refractory to mild therapy
Uncontrolled infection despite proper antibiotic therapy
Recurrent large vessel emboli after treatment has begun
Fungal endocarditis
Suppurative pericarditis
Unstable prosthetic valve

**Relative Indications**

Infection with gram-negative organism
*S. aureus* infection of a left-sided valve (particularly aortic)
Relapse after apparent cure
Evidence of intracardiac extension of infection:
   New cardiac conduction abnormality
   Abscess demonstrated by echocardiography or catheterization
   Rupture of sinus of Valsalva or of ventricular septum
Early prosthetic valve endocarditis
New periprosthetic leak
Nonstreptococcal prosthetic valve endocarditis

aortic insufficiency can often be temporarily stabilized by intense therapy with a diuretic, intravenous nitroprusside (Nipride) (for afterload reduction), and digoxin.

Patients with congestive heart failure and aortic insufficiency or acute severe aortic insufficiency require prompt valve replacement. Patients with mild congestive heart failure and mitral regurgitation may be initially managed medically with diuretics and therapy for afterload reduction. If they deteriorate hemodynamically, surgery is required. Patients who initially present with moderate to severe congestive heart failure and mitral regurgitation require valve replacement. Even if patients with congestive heart failure initially respond to medical management, decompensation can occur over the next 3 to 12 months. Patients who are treated medically should be followed closely and monitored for volume overload with repeat chest x-rays and echocardiograms at regular intervals. If there is progression of heart failure, left ventricular dysfunction, or poor control of symptoms, surgery should be performed.

### Resistant Infection

Resistant infection can be defined as continued positive blood cultures despite appropriate antibiotic treatment, and it occurs in 5 to 10% of cases. Persistent fever with negative blood cultures and improving clinical condition does not necessarily mean resistant infection since it may take a week for patients to become afebrile. However, if there is persistent fever after 1 week of appropriate antibiotic therapy, one should assess for emboli, resistant infection, or abscess formation. The portal of entry should be deter-

mined; if the source is found, it should be surgically drained. Other sites of abscess formation, including myocardium, metastatic foci to liver, spleen, or joints, should be searched for and drained. Resistant infection (often found with staphylococcal infection) can also be caused by inadequate bactericidal levels of antibiotic since bactericidal agents are required to adequately treat the infection. This can occur with tolerant strains of organisms. Tolerance occurs when the MBC is at least 32 times greater than the MIC. Fungal endocarditis is uniformly resistant to antimicrobial therapy and requires surgical treatment.

### Intramyocardial Abscess

Deep tissue infections of the heart are serious complications of endocarditis and most commonly occur with perivalvular extension from the aortic or mitral valve. Abscesses may also occur at more distant sites in the myocardium and result from hematologic spread or embolization. Myocardial abscess formation is usually associated with virulent organisms, including staphylococci, pneumococcus, or gonococcus. Prosthetic valves in the aortic position have the highest frequency of abscess formation, which can be demonstrated by two dimensional echocardiography. More recently, transesophageal echocardiography has improved the capability of identifying valve pathology. Abscesses occur in the upper septum near the AV node or bundle branches, and heart block or bundle branch block can occur in up to one-third of cases. Prolongation of the PR interval is often followed by complete heart block, and continuous telemetry monitoring with anticipation of placing a temporary pacemaker is required when the PR interval becomes prolonged. Septal abscesses may rarely create a ventricular septal defect (VSD) with left-to-right shunt, requiring surgical treatment with placement of a patch. Although there have been case reports of patients with intramyocardial abscess being cured with medical therapy alone, surgery is usually required. Resistant infection, congestive heart failure, and development of heart block are indications for surgery in patients with intramyocardial abscess formation.

### Purulent Pericarditis

Purulent pericarditis occurs most often with the extension of an annular abscess directly into the pericardial space or rupture of a sinus of Valsalva aneurysm. The most common infective organism is *Staphylococcus aureus*.

Pericardial effusions are common with endocarditis and may be secondary to immune complex deposition, nonspecific inflammation, pneumonia, or uremia. Pericardiocentesis is required to diagnose purulent pericarditis. If purulent pericarditis is found, surgical drainage is required for cure.

### Recurrent Systemic Emboli

The incidence of systemic embolization in patients with endocarditis is approximately 30%. Systemic emboli most frequently occur with organisms that cause large vegetations, including *Haemophilus parainfluenzae,* other slow-growing gram-negative organisms, fungi, *Staphylococcus aureus,* and nutritionally deficient streptococci.

Right-sided embolization causes symptoms similar to pulmonary embolism and is associated with pulmonary abscesses. Left-sided emboli are distributed randomly throughout the circulation and are most significant when they occur in the brain, kidney, or coronary vessels. Vegetations can also embolize to the vasa vasorum and cause mycotic aneurysms in large arteries. The management of patients with large vegetations is difficult and controversial. We do not generally recommend surgery in patients with large vegetations who have not had prior embolic events. Alarming vegetations or vegetations with difficult-to-treat microorganisms, however, push us toward surgery. If patients have an embolic event and are infected with an organism associated with a higher risk of recurrent emboli, have persistent vegetation on echocardiography, or have poor clinical response, we recommend surgical intervention. Most patients with a second embolic event should have surgery, although it is unknown if patients who have one or more embolic events are at increased risk for future events. Patients should not be given anticoagulants since this does not prevent future embolization. In patients who have prosthetic valves, chronic anticoagulation should be continued but at a carefully monitored, lower therapeutic range. If patients have an acute embolic event to the central nervous system (CNS), anticoagulation should be stopped until patients are stable and without evidence of CNS hemorrhage for at least 48 hours.

### Special Situation: Culture-Negative Endocarditis

Culture-negative endocarditis occurs in approximately 5% of cases. The prognosis is similar to that of culture-positive endocarditis if patients become afebrile in the first week of therapy. In patients who remain febrile after 1 week, the mortality has been reported to be as high as 50%.

The evaluation of patients with culture-negative endocarditis includes reviewing the history for previous antibiotic treatment and exposure to gonococcal or chlamydia infection. Other potential infections include brucellosis, psittacosis, Q fever, or fungi. Serologic tests should be performed for these organisms. As previously mentioned, the microbiology laboratory should be alerted to the possibility of fastidious, slow-growing organisms in order to set up special culture media. Patients with culture-negative endocarditis who remain febrile but are otherwise clinically stable should have antibiotics discontinued, and cultures should be repeated every 2 to 3 days for a week. Empiric therapy should then be started with penicillin, a penicillinase-resistant penicillin, and an aminoglycoside. If the patient becomes afebrile, therapy should be maintained for 6 weeks. If there is no clinical response, an evaluation should be undertaken for possible fever of unknown origin and a different antibiotic regimen started or surgery performed, depending on the clinical situation.

### Prosthetic Valve

Prosthetic valve endocarditis has a frequency of 1% a year. It is separated into early onset infections that occur within 60 days of surgery and late onset infections. Late onset infections are caused by organisms similar to native-valve infection with the most common organism being streptococci, but there is also an increased incidence of *Staphylococcus epidermidis*. With early onset infection, the most common organisms are *Staphylococcus epidermidis* and gram-negative organisms. Since *Staphylococcus epidermidis* is often methicillin-resistant, we recommend treating patients empirically with vancomycin and gentamicin. Further treatment should be guided by culture results. The mortality from early prosthetic valve endocarditis is greater than 70%, and from late prosthetic valve endocarditis is approximately 40%. Mortality may be decreased with early surgical intervention. Early onset prosthetic endocarditis requires surgery. Patients with late onset endocarditis caused by a streptococcal agent who are hemodynamically stable deserve a trial of medical management. Patients with late onset infection caused by a nonstreptococcal agent usually require surgery. A malfunctioning or unstable prosthesis or new congestive heart failure requires surgical intervention.

### Intravenous Drug Abusers

Endocarditis among intravenous drug abusers differs from that among nonintravenous drug

TABLE 4. **American Heart Association—Recommended Antibiotic Regimens for Endocarditis Prophylaxis***

**For Adults Having Dental or Respiratory Tract Procedures**

Standard regimen

| | |
|---|---|
| For dental procedures that cause gingival bleeding, and oral or respiratory tract surgery | Penicillin V 2.0 grams PO, 1 hr before, then 1.0 gram 6 hr later. For patients unable to take oral medications, $2 \times 10^6$ U of aqueous penicillin G IV or IM 30 to 60 min before a procedure and $1 \times 10^6$ U 6 hr later may be substituted. |

Special regimens

| | |
|---|---|
| Parenteral regimen for use when maximal protection is desired, for example, for patients with prosthetic valves | Ampicillin, 1.0 to 2.0 grams IM or IV, plus gentamicin, 1.5 mg/kg body weight IM or IV, 0.5 hr before procedure, followed by 1.0 g of oral penicillin V 6 hr later. Alternatively, the parenteral regimen may be repeated once 8 hr later. |
| Oral regimen for patients allergic to penicillin | Erythromycin, 1.0 gram PO, 1 hr before, then 500 mg 6 hr later. |
| Parenteral regimen for patients allergic to penicillin | Vancomycin, 1.0 gram IV, slowly over 1 hr, starting 1 hr before. No repeat dose is necessary. |

**For Adults Having Gastrointestinal or Genitourinary Tract Procedures**

Standard regimen

| | |
|---|---|
| For genitourinary and gastrointestinal tract procedures listed in Table 6 | Ampicillin, 2.0 grams IM or IV, plus gentamicin, 1.5 mg/kg body weight IM or IV, given 0.5 to 1 hr before the procedure. One follow-up dose may be given 8 hr later. |

Special regimens

| | |
|---|---|
| Oral regimen for minor or repetitive procedures in low-risk patients | Amoxicillin, 3.0 grams PO, 1 hr before procedure and 1.5 grams 6 hr later. |
| Regimen for patients allergic to penicillin | Vancomycin, 1.0 gram IV, given slowly over 1 hr, plus gentamicin, 1.5 mg/kg body weight IM or IV, given 1 hr before procedure. May be repeated once 8 to 12 hr later. |

*Adapted from Shulman ST, et al: Prevention of bacterial endocarditis. Circulation *70*:1123A, 1984. By permission of the American Heart Association, Inc.

abusers. It is more commonly seen in patients without underlying heart disease and more commonly involves the tricuspid valve. It also has a higher recurrence rate. The most common organism is *Staphylococcus aureus,* but polymicrobial, gram-negative, and fungal infections are also occurring with increased frequency. Right-sided endocarditis presents as acute onset with high fever, hemoptysis, shortness of breath, pulmonary infiltrates, and respiratory insufficiency in

severe cases. The decision to place a prosthetic valve must be governed by the clinical situation, as a patient who continues to use intravenous drugs will have a high recurrence rate with a high late mortality. Patients with tricuspid valve disease may avoid valve replacement, as adequate results have been obtained with surgical excision or valve débridement alone. If a prosthetic valve is required, a bioprosthesis is preferred to minimize the requirement for anticoagulation.

TABLE 5. **Cardiac Conditions for Which Endocarditis Prophylaxis Is Recommended***

**Prophylaxis Recommended**

Prosthetic heart valves (mechanical or bioprosthesis)
Surgically constructed systemic-pulmonary shunts
Rheumatic or other acquired valvular dysfunction
Prior history of infective endocarditis
Most congenital cardiac malformations
Idiopathic hypertrophic subaortic stenosis
Mitral valve prolapse with mitral insufficiency

**Prophylaxis Not Recommended**

Isolated secundum atrial septal defect
Secundum atrial septal defect repaired without a patch 6 or more months earlier
Patent ductus arteriosus ligated and divided 6 or more months earlier
Postoperatively after coronary artery bypass graft surgery

*Adapted from Shulman ST, et al: Prevention of bacterial endocarditis. Circulation *70*:1123A, 1984. By permission of the American Heart Association, Inc.

## PROPHYLAXIS

It is estimated that only 10% of cases of endocarditis develop following a procedure in which prophylaxis could have prevented infection. However, antimicrobial prophylaxis is of low risk to the patient and is recommended for certain procedures associated with a high risk of bacteremia. Patients with prosthetic cardiac valves and cardiac structural abnormalities that cause turbulent flow are at risk for developing endocarditis. The conditions for which prophylaxis is recommended and the procedures for which endocarditis prophylaxis is indicated are shown in Tables 4 and 5. We recommend treatment of mitral valve prolapse only if there is a holosystolic murmur

## TABLE 6. Procedures for Which Endocarditis Prophylaxis Is Indicated*

**Oral Cavity and Respiratory Tract**
All dental procedures likely to induce gingival bleeding (not simple adjustment of orthodontic appliances or shedding of deciduous teeth)
Tonsillectomy or adenoidectomy
Surgical procedures or biopsy involving respiratory mucosa
Bronchoscopy, especially with a rigid bronchoscope
Incision and drainage of infected tissue

**Genitourinary and Gastrointestinal Tracts**
Cystoscopy
Urethral catheterization (especially in the presence of infection)
Prostatic surgery
Urinary tract surgery
Vaginal hysterectomy
Gallbladder surgery
Colonic surgery
Esophageal dilatation
Sclerotherapy for esophageal varices
Colonoscopy
Upper gastrointestinal tract endoscopy with biopsy
Proctosigmoidoscopic biopsy

*Adapted from Shulman ST, et al: Prevention of bacterial endocarditis. Circulation 70:1123A, 1984. By permission of the American Heart Association, Inc.

or a redundant or floppy valve on echocardiography.

The new American Heart Association recommendations for prophylaxis are simplified with shorter durations of treatment and less parenteral treatment. They are shown in Table 6.

# HYPERTENSION

method of
DONALD G. VIDT, M.D.
*The Cleveland Clinic Foundation*
*Cleveland, Ohio*

The first effective therapy for arterial hypertension was introduced in the 1950s. At that time, only patients with severe and complicated hypertension were routinely treated because of the toxicity and adverse effects associated with early agents. During the subsequent 4 decades, there have been remarkable advances in the understanding of the varied hemodynamic and neurohumoral mechanisms associated with high blood pressure, as well as in new drug development. Yet, the pathogenesis of the disease remains unclear in 90 to 95% of all hypertensives, who have what is termed essential, or primary, hypertension. A role of heredity in the etiology of essential hypertension has been recognized from population studies demonstrating the tendency for hypertension to aggregate within family groups. Racial influences on the prevalence of high blood pressure have also been recognized, as well as associations with other factors, such as obesity, physical inactivity, socioeconomic status, environment, cigarette smoking, and alcohol consumption.

The definition of hypertension has been modified periodically as ongoing epidemiologic surveys and controlled clinical trials have continued to provide new information relative to the risks associated with an elevated blood pressure and the potential benefits derived from treatment. National survey data suggest that approximately 60 million Americans have hypertension, defined as blood pressure measuring 140/90 mmHg or greater or reported taking of antihypertensive medication. Thus, approximately one in four Americans is at increased risk for morbidity and premature mortality associated with high blood pressure and warrants some level of evaluation, followed by therapy or systematic tracking of blood pressure measurements.

Cardiovascular risks rise progressively with blood pressure; likewise, the higher the pressure, the greater is the potential benefit from antihypertensive therapy. Prospective clinical trials have demonstrated that reduction of blood pressure with antihypertensive therapy protects against major cardiovascular diseases, such as stroke, congestive heart failure, progressive renal failure, dissecting aneurysm, and, in some studies, coronary artery disease. In addition, adequate therapy prevents progression of hypertension to higher levels of pressure with its associated complications. Although much of the available risk/benefit information is based on levels of diastolic blood pressure (DBP), systolic blood pressure (SBP) may be an even more important indicator of cardiovascular risk and ultimate prognosis.

## DIAGNOSIS

Hypertension should never be diagnosed on the basis of a single blood pressure measurement. At each determination of blood pressure, two or more readings should be averaged as the reading for that visit. Initial elevated readings should be confirmed on at least two subsequent visits if the average DBP is 90 mmHg or greater or the SBP is 140 mmHg or greater. Criteria for initial blood pressure measurement for adults are listed in Table 1. Subsequent blood pressure measurements enable confirmation of initial elevations, whereas the degree of elevation dictates the urgency of needed follow-up. Although there are no data yet to support treatment of isolated systolic hypertension (SBP ≥160 mmHg, DBP <90 mmHg), patients with persistent elevations of SBP deserve evaluation, simple nonpharmacologic treatment measures, and possibly drug treatment.

In 1972, the National High Blood Pressure Education Program first offered recommendations for a stepped-care approach to hypertension therapy. Any appearance of rigidity in this approach was due to the limited number of agents available for treatment at the time that stepped care was introduced. Subsequent reports have broadened the "menu" for initial and subsequent therapy as new classes of agents have been developed and approved for use. Essentially all of the early clinical trials utilized this approach and relied

TABLE 1. **Classification of Blood Pressure In Adults Age 18 Years or Older***

| Range (mmHg) | Category† |
|---|---|
| *Diastolic* | |
| <85 | Normal blood pressure |
| 85–89 | High-normal blood pressure |
| 90–104 | Mild hypertension |
| 105–114 | Moderate hypertension |
| ≥115 | Severe hypertension |
| *Systolic, When Diastolic Blood Pressure is < 90* | |
| <140 | Normal blood pressure |
| 140–159 | Borderline isolated systolic hypertension |
| ≥160 | Isolated systolic hypertension |

*Adapted from Chobanian AV: The 1988 report of the Joint National Committee on Detection, Evaluation, and Treatment of High Blood Pressure. Arch Intern Med *148:* 1023, 1988.

†Classification based on the average of two or more readings on two or more occasions.

A classification of borderline isolated systolic hypertension (SBP 140–159 mmHg) or isolated systolic hypertension (SBP ≥160 mmHg) takes precedence over one of high-normal blood pressure (DBP 85–89 mmHg) when both occur in the same person. High-normal blood pressure (DBP 85–89 mmHg) takes precedence over a classification of normal blood pressure (SBP <140 mmHg) when both occur in the same person.

heavily on the thiazide diuretics and beta-adrenergic blockers. Evidence during the past 15 years that reductions in heart disease mortality have not kept pace with declines in stroke mortality have raised questions about electrolyte abnormalities and cardiac ectopy induced by diuretics, along with abnormalities in both carbohydrate and lipid metabolism associated with both diuretics and beta blockers. It has long been recognized that adverse effects associated with antihypertensive therapy represent the leading cause of patient nonadherence and failure to control blood pressure in a high percentage of hypertensive patients. Nonadherence to therapy is particularly noted with agents that impair cognitive function or sleep or that cause fatigue and decreased exercise tolerance. The emphasis in selecting antihypertensives is no longer on efficacy and safety of drugs, but rather has shifted to issues dealing with maintaining the quality of life of the treated hypertensive patient, a primary requirement for optimal long-term patient adherence to treatment.

## Objectives of the Hypertension Evaluation

The large numbers of hypertensive patients currently recognized have necessitated a reordering of clinical priorities during hypertension evaluation. Evaluation should preferably be accomplished before initiation of therapy, unless the hypertension is severe and the function of target organs is threatened. The objectives of pretreatment evaluation can be given priority as follows:

1. *To ascertain the presence of a sustained elevation of blood pressure (systolic and/or diastolic).* As yet, there are no convincing data to show that patients with labile, casual elevations of blood pressure benefit from drug therapy, nor is there evidence to suggest an increased risk of cardiovascular complications when blood pressure elevations are not sustained. Physicians must be aware of variability in office determinations of blood pressure and should recognize that serial blood pressure measurements obtained over a period of days or weeks may be necessary to confirm the presence of sustained hypertension. When questions persist regarding the appropriateness of office blood pressure readings as a reflection of hypertension, ambulatory blood pressure determinations may be extremely helpful in determining the significance of blood pressure elevations in the office, their relation to the patient's overall daily activity, and future risks. With proper patient training and calibration of equipment, reliable patient-determined blood pressure levels or 24-hour ambulatory monitoring can be extremely helpful, because they may provide a better predictor of cardiovascular risk than repeated measurements made in the office setting.

2. *To evaluate the target organs affected by hypertension (brain, heart, eyes, and kidneys) and to discover other complications or coexisting diseases.* Evidence of target organ complications at the time of initial evaluation worsens the prognosis and has an important bearing on the choice of antihypertensive agents. Careful visualization of optic fundi can provide an estimate of the duration and severity of hypertension, and the Framingham study has demonstrated that electrocardiographic evidence of left ventricular hypertrophy (LVH) is associated with higher morbidity and mortality. The coexistence of congestive heart failure or renal insufficiency not only has prognostic importance but also affects the choice of antihypertensive agents.

3. *To identify other cardiovascular risk factors.* The importance of multiple risk factors in cardiovascular morbidity and mortality is well recognized, and the clinical approach to the treatment of hypertension today cannot be limited to control of blood pressure, but must address all other manageable risk factors as well.

4. *To discover curable causes.* Priorities in the evaluation of hypertension have changed significantly in the past 2 decades. Although it is certainly considered desirable to identify those patients with remediable causes for their hypertension, the infrequent occurrence of potentially curable hypertension (<5%) makes an intensive, expensive evaluation impractical. A thorough but cost-effective pretreatment evaluation uncovers clues to justify further evaluation in most patients with potentially curable hypertension.

## Evaluation of the Hypertensive Patient

The *medical history* must include any family history of hypertension or premature cardiovascular disease, as well as diseases associated with hypertension, such as diabetes or renal disease. If the patient is known to be hypertensive, the duration of disease must be established, as well as prior antihypertensive therapy, the response to that therapy, and adverse effects, if any, to treatment. Both prescription and over-the-counter medications may interact with antihypertensive drugs to raise blood pressure or block their effects. The presence or absence of other cardiovascular risk factors, such as smoking, obesity, hyperlipidemia, or carbohydrate intolerance, and any established psychosocial or environmental factors, such as emotional stress, socioeconomic status, or specific cultural food practices, which may have a bearing on blood pressure control and on subsequent adherence to the medication regimen, should be established. In particular, the use of oral contraceptives in young women and excessive alcohol intake in both men and women represent the two most common causes of reversible hypertension. An estimate of the daily sodium intake is helpful to assess the need for subsequent dietary restriction. Symptoms obtained in the course of a careful history may alert the physician to the likelihood of specific target organ involvement or possibly secondary hypertension.

The *physical examination* helps to verify any evident target organ involvement and may provide additional clues to causes of secondary hypertension. Careful funduscopic evaluation provides evidence of arteriolar narrowing, arteriovenous compression, hemorrhages, exudates, or papilledema. Auscultation and palpation of the neck identifies carotid bruits, distended neck veins, or an enlarged thyroid gland. Examination of the heart should establish not only its size and the rate and rhythm, but also the presence of murmurs or gallop sounds. Careful auscultation of the lungs for rhonchi, rales, or wheezes, as well as respiratory excursion, helps to establish the presence of congestive heart failure or, possibly, chronic obstructive pulmonary disease. Examination of the abdomen should include both auscultation and palpation for evidence of bruits, large kidneys, abdominal masses, or dilation of the abdominal aorta. Examination of the extremities should reveal diminished or absent peripheral arterial pulses, vascular bruits, or edema; careful neurologic assessment establishes the presence of fixed neurologic deficits.

*Baseline Laboratory Tests*

Recognition that fewer than 5% of hypertensive patients have an identifiable and potentially curable cause of hypertension has led to the recommendation of a simplified and cost-effective initial laboratory evaluation, preferably performed before initiating therapy. The minimal laboratory examination should include hemoglobin and hematocrit determinations and urinalysis with microscopic examination. The latter is best performed on a midstream urine specimen to avoid contamination by vaginal, prostatic, or urethral secretions. An automated battery of blood chemistry determinations should provide creatinine, serum potassium, uric acid, calcium, and blood glucose (preferably fasting) determinations. A lipid profile should be included to provide levels of both total and high-density lipoprotein (HDL) cholesterol, serum triglycerides, and low-density lipoprotein (LDL) cholesterol (calculated). An electrocardiogram is considered cost effective for initial cardiac evaluation, although an echocardiogram is occasionally indicated, particularly in patients with multiple risk factors and borderline or mild hypertension. A chest x-ray film may be obtained in patients with a long history of cigarette smoking or prior pulmonary disease.

Proper interpretation of carefully obtained historical data, a thorough physical examination, and these simple laboratory studies provide valuable clues to the presence of curable hypertension. An extensive search for curable causes when preliminary examination affords no clues is unproductive, adds unnecessarily to the cost of evaluation, and, on occasion, may be hazardous. However, when diagnosis of a potentially curable form of hypertension is suggested, selected specific studies are recommended for confirmation (Table 2).

## TREATMENT

### Approach to Therapy

After establishing the diagnosis and severity of hypertension, the degree of target organ involvement, and the presence of coexisting disorders, therapeutic priorities can be determined. Each patient must be given access to a system of continuing care that ensures periodic assessment of blood pressure control, detects any treatment-related adverse effects, and provides opportunities to reinforce treatment goals and objectives. The key to successful treatment and prevention of late complications is the physician's ability to ensure long-term adherence to treatment. Specific attention must also be focused on other cardiovascular risk factors, which, if left untreated, can affect the subsequent response to pharmacologic therapy, as well as increase the patient's risk of cardiovascular disease and death. For healthy patients with uncomplicated hypertension, the use of nondrug therapies as initial treatment for the first 3 to 6 months after recognition of hypertension is appropriate and may effectively control blood pressure, particularly in those with diastolic pressures below 95 mmHg. Selected nonpharmacologic interventions can also be of adjunctive value in patients with more severe hypertension who are receiving pharmacologic therapy.

**Restricted Sodium Intake.** A reduction of daily sodium intake to 2 grams of sodium or 5 to 6 grams of salt may be sufficient to normalize blood pressure in some patients with mild hypertension. A high sodium intake (>100 mEq per day) may impair the effectiveness of some antihypertensive agents. Appropriate counseling regarding the sodium content of frequently purchased foods is important, because a high proportion of daily sodium intake comes from processed foods.

**Supplements.** The role of other cations, such as potassium, calcium, and magnesium, in the genesis of hypertension remains unclear. In hypertensive patients rendered hypokalemic by diuretics, potassium supplementation may have a modest beneficial effect on blood pressure. Cal-

## TABLE 2. **Identification of Curable Forms of Hypertension**

**Coarctation of Aorta**

*Suggests diagnosis*—History: little help. Physical examination: absent or reduced pulses in lower extremities; palpable pulsations over intercostal arteries in posterior thorax. Bruits over intercostal arteries. Laboratory screening: Chest x-ray film reveals notching along inferior border of the ribs, absent aortic knob.

*Confirms diagnosis*—Angiography.

*Localizes lesion*—Angiography.

**Cushing's Syndrome**

*Suggests diagnosis*—History: recent change in appearance and weight gain, extreme weakness with muscle wasting, bruising, impotence, amenorrhea. Physical examination: typical body habitus, moon facies, red stria, truncal obesity, ecchymoses, hirsutism, acne, keratosis pilaris. Laboratory screening: glucose intolerance.

*Confirms diagnosis*—Urinary 17-ketosteroids and 17-hydroxycorticosteroids, increased serum and urinary cortisol levels, dexamethasone suppression, and increased cortisol secretion rate.

*Localizes lesion*—Angiography, computed tomography.

**Pheochromocytoma**

*Suggests diagnosis*—History: symptomatic paroxysms of hypertension, including headache, tachycardia, palpitations, tremor, excessive sweating. History of labile blood pressure, substandard weight or recent weight loss, short history (<2 yr) of hypertension, pressor response to antipressor drugs or induction of anesthesia, occasional occurrence as part of multiple endocrine neoplasia syndrome (MEN Type II or Sipple's syndrome)

*Confirms diagnosis*—Plasma catecholamines or 24-hr urinary metanephrine, vanillylmandelic acid, and catecholamines. Clonidine suppression test. Glucagon provocative test.

*Localizes lesion*—Computed tomography or $^{131}$I metaiodobenzylguanidine scintiscan.

**Primary Aldosteronism**

*Suggests diagnosis*—History: inordinate weakness, periodic paralysis, paresthesia, tetany (rare). Polyuria and polydipsia (rare). Physical examination: positive Chvostek's and/or Trousseau's signs (rare). Laboratory screening: hypokalemia.

*Confirms diagnosis*—Increased urinary excretion of aldosterone (not suppressed by high sodium intake). Exaggerated kaliuresis with sodium loading or with diuretic administration. Correction of hypokalemia by sodium deprivation. Suppressed plasma renin activity after sodium deprivation.

*Localizes lesion*—Computed tomography or radioiodocholesterol scanning, aldosterone secretion rates from adrenovenous effluent.

**Renovascular Hypertension**

*Suggests diagnosis*—History: abrupt onset of moderate to severe hypertension at any age, hypertension resistant to a three-drug regimen, onset of hypertension before age 30 or after age 50 years, or accelerated or malignant hypertension. History of symptomatic carotid, coronary, or peripheral arteriosclerosis obliterans occlusive disease. Physical examination: epigastric bruit (particularly systolic-diastolic), advanced hypertensive retinopathy (severe constriction, hemorrhages, or exudates), and evidence of atherosclerotic occlusive disease of lower extremities and/or carotids, abdominal aortic aneurysm. Laboratory screening: unexplained azotemia.

*Confirms diagnosis*—Renal angiography, renal vein renin ratio >1.5, favoring the side with stenosis, digital substraction angiography (intravenous or intra-arterial), computerized renal flow scan, captopril renography.

*Localizes lesion*—Renal angiography or digital subtraction angiography.

---

cium supplementation has also been demonstrated to lower blood pressure in selected hypertensive patients and may be of particular value for those patients whose intake of dairy products is low or has been restricted for control of hyperlipidemia. Diuretic therapy may induce hypomagnesemia, along with hypokalemia, and, if these are documented, supplementation should be considered.

**Weight Reduction.** Weight reduction to within 15% of ideal weight should be recommended for all obese patients. It has become apparent that obesity risks may not be due to the weight alone, but also to the distribution of that increased weight. Upper body obesity correlates with increased risk of hypertension, impaired glucose tolerance, hypertriglyceridemia, and heart disease. Suitable weight control may also reduce dosage requirements of selected antihypertensive drugs.

**Cessation of Smoking.** Although smoking does not induce chronic hypertension, smokers clearly have increased risks of cancer and chronic pul-

monary disease; they double their risk of coronary artery disease and sudden death and increase their risk of stroke from 2- to 10-fold. Avoidance of smoking must be strongly encouraged, regardless of the patient's age.

**Exercise.** In addition to modestly reducing blood pressure, a regular aerobic exercise program can facilitate weight reduction and ensure better cardiovascular conditioning. Additional benefits may be reflected in favorable changes in the lipid profile. Isometric exercise (weightlifting) should be discouraged because it induces exaggerated rises in both SBP and DBP.

**Restriction of Alcohol.** Hypertensive patients who drink should be encouraged to moderate their ethanol intake to 1 ounce daily of ethanol, as higher intakes have been demonstrated to elevate arterial pressure. One ounce of ethanol is contained in 2 ounces of 100-proof whiskey, 8 ounces of wine, or 24 ounces of most beers.

**Caffeine.** There is no evidence to support a long-term pressor effect from the chronic ingestion of caffeine. Moderation of caffeine ingestion would seem appropriate, however, because high dosages may induce tachycardia or even cardiac arrhythmias.

**Relaxation.** Modest, long-term reductions in blood pressure have been demonstrated in selected patients with a variety of relaxation and behavior modification methods. Long-term, carefully controlled, comparative clinical trials are needed before relaxant drugs or behavior modification techniques can be considered effective primary therapy in the treatment of hypertension.

### Pharmacologic Therapy

The first factor to be considered in the selection of specific drug therapy should be evidence of favorable drug effects on cardiovascular morbidity and mortality. All of the currently available classes of antihypertensive agents are efficacious in lowering blood pressure when used in recommended dosages, and most of the older classes of agents have the added advantage of having been utilized in major clinical trials that assessed the beneficial effects of blood pressure treatment on morbid and fatal events. The propensity of some antihypertensive agents to induce both subjective and metabolic or electrolyte adverse effects should be considered, and awareness of the more common adverse effects of the different classes of antihypertensive drugs is critical to enable optimal tailoring or individualization of both initial and subsequent therapy. The majority of patients who discontinue medication and are lost from therapy do so as a result of adverse drug effects. Patients do not tolerate undesirable symptoms, a particular problem with some centrally acting agents, and beta blockers may reduce exercise tolerance. Newer classes of drugs may offer the opportunity to optimize the quality of life of the hypertensive patient by minimizing adverse effects, thus ensuring long-term compliance with the medication regimen. These favorable features have clearly contributed to the rapidly increasing acceptability of newer classes of drugs to both patients and physicians, despite the absence of long-term morbidity or mortality data with these agents. A thorough clinical appreciation of the beneficial and adverse effects of each class of antihypertensive drugs is important in efforts to tailor treatment for individual patients.

The presence of coexisting conditions is an important determinant when choosing therapy. Some antihypertensive drugs may worsen some diseases, while improving other conditions. For example, drugs with beta-adrenergic blocking properties may worsen asthma and arteriosclerosis obliterans of the lower extremities, but may improve symptoms of angina pectoris, certain migraine or vascular headaches, and essential tremor. The ability to select a drug that may offer benefit for an associated illness or condition represents a true bonus in the selection of therapy.

The cost of therapy must be considered and represents a significant barrier to treatment and long-term control of hypertension in many patients. For patients with limited resources, cost may outweigh other factors in the selection process. Agents with a longer duration of action help simplify dosing regimens and can have a positive effect on compliance with long-term treatment. In considering the cost-effectiveness of therapy, it is important to include not only the cost of the medication, but also the cost of any laboratory studies to monitor potential adverse effects, the frequency of office visits, and costs associated with uncontrolled or inadequately controlled hypertension.

Several reports have documented that reduction of DBP below 85 to 90 mmHg in patients with clinical evidence of coronary artery disease is associated with increased heart disease mortality. This may represent an important issue in determining the initial goal of treatment for older hypertensive patients.

Race and age, but not gender, may be factors in the response of patients to therapy with specific classes of agents. Of increasing interest to clinicians is the mechanism by which different classes of agents lower blood pressure, particularly those that reduce peripheral vascular resistance and induce regression of LVH. Current evidence clearly shows that LVH is a strong predictor of subsequent myocardial infarction and coronary mortality.

As the different classes of antihypertensive agents are reviewed, emphasis is placed on class-specific or drug-specific advantages or disadvantages that may be important to tailor therapy to the individual patient. Although different classes of agents are usually identified by their mechanism of action, this discussion does not review the pharmacology of the antihypertensive agents under consideration. Table 3 lists currently available agents with brand names and recommended dosages.

Although several classes of agents have been considered most appropriate as initial therapy for the majority of hypertensive patients, it should be noted that agents in each of the approved classes of drugs can be effective when used as monotherapy in selected patients and offer additive effects when used in combination. In this regard, all of the currently available classes of agents control blood pressure in approximately one-half of those with mild hypertension. Fur-

TABLE 3. **Currently Available Antihypertensive Drugs**[1]

| Agent | Trade Name | Usual Daily Dosage[2] (mg) | Precautions and Special Considerations |
|---|---|---|---|
| *Thiazides and Related Sulfonamide Diuretics* | | | |
| Bendroflumethiazide | Naturetin | 2.5–5 | May be ineffective in renal fail- |
| Benzthiazide | Exna, Aquatag | 12.5–50 | ure; hypokalemia increases |
| Chlorothiazide | Diuril | 125–500 | digitalis toxicity; may cause |
| Chlorthalidone | Hygroton | 12.5–50 | an increase in blood levels of |
| Hydrochlorothiazide | HydroDIURIL, Esidrix | 12.5–50 | lithium |
| Hydroflumethiazide | Saluron | 12.5–50 | |
| Indapamide | Lozol | 2.5–5 | |
| Methyclothiazide | Enduron | 2.5–5 | |
| Metolazone | Zaroxolyn, Diulo | 1.25–10 | |
| Polythiazide | Renese | 2–4 | |
| Quinethazone | Hydromox | 25–100 | |
| Trichlormethiazide | Naqua | 1–4 | |
| *Loop Diuretics*[3] | | | |
| Bumetanide[4] | Bumex | 0.5–5 | Effective in chronic renal fail- |
| Ethacrynic acid[4] | Edecrin | 25–100 | ure |
| Furosemide[4] | Lasix | 20–320 | |
| *Potassium-Sparing Agents* | | | |
| Amiloride | Midamor | 5–10 | Danger of hyperkalemia or |
| Spironolactone | Aldactone | 25–100 | renal failure in patients |
| Triamterene | Dyrenium | 50–150 | treated with an ACE inhibi- |
| | | | tor or a nonsteroidal anti-in- |
| | | | flammatory drug. May in- |
| | | | crease blood levels of lithium |
| *Beta Blockers*[5] | | | |
| Acebutolol | Sectral | 200–1200 | Should not be used in patients |
| Atenolol | Tenormin | 25–150 | with asthma, chronic obstruc- |
| Carteolol | Cartrol | 2.5–10 | tive pulmonary disease, |
| Labetalol[4,6] | Normodyne, Trandate | 200–1800 | congestive heart failure, |
| Metoprolol | Lopressor | 50–200 | heart block (greater than |
| Nadolol | Corgard | 40–320 | first degree), and sick sinus |
| Penbutolol | Levatol | 20–80 | syndrome. Use with caution |
| Pindolol[4] | Visken | 10–60 | in insulin-treated diabetics |
| Propranolol[4] | Inderal | 40–320 | and patients with peripheral |
| Propranolol, long-acting (LA) | Inderal LA | 60–320 | vascular disease. Should not |
| Timolol maleate[4] | Blocadren | 20–80 | be discontinued abruptly in |
| | | | patients with ischemic heart |
| | | | disease |
| *ACE Inhibitors* | | | |
| Captopril[4] | Capoten | 25–300 | Can cause reversible, acute |
| Enalapril | Vasotec | 2.5–40 | renal failure in patients with |
| Lisinopril | Zestril, Prinivil | 5–40 | bilateral renal arterial steno- |
| | | | sis or unilateral stenosis in a |
| | | | solitary kidney. Proteinuria |
| | | | may occur (rare at recom- |
| | | | mended dosages). Hyperkale- |
| | | | mia can develop, particularly |
| | | | in patients with renal insuffi- |
| | | | ciency. Rarely can induce |
| | | | neutropenia; hypotension has |
| | | | been observed with initiation |
| | | | of ACE inhibitors, especially |
| | | | in patients with high plasma |
| | | | renin activity or in those re- |
| | | | ceiving diuretic therapy |
| *Calcium Antagonists* | | | |
| BENZOTHIAZEPINE DERIVATIVE | | | |
| Diltiazem[7] | Cardizem | 60–360 | Relatively contraindicated for |
| Diltiazem SR[4] | Cardizem SR | 90–360 | congestive heart failure, sick |
| | | | sinus syndrome, or greater |
| | | | than first degree heart block. |
| | | | May cause liver dysfunction |
| DIPHENYLALKYLAMINE DERIVA- TIVE | | | |
| Verapamil[7] | Calan, Isoptin | 120–480 | As above |
| Verapamil SR | Calan SR, Isoptin SR | 120–480 | |

TABLE 3. **Currently Available Antihypertensive Drugs[1]** *Continued*

| Agent | Trade Name | Usual Daily Dosage[2] (mg) | Precautions and Special Considerations |
|---|---|---|---|
| DIHYDROPYRIDINES | | | |
| Nifedipine[7] | Procardia, Adalat | 30–180 | As above |
| Nifedipine XL | Procardia XL | 90–120 | |
| Nicardipine[7] | Cardene | 60–120 | |
| Isradipine[4,8] | DynaCirc | 5–20 | |
| Nitrendipine[8] | Baypress | 5–40 | |
| *Adrenergic Inhibitors* | | | |
| CENTRALLY ACTING ALPHA AGONISTS | | | |
| Clonidine[4] | Catapres | 0.1–1.2 | Rebound hypertension may occur with abrupt discontinuance, particularly with prior administration of high doses or with discontinuation of concomitant beta-blocker therapy |
| Clonidine TTS (patch)[9] | Catapres-TTS | 0.1–0.3 | |
| Guanabenz[4] | Wytensin | 4–64 | |
| Guanfacine | Tenex | 1–3 | |
| Methyldopa[4] | Aldomet | 250–2000 | May cause liver damage and Coombs-positive hemolytic anemia. Use cautiously in elderly patients because of orthostatic hypotension. Interferes with measurements of urinary catecholamine levels by fluorimetric methods |
| ALPHA[1]-ADRENERGIC BLOCKERS | | | |
| Prazosin[4] | Minipres | 1–20 | Use cautiously in elderly patients because of orthostatic hypotension |
| Terazosin | Hytrin | 1–20 | |
| PERIPHERALLY ACTING ADRENERGIC ANTAGONISTS | | | |
| Guanadrel sulfate[4] | Hylorel | 10–100 | Use cautiously because of orthostatic hypotension |
| Guanethidine | Ismelin | 10–150 | |
| Rauwolfia alkaloids | | | |
| Whole root | Raudixin | 50–100 | Contraindicated in patients with history of mental depression; use with caution in patients with history of peptic ulcer |
| Reserpine | Serpasil, Sandril | 0.1–0.25 | |
| *Vasodilators* | | | May precipitate angina pectoris in patients with coronary artery disease |
| Hydralazine[4] | Apresoline | 50–300 | Lupus syndrome may occur (rare at recommended doses) |
| Minoxidil[4] | Loniten | 2.5–80 | May cause or aggravate pleural and pericardial effusions |

[1]Adapted from Chobanian AV: The 1988 report of the Joint National Committee on Detection, Evaluation, and Treatment of High Blood Pressure. Arch Intern Med *148:* 1023, 1988.

[2]The dosage range may differ slightly from recommended dosage in *Physicians' Desk Reference* or package insert. Given once daily unless otherwise indicated.

[3]Larger doses of loop diuretics may be required in patients with renal failure.

[4]This drug is usually given in divided doses twice daily.

[5]Atenolol, metoprolol, and acebutolol are cardioselective; pindolol, carteolol, penbutolol, and acebutolol have partial agonist activity (ISA).

[6]Combined alpha and beta blocker.

[7]This drug is usually given in divided doses three or four times daily.

[8]Investigational drug in the United States.

[9]This drug is administered as a skin patch once weekly.

ther, two drugs in combination, as long as they are not from the same class, control blood pressure in greater than 85 to 90% of patients with mild to moderate hypertension. Because most hypertension can be controlled with available therapy, the focus of attention has shifted to the skill of the individual physician to take advantage of the above-noted clinical variables that enable skillful individualization or tailoring of treatment.

## Diuretics

It is convenient to discuss the diuretics in three categories: the thiazides and related sulfonamide diuretics; the loop diuretics; and the potassium-sparing agents (triamterene, spironolactone, and amiloride).

**Thiazide and Related Sulfonamide Diuretics.** The many available congeners of this subclass of natriuretic agents have comparable efficacy when used in recommended dosages. Intermediate to long duration of action of these agents enables once-daily administration. The natriuretic effects of thiazide diuretics are accompanied by increased urinary losses of potassium and magnesium as well. The major concern in the hypokalemic hypertensive patient relates to a possibly increased risk of ventricular arrhythmias and sudden death in the setting of intrinsic heart disease or administration of digitalis glycosides. Hypomagnesemia, associated with weakness, tremors, and anorexia, is a complication of thiazide therapy that is often overlooked unless magnesium levels are checked periodically in the course of long-term therapy. It is prudent to maintain serum potassium concentrations above 3.5 mEq per liter in the course of diuretic therapy. The most effective way to prevent significant hypokalemia is to ensure that the patient adheres to a modest sodium restriction in the diet, which minimizes sodium-for-potassium exchange in the distal renal tubule. Oral potassium supplements, potassium-sparing agents, and concurrent therapy with an angiotensin-converting enzyme (ACE) inhibitor also minimize the risks of hypokalemia.

The observation that therapeutic efficacy with thiazides is obtained with once-daily administration of lower doses than previously used (12.5 to 50 mg of hydrochlorothiazide or chlorthalidone currently used in most patients) has resulted in fewer problems with symptomatic hypokalemia and concurrent hypomagnesemia.

Thiazides increase the tubular reabsorption of uric acid, and increases approximating 1 gram per dl in the serum uric acid concentration are regularly observed. Symptomatic gout seldom occurs unless a family or personal history of acute podagra is present. In the patient with a history of gout in whom thiazides are deemed necessary for control of hypertension or hypervolemia, hyperuricemia can usually be controlled by the concomitant administration of the xanthine oxidase inhibitor allopurinol. In this setting, alternative antihypertensive agents can also be considered for initial therapy.

The major current concern regarding the use of thiazide diuretics centers on their potential adverse effects on carbohydrate and lipid metabolism. The mechanism of thiazide-induced impaired glucose tolerance probably relates to impaired insulin release and/or peripheral insulin resistance and may result in overt diabetes mellitus in some patients. The risk of impaired glucose tolerance appears to be enhanced by diuretic-induced hypokalemia. The use of a diuretic is often mandatory in the hypertensive diabetic with established nephropathy and edema. In this setting, the risk of deterioration in hyperglycemia control is probably small if obesity and caloric intake can be carefully controlled, along with the prevention of hypokalemia. Clinical observations have suggested a potentially important role for the ACE inhibitors in reducing proteinuria and in preventing progressive renal function loss in diabetics (see later discussion of ACE inhibitors).

Thiazide administration is regularly accompanied by elevations of total cholesterol, LDL cholesterol, and triglyceride levels. Although there is no direct evidence to confirm that thiazide-induced lipid changes increase coronary artery disease risk in the hypertensive patient, many clinicians remain concerned that these lipid changes may blunt the expected reductions in coronary artery disease mortality despite improved control of high blood pressure. These concerns have influenced the choice of initial therapy for many patients with mild to moderate hypertension, and it would seem prudent to avoid diuretics as initial therapy in patients with hypertension and hyperlipidemia, particularly those with LDL cholesterol levels greater than 160 mg per dl. When a diuretic is indicated, the lowest effective dosage should be utilized, and careful adherence to a low-cholesterol diet should be stressed.

Other adverse effects associated with thiazides include hypersensitivity reactions, usually manifested as macular papular rashes, and, occasionally, hypercalcemia due to decreased renal clearance of calcium. This observation has prompted the use of thiazides in selected patients as prophylaxis against kidney stone formation. The observation of prolonged, significant hypercalcemia should prompt the physician to consider other causes, such as primary hyperparathyroidism. Rare complications, such as thrombocytopenia, hemolytic anemia, and pancreatitis, have been observed.

INDAPAMIDE. Although considered with the thiazides, indapamide contains only one sulfonamide group and no thiazide ring system. The mechanism of action of indapamide is similar to that of other thiazides. A potential advantage is an apparent absence of observed effects on blood lipids, and impaired glucose tolerance has been infrequently observed. On the other hand, adverse effects, such as hypokalemia and hyperuricemia, are similar to those observed with other thiazides.

**Loop Diuretics.** The superior dose-related response to furosemide, bumetanide, and ethacrynic acid enhances the usefulness of these agents in establishing and maintaining diuresis for patients refractory to thiazide diuretics. Contrary, a short duration of action should discourage the use of loop diuretics as initial therapy in patients with otherwise uncomplicated hypertension and normal renal function. Loop diuretics represent a preferable choice in patients with refractory hypertension, congestive heart failure, or significant impairment in renal function (serum creatinine level >2.5 mg per dl). Ethacrynic acid has never attained the popularity enjoyed by furosemide or bumetanide, but may be a useful alternative for patients with known hypersensitivity to these agents. When indicated, the daily dose should be divided and administered two or three times a day for optimal effects.

Loop diuretics provide the advantage of intravenous administration, which can be extremely useful in patients with refractory edema, and can be given concurrently with other parenteral agents in the management of hypertensive emergencies. Transient deafness has been reported with furosemide and ethacrynic acid and is most common with administration of high parenteral dosages in patients with renal insufficiency. The ototoxic potential of bumetanide is significantly less, providing a potential advantage of this agent in the patient with impaired renal function.

Excessive diuresis may result in volume depletion, and excessive loss of potassium in patients receiving digitalis glycosides may precipitate digitalis toxicity. Patients with known sulfonamide sensitivity may also show allergic reactions to furosemide or bumetanide.

**Potassium-Sparing Agents.** Triamterene, spironolactone, and amiloride reduce potassium loss that results from other natriuretic diuretics and in states of increased circulating aldosterone. They may also potentiate the effectiveness of a thiazide or loop diuretic when used concurrently, but lack sufficient antihypertensive effects when used alone, making them inappropriate agents for initial therapy of patients with mild to moderate essential hypertension.

Hyperkalemia is the most common adverse effect of potassium-sparing agents, and the danger of hyperkalemia is enhanced in patients with renal insufficiency. Concurrent therapy with potassium-sparing agents, oral potassium supplements, and ACE inhibitors should be avoided because of the risk of hyperkalemia. Spironolactone and amiloride have been particularly useful when combined with thiazides in the treatment of primary hyperaldosteronism. Spironolactone resembles progesterone in its chemical configuration and may induce gynecomastia in male hypertensive patients.

## Beta-Adrenergic Blocking Agents

Currently, nine beta-adrenergic blockers have been approved by the FDA for hypertension. When used in recommended dosages, antihypertensive effects are comparable. Beta blockers reduce cardiac output and heart rate by as much as 25%, and their administration is associated with variable increases in peripheral vascular resistance. They may aggravate congestive heart failure in patients with pre-existing cardiac disease.

All beta blockers, including those with cardioselectivity and partial agonist activity, may induce bronchoconstriction in patients with poorly controlled asthma and can aggravate claudication in hypertensives with arteriosclerosis obliterans. Differences in the clinical pharmacology of these agents may affect their use if associated diseases are present and may contribute to specific adverse effects (Table 4). Beta blockers appear to be more effective in younger patients, in whom the hallmark of hypertension is an elevated cardiac output with essentially normal peripheral resistance. Black hypertensives appear to respond less well to beta blockers than caucasians do. Following initiation of beta-blocker therapy, a full week may be required before optimal effects of initial dosing are observed; this is true for dosage increments as well. Cardioselective beta$_1$ blockers may have a marginal advantage in the hypertensive patient with peripheral vascular insufficiency, and those with intrinsic sympathomimetic properties (ISA) may have an advantage in the patient with pre-existing bradycardia. With the exception of some observed effects with propranolol, beta blockers do not appear to have deleterious effects on renal excretory function.

All beta blockers cross the blood-brain barrier to some degree, with increased penetration being noted with more lipophilic agents. Fatigue; sleep disturbances, including nightmares; and depression have been observed with this class of agents. Excessive bradycardia has been reported in patients receiving beta blockers concomitantly with digitalis glycosides.

As with the diuretics, the effects of beta blockers on glucose and lipid metabolism have caused concern among clinicians. Prolonged therapy with beta blockers, particularly with nonselective agents, may impair carbohydrate tolerance, and, in insulin-dependent diabetics prone to hypoglycemia, premonitory symptoms may be masked by

TABLE 4. **Pharmacokinetics and Elimination Characteristics of Beta-Adrenergic Blockers**

| | Relative Beta$_1$ Selectivity | Partial Agonist Activity | Membrane-Stabilizing Activity | Lipid Solubility | Predominant Route of Elimination | Active Metabolites | Drug Accumulation in Renal Disease |
|---|---|---|---|---|---|---|---|
| Acebutolol | + | + | + | Weak | HM/RE (15% unchanged) | Yes | Yes |
| Atenolol | + + | 0 | 0 | Weak | RE | No | Yes |
| Carteolol | 0 | + | 0 | Moderate | HM/RE (60% unchanged) | Yes | Yes |
| Esmolol* | + + | 0 | 0 | — | HM | No | No |
| Labetalol | 0 | + | 0 | Weak | HM | No | No |
| Metoprolol | + + | 0 | 0 | Moderate | HM | No | No |
| Nadolol | 0 | 0 | 0 | Weak | RE | No | Yes |
| Penbutolol | 0 | + | 0 | High | HM | Yes | Yes |
| Pindolol | 0 | + + | + | Moderate | HM/RE (40% unchanged) | No | No |
| Propranolol | 0 | 0 | + + | High | HM | Yes | No |
| Timolol | 0 | 0 | 0 | Weak | HM/RE (20% unchanged) | No | No |

*Esmolol is an ultra-short-acting beta blocker, which is rapidly metabolized by blood, tissue, and hepatic esterases.
*Abbreviations:* HM = hepatic metabolism; RE = renal excretion. + = moderate activity; + + = marked activity.

beta blockade. Nonselective beta blockers increase plasma triglycerides and very-low-density lipoprotein (VLDL) cholesterol and suppress the HDL cholesterol levels. The concerns regarding these lipid changes and possible blunting of expected reductions in mortality from cardiovascular disease have reduced their use as initial therapy in mild hypertension. It appears that the propensity for these adverse lipid changes is lessened in the presence of cardioselectivity or partial agonist activity.

Beta blockers are the only class of antihypertensives that have been demonstrated to reduce the risk of recurrent myocardial infarction or sudden death in patients with ischemic heart disease. They have also proved efficacious in treatment of associated conditions, such as migraine headache, essential tremor, and glaucoma. A recently approved cardioselective beta$_1$ blocker, esmolol, can be used parenterally for the treatment of supraventricular tachycardia, is ultra-short acting, and has demonstrated efficacy for control of perioperative hypertension. Usage should be avoided in patients with asthma, chronic obstructive pulmonary disease, or heart block greater than first degree. The effectiveness of beta blockers as monotherapy in the treatment of mild hypertension can occur, in part, because they do not generally induce fluid retention.

**Combined Alpha and Beta Blocker.** Labetalol is a nonselective beta-adrenergic blocker that also blocks postsynaptic alpha$_1$ receptors. Unlike pure beta-blocking agents, labetalol reduces systemic vascular resistance, while the heart rate is unchanged or slightly suppressed and cardiac output is generally well maintained. Mild intrinsic agonistic activity for beta$_2$-adrenergic receptors probably plays a small role in this agent's blood pressure–lowering effects, but may help explain its improved tolerance in patients with asthma or chronic obstructive pulmonary disease. Clinical studies have demonstrated labetalol to be more effective as monotherapy in black and elderly hypertensives than other beta blockers.

Labetalol has proved reliable by intravenous infusion or intermittent pulse administration in the treatment of perioperative hypertension or hypertensive emergencies, including pheochromocytoma.

The most common adverse effect observed with oral administration of labetalol is postural hypotension, a manifestation of the drug's alpha-blocking properties. As with other beta-adrenergic blockers, labetalol should be avoided or used with caution in patients with uncontrolled asthma, heart block greater than first degree, severe sinus bradycardia, or congestive heart failure. It is notable that labetalol has no apparent adverse effects on carbohydrate or lipid metabolism.

### Angiotensin-Converting Enzyme Inhibitors

The ACE inhibitors exert their primary effect on blood pressure through inhibition of the renin-angiotensin-aldosterone system. By inhibiting the conversion of angiotensin I to the potent vasoactive peptide angiotensin II, vasodilation and blood pressure reduction are accomplished without reflex cardiac stimulation. This latter effect may result from a parasympathomimetic action of these agents. A secondary decrease in aldosterone secretion prevents sodium and water retention and adds to the utility of the ACE inhibitors as monotherapy in managing mild and moderate hypertension. Other possible mechanisms of action include accumulation of vasodilator bradykinins and prostaglandins and interactions within the central nervous system and the peripheral sympathetic nervous system to blunt baroreceptor responses. The identification of tissue-specific renin-angiotensin systems, including vascular endothelium, raises the possibility that future development of this drug class may offer more tissue-specific effects.

Because of significant renal excretion of ACE inhibitors, adjustments in dosage are required in patients with renal impairment. A potential advantage of this class of agents is the absence of adverse effects on lipid metabolism, pulmonary function, or carbohydrate tolerance. Clinical experience suggests greater efficacy as monotherapy in caucasians and younger hypertensive patients than in blacks or older individuals. These age and racial differences disappear when a diuretic is added to the regimen, and favorable additive effects are observed.

Potentially hazardous hypotension may follow the initial dose of an ACE inhibitor if it is administered to a volume-depleted patient. Diuretics should be discontinued for several days before initiating ACE inhibitor therapy. An ACE inhibitor administered unknowingly to a patient with bilateral renal artery stenosis or high-grade stenosis to a solitary kidney may cause acute and progressive renal insufficiency. Caution should be observed in considering an ACE inhibitor for the older hypertensive patient with generalized arteriosclerosis and azotemia, in whom renal artery occlusive disease may be present. Hyperkalemia is routinely observed with ACE inhibitors and may be worsened by concomitant administration of potassium supplements or potassium-sparing agents. A dry, nonproductive cough is clearly the most common adverse effect and may be observed in as many as 10% of patients. Although rarely observed, angioedema is a potentially life-threatening adverse effect. Earlier described adverse effects such as leukopenia, nephrotic-range proteinuria, dysgeusia, and rashes are infrequently observed with currently recommended therapeutic dosages of these agents, including captopril. The perceived favorable quality of life and paucity of intolerable adverse effects seen with the ACE inhibitors have clearly contributed to the rapid growth in physician prescription and patient acceptance of this class of agents.

A parenteral form of enalaparil (enalaprilat) is now available for clinical use. The recommended dosage is 1.25 mg administered at approximately 6-hour intervals. Although its efficacy in the management of hypertensive emergencies is yet to be determined, this agent may be useful postoperatively for the patient who is unable to take an oral ACE inhibitor for several days.

### Calcium Channel Blockers

Although they are a chemically diverse group of compounds, calcium blockers all act by selective inhibition of calcium influx through cell membranes. Yet, the clinical effects of various subgroups of calcium channel blockers are quite different, particularly as they relate to effects on vascular and cardiac contractile tissue and cardiac nodal conduction tissue. These variations appear to be related to differences in relative specificity of selected calcium channel blockers for effector tissues. The dihydropyridine calcium blockers, such as nifedipine (Procardia) and nicardipine (Cardene), are more vasoselective and effects on vascular smooth muscle predominate, whereas agents such as verapamil (Isoptin) and diltiazem (Cardizem) are less vasoselective and demonstrate significant inotropic effects on cardiac contractile or conduction tissue.

The availability of long-acting preparations of verapamil, diltiazem, and nifedipine now enables once- or twice-daily administration in most patients. Most calcium channel blockers have demonstrated a natriuretic effect, at least acutely, and fluid retention and weight gain do not generally occur with long-term administration. The pedal edema associated with nifedipine and nicardipine apparently represents a redistribution of fluid into extravascular tissues and is not associated with weight increase. All of the calcium channel blockers appear to demonstrate comparable efficacy in long-term control of blood pressure when used in recommended daily dosages.

Calcium blockers have no adverse effects on lipid or carbohydrate metabolism, and they are safely administered to patients with asthma or obstructive pulmonary disease. Antihypertensive effects appear to be comparable regardless of race or the age of patients treated. The predominant vasodilator effects of nifedipine and nicardipine may cause headache, reflex tachycardia, and dizziness, particularly with use of the shorter-acting agents. Extensive first-pass hepatic metabolism of these agents negates drug accumulation and dosage adjustments in patients with impaired renal function. Constipation is the most prominent side effect of the calcium blockers and is more commonly observed with verapamil and diltiazem than with the dihydropyridine derivatives. Beneficial effects may also be noted in hypertensive patients with concomitant conditions such as migraine headache or esophageal spasm. As with the ACE inhibitors, the paucity of troublesome adverse effects and the favorable quality of life of patients taking calcium channel blockers have contributed to their high rate of acceptance. Experimental observations suggesting a potential antiatherogenic effect and an ability to mitigate renal ischemia may significantly expand future utilization of this class of agents.

### Centrally Acting Alpha Agonists

The four agents in this class, methyldopa (Aldomet), clonidine (Catapres), guanabenz (Wytensin), and guanfacine (Tenex), effectively stimulate postsynaptic alpha-receptor sites in the brain (vasomotor receptors). Sympathetic outflow from the central nervous system is decreased, resulting in decreased peripheral vascular resistance and decreased blood pressure, whereas cardiac output is generally well maintained.

Dryness of the mouth and drowsiness are the most common adverse effects observed; side effects such as bradycardia, postural hypotension, and sexual dysfunction can also be attributed to their central action. Methyldopa occasionally induces a positive Coombs' test result and, rarely, hemolytic anemia. A pronounced withdrawal reaction has been observed within 12 to 48 hours after sudden discontinuation of clonidine or guanabenz therapy; it is observed most commonly in patients receiving larger dosages of either agent and is associated with irritability, tachycardia, restlessness, marked rebound hypertension, and markedly increased plasma and urinary catecholamine levels. A longer duration of action of guanfacine enables once-daily administration, whereas other agents in this class are administered twice daily.

Clonidine may be administered transdermally by an adherent patch (Catapres-TTS) that delivers the equivalent of 0.1 to 0.3 mg of clonidine daily. Dry mouth and drowsiness occur less frequently with transdermal administration, but localized skin reactions with pruritus have presented a problem with long-term use.

The central alpha agonists have proved useful in treating hypertensive patients with renal insufficiency, asthma or chronic obstructive pulmonary disease, and diabetes mellitus. They have no significant adverse effects on either carbohydrate metabolism or blood lipid concentrations; in fact, clinical trials have suggested that guanabenz may reduce total cholesterol and triglyceride levels. Administration as monotherapy may be associated with increased sodium and water retention and pseudotolerance.

### Alpha-Adrenergic Blocking Agents

Phentolamine (Regitine) and phenoxybenzamine (Dibenzyline) are nonselective antagonists of both alpha$_1$ and alpha$_2$ receptors. Intravenous administration of phentolamine concomitantly with oral administration of phenoxybenzamine is used primarily in the management of patients with pheochromocytoma or high circulating levels of catecholamines associated with clonidine- or guanabenz-induced rebound hypertension. They are both short-acting agents, and significant cardiac stimulation, with tachycardia and cardiac arrhythmias, may be associated with their use.

Two selective postsynaptic alpha$_1$ blockers, prazosin (Minipress) and terazosin (Hytrin), have proved more useful in the treatment of essential hypertension. They reduce arterial blood pressure by decreasing peripheral resistance, generally without a reflex increase in heart rate or cardiac output. They may induce significant postural hypotension and should therefore be used with caution in patients with autonomic impairment, including elderly persons with hypertension in whom baroreceptor responses are often impaired.

The selective alpha$_1$ blockers have no detrimental effects on pulmonary function, nor do they adversely affect carbohydrate or lipid metabolism. In fact, clinical studies have suggested a slight decrease in total cholesterol and a rise in the HDL cholesterol fraction with long-term therapy, making prazosin and terazosin suitable treatment choices for high-risk hypertensive patients with hyperlipidemia. Further, prazosin has proved to be a suitable alternative to the nonselective alpha blockers in the preoperative management of patients with pheochromocytoma.

Recent observations suggest that alpha$_1$ blockers may benefit the middle-aged hypertensive male with prostatic hypertrophy. Inhibitors of alpha$_1$ receptors in the base of the bladder and prostate decrease obstructive voiding symptoms. Conversely, in the female, symptoms of stress incontinence may be aggravated. Terazosin offers more predictable absorption and better bioavailability than prazosin, and terazosin's longer duration of action enables once-daily administration. A sustained-release form of prazosin is currently under development.

### Rauwolfia Alkaloids

The use of rauwolfia alkaloids, including reserpine, has declined progressively over the past 20 years with the emergence of many new classes of effective and better tolerated agents. A significant adverse effect profile that includes both sedation and depressive effects has been observed with dosages exceeding the equivalent of 0.25 mg of reserpine daily. Early concerns regarding prolonged rauwolfia alkaloid administration and malignancy appear unfounded. It is expected that usage of these agents will continue to decline.

## Postganglionic Sympathetic Inhibitors

Two agents, guanethidine (Ismelin) and guanadrel (Hylorel), inhibit the function of postganglionic sympathetic neurons by accumulation and displacement of norepinephrine from neuronal storage granules. The subsequent blood pressure reduction is associated with decreased cardiac output, owing primarily to pooling of blood in capacitance vessels and decreased venous return to the heart.

Although guanadrel has a potential advantage over guanethidine in its shorter duration of action, the potential for adverse effects and drug interactions is similar. These agents are reserved for patients with severe or refractory hypertension (step 4 agents), and, consequently, they are rarely required in the therapy of hypertension today. Additional side effects include postural hypotension, increased gastrointestinal motility and diarrhea, and retrograde ejaculation. Concomitant use of tricyclic antidepressants can antagonize the antihypertensive action of these agents by inhibiting their re-uptake in place of norepinephrine into postganglionic nerve endings.

## Ganglion-Blocking Agents

Only one ganglion blocker, trimethaphan (Arfonad), is currently available in the United States. Usage is generally restricted to treatment of selected hypertensive emergencies by a continuous, monitored intravenous infusion. Trimethaphan induces both arterial and venous dilation, with the latter promoting venous pooling and decreased venous return. Cardiac output is reduced and antihypertensive effects may be accentuated when the patient is in the upright position.

Annoying side effects include visual disturbances such as mydriasis, urinary hesitancy, impotence, and constipation. On occasion, paralytic ileus or acute urinary retention can occur and must be kept in mind when trimethaphan is utilized in the management of a hypertensive emergency such as aortic dissection.

## Vasodilating Agents

**Hydralazine.** Hydralazine (Apresoline) effectively reduces blood pressure by direct relaxation of arteriolar smooth muscle, leading to a reduction of total peripheral resistance. Hydralazine has little effect on venous capacitance, and reduction in arterial pressure is associated with reflex increases in heart rate, stroke volume, and cardiac output. The increased cardiac work may precipitate anginal symptoms in patients with coronary artery disease, and sodium and water retention often lead to pseudotolerance unless prevented by concomitant administration of an effective diuretic. The reflex increases in cardiac activity may be blunted by concomitant administration of a beta-adrenergic blocker. Stimulation of the renin-angiotensin-aldosterone system contributes to sodium and water retention and to the subsequent pseudotolerance.

Metabolism of hydralazine occurs in the liver by ring hydroxylation, subsequent conjugation with glucuronic acid, and acetylation. Slow acetylators are more likely to develop adverse effects from hydralazine such as drug fever and antinuclear antibodies with rheumatoid or lupuslike symptoms. Patients with renal failure acetylate hydralazine poorly, and dosage adjustments may be required because of decreased renal clearance of unchanged drug.

Hydralazine can be administered intramuscularly or intravenously in the treatment of hypertensive emergencies and is still a favorite of many obstetricians for the management of eclampsia of pregnancy.

**Minoxidil.** Minoxidil (Loniten) is a potent vasodilating agent with hemodynamic actions similar to those of hydralazine. Minoxidil plus a beta blocker to control reflex cardiac stimulation and a loop diuretic to control fluid retention provides a potent combination in the management of refractory or accelerated hypertension. The most common adverse effects observed are headache, tachycardia, palpitations, and aggravation of anginal symptoms. An adverse effect associated with prolonged usage, hirsutism, can be of considerable cosmetic concern to some patients. Use of topical minoxidil in the treatment of pattern baldness has not been associated with any adverse effects on blood pressure.

**Diazoxide.** Diazoxide (Hyperstat IV) is a parenteral antihypertensive reserved for the treatment of hypertensive emergencies. This agent reduces arterial pressure rapidly by a direct relaxing effect on vascular smooth muscle. Maximal hypotensive effects are usually reached within 3 to 5 minutes and may persist for 1 to 12 hours or longer following intravenous injection. A gradual, controlled reduction in blood pressure can be obtained by the repeated injection of small pulse doses of 50 to 75 mg or by a continuous intravenous infusion of 15 to 30 mg per minute until the desired blood pressure response is achieved. Concomitant administration of a beta-adrenergic blocker can prevent the reflex tachycardia that is frequently associated with diazoxide administration, and administration of a loop diuretic is recommended to prevent sodium and water retention with repeated dosages. In diabetics, diazoxide can exacerbate hyperglycemia, requiring adjustments in insulin dosage.

**Sodium Nitroprusside.** Sodium nitroprusside (Nipride) differs from other vasodilators in that both resistance and capacitance vessels are affected; thus, decreases in both arterial pressure and central venous pressure accompany its use. Because of its ability to improve left ventricular function without inducing reflex tachycardia, it has been particularly useful in management of hypertensive crises complicated by congestive heart failure or following acute myocardial infarction. Rapid onset and disappearance of effect following discontinuation necessitate carefully controlled parenteral infusion with constant nursing supervision.

The most common adverse effects relate to excessive vasodilation and hypotension, which disappear promptly when the infusion is stopped or slowed. Nitroprusside is metabolized to cyanogen in the presence of sulfhydryl groups in red blood cells and other tissues, and subsequently is converted to thiocyanate, which is excreted by the kidneys. Accumulation of thiocyanate may produce manifestations of toxicity, ranging from weakness, nausea, and tinnitus to overt psychosis, and is increased in patients with renal failure. Free cyanide ions, an intermediate step in the conversion of sodium nitroprusside to thiocyanate, may accumulate in patients with refractory heart failure and poor tissue perfusion and may induce overt cyanide toxicity. Rapid decomposition of nitroprusside on exposure to light necessitates the use of opaque wrappings during administration and periodic replacement with fresh solutions.

**Nitroglycerin.** Now available for intravenous administration, nitroglycerin has been used selectively in the treatment of hypertensive urgencies or emergencies. At low infusion rates, venous dilation predominates, whereas arteriolar dilation also occurs at higher infusion rates. By reducing left ventricular filling pressure and mean arterial pressure, diastolic volume and pressure and myocardial oxygen demand are reduced. Collateral coronary blood vessels are also dilated, and improved perfusion to ischemic areas of myocardium can be expected.

Headache, flushing, and dizziness are the common symptoms observed, although postural hypotension and paradoxic bradycardia may occur. Variable absorption by plastic containers and tubing necessitates the use of glass containers and special administration sets. Nitroglycerin shares several of the advantages of sodium nitroprusside, including its rapid onset and offset of action and the ability to titrate the drug to desired goal blood pressures under supervision. This agent may be particularly efficacious in the patient with coronary ischemia in whom hypertension is not severe and in the management of hypertensives following coronary artery bypass surgery.

## Reasoned Approach to Treatment

The most recent Joint National Committee Report on the Detection, Evaluation, and Treatment of High Blood Pressure (JNC IV) recommended that clinicians consider four classes of antihypertensive agents for initial therapy, based on clinical experience with those agents (Fig. 1). If, after several months of initial therapy, blood pressure has not been controlled, several options for subsequent therapy are offered: (1) increase the dosage of the initial drug, (2) add an agent from another class, and (3) discontinue the initial choice and substitute a drug from another class as monotherapy. In fact, when used in appropriate dosages, an agent from any currently available class of antihypertensives effectively controls blood pressure in selected patients. If a diuretic is not chosen as the initial drug, it is often advisable as a second agent because fluid retention may be responsible for the suboptimal response to some nondiuretic agents.

Before proceeding to each subsequent treatment step, it is important to look for possible reasons for nonresponsiveness to the current therapy, such as poor patient compliance, inappropriate drug dosages, failure to moderate salt intake, or interactions with other pharmacologic agents. Recognizing that hypertension can be controlled in most patients with the expanded menu of currently available therapies, it becomes increasingly important to utilize the practical clinical pharmacology of available agents and selected clinical variables to enable individualizing or tailoring of treatment to each hypertensive patient.

The choice of initial therapy, as well as subsequent choice of drugs, can be determined by practical, clinical considerations already reviewed for each class of available agents. These simple demographic and clinical considerations enable establishment of priorities of choices for initial and subsequent therapy in individual patients.

Racial differences in response to therapy have been noted with a number of agents. Black hypertensives appear to respond better to diuretics, calcium channel blockers, or agents with alpha$_1$-blocking properties, whereas caucasians reportedly show better response to ACE inhibitors and beta-adrenergic blockers. It is important to note that the addition of a diuretic to the regimen usually negates racial differences in response. Gender does not appear to play a significant role in the response to antihypertensive therapy.

The presence of other risk factors affects drug selection. As noted earlier, there is increasing concern that the use of diuretics or beta blockers causes or exacerbates carbohydrate intolerance

Figure 1. Individualized stepped-care therapy for hypertension. (*For some patients, nonpharmacologic therapy should be tried first. If goal blood pressure is not achieved, add pharmacologic therapy. Other patients may require pharmacologic therapy as initial treatment. In these instances, nonpharmacologic treatment may be a helpful adjunct.) (From Chobanian AU: The 1988 report of the Joint National Committee on Detection, Evaluation, and Treatment of High Blood Pressure. Arch Intern Med *148*:1023, 1988.)

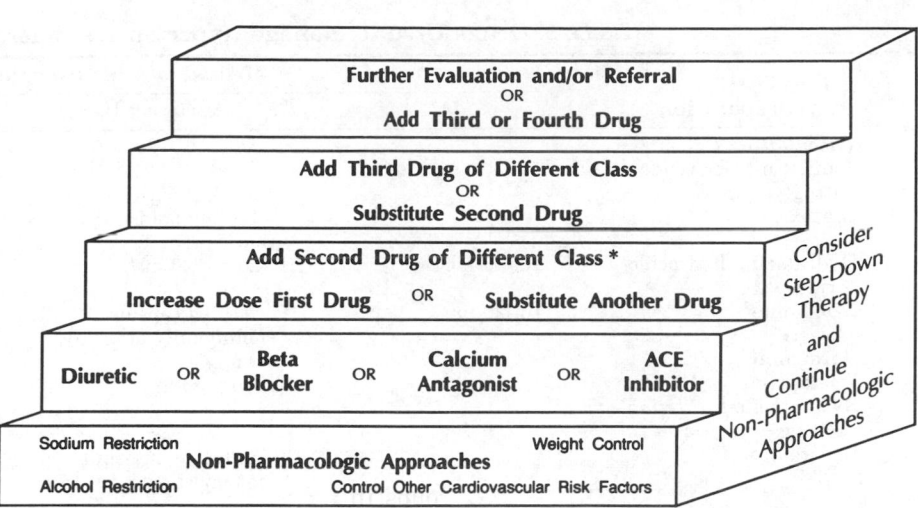

or hyperlipidemia. Many of the newer classes of agents do not adversely affect these variables. On the other hand, beta-adrenergic blockers may have a special indication in the patient who has survived a myocardial infarction. Current experimental data suggest that ACE inhibitors may preserve renal function in the diabetic with early nephropathy. Obese hypertensives usually require an oral diuretic, as excessive sodium intake usually accompanies caloric intake in these individuals.

Associated or concomitant diseases play a significant role in drug selection. Any drug with beta-adrenergic activity should be used with extreme caution in the patient with asthma or obstructive pulmonary disease. Diuretics may precipitate acute podagra in the patient with a history of gout, whereas beta blockers and calcium channel blockers have demonstrated efficacy in patients with hypertension and migraine headaches. Early symptoms of prostatism may be ameliorated in hypertensive males with the use of alpha$_1$ blockers, such as prazosin or terazosin.

Drug treatment for concomitant diseases may induce significant drug interactions with antihypertensive agents. Among the most common are the tendency for over-the-counter sympathomimetic agents to increase blood pressure, whereas nonsteroidal anti-inflammatory agents may blunt the effectiveness of several antihypertensive agents, including diuretics. A classic interaction is that between tricyclic antidepressants and selected adrenergic inhibiting agents, such as guanethidine, guanadrel, and possibly clonidine.

Finally, the quality of life aspects of therapy for the individual patient must be addressed. Those whose daily activity requires a high degree of mental acuity may not function well while taking agents that enter the central nervous system and induce drowsiness or decrease cognitive function. Beta blockers may be undesirable for physically active hypertensives. The inveterate smoker should not be treated with beta-adrenergic blockers because smoking may blunt the effectiveness of this class of drugs.

Simple clinical factors revealed in the course of a careful history and pretreatment evaluation enable establishment of priorities and individualization of initial and subsequent therapy for most patients. If appropriate dosage titration with the initial agent does not provide optimal control or induces adverse effects, a drug from another class may be substituted or may be added to the initial drug. The use of two drugs from different classes usually provides an additive effect, and many potential combinations are available.

The physician should not feel compelled to titrate an initial agent or subsequent drugs to maximal recommended dosages before considering changes in or additions to therapy. If optimal compliance is to be attained, it is important that the patient tolerate the agents and dosages prescribed. Increasingly, clinical experience has shown that small dosages of two synergistic agents may offer better control and fewer adverse effects than larger dosages of single drugs. Fixed combinations of antihypertensive drugs are best considered after optimal control has been attained with appropriate titration of single-drug preparations. If at that point a fixed combination providing the same daily dosages of individual agents is available, it may help simplify the regimen and offer cost savings.

The costs of antihypertensive therapy should never be underestimated. Studies have clearly shown that a significant percentage of the hypertensive population perceives current costs of drugs as a significant barrier to long-term ther-

TABLE 5. **Drugs Used to Manage Hypertensive Emergencies**

| Preparation | Method of Administration | | |
| --- | --- | --- | --- |
| | IM | Intermittent IV | Continuous IV |
| *Vasodilating Drugs*\* | | | |
| Sodium nitroprusside | | | 0.5–10 µg/kg/min |
| Nitroglycerin | | | 5–200 µg/min |
| Diazoxide | | 50–100 mg bolus injection | 15–30 mg/min until the desired effect is achieved |
| Hydralazine hydrochloride | 10–50 mg† | 10–20 mg/20 ml‡ | 100–200 mg/L |
| Nifedipine | 10–20 mg | (Perforated capsule sublingually or orally) | |
| Verapamil | | 5–10 mg | 3–25 mg/hr |
| Enalaprilat | | 1.25 mg q 6 hr | |
| *Sympathetic Inhibiting Drugs*\* | | | |
| Labetalol | | 20–80 mg by intermittent injection q 10–15 min | 0.5–2.0 mg/min |
| Trimethaphan camsylate | | | 0.8–6 mg/min |
| Phentolamine | 5–10 mg† | 5–10 mg bolus injection | 0.1–100 µg/kg/min |
| Reserpine | 1–5 mg†·§ | 1–5 mg from syringe over 3–5 min | |
| Methyldopa | | 250–500 mg in 100 ml over 30–60 min§ | |
| Esmolol | | 500 µg/kg bolus injection over 1 min | 25–200 µg/kg/min‖ |

\*In most cases, a rapidly acting diuretic should be given intravenously at the beginning and at appropriate intervals throughout the treatment.

†Start with smallest dose listed.

‡Inject from syringe at rate of 1 mg/min until the desired effect is obtained.

‖Titration every 5 min with reboluses each time.

§Exceeds dosage recommended by the manufacturer.

apy. For some patients, the use of relatively inexpensive antihypertensive drugs, such as oral diuretics or beta-adrenergic blockers, must be weighed against the potential benefits of newer, more expensive classes of agents.

For the occasional patient whose blood pressure cannot be controlled with optimal dosages of a two- or three-drug regimen, a search for possible causes of refractory hypertension must be considered. Again, it is appropriate to look first at issues such as compliance, appropriateness of the agents and dosages used, dietary indiscretion, and potential drug interactions. If none of these factors can be identified, appropriate additional testing may be warranted in the search for a previously unrecognized secondary cause of hypertension.

The ultimate goal of treatment is to normalize blood pressure while maintaining optimal patient compliance and quality of life. A thorough clinical appreciation of the beneficial and adverse effects of each class of antihypertensive agent can be extremely useful in efforts to tailor the selection of antihypertensive drugs to the individual patient. JNC IV also emphasized the importance of step-down therapy for patients with mild hypertension whose blood pressure has been adequately controlled for periods of 1 year or longer.

## Hypertension in the Elderly

Supportive evidence from clinical trials for treatment of hypertension in elderly patients is limited, but the information available would suggest that therapy is appropriate. It is suggested that diastolic blood pressures be controlled to less than 90 mmHg in the elderly, as with younger hypertensive individuals. Reduction of systolic blood pressure to the range of 140 to 160 mmHg appears appropriate. Treatment decisions must be based on careful assessment, as with younger patients, to address problems with concomitant diseases and medications and the quality of life. It is notable that adverse effects of diuretics on carbohydrate metabolism and blood lipids in the elderly appear to be minimal and transient, possibly owing to metabolic differences with age or to the lower dosages of diuretics currently in use. Beta blockers and ACE inhibitors can be useful in the presence of angina pectoris or congestive heart failure, respectively, particularly when combined with a small dose of a diuretic. Care must be taken to evaluate mentation and cognitive function before and during treatment in view of the central adverse effects associated with many agents. Although compliance of older patients appears comparable with that observed in

**TABLE 6. Oral Agents for Initial Management of Hypertensive Urgencies**

| Drug | Recommended Dosage | Frequency |
|------|--------------------|-----------| 
| Captopril | 25–50 mg | Repeat after 1–2 hr |
| Clonidine | 0.1–0.2 mg | Every hr as required |
| Minoxidil | 2.5–5 mg | Repeat after 2–3 hr |
| Nifedipine | 10 mg | Repeat after 30 min |
| Labetalol | 200–400 mg | Repeat after 2–3 hr |

younger hypertensives, care should still be taken to simplify the regimen, ensure regular and frequent review of medication and dosing schedules, and provide periodic assessment to search for adverse effects or potential drug interactions. Drugs that induce or exaggerate postural hypotension should be avoided in the elderly whenever possible. Finally, therapy should be initiated with half the usual recommended adult starting dosages, and drug titration should be accomplished more slowly to optimize acceptance and minimize adverse effects.

### Hypertensive Emergencies and Urgencies

Although less common in today's practice, hypertensive emergencies and urgencies still arise as a result of unrecognized or inadequately controlled chronic hypertension of primary or secondary etiology. A true hypertensive emergency is a life-threatening condition in which blood pressure should be lowered to a safer level within minutes to 1 hour. Hypertensive urgencies are those situations in which the immediate risk to the integrity of the cardiovascular system is less, but blood pressure should be reduced over several hours to 24 hours with prompt institution of appropriate oral drug therapy.

There is no single hypertensive emergency, nor is there a single generic or specific approach to initial therapy. Many conditions associated with hypertension, if inadequately controlled, can lead to excessive elevations in blood pressure that constitute a hypertensive emergency. A number of pharmacologic agents, usually administered parenterally, can be selected for treatment of emergent hypertension. These agents fall into two general categories: direct vasodilating drugs and agents that inhibit various sites in the sympathetic nervous system (Table 5). Nifedipine, although not administered intravenously, has been included in this table because its ready availability, rapid onset of action (within 15 to 30 minutes), and demonstrated efficacy in a variety of hypertensive emergencies has been established.

Several agents have been successfully used by repeated administration or loading doses for con-trolled reduction of blood pressure in hypertensive urgencies (Table 6). The acute reduction of blood pressure, whether by parenteral or oral dosing of selected agents, is usually associated with at least transient sodium and water retention, which may lead to pseudotolerance with subsequent dosing. Concomitant administration of a loop diuretic is usually desirable to maintain urinary flow and ensure continued responsiveness to the antihypertensive agent.

In managing the hypertensive emergency or urgency, prompt initiation of therapy should take precedence over time-consuming diagnostic studies. When blood pressure has been reduced to a safer level, usually a diastolic pressure in the range of 100 to 110 mmHg, additional diagnostic studies can be undertaken if considered necessary. As with the treatment of mild to moderate hypertension, thorough knowledge of the practical clinical pharmacology of available agents facilitates initial management and long-term control.

# ACUTE MYOCARDIAL INFARCTION

method of
PATRICK T. O'GARA, M.D., and
G. WILLIAM DEC, M.D.
*Massachusetts General Hospital*
*Boston, Massachusetts*

and

GREGORY D. CURFMAN, M.D.
*New England Journal of Medicine*
*Boston, Massachusetts*

Acute myocardial infarction continues to be one of the most common and vexing clinical problems that general physicians must confront. According to the American Heart Association, this year nearly 1.5 million Americans will have a myocardial infarction, and more than 500,000 of them will die. More than 300,000 of these deaths will occur before the patients are able to reach a hospital. By comparison, the next two most common causes of death in the United States in 1987 were cancer (477,000 deaths) and accidents (95,000 deaths).

Despite the magnitude of the problem, a steady downward trend in the age-adjusted death rate from heart attack has been observed during the past four decades. The mortality rate from this disease was 226 deaths per 100,000 population in 1950. Since that time, it has declined to 129 per 100,000 population in 1986, a decrease of nearly 43%. Although part of this decline can be attributed to technical advances in medical care, changes in lifestyle resulting in modification of coronary risk factors also appear to have made an important contribution. Most physicians would agree that prevention of myocardial infarction is a more reasonable goal than attempts to intervene at a time of crisis. Nevertheless, until our society becomes much more serious about preventing coronary disease, physicians must be prepared to deal with acute coronary events as they occur.

Our understanding of the pathogenesis of acute myocardial infarction has been increased considerably by the recognition that nearly all infarctions are precipitated by the formation of a thrombus in an epicardial coronary artery. This concept is not new, Herrick having elaborated on it as early as 1912, but serial visualization of the coronary arteries by arteriography has now documented the presence of a thrombus in a large majority of infarct-related coronary arteries. In many instances, the thrombus may arise from hemorrhage into or rupture of an unstable atherosclerotic plaque. The activation of platelets at the site of the unstable plaque undoubtedly plays an important part in the formation of a thrombus. Although focal spasm in a coronary vessel may also contribute to the obstruction of blood flow, spasm as the sole mechanism of obstruction is unusual. The ability to modify the process of coronary thrombosis with fibrinolytic and antiplatelet agents has markedly changed our therapeutic approach to acute myocardial infarction. Recent studies have also helped to clarify the role of coronary angioplasty in the management of patients with acute infarction.

In this article, we focus principally on the treatment of acute myocardial infarction, and we emphasize developments that have occurred during the past 5 years. Because the treatment of myocardial infarction is evolving rapidly, some of the information presented here may be outdated by the time of publication. Such is the price of progress.

## PREHOSPITAL MANAGEMENT

In part because of denial or misinterpretation of symptoms, delays of several hours or more are common before patients with acute myocardial infarction arrive at a hospital. Because more than 50% of patients who die of myocardial infarction succumb before they reach a hospital, the potential benefit of emergency transport systems could be substantial. Therefore, a growing number of U.S. cities have developed medical transportation systems for the rapid management of out-of-hospital cardiac emergencies, including myocardial infarction and its complications. Mobile coronary care units (CCUs) are now usually equipped for the intravenous administration of lidocaine and other cardiovascular drugs, continuous cardiac monitoring, and electrical cardioversion. Radio communication with the nearest hospital can alert the staff to the patient's arrival.

One of the most important recent additions to the mobile CCU is the automatic external defibrillator. By means of adhesive electrodes attached to the patient's chest, this device analyzes the cardiac rhythm and detects the presence of ventricular fibrillation. When this arrhythmia is identified, the defibrillator automatically delivers up to three 200-joule shocks. The survival rate, as measured by the percentage of patients with out-of-hospital ventricular fibrillation who are eventually discharged from the hospital, is approximately 30% with this device. This figure contrasts with a 19% survival rate when standard defibrillators are used. In the light of these encouraging results, the automatic external defibrillator is being used more widely in ambulances and other emergency transport vehicles.

## GENERAL TREATMENT MEASURES

### The Coronary Care Unit

All patients in whom the diagnosis of acute myocardial infarction is suspected with reasonable certainty should be admitted to a CCU. Studies performed in the late 1960s that raised questions about the efficacy of the CCU in improving the survival of patients with acute infarction are not applicable to the CCU of today. The state-of-the-art CCU should be equipped for continuous monitoring of the electrocardiogram (ECG) and for invasive hemodynamic evaluation. Equipment should be available for the delivery of supplemental oxygen, for transvenous and external thoracic emergency cardiac pacing, and for electrical cardioversion. The staff should be experienced in the intravenous administration of thrombolytic agents. Facilities should also be available for echocardiographic and radionuclide imaging studies for patients in whom these procedures are indicated.

In uncomplicated cases of acute myocardial infarction, the stay in the CCU need be no longer than 48 to 72 hours in most instances. Patients can then be transferred to an intermediate care area. Patients in whom the diagnosis of acute infarction is being entertained, but is of low probability, can be admitted directly to an intermediate care area for evaluation and monitoring.

### Relief of Pain, Fever, and Anxiety

Analgesia and sedation are important early goals of treatment because they can diminish tachycardia and thereby reduce myocardial oxygen demand. The mainstay of pain relief is morphine sulfate in a dose of 2 to 8 mg intravenously, which may be repeated at 10- to 15-minute intervals as required. Occasional patients may need larger doses for complete relief. The side effects of morphine include hypotension, respiratory depression, nausea, and vomiting. Respiratory depression can be attenuated with naloxone in a dose of 0.1 to 0.2 mg intravenously, although higher doses occasionally may be needed. Patients who cannot tolerate morphine can be treated with meperidine, 25 to 50 mg intravenously, which can be repeated at intervals of 10 to 15 minutes.

A low-grade fever may occur as a consequence of necrosis of myocardial tissue or associated pericarditis. Acetaminophen (Tylenol) or aspirin, 650 mg orally every 4 to 6 hours, is the agent of choice. In some patients, pericarditis, which is most likely to occur on days 2 to 5 after a transmural infarction, may respond better to indomethacin, 25 to 50 mg every 8 hours. Whether this agent interferes with scar formation after infarction is unknown. It is important to distinguish the pain of pericarditis, which may be exacerbated by respiration or changes in body position, from that of recurrent myocardial ischemia. Both problems can be associated with re-elevation of the ST segments on the ECG.

Relief of anxiety is best accomplished by the administration of diazepam (Valium), 2 to 10 mg orally every 6 to 8 hours, or a comparable agent. The importance of this comfort measure, which can help to reduce sympathetic stimulation of the heart and peripheral vessels, should not be underestimated.

### Diet and Activity

During the first 24 hours, the diet should consist of caffeine-free liquids and bland, soft solids. Thereafter, a 4-gram-sodium, cholesterol-lowering diet (less than 30% of total calories from fat and less than 10% from saturated fat) is recommended. Total calories should range from 1200 to 1800, depending on body weight and individual energy needs. A stool softener, such as docusate sodium, 100 mg orally, should be administered daily to prevent constipation. Before discharge from the hospital, the patient should receive dietary counseling from a registered dietitian. The principal dietary goals are to reduce the blood cholesterol level to less than 200 mg per dl and to achieve ideal body weight. Sodium restriction to 4 grams daily may be necessary if hypertension or heart failure is present.

During the first 48 hours, rigid enforcement of bedrest is neither necessary nor desirable in patients with no complications. Stable patients should be permitted to use a bedside commode within the first 24 hours, and they should be allowed to dangle their legs and sit in a chair after 24 hours. If the patient is free from complications after 48 to 72 hours, supervised walking may begin. The heart rate should be monitored by telemetry, and it should not be permitted to exceed the heart rate at rest by more than 20%.

The occurrence of ventricular arrhythmias or ST segment deviations during ambulation can also be detected with the use of telemetry.

### Oxygenation and Electrolytes

In patients who are suspected clinically of being hypoxemic because of pulmonary congestion or coexisting pulmonary disease, arterial blood gas levels should be measured while the patient is breathing room air. Although administration of oxygen has become standard practice in many CCUs, patients who are not hypoxemic do not require supplemental oxygen. Mild hypoxemia usually responds to oxygen delivered at a rate of 2 to 4 liters per minute by nasal prongs or mask. More severe hypoxemia may require more intensive evaluation and higher concentrations of inspired oxygen. In no case should hypoxemia in a patient with acute infarction be left untreated. Patients with anemia (hematocrit of 30 ml per dl or less) may be candidates for transfusion to improve the oxygen-carrying capacity.

Serum electrolyte levels should be measured on admission to the CCU, and hypokalemia should be corrected to a level above 4.0 mEq per liter. Patients who have been taking diuretics may be deficient in magnesium, and the serum concentration of this cation should be measured in such patients if ventricular arrhythmias are present.

### Anticoagulation

The purpose of systemic anticoagulation in patients with acute infarction is to prevent the formation of thrombi in the ventricular chambers (mural thrombi) and in the veins of the lower extremities (deep venous thrombosis). Standard anticoagulants, such as heparin, do not appear to be effective alone for the dissolution of coronary artery thrombi. Two-dimensional echocardiography has disclosed left ventricular mural thrombi in approximately 30% of patients with anteroapical myocardial infarction, but patients with inferior infarction appear to have a much lower incidence. Recent studies have shown that both deep venous and intraventricular thrombi can be prevented by the administration of heparin, 12,500 units subcutaneously every 12 hours beginning at the time of hospital admission. Although lower doses of heparin may prevent deep venous thrombosis, they may not be effective in preventing intraventricular mural thrombi. Early ambulation of the patient is also helpful in preventing deep venous thrombosis. In patients who have been treated with a thrombolytic agent, the combination of aspirin and intravenous heparin should be used routinely (see later), and therefore subcutaneous heparin should be omitted.

The efficacy of long-term oral anticoagulation in preventing systemic embolization after myocardial infarction is an unsettled question. On the basis of current information, the following approaches seem reasonable. If two-dimensional echocardiography performed before hospital discharge reveals the presence of a mural thrombus in a patient with an anterior infarction, the patient should be treated with warfarin (Coumadin) to maintain the prothrombin at one and one-half to two times the control value for 6 months. Some physicians prefer to treat all patients with anterior infarction with warfarin for 6 months, as long as there are no contraindications to systemic anticoagulation. Warfarin is not recommended routinely in patients with inferoposterior infarcts because they appear to be at much lower risk of mural thrombosis. Whether antiplatelet agents are effective in preventing late systemic embolization is currently unknown. Patients with persistent atrial fibrillation after myocardial infarction should be maintained on warfarin or aspirin.

## Length of Hospital Stay

The recommended length of hospitalization for patients with uncomplicated myocardial infarction has been shortened progressively during the past three decades. Patients with no complications are now frequently discharged after 7 to 10 days. A recent study has suggested that patients treated effectively with thrombolytic therapy may be safely discharged on the third hospital day. This recommendation is unrealistic for most patients, however, and our view is that most patients without complications should remain in the hospital for 1 week. Occasional patients who are clinically stable and have successfully completed a submaximal exercise test with no evidence of ischemia or arrhythmias may be discharged on day five, as long as careful outpatient follow-up is planned. Patients with important clinical complications, such as heart failure, persistent arrhythmias, or recurrent ischemia, must remain in the hospital until these problems have been successfully managed.

## EARLY TREATMENT OF ACUTE MYOCARDIAL INFARCTION

The treatment of acute myocardial infarction has changed rapidly over the past decade. Several approaches to coronary artery reperfusion have been proposed and evaluated in a vast array of studies involving thousands of patients. Although certain management issues have been resolved, many problems remain that will require further elucidation through properly designed prospective trials. The currently available reperfusion strategies include thrombolysis, percutaneous transluminal coronary artery angioplasty, and coronary artery bypass surgery, either alone or in combination. The ultimate goals of reperfusion therapy are limitation of infarct size, preservation of left ventricular function, and improvement in short- and long-term mortality.

## Thrombolytic Therapy

Thrombolysis has become the cornerstone of therapy for patients with acute myocardial infarction of relatively brief duration associated with epicardial injury. The evidence regarding the efficacy of lytic therapy with regard to reperfusion, preservation of regional and global left ventricular function, and survival is substantial. Accordingly, the administration of a thrombolytic agent should be considered immediately for those patients who present within *3 to 4* hours of the onset of pain compatible with myocardial ischemia and who display at least 0.1 mV of ST segment elevation in two or more anatomically grouped limb leads or 0.2 mV of ST segment elevation in adjacent precordial leads. As of this writing, neither patients with acute myocardial infarction associated with ST segment depressions or T wave inversions nor patients with unstable angina pectoris are considered candidates for such therapy. Thrombolytic treatment should be offered to patients with either anterior or inferior infarction.

The time frame within which thrombolytic therapy should be given merits further comment. Intuitively it would seem that the more quickly infarct vessel patency can be restored, the greater the physiologic and survival benefit. Indeed, several of the large-scale studies of acute myocardial infarction have verified this tenet. The largest such trial (International Study of Infarct Survival, ISIS-II), however, demonstrated survival benefit for those patients treated as long as 24 hours after the onset of symptoms. This finding has lent further support to the "open vessel" hypothesis—namely, that patency of the infarct-related artery, regardless of the time required to achieve such, is the critical element with respect to survival. Patency may lead to improved myocardial healing and remodelling, resulting in smaller end-systolic and end-diastolic volumes (decreased wall stress) and a diminished tendency towards ventricular arrhythmias. At least three additional multicenter trials are currently under way to assess critically the treatment of patients who present late (more than 6 hours) with myocardial infarction. Until further information is forthcoming, most investigators would be hesitant to extend the window of treatment beyond 6 hours. Some controversy still surrounds the management of patients who present within the 4- to 6-hour time frame. Yet, most would agree that lytic therapy should be given in the face of persistent pain and/or ST segment elevations. There is as yet too little information on the safety of the prehospital administration of thrombolytic agents by ambulance personnel to recommend such use routinely.

Contraindications to thrombolytic therapy include active bleeding, recent major surgery, a history of gastrointestinal or genitourinary bleeding, a previous cerebrovascular accident (intracerebral hemorrhage, thrombotic stroke, or transient ischemic attack), prolonged (longer than 5 minutes) cardiopulmonary resuscitation with external cardiac massage, uncontrolled hypertension (systolic pressure greater than 180, diastolic pressure greater than 110), and a hemorrhagic diathesis. The stool must be examined for occult blood immediately upon presentation. Relative contraindications are age greater than 75 years, diabetic retinopathy with neovascularization, and altered mental status.

Several thrombolytic agents have been studied intensively in numerous multicenter trials. They include streptokinase (Streptase), recombinant tissue plasminogen activator (rt-PA) (Activase), anisoylated plasminogen streptokinase activator complex (APSAC) (Eminase), single-chain urokinase plasminogen activator (SCU-PA, pro-urokinase),* and urokinase (Abbokinase) (Table 1). Investigations are currently proceeding with mutant forms of rt-PA, various synergistic combinations of drugs, and complexes of plasminogen activators coupled with monoclonal antifibrin antibodies. The agents used most frequently in the United States are streptokinase and rt-PA. APSAC has been recently approved by the FDA.

Streptokinase is a nonenzymatic protein derived from beta-hemolytic streptococci that complexes with plasminogen to form an active conjugate which in turn liberates plasmin from plasminogen. Relatively large initial doses are required to overcome the neutralizing effects of any circulating antibodies produced as a consequence of previous streptococcal infections. Streptokinase is not fibrin-specific, as a result of which it causes a decrease in the concentration of systemic fibrin and fibrinogen, with corresponding increases in fibrin(ogen) breakdown products, and the production of a systemic lytic state.

Streptokinase can be delivered subselectively to the site of thrombus in the coronary artery. The recommended dose for intracoronary use is a 20,000-unit bolus followed by 2000 to 4000 units per minute over 1 hour, up to a maximum of 250,000 units.* Its efficacy can then be assessed by coronary arteriography during or after the infusion. Patency of the infarct-related artery can be expected in approximately 60 to 80% of cases. Such therapy, however, is not widely applicable because of the need for a catheterization facility, highly trained operators, and skilled support staff. Intravenously administered streptokinase has been shown in several clinical trials to improve both left ventricular function and survival following acute myocardial infarction. Reperfusion has been achieved in 31 to 80% of patients studied, averaging 42%. The drug is administered as a continuous infusion of 1.5 million units over 1 hour. The resulting systemic lytic effect persists for as long as 24 hours after the infusion, and great care must be taken to minimize the risk of hemorrhage during this period of time. Particular attention should be paid to the avoidance of vascular punctures in noncompressible sites.

Tissue plasminogen activator, in contrast to streptokinase, is an endogenous, fibrin-specific protein of endothelial origin that activates plasminogen bound to a fibrin thrombus, theoretically resulting in the release of plasmin at the level of the clot. Tissue plasminogen activator does cause far less derangement of the hemostatic system than streptokinase. Because of its very short half-life (5.7 minutes), whatever systemic effects tissue plasminogen activator may have should resolve within 30 minutes of its discontinuation. Nevertheless, the risk of significant bleeding with rt-PA remains substantial and, in practice, is indistinguishable from that associated with streptokinase. Such risk is compounded by the routine use of adjunctive anticoagulant or antiplatelet therapy (vide infra) and by the frequent placement of intra-arterial and intravenous sheaths for catheterization. Bleeding is most common at the site of vascular access, although intracranial and visceral hemorrhage do occur rarely. As is the case for all other thrombolytic agents, the treating physicians must remain vigilant for any hemorrhagic complications that might occur in association with rt-PA.

The approved intravenous dose of rt-PA is 100 mg given over 3 hours. Usually, 60 mg are delivered over the first hour (6-mg bolus, 54-mg infu-

---

*Investigational drug in the United States.

*Exceeds dosage recommended by the manufacturer. (Max. labeling is 140,000 units.)

TABLE 1. **Thrombolytic Agents***

| Agent | Fibrin Selectivity | Systemic Lytic Effect | Dosage | Half-Life (min) | Adverse Effects/Comments |
|---|---|---|---|---|---|
| Streptokinase (SK) | 0 | + + + + | IC: 2000–4000 U/min for 60 min up to 250,000 U (a bolus of 20,000 U may be given) | | Bleeding, allergic reactions, hypotension, fever<br>Inexpensive ($200/1.5 million U) |
| | | | IV: 1.5 million U over 1 hr | 23 | |
| Recombinant tissue plasminogen activator (rt-PA), single chain | + + + + | + | IV: 6-mg bolus, 54 mg over 1st hour, 20 mg over 2nd hour, 20 mg over 3rd hour | 5 | Bleeding<br>Expensive ($2200/100 mg) |
| Anisoyl plasminogen streptokinase activator complex (APSAC) | + | + + + + | IV: 30 U over 2–5 min | 90 | Side effect profile similar to SK<br>No maintenance infusion necessary<br>? Lower incidence of reocclusion ($1500/30 U) |
| Single chain urokinase plasminogen activator (scu-PA, pro-urokinase) | + + + + | + | Optimal dose, either alone or in combination with rt-PA, not known | 7 | May be best used in synergistic combination with rt-PA<br>Expensive |
| Urokinase (UK) | 0 | + + + | IC: 4000–6000 U/min for 2 hr, average total dose 500,000 U | | |
| | | | IV: 1.5-million U bolus, then 1.5 million U over 90 min or ? 2.0 million U over 5–15 min† | 16 | Optimal IV dose has not been established<br>Not antigenic<br>Expensive ($2200/3 million U) |

0 = none; + + + + = highest.

*Adapted from Marder VJ, and Sherry S: Thrombolytic therapy: Current Status. Reprinted, by permission of the New England Journal of Medicine, *318:*1512, 1988.

†Exceeds dosage recommended by the manufacturer.

sion), 20 mg over the second hour, and 20 mg over the third hour. Reperfusion has been documented in 62 to 83% of patients, averaging 69%. Several studies have indicated that treatment with rt-PA can limit the size of the infarct, preserve left ventricular function, and improve mortality. When compared directly with streptokinase, rt-PA has proved to be more efficacious as regards earlier reperfusion of an occluded vessel, whether given early (within 3 hours) or late (3 to 6 hours) after the onset of ischemic pain. However, when assessed days to weeks following infarction, patency rates with rt-PA and streptokinase may be more nearly equal.

Anisoylated plasminogen streptokinase activator complex (APSAC) is chemically synthesized from a complex of streptokinase and lysine-plasminogen by placing an anisoyl group at the active site of the plasminogen molecule. This anisoyl group temporarily blocks plasminogen's fibrinolytic activity. The complex, when given in small doses, displays modest specificity for fibrin. Activation occurs by a process of gradual deacylation (over 90 to 105 minutes); the longer half-life of the complex allows for the administration of a single intravenous bolus. This agent may be associated with a slightly lower rate of reocclusion. Clinical trials, conducted largely in Europe, have

reported reperfusion rates in the 51 to 67% range. A reduction in mortality of approximately 50% has been observed in the two trials designed to assess this end-point. APSAC is given as a 30-unit bolus over 2 to 5 minutes, a dose at which systemic fibrinolysis occurs with production of a thrombolytic state for a minimum of 12 hours. A maintenance infusion is not required.

Single-chain urokinase plasminogen activator (scu-PA, pro-urokinase) is a direct plasminogen activator and is itself converted to urokinase by plasmin. Urokinase is a serine protease that also activates plasminogen directly. Single-chain urokinase plasminogen activator displays high specificity for fibrin and may eventually find its greatest use in its synergistic enhancement of the thrombolytic efficacy of rt-PA. Urokinase, when given intravenously as a bolus of 1.5 million units followed by a continuous infusion of 1.5 million units over 90 minutes*, may produce effects similar to those of 70 mg rt-PA. However, it produces a systemic lytic state like that observed with streptokinase. Urokinase has also been given by the intracoronary route in doses ranging from 4000 to 6000 units per minute for up to 2 hours, with an average dose of 500,000 units. Single-

---

* Exceeds dosage recommended by the manufacturer.

chain urokinase plasminogen activator has not yet been approved for clinical use; urokinase has thus far not enjoyed widespread use in the treatment of acute myocardial infarction.

Having decided to administer intravenous thrombolytic therapy, the physician is then left with a choice as to which agent would be preferable. There is no absolute right answer. It is fair to say that rt-PA has gained initial favor in the United States primarily because of the higher earlier reperfusion rates associated with its use. Yet, it is now clear from several studies that improved survival may derive from more than simply rapid clot dissolution per se.

Relative concerns over the choice of a thrombolytic agent include the desirability of avoiding a systemic lytic state, potential nonfibrinolytic side effects, and cost. The avoidance of a systemic lytic state would, in theory, seem a desirable goal. In clinical practice, however, the risk of serious bleeding complications has been relatively uniform across all classes of thrombolytic agents and independent of any measurable increase in the concentration of fibrin(ogen) degradation products. Streptokinase is associated with a variety of side effects, such as allergic reactions (cross-reactivity due to previous streptococcal infections), fever, nausea, vomiting, and hypotension. These problems occur, in the aggregate, with a frequency of 10 to 20%. The routine use of prophylactic antihistamines or corticosteroids is not recommended. Streptokinase is also not likely to be effective if given a second time between 10 days and 6 months of its initial administration because of the production of antistreptokinase antibodies. Similar concerns would apply to APSAC. Urokinase is not antigenic. Streptokinase is substantially less expensive than APSAC and rt-PA. Third-party reimbursement schedules may eventually dictate the choice of a thrombolytic agent. The results of two very large, ongoing trials comparing survival differences between streptokinase and rt-PA will likely spark further debate.

We cannot recommend categorically one particular agent for all patients with acute myocardial infarction. Rather, we would advise the physician to exercise individual judgment based on the exigencies of each particular case.

### Adjunctive Measures

Aspirin has achieved a central role in the treatment of acute myocardial infarction, with or without concomitant thrombolytic therapy, and should be administered to all patients (160 to 325 mg per day) unless contraindicated by active bleeding or known allergy. The use of heparin is more controversial; its role should be clarified further when the results of several active European trials are known. Although heparin may not facilitate fibrinolysis, it may help prevent acute reocclusion owing to rethrombosis. Most authorities now recommend the institution of heparin therapy at the end of the thrombolytic infusion. Heparin is begun, without the customary bolus, at a rate of 700 to 1000 units per hour and continued as a constant infusion aimed to prolong the activated partial thromboplastin time to twice control values.

Other measures to alter the balance of myocardial oxygen supply and demand are always essential. Sublingual nitroglycerin (0.4 mg) should be given immediately, as dictated by the systemic blood pressure, to ascertain whether the myocardial injury might respond to the nitrate-related changes in epicardial coronary tone, possible collateral flow, and ventricular preload. Nitroglycerin can also be administered safely as a continuous intravenous infusion (25 up to 1000 μg per min) with careful monitoring of the blood pressure. Intravenous administration of beta-blocking agents is also beneficial; they may improve survival and decrease the incidence of recurrent ischemia and reinfarction. In the United States, only the cardioselective agent, metoprolol, has been approved for such use. Metoprolol (Lopressor) is given in three equal doses of 5 mg separated by 2 to 5 minutes. Contraindications to its use include second- or third-degree atrioventricular block, first-degree atrioventricular block (PR interval longer than 0.24 second), bradycardia of less than 50 beats per minute, congestive heart failure, hypotension (systolic blood pressure less than 95 mmHg), and asthma. If the patient tolerates the full 15 mg loading dose, metoprolol should be continued orally beginning 6 to 8 hours later, first as 50 mg twice daily and advancing to 100 mg twice daily as tolerated. Other oral beta-blocking agents can be substituted if necessary. The goals of such therapy are a resting heart rate near 60 beats per minute and a systolic blood pressure in the range of 110 to 120 mmHg. Although the calcium channel antagonists have not been demonstrated to limit infarct size, they can be extremely helpful measures in controlling blood pressure or alleviating coronary vasospasm. Patients who demonstrate persistent injury, hemodynamic instability, or both may benefit from intra-aortic balloon counterpulsation.

### Post-thrombolytic Care

Under even the best circumstances, only 75% of patients will achieve reperfusion with thrombolytic therapy. Clinical noninvasive markers of reperfusion are imprecise. These indicators include resolution of chest pain, return of ST segment elevations to baseline, and the appearance of particular ventricular arrhythmias (frequent, late cycle premature ventricular beats, or accelerated idioventricular rhythms). Such ventricular arrhythmias do not presage ventricular fibrillation. Reperfusion is typically accompanied by a higher and earlier rise (8 to 12 hours) of myocardial-specific creatine kinase than is observed in patients who do not receive thrombolytic therapy. Unfortunately, 10 to 20% of patients who achieve successful reperfusion will experience early reocclusion.

Given the fact that a high-grade coronary artery stenosis remains at the site of a previous thrombotic occlusion in the vast majority of patients, and the fact that the risk of reocclusion may be most closely related to the severity of the stenosis, it seems logical to perform selective percutaneous transluminal coronary artery angioplasty (PTCA) after thrombolytic reperfusion. However, on the basis of several recently completed clinical trials, the routine, empiric use of PTCA, either early or late, following a course of thrombolytic therapy for myocardial infarction is no longer recommended. PTCA, or revascularization surgery where appropriate, should be undertaken only when recurrent ischemia, be it spontaneous or exercise-induced, intervenes during the hospital course. "Rescue" PTCA, which is performed immediately after a failed course of thrombolytic therapy, can be considered when signs of continuing myocardial injury and hemodynamic instability persist and when highly skilled operators are available. The associated risks of bleeding, ventricular arrhythmias, repeat reocclusion, vessel dissection, and death are higher under such circumstances.

### Direct or Primary PTCA

This term refers specifically to the use of PTCA, without thrombolytic therapy, as a direct, first-line intervention in the management of patients with acute myocardial infarction. PTCA under these circumstances can be performed in patients for whom thrombolysis is contraindicated and in patients who display ST segment depressions (as well as elevations) on the electrocardiogram. The procedure has compared favorably with thrombolytic therapy when performed by very highly skilled operators. Obviously, the risk of bleeding may be lower as compared with thrombolysis.

Reported success rates for establishing patency of the infarct-related artery have averaged nearly 90%, with acute reocclusion rates of 3 to 14% and in-hospital mortality rates of approximately 6 to 9%. Cross-sectional luminal diameters may be larger, coronary blood flow higher, and ventricu-

lar function better when the results of direct PTCA are compared with those of pharmacologic therapy. New mechanical devices under investigation, such as endovascular stents, atherectomy catheters, laser probes, and percutaneous cardiopulmonary bypass will expand the role of PTCA. Direct and even "rescue" PTCA may have its greatest benefit in the treatment of patients whose infarction is complicated by cardiogenic shock. In this setting, successful PTCA has been associated with an in-hospital survival of approximately 75%. Nevertheless, only a very few centers can accomplish direct PTCA within the time frame (2 to 3 hours from symptom onset) necessary for optimal results. The requirements of a dedicated, continuously available catheterization laboratory, highly skilled operators, and on-call technical personnel make such an approach inappropriate for widespread application.

### Coronary Artery Bypass Surgery

Coronary artery bypass graft (CABG) surgery in the treatment of acute myocardial infarction suffers from the same constraints as PTCA. The time required to mobilize the necessary resources for CABG surgery for patients who develop acute myocardial infarction outside the hospital is even greater than that for PTCA. Nevertheless, because of improvements in surgical and anesthetic techniques and in myocardial preservation at the time of surgery, the operative mortality for properly selected patients (less than 6 hours from onset of pain) may be as low as 2% at selected centers. CABG surgery can be undertaken urgently for those patients who develop acute coronary occlusion during the course of coronary angiography or PTCA. The safety and efficacy of surgery under these conditions can be enhanced by placement of an autoperfusion catheter across the obstruction (when feasible), insertion of an intra-aortic balloon pump for hemodynamic support, or if available, the institution of percutaneous cardiopulmonary bypass in the catheterization laboratory. The risk of perioperative myocardial infarction is higher when CABG surgery is undertaken for failed or complicated PTCA, but the risk is still acceptable. CABG surgery can also be performed after successful thrombolysis for patients who have recurrent ischemia but whose coronary anatomy is not suitable for PTCA. The optimal timing for surgery after thrombolysis is unknown; most surgeons would prefer to wait several days if possible to allow for some recovery in ventricular function and for a decrease in myocardial edema.

## POSTINFARCTION ISCHEMIC SYNDROMES

The development of signs and symptoms of recurrent ischemia after acute myocardial infarction is an ominous event. Given the associated increase in both morbidity (heart failure and arrhythmias) and mortality, an aggressive treatment approach is warranted. Ischemia can occur in many different forms; it may be accompanied by angina, or it may be silent. It may arise from the zone of the infarct or from noncontiguous myocardial segments. Reinfarction or infarct extension can ensue with the attendant risk of progressive ventricular dysfunction, heart failure, and death.

The pathogenesis of postinfarction ischemia is similar to that of the original infarct. Acute coronary artery reocclusion, usually by a platelet-rich thrombus or, less frequently, by an intimal flap created at the time of PTCA, complicates the course of 10 to 20% of patients following initially successful reperfusion with thrombolysis and/or PTCA. Reocclusion most commonly results from regrowth of a residual mural thrombus, largely because of intense platelet activation. Alternatively, the underlying atherosclerotic plaque could destabilize or rupture or epicardial coronary artery vasospasm could supervene, causing a further increase in vascular resistance. Precipitants of ischemia not related to the plaque must always be sought and corrected. These include inappropriate tachycardia or hypertension, anemia, fever, thyrotoxicosis, hypoxemia, and the use of medications that might have deleterious consequences such as sympathomimetics for bronchospasm.

Detection of postinfarction ischemia must always rely on a high index of suspicion. Chest pain must be vigorously evaluated and, when possible, distinguished from other common causes of chest pain in the postinfarction patient, especially pericarditis. New ischemic electrocardiographic changes, most frequently involving the ST segment and T wave, can aid in the diagnosis. These changes may be observed in the zone of the infarct or remote from it. The latter phenomenon has been referred to as ischemia-at-a-distance, an event that presages an even worse prognosis. Even in the absence of new electrocardiographic changes, pain of a nature and quality similar to that associated with the original infarction should be interpreted as having an ischemic origin until proved otherwise.

The absence of chest pain does not exclude the presence of recurrent ischemia. Indeed, "silent" or asymptomatic ST segment depressions are observed more frequently than painful or symptomatic ST segment depressions among postinfarction patients studied with continuous Holter ECG recordings. For this reason, the telemetry monitor tracings that are now a routine feature of both coronary care and intermediate care surveillance should be carefully screened for the presence of both arrhythmias and electrocardiographic repolarization abnormalities. Finally, in the absence of documented ischemia in the convalescent period, the potential for recurrent ischemia or reinfarction can be assessed by predischarge, submaximal exercise testing, preferably in conjunction with radionuclide imaging.

It has also been shown that patients with a non–Q-wave infarct are at high risk for recurrent ischemia. Although the hospital mortality is lower for these patients than for those with a Q-wave infarct, patients with a non–Q-wave infarct are more likely to have recurrent ischemia and reinfarction following hospital discharge. Therefore, the non–Q-wave infarct should be considered an incomplete event (concept of spontaneous reperfusion) that leaves behind susceptible myocardium. The search for ischemia, be it spontaneous or provoked with exercise testing, should be a very aggressive enterprise in patients with non–Q-wave infarctions.

Infarct extension complicates the course of as many as 10% of patients with acute myocardial infarction. It may be distinguished from postinfarction angina by the presence of prolonged pain or persistent electrocardiographic changes. Infarct extension occurs in the zone of the original infarct and depends for its diagnosis on a re-elevation of the myocardial-specific fraction of creatine kinase (CK-MB). Extension may occur more frequently in patients who display an early CK-MB rise (less than 15 hours), during the first infarction in overweight women, in diabetics, or in patients with non–Q-wave infarcts. Infarct extension may explain the progressively downhill course of many patients who develop cardiogenic shock.

## Management of Postinfarction Myocardial Ischemia

In the absence of any obvious contraindication (advanced age, underlying medical illness), the management of a patient with a postinfarction ischemic syndrome should be very aggressive, with a view toward prompt coronary angiography and revascularization. Concomitant medical therapy is also essential.

The general measures of oxygen administration, analgesia, relief of anxiety, antipyresis, correction of anemia (hematocrit greater than 30%), and withdrawal of offending medications are as vital here as they are for the initial event. Nitroglycerin should be given sublingually (0.4 mg) and the dose repeated as many as two more times over 15 minutes, as tolerated based on blood pressure, should pain or electrocardiographic changes persist. Although nitrates are not recommended for the patient with a completed infarct, they play an important role in the treatment of postinfarction ischemia. They are available in sublingual, oral, transmucosal, and transcutaneous preparations but must be administered in such a way as to avoid nitrate tolerance (Table 2). In general, nitrates remain most effective when the patient is exposed to them for the shortest time possible over the course of 24 hours. Continuous delivery of oral isosorbide dinitrate (Isordil) or transcutaneous 2% nitroglycerin ointment (Nitro-Bid ointment) every 4 to 6 hours, for example, is no longer recommended. A nitrate "holiday" is preferable. Alternative approaches include the use of sublingual isosorbide dinitrate (half-life 1 to 2 hours) at 4- to 6-hour intervals, oral isosorbide dinitrate on a three times daily basis, or 2% nitroglycerin ointment applied every 6 to 8 hours, but withdrawn for at least 6 hours during every 24-hour period.

Despite the well-documented tolerance that develops with the nonparenteral forms of nitrates, enthusiasm surrounds the intravenous use of nitroglycerin for angina or ischemic electrocardiographic changes that are refractory to more conventional medical measures. Nitroglycerin administered intravenously can promptly relieve ischemia both when first instituted and when its dose is increased even after several hours of a constant infusion. It is generally well tolerated, although it should be avoided in hypotensive patients (systolic blood pressure less than 95 mmHg), particularly those with right ventricular infarction. Intravenous nitroglycerin is usually begun at a dose of 25-μg per minute and increased thereafter in 25-μg increments. Doses of several hundred μg per minute are not uncommon. Continuous monitoring of the systemic blood pressure with an indwelling radial artery catheter is recommended when the dose of intravenous nitroglycerin exceeds 200 μg per minute. Problems with its prolonged use in large doses include methemoglobinemia and ethanol intoxication, the latter owing to the fact that most commercially available forms of nitroglycerin for intravenous use are prepared with ethanol as a diluent.

Beta blockade occupies a prominent place in the management of patients with myocardial infarction (Table 3). The use of metoprolol intravenously in the acute phase, either alone or as an adjunct to reperfusion therapy, has been discussed previously. Such therapy may limit the size of the infarct, reduce the frequency of reinfarction, and improve survival. For those patients not receiving a beta blocker who develop a postinfarction ischemic syndrome, the addition of such an agent to the medical regimen can be very beneficial. Beta-adrenoreceptor blockade can improve the ratio of oxygen supply to demand by counteracting those perturbations that lead to an increase in myocardial oxygen demand, such as tachycardia and hypertension. In general, a shorter-acting agent (propranolol [Inderal] or metoprolol [Lopressor]) is preferred in the acute setting, especially one that can be given intravenously. Pindolol (Visken), because of its intrinsic sympathomimetic activity, should be avoided. In patients with important bronchospastic lung disease, selection of a cardioselective agent ($\beta_1$-blocker) may be advisable. Infusions of the ultrashort-acting cardioselective agent esmolol (Brevibloc) may prove helpful in those situations where beta-blockade might be beneficial but also potentially dangerous, such as in patients with depressed ventricular function or bronchospasm.

The calcium channel antagonists have made a substantial contribution to the treatment of patients with ischemic heart disease (Table 4). For patients with postinfarction ischemic syndromes, the addition of a calcium channel antagonist to the medical regimen can often provide salutary effects. Diltiazem (Cardizem), for example, in a dose of 90 mg four times daily, has proved to be effective in reducing the incidence of early reinfarction in patients with non–Q-wave infarctions. It is not yet known whether nifedipine (Procardia) and verapamil (Isoptin) might have the same effect. Among the three agents, nifedipine is the most potent coronary and peripheral arterial vasodilator. It can be given orally or the contents of a capsule (10 mg) can be aspirated into a sterile syringe and administered sublingually. Nifedipine is particularly useful when systemic hypertension coexists with postinfarction ischemia. Verapamil has enjoyed its most frequent use in those instances when supraventricular tachycardia (paroxysmal supraventricular tachycardia, atrial flutter, atrial fibrillation) precipitates

TABLE 2. **Commonly Used Nitrate Preparations***

| Agent | Dosage | Onset of Effect | Duration of Effect |
|---|---|---|---|
| Sublingual NTG | 0.3–0.6 mg | 2–5 min | 10–30 min |
| Sublingual ISDN (Isordil) | 2.5–10 mg | 3–15 min | 1–2 hr |
| Oral ISDN (Isordil) | 5–40 mg | 15–30 min | 3–6 hr |
| 2% NTG ointment (Nitro-Bid) | ½–2 in | 20–60 min | 3–8 hr |

*Abbreviations:* NTG = nitroglycerin; ISDN = isosorbide dinitrate.
*Adapted from Frishman WH: Pharmacology of the nitrates in angina pectoris. Am J Cardiol 56:81, 1985.

TABLE 3. **Commonly Used Beta-Adrenoreceptor Antagonists***

| Agent | Relative B$_1$ Selectivity | Lipophilicity | ISA | Elimination Half-Life (hr) | Potency Ratio (Propranolol = 1) | Dosage |
|---|---|---|---|---|---|---|
| Propranolol (Inderal) | 0 | + + + | 0 | 3.5–6.0 | 1.0 | IV: 0.25-mg test dose then increments of 1.0 mg up to 0.15 mg/kg total<br>PO: 40–80 mg qid |
| Metoprolol (Lopressor) | + | + + | 0 | 3–4 | 1.0 | IV: 5-mg bolus q 5 min up to 15 mg total<br>PO: 50–100 mg bid |
| Atenolol (Tenormin) | + | + | 0 | 6–9 | 1.0 | PO: 50–100 mg qd |
| Nadolol (Corgard) | 0 | + | 0 | 14–25 | 1.0 | PO: 40–240 mg qd |
| Pindolol (Visken) | 0 | + + | + | 3–4 | 6.0 | PO: 5–20 mg tid |
| Timolol (Blocadren) | 0 | + | 0 | 3–4 | 6.0 | PO: 10–20 mg bid |
| Esmolol (Brevibloc) | + | + | 0 | 9 min | 1.0 | IV: 500 µg/kg bolus over 1 min, then infusion of 50 µg/kg/min. Rebolus of 500 µg/kg can be given 5 min later and infusion increased to 100 µg/kg/min. Maximum 200 µg/kg/min |

*Abbreviations:* ISA = intrinsic sympathomimetic activity; 0 = none; + = low; + + = moderate; + + + = high.
*Adapted from Frishman WH, Kaftka KR, and Meltzer AH: Anti-anginal agents, Part 2: B-blockers. Hosp Formul *21:*62, 1986.

or complicates myocardial ischemia. It is also a potent antihypertensive agent. Verapamil is given intravenously in 5- to 10-mg boluses (0.075 to 0.15 mg per kg) to treat supraventricular tachycardia. The dose can be repeated in 15 to 30 minutes as necessary.

All of the previously mentioned agents can lower the blood pressure, the nitrates least effectively. However, the nitrates can lower ventricular preload (venodilatation), and the possible subsequent fall in cardiac output can be very deleterious. The beta blockers, given in combination with diltiazem or verapamil, can produce conduction system disturbances, ranging from profound sinus bradycardia to a high-grade atrioventricular block. The beta blockers and calcium channel antagonists, especially verapamil and nifedipine, can impair ventricular contractile performance when used in combination, and caution must be exercised lest heart failure ensue.

Heparin and aspirin are standard adjunctive therapy to thrombolysis with or without PTCA. Aspirin is continued indefinitely (160 to 325 mg a day). Most experts now recommend that heparin be continued for at least 5 days following successful thrombolytic reperfusion. Should postinfarction ischemia occur thereafter, heparin should be reinstituted as a bolus of 5000 units followed by a continuous infusion to keep the activated partial thromboplastin time approximately twice control, unless contraindications to its use exist. Such contraindications include

TABLE 4. **Calcium Channel Antagonists***

| Agent | Dosage | Onset of Action | Peak Effect | Half-Life | Negative Inotropy | Bradycardia, AV Block |
|---|---|---|---|---|---|---|
| Nifedipine (Procardia) | PO: 10–40 mg tid/qid<br>SL: 10–20 mg q 4 hr | Within 20 min<br>Within 3 min | 1–2 hr | 4 hr | 0† | 0 |
| Diltiazem (Cardizem) | PO: 30–90 mg tid/qid | Within 15 min | 30 min | 4 hr | + | + |
| Verapamil (Isoptin) | IV: 5–10 mg (0.075–0.15 mg/kg) | 2 min | 3–5 min | <30 min‡ | + | + + |
|  | PO: 80–120 mg tid/qid‡ | 2 hr | 3–4 hr | 3–7 hr‡ | + | + + |

*Abbreviations:* 0 = none, + = mild, + + = moderate.
*Adapted from Singh BN: Clinical pharmacology of calcium antagonist drugs. Cornell Postgraduate Course on Calcium Antagonists. New York, Medcom, Inc., 1982, p. 5.
†Nifedipine can cause left ventricular dysfunction when used in combination with beta blockers. It also exerts negative inotropic effects on patients with pre-existent heart failure.
‡Half-life of verapamil increases with consecutive doses to 10–12 hr. Therefore, regular verapamil can be given bid.

bleeding and a previously documented heparin-induced thrombocytopenia.

For patients with postinfarction ischemia who fail to respond to these aggressive medical measures, intra-aortic balloon counterpulsation (IABP) should be instituted as quickly as possible. IABP frequently results in resolution of ischemia (pain, ST segment deviations) within minutes and allows subsequent coronary angiography and PTCA or CABG surgery to be performed under more stable conditions. Vascular access is the chief problem associated with institution of IABP. Anticoagulation with heparin and prophylactic cephalosporin (or vancomycin in the allergic patient) antibiotic coverage should be provided as long as the balloon is in place.

Coronary angiography and revascularization therapy are the next steps in the management of patients with postinfarction ischemia. The decision to proceed with these interventions must always be tempered by the expected outcome, the age of the patient, and the presence of other severe medical problems. Definition of the coronary anatomy with angiography should guide the appropriate choice for revascularization. In certain patients, for example, those with acute thrombotic reocclusion following initially successful reperfusion therapy, retreatment with a thrombolytic agent via the intracoronary or intravenous route would be reasonable.

When appropriate, PTCA should be directed at the culprit lesion; stenoses in other coronary arteries should not be approached at this time. The patient can return for elective PTCA of the other lesions, as dictated by their severity or functional importance, in several weeks. Alternatively, angiography may reveal coronary lesions that would best be treated with CABG surgery, such as left main coronary disease, three-vessel disease, or coronary lesions that would not be amenable to PTCA because of their morphologic characteristics (length or presence of residual thrombus) or location (lesions at bifurcations, angulated or tortuous position). Finally, it should be recognized that CABG surgery performed urgently for postinfarction ischemia is associated with a higher rate of perioperative infarction and death, as compared with elective operation.

## CARDIAC ARRHYTHMIAS

### Ventricular Arrhythmias

If searched for carefully, ventricular arrhythmias are ubiquitous early after acute myocardial infarction. Virtually all patients experience ventricular premature beats (VPBs). In the past, VPBs were treated with an antiarrhythmic agent only if they were considered to be harbingers of malignant ventricular arrhythmias. These so-called warning VPBs included those that were frequent, multifocal, repetitive, or early (R-on-T phenomenon). We now realize that VPBs can trigger ventricular tachyarrhythmias even if they lack these features. This fact has led to the widespread prophylactic use of antiarrhythmic agents, especially lidocaine, in patients with acute infarction. Prophylactic therapy has been shown to reduce the incidence of ventricular fibrillation, although the effect on mortality is uncertain. It is our practice to treat with lidocaine all patients under age 75 in whom infarction is strongly suspected, beginning with a loading intravenous bolus of 1.5 mg per kg, followed 10 minutes later by a second bolus of 0.5 mg per kg. A continuous intravenous infusion is then started at a dose of 2 to 4 mg per minute (approximately 50 μg per kg per minute). These dosages should be reduced by approximately 50% in patients with advanced congestive heart failure or liver disease. Because the half-life of lidocaine increases during continuous intravenous infusion, it may be necessary to reduce the rate of the infusion after several hours to avoid late toxicity. In view of the high incidence of toxicity in patients over age 75, we do not usually treat these patients prophylactically with lidocaine. Toxic manifestations include paresthesia, lassitude, somnolence, confusion, slurred speech, diplopia, and seizures. We usually continue prophylactic treatment for 48 hours and then taper the drug in the absence of breakthrough arrhythmias.

In patients who continue to have frequent or complex VPBs despite treatment with lidocaine, or in those who are intolerant of lidocaine, procainamide (Pronestyl) is a useful alternative. The average loading dose is 1000 mg intravenously, which should be given over 30 to 45 minutes. The blood pressure must be monitored carefully during the administration of the loading dose to avoid hypotension. A maintenance intravenous infusion should then be started at a rate of 2 to 4 mg per minute (approximately 50 μg per kg per minute).

The occurrence of ventricular tachycardia during the early hours after acute infarction has been reduced, but not eliminated, by the prophylactic use of antiarrhythmic agents. The treatment of this arrhythmia depends on its hemodynamic consequences. Patients who are unconscious should undergo electrical cardioversion immediately. Because this arrhythmia is often quite sensitive to electrical energy, the magnitude of the initial direct current shock should be only 10 to 50 joules. Anteroposterior placement of the electrodes may reduce the energy level required for cardioversion. If the initial shock is unsuccessful, the energy level should be increased by 25 to 50 joules for each subsequent shock. "Thumpversion," striking the patient on the sternum with the fist, sometimes terminates ventricular tachycardia, but this maneuver is not a reliable form of treatment and should generally not be performed in a patient who is awake.

If the patient is conscious, time is usually available for a trial of pharmacologic cardioversion. The drugs of choice are lidocaine or procainamide, administered intravenously in the doses indicated previously. An alternative is bretylium tosylate (Bretylol), 5 to 10 mg per kg, given by intravenous infusion over 3 to 5 minutes. If the arrhythmia is converted, a maintenance infusion of 1 to 2 mg per minute should be started. The principal side effect of bretylium is orthostatic hypotension, and this drug is usually reserved for patients with recurrent ventricular tachycardia in whom lidocaine and procainamide have failed. If drug therapy fails and electrical cardioversion is to be performed on a conscious patient, methohexital sodium (Brevital), 50 to 100 mg, or diazepam, 5 to 10 mg intravenously, should be administered first. Hypokalemia, hypomagnesemia, and hypoxemia should be searched for and corrected in all patients who have had ventricular tachycardia.

When ventricular tachycardia occurs (or recurs) 2 or more weeks after infarction, it is often an indication either that myocardial ischemia is present or that the infarct is large and that considerable hemodynamic compromise is present. In such patients, the arrhythmia may recur and may be difficult to suppress with drugs. The first step in management is to treat congestive heart failure, ischemia, hypoxemia, fever, or electrolyte imbalance if any of these problems are present. Even when these complications have been alleviated, specific antiarrhythmic therapy is often required. The selection of an effective antiarrhythmic agent or a combination of agents is often a painstaking empiric process, which can be guided in part by the use of ambulatory electrocardiographic (Holter) monitoring, invasive electrophysiologic testing, or both. Recent data suggest that effective suppression of asymptomatic ventricular arrhythmia documented by these techniques does not necessarily predict a better long-term prognosis after acute infarction. Cardiologic consultation is recommended to assist in management. Because a separate article in this volume is devoted to the treatment of tachyarrhythmias, only the high points of antiarrhythmic therapy are mentioned here.

Antiarrhythmic agents have been classified into four groups on the basis of their physiologic properties. Class I antiarrhythmic agents, which block the fast sodium channel in the myocardial cell membrane, are the mainstay of treatment of recurrent ventricular tachycardia. These agents are subdivided into Classes A, B, and C. Class IA drugs (quinidine [Quinaglute], procainamide [Procan], disopyramide [Norpace]), which prolong the duration of the action potential, are the agents used most commonly, although disopyramide has fallen into disfavor because of its troublesome side effects of urinary retention and congestive heart failure. Drugs in Class IA can worsen ventricular arrhythmias (proarrhythmia) in approximately 10% of patients. Class IB drugs (phenytoin, tocainamide [Tonocard], mexiletine [Mexitil]), which shorten the duration of the action potential, are considered to be second-line drugs because, as a general rule, they tend to be less effective than Class IA agents. The powerful new Class IC agents (flecainide [Tambocor], encainide [Enkaid], lorcainide*, propafenone*), which slow electrical conduction, show great promise, but their use may be restricted because of their prominent proarrhythmic effects. Among the Class IC agents, only flecainide and encainide have been approved for general use at the time of this writing. Recent data suggest that they should be used with caution after acute infarction because of their proarrhythmic effects (see later).

Class II agents, the beta-adrenergic receptor antagonists, are almost never used alone in the treatment of recurrent ventricular tachycardia but are sometimes used in combination with Class I agents.

Class III agents, such as amiodarone (Cordarone), block potassium channels. Amiodarone is effective in preventing recurrent ventricular tachycardia, but it is used only when all other drugs have failed because of its many serious side effects, including pneumonitis, hepatitis, corneal deposits, and thyroid disturbances. Oral dosing is complicated because of its long onset of action, variable pharmacokinetics, and long half-life. Amiodarone is seldom useful for the urgent management of ventricular arrhythmias because of its prolonged loading period.

Class IV agents (verapamil [Isoptin], nifedipine [Procardia], diltiazem [Cardizem]), the slow calcium channel antagonists, have little use in the treatment of ventricular arrhythmias.

A difficult question, recently addressed in part by the Cardiac Arrhythmia Suppression Trial (CAST), is whether patients with acute infarction followed by asymptomatic or minimally symptomatic VPBs, including unsustained (less than 15 beats) ventricular tachycardia, should receive prophylactic antiarrhythmic therapy. This trial found that the use of flecainide or encainide in

---

*Investigational drug in the United States.

such patients actually worsened the risk of death from arrhythmia or nonfatal cardiac arrest (proarrhythmia) even if the baseline arrhythmia was effectively suppressed. Whether the same results would apply to other antiarrhythmic agents is unknown. Also, patients with more severe ventricular arrhythmias, such as episodes of ventricular tachycardia longer than 15 beats, were not included in this trial, and the results may not apply to them. On the basis of the CAST data, and pending further studies, we do not currently recommend routine prophylactic antiarrhythmic therapy for patients with asymptomatic or minimally symptomatic ventricular arrhythmias after myocardial infarction. By contrast, patients with recurrent ventricular tachycardia should be treated with an appropriate antiarrhythmic drug (or drugs), but the physician should always be alert to the threat of proarrhythmia, especially with the Type IC agents.

Accelerated idioventricular rhythm is a slow form of ventricular tachycardia, with rates that vary between 60 and 110 beats per minute. This arrhythmia, which is more common in patients with inferior than anterior infarction, usually develops when the underlying sinus rate decelerates and the rate of depolarization of an ectopic ventricular focus increases. Because the arrhythmia is usually transient and intermittent, it often does not cause hemodynamic instability. If it is sustained, however, the loss of a synchronized atrial contraction may reduce the cardiac output. The arrhythmia should then be treated by suppressing the ventricular focus with standard doses of lidocaine or by increasing the sinus rate with atropine (0.5 mg intravenously). Because accelerated idioventricular rhythm is sometimes associated with more malignant forms of ventricular tachycardia, some physicians choose to treat it whenever it is detected. Whichever approach is followed, patients with this arrhythmia require careful monitoring of the cardiac rhythm.

Ventricular fibrillation, the most common cause of death in patients with acute infarction before hospitalization, is still a threat after admission to the CCU. As with ventricular tachycardia, the incidence of ventricular fibrillation has been sharply reduced, but not eliminated, by the prophylactic use of lidocaine. When this arrhythmia does occur, the treatment is immediate electrical defibrillation with 200 to 360 joules of direct current energy. The success of defibrillation depends critically on the time interval between the onset of fibrillation and delivery of the first shock. Therefore, speed is essential. "Quick-look" electrodes, which can both detect the cardiac rhythm and deliver the shock, are useful to confirm rapidly the presence of the arrhythmia

in unmonitored patients. In contrast to ventricular fibrillation, asystole does not respond to electrical defibrillation. This problem should be treated instead with epinephrine, 0.5 mg to 1 mg, administered either intravenously or via the endotracheal tube. This agent occasionally causes fine ventricular fibrillation to appear, and an attempt to defibrillate is then appropriate. External or transvenous pacing can also be attempted, but asystole is notoriously difficult to treat successfully, and the mortality rate is high.

In patients with small infarcts and good left ventricular function, the occurrence of ventricular fibrillation during the early hours after infarction does not usually portend a poor prognosis. Electrical defibrillation, if performed promptly, is usually successful, and the arrhythmia does not tend to recur as long as defibrillation is followed by treatment with standard doses of lidocaine or procainamide. By contrast, ventricular fibrillation in patients with large infarcts and pump failure is often difficult to treat and does tend to recur. Electrolyte imbalance, myocardial ischemia, and hypoxemia should be corrected, and every effort should be made to improve cardiac pump function. Bretylium tosylate, 5 to 10 mg per kg intravenously over 3 to 5 minutes, is sometimes helpful in suppressing the arrhythmia. Despite these interventions, the prognosis of these patients is often poor because of the extensive damage to the myocardium that is usually present.

## Supraventricular Arrhythmias

Sinus bradycardia occurs more commonly in patients with inferoposterior than those with anterior infarction because of the enhancement of vagal tone that may accompany infarction of the inferoposterior wall. Marked sinus bradycardia in this setting usually responds well to treatment with atropine, 0.5 to 1.0 mg intravenously. Paradoxical bradycardia and hypotension, mediated by vagal stimulation, are rare complications that have been reported in patients with acute infarction who have received nitroglycerin. Here, too, atropine is the drug of choice. Marked sinus bradycardia in a patient with an anterior infarction may be caused by ischemia or infarction of the sinus node (sick sinus syndrome). Atrial pacing may be required if severe bradycardia persists after a trial of atropine.

Sinus tachycardia is common in patients with acute infarction as a consequence of fever, pain, or anxiety, all of which may be associated with enhanced sympathetic tone. Sinus tachycardia that persists after these three problems have been treated should encourage the physician to look carefully for evidence of congestive heart failure, another common and worrisome cause of sinus tachycardia. A patient with sinus tachycardia should not be treated with a beta-adrenergic receptor blocking agent until it is certain that heart failure is not present. In patients with persistent sinus tachycardia and no evidence of heart failure, treatment with propranolol or metoprolol, 1 to 10 mg intravenously, is indicated to slow the heart rate to less than 90 beats per minute and thereby reduce myocardial oxygen demand. It should be emphasized, however, that congestive heart failure must be excluded before a beta-receptor blocking agent is administered.

The new onset of atrial fibrillation in acute myocardial infarction may be associated with congestive heart failure, pericarditis, atrial infarction, pulmonary emboli, or coexisting severe chronic obstructive pulmonary disease. The treatment of choice is digoxin, 0.5 to 1 mg intravenously, to slow the ventricular response rate to less than 90 beats per minute. Additional doses of digoxin (0.25 mg) may be given hourly until the target heart rate has been achieved or a total dose of 1.5 mg has been administered over 18 to 24 hours. Patients may occasionally, but not consistently, revert to sinus rhythm after treatment with digoxin. Verapamil, 5 to 10 mg intravenously, is an effective alternative to digoxin for rate control, but it should not be used if congestive heart failure is present. If the ventricular response rate is rapid and the patient is hemodynamically unstable, electrical cardioversion may be required to restore sinus rhythm. The patient should be premedicated with methohexital sodium, 50 to 100 mg, or diazepam, 5 to 10 mg intravenously, and supplemental oxygen should be given by face mask. The electrodes should be positioned anteriorly and posteriorly, and the countershock should be synchronized with the R wave of the electrocardiogram. The initial energy level should be 150 joules. If the first shock is not successful in restoring sinus rhythm, the energy level of each subsequent shock should be increased by 25 to 50 joules.

Atrial flutter and supraventricular tachycardia are uncommon in patients with acute infarction, and their treatment is discussed elsewhere in this volume.

### Conduction Disturbances

Complete (third-degree) atrioventricular (AV) block can occur in patients with anterior or inferoposterior infarction, but the mechanisms and prognosis of heart block are different, depending on the anatomic location of the infarct. In patients with inferoposterior infarction, heart block is usually caused by the simultaneous occurrence of ischemia of the AV node and enhancement of vagal tone. Third-degree block may alternate with periods of Mobitz Type I (Wenckebach) second-degree block and periods of sinus rhythm with first-degree block. A stable junctional or ventricular escape mechanism may be present, and the need for temporary pacing depends on the rate and stability of the escape mechanism and the hemodynamic condition of the patient. Many physicians choose to place a temporary pacemaker in all patients with inferoposterior infarction complicated by complete heart block. Heart block is often reversible in inferoposterior infarction, and AV nodal conduction may reappear spontaneously within 5 to 10 days. A permanent cardiac pacer is often not required, although patients with inferoposterior infarction complicated by complete heart block usually have larger infarcts and reduced long-term survival as compared with patients who do not have this complication.

When complete AV block complicates acute anterior infarction, the conduction disturbance is usually caused by an extensive infarct that has damaged both the right and left bundle branches. The prognosis is poor, even if temporary ventricular or AV sequential pacing is instituted immediately, because of the presence of severe pump dysfunction. The occurrence of complete AV block may be foreshadowed by periods of Mobitz Type II second-degree block, and therefore the latter conduction disturbance is considered to be an indication for the institution of temporary pacing.

The appearance of new bifascicular block also carries a substantial risk of progression to complete heart block. Bifascicular block can be manifested as right bundle branch block and left anterior fascicular block, right bundle branch block and left posterior fascicular block, or alternating right and left bundle branch block. Because complete AV block may appear suddenly in patients with bifascicular block, a temporary pacemaker should be inserted prophylactically. Alternatively, an external thoracic temporary pacing device can be kept on standby for immediate use if complete heart block appears. With recent modifications in its design, the external thoracic temporary pacer has proved effective in maintaining the cardiac rhythm until a temporary transvenous pacer can be placed. Because complete heart block occurs in no more than 30% of patients with bifascicular block, the availability of an external thoracic temporary pacer obviates the need for a prophylactic transvenous pacer in approximately two-thirds of patients with bifascicular block. Placement of a permanent ventricular pacer is indicated in patients with bifascicular block only if transient or sustained complete heart block occurs. Patients with new unifascicular block (such as right bundle branch block or left anterior fascicular block alone) have little risk of developing complete heart block, and temporary pacing is not indicated.

## HEMODYNAMIC ABNORMALITIES ASSOCIATED WITH ACUTE MYOCARDIAL INFARCTION

Hemodynamic abnormalities are the rule, not the exception, during the early phases of acute myocardial infarction. The principal determinants of cardiac performance, namely preload, afterload, and contractility, are all affected to varying degrees. Left ventricular preload, as measured by pulmonary capillary wedge pressure, may be inappropriately low because of hypovolemia, the administration of morphine sulfate, or excess vasomotor tone. Alternatively, preload may be abnormally elevated in patients with pulmonary congestion, as the failing left ventricle relies on the Starling mechanism to maintain cardiac output. Afterload may be inappropriately elevated in the setting of depressed cardiac output and high sympathetic nervous system tone. Contractility is always impaired in the infarcted zone and may be further compromised by associated myocardial ischemia in border zones between normal and infarcted tissue. The severity of the hemodynamic abnormality depends on the extent and location (anterior usually greater than inferior) of the infarction, as well as the presence or absence of mechanical complications such as acute mitral regurgitation, rupture of the interventricular septum or free wall of the left ventricle, and the extent of preexisting left ventricular dysfunction.

It is useful for the clinician to categorize patients during the early phases of acute infarction into subgroups on the basis of the degree of hemodynamic impairment. We have generally found the classification system of Forrester and associates (Table 5), which is based on the invasive measurement of cardiac index (normally greater than 2.2 liters per minute per M$^2$) and pulmonary capillary wedge pressure (normally less than 18 mmHg), to be the most useful for patient management and prognostication. While this classification scheme is useful, it must be recognized that patients often change from one category to another with therapy and sometimes even spontaneously. These four hemodynamic subgroups generally reflect clinical status and prognosis, and the aim of hemodynamic therapy is to achieve normal values for the cardiac index and pulmonary wedge pressure (as in subgroup I).

**Invasive Hemodynamic Monitoring.** Patients with clinically uncomplicated acute myocardial infarction do not need or benefit from routine invasive monitoring. These patients can be managed by careful clinical evaluation, which should consist of continuous electrocardiographic monitoring of heart rate and rhythm; frequent measurement of systemic arterial blood pressure by cuff; careful and repeated auscultation of the lung fields for evidence of pulmonary congestion; cardiac examination to detect ventricular or atrial gallops, murmurs, or pericardial rubs; assessment of the pulmonary vasculature by chest x-ray; assessment of systemic perfusion (urinary output, mental status, perfusion of extremities); and arterial blood sampling for $Po_2$, $Pco_2$, and pH when metabolic acidosis or hypoxemia is suspected.

We undertake invasive hemodynamic monitoring in the following settings: persistent low output state, unexplained hypotension, or shock; recurrent or refractory pulmonary congestion or edema; appearance of a new systolic heart murmur associated with hemodynamic instability; persistent or recurrent ischemic chest pain refractory to conventional analgesics and requiring intravenous nitroglycerin; extensive right ventricular infarction with hypotension; evaluation of the response to intravenous vasoactive drugs or intra-aortic balloon counterpulsation; or unexplained persistent sinus tachycardia. Whenever invasive monitoring is undertaken, it should be discontinued as soon as it is feasible in order to reduce the risk of infection.

### Hypotension

During the early prehospital phase of acute myocardial infarction, hypotension is common and usually associated with hypovolemia (Forrester Class III). Hypotension associated with bradycardia most commonly accompanies infarction of the inferior or inferoposterior wall and usually responds to the intravenous administration of atropine (0.5 to 1.0 mg) and elevation of the legs. Hypotension associated with tachycardia is particularly common in patients who have received diuretics before the infarction. Marked diaphoresis, reduction of fluid intake, or vomiting may all contribute to the development of hypovolemia.

Even if the effective vascular volume is normal, "relative" hypovolemia may be present, because ventricular compliance is reduced during the early stages of acute infarction and a pulmonary wedge pressure as high as 18 to 20 mmHg may be needed to provide sufficient preload for optimal ventricular performance. In the absence of pulmonary rales, the patient should be placed in the reverse Trendelenburg position. Atropine (0.5 to

TABLE 5. **Hemodynamic Classification of Forrester and Associates***

| Subgroup | Clinical Findings | Hemodynamic Definition | Mortality (%) | Suggested Intervention |
|----------|-------------------|------------------------|---------------|------------------------|
| I | No pulmonary congestion or peripheral hypoperfusion | PCW < 18 CI > 2.2 | 2.2 | Beta-adrenergic blockade if no contraindications |
| II | Isolated pulmonary congestion | PCW ≥ 18 CI > 2.2 | 10.1 | Diuretics, correction of hypoxemia |
| III | Isolated peripheral hypoperfusion | PCW < 18 CI < 2.2 | 22.4 | Repletion of vascular volume |
| IV | Pulmonary congestion and peripheral hypoperfusion | PCW ≥ 18 CI < 2.2 | 55.5 | Diuretics, vasodilators, sympathomimetic agent with positive inotropic effects, circulatory assistance |

*Abbreviations:* PCW = pulmonary capillary wedge pressure (mmHg); CI = cardiac index (L/min/m²).
*Modified from Forrester JS, et al. Reprinted, by permission of the New England Journal of Medicine, *295:*1404, 1976.

1.0 mg) should be administered if sinus bradycardia is present. If hypotension persists, crystalloid solution should be administered intravenously, beginning with a bolus of 100 ml of 5% dextrose/normal saline and followed by a maintenance infusion of 100 to 200 ml per hour. The patient should be carefully observed and the infusion discontinued when the systolic blood pressure rises above 90 to 100 mmHg, if the patient develops dyspnea, or if pulmonary congestion develops.

Recognition of hypovolemia is of particular importance in hypotensive patients because improvement in circulatory function can be so readily achieved by augmentation of vascular volume. Because of the poor correlation between pulmonary capillary wedge pressure and jugular venous pulse (JVP) or central venous pressure (CVP), hypovolemia may be frequently overlooked without invasive hemodynamic monitoring. Exclusion of hypovolemia as the cause of hypotension requires documentation of a depressed cardiac index despite a pulmonary wedge pressure of more than 18 mmHg.

Administration of vasoactive agents such as dopamine (Intropin) is indicated in the management of hypotension that persists after correction of hypovolemia and excessive vagal tone. We generally administer dopamine in doses of 2.5 to 5.0 μg per kg per minute by constant intravenous infusion and adjust the dosage depending on the blood pressure response. When there is clinical evidence for excessive vasodilatation, an uncommon occurrence in the absence of fever or sepsis, phenylephrine (Neo-Synephrine) is the agent of choice.

### The Hyperdynamic State

Patients with uncomplicated myocardial infarction often have excessive activation of the sympathetic nervous system because of pain and anxiety. The hemodynamic profile of a patient with a hyperdynamic state includes an increased heart rate, arterial hypertension, and elevation of the cardiac index in the presence of a normal or low pulmonary capillary wedge pressure. Other causes of sinus tachycardia, such as fever, infection, persistent pain, pericarditis, or congestive heart failure should be excluded before treatment with a beta-adrenergic blocking agent is undertaken. Propranolol is usually the drug of choice in this setting, beginning with 0.25 to 0.5 mg intravenously and increasing the dose to 1 mg if necessary. Additional doses can be administered every 5 to 10 minutes until the heart rate is less than 90 beats per minute or a total of 0.2 mg per kg has been given. When the heart rate and blood pressure have reached optimal levels, oral propranolol can be given at a dose ranging from 40 to 160 mg per day. Esmolol, an ultrashort-acting beta blocker, can be administered to patients in whom the use of beta-adrenergic blockade might be accompanied by adverse effects.

### Pulmonary Congestion and Acute Pulmonary Edema

A mild to moderate degree of pulmonary congestion is common in patients with acute myocardial infarction. The patient will complain of dyspnea and orthopnea, while objective findings often include tachypnea, bibasilar pulmonary rales, an audible or palpable third heart sound, mild to moderate hypoxemia on arterial blood gas examination, and radiologic evidence of mild to moderate pulmonary venous hypertension. Therapy should be aimed at ensuring adequate arterial oxygenation and relieving pulmonary venous congestion. Reduction in the pulmonary capillary wedge pressure will not only relieve pulmonary congestion but also will reduce left ventricular volume, wall tension, and myocardial oxygen consumption, and may improve subendocardial myocardial perfusion. A diuresis can often be initiated by the intravenous administration of furosemide (Lasix) 20 to 40 mg. Higher doses may be necessary in patients who have previously required diuretic therapy. Vasodilator therapy with organic nitrates or sodium nitroprusside may also be used as an adjunct to diuretics, particularly when mitral regurgitation or systemic hypertension accompanies pulmonary venous congestion. Long-acting nitrates, particularly oral isosorbide dinitrate (10 to 40 mg orally every 3 to 4 hours) or 2% nitroglycerin ointment (½ to 2 inches applied cutaneously three times daily), are useful agents. A dose-free period of at least 6 hours per day is recommended to decrease the likelihood of developing nitrate tolerance.

Acute pulmonary edema is most commonly caused by extensive damage to the left ventricle. Other causes of acute pulmonary edema include diminished compliance of the left ventricle with relatively normal systolic contraction (diastolic heart failure); persistent or intermittent acute mitral regurgitation caused by papillary muscle dysfunction or rupture; or profound left ventricular ischemia associated with a small or modest degree of myocardial necrosis. Regardless of the cause, rapid and marked elevation of the pulmonary capillary wedge pressure (exceeding 25 mmHg) characterizes acute pulmonary edema. Assessment of the left ventricular ejection fraction by radionuclide techniques is often critical in determining the cause of the acute pulmonary edema.

The principles of management of acute cardiogenic pulmonary edema should include maintenance of adequate gas exchange and a stable cardiac rhythm, correction of hypotension, if present, and rapid lowering of the pulmonary capillary wedge pressure. Frequent measurement of arterial blood gases is essential in order to ensure adequate gas exchange. High concentrations of oxygen (60 to 100% by Ventimask or rebreathing mask) should be tried initially and endotracheal intubation considered for patients who are unable to maintain the arterial $Po_2$ greater than 60 mmHg, who develop progressive elevation of $Pco_2$, or who exhibit significant respiratory or metabolic acidosis. Mechanical ventilation should be supplemented with positive end-expiratory pressure (PEEP) to maintain adequate oxygenation with the lowest possible oxygen concentration in the inspired air. Hemodynamic monitoring may be required to determine the optimal amount of PEEP.

After adequate oxygenation has been restored, the next goal of therapy should be the rapid reduction of pulmonary capillary wedge pressure. Initial treatment generally consists of nitrates, either intravenously, transdermally, or sublin-

gually. Nitrates produce pharmacologic phlebotomy through their peripheral venodilator effects, which shift blood volume to the extrathoracic space and rapidly decrease pulmonary venous return and thus pulmonary capillary wedge pressure. Improvement in left ventricular function may also result from a decrease in afterload and improved oxygenation of ischemic zones of myocardium. Morphine sulfate should also be administered in small doses (1 to 5 mg intravenously) in order to calm the agitated patient and produce moderate venodilation. Potent loop diuretics, such as intravenous furosemide (20 to 40 mg) or ethacrynic acid (Edecrin) (50 mg), should be given early in the treatment of pulmonary edema, but they may take 20 minutes to 1 hour to produce a diuresis. The dose of intravenous diuretics should be doubled if the initial response has been suboptimal after 45 to 60 minutes. Sodium nitroprusside may be of use in severely hypertensive patients or in those with significant mitral regurgitation or ventricular septal rupture. We do not use digitalis glycosides or aminophylline as a general routine. Rotating tourniquets or phlebotomy are reserved for patients with severe renal insufficiency and those whose response to high doses of intravenous diuretics remains inadequate. Inotropic and vasodilator therapy in the management of acute pulmonary edema will be discussed subsequently.

### Cardiogenic Shock (Low Output, Hypotensive Syndrome)

Cardiogenic shock is a syndrome characterized by severe and prolonged tissue hypoperfusion associated with hypotension (systolic blood pressure usually less than or equal to 90 mmHg) and marked reduction of cardiac output. Cardiogenic shock (in contrast to hypovolemic shock) results from severe impairment of left ventricular systolic function caused by a loss of muscle mass or following the development of mechanical complications, such as acute mitral regurgitation, rupture of the interventricular septum or free wall of the left ventricle, ventricular aneurysm, or right ventricular infarction. Cardiogenic shock is usually associated with damage to 40% or more of the left ventricle. This syndrome may be precipitated by a small infarction in a patient with previous myocardial damage or by a single massive infarction. At autopsy, approximately 70% of patients with cardiogenic shock demonstrate three-vessel coronary artery disease, usually including the left anterior descending artery. Almost all such patients are found to have thrombosis of the artery that supplies the region of recent infarction. Profound impairment of ventricular performance results in ongoing myocardial ischemia and necrosis as a consequence of systemic hypoperfusion and inadequate coronary artery blood flow. A vicious circle is thereby created, and mortality often exceeds 80%.

Severe underperfusion of various end organs due to depressed cardiac output often results in progressive dysfunction. Renal failure, hepatic dysfunction, gastrointestinal bleeding secondary to ischemia, and lactic acidosis are common during the terminal stages of cardiogenic shock. Cardiac arrhythmias are also frequent. Cardiogenic shock is more common in patients over age 65, in those with diabetes, in patients with previous myocardial infarction, and in those with infarction of the anterior wall of the left ventricle. Early thinning and stretching of necrotic myocardium (infarct expansion) may contribute to acute ventricular dilation and precipitation of the shock syndrome. It does not appear that the location of the infarct is an independent contributor to the development of shock beyond the extent of the myocardial damage itself. Surprisingly, in half the patients who develop shock, it appears relatively late (more than 24 hours) after hospital admission.

The clinical features of cardiogenic shock include vasoconstriction with cool, clammy skin and peripheral cyanosis; oliguria with urine output less than 30 ml per hr; mental obtundation; a systolic blood pressure less than or equal to 90 mmHg; and a narrow pulse pressure. Blood pressure determinations should be performed directly from an intra-arterial catheter since cuff pressures may underestimate the true pressure by 10 to 25 mmHg owing to intense vasoconstriction. Cheyne-Stokes respirations are particularly common in elderly patients or following the use of narcotic analgesics.

Hemodynamic findings include a low mean arterial pressure, depressed cardiac index (greater than 2.2 liters per minute per M$^2$), elevated pulmonary capillary wedge pressure (greater than 18 mmHg), elevated systemic vascular resistance (greater than 2000 dyne-sec-cm$^{-5}$), and a widened arteriovenous oxygen difference. Radionuclide ventriculography shows severe contractile dysfunction with a global left ventricular ejection fraction almost always less than 30 to 35%.

The prognosis is extremely poor, with an 80 to 90% hospital mortality. Survivors often have evidence of continued heart failure and cardiac arrhythmias, and the probability for long-term survival is low. Prognosis appears to be more favorable in patients under the age of 50, in those with single vessel coronary artery disease, and in patients in whom subsequent coronary artery revascularization is able to salvage a substantial amount of viable myocardium. The latter group of patients often has large areas of reversible thallium[201] perfusion defects on exercise testing, confirming the presence of nonfunctional, but viable, ischemic myocardium.

The management of cardiogenic shock consists of the following objectives: improve ventricular systolic contractile performance; maintain adequate systemic blood pressure and sustain perfusion to vital organs; reduce pulmonary congestion; preserve viable but ischemic areas of myocardium; and limit the size of the myocardial infarct. At times, however, these goals are at odds with one another. Frequently, it is necessary to use vasopressor agents in order to support blood pressure, which may lead to further ischemia in a zone of jeopardized myocardium and may, in fact, extend the size of the infarct. Likewise, alpha adrenergic agonists, while useful in supporting blood pressure, may further decrease left ventricular systolic performance owing to further elevation in afterload. Optimal management requires a constant balancing of the risks and benefits of therapy and continuous reassessment of hemodynamic changes following institution of new therapies.

The management of patients with cardiogenic shock should begin with general supportive measures. Relief of ongoing ischemic pain and anxiety should be accomplished with the use of small doses of analgesics such as morphine, 2 to 4 mg intravenously every 5 to 10 minutes. Electrolyte disturbances, fever, nausea and vomiting, and acid-base abnormalities (particularly acidosis) should be treated. The optimal left ventricular filling pressure should be established for each patient. The pulmonary capillary wedge pressure should usually average 18 to 20 mmHg, and "relative" hypovolemia may exist when lower values are present. A small increase in the filling pressure may help improve cardiac output by means of the Starling mechanism.

Adequate ventilation and oxygenation should be maintained and frequently re-evaluated by measurement of arterial blood gases. Oxygen should be administered by nasal cannula or face mask to maintain an arterial $Po_2$ greater than 70 mmHg. Endotracheal intubation and mechanical ventilation may be required temporarily to achieve adequate oxygenation and reduce the work of breathing.

Continuous electrocardiographic monitoring is essential because arrhythmias may contribute to the low output state. Because the ischemic ventricle is more susceptible to the myocardial depressant effects of antiarrhythmic agents, the need for administration of these drugs and their dosages must be carefully reviewed and monitored to avoid adverse effects. Transvenous ventricular pacing or, preferably, atrioventricular sequential pacing (which preserves atrial function) may be necessary in patients with persistent bradycardia or atrioventricular block.

Invasive hemodynamic monitoring using a pulmonary artery thermodilution catheter, as well as an indwelling intra-arterial catheter, is essential as an adjunct to careful clinical assessment. Accurate and up-to-date hemodynamic data permit the selection of specific pharmacologic agents and other therapeutic interventions and also facilitate the diagnosis of other causes of cardiogenic shock such as mitral regurgitation, acute ventricular septal rupture, hypovolemia, or right ventricular infarction (Table 6).

Specific therapeutic interventions may include pharmacologic agents (loop diuretics, intravenous vasodilators, vasopressor drugs, and positive inotropic agents); mechanical circulatory assistance (intra-aortic balloon pumping or, rarely, left or right ventricular assist devices); coronary artery reperfusion by thrombolysis, percutaneous transluminal angioplasty (PTCA), or coronary artery bypass grafting; and cardiac surgery for the correction of mechanical complications of the acute infarction. Vasopressors, vasodilators, and positive inotropic agents all have a role in the acute management of patients with shock. Frequently, drugs that raise systemic vascular resistance and augment left ventricular contractility are re-

TABLE 6. **Principal Causes of Shock Following Acute Myocardial Infarction***

| Pathophysiology Abnormality | Diagnostic Evaluation | | | Guides to Management | Prognosis |
|---|---|---|---|---|---|
| | *Clinical* | *Hemodynamic* | *Noninvasive* | | |
| Hypovolemia | Clear lungs on chest film | BP < 100 PCW < 18 CI < 2.2 | Vigorous left ventricular function | Rapid but cautious volume expansion until PCW = 15–18mmHg | Very good |
| Right ventricular infarction | Inferior MI on ECG, JVP elevation, minimal LV failure, Kussmaul's sign | BP < 100 RA pressure ≥PCW, reduced PA and RV pulse pressure, CI < 2.2 | Dilated RV with RVEF ≤.30, LVEF generally < 45, inferior and/or posterior LV dysfunction | Volume expansion if PCW < 15mmHg, inotropic support, maintain atrial transport | Good unless severe LV dysfunction coexists |
| Cardiogenic shock | Pulmonary rales, S₃ gallop, pulmonary congestion on CXR | BP < 90 PCW ≥ 18 CI < 2.2 Elevated SVR | LVEF ≤.40, marked regional LV wall motion abnormalities | Inotropes and/ or vasopressors to maintain BP < 90 and CI approx 2 L/min/ m², vasodilators & diuretics to keep PCW < 18 IABP support | Poor, mortality 80%; early reperfusion (PTCA, rt-PA) may improve outlook |
| Acute mitral regurgitation | Holosystolic murmur at apex, pulmonary rales, S₃ gallop, pulmonary congestion on chest film | PCW ≥ 18 with large V waves, CI < 2.2, SVR elevated, BP < 90 | LVEF may be high, normal or depressed, depending on extent of infarction | Vasodilators and inotropes, IABP, prompt MVR | Surgical mortality 30–40%, medical mortality 80% |
| Acute ventricular septal rupture | Shock syndrome, rales, S₃, holosystolic murmur at LLSB, thrill in 50% | BP < 90 O₂ "step-up" from RA to RV or PA | L to R shunts, by first-pass RVG, LVEF, and RVEF are variable. 2D echocardiography should visualize defect; Doppler confirms shunt | Vasodilators & inotropes, IABP Early VSD closure | Surgical mortality 40–50%, medical mortality 80–85%, outlook better with anterior MI |

*Abbreviations:* PCW = pulmonary capillary wedge pressure; CI = cardiac index (L/min/m²); SVR = systemic vascular resistance; BP = blood pressure; LVEF = left ventricular ejection fraction; RVEF = right ventricular ejection fraction; LV = left ventricle; RV = right ventricle; RA = right atrium; IABP = intra-aortic balloon pump; PA = pulmonary artery; JVP = jugular venous pressure; PTCA = percutaneous transluminal coronary angioplasty; rt-PA = tissue plasminogen activator; VSD = ventricular septal defect; MVR = mitral valve replacement; LLSB = lower left sternal border; RVG = radionuclide ventriculography; CXR = chest x-ray.

*Adapted from Shah PK, and Swan HJC: Complications of acute myocardial infarction. *In* Parmley W, and Chatterjee K (eds): *Cardiology.* Philadelphia, JB Lippincott, 1988. By permission.

quired in order to maintain adequate mean arterial pressure and coronary perfusion. Agents that have mixed alpha- and beta-adrenergic agonist properties, such as norepinephrine (Levophed) and moderate-to-high doses of dopamine, are particularly useful in this setting. In high doses, both agents can produce severe peripheral vasoconstriction and further impair cardiac output. Agents that have both inotropic and vasodilatory properties, such as dobutamine (Dobutrex) and amrinone (Inocor), may also be useful in the management of cardiogenic shock that has failed to respond to either dopamine or norepinephrine.

Vasodilators are assuming an increasingly important role in the acute management of cardiogenic shock. Many studies have reported hemodynamic improvement in patients who have marked elevation of systemic vascular resistance and pulmonary capillary wedge pressure. Afterload reduction may also benefit patients with shock caused by severe mitral regurgitation or ventricular septal defect. An intravenous vasodilator such as sodium nitroprusside is usually chosen and the dose titrated so that the systemic blood pressure does not fall below 90 mmHg. Vasodilators are not useful when severe hypotension is present but may be used in combination with vasopressor agents in order to balance the positive inotropic effect with an appropriate degree of peripheral vasodilatation. Systemic vascular resistance (SVR) should be calcualted frequently during the administration of these agents to maximize effectiveness.

Some progress has been made over the past decade in reducing the exceedingly high mortality associated with cardiogenic shock. Most approaches aim to decrease the size of the infarct and prevent the development of cardiogenic shock. Even when cardiogenic shock has developed, thrombolytic therapy or primary coronary angioplasty may result in improved left ventricular function and survival. While the impact of prompt reperfusion (less than 4 hours) on the incidence of cardiogenic shock has not been adequately studied, growing numbers of reports have documented the reversal of shock in patients treated with thrombolytic agents. Recent data have suggested that mortality may be decreased in patients treated with successful coronary angioplasty for cardiogenic shock. Short periods of circulatory support, both pharmacologic and mechanical using the intra-aortic balloon pump, may be required despite successful reperfusion until areas of myocardial "stunning" recover sufficiently to support adequate contractile function. Stunned myocardium is potentially viable, but temporarily nonfunctional because of acute ischemia. While the management of cardiogenic shock has improved and mortality has decreased, it is clear that prevention through early reperfusion and limitation of infarct size is far preferable to medical or surgical management once shock has occurred.

## Treatment

### Inotropic Agents

DIGITALIS GLYCOSIDES. While digitalis glycosides are known to increase myocardial contractility and oxygen consumption in hearts of normal size, they may result in a decrease in heart size, wall tension, and myocardial oxygen consumption in patients with heart failure and a dilated heart. Digitalization is relatively ineffective in treating acute heart failure following myocardial infarction, but long-term therapy has recently been convincingly demonstrated to improve exercise capacity in patients with chronic heart failure symptoms. Although the issue remains controversial, ventricular arrhythmias may be worsened by digitalis glycosides, particularly when given during the first 6 to 8 hours after acute infarction, and especially in the setting of hypokalemia, hypothyroidism, advanced age, or hypoxemia. Mortality has been shown to be greater in patients treated with digoxin following infarction, but this finding may be entirely explained by the confounding variables associated with its use, i.e., refractory supraventricular arrhythmias or progressive heart failure. When it is used, it should be administered intravenously at an initial dose of 0.5 mg. Additional doses of 0.25 mg should be given as needed until a total dose of 1.0 to 1.5 mg has been administered over an 18- to 24-hour period. The serum digoxin level should be measured and kept between 1 to 2 ng per ml. Levels greater than 2 ng per ml are frequently associated with digoxin toxicity, although lower levels do not exclude the presence of toxicity when digoxin sensitivity exists, particularly in the elderly or in patients with advanced heart failure.

DOPAMINE. Dopamine represents one of a variety of short-acting intravenous inotropic agents that have proved useful in the management of persistent heart failure and cardiogenic shock (Table 7). Dopamine has a variety of hemodynamic effects mediated through direct stimulation of cardiac beta-1-adrenergic receptors, peripheral alpha-adrenergic receptors, and dopaminergic receptors, as well as through the release of endogenous norepinephrine from sympathetic nerve endings. The type of receptor that is stimulated depends on the dose. At relatively low doses (0.5 to 2.0 $\mu$g per kg per minute), dopaminergic stimulation causes vasodilation of renal, mesenteric, coronary, and cerebral arterioles and increases in blood flow. With doses between 2 and

TABLE 7. **Comparative Effects of Vasodilators and Positive Inotropic Agents in the Treatment of Heart Failure**

| Agent | Drug Class | Dosage | Hemodynamic Effects | | | | Indications | Adverse Effects |
|-------|-----------|--------|------|------|------|------|-------------|-----------------|
| | | | HR | BP | PCW | SVR | | |
| Dopamine (Intropin) | Beta-adrenergic agonist | 2.5–5 μg/kg/min (low dose) | ↑ | ↑ | — | ↓ | Oliguria, borderline hypotension | Cardiac arrhythmias, tachycardia |
| | | 5–20 μg/kg/min (high dose) | ↑↑ | ↑↑ | ↑ | ↑ | Hypotension | Limb ischemia in patients with peripheral vascular disease, myocardial ischemia |
| Dobutamine (Dobutrex) | Beta-adrenergic agonist | 5–15 μ/kg/min | —↑ | —↓ | ↓↓ | ↓↓ | Refractory heart failure, low cardiac output | Cardiac arrhythmias, myocardial ischemia |
| Amrinone (Inocor) | Phosphodiesterase inhibitor | 0.75–1.5 mg/kg bolus 5–10 μg/kg/min maintenance infusion | —↑ | —↓ | ↓↓ | ↓↓ | Low cardiac output, refractory heart failure | Nausea, vomiting, diarrhea, thrombocytopenia (2%), increased ventricular ectopy, liver function test abnormalities |
| Nitroglycerin, intravenous | Smooth muscle relaxant | 25–1000 μg/min | —↑ | —↓ | ↓↓ | ↓↓ | Preload reduction in heart failure, ongoing myocardial ischemia | Headache, nausea, hypotension, particularly with RV infarction or hypovolemia, methemoglobinemia |
| Nitroprusside (Nipride) | Smooth muscle relaxant | 10–500 μg/min | —↑ | ↓ | ↓↓ | ↓↓↓ | Pulmonary edema with normal or hypertensive blood pressure, refractory heart failure, and low output in conjunction with dobutamine | Thiosulfate toxicity, intrapulmonary shunting, excessive hypotension |
| Captopril (oral) (Capoten) | Converting enzyme inhibitor | 6.75–50 mg | — | ↓— | ↓↓ | ↓↓ | Chronic low-output failure | Hypotension, proteinuria, skin rash, dysgeusia, deterioration in renal function |
| Enalapril (oral) (Vasotec) | Converting enzyme inhibitor | 2.5–20 mg qd | — | ↓— | ↓↓ | ↓↓ | Chronic low-output failure | Hypotension, angioedema, hyperkalemia |

5 μg per kg per minute, an increase in stroke volume and cardiac output mediated by stimulation of beta-1 receptors as well as peripheral vasodilation may be observed. At higher doses (5 to 20 μg per kg per minute), alpha-adrenergic vasoconstriction is observed. While helpful in supporting systemic blood pressure, vasoconstric-tion may cause tissue hypoxemia as well as elevation of the left ventricular filling pressure as a result of excessive afterload. Ventricular and supraventricular arrhythmias may occur when doses exceed 10 μg per kg per minute. It should be recognized that there is marked individual variation in dose response to this agent, and it is

essential that the lowest dose that produces optimal hemodynamics and clinical response be chosen.

DOBUTAMINE. Dobutamine is a synthetic catecholamine which is principally a beta-adrenergic agonist, produces minimal alpha-adrenergic stimulation, and does not cause the release of endogenous norepinephrine. It has potent positive inotropic and chronotropic effects but does not produce significant vasoconstriction even at high doses. It does not alter renal blood flow but does cause redistribution of mesenteric and renal blood flow in favor of coronary and skeletal vascular beds. Dose-related increases in stroke volume and cardiac output and decreases in left ventricular filling pressure may be seen in patients with acute and chronic heart failure. Several studies have demonstrated that dobutamine is preferable to dopamine in the treatment of patients with severe refractory heart failure owing to its favorable effects on pulmonary capillary wedge pressure and its properties as a vasodilator. While equivalent doses of dobutamine produce fewer arrhythmias and less tachycardia than dopamine, the lack of alpha-adrenergic stimulation makes this agent ineffective as a vasopressor and inappropriate as the sole treatment for systemic hypotension. Dobutamine should be administered beginning at 2.5 μg per kg per minute and the dose increased under close hemodynamic monitoring until cardiac output and pulmonary capillary wedge pressure improve. The dose should be reduced if systolic blood pressure exceeds 110 to 120 mmHg, the heart rate exceeds 110 beats per minute, arrhythmias appear, or ST segment monitoring documents further ischemia. The combination of dobutamine and dopamine has been useful in the management of patients with cardiogenic shock. Moderate doses of both agents have been shown to maintain arterial blood pressure better, with fewer deleterious effects on pulmonary capillary wedge pressure, than higher doses of either agent alone.

NOREPINEPHRINE (LEVOPHED). Norepinephrine is a potent alpha-adrenergic agonist which produces arteriolar and venous constriction. It has relatively modest beta-adrenergic agonist properties. It may be useful in transiently maintaining adequate arterial pressure in severely hypotensive patients but often results in a decrease in cardiac output and a decline in blood flow to peripheral tissues, especially during long-term use. It is particularly useful in the treatment of conditions associated with excessive vasodilation, particularly anaphylaxis and sepsis with high cardiac output. In patients with cardiogenic shock, it is useful when systemic arterial pressure is below 80 mmHg and the systemic vascular resistance is normal ($1200$ dyne-sec-cm$^{-5}$) or reduced. Dopamine is usually a better first choice, but its use may be limited by excessive tachycardia. Norepinephrine is particularly useful when combined with direct-acting vasodilators such as low intravenous doses of nitroglycerin or sodium nitroprusside. We prefer this approach because combination therapy tends to avoid excessive peripheral vasoconstriction and may lead to a decrease in left ventricular filling pressure. Norepinephrine is usually begun at a low infusion rate (1 to 4 μg per kg per minute) and increased to achieve optimal hemodynamic effects. Excessive peripheral vasoconstriction or arrhythmias often limit its use.

AMRINONE. Amrinone, like aminophylline, is a phosphodiesterase inhibitor. Amrinone is relatively specific for Type III phosphodiesterase, which is found in cardiac and vascular smooth muscle. It has powerful positive inotropic properties but is also a potent vasodilator with balanced effects on preload and afterload. It increases cardiac output, reduces left ventricular filling pressure, and decreases systemic vascular resistance, and it is particularly useful in patients with refractory heart failure. Amrinone is not a vasopressor; blood pressure is usually unaffected but may fall. In patients in whom preload falls dramatically, frank hypotension may occur, which may be treated by decreasing the dose or replacing volume. Amrinone is more effective than either dopamine or dobutamine in lowering pulmonary capillary wedge pressure and is intermediate between nitroprusside and dobutamine in its effects as a vasodilator and inotropic agent. Therapy should be initiated with a bolus of 0.75 mg per kg followed by an infusion of 5 to 10 μg per kg per minute. An additional bolus of 0.75 mg per kg may be given 15 to 30 minutes after the first in order to achieve maximum hemodynamic effects. A maximal dose of 18 mg per 24 hours is recommended. Ventricular arrhythmias are frequently exacerbated.

**Vasodilators.** Vasodilator therapy plays an important role in the management of patients whose infarction has been complicated by persistent heart failure, hypertension, or mechanical complications. Agents vary in their ability to reduce preload through venodilation and afterload through arteriolar dilation. Reduction of afterload results in improvement in forward stroke volume and cardiac output, while reduction of preload leads to decreases in pulmonary capillary wedge and right atrial pressures. By improving cardiac performance, vasodilators decrease myocardial oxygen demand, decrease heart size, and favorably improve subendocardial blood flow. Careful hemodynamic monitoring is essential when vasodilator therapy is instituted early after myocardial infarction to prevent hypotension. Vasodilators alone or in combination with intra-aortic balloon counterpulsation may help to provide the hemodynamic stability necessary to undertake cardiac catheterization in patients with mechanical complications and prepare the patient for surgical intervention. The rapidly changing hemodynamics during acute infarction requires that therapy be initiated with agents that can be administered intravenously, have a rapid onset of action (1 to 2 minutes), and have a short half-life (2 to 4 minutes). Nitroglycerin and sodium nitroprusside are the drugs of choice.

NITROGLYCERIN. Nitroglycerin is a rapidly acting vasodilator whose principal hemodynamic benefit is preload reduction through venodilation. At high intravenous doses, it also decreases afterload. Arteriolar dilation with nitroglycerin depends critically on preload, since the observed decreases in afterload diminish as pulmonary capillary wedge pressure falls. Nitroglycerin administered by the intravenous route is preferred by many clinicians in the setting of acute infarction and heart failure because of its potent anti-ischemic effects and its ability to reduce the size of the infarct. The drug has also been shown in experimental studies to limit "coronary steal," i.e., the diversion of blood flow from ischemic to nonischemic myocardium, which occurs to a greater degree with nitroprusside. The intravenous infusion of nitroglycerin should begin at 20 μg per minute and the dose increased by increments of 10 to 20 μg per minute every 5 minutes until the desired effect (either improvement in hemodynamics or relief of ischemic chest pain) has occurred or there has been a decline in arterial blood pressure to unacceptable limits. Adverse effects of nitroglycerin are listed in Table 7. Paradoxical bradycardia has also been reported but is usually responsive to atropine. Tachyphylaxis may develop during prolonged infusion.

SODIUM NITROPRUSSIDE (NIPRIDE). Sodium nitroprusside produces rapid, balanced vasodilation of both arterioles and venules. Sodium nitroprusside has been studied more than any other vasodilator during acute myocardial infarction and is helpful in the management of severe heart failure with or without cardiogenic shock. Its beneficial effects are most pronounced in patients with marked elevation of filling pressures and in those with either mitral regurgitation or ventricular septal rupture. Hemodynamic benefits include a decrease in systemic vascular resistance, pulmonary capillary wedge pressure, myocardial oxygen consumption, and improvement in left ventricular ejection fraction. Nitroprusside may improve cardiac output in patients with cardiogenic shock provided that the diastolic blood pressure and coronary perfusion pressure are

maintained—either through the concomitant use of inotropic agents, particularly dobutamine, or mechanical circulatory support. Therapy should begin with a low dose (10 to 20 μg per minute) and the dose increased every 5 to 10 minutes to a total dose of 15 μg per kg per minute. The dose should be titrated to achieve a fall in pulmonary capillary wedge pressure to 15 to 18 mmHg, but the systolic arterial pressure should generally not be permitted to drop below 90 mmHg. Adverse effects of nitroprusside therapy are listed in Table 7.

ORAL VASODILATORS. A variety of oral vasodilators are available for the treatment of patients with persistent heart failure following myocardial infarction. Oral and transdermal nitrates are useful in producing venodilation and are effective in patients with very high filling pressures and low cardiac output. They reduce pulmonary capillary wedge pressure without reducing cardiac output. Nitrate tolerance has become increasingly recognized in patients with angina pectoris and probably also occurs in patients with congestive heart failure. A drug-free period of at least 6 to 8 hours daily should be employed when nitrate preparations are used on a long-term basis.

While short-term therapy with hydralazine (Apresoline) or prazosin (Minipress) may be useful, tolerance is also a major problem with these two agents, and sustained improvement in functional capacity is uncommon with their use. It is our current recommendation to employ instead angiotensin-converting enzyme inhibitors for the treatment of chronic heart failure. Captopril (Capoten), enalapril (Vasotec), and lisinopril (Prinivil) have been extensively studied, reduce both preload and afterload, and have been shown effective in the long-term management of heart failure. We initiate therapy with captopril using a very small dose (6.25 mg twice daily) and titrate the dose upward on the basis of the patient's blood pressure. Orthostatic hypotension is particularly common in patients with impaired ventricular function and must be sought through frequent monitoring of orthostatic vital signs. The role of converting enzyme inhibitors in the prevention of left ventricular dilation late after myocardial infarction is currently being studied.

**Intra-aortic Balloon Counterpulsation.** Intra-aortic balloon counterpulsation has proved to be an effective temporizing measure in the management of cardiogenic shock. Phased balloon pulsation is synchronized with the electrocardiogram and the balloon is inflated at the time of aortic valve closure to produce augmentation of the diastolic pressure, while deflation occurs just before the onset of systole to produce systolic unloading. A 10 to 20% increase in cardiac output is generally achieved while the augmentation in diastolic coronary blood flow often results in improvement in myocardial ischemia.

The principal uses for intra-aortic balloon counterpulsation are as follows: (1) Temporary support for patients with cardiogenic shock that is unresponsive to medical management. (2) Short-term stabilization of patients in preparation for diagnostic studies such as cardiac catheterization or correction of mechanical lesions, including mitral regurgitation or ventricular septal rupture. (3) Stabilization of patients who have extensive areas of jeopardized myocardium that are nonfunctional but still viable before coronary revascularization. (4) Treatment of persistent myocardial ischemia that has failed to respond to medical therapy. (5) Refractory recurrent ventricular tachycardia. Counterpulsation unfortunately does not improve overall mortality in patients with cardiogenic shock unless a surgically correctable mechanical lesion is present or revascularization can be performed. We recommend this procedure for relatively young patients in cardiogenic shock who are free from peripheral vascular disease or aortic regurgitation and who have failed to show hemodynamic improvement following a short-term (30 to 120 minutes) trial of vasodilator and inotropic pharmacologic support. Early cardiac catheterization and surgical intervention is advised whenever possible.

Complications of intra-aortic balloon pumping may occur in up to 25% of patients using either the percutaneous or surgical insertion technique. These include limb or abdominal ischemia, damage to the femoral or iliac arteries, and aortic dissection. Infection is a risk when the device remains in place for a prolonged period of time, as are hemolysis, thrombocytopenia, and embolization. We treat all patients with heparin intravenously. Antibiotic treatment with a cephalosporin is given while the balloon is in place.

### Right Ventricular Infarction

Infarction of the free wall of the right ventricle may occur in as many as 30 to 40% of patients with acute inferior or posterior myocardial infarction but produces important hemodynamic abnormalities in only about 5% of patients. The clinical triad of findings that suggest right ventricular infarction are an acute inferior infarction, elevation of the jugular venous pressure (greater than 7 cm $H_2O$), clear lung fields, and hypotension. A Kussmaul's sign (an inspiratory fall of greater than 10 mm in systemic blood pressure) with little evidence for pulmonary congestion is present in approximately 70% of cases. The electrocardiogram, in addition to acute inferior-wall injury, will often show ST segment elevation in the right precordial leads ($V_{3R}$ or $V_{4R}$).

Whenever right ventricular infarction is suspected, the diagnosis should be confirmed by right heart catheterization, which typically shows elevation of right atrial and right ventricular end-diastolic pressures with little elevation in right ventricular systolic pressure. The pulmonary capillary wedge pressure is usually normal, or only slightly elevated, because the extent of the left ventricular damage is often not severe. Other hemodynamic findings may include a steep right atrial Y descent, a dip-and-plateau pattern during diastolic filling in the right ventricular pressure tracing, and a diminished pulse pressure in the pulmonary artery. These hemodynamic abnormalities may suggest the presence of pericardial tamponade, constrictive pericarditis, or acute massive pulmonary thromboembolism. Noninvasive assessment of right ventricular function (with use of gated blood pool imaging or echocardiography) may be helpful in differentiating these entities. In approximately 25% of patients, right atrial pressures may be near normal initially and become elevated only later in the course of the infarction or following volume infusion.

The hypotension observed with right ventricular infarction is usually caused by inadequate left ventricular filling resulting from right ventricular dysfunction. Volume expansion with crystalloid or colloid, often requiring 2 to 5 liters within 24 hours, is the initial treatment and serves to increase right ventricular preload and cardiac output. Frequently, volume expansion alone does not adequately correct the hypotension and inotropic support using dopamine or dobutamine may be required. Bradyarrhythmias and atrioventricular block are commonly observed and may further worsen the cardiac output through the loss of atrial contraction. With appropriate and aggressive therapy, survival rates in excess of 80% can be expected.

## MECHANICAL COMPLICATIONS FOLLOWING ACUTE MYOCARDIAL INFARCTION

### Acute Mitral Regurgitation

Acute mitral regurgitation may occur because of transient papillary muscle dysfunction secondary to myocardial ischemia or from rupture of the papillary muscle itself. Less commonly, rupture of one or more of the 120 chordae tendineae may occur. While the anterolateral papillary muscle receives a dual blood supply from the left anterior descending and circumflex arteries, the posteromedial papillary muscle has less reliable perfusion from the posterior descending branch of the dominant coronary artery. Consequently, dysfunction or rupture of the posteromedial papillary muscle (in association with an inferoposterior infarction) is approximately five times more common than dysfunction of the anterolateral papillary muscle.

The diagnosis of papillary muscle dysfunction may be made by physical examination or hemodynamic findings. Typically, a new systolic apical murmur is present and may be intermittent or persistent. Large V waves are seen on the pulmonary capillary wedge pressure tracing. Intermittent pulmonary edema, hypotension, or frank shock may occur rapidly and resolve quickly during periods of papillary muscle ischemia. Therapy of papillary muscle dysfunction includes anti-ischemic medications, such as intravenous nitroglycerin, beta blockers, or calcium channel blockers. In addition, the coronary anatomy should be defined through early catheterization when hemodynamically significant mitral regurgitation is present. Intravenous vasodilators or circulatory support using intra-aortic balloon counterpulsation may also be of use.

Partial or complete rupture of a papillary muscle is a rare complication occurring in approximately 1% of patients. Rupture typically occurs between 3 and 7 days after transmural infarction but occurs in up to 20% of cases within 24 hours. Unlike ventricular septal rupture, which is seen with extensive transmural infarctions, papillary muscle rupture may occur with a relatively small or subendocardial infarction, and the extent of coronary artery disease may be modest. The sudden onset of severe pulmonary congestion and a loud holosystolic apical murmur characterize the initial presentation. Pulmonary edema, hypotension, and frank cardiogenic shock often ensue, and 70% of patients will succumb within 24 hours if appropriate stabilization cannot be achieved. Occasionally, the systolic murmur may be brief, or even completely absent, when the cardiac output is markedly depressed.

Although it is often difficult to differentiate clinically acute mitral regurgitation from acute ventricular septal rupture, prompt right heart catheterization will establish the correct diagnosis and permit hemodynamic monitoring during pharmacologic therapy (see Table 6). Two-dimensional echocardiography should be promptly undertaken because it will frequently visualize a flail mitral leaflet. The presence of severe mitral regurgitation can be confirmed by Doppler study. Medical therapy has little role in the management of papillary muscle rupture other than temporary support until surgery can be undertaken. Intra-aortic balloon counterpulsation should be promptly initiated and diuretic, vaso-

dilator, and inotropic support administered. Early mitral valve replacement is successful in up to 60 to 70% of patients.

### Rupture of the Interventricular Septum

Rupture of the interventricular septum is a rare complication that generally occurs 3 to 5 days after infarction but may occur as early as 24 hours or as late as 2 weeks. Septal rupture appears to be slightly more common in anterior and anterolateral than inferior infarctions. Multivessel coronary artery disease is present in virtually all patients.

The most prominent physical finding of acute septal rupture is a new, harsh, loud holosystolic murmur, with palpable thrill in approximately 50% of cases. Findings of right ventricular volume overload, including tricuspid regurgitation, moderate to marked elevation of the jugular venous pressure, and a right ventricular heave, help to differentiate this condition from acute mitral regurgitation. Right heart catheterization should be performed as quickly as possible to confirm the diagnosis and define the magnitude of the left-to-right shunt. An oxygen "step-up" of greater than 10% from the right atrium to the right ventricle or the proximal pulmonary artery confirms the diagnosis.

Medical management of acute septal rupture should be instituted before definitive surgical repair. The mortality of patients not undergoing repair approaches 50% at 1 week and 80% by 8 weeks. Intra-aortic balloon counterpulsation should be undertaken immediately after confirmation of the diagnosis to stabilize the patient. Vasodilator therapy using nitroprusside is often effective but generally cannot be used before intra-aortic balloon pump insertion because of the presence of systemic hypotension. Whenever possible, cardiac catheterization should be performed to define the coronary anatomy, identify coexisting mitral valve disease, and assess ventricular function. Aggressive surgical treatment may result in a 50 to 75% short-term survival as long as cardiogenic shock and pulmonary or renal dysfunction are absent.

### Rupture of the Free Wall of the Left Ventricle

Rupture of the free wall of the infarcted ventricle occurs in approximately 10% of inpatient deaths following acute myocardial infarction. Transmural infarction is almost always present, and the infarct-related artery is totally occluded with little collateral circulation. Rupture of the free wall is most frequently seen in elderly patients with hypertension. The peak incidence is between days 3 and 8, but rupture may occur within 24 hours or as late as 3 weeks. Early ambulation, anti-inflammatory drugs, such as corticosteroids or indomethacin (Indocin), and anticoagulant therapy are suspected, but unproved, contributors to cardiac rupture.

Cardiac rupture usually presents with the development of sudden, profound right heart failure and shock, which rapidly proceeds to electromechanical dissociation. Most patients will experience tearing chest pain. Survival, which is unusual, depends on prompt recognition of this complication, urgent hemodynamic stabilization, and most important, immediate surgical repair. Pericardiocentesis may provide temporary relief of cardiac tamponade.

### Left Ventricular Aneurysm

A ventricular aneurysm is a circumscribed, noncontractile, outpouching of the left ventricle, which is composed of fibrous tissue as well as necrotic myocytes. Aneurysms have been reported to develop in 10 to 38% of transmural myocardial infarctions and are most frequently observed after anterior infarction when there is persistent total occlusion of the infarct-related artery and few collateral blood vessels. Early exercise may also contribute to aneurysm formation. The diagnosis should be suspected in patients with severe refractory heart failure, recurrent ventricular tachyarrhythmias, a dyskinetic displaced left ventricular impulse on physical examination, persistent ST segment elevations in an area of old infarction, or an abnormal bulge of the cardiac silhouette on chest film. Two-dimensional echocardiography or radionuclide ventriculography serves to confirm the diagnosis.

Surgical aneurysmectomy is the treatment of choice but should be reserved for those patients in whom medical management has been unable to control symptoms. A successful outcome depends upon the preservation of contractile function in the nonaneurysmal portion of the ventricle. Surgical aneurysmectomy, usually combined with coronary revascularization, may result in considerable functional improvement in carefully selected patients.

### RISK STRATIFICATION AFTER ACUTE MYOCARDIAL INFARCTION

The principal goal of risk stratification after acute infarction is the formulation of a specific management strategy for the individual patient. A low-risk status implies a risk of cardiac death of approximately 2% during the first year after discharge from the hospital with a small probability of recurrent infarction or new onset angina. Patients who are in the lowest risk category require few medications other than aspirin (300 mg orally daily) and prophylactic nitroglycerin and should be candidates for early return to work and normal physical activities. In contrast, patients in the intermediate or high risk categories, as will be defined subsequently, require more aggressive medical management and will frequently need invasive evaluation to determine the coronary anatomy and ventricular function.

The initial assessment of risk begins with the determination of whether the patient's clinical course has been complicated or uncomplicated. Approximately 15 to 30% of patients will experience congestive heart failure, ventricular arrhythmias, or postinfarction angina while they are in the hospital. These patients should be considered "high risk" on the basis of these clinical predictors. However, 70 to 85% of patients will have an uncomplicated hospitalization and should undergo further diagnostic studies before discharge to determine their risk for subsequent cardiac events.

Three characteristics have been clearly identified as predictors of increased risk during the first year following infarction: myocardial ischemia, which may be either symptomatic or silent and may occur at rest or during exercise; depression of left ventricular ejection fraction; and ventricular arrhythmias that persist beyond the initial 12 to 24 hours. Each has been identified as an independent risk factor for morbidity and mortality. Myocardial ischemia and impaired ventricular function are stronger predictors of subsequent mortality than ventricular arrhythmias.

Survival after hospital discharge is related to the presence or absence of myocardial ischemia, the frequency and magnitude of the ischemia, and the extent of underlying coronary artery disease. Accumulating evidence suggests that silent and symptomatic ischemia have a similar physiologic basis and similar prognosis. Inducible ischemia in the presence of multivessel disease has been shown to have a poorer prognosis than ischemia associated with single-vessel disease. This is not surprising since patients with multivessel disease have a higher rate of cardiac events in the first year than patients with single-vessel disease, regardless of left ventricular ejection fraction or other variables.

The value of a submaximal ("low level") exercise test before discharge in patients with uncomplicated myocardial infarction has been studied extensively over the past 15 years. Both the safety and predictive value of such testing have been conclusively demonstrated. Most clinical studies indicate that patients who demonstrate .1 mV or more ST-segment depression (either silent or with angina pectoris) during low-level exercise testing have a higher incidence of reinfarction, unstable angina, and cardiac death during the next year as compared with patients who have been able to perform at least 4 METS of exercise without ST segment depression. Although there is general agreement that ST segment depression during testing predicts a poorer prognosis, the importance of the degree of ST segment depression remains uncertain. Other predictors of high risk include a low exercise capacity, the failure of systolic blood pressure to rise during exercise, ischemic ST segment depression in leads beyond the infarct zone, and ventricular ectopy during exercise or in the recovery phase. Myocardial imaging with thallium[201] is frequently performed in conjunction with low-level exercise testing in order to enhance the sensitivity and specificity of the test. This technique is particularly useful in patients with preexisting electrocardiographic abnormalities such as left bundle branch block or left ventricular hypertrophy, in patients receiving antiarrhythmic agents or digitalis, and in patients with repolarization abnormalities on the ECG in areas beyond the area of acute infarction. In patients who are unable to exercise, thallium scintigraphy following dipyridamole (Persantine) administration may be useful in detecting ischemia. Patients whose thallium scan identifies perfusion defects in more than one region of the heart, delayed redistribution within or remote from the infarct itself, or abnormal uptake of radioisotope by the lungs on predischarge testing should be considered at risk for sudden death, recurrent infarction, and unstable angina during the next year. Patients who demonstrate myocardial ischemia beyond the original infarcted area or evidence for reversible ischemia in addition to fixed scarring in an infarcted area, particularly a subendocardial infarct, should undergo coronary arteriography. Those patients in whom no myocardial ischemia is detected on low-level exercise testing should undergo maximal exercise testing in 6 to 8 weeks in order to determine their need for antiischemic medications.

In addition to determining whether myocardial ischemia is present, a predischarge exercise test is helpful in documenting the ischemic threshold—i.e., the product of heart rate and blood pressure or workload at which ischemia is seen. Those patients with evidence for ischemia at a low workload or heart rate, or who demonstrate hemodynamic instability, such as a fall in blood pressure during exercise testing, should also undergo coronary arteriography to determine the extent of coronary artery disease. Routine coronary angiography is not indicated for every patient following uncomplicated infarction, regardless of whether thrombolytic therapy has been employed. Several studies have demonstrated that the angiographic severity of coronary stenoses was inadequate to predict the timing or location of a subsequent coronary occlusion. Thus, functional assessment of ischemic threshold is more predictive of future events than anatomic definition.

Ambulatory (Holter) monitoring has been used increasingly for the detection of silent myocardial ischemia following infarction. To date, only limited evidence has substantiated the prognostic utility of detecting silent ischemia by Holter monitoring in asymptomatic postinfarction patients. Ischemia detected by Holter monitoring will usually also be detected during exercise testing, particularly if thallium scintigraphy is employed. Only those patients in whom ischemia is observed at a low workload during exercise testing will have evidence for frequent and prolonged episodes of ischemia during Holter monitoring. Furthermore, silent ischemia detected by Holter monitoring is rarely observed when none can be produced during exercise testing. Therefore, low level exercise testing appears superior to Holter monitoring for predischarge evaluation and management of both painful and silent myocardial ischemia.

The left ventricular ejection fraction measured with the patient at rest is the single best predictor of outcome following acute myocardial infarction. The ejection fraction can be measured noninvasively by radionuclide ventriculography or two-dimensional echocardiography. Not all patients, however, need necessarily undergo such studies. Assessment of ventricular function is indicated in patients with persistent signs of heart failure on physical examination or chest x-ray, those in whom frequent premature ventricular beats are seen, patients with marked limitation of exercise capacity or a fall in blood pressure or ischemic response during low-level exercise testing, or those with a large infarct in whom beta-blocker therapy is being considered. In patients whose ejection fraction is between 25 and 45%, coronary arteriography should be performed if myocardial ischemia has been demonstrated, since these patients can ill afford to lose any remaining functional myocardium. Therapy with a converting-enzyme inhibitor should also be considered, regardless of the presence or absence of symptoms, in the light of the growing body of knowledge suggesting that these agents may decrease the likelihood of subsequent aneurysm formation and cardiac dilatation.

Studies have indicated that frequent or complex premature ventricular beats, occurring either at rest or during exercise, are independent risk factors for sudden death. The precise definition of what constitutes "complex" rhythm disturbances remains uncertain. Ventricular arrhythmias remain a particularly ominous finding when left ventricular dysfunction or myocardial ischemia is also present after infarction. Given the random variability of ventricular ectopy, the unproved benefits of successful suppression of ventricular arrhythmias in the postinfarction setting, and the known proarrhythmic effects of all currently available antiarrhythmic agents, routine Holter monitoring is not indicated for all postinfarction patients. It should be undertaken in those patients with a left ventricular ejection fraction below 40%, those with evidence for myocardial ischemia or ventricular ectopy during low-level exercise testing, and those with complex ventricular ectopy during the late phase of hospitalization.

The treatment of complex ventricular ectopy remains controversial. The routine use of antiarrhythmic agents for suppression of frequent unifocal premature ventricular beats or couplets following infarction is not supported by recent studies and may, in fact, contribute to a higher incidence of sudden death. Patients who demonstrate sustained or recurrent nonsustained ventricular tachycardia should usually receive antiarrhythmic therapy. Invasive electrophysiologic testing is usually not warranted when adequate suppression of nonsustained ventricular tachycardia can be documented by ambulatory electrocardiographic monitoring. However, those patients with symptomatic ectopy or ventricular arrhythmias that persist despite antiarrhythmic therapy may benefit from electrophysiologic testing. This issue remains undecided, and management must be individualized for each patient. In those patients with persistent complex ventricular arrhythmias and adequate left ventricular function, exercise testing should be undertaken to determine the presence and extent of reversible myocardial ischemia. When myocardial ischemia can be documented, coronary arteriography should be performed because coronary revascularization may result in improved survival and aid in the suppression of the arrhythmia.

## PREVENTION OF SECOND OCCURRENCE AFTER ACUTE MYOCARDIAL INFARCTION

Prevention of a second infarction and other cardiovascular events in patients who have had a first infarction has been the subject of considerable research. Both changes in lifestyle and treatment with a variety of drugs have been investigated as possible preventive measures.

The evidence is compelling that cessation of cigarette smoking promptly (within 1 to 2 years) reduces the risk of a second myocardial infarction almost to that of nonsmokers. Above all else, the physician should therefore strongly encourage current smokers who have had a first infarction to quit. Although controversy on the matter continues, patients whose blood cholesterol level is above 200 mg per dl, especially when the high-density lipoprotein level is below 40 mg per dl, are best advised to follow a cholesterol-lowering diet. The blood cholesterol level should not be measured until 4 to 6 weeks after infarction because the measurement may be spuriously low in the setting of the acute illness. If a 3- to 6-month trial of dietary therapy is not effective in reducing the blood cholesterol level below 200 mg per dl, drug therapy might be considered. Because of its efficacy and relative lack of side effects, lovastatin (Mevacor) is emerging as one of the drugs of choice. The daily dose is 20 to 80 mg orally, depending on the degree of hypercholesterolemia and the specific response to therapy. One caveat about the use of this drug is that its long-term side effects are not yet known with certainty. In addition, it is not known if lovastatin lowers cardiovascular morbidity or mortality.

Many physicians recommend that their patients engage in a structured program of physical activity after myocardial infarction, and the evidence suggests that regular exercise of a low to moderate level may prevent recurrent infarction and improve survival. Such programs should be undertaken only after the patient has completed a graded exercise test and a safe level of exercise has been defined. Walking, easy jogging, and bicycling, alone or in combination, are convenient forms of aerobic exercise for postinfarction patients. Recent evidence suggests that a program of regular exercise instituted early after a moderate or large anterior myocardial infarction may actually be harmful, by promoting expansion of the infarct and dilation of the left ventricle. An exercise program should probably be deferred in such patients.

Hypertension after acute infarction should receive appropriate drug and dietary treatment. It is worthy of note that blood pressure in hypertensive patients often decreases during hospitalization only to increase again after discharge.

Among the many drugs that have been studied for efficacy in secondary prevention after myocardial infarction, beta-adrenergic receptor blockers and antiplatelet agents have received the most attention. On the basis of a large body of evidence, many physicians choose to treat all patients after infarction with a beta-receptor blocker, usually propranolol, 20 to 80 mg orally two or three times daily, or metoprolol, 50 to 100 mg orally twice daily. Other physicians prefer to reserve beta-blocker therapy for patients at higher risk, such as those who have multivessel coronary disease or evidence of myocardial ischemia. Our practice is to treat all postinfarction patients who do not have contraindications to the use of beta-adrenergic blockers. We favor this approach in part because of recent studies showing that beta-blocker therapy is cost effective for patients at all levels of risk. However the physician must be cognizant of the various troublesome side effects of beta-receptor blocking agents.

Individual studies of antiplatelet therapy after myocardial infarction have produced mixed results. Nevertheless, a recent meta-analysis of 25 studies involving 29,000 patients suggests that antiplatelet therapy may reduce the incidence of subsequent vascular events after infarction. Aspirin is the agent of choice, but the most effective dose remains in doubt. In the absence of definitive information, we use 325 mg daily or every other day, depending on the patient's ability to tolerate the drug. We do not routinely administer dipyridamole with aspirin because of lack of evidence of an additive effect.

# REHABILITATION AFTER MYOCARDIAL INFARCTION

method of
NANETTE K. WENGER, M.D.
*Emory University School of Medicine*
*Atlanta, Georgia*

Conventional medical and surgical therapies for the patient with myocardial infarction are undertaken to decrease symptoms, restore and enhance functional status, and improve prognosis. A combination of medical, psychosocial, and behavioral factors appears to determine the extent of recovery. Rehabilitative services are increasingly incorporated into traditional medical care; these interventions are designed to limit the adverse physiologic and psychologic consequences of the acute illness and improve long-term physical, emotional, and vocational function. About 20% of the 850,000 annual survivors of myocardial infarction in the United States have some physiologic, psychosocial, or vocational disability. The major components of coronary rehabilitation include physical activity (early ambulation during hospitalization and prescriptive exercise training in the ambulatory care phase of the illness) and the provision of information and counseling designed to reduce coronary risk factors and to enhance resumption of a productive, active, and satisfying life. A position statement of the American College of Cardiology defines cardiovascular rehabilitation as "those exercise and counseling services which will reduce symptoms or improve cardiac function."

Rehabilitative care ideally begins at the onset of illness and remains a component of the long-term management of the patient. This concept highlights the responsibility of the primary physician to initiate, coordinate, and encourage rehabilitation of the patient with myocardial infarction.

The rehabilitative approach to care is aimed at reducing the physical and psychosocial invalidism associated with coronary disease. Important aspects in the rehabilitation of patients with myocardial infarction involve the behaviors and capacities to favorably alter lifestyles. The acquisition of personal skills, techniques, attitudes, and knowledge derived from participating in physical activity and educational and counseling regimens can enhance the patient's realistic adaptation to illness and ability to cope with challenges and problems in the family, workplace, and community.

## THE ACUTE PHASE: REHABILITATIVE CARE

The current abbreviated hospital stay, particularly for patients with uncomplicated myocardial infarction, has accentuated the need for early ambulation but has limited the ability to provide adequate information and counseling to the coronary patient and interested family members.

### Early Ambulation

A goal of early ambulation is to avert the deleterious consequences of protracted bedrest. The most prominent of these is a decrease in physical work capacity as much as 25% following 2 to 3 weeks of immobilization, because of a decrease in maximal cardiac output. Orthostatic hypotension and reflex tachycardia are manifestations of the hypovolemia (a decrease of 700 to 800 ml in circulating blood volume) that may be evident after 7 to 10 days of bedrest. Blood viscosity increases, owing to a greater contraction of plasma volume than of red blood cell mass. This, coupled with circulatory stasis, predisposes the patient at bedrest to thromboembolic complications. Pulmonary ventilation also decreases, as do systemic muscle mass and muscular contractile strength. Inefficient muscular contraction increases the oxygen requirement for any submaximal task.

Most patients without complications of myocardial infarction (recurrent ischemic chest pain, serious cardiac rhythm disturbances, congestive heart failure, or cardiogenic shock) can safely perform low-intensity physical activity as early as the first day after infarction. Personal care activities, use of a bedside commode, and sitting in a bedside chair are within the 1 to 2 met level appropriate for coronary care unit activities (1 met = approximately 3.5 ml $O_2$ per kg body weight per minute). Sitting in a chair two or three times daily is within the physical capability of most patients; this orthostatic challenge rather than the activity intensity, seems adequate to prevent the hypovolemia, deterioration of oxygen transport capacity, and effort intolerance of immobilization at bedrest. Patients with complications of infarction should delay initiation of physical activity until the complications are controlled and their clinical status is stable.

The current early intensive, invasive management of many patients with acute myocardial infarction, using combinations of thrombolytic therapy, coronary angioplasty, or coronary bypass surgery, is designed to salvage myocardium. The relative immobilization attendant on these procedures may evoke the unwanted manifestations of prolonged bedrest.

During the remainder of the hospital stay, progressive physical activity is designed to attain a functional level that permits usual household activities (an energy expenditure of 2 to 3 mets) to be undertaken by the time of discharge from the hospital. To accomplish this, patients perform dynamic range-of-motion warm-up exercises and progressively increase their pace and distance of walking. If stair-climbing is required at home, patients should practice this before leaving the hospital. Electrocardiographic monitoring or telemetry during early ambulation activities is required only for selected patients, such as those with high grade cardiac rhythm disturbances or asymptomatic myocardial ischemia. Supervision of early ambulation activities, however, is desirable to detect adverse responses. These may include the development of chest pain, dyspnea, undue fatigue, or palpitations; a heart rate in excess of 120 or below 50 beats per minute (for patients receiving beta-blocking drugs, heart rate increase should not exceed 20 beats per minute above resting level); the occurrence of arrhythmias; ST segment displacement compatible with ischemia; or a fall in systolic blood pressure, which usually reflects ischemic ventricular dysfunction with inadequacy of the cardiac output to meet the demand. Antihypertensive therapy should be considered when systolic blood pressure exceeds 180 mm Hg. Abnormal responses to early ambulation indicate that activity reduction and clinical reassessment are needed. Appropriate responses permit serial progression of activity intensity.

The safety of supervised early ambulation after myocardial infarction is well documented; complications of infarction are not increased. Benefits include limitation of the deconditioning effects of immobilization, lessened pulmonary atelectasis and thromboembolic complications, as well as decrease in the common emotional responses to infarction, anxiety, and depression. Early ambulation permits medically determined early discharge because of the improved functional status of the patient; it enables predischarge exercise testing and is associated, in some studies, with an earlier return to work.

Predischarge exercise testing can document the functional impact of the episode of myocardial infarction on the patient. An abnormal response to low-level exercise, preferably sign- or symptom-limited testing or alternatively testing to a predefined heart rate, helps identify patients at increased risk of proximate coronary events who require additional or more prompt diagnostic procedures to determine the requisite medical or surgical interventions. Patients at increased risk include those with a low exercise capacity (below 4 to 6 mets) and those with angina, ischemic ST segment abnormalities, or hypotension induced at low levels of exercise. Medical supervision is recommended for high-risk patients undertaking exercise rehabilitation. Predischarge exercise testing also more precisely defines safe activity levels for the minimally impaired patient who is well suited for accelerated rehabilitation and earlier return to pre-illness activities, including return to work. Further, it may lessen the common fear of physical exertion after infarction.

## Education and Counseling

The goal of this component of rehabilitative care is to provide the information, motivation, and skill training that can help patients assume responsibility for personal health care. Many psychosocial outcomes after infarction appear to be related to the patient's perception of his or her health status; this may be favorably altered by education and counseling.

The information presented in the coronary care unit is typically a brief explanation of the diagnosis and what is to be anticipated. Orientation to the procedures and equipment, with emphasis on the temporary nature of most restrictions, helps patients adjust to a life-threatening situation.

More detailed information provided during the remainder of the hospitalization enhances patients' ability to cope with the problems of illness as they plan for return home. Normal cardiac function, the development of atherosclerotic lesions, and changes of myocardial infarction (emphasizing healing) should be presented as background for subsequent therapeutic recommendations. Advice is given about resumption of activity (including sexual activity and return to work), smoking cessation, dietary modifications (of fat, sodium, and calories as needed), and control of other coronary risk factors. Reduction of conventional coronary risk factors is designed to prevent or retard the progression of atherosclerosis; a multifactorial approach has been reported to reduce the risk of reinfarction. The National Cholesterol Education Program Step 1 Diet is a reasonable recommendation, with caloric adjustment designed to attain near-ideal body weight. Control of hypertension decreases the risk of cerebrovascular complications as well as decreasing myocardial oxygen demand. Continued cigarette smoking following myocardial infarction increases the risk of reinfarction and coronary death in patients of all ages and decreases their ability to achieve physical fitness.

Since many components of care after infarction entail long-term modifications of lifestyle, education should provide insight into behaviors that may increase the risk of reinfarction and into the value of altering these habits. Acquisition of knowledge appears to favorably affect health-related behaviors. The role of behavior modification as an adjunct to effecting a change in habit is uncertain, but promising results are described. Similarly, the concept of stress management requires validation before this can be generally recommended. Counseling about return to sexual activity should involve both the patient and spouse, using the guideline that sexual intercourse can be safely resumed when other activities of daily living are reinstituted. In general, asymptomatic postinfarction patients report resumption of sexual activity within 8 weeks following infarction, although many symptomatic patients do not resume sexual activity until several months after the acute illness. Patients should be informed about their prescribed medications: purpose, dosage, and potential adverse effects. Many patients may not have previously taken medications and may be unfamiliar with problems of doing so. Recommended responses to recurrent symptoms and how to gain access to emergency medical care should be included in the teaching; identification of relevant community resources, such as home-care agencies, counseling and guidance services, vocational rehabilitation organizations, services for financial aid, and postcoronary support groups or clubs, should also be provided. Counseling of family members should address the adjustments in lifestyle to be anticipated during convalescence, while emphasizing the importance of averting unnecessary invaliding of the patient.

Inadequate or ambiguous information about coronary disease and its management (including symptoms, prognosis, planned tests or procedures, allowable activities, and return to work, among others) has been documented as a major concern for patients recovering from myocardial infarction. These aspects should be discussed before discharge from the hospital, as adequate time to address problems and receive information is often not available during subsequent office visits.

The teaching format must be flexible. A group approach often decreases anxiety, aids learning, is economical of professional time, and offers peer support. Involving the patient in planning for recovery helps return control and responsibility to the patient and enhances self-esteem. Audiovisual presentations can also facilitate learning. Written directions, take-home pamphlets, and instruction sheets provide a convenient reference for the patient and family and avoid problems related to vague or ambiguous instructions for posthospital care. Increasingly, technological advances such as home videocassettes and interactive computer educational programs facilitate the provision of information and guidance to the patient and family.

## THE CONVALESCENT OR RECOVERY PHASE

### Exercise Regimens

**Guidelines for Exercise Prescription and Surveillance.** Physical activity during convalescence is designed to improve endurance to a level that permits return to work or appropriate preinfarction activities. Activity regimens may be supervised or unsupervised. Supervised exercise currently is recommended for high-risk postinfarction patients with a low exercise capacity; significantly depressed ventricular function; angina, ischemia, or hypotension that is induced at low levels of exercise; complex ventricular arrhythmias; or who are unable to monitor their heart rate responses to activity. Ideally, unsupervised exercise for low-risk patients should follow a brief period of supervised training during which exercise guidance can be provided. Supervision may increase motivation and reassurance and enables provision of emergency care if needed. As exercise performance and fitness improve, medical supervision can be decreased. Supervised and unsupervised exercise training equally improve the functional capacity of low-risk patients after myocardial infarction.

Although fewer complications of exercise were described in supervised exercise programs with continuous ECG monitoring, it is not known whether ECG monitoring per se, closer medical supervision, or lesser exercise intensity was the major determinant. A more recent survey did not document a significant safety advantage of continuous ECG monitoring; the greater current safety of exercise for coronary patients, at least in part, relates to risk stratification and newer therapies. In supervised exercise programs without continuous ECG monitoring, intermittent pulse counting can ascertain that the heart rate response remains within the target heart rate range. Electrocardiographic surveillance need not be an all-or-none phenomenon. An ECG rhythm strip can be intermittently recorded in supervised exercise programs, using the paddles of a defibrillator as ECG leads. Patients exercising without supervision, even at a distance from a rehabilitation program, may use periodic telephone ECG transmission or a variety of inexpensive heart rate monitors during home exercise.

Individualized prescriptive exercise is the hallmark of rehabilitative physical activity, whether supervised or unsupervised. The "dosage" of exercise, determined by its frequency, intensity, and duration, is defined for each patient, as is the type of predominantly dynamic exercise that is recommended. Exercise test data provide the basis for the prescription of exercise intensity. Use of age-predicted target heart rates is inappropriate, because heart rate response may be modified by coronary disease, its therapy, the prior state of fitness, or all of these features. During exercise training, patients were traditionally recommended to attain 70 to 85% of the highest heart rate safely achieved at exercise testing. This corresponds to 57 to 78% of the peak oxygen uptake, a safe yet effective range to stimulate aerobic metabolism and develop endurance. Previously sedentary patients can improve their functional status with exercise of lesser intensity.

More recent data show an adequate training effect with a lower exercise intensity and a compensatory increase in exercise duration, particularly for unfit patients or those with a low exercise capacity. The increased comfort of exercise at 60 to 75% of the highest heart rate safely achieved at exercise testing may encourage adherence to the exercise regimen. The lower heart rate ranges also offer greater safety with unsupervised exercise. Coronary patients should exercise only within the intensity documented at exercise testing to maintain an acceptable cardiovascular response. When exercise testing is performed for exercise prescription, patients should be tested on an optimal medical regimen, taking all drugs that will be used during training. Exercise training can be accomplished in patients receiving all categories of antianginal drugs, and drug therapy may improve the ability to exercise. Two or three exercise sessions each week are recommended, preferably on nonsuccessive days. Although unfit, sedentary, or older patients may improve their exercise capacity with as few as one or two exercise sessions weekly, more than four exercise periods each week does not significantly increase maximal oxygen uptake. Exercise sessions should be 45 to 60 minutes in duration, including warm-up and cool-down periods. Although a modest increase in the frequency or duration of exercise can compensate for decreased exercise intensity, excessively long or inappropriately frequent exercise sessions engender poorer adherence to training and excessive musculoskeletal complications.

Interval training, alternating periods of high- and low-intensity exercise, can avoid an excessive oxygen debt in symptomatic coronary patients, and also permits imposition of a greater workload at each session before the occurrence of symptoms. Because the benefits of arm and leg exercise are only moderately interchangeable, both arm and leg training are required. One study identified only 50 to 70% improvement using the untrained as compared with the trained extremity, suggesting that about half of the increase in trained limb exercise response is due to a generalized training effect and half to specific changes in trained skeletal muscle.

Serial exercise testing with both supervised and unsupervised exercise training can ascertain the effects of training and help revise the exercise prescription as needed to incorporate activities of greater intensity. Documentation of functional improvement also encourages adherence to exercise training.

**Supervised Exercise Training.** Although the design of a supervised exercise program varies with the number of patients involved, the available space and equipment, and the pattern of electrocardiographic monitoring, certain common features can be recommended.

The initial 5 to 10 minutes of exercise, the warm-up period, should include stretching and range-of-motion exercises that provide musculoskeletal and cardiorespiratory readiness for exercise. The target heart rate should be attained during the 15- to 20-minute aerobic or endurance component. This may consist of walk-run sequences or exercise on a stationary bicycle or treadmill. Since these exercises train primarily the leg muscles, arm training exercises using selected calisthenics, rowing machines, or shoulder wheels should be added. Since many occupational and recreational activities involve both arm and leg work, arm training is used to improve physical performance. In the early weeks of training, activities recommended are those in which skill contributes little to the intensity of work demand, making the energy costs of exercise more predictable. The final component is a 5- to 10-minute cool-down period during which the gradual decrease in exercise intensity allows the heat load to be dissipated, the heart rate to slow, and the peripheral vasodilation of exercise to subside.

Because long-term exercise supervision is neither necessary nor feasible, most patients who attain a 7 to 8 met level can progress to unsupervised or minimally supervised exercise, usually within 3 to 6 months after infarction. At this level of exercise, combined isotonic (dynamic) and isometric training can enhance muscle strength, which then aids in dynamic exercise endurance.

**Unsupervised Exercise.** Appropriately selected low-risk patients can exercise without supervision, but they require detailed instructions to do so safely. Since both economic and logistic problems limit the availability of supervised exercise, the safety and cost-effectiveness of unsupervised exercise are currently under evaluation. Written directions for each patient should include the type of exercise; exercise intensity, duration, and frequency; the target heart rate range and methods of checking; signs and symptoms of excessive exercise; appropriate clothing and footwear; and other particulars.

Initially, most patients undertaking home exercise regimens use walking as their major activity, with gradual increases in pace and distance; warm-up exercises should precede the walking. Although predischarge exercise test results more precisely guide activity recommendations, patients whose exercise testing is deferred to several weeks after the hospitalization can use in-hospital guidelines for pulse-monitoring, i.e., a heart rate response below 120 beats per minute or not exceeding 20 beats above resting level for patients taking beta-blocking drugs.

Subsequent home exercise regimens typically involve progressive walk-jog sequences or progressive increases in the intensity and duration of exercise on a stationary bicycle, based on the results of exercise testing.

**Appropriate Expectations: Exercise Training.** The goal of prescriptive physical activity for patients recovering from myocardial infarction is improvement in cardiovascular functional capacity. This occurs in addition to the "spontaneous" functional improvement of the early weeks after infarction in patients who resume reasonable levels of activity. Aerobic capacity improves with training, with maximal oxygen uptake increasing by as much as 20%. The enhanced peripheral arteriovenous oxygen extraction by trained skeletal muscle and the improved redistribution of cardiac output decrease the demand for oxygen and thus for blood flow. Systemic vascular resistance decreases, and skeletal muscle and autonomic nervous system adaptations decrease the rate-pressure product. There is also a more rapid return to normal of the exercise heart rate. These peripheral adaptations appear to be the major factor in improved performance. The training-induced decrease in the heart rate and blood pressure response to submaximal work decreases myocardial oxygen demand. This explains the absent or lessened angina and ischemic ST electrocardiographic changes at submaximal work levels, corresponding to the patient's increased ability to perform submaximal tasks before the onset of myocardial ischemia and angina. This enables patients to function farther from their ischemic threshold when performing daily activities. Training reduces the myocardial oxygen demand for any body oxygen demand, i.e., it allows a higher level of exercise at a lessened myocardial energy cost. Training increases the exercise threshold for angina. Because usual activities require a lesser percentage of the improved physical work capacity, patients describe improved stamina or endurance. Further, the number and dosage of antianginal medications needed may decrease.

In addition to the improved physical work capacity that results from exercise training, permitting an increased intensity and duration of work, exercise also aids in weight control and favorably affects psychologic status. Serum triglyceride levels decrease with exercise training, and although the effect on total cholesterol level is inconclusive, HDL cholesterol levels increase with training. Glucose utilization and sensitivity to insulin improve. Effects on fibrinolysis and platelet function remain controversial. Participation in an exercise regimen often encourages patients to modify other more powerful coronary risk factors and aids patients in renouncing the sick role and in resuming their pre-illness lifestyle, including return to work.

There is no evidence that exercise training of moderate intensity and duration improves the coronary collateral circulation, alters coronary-obstructive lesions, or increases myocardial oxygen supply or intrinsic myocardial performance; nor do the results of individual clinical trials of exercise training show that exercise significantly alters the outcome (despite the 20 to 30% trend favoring survival in exercising patients in most intervention studies). Although meta analysis of exercise trials in postinfarction patients suggested a survival advantage, these data antedated thrombolytic therapy, contemporary pharmacotherapy, risk stratification procedures, and wide application of myocardial revascularization; extrapolation to contemporary postinfarction patients warrants caution.

### Education and Counseling

Recommendations for care must be reinforced after the patient returns home if benefits of hospital-based education are to be maintained. The patient's attitudes and beliefs about the importance of therapy influence compliance.

The current abbreviated hospital stay limits the ability to address many of the patient's and family's needs for information and advice. Continuity of in-hospital and ambulatory education and counseling is requisite as concerns not apparent in the hospital become evident when patients must make decisions about long-term care. Participation by coronary patients in community heart clubs or comparable organizations may encourage modification of risk-related behaviors and aid in reinforcing recommendations for care. Acquisition of information appears to favorably affect adoption of health-related behaviors, and improves coping behaviors as well. Technologic advances such as computer-assisted education and counseling and interactive video systems may enable teaching, reinforcement of education, and tracking of accomplishments to be performed at sites distant from a rehabilitation or hospital center—for example, at work, in the home, or in a senior citizen facility, extending the services provided by health professionals.

Recommendations should be made for progressive resumption of occupational, social, recreational, and retirement activities.

## THE MAINTENANCE PHASE

Exercise must be enjoyable, convenient, and typically social to become a long-term component of lifestyle, a feature necessary to maintain adequate physical conditioning and fitness. The ultimate goal for most patients is independence in exercising.

Exercise recommendations vary with the patient's needs and goals, general health status and musculoskeletal competence, desired occupational and recreational activities, skills, and likes and dislikes, as well as accessibility of exercise facilities and availability of exercise equipment. For example, the rationale of exercise training of many younger patients is improvement in functional status to enable a return to and maintenance of remunerative employment. Many elderly patients adhere to a low-intensity regimen to help them maintain their independent lifestyle.

In supervised or group exercise programs, aerobic games such as volleyball, basketball, handball, and tennis are limited early in exercise training because variations in skill, excitement, and competitiveness vary the oxygen cost of these activities. However, they add variety to an exercise program and improve adherence, as well as providing arm and torso exercise. The initial walk-jog-run sequences in unsupervised or super-

vised programs can subsequently be replaced by endurance activities such as swimming, bicycle riding, skating, rope jumping, rowing, and aerobic dancing.

Serial exercise testing at longer intervals can document maintenance of functional improvement and encourage adherence.

As exercise supervision decreases, alternate ways to monitor and encourage risk reduction must be devised, so that necessary reinforcement can be provided for adherence to healthy lifestyles.

## SUMMARY

Current rehabilitative care is designed to reduce the physical, psychologic, and vocational invalidism and limit medical care costs following MI. The trend is toward delivery of the specific rehabilitative services required by each patient, rather than requiring patient adherence to a highly structured and relatively inflexible regimen of rehabilitative care.

# PERICARDITIS

method of
P. SUDHAKAR REDDY, M.D.
*University of Pittsburgh School of Medicine*
*Pittsburgh, Pennsylvania*

The treatment of pericarditis entails the treatment of: (1) the underlying cause; (2) pain; (3) cardiac tamponade; and (4) constrictive pericarditis.

## TREATMENT

### The Underlying Cause

Whenever possible, the underlying cause, particularly an infectious cause, should be identified and treated with specific therapy (Table 1). However, in many cases, the cause will not be known.

### Pain

Pain can occur with or without significant pericardial effusion. Pain should be treated with aspirin, every 4 to 6 hours. If it fails, indomethacin (Indocin) 25 to 75 mg four times a day should be used. If the pain is severe and not relieved by nonsteroidal anti-inflammatory agents (NSAID), more powerful analgesics like meperidine (Demerol) may be used intravenously for a day or two. The dose should be titrated to relieve the

## TABLE 1. **Etiologic Classification of Pericardial Disease***

Acute idiopathic or nonspecific pericarditis
Acute myocardial infarction
Postmyocardial infarction syndrome (Dressler's syndrome)
Post-traumatic pericarditis (penetrating or nonpenetrating)
Post-thoracotomy syndrome or postcardiotomy syndrome
Connective tissue diseases: rheumatoid disease, rheumatic fever, systemic lupus erythematosus, scleroderma; Takayasu's arteritis
Specific infections
   Bacterial infections; infective endocarditis
   Tuberculosis
   Fungal infections: histoplasmosis, nocardiosis, blastomycosis
   Viral (Coxsackie B, influenza, ECHO)
   Amebiasis
   Toxoplasmosis
   Meningococcal disease
   Gonococcal disease
Primary or metastatic neoplasm, including lymphoma and leukemia
Postradiation pericarditis
Aortic aneurysm: rupture or leakage of dissecting or nondissecting aneurysm into the pericardial sac
Drugs: hydralazine, psicofuranine, procainamide, anticoagulant therapy, isonicotinic acid hydrazide, penicillin, minoxidil
Chylopericardium
Uremia, and in association with hemodialysis
Miscellaneous: sarcoidosis, myxedema, amyloid disease, multiple myeloma

*Adapted from Fowler, Noble O. Etiology of pericarditis. *In* Hurst JW, (ed): The Heart, 4th ed. New York; McGraw-Hill, 1978, p. 1643. Reproduced with permission.

pain with the least amount of drug, starting with 25 mg every 15 minutes. If continued treatment with narcotic analgesics is required, prednisone should be started in doses of 20 mg thrice daily for a week and then tapered slowly: 20 mg twice daily for one week, 10 mg twice daily for one week, 5 mg twice daily for one week, and then discontinued. However, in some patients, symptoms recur when the dosage is reduced to 15 mg daily or below. If the symptoms recur, the dose is increased to 60 mg and gradually tapered as outlined above until the dose reaches 5 mg above the level at which the recurrence occurred. Then it should be tapered more slowly (1 mg per week) to the level at which symptoms recurred. The dose is then reduced even more gradually 1 mg per month. If the dose can be reduced to 7.5 mg per day without recurrence, it may be maintained for a few months (approximately 6 months). After a few months, the same dose can be administered on alternate days (for 1 year). If the recurrence cannot be controlled with doses of less than 10 mg per day, pericardiectomy should be performed.

## Tamponade

Accumulation of pericardial fluid stiffens the ventricles, requiring higher ventricular filling pressure to maintain cardiac output. This is reflected in a higher venous pressure which can be estimated from the neck veins. When the compensatory rise in venous pressure fails to maintain the cardiac output, decompensation ensues. This is usually associated with pulsus paradoxus (12 mmHg or greater than or equal to a 10% fall in arterial systolic pressure with inspiration). However, in patients with left ventricular dysfunction, such as chronic renal insufficiency, cardiac output may be compromised without associated pulsus paradoxus.

When cardiac output is not compromised, pericardiocentesis is required for diagnostic purposes only.

When cardiac output appears to be compromised, pericardiocentesis should be performed urgently if the pulsus paradoxus is 20 mmHg or more and semiurgently if it is between 12 and 20 mmHg. Therapeutic pericardiocentesis should also be performed in patients with large effusions and significant elevations of venous pressure (greater than or equal to 10 mmHg), even in the absence of pulsus paradoxus.

Pericardiocentesis should be performed preferably in a cardiac catheterization laboratory by experienced physicians or under their supervision. In uremic pericarditis, recurrence is common. If it recurs, the pericardial catheter should be left in situ and the pericardial cavity drained for a day or two. Most of the patients respond to repeated pericardiocentesis with continuous drainage. If it fails, pericardiectomy is recommended. I do not recommend instillation of any steroidal agents. Of course, effective dialysis is a must in all such patients.

Although my hematology/oncology colleagues prefer to instill sclerosing agents like nitrogen mustard (mechlorethamine) [Mustargen] to prevent reaccumulation in malignant pericardial effusions, I am not convinced of their usefulness. Alternatively, a pericardial window or resection, depending on the prognosis of the patient's malignancy, is recommended. Many patients with pericardial effusion secondary to malignancy or radiation therapy tend to have effusive constrictive pericarditis. Recognition of this syndrome is important. Removal of pericardial effusion alone does not cure the patient of "stiffened heart" syndrome. Elevation of venous pressure and compromised cardiac output may persist in spite of effective pericardiocentesis; such a circumstance requires pericardiectomy.

## Constrictive Pericarditis

Pericardial thickening, parietal, epicardial, or both, may also cause stiffening of the ventricles, requiring higher filling pressures. The severity of constriction should be assessed by the degree of venous pressure elevation and decrease in cardiac output.

All patients with severe elevation of venous pressure, with or without compromise in cardiac output, should be surgically relieved of their constriction.

In patients with very mild elevation of venous pressure, surgery is optional, particularly in elderly patients or in patients with poor prognosis because of an underlying disease such as malignancy.

In my practice, I do not attempt either to unmask occult constriction or to treat it.

# PERIPHERAL ARTERIAL DISEASE

method of
JOHN D. EDWARDS, M.D., and
DAVID C. BREWSTER, M.D.
*Massachusetts General Hospital and Harvard
  Medical School
Boston, Massachusetts*

## ARTERIAL INSUFFICIENCY OF THE LOWER EXTREMITY

Vascular occlusive disease of the lower extremities is becoming a more frequent problem as the patient population ages and as atherosclerosis becomes more prevalent. The severity of the disease process at presentation can range from functional ischemia (claudication) to limb-threatening ischemia (rest pain, ischemic ulceration, or gangrene). Proper diagnosis and management of chronic lower extremity ischemia require a knowledge of the clinical manifestations and natural history of the disease.

Functional ischemia is manifested by intermittent claudication or muscular pain in the leg that occurs with exercise. This occurs when blood flow is adequate for local metabolic demands at rest but cannot increase sufficiently to meet the increased oxygen requirements of the muscle tissue during exercise. The pain of claudication is usually described as a cramp or ache in the calf or thigh that occurs after walking a predictable distance. Three characteristics differentiate it from other causes of exertional limb pain. The pain arises in a functional muscle group, is reproducible by walking a certain distance, and is relieved with only several minutes of rest. If these salient features are not present, nonvascular causes of the pain should be considered. Cauda equina compression by disk, tumor, or spinal canal stenosis produces a well-known syndrome of pseudoclaudication. In the patient with vascular disease, physical examination will usually reveal diminished or absent femoral, popliteal, or pedal pulses, depending on the level of the occlusive disease. Claudication may occur, however, even with palpable pulses at rest. In this instance, one or more proximal stenotic lesions can cause claudication but not obliterate distal pulses. Examination after exercise may reveal a diminution in or loss of pulses or the development of a bruit or thrill over the iliac or femoral vessels. Noninvasive vascular laboratory tests including Doppler velocity waveform analysis, Doppler ultrasound segmental pressures, and segmental plethysmography may be extremely helpful both in confirming the diagnosis of peripheral vascular disease and in quantitating the severity of arterial insufficiency. Treadmill exercise testing is an essential component of such evaluation.

Limb-threatening ischemia occurs when blood flow becomes inadequate for even resting tissue metabolic requirements. Ischemic rest pain (resting metatarsalgia) typically involves the toes or forefoot and is usually relieved by dependency of the limb and therefore usually occurs at night. Physical findings of dependent rubor, elevation pallor, and prolonged capillary refill are common at this stage. Foot and ankle edema is also a common finding since the patient tends to keep the foot in a dependent position. Ischemic ulcers and gangrene may be seen at this stage.

### Treatment

Seventy-five per cent of claudicants will remain stable or improve slightly without specific therapy while 25% will have progressively worsening symptoms and require surgery. Only 3 to 5% will come to require amputation. Most of these amputations occur in patients who present initially with more severe claudication (i.e., less than 1 block claudication and ankle brachial indices [ABIs] of less than .5). This generally benign limb prognosis justifies conservative management, and goals are to limit disease progression and stimulate the development of collateral circulation. The cessation of smoking and a daily exercise regimen are the main components of this management. (In one study 11% of claudicants who failed to quit smoking eventually required amputation.) Surgical treatment for claudication should be considered only in those whose disability is so severe that it limits their ability to earn a living or intolerably limits their desired lifestyle. In the future, laser technology and various atherectomy devices may expand the indications for intervention in claudicants, but at present these techniques should be considered only in patients who are truly surgical candidates.

Limb-threatening ischemia (rest pain, ischemic ulceration, or gangrene) is an indication for urgent surgical referral. These patients should be fully evaluated for possible arterial reconstruction for purposes of limb salvage. The morbidity and mortality of revascularization procedures is often less than that associated with major amputations.

It is important to remember that atherosclerosis is a systemic disease process and the majority of patients with claudication have coronary arterial disease and are at increased risk for myocardial infarction, stroke, and premature death.

## CAROTID ARTERY DISEASE

Stroke remains the third leading cause of death in the United States today. Extracranial carotid atherosclerotic disease is one of the major causes of stroke, and therefore, its treatment is an important subject. There are two mechanisms by which carotid atherosclerotic plaque can cause stroke. The plaque can result in hemodynamically significant narrowing of the carotid artery, resulting in inadequate cerebral perfusion, or the plaque may ulcerate forming a source for fibrin and platelet deposition and subsequent embolization.

Carotid duplex scanning, oculoplethysmography, and supraorbital and transcranial Doppler tests provide highly reliable noninvasive means of evaluating the carotid artery. The studies can quantitate the degree of carotid stenosis and its hemodynamic significance, and the B mode ultrasound capability of the duplex scan will define important physical characteristics of the plaque, such as the presence of ulceration. These studies should be obtained on all patients at increased risk for stroke to identify those that might benefit from carotid endarterectomy. Patients at risk include those with prior stroke, transient ischemic attacks and asymptomatic carotid bruit.

There is current controversy over the efficacy of carotid endarterectomy (CEA) vs. antiplatelet therapy in reducing the incidence of stroke in the population at risk. TIAs (transient focal neurologic deficit usually consisting of contralateral hemiparesis, paresthesias, aphasia, or ipsilateral monocular blindness [amaurosis fugax]) with an appropriate carotid stenosis are widely accepted as an indication for surgery. Patients with TIAs have a 5 to 9% risk of stroke per year. Following uncomplicated carotid endarterectomy, the risk is reduced to less than 1% per year. Prior stroke carries a risk of recurrent stroke of 10% in the first year. Antiplatelet therapy does not appear to reduce this risk. CEA may reduce this to less than 2%. The greatest controversy exists over the treatment of patients with asymptomatic carotid bruit. Several studies suggest that asymptomatic carotid stenoses of greater than 80% diameter reduction carry a 5 to 8% risk of stroke per year. Therefore, if CEA can be performed with less than 2% combined perioperative morbidity and mortality (as currently reported in many experienced medical centers), it will have a positive impact on stroke reduction in this subset of patients.

Antiplatelet agents (aspirin, ticlopidine [Ticlid]*) have been shown to have some efficacy in the reduction of stroke in patients with TIAs and minor strokes. Prospective studies comparing antiplatelet therapy and carotid endarterectomy are ongoing at this time.

## ABDOMINAL AORTIC ANEURYSM

The incidence of aortic aneurysm appears to be increasing. This is due in part to improved surveillance and in part to the increased incidence of atherosclerosis in and aging of the population. In 75%, abdominal aortic aneurysms (AAAs) are asymptomatic and found unexpectedly at the time of routine physical examination on abdominal x-rays or imaging studies (e.g., MRI, CT) performed for some other purpose, or at laparotomy. In 25%, aneurysms are symptomatic at the time of presentation. The most common presenting symptom is abdominal or back pain. Less commonly, patients may present with flank or groin pain (usually on the left). Identification of a symptomatic AAA should be considered an urgent indication for surgery whether or not there is evidence of aneurysmal expansion or rupture.

The most common and dangerous complication of AAA is rupture. Other less common complications include thrombosis, distal atheromatous embolization (AAA should be in the differential diagnosis of "blue toe syndrome"), duodenal obstruction, ureteral obstruction, and aortocaval and aortoduodenal fistulas. The risk of rupture is by far the greatest risk of AAA.

The natural history of AAA has been well defined. The risk of rupture correlates directly with the diameter of the aneurysm. AAAs with a diameter greater than 8 cm have 75% chance of rupture within 5 years, while those less than 4 cm have less than a 15% chance of rupture within 5 years. However, small aneurysms do rupture. Several studies have suggested that aneurysm rupture may account for 15 to 20% of the deaths in patients with small aneurysms.

---

*Investigational drug in the United States.

### Treatment

Despite advances in critical care and surgical technique the mortality for ruptured AAA remains in excess of 50% in most centers. The mortality for elective repair of asymptomatic aneurysms is less than 3%. The standard indication for surgical repair is AAA of 5 cm or greater in size or a symptomatic aneurysm of any size. Patients with smaller aneurysms may be followed with serial abdominal ultrasound or CT scan every 6 months. The average AAA will increase at a rate of 0.4 cm per year. A more rapid rate of expansion should be an indication for surgery.

# DEEP VENOUS THROMBOSIS OF THE LOWER EXTREMITIES

method of
ROBERT A. GRAOR, M.D.
*The Cleveland Clinic Foundation*
*Cleveland, Ohio*

Leg scanning with $^{125}$I-fibrinogen has shown that venous thrombosis is common in hospitalized patients. The frequency of venous thrombi in ambulatory patients is more difficult to estimate, but recent studies indicate that this disorder is also common, particularly if patients have been exposed to risk factors within the preceding 3 months.

## CLINICAL PRESENTATION

Patients with deep venous thrombosis (DVT) usually do not develop symptoms until the thrombus has become large and occlusive. The clinical presentation is generally associated with risk factors such as surgery or trauma, stroke, advancing age, associated malignancies, heart failure, patients with previous venous thrombosis, obesity, pregnancy, or other miscellaneous risk factors that may lead to an increased tendency to produce thrombosis. When the signs or symptoms of DVT occur, they are caused by either obstruction of venous flow, resulting in edema or inflammation of the vessel wall, or perivascular tissue, resulting in pain and discomfort. Extension of the thrombus most commonly occurs if the original thrombogenic stimulus persists. Venous thrombi usually organize and occlude veins or recanalize over time. Thrombi limited to the calf veins are known to extend into the popliteal vein in approximately 20% of cases. If extension has occurred, there is a 40 to 50% risk of clinically detectable pulmonary emboli.

## DIAGNOSIS

The clinical diagnosis of DVT is difficult owing to two problems: The symptoms of venous thrombi can also be caused by many nonthrombotic disorders, and many potentially dangerous DVTs are clinically silent because they are not obstructive and are not associated with the inflammatory changes of the perivascular and vascular wall tissues. Therefore, the sensitivity of our clinical exam remains very low. Studies have shown that the clinical sensitivity is less than 50%. The most common clinical symptoms are pain (50%), tenderness (75%), and swelling (50%). Other clinical features include cramps, redness or cyanosis, dilated veins, and an increase in temperature of the affected lower extremity. Swelling and other symptoms tend to increase as the volume of thrombus increases. Homans' sign, which is discomfort in the upper calf on forced dorsiflexion of the foot, is a time-honored diagnostic sign of DVT, but it is very insensitive and nonspecific.

### Confirmatory Diagnosis

Under perfect circumstances, the presence of an intraluminal filling defect on venography is accepted as the "gold standard" for the diagnosis of DVT, but it is currently being challenged by venous duplex (Doppler ultrasound) imaging. The venous Doppler ultrasound technique appears to be an accurate noninvasive study and actually has been shown to be equally accurate with ascending venography in some centers. Both studies are reliable methods for the diagnosis of DVT when the most reliable diagnostic criteria are used. For venography, less reliable criteria include nonfilling of segments of the deep venous system and abrupt termination of the contrast media.

It is generally agreed that patients with proximal venous thrombosis should be treated, since they are at high risk of developing pulmonary emboli. Considerable controversy exists surrounding the treatment of calf vein thrombosis. If nonanticoagulant therapy is entertained, the risk of propagation has to be considered, and follow-up of patients is mandated in an attempt to identify those who have extension of their DVT and may be at risk for fatal pulmonary embolism.

Superficial venous thrombosis is generally accurately diagnosed clinically and requires very little therapy. Only in the situation in which the superficial thrombus extends to the level of the confluence with the deep system (i.e., greater saphenous vein thrombus in the proximal thigh) is anticoagulation therapy required.

## THERAPEUTIC GOALS

Two important considerations enter the decision for treatment of deep vein thrombosis: eliminating a thrombus to prevent the sequelae of venous insufficiency and stopping additional thrombus formation to prevent pulmonary emboli. In general, anticoagulation therapy is used to prevent extension and embolization of the venous thrombi. Ideally, a thrombolytic agent could be used to eliminate the thrombus from the deep venous system, but unfortunately, not all patients who develop DVT are candidates for this therapy. Surgical extraction of the clot has not led to favorable results in the past and is not widely done. If a patient cannot receive an anti-coagulant or a thrombolytic agent, mechanical interruption of the inferior vena cava, generally with an inferior vena caval filter, is indicated to prevent potentially large pulmonary emboli. It must be kept in mind that this does not restrict the formation of the clot, nor does it prevent or reduce the incidence of serious venous insufficiency.

The choice to use thrombolytic agents to eliminate the clot from the venous system and restore normal venous hemodynamics is a complicated interplay between the clinical presentation, the natural history of the disease, and the risks associated with this type of therapy. It has been shown that from 60 to 80% of patients with fresh thrombi can undergo complete clot lysis using a thrombolytic agent such as urokinase. The risks associated with urokinase appear to be significantly less than those associated with streptokinase. Although the cost of this therapy includes one to two extra hospital days and the cost of the thrombolytic agent, this represents a small fraction of total costs if one considers the sequelae of venous insufficiency as being an expensive continuous outcome. Definitive data regarding the prevention of venous insufficiency associated with the use of thrombolytic agents are not available at present. A few small studies have demonstrated normal venous hemodynamic function 5 and 10 years following elimination of venous thrombi using thrombolytic agents. The same outcome has not been achieved with standard anticoagulation therapy.

## TREATMENT

**Heparin Therapy.** Heparin is an anionic muco-polysaccharide that binds to a plasma protein, antithrombin III, thereby enhancing the ability of antithrombin III to neutralize factors XIIa, IXa, Xa, and thrombin itself. The half-life of heparin therapy varies from 20 minutes to 2 hours and can be monitored using the activated partial thromboplastin time (APTT). Adequate prolongation of the APTT varies among laboratories, but in most, 1.5 to 2.0 times the laboratory control is considered therapeutic.

The safest and most convenient route of administration of heparin is intravenous continuous infusions following an initial bolus injection. The APTT should be performed approximately 4 to 6 hours after the bolus injection and then at least once every 24 hours. Owing to the associated uncommon yet devastating problem of heparin-associated thrombocytopenia and heparin-associated platelet aggregation, a platelet count should be ordered every other or every third day while using heparin therapy.

**Warfarin Sodium (Coumadin).** After heparin therapy has been instituted, anticoagulation using oral warfarin (Coumadin) should be begun. The initial dose of warfarin should be 10 mg, repeated daily until the prothrombin time is 1.25 to 1.5 times the control value. Following stabilization of the warfarin dose, weekly prothrombin times should be determined and the warfarin dose adjusted according to the patient's requirements. With this regimen of warfarin adjustment according to the prothrombin time, bleeding complications can be minimized.

It should be noted that warfarin affects the vitamin K–dependent clotting factors, VII, IX, X, and II. The half-life of factor VII is quite short and provides an early effect on the PT. Therefore, the initial increase in the prothrombin time is due solely to factor VII depletion, at which time the other factors, especially factor II (prothrombin), may still be at adequate levels to produce further thrombosis. Therefore, concurrent heparinization during the first 4 days of warfarin therapy is required. Only then can one consider the patient therapeutically anticoagulated on oral warfarin.

Patients should be maintained on warfarin for 3 to 6 months following the development of deep vein thrombosis. Bleeding problems associated with anticoagulation therapy are related to the length of time on therapy as well as the prolongation of the prothrombin time.

**Thrombolytic Therapy.** Streptokinase and urokinase are the two currently available agents that appear to be effective for the treatment of deep vein thrombosis. Recombinant tissue plasminogen activator for the treatment of DVT does not appear to be effective at the doses currently studied. Urokinase appears to be the preferred lytic agent owing to its equal efficacy with streptokinase but improved safety profile. Intravenous administration of urokinase can be conducted without significant side-effects or the allergic reactions that are seen with streptokinase. Urokinase is administered as an intravenous bolus initially, calculated at 4400 U per kg over 10 minutes, followed by a continuous infusion of 4400 U per kg per hour.

If streptokinase is chosen, an intravenous bolus of 250,000 IU is given followed by a continuous infusion of 100,000 IU per hour. Because of its antigenic effects, some prefer to administer hydrocortisone, 100 mg, prior to the streptokinase infusion and 100 mg every 8 hours during the first 24 to 48 hours of therapy. The pyretic response commonly associated with this medication can be controlled with acetaminophen.

The appropriate duration of infusion of a fibrinolytic agent correlates with the quantity of the thrombus. With duplex scanning, one can monitor the dissolution of a clot noninvasively. Patients selected for this therapy generally should have a symptom duration of less than 7 days.

**Venous Thrombectomy.** Venous thrombectomy is indicated for patients presenting with acute iliofemoral venous thrombosis producing phlegmasia cerulea dolens or phlegmasia alba dolens. Optimal therapy for this disease entity is unknown, but the choices include venous thrombectomy surgically and thrombolysis.

Venous thrombectomy has fallen into disfavor because of early reports documenting the high incidence of postoperative rethrombosis and no particular improvement in long-term results. With recently improved techniques of operative phlebography and the use of arteriovenous fistula, the choice of venous thrombectomy once again becomes a viable option.

**Inferior Vena Caval Devices.** The indication for placement of inferior vena caval filters include a contraindication to anticoagulation therapy, recurrent pulmonary emboli despite adequate anticoagulation, or possibly patients who are at a very high risk for the development of pulmonary emboli where anticoagulation cannot be used and therefore a prophylactic filter may be required.

# The Blood and Spleen

## APLASTIC ANEMIA

method of
RICHARD CHAMPLIN, M.D.
*M. D. Anderson Cancer Center*
*Houston, Texas*

Aplastic anemia is a life-threatening hematologic disorder characterized by pancytopenia and absent or markedly diminished hematopoietic precursors in the bone marrow. Aplastic anemia encompasses a heterogeneous group of disorders that may result from a number of potential pathophysiologic mechanisms. The incidence of aplastic anemia in the United States is estimated as 2 to 10 cases per million population per year. Males and females are equally affected. Aplastic anemia is usually an acquired disease, although congenital forms also occur. A large number of etiologic agents can cause aplastic anemia (Table 1). Various drugs, chemicals, and toxins have been implicated. Radiation and certain infections can also produce aplastic anemia. Aplastic anemia may rarely occur in association with pregnancy or thymoma. Drugs reported to cause aplastic anemia are listed in Table 2. Drugs may produce marrow failure as a predictable dose-related effect, such as with cytotoxic cancer chemotherapeutic agents. More frequently, aplastic anemia occurs as an unpredictable idiosyncratic reaction. Chemicals and toxins may also cause aplastic anemia. Benzene and related hydrocarbons and pesticides are the most commonly implicated agents. Aplastic anemia may develop following infections with a number of viruses. Hepatitis-associated aplastic anemia generally develops in adolescent males within several months of a clinical episode of non-A, non-B hepatitis and has a particularly poor prognosis. Despite a thorough personal and occupational history, a likely etiologic agent can be identified in less than 25% of patients with acquired aplastic anemia. The remaining cases are termed idiopathic.

Aplastic anemia could potentially result from a number of pathophysiologic mechanisms. The disease may be related to a primary abnormality in hematopoietic stem cells resulting in defective growth or differentiation. Aplastic anemia could also be due to abnormalities in the hematopoietic microenvironment or to abnormal regulatory cells or humoral factors. Lastly, aplastic anemia could result from immune-mediated suppression of hematopoiesis.

Supported by grant CA 23175 from the National Institutes of Health.

## DIAGNOSIS AND LABORATORY FEATURES

Aplastic anemia is characterized by reduction in production of erythrocytes, granulocytes, and platelets. Some patients present with deficiencies in only one or two lineages, but the disease usually progresses to produce pancytopenia. Aplastic anemia is commonly defined as leukocytes less than $2.0 \times 10^9$ per liter, hemoglobin less than or equal to 10 grams per dl, and platelets less than $100 \times 10^9$ per liter in the presence of a hypocellular bone marrow with less than 50% of normal cellularity. Reticulocytes are usually less than or equal to $40 \times 10^9$ per liter. Low numbers of lymphocytes and monocytes have been reported in one-third of patients with aplastic anemia. The presence of splenomegaly or immature myeloid or erythroid cells in the peripheral blood or an increase in monocytes is unusual in aplastic anemia and should suggest other disorders such as the myelodysplastic syndromes.

Careful examination of the bone marrow biopsy specimen is critical for the accurate assessment of marrow cellularity and the diagnosis of aplastic anemia. Characteristic features include markedly decreased cellularity with replacement by fat. Residual areas of hematopoiesis (hot pockets) are occasionally seen. Most residual cells are lymphocytes, plasma cells, eosinophils, and stromal cells. Granulocytes, erythrocytes, and megakaryocytes comprise less than 30% of the marrow. Marrow lymphocytes may be increased in some patients. Myelofibrosis may be present and is usually due to increased reticulin. Moderate dysplastic features may be present, but the proportion of blasts is not increased.

TABLE 1. **Etiologic Agents in Acquired Aplastic Anemia**

Drugs
  Antibiotics, anti-inflammatory drugs, anticonvulsants, phenothiazines
Chemicals and toxins
  Pesticides, aromatic hydrocarbons
Infections
  Non-A, non-B hepatitis, Epstein-Barr virus, Venezuelan equine encephalitis, cytomegalovirus, military tuberculosis
Rheumatologic and autoimmune diseases
  Systemic lupus erythematosus (SLE), rheumatoid arthritis, cytoglobulinemia, graft-versus-host disease
Paroxysmal nocturnal hemoglobinuria
Radiation
Thymoma
Pregnancy
Idiopathic

TABLE 2. **Major Drugs Causing Aplastic Anemia**

Antibiotics
   Chloramphenicol, rarely penicillins, cephalosporins, sulfonamides
Anti-inflammatory drugs
   Phenylbutazone, indomethacin, gold compounds, penicillamine, other nonsteroidal anti-inflammatory drugs
Antiepileptic Drugs
   Phenytoin, ethosuximide and other minor anticonvulsants, carbamazepine
Antithyroid drugs
Hypoglycemics
   Chlorpropamide
Antimalarials
Phenothiazines

## CLINICAL FEATURES

The clinical features of aplastic anemia are a direct consequence of the underproduction of granulocytes, erythrocytes, and platelets. Patients typically present with opportunistic infection, fatigue due to anemia, or thrombocytopenic bleeding. The prognosis primarily depends on the severity of pancytopenia. The reticulocyte count is the best single prognostic indicator. *Severe* aplastic anemia is commonly defined as two or more of the following: granulocytes less than $0.5 \times 10^9$ per liter, platelets less than $20 \times 10^9$ per liter, and reticulocytes less than $20 \times 10^9$ per liter. The other major prognostic factor is the interval of time from the patient's first symptoms to diagnosis; patients with a brief interval have a poorer prognosis than those with a gradual onset of the disease.

## TREATMENT

The treatment of aplastic anemia has three major components: (1) identification and withdrawal of potential etiologic factors, (2) supportive care with blood product transfusions and management of infections, and (3) therapy to restore normal hematopoiesis.

The most direct approach to the treatment of aplastic anemia is to identify and eliminate the causative factor(s). Unfortunately, a correctable etiologic factor can be identified in less than 25% of cases and most patients do not recover despite withdrawal of all potential etiologic agents.

A number of therapeutic measures have been proposed to restore hematopoiesis in these patients. Androgens have been extensively studied for the treatment of aplastic anemia. These agents may enhance hematopoiesis in patients with relatively mild pancytopenia, but controlled trials have failed to show any benefit of androgens versus supportive care alone. Androgen treatment may be associated with undesirable side effects, and androgens are not recommended for patients with severe aplastic anemia.

Recent data suggesting a role of the immune system in the regulation of hematopoiesis and the possibility of abnormal immunity contributing to the pathogenesis of aplastic anemia have led to evaluation of immunomodulatory treatment for this disorder. The most encouraging data have been reported with the use of antilymphocyte globulin (ALG) or antithymocyte globulin (ATG). Hematopoietic improvement and prolonged survival occur in 40 to 65% of treated patients. The efficacy of ATG and ALG has been documented by two randomized controlled trials. Following ATG or ALG therapy, peripheral blood counts typically remain unchanged for 1 to 3 months before hematologic improvement can be detected. Responding patients have slow improvement in all cell lineages, becoming independent of transfusions over several months.

### Bone Marrow Transplantation

Bone marrow transplantation is the preferred treatment for young patients with severe aplastic anemia who have an HLA-identical sibling donor. Because aplastic anemia is characterized by a marked deficiency of hematopoietic stem cells, transplantation of normal bone marrow is a logical approach for definitive treatment of this disease. Marrow transplantation has generally been restricted to patients who have an HLA-identical sibling donor. Transplantation of marrow from partially matched donors has usually been unsuccessful in patients with aplastic anemia, primarily owing to a high rate of graft rejection. Recently, registries have been established to identify unrelated histocompatible donors for bone marrow transplantation. Preliminary data indicate a higher risk of graft failure and acute graft-versus-host disease than with HLA-identical sibling donors, but many successful transplants have been performed.

Bone marrow transplantation from an HLA-identical sibling has been shown to be superior to supportive care alone or to management with androgens in prospective controlled trials. With current techniques, more than 90% of patients will achieve sustained engraftment and recovery of hematopoiesis. Overall survival is 60 to 80%, with most deaths attributable to infections or transplant-related complications. Results of bone marrow transplantation are most favorable in previously untransfused patients, since blood product transfusions may sensitize the patient to transplantation antigens of the transplant donor and increase the risk of rejection. In general, patients over 50 years of age should not be considered for transplantation because of a substantially higher mortality rate following bone marrow transplantation when compared with younger patients.

Bone marrow transplantation is an intensive

procedure requiring hospitalization for approximately 5 weeks. A number of serious and potentially fatal complications may occur. Intensive immunosuppressive conditioning treatment involving high-dose cyclophosphamide with or without total lymphoid irradiation is required prior to transplantation to prevent rejection of the bone marrow. Use of cyclosporine alone or with methotrexate post transplant has been associated with a decreased rate of graft failure and improved survival compared with other post-transplant immunosuppressive therapies.

The major complications following bone marrow transplantation relate to infections as a result of the prolonged period of immunodeficiency following the transplant and to the problems of acute and chronic graft-versus-host disease.

### Investigational Therapies

A number of other drugs have been proposed as treatments for patients with aplastic anemia. Cyclosporine has been utilized as an immunomodulatory therapy for aplastic anemia without transplantation. Anecdotal reports have claimed responses in approximately 20% of patients, but controlled studies have not been reported and clear recommendations regarding the efficacy of cyclosporine cannot be made at this time. Prospective studies are at present in progress to compare the results of cyclosporine with antithymocyte globulin therapy.

Hematopoietic growth factors are investigational agents that are likely to have a major therapeutic role in the future. A family of glycoprotein hematopoietic factors are important regulators of hematopoiesis. Recently, a number of these growth factors, termed colony-stimulating factors because of their ability to induce the growth of hematopoietic colonies in vitro, have been identified, cloned from human cells, and produced for clinical trials. Granulocyte-macrophage colony-stimulating factor (GM-CSF) and granulocyte colony-stimulating factor (G-CSF) enhance granulopoiesis in humans. Many patients with otherwise refractory aplastic anemia have had substantial increases in circulating granulocytes, monocytes, and eosinophils associated with myeloid and eosinophilic hyperplasia in the bone marrow following GM-CSF treatment. G-CSF has more limited effects, stimulating granulocyte proliferation. Unfortunately, neither G-CSF nor GM-CSF typically affects anemia or thrombocytopenia. It is not established that G-CSF or GM-CSF therapy will reduce morbidity or improve survival.

These studies are significant, however, in demonstrating that many patients with severe aplastic anemia have hematopoietic progenitors that are capable of responding to therapeutic administration of growth factors. These studies must be viewed as the beginning of a new therapeutic approach to the treatment of aplastic anemia, and other, more broadly acting growth factors may have greater efficacy. Interleukin-3 (IL-3), which stimulates earlier multipotent myeloid progenitors, is entering clinical trials. Multiple hematopoietic growth factors act synergistically to regulate hematopoiesis at multiple levels. Interleukin-1, interleukin-6, erythropoietin, G-CSF, and GM-CSF have synergistic effects with interleukin-3 *and other factors*. Combinations of growth factors will likely be necessary for optimal effects on myeloid, erythroid, and megakaryocytic cells. The use of hematopoietic growth factors holds great promise for the future treatment of aplastic anemia and other bone marrow failure states but must be presently considered investigational.

In conclusion, patients less than 45 years of age with severe aplastic anemia should be immediately referred for bone marrow transplantation as optimal therapy of this disease. The remaining patients should receive antithymocyte globulin treatment. Patients failing to respond to ATG should be considered for unrelated donor bone marrow transplantation or for clinical trials of hematopoietic growth factors or other investigational therapies.

# IRON DEFICIENCY

method of
DAVID A. SEARS, M.D.
*Baylor College of Medicine*
*Houston, Texas*

In the usual clinical circumstances, iron deficiency is diagnosed after the discovery of anemia. Anemia is found because of symptoms it produces or as a result of screening laboratory tests. In slowly developing anemia, such as that due to iron deficiency, signs and symptoms do not usually occur until the anemia is severe. Symptoms of anemia are most often nonspecific and may include increased ease of fatigue, decreased exercise capacity, lassitude, palpitations with exertion, and disturbed mentation. Signs of chronic anemia include pallor, tachypnea, hyperpnea, and tachycardia. Certain signs and symptoms may be more specific for iron deficiency anemia, such as epithelial abnormalities involving the mouth and tongue, esophagus, and nails, but these are rare. On the other hand, a history of pica, the compulsive eating of a certain food or nonfood substance, may be elicited with sufficient frequency in iron-deficient patients that it is a useful diagnostic clue. The variety of unusual substances reported to have been consumed by patients with iron deficiency ranges from croutons to cigarette ashes, but most common are starch, dirt or clay, and particularly ice. It has been debated whether iron deficiency produces clinical manifestations in the absence of anemia. Experimental data have suggested impaired muscle function, but their applicability to humans is uncertain.

Certain groups of people are in a precarious state of iron balance. In these people, regular screening for iron deficiency or routine administration of supplemental iron is warranted. Such groups include rapidly growing infants and adolescents, menstruating women, and pregnant women. Infants should receive iron supplementation beginning at 4 months of age for term infants and 2 months for preterm infants. Doses are 1 mg per kg per day for term infants and 2, 3, and 4 mg per kg per day for preterm infants weighing greater than 1500 grams, 1000 to 1500 grams, and less than 1000 grams at birth, respectively. Iron-fortified formulas and cereal are convenient sources of supplemental iron. Term infants who are breast-fed for 6 months are not at risk for iron deficiency, but preterm infants fed breast milk need iron supplementation. Ingestion of fresh cow milk may increase gastrointestinal blood loss in the infant and aggravate iron deficiency. Adolescents are not usually given supplemental iron, but attention to good sources of dietary iron is important during this period of increased iron requirement due to rapid growth. In pregnancy the iron requirement increases as pregnancy progresses. Taken over the 9-month period, the requirement is about 2.5 times the nonpregnant requirement. Thus, prenatal iron supplementation is a necessity. Many prenatal vitamin capsules or tablets contain 60 mg of elemental iron and are given in a dose of one per day. Most also contain vitamin C, which enhances iron absorption. Lactating women lose iron in their breast milk, but this loss is approximately balanced by the absence of menstrual loss. Iron deficiency is common in menstruating women, since their iron loss is twice that of men and nonmenstruating women. Routine supplementation is not recommended for all menstruating women but only for those demonstrated to have iron deficiency. The potential hazard of indiscriminate iron supplementation is iron overload and organ siderosis in susceptible populations, such as Caucasians in the United States, in whom there is a high incidence of the gene for hemochromatosis.

The sequence of events in the development of iron deficiency anemia is as follows: depletion of reticuloendothelial stores of iron and decline in the serum ferritin value, decreased saturation of the serum iron-binding protein transferrin, and finally hypochromic, microcytic anemia.

Confirmation of the diagnosis of iron deficiency depends on laboratory studies. If the anemia is microcytic (mean red cell volume [MCV] less than 80 fl), iron studies are warranted. Three laboratory tests on the patient's serum are useful: iron, total iron-binding capacity (TIBC), and ferritin. From the first two, the per cent saturation may be calculated (100 × serum iron/TIBC). Pure iron deficiency anemia is associated with a low serum iron, a low per cent saturation (less than 15%), and a low serum ferritin. In the anemia of chronic disease, the serum iron and per cent saturation are low, but the serum ferritin level, which reflects storage iron, is normal or elevated. A serum ferritin value greater than 100 ng per ml virtually excludes iron deficiency. In an anemic patient with a normal MCV, iron deficiency is not the sole etiology of the anemia but may coexist with another disorder, such as the anemia of chronic disease or folic acid deficiency. In such cases the diagnostic work-up is more complex.

Observation of the response to a trial of iron therapy may be a valid diagnostic undertaking in some cases. A therapeutic trial, as contrasted to thoughtless "shotgun" therapy, is characterized by thorough baseline and follow-up clinical observations and laboratory tests and careful consideration of what constitutes a positive result.

Whenever iron deficiency is diagnosed, it is essential that the etiology be identified. Blood loss is, of course, the most common cause. Occult gastrointestinal bleeding must always be excluded, even in the patient with heavy menses, poor diet, or other possible reasons for deficiency.

## TREATMENT

There are three ways iron deficiency anemia may be treated: red blood cell transfusion, oral iron, and parenteral iron. The first of these, transfusion, is rarely necessary because iron deficiency anemia develops slowly, and even severe anemia is usually tolerated well. An aphorism of the National Research Council Subcommittee on Transfusion Problems bears repeating: "When anemia may be treated by specific agents such as iron, $B_{12}$, or folic acid, blood transfusion is usually not justified."

### Oral Iron

The easiest, safest, and cheapest way to treat iron deficiency is with an orally administered iron salt. The iron should be in the reduced (ferrous) state for optimal absorption. Absorption occurs primarily in the proximal small intestine. It is enhanced by gastric acidity and by reducing substances, such as vitamin C. It is diminished by administration of the iron with a meal, rapid intestinal transit, surgical bypass of absorptive sites, and substances forming insoluble complexes, such as may be found in tea and coffee.

Numerous iron preparations are available. They vary in nature of the iron salt, content of elemental iron, presence of other additives (such as vitamin C), and, of course, cost. A standard therapy for adults is a 300 mg tablet of ferrous sulfate (60 mg of elemental iron) given three or four times a day on an empty stomach. Ferrous gluconate is a satisfactory alternative. It is commonly available in a 320 mg tablet containing 36 mg of elemental iron.

The major side effects ascribed to oral iron therapy are upper gastrointestinal symptoms, such as epigastric distress, heartburn, nausea, and occasionally vomiting and cramping. These seem to be dose related and can be ameliorated by reducing the dose of iron or by prescribing the iron with, rather than between, meals. The dose can be reduced by using ferrous gluconate tablets or liquid preparations of ferrous sulfate or gluconate. Both of these measures, dose reduction and giving iron with meals, will reduce the amount of iron absorbed and may therefore decrease the rate of response, but this is rarely a significant problem. Addition of vitamin C to an iron preparation enhances absorption but also increases the gastrointestinal side effects. Sustained or delayed release formulations of iron may produce fewer side effects but may also be absorbed less well.

Reasons for failure of iron therapy include incorrect diagnosis, complicating illness such as the anemia of chronic disease, failure of the patient to take the medicine, improper dose or form of the medicinal iron, continuing iron loss (e.g., occult gastrointestinal bleeding), and malabsorption of iron. Failure of the patient to take the medication should always be considered. Compliance is enhanced by explanation and encouragement by the physician. Iron malabsorption is quite rare but, if suspected, can be tested for by a simple absorption test. A baseline serum iron level is obtained, and 100 mg of iron in the form of liquid ferrous sulfate is administered to the fasting patient. The serum iron is then measured at 1 and 2 hours. In a patient whose basal level of serum iron is below normal, an increase of 200 $\mu$g per dl is common. An increase of less than 100 $\mu$g per dl suggests malabsorption. Patients for whom iron is prescribed should be warned to keep their medication out of the reach of children. Iron tablets are a common offender in accidental overdose, which can lead to the severe consequences of acute iron toxicity.

The response to oral iron therapy can be recognized earliest by a rise in the percentage of circulating reticulocytes at about 4 days, reaching a maximum at 7 to 10 days. A rise in the hematocrit and hemoglobin level will follow, and these values should return to normal over a period of several weeks. The iron therapy should be continued for an additional period of 4 to 6 months to replenish iron stores.

### Parenteral Iron

Iron for intramuscular or intravenous administration is available in the form of iron-dextran (Imferon). Solutions contain 50 mg of elemental iron per ml. Parenteral iron does not produce any more rapid response than optimally administered oral iron. It has potential severe side effects, is more expensive, and requires more medical supervision. Thus its use should be reserved for those few situations when oral iron is unsatisfactory. Such situations include intractable side effects of oral iron, malabsorption, and psychologic or social situations that render adequate treatment with oral iron impossible.

When parenteral iron is used, the total required dose should be calculated since, in the absence of bleeding, all the administered iron will be retained by the patient. The iron deficit can be simply estimated by calculating the total body hemoglobin deficit and the corresponding amount of iron. For example, assume a 70-kg man with a hemoglobin of 8 grams per 100 ml. His hemoglobin deficit is 6 grams per 100 ml. His blood volume (70 ml per kg) is 4900 ml. Thus his hemoglobin deficit is 6 grams per 100 ml $\times$ 4900 ml = 294 grams. Iron comprises 0.34% of hemoglobin. Thus the hemoglobin iron deficit is 294 grams $\times$ 0.0034 = 0.9996 grams, or approximately 1000 mg. Add 500 mg of iron to replenish stores, and the total dose is 1500 mg.

Intramuscular Imferon should be given in the upper outer quadrant of the buttock. Because the solution can stain the skin, a Z-shaped injection technique is used. Allergic reactions, including anaphylaxis, may occur. Therefore, it is prudent to administer a test dose of 0.5 ml and wait an hour before giving more. In any event, therapy for anaphylactic reactions must be available whenever parenteral iron-dextran is given. Full intramuscular doses are 1 to 5 ml (50 to 250 mg) in each buttock. The patient may experience pain at the injection site. Most of the iron is mobilized within a few days, but some may remain at the injection site for a long period.

Intravenous iron-dextran can be given in multiple small doses over a period of time or administered as a single total dose. For total-dose therapy the calculated dose is diluted in saline to a concentration of less than 5%. A test dose should be administered slowly, e.g., 10 drops per minute for 10 to 15 minutes. If no reaction occurs, the rate may be increased so as to give the total dose over 2 to 3 hours. The major concern is anaphylaxis, and resuscitative materials must be at hand. Delayed serum sickness–like symptoms may occur and may be treated with nonsteroidal anti-inflammatory agents. Synovitis may be exacerbated in patients with rheumatoid arthritis.

# AUTOIMMUNE HEMOLYTIC ANEMIA

method of
CAROL COLA, M.D., and
JACK ANSELL, M.D.
*University of Massachusetts Medical Center*
*Worcester, Massachusetts*

Immune hemolytic anemias are characterized by the premature destruction of red blood cells (RBCs) mediated by antibodies to these cells. When an individual forms antibodies directed against his or her own RBCs (autoantibodies), the term "autoimmune hemolytic anemia" (AIHA) is applied, in contrast to conditions in which alloantibodies develop against foreign RBC antigens in hemolytic transfusion reactions, or that are transferred across the placenta from mother to fetus in hemolytic disease of the newborn. Autoantibodies may be formed without apparent provocation, leading to primary, or idiopathic, AIHA. Alternatively, they may occur as a secondary phenomenon in response to antigenic stimulation by a drug or an infectious agent, in association with a lymphoproliferative disorder, or as a feature of a global derangement of the immune system in immunodeficiency syndromes and certain collagen vascular disorders (Table 1).

A shortened RBC survival results in anemia if the bone marrow is unable to compensate with increased RBC production, as evidenced by an elevated reticulocyte count. When hemolysis outstrips the marrow's ability to compensate, anemia develops. Although the reticulocyte count is the best initial indicator of hemolysis, other studies may be needed to document a hemolytic process. These include a review of RBC morphology; an analysis of hemoglobin metabolites, such as bilirubin or urinary hemosiderin; and evaluation of hemoglobin-binding proteins, such as haptoglobin. The likelihood that the results of these tests are positive depends on the briskness of hemolysis and whether the process takes place within the vascular system or extravascularly.

After hemolysis is confirmed, a search for its cause is required. The direct antiglobulin test (AGT), or direct Coombs' test, is the basis on which immune hemolysis is identified. Antibody or complement coating the surface of RBCs is detected by incubating the patient's RBCs with anti-IgG or anticomplement antibody and looking for agglutination. RBC antibody in the patient's serum (the indirect test) is detected by incubating the patient's serum with normal RBCs and then applying the direct antiglobulin test to the normal cells.

Patients with evidence of hemolysis should be evaluated for AIHA. The spectrum of hemolysis may be quite variable in AIHA. The rate of hemolysis may be so slow that anemia fails to develop, and an increased reticulocyte count provides the only clue that erythroid hyperplasia in the bone marrow is compensating for a state of accelerated RBC destruction. Alternatively, hemolysis may be fulminant and life-threatening, marked by hemoglobinemia, hemoglobinuria, and cardiovascular compromise.

Autoantibodies may be classified as either warm reactive or cold reactive. Warm-reactive antibodies are usually IgG, are theoretically most active at body temperature, and typically do not activate complement. Cold-reactive antibodies are typically IgM, are most active at temperatures below 10° C, but often have a wide thermal range of reactivity, and frequently cause agglutination and activation of the classic complement pathway.

## TABLE 1. Classification of Immune Hemolytic Anemias

**Autoimmune Hemolytic Anemia**
*Warm-Reactive Antibody*
  Primary (idiopathic)
  Secondary
    Lymphoproliferative disorders (chronic lymphocytic
      leukemia, non-Hodgkin's lymphoma, etc.)
    Collagen vascular disorders (systemic lupus,
      scleroderma, etc.)
    Infections
    Nonlymphatic malignancies
    Immunodeficiency syndromes
*Cold-Reactive Antibody*
  Primary (idiopathic) cold agglutinin disease
  Secondary
    Infections (*Mycoplasma* pneumonia, infectious
      mononucleosis, other viral infections)
    Lymphoproliferative disorders
  Paroxysmal cold hemoglobinuria
    Idiopathic
    Secondary (syphilis, viral infections)

**Drug-Induced Immune Hemolytic Anemias**
**(Warm-Reactive Antibody)**
  Drug absorption type
  Immune complex type
  Autoantibody type
  Membrane modification type

**Alloantibody-Induced Immune Hemolytic Anemia**
  Hemolytic transfusion reaction
  Hemolytic disease of the newborn

## WARM-REACTIVE (IgG-MEDIATED) AUTOIMMUNE HEMOLYTIC ANEMIA

Warm-reactive antibodies cause the majority of AIHA cases. They are typically IgG antibodies, but they may be IgA or IgM. Approximately 50% of cases are idiopathic, and 25% are drug induced; 15 to 20% are associated with lymphoproliferative disorders, and the remaining 5 to 10% are associated with miscellaneous diseases, including infections and collagen vascular disorders.

IgG-coated RBCs are cleared primarily by the spleen. Splenic macrophages bear Fc receptors for the IgG molecules and destroy the coated RBCs by phagocytosis. The Kupffer cells of the liver are far less sensitive to IgG-coated cells. Thus, hepatic clearance is not usually significant, unless antibody coating is extremely heavy (>10,000 molecules per cell) or unless the spleen is absent.

The clinical features of primary and secondary AIHA may be identical. Thus, a search for an underlying cause should always be undertaken. The presence of a lymphoproliferative disorder should be excluded by careful physical examination, and, if indicated, imaging of the chest, the abdomen, and the pelvis by computed tomography or magnetic resonance imaging and bone marrow examination. Likewise, collagen vascular disorders should be excluded by careful examination and serologic studies, and a careful drug history must be elicited.

The clinical onset of AIHA is variable, tending to be fulminant in some drug-induced types, when associated with infection, or in idiopathic forms. It is more indolent in cases associated with lymphoproliferative and collagen vascular disorders.

The presenting symptoms are those associated with anemia of any cause, notably weakness, dizziness, dyspnea, and decreased exercise tolerance. Examination reveals pallor and sometimes jaundice, depending on the extent of hemolysis and the level of bilirubin. Unexplained fever accompanies the hemolytic episode in about a third of patients. Mild to moderate splenomegaly typically develops within days to a few weeks. Massive splenomegaly should increase the suspicion of an underlying lymphoproliferative disorder. Likewise, lymphadenopathy should not be seen in idiopathic AIHA.

The blood smear in these cases frequently displays microspherocytes and large polychromatophilic cells representing reticulocytes. Although hemolysis is typically extravascular, brisk hemolysis may produce hemoglobinemia, hemoglobinuria, and a reduced haptoglobin level owing to its binding to free hemoglobin and subsequent clearance from the blood. The hemoglobin level may fall to as low as 5 grams per dl, and the reticulocyte count may range from 25 to 40%. The result of the direct AGT using anti-IgG is almost always positive, whereas the indirect test result is positive in a smaller percentage of cases.

Rarely, cases of apparent warm-reactive AIHA show a negative direct AGT result on routine analysis, possibly because of too few immunoglobulin molecules bound to the RBC. More sensitive assays, such as the antiglobulin consumption complement fixation assay, the enzyme-linked AGT, and the radiolabeled AGT, are available for these situations. These tests may detect a much smaller number of IgG molecules per cell and thus allow the correct diagnosis to be established. Marked erythroid hyperplasia is typically seen on marrow examination, but, in rare cases, erythroid hypoplasia and even an aplastic marrow can be seen. In cases characterized by reticulocytopenia, uncompensated hemolysis may lead to profound life-threatening anemia. To account for the latter, some investigators have postulated that reticulocytes express more anti-

gens and are selectively destroyed, but case reports to the contrary have been published. Maturing normoblasts have also been demonstrated to react with autoantibodies, and this interaction may impair RBC egress from the bone marrow.

## Therapy (Table 2)

**Transfusions.** Patients with fulminant hemolysis and cardiovascular compromise should be transfused. The autoantibody present in the patient's serum typically reacts with donor RBCs, destroying them at the same rate as autologous cells, but this should not deter the decision to transfuse. More important, the autoantibody frequently causes panagglutination of all donor RBCs when cross-matching is attempted. Thus, it may obscure the detection of an alloantibody that would have the potential of causing a severe hemolytic reaction. A careful history of prior pregnancies and prior transfusions should be elicited, because patients with negative histories are unlikely to harbor masked alloantibodies.

Special techniques are now available to allow the detection of these antibodies. ABO typing can generally be accomplished by using prewashed blood cells. The Rh phenotype can be determined by using agglutinins in saline. Alloantibodies directed against antigens of the Kell, Duffy, and Kidd blood groups can also produce major hemolytic reactions. These may be detected by first eluting autoantibody from the patient's RBCs, using special reagents, and then employing these RBCs to detect alloantibodies by the differential absorption technique.

If emergency transfusion is required as a life-

TABLE 2. **Therapy of Warm Antibody–Type Autoimmune Hemolytic Anemia\***

| | |
|---|---|
| Corticosteroids | Prednisone, 1.0 to 1.5 mg/kg/day; if initial response, slowly taper over several months |
| Splenectomy | For corticosteroid failures or relapses; good response in ~50% of patients |
| Transfusions | If needed for severe anemia; cross-matching can be problematic |
| Immunosuppressant agents | For corticosteroid and/or splenectomy failures; <50% response |
| Danazol | May be effective in small number of patients |
| Gamma globulin infusion | 0.4–1.0 gram/kg over 1–5 days; may temporarily improve hemolysis |
| Exchange plasmapheresis | Limited utility in warm-reactive AIHA, but may have short-term benefit |

\*See text for detailed information.

saving measure before definitive cross-matching has been accomplished, ABO-compatible Rh-negative blood should be given.

Patients whose AIHA follows a relapsing course can have extended RBC phenotyping performed during periods of remission. These patients should also be considered for autologous donation.

**Corticosteroids.** Corticosteroids constitute the mainstay of therapy for warm-reactive AIHA. Their initial effect is seen within a few days and is thought to represent a dampening of the ability of tissue macrophages to clear IgG-coated cells. After several weeks of treatment, corticosteroids may also decrease antibody production.

Prednisone (Deltasone) should be started at a dosage of 1.0 to 1.5 mg per kg per day. The reticulocyte count usually begins to rise to even higher levels in a few days; the hemoglobin level, in approximately 1 week. About 80% of patients respond to corticosteroids, but, if no response is seen after 3 weeks, the patient should be considered steroid refractory.

If a response is achieved, prednisone should be tapered to 30 mg per day over a period of about 6 weeks. Subsequent tapering should be more gradual, with the daily dosage decreased by 5 mg every 2 to 4 weeks until a dosage of 15 mg per day is achieved. After that, alternate-day therapy may be employed. If the dosage cannot eventually be decreased to less than 15 mg per day without causing a relapse, the long-term side effects mandate consideration of an alternative therapy.

**Splenectomy.** Splenectomy initially yields a good response in 50 to 60% of patients, although permanent remission is achieved in less than 50%. Relapses may occur late, months to years after the operation. Patients with splenomegaly are more likely to respond to splenectomy. $^{51}$Cr-labeled RBC splenic sequestration studies have been used to predict response to splenectomy, but results may be variable; thus, this technique is of questionable clinical utility.

**Other Therapies** Cytotoxic immunosuppressive agents have also been employed with some success. Azathioprine( Imuran),* 125 mg per day, or cyclophosphamide (Cytoxan),* 100 mg per day, can be given to patients who have experienced treatment failure or are not candidates for corticosteroids or splenectomy. A response is achieved in 40 to 50% of patients. Treatment should be continued for 4 to 6 months, if it is tolerated, and then slowly tapered over the subsequent 6 months.

The modified androgen danazol (Danocrine)* may also be effective in AIHA. Danazol should be started at a dosage of 200 mg four times per day and continued for at least a 2-month trial. A rise in hemoglobin concentration is usually seen within 3 weeks. If hemolysis is severe, high-dose corticosteroids should be administered concurrently. After remission is obtained, the steroids can be tapered. If remission is sustained on danazol alone for a month, the dosage can be gradually tapered to 200 to 400 mg per day. Treatment should be continued for 1 year, as shorter courses are more likely to result in relapse.

Gamma globulin (Gammagard, Sandoglobulin)* infusion may also be efficacious as a temporizing measure. Infusions of 400 mg per kg per day for 5 days may produce a sustained response. In some cases, a dosage of 1 gm per kg once weekly or less often may be similarly beneficial. If relapse occurs, infusions may be repeated to sustain remission for a few months, while awaiting a spontaneous remission or the benefits of immunosuppressive therapy. Gamma globulin may inhibit phagocytosis by splenic macrophages by binding to and blocking their Fc receptors. Long-term therapy produces a decrease in the antiglobulin titer, suggesting an alternative mechanism. Another postulated mechanism would be the formation of anti-idiotype–idiotype complexes on the RBC surface.

Exchange plasmapheresis offers another means of temporizing. Its utility in warm-reactive AIHA is limited, however, because of the continuous production of autoantibodies and the large extravascular distribution of IgG.

## DRUG-INDUCED AUTOIMMUNE HEMOLYTIC ANEMIA

Drugs are an uncommon but well-documented cause of AIHA. A variety of drugs have been implicated, but only a few have been thoroughly investigated with regard to their pathophysiologic mechanisms. Whenever an immune hemolytic anemia is suspected, a detailed medication history must be obtained and all nonessential medications discontinued. Four pathophysiologic mechanisms have been described to account for drug-induced autoimmune hemolytic anemia:

**Drug Adsorption (Hapten) Mechanism.** This type of drug-induced AIHA may be seen with the use of high dosages of intravenous penicillin ($>10 \times 10^6$ u per day). The drug is adsorbed onto the RBC membrane, and drug-induced IgG antibody reacts with membrane-bound penicillin. The direct AGT result is strongly positive against IgG on the patient's RBCs, although complement components can rarely be found. Acute intravascular hemolysis is uncommon, and the onset is gradual. Cessation of the drug leads to a gradual resolu-

---

*This indication is not listed in manufacturer's directive.

*This indication is not listed in manufacturer's directive.

tion of the hemolysis over several days to a week or two. The direct AGT may remain weakly positive for several weeks.

**Immune Complex Mechanism.** Quinidine (Quinaglute) is the prototypic drug that may induce an immune hemolytic anemia by an immune complex mechanism. Serum IgG or IgM antibody is formed against the drug, and the immune complex attaches to the RBC membrane, frequently leading to complement activation and acute intravascular hemolysis. The direct AGT result is positive, often because of complement components on the RBC membrane. Hemolysis often develops suddenly and may be life-threatening. Patients who have been previously sensitized need only small amounts of drug to precipitate acute hemolysis. Hemolysis rapidly abates when the drug is discontinued.

**Autoantibody Mechanism.** This third type of drug-induced AIHA is typified by the response to alpha-methyldopa (Aldomet). The immune hemolytic anemia that develops is similar to primary (idiopathic) AIHA, and the precise mechanism of antibody stimulation by the drug is unclear, but may be due to an alteration, or an unmasking, of RBC antigens that are no longer seen as self-antigens, or to an alteration of the immune system's response to self-antigens. The development of an IgG autoantibody is dose related, occurring in approximately 10 to 20% of patients 3 to 12 months after starting methyldopa, but only a small percentage (about 1%) develop clinical hemolysis. If hemolysis occurs, it does so gradually, without evidence of acute intravascular hemolysis. The direct AGT result is positive to a varying degree, with or without hemolysis. Cessation of the drug leads to eventual resolution of hemolysis during a few weeks, but a positive AGT result may take months or longer to normalize. Prednisone may bolster the RBC counts until spontaneous recovery occurs.

**Membrane-Modification Mechanism.** This last mechanism of drug-induced immune hemolysis has been attributed to cephalosporin analogues. The drug is thought to alter the RBC membrane, leading to nonspecific and nonimmunologic adsorption of serum proteins that may induce a positive direct AGT result. Hemolysis in this setting is rare. Cephalosporins have also been implicated in hemolytic anemias by other mechanisms noted earlier.

## COLD-REACTIVE (IgM-MEDIATED) AUTOIMMUNE HEMOLYTIC ANEMIA

Cold-reactive AIHA is typically mediated by IgM autoantibodies. Because these are most active at temperatures below 10° C, agglutination and complement activation occur while blood is coursing through peripheral blood vessels. After the blood is rewarmed centrally, the IgM molecules dissociate from the RBC membrane, leaving behind a residue of complement activation. This intrinsic difference in activity usually precludes the development of fulminant hemolysis.

Cold antibodies may produce mild chronic or seasonal hemolytic anemia. Severe hemolytic anemia occurs less frequently, usually in the setting of a cold-reactive antibody with an unusually broad thermal range. IgM cold agglutinins can produce agglutination of RBCs intravascularly and such massive agglutination may produce veno-occlusive disease manifested as painful cyanosis of the peripheral tissues of the nose, the ears, and the digits.

Cold antibody–induced hemolysis is mediated through activation of the classic complement pathway. During activation, C3 is cleaved to C3a and C3b. The latter binds to the RBC surface, and the RBCs are cleared by the reticuloendothelial system via the interaction between C3b and C3b receptors. This interaction is most effectively mediated by the Kupffer cells of the liver; splenic macrophages contribute less. After they are captured, either the RBCs are consumed by phagocytosis or C3b may be cleaved further into C3c and C3d by C3b inactivator. If this latter process occurs, the C3d remains cell bound, and the RBC is regurgitated back into the circulation. C3d on the RBC membrane blocks potential sites of C3b attachment, thereby protecting these cells from future immunologic clearance. These AGT-positive C3d-bearing cells actually survive longer in the circulation of patients with cold agglutinin disease than transfused normal cells do.

Cold-reactive AIHA can occur in a primary, or idiopathic, form or may be associated with various infectious agents or certain lymphoproliferative disorders. The IgM autoantibody in primary cold agglutinin disease is monoclonal with specificity for the I antigen on RBCs. The antibody accompanying certain infections is polyclonal, also with I specificity, except with infectious mononucleosis (Epstein-Barr virus), in which the antibody has i specificity.

**Primary Cold Agglutinin Disease.** Idiopathic cold agglutinin disease is primarily a disease of the elderly. It occurs clinically with cold-induced acrocyanosis, typically with an episodic relapsing course. With prolonged exposure to low temperatures, dry gangrene may develop. The associated hemolysis is usually mild to moderate, but may be severe.

Conservative therapy includes decreasing the patient's exposure to cold, with either protective clothing or a move to a warmer climate. When cardiovascular compromise mandates transfusion, cross-matching must be performed at 37° C, and blood must be warmed prior to transfusion. Plasmapheresis provides the most effective therapeutic modality available. Splenectomy and immunosuppressive therapy are generally not beneficial. Likewise, steroids are not usually effective in managing cold-reactive AIHA. They are of benefit in occasional cases when the antibody has a high thermal amplitude, but is present in low titer, or when an IgG cold-reactive antibody is the culprit.

**Secondary Cold Agglutinin Disease.** Several infectious diseases are capable of invoking an increase in polyclonal cold agglutinins. The most common cause of high-titer cold agglutinins is *Mycoplasma pneumoniae*. Anti-I agglutinins appear during convalescence in more than 80% of patients with *Mycoplasma* pneumonia. Infectious mononucleosis elicits synthesis of anti-i antibodies. Other infectious conditions associated with cold agglutinins include influenza, mumps, syphilis, and malaria. Infection-induced cold antibodies usually appear from 1 to 3 weeks after the onset of the infectious illness. Their presence is self-limited, usually abating within a month.

Monoclonal cold-reactive antibodies of the IgM-κ type may be seen in association with lymphoproliferative disorders. Therefore, all patients with chronic cold agglutinin disease should be screened for these disorders by the methods described earlier. Lymphomas are diagnosed in up to a third of such cases.

## PAROXYSMAL COLD HEMOGLOBINURIA

Paroxysmal cold hemoglobinuria (PCH) is a rare, acquired hemolytic disorder caused by cold-reactive antibodies directed against antigens of the P blood group system. It is usually seen in individuals with a history of tertiary syphilis or a recent viral infection. Now that syphilis is uncommon, PCH is primarily seen in the pediatric population.

The anti-P antibody has been termed "Donath-Landsteiner antibody." It is an IgG antibody that activates complement. In this disorder, the anti-C3 direct AGT result turns positive. IgG is not detected on the RBC surfaces, however, because the cold-reactive IgG dissociates at body temperature. The Donath-Landsteiner test is performed by adding patient serum to test RBCs on ice for 30 minutes, followed by incubation at 37° C for 30 minutes. Evidence of hemolysis constitutes a positive test result.

On exposure to cold, patients with PCH may develop fulminant intravascular hemolysis with resultant hemoglobinemia. They frequently develop abdominal or back pain, appear apprehen-

sive, and may exhibit tachypnea. Anaphylactoid manifestations, such as urticaria, may also be seen. Subsequently, frank rigors and fever occur. Hemoglobinuria develops and may persist for 1 to 2 days.

The acute postinfectious form of PCH is self-limited, with spontaneous recovery occurring within a few days. The less common idiopathic form is managed by the avoidance of cold. If transfusional support is necessary, the transfusion of p or p$^k$ blood types may be performed, as these types lack the P antigen and are thus not susceptible to the offending antibody. These blood types are rare, however. If they are not available, cross-matched blood may be given using a blood warmer.

# NONIMMUNE HEMOLYTIC ANEMIA

method of
WILLIAM N. VALENTINE, M.D.
*Center for Health Sciences*
*University of California, Los Angeles*
*Los Angeles, California*

Although moderate shortening of the normal life span of red blood cells occurs in many patients, the term "hemolytic anemia" is usually reserved for syndromes in which hemolysis is substantial and plays a meaningful role in the pathogenesis of clinical and hematologic manifestations. In actuality, anemia is not always present because normal bone marrow can compensate for premature destruction of erythrocytes by increasing the production of red cells about six to eight times. If hemolysis exceeds the capacity for compensation, anemia is inevitable.

The nonspecific hallmarks of hemolysis are persistent reticulocytosis, polychromasia of red blood cells on stained blood films, erythroid hyperplasia of marrow, and sometimes an increase in plasma lactate dehydrogenase level and jaundice. The latter, when present, is caused by increased catabolism of hemoglobin and the resultant increase in indirectly reacting bilirubinemia. Purely hemolytic jaundice is never associated with bilirubinuria or with elevation of the directly reacting fraction of serum bilirubin. The latter may occur, of course, as a concomitant of hemolytic syndromes from causes other than hemolysis per se (e.g., biliary obstruction with pigment stones, transfusion-induced hepatitis, microinfarcts of liver in sickle cell anemia). Splenomegaly is a common, but not universal, accompaniment of chronic hemolysis. One notable exception occurs in the adult with sickle cell anemia. Although infants and young children present with splenomegaly, repeated splenic infarction commonly results in what may be termed an "autosplenectomy" by the time of adulthood. In a subset of hemolytic syndromes, hemolysis may be largely intravascular. If it is sufficiently marked, hemoglobinemia and overt hemoglobinuria may be present. The latter must be clearly differentiated from hematuria. The nonspecific hallmarks of hemolysis may be mimicked during a regenerative response to anemia of other etiology (e.g., hemorrhage, hematinic therapy). If the hemorrhage is internal, overt bleeding may be absent and resorption of hematomas may be accompanied by hyperbilirubinemia and jaundice. Ineffective erythropoiesis, such as that accompanying a variety of refractory anemias with cellular bone marrow, including pernicious anemia, folate deficiency, and the thalassemia syndromes, may also, when marked, be associated with jaundice, anemia, and elevation of the plasma lactate dehydrogenase level. These manifestations are secondary to intramarrow death of partially hemoglobinated, nucleated erythroid precursors never destined to reach the circulation, a form of intramarrow red blood cell precursor hemolysis. Other clinical and laboratory features point to the correct diagnosis.

## CLINICAL EVALUATION

Hemolytic anemia whose pathogenesis lies in immunologic mechanisms is described elsewhere and will not be discussed further here. Management of the nonimmune hemolytic anemias rests squarely on their expeditious and correct diagnosis, and the latter is directed by answers to several pertinent questions.

*Is the hemolysis of infectious or toxic origin?* Life-threatening sepsis with hemolytic organisms such as *Clostridium perfringens* obviously requires prompt diagnosis and heroic measures. Hemolysis accompanies red blood cell parasitism with plasmodia in malaria. Severe lead poisoning is associated with marked hemolytic anemia, as is the much rarer exposure to arsine gas. Hemolysis also may result from spider and snake bites and, more rarely, from bee stings. However, in all of these situations, the clinical picture is dominated by systemic and local manifestations, and in most instances the history, physical examination, and pertinent laboratory findings point early to the correct diagnosis. The diagnosis of red blood cell parasitism may, however, be obscure, particularly in areas where its incidence and the index of suspicion are low.

*Is the hemolysis predominantly intravascular, or is it mediated by the reticuloendothelial system?* If the hemolysis is ongoing, the serum haptoglobin, a protein binding free hemoglobin, is essentially undetectable. If the hemolysis is sufficiently marked, frank hemoglobinuria is noted; if it is milder, hemoglobin passing the renal filter is taken up by tubular epithelium, whose shed cells in centrifuged urinary sediment stain positively for iron. Hemosiderinuria and hemoglobinuria both reflect intravascular hemolysis. Intravascular hemolysis occurs in microangiopathic syndromes with diffuse lesions in the microvasculature, with defective cardiac prostheses, in patients with glucose-6-phosphate dehydrogenase (G6PD) deficiency during hemolytic episodes, in the comparatively rare syndrome of paroxysmal nocturnal hemoglobinuria, and in certain rare, unstable hemoglobinopathies.

In reticuloendothelial-mediated hemolysis, red blood cells are prematurely destroyed by phagocytic macrophages. The serum haptoglobin level may be moderately low, but the haptoglobin does not disappear.

Hemoglobinuria, hemosiderinuria, and iron deficiency are not part of the picture. This is the case in sickle cell disease and other major hemoglobinopathies; in hereditary spherocytosis, elliptocytosis, and other syndromes caused by defective erythrocyte membranes; in hemolysis associated with most red blood cell enzymopathies other than G6PD deficiency; and in the rare abnormality of hereditary acanthocytosis.

*Is the syndrome hereditary or acquired?* A family history of anemia, jaundice, early cholelithiasis, painful crises, red urine, splenomegaly, or splenectomy may direct the diagnostic regimen toward the hereditary syndromes. Ethnic derivation and a history of lifelong symptoms have obvious implications.

*Is the pathogenic abnormality intracorpuscular or extracorpuscular?* In all hereditary syndromes with the exception of the abetalipoproteinemia of hereditary acanthocytosis, the pathogenic defect is intracorpuscular; in all acquired hemolytic anemias with the exception of paroxysmal nocturnal hemoglobinuria, it is extracorpuscular.

*Is the hemolysis episodic or chronic?* In many of the manifold variants of G6PD deficiency, hemolytic episodes occur only with oxidant stresses such as ingestion of certain antimalarial drugs, nitrofurantoin, sulfanilamide, or, with some variants, fava beans. Infections and surgical stress may also produce episodic hemoglobinuria in deficient persons. In other syndromes, such as hereditary spherocytosis, jaundice may wax and wane, and anemia occasionally worsens rapidly as a result of transient marrow failure during certain myelosuppressive viral infections (the so-called self-limited aregenerative or aplastic crises).

*Are there telltale morphologic abnormalities on the stained blood film?* Although sophisticated evaluation of red blood cell morphology may require consultative assistance, its importance in directing diagnosis and management renders it mandatory that the necessary evaluation be obtained from the laboratory or a specialist. The stained blood film, properly evaluated, yields more valuable clues than any other single laboratory procedure. The small, round, densely staining "spherocyte," lacking the normal zone of central pallor, when present in substantial numbers and in the absence of a positive Coombs' test strongly suggests hereditary spherocytosis. The spherocyte, a cell whose surface area is relatively small for its volume, lyses at concentrations of hypotonic saline, leaving normal erythrocytes intact. The osmotic fragility test therefore provides laboratory confirmation of spherocytosis. The test is rendered more sensitive in doubtful cases if whole blood is sterilely incubated at 37° C for 24 hours before testing. Small numbers of spherocytes may be present in clostridial sepsis, in hemolytic episodes occurring in G6PD-deficient persons, and together with elliptocytes in certain hemolytic forms of hereditary elliptocytosis.

Cells appearing as targets on stained blood films are present in all the major hemoglobinopathies. Hemoglobins S, C, D, and E are mutants found in large numbers of persons. Hemoglobins S and C are encoded by genes arising in Africa, the latter having a much more circumscribed distribution in West Africa. Hemoglobin D$^{Punjab}$ is found in large numbers in persons from Pakistan and northwest India. Hemoglobin E has a wide distribution in Burma and parts of Southeast Asia. "Target cells" are also common in thalassemia; in certain forms of liver and biliary disease; and, to a lesser extent, after splenectomy and in marked iron deficiency.

Irreversibly "sickled cells" on the stained blood film indicate sickle cell anemia or syndromes involving the simultaneous inheritance of hemoglobins S and C (SC disease), S and D$^{Punjab}$ (SD disease), or S and beta-thalassemia. They are not seen in persons heterozygous for hemoglobin S.

"Schistocytes" are fragmented, traumatized red cells. When present, they suggest microangiopathic anemia or the "Waring Blender" syndrome occurring with defective cardiac prostheses.

"Heinz bodies" are inclusions of denatured hemoglobin. They occur particularly in hemolysis accompanying G6PD deficiency and in certain rare, unstable hemoglobinopathies. Because of the efficiency of the pitting function of the normal spleen, they are often inconspicuous except in splenectomized subjects.

"Acanthocytes" are irregularly shaped cells with pseudopod-like or finger-like projections. They are seen most prominently in hereditary acanthocytosis, a rare syndrome caused by genetically determined abetalipoproteinemia.

"Stomatocytes" appear on stained blood films to have a slit, or mouth-like, zone of central pallor. They can be artifacts of preparation, but they occur in a subset of hemolytic syndromes caused by defective cell membranes and grossly abnormal fluxes of the cations Na$^+$ and K$^+$.

"Elliptocytes" are oval or sausage-shaped red blood cells. They are associated with both a benign abnormality lacking hemolysis and an overtly hemolytic disorder.

*Is the hemolysis caused by direct red blood cell trauma?* Red blood cells may be severely damaged and fragmented when passing through a damaged microvasculature. In the latter case, the erythrocyte may be forced through partially occluded areas where endothelium is disrupted and fibrin networks abound. Diffusely damaged microvasculature is associated with the syndrome of thrombotic thrombocytopenic purpura and, at times, with malignant hypertension, acute glomerulonephritis, and widespread metastatic, neoplastic emboli. Trauma may likewise accompany defective valvular prostheses in the heart and other surgical complications such as incomplete epithelialization of repaired septal defects. The intracardiac battering of red blood cells that can be associated with these abnormalities may cause hemolysis in the "Waring Blender" syndrome.

## MANAGEMENT

**Syndromes Secondary to Infections and Toxins.** Treatment is focused on the underlying disease: administration of appropriate antibiotics and/or antimalarials, support of blood pressure, maintenance of fluid balance, and prompt therapy of special complications. Transfusions may or may not be necessary in individual cases. The diag-

nosis of lead poisoning mandates removal of the patient from the toxic environment and may require treatment with lead-chelating agents.

**Prevention of Hemolytic Episodes.** When clinically significant G6PD deficiency is present, the patient should be advised to avoid medications and agents known to produce oxidant stress and to precipitate hemolysis. Although many medications have been doubtfully or even erroneously incriminated in the production of hemolytic episodes, a number of them are firmly established. These include sulfanilamide (but not all sulfa-containing medications), furadantin, acetanilid, the antimalarials primaquine and pamaquine, and trimethoprim-sulfamethoxazole (Bactrim). Ingestion of fava beans provokes hemolysis in some G6PD deficiency syndromes but not in others. There are more than 300 reportedly different G6PD variants (some may prove to be identical), and their phenotypic clinical manifestations differ widely in different genotypes. Hemolytic episodes may be precipitated by oxidant stress in patients with certain rare, unstable hemoglobinopathies and rare erythroenzymopathies other than G6PD deficiency. When drug-induced hemolysis is suspected, prompt withdrawal of all potentially involved medications is indicated.

**Transfusions.** Transfusions are overused and should be avoided except for specific indications. The latter include rapidly worsening anemia, clinical or electrocardiographic evidence of myocardial ischemia, obtundation believed to be related to anemia, infectious complications, the possibility of surgery, and, at times, pregnancy. The well-known potential complications of transfusion—hepatitis and other viral infections, transfusion reactions, development of alloantibodies after repeated transfusions, and ultimately iron overload—constitute contraindications if the patient is stable and if a reasonable quality of life is being maintained. In short, the patient, and not an arbitrary hemoglobin level, is the object of treatment. Exchange transfusion may prove necessary in newborns with kernicterus-threatening hyperbilirubinemia secondary to hemolysis. The use of exchange or other transfusions in the management of painful crises or the acute chest syndrome in patients with sickle cell syndromes also requires sophisticated evaluation and is frequently controversial. Transfusion in the splenic sequestration syndrome sometimes encountered in young children with sickle cell anemia is an emergent and potentially life-saving measure. In general, when transfusion is indicated, packed red blood cells are the modality of choice. Transfusions in patients with paroxysmal nocturnal hemoglobinuria may present a special problem. Reactions caused by transfused plasma that contains components of the complement system may occur in some patients with this disorder. In this case, recipient (not donor) cells undergo lysis. When it occurs, all subsequent transfusions should be with saline-washed red blood cells. (Recipient cell lysis is one of the few indications for this procedure.) Such cells must be administered shortly after washing to ensure viability.

**Splenectomy.** Splenectomy as an emergency procedure may be lifesaving in splenic sequestration crises occurring in young children with sickle cell anemia. Although the morphologic abnormalities persist, splenectomy is clinically curative in the great majority of patients with hereditary spherocytosis. Jaundice abates, reticulocyte counts markedly decrease, and the erythrocyte life span measured with $^{51}$Cr labeling of red blood cells is nearly normal. In a subset of these patients, some evidence of hemolysis persists. Although this has often been ascribed to residual accessory spleens, only rarely does it appear to be the case. Whether or not splenectomy is recommended in the mildest compensated cases is controversial. It is the author's belief that in the absence of contraindications, the procedure has genuine benefit chiefly in ameliorating the likelihood of later cholecystitis and cholelithiasis. The patient must share in the decision. If it is not contraindicated, when cholecystectomy is necessary in patients with this disorder, splenectomy may simultaneously be performed. Results of splenectomy are gratifying in most cases of hemolytic elliptocytosis and in certain cases of hemolytic syndromes characterized by stomatocytosis. The procedure is usually ineffective in the G6PD deficiency syndromes and in microangiopathic hemolytic anemias. In patients with pyruvate kinase deficiency, and probably in other hemolytic erythroenzymopathies involving anaerobic glycolysis, splenectomy is indicated only when comfortable existence requires frequent transfusions. After the procedure, hemolysis remains severe and reticulocytosis may often be increased, but a partial benefit in the form of diminished or eliminated transfusion requirements and an increase of 1 to 3 grams per dl in hemoglobin may be distinctly worthwhile. In the most severe syndromes, splenectomy may be lifesaving.

**Cholelithiasis and Cholecystectomy.** In all chronic hemolytic anemias, the increased amount of bilirubin continuously presented to the liver and excreted in bile sharply increases the incidence of pigment stone formation, cholecystitis, and biliary obstruction, all of which may appear at an early age. Surgical management is frequently indicated. Simultaneous splenectomy should be considered only in those syndromes where its value is substantiated. In patients with sickle cell syndromes, avoidance of hypoxia during and after surgery is of great importance.

**Iron, Folate, and Corticosteroids.** Iron administration is contraindicated except where iron deficiency is documented. Normally there is no deficiency, and especially when transfusions have been necessary, iron stores are replete and perhaps excessive. Exceptions are the hemolytic syndromes characterized by intravascular hemolysis, hemoglobinemia, hemoglobinuria, and/or hemosiderinuria. Renal loss of hemoglobin in these circumstances is often a cause of associated iron deficiency that requires appropriate treatment (300 to 900 mg of ferrous sulfate per day). Corticosteroids have no place in the management of the syndromes discussed here, with the possible exception of the rare syndrome of thrombotic thrombocytopenic purpura.

Chronic hemolysis increases folate requirements, and folate in doses of 1 mg per day is a rational supplement. This may modestly increase the hemoglobin level and may provide some protection against the aregenerative crises discussed in the next section. We favor the routine administration of such supplements in patients with ongoing hemolysis of any etiology.

**The "Aplastic" or "Aregenerative" Crisis.** In any chronic hemolytic syndrome, transient acute marrow suppression may occur in the course of an illness that is usually attributed to a parvovirus. Marrow temporarily becomes hypoplastic, reticulocytopenia intervenes, the serum bilirubin level falls, and cytopenia becomes evident. Neutropenia and thrombocytopenia rarely become sufficiently severe to cause clinical manifestations, but in the presence of substantial hemolysis, anemia rapidly worsens and often becomes symptomatic. The crisis is self-limited, ordinarily lasting for 7 to 12 days. Afterward, marrow activity surges back, heralded by returning reticulocytosis and correction of cytopenia. During the period of marrow suppression, transfusion may or may not be required.

**Special Considerations.** Certain hemolytic syndromes have prominent accompaniments of clinical significance. Paroxysmal nocturnal hemoglobinuria may be associated in some patients with marrow hypoplasia, with a hypercoagulable state and widespread thrombotic phenomena, and sometimes with a variety of underlying myeloproliferative syndromes. Hemolysis in thrombotic thrombocytopenic purpura accompanies a greatly diminished platelet count, bleeding, and fluctuating, often severe, neurologic manifestations. The sickle cell syndromes are not only hemolytic but manifest a large array of vaso-occlusive problems discussed elsewhere. The patient with microangiopathic anemia has underlying diffuse disease of the microvasculature and sometimes metastatic neoplasia. The presence of marked intra-cardiac red blood cell trauma with defective prostheses may require replacement of the latter by the cardiac surgeon.

# PERNICIOUS ANEMIA AND OTHER MEGALOBLASTIC ANEMIAS

method of
A. MAJID SHOJANIA, M.D.

*Medical School of the University of Manitoba
and St. Boniface General Hospital
Winnipeg, Manitoba, Canada*

Pernicious anemia (PA) is a disorder caused by a deficiency of vitamin $B_{12}$ which in turn is due to idiopathic or immune-mediated deficiency of the gastric intrinsic factor (IF). IF is required for vitamin $B_{12}$ absorption. Pernicious anemia was, for many years, the only known disease to cause megaloblastic anemia, and consequently, the terms "pernicious anemia" and "megaloblastic anemia" were used interchangeably. Even today, the term "pernicious anemia" is sometimes erroneously applied to other diseases that cause megaloblastic anemia.

Megaloblastic anemias are a group of disorders in which the characteristic morphologic changes of hematopoietic cells are produced as the result of impaired DNA but normal RNA synthesis. The abnormality in these disorders is not limited to hematopoietic cells. Any cell that has to undergo DNA synthesis may show similar "megaloblastic" changes.

The diagnosis of megaloblastic anemia is rewarding because the disease can usually be easily treated to the great satisfaction of the symptomatic patient. Hematologic abnormalities, no matter how severe and advanced, can be treated with full recovery, whereas neurologic abnormalities that may be present, if not treated early, may become irreversible.

When megaloblastic anemia is diagnosed, it should be considered to be due to folate or vitamin $B_{12}$ deficiency unless proved otherwise. Many chemotherapeutic agents do produce megaloblastic anemia, but this possibility is generally evident in patient's history; moreover, physicians who prescribe chemotherapeutic agents are quite familiar with this complication of chemotherapy. Inborn errors of metabolism causing megaloblastic anemia are many by name, but their occurrence is extremely rare.

When megaloblastic anemia is suspected on the basis of the patient's history, the physical examination findings, or observation of the existence of macrocytic anemia, one needs first to establish that megaloblastic changes are indeed present in the peripheral blood or in the bone marrow. One must then establish the cause and treat the deficiency of the vitamin, and, if possible, determine and treat the underlying cause of the deficiency. Omitting the first step may lead to erroneous diagnosis with sometimes serious consequences. Anemia should not be attributed to folate or vitamin $B_{12}$ deficiency on the basis of low serum folate or serum vitamin $B_{12}$ levels, unless there are also megaloblastic changes in the blood or in the bone marrow. Low serum folate or low serum vitamin $B_{12}$ levels may be seen in many conditions that may also cause anemia, but not megaloblastic anemia.

## DEMONSTRATION OF THE EXISTENCE OF MEGALOBLASTIC ANEMIA

In fully developed megaloblastic anemia, the complete blood count (CBC) demonstrates the existence of macrocytic anemia, leukopenia with neutropenia, and thrombocytopenia. An examination of the blood smear shows macrocytes and an increased number of hypersegmented neutrophils. However, in the early stages, many of these features may be absent. The earliest change in CBC that suggests the presence of megaloblastic anemia is the rise of mean corpuscular volume (MCV), as determined by the same equipment as for the automated CBC test. Macrocytosis (an increase in MCV) generally appears before the anemia develops. However, when megaloblastic anemia is associated with conditions that cause microcytosis (such as iron deficiency, thalassemia, or anemia of chronic disease), the MCV may be normal. Not all macrocytic anemias are megaloblastic; other conditions that may cause macrocytosis without megaloblastic changes are liver disease, chronic alcoholism, obstructive jaundice, aplastic or hypoplastic anemias, myelophthisic conditions, bone marrow infiltration with malignant cells, chemotherapy, myelodysplasias, hypothyroidism, sideroblastic anemias, chronic obstructive pulmonary disease, absence of spleen, and rapid red blood cell (RBC) production (high reticulocyte count). Similarly, an increased number of hypersegmented neutrophils may also be found in several other conditions, such as chronic infection, myeloproliferative disorders, severe iron deficiency anemia, uremia, and hereditary hypersegmentation of neutrophil nuclei. However, when macrocytosis is associated with an increased number of hypersegmented neutrophils, there is a strong possibility that megaloblastic anemia is present.

Bone marrow examination is generally required for the proper diagnosis of megaloblastic anemia. Unless the peripheral blood picture is clear-cut and there is no suggestion of associated problems in the patient's history or in the physical examination, I generally prefer to examine the bone marrow, even if the peripheral blood picture shows megaloblastic features, because these changes in the blood may be secondary and the primary disorder may be a malignancy involving the bone marrow, or the changes may be due to myelodysplasia.

The results of several other biochemical tests may be abnormal in megaloblastic anemias. These tests are not needed for the diagnosis of megaloblastic anemias, but one should be aware of these changes to avoid erroneous diagnosis or unnecessary additional investigations. In megaloblastic anemias, there may be an increase in levels of serum unconjugated (indirect) bilirubin, uric acid, and aspartate aminotransferase (serum glutamic-oxaloacetic transaminase); serum lactate dehydrogenase levels may be markedly elevated and serum iron and serum ferritin concentrations may be high. Serum haptoglobin levels may be low, and methemalbuminemia may be present.

## DEMONSTRATION OF THE CAUSE OF MEGALOBLASTIC ANEMIA

Both folate deficiency and vitamin $B_{12}$ deficiency cause identical hematologic changes in the peripheral blood and in the bone marrow. The history and the physical examination may suggest the likely vitamin deficiency, but the definitive diagnosis generally necessitates laboratory testing. A detailed history, with special attention to diet, gastrointestinal and neuropsychiatric symptoms, medications, and the history of any previous surgery on the gastrointestinal tract, may help to suggest the most likely diagnosis. Green leafy vegetables and fresh fruits are good sources of dietary folate (cooking destroys much of the food folate); decreased dietary intake is the most common cause of folate deficiency. In contrast, dietary vitamin $B_{12}$ is present only in animal products. Because the daily requirement of vitamin $B_{12}$ is quite small, most diets provide adequate vitamin $B_{12}$ with the exception of long-standing strict vegetarians who may develop vitamin $B_{12}$ deficiency owing to low dietary intake. The main cause of vitamin $B_{12}$ deficiency is vitamin $B_{12}$ malabsorption, either due to lack of IF (with PA or after gastrectomy) or due to ileal conditions (after ileal resection, Crohn's disease, or lack of vitamin $B_{12}$ receptors). The minimal daily requirement for folate is 100 to 200 µg, and that for vitamin $B_{12}$ is 1 to 2 µg. When no vitamin $B_{12}$ is being absorbed, it may take 2 to 10 years for an adult to develop vitamin $B_{12}$ deficiency megaloblastic anemia. On the other hand, when no folate is being absorbed or provided in the diet, folate deficiency megaloblastic anemia may develop in a few months. Consequently, in conditions in which the intake or absorption of both vitamins is decreased (malabsorption syndrome or alcoholism) or when the requirement for both vitamins is increased, such as during rapid growth (prematurity and infancy, adolescence, and pregnancy) or in the cases of increased cell production (malignancy, hemolytic anemia, and myeloproliferative disorders), the patient experiences folate deficiency megaloblastic anemia and seeks medical advice long before vitamin $B_{12}$ deficiency megaloblastic anemia has had the chance to become established.

Many drugs may also cause folate deficiency megaloblastic anemia by interfering with metabolism or absorption of folate or by increasing the body requirement for folate. These include folate antagonists (methotrexate, trimethoprim [Proloprim], triamterene [Dyrenium], pyrimethamine [Daraprim], and pentamidine [Pentam]), anticonvulsants (phenytoin [Dilantin], phenobarbital, and primidone [Mysoline]), oral contraceptives, antituberculous medications (cycloserine and isoniazid), alcohol, and salazopyrine. Many other drugs may also interfere with vitamin $B_{12}$ absorption or metabolism (colchicine, potassium chloride, para-aminosalicylic acid, neomycin, alcohol, metformin,* phenformin,* and high-dose ascorbic acid). However, the long-lasting body store of vitamin $B_{12}$ generally prevents the development of vitamin $B_{12}$ deficiency megaloblastic anemia. The exception to this rule is prolonged nitrous oxide anesthesia, which can cause acute megaloblastic changes within 1 to 2 days by destroying biologically active vitamin $B_{12}$. The presence of paresthesia, decreased vibration sense, or other neurologic signs of subacute combined degeneration of the spinal cord favors the diagnosis of vitamin $B_{12}$ deficiency.

### Diagnosis of Vitamin $B_{12}$ and Folate Deficiency

**Serum Folate and Serum Vitamin $B_{12}$ Assay.** In the presence of megaloblastic anemia, levels of both serum folate and serum vitamin $B_{12}$ have to be determined because a deficiency of either vitamin may cause a subnormal serum level of the other vitamin. In the presence of megaloblastic anemia, low serum folate and normal serum vitamin $B_{12}$ levels establish the diagnosis of folate deficiency anemia. Low serum vitamin $B_{12}$ and normal serum folate levels establish the diagnosis of vitamin $B_{12}$ deficiency anemia. However, if both serum folate and serum vitamin $B_{12}$ levels are low, one has to demonstrate whether this is due to combined deficiency or whether only one is the true deficiency. In the latter situation, if the patient is not a long-standing vegetarian, I check the Schilling test. If the Schilling test result is abnormal, the need for vitamin $B_{12}$ therapy is established and I would continue with the vitamin $B_{12}$ therapy and repeat the serum folate determination in 3 to 4 weeks. If the serum folate level is still low, I assume that the patient is also folate deficient. If the Schilling test result is normal, and, again, if the patient is not a vegetarian, I assume that the patient is not vitamin $B_{12}$ deficient and the true deficiency is folate deficiency. (On rare occasions, patients with gastric achlorhydria may develop vitamin $B_{12}$ deficiency megaloblastic anemia associated with a normal standard Schilling test result, but if a modified Schilling's test is used with radioactive vitamin $B_{12}$ bound to egg albumin or chicken serum, the Schilling test would show vitamin $B_{12}$ malabsorption.)

Familiarity with the laboratory's method for determination of serum folate and vitamin $B_{12}$ levels is necessary for a proper interpretation of serum folate and vitamin $B_{12}$ results. For example, if a microbiologic assay is being used, some antibiotics and antimetabolites may interfere with the growth of microorganisms and produce falsely low results. On the other hand, if a radioisotope method is being used, the serum folate level may be normal in a patient who has megaloblastic anemia owing to the use of a folate antagonist.

**Red Blood Cell Folate.** Red blood cell folate is a better representative of the body store of folate than is serum folate. However, after the diagnosis of megaloblastic anemia is made, the tests for serum folate and serum vitamin $B_{12}$ are more likely to provide an accurate diagnosis than the tests for RBC folate and serum vitamin $B_{12}$. This occurs because more patients with vitamin $B_{12}$ deficiency anemia have low RBC folate

---

*Not available in the United States.

*Investigational drug in the United States.

than have low serum folate levels. The RBC folate assay may be more informative than the serum folate assay if microbiologic assay is being used and the patient is taking antibiotics, in which case, the serum folate determination may be falsely low, but the RBC folate would provide the true folate level. This is because the high dilution of blood required for the RBC folate assay reduces the concentration of antibiotic enough so that it does not inhibit the growth of the microorganism used in the assay. Similarly, the RBC folate would be more informative than serum folate level if blood for the assay is taken a couple of days after the initiation of folate therapy. In this case, the serum folate would be normal but the RBC folate level would still be low if the patient were folate deficient.

**Urinary Formiminoglutamic Acid and Methylmalonic Acid Excretion.** These tests have been proposed for the diagnosis of folate and vitamin $B_{12}$ deficiency, respectively. However, they are not available in most of the laboratories, and they do not provide extra information, except in some unusual cases or if an inborn error of metabolism of folate or vitamin $B_{12}$ is suspected.

**Therapeutic Trial.** It should be remembered that the deficiency of either vitamin may show hematologic response if treated with large doses of the other vitamin. Therapeutic trial have diagnostic value only if a minimal daily dosage of the vitamine is used (1 μg of vitamin $B_{12}$ intramuscularly daily for 10 days or 100 μg of folic acid orally daily for 10 days). In such cases, good hematologic response (reticulocytosis in 6 to 10 days) is noted only if the patient were deficient in the vitamin used. However, therapeutic trial is time consuming and requires prolonged hospitalization and careful observation. Given the availability of other tests (mentioned earlier), it is rarely indicated, except for investigation of unusual cases or if there is no access to serum folate and vitamin $B_{12}$ assay or the Schilling test.

**Deoxyuridine Suppression Test.** This test has been promoted as a sensitive and rapid test to differentiate between folate and vitamin $B_{12}$ deficiency. However, the test is more valuable in research than in diagnostic laboratories. The test is not available in most laboratories, except for research centers, but even in an ideal situation its ability to provide rapid diagnosis is hardly an advantage.

*Diagnosis of Underlying Cause of Folate or Vitamin $B_{12}$ Deficiency*

**Schilling's Test.** Any patient with vitamin $B_{12}$ deficiency must have vitamin $B_{12}$ malabsorption (except for strict vegetarians, breast-fed infants of vitamin $B_{12}$–deficient mothers, or someone who has undergone nitrous oxide anesthesia). Consequently, the Schilling test, which determines the adequacy or inadequacy of vitamin $B_{12}$ absorption, is useful in the work-up of a patient with confirmed or suspected vitamin $B_{12}$ deficiency. Furthermore, if the Schilling test proves the presence of vitamin $B_{12}$ malabsorption, the subsequent test with provision of IF can help to differentiate between vitamin $B_{12}$ malabsorption due to lack of IF (with PA or after gastrectomy) and that due to condi-

tions of the terminal ileum (postresection, Crohn's disease, or lack of vitamin $B_{12}$ receptors). A proper 24-hour urine collection and a proper renal function are necessary for the interpretation of the Schilling test. Abnormal test results may be obtained if the urine collection is incomplete or if the patient has uremia. In such cases, arrangements should be made with the laboratory to use some other method of determining vitamin $B_{12}$ absorption—e.g., measuring the plasma radioactivity or the radioactive count over the liver. The Schilling test is best performed after megaloblastic anemia is corrected; otherwise, the presence of megaloblastic changes in the gut mucosa may cause vitamin $B_{12}$ malabsorption, even if the megaloblastic anemia is not due to vitamin $B_{12}$ malabsorption.

**Gastric Analysis** This test is rarely indicated now. The adult form of PA is associated with histamine-fast achlorhydria. The test causes significant discomfort for the patient, and the achlorhydria, if found, is not specific for PA. If gastric analysis is used, the gastric juice could also be used for the assay of gastric IF, which is absent or markedly decreased in adult form of PA.

**Intrinsic Factor Antibody.** IF antibody may be present in the serum of some patients with PA or other immune-mediated disorders, but it is rare in normal people. If the serum vitamin $B_{12}$ level is low, the presence of IF antibody in serum supports the diagnosis of PA. However, if the serum vitamin $B_{12}$ assay and Schilling's test are available, this test is rarely needed.

## TREATMENT

### Initial Therapy

After the diagnosis of megaloblastic anemia is established, I make certain that blood is drawn for serum folate and serum vitamin $B_{12}$ determinations and I start the patient on a regimen of the vitamin that I think is most likely to be deficient in the patient. If one has access to laboratories that are able to perform serum folate, serum vitamin $B_{12}$, and Schilling's tests, I do not see that anything is gained by waiting for the results of serum folate and vitamin $B_{12}$ determinations before starting therapy, unless the patient's history suggests an unusual form of megaloblastic anemia. Even if something goes wrong with the serum folate and vitamin $B_{12}$ assay, one can usually arrive at the proper diagnosis with the Schilling test at a later date. When I suspect that vitamin $B_{12}$ deficiency is the most likely possibility and that the patient is not sick enough to justify hospitalization, I give the patient 1000 μg of vitamin $B_{12}$ (cyanocobalamin) intramuscularly and ask the patient to return in 1 week, by which time the results of serum folate and vitamin $B_{12}$ determinations are available and I can also check the CBC and reticulocyte response. If the diagnosis of vitamin $B_{12}$ deficiency is confirmed, I continue with weekly vitamin $B_{12}$

injections, 1000 μg for 7 to 8 weeks, and then, if needed, I do the Schilling test and start the patient on maintenance therapy. If the test results indicate folate deficiency, I discontinue vitamin $B_{12}$ therapy and start the patient on a regimen of folic acid, 5 mg orally daily. If the patient has severe anemia and needs hospitalization or is already in the hospital with megaloblastic anemia and I suspect vitamin $B_{12}$ deficiency, I give a vitamin $B_{12}$ injection, 1000 μg daily for 7 to 8 days. After the serum folate and vitamin $B_{12}$ assay results are available, I then proceed with therapy as stated earlier for outpatients. When I suspect that the most likely diagnosis is folate deficiency, I start the patient on a regimen of oral folic acid, 5 mg daily for 4 weeks, and ask the patient to return in 1 week. If the serum folate result confirms the diagnosis, I continue the therapy. If the serum folate is normal and the serum vitamin $B_{12}$ level is low, I stop folic acid and treat the patient as vitamin $B_{12}$ deficient. If both serum folate and serum $B_{12}$ concentrations are low, I continue with folic acid, and I would also give one dose of vitamin $B_{12}$, 1000 μg intramuscularly, until I can do the Schilling test and either rule out or establish vitamin $B_{12}$ deficiency. Physicians are taught not to treat vitamin $B_{12}$ deficiency megaloblastic anemia with folic acid because the patient may show a hematologic response to folic acid, but go on to experience neurologic complications of vitamin $B_{12}$ deficiency, which may become irreversible. This is true; however, this does not occur rapidly and if one can make sure that the patient is seen within 1 to 2 weeks to correct a mistake, if the diagnosis was incorrect, no real harm is done to the patient.

Blood transfusion in megaloblastic anemia is rarely indicated, unless the patient is critically ill and has severe anemia with cardiopulmonary distress. In such cases, the transfusion of packed RBCs should be given with great caution and with the use of diuretics to prevent cardiac overload and heart failure.

Following the initiation of therapy in cases of severe megaloblastic anemia, transient hypokalemia may develop as the result of a shift of potassium into the cells and newly formed cells. Some researchers have attributed cases of sudden death after initiation of therapy to this hypokalemia. Although a dangerously low serum potassium level is rare in treated megaloblastic anemia, it is prudent to use temporary potassium supplementation if the serum potassium concentration is low.

Following the initiation of the proper vitamin therapy in megaloblastic anemia, mild reticulocytosis begins to appear after 3 days, and peak reticulocyte response occurs within 6 to 10 days after the initiation of therapy. During the first week of therapy, the hemoglobin concentration of blood may continue to go down; however, the patient generally begins to feel much better within 1 to 2 days of therapy.

### Maintenance Therapy of Vitamin $B_{12}$ Deficiency

Vitamin $B_{12}$ deficiency due to lack of dietary intake (in vegetarians) can be treated with vitamin $B_{12}$, 2 to 3 μg per day orally. But vitamin $B_{12}$ deficiencies that are due to vitamin $B_{12}$ malabsorption (with PA, postgastrectomy, or with diseased or resected terminal ileum) should be treated with monthly injections of vitamin $B_{12}$ after completion of the initial therapy of seven or eight injections. Maintenance therapy is possible with large oral daily doses of vitamin $B_{12}$ or with a daily dose of vitamin $B_{12}$ plus intrinsic factor, but there is nothing to recommend these methods except for extremely rare instances of patients who are allergic to parenteral vitamin $B_{12}$. Parenteral $B_{12}$ therapy ensures adequate maintenance and compliance with therapy and is cheaper. Although therapy can be satisfactorily maintained with an injection of 100 μg of vitamin $B_{12}$ once a month, I prefer to use 1000 μg of vitamin $B_{12}$ monthly. Despite a large urinary loss following the use of the larger dose, more vitamin $B_{12}$ is retained after therapy with 1000 μg than after 100 μg, and the difference in cost between the two doses is only a few cents. After the vitamin $B_{12}$ malabsorption is documented, the need for lifelong monthly maintenance therapy should be explained to the patient. Recurrence of vitamin $B_{12}$ deficiency should not occur at all, but it is not uncommon because sometimes the physicians discontinue the therapy after hematologic recovery is complete; sometimes, when patients miss one or two injections and do not notice any difference, they assume that continued therapy is no longer necessary. After initial therapy of vitamin $B_{12}$ deficiency, parenteral vitamin $B_{12}$ should not be given more often than once a month. Some patients develop a sort of psychologic dependence on vitamin $B_{12}$ and begin feeling tired or unwell a few days before they are due to receive their next monthly injection of vitamin $B_{12}$ and talk their physicians into giving the injections earlier and earlier. On the other hand, sometimes the physician gives the vitamin $B_{12}$ injections more often because the patient has become anemic. This is an improper practice because the patient who has been receiving monthly vitamin injections cannot possibly be vitamin $B_{12}$ deficient. Accordingly, such a patient requires proper investigation to establish the cause of anemia.

## Maintenance Therapy of Folate Deficiency

Folate deficiency can generally be treated with oral folic acid even if the cause of deficiency is malabsorption of dietary folate (unless the patient has severe gastroenteritis with vomiting and diarrhea or the patient is unconscious, in which case the initial doses should be given parenterally). Folic acid, 5 mg daily for 2 to 4 weeks, is adequate for the initial therapy of folate deficiency. If the deficiency was due to a deficient diet, and the diet or underlying cause of the deficiency can be corrected, no maintenance therapy with folic acid is needed. If the underlying cause or the diet cannot be corrected, however, maintenance therapy with a daily oral dose of 0.5 to 1 mg of folic acid should be continued.

### Prophylaxis

In patients who have had a total gastrectomy or a resection of terminal ileum, the prophylactic use of vitamin $B_{12}$, 1000 μg intramuscularly once a month, is recommended. If the patient has had a partial gastrectomy or a diseased ileum or a low serum vitamin $B_{12}$ level, a Schilling's test should be performed; if the Schilling test indicates vitamin $B_{12}$ malabsorption, prophylactic monthly vitamin $B_{12}$ therapy should be started. It is safer (and cheaper) to treat vitamin $B_{12}$ malabsorption prophylactically than to wait until vitamin $B_{12}$ deficiency megaloblastic anemia develops before starting the therapy. It should be noted that some vitamin $B_{12}$–deficient patients may have neuropsychiatric symptoms without any significant changes in the peripheral blood; follow-up of the patients who have vitamin $B_{12}$ malabsorption with repeated CBCs, but without vitamin $B_{12}$ therapy, is not a safe practice.

Prophylactic folic acid therapy, 1 to 5 mg daily, is commonly used, with some justification, in conditions that are associated with increased folate requirement (pregnancy, chronic hemolytic anemia, or long-term hemodialysis). Some centers also use folic acid prophylactically in the first few months for small premature infants and periconceptually in women who have previously given birth to an infant with a neural tube defect.

In malignancies and in myeloproliferative disorders, folate deficiency is not uncommon. However, folate deficiency should not be corrected, unless it is believed that the advantage of correcting the deficiency outweighs the disadvantage of providing folic acid and enhancing the growth of the malignant cells or hematopoietic cells, which may be partially suppressed by folate deficiency.

# THALASSEMIA

method of
GEORGE F. ATWEH, M.D.
*State University of New York*
*Brooklyn, New York*

The thalassemias are a group of disorders characterized by imbalanced synthesis of the different polypeptide chains that make up the hemoglobin (Hb) molecules. As a group, they account for some of the commonest and best studied single-gene disorders of humankind. The heterogeneity of these disorders at the clinical level has been recognized by hematologists for many decades. More recently, molecular genetics provided the tools to explain the molecular pathologic changes and pathophysiology that are responsible for this wide variability in the clinical spectrum of these disorders. These biologic insights have already revolutionized the approaches to prenatal diagnoses of thalassemia and other related disorders. In addition, a totally new approach to the treatment of these single-gene disorders based on gene therapy seems to be an attainable goal in the not-too-distant future.

The vast majority of hemoglobin in adult blood is Hb A, which consists of two alpha chains and two beta chains. The remaining hemoglobin is divided between a minor adult component known as Hb $A_2$ (two alpha and two delta chains) and a small amount of fetal hemoglobin known as Hb F (two alpha and two gamma chains). The production of alpha-like globin chains (zeta and alpha) is roughly equivalent to the production of non–alpha-globin chains (epsilon, gamma, delta, and beta) at all stages of development. This leads to balanced association with heme to make up the different hemoglobin molecules. When the production of one or more of these polypeptide chains is perturbed, this results in one of several disorders, which are collectively referred to as the thalassemias.

## PATHOPHYSIOLOGY

Beta-thalassemia results from decreased synthesis of the beta-globin chains. When a mutation leads to complete loss of activity of a beta-globin gene, the mutant gene is designated a beta⁰-thalassemia gene. On the other hand, when a mutation leads to partial loss of activity, the mutant gene is designated a beta⁺-thalassemia. When either a beta⁰- or a beta⁺-thalassemia gene is inherited in a simple heterozygous state, a minor imbalance between alpha- and beta-globin chain synthesis occurs. The resulting anemia is mild and the affected individuals usually lead a normal healthy life. The spleen may be slightly enlarged owing to chronic sequestration of red blood cells. This condition is known as *beta-thalassemia trait,* or *beta-thalassemia minor.*

When two mutant beta-globin genes are inherited together, the result is a more profound imbalance between alpha-like and beta-like globin chains. This leads to precipitation of the excessive insoluble alpha-globin chains, destruction of red blood cells in the bone marrow and reticuloendothelial cells, and a severe clinical disorder. Because the switch from fetal to adult hemoglobin production starts at about birth and is virtually completed by the sixth month of life, the disease usually does not manifest clinically before the age of 6 months. Infants who inherit either two beta$^0$-thalassemia genes or one beta$^0$- and one beta$^+$-thalassemia gene are usually transfusion dependent beginning at the age of 6 to 12 months. This condition is known as *beta-thalassemia major*. In the past, when these patients were transfused to a level that merely sustained life, they developed massive erythroid expansion in the bone marrow with extramedullary hematopoiesis. This leads to bony deformities, osteoporosis, pathologic fractures, and growth retardation. Massive splenomegaly and hypersplenism in this setting occurs in the first decade of life as a result of chronic hemolysis. This in turn leads to leukopenia, thrombocytopenia, and increased transfusion requirement. The most serious complication of beta-thalassemia, however, is iron overload as a result of transfusional iron and excessive iron absorption from the gastrointestinal tract. Because the human body does not have an intrinsic mechanism for excreting excessive iron, this iron would accumulate and lead to end-organ damage.

The most serious of the toxicities of iron is its effect on the heart. Cardiac hemochromatosis usually develops in the second decade of life. This can manifest as episodes of pericarditis, atrial and ventricular arrhythmias, and eventually intractable congestive heart failure. The deposition of iron in parenchymal cells of the liver leads to hepatic fibrosis and ultimately cirrhosis. Iron accumulation in the pancreas may lead to glucose intolerance and even insulin-dependent diabetes mellitus in some cases. Other endocrine abnormalities are also prevalent in these patients as a result of iron toxicity to the hypothalamus and pituitary, leading to partial hypopituitarism. All of these toxicities are being averted now that iron chelation therapy is being started at an early age in patients with transfusion-dependent beta-thalassemia.

*Beta-thalassemia intermedia* is defined as homozygous beta-thalassemia in which tranfusions are not required to sustain life. The anemia is considerably less severe than in beta-thalassemia major, and consequently, the complications described earlier are, for the most part, averted. The molecular basis of these conditions is quite heterogeneous. The majority of these patients inherit beta$^+$-thalassemia genes in which the decrease in beta-globin synthesis is quite mild. In other patients, the mild phenotype is a result of the inheritance of a genetic determinant of high fetal hemoglobin synthesis along with the two beta-thalassemia genes. The increased production of gamma-globin chains in these patients results in decreased imbalance between alpha- and non–alpha-globin chains and less precipitation of free alpha-globin chains. In addition, the increased gamma-globin chains associate with alpha-globin chains to form fetal hemoglobin. This fetal hemoglobin contributes to the total oxygen-carrying capacity of blood and ameliorates the anemia. In yet another group of patients with beta-thalassemia intermedia, homozygous beta-thalassemia coexists with alpha-thalassemia. This also decreases the imbalance between alpha- and non–alpha-globin

chains and results in less red blood cell destruction. As a result of all these factors, beta-thalassemia intermedia is more common in populations in which the beta$^+$-thalassemia mutations are generally mild and alpha-thalassemia is prevalent. This is the case in the American black population.

Each diploid set of human chromosomes contains four alpha-globin genes on chromosome 16 as opposed to two beta-globin genes on chromosome 11. Consequently, there is more clinical heterogeneity of the alpha-thalassemia syndromes as a result of partial or complete dysfunction of one, two, three, or four alpha-globin genes. When a single alpha-globin gene is inactivated, the condition is known as a "silent carrier" state. This is characterized by the absence of anemia and a slight microcytosis. When two alpha-globin genes are dysfunctional, the condition is known as an alpha-thalassemia trait. This is characterized by a low-grade anemia and microcytosis. When three alpha-globin genes are inactivated, the disorder is known as hemoglobin H disease. Hemoglobin H consists of four beta-globin chains and can be detected by standard hemoglobin electrophoresis. These patients have mild transfusion-independent anemia and a clinical syndrome essentially identical to beta-thalassemia intermedia. Finally, when all four alpha-globin genes are deleted, the condition is incompatible with life and results in death in utero. This occurs because fetal hemoglobin, which is crucial for the survival of the fetus, cannot be formed in the absence of alpha-globin chains. This condition is known as hydrops fetalis.

It has been recognized for many years that a high level of fetal hemoglobin can ameliorate the clinical severity of thalassemia and sickle cell anemia. This has generated a lot of interest in the study of the genetic determinants that result in increased expression of the gamma-globin genes. Some of these determinants result in a profound increase in fetal hemoglobin levels, approaching 30% in the heterozygous states, whereas others result in a moderate but consistent increase in fetal hemoglobin in the 1 to 3% range. The best studied of these conditions are known as hereditary persistence of fetal hemoglobin (HPFH) and delta-beta-thalassemia.

HPFH has been described in the heterozygous and homozygous states. It should be called a disorder and not a disease, because it is not associated with any morbidity or mortality. The majority of these cases result from big deletions that remove the delta- and beta-globin genes. These deletions, however, activate the synthesis of gamma-globin chains and result in an almost balanced ratio of alpha-globin/non–alpha-globin chains with no anemia. Some patients with HPFH have increased expression of one of the two gamma-globin genes in the absence of a deletion in the beta-globin gene cluster. These are usually associated with point mutations in the promoters of the affected gamma-globin genes, which increase their activity in adult life. The delta-beta-thalassemias are related conditions also characterized by big deletions, which remove the delta- and beta-globin genes and activate the remaining gamma-globin genes. In these conditions, however, the increased synthesis of gamma-globin chains does not completely compensate for the absent synthesis of the deleted delta- and beta-globin chains.

Thus, unlike HPFH, they are associated with mild anemia and microcytosis. Whereas in deletion HPFH every red blood cell contains some fetal hemoglobin (i.e., pancellular), in delta-beta-thalassemia, some red blood cells contain fetal hemoglobin and others do not (i.e., heterocellular). It is still not clear why some deletions result in an HPFH phenotype, whereas others result in a delta-beta-thalassemia phenotype.

## LABORATORY DIAGNOSIS

As in the diagnosis of most clinical disorders, a high index of suspicion is essential to making the correct diagnosis. Thalassemic disorders should be suspected in any individual of certain ethnic backgrounds (e.g., African, Mediterranean, and Southeast Asian) with anemia. Microcytosis (low mean corpuscular volume), a useful clue to the existence of a hemoglobin synthesis disorder, is by no means diagnostic. The alpha-thalassemia trait, the beta-thalassemia trait, and the delta-beta-thalassemia trait all present with a mild anemia and microcytosis. Peripheral blood film inspection usually confirms the microcytosis and shows marked anisopoikilocytosis, target cells, cigar-shaped cells, and some basophilic stippling. The reticulocyte count is usually minimally elevated, and serum iron and ferritin levels are in the normal range. The hemoglobin electrophoresis does not show any abnormal hemoglobins. Quantitation of Hb $A_2$ and Hb F should be performed in every patient suspected of having a thalassemic disorder. The level of Hb $A_2$ is elevated in the vast majority of individuals with the beta-thalassemia trait. It may be normal, however, if iron deficiency coexists with beta-thalassemia and in a condition known as the "silent" beta-thalassemia trait, which is prevalent in the Ferrara region of Italy. Hb F elevations in the 1 to 5% range are also seen in the beta-thalassemia trait. In delta-beta-thalassemia trait, Hb $A_2$ level is usually low to normal, whereas the percentage of Hb F is markedly elevated (in the 10 to 20% range). If the peripheral blood film is stained for fetal hemoglobin, the distribution is usually heterocellular.

The diagnosis of the alpha-thalassemia syndromes is a little more difficult. Hb $A_2$, which is helpful in the diagnosis of the beta-thalassemias, is normal in alpha-thalassemia. Thus, the diagnosis is usually made by excluding beta-thalassemia and iron deficiency in a patient from certain ethnic backgrounds and with a supportive family history. Southern blotting can easily detect the vast majority of the alpha-thalassemias, because, for the most part, alpha-thalassemia results from gene deletions rather than subtle small mutations. This technique, however, is not widely available in the clinical setting.

The diagnosis of homozygous beta-thalassemia is made when a patient has profound anemia early in life. The blood film findings are similar to those with the trait, but more severe, with many nucleated red blood cells, which suggest extramedullary hematopoiesis. Hemoglobin analysis shows the majority of the hemoglobin to consist of the fetal variety with small elevations of Hb $A_2$. Hb A may be present, when one or both of the inherited thalassemia genes are of the beta$^+$ variety. The diagnosis of Hb H disease is perhaps the easiest of all the thalassemic disorders because a characteristic abnormal hemoglobin band is seen on hemoglobin electrophoresis. Supravital staining of the peripheral blood with brilliant cresyl blue also demonstrates classic inclusions in Hb H disease.

## THERAPY

**Transfusions.** Because no specific therapy is currently available that can correct the basic defects that result in anemia, supportive therapy with blood transfusions must be relied on to sustain life. In the early days of treatment of these conditions, it was common practice to transfuse patients to an acceptable level that would merely sustain life. In practical terms, blood transfusions were given to maintain the hemoglobin level between 6 and 8 grams per dl. More recently, the trend has been to follow a "hypertransfusion" regimen in these cases, maintaining a hemoglobin level between 10 and 12 grams per dl. The rationale for this approach is that this more "physiologic" hemoglobin level will avert the complications of ineffective erythropoiesis by correcting the anemia and suppressing its stimulus to the bone marrow. Thus, growth is improved, bone deformities and hepatosplenomegaly are avoided, and the quality of life is significantly enhanced. The main argument against such programs is that they may aggravate the iron overload by the more liberal use of blood transfusions. It has been convincingly demonstrated, however, that this is not the case, even in the absence of a chelation therapy program. This is probably a result of decreased dietary iron absorption from the gut owing to decreased anemia and ineffective erythropoiesis.

Several other approaches to transfusion therapy have also been advocated. "Supertransfusion" therapy is one such approach in which the aim is to maintain the hemoglobin level above 12 grams per dl. The rationale is that with chronic use of such a program, the number of transfusions needed to maintain this high hemoglobin level is not greater than what would be needed in a classic hypertransfusion program. This is presumably a consequence of a decrease in the blood volume, which results from decreased blood circulation to the expanded bone marrow and reticulendothelial tissues. Another highly experimental approach is neocyte transfusion therapy. This is based on the hypothesis that young red blood cells, which can be separated from older cells by differences in their buoyancy, may have a longer survival in the circulation and thus help to decrease the transfusion requirements. Neither of these approaches, however, has been shown to be more effective than the hypertransfusion program that is in wide clinical use.

Alloimmunization in frequently transfused patients may pose some difficulties. In the vast majority of cases, however, careful blood typing for the less common blood antigens allows proper cross-matching and successful transfusions. Red blood cell survival, however, may be shortened when the transfused cells are not fully compatible. Febrile transfusion reactions, usually directed against white blood cell antigens, can be averted by using in-line white blood cell filters. Occasionally, the use of frozen and washed packed red blood cells is necessary to avoid these febrile reactions.

**Iron Chelation.** Because most of the morbidity and mortality in transfusion-dependent patients with thalassemia can be directly attributed to iron toxicity, there has been an intensive search for means of removing the excessive iron from the body. Because phlebotomy is not an option in these patients, as it is in patients with hemochromatosis, the only available approved method is iron chelation with the parenteral drug deferoxamine mesylate (Desferal). This drug is inactive as an oral agent and has a short half-life when given parenterally. Thus, the most effective way of administering this compound is as a slow subcutaneous continuous infusion by means of a pump attached to a narrow-gauge (butterfly) needle. Negative iron balance can be effectively achieved by administering 20 to 40 mg per kg per day for 8 to 12 hours overnight. This would allow the affected child to be fully mobile and active during waking hours. The current recommendations are to start the chelation therapy at the age of 4 to 5 years before significant toxicity of iron overload starts to manifest. Compliance may be particularly difficult in adolescence owing to the inconvenience of the route of administration. Rotation of the subcutaneous infusion sites on the abdominal wall and the thighs or mixing 5 mg of hydrocortisone with the administration mixture may help alleviate the local burning and irritation. The cost of treatment with such a program may be prohibitive, particularly in poor countries where these conditions are prevalent. Obviously, the development of oral chelating agents would be a major milestone in improving the care of these patients.

**Other Measures.** A properly timed splenectomy may be one of the more important decisions to be made in the overall management of patients with these disorders. When the spleen causes symptoms, such as pain and early satiety, by its sheer size, there are few who contest the usefulness of splenectomy. One of the responsibilities of the physician managing a patient with thalassemia major is to keep accurate records of the volume of packed red blood cells needed to maintain the hemoglobin level above 10 grams per dl. Most experts would recommend splenectomy when more than 250 ml per kg per year is needed. With this high transfusion requirement, it is extremely difficult to maintain the patient in negative iron balance by iron chelation therapy. When hypersplenism develops (leukopenia and thrombocytopenia are present), the surgical removal of the spleen becomes essential. If the spleen is removed at an early age (<5 years), the risk of infection may be unacceptably high. Even in older patients, the increased risk of infection is still significant. These patients should be immunized with a polyvalent pneumococcal vaccine preoperatively and should be given prophylactic penicillin, 250 mg per day orally, to decrease the risk of pneumococcal and meningococcal sepsis. They should also be treated with broad-spectrum antibiotics, after obtaining appropriate cultures, whenever they develop fever or other signs of infection.

Patients whose hyperactive bone marrow is not suppressed by the use of a hypertransfusion program have an increased demand for folate and should be given supplements of 1 mg of folic acid daily. Deficiencies of vitamins C and E are also common in these patients and the use of 100 mg per day of the former and 200 IU per day of the latter is advisable. The diabetes, cirrhosis, and cardiac dysfunction that may develop as a result of iron toxicity should be managed according to the same principles that are used when these disorders arise de novo. Finally, the value of a close relationship between the patient and the family and the caring physician cannot be overemphasized in the management of these chronic, debilitating disorders.

## FUTURE GOALS

None of the measures described earlier for the treatment of thalassemic disorders are curative. It is encouraging, however, that a significant number of children are alive and apparently cured of their disease today as a result of bone marrow transplantations from an allogeneic nonthalassemic donor. The rationale for bone marrow transplantation is to totally ablate the thalassemic bone marrow stem cells and replace them with donor stem cells that can support normal erythropoiesis. The rate of success has been highest in the young who are not yet alloimmunized by multiple transfusions and who do not have significant iron overload. However, this modality of treatment remains highly experimental and ethically controversial as long as it carries a high risk of mortality (20 to 30%). It is difficult to justify wide use of a procedure that carries such a high mortality in the treatment of a chronic disorder with a life expectancy of more than 20 years, and possibly much longer with the aggressive use of chelation therapy at an early age.

Another modality of treatment that offers the possibility of cure in the thalassemias is somatic gene therapy. This involves the introduction of a normal beta-globin gene into the bone marrow of a thalassemic individual. Considerable progress has recently been made in defining some of the regulatory elements that are essential to drive a high level of expression of an exogeneous beta-globin gene introduced into erythroid cells. This had been a major hurdle to the success of such a modality of treatment. The remaining major technologic hurdle is the difficulty of introducing the normal gene into the elusive bone marrow stem cell with a high efficiency using a delivery system that does not pose a significant risk to the function of other genes in the bone marrow cells. Most experts believe that it is only a question of time before such a system is developed and the long awaited hope of somatic gene therapy becomes a reality for patients with thalassemic disorders.

Finally, it should be mentioned that an active search for pharmacologic agents that can delay or reverse the switch from fetal to adult hemoglobin production is under way. The first such agent to be used in patients was 5-azacytidine, which can hypomethylate fetal genes and reactivate their expression. Hydroxyurea was also used in a larger number of patients, and it showed some promise. More recently, recombinant erythropoietin has been shown to increase fetal hemoglobin production in baboons. Human experiments are planned in the near future. None of these agents can be recommended for general use at this stage, but the results of these studies are awaited with great interest.

# SICKLE CELL DISEASE

method of
MABEL KOSHY, M.D.
*University of Illinois at Chicago*
*Chicago, Illinois*

Sickle cell disease is encountered in many parts of the world and is found in people of African, Mediterranean, Indian, and Middle Eastern heritage. In the Western Hemisphere, it is common among blacks and Hispanics in the Caribbean, Central America, United States, and other parts of South America.

Sickle cell disease refers to a group of genetic disorders characterized by the predominance of hemoglobin S. Sickle cell anemia (SS) defines the homozygous state with the inheritance of hemoglobin S from both parents. Other disorders include sickle hemoglobin C disease (SC), sickle beta-thalassemia plus (SB$^+$), sickle beta-thalassemia zero (SB$^0$), sickle with alpha-thalassemia (SS$\alpha$ thal), and rarer combinations of sickle hemoglobin with D and O (SD, SO).

Sickle trait or carrier state has both hemoglobin A and S. The ratio of hemoglobin S varies from 30 to 45%. Sickle trait is not associated with major medical complications and will not be discussed here.

The major normal hemoglobin is made up of two alpha and two beta chains. Sickle hemoglobin differs from normal hemoglobin by a single amino acid substitution of valine for the normally occurring glutamic acid at the sixth position of the beta chain. This amino acid substitution causes hemoglobin S to be insoluble within the red cell upon deoxygenation. Deoxygenation results in polymerization, the formation of tactoids within the red cells, causing their abnormal sickle shape.

The fundamental cause of sickle cell disease is the decreased deformability of the sickle red cell produced by gelation of hemoglobin S. The cardinal pathophysiologic features of sickle cell disorders include chronic hemolytic anemia and vaso-occlusion by the abnormal sickle cells resulting in ischemic tissue injury. The hemolytic anemia is caused by sickling and unsickling of these abnormally shaped red cells, which result in shortened red cell survival, jaundice, formation of gallstones, and a hyperactive marrow. Tissue injury is produced by the accumulation of sickled erythrocytes in blood vessels causing obstruction of flow. Gelation and co-polymerization occur as a direct relationship of the hemoglobin S concentration in the red blood cell and oxygen tension. Hemoglobin S polymers occur within the intact erythrocyte even at physiologic oxygen tensions. Such polymerization has not been detected in sickle trait, and sickle trait individuals develop problems only when oxygen tensions are lowered below physiologic levels.

In sickle cell disease, almost all tissues and organs are at risk for ischemic injury. The organs most at risk are those with venous sinuses, i.e., the spleen and bone marrow; or those with limited terminal arterial supply, such as the eyes and head of the femur. Symptoms of hypoxic injury may be acute, as exemplified by painful episodes; or insidious in onset, as in aseptic necrosis or sickle retinopathy. The combination of both acute and chronic tissue injury results in organ failure as the patient advances in age. Multiple organ involvement is common with sickle cell disease.

The clinical problems of sickle cell disease include acute, chronic, and other inter-related events. Acute events include painful episodes, chest syndrome, worsening of anemia, and neurologic effects. Chronic events are those that are non–life-threatening but disabling to the patient—e.g., avascular necrosis of the femoral head, chronic eye changes, renal disease, and leg ulcers. The use of general anesthesia for surgery, pregnancy, and other clinical events may exacerbate sickle cell disease.

Recently it has been reported that mutational events gave rise to the beta S gene in different locations in the African continent, Saudi Arabia, and India. These resulted in four haplotypes containing the beta S gene with clinical and hematologic findings that differ from one another. The types include (1) the Central African Republic, Carr haplotype, with severe clinical disease; (2) the Atlantic West African, Senegal haplotype, with mild disease; (3) the Central West African, Benin haplotype, with intermediate severity; and finally (4) the sickle cell anemia that has been described among Saudi Arabians, Iranians, and Indians with a very mild form due to the high fetal hemoglobin.

There is, at present, no definitive treatment for sickle cell disease. Treatment is mainly symptomatic. Several drugs have been used to treat sickle cell disease. Drugs, like sodium cyanate, were tried because they had properties to inhibit gelation of hemoglobin S but were discontinued because of toxicity. The use of low sodium diet and desmopressin (DDAVP) to decrease the concentration of hemoglobin S was unsuccessful because of poor response and side effects. The first drug to increase fetal hemoglobin was 5-azacytidine through hypomethylation, but it was not used for treatment because of the toxic side effects. Hydroxyurea (Hydrea) was subsequently used to increase fetal hemoglobin. Currently a National Institute of Health (NIH)–funded cooperative study is in progress to evaluate the role of hydroxyurea in the treatment of sickle cell disease. Preliminary reports appear promising and are awaiting double-blind randomized trials. Other drugs to alter sickle membrane effect (cetiedil*) and other compounds that interfere with oxygen dissociation have had inconclusive results. Vasodilators and lubricants to decrease the microvascular entrapment have been tried. To date, none of these methods have been successful in treating sickle cell disease or preventing sickle cell crises.

At birth, the infant's sickle cell blood contains sufficient fetal hemoglobin to prevent clinical symptomatology until about the age of 3 months. After about 3 months, the adult hemoglobin replaces fetal hemoglobin, and this results in co-polymerization, gel formation, and the abnormal stiff red cells that cause anemia and vaso-occlusion. In children, the early findings include the hand-foot syndrome or dactylitis, infections (e.g., meningitis, pneumonia), acute febrile events, and splenic sequestration. Penicillin prophylaxis is recommended for children from the age of 3 months until 5 years of age, and at 18 months of age the pneumococcal and Haemophilus influenzae vaccines are advocated. Children diagnosed at birth should be referred to a pediatrician, and pediatricians are recommended to review the supplement to *Pediatrics,* May 1989, Vol. 83: "Newborn Screening for Sickle Cell Disease and Other Hemoglobinopathies."

## DIAGNOSIS

An evaluation of a patient with sickle cell disease includes the establishment of the diagnosis by hemoglobin electrophoresis and the documentation of the baseline steady state, complete blood count, biochemical laboratory tests, and a thorough physical examination. Diagnosis of the specific sickle cell disorder can be established by analysis of the beta chain complex

*Not available in the United States.

using DNA techniques. In the absence of availability of this technology, reliance is placed on clinical history; peripheral blood counts; red cell indices; inspection of the peripheral smear; and hemoglobin electrophoresis with measurements of the major and minor hemoglobins on cellulose acetate, citrate agar electrophoresis, and solubility testing. Macrocytic anemia (Hb 6 to 8 grams per dl) and high reticulocyte count with sickled cells on peripheral blood smear are common in sickle cell anemia. The presence of microcytosis is associated with the presence of the thalassemia gene, $SB^+$, $SB^0$, SS thal, or rarely iron deficiency. Patients with SC or $SB^+$ may have less anemia (Hb 11 to 13 grams per dl), but those with $SB^0$ may have severe anemia with microcytosis.

The antenatal diagnosis of sickle cell disease can be determined by DNA technology either of amniotic fluid cells estimated at about 16 weeks of pregnancy or by chorionic villus sampling from 9 weeks of pregnancy. At birth, examination of the cord blood by hemoglobin electrophoresis can be utilized in the absence of DNA technology for newborn screening of abnormal hemoglobin. Prenatal diagnosis is usually a very sensitive issue, as termination of pregnancy will be discussed. Therefore, counselling of both parents prior to any prenatal testing should be considered important. Once an infant is diagnosed by either technique to have sickle cell anemia or sickle cell disease, the child should be referred to a pediatric hematologist for long-term care.

## CLINICAL PRESENTATION

Many factors alter the clinical manifestation of sickle cell disease, and these include climatic and socioeconomic conditions. Additional factors that alter clinical presentation include the presence of other abnormal hemoglobin besides hemoglobin S, the presence of alpha thalassemia, the amount of fetal hemoglobin, and the four known haplotypes.

## TREATMENT

### Painful Episode

The episodes referred to as "pain crises" are thought to result from microscopic areas of infarction in bones or tissues. Clinically the patient may present with physical evidence of pain, which may be localized or generalized, and low-grade temperatures. Fever and leukocytosis are accompanying findings. Mild elevations of liver enzymes and of bilirubin have also been described. The acute painful episode (or painful crisis) is more common in patients with sickle cell anemia, but it can also be seen in patients with sickle C and sickle beta-thalassemia. Many precipitating factors have been associated with the onset of painful episodes, and these include dehydration, infection, physical exertion, and psychosocial problems. The painful event may occur anytime during the day and may most often occur spontaneously without any provoking factors. The onset of pain crisis varies from individual to individual. In the large cooperative study conducted by the NIH, it was evident that two-thirds of the patients have infrequent pain crises, whereas one-third of the patients have very severe and repeated attacks of painful episodes. Ameliorating factors include high fetal hemoglobin levels and presence of alpha- or beta-thalassemia.

Treatment includes making the patient comfortable and reassuring the patient that the painful episode is a transient event. Once the decision is made that it is an uncomplicated pain crisis, the individual should be treated with fluids and appropriate analgesics. Patients with an unrelenting pain crisis should be admitted for fluids and parenteral narcotics and be evaluated for other associated complications.

Optimal treatment for pain control includes identifying patients with chronic pain syndrome and elimination or control of the inciting event. Any number of narcotics are available for use in pain control, and the primary care physician should be able to provide adequate analgesia at fixed schedules for the acute phase for 3 to 4 days. Drug dependence and other complicating events must be considered in patients who have repeat admissions for painful episodes.

Most patients will respond to oral fluids and analgesics in mild pain crisis. Analgesics could include medications such as aspirin, acetaminophen, and codeine; in the more severe cases, parenteral narcotics may be required to relieve the pain. If home therapy does not give any relief, it is recommended that the patient report to the local clinic or the hospital. Some patients may require hospitalization for 3 to 4 days, requiring intravenous fluids and analgesics.

Children and young adults should be encouraged to lead normal lives and attend college. Teachers should be made aware of the illness so that schoolwork may be made available for the student during the illness. Participation in physical activities should be encouraged to tolerance. Transfusions are usually not required for the management of painful episodes.

## Aplastic Crisis

Aplastic crisis is heralded by the presence of severe anemia associated with reticulocytopenia. Most often viral infections, especially parvovirus, have been reported to cause temporary arrest of the red cells. Blood transfusion is often required for severe anemia, until the bone marrow recovers from the transient aplasia. Transfusion to maintain hemoglobin to the normal levels (steady-state level) is sufficient. Definitive diagnosis could be made by bone marrow analysis and titers for parvovirus.

## Hepatic Sequestration

Hepatic sequestration is an uncommon event, and patients present with fever, worsening anemia, increasing jaundice, and elevation of liver enzymes. Physical examination shows the presence of enlargement of the liver and sudden drop in hemoglobin. Treatment is symptomatic, and blood transfusion therapy may be necessary.

## Splenic Sequestration

This event is seen more commonly in children, but a small percentage of adults have persistent splenomegaly and have been known to demonstrate a sudden enlargement of the spleen, resulting in entrapment of a significant portion of the red cell mass and precipitating a sudden drop in hemoglobin and risk for other complications. Blood transfusion therapy to maintain hemoglobin levels between 10 and 11 grams is recommended. Repeated and life-threatening splenic sequestration may require splenectomy. Pneumococcal vaccine prior to the procedure is recommended.

## Acute Chest Syndrome

This acute event presents with fever, cough, pleuritic-type chest pain, and pulmonary infiltrate. This syndrome must be evaluated by blood and sputum cultures; chest x-ray; ventilation-perfusion scan and pulmonary arteriogram when necessary; and arterial blood gases.

The etiology and pathology of acute chest syndrome are poorly understood. Yet, this is the most frequent cause of hospitalization in both pediatric and adult age groups. Fever, leukocytosis, tachycardia, and tachypnea are constant findings. Occasionally patients present with cyanosis. Chest x-ray usually demonstrates pulmonary infiltrates that may be patchy or localized and affecting one lobe or multiple lobes. Blood gases show evidence of hypoxia. The differential diagnosis should include pneumonia (with positive sputum and blood cultures), pulmonary infarct, pulmonary emboli, and bone marrow embolization. The organisms for pneumonia include *Streptococcus pneumoniae* and *Haemophilus influenzae,* and in adults one must consider gram-negative organisms and *Staphylococcus* besides *S. pneumoniae.* Patients should be treated with fluids, antibiotics, analgesics, oxygen supplementation, and blood transfusion therapy. Blood transfusion therapy should be provided to maintain the hemoglobin S level less than 50%.

### Neurologic Complications

Acute neurologic complications are reported in 6 to 20% of children and in approximately 10 to 15% of adults. Coma, convulsions, stupor, transient ischemic attacks, and clearly defined strokes can occur in any age group. Focal neurologic manifestations include hemiparesis, hemianesthesia, visual field defects, aphasia, and cranial nerve palsies. Generalized lesions include seizure disorder and coma. Diagnosis of a neurologic event includes computed tomography, magnetic resonance imaging, lumbar puncture, and arteriography for all patients with subarachnoid hemorrhage to detect a surgically correctable lesion. Blood transfusion prior to arteriography is recommended. Exchange blood transfusion and chronic transfusion therapy is recommended in children with acute neurologic events. Most clinics maintain patients with strokes on chronic transfusion therapy for 3 years, sustaining hemoglobin levels between 10 and 11 grams per dl and hemoglobin S percentage less than 30%. The approximate duration of prophylactic blood transfusion after a cerebrovascular accident is not known. In adults, cerebral infarction and hemorrhages occur with equal frequency. Blood transfusion therapy for the acute phase is recommended. Chronic transfusion therapy has to be decided on an individual base.

Eye changes and proliferative retinopathy have been described in sickle cell disease, the highest incidence occurring among patients with sickle C disease. Routine eye examination by the ophthalmologist is important. Early proliferative retinopathy may be treated with laser or cryotherapy and photocoagulation. Retinal detachment needs surgical treatment after partial exchange transfusion to suppress hemoglobin S to less than 35%.

### Infection

Patients with sickle cell disease are at a high risk for infection, owing to impaired splenic function, deficiency in serum opsonin, and poor clearance of organisms due to overloading of the reticuloendothelial system. *Streptococcus pneumoniae* and *H. influenzae* remain the predominant pathogens in children under the age of 6. Penicillin prophylaxis and use of pneumococcal vaccine are encouraged in children. Gram-negative organisms, *Staphylococcus,* and *Mycoplasma* must be considered in addition in the adult. There is also increased incidence of *Salmonella* septicemia and *Salmonella* osteomyelitis in sickle cell anemia.

Parvovirus has also been incriminated as a cause of infection, particularly in patients presenting with aplastic crisis.

### Priapism

Priapism is persistent, painful penile erection. It may be an acute reversible painful erection lasting for a few hours, an acute but prolonged episode lasting for days, or chronic persistent but painless or acute chronic priapism. Therapy should be planned at relieving pain and emptying the corpora cavernosa. Treatment would include hydration, pain control, and exchange blood transfusion therapy. If detumescence does not occur by 24 hours in spite of the preceding treatment, a Winter procedure or its modification under local anesthesia is encouraged.

### Hematuria

Gross and painless hematuria is a complication most often seen with sickle trait and sickle cell disease. Hematuria can be treated symptomatically. Infection, renal calculi, or arteriovenous malformation must be ruled out. Painless hematuria secondary to sickle hemoglobin is thought to be caused by sickling in the vasa recta, resulting in stasis and ischemia with seepage of blood into the renal parenchyma and collecting system. Papillary necrosis is a common finding. Treatment may include fluids, bed rest, alkalinization of the urine, and epsilon aminocaproic acid (Amicar*), at a dose of 2 to 8 grams a day. Occasionally hematuria is so profound that the patient requires blood transfusion therapy. The use of this drug can be associated with clot formation in the renal pelvis and ureter. Thus, patients to receive Amicar should be hospitalized for bed rest and intravenous fluid therapy.

### Chronic Renal Failure

This is seen in a small number of patients with sickle cell disease. Etiology of renal disease should be pursued before labeling chronic renal failure secondary to sickle nephropathy. Conservative management is advised in early stages. As renal failure progresses, patients should be referred for renal dialysis or kidney transplantation.

### Growth and Development

A constitutional rather than primary endocrine cause of delayed onset of puberty in sickle cell

---

*This use is not listed in the manufacturer's official directive.

disease patients was noted in the NIH's Cooperative Study of Sickle Cell Disease. Growth and maturation were significantly delayed for all sickle cell disease patients compared with controls. Subjects with SS and SB⁰ were slightly smaller and less sexually developed than those with SC and SB⁺ thalassemia. Infertility does not appear to be a problem related to sickle cell disease.

### Skeletal System

The skeletal system is a frequent site of abnormal findings due to bone marrow hyperplasia, infarction, and avascular necrosis of the femoral heads and other articular bones. Avascular necrosis of the bones occurs in a high frequency of SS patients and less frequently in those with SC, SB⁺, and SB⁰ thalassemias. Diagnosis of avascular necrosis is made when the patient has pain and radiographically detectable joint deformity late in the disease. Prosthetic joint replacement is recommended in patients who have severe debilitating pain. Exchange transfusion prior to the procedure is recommended. Early lesions may be diagnosed by magnetic resonance imaging. Symptomatic treatment; avoidance of weight bearing; and use of crutches, splints, and analgesics are usually suggested. Prosthesis is not advised for these early cases. Surgical decompression of increased intraosseous pressure is being evaluated.

### Leg Ulcers

Leg ulcers are common in patients with sickle cell anemia and are rare in patients with SC and SB⁺ thalassemias. The incidence rates are higher in males than females, and leg ulcers occur more frequently after the age of 20 years. The ulcers appear as simple or multiple lesions on both lower extremities. Local therapy is recommended for newly formed ulcers.

Chronic nonhealing ulcers of long duration are seen in 10 to 20% of patients with sickle cell anemia. Multiple methods of treatment, local care, blood transfusion therapy, and skin grafting are associated with similar recurrence rates. Meticulous attention to enhance healing of newly formed ulcers must be stressed to the patient. Cleaning the ulcer with mild soap and water, removing slough, and applying wet to dry saline dressings several times a day are urged. Local infection and inflammation may need evaluation to exclude osteomyelitis. Silver sulfadiazine (Sil-

vadene) cream applied before returning to saline dressing may be helpful if slough persists.

### GI System

Abdominal colic is reported more frequently in infants with SS than in other syndromes. It is important to evaluate the presence of gallstones or bowel infarct. Gallstones are known to be a complication of all patients with hemolytic anemia and occur in about 70% of patients by the age of 20 years. The presence of cholelithiasis does not necessitate the need for surgery. Patients may be treated with fluids and analgesics, and elective surgery is recommended if they have repeated episodes.

### Blood Transfusion

There is still controversy about the use of transfusion in the management of sickle cell disease. At present, there is no definite recommendation for the use of prophylactic transfusion. Transfusions are reserved for acute events—i.e., acute chest syndromes, hypoxia, new neurologic events, and severe anemia—and in preparation for surgery and anesthesia. Transfusion may be given by either simple or exchange blood transfusion therapy, maintaining hemoglobin levels at 10 to 11 grams per dl and hemoglobin S less than 50%.

### Pregnancy

There is no proof that prophylactic transfusion alters the outcome of pregnancy. Pregnant patients with sickle cell anemia and their infants are at increased risk. They require meticulous prenatal care and early detection of complications. Transfusion therapy during pregnancy is reserved for those patients with previous perinatal mortality, for complications including preeclampsia and severe anemia, and in preparation for surgical intervention (cesarean section). Complications of transfusion include development of alloimmunization, iron overload, transfusion-related hepatitis, and human immunodeficiency virus (HIV) infection.

### CONCLUSION

The clinical presentation of patients with sickle cell disease varies; one cannot predict which patient will and will not develop major complications. Therefore, each patient must be evaluated as an individual.

# NEUTROPENIA

method of
JANICE LYNN GABRILOVE, M.D., and
MICHAEL S. GORDON, M.D.
*Memorial Sloan-Kettering Cancer Center*
*New York, New York*

The neutrophil granulocyte serves as an important component of the immune system. Through its ability to identify and destroy foreign pathogens, it serves as a general and primary defense mechanism against various organisms, particularly bacteria. Neutrophils function predominantly via phagocytosis. Intracellular organisms are destroyed by lysosomal enzymes and the production of toxic oxygen radicals.

Neutrophils are produced by the bone marrow at a baseline rate of 850 million cells per kg per day. Mean survival of a mature neutrophil in the circulation is approximately 7 hours. Neutrophils migrate out of the circulation and into tissues in response to various chemotactic factors, most commonly produced in the setting of infection. Those neutrophils that do not migrate out of the circulation are cleared by the splenic reticuloendothelial system as their life span nears an end.

There can be some variation in the normal value for neutrophil number. Values of greater than 1500 cells per μl are considered the minimum acceptable level in a normal host. In some racial and ethnic groups, values may be lower. For example, blacks often have neutrophil counts as low as 1000 cells per μl in otherwise normal hosts. These variations in neutrophil number are felt to be secondary to differences in the distribution between the circulating and marginated pools of cells, and not a deficiency in production.

A deficiency in the number of neutrophils is termed neutropenia. The primary complication of neutropenia is infection. The relative risk of infectious complications is highly dependent upon the circulating number of neutrophils at the time in question. Data extracted by Bodey and colleagues from patients receiving cytotoxic marrow suppressive chemotherapy for myeloid leukemia indicate a 20% rise in infectious complications as the neutrophil count drops to below 1000 cells per μl. As the count falls below 500 cells per μl, the risk of infection rises to 50%, and reaches 100% with neutrophil counts below 200 cells per μl. In addition to the level of neutropenia, the duration of neutropenia plays a role in the likelihood of infection. Concomitant mucositis may further increase the rate of infection by providing additional portals of entry for infectious organisms.

Abnormalities of neutrophil function, regardless of the absolute number, may occur in some diseases, yielding a state of "relative neutropenia." Dysfunction can involve defects in degranulation (Chédiak-Higashi disease), superoxide production (chronic granulomatous disease), or chemotaxis (thermal burns, diabetes mellitus, or drugs such as ethanol or steroids).

## COMPLICATIONS

Infections in a patient with neutropenia require prompt antibacterial therapy. Cultures of blood, sputum, and other indicated body fluids should be sent to the laboratory prior to the start of antibiotics. Antibiotic choices should be made with the intent to cover a broad spectrum of bacteria. Included among these are streptococci and staphylococci from the skin, as well as gram-negative enterics. In general, the combination of an aminoglycoside with a third generation cephalosporin or an antipseudomonal penicillin is considered first line therapy. Patients who do not respond to broad-spectrum antibiotics and continue to be febrile are candidates to begin amphotericin B to cover fungal pathogens.

## CLINICAL SYNDROMES (Table 1)

There are a variety of disorders that can cause neutropenia. These can be subdivided into three major categories.

**Primary Disorders.** Three primary disorders of neutropenia have been described. The first of these is congenital neutropenia, which can principally be divided into two major syndromes: Kostmann's syndrome and Shwachman-Diamond syndrome. In Kostmann's syndrome (infantile agranulocytosis), an autosomally recessive disease, patients present with profound neutropenia (less than 500 cells per μl), eosinophilia, monocytosis, and hypergammaglobulinemia. It is associated with a maturation arrest in the bone marrow at the promyelocyte-myelocyte stage, recurrent bacterial infections, and oral ulcerations.

Shwachman-Diamond syndrome, inherited as an autosomal recessive trait, is characterized by chronic neutropenia in the first decade of life, normal monocyte counts, bone marrow granulocyte hyperplasia, hypergammaglobulinemia, and exocrine pancreatic insufficiency.

Cyclic neutropenia may be congenital or acquired. The congenital type is of autosomal dominant transmission with varying penetrance. Both types are characterized by oscillations of the absolute neutrophil count (ANC) from low-normal ranges to nadir values of 0 to 200 cells per μl. The periodicity of the cycling phenomenon is 14 to 21 days. Review of peripheral blood displays a monocytosis during the period of greatest neutropenia. Coincident with this, bone marrow examination usually indicates a myeloid maturation arrest. Many of these patients have mild cycling of erythroid and megakaryocytic lines in conjunction with the neutropenia. In addition to experiencing chronic, recurring bacterial infections, these patients frequently demonstrate a high incidence of mucosal ulceration involving the oropharyngeal, anorectal, and vaginal region. The occurrence of these ulcers is linked to the cycling of the neutrophils—worsening as neutropenia becomes more severe and clearing as neutrophil counts improve. As in some of the congenital neutropenias, there is a compensatory hypergammaglobulinemia. There have been occasional spontaneous remissions in both types of cyclic neutropenia.

Idiopathic neutropenia presents with mild to moderate neutropenia (ANC values of 500 cells per μl or less). This disorder probably represents a spectrum of etiologies and is characterized by a normocellular or hypocellular bone marrow with decreased mature mye-

TABLE 1. **Clinical Syndromes of Neutropenia**

I. Absolute neutropenia
  A. Primary disorders
    1. Congenital
      a. Kostmann's syndrome
      b. Shwachman-Diamond syndrome
    2. Cyclic
      a. Congenital
      b. Acquired
    3. Idiopathic
  B. Secondary disorders
    1. Malignant
      a. Lymphoid
        (i) Hairy cell leukemia
        (ii) Chronic lymphocytic leukemia
        (iii) Hodgkin's disease
        (iv) Non-Hodgkin's lymphoma
        (v) Multiple myeloma
        (vi) Acute lymphoblastic leukemia
      b. Myeloid
        (i) Acute myeloid leukemia
        (ii) Myelodysplastic syndrome
          Refractory anemia
          Refractory anemia with excess blasts
          Refractory anemia with excess blasts in
            transformation
    2. Non-malignant
      a. Autoimmune diseases
        (i) Felty's syndrome
        (ii) Systemic lupus erythematosus
        (iii) Rheumatoid arthritis
      b. T8 lymphocytosis (T-gamma disease)
      c. AIDS/HIV infection
      d. Aplastic anemia
  C. Drug Related
    1. Chemotherapy
    2. Antibiotics
      a. Penicillin
      b. Sulfas
      c. Chloramphenicol
    3. Antithyroid drugs
    4. Antidepressants
    5. Anticonvulsants
      a. Carbamazepine
      b. Phenytoin
    6. Radiation therapy
    7. Organic solvents
II. Functional neutropenia
  A. Drugs
    1. Steroids
    2. Ethanol
  B. Chédiak-Higashi disease
  C. Chronic granulomatous disease
  D. Autoimmune disease
  E. Thermal damage
  F. Diabetes mellitus

to have an inhibitory effect on normal myeloid progenitor growth. Such "inhibitory factors" may play an etiologic role in the neutropenia seen in the setting of ALL, hairy cell leukemia (HCL), chronic lymphocytic leukemia (CLL), non-Hodgkin's lymphoma and Hodgkin's disease, multiple myeloma (MM), myeloid malignancies such as acute myeloid leukemia (AML), and myelodysplastic syndromes (MDS) (including refractory anemia [RA], refractory anemia with excess blasts [RAEB], and refractory anemia with excess blasts in transformation [RAEB-t]). In the latter two disorders, neutropenia also results from a relative maturation arrest of myeloid elements.

Autoimmune diseases such as systemic lupus erythematosus (SLE) and rheumatoid arthritis are the most frequently encountered nonmalignant disorders associated with neutropenia. Felty's syndrome, with its constellation of arthritis, neutropenia, ulcers, and splenomegaly, is a major treatment problem. These patients often have high titers of antineutrophil antibodies.

T8 lymphocytosis or T gamma disease is a disorder characterized by a true peripheral blood and bone marrow lymphocytosis (greater than 5000 cells) due to an increase in peripheral blood large granular lymphocytes (greater than 50% of the total lymphocyte count), with T suppressor–natural killer phenotype. These cells have a potentially suppressive effect on myeloid maturation associated with the marrow lymphocytosis. The disease is characterized by mild neutropenia with few infectious complications except a slight increase in viral syndromes.

Neutropenia associated with human immunodeficiency virus (HIV–1) infection is felt to be secondary to viral suppression of normal myeloid progenitor growth or an immune etiology. Infectious complications, however, are predominantly with nonbacterial opportunistic infections, secondary to the overall immunocompromised state and not the neutropenia.

Aplastic anemia is a state of hypoproduction of all hematopoietic cell lines. Its precise etiology is unknown, but alterations in the marrow microenvironment, loss of stem cells, and constitutive production of negative regulators by polyclonal populations of suppressor cells in response to unknown antigens are several hypotheses. In this condition, severe neutropenia is one component of pancytopenia.

Infections such as viral (e.g., hepatitis), rickettsial, and gram-negative sepsis have been known to cause transient neutropenia. In the case of endotoxemia, bone marrow suppression may be due to production of negative regulators such as tumor necrosis factor (TNF).

**Drug-Related Disorders.** The final group of neutropenic syndromes are those related to various drug therapies. Chemotherapy characteristically causes neutropenia 10 to 14 days after infusion of the drugs. In some circumstances, nadir of blood counts occurs 3 to 4 weeks after administration. The extent and duration of neutropenia are dependent upon the dose of the drug, the presumed marrow progenitor level upon which the drug acts, and concomitant administration of other chemotherapeutic agents.

A variety of medications have been implicated in the development of neutropenia. Among these, antithyroid drugs, antidepressants (tricyclics), anticonvul-

loid cells, occasional peripheral monocytosis, hypergammaglobulinemia, and a usually slight increase (although sometimes frequent) in infectious complications.

**Secondary Disorders.** The secondary disorders of neutropenia are most often the result of an underlying malignant or nonmalignant disease. Among the malignant disorders, the majority are of hematologic origin.

Lymphoid malignancies such as acute lymphoblastic leukemia (ALL) have been shown to produce transforming growth factor beta (TGF-B), which is known sants (carbamazepine and phenytoin), and antibiotics (penicillins, sulfas, and chloramphenicol) are prime examples. Mechanisms include antibody production (e.g., cephalosporins) and presumed progenitor cell injury (chloramphenicol). Resolution of neutropenia varies. For cephalosporins, this occurs classically within 7 days; for other drugs, recovery occurs gradually after the drug is withdrawn.

Radiotherapy, particularly gamma radiation, can cause suppression of peripheral blood counts. This is on the basis of toxicity to hematopoietic progenitors both circulating and intramedullary. Exposure to radiation in large enough doses (greater than 200 cGy of total body irradiation) can cause syndromes of pancytopenia related to marrow aplasia.

## PATIENT EVALUATION (Table 2)

Evaluation of patients with neutropenia begins with a thorough history and review of data. In particular,

TABLE 2. **Evaluation of Neutropenia**

A. Review of previous blood counts
B. History
  1. Exposure
    a. Radiation
    b. Organic solvents
  2. Drug/medication history
  3. Infectious complications
  4. Periodicity of symptoms
C. Physical examination
  1. Ulcers (oropharyngeal, anorectal, vaginal)
  2. Lymphadenopathy
  3. Splenomegaly
  4. Signs of infection
D. Review of peripheral smear
  1. Evidence of dysmyelopoiesis
    a. Pelger-Huët neutrophils
  2. Lymphocytosis
    a. Large granular lymphocytes
  3. Abnormal cells
    a. Hairy cells
    b. Myeloblasts
    c. Lymphoblasts
E. Bone marrow aspiration and biopsy
  1. Morphology
  2. Cytogenetics
  3. Cell surface markers
    a. Lymphoid vs. myeloid
  4. Special stains
    a. Sideroblast
    b. PAS, Sudan black, alpha naphthyl esterase
F. Complete blood counts every other day × 1 mo
  1. Rule out cyclic component
G. Peripheral blood studies
  1. Antineutrophil antibody
  2. HIV antibody
  3. Autoimmune work-up
    a. Rheumatoid factor
    b. Antinuclear antibody
    c. Complement (C3, C4, CH50)
  4. Vitamin $B_{12}$ and folate
  5. Chemistries
    a. Liver function tests including lactate dehydrogenase
    b. Renal function
    c. Uric acid
  6. Serum and immunoelectrophoreses

previous blood counts can aid in defining the duration of the abnormality in question. History-taking must concentrate on any previous exposure to radiation or organic solvents as well as a full drug and medication screening. Previous infectious signs or symptoms should be elicited and their periodicity noted. Any possible related illnesses such as infections (previously noted) must be elaborated. A complete physical examination, paying particular attention to mucosal ulcerations, lymphadenopathy, splenomegaly, or any signs of infection, should be performed.

Hematologic evaluation should begin with a review of the peripheral blood smear, paying particular attention to abnormal cells that may be indicative of disorders such as HCL, CLL, the acute leukemias, and other hematologic disorders. Complete blood count with differential count should be obtained every other day for a period of 1 month to rule out a cyclic component. Bone marrow aspiration and biopsy must be performed with special studies for cytogenetics, cell markers (lymphoid and myeloid), sideroblast stain, and as standard morphology.

Peripheral blood should be sent for antineutrophil and HIV antibodies, autoimmune work-up (including rheumatoid factor, antinuclear antibody, and complement studies), vitamin $B_{12}$, folate, liver and renal function tests, lactate dehydrogenase, uric acid, and serum and immunoelectrophoreses.

## TREATMENT

Treatment of neutropenia remains dependent upon the proposed etiology. Development of acute neutropenia must provoke a search for possible offending drugs or signs and symptoms of infection. In general, these types of neutropenia require either the cessation of implicated drugs or the prompt identification of complicating disorders. Resolution of neutropenia in these instances frequently is rapid.

Among the primary neutropenic disorders, various therapies have been tried. In the congenital disorders, minimal response has been noted to steroids, gamma globulin, lithium salts, splenectomy, or plasmapheresis. Allogeneic bone marrow transplantation has resulted in partial as well as complete remissions. Most recently, therapy with growth factors has yielded varying responses. Granulocyte colony-stimulating factor (G-CSF) has resulted in improved neutrophil counts associated with decreased infectious episodes. On the other hand, granulocyte-macrophage colony-stimulating factor has shown no clinical benefit.

Cyclic neutropenia, both congenital and acquired, may exhibit spontaneous clinical remissions. Various therapies such as gammaglobulin, plasmapheresis, splenectomy, and corticosteroids have proved to be without benefit. Lithium carbonate has resulted in some increases in neutrophil counts, though its exact mechanism of action is unknown.

The grey collie model for cyclic neutropenia has allowed studies to explore the therapeutic role of hematopoietic growth factors. Based upon benefits seen with G-CSF, this growth factor has now been studied in patients with this disorder. Initial studies by Dale and associates indicate significant improvement in neutrophil counts and cycling periodicity.

Results of therapy for idiopathic neutropenia are essentially the same as noted for the cyclic states, with the exception that recent reports indicate that GM-CSF as well as G-CSF may produce increases in neutrophil counts and clinical improvement.

Neutropenia secondary to underlying illnesses responds best to treatment of the primary disorder. Among the malignant states, CLL, ALL, MM, non-Hodgkin's lymphoma, and Hodgkin's disease are best managed with appropriate combination chemotherapy regimes. In HCL, the interferons and pentostatin appear to be the most effective agents for inducing clinical remission. Recent studies with G-CSF in HCL have resulted in improvement in neutrophil counts and concomitant infections previously unresponsive to antibiotic therapy without significant effect on the underlying disease. Clinical trials of G-CSF in combination with alpha-interferon are at present underway.

Standard chemotherapy for patients with myeloid leukemia remains the "gold standard" for its treatment. Studies with G-CSF and GM-CSF are ongoing to evaluate the ability of these cytokines to either cycle leukemia cells into S-phase to improve cell kill of chemotherapy or, in the case of G-CSF, to evaluate the potential differentiating effect on myeloid blasts.

In the myelodysplastic syndromes, low-dose cytosine arabinoside (ara-C) has resulted in approximately 30% complete response rates. Intensive chemotherapy and vitamins have yielded lesser response rates. Allogeneic bone marrow transplantation has a high rate of complete response and is the therapy of choice in patients with an HLA-matched donor. Recent attempts at differentiation therapy with hexamethylbisacetimide (HMBA)* and cis-retinoic acid have resulted in few significant responses. Because the major complications of these disorders are the cytopenias that accompany them, treatment with various growth factors has been studied. Trials with G-CSF and GM-CSF have both resulted in significant improvements in both total white blood count and neutrophil counts.

In secondary neutropenia associated with autoimmune disorders, gamma globulin and plasmapheresis have been used without success. Corticosteroids have been effective in SLE, and in conjunction with other appropriate medications have yielded responses in the rheumatoid arthritides. Splenectomy in patients with Felty's syndrome has resulted in transient rises in neutrophil counts, with subsequent declines to preoperative levels.

T8 lymphocytosis has been noted to respond to gamma globulin with partial but no complete responses. Alternative treatment with steroids and plasmapheresis has been ineffective.

In patients with neutropenia associated with HIV-1 infection, G-CSF and GM-CSF have been used alone and in conjunction with antiviral therapy (zidovudine [AZT, Retrovir]), with improvement of neutrophil counts.

Various therapies have been utilized in aplastic anemia. Corticosteroids, androgens, antithymocyte globulin (ATG), and allogeneic bone marrow transplantation have become the mainstay of therapeutic interventions. Most recently, various cytokines and growth factors, including G-CSF, GM-CSF, and, in one study, interleukin-3, have shown some initial promise in improving neutrophil counts in selected patients.

Neutropenia due to drugs or medications is best treated by removal of the offending agent, with resolution of neutropenia most often occurring within 48 hours. Both G-CSF and GM-CSF have been used on a compassionate basis in drug-related neutropenia, with an acceleration of recovery noted.

Prospects in the treatment of neutropenia secondary to chemotherapy have been bouyed by favorable results in trials using both G-CSF and GM-CSF. Other cytokines (interleukin-1 and interleukin-3), whose actions occur in earlier stages of hematopoiesis, are currently being studied with the hope of impacting upon the deficiencies of other cell lineages associated with chemotherapy as well as further augmenting myeloid reconstitution.

Granulocyte transfusion must be reserved for those patients with documented life-threatening bacterial or fungal infections in the presence of neutropenia. The transfusion must be ABO compatible and should be administered for a maximum of 7 to 10 days or until the infection resolves. Risks associated with granulocyte transfusion include ABO incompatibility as well as reports of leukoagglutination associated with coadministration of amphotericin B.

---

*Available only as an investigational drug in the United States.

# HEMOLYTIC DISEASE OF THE FETUS AND NEWBORN

method of
C. R. HARMAN, M.D.
*The University of Manitoba*
*Winnipeg, Manitoba, Canada*

## ETIOLOGY

In serious hemolytic disease at birth, the diagnosis is *alloimmunization,* until proved otherwise. *Bacterial sepsis* cannot be ignored as a possible cause, because of the high associated mortality. These two causes are differentiated readily, but both must be given careful attention in the acutely ill newborn. Later in neonatal life, a long list of differential diagnoses becomes possible, but alloimmunization remains the most likely process causing severe hyperbilirubinemia and risk of kernicterus. Most *chronic infections,* especially the STORCH group, involve combined deficits of hemolysis and decreased hepatic function, with decreased bilirubin clearance. Recently, parvovirus has been implicated, as it causes bone marrow failure *and* hemolysis, resulting in severe hydropic disease.

Several hereditary disorders predispose to red blood cell (RBC) deformation, with splenic or microangiopathic hemolysis. These include *hereditary RBC membrane defects*—spherocytosis is the most common. Usually milder than other hemolytic anemias, they may be aggravated by superimposed infection, asphyxia, trauma, or other biologic stress, with rapid fall in hemoglobin level and progressive jaundice, requiring exchange transfusion to prevent kernicterus. *Hereditary RBC enzyme defects* are susceptible to similar stresses. The most serious of these, glucose-6-phosphate dehydrogenase (G6PD) deficiency, may also be triggered by oxidant agents (acetylsalicylic acid, sulphonamides, antimalarials, fava beans, mothballs, etc.). Owing to its potential for a rapid course, with serious hyperbilirubinemia of a level requiring exchange transfusion to prevent kernicterus, G6PD deserves attention in nonalloimmune (Coombs-negative) hemolytic situations.

Finally, newborns with *chronic fetal-maternal hemorrhage* may have all the physical manifestations of hydrops fetalis, including severe anemia and erythroblastosis, but without *any* hemolysis.

### Alloimmunization

Specific cross-matching, Rh prophylaxis (antepartum, as well as postpartum), and better prenatal care have combined with the declining pregnancy rate to lower the frequency of Rh disease. "Atypical" blood group antigens and nonalloimmune hemolytic disorders have thus attained more relative importance statistically. Alloimmunization remains the major cause of hemolytic disease of the fetus and newborn (HDFN), however, especially in early or rapidly progressive neonatal disease and most cases of hydropic fetal disease.

**Blood Group Incompatibility.** The tremendous variety

TABLE 1. **Major Non-D Antigens Associated with Clinical Hemolytic Disease of the Fetus and Newborn**

| Blood Group | Frequent | Uncommon |
|---|---|---|
| Rh | c, E, C$^w$ | e, C, Ce, cE |
| Kell | K | Kp$^a$, Kp$^b$, k |
| Duffy | | Fy$^a$ |
| MNS | | s |
| Private | | Wr$^a$ |
| ABO | A, B | AB |

of human blood group antigens gives unlimited possibility for differing blood types between mother and fetus in a given pregnancy. Clinical manifestations of incompatibility are restricted, however, to a smaller group of antigens. Some antigens (e.g., Lewis) are not expressed by fetal blood, whereas others are so relatively nonantigenic that even serious sensitization as the result of maternal incompletely matched transfusion has limited potential for disease. Others cause disease rarely and have been ignored, but when sensitization develops, they are as capable of producing severe hydrops as the Rh group. These have been termed the "atypical" blood group antigens (Table 1). No antibody detected in a pregnant woman should be ignored: when in doubt, one should investigate.

True Rh disease remains responsible for 80 to 90% of all alloimmune forms. It is readily preventable—that is the only factor which separates it from disorders of other blood group antigens—and the discussion of classic Rh disease is fully applicable to that of the so-called atypical blood groups.

**Pathogenesis of Alloimmune Disease** (Figure 1). Fetal genetic content (blood type) is determined by parental blood groups, in mendelian fashion. Rh negativity occurs in 15% of Caucasians (D-antigen negative, denoted dd). Of the remaining 85%, 44% are homozygous DD, and 56% are Dd. An Rh-negative woman has a 61% chance of having an Rh-incompatible fetus (on

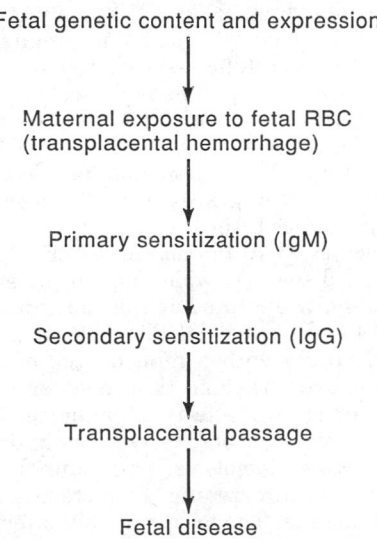

Fetal genetic content and expression

↓

Maternal exposure to fetal RBC (transplacental hemorrhage)

↓

Primary sensitization (IgM)

↓

Secondary sensitization (IgG)

↓

Transplacental passage

↓

Fetal disease

**Figure 1.** Pathogenesis of alloimmunization.

the basis of general statistics), rising to 72% if the father is known to be Rh positive. Rh negativity occurs in 4 to 5% of American blacks and less than 1% of Orientals.

Maternal exposure to fetal red blood cell antigen may occur by many routes. The most common is *transplacental hemorrhage* (TPH), leakage of small amounts of fetal blood (< 2 ml in 95% of cases) into the maternal circulation. This commonly occurs at delivery, but also may happen at any time antenatally. Up to 70% of pregnancies may show evidence of TPH, readily detectable in maternal blood with the Kleihauer technique. An acid buffer elutes the adult hemoglobin from the maternal blood sample, leaving the intact fetal red blood cells detectable with light microscopy. TPH is usually late in pregnancy, provoking sensitization which affects subsequent siblings bearing the antigen in question. Rarely, antenatal TPH may be early enough for sensitization and transmission of disease to occur in the same pregnancy. *Blood transfusion* remains a source of alloimmunization, as current cross-matching ensures compatibility for ABO type, and for D in the Rh system, only. Exposure to other antigens (see Table 1) may occur at transfusion; combined with an antigen-positive father, this may lead to serious alloimmune disease. With the first exposure of an Rh-negative woman to D-positive cells, D antigen is processed in a competent fashion and the preliminary response, anti-D IgM antibody, follows in a few months. IgM does not cross the placenta and does not cause fetal disease. When sensitization has reached this point, however, disease can no longer be prevented. The smallest subsequent exposure to D antigen causes a full-blown IgG response in a matter of weeks. IgG is the agent of fetal disease. It crosses the placenta by facilitated transport and attains fetal concentrations equivalent to those in the mother.

Variations abound. Up to 30% of women are not sensitized despite proven exposure to D antigen ("nonresponders"). If fetal-maternal ABO incompatibility exists, fetal cells are hemolyzed rapidly by AB antibodies already in maternal circulation, precluding processing of the D antigen. Other protective effects include the following: 90% of TPH occurs at delivery—i.e., there is no risk for that pregnancy; most TPH is of small volume—sensitization occurs less often; and nonspecific pregnancy effects may protect against sensitization to some degree. After sensitization is complete, however, transmission of IgG to the fetus is inevitable. Various means have been tried to reduce the strength of IgG response; these are regarded as temporary and/or futile.

**Fetal Responses to Alloimmunization** (Figure 2). The range of fetal disease is wide and, in general, varies with the strength and duration of maternal antibody production. In untreated HDFN, 50% of pregnancies are affected mildly with a mild degree of anemia at birth and require either no treatment or only phototherapy to reduce the effects of jaundice. Of the remainder, half will be born alive (nonhydropic), but experience severe hemolysis, with jaundice and the potential for life-threatening kernicterus, associated with severe anemia. The most severely affected group, about 25% of the total, result in stillbirth or neonatal

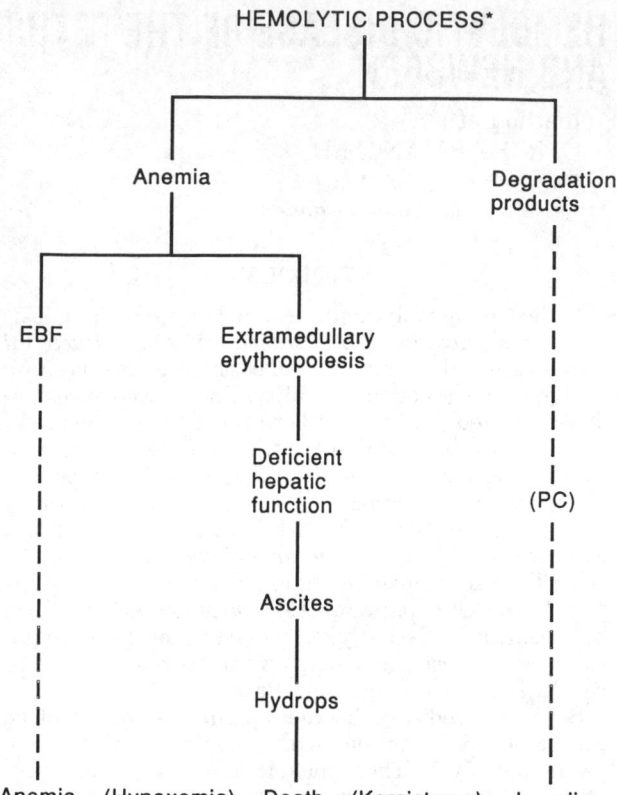

EBF = erythroblastosis fetalis; PC = placental clearance.
*In the case of Rh disease, transplacental passage of anti-D IgG

**Figure 2.** Pathophysiology of HDFN.

death before term, 50% dying of hydropic disease before 34 weeks' gestation.

Variations in disease severity among fetuses are poorly understood. The underlying mechanism is IgG-mediated hemolytic destruction of fetal RBCs in the fetal reticuloendothelial system (RES). Anti-D IgG does not activate complement, but by the Fc fragment does identify bound fetal RBC to the RES. The fetal RBCs are then deformed by digestion, removed by the RES, and destroyed by phagocytosis and extravascular hemolysis. The ultimate results of extravascular hemolysis are degradation products and progressive anemia. The responses to hypoxic effects of anemia lead to extramedullary erythropoiesis, in the liver, the spleen, the intestines, and the skin, displacing normal functions. For example, as islands of hematopoiesis distend the liver, hepatic function falls, serum albumin level drops, and portal and systemic venous pressure rise, leading to ascites, further protein loss, and ultimately to universal edema (anasarca). At the same time, the anemia is not effectively countered—newly released RBCs and precursors are hemolyzed rapidly. This results in a circulating blood picture of only immature RBC precursors (erythroblastosis fetalis). Parallel events occur in the placenta, compromising gas exchange and other functions owing to massive edema. The result is fetal death due to hydrops fetalis;

massive hepatosplenomegaly, deficient liver function and hypoalbuminemia, gross anasarca, pleural and pericardial effusions, deficient cardiac function, impaired placental function, and gross hydramnios occur.

Liveborn hydropic infants are in grave danger owing to cardiovascular insufficiency with severe venous hypertension, grossly distended liver and intra-abdominal circulatory compromise, ventilator difficulties due to pleural effusions and chest wall edema, and airway obstruction by gross edema. Anti-D remains in circulation for up to 6 weeks, so even the nonhydropic newborn may be threatened. If untreated, IgG-mediated hemolysis may continue rapidly, and, because the maternal-placental link no longer removes the resulting bilirubin, disease may progress to severe jaundice and kernicterus. Deposition of unconjugated bilirubin, which is lipid soluble, in the neurons of the central nervous system results in neuronal death with yellow staining of the dead areas. This severe consequence of untreated neonatal disease carries an 80% mortality, with extreme morbidity in survivors. There is virtually no clinical reason why kernicterus should occur with modern neonatal management.

## SURVEILLANCE

### Screening of the Rh-Negative Woman (Figure 3)

*All* pregnant women should be screened in *all* pregnancies, regardless of Rh type. An antibody identified on general screening should be characterized by a competent serology laboratory. This identification may include (1) indirect antiglobulin test (indirect Coombs'

test), (2) albumin titration of combined IgG and IgM, and (3) direct measurement of absolute IgG concentration. The clinician must know the source and type of testing: 1:64 by indirect Coombs' test, 1:16 by albumin suspension, and 1 μg per ml by autoanalyzer are roughly equivalent. The levels cited are critical antibody strengths, indicating a need for invasive testing. When antibody strength has reached this level, maternal antibody titers may no longer reflect disease severity; direct fetal testing is mandatory.

With a posterior placenta, at early gestations, or if previous disease does not indicate extreme likelihood of hydrops, amniocentesis may be the procedure of choice. It carries a low risk of TPH, which would aggravate maternal sensitization, when the above conditions are met. When the placenta is anterior, or when severe fetal anemia is likely on the basis of history or markedly elevated antibody titers, the patient should be referred to a tertiary center capable of the appropriate fetal blood sampling and fetal management.

### Amniocentesis

Under real-time ultrasound direction, this procedure ideally obtains an uncontaminated sample of amniotic fluid, which is protected from exposure to light and analyzed by spectrophotometry. Absorption at 450 nm produces a typical rise, reflecting the yellowness (presence of bilirubin) of the fluid. Measured vertically and plotted on semilogarithmic paper, optical density difference at 450 nm (delta $OD_{450}$) indicates the cumula-

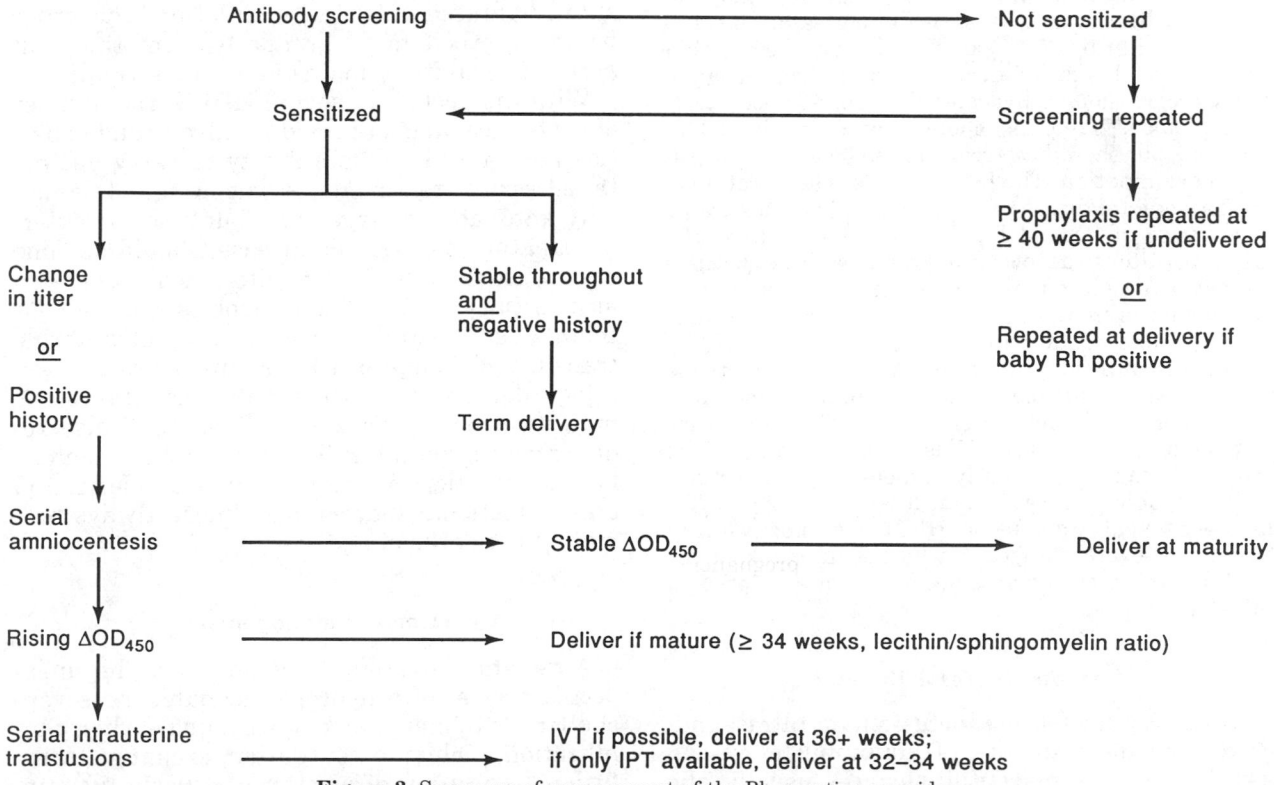

**Figure 3.** Summary of management of the Rh-negative gravida.

TABLE 2. **Ultrasound Classification of Alloimmune Disease**

| Class | Ultrasound Appearance | | | | Abnormal BPS (<4/10) |
|---|---|---|---|---|---|
| | Placenta | Ascites | Effusion | Anasarca | |
| I | + | − | − | − | − |
| II | + | + | − | − | − |
| III | + | + | + | + | − |
| IV | + | + | + | + | + |

*Abbreviations:* BPS = biophysical profile score.

tive amount of hemolysis. The delta $OD_{450}$ plotted against gestational age indicates subsequent action. This management should not be entertained without consultation with a tertiary center, but the recommendations may be summarized as follows: If the fluid remains in Liley's Zone 1 (with no acute antibody rise in the interim), it can be repeated every 2 to 4 weeks, depending on history and antibody level. In Zone 2, frequent repetition as often as weekly may be necessary to ensure that the trend is downward and parallel to the zone lines, indicating a low risk of severe disease. If the delta $OD_{450}$ remains static (in effect rising against the normal downward slope of the zone lines) or if there is frank increase in delta $OD_{450}$, the patient should be referred for intrauterine treatment.

*Fetal Blood Sampling*

Many tertiary centers managing severe HDFN now offer ultrasound-directed cordocentesis to determine fetal hemoglobin level, as early as 17 to 18 weeks. Normally, fetal hemoglobin level rises throughout pregnancy; in 95% of fetuses it is greater than 90 grams per liter at 20 weeks, rising to greater than 120 grams per liter by 40 weeks. Fetuses with hemoglobin levels below this fifth percentile require transfusion to avoid progression to hydropic disease. Amniocentesis or fetal blood sampling should not be performed in isolation, but should be accompanied by detailed ultrasound examination. The latter enables classification of severity of fetal disease (Table 2). In Class I disease, a wide range of hemoglobin levels is found (from 100 grams per liter to as low as 40 grams per liter). Fetuses already hydropic on ultrasound examination always are anemic, with hemoglobin levels as low as 20 grams per liter, and require immediate transfusion. Ultrasound classification of disease is not used to postpone appropriate management, but may indicate the absolute urgency of such intervention. The fetus with moribund hydrops (Class IV) is in extreme danger and should be managed virtually immediately in a tertiary center capable of intravascular fetal transfusion (IVT). Intraperitoneal transfusion (IPT) does not work in fetuses so severely affected, who are incapable of the fetal breathing movements necessary for absorption of the blood.

### Intrauterine Fetal Therapy

Intravascular fetal transfusion via ultrasound-guided needle puncture of an umbilical vessel, usually on the placental surface, usually the umbilical vein, is now the management of choice in many centers for intrauterine treatment of fetal disease. This therapy has produced revolutionary improvement in the outlook for such severely affected infants. The aim of modern IVT is to produce healthy, nonanemic, nonhydropic, mature infants. Survival of up to 95% in nonhydropic disease and more than 80% in hydropic disease is now attained. There is a realistic chance of intact survival, provided therapy is initiated before the fetus becomes hypoxemic and acidotic. This places the onus on the referring physician even more strongly: there is virtually no excuse for voluntary nontreatment of even severe disease.

Intraperitoneal fetal transfusion (IPT), once the management standard, has now assumed an adjunctive role. IPT is used only in nonhydropic disease, when fetal position is unsuitable for IVT, and *ideal* for IPT. Risks of premature labor and/or premature rupture of membranes (30%) and of traumatic fetal death (3% for posterior placenta, 7% for transplacental procedures) mean that it is used only in selected situations. Beyond 32 weeks gestation, for example, delivery is chosen, rather than risking traumatic fetal death at IPT. On the other hand, IVT is apparently so safe that it may be used up to 34 to 35 weeks' gestation, achieving term delivery of a nonanemic fetus. Combining IVT and IPT at the same time, delivering a larger volume of blood, one being instantly infused into the circulation, the other being absorbed more gradually from the fetal peritoneal cavity, remains under investigation.

With the decline in severe HDFN, the number of centers capable of providing ultrasound expertise and procedural familiarity to carry out detailed serial treatments is shrinking. Thus, not only antenatal management, but also intrauterine treatment of serious disease, should be done only in close collaboration with a dedicated team at a tertiary center. The outlook is excellent for infants successfully treated by intrauterine transfusion. Long-term follow-up shows no neurologic deficits and, although the neonatal course may occasionally be stormy (and thus also requiring the special skills of a tertiary center), hepatic function, subsequent hematopoiesis, and other functional indices are almost always normal by 6 months of age.

### Neonatal Management

Antenatal ultrasound should avert the unexpected arrival of a hydropic neonate; the severe challenges in management are noted earlier. Stabilization, including ventilation, exchange transfusion, aspiration of ascites, and basic life sup-

TABLE 3. **When Should Prophylaxis Be Given?**

In an unsensitized Rh-negative woman, *any* significant obstetric event when the fetus/newborn is not *proven* Rh negative

**All Cases**
Spontaneous abortion
Therapeutic abortion
Chorion villus sampling
Genetic amniocentesis
Lung profile amniocentesis

**Dose Depends on Kleihauer's Test**
Antepartum hemorrhage
Obstetric manipulation
Manual removal of placenta
Molar pregnancy
Large transplacental hemorrhage

**Routine Prophylaxis**
(none of the above events)
28 weeks gestation *and*
40 weeks if undelivered, or
Delivery of Rh-positive infant

port, must be aggressive and early to maximize survival. If neonatal care is superlative, outlook depends on the degree of prematurity.

In nonhydropic infants with serious hemolysis, diagnosis is critical. Blood is obtained, pretransfusion, for Coombs' test, complete blood count and smear, bilirubin studies, blood gases and pH determinations, blood cultures, and other studies (an extra tube). Life-threatening bacterial sepsis, congenital infection, or hemorrhage is easily identifiable and may require urgent simple transfusion. Immediate exchange transfusion at birth is indicated by hemoglobin level of less than 90 grams per liter and bilirubin concentration of greater than 100 μmol per liter. Double-volume exchange transfusion ($2 \times 80$ ml per kg) with Group O, maternally compatible fresh blood should be done by an experienced team with full laboratory back-up. Moderate disease with significant hemolysis, but with cord blood hemoglobin level of greater than 100 grams per liter and bilirubin concentration of less than 100 μmol per liter, may be managed with phototherapy. If bilirubin rises to greater than 300 μmol per liter on phototherapy, exchange transfusion is needed.

TABLE 4. **ABO Versus Rh Alloimmunization**

| Factor | Rhesus | ABO |
|---|---|---|
| Incompatible pregnancy | 9–11% | 25–30% |
| Fetal antigen expressed | + + + | ± |
| Maternal antibody response | IgG | IgM >> IgG |
| Fetal targets | Red blood cells only | Multiple tissue sites |
| Placental targets | Uncertain | Definite |
| Antibody-antigen binding | Strong to very strong | Weak to moderate |

Careful infant follow-up is indicated, as simple transfusion may be needed (hemoglobin less than 70 grams per liter) for anemia due to ongoing mild hemolysis and the relative bone marrow inactivity of the 1- to 4-month-old infant. These babies usually are not iron deficient. Recurring anemia or jaundice suggest an intrinsic cause, such as hereditary RBC disorders, primary hepatic disorders, and so on.

### Rh Prophylaxis

Small amounts of anti-D immune globulin (intramuscular RhoGAM; intravenous or intramuscular WinRho) protect against sensitization of Rh-negative women exposed to Rh-positive fetal blood. The standard 300-μg dose (WinRho, pure anti-D IgG prepared by column fractionation) protects against TPH of up to 15 ml. Provided none of the events in Table 3 occurs, prophylaxis given at 28 weeks and again at delivery (or at due date if undelivered) prevents 99.5% of sensitization, reducing the population sensitized to less than 2 per 10,000. How this passive immunity works is not fully clear. It carries no benefit to the woman already sensitized. The primary physician is directly responsible for this detailed prophylaxis, usually coordinated through a centralized program.

### ABO Incompatibility

This is *not* analogous to other incompatibilities. ABO antibodies are in constant, low-grade concentration, but are usually *IgM*. About 50% of Group O women produce anti-A and anti-B *IgG*, which can cross the placenta. Several factors (Table 4) combine to make ABO incompatibility (which happens in 20 to 30% of pregnancies) of reduced impact. By itself, ABO hemolysis does not cause hydrops or stillbirth. If severe neonatal jaundice occurs, compounding factors, such as infection, gastrointestinal anomalies, or drugs, should be suspected.

# HEMOPHILIA AND VON WILLEBRAND'S DISEASE

method of
CRAIG S. KITCHENS, M.D.
*VA Medical Center*
*Gainesville, Florida*

Patients with heritable disorders of coagulation may present as "free bleeders," a term sensitive enough to include most persons with von Willebrand's disease or a deficiency of one of the plasma coagulation proteins but not specific enough for modern medicine. Current therapy of these disorders is based on the establishment of a precise diagnosis that dictates the specific therapy in specific clinical conditions for a specific patient. In addition, as these disorders are heritable, the correct diagnosis assists the care of the patient throughout life and confirms or denies that diagnosis in his or her kindred.

Precise diagnosis depends in part on evidence garnered by the history and physical examination but is confirmed by specific laboratory tests. The history and physical examination justify the practitioner's decision as to which patients should be subjected to further laboratory testing. This chapter is limited to a discussion of von Willebrand's disease and a congenital deficiency of Factor VIII (hemophilia A), Factor IX (hemophilia B), or Factor XI (hemophilia C) (Table 1). Congenital deficiencies of Factor I (fibrinogen), Factor II (prothrombin), Factors V, VII, X, XII, and XIII, and acquired deficiency of any factor, although each just as precise a diagnosis with its specific therapy, are beyond the scope of this review.

Clinical suspicion is key in leading the primary care physician to the correct diagnosis. Table 2 gives clues as to which patients and their clinical manifestations should cause suspicion. Hemorrhagic events are clearly linked to the degree of deficiency in persons lacking Factors VIII or IX. Ironically, the *lack* of hemorrhagic manifestations, absence of joint destruction, and a seemingly negative family history in the milder forms of hemophilia may prove to be dangerous because of the occult nature of this disorder. Lack of clinical suspicion of an underlying heritable coagulation disorder can lead to either an operation, with resultant massive postoperative hemorrhage, or, in an actively hemorrhaging patient, the failure to consider such a

diagnosis. Indeed, in my professional experience, fatal or serious hemorrhage is more common in mild forms than in severe forms. The patient, family, and practitioner are aware of the hemorrhagic potential of the severe types; that of the milder types is rarely suspected. In addition, it appears that the combined frequency of all the milder forms is about the same as that of the severe types, namely, approximately 1:10,000. Factor levels in Factor VIII deficiency and Factor IX deficiency are constant (within the degree of laboratory variability), both in an individual patient over time and in his or her kindred. Accurate diagnosis and all the events that hinge on it depend on the primary care physician's suspicion and confirmation of the diagnosis.

Although the severity of symptoms and the degree of deficiency of either Factor VIII or Factor IX correlate well, such is not the case in Factor XI deficiency. A patient experiencing a slight hemorrhage may have 1 per cent of normal Factor XI levels, whereas another patient having a major postoperative hemorrhage may have 20 per cent of normal activity.

Attempts to correlate clinical manifestations with laboratory parameters in von Willebrand's disease are even more surely doomed to failure. I expect and prepare for the worst in an attempt to deal with this fact. With the exception of those rare patients with homozygous von Willebrand's disease (Type III, Factor VIII levels, and von Willebrand's factor levels 0 to 3 per cent of normal and having very long bleeding times; see Table 3), there is no correlation between hemorrhagic manifestations and laboratory findings. In fact, the consistency of these test results over time in an individual with von Willebrand's disease is poor. Any of these test results may change, even though the hemorrhagic potential may not. The consistency among family members is even poorer. Accordingly, there is no laboratory test or tests that are pathognomonic for

TABLE 1. **Characteristics of Hemophilia and von Willebrand's Disease**

| Disorder | Degree | Activity of Factor* (%) | Prolonged PTT | Prolonged BT | Genetics | Comments |
|---|---|---|---|---|---|---|
| Factor VIII deficiency | Severe | <1 | Always | No | Sex-linked | Lifelong, obvious disease |
| | Moderate | 1–5 | Usually | No | Sex-linked | Bleeding and hemarthrosis with trauma |
| | Mild | 5–25 | Usually | No | Sex-linked | Bleeding usually only with trauma or surgery; disease process often occult |
| Factor IX deficiency | Severe | <1 | Always | No | Sex-linked | Lifelong, obvious disease |
| | Moderate | 1–5 | Usually | No | Sex-linked | Bleeding and hemarthrosis with trauma |
| | Mild | 5–25 | Usually | No | Sex-linked | Bleeding usually only with trauma or surgery; disease process often occult |
| Factor XI deficiency | | 1–70 | Usually | No | Autosomal | Highly variable; often precipitated by surgery or aspirin administration |
| von Willebrand's disease, common variety (Type I) | | 30–70 | Occasionally | Usually | Autosomal | Mucocutaneous bleeding; hemarthrosis rare |

*Activity of the patient's factor compared with normal pooled plasma, which is defined as 100% activity.
*Abbreviations:* PTT = partial thromboplastin time; BT = bleeding time.

TABLE 2. **Clinical Manifestations Helpful for Diagnosis of Hemophilia and von Willebrand's Disease**

**Manifestations of Severe Deficiency of Either Factor VIII or Factor IX**

Positive family history 75% of the time; spontaneous mutation in 25%

Diagnosis established by age 2 yr

Spontaneous hemarthroses: knee, elbow, ankle, wrist, shoulder, hip

Destruction of these joints, resulting in limp or other dysfunction

Family history of bleeding in a sex-linked pattern (e.g., maternal uncles, maternal grandfathers, and male siblings)

Extensive medical history and frequent emergency room visits

Frequent soft tissue hemorrhage; bleeding after circumcision

Extensive bleeding after trauma or surgery

**Manifestations of Moderate Deficiency of Either Factor VIII or Factor IX**

Family history typically negative, except under close scrutiny

Diagnosis may be delayed until second or third decade

Hemarthrosis rare and usually occurs only with trauma; joint deformity rare

Soft tissue hemorrhage frequent

Postoperative bleeding severe; frequently delayed 24–72 hr

Bleeding after dental extractions

**Manifestations of Mild Deficiency of Either Factor VIII or Factor IX**

Family history typically appears negative; disease occult

Diagnosis may be made at any age

Joint disease and joint deformity rare

Hemorrhage after trauma or surgery, usually delayed 24–72 hr

Bleeding after dental extractions, particularly if aspirin prescribed

**Manifestations of Factor XI Deficiency**

50% of patients are of European Jewish extraction

Family history may be positive in an autosomal dominant fashion

Diagnosis may be made at any age

Hemorrhage often follows surgery, dental extractions, or trauma; often precipitated by aspirin administration

**Manifestations of von Willebrand's Disease (Type I)**

Family history usually positive in autosomal dominant fashion (e.g., equal number of males and females and no skipped generations)

Diagnosis may be made at any age

Frequent childhood epistaxis

Bleeding after dental extractions, particularly if aspirin is prescribed

Bleeding after shaving and with minor cuts and abrasions

Serious or fatal bleeding unusual

either the presence or absence of von Willebrand's disease.

Factor VIII serves as a cofactor and Factor IX serves as an enzyme in the coagulation cascade. Deficiency of either results in slow and defective generation of thrombin and, hence, impaired hemostasis. The greater the deficiency, the more severely impaired is coagulation, which can be manifested clinically by hemorrhage and, in the laboratory, by a prolonged partial thromboplastin time (PTT). However, because the PTT is not extremely sensitive to levels of either Factor VIII or Factor IX, and because reagents used in the PTT vary in their ability to detect a partial deficiency of either

of these factors, the PTT should *not* be depended on to exclude hemophilia as a diagnostic possibility: A normal PTT does not exclude mild hemophilia A or B. In addition, the PTT cannot be relied on to follow therapeutic replacement levels of these factors. Rather, specific measurement of plasma levels of these factors is in order for both diagnostic and therapeutic purposes.

## TREATMENT

Treatment principles are based on the fact that if bleeding is caused by the deficiency of a given

TABLE 3. **Types of von Willebrand's Disease**

| Type | Abnormality | Occurrence | Factor VIIIc* | Factor VIII$_{RAg}$† | Bleeding Time | Multimeric Analysis of Factor VIII |
|------|-------------|------------|---------------|---------------------|---------------|-----------------------------------|
| I | Heterozygous deficiency of Factor VIII molecule | Common | 30–70% | 30–70% | 6–20 min | Normal distribution |
| II | Heterozygous abnormality of Factor VIII molecule | Rare | 70–150% | 70–150% | >20 min | Absence of high-molecular-weight forms |
| III | Homozygous deficiency of Factor VIII molecule | Rare | <3% | <3% | >20 min | Absence of all forms |

*Factor VIIIc refers to that part of the Factor VIII molecule involved in blood coagulation.

†Factor VIII$_{RAg}$ (also known as von Willebrand's factor) refers to the part of the Factor VIII molecule measured by immunologic methods.

coagulation factor, replacement of that factor leads to improved or even normal hemostasis. Factor replacement is typically achieved by infusion of plasma products, either cryoprecipitate or Factor VIII concentrate in Factor VIII deficiency; Factor IX concentrate in Factor IX deficiency; fresh-frozen plasma (FFP) in Factor XI deficiency; and cryoprecipitate in von Willebrand's disease. A new product not derived from blood or blood products, 1-deamino-8-D-arginine vasopressin (DDAVP) (Stimate), a vasopressin analogue, is probably the agent of choice in the common type (Type I) of von Willebrand's disease and mild Factor VIII deficiency; it is not efficacious in Type II or Type III von Willebrand's disease, in severe deficiency of Factor VIII, or in any deficiency of either Factor IX or Factor XI.

The *degree of factor replacement* is dictated by the seriousness of the clinical situation. One may not wish to replace totally (i.e., to 100 per cent level of activity) the deficient factor because (1) excessive factor is no more hemostatic than sufficient factor, (2) the cost is excessive, and (3) these products are limited worldwide so their use must be distributed among all patients.

A unit of Factor VIII, IX, or XI is defined as the amount of that factor in 1 ml of normal human plasma. In clinical medicine, I assume that an adult patient has a plasma volume of 3000 ml. If the baseline level of Factor VIII is 0 per cent, infusion of 1500 units of Factor VIII should result in an initial therapeutic level of 50 per cent, whereas infusion of 3000 units would increase the Factor VIII level from 0 per cent to 100 per cent. Because the volume of distribution of Factor VIII appears to be the plasma volume, calculation (which is actually an estimate) of the amount of Factor VIII to be infused is simple. The volume of distribution for Factor IX behaves more like twice the plasma volume, so roughly twice as much Factor IX is needed to achieve a desired level. For instance, 3000 units of Factor IX infused into a patient with 0 per cent Factor IX results in a therapeutic plasma level closer to 50 per cent than to 100 per cent. The volume of distribution of Factor XI is roughly the plasma volume.

The *frequency of infusion* is determined by the half-life of the factor. For Factor VIII, this is approximately 8 to 12 hours, and for Factor IX it is 12 to 24 hours. For Factor XI, the half-life is 60 to 80 hours, long enough that it allows Factor XI levels to accumulate from therapeutically infused FFP. This is fortunate because FFP is the only therapeutic source of Factor XI. Aggressive treatment with FFP is more cumbersome than the infusion of concentrates that are available for replacement of either Factor VIII or Factor IX.

The *duration of infusion* is difficult to determine with certainty. For some events, such as early treatment of a simple hemarthrosis, a single infusion suffices. In contrast, infusion may be needed for 10 to 14 days after a complicated surgical procedure.

Infusion of DDAVP typically doubles or triples the native Factor VIII level in patients with moderate hemophilia; for instance, the Factor VIII level can be raised from 8 per cent to approximately 20 per cent after such infusion. If such levels are thought to be sufficient for the clinical situation, the use of DDAVP is strongly encouraged. DDAVP is administered intravenously, at a dose of 0.3 microgram per kg in 50 ml of saline over 30 minutes every 12 to 24 hours.

These therapeutic guidelines are just that; factor levels, both peak and trough, must be determined by precise factor assay. Based on the results, the dosage, frequency, and duration of therapy can be monitored and modified accordingly.

Therapeutic decisions are less clearly made in von Willebrand's disease, as there is no good correlation between clinical bleeding and either Factor VIII levels or bleeding times, although both usually improve after successful therapy. Most available Factor VIII concentrate, although highly effective in hemophilia A, is not as effective in von Willebrand's disease. Cryoprecipitate is thought to be the superior source of von Willebrand's factor, the absence of which is probably more important than the modest degree of Factor VIII clotting activity seen in the common type (I) of von Willebrand's disease. Usually 5 to 10 bags (1 bag being defined as the cryoprecipitate prepared from 1 unit [300 ml] of FFP) of cryoprecipitate are administered every 8 to 12 hours. DDAVP is efficacious and safe to use in Type I von Willebrand's disease. It is administered as previously described.

Although patients with heritable disorders of coagulation are at risk for bleeding in almost any conceivable fashion, place, or time, certain hemorrhagic events are characteristic of these disorders. These will be addressed separately.

### Hemarthrosis

Bleeding into joint spaces is characteristic of severe classic deficiency of either Factor VIII or Factor IX. It is the most common hemorrhagic event in hemophiliacs. When it occurs spontaneously (or with trauma so minimal that it is not recalled by the patient), deficiency of the factor is usually total. Hemarthrosis is extremely rare in von Willebrand's disease and Factor XI deficiency. The joints most commonly involved include (in descending order) the knee, elbow, ankle, wrist, shoulder, and hip. Other joints bleed far less often. In my experience, ankle bleeds can be almost totally eliminated by the use of boots. Repeated bouts of either untreated or undertreated hemarthroses lead to the joint destruction (hemarthropathy) characteristic of severe hemophilia. Individuals with moderate and mild hemophilia bleed in the joints only after trauma or overusage, such as with jumping or falls.

Because joint bleeds are common, patients become knowledgeable about their nature. They initially perceive bleeding in the joint by a peculiar warm, tingling sensation rather than pain. It is axiomatic that early bleeds can be treated more easily than established bleeds. Accordingly, patients who direct their own care often promptly infuse themselves with factor at home, at the job site, or even in school to stop the joint bleed and to alleviate the progression of pain. This can be done so rapidly and easily that little productive time is lost. Patients have taught me how little factor may be required for hemostasis. If their bleeds are treated promptly, some patients can control a hemarthrosis with as little as 300 to 400 units of factor, which raises their plasma factor level to only 10 per cent. Such infusion obviously is not only less expensive for the patient, society, or both but also makes good medical sense. Factor replacement is the mainstay of therapy for joint bleeds. Splints, joint aspiration, and casts have no place in the modern treatment of acute hemarthrosis. With proper training, the patient can treat the vast majority of hemarthroses without consultation with the physician. The frequency of hemarthrosis varies enormously even within a given patient. Some patients experience spontaneous hemarthrosis twice a week for months for some time and then experience it once every month or so. The reason for this disparity in frequency is unknown.

Most joint bleeds respond to a single infusion of factor sufficient to raise the level to 10 to 20 per cent. The notable exception is hemarthrosis of the hip joint, which is rather rare but does require several days of aggressive replacement therapy.

Chronic joint bleeds lead to joint destruction. Definitive surgical management of chronic hemarthropathy is outside the scope of this review. Occasionally, rather than having a random distribution of joint bleeds, a patient may experience repeated bleeds in a single joint. Synovium in the affected joint may become extremely hypertrophic, inflamed, and boggy. In addition, because of the hypervascularity of the synovium, the bleed may become more frequent, perpetuating a vicious cycle. These joints often respond favorably to surgical synovectomy.

## Soft Tissue Bleeds

These bleeds are the second most common bleeding manifestation and, again, are limited generally to hemophiliacs rather than affecting patients with von Willebrand's disease. Key to the management of soft tissue bleeds is recognition of potential damage from the bleed. For instance, an abdominal or chest wall bleed may be spectacular but is not dangerous to the patient. By contrast, a much smaller bleed in the neck could compromise the airway. Soft tissue bleeds are often initiated by trauma but can be spontaneous. Bleeding often occurs between fascial planes. Three types of soft tissue bleeds require special discussion. The first of these is the *retropharyngeal hematoma,* which can dissect between fascial planes in the retropharyngeal area, with resultant obstruction of the airway. This hemorrhage is rather rare but is important because of its danger. A sore throat or difficulty in breathing in a hemophiliac should raise this possibility. Replacement therapy should be aggressive, with peak levels of 100 per cent and trough levels of 50 per cent maintained for a minimum of 5 to 7 days. Prompt therapy obviates the need for surgical manipulation. The second soft tissue hemorrhage of importance is *other hemorrhages in the mouth and throat area.* These can occur in the tongue, floor of the mouth, or anterior neck. They should be treated as aggressively as retropharyngeal bleeds. The third important soft tissue bleed is the *gastrocnemius bleed,* which is extremely painful, as it dissects between the two heads of the gastrocnemius muscle into the leg as a result of the forces of gravity and pressure. Because of the pain, the patient hyperextends the ankle to shorten the length of the gastrocnemius. If this bleed is not aggressively treated, the muscle deformity becomes chronic and the patient walks on the toes of the affected leg, the classic equine gait. In my experience, the development of equine gait is often the first major orthopedic event in a downhill, domino-type progression of joint disease. Accordingly, gastrocnemius bleeds should be aggressively identified by the painful swelling of the leg and the characteristic posture that the patient assumes. I treat this bleed with peak and trough levels of 80 per cent and 40 per cent, respectively, for at least a week, during which time aggressive physical therapy is provided to allow the patient to walk with the heel flat, bearing the body's full weight.

## Genitourinary Bleeding

Menometrorrhagia, and especially menorrhagia, may occur in patients with bleeding disorders. Because most hemophiliacs are males, excessive menstrual bleeding is unusual in hemophilia except in patients with deficiency of Factor XI. Such symptoms may be bothersome in females with von Willebrand's disease and may, in fact, be a presenting feature leading to a hemostatic diagnosis. Excessive menstrual bleeding often responds to hormonal treatment, such as with birth control pills. Pregnancy ameliorates bleeding in von Willebrand's disease, so routine delivery is rarely a hemostatic problem even without specific therapy.

Spontaneous, nontraumatic urinary bleeding of renal origin is frequently encountered in hemophiliacs and occasionally in patients with von Willebrand's disease. It is almost never associated with structural lesions such as those seen in nonhemophiliacs. Accordingly, exhaustive examinations for neoplastic growths, stones, or abscesses are rarely productive. This is one hemorrhagic episode for which epsilon-aminocaproic acid is contraindicated for fear of causing obstructive uropathy from clotted blood. If hematuria is spontaneous, it may be treated with aggressive factor replacement, although in my experience this rarely shortens the natural history of the event. Often no therapy is just as effective; the bleeding stops in about 1 week.

### Retroperitoneal Hemorrhage

This is a rare but classic hemorrhagic event in hemophiliacs, representing the second leading cause of hemorrhagic death. It is unusual in von Willebrand's disease. This hemorrhage should always be considered in the hemophiliac who is hypotensive and tachycardic and has mild abdominal pain. Because of the almost limitless size of the retroperitoneal area, patients can bleed to death internally before any physical findings direct the unsuspecting clinician to retroperitoneal bleeding. If the diagnosis is entertained, prompt, aggressive replacement therapy should be given, aiming for peak levels of 100 per cent. After full replacement, radiographic examination with either computed tomography or ultrasound establishes the diagnosis. Full replacement therapy for approximately 1 week is in order. Surgical exploration is not indicated.

### Gastrointestinal Bleeding

In contrast to genitourinary bleeding, gastrointestinal bleeding is usually associated with a structural lesion. This bleeding is common in both hemophiliacs and patients with von Willebrand's disease. More often than not, peptic ulcer disease, neoplastic growths, or the like underlie this hemorrhagic manifestation. Replacement

therapy should be given, aiming for peak levels of 50 per cent. During replacement therapy, diagnostic radiography or endoscopic procedures should be performed, as in other patients.

### Epistaxis

Epistaxis is rare in hemophiliacs without trauma but is characteristic of von Willebrand's disease, particularly in the first two decades of life. Epistaxis in patients with von Willebrand's disease can be easily corrected with administration of either cryoprecipitate or DDAVP. Surgical treatment is rarely, if ever, of benefit.

### Central Nervous System Bleeding

This is the rarest of the classic bleeds of hemophilia or von Willebrand's disease but is the leading cause of hemorrhagic death. It may be spontaneous but more often is associated with trauma, including that which appears trivial. At the first suspicion of an ongoing central nervous system hemorrhage, full replacement to 100 per cent factor levels is mandatory before further investigation. After full replacement, radiographic or other investigations to establish the presence or absence of central nervous system bleeding should take place. At no time should these investigations take place before the prompt replacement of 100 per cent factor levels in these patients. The clinician and patient must have a high suspicion of, appreciation of, and respect for central nervous system bleeding.

### Other Special Considerations

**Trauma.** The hemophiliac who has sustained significant trauma should immediately receive total factor replacement. No lesion, whether a fracture or a gunshot wound, or one from an automobile accident, can improve until factor replacement has been done. After factor replacement and other acute resuscitative measures, the patient should be treated like any other trauma patient. The patient is at such high risk for bleeds from multiple sites that replacement should be done based on suspicion alone. The physician must *not* insist on waiting for hemorrhage to become so established that the physical or radiographic examination detects an advanced hemorrhage, which is then far more dangerous and resistant to therapy.

**Surgery.** Modern aggressive replacement therapy for hemophiliacs has enabled these patients to enjoy the full benefits of modern surgery. Far too often in the past, surgical procedures were performed on hemophiliacs too late and too emergently to achieve acceptable results. It is our belief that hemophiliacs or patients with von Willebrand's disease without an inhibitor can undergo any surgical procedure, and the decision to perform these procedures should be based on the same indications or contraindications used in other patients. Patients prepared appropriately before surgery experience no more morbidity and mortality than otherwise normal patients undergoing a similar operation. Surgical hemostasis is perfectly normal with appropriate aggressive control of the underlying disease. Recent consecutive clinical series have demonstrated no excessive morbidity and mortality in hemophiliacs undergoing the full gamut of modern surgical procedures.

**Dental Procedures.** These procedures can be performed in patients with hemophilia or von Willebrand's disease as simply as in other patients. Preventive dentistry and restorative work should be aggressively maintained. Usually, only minimal amounts of factor replacement are necessary, aiming for peak and trough levels of approximately 20 per cent and 10 per cent, respectively. Some authorities have combined this low-level replacement with administration of epsilon-aminocaproic acid; I have found that this adds little more than the variability of another drug. Partial replacement therapy should be continued for 4 or 5 days after the procedure.

**General Medical Care.** As in any chronic condition, the maintenance of optimal health is beneficial. Accordingly, patients should receive good dental care, be kept up-to-date on immunizations, and keep themselves in trim physical condition.

**Safety of Replacement Therapy.** Before the availability of modern replacement therapy, the length and quality of life of the hemophiliac or patient with von Willebrand's disease were severely compromised. Some studies indicated that the average age at death in severe hemophilia was 8 years. Because surgical therapy was im-

TABLE 4. **Impact of Comprehensive Health Care on Hemophiliacs\***

| Outcome Data | Before | After | % Change |
|---|---|---|---|
| Patients performing self-infusion (home care) | 514 | 2517 | +390 |
| Average days/yr lost from work or school | 14.5 | 3.9 | −73 |
| Average hospital admission/yr | 1.9 | 0.22 | −88 |
| Average days/yr spent as inpatient | 9.4 | 1.6 | −83 |
| Percentage of unemployed adults | 36 | 9.4 | −74 |

\*Modified from data from the National Hemophilia Foundation.

possible, patients were also at risk of dying of processes that usually do not lead to death in this century, such as appendicitis or mild trauma. In the second half of this century, with the advent of better diagnostic and therapeutic resources, patients who have a heritable bleeding disorder expect a nearly normal life span. However, confounding factors have recently appeared. The first of these is the unacceptably high incidence of transfusion-associated hepatitis, mostly caused by hepatitis B and non-A, non-B (C) hepatitis. Nearly all multiply transfused patients have a mild, persistent form of liver disease characterized by chronic, stable, but mild elevations of serum transaminase levels. The vast majority do not progress to chronic active hepatitis. About 10 per cent of these patients develop cirrhosis and hepatic failure. More recently, of course, has been the specter of acquired immunodeficiency syndrome (AIDS) associated with administration of contaminated blood product concentrates prepared approximately between 1979 and 1983. The vast majority of patients transfused with these products during that time now test positive for human immunodeficiency virus, and many will develop AIDS, with its attendant prognosis. Safer blood products are now either commercially available or being prepared. Such progress will no doubt brighten the future of hemophiliacs, as will further therapeutic developments for AIDS.

**Comprehensive Care.** The concept of comprehensive care for the patient with a heritable bleeding disorder has had a great positive impact on these patients and their families (Table 4). Health care providers attuned to the hemophiliac's needs are quick to offer prophylactic care and psychosocial support and have become accustomed to easing the socioeconomic burden of the disorder. For instance, health insurance or employment may pose difficulties for a hemophiliac. However, support groups, including lay organizations such as the National Hemophilia Foundation, have proved effective in combating not only the medical aspects of the disease but also its socioeconomic and psychologic impacts on the patient and the family. Health care providers should help patients with heritable bleeding disorders to make contact with such support organizations.

**Inhibitors.** Inhibitors directed against a factor develop in approximately 7 to 10 per cent of patients with hemophilia A and in a smaller number of those with hemophilia B. This dreaded situation makes replacement therapy with factor concentrate either impossible or extremely difficult. Appropriate therapy for this unfortunate situation is beyond the scope of this review. Most such patients should receive expert consultation for further assistance.

# PLATELET-MEDIATED BLEEDING DISORDERS

method of
MARY ELLEN M. RYBAK, M.D., and
PAUL MARCOUX, M.D.
*University of Massachusetts*
*Worcester, Massachusetts*

Platelet-mediated bleeding disorders are potential causes of morbidity and mortality. These hemorrhagic diatheses are commonly due to severe thrombocytopenia, but bleeding may also be secondary to platelet function defects. Thrombocytopenia may be due to decreased platelet production, increased platelet destruction, excessive splenic pooling, or dilution. Qualitative platelet function abnormalities occur in acquired states such as uremia, liver disease, and chronic myeloproliferative disorders; in association with drug administration; and, less frequently, in congenital disorders.

In the evaluation of the patient with a suspected platelet disorder, it is essential to determine the primary etiology of the thrombocytopenia or functional platelet defect so that therapy can be appropriately directed. A thorough history with regard to age of onset, duration and type of bleeding, and hemorrhage with previous surgery or trauma can help distinguish between inherited and acquired platelet disorders and determine the severity of the problem. Patients should be questioned specifically about all medications as well as alcohol and illicit drugs, exposure to toxins and radiation, antecedent illnesses, and symptoms suggestive of an underlying malignancy or connective tissue disease. Patients with thrombocytopenia should be questioned about risk factors for human immunodeficiency virus (HIV) infection. Physical examination may reveal signs suggesting a platelet-mediated bleeding diathesis: petechiae, ecchymoses, epistaxis, gingival bleeding, gastrointestinal bleeding, hematuria, or menometrorrhagia. Lymphadenopathy, hepatosplenomegaly, rashes, or neurologic defects may provide clues to an associated illness. Laboratory examination should include a complete blood count and peripheral blood smear morphology. Bone marrow aspiration and biopsy are generally well tolerated and provide essential diagnostic information in thrombocytopenia. In the case of severe (less than 5000 platelets per µl) thrombocytopenia, bone marrow aspiration alone is initially sufficient.

## TREATMENT

General measures in the management of all patients with platelet disorders include the avoidance of intramuscular injections, rectal temperatures, or invasive procedures unless absolutely necessary. All aspirin and other drugs that inhibit platelet function should be discontinued. Long term, estrogens or progesterone may be necessary to suppress menses in patients with menometrorrhagia. Platelet transfusions (described later) should be given to patients with active bleeding, especially in cases of intracranial hemorrhage or gastrointestinal bleeding. Patients with abnormalities of platelet function with or without thrombocytopenia may require transfusions even at platelet counts generally considered sufficient to prevent spontaneous bleeding.

## Thrombocytopenia Secondary to Decreased Platelet Production

Rarely, thrombocytopenia may be due to congenital syndromes with decreased platelet production such as Fanconi's syndrome, amegakaryocytic thrombocytopenia, Wiskott-Aldrich syndrome, and May-Hegglin anomaly. More often, decreased platelet production is acquired. Drugs such as myelosuppressive chemotherapy and interferons consistently decrease platelet production; other drugs such as thiazide diuretics, estrogenic hormones, and prednisone can occasionally suppress platelet production. Thrombocytopenia is common in chronic alcoholism; this bleeding problem is exacerbated by coexistent cirrhosis, splenomegaly, and malnutrition. Platelet counts usually rise within 3 to 5 days of discontinuing alcohol. Megaloblastic anemia and thrombocytopenia are seen in vitamin $B_{12}$ and folate deficiency; platelet counts normalize within 1 to 2 weeks of vitamin supplementation. Viral infections including measles, varicella, infectious mononucleosis, cytomegalovirus (CMV) infection, and hepatitis may lead to both decreased thrombopoiesis and shortened platelet survival. Thrombocytopenia is usually moderate and self-limited, but bleeding may be disproportionate as a result of secondary functional platelet defects. Marrow replacement by tumor, fibrosis, or leukemia may also cause thrombocytopenia. General supportive measures described earlier should be employed. Platelet transfusions are indicated when the platelet count falls below 20,000 per µl or for invasive procedures if platelets are less than 50,000 per µl.

## Thrombocytopenia Secondary to Decreased Platelet Survival

*Increased platelet destruction* occurs in immune-mediated thrombocytopenia and in non-immune-mediated platelet consumptive disorders. Platelet destruction should be suspected in patients with significant thrombocytopenia and normal to increased numbers of megakaryocytes in the bone marrow. Immune thrombocytopenic purpura (ITP) and drug-induced immune thrombocytopenia are the two most common causes of immunologic destruction of platelets. HIV infection is emerging as a frequent cause of thrombocytopenia. Less common causes include post-transfusion purpura and underlying conditions such as connective tissue disorders, lymphoproliferative disorders, solid tumors (especially ovarian and renal cell carcinoma), and infection. Nonimmune platelet consumption is seen in a number of situations, including thrombotic thrombocytopenic purpura (TTP), disseminated intravascular coagulation (DIC) (discussed elsewhere in this text), and sepsis, and in patients on cardiopulmonary bypass and those receiving massive red blood cell transfusions.

### Immune Thrombocytopenic Purpura (ITP)

*Acute immune thrombocytopenic purpura,* ITP of abrupt onset, occurs most often in children but also occurs in adults, frequently following a viral infection or viral immunization. Spontaneous remissions within 1 to 6 months are seen in 80 to 90% of children but are less common in adults. Because the disease is often self-limited, specific therapy is not always indicated. Restriction of strenuous physical activity and avoidance of platelet inhibitors (e.g., aspirin) decrease the risk of dangerous bleeding. When evidence of active bleeding from the skin, mucosa, or the gastrointestinal or urinary tracts exists, the degree of thrombocytopenia is usually severe (less than 10,000 platelets per μl) and therapy is required. High-dose intravenous gamma globulin (IV-IG) (200 to 400 mg per kg per day for 5 days or a single dose of 1 gram per kg) will improve platelet counts in 80% of patients. IV-IG may alter autoantibody production or produce reticuloendothelial Fc receptor blockade, resulting in decreased platelet destruction. Glucocorticoids (e.g., prednisone, 1 mg per kg per day) are used infrequently in children with acute ITP but are recommended in the treatment of adults. Platelet transfusions may provide temporary protection in cases of active bleeding, especially if given after IV-IG, but should not be routinely administered. Emergency splenectomy is reserved for cases in which life-threatening bleeding continues despite IV-IG, prednisone, and platelet transfusion therapy.

*Chronic ITP* is primarily a disease of adults, with peak incidence between the ages of 20 and 40 years and with females affected three times more often than males; it is a common manifestation of HIV infection. The onset is insidious, and the degree of thrombocytopenia is usually less severe than in acute ITP. In 90 to 95% of patients with chronic ITP, there is evidence of antiplatelet antibodies, usually of the IgG class,

which are frequently directed against specific platelet membrane glycoproteins (e.g., GPIIIa, Ib, or IX). History, physical examination, and laboratory evaluation should exclude diseases associated with immune thrombocytopenia such as systemic lupus erythematosus, lymphoproliferative disorders, and HIV infection before the diagnosis of primary ITP is made.

Treatment of chronic ITP is initiated for bleeding or for platelet counts below 40,000 per μl. Platelet transfusions have a very limited role in the treatment of ITP because of immune destruction of transfused platelets. Glucocorticoids; prednisone, 1 to 2 mg per kg per day; or the equivalent dose of intravenous hydrocortisone or methylprednisolone sodium succinate (Solu-Medrol) is the initial treatment of choice. Platelet counts begin to rise within 7 days in most patients but may not peak for several weeks. Improvement in hemostasis generally occurs within 48 hours of treatment. Delayed responses occur; therefore, therapy should be continued for a minimum of 4 to 6 weeks if partial but inadequate improvement in the platelet count is seen. In rare cases, a dose of 2 mg of prednisone per kg may be necessary to induce remission. Once an adequate and stable platelet count is achieved, prednisone is gradually tapered. Relapses are seen in greater than 75% of patients, necessitating a return to higher maintenance doses. If maintenance therapy is required, the lowest dose of prednisone, ideally every other day, should be used to minimize steroid side effects. For patients with initial platelet counts over 40,000, a short trial of corticosteroids may be given; however, long-term steroids are rarely indicated.

Splenectomy should be considered in patients with chronic ITP who fail to respond to steroids or who require unacceptable prednisone maintenance doses (e.g., greater than 10 mg per day). Emergency splenectomy may be necessary in cases of severe active bleeding when other modalities of therapy in ITP have failed to achieve hemostasis. Pneumococcal and *Haemophilus influenzae* vaccines should be administered 2 to 3 weeks prior to elective splenectomy. Approximately 50 to 80% of patients achieve partial or complete remissions with splenectomy. However, up to 30% of patients responding to splenectomy suffer relapse within 18 months, requiring resumption of glucocorticoid therapy or other agents generally reserved for patients with refractory ITP. As in patients with acute ITP, patients with chronic ITP respond to IV-IG. Prolonged remissions have been achieved, but responses are often transient (2 to 3 weeks). IV-IG may have utility in managing patients with ITP who present with life-threatening hemorrhage, since the platelet count may rise within hours of administration. In addition, transfused platelets may have improved survival after IV-IG administration. Plasmapheresis with or without a *Staphylococcus* protein A column may remove antibodies and is effective in up to 50% of patients with chronic ITP.

Alternate therapeutic modalities include danazol (Danocrine)*, 400 to 800 mg daily, which has been reported to induce remissions in approximately 50% of patients. Cyclophosphamide (Cytoxan)†, 50 to 100 mg daily, or azathioprine (Imuran)‡ when combined with prednisone therapy produces favorable responses in 30 to 40% of patients with refractory ITP but have potentially serious side effects. Intravenous vinblastine§ (10 mg) or vincristine (2 mg)‖ may transiently improve the platelet count, but these agents are limited by myelosuppression and neurotoxicity, respectively. Colchicine and alpha interferon have limited efficacy but have also been used.

### Drug-Induced Immune Thrombocytopenia

A large number of medications cause immunologic destruction of platelets by immune-complex formation or direct drug interaction with the platelet membrane. The most frequently implicated drugs include quinidine and other antiarrhythmics, quinine, sulfonamide derivatives, gold salts, and heparin. Mucocutaneous bleeding and thrombocytopenia may develop within 24 hours of exposure to the offending agent. Drug-dependent antibody can be detected by in vitro assays with normal platelets, patient serum, and suspected drug. In vivo challenge with a drug suspected of causing immune thrombocytopenia is very dangerous and should only be considered if the drug is irreplaceable and deemed absolutely essential. Treatment consists of immediate discontinuation of the drug. Transfused platelets are quickly destroyed and are used only for active hemorrhage. Corticosteroids do not improve the rate of recovery but may ameliorate bleeding, owing to their effects on the microvasculature.

Heparin induces thrombocytopenia by two different mechanisms. Mild transient nonimmune thrombocytopenia occurs within a few days of initiating heparin in 15 to 30% of patients. Less commonly, heparin-induced platelet antibodies cause thrombocytopenia within 5 to 14 days of initiating heparin therapy. In approximately 10% of cases, heparin-antibody complexes may cause platelet aggregation leading to thromboembolic arterial occlusions. In immune heparin thrombocytopenia, immediate discontinuation of heparin therapy is mandated. Dextran and pneumatic boots may be used when continued anticoagulation or deep venous thromboses prophylaxis is desired until full anticoagulation with warfarin (Coumadin) is achieved.

### Post-transfusion Purpura (PTP)

PTP is a rare disorder in which patients develop an abrupt and profound thrombocytopenia and bleeding 5 to 12 days after a blood transfusion containing platelets. Most afflicted patients are females with a history of pregnancy or patients with prior transfusions. Most of those patients lack the $PLA_1$ platelet antigen, which is present on GPIIIa in 97% of the general population. Upon exposure to the $PLA_1$ antigen by transfusion or pregnancy, these patients develop anti-$PLA_1$ antibodies. Upon repeat exposure, both transfused and autologous platelets are destroyed.

Plasma exchange is the most effective therapy available. In most instances, hemorrhagic symptoms subside and platelet levels rise significantly within 1 to 5 days following one to four plasma exchanges of 5 to 10 units of plasma per exchange. When plasmapheresis is unavailable or not successful, intravenous gamma globulin, 400 mg per kg for 2 to 5 days, may be efficacious.

### Thrombocytopenia Secondary to Increased Platelet Consumption: Thrombotic Thrombocytopenic Purpura (TTP)

TTP is characterized by the pentad of consumptive thrombocytopenia, microangiopathic hemolytic anemia, fluctuating neurologic deficits, fever, and renal dysfunction. Generalized mucocutaneous bleeding is common, and the thrombocytopenia is often severe. The manifestations of this syndrome are caused by deposition of platelet microthrombi in the microvasculature. Idiopathic TTP, comprising 90% of cases, may have an acute, relapsing, or chronic course and is rarely familial. TTP may also occur in association with a variety of conditions, including connective tissue disorders, pregnancy, drug exposure, infections, and malignancies. Although the exact pathogenic mechanisms leading to microthrombi formation are unknown, endothelial damage with decreased $PGI_2$ production and release of large von Willebrand's factor (VWF) multimers that interact with a circulating platelet aggregatory factor and altered fibrinolysis may be involved.

TTP is 90% fatal without treatment. Intensive

---

*This use of danazol is not listed in the manufacturer's official directive.

†This use of cyclophosphamide is not listed in the manufacturer's official directive.

‡This use of azathioprine is not listed in the manufacturer's official directive.

§This use of vinblastine is not listed in the manufacturer's official directive.

‖This use of vincristine is not listed in the manufacturer's official directive.

plasma exchange of at least one to two plasma volumes with fresh-frozen plasma is the initial treatment of choice and should be initiated immediately. Favorable responses are seen in 70 to 90% of cases. If plasma exchange is unavailable or delayed, infusions of fresh-frozen plasma, 6 to 8 units daily, can be given with approximately 60 to 70% of patients showing improvement in symptoms and elevations of platelet counts within several days of therapy. TTP is discussed in detail elsewhere in the text.

### Thrombocytopenia Secondary to Dilution and Loss

Patients receiving massive blood transfusions may develop multiple defects in hemostasis. Patients receiving 12 to 20 units of blood have decreases in the platelet count to approximately 100,000 per μl. In addition, most cases of massive transfusion are associated with trauma or surgical complications and platelets are consumed at sites of injury. Prophylactic transfusion of platelets following massive transfusions may not reduce further blood loss but is still generally recommended when platelet counts fall below 60,000 to 80,000 per μl or when evidence of microvascular hemorrhage exists.

### Qualitative Disorders of Platelet Function

Qualitative platelet disorders should be suspected in patients with a history of mucocutaneous hemorrhage, elevated bleeding time, and normal or mildly reduced platelet counts. The rare congenital disorders of platelet function involve platelet membrane defects: Bernard-Soulier syndrome, Glanzmann's thrombasthenia; storage pool deficiencies; and defects in thromboxane synthesis. Acquired disorders are more common and occur in uremia, myeloproliferative disorders, dysproteinemias, and liver disease and with administration of a number of drugs.

**Uremia.** Bleeding is a common complication of uremia and is related to multiple platelet defects. The bleeding time is the best diagnostic test to assess bleeding tendency. There is no direct correlation between prolongation of the bleeding time and serum creatinine concentration. Dialysis may partially correct the bleeding diathesis but does not always correct in vitro platelet dysfunction. Administration of desmopressin* (DDAVP) (0.3 μg per kg intravenously) shortens the bleeding time for up to 8 hours and may prevent bleeding after invasive procedures. DDAVP causes the release of high-molecular-weight VWF from endothelial cells, but this re-

lease may not be entirely responsible for the improvement of hemostasis. Cryoprecipitate, 10 to 12 units intravenously, also temporarily reduces bleeding times and clinical bleeding. Transfusion of red cells to a hematocrit above 30% shortens the bleeding time. Conjugated estrogens (Premarin)* given as intravenous infusions of 0.6 mg per kg for 5 days† shorten bleeding times, with maximum effects at 5 to 7 days and benefit for 14 days.

**Drugs.** The possible exposure to antiplatelet drugs must be considered in any patient with abnormal bleeding and evidence of a qualitative platelet defect. The most commonly implicated drugs include aspirin and other nonsteroidal anti-inflammatory agents; high doses of penicillins and other antimicrobials, phosphodiesterase inhibitors, adenylate cyclase activators, tricyclic antidepressants, phenothiazines, and some sympathetic blocking agents also cause platelet dysfunction. In all cases, the offending drug should be discontinued if bleeding occurs.

**Other Platelet Defects.** Qualitative platelet defects have been recognized in association with *myeloproliferative disorders,* including essential thrombocythemia, polycythemia vera, and chronic myelogenous leukemia. Platelet defects vary, as does the incidence of clinical bleeding and thromboembolic complications. Platelet dysfunction and the bleeding tendency can be corrected by myelosuppressive therapy in some patients. Occasionally, platelet transfusions are necessary at times of active bleeding. Antiplatelet drugs should be avoided except in syndromes of microvascular arterial thrombosis.

Platelet defects occur commonly in *dysproteinemias* and are related to the concentration of the paraprotein. Plasmapheresis with removal of the paraprotein is effective in managing patients with acute hemorrhagic episodes. Chronic bleeding can usually be controlled by chemotherapy of the primary disease.

Patients with *chronic liver disease* often have a bleeding diathesis related to multiple defects including deficiencies in coagulation factors, increased fibrinolysis, low-grade DIC, and variable qualitative platelet defects. At times of active bleeding, platelet transfusions are generally considered, with fresh-frozen plasma and DDAVP, as described earlier.

*Cardiopulmonary bypass* is associated with both qualitative and quantitative platelet defects. Platelet transfusion and/or DDAVP may be given for bleeding and platelet counts less than 50,000

---

*This use of desmopressin is not listed in the manufacturer's official directive.

*This use of conjugated estrogens is not listed in the manufacturer's official directive.
†Exceeds dosage recommended by the manufacturer.

per μl, although the efficacy of DDAVP in this situation is controversial.

### Platelet Transfusion Therapy

The objective of platelet transfusion therapy is to restore sufficient numbers of platelets to stop or prevent bleeding in patients with thrombocytopenia or functional platelet defects. In general, platelet transfusions are indicated in all patients with thrombocytopenia or functional platelet defects or both who have active bleeding. When thrombocytopenia is the only abnormality, a platelet count of greater than 50,000 platelets per μl is adequate for hemostasis. Improvements in hemostasis may occur below this level, but transfusion is unlikely to be of added benefit once platelet counts are greater than 50,000 per μl. If a disorder of platelet function exists, the bleeding time may be useful in determining when platelet transfusion would be beneficial. A bleeding time less than twice the upper limits of normal is generally not considered an indication for platelet transfusion unless other conditions are interfering with hemostasis or a surgical procedure is contemplated.

The indications for the prophylactic administration of platelets are more controversial. Generally, platelets are transfused prophylactically when counts fall below 20,000 platelets per μl because spontaneous hemorrhage is more likely to occur below this level. Prophylactic transfusions at platelet levels less than 20,000 per μl are recommended in patients with temporary thrombocytopenia related to myelosuppressive therapy. Patients with chronic thrombocytopenia may tolerate platelet counts below this level if their clinical course is closely monitored. The risk of bleeding increases when there are precipitous declines in the platelet count. Platelets are generally administered prior to surgery or invasive procedures when platelet counts are less than 50,000 per μl or when functional platelet defects are documented. Thrombocytopenia, per se, resulting from immune destruction of platelets, massive blood transfusion, splenic pooling, or cardiopulmonary bypass is not considered an indication to transfuse platelets unless there is evidence of clinical bleeding.

Several different types of platelet products are available. Platelets are separated from whole blood donation then pooled into therapeutic concentrates. Single-donor platelets are obtained by plateletapheresis with the number of platelets harvested per apheresis equal to the number of platelets from 5 to 10 units of blood. Single-donor platelets are obtained from either random or HLA-matched donors. Pooled-donor platelets are currently recommended initially for most recipients. The usual therapeutic dose is 1 unit per 10 kg body weight, infused over 10 to 20 minutes, which ideally raises the platelet count 6000 per μl per unit. Acetaminophen, 650 mg, and diphenhydramine (Benadryl), 25 to 50 mg, orally administered one-half hour prior to transfusion may lessen the minor pyogenic reactions during platelet infusion.

Single-donor platelets should be reserved for those patients who are alloimmunized to platelet antigens. Alloimmunization should be suspected when platelet counts measured 1 hour post transfusion fail to show the expected rise. Owing to the difficulty and cost involved in obtaining HLA-matched single-donor platelets, nonmatched single-donor platelets are used initially. About 50 to 75% of patients refractory to random single-donor platelets will have beneficial responses to HLA-matched transfusions. ABO compatibility is not usually important between platelet donor and recipient. Platelet cross-matching techniques, other than HLA typing, are currently investigational but hold promise for use in the near future. Rh immunization by red cells contained in platelet concentrates is possible, and Rh-positive products should be avoided in Rh-negative recipients or at least followed by Rh immunoglobulin (RhoGAM) (300 μg intramuscularly). UV irradiation of platelets prior to administration may decrease alloimmunization; x-irradiation of platelets may be necessary to prevent graft-versus-host disease in severely immunosuppressed recipients.

Patients receiving platelet transfusions are at risk of contracting blood infections—most importantly hepatitis, HIV, and CMV despite stringent screening techniques—and very rarely bacterial infections. The benefits of platelet transfusion therapy should clearly outweigh the risks of alloimmunization and infection before transfusion is considered.

# DISSEMINATED INTRAVASCULAR COAGULATION

method of
STEVEN W. ANDRESEN, D.O., and
RONALD M. BUKOWSKI, M.D.
*Cleveland Clinic Foundation*
*Cleveland, Ohio*

Disseminated intravascular coagulation (DIC) is an often fulminant, potentially catastrophic coagulopathy associated with a multitude of primary medical or surgical illnesses. Conditions associated with DIC include obstetric complications, such as abruptio placentae, amniotic fluid embolism, and retained dead fetus syndrome. Sepsis related to either a bacterial or a viral etiology may also produce this entity. Malignancy, liver disease, burns or other causes of tissue injury, vascular disorders such as Kasabach-Merritt syndrome, intravascular hemolysis, connective tissue diseases, and prosthetic devices such as the intra-aortic balloon pump may all be associated with the development of DIC.

Whatever the precipitating cause, when coagulation mechanisms are activated, intravascular fibrin is produced, microvascular thrombosis occurs, and ischemic end-organ damage results. With the continued consumption of coagulation factors and platelets and the development of secondary fibrinolysis, a hemorrhagic diathesis may result.

The most common causes of DIC likely produce endothelial cell damage with subsequent activation of Factor XII, release of platelet factor 3, and/or the production and release of tissue thromboplastin.

Clinical findings in patients with DIC are most commonly related to the underlying disorder. Hemorrhagic or thrombotic manifestations lead to the consideration of the diagnosis of DIC. Most patients with acute, severe DIC bleed from several unrelated sites. Although bleeding from a surgical wound is common, this in concert with bleeding from venipuncture sites, gastrointestinal or pulmonary bleeding, and/or petechiae and purpura is the hallmark of the condition. In addition to hemorrhage, ischemic injury to lung, kidney, and heart may occur from microvascular thrombosis.

In the appropriate clinical setting, when signs of DIC are present, laboratory confirmation is needed. The prothrombin time (PT) and activated partial thromboplastin time (APTT) are usually prolonged. These test systems are prolonged by fibrinogen levels that are less than 100 mg per dl. In addition, fibrinogen degradation products (FDP) inhibit fibrin monomer polymerization, which may also prolong the tests. However, abnormalities of the PT and APTT are not universal and normal times do not exclude the diagnosis of DIC. The thrombin time is also prolonged by the presence of hypofibrinogenemia and FDP. Hypofibrinogenemia is commonly present in acute DIC. Although fibrinogen is an acute phase reactant and may be elevated secondary to the primary disease, in DIC associated with hemorrhage, one would expect it to be decreased. Platelets are also consumed in the production of intravascular thrombi, and significant thrombocytopenia is usually present. Platelet functional abnormalities also exist, which may result from the coating of platelet surfaces with FDP. If the fibrinogen level is depressed, evidence for activation of thrombin and plasmin should be sought. Plasmin digests fibrinogen and fibrin into degradation products. Tests for degradation products are straightforward and when their presence is detected indicate that plasmin has been present. Evidence for the activation of thrombin is the fibrin monomer, which may be assayed with the protamine sulfate test. However, false-negative results with this test system are frequent.

A recent development from the coagulation laboratory is the D-dimer assay. This is a direct approach for determining the presence of both thrombin and plasmin. When thrombin forms fibrin, which is subsequently degraded by plasmin, previously fused regions known as the D-dimer are released. Monoclonal antibodies that react to this area and do not cross-react with fibrinogen or FDP have been produced. This assay is very helpful in the laboratory evaluation of DIC and is a simple test to perform.

Many of the activated coagulation factors generated during the process of DIC are irreversibly complexed to antithrombin III. This results in a significant decrease of functional antithrombin III levels. In some hands, a correlation exists between antithrombin III levels and the severity of DIC. In addition, antithrombin III levels may be useful in monitoring anticoagulant therapy in DIC.

A distinct entity known as chronic DIC exists. In this disorder, there is increased production and decreased survival of platelets, fibrinogen, and coagulation factors. However, a "compensated" state may exist with the usual laboratory parameters being near normal. In this disorder, thrombotic manifestations may predominate; however, bleeding is also seen. A chronic or compensated DIC may be unmasked by any additional stress such as a surgical procedure that causes further consumption of fibrinogen and coagulation factors with resultant serious hemorrhage.

## TREATMENT

The treatment of DIC revolves around the correction of the precipitating pathologic process. Interventions designed to interrupt the coagulopathy are only temporizing measures until the underlying disease process can be corrected. For example, the evacuation of the uterus in the setting of an obstetric complication and aggressive antibiotic therapy in the case of septicemia are the pivotal points of treatment. Careful attention to the patients' cardiopulmonary and acid-base status are not only necessary for their overall well-being, but are also helpful in potentially diminishing the ongoing coagulopathy.

In patients who have a rapidly reversible underlying process, attention to this and, if hemorrhage is present, transfusion of fresh-frozen plasma as a source of coagulation factors, cryoprecipitate as a source of fibrinogen and Factor VIII complex, and platelets may be used as necessary to control bleeding. If the precipitating process is not readily controllable and/or bleeding continues after the initiation of therapy, anticoagulation is indicated. Heparin may be given at a dosage of 80 U per kg every 4 to 6 hours subcutaneously or at a dosage of 20,000 to 30,000 U over a 24-hour period by continuous intravenous infusion. Either route is capable of controlling DIC. The goal of therapy is the cessation of clinical bleeding and from a laboratory standpoint the attainment of a fibrinogen level above 100 to 150 mg per dl. Contraindications to the use of heparin in this situation include central nervous system lesions or severe thrombocytopenia. In addition, some groups have used the measurement of antithrombin III levels as a guide to the efficacy of therapy. In fact, on an experimental basis, infusions of concentrates of antithrombin III have been helpful in the treatment of DIC. If hemorrhage persists and anticoagulant therapy has been successful in interrupting DIC as demonstrated by an increasing fibrinogen and/or antithrombin III level, specific component therapy with fresh-frozen plasma and/or cryoprecipitate may be considered. It may be hazardous to infuse clotting factors if ongoing consumption is present.

As noted earlier, secondary fibrinolysis is a physiologic mechanism attempting to deal with the ongoing deposition of intravascular fibrin. Rarely, this secondary fibrinolysis continues despite the therapy of the initial inciting event and successful anticoagulation. In this setting, therapy with aminocaproic acid (Amicar) may be considered at a dose of 0.5 to 1.0 gram per hour as a 24-hour continuous infusion. Aminocaproic acid should not be used unless the DIC has been interrupted with successful anticoagulant therapy (i.e., heparin), in that blockade of fibrinolysis may aggravate an ongoing thrombotic process.

Patients with chronic or compensated DIC rarely present with a hemorrhagic diathesis. More commonly, thrombotic events predominate. In the chronic DIC associated with malignancy and multiple thrombotic events, the response to oral anticoagulation with sodium warfarin (Coumadin) derivatives is poor. Thus, should anticoagulation be needed, chronic administration of heparin is more useful. It should be remembered, however, that a "compensated" chronic DIC may be unmasked with an additional stress such as an operation with clinical hemorrhage resulting.

# THROMBOTIC THROMBOCYTOPENIC PURPURA

method of
STEVEN W. ANDRESEN, D.O., and
RONALD M. BUKOWSKI, M.D.
*Cleveland Clinic Foundation*
*Cleveland, Ohio*

Thrombotic thrombocytopenic purpura (TTP) is a rare, potentially fulminant, multisystem disorder produced by microvascular thrombotic events. It is best considered under the broader category of thrombotic microangiopathies, which in addition to TTP include the hemolytic uremic syndrome and the eclampsia–pre-eclampsia syndrome.

The characteristic presentation of patients with TTP consists of the clinical triad of microangiopathic hemolytic anemia, thrombocytopenia, and fluctuating neurologic signs and symptoms. Renal disease and fever complete the classic pentad. Other common findings include constitutional symptoms, nausea and vomiting, abdominal pain, and arthralgias. Neurologic manifestations include altered mental status, confusion, headache, aphasia, seizures, and coma. Motor and sensory deficits may be evanescent.

The anemia is microangiopathic in nature and thus associated with schistocytosis, elevated lactate dehydrogenase (LD), indirect bilirubin, and reticulocyte count. The direct Coombs' test is negative. The degree to which LD is elevated is an excellent indicator of the severity of hemolysis.

Thrombocytopenia is often severe and is thought to be secondary to platelet agglutination. Bleeding complications such as purpura and oropharyngeal, pulmonary, gastrointestinal, retinal, and cerebral hemorrhage may occur. Mild abnormalities in renal function tests, hematuria, and/or proteinuria are the usual renal manifestations. The etiology of the frequently seen fever is uncertain. In the absence of a secondary problem such as sepsis or respiratory failure, biochemical evidence of disseminated intravascular coagulation is not seen. Heart failure or arrhythmias may be present and are associated with the same underlying process that produces the various other manifestations of the disease.

The characteristic pathologic finding is hyaline thrombi partially obstructing blood flow in the microvasculature. These intraluminal thrombi are composed of platelet aggregates and fibrin. Endothelial cell hyperplasia is often also detected, depending on the age of the lesion. Thrombi are widespread and involve virtually all organ systems. This process and the resultant ischemia that it produces are responsible for the clinical manifestations of the disease.

The etiology and pathogenesis of these vascular lesions remain unclear. Most authorities agree that platelet agglutination plays a dominant role in this process. Whether this process results from a primary platelet problem or as a result of perturbation of endothelial cell function remains an area of intense interest. Plasma from patients with TTP has been demonstrated to show an increase in platelet aggregating activity. This may be secondary to a specific agent termed platelet activating factor (PAF). In addition, unusually large Factor VIII:vWF multimers have been described in patients with chronic relapsing TTP. It is possible that these abnormal Factor VIII:vWF multimers also participate in platelet agglutination. Potentially, the underlying etiology of the process is an absent plasma inhibitor to either or both of these factors.

The differential diagnosis of TTP includes other thrombotic microangiopathies such as the hemolytic uremic syndrome, the vasculitides, disseminated intravascular coagulation, and critically ill patients with sepsis or disseminated malignancy. In TTP the neurologic symptoms predominate, whereas in the hemolytic uremic syndrome renal manifestations are the major problem. In TTP uncomplicated by a secondary process, there should not be evidence of disseminated intravascular coagulation. Distinguishing between TTP and a severe vasculitis may be difficult.

Historical reports have documented a mortality rate in this disease of approximately 80%. In recent years survival has improved to approximately 60%, likely as a result of better supportive care; increasing clinician awareness of the disease, which has resulted in earlier diagnosis; and improvement in therapeutic approaches to the disorder, best exemplified by plasma exchange.

## TREATMENT

Considerable data exist that once the diagnosis is made, prompt institution of plasma exchange by plasmapheresis may be lifesaving. Therapy should be instituted despite the severity of the symptoms and the overall status of the patient. Generally, 2- to 4-liter exchanges are undertaken and replacement must be with fresh-frozen plasma. This is continued daily until significant improvement has been achieved or the patient expires. If pheresis is not immediately available, infusion of fresh-frozen plasma at 30 to 50 ml per kg daily should be started until pheresis becomes available. There is information that suggests that the use of vincristine with plasmapheresis may increase response rates and subsequent survival. This concept is under study at present. Some authorities recommend the institution of therapy with corticosteroids and/or antiplatelet agents, yet this remains controversial. If steroids are used, the administration of methylprednisolone at 1 mg per kg intravenously daily is acceptable. The goal of therapy is normalization of the neurologic signs and symptoms and LD levels, and the achievement of a platelet count greater than 100,000. If the patient does not respond to exchange within 3 to 5 days, other options should be investigated. If vincristine (Oncovin) has not been used initially, 1 mg may be given intravenously every 4 to 5 days for approximately four doses. Recent evidence suggests that infusion of high doses of immunoglobulins may produce responses in TTP. As is the case with infusion of fresh-frozen plasma, this may be helpful by supplying normal immunoglobulin inhibitors to PAF and/or Factor VIII:vWF. Other options include the use of antiplatelet agents such as aspirin, dipyridamole (Persantine), or dextran; splenectomy; infusion of cryosupernatant; infusion of prostacyclin; and immunosuppression. When alternative therapeutic measures are considered, they should be used in addition to rather than in place of continued plasmapheresis.

Aggressive cardiopulmonary supportive care is often needed, as are red cell transfusions. Platelet transfusions should be avoided because they in-deed may aggravate the underlying pathologic process.

As more patients survive the initial episode of TTP, a distinct entity known as chronic relapsing TTP has been described. Hematologic aberrations predominate in this entity rather than those of neurologic or renal disease. The therapeutic approaches to these relapses remain the same as for those of the initial episodes. In addition, prophylactic measures such as plasma infusion may be needed to prevent future relapses. Monitoring of the very large Factor VIII:vWF multimers may be useful in following patients with the chronic relapsing variety. In those patients responding to therapy, careful follow-up is needed in order that relapse may be detected early.

# HEMOCHROMATOSIS

method of
MARK L. BASSETT, M.D.
*Australian National University*
*Canberra, Australia*

The term "hemochromatosis" refers to iron overload of parenchymal cells of the liver and other organs. Idiopathic, hereditary, or genetic hemochromatosis (GH) refers to the autosomal recessive disorder in which there is a lifelong increase in iron absorption of unknown cause, leading eventually to iron-induced damage to tissues. In time, this results in cirrhosis, cardiac failure, diabetes, pituitary dysfunction, hypogonadism, and arthritis. In secondary hemochromatosis there is also iron overload of parenchymal cells (e.g., hepatocytes), usually secondary to increased iron absorption from hemolytic anemias associated with ineffective erythropoiesis (e.g., thalassemia major). Some authorities distinguish the latter disorder from transfusional siderosis in which iron is deposited predominantly in phagocytic cells. However, there is considerable overlap because many patients with hemolytic disorders have excess iron stores from both increased absorption and blood transfusions, and with time, there is redistribution of iron. In practice, one can regard excess iron as potentially toxic, regardless of the type of cell in which the iron is deposited.

### DIAGNOSIS OF IRON OVERLOAD

The diagnostic tests for increased body iron stores are the same regardless of the cause of iron overload. Simple tests can be used to detect the presence of increased iron stores whereas more sophisticated tests are required to quantitate the magnitude of iron overload. Measurement of the serum iron concentration alone is unsatisfactory; however, the ratio of the serum iron to the iron-binding capacity (per cent saturation of transferrin) reliably indicates the presence of iron overload, especially when screening young asympto-

## TABLE 1. Diagnosis of Hemochromatosis

**Screening Tests**
Transferrin saturation greater than 55%
Serum ferritin greater than age-related normal range
Urinary iron excretion greater than 2 mg/24 hr following
  0.5-gram deferoxamine IM

**Tests to Confirm Iron Overload**
Liver biopsy—Perls' stain for iron
Liver biopsy—iron quantitation by chemical assay
Hepatic density by computed tomography (less reliable)

matic family members for GH (Table 1). The serum ferritin concentration is also a useful test and correlates better with the level of body iron stores than either the serum iron concentration or transferrin saturation. However, it is affected by other factors such as inflammation, malignancy, and hepatic necrosis, resulting in elevated levels out of proportion to body iron stores. It is less sensitive than the transferrin saturation in screening for GH, even when an age-related normal range is used. Iron overload can also be assessed by measurement of urinary iron excretion following injection with deferoxamine, although this technique is cumbersome.

Confirmation of increased body iron requires a tissue biopsy, usually liver biopsy, with staining for iron (Perls' Prussian blue stain) and preferably chemical quantitation of iron. In some patients liver biopsy may not be possible (e.g., because of an uncorrectable coagulation disorder), and an alternative method is to quantitate the degree of hepatic iron overload by computed tomography (CT), although this method lacks sensitivity at marginally elevated iron levels. Bone marrow quantitation of iron is not helpful in assessing the degree of iron overload. An additional useful method of diagnosing GH is demonstration of HLA-association. The gene coding for GH is linked to the human leucocyte antigen (HLA) system. Once the diagnosis is firmly established in one family member, the HLA status of that person can be compared with that of the siblings. Subjects with GH will almost always have two HLA haplotypes in common (homozygotes), whereas heterozygotes will have only one HLA haplotype in common.

## GENETIC HEMOCHROMATOSIS

This disorder often presents insidiously with lethargy, skin pigmentation, and weight loss. Many patients are asymptomatic or have mild symptoms. Physical findings may be few (e.g., hepatomegaly, skin pigmentation). Relatives of the proband frequently have no physical findings, but it is just as important to make the correct diagnosis and commence treatment. Without treatment, most patients with GH will accumulate excessive amounts of iron, although in women and in some male patients this may not reach toxic levels until later in life. With treatment, patients usually feel more energetic, appetite and weight improve, skin pigmentation lessens, liver and cardiac function improve, and

insulin requirements may diminish if the patient has diabetes. Despite iron removal, patients who have cirrhosis have a high risk (about 20 to 30%) of hepatocellular carcinoma at some stage in their lives. This complication does not occur (or is exceedingly rare) in precirrhotic patients who are iron depleted.

### Treatment

The aim of treatment is to remove excess body iron by repeated phlebotomies (Table 2). Because 500 ml of blood contains approximately 250 mg of iron, about 1 gram of iron can be removed per month by weekly phlebotomies. Patients with advanced GH may have 20 to 40 grams of excess iron, whereas young asymptomatic patients usually have excess body iron stores in the 5- to 10-gram range (normal less than 1.5 grams).

Patients usually tolerate weekly phlebotomies of 450 to 500 ml well, although patients in the older age group should have a smaller volume removed (e.g., 350 ml). In very severe iron overload two phlebotomies per week are recommended. It is important for patients to rest for a few minutes following the procedure and to keep firm pressure on the venipuncture site for 5 minutes. Patients often notice tiredness for 24 hours following the phlebotomy, followed by a feeling of increased well-being. This is not related to iron removal but probably is due to increased erythropoiesis. The hemoglobin concentration should be determined prior to each phlebotomy. In some patients it falls in the first few weeks until the rate of erythropoiesis stabilizes at a higher level. Such patients may require temporary suspension of phlebotomy as well as folate therapy. A small proportion of patients with GH will not tolerate phlebotomy therapy, for instance, those with cardiac failure or difficult venous access. In these patients, chelation therapy should be considered (see below).

### Monitoring Treatment

Removal of excess body iron by phlebotomy is best monitored by measurement of the serum

## TABLE 2. Treatment of Hemochromatosis

**Initial Treatment**
Weekly phlebotomy (400–500 ml)
Monitor hemoglobin concentration and serum ferritin concentration
Continue treatment until serum ferritin is in the low-normal range
Treat complications of the disease (e.g., diabetes)

**Maintenance Treatment**
One phlebotomy every 3–4 months
Maintain serum ferritin in the low-normal range

ferritin concentration. In the early stages of treatment there may be wide fluctuations, but these usually settle and the serum ferritin gradually falls with each treatment. The aim is to remove all excess iron, reducing the serum ferritin to the low normal range. There is no logic in making the patient iron deficient. In some patients (e.g., in whom the serum ferritin concentration is elevated due to arthritis or other inflammatory disease), it may be necessary to perform a repeat liver biopsy to establish that all excess iron has been removed.

### Maintenance Therapy

Once body iron stores have been reduced to normal (or low normal), weekly phlebotomies can be discontinued and replaced by one phlebotomy every 3 or 4 months. The precise frequency varies, and in the individual patient this can only be determined by monitoring the serum ferritin concentration over the course of several years. There is no role for a low iron diet in the management of GH since iron is ubiquitous in food. However, patients should avoid iron-containing medications such as vitamin preparations. Pharmacologic doses of ascorbic acid (vitamin C) should be avoided since this increases the level of iron absorption and promotes iron toxicity.

### SECONDARY IRON OVERLOAD

Iron overload may occur secondary to increased erythropoiesis (e.g., chronic hemolytic anemias such as thalassemia major), repeated blood transfusions, oral and parenteral iron therapy, and (in a milder form) in liver disease, especially alcoholic cirrhosis. The latter disorder is known as alcoholic siderosis and is distinguished from GH by the relatively low levels of excess iron and the presence of histologic features of alcoholic liver disease. In practice, measurement of the hepatic iron concentration (HIC) on a liver biopsy specimen is the most reliable method for distinguishing this disorder from GH. If the ratio of HIC (in μM per gram dry weight) to age of the patient is greater than 2.0, this is strong evidence in support of GH, whereas normal subjects and patients with alcoholic siderosis have HIC to age ratios of less than 2.0. This ratio reflects the fact that iron stores increase progressively with age in GH.

### Treatment

For obvious reasons, chronic anemia prohibits phlebotomy as a treatment modality. Chelation therapy using deferoxamine (DFO) (Desferal) is currently the most widely used treatment, al-though there are newer chelation agents undergoing clinical trials. The disadvantage of DFO is that it is expensive and requires parenteral administration; newer agents (e.g., 1,2-dimethyl-3-hydroxypyrid-4-one) under investigation are effective with oral administration.

Treatment of secondary iron overload should commence before there is evidence of grossly increased iron stores and tissue damage. DFO can be administered by intravenous or subcutaneous infusion. The latter is more convenient, since it requires an infusion pump rather than long-term placement of an indwelling intravenous catheter. Intravenous infusion should not exceed 10 mg per kg per hour. Subcutaneous infusion of approximately 2 grams of DFO per 24 hours results in a urine iron output of 30 mg or more. Urinary iron excretion on DFO should be measured and compared with estimated iron intake (blood transfusions and diet) to confirm that negative iron balance is achieved.

Side effects of DFO are occasionally a problem, but the benefits of iron removal usually outweigh the risks. The most common problem with subcutaneous DFO is the development of local pain and erythema at the injection site. The site of needle insertion should be rotated, and if the problem persists, hydrocortisone cream may be applied to the skin following the injection. Anaphylaxis or urticarial reactions from DFO are rare. There is concern about possible long-term toxicity to the optic and otic nerves, and patients on long-term treatment should have regular auditory and visual examinations. Ascorbic acid may be administered to boost iron excretion in patients who achieve only marginal negative iron balance on DFO. Ascorbic acid administration should be limited to 250 to 500 mg per day, and chelation therapy should commence before the introduction of ascorbic acid. Care should be taken in patients with cardiac disease, and the patient should be monitored for evidence of arrhythmias or impaired cardiac function.

While chelation therapy has been of considerable benefit in many patients with secondary iron overload, particularly younger patients with chronic hemolytic anemias, it is usually only indicated in patients who otherwise have a good life expectancy. It is also inappropriate to treat secondary iron overload in patients with alcoholic liver disease, unless the iron stores are in the range seen in GH. Such patients probably have both diseases and should be treated no differently from a patient with GH. In alcoholic siderosis neither phlebotomy nor chelation therapy is indicated, and both are usually poorly tolerated if attempted. However, phlebotomy therapy may be used to assess iron stores (as a diagnostic test) by estimating the amount of iron removed to produce borderline iron deficiency. Patients with alcoholic siderosis usually have iron stores of less than 3 grams (estimated by phlebotomy), whereas patients with GH usually have iron stores in excess of 5 or even 10 grams, depending on age. If there is doubt about the precise diagnosis, it is preferable to remove the excess iron and, in the process, quantitate body iron stores.

# HODGKIN'S DISEASE: CHEMOTHERAPY

method of
JAY MARION, M.D.
*Missouri Baptist Medical Center*
*St. Louis, Missouri*

Hodgkin's disease is a lymphoreticular malignancy that usually presents with painless lymphadenopathy. Preceding the diagnosis, the patient may also be aware of systemic symptoms such as generalized malaise, fatigue, and anorexia. Three such constitutional symptoms have been associated with a reduction in survival and thus have special significance. These have been titled "B symptoms" and include

1. Unexplained weight loss of more than 10% of the body weight in 6 months
2. Night sweats
3. Unexplained increases in temperature above 38° C

It is essential to document the presence or absence of B symptoms and to include the appropriate suffix to the numerical stage when discussing a patient with Hodgkin's disease. This anatomic staging system, which was developed at the Ann Arbor Conference in 1971, is widely accepted by clinicians who treat Hodgkin's disease (Table 1). It is a functional staging system because the usual pattern of spread in Hodgkin's disease is predictable and nonrandom. There is usually orderly spread via lymphatic channels to contiguous lymph node chains. Hematogenous spread does not usually occur until the disease has involved the spleen.

Approximately 70% of all patients with Hodgkin's disease can be cured. Radiation therapy has curative potential in early-stage disease, and combination chemotherapy is similarly effective in advanced-stage disease. Because the initial therapy chosen depends on the stage of the disease, the outcome is affected by the accuracy of the staging process. Thus, after a diagnosis of Hodgkin's disease is made, further studies are usually indicated to allow for the appropriate staging of the patient. Exhaustive staging studies, however, should not be undertaken in all patients as a matter of routine. Invasive staging studies, such as laparotomy, should be performed only in patients in whom a change in stage would result in a change in initial therapy. There remains much controversy regarding the role of aggressive staging procedures in various subsets of patients.

## TREATMENT

Patients with early-stage Hodgkin's disease (Stages I and II) are usually managed with radiotherapy alone. Stage IIIA patients who have only minimal disease in the upper abdomen at laparotomy may also be managed primarily with radiotherapy. Some Stage I and II patients who have bulky adenopathy or multiple sites of disease are best managed with a combination of radiotherapy and chemotherapy. Patients with more advanced disease (Stages IIIB and IV) are usually offered chemotherapy for primary management. Such treatment is almost always given with curative intent.

### Chemotherapy

Effective chemotherapeutic regimens in Hodgkin's disease include combinations of drugs that have different mechanisms of action, nonoverlapping toxicity, and proven efficacy in that disease. The landmark studies at the National Cancer Institute (NCI) in the late 1970s demonstrated that more than 50% of patients with advanced Hodgkin's disease could be cured with a combination of four chemotherapeutic agents: nitrogen mustard, vincristine, procarbazine, and prednisone (MOPP) (Table 2). It remains the standard with which all other regimens are compared. A recently published 20-year update of the NCI data demonstrated an 84% complete response rate with MOPP. Sixty-six per cent of the com-

TABLE 1. **Hodgkin's Disease: Ann Arbor Staging System**

| Stage | Characteristics |
|-------|-----------------|
| I | Involvement of a single lymph node region (I) or of a single extralymphatic organ or site ($I_E$). |
| II | Involvement of two or more lymph node regions on the same side of the diaphragm (II) or localized involvement of an extralymphatic organ or site and of one or more lymph node regions on the same side of the diaphragm ($II_E$). |
| III | Involvement of lymph node regions on both sides of the diaphragm (III), which may be accompanied by localized involvement of an extralymphatic organ or site ($III_E$), or by involvement of the spleen ($III_S$), or both ($III_{SE}$). |
| IV | Diffuse or disseminated involvement of one or more extralymphatic organs or tissues, with or without associated lymph node enlargement. Involvement of the liver or bone marrow is always considered Stage IV. |
| Note: | Unexplained increase in temperature > 38° C (>100.5° F), night sweats, and/or weight loss > 10% of body weight in 6 mo preceding diagnosis are defined as systemic symptoms and denoted by the suffix letter B. Asymptomatic patients are denoted by the suffix letter A. |

TABLE 2. **Chemotherapy Regimens for Hodgkin's Disease**

| Agent | Dose (mg/M²) | Days and Route |
|---|---|---|
| **MOPP** | | |
| Nitrogen mustard | 6 | 1 and 8 IV |
| Vincristine (Oncovin) | 1.4 | 1 and 8 IV |
| Procarbazine | 100 | 1–14 PO |
| Prednisone | 40 | 1–14 PO |
| *Repeat every 28 days* | | |
| **BVCPP** | | |
| Carmustine (BCNU) | 100 | 1 IV |
| Vinblastine | 5 | 1 IV |
| Cyclophosphamide | 600 | 1 IV |
| Procarbazine | 100 | 1–10 PO |
| Prednisone | 60 | 1–10 PO |
| *Repeat every 28 days* | | |
| **ABVD** | | |
| Doxorubicin (Adriamycin) | 25 | 1 and 15 IV |
| Bleomycin | 10* | 1 and 15 IV |
| Vinblastine | 6 | 1 and 15 IV |
| Dacarbazine (DTIC) | 375 | 1 and 15 IV |
| *Repeat every 28 days* | | |
| **MOPP-ABV Hybrid** | | |
| Nitrogen mustard | 6 | 1 IV |
| Vincristine (Oncovin) | 1.4 | 1 IV (maximal dose 2.0 mg) |
| Procarbazine | 100 | 1–7 PO |
| Prednisone | 40 | 1–14 PO |
| Doxorubicin (Adriamycin) | 35 | 8 IV |
| Bleomycin | 10* | 8 IV |
| Vinblastine | 6 | 8 IV |
| *Repeat every 28 days* | | |

*Dose in U/M².

plete responders have remained free of disease for more than 10 years after treatment. However, although MOPP has revolutionized the management of advanced Hodgkin's disease, it has not turned out to be a panacea. At least 15% of patients do not achieve a complete remission, and approximately 30% of complete responders ultimately relapse. MOPP is also associated with significant and sometimes lasting toxicity. This acute toxicity almost always includes nausea and vomiting, which can be variably controlled with antiemetic regimens. Myelosuppression is also common; a sliding scale of dose reduction for cytopenias that is built into the regimen must be strictly followed. Potential delayed toxic complications of MOPP include infertility and secondary malignancy.

**Infertility.** Infertility is a well-defined, long-term complication of MOPP chemotherapy. Because many patients with Hodgkin's disease are of reproductive age, this is not a minor toxicity. MOPP has been shown to produce profound, lasting impairment of fertility in the majority of men. This regimen also induces ovarian failure in the majority of premenopausal women. The closer a woman is to natural menopause, the more likely it is that she will develop premature ovarian failure. Women who retain fertility after MOPP chemotherapy appear to have normal pregnancies and normal children.

**Secondary Malignancy.** Patients with cured Hodgkin's disease have a small but increased risk of developing acute leukemia. This is usually a myeloid leukemia and is often preceded by a refractory anemia or another myelodysplasia. Chromosomal abnormalities are commonly found in the leukemic cell lines. The interval between completion of treatment and the appearance of leukemia is approximately 5 to 8 years. The overall incidence of acute leukemia in patients with cured Hodgkin's disease is approximately 3 to 4%. The subgroup of patients who are treated with both radiotherapy and MOPP chemotherapy are at higher risk than those who are treated with either modality alone. The incidence of solid tumors in cured Hodgkin's disease patients does not appear to be increased.

**Alternative Chemotherapeutic Regimens.** Because MOPP alone is unable to cure approximately 40% of patients with Hodgkin's disease and is associated with significant toxicity, there has been an impetus to develop alternative chemotherapeutic regimens. Several other drugs with proven efficacy in Hodgkin's disease are theoretically non–cross-resistant with the agents in MOPP. Such drugs (doxorubicin, bleomycin, carmustine, dacarbazine, lomustine, and vinblastine) have been used in various combinations as initial and salvage therapies in Hodgkin's disease (Table 2). The combination of doxorubicin (Adriamycin), bleomycin, vinblastine, and dacarbazine (ABVD) has been shown to produce complete remissions in approximately 30 to 60% of patients who fail to respond to MOPP. Acute toxicity with ABVD is similar to that experienced with MOPP (nausea, vomiting, alopecia, and cytopenias). ABVD, however, is less often associated with infertility and the induction of secondary malignancies, and thus has been used as an alternative to MOPP for initial therapy. Comparative trials suggest that it is therapeutically equivalent to MOPP. ABVD may thus be the therapy of choice in patients with advanced Hodgkin's disease who desire to maintain fertility. However, this regimen must also be given with caution because it is associated with long-term cardiac toxicity (doxorubicin) and pulmonary toxicity (bleomycin).

**Guidelines for Administration.** The optimal number of chemotherapy cycles required to attain a durable, complete remission varies from patient to patient. The usual practice is to offer a minimum of six cycles of MOPP, or its equivalent, to patients with advanced Hodgkin's disease. The response to therapy should be monitored during treatment, and patients should receive two cycles after the documentation of a clinical complete remission. Maintenance therapy after these additional two cycles has not been shown to improve survival. The importance of administering full doses of chemotherapy in a timely fashion cannot be overemphasized. Dose reductions, if necessary, should follow the established protocol guidelines.

**New Directions.** Attempts are under way to improve both the initial and salvage therapies available to patients with advanced Hodgkin's diseases. The goal is to provide more effective and less toxic chemotherapeutic regimens. Alternating the use of MOPP and ABVD as initial therapy in selected patients with advanced disease is common but has not been clearly demonstrated to be superior to using MOPP alone. Other "hybrids" of MOPP and ABVD regimens are also being investigated as primary therapy. Autologous and allogeneic bone marrow transplantation has been demonstrated to be an effective salvage therapy for a small percentage of patients with refractory disease. The role of bone marrow transplantation in these patients is presently being defined through cooperative trials.

# HODGKIN'S DISEASE: RADIATION THERAPY

method of
ANDREW RAUBITSCHEK, M.D., and
ELI GLATSTEIN, M.D.
*National Cancer Institute*
*Bethesda, Maryland*

Hodgkin's disease spreads to involve contiguous nodal groups and presents primarily in the cervical and supraclavicular regions. The majority of patients with supradiaphragmatic disease will also have mediastinal disease. Spread to subdiaphragmatic locations is less common, although disease can be missed by clinical evaluation alone.

## STAGING

The procedures used for staging Hodgkin's disease are presented in Table 1 along with their indications and diagnostic yields.

### Laparotomy

Staging laparotomy was introduced in the early clinical studies of Hodgkin's disease and still has a place in its evaluation today. Laparotomy should be performed whenever the results of the pathologic eval-

**TABLE 1. Procedures Used for Staging Hodgkin's Disease**

| Procedure | Indications | Diagnostic Yield |
|---|---|---|
| History | All patients | Night sweats with fever, weight loss >10% |
| Physical examination | All patients | Involved lymph nodes, extranodal sites, pericardial rubs, pleural effusions, hepatosplenomegaly |
| Chest x-ray | All patients | Mediastinal, hilar disease; pericardial effusion or mass; pleural effusion, cardiophrenic adenopathy |
| Lymphangiogram | All patients, unless contraindicated by pulmonary dysfunction or allergy | Periaortic, common iliac, external iliac, or femoral lymphadenopathy |
| CT scan of the chest | Suspected mediastinal, hilar, or pulmonary parenchymal disease | Mediastinal, hilar, or pulmonary parenchymal disease |
| Liver/spleen scan | All patients | Hepatic/splenic involvement |
| Bone scan | Symptomatic or elevated alkaline phosphatase | Osseous involvement (correlate with bone x-rays) |
| CT scan of the abdomen | Equivocal lymphangiogram or liver/spleen scan | Enlarged lymph nodes, splenomegaly, filling defects in liver or spleen |
| Bone marrow biopsy | All patients | Marrow involvement with Reed-Sternberg cells |
| Gallium scan (optional) | General screening for areas of lymphomatous involvement | Increased uptake in areas of adenopathy |
| Laparotomy | See text | Pathologic evidence of subdiaphragmatic disease |

uation of the spleen, liver, and lymph nodes in the subdiaphragmatic area could influence the choice of treatment options. Usually this involves patients with supradiaphragmatic presentation who do not have unequivocally positive lymphangiograms or computed tomography (CT) of their abdomens and therefore may be eligible for radiation treatment.

Staging laparotomy ideally includes splenectomy with the placement of radiopaque clips at the point of ligation of the splenic vessels close to their origin. Clips should also be placed on the nodes that are sampled. In addition, young female patients can have their ovaries moved to the midline either in front of or behind the uterus as low down in the pelvis as possible and their location marked with radiopaque clips. This will help to preserve fertility in up to 70% of the young females who undergo high-dose irradiation of the pelvis.

*Modified Ann Arbor Staging Classification*

Stage I    Involvement of a single lymphatic region or a single extralymphatic site (1E)

Stage II   Involvement of two or more lymphatic sites on the same side of the diaphragm

Stage III  Involvement of lymphatic regions on both sides of the diaphragm

Stage IV   Disseminated extralymphatic involvement (bone marrow, liver, pleura, skin)

A = asymptomatic; B = fever, sweats, unexplained weight loss greater than 10% body weight (A and B apply to all stages).

## TREATMENT

Radiation techniques are specialized for each treatment field. Linear accelerators are used to provide high energy beams with large field sizes so that adjacent nodal groups can be treated in contiguity. Most patients can be treated using an isocentric technique with the patient positioned supine. An occasional patient will need to be treated at extended distance in order for adjacent lymph node areas to be encompassed within the same field.

Radiation portals are designed carefully by simulating the treatment field on a machine capable of producing diagnostic x-ray films. In addition, most patients are also scanned on a CT machine in the treatment position to ensure adequacy of the treatment volume. The therapeutic radiologist works in conjunction with the dosimetrist to outline the volume to be treated. Individualized blocks are then drawn on the simulator films and their accuracy verified using a computerized treatment planning system that allows for the entry of the CT data in addition to the blocking information.

The mantle field is used to encompass all the lymph node areas above the diaphragm including cervical, supra- and infraclavicular, mediastinal, hilar, and axillary nodes. The inferior border should cover the cardiac silhouette, approximately at the T10 to T11 vertebral body interspace. The superior border is set to skim the bottom edge of the mandible in order to cover the cervical nodes. In patients with cervical disease above the thyroid notch, an additional preauricular field adjacent to the superior edge of the mantle field is required to ensure adequate coverage. This preauricular field can be set up on the involved side only and partially treated with electrons to avoid treating the contralateral parotid gland.

In order to prevent unnecessary radiation of sensitive tissues, blocks are placed within the field to shield the lungs and humeral heads. The posterior cervical spine and the larynx are also blocked if there is no midline or bulky disease in this area. The entire cardiac silhouette is treated with 1500 centigray (cGy) if mediastinal disease is present. A pericardial block is then placed in the field, ensuring that it does not block any sites of known disease. At 2500 to 3000 cGy a subcarinal block is placed approximately 5 to 6 cm beneath the carina. Some institutions have recommended a posterior thoracic cord block after 2000 cGy. At the National Cancer Institute (NCI), we recommend a midplane dose of 4500 cGy to the mantle field unless the patient has received chemotherapy as part of a planned combination therapy program, in which case the dose is decreased. The abdominal field is gapped to the lower part of the mantle field and includes the para-aortic nodes, the splenic hilum, and the spleen if still present. The lower limit of the field extends to the beginning of the common iliac nodes, usually at L4 level. The liver is not usually treated unless there is splenic involvement. We do not treat the common iliac chains in pathologically staged patients with disease above the diaphragm, unless the patient has stage IIB disease. In this clinical situation, we recommend treating the common and external iliac chain in conjunction with the femoral area in a separate pelvic field.

The pelvic field is set up to cover the common iliac, the external iliac, and the femoral nodes. A midline block is placed to shield the central part of the pelvis up to the sacrum. The position of the blocks is otherwise determined by the outline of the lymph nodes on lymphangiogram. Although CT can be useful for setting up other fields, the lymphangiogram is essential for ensuring adequate coverage in this area because a lymph node outside the standard location is often visualized that should be included in the field. For males we use a separate testicular shield to decrease the scattered and transmitted doses to this sensitive organ. In females we recommend an oophoropexy at the time of laparotomy to place the ovaries midline behind the uterus, with metal staples to mark their location. The bottom of the field is placed beneath the visualized femoral nodes on the lymphangiogram. Care should be taken to irradiate as little of the hip joint as possible. It is possible to treat the femoral area by electrons given only anteriorly as a supplement to an anterior photon field. This reduces the dose to the femurs and provides good coverage for the anterior structures. (When this treatment regimen is used, the posterior field is blocked beneath the inguinal ligament, and the electron field is set up only anteriorly.)

### Radiotherapeutic Management of Hodgkin's Disease

In general, treatment with radiation alone is reserved for those patients with pathologic Stage

I or II disease. As discussed earlier, patients with supradiaphragmatic presentation should undergo pathologic staging to verify absence of disease below the diaphragm. For those patients with Stage I disease with subdiaphragmatic presentation, no pathologic staging is indicated if CT of the chest is negative. However, if para-aortic nodes are positive on lymphangiogram or physical examination raises the question of supraclavicular adenopathy, a scalene node biopsy can be performed to rule out disease. An intrathoracic procedure is rarely, if ever, required.

For those patients with subdiaphragmatic Stage I/II disease whose physical examination or radiographic studies indicate an enlarged spleen, liver biopsy may be considered, since patients with significant splenic disease run an increased chance of having hepatic involvement.

Stage I patients who have neck disease above the hyoid bone or in the axilla represent an extremely favorable group and mandate different evaluation. Because this group has a low incidence of occult disease in the mediastinum or subdiaphragmatic area, they are not pathologically staged beneath the diaphragm but merely subjected to a scalene node biopsy of the involved side to rule out occult contiguous nodal disease. If this biopsy is negative, they are treated with a minimantle field only, which does not include the mediastinum and subdiaphragmatic areas.

Stage I patients with disease limited to the mediastinum are treated similarly in regard to staging; however, their radiation portals necessarily include the mediastinum.

Patients with massive mediastinal disease (greater than one-third the largest thoracic diameter) generally do not require surgical staging because most treatment programs involve combined modality therapy. Some patients may be candidates for radiation therapy if their disease does not overlie too much lung and does not expand in the recumbent position. Over the past 2 years we at the NCI have begun to treat some of these patients in a specially designed chair to minimize the volume of lung irradiated. If patients are being considered for treatment with radiation alone, a staging laparotomy may be desirable.

For those patients who are going to be treated with combined modality therapy, clinical staging of the abdomen is probably sufficient and no radiation therapy in this area is warranted unless the patient has extensive bulky adenopathy or fails to respond completely to chemotherapy.

Current studies throughout the world are defining other Stage II patients who should be considered for more aggressive approaches than radiotherapy alone. These probably include patients with five or more sites of disease and significant B symptoms.

Stage III patients are most often treated with chemotherapy, although excellent results can be achieved with radiation alone in carefully selected patients, i.e., those with minimal amounts of disease on both sides of the diaphragm and minimal splenic involvement.

In those patients with more extensive Stage III disease, combined modality therapy has been used, but most authors consider the risk of secondary neoplasia to outweigh the improved initial complete response rate. Stage IV patients are treated with combination chemotherapy alone.

Although there are some reports of successful long-term remissions induced by radiation following relapse, it is generally accepted that radiation therapy has a minimal role in the management of patients who relapse after initial chemotherapy.

# ACUTE LEUKEMIA IN ADULTS

method of
RICHARD A. LARSON, M.D.
*The University of Chicago*
*Chicago, Illinois*

Acute leukemia is a malignant proliferation of bone marrow cells that is uniformly fatal when left untreated. However, with the use of intensive chemotherapy regimens and skillful supportive care, many patients may be cured of this devastating disease, particularly younger adults. Because the best opportunity to cure acute leukemia requires appropriate diagnosis and optimal initial treatment, it is highly desirable to refer newly diagnosed patients to regional oncology centers where appropriate expertise and resources are readily available.

## ETIOLOGY OF LEUKEMIA

Leukemia and other cancers result from genetic mutations in somatic cells. When mutational damage alters normal growth regulatory mechanisms in a hematopoietic stem cell, a clone of neoplastic cells may proliferate, overwhelming the normal bone marrow through a selective growth advantage. Leukemia cells usually retain characteristics of their original cell lineage, allowing subclassification (Table 1). However, because these are neoplastic cells, aberrant expression of proteins not usually manifested by normal cells of a particular hematopoietic lineage may be detected, yielding a "mixed cell" phenotype.

## PRESENTATION AND DIAGNOSIS

Symptoms may occur with an abrupt onset or in a more insidious manner. This is related to the rate of

TABLE 1. **French-American-British (FAB) Classification of Acute Leukemias**

| FAB Subtype | |
|---|---|
| | **Lymphoblastic (ALL)** |
| L1 | Small cells; homogeneous |
| L2 | Large cells; heterogeneous |
| L3 | Large cells; homogeneous (Burkitt type) |
| | **Myeloid-Nonlymphoblastic (AML-ANLL)** |
| M1 | Acute myeloblastic leukemia without maturation (AML) |
| M2 | Acute myeloblastic leukemia with maturation (AML) |
| M3 | Acute promyelocytic leukemia—hypergranular (APL) |
| M3V | Acute promyelocytic leukemia—microgranular (APL) |
| M4 | Acute myelomonocytic leukemia (AMMoL) |
| M4Eo | Acute myelomonocytic leukemia with abnormal eosinophils (AMMoL-M4Eo) |
| M5a | Acute monoblastic leukemia—poorly differentiated (AMoL) |
| M5b | Acute monocytic leukemia—well differentiated (AMoL) |
| M6 | Erythroleukemia (EL) |
| M7 | Acute megakaryoblastic leukemia (AMegaL) |

proliferation of the malignant clone, the degree of suppression of normal blood elements, and the extent of infiltration into normal tissues. Most commonly, patients seek medical attention with fatigue and malaise due to anemia. Fever is often present and usually indicates an underlying infection. Bleeding and easy bruisability are common. Occasionally, patients may present with leukemic infiltrates in the skin or seek dental care because of symptoms due to gum hypertrophy. Patients may be gravely ill or may appear remarkably well except for pallor, ecchymoses, or petechiae. Lymphadenopathy is relatively uncommon in adults and then is seen mostly with acute lymphoblastic leukemia (ALL). Mild splenomegaly is present in a small fraction of patients.

Acute leukemia almost always causes marked abnormalities in the peripheral blood counts. Anemia may be mild, moderate, or severe, and the red blood cells may be mildly macrocytic. Most patients will have moderate to severe thrombocytopenia. Although an elevated white blood cell count and readily recognizable circulating blast cells are frequently present, not all patients have leukocytosis. Some patients actually present with leukopenia, and malignant cells may not be observed in the peripheral blood. A careful review of a blood smear often demonstrates dysplasia in one or more cell lines. In elderly patients, acute leukemia frequently evolves from a myelodysplastic syndrome; mature granulocytes are often hypogranular with poorly condensed nuclear chromatin, and platelets may be large in size but lacking normal granulation. The most common biochemical abnormality associated with acute leukemia is hyperuricemia, which can be so elevated as to contribute to renal failure. Occasionally, an abnormal coagulation profile will demonstrate disseminated intravascular coagulation (DIC), owing in part to the release of thromboplastic material from degenerating malignant cells. This is most common in acute promyelocytic leukemia

but may accompany any type of leukemia or may be due to infection. The chest radiograph may show evidence of an interstitial infiltrate due to hyperleukocytosis or infection. Mediastinal or hilar lymphadenopathy may also be detected, particularly in T cell ALL. Leukemia cells are occasionally found in the spinal fluid at diagnosis, but a lumbar puncture should be deferred in asymptomatic patients with high numbers of circulating blast cells. It is relatively uncommon for acute myeloid leukemia (AML) to cause neurologic symptoms, whereas ALL more commonly infiltrates the arachnoid membranes surrounding the brain, causing cranial neuropathy.

The diagnosis and subclassification of acute leukemia rest upon the interpretation of an adequate bone marrow sample. A marrow aspiration specimen together with a bone marrow core biopsy sample provides important information. Auer rods are often observed in malignant myeloblasts. Cytochemical reactivity detects myeloperoxidase or nonspecific esterase activity in myeloid leukemias, whereas such activity is absent in lymphoid leukemias. Immunophenotypic analysis by flow cytometry or immunohistochemical techniques detects cell surface antigens that corroborate the diagnosis. Cytogenetic analyses of bone marrow specimens provide important diagnostic and prognostic information in acute leukemia. Metaphase cells are karyotyped after direct preparation or short-term (24 to 48 hours) unstimulated cultures. Characteristic recurring chromosomal abnormalities include the gain of extra chromosomes; the loss of certain chromosomes; and structural rearrangements such as translocations, deletions, insertions, and inversions. Several distinct subtypes of acute leukemia can now be defined according to their characteristic morphologic, cytochemical, immunophenotypic, and cytogenetic features. These disorders have a more predictable clinical course than less well-defined leukemias.

## TREATMENT

### Prophylactic Measures

The success of remission induction chemotherapy for acute leukemia depends not only upon the drug susceptibility of an individual patient's particular leukemia but also upon the ability of that patient to survive the rigors of treatment. Significant advances have been made in the supportive care of patients undergoing intensive cytotoxic therapy. Prevention and early treatment of infection have been of foremost importance. Prior to treatment, all patients should have a thorough dental evaluation to rule out oral sources of potential infections. Patients are placed in protective isolation within single rooms; in this way, immunocompromised patients are protected from common infectious agents in the hospital environment. Laminar airflow rooms are not necessary for successful treatment, but patients are generally restricted from eating fresh fruits and vegetables to decrease their enteric bacterial flora. Strict attention to thorough hand-washing by all medical and nursing personnel and visitors is necessary. Prophylactic antibiotic therapy has limited use; it is often poorly tolerated and may lead to the emergence of resistant organisms. Oral trimethoprim-sulfamethoxazole (Bactrim) is routinely used in childhood ALL to decrease the risk of *Pneumocystis carinii* pneumonia. Patients who are neutropenic (less than 500 granulocytes per μl) and who become febrile (greater than 38.5° C) should be examined thoroughly for evidence of bacterial, fungal, or viral infections. Blood, sputum, throat, urine, and stool cultures should be obtained. Broad-spectrum antibiotics should be started empirically because the risk of septic shock is very high in granulocytopenic, febrile patients. Infections by either gram-positive or gram-negative bacteria are common. Many antibiotic regimens have proved useful in this setting. We use mezlocillin (Mezlin), cefazolin (Kefzol), and tobramycin (Nebcin) as a standard empiric regimen or ceftazidime IM or IV as a single agent for any patient with renal dysfunction. Amphotericin B (Fungizone) (0.5 mg per kg) is added empirically after 72 to 96 hours if a patient remains febrile on appropriate antibacterial therapy. Granulocyte transfusions are rarely needed but can be lifesaving if bacteremia persists despite appropriate antibiotic treatment.

Bleeding is a common problem at diagnosis and during therapy for acute leukemia; the risk rises as the platelet count decreases. Platelets should be transfused prophylactically to maintain a platelet count greater than 20,000 per μl in order to decrease the risk of spontaneous hemorrhage such as stroke or gastrointestinal bleeding. No salicylates or other drugs that interfere with platelet function should be given, nor should intramuscular injections be given to a thrombocytopenic patient. DIC may be successfully treated with low doses of continuous intravenous heparin (5 to 10 U per kg per hour). The fibrinogen level should be maintained at greater than 100 mg per dl using cryoprecipitate infusions. Once heparin therapy has been initiated, fresh-frozen plasma may be safely transfused in patients with active DIC to replete the clotting factors rapidly to normal. Vitamin K should be given by mouth or parenterally, particularly to patients on broad-spectrum antibiotics who may become vitamin K deficient. The use of single-donor platelets collected by apheresis will decrease the rate of alloimmunization in leukemia patients. Patients who become alloimmunized may require HLA-matched platelets or cross-matched platelets in order to achieve an adequate post-transfusion platelet count. Techniques to remove leukocytes by filtration or centrifugation from red cell or platelet transfusion units may slow the rate of alloimmunization. Red blood cell transfusions should be used to maintain a hematocrit of approximately 30%.

Soft Silastic central venous catheters (e.g., Hickman or Groshong) that tunnel under the skin and enter the brachiocephalic vein are widely used. They allow direct access to a large vein for infusion of chemotherapy, antibiotics, and blood transfusions and also allow painless blood sampling for laboratory monitoring. Parenteral hyperalimentation can be easily administered through these catheters if necessary.

A blood chemistry panel will identify organ dysfunction from leukemic infiltration into the liver or kidneys or metabolic abnormalities due to tumor cell lysis syndrome. Renal and hepatic function may actually improve after chemotherapy has begun, but until this happens these patients must be observed very closely because both chemotherapy drugs and the products of tumor cell lysis are cleared through the biliary system and the kidneys. The tumor cell lysis syndrome results from the rapid destruction of tumor cells and occurs most commonly in ALL patients, especially those with T cell or mature B cell phenotypes. Serum levels of potassium, phosphate, and uric acid can rise rapidly, causing serious cardiac arrhythmias or a decline in serum calcium levels so that tetany results. Acute renal failure may occur, requiring hemodialysis. Pretreatment with allopurinol (Zyloprim) (300 mg per day) plus alkalinization of the urine with oral or intravenous sodium bicarbonate and acetazolamide (Diamox) can diminish the risks of hyperuricemia. A good urine flow should be induced, but care must be taken not to overhydrate patients.

### Emergency Treatment

Hyperleukocytosis (greater than 100,000 blast cells per μl) is a true medical emergency. Leukostasis and hypoxemia in the capillary beds can induce respiratory distress, cardiac arrhythmias, and central nervous system symptoms, leading to coma. Death follows rapidly unless the circulation can be restored. Emergency measures include leukapheresis to remove a large mass of tumor cells directly from the blood stream combined with oral hydroxyurea (Hydrea) (1 gram every 4 hours).* A single dose of cranial irradiation (200 to 400 cGy) can ameliorate CNS symptoms due to leukostasis. Once the circulation through the capillaries has been restored, systemic chemotherapy should be initiated rapidly. Prophylactic platelet transfusions should be

---

*Exceeds dosage recommended by the manufacturer.

given to prevent bleeding as the circulation is restored to hypoxemic tissues. Red cell transfusions can precipitate a hyperviscosity syndrome in a patient with hyperleukocytosis and should be delayed if possible until the white blood cell count falls.

### Acute Myeloid Leukemia

The optimal chemotherapy for adults with AML has not yet been determined. Recent clinical trials suggest different risk groups of patients who are more or less likely to respond to standard intensive remission induction chemotherapy programs. Treatment is given in two or three phases: induction and consolidation with or without maintenance. Our current induction regimen for standard-risk patients consists of cytarabine (Cytosar-U) (100 mg per $M^2$ per day) for 7 days with daunorubicin (Cerubidine) (50 mg per $M^2$ per day) for 3 days. Both drugs are given by continuous intravenous infusion. Patients older than 60 years receive a reduced dose of daunorubicin (35 mg per $M^2$). A bone marrow examination is repeated after 6 complete days of chemotherapy, and those patients whose marrow is already extremely hypocellular receive no further therapy for the first treatment cycle. In contrast, patients with residual leukemia in a cellular marrow on day 7 receive 3 additional days of cytarabine but no additional daunorubicin. Alternatively, young patients with residual leukemia in a cellular marrow on day 7 may benefit from six doses of high-dose cytarabine (2 grams per $M^2$ every 12 hours*) starting on day 8 in lieu of continuous infusion cytarabine at more standard doses. One week after the completion of chemotherapy, the bone marrow is examined once again. Any patient with residual leukemia in a cellular marrow receives a second induction course identical to the first. Those patients with marrow hypocellularity are followed weekly with repeat marrow examinations for evidence of normal regeneration. Patients in whom leukemia regenerates require a second induction course. It must be kept in mind that normal myeloid regeneration may appear first as a proliferation of myeloblasts and promyelocytes and this may be confused with residual or recurrent AML. In such cases, another bone marrow examination should be performed several days later prior to instituting any further chemotherapy. If the immature myeloid elements reflected early regeneration, clear evidence of differentiation to more mature granulocytes should now be present as well as some erythroid and megakaryocyte recovery. Approximately 70

to 80% of patients with AML achieve a complete remission with one or two induction courses. Mortality during treatment should be less than 10 to 15%.

Alternative remission induction regimens may utilize 6-thioguanine in conjunction with cytarabine and daunorubicin (TAD). For young patients, high-dose cytarabine (2 to 3 grams per $M^2$ every 12 hours*) for 12 doses followed by 3 days of daunorubicin (30 mg per $M^2$ per day) can be useful. Patients whose AML is refractory to standard induction chemotherapy regimens are certainly candidates for Phase II chemotherapy trials. Effective agents include mitoxantrone (Novantrone), amsacrine,† diaziquone (AZQ),‡ etoposide (VePesid), and high-dose cyclophosphamide (Cytoxan), either alone or in combinations.

The term "complete remission" is defined by the absence of detectable leukemia in the bone marrow and blood, the regeneration of normal marrow elements, and the return to normal levels of all three blood cell lines. Nevertheless, as many as $10^8$ leukemia cells may remain at this point. If no postremission therapy were given, most patients with AML would relapse within 2 to 4 months. Thus, consolidation chemotherapy is directed at destroying the small numbers of clonogenic leukemia cells that remain undetected. Again, the optimal therapy has not yet been determined. We use three or four courses of cytarabine (100 mg per $M^2$ for 7 days) plus daunorubicin (50 mg per $M^2$ for 3 days), alternating with high-dose cytarabine (2 grams per $M^2$ every 12 hours for eight doses*). Each course begins within 1 week of recovery of peripheral blood granulocytes and platelets. Each consolidation course is followed by bone marrow hypoplasia and peripheral blood pancytopenia. Thus, the risk of bleeding or infection continues, and all patients require blood transfusion support. Mortality during this phase is usually 5% or less.

It has not been proved that low-dose outpatient maintenance chemotherapy increases the fraction of patients with AML who can be cured. We administer no further therapy once the consolidation sequence has been completed. Should patients have a relapse of AML, a second remission can frequently be induced using the same chemotherapy regimens discussed earlier. Alternatively, such patients should be considered for investigational agents or marrow transplantation protocols.

Some patients are not good candidates for in-

---

*Exceeds dosage recommended by the manufacturer.

---

*Exceeds dosage recommended by the manufacturer.
†Investigational drug in the United States (available from the National Cancer Institute on protocol).
‡Investigational drug in the United States (orphan drug: inquiries can be made to 1–800–336–4797).

tensive chemotherapy for AML because they are too elderly or debilitated. In addition, patients whose disease is refractory to two or three courses of intensive remission induction chemotherapy are not likely to be cured. In these circumstances, palliative chemotherapy is frequently used to slow the proliferation of malignant myeloblasts, preferably as an outpatient treatment, with relatively little toxicity. Several oral chemotherapy drugs are effective in this regard, including hydroxyurea, busulfan, and 6-thioguanine. Unfortunately, all of these agents induce relatively nonselective myelosuppression, so that thrombocytopenia and anemia may worsen even as the white blood cell count is reduced.

### Acute Lymphoblastic Leukemia

The treatment of ALL in children is quite successful, but the prognosis for adults with ALL is not yet as optimistic. This may be in part due to the fact that certain high-risk subgroups of ALL, such as those with the Philadelphia chromosome or with myeloid antigens, are more commonly present in the adult populations. Currently, we are testing a very intensive five-drug induction regimen in adults (CALGB [Cancer and Leukemia Group B] protocol 8811) that has proved successful in children with high-risk ALL. Cyclophosphamide (Cytoxan) (1200 mg per $M^2$) is given on day 1 together with daunorubicin (45 mg per $M^2$ per day) on days 1, 2, and 3. Vincristine (Oncovin) (2 mg) is given on days 1, 8, 15, and 22. Prednisone is given for 21 days at 60 mg per $M^2$ per day, and L-asparaginase (Elspar) is given subcutaneously (6000 U per $M^2$) twice per week during the first 3 weeks. Doses of cyclophosphamide and daunorubicin are reduced by one-third and the prednisone is reduced to 7 days in patients older than 60 years. Serious infections are common, but most patients have achieved a complete or partial remission by day 29 using this induction regimen. The consolidation sequence uses intravenous cyclophosphamide and vincristine plus subcutaneous cytarabine and L-asparaginase plus oral 6-mercaptopurine over the next 2 months. The central nervous system prophylaxis course employs cranial irradiation (2400 cGy to the whole brain) plus five weekly injections of intrathecal methotrexate (15 mg). Throughout this period, daily oral 6-mercaptopurine (Purinethol) (60 mg per $M^2$) is given. A short maintenance program continues for the next 5 weeks using oral 6-mercaptopurine plus weekly oral methotrexate (20 mg per $M^2$). The fourth course is a late intensification treatment using doxorubicin (30 mg per $M^2$) weekly for 3 weeks together with weekly vincristine (2 mg)

and daily dexamethasone (Decadron) (10 mg per $M^2$). Finally, cyclophosphamide (1000 mg per $M^2$) is given intravenously along with eight doses of subcutaneous cytarabine (75 mg per $M^2$) and daily oral 6-thioguanine (60 mg per $M^2$) over 2 weeks. In common with childhood ALL treatment programs, most adults also receive prolonged maintenance treatment extending for 18 to 24 months from the time of diagnosis. We currently use oral 6-mercaptopurine (60 mg per $M^2$ per day) with weekly oral methotrexate (20 mg per $M^2$ per week) plus monthly pulses of vincristine (2 mg intravenously) with 5 days of prednisone (60 mg per $M^2$ per day). Other agents useful in remission induction or consolidation treatment of ALL include high-dose cytarabine, high-dose methotrexate with leucovorin, and mitoxantrone.

Patients who suffer a relapse of ALL after completion of therapy can usually achieve a second remission with reinstitution of the original induction chemotherapy regimen. However, patients who relapse in the midst of initial treatment or maintenance are far less likely to achieve a second remission or long survival. These patients are candidates for investigational chemotherapy programs or marrow transplantation protocols.

### Bone Marrow Transplantation for Acute Leukemia

Bone marrow transplantation allows the use of high doses of marrow-ablative chemotherapy for the treatment of patients with leukemia. The objective here is to destroy in a single treatment course all of the residual leukemia cells in a patient's body using high-dose chemotherapy with or without total body irradiation. As a consequence of such intensive treatment, the patient's normal bone marrow is also destroyed, as is the immune system. Thus, genetically identical or closely matched bone marrow must be transfused in order to rescue such a patient from otherwise fatal marrow aplasia. Both the medical risks and the financial costs of bone marrow transplantation are high, creating controversy as to when this technique should best be employed for patients with acute leukemia. Mortality or significant long-term disability can be due to infection, normal tissue damage following intensive cytotoxic treatment, or the immunologic reaction called graft-versus-host disease (GVHD).

One general strategy advocates not employing transplantation in patients with acute leukemia in first remission unless there are poor-risk features predicting a short remission duration and a very-well-matched donor is available. However, if a patient relapses after having received an intensive initial treatment program, disease-free survival is generally (but not always) short. Thus, the risks and costs of marrow transplantation are more easily justified for patients who have had a relapse of leukemia. Patients who are less than 40 years old and have an HLA-identical sibling are good candidates for allogeneic transplantation. It may be possible to extend the upper limit on age with the use of T cell depletion from the donor marrow to diminish the incidence and severity of GVHD. The use of marrow from a matched but unrelated donor may also be feasible.

Our preparative regimen prior to allogeneic marrow transplantation for patients with myeloid leukemia uses high-dose busulfan (16 mg per kg) and high-dose cyclophosphamide (120 mg per kg). For patients with ALL, we use hyperfractionated total body irradiation (1200 cGy) plus high-dose cyclophosphamide (120 mg per kg). All patients receive prophylaxis against GVHD using cyclosporine and methylprednisolone or methotrexate. Evidence of engraftment usually occurs within 14 days, although complete maturation of the new marrow and the immune system requires several months or longer.

For patients who lack an HLA-identical sibling, techniques have been developed using high-dose chemotherapy followed by reinfusion of autologous bone marrow collected during remission. This technique avoids the immunologic reaction of GVHD but has the disadvantage of potentially reinfusing small numbers of residual leukemia cells that were present during the marrow harvest. For this reason, various methods of "purging" the marrow of residual malignant cells have been developed. These include incubation with chemotherapeutic drugs or monoclonal antibodies and complement or differential density centrifugation or elutriation. The ability of any of these techniques to remove all contaminating malignant cells remains to be proved, but some patients have had long-term disease-free survival when treated in this fashion following a relapse of acute leukemia. The autologous bone marrow harvest is usually performed soon after completion of initial intensive chemotherapy, and the patient's remission marrow is stored at −70° C. Should the patient suffer relapse, high-dose chemotherapy similar to that used for allogeneic marrow transplantation is administered over 6 to 8 days. Then the patient's marrow is thawed and reinfused; blood counts usually recover within several weeks' time. Autologous bone marrow reinfusion is now being tested as an alternative to intensive consolidation regimens for patients in first remission.

## CONCLUSIONS

The successful treatment of adults with acute leukemia requires a multidisciplinary approach.

It is important that the patient and family be provided with emotional support during the initial diagnosis and subsequent treatment. Teamwork among physicians, nurses, dieticians, pharmacists, social workers, and the blood bank is critical. Twenty-four hour housestaff coverage is necessary to respond to emergencies that could otherwise lead to rapid deterioration of a patient in the midst of chemotherapy. Although major challenges remain to be overcome, the majority of young and middle-aged adults can today be successfully treated for acute leukemia.

# ACUTE LEUKEMIA IN CHILDHOOD

method of
CAROLA A. S. ARNDT, M.D., and
GERALD S. GILCHRIST, M.D.
*Mayo Clinic*
*Rochester, Minnesota*

There are two major forms of acute leukemia in childhood—lymphocytic and nonlymphocytic. It is possible to cure children with acute leukemia, especially those with the lymphocytic form. At present, there is no one standard method of treatment; most children in the United States are treated on research protocols that incorporate the best known therapy but also include innovative therapy that can be evaluated in a research setting. The treatment programs we utilize are based on those developed over the past 25 years in the Children's Cancer Study Group. They may vary in some details from those employed by other cooperative groups or pediatric cancer centers, but the same basic principles underlie all the treatment regimens currently in use. All children with acute leukemia will die if not treated.

## ACUTE LYMPHOCYTIC LEUKEMIA (ALL)

Lymphocytic leukemia is subclassified in four ways: (1) by the findings on physical examination and routine laboratory values, (2) by morphologic criteria using standard microscopic techniques, (3) immunologically, and (4) cytogenetically. Cytogenetic findings are emerging that may identify children with greater and lesser chances of long-term survival.

At the present time, patients are classified into poor-, intermediate-, or good-prognosis groups based on an algorithm incorporating variables of age, sex, physical findings, peripheral blood count at presentation, and immunophenotypic and cytogenetic analysis of blasts. Intensity of treatment depends on assignment to a particular prognosis group.

### Induction

Standard treatment for children with ALL begins with induction of remission with intravenous vincristine (Oncovin), oral prednisone, intramuscular L-asparaginase (Elspar), and intrathecal methotrexate. Daunorubicin (Cerubidine) may be included in high-risk patients. Renal function and serum uric acid should be normal or improving before treatment is started. Correction of anemia and treatment of infection should also be well under way before specific antileukemic therapy begins. Prednisone in a dosage of 40 mg per $M^2$ per day in three divided doses is given by mouth for 28 days; vincristine, 1.5 mg per $M^2$ (maximal dose, 2 mg) intravenously every 7 days for four doses; and L-asparaginase, 6000 IU per $M^2$ intramuscularly beginning on the third day of treatment and continuing at three doses per week for a total of nine doses. If daunorubicin is included, the dosage is 30 mg per $M^2$ intravenously weekly for three doses. The dose of intrathecal methotrexate is adjusted according to the age of the child: less than 2 years, 8 mg; 2 to 3 years, 10 mg; and 3 years and over, 12 mg. This is given on the first day of treatment and again on day 14.

### Consolidation

Remission is achieved when the bone marrow no longer contains leukemic blasts, extramedullary involvement has resolved, and peripheral blood counts are normalizing. At this point, treatment is directed at eradicating occult disease of the central nervous system, which is assumed to be present in most children. Intrathecal methotrexate is given weekly for four additional doses. All children in the poor-risk group and those over 10 years with intermediate-risk characteristics receive cranial radiation (1800 rad in 10 fractions), whereas children in the good-prognosis group and younger than 10 years in the intermediate group do not. Attempts are being made to eliminate cranial radiation without an unacceptable increase in the incidence of CNS relapse. Younger children (under 3) are thought to be at greater risk for central nervous system toxicity related to the radiation.

### Maintenance

Maintenance chemotherapy is part of every ALL protocol. A standard program includes vincristine, 1.5 mg per $M^2$ (maximal dose, 2 mg) administered intravenously once every 4 weeks. Prednisone, 40 mg per $M^2$ orally in three divided doses, is given for 5 days starting the day the vincristine is administered. 6-Mercaptopurine

(Purinethol), 75 mg per $M^2$ orally, is given once daily and methotrexate, 20 mg per $M^2$ orally, once weekly. Intrathecal methotrexate is administered every 12 weeks if children have not received cranial irradiation. Treatment is continued for 2 to 3 years from the time of diagnosis. Routine bone marrow studies during remission are not absolutely indicated because most relapsing children will exhibit changes in the peripheral blood count or show some other indication of relapse. Treatment of relapse is not jeopardized by delay of a few weeks in diagnosis.

Routine examination of the cerebrospinal fluid after cytocentrifugation is indicated every 12 weeks, since central nervous system leukemia is best treated before it becomes symptomatic.

### Additive Therapy

Children with an intermediate or poor prognosis are usually treated in clinical trials that attempt to identify therapy that represents an improvement over standard treatment. These protocols are characterized by the addition of drugs such as cytosine arabinoside (Cytosar-U), daunorubicin (Cerubidine), doxorubicin (Adriamycin), and cyclophosphamide (Cytoxan). In induction, consolidation, and remission, these drugs produce greater toxicity and are associated with an increased likelihood of infectious and other complications, particularly during induction. Whether an individual child should be treated on such a protocol and randomly assigned to a standard or innovative regimen is a difficult issue that should be thoroughly explored with the family. We are currently utilizing additive therapy with reintensification and reconsolidation after achievement of remission in all patients identified as having high-risk characteristics.

Infants have had a very poor prognosis with standard therapy, and all are treated in a more intensive fashion. Children with lymphomatous features are currently being treated with innovative programs that should be undertaken in a research setting. Burkitt's cell leukemia (i.e., B cell leukemia, L3) is treated in the same way as Burkitt's lymphoma.

### Relapse During Treatment

**Bone Marrow Relapse.** If bone marrow relapse occurs while the child is on maintenance therapy, the prognosis is very poor. A variety of chemotherapeutic approaches have produced few long-term survivors following relapse on therapy. One of the best reported regimens utilizes a standard reinduction with the addition of daunorubicin, 30 mg per $M^2$ intravenously weekly for three doses.

Maintenance treatment is given utilizing chemotherapeutic agents and/or regimens to which the patient has not previously been exposed.

Central nervous system prophylaxis should be repeated after relapse because the CNS is a frequent site of subsequent relapse. If there is a suitable donor, bone marrow transplantation following reinduction of remission is indicated for the child who relapses while on therapy, since this has produced long-term survival in approximately 30% of children so treated. Autologous bone marrow transplantation with monoclonal antibody–purged marrow is also a consideration for those patients without a histocompatible donor who have already received intense therapy with many agents.

**Central Nervous System Relapse.** This should be treated with intrathecal methotrexate until clearing of the CSF, followed by craniospinal irradiation. Systemic reinduction therapy is mandatory in patients with CNS relapse, which is a harbinger of bone marrow relapse. The entire treatment period must be prolonged following CNS relapse, and intrathecal chemotherapy must be included in the maintenance phase. Repeated CNS relapse is an indication for addition of cytosine arabinoside and hydrocortisone to intrathecal therapy. A second course of cranial irradiation should be avoided if the child is a marrow transplant candidate.

**Testicular Relapse.** This is treated with radiation to the scrotum (usually 2400 rad), systemic reinduction, and prolongation of the period of treatment.

### Relapse Off Treatment

Relapse after the child has finished a standard period of maintenance therapy has a better prognosis. It is treated in substantially the same manner as relapse occurring on treatment except that bone marrow transplantation is not currently recommended for children who relapse after being off treatment more than 1 year.

### ACUTE NONLYMPHOCYTIC LEUKEMIA (ANLL)

Standard therapy for nonlymphocytic leukemia has produced far fewer cured patients than treatment for lymphocytic leukemia. Prognostic factors have not been clearly defined. Almost all children with nonlymphocytic leukemia are treated in a similar fashion. This situation will probably change soon because of the emerging differences based on French-American-British (FAB) morphologic classification and cytogenetic analysis.

The standard induction therapy consists of cytosine arabinoside (Cytosar-U), 100 mg per $M^2$ per day by continuous intravenous infusion for 7 days; daunomycin (Cerubidine), 45 mg per $M^2$ is given by intravenous push daily for the first 3 days. Cytosine arabinoside is given intrathecally on day 1 to treat occult central nervous system disease, which is recognized with approximately the same frequency as in lymphocytic leukemia. The dose of intrathecal cytosine arabinoside is 20 mg for children under 1 year of age, 30 mg for children 1 to 2 years old, 50 mg for children 2 to 3 years old, and 70 mg for children over age 3 years. Following successful induction, intensification therapy with multiple agents is given. Total duration of therapy for ANLL is approximately 6 months.

We are currently evaluating a more intensive induction regimen that adds etoposide (VP-16), ara-C, 6-thioguanine, and dexamethasone to the "standard drugs." To date, the best long-term survival in children with ANLL has been achieved in patients who undergo bone marrow transplantation from a histocompatible donor following successful induction. The majority of patients, however, do not have a histocompatible donor. These patients currently undergo very intense chemotherapy with the inclusion of high-dose ara-C, for a short period of time. This type of treatment is being compared with autologous bone marrow transplantation in patients who do not have a compatible donor.

After successful bone marrow transplantation or intensification with high-dose chemotherapy, maintenance therapy in ANLL does not improve disease-free survival.

The intense treatment that is required for ANLL is associated with significant morbidity and mortality, especially related to sepsis. The treatment for ANLL should be carried out in a center capable of providing all components of intense supportive care.

Relapse of ANLL in the bone marrow is virtually always fatal when treated with conventional chemotherapy. It is a definite indication for bone marrow transplantation if possible.

### INITIAL MANAGEMENT OF ALL AND ANLL

This section applies to both types of acute leukemia (Table 1).

### Venous Access

Insertion of a permanent indwelling venous access device (Broviac, Hickman, Port-a-cath, etc.) should be considered as soon as possible in patients who will receive intensive therapy.

TABLE 1. **Initial and Emergency Measures for Acute Lymphocytic Leukemia (ALL) and Acute Nonlymphocytic Leukemia (ANLL)**

| Finding | Management |
|---|---|
| Diagnosis of leukemia | Inform family and reassure (see text) |
| WBC >100,000 ANLL WBC >200,000 ALL | Leukapheresis |
| Congestive heart failure and/or anemia | Transfuse packed red cells, 10 ml/kg (if WBC <100,000) |
| Bleeding | Transfuse platelets, 1 unit/M²/ 10,000 increment desired; determine whether disseminated intravascular coagulation is present |
| Infection | Blood cultures. Antibiotics for both gram-negative and gram-positive organisms |
| Hyperuricemia Hyperkalemia Renal failure | Allopurinol Hydration Urinary alkalinization |

### Anemia

In transfusing packed red cells to correct anemia, we use the same criteria for transfusion as in other patients. In the presence of cardiovascular compromise, fever, and a hemoglobin level less than 6 grams per dl, more urgent transfusion will be required. Blood products should be irradiated to 2000 rad to prevent graft-versus-host disease. Red cells should be given only to correct symptomatic anemia in children with hyperleukocytosis. For other children, packed cells in a volume of 10 ml per kg over 1 to 2 hours are usually tolerated without cardiovascular compromise. Several small transfusions may be necessary to raise the hemoglobin level to 8 to 9 grams per dl.

### Fever

Fever in the newly diagnosed child may be secondary to the leukemia or to infection. If the child is febrile, blood for cultures should be drawn. One should culture all local sites of infection, since even a small skin infection may lead to sepsis in these immunocompromised children. At this stage, if the child is not clinically septic and if the absolute neutrophil count (ANC) is above 500 per μl, antibiotics can be withheld pending culture results. Fever often resolves within hours of starting specific antileukemic therapy. However, if the patient is absolutely neutropenic (ANC less than 500 per μl) and febrile, antibiotic therapy should be initiated rapidly following obtainment of cultures.

If antibiotics are started, coverage for gram-negative organisms and penicillin-resistant staphylococci should be included. We use ceftazidime (Fortaz) at a dosage of 150 mg per kg per day intravenously in three divided doses and oxacillin (Prostaphlin) in a dosage of 150 to 300 mg per kg per day intravenously in three to four divided doses. Vancomycin (Vancocin) at 25 to 40 mg per kg per day intravenously is substituted if oxacillin-resistant organisms are suspected or identified. Fungal and other opportunistic infections are less likely to occur, and infections with common bacterial pathogens are more common at the time of diagnosis. If patients are still febrile on the seventh day of antibacterial therapy, amphotericin B (Fungizone) at a dosage of 0.5 mg per kg per day intravenously should be added empirically to the treatment program and continued until the ANC is above 500 per μl.

### Bleeding

Bleeding is usually caused by thrombocytopenia, although disseminated intravascular coagulation may be a contributing factor. One unit of platelets per M² produces an average increment of 10,000 per μl. Platelet counts of 50,000 per μl will usually produce normal hemostasis. In parallel with platelet transfusion, local measures to stop bleeding are usually indicated (for example, packing the nose for control of epistaxis).

### Hyperleukocytosis

Hyperleukocytosis (total white cell count over 100,000) occurs in 9 to 13% of children with ALL and in 5 to 22% of children with ANLL. Hyperleukocytosis increases blood viscosity by leading to blood cell aggregates and thrombi in the microcirculation. Immediate measures should include hydration, alkalinization, and allopurinol administration. Platelet transfusions should be instituted to maintain a platelet count over 20,000 per μl in order to minimize the risk of intracerebral hemorrhage. Red cell transfusion to achieve a hemoglobin concentration above 6 grams per dl should be avoided until the blast count is subsiding because the increased hematocrit will increase blood viscosity and the danger of hemorrhagic infarction. The role of leukapheresis to decrease the tumor burden and the white count is controversial. Patients with ANLL seem to be at higher risk for thrombotic and hemorrhagic complications secondary to hyperleukocytosis than patients with ALL. Therefore, leukapheresis should be considered if the white blood cell count is over 100,000 in ANLL and over 200,000 in ALL.

### Metabolic Stabilization

Newly diagnosed children are at risk for developing hyperuricemia, which can result in renal failure, hyperkalemia, and hypocalcemia. Measurements of uric acid, creatinine, sodium, potassium, calcium, and phosphorus should be obtained immediately and monitored closely during the initial management period. Allopurinol (Zyloprim), in a dosage of 100 mg per $M^2$ orally three times daily, should be started as soon as diagnosis is made. Hydration should be maintained with intravenous fluids. In the absence of renal failure, we use fluid containing 5% dextrose, 0.2% sodium chloride, 10 to 40 mEq per liter of potassium chloride, and sodium bicarbonate in a dosage of 40 to 60 mEq per $M^2$ per day. The goals of this hydration are to keep the body weight stable, urine output up to 100 ml per $M^2$ per hour, urine pH above 7.0, and serum sodium and potassium concentrations within normal limits. Usually, 3000 ml per $M^2$ per day is adequate. The goal of alkalinization is to prevent uric acid from precipitating in the renal tubules resulting in uric acid nephropathy. Once treatment with chemotherapy is begun, alkalinization should be discontinued because of the risk of hypocalcemia and hyperphosphatemia (the latter resulting from tumor cell lysis) leading to calcium and phosphorus precipitation in the kidney. Electrolytes, calcium, phosphorus, and uric acid should be frequently monitored, and allopurinol should be continued during induction. Rarely, renal dialysis may be indicated for uncontrollable tumor lysis syndrome and renal failure.

### Psychosocial Stabilization

The family and child with the diagnosis of leukemia are extremely vulnerable. The physician can offer realistic support by assuring the family that every child with the diagnosis has the potential for cure (the actual percentage in numerical terms ranges widely and can be predicted more accurately when other clinical features are taken into account). In addition, it is reassuring to families to know that most children will enter a period of remission (70 to 95%, depending on the type of leukemia). Assuring the family that they have done nothing to cause the disease, that it will not likely affect siblings, and that it could not have been prevented helps allay much of their anxiety. We point out that other family members should not be neglected in spite of the enormous attention that will be directed to the child with leukemia. Referral to a social worker and early identification of the need for financial assistance should be done during the first week. Published material, such as the book by Lynn S. Baker, *You and Leukemia: A Day at a Time* (revised ed., W. B. Saunders Co. , 1988), provides accurate information in understandable language and can enable the family to begin to frame their questions about how this disease will affect them. Other materials are available from the National Cancer Institute and the American Cancer Society. After the initial interview, further conferences with the parents will be necessary to reinforce material discussed earlier. Most parents are unable to assimilate all the facts while still coming to grips with the diagnosis of a potentially fatal disease in their child.

It is our policy to explain the diagnosis, the nature of the disease, and the prognosis to both patient and parents. We ensure that the child feels comfortable asking questions of parents, nurses, social workers, and physicians. Principles of treatment are also covered in an early session. Answers to questions always start with an assessment of the child's information level in asking it. The reaction of some parents to "protect" their child from this type of information must be resisted. However, the child can be protected from details he or she is not ready to handle by answering questions directly and concretely after first assessing what the patient already knows.

## MANAGEMENT DURING REMISSION

If leukemia remains under control, the result should be a child emotionally and physically capable of participating in a full range of normal activities in a healthy family environment. Prevention and therapy should be available for most problems that could endanger this outcome.

### Psychosocial Management

Children in remission will usually be in school and enjoying the normal activities of childhood. Athletics and other extracurricular activities are to be encouraged. Discipline both at school and at home should not be different for the child with leukemia. Siblings of the patient should receive adequate recognition to prevent those problems that occur when children feel they are secondary in the family's concerns.

A social worker familiar with the psychosocial effects of childhood cancer is an important member of the treating team. In addition to evaluating the child's and family's emotional resources, the social worker can assist in determining whether the family is eligible for assistance through various state or federal programs. Other support from the Leukemia Society of America and the American Cancer Society is available. Nonmedical expenses incurred by the family are often a greater burden because they are not covered by medical insurance. Facilities such as the Ronald McDonald Houses are available to reduce the cost of living away from home. The Leukemia Society of America may pay some travel costs. Car pooling may be possible. Certain costs are tax deductible.

Local support groups assist many families in dealing with problems associated with diagnosis of a potentially fatal disease. Many groups are affiliated with the Candlelighters Foundation (1312 18th Street NW, Suite 200, Washington DC 20036; telephone (202) 659–5136 or (800) 366-CCCF).

Some couples may need referral for marriage counseling. Every relationship in the family will be strained by the occurrence of leukemia in a child, and asking about these problems should become a routine part of medical care.

### Infection During Remission

**Fever.** Infection when the neutrophil count is over 1000 per µl may be handled just as it would be for a child without leukemia. That is, specific infections are treated whereas undifferentiated illnesses may be assumed to be viral and self-limited unless they take a different course. However, if a child has an indwelling central venous catheter (Broviac, Hickman or Port-a-cath), catheter-related sepsis must be ruled out and consideration given to administration of intravenous antibiotics (to cover gram-negative organisms as well as staphylococci) through the catheter until culture results are known.

If there is neutropenia (particularly if the count is under 500 per µl), fever alone is an indication for blood cultures and initiation of antibiotics as described above.

***Pneumocystitis carinii* Pneumonia.** This formerly fatal complication can be largely prevented by administration of prophylactic trimethoprim-sulfamethoxazole (Bactrim, Septra), orally 5 mg per kg (as the trimethoprim component) per day in two divided doses administered on 3 consecutive days each week. If the disease occurs, it should be treated with trimethoprim-sulfamethoxazole intravenously at a dosage of 10 to 20 mg per kg per day given in two to three doses. If this fails, pentamidine should be used. Respiratory failure is often a complication of this type of pneumonia, so that a child should be treated in a facility capable of ventilatory support. Pneumocystitis should be suspected in any child with a cough with or without fever and a chest radiograph that shows a diffuse interstitial process.

**Varicella.** If patients have had chickenpox prior to the diagnosis of leukemia, they will remain immune. If they have not had chickenpox and are exposed through a sibling or playmate (phys-

### TABLE 2. Drugs Used to Treat Acute Lymphocytic Leukemia

| | Commonly Encountered Adverse Reactions |
|---|---|
| Vincristine (Oncovin) | Alopecia, neuritic pain, constipation, difficulty in walking, peripheral neuropathy, leukopenia, severe cellulitis if extravasated |
| Prednisone (Deltasone) | Immunosuppression, increased appetite and weight gain, Cushing's syndrome, myopathy, mood changes, diabetes mellitus, relative adrenocortical insufficiency in times of stress |
| L-Asparaginase (Elspar) | Anaphylactic reactions, decreased protein synthesis (including coagulation factors), pancreatitis and diabetes mellitus |
| 6-Mercaptopurine (Purinethol) | Myelosuppression, hepatotoxicity, immunosuppression |
| Methotrexate (low dose, oral) | Stomatitis, myelosuppression, immunosuppression, photosensitivity, hepatic fibrosis |
| Doxorubicin (Adriamycin) | Myelosuppression, cardiac toxicity, alopecia, nausea and vomiting, stomatitis, gastrointestinal ulceration, severe cellulitis if extravasated, hypersensitivity reactions |
| Daunorubicin (Cerubidine) | Myelosuppression, cardiac toxicity, alopecia, nausea and vomiting, stomatitis, gastrointestinal ulceration, severe cellulitis if extravasated, hypersensitivity reactions |
| Cyclophosphamide (Cytoxan) | Myelosuppression, nausea and vomiting, hemorrhagic cystitis, decreased gonadal function, alopecia |
| Cytosine arabinoside (Cytosar) | Myelosuppression, nausea and vomiting, stomatitis |

ical contact), they are at risk for fatal complications of chickenpox. Varicella-zoster immune globulin (VZIG) in a dose of 1 vial per 10 kg is given intramuscularly within 96 hours of exposure. This product is available through Red Cross blood banks. VZIG may attenuate chickenpox and not prevent it completely. If either primary varicella or varicella-zoster occurs in a patient being treated for leukemia, all chemotherapy should be stopped and the patient hospitalized and treated with intravenous acyclovir. Treatment is continued until all lesions are crusted over to prevent potentially fatal systemic dissemination of infection.

**Immunization.** All live virus vaccines (measles, mumps, rubella, and polio) should be avoided while a child is on treatment and for 6 months thereafter. Diphtheria, pertussis, and tetanus (DPT) immunizations may be given safely and have recently been shown to give effective antibody levels, even while chemotherapy is continued. Immunizations may be administered on schedule to siblings, although they should receive killed polio vaccines.

TABLE 3. **Treatment of Chemotherapy Extravasations**

**Vincristine (Oncovin)**
1. Stop administration of drug immediately if extravasation is suspected.
2. If possible, gently withdraw 2–3 ml of blood or any extravasated solution.
3. Remove the needle.
4. Inject hyaluronidase (Wydase) locally. Use a 27-gauge needle and multiple injections subcutaneously to include the entire erythematous area. Amount of hyaluronidase will vary depending on the size of the infiltration.
5. Apply moderate heat to the area to help disperse the drug and decrease local tissue destruction.
6. Notify responsible MD.

**Steps for Other Vesicant Antineoplastic Agents**
1. Stop administration of drugs immediately if extravasation is suspected.
2. If possible, gently withdraw 2–3 ml of blood or any extravasated solution.
3. Remove the needle.
4. Inject hydrocortisone sodium succinate (Solu-Cortef), 50–100 mg subcutaneously. Use a 27-gauge needle and multiple injections, being sure to include the entire erythematous area. Dosage of Solu-Cortef will vary depending on the size of the infiltration.
5. Apply a film of steroid cream, cover the skin with sterile gauze, and secure with paper tape.
6. Apply ice packs to the area q 20 min for 24 hr.
7. Have the patient apply steroid cream bid until all the erythema has disappeared, more often if tension in the area. Encourage exercising the affected hand or arm; do not allow pain to restrict full range of motion.
8. Notify responsible MD.

## Myelosuppression

During remission on standard treatment, it is unusual for major myelosuppression to occur in other than the granulocyte series. The more intensive regimens currently in use, however, may produce significant thrombocytopenia and anemia. These complications should be managed with appropriate transfusion support. Persistent pancytopenia may herald the onset of relapse, and a bone marrow examination is indicated if recovery is not prompt. Modification of doses of maintenance drugs may be necessary to prevent severe myelosuppression.

## Drug-Related Toxicities

The institution where therapy is planned should provide the treating physician with information about the toxicities of the specific drugs a patient is to receive. Problems of alopecia, constipation, hypercortisonism, and myelosuppression are common to all treatment programs. Most of the drugs used in childhood leukemia treatment are reviewed in the *Physicians' Desk Reference* (Medical Economics Co., Oradell, NJ, 1990). Table 2 is a partial list of drug toxicities; Table 3 outlines a method for treating extravasation of vesicant drugs.

# THE CHRONIC LEUKEMIAS
method of
**KENNETH A. FOON, M.D.**
*Roswell Park Cancer Institute*
*Buffalo, New York*

and

**ROBERT PETER GALE, M.D., PH.D.**
*UCLA School of Medicine*
*Los Angeles, California*

### CHRONIC MYELOGENOUS LEUKEMIA

Chronic myelogenous leukemia (CML) is a hematologic neoplasm characterized by the proliferation and accumulation of mature myeloid cells and their progenitors, including granulocytes, red blood cells, monocyte-macrophages, megakaryocytes, and some B lymphocytes.

CML is a clonal disorder caused by a somatic mutation in a pluripotent hematopoietic stem cell. Studies of polymorphic genetic systems such as glucose-6-phosphate dehydrogenase in heterozygous individuals with CML indicate the presence of a single allele in the malignant cells. Additional markers of clonality include the presence of the Philadelphia (Ph[1]) chromosome and other clonal cytogenetic markers as well as quinacrine fluorescence staining of chromosomes.

CML represents 30% of adult leukemia. The median age is 50 years, with a slight male predominance. The etiology of CML is unknown. The incidence of CML increased substantially in Japanese atomic bomb survivors; most patients had the Ph[1] chromosome. This effect was greatest in young individuals and occurred relatively rapidly. This increase in CML was not specific; incidences of acute myelogenous leukemia (AML) and acute lymphoblastic leukemia (ALL) were also elevated. However, there is no identifiable etiologic factor in most cases of CML. CML is an acquired disorder; there is no concordance for CML between monozygotic, identical twins. Furthermore, the Ph[1] chromosome, characteristic of the malignant clone, is not present in unaffected cells such as fibroblasts nor in residual normal hematopoietic stem cells.

### Chronic and Acute Phases

An understanding of several clinical features of CML is essential to a critical consideration of the underlying molecular events. CML is characterized by two discrete phases: a chronic phase, typically of 3 years duration; and an acute phase, which lasts from one-half to 1 year. In 50% to 75% of individuals, there is an intervening accelerated phase associated with increased myelopoiesis and resistance or inability to tolerate therapy.

During the chronic phase of CML, increased myelopoiesis is restricted predominantly to granulocytes, monocyte-macrophages, and platelets; increased erythrocyte production is rare. In most instances, the affected cells retain the ability to mature normally and have a normal or slightly increased life span. The acute phase of CML, in contrast, is characterized by loss of differentiation; the cells fail to mature but retain the ability to divide, characteristics of myeloblasts and less differentiated myeloid cells.

## The Philadelphia Chromosome

In 1960, Nowell and Hungerford described a minute G group chromosome in bone marrow cells from two patients with CML; they designated this the Ph[1] chromosome. The Ph[1] chromosome is a shortened chromosome 22 arising from a reciprocal translocation between chromosome 9 and 22, designated t(9;22). Cell synchronization and high-resolution banding techniques have identified the chromosome breakpoints as t(9;22) (q34.1;q11.21). The Ph[1] chromosome is present in hematopoietic cells from 95% of individuals with CML. In most cases of CML, most or all of the ABL proto-oncogene located on chromosome 9 is translocated into a gene designated BCR (for breakpoint cluster region) on chromosome 22.

## Clinical Manifestations

Typical presenting symptoms in CML include fatigue, malaise, headache, and weight loss. Infections and bleeding are uncommon at presentation. Rare patients will present with leukostasis with cerebral vascular accidents, infarctions, venous thrombosis, and pulmonary insufficiency. Physical examination may demonstrate splenomegaly; hepatomegaly is unusual at diagnosis. Lymphadenopathy is very infrequent. Many patients, of course, are diagnosed from routine white blood counts performed for other reasons.

With disease progression, there are increasing problems with fevers, weight loss, infections, bone and joint pains, bleeding, and increasing hepatosplenomegaly. Extramedullary disease may herald transformation to the blast or acute phase. Frequent sites of extramedullary disease include soft tissue, skin, central nervous system, lymph nodes, and bone.

The hallmark of CML is leukocytosis with immature myeloid cells in the peripheral blood;

blasts are less than 5%. Typically, there are an elevated serum lactate dehydrogenase, uric acid, vitamin $B_{12}$, and $B_{12}$ binding capacity. The latter reflect the increased granulocytic pool. The granulocytic character still has a low leukocyte alkaline phosphatase score. There may be eosinophilia, basophilia, and monocytosis.

The bone marrow is hypercellular with myeloid and megakaryocytic hyperplasia and high myeloid erythroid ratios. The percentage of blasts is normal or minimally increased. Basophilia, eosinophilia, and monocytosis are common.

With acceleration, there is increasing anemia, thrombocytopenia, blasts, and cytogenetic evolution. Collagen fibrosis in the bone marrow may be associated with megakaryocytopenia, thrombocytopenia, and marrow failure, which is the terminal event in a minority of patients.

CML blast crisis is defined by the presence of 30% or more blasts in the peripheral blood or bone marrow. Sixty per cent of cases are myeloid blast crisis with myeloperoxidase-positive blast cells; and 20% are lymphoid blast crisis, which is myeloperoxidase negative and terminal deoxynucleotidyl transferase (TdT) positive. Most cases of lymphoid blast crisis are also positive for the common acute lymphoblastic leukemia antigen (CD10). The remaining cases are either undifferentiated blast crisis, megakaryocytic, or erythroid.

## Therapy

### Chronic Phase

Two drugs commonly used to treat CML are busulfan (Myleran) and hydroxyurea (Hydrea). Busulfan is an alkylating agent. Busulfan appears to affect early progenitor cells. The usual dose is 2 to 8 mg daily. Busulfan should be discontinued when the white count is less than $20 \times 10^9$ U per liter, because of its protracted effect.

Hydroxyurea is a ribonucleotidase inhibitor. It differs from busulfan in that it induces rapid disease control for a short duration. The initial dose is 1 to 3 grams daily. The dose is reduced in half with each 50% reduction of the white blood cell count. A white blood cell count of 20 to $30 \times 10^9$ per liter is a reasonable goal. Busulfan is favored by many physicians because it requires less frequent monitoring. However, it is associated with more serious side effects, which include severe myelosuppression; pulmonary, endocardial, and bone marrow fibrosis; and an Addison-like wasting syndrome.

There is no obvious survival advantage to either busulfan or hydroxyurea. High-dose intermittent therapy appears equivalent to daily therapy. It is rare for patients treated with these drugs to have disappearance of the Ph[1] chromosome.

Other drugs used in CML include chlorambucil (Leukeran), melphalan (Alkeran), 6-mercaptopurine (Purinethol), and cyclophosphamide (Cytoxan). These offer no advantage except in circumstances in which the side effects of busulfan or hydroxyurea are unacceptable or they are no longer effective for disease control.

Intensive leukapheresis may control the blood counts; however, it is expensive and cumbersome. Leukapheresis is useful in emergencies in which leukostasis-related complications such as pulmonary failure or cerebrovascular accidents are likely. It may also have a role in pregnant females, in whom it is important to avoid potentially teratogenic drugs.

Splenectomy was used in CML because of the suggestion that evolution to acute phase might occur in the spleen. However, splenectomy is not effective in controlled trials and is reserved for symptomatic painful splenomegaly unresponsive to chemotherapy or for significant anemia or thrombocytopenia associated with hypersplenism. Splenic radiation is also used to reduce the size of the spleen in some instances.

The goal of intensive combination chemotherapy in CML is eradication of the Ph[1] chromosome–positive clone. Combination chemotherapy includes cytarabine (Cytosar-U), 6-thioguanine (Thioguanine), and an anthracycline (Adriamycin), similar to AML treatment regimens. Typically, 30 to 50% of patients have had suppression of the Ph[1] chromosome–positive clone. In some studies, median survival is increased (50 to 60 months versus 30 to 40 months). These differences might be explained by patient selection; none of these studies was randomized. Most attempts at intensive chemotherapy were abandoned.

Interferons are naturally occurring proteins classified into three major classes: alpha, beta, and gamma. They have antiviral, antiproliferative, immunomodulating differentiating and oncogene regulatory properties. Alpha and beta interferons have structural and biologic similarities and bind to the same receptor. Gamma interferon differs structurally and biologically and binds a different receptor.

Interferons have a direct antiproliferative effect on the leukemia clone in CML. Interferon-gamma suppresses Ph[1] chromosome–positive cells following in vitro culture. Early studies in 51 patients with chronic phase CML treated with interferon-alpha* (Intron-A, Roferon-A) at 3 to

$9 \times 10^6$ U intramuscularly daily led to 36 complete hematologic remissions. Twenty patients demonstrated a decrease in the proportion of Ph[1]-positive cells. There was no evidence of BCR rearrangement in persons with complete disappearance of Ph[1] chromosome–positive cells. In another study, 44 persons with chronic phase CML received interferon-alpha $5 \times 10^6$ U per $M^2$ intramuscularly daily; 27 achieved a complete hematologic remission and 17 showed a decrease in the Ph[1] chromosome–positive cells. Early treatment in chronic phase (within 12 months of diagnosis) resulted in higher hematologic and cytogenetic response rates. Recombinant interferon-gamma is also active in CML but seems inferior to interferon-alpha. Because of nonpartial cross-resistance, IFN-gamma and -alpha are being studied in combination.

Side effects of interferons include fever, chills, flu-like symptoms, headache, nausea, diarrhea, and anorexia; these are rarely dose limiting. Serious toxicities include severe anorexia, weight loss, neurotoxicity, thrombocytopenia, anemia, cardiac and renal abnormalities, and bone marrow hypoplasia.

Combinations of chemotherapy with interferon-alpha have also been investigated. This is based on the rationale that intensive chemotherapy improved survival in intermediate- and high-risk patients, whereas interferon-alpha had its best results in low-risk groups. Ph[1] suppression occurred rapidly and was of short duration with intensive chemotherapy and developed slowly with interferon-alpha therapy and was longer lasting. In one study, 32 patients were treated with three cycles of intensive chemotherapy with daunorubicin (Cerubidine), vincristine (Oncovin), cytarabine, and prednisone, which were followed by interferon-alpha, $3 \times 10^6$ U intramuscularly daily. Over half of these patients had a greater than 65% suppression of the proportion of Ph[1] chromosome–positive cells. The projected 3-year survival is 82%.

The goal of bone marrow transplantation is to cure CML. Transplants are typically from HLA-identical siblings or identical twins. Sometimes autologous transplants using bone marrow stored in the chronic phase are performed. Results of twin transplants in the chronic phase indicate 70 to 80% 3-year disease-free survival with a 20% relapse rate. Results are considerably less favorable in the accelerated and acute phase.

Results of HLA-identical sibling transplants in CML indicate a 3-year disease-free survival rate of 40 to 70%. Transplant results are best in the chronic phase—about 60% 5-year disease-free survival with a 10% relapse rate. Results are best in persons less than 30 years of age. Transplants in more advanced CML result in about 20 to 30%

---

*This use of interferon-alpha is not listed in the manufacturers' official directives.

5-year disease-free survival and about 50% relapse. Most data suggest that transplantation should be performed in the chronic phase. Although some patients receive transplants at the time of diagnosis, others prefer to wait 1 to 2 years. Sometimes this decision is based on analysis of risk factors for duration of the chronic phase.

Typical conditioning regimens include high-dose cyclophosphamide and total body radiation. Modifications such as adding high-dose cytarabine, anthracycline, etoposide (VePesid), or busulfan produce similar results. Recently busulfan and cyclophosphamide without radiation were reported to also be effective.

T cell depletion has been used in CML to decrease the incidence and severity of graft-versus-host disease. Although effective, it appears that this benefit is offset by increased graft failure and leukemia relapse; disease-free survival is not improved.

Splenectomy pre-transplantation was suggested to decrease relapse post-transplantation. It is associated with a more rapid engraftment and decreased platelet transfusions. However, no decrease in relapse was observed.

### Accelerated and Acute Phase

The myeloid form of acute phase CML is usually resistant to chemotherapy. Nevertheless, it is typically treated with regimens similar to those used for AML. Induction of bone marrow aplasia to allow CML or chronic phase cells has been attempted. Drugs such as anthracycline and cytarabine are often used in the myeloid acute phase. Remission rates of 20 to 30% are reported, but these are generally short lived and median survival is 2 to 12 months. High-dose cytarabine may result in more remissions but no significant benefit in survival. Remission in myeloid acute phase CML is characterized by persistence of the Ph chromosome and is therefore regarded as reinduction of chronic phase.

Use of differentiation agents in myeloid acute phase CML was also attempted. Several agents induce differentiation of leukemia cells in vitro including retinoids, homoharringtonine, interferons, and cytarabine. In one trial, mithramycin (Mithracin*), 1 mg per $M^2$ two to three times weekly, and hydroxyurea reinstated the chronic phase in six of nine patients in the myeloid acute phase.

Therapy of lymphoid acute phase is more successful, with a median survival of 9 to 12 months. Remissions are achieved in up to 70% of persons treated with vincristine, prednisone, and an anthracycline. Unfortunately, all eventually relapse. Although a second remission is sometimes achieved, none of these patients are cured.

The results of bone marrow transplantation in the accelerated and acute phase of CML are less favorable than in the chronic phase. Relapse rates as high as 60% are reported. Five-year disease-free survival is reported in 10 to 20% of recipients. Because there are no cures with chemotherapy, bone marrow transplantation is the therapy of choice.

Recently, there has been interest in autotransplantation in CML. Results of autotransplantation in advanced CML are disappointing. Approximately 50% of patients obtain a second chronic phase; it is typically short lived, and less than 25% of patients survive 1 year.

## CHRONIC LYMPHOID LEUKEMIAS

### Chronic Lymphocytic Leukemia

Chronic lymphocytic leukemia (CLL) is characterized by proliferation and accumulation of mature-appearing but biologically immature B lymphocytes. The National Cancer Institute Sponsored Working Group and the International Workshop on Chronic Lymphoid Leukemia have proposed similar criteria for the diagnosis of CLL, which include (1) phenotypic B cells bearing the CD5 antigen, (2) absolute lymphocytosis (greater than $5 \times 10^9$ per liter) sustained for 4 weeks, (3) mature lymphocytes with no more than 55% atypical and immature lymphoid cells, (4) greater than 30% bone marrow involvement.

CLL typically occurs in persons over 50 years of age (median age, 60 years). Less than 10% of cases occur in adults under 40 years of age; rare cares are reported in children. The cause(s) of CLL is unknown. Unlike CML and acute leukemias, CLL is not induced by radiation, chemicals, or alkylating agents. CLL represents 30% of leukemias in the West. Ten thousand new cases are diagnosed annually in the United States. In contrast, CLL is rare in the Orient, representing less than 5% of all leukemias.

CLL results from malignant transformation of a B lymphocyte; the small proportion of reported cases involving T lymphocytes most likely represent misdiagnosed cases of one of the chronic T lymphoid leukemias (mentioned later) or yet unidentified T cell malignancies. CLL is clonal; the cells express a single immunoglobulin light chain, either kappa or lambda on the cell surface. More sophisticated techniques confirm clonality by unique immunoglobulin idiotype, a single pattern of glucose-6-phosphate dehydrogenase (G6PD) activity in heterozygotes, clonal chromo-

*This use of mithramycin is not listed in the manufacturer's official directive.

somal abnormalities, and clonal immunoglobulin gene rearrangement.

Hypogammaglobulinemia occurs in about one-half of persons with CLL. This incidence is time dependent; eventually almost all develop hypogammaglobulinemia. Infections, particularly with encapsulated organisms and more recently with gram-negative bacteria, are a frequent cause of morbidity and mortality.

Many persons with CLL may develop features of autoimmunity of the hematopoietic system. For example, autoimmune hemolytic anemia occurs in about 20% of cases sometime during the course of the disease. This usually results from IgG antibodies against Rh blood group antigens. These autoantibodies are polyclonal and are therefore not produced by the malignant B cell clone of CLL. Also, about 10% of persons with CLL develop thrombocytopenia or neutropenia from autoantibodies to platelets or neutrophils. Rarely, patients develop a syndrome resembling pure red cell aplasia.

Important clinical correlations have been gleaned from recent studies. The first important correlation is that an abnormal karyotype is a poor prognostic sign and that trisomy 12 and possibly 14q+ are the least favorable abnormalities. In addition, those with increasing numbers of chromosomal abnormalities do more poorly. Unlike CML and follicular lymphomas, in most cases the karyotype is unchanged in an individual patient.

### Clinical Features

One of the major challenges in CLL is to individualize therapy. The course of CLL is variable. Some persons are older (median age, 60 years), or have only elevated lymphocytes, asymptomatic lymphadenopathy, or splenomegaly. Others have age-related medical complications. These older persons are unlikely to die of CLL and may require no specific treatment. In contrast, some young persons with CLL present with severe bone marrow failure including anemia and thrombocytopenia. They may have a rapid, progressive course with median survival of less than 2 years. Most persons with CLL have an intermediate prognosis and do reasonably well for several years without therapy but eventually require treatment. Very rarely, spontaneous remissions are observed in persons with well-documented CLL.

Ideally, one would use prognostic factors to select optimal therapy. Several staging systems that reflect grouping of prognostic variables are proposed. The Rai classification originally included five stages based on lymphocyte levels, lymphadenopathy, splenomegaly or hepatomeg-

aly, and nonimmune-related anemia (less than 11 grams per dl) and thrombocytopenia (less than $100 \times 10^9$ per liter). This system was simplified into three stages: low (Stage 0), intermediate (Stages I and II), and high (Stages III and IV) (Table 1). These groups constitute approximately 25%, 50%, and 25% of patients, respectively.

The Binet classification also has three stages (Table 1), which are distinguished based on bone marrow failure and the number of abnormal lymphoid areas. Stages A, B, and C account for 50%, 30%, and 20%, respectively.

### Therapy

Persons with CLL commonly develop hypogammaglobulinemia, which may be severe. The etiology is complex and is probably related to both intrinsic and extrinsic abnormalities of B and T lymphocyte function. These persons also respond abnormally to immunization. Intramuscular immunoglobulin therapy has been evaluated; no benefit was seen, but most investigators consider the dose and schedule inadequate. A prospective randomized study suggests that intravenous immunoglobulin (400 mg per kg given every 3 weeks) reduces bacterial infections of moderate

TABLE 1. **Staging Systems for Chronic Lymphocytic Leukemia**

| | **Rai Staging System** | |
|---|---|---|
| Stage* | Criteria | Median Survival (yr) |
| 0 | Lymphocytes >15 × 10⁹/L Bone marrow >40% lymphocytes | >10 |
| I and II | Blood and bone marrow lymphocytosis plus lymphadenopathy and/or liver and/or spleen enlarged | 5 |
| III and IV | Blood and bone marrow lymphocytosis plus anemia (Hgb <11 grams/dl) and/or thrombocytopenia (platelets <100 × 10⁹/L) | 2 |

| | **Binet Staging System** | |
|---|---|---|
| Stage* | Criteria | Median Survival (yr) |
| A | No anemia or thrombocytopenia, less than three of the following five areas involved: axillary, inguinal-cervical (unilateral or bilateral), lymphadenopathy, liver, spleen | 9 |
| B | No anemia or thrombocytopenia; three or more involved areas | 4 |
| C | Anemia (Hgb <10 grams/dl) and/or thrombocytopenia (platelets <100 × 10⁹/L) | 2 |

*Autoimmune hemolytic anemia and thrombocytopenia are independent of stage or group.

severity. Also, the probability of remaining infection-free was increased, as was the time to first infection. Other infections were not affected, nor were autoimmune complications. The major issue in this situation is detecting which persons with CLL should receive this treatment. Presumably, these are likely to be those with severe hypogammaglobulinemia or with a prior history of serious infections.

Immune-mediated hemolytic anemia, thrombocytopenia, and neutropenia are generally treated with prednisone. Persons who fail to respond may require splenectomy. Chemotherapy may be required to control the underlying disease. Intravenous gammaglobulin is also being studied in immune thrombocytopenia and anemia that develop in CLL.

One unresolved question in the treatment of CLL is when to initiate therapy. There is no evidence that therapy of persons with only elevated leukocytes and lymphadenopathy prolongs survival. When limited lymph node enlargement causes symptoms, local or systemic therapy may be initiated. Most physicians initiate systemic therapy when patients develop anemia, thrombocytopenia, or massive splenomegaly.

Chlorambucil (Leukeran) is the drug most commonly used to treat CLL. It is an aromatic derivative of nitrogen mustard that is absorbed orally. The standard dose of chlorambucil is 0.08 to 0.12 mg per kg of body weight per day; it may also be given at a dose of 0.4 to 1 mg per kg once every 2 to 4 weeks. Response rates to chlorambucil are about 60%, with 10 to 20% complete remissions. Responses may take several months to achieve. Cyclophosphamide (Cytoxan), 50 to 100 mg per $M^2$ orally daily or 300 mg per $M^2$ orally for 5 days every month, is probably as effective as chlorambucil and can be given intravenously or orally. Corticosteroids are used to control leukocytosis and to treat immune-mediated hemolytic anemia and thrombocytopenia. The usual dosage is 30 to 60 mg per $M^2$ of body surface area per day. Corticosteroids should not be used alone to treat CLL except for autoimmune hemolytic anemia and thrombocytopenia, or in advanced disease unresponsive to other therapies. Prednisone is often given with chlorambucil. Fludarabine monophosphate is also effective in CLL. The dosage is 25 to 30 mg per $M^2$ intravenously per day on days 1 through 5 monthly. In recent studies, partial and complete responses were reported in almost 50% of patients resistant to standard therapies. 2'-Deoxycoformycin (pentostatin), an adenosine deaminase inhibitor, also has activity in CLL (4 mg per $M^2$ intravenously every 2 weeks), as does chlorodeoxyadenosine (0.1 mg per kg daily by continuous intravenous infusion days 1

through 7 monthly). These latter three drugs are investigational.

The role of multidrug chemotherapy in CLL is controversial. As indicated, corticosteroids are often included in combination with chlorambucil, but convincing data that this combination increases the response or improves survival are not available. Combination therapy with cyclophosphamide (300 mg per $M^2$ orally on days 1 to 5 every month or 800 mg per $M^2$ on day 1 every month intravenously), vincristine (1 mg per $M^2$ intravenously on day 1 every month), and prednisone (40 mg per $M^2$ orally on days 1 to 5 every month) (CVP) is used in advanced disease. Response rates are comparable with those of chlorambucil or chlorambucil with or without prednisone; there may be a role for this combination in persons resistant to chlorambucil. Recent reports suggest that adding doxorubicin (Adriamycin) on day 1 at 25 mg per $M^2$ to CVP improves survival. Other chemotherapy combinations are being investigated but cannot be recommended at present.

Whole-body irradiation is proposed as a therapy for advanced CLL. This approach has severe hematologic toxicity, and responses are no better than those achieved with chemotherapy. Despite these limitations, whole-body irradiation may be useful in persons resistant to chemotherapy. Local irradiation is used to treat lymphadenopathy compromising vital organs and for painful bone lesions. Splenic irradiation is also used to treat painful splenomegaly, progressive lymphocytosis, anemia, and thrombocytopenia.

There is no role for splenectomy in the routine therapy of CLL. However, it may be useful for hemolytic anemia, thrombocytopenia, pancytopenia, and painful splenomegaly. Splenectomy may lead to a sustained improvement in previously depressed hematologic parameters in persons with hypersplenism.

In summary, persons with low-stage disease (Stage 1 or A) have not been convincingly shown to benefit from treatment. Initial therapy for persons requiring treatment is usually chlorambucil or cyclophosphamide, with or without prednisone, given as pulse therapy every 2 to 4 weeks. Combinations of other chemotherapeutic agents should be reserved for more advanced disease. Persons with intermediate-stage disease (Stage I, II, or B) have comparable response rates with chlorambucil and CVP. Persons with advanced disease (Stage III, IV, or C) respond favorably to CVP with low-dose doxorubicin, but this combination cannot be recommended until these data are confirmed.

Another unanswered question in the therapy of CLL is whether maintenance chemotherapy is useful. Currently, there is little evidence that maintenance chemotherapy in CLL improves survival, although one large study suggested that 18 months of treatment prolonged survival in persons with Stages III and IV CLL.

### Prolymphocytic Leukemia

Prolymphocytic leukemia (PLL) was first described by Galton and coworkers in 1974. The white blood cell count is typically greater than $100 \times 10^9$ per liter and consists predominantly of prolymphocytes. Extensive spleen involvement is common, as are hepatomegaly and bone marrow infiltration; lymphadenopathy is usually absent or minimal. The disease is typically aggressive and responds poorly to therapy. PLL may be a disease of B or T lymphocytes.

The median age of persons with PLL (both B and T cell types) is approximately 60 years, with a strong male predominance. The etiology is unknown.

#### Clinical Features

Typical presenting features of B-PLL are fatigue, weakness, and weight loss. Fever unassociated with infection is also common. Some persons experience abdominal pain and early satiety from massive splenomegaly. The outstanding physical sign is splenomegaly; hepatomegaly may also be prominent. Lymphadenopathy is absent or modest. Rare persons have petechiae and purpura from thrombocytopenia. T-PLL has similar features, with the addition of skin involvement in 25% of cases.

Leukocytes often exceed $100 \times 10^9$ per liter and are composed predominantly of prolymphocytes. The hemoglobin is less than 12 grams per dl, and platelets are less than $150 \times 10^9$ per liter; some persons have granulocytopenia.

#### Therapy

PLL typically exhibits a rapid downhill course. Combination chemotherapy with cyclophosphamide (750 mg per $M^2$ on day 1, intravenously), doxorubicin (50 mg per $M^2$ on day 1, intravenously), vincristine (2 mg on day 1, intravenously), and prednisone (100 mg per day, on days 1 to 5, orally) at 3- to 4-week intervals is often used. Some complete remissions are reported. Splenic radiation is also used to treat PLL. In one study, 12 patients were treated with weekly doses of 100 cGy to a maximum total of 1000 cGy; there was little morbidity, and 7 patients responded. Splenectomy is reported to be successful in some instances.

### Hairy Cell Leukemia

Hairy cell leukemia ("leukemic reticuloendotheliosis") was first described by Borouncle and coworkers in 1958. Remarkable progress in the diagnosis, biology, immunology, and therapy of this disease has occurred over the past 15 years. Hairy cell leukemia is a B cell disease; a rare T cell variant is reported (less than 1% of cases).

Hairy cell leukemia accounts for 1 to 2% of leukemias. It affects predominantly males in a ratio of 5:1. The median age of affected persons is approximately 50 years. In the U.S., most patients are white.

Human T cell leukemia virus-II (HTLV-II) has been isolated from cells of rare patients with T cell hairy cell leukemia. Thus far, a viral etiology for typical hairy cell leukemia cannot be implicated.

#### Clinical Features

The most common presenting complaints are weakness and fatigue. One-third of persons have a bleeding tendency with easy bruising; one-third have recurrent infections. Abdominal discomfort from an enlarged spleen is present in 25%. A few persons have weight loss, fever, and night sweats. Splenomegaly is the most common physical finding at diagnosis and is found in virtually all patients, over 80% of persons having massive enlargement. Approximately 10% of patients have lymphadenopathy and 20% hepatomegaly with abnormal liver function tests. The serum protein electrophoresis is abnormal in 25%, but a monoclonal pattern is rare. However, recent data suggest that a monoclonal pattern is commonly detected by immunofixation. Most persons present with mild to moderate normochromic normocytic anemia secondary to replacement of the bone marrow by leukemia cells and to hypersplenism. Approximately 20% of cases have a leukemia phase. Eighty per cent of affected persons have neutropenia, and 50% have platelets less than $100 \times 10^9$ per liter. Qualitative platelet abnormalities are common.

One-third of persons with hairy cell leukemia develop infections during the course of their disease; over half of these involve gram-negative organisms. Atypical mycobacteria is common and may require an open lung biopsy. Disseminated fungal diseases may occur, whereas *Pneumocystis carinii* infection is rare.

Other complications of hairy cell leukemia include vasculitis and bone lesions. Systemic vasculitis is documented by biopsy of skin lesions. The management usually requires high-dose steroids. Long-bone involvement, usually of the femur, can result in lytic lesions and associated pain and pathologic fractures.

#### Therapy

Approximately 10% of persons with hairy cell leukemia never require treatment. They are usually elderly, have only modest splenomegaly, and have granulocytes greater than $1 \times 10^9$ per liter. The remainder ultimately require therapy. Initial therapy for hairy cell leukemia is usually splenectomy. Spleen size does not predict response to splenectomy. Approximately 50% of cases have normalization of blood counts; this response does not correlate with spleen size but rather with the degree of bone marrow replacement by hairy cells. Usually a low percentage of hairy cells persists in the peripheral blood. It is suggested that persons with extensive replacement of bone marrow by hairy cells might benefit from alternate therapies. Post splenectomy, approximately one-half show disease progression from several months to greater than 10 years later. Approximately one-half develop a leukemia phase. In the remaining one-half, bone marrow failure is the rule. In both groups, the bone marrow is densely infiltrated by hairy cells. Until recently, persons with progressive disease received chlorambucil. This improves erythrocytes and platelets but does not improve granulocytes. Other putative therapies such as halotestin and oxymetholone are not effective. Intensive combination chemotherapy is toxic and rarely effective.

Newer therapies are active in hairy cell leukemia. Interferon-alpha at low doses ($2 \times 10^6$ U per $M^2$ three times weekly with interferon-alfa-2b [Intron-A] or $3 \times 10^6$ U daily with interferon-alfa-2a [Roferon-A]) induces complete or partial remissions in 90% of patients. Because less than 5% of persons become resistant to interferon and 90% have normalization or near-normalization of blood counts, most patients live normal lives without transfusions, bleeding, or infections. Recent data suggest that approximately 5% of patients develop neutralizing antibody to the interferon-alpha. Toxicity is usually restricted to mild fatigue and malaise. Many persons with good partial remissions or complete remissions can discontinue interferon for periods of 1 to 3 years; they respond again when the disease progresses.

2'-Deoxycoformycin* or pentostatin,* an adenosine deaminase inhibitor, is also effective in hairy cell leukemia. Treatment with 4 mg per $M^2$ every 2 weeks produces complete and partial remissions in over 90% of cases. 2'-Deoxycoformycin leads to a more rapid response than interferon-alpha and provides more complete responses. Toxicities include rash, diarrhea, nausea, and vomiting; these are generally mild at the doses cited. Recent data suggest that treatment with 2'deoxycoformycin causes a profound decrease in all lymphocyte subsets associated with a marked decrease in proliferative responses

*Investigational drug in the United States.

to mitogens and alloantigens. Six of 21 patients treated with 2'deoxycoformycin developed localized herpes infections. A randomized trial of 2'deoxycoformycin versus interferon-alpha is under way.

Recently, another investigational drug, chlorodeoxyadenosine, 0.1 mg per kg daily by continuous intravenous infusion on days 1 through 7 monthly, demonstrated complete and durable responses in 11 of 12 patients after one course of therapy.

In summary, splenectomy is recommended in persons who are good surgical candidates and whose bone marrow is not diffusely replaced by hairy cells. Interferon-alpha (2 to $4 \times 10^6$ U thrice weekly intramuscularly or subcutaneously) is recommended if a splenectomy is not chosen or fails. 2'-Deoxycoformycin (4 mg per $M^2$ every 2 weeks intravenously) and chlorodeoxyadenosine are available only for experimental studies.

## Adult T Cell Leukemia-Lymphoma

Adult T cell leukemia-lymphoma (ATL) is a T cell lymphoproliferative syndrome first described in Japan in 1977 and later identified in the United States, the Caribbean, and other areas. ATL is characterized by pleomorphic neoplastic cells with membrane features of mature T helper lymphocytes.

Epidemiologic studies of HTLV-I focus on serologic studies of normal populations that might elucidate the distribution of HTLV-I infection. Based on such studies, it is clear that ATL is correlated with HTLV-I infection. Additional data in the United States suggest that persons with the acquired immune deficiency syndrome (AIDS) and hemophiliacs are often exposed to HTLV-I via blood or blood products.

### Clinical Features

The median age of persons with ATL is approximately 40 years. They typically present with an elevated leukocyte count ranging from 5 to $100 \times 10^9$ per liter with circulating malignant lymphocytes in most cases. Anemia and thrombocytopenia are uncommon. Onset of symptoms is typically acute, with rapidly developing cutaneous lesions, hypocalcemia, or both. Skin lesions are variable. Some persons have discrete tumor nodules, and others have confluent smaller nodules. Some persons present with plaques, papules, and nonspecific erythematous patches and erythroderma. Persons with hypercalcemia typically have weakness, lethargy, confusion, polyuria, and polydypsia. Radionuclide bone scans show diffusely increased uptake throughout the skeleton, most prominent in the joints and skull. These scans are referred to as "super scans" and are unusual in other persons with malignant lymphomas. Isolated lytic bone lesions may also occur; alkaline phosphatase is typically elevated.

Lymph node enlargement occurs in all patients although the nodes are initially small in some. Many patients have generalized lymphadenopathy, and most have retroperitoneal adenopathy. Hilar adenopathy is common, but a mediastinal mass is rare. Bone marrow is also typically infiltrated with leukemia cells. Additional sites of disease include the lung, liver, and central nervous system.

Opportunistic infections are common in persons with ATL even though most have normal serum immunoglobulin levels. *Pneumocystis carinii* infection is common, as is cryptococcal meningitis. Bacterial and fungal infections are also common. A variety of pulmonary problems develop, including infections and leukemic infiltrates.

A variant of ATL termed "smoldering ATL" is described. These patients have an indolent course except for opportunistic infections. They typically have a long survival without therapy and without hypercalcemia. Skin lesions are characteristic and occur as erythema, papules, or nodules. The proportion of ATL cells in the blood is quite low (less than 5%), with minimal lymphadenopathy, hepatosplenomegaly, and bone marrow infiltration. One patient developed aggressive ATL after more than 5 years of illness and another after 13 years. Persons with smoldering ATL are more likely to have a normal karyotype.

### Therapy

Treatment with combination chemotherapy including doxorubicin (as described in the PLL section) results in complete clinical remission in many persons. However, response duration is typically less than 1 year. Relapses often occur at sites of initial disease, but new sites can include the skin, liver, and central nervous system.

## Cutaneous T Cell Lymphoma

Cutaneous T cell lymphoma (CTCL) consists of mycosis fungoides and the Sézary syndrome. These disorders are malignant proliferations of T lymphocytes of the "helper" phenotype in which the initial clinical presentation is in the epidermis.

CTCL is an uncommon malignancy in the U.S., with approximately 1500 new cases per year. The average annual adjusted mortality rate is approximately 400 to 500 deaths per year. CTCL occurs most commonly in males with a 2:1 ratio;

it is less frequent in blacks. The median age at diagnosis is 55 years. Initial skin lesions are clinically and histologically nonspecific, and it may be many years before the diagnosis is confirmed. Median survival after histologic diagnosis is approximately 10 years.

### Clinical Features

Most cases of CTCL progress through distinct stages of skin involvement. These stages begin with a "premycotic," erythematous, or eczematoid stage; progress to an infiltrative "plaque" stage; and eventuate in the "tumor" stage. Progression is variable but commonly occurs over several years.

In 1938, Sézary and Bouvrain described a syndrome of pruritus and generalized exfoliative erythroderma with abnormal hyperconvoluted lymphoid cells in the blood; this is referred to as Sézary's syndrome. Sézary's syndrome has biologic features similar to the other forms of mycosis fungoides. These diseases are collectively referred to as CTCL. Most patients with generalized erythroderma have varying numbers of circulating "Sézary" cells; 25% of those with plaque or tumor stage also have circulating Sézary cells.

### Therapy

Four therapeutic modalities produce remissions in most persons with CTCL, including topical nitrogen mustard, photochemotherapy with psoralen and ultraviolet A light (PUVA), radiotherapy (particularly total body electron beam therapy), and systemic chemotherapy. Each induces remissions, but cure is uncommon and possible only in early disease.

Topical nitrogen mustard is used predominantly in persons with early cutaneous stages. In more advanced stages, this approach is used to supplement other therapies. The major advantage of topical therapy is that it is relatively nontoxic. Disadvantages include the inconvenience of daily application to large skin surfaces, the allergic reactions in up to half of cases, the potential for skin cancer, and the inability to cure the disease. Nitrogen mustard (Mustargen) (10 mg diluted in 60 ml of tap water or 60 grams of a water-miscible cream) is administered daily using a cotton swab or small paint brush. Therapy is continued for up to 12 months in responders. Frequency is then reduced to every other day for an additional 1 to 2 years. Therapy is discontinued after 3 years or when cutaneous lesions disappear completely.

Psoralen is a phototoxic furocoumarin activated by ultraviolet A light. In its active form, it binds covalently and reversibly to DNA. Ultraviolet A light penetrates only the upper part of the dermis. Therefore, psoralen activated by ultraviolet A light (PUVA) affects cells primarily in the epidermis and papillary dermis. A 60% complete remission rate is reported with psoralen; persons with generalized erythroderma and tumors have lower response rates than those with plaques. Psoralen (Oxsoralen) is usually given at a dose of 0.6 mg per kg orally, 2 hours prior to the ultraviolet A light therapy. Treatments are initially given three times weekly. Maintenance therapy may be given every 2 to 4 weeks indefinitely. Adverse effects of PUVA therapy include mild nausea, pruritis, and sunburn-like changes with atrophy and dry skin. PUVA is noncross-resistant with other treatment modalities. Disadvantages are the inability to cure CTCL and expense. Long-term side effects are not yet reported.

Electron beam therapy penetrates only into the upper dermis, and there are minimal systemic effects with an 80% complete remission rate. Twenty per cent of persons remain relapse-free at 3 years, and few experience relapse. Typically, treatment is 40 cGy per week to a total dose of 3600 cGy in 8 to 9 weeks. The advantage of electron beam therapy is a high frequency of durable complete responses without systemic toxicity. Disadvantages are alopecia, atrophy, edema, dermatitis, and cost.

The largest experience with single-agent chemotherapy is with alkylating agents, including nitrogen mustard (mechlorethamine or Mustargen) (0.4 mg per kg every 4 to 6 weeks, intravenously), cyclophosphamide (300 mg per $M^2$ orally for 5 days every month), and chlorambucil (0.4 to 1.0 mg per kg once every 2 to 4 weeks). Response rates of 60% with 15% complete remissions are reported. Similar results occur with methotrexate (2.5 to 10 mg daily, orally), bleomycin (Blenoxane) (7.5 to 15 U twice weekly, intramuscularly), and doxorubicin. Single-agent therapy does not cure CTCL. Combination therapy with these and other drugs produces objective responses in greater than 80% of persons and complete responses in approximately 25%. Duration of remission varies, with a median of about 1 year and with no long-term disease-free survival reported.

Randomized trials with whole-body electron beam therapy as a single modality compared with electron beam therapy followed by topical nitrogen mustard suggest a benefit of combined therapy. Studies of electron beam therapy combined with chemotherapy suggest an advantage over either treatment alone. However, cutaneous and hematologic toxicity is increased.

There are many experimental approaches to therapy of CTCL. One study reported a 50% response with high-dose interferon-alpha (50 × $10^6$ U per $M^2$ thrice weekly*). In another study, three of four persons receiving 13 cis-retinoic acid improved. Some studies use leukapheresis to treat persons with CTCL; success is claimed. In other studies, subjects receive oral psoralen followed by leukapheresis. The lymphocyte-enriched blood fraction is exposed to ultraviolet A light and returned. Treatment of four persons with advanced CTCL with 2'deoxycoformycin resulted in two complete and two partial responses. Finally, therapy with monoclonal antibodies was also studied. Unlabeled monoclonal antibodies had only a minimal transient effect. In one study, [131]I-labeled monoclonal antibody produced more prolonged and consistent responses.

## Large Granular Lymphocytic Leukemia

Large granular lymphocytes (LGL) are a heterogeneous group of thymus-independent cells that are largely responsible for most, if not all, natural killer (NK) activity and have an important role in antibody-dependent cell-mediated cytotoxicity (ADCC).

Recently, a T cell lymphoproliferative disorder referred to as LGL leukemia or "chronic T gamma lymphoproliferative disease" was recognized. This disease typically follows a chronic course characterized by lymphocytosis with bone marrow infiltration, neutropenia, and recurrent infections.

Median age of affected persons is 60 years; there is a 2:1 male to female ratio, and virtually all are Caucasian. Attempts to isolate viruses from cases are negative.

### Clinical Features

The typical presentation is that of recurrent bacterial infections, usually a consequence of granulocytopenia. Fatigue from anemia is also common. Bleeding is rare; platelet levels are usually normal. One-half of patients have mild to moderate splenomegaly; approximately 20% have hepatomegaly, and less than 10% have lymphadenopathy. A small proportion have hypogammaglobulinemia, and approximately one-third have hypergammaglobulinemia. Skin infiltration is rare.

In this disease, the malignant cells infiltrate the bone marrow, blood, spleen, and liver. In one-half of cases, lymphocytes are greater than $10 \times 10^9$ per liter. Bone marrow lymphocytosis ranges from 30 to 75%; some persons have reduced myelopoiesis. Approximately one-half of patients have severe granulocytopenia with lev-

*Exceeds dosage recommended by the manufacturer.

els less than $0.5 \times 10^9$ per liter. At least one-half of persons with this disorder have anemia with hemoglobin levels less than 12 grams per dl.

### Therapy

Most persons do not require therapy save for transfusions for anemia and antibiotics for infections. Chemotherapy with single alkylating agents such as chlorambucil or cyclophosphamide, or combination chemotherapy with alkylating agents, vincristine, and prednisone is used to treat progressive disease. Although chemotherapy is usually not effective, some patients benefit. Some persons were treated by splenectomy or by spleen radiation without benefit. Because this disease appears to represent a spectrum from almost benign to a more aggressive malignancy, it is not possible to recommend a specific therapeutic approach. Clearly, many persons will not require chemotherapy and can be followed for many years.

We recently studied recombinant interferon-alpha in persons with LGL leukemia. No benefit was demonstrated. One person with pure red cell aplasia associated with this disorder had normalization of hemoglobin without an apparent effect on the underlying disorder. Studies with 2'-deoxycoformycin are in progress. Two patients treated with cyclosporine had a dramatic increase in their absolute neutrophil count. Hematopoietic growth factors such as granulocyte-colony stimulating factor (G-CSF), might benefit patients with granulocytopenia.

# NON-HODGKIN'S LYMPHOMAS

method of
ALEXANDRA M. LEVINE, M.D., and
JOAN ESPLIN, M.D.
*University of Southern California School of
   Medicine*
*Los Angeles, California*

The past 20 years has brought new insights into the biology of lymphoma, as well as its natural history, pathogenesis, and therapy. These changes have translated into new therapeutic modalities and the potential for long-term, disease-free survival, or even cure.

The classification of lymphomas has been controversial and complex. The Rappaport system, used since the 1950s, has now been replaced by other systems, such as that of Lukes and Collins, based upon modern concepts of immunology and the understanding that lymphomas are malignancies of T or B lymphocytes in various stages of maturation and transformation. These newer concepts have been translated into the "Working Formulation for Clinical Usage," in which lymphomas have been subdivided into three broad categories: low-grade, intermediate-grade, and high-grade, as demonstrated in Table 1.

The initial evaluation of a patient with lymphoma should include the following: a careful history and physical examination; complete blood counts; chemistry panel; serum lactate dehydrogenase (LDH); chest x-ray; computed tomography of the chest, abdomen, and pelvis (CT scan); and bilateral bone marrow biopsies. A gallium scan should also be included in patients with intermediate- or high-grade lymphoma. Additional studies may also be indicated in selected patients, such as bone scan, magnetic resonance imaging (MRI) or CT scan of brain, and/or lumbar puncture. At the conclusion of these studies, a specific designation is made regarding the Ann Arbor stage of disease (Table 2). The purpose of this staging evaluation is twofold: (1) to determine the precise extent of disease in order to plan appropriate therapy, and (2) to document all sites of initial disease so that accurate conclusions may be drawn regarding the results of therapy. The specific therapeutic regimen to be used is based upon the pathologic type of disease as well as the extent of disease in a given patient.

## LOW-GRADE LYMPHOMAS

Low-grade lymphomas include small-cleaved lymphoma; lymphoma-leukemia of small B lymphocytes; and follicular mixed lymphoma. The median age at diagnosis is 55 to 60 years, with an equal sex distribution. Approximately 80 to 90% of patients present with advanced Stage III or IV disease; systemic "B" symptoms, such as fever, night sweats, and/or weight loss; or bulky (over 10 cm) tumor masses. Despite the widespread nature of the disease, however, patients with low-grade lymphomas typically have an indolent course, with a median survival of 8 to 10 years, despite the fact that the disease is not curable in the traditional sense. In fact, if initially asymptomatic and left untreated, 20 to 30% of patients may undergo a spontaneous remission of disease, lasting an average of 15 months.

Approximately 10% of patients with low-grade lymphoma have localized Stage I or minimal bulk Stage II disease. These patients are the only subset of low-grade disease that may be curable, using involved or extended field radiotherapy (4000 cGy). Approximately 50 to 80% of these patients will experience long-term disease-free survival, or "cure."

The majority of patients with low-grade lymphoma present with advanced disease. Because modern chemotherapy depends upon agents that inhibit DNA synthesis, and since such a small percentage of malignant cells are actually dividing at any one time (1 to 3%), these patients are probably not curable at the present time using multiple-agent chemotherapy. Notably, however, they may live for extended periods with relatively

TABLE 1. **Pathologic Classification of Non-Hodgkin's Lymphomas***

| Rappaport Classification | Working Formulation Classification |
| --- | --- |
| **Low-Grade** | |
| Diffuse lymphocytic, well differentiated | Small lymphocytic |
| Nodular, poorly differentiated lymphocytic | Follicular, predominantly small cleaved cell |
| Nodular, mixed lymphocytic-histiocytic | Follicular, mixed small cleaved and large cell |
| **Intermediate-Grade** | |
| Nodular histiocytic | Follicular, predominantly large cell |
| Diffuse lymphocytic, poorly differentiated | Diffuse, small cleaved cell |
| Diffuse mixed lymphocytic-histiocytic | Diffuse, mixed small and large cell |
| Diffuse histiocytic | Diffuse, large cell |
| **High-Grade** | |
| Diffuse histiocytic | Large cell, immunoblastic |
| Lymphoblastic convoluted/nonconvoluted | Lymphoblastic |
| Undifferentiated, Burkitt's and non-Burkitt's | Small noncleaved cell |

*From Bierman P, and Armitage JO: Non-Hodgkin's lymphomas. *In* Rakel RE (ed): Conn's Current Therapy 1989. Philadelphia, WB Saunders Co., 1989, pp. 368–373.

minimal therapy, in the presence of known disease.

If the patient is asymptomatic at presentation, a viable option is to "watch and wait," withholding specific therapy until such a time that symptoms or signs develop. This approach also allows the physician to gauge the pace of disease in an individual patient. With such an approach of watchful waiting, the group at Stanford has found that the majority of asymptomatic patients will not require therapy for 3 to 4 years. The most common cause of initiating therapy was development of a large mass that was cosmetically unacceptable to the patient or development of anemia in a patient with known marrow involvement. Other reasons to begin therapy include development of systemic "B" symptoms and organ dysfunction due to lymphomatous infiltration.

Once therapy is deemed necessary, the regi-

TABLE 2. **Ann Arbor Staging Classification for Non-Hodgkin's Lymphoma***

| | |
| --- | --- |
| **Stage I:** | Involvement of a single lymph node region (I) or of a single extralymphatic organ or site (I$_E$). |
| **Stage II:** | Involvement of two or more lymph node regions on the same side of the diaphragm (II) or localized involvement of an extralymphatic organ or site and of one or more lymph node regions on the same side of the diaphragm (II$_E$). |
| **Stage III:** | Involvement of lymph node regions on both sides of the diaphragm (III), which may also be accompanied by localized involvement of an extralymphatic organ or site (III$_E$) or by involvement of the spleen (III$_S$), or by involvement of both (III$_{SE}$). |
| **Stage IV:** | Diffuse or disseminated involvement of one or more extralymphatic organs or tissues with or without associated lymph node enlargement. |

*From Bierman P, and Armitage JO: Non-Hodgkin's lymphomas. *In* Rakel RE (ed): Conn's Current Therapy 1989. Philadelphia, WB Saunders Co., 1989, pp. 368–373.

mens used most commonly have included the CVP regimen or single-agent chlorambucil (Leukeran) (Table 3). Complete remissions are achieved in approximately 70 to 80% of patients, although these remissions are not durable. When relapse does occur, treatment may be repeated using the same agents, and second or even third remissions are commonly achieved. It is important to understand that although therapy may not be initiated at presentation, when the decision is made to treat, the goal should be attainment of complete response, as these patients live longer than those who achieve only partial or no response to therapy. Specific response rates and duration of response also vary with the specific type of low-grade lymphoma being considered. Thus, although complete remission is expected in the majority of patients with follicular small cleaved or follicular mixed lymphoma, it is unusual to achieve complete remission in the patient with lymphoma-leukemia of small B lymphocytes. Patients with follicular mixed lymphoma may experience a longer duration of response when compared with those with follicular small cleaved disease.

New approaches have been suggested in recent years for patients with low-grade lymphoma. In an attempt to ascertain if watchful waiting will ultimately lead to longer survival times, the group at the National Cancer Institute (NCI) has embarked upon a large study that randomizes patients to either watchful waiting ("expectant therapy") or the ProMACE-MOPP (see Table 4) regimen, with total nodal radiotherapy. Results will require many years of follow-up. Further, very intensive chemotherapy with bone marrow transplantation is also being studied at some centers in an attempt to ascertain if these patients may, in fact, be curable when such large doses of chemotherapy are employed. A third new area of investigation involves the biologic response modifiers, such as interferon-alpha (Ro-

TABLE 3. **Chemotherapy Regimens for Low-Grade Lymphomas**

**CVP**
Cyclophosphamide (Cytoxan), 400 mg/M$^2$ PO, days 1–5
Vincristine (Oncovin), 1.4 mg/M$^2$ IV, day 1
Prednisone, 100 mg/M$^2$ PO, days 1–5
(21-day cycles)

**CHLOP**
Chlorambucil (Leukeran), 12 mg/M$^2$ PO (maximum 20 mg), days 1–5
Vincristine (Oncovin), 1 mg/M$^2$ IV, day 1
Prednisone, 100 mg PO, days 1–5
(21- to 28-day cycles)

**CHLORAMBUCIL**
16 mg/M$^2$ PO, days 1–5 q mo
*or:* 2–10 mg PO daily

**ABP**
Doxorubicin (Adriamycin), 75 mg/M$^2$ IV, day 1
Bleomycin (Blenoxane), 15 mg/M$^2$ IV, days 1, 8
Prednisone, 100 mg/M$^2$ PO, days 1–5
(21-day cycles)

**HOP**
Doxorubicin, 80 mg/M$^2$ IV, day 1
Vincristine (Oncovin), 1.4 mg/M$^2$ IV (maximum 2 mg), day 1
Prednisone, 100 mg PO, days 1–5
(21-day cycles)

**C-MOPP**
Cyclophosphamide, 650 mg/M$^2$ IV, days 1, 8
Vincristine (Oncovin), 1.4 mg/M$^2$ IV (maximum 2 mg), days 1, 8
Procarbazine (Matulane), 100 mg/M$^2$ PO, days 1–14
Prednisone, 40 mg/M$^2$ PO, days 1–14
(28-day cycles)

**CHOP**
Cyclophosphamide, 750 mg/M$^2$ IV, day 1
Doxorubicin, 50 mg/M$^2$ IV, day 1
Vincristine (Oncovin), 1.4 mg/M$^2$ IV (maximum 2 mg), day 1
Prednisone, 100 mg PO, days 1–5
(21- to 28-day cycles)

feron-A) (IFN-alpha). Although response rates of approximately 40% have been achieved with IFN-alpha in patients with follicular small cleaved cell disease, response is unlikely in patients with lymphoma-leukemia of small B lymphocytes. Additional new agents, such as monoclonal antibodies, conjugated with toxins or with radioisotopes are also under investigation, with promising early results.

Although the low-grade lymphomas are usually indolent diseases, approximately 5% of untreated patients will experience spontaneous transformation of their disease to a more aggressive high-grade lymphoma; approximately 30% of all patients experience such transformation at some time during the course of illness, and a much higher percentage may have foci of transformation noted at the time of autopsy. Therefore, if a patient with underlying low-grade lymphoma experiences a change in disease pattern over time, such as development of new "B" symptoms, or if a new rapidly growing mass is detected, the affected area should be biopsied in an attempt to ascertain if transformation has occurred, which would mandate a change in therapy and therapeutic philosophy. When transformation does occur, prognosis is poor.

## INTERMEDIATE-GRADE LYMPHOMAS

The introduction of combination chemotherapy for patients with intermediate-grade lymphomas has made even advanced-stage disease "curable." As in low-grade lymphomas, however, Stage I or nonbulky Stage II disease requires a different approach. The most important concept in deciding upon therapy for patients with localized intermediate-grade lymphoma is that of accurate staging. Because the vast majority of patients do have extensive disease (II, III, or IV), it must be remembered that patients with truly localized lymphoma will be unusual. In a study published from the University of Chicago, all patients underwent surgical laparotomy in order to prove the presence of pathologic Stage I or II disease and were then treated with extended field radiation (4000 cGy). Seventy per cent of patients with pathologic Stage I disease experienced continuous disease-free survival at 10 years (i.e., "cure"), whereas only 31% of patients with pathologic Stage II disease experienced long-term disease-free survival. Thus, the patient with truly localized, Stage I disease may be curable with radiation. However, patients with Stage II disease should receive chemotherapy. Another approach is the use of chemotherapy (CHOP regimen, Table 3) with or without additional radiation to patients with clinically staged I and II disease. Using multiple-agent chemotherapy as the major treatment modality, approximately 70 to 80% of patients have been found to experience long-term disease-free survival, or "cure," indicating that the physician has several options in patients with apparently localized disease. Either "aggressive" staging can be employed with laparotomy, in the hopes of proving localized Stage I disease, with subsequent use of radiation therapy; or, alternatively, less intensive staging can be accomplished, withholding laparotomy, with subsequent use of CHOP, either with or without the addition of local radiation. The value of radiation added at the completion of chemotherapy has not yet been fully elucidated.

Combination chemotherapy is the treatment of choice for patients with intermediate-grade lymphoma of advanced stage (bulky II, III or IV). As shown in Table 4, many different regimens have been employed since the 1970s and have been

TABLE 4. **Chemotherapy for Intermediate-Grade Lymphomas***

**First-Generation Regimens**

C-MOPP†

CHOP†

BACOP
  Cyclophosphamide, 650 mg/M² IV, days 1, 8
  Doxorubicin (Adriamycin), 25 mg/M² IV, days 1, 8
  Vincristine (Oncovin), 1.4 mg/M² IV, days 1, 8
  Bleomycin, 5 mg/M² IV, days 15, 22
  Prednisone, 60 mg/M² PO, days 15–29
  (28-day cycles)

COMLA
  Cyclophosphamide, 1.5 grams/M² IV, day 1
  Vincristine, 1.4 mg/M², days 1, 8, 15
  Methotrexate, 120 mg/M² IV, days 22, 29, 36, 43, 50, 57, 64, 71; beginning 24 hr after methotrexate infusion, leucovorin, 25 mg/M² PO q 6 hr for four doses
  Cytarabine, 300 mg/M² IV, days 22, 29, 36, 43, 50, 57, 64, 71
  (Three cycles with 2-week rest between cycles)

**Second- and Third-Generation Regimens**

COP-BLAM
  Cyclophosphamide, 400 mg/M² IV, day 1
  Vincristine (Oncovin), 1 mg/M² IV, day 1
  Doxorubicin, 40 mg/M² IV, day 1
  Prednisone, 40 mg/M² PO, days 1–10
  Procarbazine, 100 mg/M² PO, days 1–10
  Bleomycin, 15 mg IV, day 14
  (21-day cycles with escalation of cyclophosphamide and doxorubicin doses)

CAP-BOP
  Cyclophosphamide, 650 mg/M² IV, day 1
  Doxorubicin (Adriamycin), 50 mg/M² IV, day 1
  Procarbazine, 100 mg/M² PO, days 1–7
  Bleomycin, 10 mg/M² subcutaneously, day 14
  Vincristine (Oncovin), 1.4 mg/M² IV (maximum 2.0 mg), day 14
  Prednisone, 100 mg PO, days 14–20
  (21- to 28-day cycles)

M-BACOD
  Bleomycin, 4.0 mg/M² IV, day 1
  Doxorubicin (Adriamycin), 45 mg/M² IV, day 1
  Cyclophosphamide, 600 mg/M² IV, day 1

  Vincristine (Oncovin), 1.0 mg/M², day 1
  Dexamethasone, 6.0 mg/M² PO, days 1–5
  Methotrexate, 3.0 grams/M² IV, day 14; beginning 24 hr after methotrexate is completed, leucovorin, 10 mg/M² IV; then 10 mg/M² PO q 6 hr for 72 hr
  (21-day cycles)

ProMACE-MOPP
  Etoposide (VePesid), 120 mg/M² IV, days 1, 8
  Cyclophosphamide, 650 mg/M² IV, days 1, 8
  Doxorubicin, 25 mg/M² IV, days 1, 8
  Methotrexate, 1.5 gm/M² IV, day 14; beginning 24 hr after methotrexate infusion is initiated, leucovorin, 50 mg/M² IV, q 6 hr for five doses
  Prednisone 60 mg/M² PO, days 1–14
  (28-day cycles with cycle number determined by rate of tumor regression.) Later MOPP given, with number of cycles determined by rate of tumor regression; additional ProMACE given for patients in remission.

ProMACE-CytaBOM
  Cyclophosphamide, 650 mg/M² IV, day 1
  Doxorubicin (Adriamycin), 25 mg/M² IV, day 1
  Etoposide, 120 mg/M² IV, day 1
  Prednisone, 60 mg/M² PO, days 1–15
  Cytarabine, 300 mg/M² IV, day 8
  Bleomycin, 5 mg/M² IV, day 8
  Vincristine (Oncovin), 1.4 mg/M², day 8
  Methotrexate, 120 mg/M², day 8; beginning 24 hr after methotrexate infusion is initiated, leucovorin, 25 mg/M² PO, q 6 hr for four doses
  (21-day cycles)

MACOP-B
  Methotrexate, 400 mg/M² IV, weeks 2, 6, 10; beginning 24 hr after methotrexate infusion is initiated, leucovorin, 15 mg PO, q 6 hr for six doses
  Doxorubicin (Adriamycin), 50 mg/M² IV, weeks 1, 3, 5, 7, 9, 11
  Cyclophosphamide, 350 mg/M² IV, weeks 1, 3, 5, 7, 9, 11
  Vincristine (Oncovin), 1.4 mg/M² (maximum 2 mg) IV, weeks 2, 4, 6, 8, 10, 12
  Bleomycin 10 mg/M² IV, weeks 4, 8, 12
  Prednisone, 75 mg PO daily with taper over last 2 wk
  (whole regimen delivered in 12 weeks)

*From Bierman P, and Armitage JO: Non-Hodgkin's lymphomas. *In* Rakel RE (ed): Conn's Current Therapy 1989. Philadelphia, WB Saunders Co., 1989, pp. 368–373.
  †See Table 3 for drugs and dosage schedules.

termed "first-," "second-," or "third-generation" regimens. The prototype of the first-generation regimen is CHOP. Employing CHOP in over 300 patients, the Southwest Oncology Group (SWOG) has recently published 12-year follow-up data, indicating that although the complete remission rate is approximately 50 to 60%, half of these responders will eventually relapse, leaving 30% of all patients treated who have presumably been cured of disease.

The second-generation regimens added additional agents, such as high-dose methotrexate with leucovorin rescue at mid-cycle, interspersed

with other, first-generation agents. Examples would include the M-BACOD regimen and others (Table 4). In subsequent years, yet additional agents were added, the time between cycles was decreased, the marrow toxic agents were alternated with marrow sparing agents. Examples of these regimens include ProMACE-MOPP and the MACOP-B regimen. As initially published, these newer, more intensive regimens have been associated with higher complete remission rates and a greater proportion of long-term disease-free survivors. They have also been associated with greater toxicity, as might be expected. Recently,

TABLE 5. **Chemotherapy Regimens for High-Grade Burkitt's and Convoluted T Lymphoblastic Lymphomas**

**Regimen I (COMP)**

*Induction*
Cyclophosphamide, 1.2 grams/M$^2$ IV, day 1
Vincristine, 2.0 mg/M$^2$ (maximum dose, 2.0 mg) IV, days 3, 10, 17, 24
Methotrexate, 6.25 mg/M$^2$ intrathecally, days 5, 31, 34
Methotrexate, 300 mg/M$^2$ IV (60% of dose as IV push, 40% as 4-hr infusion), day 12
Prednisone, 60 mg/M$^2$ (maximum dose, 60 mg), PO, daily in four divided doses, days 3–30, with doses decreasing to 0 on days 31–37

*Maintenance Cycle*
Cyclophosphamide, 1.0 g/M$^2$ IV, day 1
Vincristine, 1.5 mg/M$^2$ IV (maximum dose, 2 mg), days 1, 4
Methotrexate, 6.25 mg/M$^2$ intrathecally, day 1 (excluded from first maintenance cycle)
Methotrexate, 300 mg/M$^2$ IV (60% of dose as IV push, 40% as 4-hr infusion), day 15
Prednisone, 60 mg/M$^2$ (maximum dose, 60 mg) PO, days 1–5 (excluded from first maintenance cycle)
Repeat maintenance cycle every 28 days

**Regimen II (Modified LSA$_2$-L$_2$)**

*Induction (Weeks 1–4)*
Mediastinal radiotherapy, 2000 rad, week 1
Cytoxan, 1200 mg/M$^2$ IV, day 1
Vincristine, 2 mg IV, days 1, 8, 15, 22
Prednisone, 60 mg/M$^2$ PO, days 1, 8, 15
Methotrexate, 6 mg/M$^2$ intrathecally, days 1, 15, 22
Adriamycin, 60 mg/M$^2$ IV, day 15

*Consolidation (Weeks 5–12)*
Ara-C (cytarabine), 150 mg/M$^2$ IV or subcutaneously q 12 hr × 10 doses, day 29
6-Thioguanine, 75 mg/M$^2$ PO q 12 hr × 10 doses, day 29
Cranial radiation, 2400 rad, days 29–43
L-Asparaginase (Elspar), 10,000 U IV, daily × 10 days, day 71 (week 10)
CCNU (CeeNu), 100 mg/M$^2$ PO, day 169 (day 1 of week 12)
Methotrexate, 6 mg/M$^2$ intrathecally, day 169 (day 1 of week 12)

*Maintenance (Weeks 13–156)*
6-Thioguanine, 300 mg/M$^2$ × 4 days PO
Cytoxan, 600 mg/M$^2$ IV, day 5
*Rest 2 weeks*
Hydoxyurea (Hydrea), 1000 mg/M$^2$ PO × 4 days
Adriamycin, 45 mg/M$^2$ IV, day 5
*Rest 2 weeks*
Methotrexate, 10 mg/M$^2$ PO × 4 days
CCNU, 50 mg/M$^2$ PO, day 5
*Rest 2 weeks*
Ara-C, 150 mg/M$^2$ daily × 4 days
Vincristine, 2 mg IV, day 5
*Rest 2 weeks*
Methotrexate, 6 mg/M$^2$ intrathecally
Recycle maintenance

**Regimen III (I.T. Magrath Protocol 77-04)**

*Cycle 1*
Ara-C, 30 mg/M$^2$, intrathecally, days 1, 2, 3, 7
Cytoxan, 1200 mg/M$^2$ IV, day 1
Methotrexate, 12.5 mg/M$^2$ intrathecally (max. 12.5 mg), day 10
Methotrexate, 300 mg/M$^2$ first hour, 60 mg/M$^2$ hours 2–42; leucovorin rescue, days 10, 11, 12

*Cycle 2–6*
Ara-C, 45 mg/M$^2$ intrathecally, days 1, 2, (delete day 2 for Cycle 4–6)
Methotrexate, 12.5 mg/M$^2$ intrathecally (max. 12.5 mg), days 3, 10 (delete day 3 for Cycle 4–6)
Prednisone-prednisolone, 40 mg/M$^2$ IV or PO, days 1–5
Vincristine, 1.4 mg/M$^2$ IV (max. 2 mg), day 1
Adriamycin, 40 mg/M$^2$ IV, day 1
Cytoxan, 1200 mg/M$^2$ IV, day 1
Methotrexate 300 mg/M$^2$ first hour, 60 mg/M$^2$ hours 2–42; leucovorin rescue, days 10, 11, 12

*Cycle 7–15*
Prednisone, vincristine, Adriamycin, Cytoxan as in Cycle 2–6
Methotrexate, 300 mg/M$^2$ first hour, 60 mg/M$^2$ hours 2–42; leucovorin rescue, days 13, 14, 15

these newer regimens have been compared prospectively with the first-generation regimens, such as CHOP. Although several large, cooperative national trials are still in process, early comparisons have indicated that the more intensive regimens may not, in fact, be superior to CHOP. The current SWOG study, which prospectively randomizes patients to receive CHOP, M-BACOD, ProMACE-MOPP, or MACOP-B, is awaited with much interest and is expected to resolve the existing controversy in this area. It is also important to remember that not all patients are the same, with prognosis depending upon the extent of tumor burden, as measured by mass size (greater or less than 10 cm), elevated LDH; and more than two extranodal sites of disease; and upon the underlying vigor of the patient, as measured by performance status. Thus, the choice of any particular regimen will also depend upon the precise characteristics of the patient.

## HIGH-GRADE LYMPHOMAS

Although the Working Formulation for Clinical Usage has only recently been published, difficulties with the classification have already become apparent, as exemplified by the "high-grade lymphomas," which include immunoblastic lymphoma, small noncleaved lymphoma, and T cell lymphoblastic lymphoma. These diseases are each unique, and specific therapy will depend upon which type of lymphoma is present.

The "immunoblastic" lymphomas, although designated within the "high-grade" category, seem to behave and respond very much like the intermediate-grade lymphomas. Therapy for the patient with immunoblastic lymphoma, then, will be similar to that discussed for intermediate lymphomas.

Small noncleaved lymphoma is truly high-grade disease, with rapid tumor growth and early dissemination to the central nervous system, especially in the setting of bone marrow involvement. Several regimens for this specific tumor type have been described (Table 5) and seem to be efficacious. Interestingly, this tumor is relatively more common in children, in whom a much higher rate of long-term disease-free survival is found when compared with adults with the same pathologic type of disease.

T cell lymphoblastic lymphoma is most commonly seen in young male adults. The disease usually begins in the thymus and presents with a large mediastinal mass. Rapid dissemination into the central nervous system and the bone marrow is expected, and circulation of abnormal cells in the blood is not unusual, appearing similar to acute lymphoblastic leukemia, or T cell ALL. Localized therapy is never indicated in these patients, even when the extent of disease appears to be localized. Prophylactic therapy to the central nervous system, employing radiation, as well as intrathecal chemotherapy is mandatory. Several successful therapeutic regimens have been described, as given in Table 5.

## AIDS-RELATED LYMPHOMAS

The AIDS-related lymphomas are of the high-grade B cell type, including small noncleaved and B immunoblastic lymphomas. Widespread, extranodal disease is expected in approximately 80 to 90% of patients at presentation, and either initial involvement or relapse of disease in the central nervous system (CNS) is seen in 30 to 50%. With the use of the second- or third-generation regimens (see Tables 4 and 5), median survival has been approximately 6 months in all reported series. Prognostic factors associated with short survival include history of AIDS prior to the lymphoma; CD4 lymphocyte count less than 200 per dl at diagnosis; poor performance status; and Stage IV disease (especially with marrow involvement). Recently, the use of lower-dose chemotherapy, with early CNS prophylaxis, and maintenance therapy with zidovudine (AZT, Retrovir) has shown promising results, with complete response in approximately 50%, lasting in excess of 12 months. Inhaled pentamidine should be used in an attempt to prevent *Pneumocystis carinii* pneumonia, the most common opportunistic infection in the setting of AIDS.

Aside from disseminated lymphomatous disease, patients with infection by the human immunodeficiency virus (HIV) may also present with lymphoma primary to the CNS, in the absence of systemic lymphoma. Although radiotherapy has been employed in these patients, short survival has been uniformly experienced, with death often due to intercurrent opportunistic infections.

## SALVAGE THERAPY

Patients with intermediate- or high-grade lymphoma who experience relapse after multiple-agent combination chemotherapy have a poor prognosis. Cure rates with salvage regimens are low, with less than 10% long-term disease-free survival. About 50% of patients will respond to regimens such as DHAP, including complete remission in 10 to 30% (dexamethasone [Decadron], 40 mg intravenously or orally daily, for four days; cisplatin [Platinol], 100 mg per $M^2$ via continuous infusion over 24 hours on day 1; and cytosine arabinoside [cytarabine, Cytosar-U] 2 grams per M² intravenously following the cisplatin infusion, and then repeated in 12 hours). Another approach would be the use of very-high-dose chemotherapy and/or radiotherapy, followed by bone marrow transplantation (autologous or allogeneic). In the best of circumstances, when the patient is given a transplant at the time of minimal tumor burden and is still sensitive to chemotherapy, 35 to 50% long-term disease-free survival is expected.

# CUTANEOUS T CELL LYMPHOMA
## (Mycosis Fungoides and Sézary's Syndrome)

method of
HERSCHEL S. ZACKHEIM, M.D.
*University of California, San Francisco*
*San Francisco, California*

Cutaneous T cell lymphoma (CTCL) is a neoplasm of T lymphocytes. The major forms of CTCL are mycosis fungoides (MF), which comprises about 90%, and Sézary's syndrome, the leukemic form, about 10% of cases.

The annual incidence in the United States is approximately 3 to 4 per million. CTCL is primarily a disease of older persons. About two-thirds of cases are diagnosed by histology between ages 40 and 69. However, it may begin in adolescence. Men outnumber women by about 2:1.

The etiology is unknown. Some evidence suggests a retrovirus, such as the human T cell lymphotropic viruses HTLV-1 and/or HTLV-5, but the data are not conclusive. Exposures to physical agents, toxins, and chemicals have also been proposed as etiologic factors, but this has not been confirmed.

The neoplastic T cells in CTCL are primarily of the helper-inducer type. Helper-inducer T cells cooperate with B lymphocytes in the process of antibody formation.

## CLINICAL FEATURES

### Mycosis Fungoides

The principal stages in the evolution of the cutaneous lesions of MF are patch, plaque, and tumor.

Patch stage lesions may be nonatrophic or atrophic.

Nonatrophic patches are erythematous, slightly scaly, thin lesions, usually 2 to 8 cm in diameter or larger. They may appear anywhere on the body surface but have a predilection for the bathing trunk area—i.e., the hips, buttocks, lower abdomen, and groin.

Atrophic patches are very thin, mildly scaly, often wrinkled lesions ranging from a few centimeters to over 12 cm in diameter. These often exhibit telangiectasia and a reticulated pigmentation. They appear predominantly in the bathing trunk area, breasts, inner arms, and inner thighs.

Patch stage lesions are usually only mildly pruritic, if at all. Adenopathy is uncommon.

As the cutaneous infiltrate deepens, palpable plaques appear. These are sharply defined, scaly or lichenified, slightly elevated lesions that are usually red, reddish brown, or dusky in color. They are usually 2 to 4 cm in diameter but may be much larger, and may appear in any location. Pruritis is more common than in patch stage lesions. Plaque stage lesions may also present as papules. Patients with extensive plaques often have palpable lymph nodes. These are generally discrete, movable, and nontender. In the plaque stage, the nodal histologic appearance is predominantly a nondiagnostic dermatopathic lymphadenitis.

With disease progression, tumors develop. They are usually moderately firm, elevated, dusky, red or purple-colored nodules, 1 to 3 cm in diameter or larger. They may occur on any part of the body but are often seen on the face and scalp. Tumor stage lesions may also appear as deeply infiltrated ulcers.

### Sézary's Syndrome

Sézary's syndrome is the leukemic form of CTCL. There is universal, or almost universal, erythroderma. Pruritus is almost always intense. Adenopathy is usually present. The erythroderma is mostly exfoliative but may be lichenified or purely macular. The palms and soles are commonly red, scaly, hyperkeratotic, and often painfully fissured. Sézary's syndrome may evolve gradually from a long-standing dermatitis or develop rapidly de novo. Disease progression may lead to internal involvement.

### Systemic Involvement

Palpable adenopathy is usually the first sign of systemic disease. Histologic definite lymphoma is most likely to occur in patients with tumor stage disease or Sézary's syndrome. The liver and spleen may be palpable in advanced cases.

Almost any organ of the body may be involved with metastatic disease. The lymph nodes, lungs, spleen, liver, and kidneys are most often affected. Approximately 70% of all patients autopsied show evidence of extracutaneous disease, although this is often not suspected clinically.

## LABORATORY DIAGNOSIS

### Mycosis Fungoides

The essential feature in the histologic diagnosis of patch and plaque stage MF is epidermotropism, i.e., infiltration of the epidermis by lymphocytes. A variable proportion of these lymphocytes are atypical, having hyperconvoluted hyperchromatic enlarged nuclei. They may be present singly or in clusters, or form discrete, sharply defined clusters surrounded by a halo (Pautrier's microabscesses).

There is a polymorphous, predominantly lymphocytic infiltrate in the upper dermis, usually in close apposition to the epidermis, containing varying proportions of atypical lymphocytes. This tends to be light, patchy, and mildly to moderately atypical in patch stage lesions, whereas in plaque stage lesions the infiltrate is heavy, band-like, deeper, and more frankly malignant. In tumor stage lesions, a highly malignant massive infiltrate often containing huge atypical hyperchromatic "mycosis cells" or blast forms extends to the lower dermis or subcutis.

In early stage disease, diagnosis is often difficult and multiple biopsy specimens are usually required. Shave biopsy specimens are generally preferred because the infiltrate is mostly in the upper dermis and a greater area of epidermis is provided. Punch specimens are more appropriate for deeply infiltrated plaques and tumors.

### Sézary's Syndrome

The diagnosis of Sézary's syndrome requires the presence of atypical lymphocytes in the blood (Sézary cells). The Sézary cell is a hyperconvoluted lymphocyte identical to that found in the skin in MF. It is usually considerably larger than a normal lymphocyte, but a small cell variant is recognized. It can be found in buffy coat and routine blood smears but is best identified by electron microscopy or in plastic-embedded thin (1 to 2 $\mu$m) sections of the mononuclear cell layer. With most techniques, the presence of 5% or 10% Sézary cells (as a percentage of lymphocytes) is considered abnormal.

### PATIENT WORK-UP

Once the diagnosis of CTCL has been established, further studies are indicated to determine the extent of the disease. A minimum work-up should include a complete history and physical examination, whole-body mapping of skin lesions, estimation of percentage of skin surface involved by MF, complete blood count with differential, blood chemistry panel, chest x-ray, and lymph node biopsy in the presence of clinical adenopathy. In the event of nodal involvement by MF, computed tomography of the abdomen and pelvis is indicated. Suspected visceral involvement should be confirmed by biopsy. The most common sites are the lungs, spleen, and liver. The blood of patients with over 10% of skin surface involvement, palpable ade-

### TABLE 1. TNM Classification of Mycosis Fungoides (MF)

| | |
|---|---|
| T1 | Limited plaque. Patches or plaques involving <10% of the skin surface |
| T2 | Generalized plaque. Patches or plaques involving ≥10% of the skin surface |
| T3 | Tumor stage. One or more tumors |
| T4 | Erythroderma. Total skin erythema, with or without tumors |
| N0 | No palpable lymph nodes |
| N1 | Palpable adenopathy. Histologic findings not diagnostic of MF |
| N2 | Palpable adenopathy. Histologic findings diagnostic of MF |
| M0 | No visceral involvement |
| M1 | Visceral involvement. Confirmed by biopsy |

### TABLE 2. Staging Classification of Mycosis Fungoides

| Stage | T | N | M |
|---|---|---|---|
| IA | 1 | 0 | 0 |
| IB | 2 | 0 | 0 |
| IIA | 1–2 | 1 | 0 |
| IIB | 3 | 0–1 | 0 |
| III | 4 | 0–1 | 0 |
| IVA | 1–4 | 2 | 0 |
| IVB | 1–4 | 0–2 | 1 |

nopathy, tumors, or generalized erythroderma should be examined for Sézary cells.

### STAGING

Following the work-up, the patient's disease should be staged. Important factors include the extent and character of skin involvement, presence and histologic diagnosis of lymph node enlargement, and visceral involvement. Table 1 presents the TNM classification of MF. Table 2 presents the staging system based on the TNM classification recommended by the 1978 National Cancer Institute–MF Cooperative Group Workshop.

### TREATMENT

#### Treatment Modalities for CTCL

Treatment modalities effective in cutaneous MF include PUVA, topical mechlorethamine (Mustargen), topical carmustine (BiCNU), total skin electron beam therapy, low-dose methotrexate, interferon-alpha-2a (Roferon A),* etoposide (VePesid), and isotretinoin (Accutane).†

**Psoralens Plus Ultraviolet Light A.** Psoralens plus ultraviolet light A (PUVA) therapy consists of an oral psoralen followed (2 hours later) by exposure to long ultraviolet light. PUVA causes selective killing of T cells. Treatments are given two or three times weekly until clearing occurs. This usually takes about 2 to 6 months. Treatments are then gradually tapered to once weekly and then once monthly depending on the clinical course. Approximately half the patients will experience complete clearing and another third partial clearing. Most patients experience relapse upon discontinuance of therapy. Prolonged use of PUVA is associated with an increased risk of skin cancer, especially squamous cell carcinoma. PUVA is effective in patch stage MF, but because of the limited penetration of UVA it cannot be relied upon to clear infiltrated plaques.

**Topical Mechlorethamine.** Topical mechlorethamine (nitrogen mustard) is used either in an

---

*This use of Roferon is not listed in the manufacturer's official directive.
†This use of isotretinoin is not listed in the manufacturer's official directive.

aqueous solution or in an anhydrous ointment base in concentrations of 10 to 20 mg per dl. This is applied daily to the entire body surface except the genital area, unless involved. The intertiginous areas are treated cautiously. Clearing commonly takes 6 to 12 months, although some patients treated with the aqueous solution experience clearing within a few months. Following clearing, daily maintenance treatment for 6 to 12 months is often used. The principal disadvantage of the aqueous solution is the development of allergic or irritant contact dermatitis in about two-thirds of the patients. However, some of the patients can be desensitized by using very dilute solutions, such as 10 mg mechlorethamine in 1200 ml of water, and gradually increasing the strength as tolerated.

Topical mechlorethamine is usually effective in patch and upper dermal plaque stage disease. However, it is generally ineffective for deeply infiltrated plaques or tumor stage lesions. Prolonged use poses an increased risk of skin cancer, especially squamous cell carcinoma, formation.

**Topical Carmustine.** Topical carmustine (BiCNU) is used in a concentration of 10 mg per 60 ml dilute alcohol for daily total body applications for 6 to 12 weeks as tolerated. Residual lesions are treated locally with a 0.2% solution in 95% ethanol daily for 4 to 6 weeks. Patients who have an inadequate response to the 10-mg dose are retreated, after a rest period of 4 to 6 weeks, with 20 mg daily. Patients who present with limited disease (less than 5% surface involvement) are often treated only locally with a 0.1% or 0.2% solution.

BCNU is absorbed through the skin and can cause bone marrow depression, although this occurs in less than 10% of the patients. Therefore, blood counts are obtained every 2 weeks during and for up to 6 weeks after treatment. The latter is necessary because a single intravenous dose of BCNU causes delayed bone marrow depression after 4 to 6 weeks.

Topical BCNU is effective in clearing lesions of patch and medium-depth plaque stage disease, and in some patients has cleared deep infiltrates. It is only weakly allergenic but commonly produces erythematous reactions, often accompanied by tenderness. This may be followed by telangiectasia, which usually disappears within a few months, although it may be more persistent. BCNU can be used in patients who are allergic to mechlorethamine. Maintenance therapy in the absence of active lesions is not used.

**Electron Beam Therapy.** The total skin surface is irradiated with electrons produced by a linear accelerator. At the University of California, San Francisco (UCSF), patients are treated four times weekly to six fields for 9 weeks with electrons generated at 6 megavolts for a total of 3600 cGy (centigrays). Electron beam therapy is effective in clearing deep infiltrates. Thus it is particularly useful for patients with extensive thick plaques or tumors. Booster doses are usually given to tumor stage lesions. Complications include temporary alopecia, erythema, telangiectasia, hyperpigmentation, leg edema, skin dryness, and nail dystrophy.

**Methotrexate.** Low-dose methotrexate is of considerable value in the management of patients not satisfactorily controlled by any of the previously described modalities. Assuming that the baseline blood count and blood chemistries, particularly the creatinine and transaminase levels, are within normal limits, an initial dose of 10 mg is given orally or intramuscularly and gradually escalated once weekly to 50 mg or 75 mg as needed and tolerated. Most patients require less than 50 mg. Blood counts should be obtained weekly and blood chemistries every 2 to 4 weeks. Methotrexate can be given in combination with topical chemotherapy.

**Other Agents.** Recent reports indicate that interferon-alpha-2a* is of value in some patients with resistant plaque or tumor stage disease. Dosages vary widely from 3 million to 36 million IU given intramuscularly daily, thrice or once weekly. The most common side effects are fatigue, fever and/or chills, and anorexia. Oral etoposide may be effective in some patients with resistant plaque or tumor stage disease. However, it can cause severe bone marrow depression and must be given with considerable caution. The oral retinoid isotretinoin,† may also be helpful in some patients with difficult cutaneous disease. The most common side effects are skin and mucosal dryness and alopecia.

**Extracorporeal Photopheresis.** Extracorporeal photopheresis (photochemotherapy) is a relatively new technique that has shown promise in the treatment of Sézary's syndrome. Two hours after ingestion of the psoralen methoxsalen, a lymphocyte-enriched blood fraction is passed through a sterile cassette, exposed to ultraviolet A, and then returned to the patient. There have been no major side effects. The long-term value of this technique has yet to be determined.

### Patient Management

At UCSF, patients with less than 10% surface involvement by patches or plaques are treated initially with topical BCNU. If lesions are fairly

---

*This use of interferon is not listed in the manufacturer's official directive.

†This use of isotretinoin is not listed in the manufacturer's official directive.

well localized, applications are made only to involved areas. If they are widely scattered, the total skin surface is treated. Patients with over 10% involvement with patches or superficial plaques are also treated topically with BCNU. However, if there are generalized, deeply infiltrated plaques, total skin electron beam therapy is preferred. Recurrent lesions are treated locally with topical BCNU. If this is inadequate, combined BCNU and low-dose methotrexate or methotrexate alone is used.

Patients with tumor stage disease usually also have infiltrated plaques and are treated with total skin electron beam radiation. Booster doses are given to individual tumors. Recurrent plaques are common after 6 to 12 months and are treated with topical BCNU and/or low-dose methotrexate.

Patients with Sézary's syndrome are treated initially with low-dose methotrexate. Failing this, interferon-alpha-2a, topical BCNU, and extracorporeal photopheresis are tried. Recent experience at UCSF with low-dose methotrexate has been favorable. Ten of seventeen patients achieved either a complete or a partial (over 50% improvement) response. The estimated 5-year survival rate of 71% was higher than in other published reports.

Patients with systemic involvement are usually treated with combination chemotherapy such as is used for other systemic lymphomas. Such combinations include cyclophosphamide (Cytoxan), vincristine (Oncovin) and prednisone (COP); or cyclophosphamide, doxorubicin (Adriamycin), vincristine, and prednisone (CHOP); and others. However, in general, responses are short lived and survival is poor. The median survival for patients with visceral involvement is approximately 15 months.

## PROGNOSIS

Prognosis worsens with increasing stage (see Table 2) and is also influenced by type of treatment, age, and presence of other disease. Nevertheless, overall, CTCL is a relatively indolent lymphoma. The median survival for all cases in

TABLE 3. **Five-Year Results of Treatment of Cutaneous Disease**

| | Survival (%) | Freedom from Relapse (%) | Treatment |
|---|---|---|---|
| Limited patch-plaque | 98 | 37 | BiCNU |
| Generalized patch-plaque | 77 | 12 | BiCNU |
| Tumor stage | 55 | 0 | EB + BiCNU |

Abbreviations: EB = total skin electron beam therapy; BiCNU = topical carmustine.

several large series is approximately 10 to 14 years, and this is in a predominantly older age group. Results of treatment with topical BCNU for patients with cutaneous disease are presented in Table 3.

# MULTIPLE MYELOMA
method of
MALCOLM R. MACKENZIE, M.D.
*University of California, Davis*
*Davis, California*

Multiple myeloma is a neoplastic disease of B cells, primarily manifested by an expansion of the plasma cell in the bone marrow compartment. Symptoms are caused by both local expansion of the plasma cells and remote effects of the biologic material secreted by the plasma cell. The disease has an incidence of 5 per 100,000 individuals and reaches a peak in the sixth decade of life. The disease is uncommon before the age of 40. It is characterized by the secretion of a single (i.e., monoclonal) immunoglobulin species in serum, urine, or both. In only extremely rare instances do the plasma cells fail to secrete immunoglobulin molecule. The local effects of plasma cell expansion include the development of multiple osteolytic lesions, best appreciated by routine x-rays or computed tomography, but rarely by bone scan; and localized pressure, by an expanding mass of plasma cells, of most concern involving the spinal cord or the roots of peripheral nerves. The erosion of bone, which is mediated by a set of materials known as osteoclast activating factors, which include some of the tumor necrosis factor family, results in unopposed activity of osteoclasts and the frequent production of hypercalcemia. Unrestrained hypercalcemia for a prolonged period of time will produce renal lesions. The secretion of the immunoglobulin molecule, particularly of the light chain component—i.e., Bence-Jones proteins, which are then secreted by the kidney—produces a varied amount of renal (i.e., glomerular and tubular) damage, providing further insults to the kidneys. Secretion of products either by the plasma cell or by lymphocytes and macrophages in response to plasma cell proliferation results in a suppression of normal primary immune responses and leaves the patient particularly vulnerable to recurrent infections.

Finally, the suppression of normal hematopoiesis by the plasma cells residing within the bone marrow compartment leads to anemia, and thrombocytopenia and granulocytopenia.

The mere presence of a monoclonal peak in serum or urine is insufficient to base the diagnosis of multiple myeloma. There is a wide spectrum of disorders that must be differentiated by the physician. Second, the disease myeloma itself also has a wide spectrum of stages in which symptoms develop, and there is a variable rate of progression in an individual patient. It is important, then, that the clinician adhere to diagnostic criteria for the various conditions described later, and once one has decided the patient has myeloma, to stage them. Major diagnostic criteria for multiple myeloma are the identification of a plasmacytoma on tissue biopsy, a bone marrow plasmacytosis with greater than 30% plasma cells, and the presence of a monoclonal immunoglobulin peak on serum or urine electrophoresis that exceeds 3.5 grams per dl for IgG or 2.0 grams for IgA and greater than 1 gram per 24 hours of light chain excretion in the urine. At times, a patient will not fulfill these criteria. Minor criteria are considered a bone marrow plasmacytosis with 10 to 30% plasma cells, documented to be monoclonal, preferably by immunoperoxidase studies; a monoclonal globulin peak present less than the values given earlier; the presence of multiple lytic bone lesions; and finally the depression of normal immunoglobulin values—i.e., of those immunoglobulins not represented in the monoclonal peak, with IgM less than 50 mg, IgA less than 100 mg, or IgG less than 600 mg per dl. The diagnosis of myeloma requires a minimum of one major criteria and one minor criteria, or all of the minor criteria present in obviously symptomatic patients. Once the diagnosis of myeloma is established by the criteria listed earlier, the patient's disease should be staged.

A patient in Stage I, thought to represent a low tumor cell mass group, should have all of the following criteria: hemoglobin greater than 10 grams per dl, serum calcium less than 12 mg per dl, and normal skeleton roentgenograms or a solitary lytic lesion. If there is an IgG peak, the component should be less than 5 grams per dl, if IgA should be less than 3 grams per dl, and urine light chain M component should be greater than 4 grams per 24 hours. The patient with a high tumor mass, in essence one in a poor-risk group, should have one or more of the following characteristics (note the difference between Stage I and Stage III criteria): Stage I requires all of the criteria to be fulfilled; Stage III requires only one of the criteria to be filled—i.e., hemoglobin less than 8.5 grams per dl, serum calcium above 12 mg per dl, advanced and multiple lytic bone lesions, an IgG protein greater than 7 grams per dl, an IgA protein greater than 5 grams per dl, and a urine light chain immunoglobulin peak greater than 12 grams per 24 hours. Patients who do not fulfill either low-stage or high-stage group criteria are considered to be in Stage II.

There is a further important modification of the staging dividing into A or B with individuals who clearly have normal renal function as A, and those with abnormal function who have a blood urea nitrogen greater than 30 mg per dl or a serum creatinine greater than 2 mg per dl as B. Once it has been determined that a patient has Stage I myeloma, one must be sure than one is not dealing with two entities that have been described in recent years: indolent myeloma and smoldering myeloma. Indolent myeloma criteria are the same as for myeloma, but with the following modifications. There are either no bone lesions or only limited bone lesions (i.e., less than three lytic lesions), there are no compression fractures, there should be no symptoms, the hemoglobin should be greater than 10 grams per dl, and there should be normal renal function. Smoldering myeloma should have a similar criteria, except there should be no demonstrable bone

lesions and the bone marrow plasma cells should be between 10 and 30%. These individuals can be followed closely, with determination of their hemoglobin and renal function, and serum M component performed on bimonthly intervals during the first 6 to 12 months, and perhaps every 3 months as long as the situation remains stable. Individuals with Stage I myeloma have a median survival of at least 5 years, and frequently no therapeutic intervention is required. These patients must be differentiated from the individuals with the situation known as monoclonal gammopathy of undetermined significance (MGUS). These individuals are asymptomatic; have an M component level with an IgG less than 3 grams per dl, an IgA less than 2 grams per dl, and a Bence-Jones protein less than 1 gram per 24 hours; bone marrow plasma cells less than 10%; and no bone lesions. These individuals' M components are usually found as an incidental finding. Only about 20% of patients initially felt to have MGUS will progress to overt myeloma. MGUS requires evaluation and follow-up but no therapy.

Prognosis in myeloma is related to stage and to two other simple measurements: (1) the serum albumin level at presentation; (2) the serum beta$_2$ microglobulin level. Individuals with serum beta$_2$ microglobulin levels less than 6 μg per ml and a concomitant serum albumin greater than 3 grams per dl have an excellent prognosis. Patients with beta$_2$ microglobulin levels greater than 6 μg per ml and with a serum albumin less than 3 grams per dl have an exceedingly poor prognosis without intervention. Serial determinations of beta$_2$ microglobulin levels appear not to add any information to this classification.

## TREATMENT

Once the decision is made to treat a myeloma patient, the following principles should be kept in mind: (1) Although it is a readily treatable malignant disease, it is not (with our current methodologies) a curable malignant disease. (2) It is almost always a disseminated malignant disease, so that local measures should only be used to alleviate local and severe problems, such as (a) bones that are in immediate danger of fractures, such as the femur or humerus; (b) significant impingement upon the spinal cord; or (c) painful lesions that appear to be relatively refractory to systemic chemotherapy. Younger individuals with this disease—i.e., under the age of 50—should be considered for more radical therapies such as allogeneic bone marrow transplant, if a suitable donor is available, or autologous bone marrow or peripheral stem cell transplant with high-dose radiation and combination chemotherapy, as is being explored at various centers.

### Chemotherapy

Chemotherapy can be divided basically into two major categories: induction and maintenance.

The choice of agents for induction, despite 2 decades of systematic studies, remains moderately controversial. The standard care during the 1970s was the administration of oral melphalan (Alkeran) in combination with oral prednisone. Although a variety of schedules have been published, the author prefers an intermittent schedule giving melphalan at 0.25 mg per kg per day for 4 days, in association with prednisone, 1 mg per kg per day for the same 4 days, with the cycle repeated every 4 to 6 weeks, depending upon the patient's hematologic toxicity. It is important when administering oral melphalan to recognize that it is inconsistently absorbed and that in the early cycles, it is important to document that there has been a drop in the white blood cell count to 2000 to 3000 per mm$^3$ at approximately 2 weeks after the initiation of therapy. If the count fails to demonstrate drug action, the drug should be increased. Conversely, if there is an excessive induction of leukopenia—i.e., white counts below 1000 to 1500 per mm$^3$ or granulocyte count dropping below 500 to 750 per mm$^3$ the dose should be lowered. A response is defined by the diminishment of the serum protein electrophoretic and monoclonal spike to 50% of the pretreatment value, as defined by the Myeloma Task Force in 1973. A more stringent criterion has been suggested by the Southwest Oncology Group of 75% in the serum and/or urine abnormality, but it is not clear that this standard has yielded substantial therapeutic benefit. Both criteria are clearly partial responses, with a complete response being defined as the diminishment of all protein abnormalities to a normal baseline and the correction of anemia to normal values. In patients who have achieved a response, investigative studies with anti-idiotype reagents indicate that there still is residual disease; thus, it is doubtful that a complete response has even been achieved with our current agents. In a series of studies during the late 1970s, the Southwest Oncology Group presented evidence that the more complicated regimens that included alternating cycles of multiple-agent chemotherapy were more effective. These include vincristine (Oncovin), 1.0 mg intravenously on day 1; melphalan, 6 mg per M$^2$ orally on days 1 through 4; cyclophosphamide (Cytoxan), 125 mg per M$^2$ orally on days 1 through 4; and prednisone, 60 mg per M$^2$ orally on days 1 through 4; alternating with vincristine, 1 mg intravenously on day 1; BCNU (carmustine), 30 mg per M$^2$ intravenously on day 1; doxorubicin (Adriamycin), 30 mg per M$^2$ intravenously on day 1; and prednisone, 60 mg per M$^2$ orally on days 1 to 4. Each cycle is repeated at 3- to 4-week intervals for 6 to 12 cycles. Maximum lifetime dose of Adriamycin is 480 mg per M$^2$.

A second intensive regimen that has been suggested is the use of melphalan, 0.2 mg per kg per day, days 1 through 4; prednisone, 1 mg per kg per day, days 1 through 7; vincristine, 0.03 mg per kg, Day 1; BCNU, 1.0 mg per kg per day, day 1; and cyclophosphamide, 10 mg per kg per day on day 1; the last three all being given intravenously. This cycle is repeated every 5 weeks. American studies of these combination agents in head-to-head trial with melphalan and prednisone have indicated substantial increase in response rate and survival statistics. This has not been true in European trials with similar or identical regimens, thus raising the question, "Is the substantial increase in expense and morbidity that the multiple-agent regimens inevitably require justified over standard melphalan and prednisone?" Now that these studies have had a chance to "mature"—i.e., have long-term follow-up, it is clear that with the more intensive regimen, although the median survivals may not be substantially different worldwide, in those individuals who do respond, a substantial number (20 to 25%) demonstrate a prolonged survival over those patients treated with melphalan and prednisone alone. The survival rates of 8 to 10 years are now being seen in this treated group, a phenomenon that was rare in the 1960s and 1970s. It also appears that those patients with high-burden (i.e., Stage III) disease have considerably better response rate and survival times with the multiple-agent regimens over standard melphalan or prednisone.

The author's approach to therapy is as follows: Individuals under the age of 70 who have Stage III disease should receive a multiple-agent regimen. Individuals under the age of 70 with Stage II and/or symptomatic Stage I disease should be considered for melphalan and prednisone, with careful monitoring of the white blood cell counts to make sure that an adequate dose of melphalan is being administered. For individuals over the age of 70, one should make an assessment of the physiologic age of the individual and the presence of concomitant disorders before selecting which regimen to administer. It is important to note that individuals who have renal disease—i.e., with blood urea nitrogen (BUN) concentrations of 30 to 49 mg per dl and creatinine levels of 2.0 to 2.9 mg per dl—should only receive 50% of their theoretical calculated alkylating agent dose. For patients with more severe impairment of renal function (i.e., BUN of greater than 50 or creatinine greater than 3), only 25% of the calculated dose will be given initially. As the individual's tolerance for this chemotherapy is assessed, the doses can be adjusted upward toward the full dose. It is clearly important to get adequate doses of these therapeutic agents to the patient to get maximum results.

## Maintenance Therapy

Several studies have now shown that once maximum tumor reduction has been achieved, continuing with the induction regimen provides little survival value. Such patients, however, should be monitored closely and if an increase in their monoclonal abnormalities should increase to greater than 25 to 30% of the nadir value, reinstitution of therapy should be considered. An alternate possibility is the introduction of a biologic response modifier. Current research suggests these drugs prolong remissions. Hence, one should seriously consider the use of interferon-alpha–2a (Roferon-A) or interferon-alpha–2b (Intron-A) in doses of 3 million IU per $M^2$, administered subcutaneously three times a week. Because this is rapidly evolving area, it would be important to keep abreast of the medical literature as to whether or not additional agents such as dexamethasone provide additional benefit.

## Relapse in Patients

The problem of patients with refractory disease and those who experience relapse is severe with only limited options. If the patient has received only melphalan and/or prednisone, responses have been achieved by the use of the vincristine, carmustine, doxorubicin, and prednisone regimen outlined earlier. If the patient is refractory to initial therapy or has received other combination drugs, one can use a regimen of infusional (i.e., a continuous infusion over 4 days) vincristine (Oncovin), 0.4 mg per day, and Adriamycin, 9 mg per $M^2$ per day, with dexamethasone given orally, 40 mg a day times four, and then again on day 9 and day 17 of a 28-day cycle. About 25% of patients previously refractory to other regimens will respond to this therapy, and 50 to 60% of patients with relapse have been noted to respond. Because these agents (vincristine and Adriamycin) are highly toxic if given outside the venous system, such therapy requires a central indwelling catheter. It is the author's preference to use a single-lumen Hickman catheter because of the potential danger of a needle being dislodged from a subcutaneously placed catheter system during the period of the 4-day infusion. Infusion may be given as an outpatient procedure using infusion pumps and is exceedingly well tolerated by most patients. With patients with very refractory disease, particularly those with severe bone pain, one may consider giving sequential hemibody or even total body irradiation. These maneuvers have been successful in relieving pain in carefully selected patients. As indicated earlier, local irradiation can be utilized to relieve areas of obvious plasmacytoma involvement, particularly those threatening neurologic catastrophes, but it is important to limit, at least early in the course of patients with myeloma, their radiation exposure, owing to the substantial damage to bone marrow with subsequent inability to provide adequate doses of systemic chemotherapy.

## Supportive Therapy for Complications

**Hypercalcemia.** Hypercalcemia should be treated with initial isotonic saline diuresis, furosemide (Lasix) in doses of 40 to 80 mg or higher, as required, and prednisone, 40 mg per $M^2$ per day. Obviously, if this is an initial presentation, specific chemotherapy should be started as soon as possible. Unresponsive patients may require mithramycin (Mithracin), 15 to 20 μg per kg over 4 to 6 hours, in 1 liter of isotonic saline given at 7- to 10-day intervals. Calcitonin has only given transient benefit and is not regularly employed. Acute renal failure can be managed aggressively with interim dialysis while one awaits a response to systemic chemotherapy. As indicated earlier, life-threatening infections with pneumonia, septicemia, etc. are markedly increased with patients with myeloma. They are due to gram-positive encapsulated organisms but with a substantial contribution of gram-negative bacteria. Appropriate cultures should be obtained and patients treated with broad-spectrum antibiotics. Prophylactic gammaglobulin administration has not been demonstrated to be helpful in these patients.

**Hyperuricemia.** Hyperuricemia, owing to either tumor proliferation or induction chemotherapy, can be reduced or prevented by the use of allopurinol (Zyloprin), 300 to 600 mg per day, and if the hyperuricemia is severe, urine should be alkalinized with sodium bicarbonate, 1 to 2 grams orally every 6 hours.

**Neurologic Defects.** As indicated earlier, patients with spinal cord involvement should be evaluated promptly. Extradural compression of the spinal cord is common from vertebral collapse. Prompt evaluation with either CT or MRI scanning should be undertaken to ascertain whether or not there is bone involvement, secondary to vertebral collapse, or plasmacytoma. Plasmacytomas should then be treated with radiation therapy, and on some occasions, neurosurgical intervention to relieve bone compression may be required.

**Hyperviscosity.** Hyperviscosity is relatively uncommon in multiple myeloma, though it does occur more frequently in patients with increased levels of IgA or in those individuals with very high concentrations of IgG—i.e., 12 to 14 grams per dl. It should be suspected in patients with visual difficulty, severe bleeding diathesis, or altered mental status when the physical finding is of "box-car" or sausage-shaped abnormalities of the retinal veins. Plasmapheresis is highly effective in temporary relief of these symptoms and should be combined with systemic chemotherapy.

**Amyloidosis.** Amyloidosis may occur in 10 to 20% of patients with myeloma, and should be considered in individuals with carpal tunnel syndrome, peripheral neuropathy, or unexplained nephrotic syndrome. Unfortunately, this complication does not respond well to therapy, so it is important that patients be so informed.

**Newer Developments.** More vigorous regimens of high-dose chemotherapy combined with radiation therapy and autologous bone marrow or peripheral stem cell transplantations are being explored and may yield benefits, particularly for the younger individuals with this disease.

# POLYCYTHEMIA VERA

method of
STEVEN M. FRUCHTMAN, M.D.
*Mount Sinai School of Medicine*
*New York, New York*

The pathogenesis of polycythemia vera (PV) is not known. However, on the basis of prospective, randomized trials, the optimal management for patients with PV is being elucidated, although it is still controversial. Treatment strategy for patients with PV demands careful attention to (1) diagnostic classification to ensure correct diagnosis, and (2) familiarity with the natural history of the disease.

PV is a chronic, slowly progressive disorder characterized by panhyperplasia of the bone marrow involving the erythroid, myeloid, and megakaryocyte series. The hyperplastic marrow leads to elevation of the red cell mass, considered essential for the diagnosis of the disease, and varying degrees of leukocytosis and thrombocytosis. Sites with the potential for hematopoiesis, such as the liver and spleen, can be activated with enlargement of these organs owing to extramedullary hematopoiesis. The hemorrhagic and thrombotic complications of the disease may be due to the hyperplastic marrow with an increased number of circulating elements, causing mechanical obstruction of the microcirculation. Abnormalities in function of the circulating elements and vascular endothelium may also play a role.

PV is a hematologic malignancy involving an abnormal clone of the pluripotent marrow stem cell. The neoplastic nature of the disease was confirmed by using glucose-6-phosphate dehydrogenase (G6PD) and cytogenetic analysis. Female patients with PV who were heterozygous at the X chromosome–linked locus for G6PD were studied. In nonhematopoietic tissue, such as skin fibroblasts, as predicted by Lyon's hypothesis of random inactivation of one X chromosome, equal amounts of Type A and Type B isoenzymes are found. In PV patients who are heterozygous for G6PD, when red cells, granulocytes, platelets, and B lymphocytes are studied, only one G6PD isoenzyme is found. This suggests the presence of an abnormality in the pluripotent stem cell giving rise to a clone that replaces the bone marrow and peripheral blood, resulting in PV. Stem cells from these patients are capable of forming in vitro erythroid colonies without the addition of erythropoietin to the culture system. These "endogenous" erythroid colonies arise from the abnormal clone and suggests autonomous cell growth.

Clinical evaluation has confirmed the biochemical findings that PV behaves as a malignant process. Patients with PV left untreated do poorly; 50% are reported to die within 18 months of the first sign or symptom. Untreated PV patients are at an especially high risk of developing both thrombotic and hemorrhagic complications. Death is frequently due to thrombosis, especially of the cerebral, coronary, and pulmonary circulations. Unusual sites for thrombosis, such as the hepatic veins, femoral artery or vein, and mesenteric thrombosis are also seen. With appropriate therapy a dramatic improvement in survival has been reported, with most studies citing median survivals of 8 to 15 years.

The pathogenesis of the increased frequency of thrombosis in these patients is not completely understood. However, the increase in blood viscosity secondary to the elevated hematocrit plays an important role. Thus, phlebotomy to normalize the red cell mass is an integral part of clinical care. Studies have shown that cerebral blood flow decreases in individuals with hematocrits above 53% and returns to normal with hematocrit reduction. Cerebral function is also improved by the reduction of the hematocrit to levels below 45%. However, these patients are still prone to thrombotic and hemorrhagic complications even when the blood volume is normalized by phlebotomy. Thus, in addition to whole blood viscosity, it is believed that qualitative abnormalities of the circulating elements and vascular endothelium may play a role. Typically, patients with PV have an elevated platelet count and in vitro abnormalities in platelet function.

Because of the potentially malignant nature of PV, close monitoring and appropriate therapy are of great importance. Before therapy can be initiated, the clinician must be certain that PV is the correct diagnosis. One must be able to differentiate among the various conditions that cause an increased concentration of packed red cells per unit volume of peripheral blood. Relative or spurious polycythemia must be differentiated from absolute polycythemia, and secondary erythrocytosis from primary. Treatment designed to suppress the bone marrow would be harmful in situations in which increased erythropoietic activity reflects the marrow's physiologic response to a hypoxemic state. In the secondary polycythemias, one must find the underlying cause and attempt to correct it. Therefore, it is essential that the clinician understand the mechanism of erythrocytosis before initiating therapy.

TABLE 1. **Parameters for the Diagnosis of Polycythemia Vera***†

| | |
|---|---|
| A1. Increased red cell mass<br>    Males ≥ 36 ml/kg<br>    Females ≥ 32 ml/kg | B1. Thrombocytosis: platelet<br>    count >400,000/µl |
| A2. Normal arterial O$_2$<br>    saturation (≥92%) | B2. Leukocytosis:<br>    WBC >12,000/µl<br>    (no fever or infection) |
| A3. Splenomegaly | B3. Leukocyte alkaline<br>    phosphatase: >100<br>    (no fever or infection) |
| | B4. Serum B$_{12}$: (>900 pg/ml)<br>    or unbound B$_{12}$ binding<br>    capacity (>2200 pg/ml) |

*Diagnosis acceptable if following combinations are present: A1 + A2 + A3; A1 + A2 + any from category B.

†Modified from Berlin NI: Diagnosis and classification of the polycythemias. Semin Hematol *12*:343, 1975.

## DIAGNOSIS

In the patient who presents with an elevated hematocrit, hemoglobin concentration, or red blood cell (RBC) count, a diagnosis of PV can be rapidly established. However, it is of utmost importance that the clinician understand the mechanism of erythrocytosis so that secondary causes of polycythemia and relative erythrocytosis can be excluded. By using the criteria of the Polycythemia Vera Study Group (PVSG) shown in Table 1, the diagnosis of PV can be made with great confidence.

Hypoxemia, a common problem in patients with chronic lung disease and right-to-left shunts, should be excluded. Hypoxemia and elevated carboxyhemoglobin levels seen in smokers are common causes of secondary erythrocytosis in response to decreased tissue oxygenation. These patients are managed by cessation of smoking and attempts to improve blood oxygenation, if possible. The finding of splenomegaly due to extramedullary hematopoiesis is important to help confirm the diagnosis of PV; however, splenomegaly can also be found in the setting of alcoholic liver disease and portal hypertension. Many patients with alcoholism may smoke or be prone to hemoconcentration due to the development of ascites or the use of diuretics. It is important to differentiate these patients from those with PV.

Measurement of the $^{51}$Cr* erythrocyte mass is essential in confirming the existence of true erythrocytosis. A hematocrit above 60% almost invariably predicts an elevated erythrocyte mass, but at hematocrits below 60%, the erythrocyte mass may be elevated, normal, or even low, depending on the extent to which the elevated hematocrit reflects a reduced plasma volume rather than an expanded erythron. By following the algorithm outlined in Figure 1, patients with an elevated hematocrit can be categorized as having relative, secondary, or primary polycythemia. Relative polycythemia, also known as Gaisböck's syndrome or spurious or "stress" erythrocytosis, is characterized by an elevated hematocrit but normal erythrocyte mass. Therefore, this syndrome is not an example of true erythrocytosis. Patients with relative polycythemia are usually middle-aged men who are obese and hypertensive. There are two subsets of patients with relative

erythrocytosis: those with a high-normal erythrocyte mass and low-normal plasma volume, and those with a normal erythrocyte mass and a low plasma volume. This latter group is at increased risk for thromboembolic complications. The relationship of this syndrome to "smoker's polycythemia" is uncertain because many reports on relative polycythemia have not included smoking histories or carboxyhemoglobin levels. Carboxyhemoglobinemia is associated with a reduction in plasma volume and an increase in erythrocyte mass.

Secondary erythrocytosis results either from physiologically appropriate stimuli to compensate for inadequate tissue oxygenation or from physiologically inappropriate stimulation of erythropoiesis. The kidney regulates erythropoietin secretion by monitoring tissue oxygen delivery. Tissue oxygen delivery can be compromised by hypoxemia, an abnormal hemoglobin with increased affinity for oxygen (P-50), or reduced tissue blood flow. Erythrocytosis may be found in each case of decreased oxygen delivery mentioned as a compensatory mechanism. The increased erythrocyte mass may eliminate the deficit in tissue oxygenation and enable a new equilibrium to be established at a higher hematocrit value. An excessive rise in erythrocyte mass can impair tissue oxygen delivery as a result of increasing blood viscosity. A balance exists between the benefits of an increased hematocrit and the decrease in blood flow with increased viscosity. Thus, phlebotomy may be required for these patients.

Inappropriate secondary erythrocytosis can be seen in association with autonomous erythroid stimulation by substances from certain neoplasms or cysts, for example, uterine tumors, renal cell carcinoma, or renal cysts. Renal ischemia produced by renal mass lesions, hydronephrosis, or after renal transplantation can lead to increased erythropoietin secretion and erythrocytosis. The cause of erythrocytosis in patients with secondary polycythemia must be sought by the clinician and, if possible, its cause corrected. Most causes of polycythemia can be elucidated by using the criteria outlined in Table 1 and Figure 1; rarely, specialized tests such as erythropoietin levels or studying the erythropoietin requirements of erythroid precursors in tissue culture are helpful.

## THERAPY

### Phlebotomy

Once the diagnosis of PV is established, it is important to reduce the increased blood volume by repeated phlebotomy to prevent thrombotic or hemorrhagic complications in patients at risk. This is best accomplished by phlebotomies of 250 to 500 ml every other day until a hematocrit of between 40 and 45% is obtained. In the elderly or those with a compromised hemodynamic status, blood should be withdrawn only twice weekly, and only 250 to 300 ml should be removed at each session. Once control has been established, phlebotomy is useful in indolent cases of PV in which only occasional blood removal is sufficient to control the erythrocytosis. Once a

---

*$^{51}$Cr = radioactive sodium chromate.

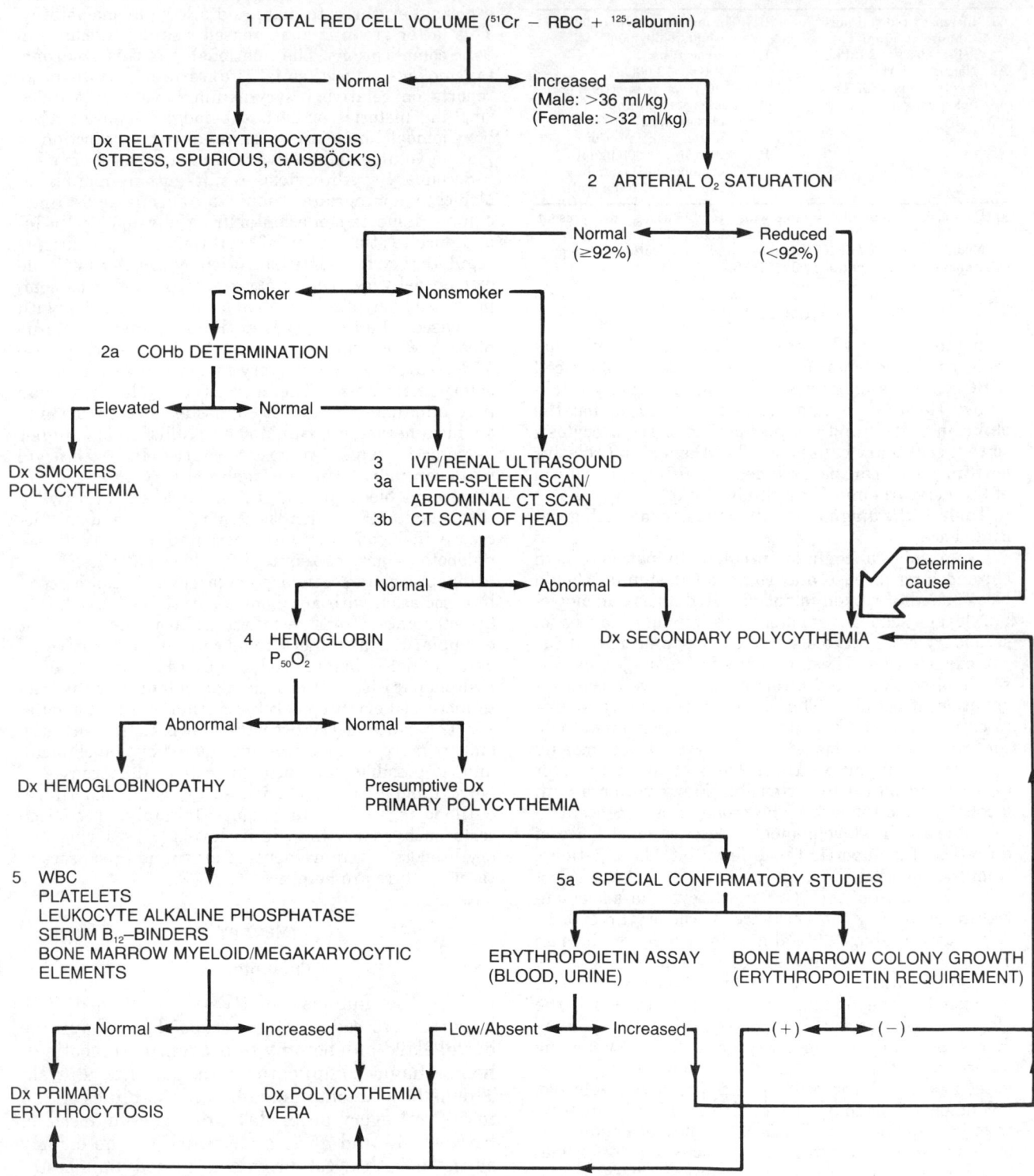

**Figure 1.** Algorithm for evaluation of an elevated hematocrit. (Modified from Berlin NI: Diagnosis and classification of the polycythemias. Semin Hematol *12*:343, 1975.)

normal hematocrit has been reached, blood counts should be obtained every 4 to 8 weeks to determine the frequency of phlebotomies. A phlebotomy should be performed whenever the hematocrit is equal to or greater than 45%. When a state of sufficient iron deficiency has been reached, the frequency of phlebotomies will decrease. Iron supplementation should be avoided because this will stimulate erythropoiesis and increase the hematocrit and red cell mass. Iron deficiency is reported to produce symptoms unrelated to anemia, such as dysphagia, soreness of the tongue, koilonychia, and pica. However, these problems are extremely rare, and patients invariably feel better following phlebotomy and after adjustment to their normal red cell mass has occurred.

Phlebotomy is the treatment of choice in young patients, to avoid the possibility of an increased incidence of neoplastic transformation associated with the long-term use of myelosuppressive therapy or radioactive agents. However, patients treated solely with phlebotomy therapy do have a significant, but low, incidence of developing acute leukemia, especially those who develop "spent" PV. Patients under the age of 50 and all women in the childbearing years should be managed with phlebotomy unless there are specific thrombosis-related risk factors. The most significant risk factor is a prior thrombotic event (including myocardial infarction, peripheral arterial occlusion, pulmonary infarction, and venous thrombosis other than thrombophlebitis); one-third of individuals who survive an initial thrombotic event have a second or subsequent thrombosis with a case fatality rate of approximately 35%. In such cases, myelosuppression with hydroxyurea (HU) may be required. The rare patient with PV who is pregnant should be treated with phlebotomy, although in such patients, the hematocrit often declines to normal or anemic levels as a result of changes in blood volume.

Based on studies reporting fewer vascular occlusive complications in PV patients when the hematocrit is maintained below 45% than when it is in the higher normal range, the value of 45% is the therapeutic objective. In patients who are placed on myelosuppressive therapy, phlebotomy is used to bring the hematocrit into the therapeutic range until the effect of bone marrow suppression influences the peripheral blood count. Intermittent phlebotomy is used as adjuvant therapy in patients requiring myelosuppression whenever the hematocrit is above 45%, in order to help control the blood and minimize the amount of myelosuppression used.

## Myelosuppression

Phlebotomy will not control the thrombocythemia, leukocytosis, hyperuricemia, hyperme-tabolism, pruritus, and complications of splenomegaly seen in PV patients. Patients treated with phlebotomy alone have a higher incidence of serious thrombotic complications during the first 3 years of therapy compared with patients treated with myelosuppressive agents. Thrombosis is the cause of 47% of deaths in patients treated with phlebotomy, compared with 28% in a chlorambucil-treated group and 31% in patients treated with radioactive phosphorus. Thrombosis is especially common in patients over 70, in patients with a prior history of thrombosis, or in those with a high phlebotomy requirement. Myelosuppression with radioactive phosphorus or oral chemotherapeutic agents will control the leukocytosis and thrombocythemia seen in these patients. Sense of well-being, control of hypermetabolism as manifested by weight loss and fatigue, hyperuricemia, and pruritus can be improved with marrow suppression. Hepatosplenomegaly and complications from massive splenomegaly, such as early satiety, recurrent splenic infarctions, and mechanical bowel syndromes, can be decreased.

Chlorambucil (Leukeran) was a commonly used alkylating agent for the treatment of PV. However, the PVSG has shown that the risk of developing acute leukemia in patients given chlorambucil was two to three times that in patients given radioactive phosphorus ($^{32}$P), and 13 times that in patients treated with phlebotomy alone. As a result of these studies, the PVSG no longer recommends the use of chlorambucil in the treatment of PV. Other groups have used melphalan, cyclophosphamide, and busulfan as myelosuppressive agents. The fear remains that these alkylating agents are not free of leukemogenic potential after long-term use. PVSG recommends the use of HU or $^{32}$P for patients who require myelosuppressive therapy.

### Hydroxyurea

Hydroxyurea (Hydrea) is a nonalkylating myelosuppressive agent with specificity for cells in the synthetic phase of the cell cycle. It inhibits ribonucleoside diphosphate reductase and it effectively controls the hematocrit and platelet count in 90% of patients within 12 weeks of initiation of therapy. However, it must be used with caution and the peripheral blood monitored frequently to avoid excessive marrow suppression. Dose requirements can vary widely, and some patients require only minimal doses of the drug. After the hematocrit has been normalized with phlebotomy, HU is given orally at an initial dose of 15 mg per kg per day. The patient is followed with weekly blood counts for 1 month. If at any time during therapy the white blood cell count falls below 3500 cells per mm³ or the platelet count falls to less than 100,000 platelets per mm³, HU is withheld until these elements normalize and then is reinstituted at 50% of the prior dose (Fig. 2). When the peripheral blood is maintained within an acceptable range on a stable dose of HU, the interval between blood counts is lengthened to 2 weeks and then to every 4 weeks. If these recommendations are followed closely, significant drug toxicity can be avoided.

For patients who require frequent phlebotomies or have platelet counts greater than 600,000 per mm³, the dose of HU can be increased by 5 mg per kg per day at monthly intervals, with frequent monitoring until control is achieved or a maximum dosage of 2 grams per day has been reached. The majority of patients will be controlled with doses between 500 and 1000 mg per day, but in rare patients 500 mg three times weekly is adequate. Supplemental phlebotomy is preferable to increased myelosuppression to control the hematocrit.

In emergency situations, particularly those presenting with signs of decreased cerebral perfusion in the setting of an elevated hematocrit or marked thrombocytosis, more rapid control of disease may be crucial. Daily phlebotomy to a hematocrit of 45% should be accompanied by a loading dose of HU of 30 mg per kg per day for 7 days, followed by the maintenance dose of 15 mg per kg per day. Platelet counts into a safer range can be expected within 2 weeks using this regimen. Using this more intensive protocol patients may develop cytopenias. Platelet pheresis, in addition to HU, has been used in situations in which rapid reduction in the platelet count is required until adequate marrow suppression is obtained.

Besides the requirement for close observation to prevent excessive marrow suppression, acute toxicity is rare; occasionally, a rash, nausea, or oral ulcerations may be seen. To date, patients with PV treated with HU have no greater incidence of leukemic transformation than a cohort of patients followed by the PVSG and treated solely with phlebotomy.

### Radioactive Phosphorus (³²P)

The beta particle released by ³²P will deliver local irradiation to the hyperplastic marrow and sites of extramedullary hematopoiesis. ³²P will control the clinical symptoms of PV, such as fatigability, headache, bone pain, weight loss, and pruritus. In about two-thirds of cases hepa-

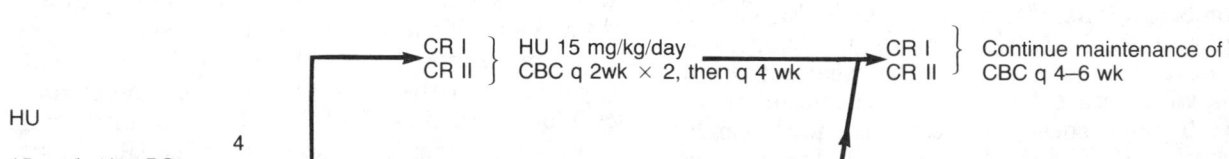
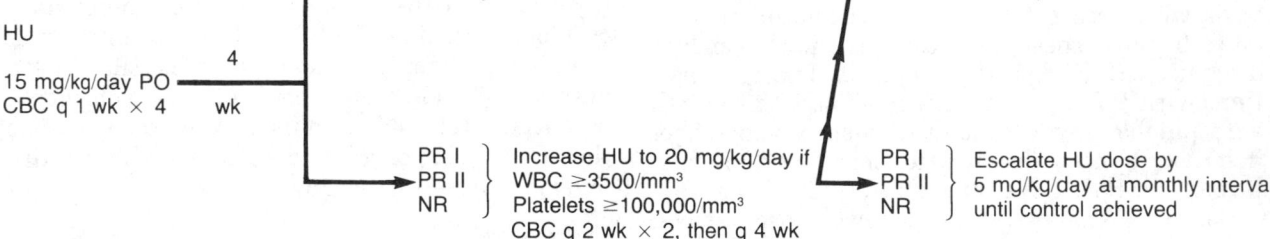

**Induction**                                                                    **Maintenance**

1. Hematocrit to be maintained between 40 and 45% by supplementary phlebotomy if necessary.
2. If WBC <3500/mm³ and/or platelet count <100,000/mm³, stop therapy. Patient to be managed with phlebotomy alone. When WBC >3500/mm³ and/or platelets >100,000/mm³, HU can be restarted at 50% of maintenance dose.
3. After dose of HU is increased, obtain CBC q 2 wk × 2, then q 4–6 wk during maintenance.
4. Patients unable to achieve CR I or CR II despite escalation of HU dose because of WBC <3500/mm³ or platelets <100,000/mm³ should be placed on optimum HU dose and phlebotomized.

#### Classification of Response to Therapy

| Hematocrit (%) | Platelets/mm³ | Classification* |
|---|---|---|
| 42–47 | ≤600,000 | CR I |
| <42 | ≤600,000 | CR II |
| 42–47 | >600,000 | PR I |
| <42 | >600,000 | PR II |
| >47 | >600,000 | NR |

*Key to abbreviations: CR = complete remission. PR = partial remission. NR = no response.

**Figure 2.** Management of polycythemia vera with hydroxyurea (HU).

tosplenomegaly will decrease in size and become nonpalpable. Therapy with $^{32}$P is convenient for the patient and is not associated with radiation sickness. A single intravenous injection may suppress the marrow adequately for many months or years without the requirement for additional therapy or repeated phlebotomy. However, the total dosage must be limited to avoid potential toxicities. The dosage schedule is 2.3 mCi per square meter of body surface area intravenously, not to exceed 5 mCi for the first dose. Supplemental phlebotomy may be required until adequate marrow suppression ensues. If the response is inadequate in 3 months, a second injection is given and the dose increased by 25%. After an additional 3 months, if remission is still not achieved, a third injection at a further 25% increase in dose can be given, not to exceed 7 mCi. Retreatment is restricted to 6-month intervals thereafter and is required only if the peripheral blood is no longer controlled. Total yearly dose is not to exceed 15 mCi. Complete blood counts should be followed every 2 to 3 months and phlebotomy used as necessary before and during $^{32}$P therapy. If there is minimal response to $^{32}$P, other therapy, such as HU, must be used.

Although $^{32}$P is effective therapy, like chlorambucil, this agent is leukemogenic. Therefore $^{32}$P should not be used in young patients with potentially long life spans and is restricted for use in the elderly (patients over 70) who require myelosuppression. HU, although effective in this age group, requires very careful monitoring and follow-up, which in the elderly may lead to problems with compliance. The agent of choice in patients under age 70 requiring myelosuppression, i.e., those with previous thrombosis, painful splenomegaly, or a high phlebotomy requirement, is HU.

### Adjuvant Therapy

Hyperuricemia and its complications, such as acute gout and nephrolithiasis, result from excessive nucleoprotein breakdown secondary to increased hematopoiesis and are controlled with myelosuppression if this modality of therapy is indicated. For phlebotomy-treated patients, allopurinol 300 mg per day given orally will control the hyperuricemia or hyperuricosuria. Acute attacks of gout can be managed with colchicine or nonsteroidal anti-inflammatory agents as required.

Pruritus can be problematic and is seen in 50% of patients. It is generalized and made worse after bathing or showering. Antihistamines may be helpful (cyproheptadine [Periactin] 4 mg orally three times daily) alone, or in combination with cimetidine (Tagamet)* (300 mg orally four times daily). If myelosuppression is required, pruritus usually subsides.

Because of the expanded blood volume and platelet abnormalities in PV, surgical intervention can be dangerous. Elective surgery or dental extractions should not be contemplated unless hematologic control has been achieved for several months. If emergency surgery is necessary, the patient should be phlebotomized until a normal hematocrit is achieved with maintenance of the intravascular volume with intravenous fluids. Postoperatively, patients should be mobilized as soon as possible to help prevent thrombosis.

---

*This use of cimetidine is not listed in the manufacturer's official directive.

# THE PORPHYRIAS

method of
KARL E. ANDERSON, M.D.
*The University of Texas Medical Branch at Galveston*
*Galveston, Texas*

The porphyrias result from deficiencies of specific enzymes of the heme biosynthetic pathway and are characterized by typical patterns of accumulation and excretion of intermediates (or oxidized intermediates) of this pathway. Treatment requires an accurate diagnosis of the type of porphyria present and an understanding of factors in addition to the underlying genetic defects that contribute to clinical expression of these metabolic diseases. Such factors include hormones, drugs, nutrition, and sunlight.

Each of the seven types of human porphyria has been associated with deficient activity of one of the eight enzymes in the heme biosynthetic pathway (Table 1). Symptoms of porphyria are nonspecific and can mimic other, more common diseases. Therefore, diagnosis rests on a high index of suspicion and appropriate laboratory testing. Unfortunately, correct diagnosis is often delayed in patients with porphyria. Conversely, a diagnosis of porphyria is often made incorrectly in patients who do not have these disorders.

Major clinical manifestations of the porphyrias consist of cutaneous photosensitivity, caused by excitation of excess tissue porphyrins by long-wave ultraviolet light, and poorly understood effects on the nervous system. The latter can be life-threatening and occur only in the types of porphyrias in which porphyrin precursors accumulate. Because only treatment is discussed here, the reader should consult another source for a more complete description (Anderson KE: The porphyrias. *In* Williams WJ, Beutler E, Erslev AJ, and Lichtman MA (eds.): Hematology, 4th ed. New York, McGraw-Hill, 1990, pp 722–742).

TABLE 1. **Major Human Porphyrias**

| Disease | Deficient Enzyme | Autosomal Inheritance | Photosensitivity | Neurologic Symptoms |
|---|---|---|---|---|
| ALA-D porphyria | Delta-aminolevulinic acid dehydratase | Recessive | − | + |
| Acute intermittent porphyria | Porphobilinogen deaminase | Dominant | − | + |
| Congenital erythropoietic porphyria | Uroporphyrinogen III cosynthase | Recessive | + | − |
| Porphyria cutanea tarda | Uroporphyrinogen decarboxylase | Dominant | + | − |
| Hereditary coproporphyria | Coproporphyrinogen oxidase | Dominant | + | + |
| Variegate porphyria | Protoporphyrinogen oxidase | Dominant | + | + |
| Erythropoietic protoporphyria | Ferrochelatase | Dominant | + | − |

## TREATMENT

### Porphyria with ALA Dehydratase Deficiency

"ALA-D porphyria" is the most recently described form of porphyria and has been reported in only three unrelated males in Europe. Symptoms resembled acute intermittent porphyria. There is insufficient experience to recommend a specific regimen of treatment.

### Acute Intermittent Porphyria

The genetic defect in acute intermittent porphyria results in an approximately 50% deficiency of porphobilinogen deaminase. Clinical expression is highly variable and is related to factors in addition to the enzyme deficiency, including drugs, steroid hormones, and nutrition. Multiple precipitating factors are probably the rule in this disease. Symptoms are always associated with increased urinary excretion of the porphyrin precursors delta-aminolevulinic acid and porphobilinogen. The great majority of subjects with porphobilinogen deaminase deficiency remain clinically asymptomatic and may never display increased delta-aminolevulinic acid and porphobilinogen. Acute intermittent porphyria, variegate porphyria, and hereditary coproporphyria are referred to collectively as the acute porphyrias because symptoms of acute attacks of these diseases are indistinguishable.

Abdominal pain is the most common symptom of an acute attack. Others include nausea, vomiting, constipation, tachycardia, hypertension, mental symptoms, pain in the limbs, head, neck, or chest, muscle weakness, and sensory loss.

Signs of ileus and tachycardia, hypertension, restlessness, fine tremors, and excess sweating are common. Peripheral neuropathy may occur and is primarily motor. The central nervous system (CNS) can be involved, as manifested by mental involvement or seizures. Hyponatremia may be due to inappropriate antidiuretic hormone (ADH) secretion or may result from vomiting, diarrhea, poor intake, or excessive renal sodium loss. The disease may predispose to chronic hypertension and impaired renal function.

Endogenous steroid hormones are probably the most important precipitating factors. This is indicated, for example, by the rarity of symptoms and excess porphyrin precursor excretion before puberty, more frequent clinical expression in women than men, premenstrual attacks in some women, and exacerbations after administration of sex steroid preparations. Cyclical attacks of porphyria are most common during the luteal phase when progesterone levels are highest.

Attacks of porphyria can occur during pregnancy. However, pregnancy is usually well tolerated. Worsening of symptoms during pregnancy may sometimes result from hyperemesis gravidarum and impaired nutrition.

Drugs remain important as causes of acute porphyric attacks. Patients may do well after the diagnosis is established and harmful drugs are avoided. However, drug-related attacks are less common than in the past and are probably seldom related to drugs alone. Endogenous hormones and nutritional factors commonly play an additional role.

The major drugs known or strongly suspected to be harmful in the acute porphyrias as well as drugs that are known to be safe are listed in Table 2. Barbiturates are most notorious. Advanced motor neuropathy and paralysis are more likely after barbiturate intake than when an attack occurs without such exposure. Benzodiazepine sedative-hypnotics have been suspected to cause attacks but appear to be much less hazardous, particularly with small doses. There is insufficient published information to allow most drugs to be classified as definitely harmful or safe.

A low caloric intake instituted in an effort to lose weight is a common contributing cause of attacks of porphyria. Intercurrent infections, other illnesses, and major surgery may also provoke attacks. The mechanisms may involve metabolic stress, impaired nutrition, and the increased production of steroid hormones and certain of their metabolites.

Acute attacks usually require hospitalization for treatment of severe pain, nausea, and vomiting and for administration of intravenous glucose

TABLE 2. **Major Examples of Safe and Unsafe Drugs in Acute Intermittent Porphyria, Hereditary Coproporphyria, and Variegate Porphyria**

| Unsafe | Safe |
|---|---|
| Barbiturates | Narcotic analgesics |
| Sulfonamide antibiotics | Aspirin |
| Meprobamate | Acetaminophen |
| Glutethimide | Phenothiazines |
| Methyprylon | Penicillin and derivatives |
| Ethchlorvynol | Streptomycin |
| Phenytoin | Glucocorticoids |
| Mephenytoin | Propranolol |
| Succinimides | Bromides |
| Carbamazepine | Insulin |
| Valproic acid | Atropine |
| Pyrazolones | |
| Griseofulvin | |
| Ergots | |
| Synthetic progestins and estrogens | |
| Danazol | |
| Alcohol | |

and hematin. Hospitalization also facilitates close monitoring of nutritional status, investigation of the precipitating cause or causes of an attack, and observation for neurologic complications and electrolyte imbalances. Narcotic analgesics are usually required for abdominal pain. Nausea, vomiting, anxiety, and restlessness generally respond well to chlorpromazine or other phenothiazines. Large doses of phenothiazines are usually not required and may produce unpleasant side effects. Chloral hydrate can be employed for insomnia. Diazepam in low doses is probably safe if a minor tranquilizer is required.

Carbohydrate administration is beneficial in treating attacks of acute intermittent porphyria because it represses hepatic delta-aminolevulinic acid synthase, the initial and rate-limiting enzyme of the heme biosynthetic pathway in liver. Carbohydrate can be given orally as sucrose, glucose polymers, or carbohydrate-rich foods. However, oral intake may be poorly tolerated and may contribute to distention and ileus. Therefore, intravenous administration of glucose (at least 300 grams daily) is usually indicated. Use of a central venous catheter facilitates more complete parenteral nutrition support. The administration of concentrated glucose solutions through a central venous catheter, rather than giving more dilute solutions peripherally, also helps avoid excess fluid volumes.

Heme given by intravenous infusion as hematin or heme arginate is more effective than glucose in reducing porphyrin precursor excretion and is probably also more effective in terminating an acute attack. Although it has been recommended that glucose infusions be employed for

initial treatment, heme therapy should probably be given initially because its effectiveness is reduced when treatment is delayed. A lyophilized preparation of hemin (Panhematin) is approved for treatment of this disease. After reconstitution with sterile water, the drug is unstable and should be infused promptly. The usual recommended dose is 4 mg per kg infused intravenously once or twice daily, but lower doses (e.g., 1 to 1.5 mg per kg once daily) may be equally effective. A clinical response to hematin is dependent upon the degree of neuronal damage and may not be observed for at least 48 hours. Severe neurologic damage and subacute or chronic symptoms are unlikely to respond to hematin. The only common side effects with recommended doses are phlebitis at the site of infusion and a transient anticoagulant effect. Excessive doses of hematin may produce acute renal tubular damage. Heme arginate (an incompletely characterized complex of hematin and arginine) has been studied in Europe. It is more stable and less likely than hematin to cause phlebitis and anticoagulation but is not available in the United States except as an investigational drug.

Treatment with hematin should be instituted only after the diagnosis of an attack of one of the acute porphyrias has been confirmed at least by a marked increase in urinary porphobilinogen. Diagnosis is more difficult after hematin administration because it can normalize porphyrin precursor excretion.

Beta-adrenergic blocking agents may control tachycardia and hypertension in acute attacks of porphyria but probably do not hasten recovery. Propranolol may even be hazardous in patients with hypovolemia and incipient cardiac failure because in this situation increased catecholamine secretion may be an important compensatory mechanism.

An attack of porphyria may resolve quite rapidly, with abdominal pain disappearing within a few hours and paresis within a few days. Even advanced neuropathy is potentially reversible. After a severe attack, motor function and mental health may continue to improve for several years but may leave some residual weakness.

Treatment should include identifying and removing inciting factors such as harmful drugs and nutritional restitution. Symptoms during the luteal phase of the menstrual cycle usually resolve with the onset of menses.

Measures in addition to avoiding harmful drugs can be considered to prevent further exacerbations. Patients who wish to lose excess weight should do so gradually and when they are clinically stable. Consultation with a dietician is recommended. The patient may be prescribed a diet containing at least 60 to 70% of energy in the form of carbohydrate and an amount of energy approximately 10% less than that calculated (using the Harris-Benedict equation) to maintain body weight at a constant level. Such a weight loss regimen requires considerable patience but is unlikely to contribute to activation of porphyria.

Prevention of premenstrual attacks by administration of a luteinizing hormone releasing hormone (LHRH) analogue is a promising new and still investigational approach (Anderson KE: LHRH analogues for hormonal manipulation in acute intermittent porphyria. Semin Hematol 26: 10, 1989). Exogenous estrogens, progestins, and androgens have prevented acute cyclical attacks in some women. However, such steroids sometimes worsen the disease. In contrast, LHRH analogs are peptides which appear not to have detrimental effects on heme metabolism. Ongoing studies with these agents suggest that ovulatory suppression is seldom needed for more than several years in women with frequent cyclical attacks of porphyria. Oophorectomy is irreversible and is not an acceptable option for preventing cyclical attacks.

Prophylactic hematin infusions have been effective in some patients in whom attacks could not be prevented by other means. However, frequent phlebitis at the infusion sites has been limiting. Heme arginate, which seldom produces phlebitis, may be useful for this purpose in the future.

The prognosis of patients with acute attacks of porphyria is generally good. Indeed, there has recently been a decrease in the frequency of acute attacks, owing in part to decreased use of barbiturates. Avoiding or interrupting pregnancy should not be recommended because of risk of porphyria in an offspring, because acute intermittent porphyria remains latent in most individuals who inherit it and the outlook is good even in those who do develop symptoms. Similar considerations apply in variegate porphyria and hereditary coproporphyria.

### Congenital Erythropoietic Porphyria

This condition, also known as Günther's disease, is an autosomal recessive disorder due to a deficiency of uroporphyrinogen III cosynthase. Only about 100 cases have been reported. Reddish urine may be noticed shortly after birth. Severe cutaneous photosensitivity usually begins in early infancy. Recurrent vesicles and secondary infection can lead to cutaneous scarring and deformities and loss of digits and facial features. Variability in clinical expression is illustrated by onset of symptoms in adult life in some cases.

Sunlight, other sources of ultraviolet light, and minor skin trauma are the major environmental influences in this disease. Hemolysis is almost always present but is variable in degree and is an important endogenous influence on disease severity. Splenomegaly is found in almost all cases. Neurologic manifestations do not occur. Life expectancy is often shortened by infection or hematologic complications.

Protection of the skin from sunlight and minor trauma is highly important. Sunscreen lotions may be helpful. Prompt treatment of bacterial infections, which are common, may help in preventing scarring and mutilation. Hospitalization for treatment of severe and systemic infections is sometimes required. Such measures are usually only partially successful.

Blood transfusions given in sufficient amounts to significantly suppress erythropoiesis may represent the most effective form of treatment. Improvement with splenectomy may have been due in some cases to blood transfusions given at the time of surgery. Oral charcoal may be helpful by increasing fecal excretion of porphyrins. Beta-carotene may provide some cutaneous protection.

### Porphyria Cutanea Tarda

Porphyria cutanea tarda is the most common type of porphyria, occurs primarily in adults, and is due to a deficiency of uroporphyrinogen decarboxylase in the liver. Cutaneous photosensitivity is the major clinical feature. Neurologic effects are not observed. It is most common in men but has become more frequent in women in association with alcohol and estrogen use. Studies of uroporphyrinogen decarboxylase indicate that there are at least three forms of this disease, although they do not differ substantially in terms of clinical presentation or treatment. In the familial (autosomal dominant) form of porphyria cutanea tarda, uroporphyrinogen decarboxylase is deficient in erythrocytes and other tissues in addition to the liver. In the "sporadic" form of the disease, the enzyme activity is normal in erythrocytes and is deficient only in the liver. Recently, a familial form of porphyria cutanea tarda in which only the hepatic enzyme activity is reduced has been described. The family history is often negative even in familial forms of the disease.

Associated factors that clearly contribute to the pathogenesis of porphyria cutanea tarda include liver damage, alcohol intake, excess iron, and estrogens. Most patients have a history of moderately heavy or heavy alcohol intake but are usually not frank alcoholics. Liver function tests usually reveal mild to moderate hepatocellular damage. Liver histopathology is almost always evident, but it is usually not diagnostic of alcoholic liver disease. Iron stores may be normal or increased. Increased serum iron and ferritin levels are common. Mild to moderate erythrocytosis is also common and is unexplained. Patients with this disease are at risk to develop hepatocellular carcinoma.

Ferrous iron inhibits hepatic uroporphyrinogen decarboxylase in vitro. Studies in cultured hepatocytes and intact animals provide further evidence that iron is important in contributing to inhibition of this enzyme. In patients with porphyria cutanea tarda, an acquired iron-dependent process inactivates the enzyme activity. Iron removal by therapeutic phlebotomies (see later discussion) may not immediately normalize hepatic uroporphyrinogen decarboxylase. However, the enzyme activity does return to normal after a prolonged clinical remission.

Porphyria cutanea tarda may develop in men treated with estrogens for prostate cancer and in some women treated with oral contraceptives or estrogens. Barbiturates and other drugs that are harmful in acute intermittent porphyria, hereditary coproporphyria, and variegate porphyria are seldom reported to exacerbate porphyria cutanea tarda but should be avoided as a precaution. The mechanisms by which alcohol and estrogens contribute to activation of this form of porphyria are not well defined.

Porphyria cutanea tarda is the most readily treated form of porphyria. Treatment approaches include phlebotomy, low-dose chloroquine, and avoidance of alcohol, estrogens, iron supplements, or other contributing factors. Improvement after cessation of alcohol can be unpredictable or slow, and it is usually advisable to begin a course of phlebotomies or low-dose chloroquine.

Repeated phlebotomy can gradually reduce the excess hepatic iron and produce remissions in almost all patients. About 450 ml of blood can be removed every 1 to 2 weeks. The most useful laboratory parameters to follow are serum ferritin levels and plasma or urine porphyrin levels. Ferritin levels commonly begin to decrease somewhat before porphyrin levels. The intervals between phlebotomies can be lengthened when there is evidence of improvement. It is important also to follow hemoglobin levels or the hematocrit in order to avoid a symptomatic degree of anemia. After a remission is obtained, further phlebotomies may not be needed even if ferritin levels later return to normal. Plasma or urine porphyrins can then be followed at 3- to 6-month intervals. Even cutaneous scarring and pseudoscleroderma can improve with phlebotomies. Abnormal liver function tests and histology may improve but not completely resolve. Because iron overload in this disease is seldom massive, a remission can occur after only a few phlebotomies (an average of 5 to 6 phlebotomies was required in one series). Long-standing remissions may be achieved even after several relapses.

Chloroquine concentrates in the liver, and especially in lysosomes and mitochondria. The drug may complex to excess porphyrins in the liver in porphyria cutanea tarda and promote their removal. Alternatively, the drug may act primarily by damaging or destroying hepatocytes containing most of the stored porphyrins. Chloroquine given in usual doses to patients with porphyria cutanea tarda produces a marked increase in porphyrin excretion, nausea, malaise, and fever, and increased serum transaminase and ferritin levels. Photosensitivity may also increase. However, these adverse effects are generally transient and are followed by complete remission of the disease. However, because of the substantial side effects, usual doses of chloroquine are not recommended in porphyria cutanea tarda.

Courses of low-dose chloroquine (e.g., 125 mg twice weekly for several months or as needed) or hydroxychloroquine have been reported to be effective in producing remissions of this condition and are associated with minimal or no side effects. This represents a useful treatment alternative when repeated phlebotomies are contraindicated.

Treatment may reduce the risk of developing hepatocellular carcinoma, although this is not established. It may be useful to carry out hepatic imaging as a basis for follow-up in patients with porphyria cutanea tarda.

A severe and intractable form of porphyria cutanea tarda sometimes occurs in association with end-stage renal disease. Iron overload is a major contributing factor in these patients, but phlebotomy is usually contraindicated by anemia. Chloroquine is also not effective because the renal route for porphyrin excretion is absent and the excess porphyrins are not dialyzable. Genetic recombinant erythropoietin represents a therapeutic advance in this disorder. Initial studies indicate it can mobilize excess iron and support phlebotomies in such patients (Anderson KE, Goeger DE, Carson RW, Lee S-M, and Stead RB: Erythropoietin for the treatment of porphyria cutanea tarda in a patient on long-term hemodialysis. N Engl J Med, *322*:315, 1990.)

## Hereditary Coproporphyria

Hereditary coproporphyria is due to a deficiency of coproporphyrinogen oxidase. It is clinically very similar to acute intermittent porphyria, although generally somewhat milder.

Photosensitivity sometimes occurs. Clinical expression of this disease is influenced by many of the same factors that are important in acute intermittent porphyria.

Exacerbations of this disease are treated in the same manner as acute intermittent porphyria. Cholestyramine (Questran) may be of some value for photosensitivity. Phlebotomies and chloroquine are not effective.

## Variegate Porphyria

This disease is due to a deficiency of protoporphyrinogen oxidase. Neurovisceral manifestations are indistinguishable from those of acute intermittent porphyria or hereditary coproporphyria. Skin manifestations usually occur apart from the neurovisceral symptoms. They are very similar to those of porphyria cutanea tarda and hereditary coproporphyria. Drugs, steroids, and nutritional factors that are detrimental in acute intermittent porphyria can also provoke exacerbations of variegate porphyria. This disease is particularly common among the white population in South Africa.

Treatment of acute attacks of variegate porphyria with hematin and glucose and other measures employed in acute intermittent porphyria is usually effective. Phlebotomy and chloroquine are not effective. Measures that protect the skin from sunlight including gloves, a broad-brimmed hat, other clothing, opaque sunscreens, and exposure to short-wave ultraviolet light (which increases skin pigment but does not excite porphyrins) may be helpful.

Striking decreases in acute attacks and deaths from variegate porphyria have been noted recently in South Africa. This is due to screening for and identifying latent cases, avoiding harmful drugs, and better treatment of acute attacks with intravenous glucose and respiratory support.

## Erythropoietic Protoporphyria

This disease results from a deficiency of ferrochelatase. Excess protoporphyrin is found in erythroid cells, plasma, bile, and feces of patients in whom the disease is clinically expressed. This is the most common form of erythropoietic porphyria and is perhaps the second most common human porphyria. The considerable variation in degree of clinical expression is not well explained.

The cutaneous manifestations of this disease are distinct from those of other porphyrias. Photosensitivity is characterized by burning, itching, erythema, and swelling, which can occur within minutes of sun exposure. Vesicles, pigment changes, and scarring are uncommon. There are no neuropathic manifestations. Drugs that exacerbate hepatic porphyrias are not known to worsen erythropoietic protoporphyria, although they are generally avoided as a precaution.

Hemolysis is uncommon or very mild in uncomplicated cases of erythropoietic protoporphyria. Depletion of iron stores may be relatively common even in the absence of iron deficiency anemia. Mild anemia with hypochromia and microcytosis is noted in some cases and, for unknown reasons, may respond poorly to oral iron.

Patients with this condition seem predisposed to develop gallstones. These stones may produce symptoms at an unusually young age, are fluorescent, and are composed at least in part of protoporphyrin.

Beta-carotene (Solatene) is marketed for treating erythropoietic protoporphyria. Its clinical benefits have been substantiated in large series of patients. Its mechanism of action may involve quenching of singlet oxygen or free radicals. Doses of 120 to 180 mg daily in adults generally maintain serum carotene levels in the recommended range of 600 to 800 μg per dl. Tolerance to sunlight is improved in most patients 1 to 3 months after beginning treatment. The only expected side effect is a mild and dose-related skin discoloration due to carotenemia. The drug is less effective in other forms of porphyria associated with photosensitivity. Dihydroxyacetone (Vitadye, Chromelin) and lawsone (napthoquinone)* may darken the skin when applied topically and benefit some patients.

Cholestyramine may interrupt the enterohepatic circulation of protoporphyrin and improve cutaneous symptoms in some patients with protoporphyria. Splenectomy may be beneficial when the disease is complicated by hemolysis and splenomegaly. Iron deficiency, caloric restriction, and drugs or hormone preparations that impair hepatic excretory function should be avoided.

Liver function is usually normal in erythropoietic protoporphyria. However, a minority of patients develop liver disease, which can progress rapidly to death from liver failure. Intercurrent factors such as viral hepatitis, alcohol, iron deficiency, fasting, and oral contraceptive steroids have played a role in some patients. Hepatic complications may be preceded by progressively increasing levels of erythrocyte and plasma protoporphyrin, abnormal liver function tests, marked deposition of protoporphyrin in liver cells and bile canaliculi, and increased photosensitivity. Other early indications include an increasing ratio of erythrocyte to fecal protoporphyrin and an increasing ratio of biliary protoporphyrin to

---

*Not available in the U.S.

biliary bile acids. An enterohepatic circulation of protoporphyrin may favor its retention in the liver when liver function is impaired. Liver damage probably results at least in part from protoporphyrin accumulation itself. Hepatic complications and hemolysis in one reported case improved greatly after splenectomy, suggesting that the bone marrow was the major source of protoporphyrin.

Treatment of the hepatic complications of this disease is difficult. Resolution may occur spontaneously if a reversible cause of liver dysfunction, such as viral hepatitis or alcohol, is contributing. Transfusions or intravenous hematin to suppress erythroid and hepatic protoporphyrin production, correction of iron deficiency, and cholestyramine or activated charcoal may be beneficial. Some patients have undergone liver transplantation.

# THERAPEUTIC USE OF BLOOD COMPONENTS

method of
MELANIE S. KENNEDY, M.D., and
JANICE F. BLAZINA, M.D.
*The Ohio State University Hospitals*
*Columbus, Ohio*

Blood and blood components are considered drugs and are regulated by the Food and Drug Administration (FDA). The collection and preparation of blood components for storage and transfusion are considered manufacturing. The FDA closely monitors blood banks for adherence to good manufacturing practices.

Blood and blood components have significant risks of transmissible diseases and other untoward effects. The criteria for transfusion have been re-examined by several groups, leading to revised guidelines for transfusion. In addition, the use of autologous transfusion has increased because of its decreased risks.

## BLOOD COMPONENTS

### Whole Blood

Whole blood has limited indications. Whole blood should be reserved for those patients who require replacement of both red blood cell mass and blood volume and who require coagulation factor replacement. Thus, patients undergoing exchange transfusion, both adults and neonates, and rapidly hemorrhaging patients can receive whole blood (Table 1). In some patients, the use of packed red blood cells and fresh-frozen plasma is preferred because of the need for all coagulation factors in optimal amounts.

Whole blood is contraindicated in severe

TABLE 1. **Blood Components for Red Blood Cell Therapy**

| Component | Hematocrit (%) | Indications |
|---|---|---|
| Whole blood | 35–45 | Rapid hemorrhage Exchange transfusion |
| Red blood cells | 70–80 | Chronic anemia Hemorrhage |
| Leukocyte-poor red blood cells | 60–80 | Febrile transfusion reactions Prevention of alloimmunization |
| Washed red blood cells | 50–70 | Allergic transfusion reactions |
| Frozen red blood cells | 50–70 | Rare blood types |

chronic anemia. These patients have normal blood volumes and may be unable to tolerate the extra oncotic pressure of the plasma in whole blood.

In the "typical" 70-kg human, each 500-ml unit of whole blood should increase the hematocrit 3 to 5% and the hemoglobin 1.0 to 1.5 grams per dl. This increase may not be apparent for 48 to 72 hours while the blood volume re-equilibrates.

### Red Blood Cells

Increase in red cell mass, and thus oxygen carrying capacity, is the primary indication for red blood cell transfusions. The need for red blood cell transfusion is not determined by preset hemoglobin levels. Recommendations in 1985 included a hemoglobin level of 8.0 grams per dl for chronic anemia; more recent recommendations mention a hemoglobin concentration of 7.0 grams per dl. Transfusion should be determined by the signs and symptoms of the patient: pulse rate, mentation, angina, and ability to carry out the tasks of daily living.

Red blood cells are contraindicated in well-compensated anemia and nearly all nutritional anemias.

The increment in the patient's hemoglobin and hematocrit is the same for red blood cells as for whole blood. However, the increase will be evident more quickly with red blood cells, because the blood volume to equilibrate is less.

Most blood centers prepare red blood cells with additive solutions. In this method, nearly all the plasma is removed from whole blood, and then a solution is added to the red blood cells for improved preservation during storage. The final product volume is 50 to 75 ml more than packed red blood cells, but the plasma volume is less. The oncotic load is similar in that a small amount of mannitol is in the additive solutions.

Deliberately transfusing transplantation candidates with organ donor blood has been shown to improve graft survival. This effect is also seen with transfusion of random donor blood to a lesser extent. Also, there are several reports that transfusion can increase the risk of metastatic and recurrent malignancy and the risk of postoperative infections. These findings need to be confirmed with carefully controlled studies. Nevertheless, the implications are serious and should dictate careful consideration of necessity for each transfusion.

This immunosuppressive effect in transplantation has been reported to be less with washed red blood cells and not to occur with cell-free plasma products. Whether this is also true for malignancy and infection has yet to be determined.

**Leukocyte-Poor Red Blood Cells.** Until recently, leukocyte-poor red blood cells were reserved for those patients having a history of repeated and/ or severe febrile transfusion reactions. However, interest is now in another area: prevention of alloimmunization to leukocyte antigens. Prevention of alloimmunization is important for patients who are likely to need support by platelet transfusions. About 50% or more of patients will become refractory to platelet transfusions through alloimmunization. This has been shown to be reduced, but not eliminated, by the use of leukocyte-poor red blood cells and platelet concentrates. Recently, filters have become available that can be used at the bedside to remove more than 95% of leukocytes from the blood products. The filters have several advantages over earlier methods, allowing more red blood cells to be available for transfusion, reducing logistic problems, and removing more leukocytes.

**Washed Red Blood Cells.** The use of washed red blood cells as leukocyte-poor has no advantage over filtered red blood cells. However, washed red blood cells can be used for patients who have severe allergic reactions to blood components. Allergic reactions are due to plasma proteins in the transfused blood. Nearly all the plasma protein is removed in washing procedures.

**Frozen Red Blood Cells.** Frozen red blood cells should be reserved for providing rare blood units to patients with red cell incompatibility problems and for storing autologous units in unusual circumstances. The process is expensive, time consuming, and logistically difficult, with a 24-hour outdate after thawing and washing.

### Platelets

Platelets are indicated for patients with very low platelet counts (less than 10,000 to 20,000 per µl) to prevent life-threatening hemorrhage,

TABLE 2. **Indications for Platelets**

| Indication | Platelet Count (per µl) |
|---|---|
| Prophylaxis, medical patient | <10,000–20,000 |
| Prophylaxis, surgical patient | <50,000 |
| Hemorrhage | <50,000–100,000 |

patients undergoing invasive procedures with platelet counts less than 50,000 per µl, and patients who are bleeding with thrombocytopenia (with or without additional coagulation defects) or platelet dysfunction (Table 2). Although platelet functional abnormalities are theoretically important, in actual practice they are uncommon indications for platelet transfusion. Platelet transfusions are not indicated prophylactically for cardiovascular surgery patients; these patients should receive transfusion for abnormal hemorrhage.

Platelets can be prepared from whole blood or by apheresis. Platelets prepared from whole blood represent the majority of platelet transfusions. The recommended dose is 6 units (bags) of platelets for adults and fewer units for children. Each unit should increase the platelet count 5000 to 10,000 per µl in the "typical" 70-kg human. Less than expected platelet count increment and platelet survival can be caused by massive splenomegaly, high fever, sepsis, disseminated intravascular coagulation (DIC), and platelet-HLA antibodies. The 1-hour post-transfusion platelet count increment is more affected by platelet-HLA antibodies than by splenomegaly, fever, or DIC. If the 1-hour increment is less than 50% of expected, the patient may be refractory due to HLA and/or platelet antibodies. In this case, the patient should be HLA typed and screened for antibodies. In the presence of antibodies, compatible donors can be selected for harvesting of platelets by apheresis.

The platelet count increment can be corrected for body surface area for more accurate comparisons of increments to expected increment of 10,000 per µl per $M^2$. The formula widely used is as follows:

$$\frac{\text{Absolute platelet increment per µl} \times \text{body surface area (M}^2)}{\text{Number of platelets transfused (10}^{11})}$$

in which the absolute platelet increment is post-transfusion minus the pre-transfusion platelet count and the number of platelets transfused is the number of units multiplied by 0.55 (minimum number of platelets expressed in $10^{11}$). For apheresis platelets, the number is 3.0 platelets transfused. A corrected increment of less than 5000 per µl indicates refractoriness.

TABLE 3. **Indications for Fresh-Frozen Plasma and Cryoprecipitate**

| Component | Indications |
|---|---|
| Fresh-frozen plasma | Coagulation factor deficiencies<br>    Single<br>    Multiple<br>    Warfarin (Coumadin) reversal<br>Thrombolytic factor deficiencies |
| Cryoprecipitate | von Willebrand's disease<br>Hypofibrinogenemia |

## Fresh-Frozen Plasma

Fresh-frozen plasma should only be used to increase the level of coagulation or thrombolytic factors in patients with demonstrated deficiencies (Table 3). Fresh-frozen plasma contains all the coagulation factors but is not a concentrate. Therefore, each unit (bag) of fresh-frozen plasma increases each coagulation factor only 2 to 3%. Fresh-frozen plasma is rarely indicated if the prothrombin time (PT) and/or partial thromboplastin time (PTT) is less than 1.5 times normal.

Fresh-frozen plasma may be used for patients who require correction of warfarin-induced deficiency of vitamin K–dependent coagulation factors II, VII, IX, and X. These patients may require emergency surgery or may be bleeding with or without overdose. Patients anticipating elective surgery should have their deficiency corrected by discontinuing the drug or administering vitamin K.

Patients with severe liver disease and hemorrhage or undergoing surgery may receive fresh-frozen plasma for partial correction of their multiple coagulation factor deficiencies. Because fresh-frozen plasma is not a concentrate, other blood products, such as cryoprecipitate or factor concentrates, may be needed to increase functional fibrinogen and other coagulation factors to therapeutic levels.

Fresh-frozen plasma may be indicated for antithrombin III deficiency and thrombotic thrombocytopenic purpura.

Fresh-frozen plasma should not be used for volume expansion or nutritional supplementation, as safer products are available. Prophylactic fresh-frozen plasma is not recommended in massive transfusion or cardiopulmonary bypass; rather, a coagulation deficiency should be documented.

## Cryoprecipitate

Cryoprecipitate contains Factor VIII, von Willebrand's factor, fibrinogen, and Factor XIII and is indicated for deficiencies of these coagulation factors. Cryoprecipitate, prepared from fresh-frozen plasma, contains about half of the harvested coagulation factors in about one-fifteenth the volume. Thus, large amounts of coagulation factor(s) may be given without danger of volume overload.

Although cryoprecipitate was the first concentrate available for Factor VIII deficiency or classic hemophilia, the lyophilized Factor VIII concentrates are now preferred because they are treated to prevent infectious disease transmission. Thus, cryoprecipitate is reserved for treatment of von Willebrand's disease, hypofibrinogenemia, and dysfibrinogenemia (see Table 3).

A pool of six bags of cryoprecipitate contains about 1500 mg of fibrinogen. To increase a patient's fibrinogen level from 50 to 100 mg per dl, assuming a 3-liter (30-dl) plasma volume, 6 bags would be required.

## AUTOLOGOUS TRANSFUSION

Autologous donation-transfusion is the collection of blood from an individual for intended reinfusion. The use of autologous blood is strongly recommended because the patient's own blood is the safest blood—safest in avoiding transfusion-transmitted diseases, alloimmunization, and most transfusion reactions. Four types will be discussed (Table 4).

### Predeposit Autologous Blood Donation-Transfusion

Predeposit, or preoperative, autologous blood donation involves drawing a unit or units of blood from a donor-patient before scheduled surgery. Patients for whom transfusion is not expected (e.g., pregnant women undergoing normal delivery) are discouraged from donating, for two reasons. First, there is low likelihood that blood will be needed at all; second, in situations in which blood is required, a single unit is unlikely to be sufficient. On the other hand, patients who are scheduled for procedures such as orthopedic surgery that usually require blood transfusion are encouraged to donate sufficient units to meet their needs. The attending physician should discuss the likelihood of blood usage with each patient and assist the patient in the decision to

TABLE 4. **Autologous Donation and Transfusion**

| Technique | Method |
|---|---|
| Predeposit (preoperative) | Donation of 1 or more units days to weeks before need |
| Perioperative hemodilution | Donation of 1 or more units with infusion to maintain normovolemia |
| Intraoperative blood salvage | Collection of shed blood for immediate reinfusion |
| Postoperative blood salvage | Collection of blood from operative sites for reinfusion |

use autologous blood. For those patients who can benefit from autologous transfusion, the attending physician should prescribe the number of units to be drawn and give the patient the written request to present to the blood collection facility.

Depending upon the anticoagulant-preservative used, patients may donate blood up to 35 or 42 days before the scheduled date of surgery. Although blood may be collected as often as every 3 days and up to 72 hours before surgery, donations are more commonly scheduled weekly with the last donation 1 week before surgery. At the time the decision is made for autologous donation, the patient should be started on oral iron, such as ferrous sulfate or gluconate, 325 mg three times a day, to build total body iron reserves and to replenish the iron that is removed with each phlebotomy. Iron therapy should be continued daily throughout the donation period and for several weeks after surgery.

The criteria for predeposit autologous donation are much less rigid than those for homologous (regular) blood donation. Standards of the American Association of Blood Banks (AABB) recommend the minimum hemoglobin for acceptance of autologous donors to be 11 grams per dl (110 grams per liter) or the hematocrit to be 33% (0.33). There are no age limits, so that children and the elderly, who might be excluded as homologous donors, are acceptable in many instances. Likewise, the weight requirement for homologous donors is not applicable to autologous donors, and individuals weighing less than 110 pounds may donate reduced amounts of blood, not to exceed 10% of blood volume. The blood is collected into the proportionately reduced amount of anticoagulant solution. As a practical matter, collection from children can be performed in those as young as 8 years of age and as small as 50 pounds. However, the parent and child must agree to the procedure and the child must be able to cooperate.

Contraindications to predeposit autologous donation are few. Bacteremia is an important contraindication; donation is deferred to avoid the possibility of bacterial contamination of the unit of blood. Some severe cardiac conditions, such as aortic stenosis and severe angina with hypotension, may also preclude donation. However, many patients with stable coronary artery disease or stable valvular disease can donate without difficulty.

All autologous donors should be given the informational materials describing high-risk groups for acquired immune deficiency syndrome (AIDS) and the opportunity to self-exclude themselves confidentially—i.e., indicate that the donated blood should not be used for transfusion to others. The blood must be tested for ABO, Rh, antibody to human immunodeficiency virus, and hepatitis B surface antigen.

The blood units are labeled "Autologous Donor," and those that come from individuals who do not meet homologous blood criteria, either by history or by laboratory testing, are additionally labeled "For Autologous Use Only." These latter units may be transfused only to the donor.

The autologous blood units may be processed into red blood cells and other components or left as whole blood. Facilities may decide to cross-over—that is, place into inventory either unused autologous units or components from autologous donors who meet all homologous criteria. Crossover has been a matter of considerable controversy.

Those opposed to cross-over cite the small number of units actually available for homologous use, the complexity of record keeping, the logistics of tracking units, and the possibility that predeposit donors may conceal facets of their lives that could be potentially harmful to others receiving their blood. Those in favor of cross-over see an increased inventory and the use rather than wastage of a precious resource.

When autologous blood units are received at the hospital, they must be kept physically separate from the homologous inventory. An inventory system must be in place to ensure that the unit(s) will be available when the donor-patient actually goes to surgery. Safeguards must be in place to ensure that the autologous units are transfused first and that any additional homologous units required are transfused afterwards.

The transfusion trigger for reinfusing autologous units to the donor-patient is another area of controversy. For example, a patient who has not donated autologous blood may not receive transfusion until the hemoglobin falls below 8 grams per dl, but a patient with autologous units may receive transfusion at a higher level. Each hospital transfusion committee should establish guidelines for the use of autologous blood, including whether deviations from criteria for homologous blood transfusion are acceptable.

Yet another decision regards the length of storage for autologous units. Some facilities, such as our own hospital, do not cross-over unused units and instead store them until they expire. Other choices are to release for cross-over or discard units at discharge of the patient, at a specified time interval following surgery, or upon release by the attending physician. Whatever the choice, the donor-patient must be made aware of how long the blood will be available.

### Perioperative Hemodilution

Perioperative hemodilution, or acute normovolemic hemodilution, involves the collection of

1 or 2 units of blood from a patient immediately before or after induction of anesthesia with infusion of a crystalloid or colloid solution to replace the blood volume. Usually this technique is carried out by anesthesia personnel. The procedure is used primarily for cardiac and orthopedic patients, including those who have had insufficient time to predeposit the required number of blood units. The blood is collected into standard blood collection bags and stored up to 6 hours at room temperature. If reinfusion cannot be accomplished in that length of time, the blood should be placed into a monitored refrigerator at 4° C and transfused within 24 hours of collection.

Among the advantages of this procedure are the lowered hematocrit during surgery that leads to lowered blood viscosity and potentially improved tissue perfusion. Blood lost during surgery is dilute, so that the actual red cell mass lost is smaller than it would be without hemodilution. Fresh blood is available for reinfusion at completion of the surgery.

### Intraoperative Blood Salvage

Intraoperative blood salvage involves collection of blood from the operative site during surgery and is usually more costly than either of the preceding types of autologous donation-transfusion. Circulation technologists or anesthesiologists most commonly perform the procedure, usually using specialized equipment dedicated to that purpose. The types of machines in use are similar in that blood is suctioned into a reservoir with anticoagulant and the collected blood is reinfused during or at completion of surgery. All equipment used must be aseptic and pyrogen free and designed to prevent air embolism. The blood may be washed to remove tissue debris or concentrated before reinfusion through a filter.

Candidates for intraoperative salvage should be limited in most cases to those patients who are expected to require at least 2 or more units of blood. The disposables, cost, and time involved in setting up and using the salvage machine make this technique prohibitively expensive for collection of a single unit. In general, one of the other forms of autologous donation-transfusion is preferable when less than 1000 ml of blood loss is anticipated. Frequent users, therefore, include many cardiac and orthopedic surgery patients. Collection of blood contaminated with bacteria, such as in cases of intra-abdominal abscesses or spillage of intestinal contents, is contraindicated. The procedure is also contraindicated if malignant cells would be salvaged along with the blood.

Blood collected by intraoperative salvage may not be transfused to any other individual. Blood that is processed or stored at a site outside the operating room must be labeled with patient identification. The salvaged blood should be reinfused within 6 hours if stored at room temperature; the expiration time is 24 hours if stored at 4° C.

### Postoperative Salvage

Postoperative salvage refers to the collection of shed blood from body cavities or other closed operative or traumatic sites. Most commonly, patients who have undergone cardiothoracic or orthopedic surgery are candidates for the procedure. Chest tube drainage may be collected into a closed container without an anticoagulant; the blood is defibrinated in the chest cavity. The blood is then reinfused through a filter within 6 hours of beginning the collection or discarded. Blood salvaged postoperatively may not be transfused to any other individual.

### DIRECTED DONATIONS

Directed donations involve the selection of donors for personal use by a patient in preference to blood from the general supply of community volunteer donors. Although autologous donations have been hailed for their many benefits, directed, or designated, donations have been only reluctantly accepted and offered, often in response to perceived legal ramifications.

The safety of the blood from directed donors versus community donors has been a much-debated issue. It was feared that directed donors would conceal personal information that would otherwise exclude them. Also viewed as a problem was the lack of confidentiality when a directed donor is unsuitable due to an infectious disease marker. Many directed donors, as first-time donors, have a higher rate of infectious disease markers than repeat donors. A number of studies have shown higher rates of positive infectious disease markers in directed donors than community donors. However, other studies have concluded that directed donors are not less safe nor more safe than community donors.

The attending physician should be aware of the patient's wishes and specify in writing the number of units required. The decision for directed donations should be made in sufficient time to allow completion of regular processing and testing of the blood before release. An understanding should be reached with the collecting facility regarding the use of compatible rather than strictly identical ABO groups and Rh types. Patients requesting directed donations may fail to realize that family members, friends, or others they enlist as donors may have blood types incompatible with their own. For example, a group O Rh negative patient will have greater difficulty in locating individuals of the same type than someone group A Rh positive, who could potentially have donors of group A or group O, Rh positive or Rh negative.

Policies should be established to exclude certain individuals as directed donors. We recommend the husband (and his blood relatives) not donate for a woman of childbearing age due to the risk of alloimmunization and possible threat to later pregnancies. We also recommend blood relatives of a potential bone marrow transplant patient not be directed donors because of the increased risk of failure of engraftment or rejection. Additionally, all blood components from first-degree relatives of a patient should be irradiated to prevent graft-versus-host disease in the event of shared histocompatibility loci.

The time and administrative complexities involved in directed donations are similar to those of autologous donations, both at the collecting facility and at the transfusion service. The issues about cross-over of unused directed donor units or the components are similar to those of autologous donations. Some hospitals, such as our own, may choose to allow directed donor units to expire if unused by the intended recipient.

For directed donor units, physicians should use the same criteria for transfusion as for any homologous blood unit. If a given patient has both autologous and directed units available, the autologous units should be transfused first, then the directed units, and last, if necessary, any homologous units.

# ADVERSE EFFECTS OF BLOOD TRANSFUSION

method of
CAROL A. BELL, M.D.
*Brotman Medical Center*
*Culver City, California*

Transfusion of blood or blood components is intended to correct deficits in red cells, white cells, platelets, or coagulation factors. These therapies are effective but temporary, and although they are generally safe there is always unavoidable risk of either immune- or non-immune-mediated adverse consequences (Table 1). These consequences vary from mild to fatal or may have long-term morbidity. Increasingly the risk of infection outweighs the danger of immune reactions. Because there is no zero-risk transfusion, the risk/benefit ratio must strongly favor the benefit. The risks of transfusion and alternatives to transfusion should

TABLE 1. **Classification of Transfusion Reactions**

**Immune Mechanisms**
1. Acute catastrophic intravascular hemolysis
2. Delayed hemolysis
3. Nonhemolytic febrile
   a) Leukoagglutinin
4. Allergic
   a) Urticaria
   b) Asthma
   c) Noncardiogenic pulmonary edema (leukoagglutinins)
5. Graft-versus-host

**Nonimmune Mechanisms**
1. Vascular overload
2. Embolism
   a) Air
   b) Tissue particles and fat
3. Infections
   a) Bacterial sepsis
   b) Syphilis
   c) Parasitic infections
      i. Malaria
      ii. Chagas' disease
      iii. Babesiosis
      iv. Lyme disease
   d) Viral infection
      i. Hepatitis B
      ii. Non-A, non-B hepatitis (hepatitis C)
      iii. CMV or EB virus
      iv. HIV-1
      v. HTLV I

be discussed with the patient, and these discussions should be documented.

Transfusion of red cells is used to increase the oxygen carrying capacity of the blood. However, the red cell normally functions far below its potential. There is increasing scientific evidence that tissue oxygen perfusion is adequate at hemoglobin levels of 7 grams per dl in many patients. Hypovolemia may be treated with other volume expanders such as crystalloids, synthetic colloids, albumin, or plasma protein fraction that do not have the same risk of infection and can reduce the red cells needed. Before elective surgery, consideration should be given to autologous blood transfusion. With current anticoagulants, blood may be stored in a refrigerator for 42 days, which may allow the patient to donate as many as 3 or 4 units for his or her own surgery. In addition, using preoperative hemodilution or intraoperative salvage of shed blood further reduces dependence on homologous donor red blood cells. Conservative use of blood products reduces the potential for transfusion reactions.

Acute transfusion reactions can be defined as any untoward reaction occurring while blood or its components are being infused or in the 2 to 3 hours following transfusion. Delayed reactions occur days to weeks or months later and, in the case of human T cell lymphotrophic virus I (HTLV I) infection, years later.

## ACUTE REACTIONS TO BLOOD TRANSFUSION

The symptoms of acute transfusion reaction can be quite variable and may not correlate with the actual clinical severity of the reaction. Therefore, it is prudent to assume that every immediate reaction may be caused by acute intravascular hemolysis and to stop the infusion immediately and keep the intravenous line open with normal saline so that further therapy may be given if necessary.

### Acute Catastrophic Intravascular Hemolysis

Acute catastrophic transfusion reactions are almost always due to ABO incompatability resulting from human error in identification of the blood specimen drawn for cross-match or in identification of the patient at the time of infusion. These reactions account for the majority of the transfusion fatalities—approximately 15 to 20 per year. The ABO blood group is unique because of the obligatory antibodies—anti-A, anti-B, or both—present in the recipient's plasma. These antibodies are hemolytic because they activate the classic complement pathway. Red cell lysis is massive, producing hemoglobinemia and hemoglobinuria. The antigen containing stroma from the lysed, incompatible red cells produces renal cortical necrosis with oliguria or anuria. Less commonly, other red cell antibodies such as anti-C, anti-S, anti-Kell, or anti-Duffy[a] may cause intravascular hemolysis. These antibodies, unlike anti-A or anti-B, are present in patients who have previously received tranfusions and who have been immunized after one or more transfusions; for that reason, acute hemolytic reactions to these antibodies are less common.

Acute intravascular hemolysis is usually heralded by fever and chills, followed by hypotension, disseminated intravascular coagulation (DIC), renal failure, shock, and death. DIC produces generalized oozing from mucous membranes, venipunctures, and operative wounds. Other symptoms of acute hemolysis include pain at the site of the infusion, chest or flank pain, nausea, vomiting, and dyspnea.

Not all patients exhibit all the signs or symptoms listed in Table 2, but fever occurs in 80% of cases. Unfortunately, the patient who is under anesthesia does not show the early symptoms of fever or chills nor feel pain, so that the first signs of a major transfusion reaction are hypotension,

TABLE 2. **Signs and Symptoms of Acute Hemolytic Transfusion Reactions**

| Mild, Early | Major, Late |
| --- | --- |
| Fever | Chest pain |
| Chills | Dyspnea |
| Flank pain | Hemoglobinuria |
| Hypotension | Oliguria, anuria |
| Impending sense of doom | Generalized oozing |
|  | Shock |

generalized oozing from the surgical field, and hemoglobinuria. For this reason, transfusion during general anesthesia should be kept to a minimum. Because shock is a frequent symptom of serious reactions, the unwary may compound the disaster by administering more incompatible blood in the mistaken belief that the shock is hypovolemic shock.

Acute hemolytic reactions are dose related and are more likely to be fatal if not recognized promptly and the transfusion stopped. The blood filter and intravenous tubing should be changed because they contain a further 50 ml of incompatible blood. The volume of incompatible blood that may be fatal can be as little as 200 ml. Children can be seriously affected by even smaller volumes.

When a transfusion reaction is suspected, the blood must be stopped but the intravenous line kept open with normal saline (0.9% NaCl). The paperwork identifying the blood and the patient should be immediately checked because clerical error is the most common cause of ABO incompatible transfusion. A blood specimen is taken to check for hemoglobinemia, and a urine specimen is obtained to document urinary output and to check for hemoglobinuria. A direct antiglobulin test (DAT) is performed to detect sensitized donor cells. However, after massive hemolysis, this test may be negative because all the incompatible cells have been destroyed. Therapy is summarized in Table 3. The most important goal is to keep the patient well hydrated, while avoiding congestive heart failure, to preserve renal function. Hypotension should be treated with 5% albumin and intravenous crystalloids to maintain renal perfusion.

Increased hydration and diuresis should be maintained until hemoglobinuria is cleared, which may require as long as 24 hours depending on the volume of incompatible blood. Diuretics that promote renal blood flow, such as furosemide (Lasix) or ethacrynic acid (Edecrin), are preferred over older osmotic diuretics such as mannitol. The volume of saline administered must be adequate to support the diuretic agent and the amount of concurrent albumin infused so that urine flow is 100 ml per hour yet congestive heart failure is avoided. Vasopressors such as dopamine (Intropin) are to be avoided, since they cause vasoconstriction and may diminish renal blood flow. If DIC is present, treatment requires cryoprecipitate, which replaces Factor VIII and fibrinogen, fresh-frozen plasma (FFP) to replace other coagulation factors, and platelets. Treatment of DIC with heparin is fraught with hazard in the already bleeding patient. When DIC appears, the consumption of coagulation factors is beyond the point of heparin therapy, and replacement of

TABLE 3. **Treatment of Intravascular Hemolytic Transfusion Reaction**

| Symptoms | Treatment |
|---|---|
| Hemoglobinuria, oliguria | 1. Prevention of renal failure<br>  a) 1000 ml 0.9% NaCl/hr for 2–3 hr<br>  b) Diuretic:<br>    Furosemide   40 mg IV *or*<br>    Ethacrynic acid   50 mg IV<br>  c) Maintain urine flow   100 ml/hr for 6–8 hr or until hemoglobinuria clears |
| Generalized diffuse bleeding | 2. Treatment of DIC<br>  a) Cryoprecipitate—6 units with 6 platelet concentrates as needed for prolonged PTT<br>  and thrombocytopenia. Repeat in 30 minutes if clotting not achieved. |
| Hypotension, shock | 3. 5% albumin with adequate saline infusion to maintain systolic pressure above 100 mmHg. |

coagulation factors is necessary to replace those already consumed. For the adult, 6 units of cryoprecipitate administered in conjunction with 6 platelet concentrates is often effective. The dose of each can be repeated in 30 minutes if bleeding persists, and this therapy is usually satisfactory. Although the platelet count and partial thromboplastin time (PTT) can be monitored, the cessation of clinical bleeding is the important indicator of the adequacy of therapy.

### Delayed Hemolytic Reactions

Red cell antibodies may fade with time, so that pretransfusion screening or the cross-match will not show incompatibility. For that reason, it is advisable to provide patients with a card listing the identified antibody. Red cell antibodies that are weak may increase in titer after transfusion of antigen-positive red blood cells. The secondary immune response occurs in 24 hours to 10 days, and with the increase in titer the incompatible cells are coated with antibody and sequestered in the reticuloendothelial system, usually in the spleen. This extravascular red cell destruction is slow and may be asymptomatic except for failure to achieve and maintain expected elevations in hemoglobin (1 gram per unit of packed red cells) in the absence of bleeding. Antibodies in the Rh system (anti-E and anti-c) are commonly involved. If destruction is more rapid, there may be mild transient elevations in bilirubin (1.5 mg to 3 mg per dl) in the first 6 to 8 hours post transfusion, with an increase in the indirect fraction. In some cases, as with anti-Kidd, there may be abrupt intravascular hemolysis at 7 to 10 days post transfusion of all the Kidd-positive units given. The hemoglobinura is alarming but often asymptomatic, although oliguria can occur. Increased hydration should be maintained to clear the urine hemoglobin rapidly.

### Hemolysis due to Transfused Antibody

The previous discussion has described hemolysis of donor red cells by patient antibody. Of lesser importance is the hemolysis of *patient* red cells by anti-A or anti-B found in ABO group–incompatible frozen plasma or cryoprecipitate. (Donors of these products are screened for other immune antibodies, so that they are usually not a consideration.) The relative volume of frozen plasma or cryoprecipitate to the patient's blood volume makes these reactions of somewhat less clinical significance. However, in infants or children under 5 years, these reactions can produce mild to moderate intravascular hemolysis and fever or chills. The reactions are usually immediately recognized and should be treated by adequate hydration.

### Nonhemolytic Febrile Reactions Caused by Leukocyte Antibodies

The most common transfusion reaction symptom is fever, with or without chills. Because it is a symptom of intravascular hemolysis, it cannot be ignored, but in many cases no direct cause will be identified. Fever that begins 45 minutes into the transfusion or in the first hour post transfusion is characteristic of a leukoagglutinin reaction caused by antibodies to granulocytes. This type of reaction is often preceded by severe chilling before the abrupt rise in temperature to 104° or 105° F. Leukoagglutinins are seen in patients receiving multiple transfusions or following pregnancies. They may be present without prior transfusion or pregnancy in patients with acute myelogenous leukemia. Treatment consists of acetaminophen (Tylenol), 650 mg orally, repeated in 3 to 4 hours. Future blood components may need to be saline washed or filtered to decrease leukocyte exposure. If the antibody titer is high, frozen deglycerolized red cells should be given to minimize the granulocyte exposure. These products increase the cost of transfusion three to five times. In 50% of cases, a single febrile reaction is not repeated, so that it is not necessary to provide these more expensive components. For patients with strong leukoagglutinins, transfusion of platelet concentrates with the included buffy coat is a serious problem. Filters that remove granulocytes are now available for both red cell products and platelets. The negatively charged fibers in these filters attract granulocytes (but not lymphocytes) to them. The decrease in granulocytes is frequently efficient enough to prevent further febrile reactions. For patients who continue to have leukoagglutinin reactions, premedication with acetaminophen may be necessary. In general, premedication is avoided because it may obscure the very symptoms used to recognize a transfusion reaction (Table 4).

In rare cases, patients receiving multiple transfusions (e.g., thalassemics) develop leukoagglutinates that aggregate in the pulmonary circulation causing noncardiac pulmonary edema and acute respiratory distress. The chest x-ray may show interstitial infiltrates. These reactions may respond to high doses of steroids (e.g., prednisolone [Hydeltrasol], 80 to 160 mg intravenously) in addition to acetaminophen, 650 mg orally. Symptoms usually clear in 12 to 24 hours, and the chest x-ray is clear in a few days. Further transfusion should be given slowly and the patient premedicated with steroids. Fevers that persist for many hours to days post transfusion are not likely to be caused by transfusion, and some other source should be identified.

### Reactions due to Platelet Antibodies

Antibodies to platelets occur in patients immunized to platelet antigens by previous transfusion or pregnancy. Allo-anti-Pl$^{A1}$ in a patient negative for this antigen destroys infused platelets approximately 1 week post transfusion, resulting in thrombocytopenic purpura. In infants, reactions are severe and death from intracranial hemorrhage is common. Plasma exchange that reduces the amount of platelet alloantibody is occasionally successful. The plasma exchanged is 1 to 1.5 plasma volumes, and the exchange is repeated two to three times over several days. Because anti-Pl$^{A1}$ is usually IgG antibody, which easily re-enters the vascular space from the extravascular compartment, plasma exchange is often of limited benefit. The half-life of IgG antibody is 45 days, so that the antibody usually fades if not re-stimulated. Donors with high-titer anti-Pl$^{A1}$ in their plasma can provoke an immediate response of fever, rash, or purpura in the transfusion recipient who is Pl$^{A1}$ positive.

### Complications of Massive Transfusion

In addition to the known risks of post-transfusion infection and hemolysis, massive transfusion has additional risks related to volume. Large volumes of refrigerated blood with core temperature of 10° C infused rapidly may provoke arrhythmias, particularly if administered through a central line. Inline blood warmers reduce this risk. Massive amounts of citrate anticoagulant have a theoretical potential of causing citrate toxicity and metabolic acidosis. However, if the patient can be kept warm, citrate has minimal risk. The patient in hypovolemic shock is initially in metabolic acidosis; as the patient is resuscitated with fluids and transfusion, he or she usually develops compensatory respiratory alkalosis. Citrate-induced hypocalcemia is uncommon, although the risk is greater in exchange transfusion of infants because of their small blood volumes. Treatment with calcium gluconate often creates more problems than it solves. For infants, it is wise to remove some of the anticoagulant from the blood bag before the exchange or to use saline-washed red cells.

When more than one blood volume of blood and components is infused, there is potential dilution of labile coagulation factors and platelets by the stored blood. Based on prolongation of the prothrombin and partial thromboplastin times (PTT), a platelet count less than 50,000 per mm³, and clinical bleeding or generalized oozing, therapy with fresh-frozen plasma (FFP), cryoprecipitate, and platelets should be instituted. Stored bank blood has decreased labile Factors VIII and V and no functional platelets. Stable Factors VII, IX, X, XI, XII, and fibrinogen remain in adequate amounts even with storage. Thus massive transfusion with stored blood reduces levels of the labile factors. The differential diagnosis of dilution coagulopathy and DIC in the patient with massive transfusions is frequently a problem and may be resolved by measuring patient plasma fibrinogen. Transfused components contain and therefore provide fibrogen, whereas DIC consumes it. In addition, where platelet counts are below 30,000 per mm³, DIC is more likely. In the

### TABLE 4. Treatment of Nonhemolytic Febrile Reactions

| | |
|---|---|
| Leukoagglutinins | Acetaminophen, 650 mg PO to 3–4 hr. Repeat once |
| Noncardiac pulmonary edema | Prednisolone, 80–200 mg IV<br>Acetaminophen, 650 mg suppository |
| Bacteremia | Cefoxitin, 1–2 grams IV q 6 hr |

patient with prolonged hypovolemic shock, both dilution coagulopathy and DIC may be present, one superseding the other. Coagulation factors may be replaced with FFP, but the 250-ml volume for each unit limits the amount that can be given without inducing congestive heart failure and pulmonary edema. Cryoprecipitate contains Factor VIII and fibrinogen and is 50 ml per unit. Four cryoprecipitate units provide 1 gram of fibrinogen. Initial therapy for either dilutional coagulopathy or DIC is 8 cryoprecipitates with 6 to 8 platelet concentrates repeated in 30 to 60 minutes until bleeding is controlled. The PTT and the platelet count can be monitored to assess therapy.

### Allergic Reactions

*Urticaria* is the mildest reaction. Hives, skin blotches, or generalized itching appear after the patient is exposed to the donor plasma containing specific IgE antibody to a substance to which the recipient is allergic. These reactions are much less likely when packed red blood cells with the diminished plasma volume are transfused.

Although urticarial reactions may be mild, the unit should be discontinued because of the potential for producing an asthma attack in the atopic patient. Antihistamines are given, such as diphenhydramine (Benadryl), 50 mg intravenously or orally, or tripelennamine (PBZ), 50 mg orally. An urticarial response is seldom repeated with subsequent transfusions. However, urticaria associated with fever often heralds a leukoagglutinin reaction, which requires treatment as previously described.

*Anaphylactic reactions* may occur in patients who are IgA deficient (1 in 800 of the population) and who have developed anti-IgA antibodies. These patients may have anaphylactic reactions not only to red blood cells but also to platelets, FFP, cryoprecipitate, and albumin. Symptoms include flushing, dyspnea, hypotension, or retrosternal pain 10 to 15 minutes after the transfusion has begun. In the mildest form, only hives appear. Reactions become progressively worse with further transfusions. Treatment includes prednisolone, 80 mg intravenously; epinephrine, 1:1000, 0.4 ml given subcutaneously or intravenously; and antihistamines (Table 5). Future transfusions require saline-washed or frozen deglycerolized red blood cells, which have no remaining plasma. If plasma products are required, specific donors who are themselves IgA deficient are available in many large blood centers, through the American Association of Blood Banks, or through American Red Cross rare donor files.

## NONIMMUNE TRANSFUSION REACTIONS

### Vascular Overload

Vascular overload is the most common nonimmune reaction, occurring in 10 to 15% of patients receiving transfusions. The margin for venous vascular expansion is only 10%, which is critical in the chronically anemic patient or the patient with a small blood volume. Even packed red blood cells can produce congestive heart failure. Patients with compensated anemia receiving transfusions immediately prior to surgery may develop congestive heart failure with positioning (e.g., elevation of the legs, as in pelvic surgery).

Symptoms of vascular overload in the monitored patient consist of premature ventricular contractions or frank arrhythmias, which can progress to ventricular tachycardia and death. There may be abrupt rises in systolic blood pressure of 50 to 100 mmHg, dyspnea, and overt congestive heart failure. Treatment is diuresis using furosemide, 40 mg intravenously, repeated in 2 hours if necessary. If pulmonary edema is not controlled, phlebotomy and rotating tourniquets may be necessary. Symptoms may be relieved within 3 to 4 hours by aggressive treatment but tend to recur within hours. Therefore, the patient should be monitored for 6 to 8 hours after the transfusion, and further furosemide given if necessary.

### Embolism

Embolic phenomena are uncommon complications with transfusion because all blood products, including platelets, plasma, or cryoprecipitate, must be administered through a 170-μm blood filter. Leukoagglutinates that form with storage of red blood cell products have not been proved to cause pulmonary perfusion problems, and 40-μm filters are not necessary for routine transfusion. Microfilters are necessary in surgical procedures that bypass the lungs because these microemboli may produce small strokes.

There is increasing emphasis on intraoperative salvage of blood. With some equipment, there is the potential for air embolus because the suction device is in direct communication with the circulation. Such salvage pumps are no longer manufactured, but this older equipment may be still in use. In most cases, a collecting canister is between the environment and the circulation, and therefore traps potential air emboli. Air embolism under anesthesia may produce hypotension and cardiac arrest. In the conscious patient, air embolism produces chest pain and ill-defined anxiety. It is treated by placing the patient in Trendelenburg's position on the left side so that

TABLE 5. **Treatment of Allergic Reactions**

| Symptom | Therapy |
|---------|---------|
| Urticaria | Diphenhydramine, 50 mg IV or PO, *or* tripelennamine 50 mg PO |
| Asthmatic attack | Diphenhydramine, 50 mg IV |
| Anaphylaxis | Epinephrine, 1:1000 0.4 ml subcutaneously, prednisolone 80 mg IV; in IgA anaphylaxis, use negative donors |

the air bubble remains in the right ventricle until the heart beat reduces the bubble to microscopic particles.

### Nonimmune Hemolysis

Nonimmune cases of hemolysis are caused by mechanical injury to red cells such as by addition of medications to blood bags, fragmentation of cells by extracorporeal pump oxygenators, injury of red cells by microwave blood warmers, or warming with water temperatures above 40° C. The symptoms are hemoglobinemia and hemoglobinuria. Mechanical destruction of red cells, as with pump oxygenators, may produce marked hemoglobinemia and hemoglobinuria, but rarely with renal shutdown, DIC, and shock as seen in immune hemolysis. These reactions are easily avoided by not adding medications to blood and by using in-line blood warmers with sensor-alarm systems. If mechanical hemoglobinuria occurs, the patient should be hydrated to maintain urine flow rates of 100 ml per hour until hemoglobinuria clears. Hemoglobin alone does not cause cortical necrosis, whereas the stroma with foreign antigen, as seen in immune hemolysis, does produce such necrosis.

### Infection

The blood donor's skin is prepared with povidone-iodine (Betadine) and although the procedure is aseptic, it is not sterile, and bacteria are potentially present in the collected blood. Blood and its components are natural media for bacterial growth. This unhappy event is prevented by storage of these components in properly monitored refrigerators that can keep the temperature at 1 to 6° C. Contamination of the blood product can also occur at the time that blood is hooked to the intravenous tubing. FFP cryoprecipitate can be contaminated during thawing by the water in the warming bath, a natural source for *Pseudomonas*. Platelets stored at room temperature must be transfused within 5 days; longer storage periods have produced several incidents of transfusion sepsis with death.

To reduce the opportunity for bacterial growth,

blood products should be infused within 4 hours, limiting the time the bag is at room temperature. If vascular overload is a clinical problem, so that blood must be infused over a longer time, the unit should be aliquotted so only a small volume is allowed to be at room temperature and the remainder of the blood is kept properly refrigerated.

Postoperative drainage devices are available with suction tubing that drains surgical areas into collection bags that are then inverted and reinfused into the patient. These collection containers should not be allowed to remain at room temperature for more than 6 to 8 hours, and the blood reinfused rapidly to prevent potential transfusion sepsis. It is desirable to wash red cells collected in this manner in order to remove fat and other cellular or surgical debris.

Transfusion sepsis produces a fulminant reaction that is usually rapidly fatal. Severe hypotension, chills, and dyspnea often precede the development of fever, nausea, and vomiting. Bacterial reactions must be prevented because treatment is seldom successful. Blood should never be stored in medicine refrigerators on the ward because the interior temperature is often warmer than the 1 to 6° C required and bacterial growth can occur. If a bacterial reaction is suspected, the unit is stopped immediately. The blood bank should immediately prepare and read a Gram's stain, culture the blood or platelet bag, and take blood cultures from the patient. A positive Gram's stain indicates significant bacterial contamination. Therapy should be immediately instituted; therapy consists of an intravenous antibiotic such as cefoxitin, if the organism is unidentifiable, and high-dose steroids. Blood pressure should be maintained with dopamine.

## TRANSFUSION-TRANSMITTED DISEASE

Infection following transfusion can never be totally prevented despite rigid interviewing of donors and an increasing array of tests performed on the donated blood.

### Hepatitis

Prior to 1972, the major post-transfusion infection was hepatitis B, but with uniform testing of blood for hepatitis B surface antigen, hepatitis B infection has been reduced to 10% of cases. Ninety per cent of cases of transfusion-transmitted hepatitis are due to non-A, non-B (NANB) hepatitis, now called hepatitis C (HCV). Approximately half of patients with NANB hepatitis develop chronic active hepatitis, which ends in cirrhosis in 10%. In an effort to exclude potential carriers of HCV, so-called surrogate tests were instituted in 1987.

These tests are anti–hepatitis B core and alanine aminotransferase (ALT). Although 5 to 8% of donated blood is therefore discarded, these two tests were expected to decrease NANB by only 30%. The incidence of NANB hepatitis, which was 8%, was expected to decrease to 2%, or 1 in 50 transfusions. This decrease has been slow to be documented. In 1990, tests for anti-HCV became available for screening donor blood. It is postulated that post-transfusion hepatitis incidence will be reduced to less than 1%. Still other viruses that are non-A, non-B, non-C may be responsible for post-transfusion hepatitis. Additionally, carriers of HCV may have a window period of 5 to 12 months before they exhibit seroconversion and the donation is discarded, thus permitting some tainted units to be transfused.

NANB hepatitis may produce only mild malaise and the patient is not jaundiced in 90% of cases, so that the diagnosis may be difficult to make. Treatment of the acute illness, if recognized, is supportive. The patient should be followed with periodic ALT determinations for 1 or 2 years. If liver enzymes remain intermittantly elevated, the patient should be referred for long-term follow-up.

### Cytomegalovirus

Cytomegalovirus and Epstein-Barr virus are widespread in the population, with over 50% of people having antibodies by their twentieth year. These viruses are so common that they are almost normal flora. The viruses are carried in the monocytes and lymphocytes of whole blood. Rarely they produce postperfusion syndrome, a serum sickness–type illness originally noted after open heart surgery.

Immunosuppressed patients or premature infants of less than 1200 grams may develop clinically significant CMV illness post transfusion. In the case of adults, this may be reactivation of their latent virus infection. CMV infection in neonates may be received from their seropositive mothers rather than from blood transfusion. Although seroconversion may occur, it does not always indicate disease. Symptoms in these premature children may include respiratory distress, pallor, and, rarely, death. In the immunosuppressed adult, CMV pneumonia or hepatitis may prove fatal. For these patients, blood products from previously screened CMV-negative donors are available. Leukocyte filtration of cellular products (red blood cells, or platelet concentrates) may decrease the viral dose. Filtered products may supplement CMV-negative donors.

### Post-transfusion Syphilis

Syphilis is almost never transmitted by transfusion in this era because the current complex testing of donated blood results in refrigeration of blood products for 36 to 48 hours before release, and the treponeme does not survive. Although donor blood is tested for reaginic antibodies to syphilis, 80 to 90% of positive results are biologic false reactions.

### Malaria

Malaria is occasionally transmitted in whole blood or red cells because the parasite is intracellular. Persons who are at high risk because of place of origin or who are on suppressive therapy are excluded from donating. In areas of the world where malaria is endemic, a chemoprophylactic agent is often added to the blood bag to kill the parasite. The incubation period depends on the type of malaria but is usually 2 to 3 weeks, followed by paroxysmal fevers. Treatment for most types of malaria is chloroquine (Aralen) for 3 days. Falciparum malaria is frequently resistant to chloroquine and should be treated with sulfadoxine-pyrimethamine (Fansidar), three tablets as a single dose.

### Other Uncommon Post-transfusion Infections

Chagas' disease is rarely transmitted in the United States; however, many donors from South and Latin America have antibodies to the causative organism, suggesting that they have been infected. The risk to recipients is considered to be limited at the present time. Babesiosis has been transmitted by donors from Cape Cod, where the disease is passed by mosquitoes. Lyme disease, caused by *Borrelia burgdorferi,* can potentially be transmitted by transfusion. In endemic areas, individuals with recent tick exposure are deferred from donating blood.

### Human Immunodeficiency Virus

Human immunodeficiency virus (HIV) can be transmitted through blood transfusion from high-risk individuals or their sexual partners. Serologic testing for anti-HIV, which began in Spring 1985, is 99% effective in excluding infectious donors. This test, combined with intensive interviews of potential donors, further diminishes the risk by excluding donors with high-risk behavior who have not developed the antibody as yet—the so-called window period of 6 to 12 weeks. Although more than 100,000 cases of AIDS have been reported by the beginning of 1990, only 1.8% of cases have been associated with transfusion. Almost all exposures are due to transfusions given before 1985. Published estimates of the risk of disease transmission by transfusion vary from 1:100,000 to 1:150,000. Eighty per cent of hemophiliacs are HIV positive owing to exposure by coagulation factors. Use of Factor VIII, heat treated in solution (pasteurized), has begun to diminish this percentage. Clinical trials of recombinant Factor VIII, which does not have the infectious potential, are now in progress.

## Anti–HTLV I

The major blood banking organizations—American Association of Blood Banks, American Red Cross, and Council of Community Blood Centers—have instituted testing of blood components for the retrovirus HTLV I (human T cell lymphotropic virus I). In southern Japan, where the virus is endemic, there has been a high incidence of adult T cell leukemia in people with antibodies to HTLV I. In the Carribbean, there has been an association of anti–HTLV I with tropical spastic paraparesis. Until recently, no direct transmission by transfusion has been demonstrated, although in Japan, when blood donations were screened to exclude HTLV I positive individuals, the incidence of post-transfusion seroconversion also declined. However, seroconversion was not associated with either T cell lymphoma or spastic paresis. Initial studies of the donor population in the United States indicate that 6 in 10,000 donors have confirmed antibody. Anti–HTLV I is usually associated with intravenous drug abuse. It is expected that only red cell products and platelets carry the virus and that FFP and cryoprecipitate do not, since the hemophiliac population in the United States has not been shown to have the antibody. Because the incubation period for T cell leukemia or lymphoma is as long as 30 years, it may be difficult to prove that the disease has been prevented by anti–HTLV I screening. Post-transfusion paresis has been reported in two patients who received blood from HTLV I–positive donors before screening was instituted.

## Creutzfeldt-Jakob Disease

This slow viral disease has been transmitted with corneal transplants from patients who had received human growth hormone. No cases of post-transfusion Creutzfeldt-Jakob disease have been reported, but persons who have received human growth hormone are permanently prevented from donating blood.

## Graft-Versus-Host Disease

Cellular blood products, red cells, platelets, and granulocytes contain immune competent lymphocytes that have the potential of producing graft-versus-host (GVHD) disease in the immunosuppressed adult or premature infant. GVHD is usually fatal, either acutely or in the long term. Recently, post-transfusion GVHD (PT-GVHD), or fatal erythroderma, has been reported in *immunocompetent* recipients. The disease is believed to be caused by receiving lymphocytes from a donor sharing one or more HLA haplotypes with the recipient, which permits engraftment. The differences in HLA haplotype then induces rejection of the recipient tissues by the engrafted lymphocytes. Symptoms of PT-GVHD include onset in 10 to 30 days of erythroderma, marrow aplasia with pancytopenia, diarrhea, fever, sepsis, and death. Cases have been reported in newborns receiving exchange transfusions, cardiac surgery patients, and sporadic patients undergoing other surgical procedures. Shared HLA haplotypes are more likely to occur when the donors are closely related to the recipient, as is often the case in directed blood donations. It is now recommended that cellular blood components from parents, children, or siblings be irradiated before transfusion. GVHD in both immunosuppressed and immunocompetent recipients can be prevented by irradiating blood products with a dose of 1500 to 3000 rad before transfusion. Irradiation may shorten the storage of these components. There has been no successful treatment of PT-GVHD.

## SUMMARY

Adverse immune consequences of transfusion can often be treated successfully. Infectious consequences can be treated in some cases, but in the case of AIDS, HTLV I infection, or PT-GHVD, prevention is the only course: prevention by serologic screening of the donated blood and by reducing utilization of blood products in general and from related donors in particular.

# Section 6

# The Digestive System

## BLEEDING ESOPHAGEAL VARICES

method of
ALAN S. LIVINGSTONE, M.D.
*University of Miami*
*Miami, Florida*

Few events in clinical medicine are more impressive or more lethal than bleeding from esophageal varices. The relationship between portal hypertension and variceal hemorrhage has been recognized for almost a century, stimulating medical, endoscopic, and surgical therapeutic approaches. The numerous and widely disparate management options underline the lack of consensus as to the optimal treatment algorithm.

### PROPHYLAXIS

Bleeding from esophageal varices is a highly lethal event, with the mortality from the first episode ranging between 20 and 60%. This has prompted the legitimate question of whether this initial hemorrhage can be prevented. Twenty years ago, four prospective randomized studies comparing prophylactic portacaval shunts and medical therapy were undertaken. The patients all had cirrhosis and esophageal varices, but had never bled. The group with shunts had an immediate operative mortality of almost 10%, and no increased five-year survival. Further, one third manifested varying degrees of hepatic encephalopathy. Accordingly, prophylactic shunting was abandoned.

In the past decade, with increasing experience with endoscopic variceal sclerotherapy, there has been a resurgence of interest in the prophylaxis of esophageal bleeding. A limiting factor in all prophylactic protocols has been the inability to identify the patients who are going to bleed. Overall, perhaps only a third of patients with cirrhosis and varices will eventually hemorrhage. Therefore, without accurate screening criteria, two-thirds of patients would be unnecessarily treated. Numerous ongoing trials are attempting to resolve this dilemma by looking at the endoscopic appearance of the varices and the Child's classification of the cirrhotic.

Trials of prophylactic endoscopic sclerotherapy in cirrhotics with varices who have never bled have produced contradictory results. Some initial European studies suggested a reduction in bleeding and mortality with sclerotherapy. However, these trials had extremely high incidences of bleeding in the control groups. In the United States, the Veterans Administration Cooperative Study had to be terminated prematurely because the sclerotherapy group not only had a higher incidence of bleeding but also an increased mortality of 29% versus 16% in the control patients. A similar experience at Parkland Hospital suggested that prophylactic sclerotherapy produced more frequent bleeding and no improvement in survival. Widespread use of prophylactic sclerotherapy is not justifiable and should be reserved for patients in controlled clinical trials.

Pharmacologic prophylaxis is actively being investigated. A recent prospective randomized trial of patients with predominantly alcoholic cirrhosis and large varices that had never bled was conducted using propranolol (Inderal). The propranolol-treated group not only had a lower incidence of bleeding, but also a significantly improved survival. Further trials are necessary to define the ultimate role of pharmacologic management.

### MANAGEMENT OF ACUTE BLEEDING

The goal is to accurately diagnose the source of bleeding and to rapidly control it. Massive transfusions with ongoing instability produce a jaundiced, encephalopathic patient with tense ascites, a marked coagulopathy, and a hepatorenal syndrome—and death.

#### Diagnosis

Clinical evaluation commonly identifies the cirrhotic patient and raises the suspicion of esophageal varices. However, up to 50% of cirrhotics who are hemorrhaging do so from a source other than their varices or from a source in addition to their varices. Upper gastrointestinal endoscopy is mandatory for the optimal management of these bleeding patients. Identification of a Mallory-Weiss tear or a bleeding duodenal ulcer distinctly alters the therapy. If a bleeding varix is

411

visualized, it can be sclerosed acutely. Demonstration of a diffuse bleeding gastritis may reflect a hypertensive gastropathy. This is just another manifestation of portal hypertension and should be managed as one treats bleeding varices, except that endoscopic sclerotherapy is not an option.

### Resuscitation and Monitoring

The general principles governing the management of any unstable bleeding patient apply, but there are some notable exceptions. These patients are ideally managed in an intensive care unit. Large-bore peripheral intravenous catheters should be placed, as well as a central venous line for the administration of vasopressin (Pitressin). An unobstructed airway must be maintained and aspiration pneumonia avoided. If there is any doubt, these encephalopathic, vomiting patients should be intubated prior to endoscopy or placement of a Sengstaken-Blakemore tube. A Swan-Ganz catheter is most helpful in the elderly patient with pre-existing heart disease who developed cirrhosis after transfusions. The majority of younger, alcoholic cirrhotics have a hyperdynamic circulation, and the cardiac output is invariably elevated even when the patient is relatively hypotensive. Further, cirrhotics typically have low wedge pressures and attempts to raise the wedge pressure to the 12 to 14 cm $H_2O$ range result in over-resuscitation, increased bleeding, and massive ascites formation. Oftentimes, the experienced clinician can adequately adjust treatment of the patient using the measurement of blood pressure, pulse, and urinary output.

Typically, patients in shock can be supported with large volumes of crystalloids, but in cirrhotics these must be avoided. Lost blood should be replaced with red blood cells to maintain the hematocrit at approximately 30%. Although it sounds heretical, volume resuscitation with a 5% dextrose solution, and albumin, is preferable to crystalloid solutions as long as profound hyponatremia does not develop. Clinically significant hyponatremia in a cirrhotic is rarely a problem if the serum sodium is greater than 125 mEq per liter. In stable patients with marginal urinary output, the use of small doses of diuretics is preferable to volume loading. The consequence of injudicious crystalloid resuscitation is massive ascites that may be extremely difficult to treat.

Even stable cirrhotics may have prolongations of their prothrombin and partial thromboplastin times, as well as thrombocytopenia. In the actively hemorrhaging cirrhotic, fresh-frozen plasma and platelets may be necessary to correct the coagulopathies.

Hepatic encephalopathy often follows an acute bleeding episode. This can be treated with gentle purging of the gastrointestinal tract, either from above or with saline enemas. Lactulose (Chronulac), 15 to 30 ml every 4 to 6 hours, or neomycin, 2 to 4 grams a day in divided doses, may also be useful. Along with the blood in the gastrointestinal tract, other factors producing hepatic coma include hypokalemic alkalosis, sepsis, and numerous medications. In general, sedatives and narcotics should be used sparingly in cirrhotics. Of course, if delirium tremens is suspected, chlordiazepoxide (Librium) or other suitable medications must be employed.

### Pharmacologic Agents

Vasopressin (Pitressin) has been widely used to control acutely bleeding varices.* The salutary effects are a result of the marked splanchnic arterial vasoconstriction, with a secondary reduction of about 50% in portal venous blood flow. This reduces portal pressures by up to 70%; a consequent cessation of variceal bleeding occurs in about half the patients.

Vasopressin should be administered only through a central venous catheter because subcutaneous extravasation can result in skin necrosis. An initial loading dose of 20 U over 20 minutes can be given and then followed with 0.4 to 0.6 U per minute.† Higher dosages have been used but are associated with a higher incidence of side effects. Continuous infusion of vasopressin in the superior mesenteric artery has no advantages over intravenous infusion. The serious complications relate to generalized vasoconstriction and include bradycardia, hypertension, and myocardial ischemia. Nitroglycerin used in conjunction with vasopressin can reverse these coronary and systemic side effects. At the same time, it further reduces portal pressure by decreasing portal venous resistance. Nitroglycerin can be administered by a sublingual, transdermal, or intravenous route. When given intravenously, the nitroglycerin has to be titrated carefully starting at dosages as low as 15 µg per minute.* The effect is to normalize heart rate, blood pressure, and cardiac output. After bleeding has stopped, the patient can be weaned from vasopressin, by reducing the dost by 0.1 U per minute every 6 to 12 hours.

Other pharmacologic agents that have been used to manage acute esophageal bleeding include terlipressin (Glypressin), somatostatin, and nitroprusside (Nipride). The utility of these drugs has yet to be defined. The negative inotropic and

---

*This use of vasoprossin is not listed in the manufacturer's official directive.

†Exceeds dosage recommended by the manufacturer.

chronotropic effects of propranolol preclude its use in the bleeding patient.

## Balloon Tamponade

Prior to the past decade, if vasopressin did not arrest the hemorrhage, balloon tamponade would have been employed. The most popular method uses the Sengstaken-Blakemore tube, which has only three lumina and requires placement of a nasogastric tube above the esophageal balloon to aspirate secretions.

To prevent aspiration, I routinely intubate the majority of patients prior to the insertion of the Sengstaken-Blakemore tube. Balloons should be prechecked and placement can be by either the oral or the nasal route. Fifty milliliters of air should be injected into the gastric balloon, and the subdiaphragmatic position verified on x-ray film. This prevents inflating the gastric balloon in the distal esophagus and rupturing it. When the balloon is in the correct position, 250 ml of air is injected into the gastric balloon and the tube is snugged up against the gastroesophageal junction. Steady traction of 1 to 2 lb can be achieved by attaching the tube to the faceguard of a football helmet. If control of hemorrhage is not rapidly achieved, the esophageal balloon can be inflated to a pressure of 25 to 45 mmHg. The pressure in the esophageal balloon must be constantly monitored and intermittently reduced to prevent esophageal necrosis. If bleeding is controlled over a period of 24 hours, the esophageal balloon pressure can be lessened. After 48 hours, the gastric balloon can be deflated.

Balloon tamponade acutely arrests hemorrhage in about 75% of patients, but, after the balloons are deflated, 40% of the patients rebleed. Currently, it is most commonly used when sclerotherapy is unavailable or has failed. It may stabilize a patient sufficiently to allow emergency surgery. Major complications include aspiration and esophageal rupture.

## Percutaneous Transhepatic Obliteration of Varices

This modality has been largely supplanted by the more frequent use of endoscopic sclerotherapy. With percutaneous transhepatic obliteration, the portal vein was catheterized percutaneously, identifying and sclerosing the coronary vein along with any other major variceal collaterals. Patients with hepatopetal flow in their portal veins could experience short-term stabilization. However, on long-term follow-up, half the patients eventually rebled. In patients with hepatofugal flow, the results were poor owing to a high incidence of portal vein thrombosis and death.

## Emergency Endoscopic Sclerotherapy

Emergency endoscopic sclerotherapy has radically altered the sequential management of bleeding esophageal varices. Currently, if patients do not stop bleeding with administration of vasopressin, endoscopic sclerotherapy is employed. There are many variations of the sclerotherapy technique, and there is much debate about the type of sclerosant and whether the injection should be intravariceal or paravariceal. These variables appear much less important than the skill of the endoscopist. Today, almost all sclerotherapy is done through a flexible endoscope, as opposed to the rigid scopes that were initially used.

Acute sclerotherapy is effective in thrombosing a bleeding varix, but up to 50% of the patients rebleed during the initial hospitalization. These patients must undergo aggressive re-endoscopy and resclerosis. In spite of the most aggressive endoscopic regimens, some patients continue to bleed and should be operated on. The most common minor complications of sclerotherapy are esophageal ulceration and stricture formation. The major lethal complications are esophageal perforation and massive hemorrhage.

An interesting study compared sclerotherapy and portacaval shunt surgery in poor-risk Child's Class C cirrhotics. This study was designed to assess therapeutic efficacy as well as relative cost. The initial mortality in both groups of bleeders was approximately 50%. The length of hospitalization and the initial cost was greater in the shunted patients. Half of the sclerosed patients rebled in the hospital, and 75% of them rebled on follow-up. Forty per cent of the sclerosed patients eventually had to have shunts to control hemorrhage. In contrast, no patient in the portacaval shunt group rebled. Eventually, with the repeated hospitalizations, there was no difference in the health care costs in the two groups.

## Emergency Nonshunting Procedures

If the patient continues to bleed in spite of the above measures, surgery is necessary if the patient is to be salvaged. Nonshunting procedures can be contemplated when the patient's condition is so poor that he or she would not survive a more definitive operation, when the surgeon does not have the expertise to perform a more complicated shunt, or if the patient has thrombosis of the mesenteric venous system precluding a shunt operation.

Transthoracic variceal ligation carries a mortality of between 25 to 50%. Further, a second definitive operation is necessary to prevent recurrent bleeding, which otherwise occurs in about half of the patients. Similar results can be accomplished by a transabdominal route by using the EEA stapling device to transect and reanastomose the esophagus. This is a simple and rapidly performed technique, but still carries a mortality in the emergent situation of up to 50%, with eventually a 50% rebleeding rate. Further, in this era when almost all patients have first had endoscopic sclerotherapy, the thickened distal esophagus may make the application of the stapling instrument technically quite difficult.

There have been numerous, more aggressive nonshunt procedures, many of which revolve around variations of gastric devascularization. An interesting operation is the Sugiura procedure, which includes a transthoracic esophageal devascularization and transection, and a laparotomy with splenectomy, gastric devascularization, and pyloroplasty. Japanese investigators have been able to perform this operation with a mortality of only 13% and a rebleeding rate of less than 10%. However, it is important to realize that, in Sugiura's series of patients, less than 10% had alcoholic cirrhosis. The results have not been duplicated in North America.

### Emergency Shunts

There is no question that shunts are the most effective method of permanently arresting variceal hemorrhage. They fall into two broad categories, central and selective.

Central shunts totally divert all portal blood into the systemic circulation. The most commonly performed central shunts have been the end-to-side and the side-to-side portacaval shunts. The latter, by decompressing the liver as well as the portal circulation, is probably more effective in controlling ascites. Interposition shunts between the portal vein and the inferior vena cava, the superior mesenteric vein and the inferior vena cava, or the splenic vein and the renal vein have also been designed in an effort to simplify the dissection. These interposition shunts have the benefit that they can be more readily taken down if the patient develops intractable encephalopathy or eventually comes to liver transplantation. It must be remembered, however, that interposition shunts have an increased risk of thrombosis because a prosthesis is being placed in the venous circulation. The operative mortality is proportional to the Child's Class, being about 15% for Class A patients and more than 50% for C patients. The best reported results for emergency portacaval shunts are from San Diego researchers, quoting an operative mortality of 17% and a 5-year survival of 72%.

Distal splenorenal shunts maintain portal perfusion, but are not usually performed emergently because of the technical difficulties and the prolonged operative time required for this selective procedure. However, in centers with experience, this operation can be performed in an emergency situation with an operative mortality of less than 30% and control of bleeding in more than 90%.

In this modern era, prior to performing any shunt, one must consider whether the patient is a current or future candidate for a liver transplant. Operations in the hilum of the liver, such as portacaval shunts, greatly complicate or may even preclude future liver transplantation.

## ELECTIVE MANAGEMENT OF VARICES

After an initial hemorrhage, the chance of rebleeding from varices within 1 year is at least 60%. Therefore, it is reasonable to consider definitively treating this high-risk cohort of patients.

### Pharmacology

Propranolol is the only drug that has been extensively evaluated for the prevention of recurrent variceal hemorrhage. It is typically given in dosages sufficient to reduce the resting pulse rate by 25%. Although the initial studies seemed promising, subsequent studies have shown the benefits of propranolol to be equivocal, with a significant rate of rebleeding.

### Endoscopic Variceal Sclerotherapy

Repeated endoscopic sclerotherapy has become the most popular treatment for long-term control of varices. It is seductively attractive in that it can be performed in the awake patient in an outpatient setting by any experienced endoscopist. Further, in the elective situation, the mortality is low and the morbidity acceptable. However, analysis of the long-term benefits reveals conflicting information.

Most studies have compared sclerotherapy with medical treatment controls. Although rebleeding is less frequent in sclerosed patients, the long-term rebleeding rate is still about 50%, in spite of repeated sclerotherapy sessions. Effects on survival are also uncertain. Although some studies show no difference between the two groups, others demonstrate improved survival in sclerosed patients versus untreated controls. (It should be noted that the control patients were allowed to bleed to death without being provided other treatment options.)

It is apparent that repeated sclerotherapy can be effective long-term therapy in some patients.

Others, however, repeatedly bleed and must be considered for other treatment regimens.

### Elective Nonshunting Procedures

The limitations of these procedures have already been alluded to earlier. By not reducing the underlying portal hypertension, there is a long-term rebleeding rate of approximately 50%. An exception may be the Sugiura procedure. The precise role of this latter operation in North America remains to be defined.

I currently reserve these operations for patients who are not candidates for sclerotherapy or selective shunting and for salvage operations after a failed shunt.

### Elective Shunts

Elective central shunts can be performed with an operative mortality of 5 to 10%. They are effective in treating ascites and have a rebleeding rate of less than 10%. Unfortunately, they all decrease portal perfusion, are associated with a significant incidence of encephalopathy, and have a 5-year survival rate that is no different than that in medical treatment controls. Consequently, elective central shunts are best performed when there is hepatofugal flow or massive intractable ascites.

The distal splenorenal shunt is the most popular selective shunt, and in skilled hands can be performed with an operative mortality of less than 5%. Recurrent hemorrhage is averted in more than 90% of patients. It maintains portal perfusion of the liver, and the incidence of chronic, clinical encephalopathy is less than with central shunts. The 5-year survival in alcoholics is similar with selective and central shunts. However, there is a significantly higher survival in nonalcoholics with the distal splenorenal shunt.

Several studies have compared sclerotherapy with the distal splenorenal shunt. These studies have again confirmed that the rebleeding rate averages 50% with sclerotherapy and that some of these patients will bleed to death. Perhaps the best compromise may be to use sclerotherapy as an initial form of therapy, followed by a distal splenorenal shunt in those patients who rebleed. It is imperative not to allow the patient to rebleed so massively that he or she is no longer an acceptable candidate for shunting.

### Transplantation

It would be inappropriate to conclude without briefly mentioning liver transplantation. With better techniques and increased availability of organs, more and more patients with advanced liver disease and bleeding varices have transplantation. Stable cirrhotics with good liver reserve (Child's Class A or B) can still be treated with sclerotherapy and/or selective shunting. As previously mentioned, portacaval shunts should be avoided because of the technical complications they present for possible future transplantation.

# CHOLECYSTITIS AND CHOLELITHIASIS

method of
EDWARD C. SALTZSTEIN, M.D., and
LEO C. MERCER, M.D.
*Texas Tech University School of Medicine*
*El Paso, Texas*

Gallstones and diseases resulting from them are among the most common clinical entities encountered by physicians in the United States. An estimated 10% of the population, or more than 20 million Americans, have gallstones, with 800,000 new cases reported annually. The majority of patients with stones have supersaturated bile, and the precipitation of cholesterol from solution forms the nidus for stones in the gallbladder. Other factors that may cause precipitation of cholesterol are bacteria, fungi, intestinal reflux, and stasis of bile.

Anomalous anatomy is more frequent in the extrahepatic biliary ductal system than anywhere else in the body, and a thorough knowledge of the anatomy is essential to avoid operative injury, especially to the common bile duct. From a surgical standpoint, the origin of the cystic duct and cystic artery is not important in cholecystectomy; if one ligates and/or divides only those structures identified as going to the gallbladder, the incidence of injury (particularly to the common bile duct) is minimized.

## DIAGNOSIS

In many patients, gallstones are not symptomatic and are diagnosed during a general evaluation or in the course of an evaluation for other problems. When biliary tract stone disease is suspected, a history to elicit symptoms supporting the diagnosis is taken. Classically, patients present with colicky or constant right upper quadrant pain that radiates to the back. A temporal relationship between food intake and pain exists in which eating aggravates pain, and an intolerance of fatty foods may be particularly evident. Up to 80% of gallbladder patients are female, and a history of multiple pregnancies is frequent. A history of dark urine and/or light stools suggests common duct obstruction. Pertinent physical findings include varying degrees of right upper quadrant and epigastric tenderness and rebound tenderness. Bowel sounds may be depressed, and jaundice may be present.

The differential diagnosis includes other right upper quadrant inflammatory processes, particularly hepatitis, pancreatitis, and peptic ulcer disease. These possibilities should be evaluated when history and physical examination are performed.

Important x-ray and laboratory studies to establish the diagnosis are ultrasonography, radionuclide imaging, and liver function studies. When the diagnosis is not readily apparent, helpful studies are oral cholecystography, duodenal drainage analysis, and endoscopic retrograde cholangiopancreatography.

### Abdominal Roentgenography

Abdominal films are of benefit if radiopaque stones are visualized (15% of biliary calculi) or if an "air cholangiogram" is seen (pathognomonic of a biliary-enteric fistula).

### Ultrasonography

Ultrasonography is accurate in defining biliary calculi in 95% of cases, and false-positive results are rare. It is usually the only diagnostic tool required, and with ultrasonographic evidence of stones, one can proceed with cholecystectomy. Ultrasonography may also demonstrate stones in the common bile duct and can demonstrate the size of the duct as well as pancreatic abnormalities.

### Radionuclide Imaging

$^{99m}$Tc-labeled iminodiacetic acid (IDA) scanning "lights up" the liver, gallbladder, extrahepatic ducts, and duodenum in the normal person. Nonvisualization of the gallbladder strongly supports a diagnosis of acute cholecystitis, whereas visualization rules it out. Visualization of the radionuclide in the intestine rules out complete ductal obstruction (and therefore cholangitis). In general, the diagnosis of acute cholecystitis can be made by the history and physical findings, plus the demonstration of stones by ultrasonography. In this situation, radionuclide imaging may be useful to rule out other conditions, such as amebic liver abscess.

### Liver Function Studies

Because of the increased morbidity and mortality associated with delayed or untreated cholangitis, the presence of jaundice must be ascertained in patients with symptomatic biliary calculi. The combination of right upper quadrant pain, fever, and jaundice (Charcot's triad) represents cholangitis until proved otherwise. Liver function studies are indicated to assist in distinguishing between hepatitis and obstructive jaundice. Further diagnostic studies (radionuclide imaging, percutaneous transhepatic cholangiography) and subsequent prompt surgical decompression of the common duct may be required.

### Serum Amylase Level Determination

Because hyperamylasemia and/or pancreatitis complicates biliary calculi in up to 25% of cases, serum amylase level determinations should be done routinely.

## TREATMENT

### Asymptomatic Gallstones

Conflicting evidence exists regarding the likelihood that patients with asymptomatic stones will develop symptoms (10 to 50%). However, there appears to be no significant increase in mortality when treatment (cholecystectomy) is delayed until the onset of symptoms. The deaths that do occur usually involve elderly patients with known stones who develop acute cholecystitis requiring emergent surgery. Recent successful experience in managing patients with diabetes indicates that diabetes per se does not increase the complication rate of acute cholecystitis and therefore is not an absolute indication for cholecystectomy in the asymptomatic patient.

### Symptomatic Stones—Biliary Colic and Acute Cholecystitis

Biliary colic results from contraction of the smooth muscle of the gallbladder and/or extrahepatic ducts that is believed to be related to intermittent obstruction by stones. Anticholinergic drugs such as dicyclomine hydrochloride (Bentyl) or Donnatal may be tried to relieve smooth muscle spasms, and a low-fat diet may be instituted.

It is generally agreed that cholecystectomy is indicated for symptomatic biliary calculi. The risk of elective surgery is extremely low and eliminates the risk of urgent surgery for subsequent acute cholecystitis, particularly in the elderly patient. After a general evaluation to determine the operative and anesthetic risks, patients can be brought to the hospital the day of surgery. Prophylactic antibiotics are indicated in patients over age 60 years, those with choledocholithiasis, and those with diabetes. However, we routinely give perioperative antibiotics to all patients, using cefazolin (Ancef), 1 gram intravenously every 8 hours for a total of three doses. Operative cholangiography of the transcystic duct should accompany cholecystectomy to identify common duct stones (both their number and location), to prevent unnecessary duct explorations, and to identify anatomic variations and possibly avoid operative ductal injury. When common duct stones are identified by intraoperative cholangiography, common duct exploration with stone removal and large T tube drainage is indicated. A No. 14 French or larger T tube to facilitate fluoroscopically controlled basket retrieval of possibly retained stones should be used. Almost all patients have their drains removed, are afebrile, and are able to eat the day after cholecystectomy, and more than one-half of our patients are discharged home 24 hours postoperatively.

Acute calculous cholecystitis results from obstruction of the cystic duct, with subsequent edema of the gallbladder, relative vascular insufficiency, and secondary infection. Infection occurs via overgrowth of organisms in the gallbladder bile, via lymphatics, and possibly by translocation of colon organisms. Patients present with constant pain and an elevated temperature. The white blood cell count is not necessarily elevated. We start to administer antibiotics empirically (without culture) on the basis of the organisms likely to be found (enteric organisms, most commonly *Escherichia coli*), using piperacillin (Pipracil), 2 grams intravenously every 6 hours. Narcotics, such as morphine and meperidine, are contraindicated because they cause contraction of the sphincter of Oddi and mask symptoms that are important to follow in evaluating the success of therapy.

Although clinical resolution of acute cholecystitis can be obtained in more than 85% of patients with antibiotics, nasogastric suction, and possibly anticholinergic drugs, prompt cholecystectomy is generally the preferred treatment. Surgery as soon as the diagnosis is made (by ultrasonography with or without radionuclide imaging) and the patient is appropriately resuscitated is safe, greatly reduces the hospital stay, avoids observation for possible failure to respond to nonsurgical therapy, and is not associated with increased technical difficulty. Forty per cent of our patients are discharged within 24 hours and 60% within 48 hours of surgery for acute cholecystitis.

Although this practice is controversial, we also operate on patients with biliary hyperamylasemia and/or pancreatitis as soon as the diagnosis is made. Cholecystectomy, intraoperative cholangiography, and common duct exploration as necessary are performed.

## ALTERNATIVE AND NEW THERAPIES

The role of medical dissolution of gallstones, if any, has not been defined. Chenodeoxycholic acid increases the bile acid pool and slowly dissolves cholesterol gallstones. However, the treatment is prolonged (1 to 2 years) and expensive. Further, on cessation of therapy, the bile returns to its previous lithogenic state, and more than 30% of patients re-form stones in 5 years. Because cholecystectomy is such a safe and effective procedure, treatment with agents that increase the bile acid pool should probably be reserved for patients who have small stones (<2 cm) in functioning gallbladders and who are prohibitive risks for surgery.

The efficacy of extracorporeal shock wave lithotripsy (ESWL) in selected patients is becoming apparent. Early studies on patients with one to three radiolucent gallstones with a total stone mass of 30 mm or less and with functioning gallbladders showed complete disappearance of stone fragments in up to 90% at 12 months. ESWL is noninvasive and therefore of interest as an alternative to cholecystectomy. There is concern over the consequences of stone fragments passing into the extrahepatic ductal system, but there are now reports of successful treatment by ESWL of small numbers of patients with retained stones and other complex biliary tract stone disease. The data from several centers in the United States are accumulating to confirm and expand the initial reports from Germany.

Another experimental technique is the instillation, via a percutaneous catheter into the gallbladder, of a potent lipid solvent, methyl tertbutyl ether, that solubilizes the cholesterol in cholesterol stones, causing dissolution within hours. The safety of this technique has not been established. It is of interest as an alternative to cholecystectomy because it can be done on an outpatient basis under local anesthesia.

Each of these three therapies preserves the gallbladder. Of concern is the likelihood of gallstone recurrence after therapy and the unknown effects of preservation of a chronically diseased organ. In addition, none of these therapeutic options are now applicable to the nonfunctioning gallbladder (the more seriously ill patient). Cholecystectomy remains the procedure of choice for the vast majority of patients with biliary calculi. It is safe, definitive, and well tolerated, with minimal morbidity and brief hospitalization (and therefore reduced cost).

A recent technologic advance affecting surgical practice is the evolution of laparoscopic cholecystectomy. The indications have not been defined as yet, although early results suggest that the procedure may be applicable to the minimally inflamed organ. Laparoscopic cholecystectomy should be performed by surgeons who are qualified to perform an open cholecystectomy if necessary.

## ACALCULOUS CHOLECYSTITIS

Acute and chronic inflammatory disease of the gallbladder occurs without stones. Acalculous cholecystitis occurs in less than 5% of adult patients in the United States and in a somewhat larger percentage in children. It is frequently seen as a complication of burns, sepsis, cardiovascular disease, major surgery, prolonged illness, or conditions that may result in significant inactivity of the gut with biliary stasis, and especially in patients receiving total parenteral nutrition. Antomic variations causing kinking of the cystic duct may be involved.

Acalculous cholecystitis should be considered in patients who develop signs and symptoms of cholecystitis and in whom ultrasonography does not reveal stones. Ultrasonography may reveal a thickened gallbladder wall. The accuracy of radionuclide imaging is questionable in these cases, but nonvisualization of the gallbladder supports the diagnosis.

Although a small percentage of patients may respond to nasogastric suction, anticholinergic drugs, and antibiotics, prompt cholecystectomy to prevent progression to gangrene and rupture and to prevent further compromise of the underlying medical condition is indicated.

# CIRRHOSIS

method of
FRANK L. IBER, M.D.
*Loyola University and Edward Hines, Jr., VA*
   *Hospital*
*Chicago, Illinois*

Cirrhosis is a chronic, usually progressive liver disease characterized clinically by failure of liver cell function and portal hypertension. Histologic examination is valuable in establishing the etiology but is infrequently essential to diagnose cirrhosis. Portal hypertension usually can be identified by endoscopy or barium swallow (for esophageal varices) or by sonography or other imaging (to establish enlarged portal veins or collaterals).

## ETIOLOGY OF CIRRHOSIS

Common etiologies
   Alcohol
   Chemical exposure
   Medicinal agents
   Hepatitis B
   Non-A, non-B(C) hepatitis
   Schistosomiasis
   Primary biliary cirrhosis
   Chronic active hepatitis
Uncommon etiologies
   Hepatitis D
   Iron storage disease
   Copper storage disease
   Alpha$_1$-antitrypsin deficiency

Although the diagnosis of cirrhosis is relatively easy, establishing the etiology is more difficult. Removing the causes of injury (e.g., toxin or alcohol) or controlling a harmful effect (e.g., of steroid treatment of autoimmune cirrhosis) improves survival of patients.

## TREATMENT

Permanent removal of the cause of cirrhosis is the mainstay of treatment; if this is not possible, many specific therapies exist that intermittently or partially control new hepatic damage. A large number of nonspecific measures that reduce disability are useful. Many complications of cirrhosis, including ascites, malnutrition, infection, and variceal hemorrhage, can be effectively treated to avoid incapacitation and death.

### Nonspecific Treatment

The goals of this approach are to delay and reduce disability caused by cirrhosis and its complications. Diet, appropriate activity, and avoidance of new liver damage are all effective. The ultimate nonspecific therapy for the final stage of cirrhosis is *transplantation.*

**Diet.** The diet should be nutritious and contain about 20% excess of calories, protein, and most trace nutrients. Hence the inactive 70-kg person should eat at least 2500 calories daily with at least 1 gram of protein per kg. If the patient is unable to eat this amount, feeding at least one-third of the daily food as breakfast and adding evening snacks is effective. There should be no restriction of fat. All cirrhotics metabolize sodium poorly, so salty foods, condiments, and added salt should be avoided. Dietary supplements are appropriate when there is specific malnutrition, in alcoholics for 1 month after drinking stops or longer if drinking continues, and in jaundiced subjects. Alcoholics need a multivitamin with minerals and often require extra magnesium and zinc; these requirements may be identified by serum measurements. Patients with jaundice need parenteral vitamin K (5 mg menadione intramuscularly monthly) and oral supplements of 10,000 U of vitamin A, 50,000 U of vitamin D, and 400 U of vitamin E as long as the jaundice continues. Almost all patients who are taking diuretics or those with diarrhea caused by lactulose need oral potassium supplements as determined by serum potassium levels. A common dose is 40 mEq per day.

**Activity.** Activity should be undertaken daily with a goal of preserving muscle mass and exercise tolerance short of producing extreme fatigue. Regular and increasing walking or noncompetitive exercises (aerobics) often increase work tolerance even in the face of progressive liver disease. Additional rest to avoid extreme fatigue should be encouraged, with 10 hours in bed and a rest period in the middle of the day often required.

**Potential Injurious Agents.** Agents such as alcohol, new medications, health store macrosupplements of nutrients, and extensive solvents that are used in certain hobbies should be avoided. The patient should ask the physician about the possible hepatic effects of treatments, query physicians at work about agents at the work place, and avoid new chemical exposures. In alcoholic patients, blood or urine tests for alcohol at the time of routine visits to the physician have been found to be valuable in detecting and confronting the problem of surreptitious alcohol use. All patients should be tested for hepatitis B; the patients who have not acquired this infection should be immunized with recombinant vaccine. Patients who are exposed to crowds should also receive influenza and pneumococcal immunization.

**Useful Office Information.** Information should be acquired on all patients, particularly those doing well. Patients should keep a diary of weight with weekly recordings. Sudden weight gains may indicate new ascites or raised plasma volume, which increases the risk of hemorrhage. Suitable patients can be given furosemide (Lasix), 40 mg in a single dose, if weight increases by 3 lb. At a minimum, patients should visit the physician yearly. On each visit, the patient's weight and a sample of handwriting (or the trail-making test, which is provided by the manufacturers of lactulose), as well as liver chemistries, electrolytes, and creatinine, should be obtained. The blood alcohol level is also measured in alcoholic patients. A test for occult blood should be done. A barium esophagogram or endoscopy should be obtained each year; after varices appear, endoscopy is required yearly to determine the likelihood of bleeding. If these tests have been performed regularly, early complications are often identified and effectively treated without the need for hospitalization. When clinical deterioration is encountered, a prompt search for occult infection, gastrointestinal bleeding, and hepatocellular carcinoma (by alpha-fetoprotein) should be undertaken.

### Therapies for Specific Diseases

**Alcoholic Liver Disease.** This liver disease improves with total abstinence from alcohol and adequate oral nutrition; in most patients this therapy is all that is required. In severe cases of acute injury with both malnutrition and jaundice, intravenous alimentation with 1000 ml of 3 to 5% amino acids seems to be beneficial, usually continued until eating is possible or for a maximum of 1 month. In these same cases, treatment with oral oxandrolone (Anavar), 20 mg per day for 1 month, has improved survival and is used in malnourished patients. I do not currently use either propylthiouracil, 300 mg daily for 3 or 4 months, or colchicine, 1 mg daily, to treat these patients. To facilitate alcohol withdrawal, I use diazepam (Valium) as needed for a maximum of 1 week. Disulfiram (Antabuse), 250 mg per day, is occasionally used in conjunction with other therapy for alcoholism with no detrimental effects on the liver. Some form of therapy for alcoholism is essential, the most effective treatment for alcohol abstinence being the program of Alcoholics Anonymous.

**Hepatitis B.** Hepatitis B in its viral replicative stage (identified by HBs, HBe antigens, and DNA in the serum) has been arrested by treatment with interferon-alpha. A dose of 3 to 6 million units three times weekly for 16 weeks has been used.

**Hepatitis C (Non-A, Non-B Hepatitis).** Persistent active and symptomatic disease for greater than 6 months seems to be suppressed with interferon-alpha. Three to six million units three times a week is used for 6 months.

**Idiopathic Chronic Active Hepatitis.** This hepatitis, which occurs often with cirrhosis, may be discerned by immunologic markers such as antinuclear antibody and anti–smooth muscle antibody and has a typical biopsy pattern. The illness is highly responsive to prednisone, 20 mg per day, with biochemical and clinical improvement apparent in 1 or 2 months. For chronic management, azathioprine (Imuran) is added in a dose of 50 mg per day and the dose of prednisone is reduced to 10 mg per day. Treatment should be continued for 1 year after biochemical stability is achieved and then should be slowly discontinued.

**Biliary Cirrhosis.** Treatment with colchicine, 1 mg per day, and, more recently, methotrexate, 25 mg intravenously weekly, has been found to be effective. Pruritus is best treated with cholestyramine (Questran), by taking a 9-gram dose both before and after breakfast and additional doses with each subsequent meal. Bone loss is a major incapacitating problem and should be treated prophylactically with extra calcium equivalents (to 1 pint of milk daily) and sufficient oral or intramuscular vitamin D to maintain normal serum 25-hydroxyvitamin $D_2$ levels. Typically, 100,000 IU of oral vitamin D is required daily, or this dose of intramuscular vitamin $D_2$ monthly. This cirrhosis in its late stages is one of the most frequent reasons for liver transplantation.

**Hemochromatosis.** Recognized by an increased serum ferritin level and an elevated iron content of the liver, hemochromatosis is treated by repeated phlebotomies of 500 ml each. The frequency of phlebotomy is weekly or twice-weekly if the hemoglobin can regenerate this quickly.

After a few weeks, weekly or twice-monthly phlebotomy is used.

**Wilson's Disease.** Recognized by a low serum ceruloplasmin level, raised liver copper concentration, and a Kayser-Fleischer corneal ring, Wilson's disease is treated with oral penicillamine, 2 to 3 grams per day.

**Hepatic Schistosomiasis.** Biopsy and large egg loads in the stool in patients from endemic areas indicate hepatic schistosomiasis. Praziquantel is used for treatment. The Parasitic Disease Drug Service (Atlanta, GA, 404–329–3654) can provide up-to-date information on useful drugs and their availability and on newer diagnostic tests.

## TREATMENT OF COMPLICATIONS OF CIRRHOSIS

### Ascites

Ascites, or edema, in liver disease rarely requires urgent intensive treatment. Severe restriction of respiration, nonreducible umbilical hernias, and variceal bleeding are the only clear indications for urgent treatment. In such circumstances, a large (3 to 6 liters) paracentesis is the most reliable treatment, but about two-thirds of the removed volume will recur in 48 hours and require removal again. All other cases are managed with dietary sodium restriction and diuretics. Treatment of ascites is required for many months, so the diet selected should be one that can be followed at home and should include 4 grams of sodium chloride (70 mEq) per day or less. The diuretic of choice is spironolactone (Aldactone), starting at 150 mg per day in three divided doses and increasing if needed to 600 mg per day. The progress of diuresis should be followed by measuring body weight at least three times weekly; weights should be recorded in a diary. The goal of safe diuresis is a weight loss of 0.5 to 2 lbs per day and can most rapidly be predicted by obtaining urine sodium values on a single sample in the middle of the day. A negative sodium balance must be attained; if the diet includes 4 grams of sodium chloride (70 mEq), the urine loss must be at least 100 mEq per liter (about the same as per 24 hours) to attain weight loss. Values less than this require more spironolactone or addition of furosemide, 40 mg in the morning, with doubling each 2 days until the desired effect is obtained. A 2- to 4-hour period of supine rest assists diuresis. Potassium supplements are almost always required (40 mEq per day is a typical dose), and assays of serum electrolytes and creatinine levels are needed weekly during the first month and monthly thereafter. Water restriction is required if the serum sodium level is less than 125 mEq per liter and should be kept to a maximum of 1000 ml of fluid per day. Nonsteroidal anti-inflammatory drugs are to be avoided because they precipitate hepatorenal syndrome. Patients who develop elevation of the creatinine level before diuresis occurs or who are refractory may be candidates for the surgical placement of a LeVeen-type peritoneovenous shunt. A consultation with a physician who is experienced in treating chronic ascites with such devices, at least by phone, usually predicts accurately whether the treatment will be effective.

A frequent complication of ascites is spontaneous bacterial peritonitis, which should be suspected if fever, clinical deterioration, failure of diuresis, or onset of hepatic encephalopathy occurs and which is verified by diagnostic paracentesis. The characteristic finding is more than 250 polymorphonuclear cells per $mm^3$ in the fluid. Many fluids have small numbers of bacteria, pH less than 7.25, or an elevated lactate dehydrogenase level. Treatment is undertaken on the basis of the elevated ascites white blood cell count and consists of intravenous cefoxitin (Mefozin) or cefamandole (Mandol). Combinations with aminoglycosides are more toxic in the cirrhotic patient and are to be avoided.

Hepatorenal syndrome frequently occurs in patients with ascites who are undergoing diuresis or who hemorrhage. Diminishing renal output, rising creatinine levels, and absence of urine sediment are the prominent features. Treating infections, restoring blood volume, and removing diuretic and nonsteroidal anti-inflammatory drugs from treatment may lead to reversal of the syndrome. A fluid challenge of 500 ml of saline with 25 grams of albumin, while urine output is monitored, is used to identify plasma volume depletion.

### Hepatic Encephalopathy

Hepatic encephalopathy is disordered central nervous system function produced when materials from the intestine reach the brain through porto-systemic shunts. In cirrhosis, these shunts are mostly through collateral portal venous channels. Toxins that have some role include ammonia, mercaptans, eight-carbon fatty acids, and a gamma-aminobutyric acid–like material. All seem to be produced by the action of bacteria on dietary protein in the small and large intestines.

Treatment is highly effective when the hepatic encephalopathy is mild, but when the patient cannot be aroused it is disappointing. In about one-half of the cases, a precipitating cause is found, the removal of which leads to prompt improvement. Gastrointestinal bleeding, occult infection, unrecognized potassium depletions, and central nervous system depressant drugs are common precipitants; fluid and electrolyte imbalance, anoxia, and additional liver disease are precipitants less frequently associated with a dramatic response.

All patients are provided nonspecific treatment, with the intensity of each measure proportional to the severity of the encephalopathy. Some dietary protein restriction is usually used: a diet free of meat, eggs, and dairy products (i.e., a diet of approximately 20 grams of protein; fruit; and vegetables) is readily obtained and used in most patients able to eat. Lactulose, 30 ml of a 50% solution by mouth (or gastric tube if the patient cannot cooperate) three to five times on the first day and three times daily thereafter, is useful. A diarrhea will result, and the electrolyte losses, often high in potassium, need to be replaced. If these measures do not lead to improvement in 48 hours, antibiotics are added. Oral neomycin, 1 gram every 24 hours, is sufficient, but almost any antibiotic alone or in combination capable of suppressing gut flora is effective. Nutrition should be adequate, and intravenous alimentation (including protein) is given if needed, with no danger of worsening the coma. Special amino acid preparations, such as combinations with high concentrations of branched chain amino acids, are of no special benefit. Unresponsive patients should have a careful review of the diagnosis performed, including computed tomography. If the patient is unconscious for 4 days because of liver encephalopathy, cerebral edema ensues and produces death by medullary herniation. In patients who are awaiting transplantation or who are expected to recover liver function, intravenous mannitol to lessen swelling, hyperventilation, and even a cranial decompression based on monitoring intraventricular pressures have been lifesaving. Recurrent liver encephalopathy produces a permanent basal ganglion disease called non-wilsonian hepatolenticular degeneration.

### Bleeding Esophageal Varices

Bleeding esophageal varices are best treated by planning that the event may occur. Endoscopy can now predict which varices are likely to bleed (extent, size, presence of vessels on varices), and these patients are subjected to closer follow-up to avoid increased plasma volume. The weight should be monitored three times weekly and each 2 to 3 lb of weight gain should be reversed with diuretics. Prophylactic propranolol (Inderal) therapy is recommended for patients who have extensive varices with endoscopic markers of probable bleeding.

Gastrointestinal bleeding may be with hematemesis, with melena, or occult from varices, but the source must be identified, usually by endoscopy. Resuscitative measures must be promptly undertaken, and sclerotherapy to eradicate the bleeding vessel must be considered. Sclerotherapy destroys three to five varix columns with each treatment, and four to seven treatments at weekly intervals are required to eradicate the varices and the possibility of bleeding. Once eradicated, varices seldom recur for 1 year. For patients who have not bled or patients who are unwilling to undergo sclerotherapy, treatment with propranolol seems to be effective. The dose of 40 to 80 mg twice daily is used for the indefinite future. Portacaval shunts are used for patients with low operative risk (Child's A classification: no major jaundice, malnutrition, ascites, encephalopathy, or coagulopathy) and recurrent variceal hemorrhage.

# DYSPHAGIA AND ESOPHAGEAL OBSTRUCTION

method of
LAWRENCE D. BAILEY, JR., M.D., and
RICHARD W. McCALLUM, M.D.
*University of Virginia Health Sciences Center*
*Charlottesville, Virginia*

Dysphagia (difficulty swallowing) can be due to (1) oropharyngeal transfer, (2) motility and transit difficulties, or (3) mechanical obstruction. A wide variety of potential causes make a carefully designed diagnostic strategy important in order to avoid unnecessary and expensive tests while retaining the ability to make an accurate and timely diagnosis.

### DIAGNOSTIC STRATEGY

*History*

A thorough history and physical examination can categorize the type of dysphagia in over 80% of patients and direct your evaluation. Initial questions should focus on the duration of the problem, the type of food that causes dysphagia, and the location. Because patients with dysphagia from benign and malignant causes typically delay presentation, the duration of symptoms may be difficult to interpret. However, the gradual progression of symptoms indicates mechanical obstruction and rapidly progressive dysphagia increases the likelihood of a malignant cause. Intermittent symptoms are more characteristic of a motility disorder such as spasm or rings. Patients with stenosis of more than 50% (the esophageal lumen is less than 13 mm) will frequently admit to difficulty with meats (especially steak) and bread. They will often eliminate these and other solids from their diets before seeking medical attention. More difficulty with liquids than with solids is associated with oropharyngeal transfer problems. The level of obstruction may be incorrect because some patients have referral of their symptoms.

After characterization of the type of dysphagia, the history should be directed toward identifying associated symptoms and diseases. The most commonly associated symptom is heartburn. This may be accompanied by water brash, atypical asthma, hoarseness, sore throat, or a sour taste in the mouth. The absence of heartburn does not rule out reflux stricture, as some patients may be asymptomatic. Regurgitation of undigested food or halitosis may suggest a Zenker's diverticulum. A history of a recent cerebrovascular event or a neuromuscular disease (e.g., multiple sclerosis) may lead to investigation of a transfer problem. Risk factors for immunodeficiency such as the acquired immune deficiency syndrome (AIDS), corticosteroid use, or post-transplant syndromes make infectious etiologies more likely. Symptoms of Raynaud's phenomenon or tightness of skin over the fingers may suggest a previously undiagnosed case of CREST syndrome* or scleroderma. A careful medication history may reveal medicines that can cause pill-associated esophagitis. Smoking, alcohol use, previous caustic injury, and ethnic origin (e.g., Orientals, blacks) are etiologically related to carcinoma of the esophagus.

### Physical Examination

The physical examination is of limited usefulness in the characterization of dysphagia. In the patient who has difficulty with liquids, observation of the timing of the dysphagia may suggest transfer difficulties as opposed to mechanical obstruction. Immediate problems with swallowing (less than 3 seconds) often indicate transfer problems or cervical esophageal pathology, especially when associated with symptoms of aspiration. Careful examination for sclerodactyly, calcinosis, or Raynaud's phenomenon may suggest previously undiagnosed scleroderma. Oral candidal or herpetic lesions may suggest coexistent esophagitis. Some patients with severe reflux will have unexplained erosion of the tooth enamel at the gum line. Cervical lymphadenopathy may suggest metastatic carcinoma or possibly AIDS. Neurologic evaluation of the oropharynx with careful attention to the tongue and gag reflex is important in transfer dysphagia. Inspection of the teeth or dentures may also reveal the inability to chew food adequately.

### Radiology

The barium swallow should almost always be the initial diagnostic study to be performed. Studies should include both upright and recumbent positions. Utilization of a proper consistency and an adequate amount of barium is important to ensure that the esophagus is adequately distended in order to demonstrate any stenotic area. Rapid sequence or videofluoroscopic imaging provides excellent demonstration of the oropharyngeal phase of swallowing. Gross motility distur-

---

*CREST = calcinosis cutis, Raynaud's phenomenon, esophageal dysfunction, sclerodactyly, and telangiectasia.

bances of esophageal transit such as achalasia or severe diffuse esophageal spasm may be diagnosed by barium swallow, but in general, reliable determination of motility disturbances is best done by esophageal manometry.

In patients with solid food dysphagia, it is not surprising that a barium swallow may fail to demonstrate an etiology. If the liquid study fails to demonstrate a cause for dysphagia, it is necessary to employ a bolus challenge study. This is usually performed with a 13-mm barium tablet or a marshmallow. In the patient in the upright position, a tablet should traverse the esophagus in less than 20 seconds. If the tablet fails to clear the esophagus after several small sips of water, it is probable that there is obstruction at that level. A marshmallow (softened in the mouth) can be swallowed with a sip of barium. This will appear as a radiolucent bolus and may impact at an area of narrowing and reproduce the symptoms of dysphagia, which can focus future investigations.

### Endoscopy

Fiberoptic endoscopy often provides important diagnostic and therapeutic information and should usually be performed in patients with dysphagia. The most important function of endoscopy is the visualization and biopsy of strictured areas or mass lesions. A normal appearing mucosa in an area of narrowing by barium study suggests extrinsic compression or a segmental motor defect. Esophagitis can also be diagnosed by both visual and histologic criteria, and Barrett's esophagus can be diagnosed. Endoscopy can provide access to several therapeutic options including balloon dilatation, removal of fibromuscular polyps, foreign body retrieval, and laser palliation of malignant strictures. Endoscopy is *not* a reliable method of diagnosing motility disorders.

### Esophageal Manometry and Provocative Tests

In the patient in whom a cause of dysphagia is not identified with the preceding studies, esophageal manometry can be useful. Achalasia, diffuse esophageal spasm, "nutcracker" esophagus, hypertensive lower esophageal sphincter (LES), and segmental esophageal transit abnormalities are the most common diagnoses that can be found with manometry. Aperistalsis with a decreased LES pressure may also diagnose a previously unsuspected case of scleroderma. Helpful adjunctive tests to standard motility testing is the use of the Bernstein and Tensilon tests. The Bernstein test consists of dripping either hydrochloric acid or normal saline in a blind fashion to determine if the dysphagia or chest pain can be reproduced. The Tensilon test involves giving a standard dose of edrophonium chloride (Tensilon) and determining if symptoms are reproduced and if there are manometric changes.

## OROPHARYNGEAL TRANSFER DYSPHAGIA

Patients with transfer dysphagia typically present with dysphagia greater for liquids than solids. Symptoms of nasal regurgitation or aspiration are most frequently seen with oropharyngeal pathology. The basic pathologic event is discoordination of the swallowing mechanism or weakness of the tongue or hypopharyngeal muscle. Swallowing studies utilizing videofluoroscopic technique are the most useful diagnostic tool. Evaluation by a speech pathologist may also be helpful.

Neuromuscular diseases account for the vast majority of transfer dysphagia. The most common cause is cerebrovascular disease. Other diseases that may have manifestations of oropharyngeal dysphagia include multiple sclerosis, myasthenia gravis, Parkinson's disease, poliomyelitis, botulism, amyotrophic lateral sclerosis, hypothyroidism, hyperthyroidism, amyloidosis, polymyositis, and central nervous system tumors. There are also patients with isolated dysfunction of the cricopharyngeal muscles who present with symptoms of dysphagia and aspiration.

The therapy for these conditions is based on the underlying cause. Maintenance of nutritional well-being is of paramount importance. In patients with severe transfer dysfunction (especially with aspiration), the placement of a percutaneous gastrostomy may be lifesaving. This may permit time for neurologic deficits to improve. Speech pathologists may also be of assistance in "retraining" stroke victims to swallow. Altering dietary consistency to make food thicker may allow patients to be able to maintain nutrition with reduced risk of aspiration. Medical treatment of underlying conditions may provide improvement. Thyroid replacement for hypothyroidism, L-dopa for Parkinson's disease, cholinesterase inhibitors for myasthenia gravis, and steroids for polymyositis are common examples. Patients with isolated cricopharyngeal dysfunction and significant symptoms of aspiration may benefit from a myotomy. This is diagnosed by videofluoroscopic barium study and manometry.

## MOTILITY DISORDERS

### Achalasia

Achalasia is an idiopathic primary motility disorder of the esophagus manifested by a loss of primary and secondary peristalsis and a LES with poor relaxation. Pathologic examination reveals loss of the myenteric plexus cells between the longitudinal and circular layers of muscle. The idiopathic primary form of this disease must be distinguished between achalasia secondary to invasive carcinoma. Chagas' disease (South American trypanosomiasis) also has similar histologic and clinical features.

Patients with achalasia present with both solid and liquid dysphagia. They typically have had symptoms for months to years before presentation. They often have symptoms of regurgitation (often of day-old food) and aspiration. Finding food on the pillow after sleeping is characteristic of this condition. Some patients will give a history of having to swallow numerous times to relieve a substernal "full" feeling. Nutrition may be difficult to maintain, and weight loss is not uncommon. Significant weight loss makes secondary achalasia more likely. About 30% of patients will complain of substernal chest pain. A prolonged history of chest pain may be associated with so-called vigorous achalasia.

The diagnosis of achalasia is usually suggested by the preceding historical findings, although an occasional patient may present with pulmonary symptoms alone. Plain films of the chest may show an absence of the gastric air bubble and an unexplained air-fluid level in the chest. A barium swallow will classically show a dilated esophagus with a smooth distal tapering or "bird's beak." Esophageal enlargement may not occur for several years, in which case the diagnosis may be missed by radiology alone. The esophagus is often tortuous or "sigmoid," and there is usually retained food in more severe cases. An epiphrenic diverticulum may also be present. Upper gastrointestinal endoscopy is indicated to rule out gastric malignancy causing secondary achalasia.

After secondary causes of achalasia have been ruled out, esophageal manometry should be performed to establish the diagnosis of achalasia. In patients with more advanced disease, the placement of the motility catheter may be difficult, owing to the large dilated esophagus or an epiphrenic diverticulum. It is important that the LES be evaluated, and endoscopic or fluoroscopic placement should be utilized. There is an absence of peristaltic contractions in the smooth muscle portion of the esophagus. The nonperistaltic contractions are usually of low amplitude (less than 25 mmHg), but a subgroup called vigorous achalasia will have high-amplitude nonperistaltic contractions (greater than 50 mmHg). The LES will have an elevated pressure in 60% of patients and will fail to relax (normal is greater than 80% of gastric baseline) with swallows. This distinguishes achalasia from connective tissue disorders (e.g., scleroderma) that may have aperistalsis but have low LES pressures.

There are several modalities available to treat achalasia, but the primary rationale of all treatments is to reduce LES pressure. Pneumatic dilatation of the LES is the preferred initial treatment. This may be accomplished by the use of Rigiflex balloons or Browne-McHardy dilators. The Rigiflex balloon offers the advantage of having a guidewire lumen to facilitate placement and is smaller and more comfortable to the patient. The Rigiflex balloon is available in sizes of 30, 35, and 40 mm. Balloon techniques work by essentially causing a controlled tear of the esophagus and thereby interrupting the LES. There is a 2 to 10% rate of perforation associated with balloon dilation. Tears limited to the esophageal wall or mediastinum can be managed by placing the patient on antibiotics and giving nothing by mouth. Free perforation, especially with contamination of the pleural cavity, requires emergency thoracotomy for repair. Because of the need for possible thoracotomy, patients who are not surgical candidates should not undergo pneumatic dilatation.

The patient fasts for at least 12 hours, and it is prudent to have the patient on liquids for 24 to 48 hours to lessen the risk of retained foreign material. The patient's oropharynx is anesthetized with topical spray or gargle, and he or she is lightly sedated with midazolam and meperidine. Because of its guidewire capacity and less patient discomfort, the Rigiflex balloon is preferred. This is placed under fluoroscopic guidance until the midpoint of the balloon is compressed by the LES. If it is difficult to place the balloon, a guidewire is placed with either endoscopic or fluoroscopic assistance. We normally use a 30- or 35-mm balloon for our initial treatment modality. A 40-mm balloon may be used in selected cases that do not respond to the smaller balloons. The balloon is normally inflated to 12 to 15 psi for 60 seconds. The "waist" of the balloon should disappear if the treatment is successful. The patient will complain of pain, and the balloon is often blood tinged. The incidence of perforation is 2 to 8% and a water-soluble contrast study should be performed after the procedure.

After completion of the procedure, the patient should be observed overnight for fever or chest pain. If a contained perforation is diagnosed, the patient may be observed on antibiotics and acid suppression and kept fasting. If free perforation is diagnosed, especially with contamination of the pleural cavity, emergency thoracotomy is indicated. Certain patients with limited free perforations can be managed nonoperatively.

The preferred surgical procedure of choice is the modified Heller myotomy in which an anterior myotomy is performed by cutting the anterior circular muscle up to several centimeters above the LES. Success rates are 80 to 90% for the relief of dysphagia and are probably better than those of balloon dilation. The relative ease of balloon dilation has reduced the frequency of this surgery, but it still is an effective therapy in patients who do not respond to at least two attempts at balloon dilation or on whom balloon dilation cannot be performed because of technical reasons. The major complications of myotomy are reflux esophagitis and stricture. The advent of H$_2$ blocker therapy and modification of the Heller procedure to include a "loose" fundoplication have reduced the rate of these complications to less than 10%.

The role of medical therapy in achalasia is unclear. As with surgery and balloon dilation, the aim is to lower LES pressures in order to improve esophageal emptying. Calcium channel blockers (nifedipine, diltiazem, and verapamil) have been shown to lower LES pressures. Nifedipine is the drug of choice but has significant side effects, including postural hypotension and fluid retention. Nitrates have also been employed. They may be used sublingually, as a paste, or in long-acting oral preparations such as isosorbide dinitrate. Therapy is often limited by side effects, especially headache, which may limit therapy in up to 50% of patients. Anticholinergic medications such as propantheline bromide (Pro-Banthine), 10 to 20 mg four times per day, are also used. Medical therapy may be appropriate in several settings. In the patient who refuses disruption of the LES or is not a surgical candidate, medical therapy may provide palliation. Patients with early achalasia without a dilated esophagus may be treated with medical therapy and followed if their quality of life is acceptable.

## Disorders Associated with Esophageal Spasm

Spastic disorders of the esophagus are probably a diffuse collection of diseases. The most commonly described entities are diffuse esophageal spasm (DES), segmental spasm, nutcracker esophagus, and hypertensive LES. These diseases are idiopathic and there is no cure, although a variety of palliative options are available and will be discussed later. These diagnoses are suggested in a patient with chest pain symptoms also presenting with dysphagia. The diagnosis is established by esophageal manometry, Bernstein's test, and challenge testing with edrophonium (Tensilon). Tensilon provocation may bring out evidence of esophageal spasm in a patient with a normal baseline motility study.

Dysphagia occurs in up to 70% of patients with DES. However, the most common symptom is chest pain, especially with eating. Manometry shows high-amplitude contractions with a frequency of nonperistaltic swallows of up to 80%. LES pressures are usually normal, although they may be elevated in some patients. A barium swallow may show a "corkscrew" esophagus in more advanced cases. This diagnosis is most frequently made in the evaluation of noncardiac chest pain, and patients rarely come to medical attention when they have dysphagia alone.

Nutcracker esophagus is characterized by frequent high-amplitude contractions that are almost always associated with chest pain. Contractions are of variable duration and may last for several seconds. The majority of contractions are peristaltic. In some patients this disorder may be difficult to distinguish from DES, and some authors feel that this may be a continuum with DES. Nutcracker esophagus may progress to DES in about 5% of cases. Some of these patients may have marked dysphagia for solids or liquids, although most will report only a sensation of food briefly catching in their esophagus.

An isolated hypertensive LES is sometimes seen. This is distinguished from achalasia by the presence of normal peristalsis. These patients present with dysphagia and/or chest pain if symptomatic. This is usually clinically significant if there is abnormal relaxation of the LES. Diagnosis is made by manometry and is seen occasionally in normal volunteers.

The treatment of spastic disorders of the esophagus is based on decreasing the frequency and amplitude of the contractions. Because acid reflux may serve to trigger or exacerbate episodes of spasm, acid suppression with $H_2$ blockers or omeprazole (Losec) may help some patients. Sublingual nitroglycerin, 0.4 mg as needed; oral or sublingual nifedipine, 10 to 20 mg before meals; and isosorbide dinitrate (Isordil), 10 to 20 mg before meals, may be effective, especially in patients with chest pain. Nifedipine is more effective in subgroups in which the LES pressure is elevated. Anticholinergic agents such as dicyclomine hydrochloride (Bentyl) in doses of 10 to 30 mg three times per day or propantheline bromide (Pro-Banthine) in doses of 10 to 20 mg three or four times per day may also be helpful and have the added benefit of decreasing acid secretion. In patients who are not responsive to medical therapy, bougienage may give some relief of symptoms, although this is usually transient. Very rarely, pneumatic dilatation or esophageal myotomy is performed in patients with severe pain and dysphagia.

### Miscellaneous Motility Disorders

Diabetes and amyloidosis are often seen to involve the esophagus if careful manometric studies are performed; however, clinical symptoms are unusual. Short-segment aperistalsis has been described, often in the setting of food impaction. This is diagnosed by the use of a barium tablet or marshmallow challenge during a barium swallow. Then careful manometry reveals an aperistaltic segment. Treatment consists of periodic bougienage.

### Scleroderma

Patients with scleroderma present with dysphagia for two reasons. In advanced disease, there is aperistalsis with markedly diminished LES pressure. The combination of poor acid clearance and lack of resistance to reflux makes these patients very susceptible to reflux esophagitis and subsequent stricture formation. In the upright position the lack of peristalsis has a relatively minor contribution to dysphagia, and the major reason for dysphagia is due to esophagitis, transition to Barrett's epithelium, and stricture formation.

Treatment is aimed at reduction of reflux and maintenance of adequate luminal diameter. With the availability of omeprazole (Losec), gastric acid production can be reduced to essentially zero. This offers great promise in preventing acid-induced reflux strictures and progression to Barrett's esophagus. In patients with less severe reflux disease, treatment with full-dose $H_2$ blocker therapy is usually adequate. Because of the lack of peristaltic function, antireflux surgery is contraindicated. Metoclopramide (Reglan), 5 to 20 mg before meals and at bedtime, can also be of benefit. The availability of omeprazole (Losec) and the frequency of side effects make the use of metoclopramide less attractive. Dilatation of strictures is crucial to enable these patients to maintain good oral intake. Therapy is usually designed with the goal of maintaining a luminal diameter of greater than 17 mm (50 French). Various types of esophageal dilators will be discussed below. Dilation may only need to be performed once, but patients often require repeat dilation at frequencies of 1 to 12 months.

## OBSTRUCTIVE DYSPHAGIA

Esophageal obstruction may result from luminal narrowing, compression by adjacent structures or tumors, esophageal diverticula, surgical manipulation of the esophagus, and foreign bodies in the lumen. In obstructive dysphagia, evaluation is best performed by barium swallow (meglumine diatrizoate [Gastrografin] if complete obstruction is suspected) and endoscopy. A chest computed tomographic study may occasionally be necessary to define structures that compress the esophagus. Plain films of the neck, chest, and abdomen are also helpful in patients with suspected foreign body ingestion.

### Esophagitis

Severe esophagitis alone may present with dysphagia if there is enough associated edema and inflammation to compromise the esophageal lumen. Gastroesophageal reflux is associated with symptoms of heartburn or pyrosis in most but not all patients. A lack of heartburn in a patient with esophagitis requires investigation of predisposing factors. Special types of esophagitis that are more likely to be associated with dysphagia include pill-associated, infectious, and caustic ingestions. Medications that commonly may cause esophagitis include aspirin, tetracycline, potassium chloride, quinidine, and nonsteroidal anti-inflammatory agents. Elderly patients are particularly vulnerable to tablet-induced esophagitis, owing to decreased salivary output, less effective esophageal clearance, and because they ingest more medications. Infectious esophagitis usually occurs in immunocompromised patients but can occur in normals. The most common etiologic agents are *Candida albicans,* herpes simplex virus (HSV), and cytomegalovirus (CMV). Caustic ingestions may present as a medical emergency or at a later date as resultant stricture. Damage to the oropharynx cannot be used to gauge the extent of the esophageal damage.

Diagnosis and treatment should be aimed at determining the etiology and extent of the disease and providing adequate therapy. Endoscopy is clearly superior to barium swallow in the diagnosis of esophagitis. In the case of gastroesophageal reflux, endoscopy can confirm the presence of Barrett's esophagus or unsuspected neoplasm, and viral cultures and histology will establish the diagnosis of infectious esophagitis. In acute caustic ingestion, we recommend careful assessment of the extent of injury after cardiopulmonary stabilization of the patient. The main goal is to evaluate the severity of the "burn" in order to identify patients at high risk for perforation. Gastroesophageal reflux–induced esophagitis is initially treated with $H_2$ blockers; antacids; small, low-fat meals; not eating 4 hours before bedtime; elevation of the head of the bed; and stopping cigarettes. More difficult cases may require the addition of metoclopramide (Reglan), 5 to 10 mg four times per day, to increase LES pressure and increase gastric emptying. A limited course of omeprazole (Losec), 20 mg per day, may help to promote healing. Candidal esophagitis can be treated with nystatin (Mycostatin), 1 to 3 million units four times per day.* In severely immunocompromised patients, ketoconazole (Nizoral), 400 mg once daily, or intravenous amphotericin (0.3 to 0.5 mg per kg per day) is used. HSV infections are usually treated with Acyclovir (Zovirax), 200 to 400 mg five times per day. CMV infections are potentially treatable with

ganciclovir, which is currently an experimental drug.

### Strictures, Rings and Webs

Strictures secondary to gastroesophageal reflux are the most common cause of obstructive dysphagia. Affected patients have an increased number of reflux episodes and poor acid clearance from the esophagus. Strictures are most common in the distal esophagus but can occur in any part of the esophagus. They may be up to several centimeters long. Long narrow strictures are particularly characteristic of patients who have had a nasogastric tube in place for several days. Treatment is prevention of further reflux, either medically as cited earlier or surgically. Schatzki's ring, which is a mucosal ring found at the squamocolumnar junction, is a common cause of dysphagia. These rings often occur in a setting of reflux. Patients present with intermittent dysphagia or not infrequently with food impaction. Treatment consists of a single bougienage, although some patients may require repeat dilatations, especially in the setting of reflux. Esophageal webs are rare and usually occur in the upper third of the esophagus. They are associated with iron deficiency anemia in the Plummer-Vinson or Patterson-Kelly syndrome. Symptoms of dysphagia and aspiration are most commonly seen. Treatment consists of dilatation, or occasionally surgical removal is required.

### Esophageal Diverticula

Esophageal diverticula may be classified into three types: Zenker's, traction, and epiphrenic. Zenker's diverticula are found at the level of the upper esophageal sphincter (UES). The pathogenesis is controversial but may be the result of motor abnormalities of the UES. Patients present with transient cervical dysphagia with progressive regurgitation and aspiration. Some will have episodes of regurgitation of day-old undigested food. They may also present with a retropharyngeal abscess. Treatment consists of either cricopharyngeal myotomy or removal of the diverticulum. Traction diverticula usually occur in the middle third of the esophagus. The pathogenesis is unclear. These diverticula are usually asymptomatic and are detected incidentally at barium swallow. Occasionally, the patient may have dysphagia or food impaction. Treatment is usually not required. Epiphrenic diverticula occur in the lower third of the esophagus and are associated with motor abnormalities of the LES. Symptoms of dysphagia and regurgitation of large amounts of fluid are the most common symptomatic com-

---

*Exceeds dosage recommended by the manufacturer.

plaints. The associated motor abnormality is probably the major contributor to dysphagia. Treatment consists of attempts at correction of the associated motor abnormalities and resection of the diverticulum in more severe cases.

## Techniques of Esophageal Dilatation

The goal of esophageal dilatation is to maintain an esophageal lumen that allows effective swallowing. This usually requires a lumen of 50 French or greater. Once successful results are obtained, we then perform further dilatations only if symptoms recur. The perforation rate is less than 1%. There are four basic types of esophageal dilators: mercury-filled bougies (Maloney and Hurst), tapered plastic over guidewire dilators (Savary-Guillard), metal olives over guidewires (Eder-Puestow), and balloons. Each type has advantages and disadvantages. We tend to use Maloneys, balloons, and Savary-Guillards. Maloney dilators are tapered bougies that are best suited for straight uncomplicated strictures and Schatzki's rings. They do not require fluoroscopy, sedation, or special equipment. However, they can be difficult to use in complicated strictures and there is no confirmation of passage. We use balloon dilators that will pass through an endoscope and range in size from 7 to 20 mm. These balloons have the theoretical advantages of having less shear force and a lower perforation potential, although these advantages have not been well demonstrated in practice. Their main advantage is that they can be placed in difficult strictures with endoscopic guidance. The increase in luminal size has been shown to be less with balloons than with bougies. Savary-Guillard and Eder-Puestow dilators require fluoroscopic control for placement of the guidewire. They are particularly effective for long, irregular tight strictures.

Our basic approach is to examine most strictures identified by barium swallow endoscopically to exclude malignancy or Barrett's esophagus and to calibrate the stricture. If the stricture is short and straight, we will then perform Maloney dilatation at the same sitting to 56 or 60 French, usually not increasing the total size of dilators more than 12 French per session. If the patient has chest pain or there is gross blood on the dilator, we bring the patient back in 7 days. If the stricture is less than 10 mm (30 French), we will perform initial balloon dilatation followed by subsequent Maloney dilatation. For very tight, tortuous lesions, we use the wire-guided Savary-Guillard technique under fluoroscopy followed by Maloneys or balloons. By using these precautions, we can keep complications to a minimum.

## Esophageal Neoplasms

Malignant dysphagia is much less common than benign strictures. Despite this, malignancy must always be ruled out. The most common malignancies of the esophagus are squamous cell carcinoma and adenocarcinoma. Leiomyomas, leiomyosarcomas, lymphomas, and metastatic lesions are seen but are rare. The prognosis for these tumors is dismal, with less than 10% long-term survival. The major goal of therapy is palliation except in certain select, very early tumors. Esophageal lumen patency may be maintained by the use of the preceding dilation techniques, bipolar tumor probes, laser therapy, radiation therapy, or esophageal prosthesis. Palliative surgery such as blunt esophagectomy with esophagogastric cervical anastomosis is also an option. There are ongoing trials looking at combined modalities in the treatment and palliation of esophageal cancer.

## Esophageal Foreign Bodies and Impactions

The most common esophageal foreign body is meat impaction. This may occur with virtually all types of dysphagia but is most common with Schatzki's rings and reflux strictures. Meat tenderizer has been used previously, but serious complications have been reported; therefore, it should never be used. In a patient who is able to handle the secretions, removal of the impaction is not an emergency. The bolus may pass spontaneously if primary or secondary spasm is relieved. Nifedipine (10 mg sublingually), nitroglycerin (0.5 mg sublingually), or glucagon (0.5 mg intravenously) may be helpful. Often the patient will get spontaneous relief while waiting for therapy. Because impactions are quite uncomfortable, we prefer to remove them endoscopically if there is no relief with medical intervention. After the impaction is resolved, it is important to evaluate the cause of dysphagia and treat any strictures or rings in order to prevent recurrence.

Hard foreign bodies that are lodged in the esophagus should be removed immediately. If they are left in place, the risk of pressure necrosis and subsequent perforation is significant. Careful attention to the type of foreign body, location in the esophagus, and preparation of the patient (including general anesthesia if necessary) is crucial. Removal of foreign bodies should be attempted only by an experienced endoscopist.

## Compressive Disorders

Dysphagia may be caused by compression of the esophagus by any of the surrounding structures. Patients with thyroid enlargement may present with dysphagia. Mediastinal lymph node involvement by tumor can compress the esophagus. Vascular compression by an aberrant subclavian artery (dysphagia lusoria) or by the aortic arch (dysphagia aortica) in the elderly with a dilated and tortuous aorta can occur. Treatment consists of surgical decompression in severe cases.

### Miscellaneous Disorders

Patients who have had a Nissen fundoplication may have dysphagia if the "wrap" is too tight. Preoperative manometry studies will guide the surgeon in his or her technique. The dysphagia will occasionally respond to dilatation and time but may require surgical revision. Patients who have had radiation may have strictures and esophagitis acutely. Bullous and pemphigoid lesions of the skin may involve the esophagus and cause dysphagia. Congenital lesions of the esophagus such as atresia or congenital esophageal stricture are usually seen in children. Treatment is usually surgical, depending on associated abnormalities.

# DIVERTICULA OF THE ALIMENTARY TRACT

method of
FRANZ GOLDSTEIN, M.D.
*Jefferson Medical College of Thomas Jefferson
    University*
*Philadelphia, Pennsylvania*

Diverticula are outpouchings through the wall of the digestive tube and may be congenital or acquired. They can be true diverticula, containing all layers of the gut wall, or they may be false when only mucosa and submucosa herniate through the wall. Despite numerous theories of how diverticula form, with abnormalities of intestinal motility high on the list of causes, their true pathophysiology is not clear. In terms of causing illness, diverticula at any level of the gastrointestinal tract range from totally asymptomatic through severely symptomatic, with at times the need for emergency treatment.

## ESOPHAGEAL DIVERTICULA

The most important diverticula occurring in the esophagus are so-called Zenker's diverticula, first fully described by the German pathologist Zenker in 1874. They are an example of pulsion diverticula, which are acquired and occur mostly in late adult life. Increased intraluminal pressure and functional obstruction at the level of the cricopharyngeus seem to be major causes. A congenital weakness of the musculature in the hypopharynx may contribute to this mucosal herniation. Protrusion of the mucosa usually occurs between the oblique fibers of the inferior constrictor of the pharynx and the transverse muscle fibers of the cricopharyngeus. Functionally, premature contraction of the cricopharyngeus may occur during pharyngeal contraction. The upper esophageal sphincter corresponds to the cricopharyngeus and is definable manometrically as a high-pressure zone at the C5-6 level, approximately 2 cm in length. Some, but not all, studies have implicated elevated upper esophageal sphincter pressures as contributory to the production of Zenker's diverticula.

Small Zenker's diverticula may not be symptomatic and do not require treatment. These diverticula may progressively enlarge, and the sac may descend and lie between the esophagus and the vertebral column. The sac may occasionally extend to the posterosuperior mediastinum. Large diverticula tend to fill preferentially and tend to angulate or compress the esophagus and produce its partial or complete obstruction.

Symptoms of a large Zenker's diverticulum often involve noisy deglutition, foul-smelling breath, and spontaneous regurgitation of fresh and undigested food and saliva. Eating and drinking may be accompanied by regurgitation and by coughing and choking if aspiration into the airways occurs. Especially in elderly persons, respiratory complications can become critical and include hoarseness due to edema of the vocal cords, asthma, pneumonia, and even lung abscess. Malnutrition may occur, and rarely squamous cell carcinoma may supervene in long-standing cases.

On physical examination, a large diverticulum is occasionally palpable. The diagnosis can often be suspected from history alone, but confirmation is clearly needed by x-ray contrast examinations. Lateral views of the neck most clearly demonstrate the abnormality. Upper endoscopy is not recommended, as it can be hazardous and can cause perforation. When treatment is indicated for large diverticula, the preferred treatment is surgical correction, a one-stage pharyngoesophageal diverticulectomy. In some patients, cricopharyngeal myotomy is added, but this should be done only if increased pharyngeal pressures can be demonstrated.

### Midesophageal Diverticula

Diverticula arising from the midesophagus have traditionally been considered traction diverticula produced by mediastinal fibrosis resulting from inflammatory conditions such as tuberculosis. They are much less frequent now than when tuberculosis was more common. Midesophageal diverticula tend to be small and asymptomatic.

### Epiphrenic Diverticula

Diverticula of the lower esophagus frequently arise in association with hiatal hernias and motility disorders that may be primary or caused by an esophageal stricture just distal to the diverticulum. Most epiphrenic diverticula do not cause symptoms per se, but, if they are large, may aggravate nocturnal regurgitation of food and rarely can produce dysphagia and chest pain. If treatment is needed, it is often surgical and is aimed at correcting the underlying motor and anatomic abnormality by means of diverticulectomy and rarely also long esophagomyotomy. Dilation of coexistent strictures and vigorous antacid therapy, using $H_2$ receptor antagonists and, if necessary, omeprazole (Losec), may suffice in some patients.

Intramural pseudodiverticula of the esophagus are uncommon, but do occur in the form of small flask-shaped outpouchings, seen mostly in the upper third of the esophagus and usually in association with esophageal strictures. Infections, particularly with *Candida albicans,* believed to result from stasis, occur in such patients. Treatment consists of dilation of associated strictures and administration of fungicidal agents against *Candida* infection.

## DIVERTICULA OF THE STOMACH

Gastric diverticula are not common and are usually of little clinical significance. They occur most commonly on the posterior wall of the lesser curvature of the stomach just below the gastroesophageal junction and at times may simulate gastric ulcers. The differentiation between a penetrated gastric ulcer and a diverticulum may require endoscopic examination. These diverticula tend to be congenital in origin and usually contain all layers of the gastric wall. Large retentive diverticula may cause foul breath and occasionally food regurgitation. Malignancy can be excluded by cytologic and biopsy examination. Surgical treatment of gastric diverticula is rarely needed, but may be necessary for the rare complications of bleeding, perforation, or inflammation. Gastric diverticula occasionally occur in the midstomach or antrum, and again the differentiation from large gastric ulcers and tumors is of paramount importance. If the defects can be identified as diverticula, they rarely require any form of treatment.

## SMALL INTESTINAL DIVERTICULA

### Diverticula of the Duodenum

After the colon, the duodenum is the most common site of diverticula in the gastrointestinal tract. Most duodenal diverticula are solitary and occur most often in the second portion of the duodenum close to the ampulla of Vater. Most are asymptomatic and are found incidentally during barium examinations of the upper gastrointestinal tract or endoscopy. At autopsies, more than 20% of patients are found to have diverticula of the duodenum, and about 20% of these have more than one diverticulum. They usually are acquired and false. At times, they can be confused with perforated ulcers, but the presence of normal duodenal folds identifies them as diverticula.

Although the vast majority of duodenal diverticula do not produce symptoms, a few do. I first described in 1963 the association of a single large diverticulum with malabsorption, steatorrhea, and weight loss. Because of the retroperitoneal location of duodenal diverticula, their excision is difficult, and patients with malabsorption associated with diverticulosis, single or multiple, are best treated with antibiotics. Duodenal diverticula can also cause hemorrhage, which is sometimes severe; in such instances, surgical treatment may become necessary. In rare instances, diverticula can become inflamed and might even perforate. Because of the proximity to the ampulla of Vater, they can occasionally produce obstruction of the pancreatic and/or common bile duct and produce pancreatitis and/or cholangitis. Their presence can also complicate endoscopic retrograde cholangiopancreatography (ERCP) or make it more difficult.

Treatment of duodenal diverticula is reserved for patients with clearly related complications. Bacterial overgrowth is best treated with intermittent courses of antibiotics, such as tetracycline, 250 mg four times a day for 5 to 7 days, or metronidazole, in similar or slightly higher dosage. At times, a single course of therapy brings about lasting remission, but frequently courses have to be repeated when symptoms recur. When duodenal diverticula are associated with intestinal pseudo-obstruction, prokinetic drugs may be tried; at present, the only such drug available in the United States is metoclopramide, and its side effects can be troublesome. The expected approval of cisapride* should provide a better agent for the treatment of pseudo-obstruction.

The treatment of acute complications, such as obstruction, hemorrhage, diverticulitis, or perforation, is surgical and may involve resection of

---

*Not available in the United States.

the affected segment with primary anastomosis. Such surgery can be difficult. In some instances, cholecystectomy and/or choledochoduodenostomy may have to be undertaken. In some instances, a Roux-en-Y duodenojejunostomy is needed.

### Diverticula of Ileum and Jejunum

Diverticula of the small bowel below the ligament of Treitz are usually acquired and are uncommon. They occur along the mesenteric border, mostly in older age groups. They may be single or multiple and are occasionally numerous. They are incomplete diverticula and usually consist of herniated mucosa and submucosa in areas where blood vessels enter the bowel. There may be a relationship to intestinal pseudo-obstruction.

Isolated diverticula of jejunum and ileum tend to be asymptomatic. With multiple diverticula, a syndrome of macrocytic anemia due to vitamin B12 malabsorption and of steatorrhea, and at times massive malabsorption, can occur. Rarely, diverticula give rise to small bowel obstruction, possibly owing to associated inflammation, adhesions, and volvulus. Perforation is even less common, and bleeding is distinctly rare. In my experience, malabsorption in association with small bowel diverticulosis has been more common than generally appreciated and has been at times unrecognized for long periods of time. The malabsorption is caused by bacterial overgrowth associated with stasis in the diverticula and eventually in the entire small intestinal lumen, with or without antecedent or subsequent pseudo-obstruction. When available, small bowel intubation, sampling, and culture of the sample by quantitative culture methods is the most accurate way to make the diagnosis of bacterial overgrowth and gives information about the sensitivities of the recovered organisms. These tend to be predominantly coliforms with varying growth of strict anaerobic flora, which in some instances exceeds the aerobic flora. Despite the multiplicity of bacterial organisms recovered, the condition is often manageable with antibiotic treatment directed at the predominant aerobic flora, presumably because the anaerobic flora cannot thrive after the aerobic organisms are eradicated and no longer remove the oxygen toxic to strictly anaerobic species. Other methods of detecting bacterial overgrowth in the small bowel are various modifications of breath tests, such as the $^{14}$C xylose absorption test. Empiric treatment of multiple diverticula is similar to that of single diverticula with bacterial overgrowth, but repeated courses of tetracycline, metronidazole, or ampicillin are usually required to maintain patients in a clinically stable state and to maintain adequate nutrition. Surgery is rarely indicated and is limited to such complications as intestinal obstruction, volvulus, hemorrhage, diverticulitis, and perforation. In such instances, the involved segment of small bowel may have to be resected.

### Meckel's Diverticulum

Meckel's diverticula are the most common congenital abnormality of the gastrointestinal tract, occurring in about 2% of the population. They result from incomplete obliteration of the embryonic vitelline duct and are true diverticula. They arise from the antimesenteric border of the ileum, generally within 3 feet of the ileocecal valve.

The most common complication of Meckel's diverticula is bleeding and seems related to ectopic gastric epithelium that produces acid and leads to ulceration and bleeding. The bleeding can be mild or severe and, if chronic, can lead to iron deficiency anemia. Acute Meckel's diverticulitis can mimic acute appendicitis. Surgeons generally look for Meckel's diverticula when they open the abdomen for other reasons or in search of sources of bleeding or pain.

The diagnosis of Meckel's diverticula is occasionally made by a well-performed small bowel progress meal. If available, enteroclysis is preferable and more accurate. Occasionally, $^{99m}$Tc scanning is used and usually demonstrates ectopic gastric mucosa when present in the diverticulum. This technique is particularly useful when bleeding from a diverticulum is suspected. Rarely, Meckel's diverticula can give rise to intussusception and volvulus.

Asymptomatic diverticula are best left alone or removed if encountered during laparotomy for other causes. Symptomatic Meckel's diverticula are best resected, as there is no medical treatment of this condition.

In patients with gastrointestinal bleeding of obscure origin, angiography and/or nuclear bleeding scans usually suggest the approximate location of the bleeding site and may offer important clues to the presence of Meckel's diverticula. A specific bleeding site is usually not identified preoperatively, except when technetium scans identify gastric mucosa within a diverticulum.

## COLONIC DIVERTICULA

Colonic diverticula, or diverticulosis of the colon, are by far the most common diverticula of the gastrointestinal tract and occur in about 50% of Western populations older than age 60 years. Most of such diverticula are acquired pseudodiverticula resulting from herniation of mucosa and submucosa through the muscular layer of the colon, often between the mesenteric and lateral taeniae. Rarely, diverticula of the cecum and the ascending colon are congenital and are true diverticula. They can occasionally give rise to diverticulitis and mimic appendicitis. Far more commonly diverticulosis is acquired and most frequently involves the sigmoid colon, but, in decreasing order, may involve the descending, transverse, and ascending colon. A single cause of diverticulosis, the mere presence of diverticula, does not exist, and many factors may contribute to its development. Among them could be advancing age, weakness of tissues, increased intraluminal pressures, faulty bowel habits, diet, specifically deficient amounts of dietary fiber, and hypertrophy of the colonic musculature, to mention just the main ones. Some authors have classified diverticulosis into two major types—i.e., spastic diverticulosis perhaps related to antecedent spastic or irritable colon, and simple massed diverticulosis encountered in an older age group and without specific clues as to its pathogenesis.

Many patients with diverticulosis are unaware of diverticula or are made aware of them through barium enemas or colonoscopy done for various reasons. The exact percentage of patients who eventually experience symptoms is variously estimated at 5 to 25%. The wide variation in estimated symptom frequency is in part due to the inability to separate the symptoms of diverticulosis from those of the irritable bowel syndrome, whether they be considered etiologically related or simply coexistent. Colonic diverticulosis is encountered far more commonly in Western countries and has been widely recognized only in the twentieth century, the earliest complete report dating to 1925. The changes in lifestyles and diet, with particular reference to inadequate fiber intake, are believed to be important etiologic factors in the rapid increase in the incidence and prevalence of diverticulosis.

Symptoms attributed to diverticulosis include diarrhea, constipation, alternating diarrhea and constipation, intestinal distention, and abdominal pain; they are similar to those of the irritable bowel syndrome. Such patients should be free of fever, leukocytosis, and appreciable tenderness over the left lower quadrant, although tenderness can be produced by a severe spastic colon alone. However, rigidity and other findings of peritoneal irritation tend to point to diverticulitis or other inflammatory conditions.

The diagnosis of diverticulosis is made by barium enemas, with double contrast examinations preferred (except in patients with diverticulitis), and/or colonoscopy. In patients with multiple diverticula noted by x-ray film in either a segment or the entire length of colon, the recognition of coexistent polyps or carcinomas can be difficult or impossible. In such instances, colonoscopy is advised to make this important differentiation. If the diagnosis of diverticulosis was initially made by colonoscopy, there probably is not much need to confirm it by barium enema, although some value exists in obtaining a permanent visual record and a better localization of the site of diverticular disease. Computed tomography scanning is used increasingly to detect and delineate the extraluminal complications of diverticular disease, including abscesses, fistulas, and penetration of the inflammatory process into adjacent structures.

The differentiation on radiographic grounds between diverticulosis and diverticulitis is not always easy or even possible. Clearly, the demonstration of abscesses or fistulas documents the presence of diverticulitis. Fixed, eccentric subtraction defects in the barium column suggest an impinging inflammatory mass. Areas of irregular, jagged margins and mucosal distortion suggest inflammation due to diverticulitis. Other signs exist, but may not allow definitive interpretations.

In the differential diagnosis of diverticular disease, carcinoma should always be considered and colonoscopy may be the most accurate way of establishing this diagnosis. Barium enema may suggest a carcinoma in strictured areas, especially when the fold pattern is distorted or obliterated. Crohn's disease can be a treacherous diagnosis and can coexist with diverticulosis. Submucosal tracking has been seen in both diverticular disease and Crohn's disease. Ulcerative colitis can at times be difficult to recognize in patients with coexistent diverticular disease. Acute forms of colitis, including ischemic colitis, and various infectious colitides can pose difficulties in the differential diagnosis of diverticulitis or diverticulosis with bleeding.

The treatment of uncomplicated diverticulosis is not well established, but most authors would try to normalize bowel function and avoid food ingredients that might tend to increase discomfort, possibly highly seasoned foods or lactose-containing foods in patients with lactose intolerance. Efforts to increase fecal bulk are linked to increased fiber intake. My preference is to let people eat normal diets and supplement the diet with bulking agents, such as psyllium (e.g., Konsyl, Metamucil, Hydrocil) or methylcellulose (e.g., Citrucel), wheat bran, or combinations of the above. Efforts to normalize bowel function with large intake of fruits and vegetables are generally unsuccessful, and dependence on bran intake alone also tends to be frustrating. The avoidance of nuts and seeds is probably unimportant, and there is little, if any, documentation to prove the noxious character of such foods. Low-fiber diets, once recommended, are contraindicated. There is value in promoting normal eating and bowel habits, with emphasis on eating breakfast and utilizing the remnant gastrocolic reflex to evacuate the bowels in the morning. By not doing so, the urge to move one's bowels may occur at various times, mostly inconvenient, and often results in suppression of the defecatory urge with ultimate disorganized bowel function. There has long been a suspicion that impaired bowel function, particularly constipation, is conducive to the main complication of diverticulosis—i.e., diverticulitis. If bulking agents alone do not suffice to control constipation, my preference is for adding stool softeners (calcium or sodium docusate) and, if this does not suffice, add also a peristaltic stimulant, such as senna alkaloid, with dosages adjusted to patient needs.

### Complications of Diverticulosis

The major complications of diverticulosis are bleeding and diverticulitis and its complications, such as abscess formation and fistulas to adjacent organs. Because, in many patients, it is unclear at any given stage whether one deals with uncomplicated diverticulosis or any of the various complications, the term "diverticular disease" is often used to denote the difficulty in differentiating among the various phases of this disease.

In discussing the complications of diverticulosis and their treatment, an introductory comment may be in order. Contemporary medicine has been greatly influenced by the outcome of controlled randomized clinical trails (RCT). In conditions in which well-executed RCTs are available, their results are generally accepted as providing the best diagnostic or treatment options. In diverticular disease of the colon, among the most common conditions of older persons in Western societies, few RCTs are available to answer the enormous number of questions that arise concerning both diagnosis and treatment. The clinician therefore must be guided by his or her own experience, by uncontrolled clinical trials of others, and by so-called anecdotal evidence, whatever that dreaded term might denote. The spectrum of complications of diverticular disease is wide and sometimes difficult to unravel, and the differential diagnosis of diverticular disease, other colonic conditions, or those of adjacent structures can be challenging.

**Diverticular Bleeding.** Bleeding from colonic diverticulosis is fairly common, with estimates varying from 5 to 25%. Bleeding tends to be brisk and abrupt; it can be massive or exsanguinating, but can also be mild and intermittent. When colonic bleeding is massive, angiography can be of value to localize the site of bleeding. A nuclear bleeding scan can do the same in a noninvasive manner. If the bleeding is submassive, colonoscopy is the preferred and often most available diagnostic modality to identify the site and source of bleeding. At times, flexible sigmoidoscopy may be sufficient or may precede full colonoscopy. If bleeding stops spontaneously, colonoscopy is the diagnostic modality of choice, with flexible sigmoidoscopy and double contrast barium enema the next best option. Significant bleeding from diverticula is often followed by subsequent bleeding episodes, and such patients tend to require surgical resection eventually. If a definite short segment of bowel can be identified as the source of bleeding, its removal can be sufficient to prevent further hemorrhages. When multiple segments appear to be involved or the patient has extensive diverticular disease, the preferred treatment is a subtotal colectomy with an ileodistal sigmoidostomy. Angiographers occasionally have been able to stop bleeding by the infusion of vasopressin or the injection of autologous clot or absorbable gelatin sponge (Gelfoam), but these methods are not widely used or entirely safe. In the differential diagnosis of diverticular bleeding, one has to consider other sources of bleeding, including polyps and malignant tumors, the ever more widely recognized angiodysplasia, and irritable bowel disease. If a patient has bled once and stopped, and never had prior treatment directed at normalization of bowel function, it is worthwhile to institute a regimen designed to normalize bowel function and promote daily evacuations, relying on the proper use of bulking agents, with or without added stool softeners and occasionally peristaltic stimulants. Constipation has been considered to be a factor leading to both diverticular bleeding and diverticulitis and hence should be corrected if at all possible.

**Diverticulitis.** Diverticulitis, or inflammation and infection of a segment of diverticular disease, is the most common complication of diverticulosis. Its diagnosis is largely clinical and relies on the clinical findings of left lower quadrant pain and tenderness, leukocytosis, and fever. Confirmation of the diagnosis can be difficult in some cases and may require restraint because confirmatory diagnostic procedures can be risky. In most instances, diverticulitis is caused by microperforation and there are localized peritoneal signs; in more severe cases, overt bowel perforation may have occurred and peritonitis and sepsis may follow. Some patients have diverticulitis with minimal or no peritoneal signs; I have seen patients with intramural abscesses that gave rise to virtually no localized signs, yet who had distant abscesses of the liver, the subhepatic space, the lungs, and the bones. Blood cultures are clearly important in any patient with suspected diverticulitis, to ascertain if sepsis is present and to obtain antibiotic sensitivities of the major organisms causing sepsis. The simple digital rectal examination has importance and often elicits signs of induration and tenderness of an inflamed loop of sigmoid, confirming the diagnosis of diverticulitis. The use of barium enemas and endoscopy is helpful and important but requires caution and proper technique and timing for safest and best results. This is one situation in which a double contrast barium enema is not indicated. Instead, after the most acute phase of diverticulitis is overcome, a thin barium mixture can be gently infused or instilled into the colon without air insufflation, merely to demonstrate the presence of diverticular disease and the presence or absence of extraluminal barium. The presence of extraluminal barium connotes the presence of an abscess. Flexible sigmoidoscopy or colonoscopy should not be done during the most acute phase of diverticulitis, but can be done when there is no acute inflammation. Air insufflation should be held to a minimum, and caution should be exerted not to push against resistance in areas of sharp angulation frequently encountered in this condition. Endoscopic inspection of the interior of the colon can show telltale signs of inflammation of the mucosa that, in conjunction with other findings, may clinch the diagnosis of diverticulitis. In addition, the lumen tends to be rigid, and any manipulation of even a sigmoidoscope can elicit severe pain. In recent years, computerized scanning has become increasingly important in delineating extraluminal manifestations, such as abscesses, adherence to the peritoneum, and free fluid. In milder cases, it can be difficult or impossible to differentiate diverticulitis from severe spastic colon manifestations. In long-standing cases, colonic stenosis may occur, leading to pain and partial obstruction. Either barium enema or endoscopy can provide diagnostic proof.

During bouts of acute diverticulitis, dietary restrictions are usually indicated. In milder cases, it is sufficient to restrict oral intake to clear liquids for a day or two, then gradually increasing the diet toward normal but avoiding high-fiber foods until the acute condition has subsided. During more severe bouts, especially if patients require hospitalization, it is best to avoid all oral intake for several days and provide all nutrients by the intravenous route. If this should be more than a few days, peripheral or central hyperalimentation can be added to avoid nutritional depletion.

The primary treatment of diverticulitis consists of antibiotics. Here again, no unanimity of opinion exists and controlled trials are amazingly few. Part of the difficulty may reside in the highly complex colonic flora and the impossibility of culturing the organisms implicated in the infectious process unless sepsis supervenes and positive blood cultures are obtainable. Antibiotic treatment in most cases is given because most of the time the infection is mixed and is due to both strict anaerobic bacteria, such as *Bacteroides fragilis,* and facultative anaerobic coliform organisms, such as *Escherichia coli.* Because of this uncertainty, broad-spectrum antibiotics or combinations of antibiotics are usually chosen. In milder cases in which antibiotics can be given by mouth, ampicillin is often used because of its activity against *E. coli* and other coliforms. Cephalexin (Keflex) active against strains of *E. coli* can be used in patients with intolerance for ampicillin. Amoxicillin or its combination with clavulanic acid (Augmentin) is another option, though considerably more expensive. Treatment with antibiotics should be given in conventional dosages for at least 5 to 7 days, at times longer, but with caution regarding ineffectiveness, hypersensitivities, and the development of gastrointestinal intolerance, including pseudomembranous colitis.

When intravenous antibiotics need to be administered, cefoxitin (Mefoxin) has been widely used. Frequently, two drugs are given, one for anaerobes and one for aerobes, and one such combination that is relatively cost efficient consists of metronidazole (Flagyl) and cefazolin (Ancef), usually administered for periods of 5 to 14 days. If no response is obtained after appropriate time periods, other antibiotics can be tried or complications should be suspected and surgery considered. The usual side effects associated with antibiotic usage should be kept in mind.

Surgery for diverticular disease is indicated for medically unresponsive acute diverticulitis and for complications such as abscess formation, perforation, and fistulas, but also for intractable lesser complications such as diverticular stenosis or recurrent mild attacks of diverticulitis. In the latter situation, patients should be informed that the option for surgery may represent a lower risk in the long run than allowing the condition to continue and ultimately to lead to more serious complications, especially perforation of the colon. When surgery is performed, preferentially a one-stage procedure is carried out, resecting the diseased portion of bowel with primary anastomosis. When this cannot be safely accomplished, for instance, in cases of severe inflammation with or without abscess formation, a two-stage or even three-stage operation may be needed. At worst, an abscess may have to be drained and a temporary colostomy established without initial resection. Frequently, the surgeon can remove the diseased segment, leave the distal stump in the pelvis, in a so-called Hartmann's procedure, and provide a temporary protective colostomy followed by anastomosis after a few months when the acute inflammation has subsided. Drainage of abscesses can sometimes be performed by the percutaneous route and thus can spare patients one stage of more invasive surgery. The results of surgery, if done in a timely and proper manner, are generally excellent, and surgery should not be withheld from patients who clearly meet the indications for surgical treatment. For especially bad infections, such as those associated with perforation and abscess, cefoxitin with or without gentamicin, or clindamycin plus gentamicin, has been recommended.

The prognosis of patients with diverticular disease is generally favorable because some way of treatment can be found, be it medical or surgical. At the extreme, a subtotal colectomy can be performed with a relatively low risk, except in patients who are poor risks for any surgery because of concurrent systemic diseases.

# ULCERATIVE COLITIS

method of
JAMES H. BUTT, M.D.
*Harry S Truman Memorial Veterans Hospital*
*Columbia, Missouri*

Ulcerative colitis (UC) is a relatively rare, idiopathic, inflammatory disorder involving the colon and the rectum. In an established general clinical practice, it would be unusual to follow more than 3 to 5 patients with diagnosed UC and to diagnose more than 5 to 10 new cases in a lifetime of practice.

UC is socially disabling, chiefly through the symptoms of pain, frequency, urgency, tenesmus, and incontinence arising from rectal involvement. Additional disability results from the worry and expense generated by any chronic disease. The specter of cancer complicating UC has been greatly exaggerated, because only a small group of patients (3%) with UC are at risk. In this group the risk is significant, but, in the majority of patients with UC, the risk of cancer is not much different from that in the noncolitic population and can be handled by the usual cancer surveillance techniques.

### General Treatment

As in any chronic disease, the role of the physician is to foster patient independence from the physician. Patients need to be reassured that the majority of patients with a mild first attack of distal disease (70%) have no altered life expectancy and that the disease is curable by surgery.

Many patients, however, fear surgery because of the prospect of ileostomy. First, few patients (10%) undergo operation in the course of UC. Second, long-term follow-up reveals no excessive mortality related to the ileostomy. Third, 90% of patients with ileostomy have little economic or sexual dysfunction consequent to the ileostomy; this is in sharp contrast to the economic and sexual dysfunction of patients (25%) with continuous symptoms of UC before surgery. Finally, ileorectal anastomosis with or without a reservoir (Park's pouch) is now generally available. These operations obviate sexual and bladder dysfunction (15%), which may accompany proctectomy even in the most skilled hands.

An irritable bowel syndrome affects about one-third of UC patients in remission, with symptoms identical to those of active UC, except rectal bleeding. It is important to investigate this problem rather than automatically treat each episode as an exacerbation of UC. Frequent visits are unnecessary for the well-educated patient who is in remission.

### Nutrition

No evidence at present indicates that bowel rest has an important role in management, except eliminating high-residue foods during a flare of UC and eliminating oral intake of food during acute, fulminating UC with accompanying ileus, peritoneal signs, or toxic dilation of the colon.

The restoration of nutritional deficits is critical in the patient facing surgical intervention. It is rare for a patient with UC to require parenteral alimentation because the small bowel is usually functional. Parenteral hyperalimentation may be useful, however, as preoperative and postoperative adjunctive therapy, but should be used with restraint because the complication rate is increased in patients with active UC.

Supplemental feedings of low osmolality (approximately 300 mOsm per kg) are best. Overnight feedings may be given through a small-caliber, soft nasoduodenal tube, such as the Dobbhoff enteric feeding tube. The risk of aspiration should be assessed, but most patients tolerate such feedings without difficulty if there is elevation of the head of the bed and attentive nursing care. In selected patients, this can be continued at home with a great reduction in cost. Caloric demands during repletion may vary from 3000 to 5000 calories per day and in children or adolescent patients with growth retardation may approach 80 calories per kg per day to restore growth and sexual development. Caloric repletion as an alternative to surgical intervention should be attempted in developmental problems without compelling indications for surgery. Neither

TABLE 1. **Activity of Ulcerative Colitis**

| Activity (% of Patients) | Bowel Movements | Rectal Bleeding | Fever | Tachycardia | Anemia (Hb g/dl) | ESR |
|---|---|---|---|---|---|---|
| Mild ($\simeq$70) | ≤4/day | Occasional BM | 0 | 0 | ≥10.5 | ≤30 mm/hr |
| Moderate ($\simeq$25) | 4–6 day | Some BM | ± | ± | ± | ± |
| Severe ($\simeq$5) | ≥6/day | Most BM | ≥37.5 C PO | ≥90/min | ≤10.5 | ≤30 mm/hr |

*Abbreviations:* BM = bowel movements; GSR = erythrocyte sedimentation rate.

growth retardation nor undernutrition are primary indications for surgical intervention.

### Psychotherapy

The most critical factor in the psychotherapy of patients with UC is continued care by the same physician, with repetitive, detailed communication with the patient about medications and their side effects; laboratory, endoscopic, and radiologic studies; and surgical options. Physician absences should be carefully communicated to the patient, with substitution of a familiar surrogate, during active disease.

The use of tranquilizers and antidepressants should be restricted to patients with clinically evident problems that require such therapy independently of the diagnosis of UC. The anticholinergic side effects of tranquilizers and antidepressants can be dangerous in active UC. Psychiatric referral may occasionally be necessary for suicidal patients and those with steroid psychosis. Referral should be considered in those who are severely depressed or who have a change in capacity to cope with psychosocial problems discordant with UC activity. Depression may occasionally reflect development of subclinical complications masked by steroid therapy. A careful evaluation for complications prior to referral is important because most psychiatrists have limited experience with inflammatory bowel disease and are not sensitive to the potential psychologic expression of subclinical physical complications.

The National Foundation for Ileitis and Colitis (444 Park Avenue South, New York, NY 10016, 212–685–3440) can provide patient education materials and support through mutual help groups offered by many local chapters. The *Crohn's Disease and Ulcerative Colitis Fact Book* published by this foundation has proved particularly helpful in patient education. The self-help groups are designed to permit patients and family members to share their experiences with others who must cope with the disease. For patients who have had an ileostomy, similar mutual help groups are available through the United Ostomy Association (36 Executive Park, Suite 120, Irvine, CA 92714, 714–660–8624). These self-help groups bring together people who have had ileostomies and are a valuable source of information for the patient about to undergo colectomy. The patient can see young, healthy, vigorous people who have an ileostomy without limitation in their activities.

### Specific Treatment

Various factors must be assessed in new patients or patients with relapse.

AGE. There is a sharp increase in mortality in patients older than age 70 years. Relapse after induction of remission is also more likely in this age group and is least likely in those younger than age 30 years.

ACTIVITY OF DISEASE. Disease activity can be assessed clinically (Tables 1 and 2) and by proctoscopy. Proctoscopy is necessary if the history of bowel frequency or rectal bleeding is discordant with objective signs of activity. For example, a patient with inactive UC commonly may have irritable bowel syndrome with frequent bowel actions, or a patient with active UC may not report rectal bleeding

EXTENT OF DISEASE. Extent-of-disease statistics are based on radiologic rather than endoscopic determinations (Table 3). Distal colitis includes proctosigmoiditis; substantial disease extends from the rectum through part of the transverse colon; extensive disease occurs from the rectum to the hepatic flexure or beyond to the cecum. The extent of disease is difficult and dangerous to assess during active UC. Physical examination, proctoscopy (if not contraindicated by toxic dilation of the colon), and plain film of the abdomen may be the only safe ways to meas-

TABLE 2. **Activity of Ulcerative Colitis: Sequelae During 5 Years**

| Activity (% of Patients) | Mortality (%) | Resection (%) | Remission (%) | Relapse (%) |
|---|---|---|---|---|
| Mild ($\simeq$70) | 0 | 0 | $\simeq$90 | $\simeq$65 |
| Moderate ($\simeq$25) | $\simeq$3 | $\simeq$4 | $\simeq$85 | $\simeq$60 |
| Severe ($\simeq$5) | $\simeq$25 | $\simeq$30 | $\simeq$40 | $\simeq$50 |

TABLE 3. **Extent of Disease: Sequelae During 5 Years**

| Radiologic Extent* (% of Patients) | Mortality (%) | Resection (%) | Hospitalization (%) | Relapse (%) | Extension (%) |
|---|---|---|---|---|---|
| Distal ($\simeq$74) | 0 | $\simeq$5 | $\simeq$18 | $\simeq$70 | $\simeq$15 |
| Substantial ($\simeq$12) | 0 | $\simeq$3 | $\simeq$30 | $\simeq$60 | $\simeq$21 |
| Extensive ($\simeq$14) | $\simeq$5 | $\simeq$30 | $\simeq$70 | $\simeq$60 | — |

*See text.

ure the extent of involvement during a severe attack. Stool accumulates proximal to areas of inflammation, so that a rough assessment of extent of disease can be made if there is stool present on the plain film. Periodic reassessment of the extent of disease by biopsy during inactive phases is necessary to establish the risk of cancer and the need for cancer surveillance.

DURATION OF DISEASE. Mortality is highest in the first attack and first 4 years of the disease.

OTHER COLONIC DISEASES. Toxic, viral, bacterial, and parasitic causes of colonic diseases mimicking UC must be excluded by history and by laboratory test results before initiating specific therapy.

OTHER SYSTEMIC PROBLEMS. Tuberculin reactivity should be tested early in the course of UC before initiation of corticosteroid (CS) therapy because prolonged CS therapy may reactivate tuberculosis. Gastric and duodenal ulceration may become a problem with CS and sulfasalazine (SS) therapy and the stress of acute or chronic disease; prophylaxis with sucralfate (Carafate), 1 gram twice daily, may be indicated. Liver disease in UC may have an associated coagulopathy, accentuating bleeding, and may require correction with blood constituents. Iliofemoral thrombophlebitis in association with UC may require anticoagulation with heparin, which carries an obvious hazard of increased colonic bleeding. Streptokinase and urokinase are too hazardous for use in active UC. Other systemic diseases involving cardiovascular, pulmonary, and renal systems may complicate therapy and make surgical intervention both more hazardous and more urgent in the older age groups. Pregnancy compounds the problem of therapy: medical therapy with CS and SS is probably safe throughout pregnancy, whereas surgical intervention is associated with a high fetal mortality. Immunosuppressive agents (azathioprine [Imuran] and 6-mercaptopurine [Purinethol]) are contraindicated in pregnancy.

## Medical Treatment

**Topical Therapy.** Symptomatic relief of pain, incontinence, tenesmus, urgency, and frequency is achieved by topical rectal therapy no matter what the extent or severity of disease. For proctitis limited to the distal 10 cm of the rectum, 25-mg hydrocortisone suppositories twice daily are highly effective. Suppositories with local anesthetics, glycerin, and belladonna alkaloids have potential side effects in UC and should be avoided.

An effective alternative to suppositories and to enemas is hydrocortisone foam (Cortifoam), which delivers 80 mg of hydrocortisone with each application. Each aerosol container delivers approximately 14 doses into an anal applicator. Charging the applicator is an obstacle for some patients; pharmacists should demonstrate the procedure. The patient should be cautioned not to insert the aerosol container spout into the anus! Foam is equivalent in clinical efficacy to enemas and reaches the midsigmoid colon in most patients. Foam is approximately two-thirds the cost of enemas per treatment and is subjectively much more acceptable, especially to patients receiving twice-daily treatments, because it is easily retained in the upright position. Within 2 weeks, 75% of patients with disease distal to the midsigmoid improve on twice-daily therapy alone. This improvement increases to more than 90% after 4 to 6 weeks with a reduced dosage, in contrast to 60% success with enemas. CS side effects, including adrenal suppression, occur with topical applications. There is a local effect of topical therapy that is independent of any systemic effect. CS enemas given twice weekly have been ineffective in maintaining remission.

**Sulfasalazine.** Sulfasalazine (Azulfidine) is an extremely valuable drug, used for the past 40 years in the treatment of UC. In mild and moderate UC and in maintenance of remission, SS is a useful agent. There are two components with an azo linkage: 5-aminosalicylic acid (5-ASA, the active component) and sulfapyridine. The azo linkage is split by bacterial action in the colon or occasionally in the proximal ileum. Sulfapyridine is absorbed from the colon and is a cause of multiple side effects. Sulfonamides have no therapeutic effect in UC. Unsplit SS, however, may have a therapeutic effect that is independent of that of 5-ASA. Allergy to sulfonamides or salicylic acid is a contraindication to the use of SS.

GASTROINTESTINAL SIDE EFFECTS. Unfortunately, 20% of patients are intolerant of SS, experiencing unpleasant side effects consisting of nausea, vomiting, and abdominal pain. These can be minimized by initiating the medication at no more than 1 tablet three times daily for 1 to 5 days and by limiting the dosage to 3 grams per day. Gastrointestinal side effects can be further limited by using enteric-coated tablets (30% more expensive than regular tablets).

HEMATOLOGIC SIDE EFFECTS. These are common. A decrease in leukocyte count of 500 to 1200 per mm$^3$ occurs in most patients, but a drop below 4000 per mm$^3$ in approximately 3% of patients is an indication for prompt withdrawal because idiosyncratic, probably irreversible "agranulocytosis" can occur, especially in the first 12 weeks of therapy. Regular monitoring of the leukocyte count and the differential leukocyte count is advisable, adding substantially to the cost of treatment. Other adverse effects are hemolytic anemia, which may reflect a glucose-6-phosphate dehydrogenase deficiency, methemoglobinemia, and folic acid malabsorption, which rarely (2.5%) leads to anemia.

REVERSIBLE MALE INFERTILITY. Treatment with SS has resulted in oligospermia, abnormal sperm size, and abnormal motility in more than 70% of patients.

RASHES. Rashes may occur within a few days of initiating therapy and should be controlled by stopping the drug. Use of SS may be critical for patients in whom CS therapy represents a major health hazard, such as those with osteoporosis or diabetes mellitus. Some of these rashes are due to photosensitivity and can be managed by sunscreens and protective clothing.

DENSITIZATION. Desensitization to SS may be attempted for gastrointestinal symptoms of nausea, vomiting, and headache by discontinuing the drug for 1 to 2 weeks and resuming therapy at 0.125 gram per day for 1 week, then increasing by 0.125 gram every week to a maintenance dose of 2 to 3 grams per day.

Desensitization for SS-induced rash and fever has been carried out by reinitiation of therapy (with 1 mg per day) after a rest period and doubling the dosage daily with a plateau in dosage for 1 week at 10 and 100 mg until a maintenance level of 2 to 3 grams per day has been reached. Patients who have undergone desensitization for rash should be closely watched for clinical or laboratory signs of systemic toxicity, at which point SS should be stopped. Cessation of SS therapy must be followed by another program of desensitization before dosage can be renewed. Desensitization is not safe after life-threatening reactions to SS occur, such as hemolysis, leukopenia, agranulocytosis, hepatitis, pancreatitis, and exfoliative dermatitis.

MAINTENANCE THERAPY. In mild to moderate UC, a dosage of 3 to 4 grams of SS per day for 1 week followed by 2 grams per day for 2 weeks can achieve remission in more than 75% of patients without adjunctive therapy. Two grams of SS per day has maintained remission in 80% of the patients studied for up to 1 year, in sharp contrast to remission in 20% of the patients receiving placebo. The optimal duration of maintenance therapy is unknown, but is likely to be 2 to 5 years or perhaps even longer. The high relapse rates noted in Tables 2 and 3 probably reflect patient noncompliance with maintenance therapy and lackadaisical follow-up by physicians. About half of patients remain in remission after withdrawal following 1 year of successful SS maintenance therapy. Antibiotic therapy affecting intestinal bacteria may block the breakdown of SS and partially inactivate it. Relapse of UC may be precipitated by antibiotic therapy with or without toxin-producing *Clostridium difficile* overgrowth.

**Aminosalicylic Acid Derivatives.** 5-Aminosalicylic acid, or mesalamine, has been recognized for 15 years as an active component of SS. Its chemical instability made it impractical for routine clinical use until recently. An enema preparation of 5-ASA (Rowasa) has recently been released for treatment of acute, mild to moderate, distal ulcerative colitis, containing 4 grams of 5-ASA stabilized by a salt of metabisulfite and gum xanthran in a 60-ml volume. 4-Aminosalicylic acid, the familiar para-aminosalicylic acid (PAS), used for many years in antituberculosis therapy, is under study as well for use as an enema preparation, and may be more effective than 5-ASA; PAS has not been released as yet for treatment of inflammatory bowel disease.

Oral preparations include 5-ASA in two pH-dependent release preparations, Pentasa and Asacol, and diazo-5-aminosalicylic acid, olsalazine (Dipentum), a preparation like SS, with 5-ASA released by the action of enteric bacteria on the diazo bond. Olsalazine has been approved by the U.S. Food and Drug Administration (FDA) GI Advisory Committee but has not yet been released. The two mesalamine preparations are undergoing prolonged, FDA-mandated trials, despite adequate study and marketing in other countries. In general, these preparations are more effective than placebo but less effective than predicted on a stoichiometric basis with SS (400 mg of 5-ASA is equivalent to 1000 mg of SS). The oral preparations have differing characteristics: olsalazine displays an unpleasant and confusing side effect of diarrhea severe enough to warrant discontinuation of the drug in 5 to 10% of patients; Pentasa has relatively low maintenance of remission in long-term studies: 63% at 6 months and 54% at 12 months; this maintenance of remission was not different from that in the

SS controls in the Pentasa study but was quite different from published maintenance of remission for SS studied independently, 80% at 12 months; ASAcol has displayed a failure to control distal disease in some patients, reflecting dissolution of the pH-dependent coating and drug release in the right side of the colon proximal to the sigmoid colon and rectum.

In general, these agents represent an advance, but the cost of the only released preparation (ROWASA) is fivefold the cost of hydrocortisone foam and makes its use problematic except for patients intolerant of, allergic to, or refractory to SS in whom acute, mild to moderate, distal disease makes 5-ASA topical therapy an attractive alternative to systemic CS. These agents permit reversal of male infertility induced by SS.

TOPICAL THERAPY. 5-Aminosalicylic acid enemas may be used as sole therapy for patients with acute, mild to moderate, distal disease within reach of the enemas, usually 20 to 40 cm from the anus, or as adjunctive therapy with SS or CS. The clinical effect of 5-ASA enemas in association with CS is diminished. One enema should be instilled at bedtime with the patient on his or her left side and should be retained as long as possible. If the enema is promptly expelled, there is severe rectal disease and other therapy should be instituted or augmented promptly. The usual course of treatment is 6 weeks. It is likely that therapy continued beyond 6 weeks will be effective for chronic active disease and for maintenance of remission, but use for those indications is not approved; appropriate treatment and maintenance schedules have not been determined, and there is an increased risk of side effects with time. A suppository preparation has been effective in distal disease within 20 cm of the anus, but is not available in the United States.

ADVERSE EFFECTS. Twenty per cent of patients undergoing treatment with 5-ASA enemas for 2 weeks exhibited minimal side effects, but only 5% discontinued the drug, none for clear-cut effects of the drug. In sharp contrast, 8% of patients treated with CS enemas had minimal side effects and none left the study. Some patients taking the oral preparations have had major side effects.

**Corticosteroid Therapy.** Corticosteroid therapy is used in the treatment of moderate to severe disease, in initial attacks, in acute relapses, and in chronic active disease. There is also a role for CS in the maintenance of remission if the patient is intolerant of or allergic to SS and the risk/benefit ratio of CS therapy warrants its long-term use. The most common single cause of CS treatment failure is premature tapering of the drug. In the extreme, abrupt discontinuation of any medication in UC may be disastrous.

CS are hazardous drugs with significant adverse reactions in 20 to 25% of patients treated for 3 months or longer. These include sepsis, peptic ulcer, osteoporosis, fractures, psychosis, hypertension, sinusitis, urinary tract infections, glucose intolerance, acne, and myopathy. Prednisone or prednisolone is given in a single oral dose of 40 to 60 mg daily (there is no therapeutic advantage in divided doses) as 5-mg tablets (20-mg tablets may improve compliance, but seem to be clinically less effective) for 2 to 5 weeks before attempting to taper the drug in patients with moderate disease. Occasionally, once-a-day dosage is complicated by night fevers and dysentery; this is ominous and indicates relapse. Approximately 50% of patients are in remission within 2 weeks and another 40% improve. After 3 to 5 weeks of treatment, 66 to 75% are in remission and 20% improve. Tapering of drug dosage for those patients in remission should begin no later than 6 weeks after initiation of therapy and proceed at the rate of 1 mg per day in 2.5- to 5-mg increments. Attempts to taper in those who have improved but are not in remission is much more problematic, but tapering should be tried at half the rate for those in remission. The use of topical rectal therapy in such patients may be helpful. At dosages less than 15 to 20 mg per day, a flare of UC may occur, calling for more frequent clinical surveillance during tapering. The patient and physician alike should be alert for symptoms and signs of relapse. The total course of treatment may be 3 to 4 months, allowing for ample exposure to side effects of CS. In prolonged treatment with CS (longer than 25 days), gastric and duodenal ulcer prophylaxis is prudent with sucralfate, 1 gram twice daily. SS maintenance therapy should begin after a CS taper to 20 mg and continue after CS is withdrawn.

The residual 5 to 15% of patients who flare during withdrawal of CS or who have chronic symptoms despite improvement with CS should have the diagnosis of UC reassessed to look for bacterial, viral, parasitic, and toxic causes. Mucosal biopsies should be obtained. Flexible sigmoidoscopy or colonoscopy may be hazardous in active inflammatory bowel disease because of the extensive air insufflation during the procedure. Rigid sigmoidoscopy still represents a bargain, involving minimal inconvenience, cost, and preparation for the patient. Biopsies at 3 to 6 weeks into the attack should confirm the diagnosis of UC in 80% of patients and effectively exclude cases of acute, self-limited, transient colitis from prolonged and dangerous CS therapy.

Patients who have experienced flares during withdrawal of CS or who have chronic symptoms despite improvement with CS are candidates for chronic CS suppressive therapy. Efforts should be made to minimize the dosage for suppression and to attempt to give the patient alternate-day CS; the usual dosage will be twice the minimal daily dose required for suppression. Surgery should be considered as an option at this time. If the patient refuses surgery and if the dosage of CS is too high for safe, long-term maintenance (>20 mg per day), a trial of azathioprine (Imuran) or 6-mercaptopurine (Purinethol) may be helpful.* Many authorities, however, believe that immunosuppressive therapy is still experimental and should not be undertaken, except under the aegis of institutional medicine, such as a university medical center or clinic. One-third of patients have a remission when immunosuppressive therapy is added to CS and another third show improvement, marked by decreased CS requirements, within 6 months of initiating treatment. As an alternative to surgery in the poor-risk or reluctant patient, immunosuppressive therapy, despite its lack of FDA approval, seems a reasonable approach to medically recalcitrant patients. A potential problem of long-term immunosuppressive therapy is the development of malignancies.

A second residual group of 5 to 15% of patients who deteriorate during or who fail to respond to CS therapy must also be investigated for possible alternative diagnoses. Intensive CS therapy as described for severe UC can be attempted, but usually is not successful in this group, and semielective surgery should be considered. Azathioprine therapy might be thought helpful in the group who fail to respond to CS, but deteriorating patients are not appropriate candidates for azathioprine therapy.

CS therapy in severe UC is problematic. During resuscitation with intravenous fluids, electrolytes (especially K, Mg, and $PO_4$), and blood, 50 to 75 mg of methylprednisolone (Solu-Medrol) is given as a bolus, followed by 25 mg every 6 hours. If there are abdominal peritoneal signs or toxic megacolon, antibiotic therapy should be initiated with a broad-spectrum cephalosporin and metronidazole intravenously. Parenteral hyperalimentation should be initiated and the patient should be given nothing by mouth. Nasogastric suction with a small-caliber tube (No. 12–14 French) is helpful for reducing ileus. Close clinical, laboratory, and radiographic observations are necessary. Abdominal examination must be performed several times daily in conjunction with a surgeon. Laboratory monitoring for blood loss, electrolyte and acid-base imbalances (either rising or falling

$HCO_3$ levels), and falling albumin level should be performed daily to assess the response to therapy. Clinical and radiologic monitoring should be continued to determine the development of possible complications, such as extension of colitis, toxic megacolon, sepsis, subclavian or iliofemoral thrombophlebitis, and massive hemorrhage.

Serial abdominal films can reveal the horrifying rapidity of the development of toxic dilation, distinguished from simple ileus by irregular colonic margins, loss of haustrations in the involved segment, and remnants of mucosa that appear as "islands" in stark air relief in the colonic gas shadow. The development of toxic megacolon after initiation of therapy for severe colitis is an ominous sign and frequently indicates the need for surgical intervention. Perforation markedly increases the likelihood of death. Toxic megacolon precipitated by hypokalemia, hypomagnesemia, or anticholinergics and other antidiarrheals may clear rapidly as the electrolyte imbalance is corrected or the drug is metabolized. Toxic megacolon precipitated by barium enema or air insufflation during colonoscopy, on the other hand, more often may have serious consequences. Fulminating colitis may require surgical intervention, even if the toxic megacolon resolves.

Persistent symptoms and signs of severe colitis at the end of 24 hours of intravenous CS therapy—that is, temperature greater than 38° C and more than 12 bowel movements—predicts medical failure in more than 50% of patients. If decisive improvement does not occur within the first 4 days of treatment—that is, the temperature drops below 38° C and toxic dilation resolves, there is less than a 13% chance of medical therapy success. If there is no improvement within 3 to 10 days or if there is deterioration in clinical, laboratory, and radiographic variables, abdominal colectomy, sparing the rectum, must be considered. The decision to perform a total proctocolectomy remains with the surgeon, but, in general, abdominal colectomy is safer in a critically ill patient. Prolongation of medical therapy increases overall mortality about 10-fold as a consequence of both operative deaths and deaths under medical treatment. On the other hand, if remission is achieved, only 40 to 50% of patients experience relapse during 5 years of follow-up and approximately 5% require surgical intervention; surgical series suggest a much higher surgical rate in follow-up, i.e., that 50% of such patients require surgery. There is thus much to be gained from a trial of medical management; unfortunately, there is much to be lost as well!

After the attack of fulminating colitis has settled, tapering should be undertaken cautiously.

---

*Use of these agents in inflammatory bowel disease is not an approved indication.

The patient should be given a dose of oral prednisolone or prednisone equal to that being given intravenously. The intravenous dose should be reduced by approximately 25% daily after the institution of oral therapy. If there is no flare during the 4 days required for discontinuation of intravenous therapy, the patient can be handled as mentioned for a moderate colitis, with the dosage reduced by approximately 0.5 mg per day in 2.5-mg increments. Throughout this period, the possibility of relapse must be kept in mind and the patient kept in the hospital under close clinical surveillance. After the patient has reached the ordinary therapeutic dosage level of CS—that is, 40 to 60 mg per day of prednisone or prednisolone—with improved nutrition and clearing of symptoms and signs of acute colitis, discharge to follow-up as an outpatient is permitted, as described for moderate colitis.

### Cancer Surveillance

The risk of colon cancer in UC is small (3%) and restricted to 5 to 15% of patients with extensive colitis of more than 8 years' duration. Patients with lesser extent of colitis are said to have an increased risk of cancer, but the data are seriously flawed.

Patients who have had extensive UC for 8 years with continuous symptoms requiring CS therapy, placing their general health at risk and jeopardizing their socioeconomic life by frequent relapses, should be encouraged to undergo surgery. Risk of cancer only adds to the indications for colectomy.

More than half of patients with extensive UC are asymptomatic at 10 years. Such patients sensibly are reluctant to undergo surgery. In the young patient, prophylactic colectomy is a reasonable option as long as the hazards of surgery are kept in mind, including surgical mortality (occurring in less than 3% in centers specializing in colorectal disease, but in 5 to 10% in many community hospitals), alteration in body image, complications of ileostomy (occurring in approximately 10%), and sexual and bladder dysfunction (in 15%). In patients with ileorectal anastomosis without a Park's pouch, there is a reduced but continued risk of cancer that requires surveillance.

Alternatives to prophylactic colectomy are to do nothing or to proceed with continued surveillance for cancer with colonoscopy every 1 to 2 years to check for mass lesions and to perform biopsies for dysplasia. If colonoscopy is unsuccessful, air contrast barium enema is indicated. The interpretation of dysplasia is difficult and should be confirmed by a pathologist experienced with this problem. By utilizing evidence of dysplasia to monitor malignant change, most cancers are detected at the earliest stage of invasion (84% are Dukes' Stage A) with a 5-year survival much better than in groups of patients with spontaneously developing cancer, which are usually detected late in the course.

# CROHN'S DISEASE

method of
MARK A. PEPPERCORN, M.D.
*Beth Israel Hospital*
*Boston, Massachusetts*

Crohn's disease is an idiopathic, recurrent, focal inflammatory process that may affect any portion of the gastrointestinal tract. Disease limited to the small intestine occurs in about one-third of patients. Twenty per cent of patients have colitis only, whereas the remaining half have both ileal and colonic involvement. One-third of patients have perianal lesions, and up to 20% may have associated involvement of the skin, the eyes, joints, and the liver. The variable anatomic distribution of disease and the transmural nature of the pathologic process contribute to a diverse clinical presentation. The clinical course is characterized by unpredictable spontaneous exacerbations and remissions.

## MANAGEMENT

### Drug Therapy

**Sulfasalazine.** Sulfasalazine (Azulfidine) has been a mainstay of the treatment of both ulcerative colitis and Crohn's disease since its introduction to clinical medicine almost 50 years ago. Controlled trials have shown it to be efficacious in Crohn's disease involving the colon. It has been difficult to show efficacy in similar studies for patients with ileitis alone, although the experience of practitioners suggests that a subset of patients with ileitis benefit from sulfasalazine. Unlike ulcerative colitis, in which sulfasalazine is effective in preventing relapses of disease in remission, no prophylactic benefit of this drug has been shown in Crohn's disease, nor does it prevent recurrences of the disease postoperatively. The drug should be considered in any patient with Crohn's disease with mild to moderate symptoms and is given at an initial dosage of 500 mg orally twice daily, with advancement over several days to 1 gram orally three or four times daily. Folic acid, 1 mg per day, should be added, because sulfasalazine may interfere with dietary folate absorption. Responses usually occur within 3 to 4 weeks, at which time the dosage can be tapered to 2 grams per day and maintained for an additional 3 to 6 months. At that point, if the patient is in remission, the drug can be stopped. In patients who relapse quickly and then respond to reinstitution of therapy, indefinite use of sulfasalazine at a maintenance level of 2 grams per day should be considered.

The utility of sulfasalazine is limited by a high incidence of intolerance and allergic reactions. Nausea, anorexia, headache, and dyspepsia may plague up to 20% of patients receiving the drug, but often can be overcome by lowering the dosage. Mild neutropenia and hemolysis may be reversed by lowering the dosage; nonetheless, the complete blood count (CBC) should be monitored initially. Minor allergic reactions, such as rash and fever, can be mitigated in 75% of patients by a process of gradual desensitization. More severe adverse effects, such as agranulocytosis, severe hemolysis, hepatitis, pancreatitis, pneumonitis, alterations in sperm counts and morphology, and exacerbations of colitis, require stopping the drug.

Sulfasalazine consists of sulfapyridine, one of the original sulfonamides, linked via an azo bond to 5-aminosalicylic acid (5-ASA), an aspirin analogue. Pharmacologic studies show that the drug is partially absorbed from the proximal gastrointestinal (GI) tract, with part of the absorbed portion excreted unchanged in the urine. The remaining absorbed portion returns unchanged to the GI tract via the bile where, together with the unabsorbed portion, it traverses the intestine until it encounters the bacterial flora, primarily in the distal ileum and the colon. Intestinal bacteria are solely responsible for the initial stage of sulfasalazine metabolism, reduction of the azo bond with release of sulfapyridine and 5-ASA. The sulfapyridine is largely absorbed, achieving high serum levels, metabolized by the liver, and excreted in the urine. Most of the side effects noted with sulfasalazine can be attributed to the sulfa moiety. The 5-ASA portion, on the other hand, stays largely in contact with the colon and is excreted in the feces. These observations suggest that the parent (sulfasalazine) might be serving merely as a vehicle for delivery of an active component (5-ASA) to distal disease sites. This speculation, coupled with the findings of toxicity related to the sulfa portion, led to the development of a new group of agents, the aminosalicylates.

**Aminosalicylates.** The hoped-for promise of the aminosalicylates has been realized, because they have proved efficacious in patients with inflammatory bowel disease and are tolerated by 80 to 90% of patients sensitive or allergic to sulfasalazine. Topical forms of 5-ASA (known generically as mesalamine in the United States and mesalazine in Europe) or 4-aminosalicylic acid, developed because of initial problems with 5-ASA stability, are clearly effective in active distal ulcerative colitis. Although less thoroughly studied in Crohn's disease involving the rectosigmoid, a nightly 4-gram 5-ASA enema (Rowasa) may achieve similar results as in ulcerative colitis when given over a 2- to 3-week period. Administration can then be tapered to an every-other-night or every-third-night regimen, with the hope of maintaining a remission. Several oral forms of 5-ASA are under investigation. These include slow-release forms (Pentasa, Asacol, Rowasa) and a dimer, olsalazine (Dipentum),* which links 5-ASA to itself via an azo bond. Although oral 5-ASA agents are not yet available in the United States, early studies in Crohn's disease have given promising results. The slow-release forms achieve high levels of 5-ASA in the small intestine and may be especially effective in patients with Crohn's ileitis, in which sulfasalazine is often of limited benefit.

**Metronidazole.** Initially developed for the treatment of *Trichomonas* infection and effective against anaerobic bacteria, metronidazole (Flagyl) has been shown useful in controlled trials in patients with Crohn's disease involving the colon and in large uncontrolled experiences in patients with severe perianal disease. It has not been useful when only the ileum is involved. In Crohn's colitis, the drug should be considered in patients unresponsive or intolerant to sulfasalazine. The drug should be given initially at a dosage of 10 mg per kg per day. The desired benefit is usually seen within 4 weeks, and metronidazole can then be safely continued for 4 to 6 months. There are no studies of the adjunctive or prophylactic benefit of metronidazole in Crohn's disease. Although mutagenicity and carcinogenicity have never been established in humans, concerns about these possibilities make it prudent to limit the long-term use of the drug to patients in whom no obvious alternative exists. Such patients are those with refractory perianal disease. These patients often require higher dosages (in the range of 10 to 20 mg per kg per day) and flare unless maintained indefinitely at somewhat lower dosages. The use of metronidazole, especially at higher dosages, is limited by adverse effects, including nausea, anorexia, tongue discomfort, and paresthesias attributable to a reversible peripheral neuropathy.

**Corticosteroids.** Long a mainstay of therapy in patients with inflammatory bowel disease, steroid administration should be initiated in any patient with Crohn's disease in whom the above measures fail or cannot be used and in patients with

---

*Not available in the United States.

severe forms of the disease. As with topical aminosalicylate preparations, steroid enemas (hydrocortisone enema [Cortenema]) should be considered in patients with active Crohn's proctosigmoiditis. Patients should take one enema every night for 2 to 3 weeks and then taper to every other night over the subsequent 2 weeks. New, rapidly metabolized forms of topical steroid with no systemic effects, such as tixocortol pivalate, may eventually replace standard forms of therapy.

For patients with more extensive, mild to moderate Crohn's colitis and with involvement of the small bowel, prednisone, 40 to 60 mg per day, is initiated and continued for 10 days to 2 weeks. After the desired response is obtained, the dosage should then be tapered by 5 mg every 7 to 10 days. After a patient achieves remission, there is no benefit of continuing the steroid as a prophylactic agent to prevent relapses. However, some patients continue to have mild, smoldering active disease as the dosage is tapered and benefit from continued low dosages of the drug, in the range of 5 to 10 mg per day. The long-term risk of such therapy has to be weighed against the benefit and treatment alternatives.

For patients with severe and/or fulminant disease, many of whom require hospitalization, some form of parenteral corticoid is usually the treatment of choice, in concert with bowel rest, parenteral nutrition, and broad-spectrum parenteral antibiotics. For patients already receiving oral steroids, intravenous hydrocortisone (Solu-Cortef), 300 mg per day, or the less-salt-retaining preparations methylprednisolone (Solu-Medrol) or prednisolone, 48 to 60 mg per day, should be given. For patients who have not recently been given oral steroids, intravenous adrenocorticotropic hormone (ACTH), 120 U per 24 hours, may have benefit over standard steroid preparations, although such benefit has been shown only in severe ulcerative colitis and not in Crohn's disease in controlled trials. If patients with severe disease do not respond in 2 to 3 weeks, surgery is a consideration. For those who do respond, oral prednisone can be substituted for the parenteral steroid, initially in a dosage of 40 to 60 mg per day with gradual tapering.

**Immunosuppressants.** Azathioprine (Imuran) and its metabolite, 6-mercaptopurine (Purinethol), have gained increased acceptance in the treatment of difficult-to-manage patients with Crohn's disease. They should be considered in patients refractory to other drugs, those dependent on steroids, patients with nonhealing fistulas, those with refractory perianal disease, and those with early postoperative recurrence. The mean time for clinical response is about 3 months, and some patients may not show benefit for 6 to 9 months. By initiating dosage at 50 mg per day and not advancing beyond 1.5 to 2 mg per kg per day and by vigilant monitoring of the CBC, problems with bone marrow depression can be minimized. Because the long-term risk of malignancy and infertility are still not fully resolved, treatment with these agents for longer than 1 year should be approached cautiously. However, these agents can maintain remission in Crohn's disease; in certain difficult-to-manage patients, indefinite long-term therapy is justified. An unrelated immunosuppressive agent, cyclosporine, which is useful in transplant patients, has emerged as useful in uncontrolled trials with severe Crohn's disease. A rapid onset of action may give it an advantage over the slower-acting immunosuppressants. Use of this agent should be restricted to controlled trials, except in situations in which there are no acceptable alternative therapies.

**Potential New Approaches.** The finding of an atypical *Mycobacterium* in several patients with Crohn's disease has led to open trials and hopeful but preliminary results using antituberculous drugs in two- and four-drug regimens. Similarly, oxygen-free radical scavengers, superoxide dismutase and penicillamine, have been successful in a limited number of patients with Crohn's disease in open trials. Moreover, in an uncontrolled study, methotrexate induced both clinical and colonoscopic remissions in a limited number of patients with refractory Crohn's disease. Manipulations of the immune system utilizing interferon and T lymphocyte apheresis have been successfully employed in small numbers of patients with resistant Crohn's disease. Finally, hyperbaric oxygen has been reported to cause dramatic improvement in one patient with severe refractory perianal Crohn's disease. Although these approaches are promising, the results are so preliminary that their use should be restricted whenever possible to randomized placebo-controlled trials.

**Nonspecific Antidiarrheal Drugs, Cholestyramine, and Antibiotics.** Drugs such as diphenoxylate with atropine (Lomotil), loperamide (Imodium), codeine, and deodorized tincture of opium may be of use in patients with mild, well-established chronic symptoms. Their use should be limited, given the addictive potential of such agents (except for loperamide), and they should be avoided in patients with severe forms of disease because of the risk of precipitating ileus. Various forms of fiber, including bran and psyllium (Metamucil, Citrucel, Perdiem) can help decrease watery diarrhea. Similarly, cholestyramine (Questran), the bile salt–binding agent, can be of major benefit in patients with watery diarrhea following ileal resection. One packet (4 grams) in a glass of water or juice taken once or twice a day controls symptoms in most such patients. Broad-spectrum antibiotics (e.g., ampicillin and an aminoglycoside) should be considered in patients with Crohn's disease with localized peritoneal signs, because such patients usually have experienced a complication of their disease with microperforation and localized bacterial sepsis. There has been enthusiasm as well for the use of a variety of broad-spectrum antibiotics in less acute clinical presentations of Crohn's disease. In particular, patients with strictures of the small intestine and secondary bacterial overgrowth may benefit from courses of an antibiotic such as tetracycline. Finally, ciprofloxacin (Cipro) has recently proved effective in perianal Crohn's disease.

### Nutritional and Psychosocial Considerations

**General Dietary Instructions and Nutritional Supplementation.** Food is the best source of nutrition, and the emphasis for most patients should be on normalization of the diet and adequate caloric intake. Patients with intestinal strictures and partial obstruction may benefit from a low-residue diet. Moreover, patients with calcium oxalate stones associated with steatorrhea and hyperoxaluria should be instructed in a low-oxalate diet. In patients with extensive ileal resection and steatorrhea, a low-fat diet with medium-chain triglyceride supplementation should be considered. These patients need replacement of calcium, vitamin D, and vitamin K as well. Lactose intolerance can mimic the symptoms of Crohn's disease and should be documented or excluded if there is any question of its existence. A lactose-free diet with calcium supplementation can be offered if appropriate. Finally, vitamin $B_{12}$ replacement may be necessary for patients with moderate or extensive ileal resections. A Schilling's test should be performed several months postoperatively to document the need for such therapy.

**Enteral and Parenteral Diets.** Although there is some debate about their actual utility, both enteral diets and total parenteral nutrition (TPN) have been shown to be useful as primary therapy in inducing remissions in certain patients with Crohn's disease. They should be considered in particular in patients refractory to pharmacologic therapy, especially in poor-operative-risk candidates. Such diets can also be utilized in an attempt to heal fistulas, as adjuncts to drug therapy, and in helping to prepare patients for surgery. Growth failure in children with Crohn's disease can often be overcome by increasing caloric intake with elemental diets. Finally, TPN given at home is often a necessity for patients

with severe short-bowel syndrome, usually resulting from multiple resections.

**Psychologic Support.** Although there is no evidence to support the concept that psychologic factors are etiologic in Crohn's disease, there is no question that psychosocial pressures can influence the course of a patient's illness and have to be addressed. Often, a caring physician who is willing to answer questions and be available at all times is all that is needed. At other times, mild psychotropic agents in conjunction with behavior modification and support groups are of enormous benefit. In this regard, the National Foundation for Ileitis and Colitis can be extremely helpful in providing patients with emotional support and educational materials.

# IRRITABLE BOWEL SYNDROME

method of
JAMES C. REYNOLDS, M.D.
*University of Pittsburgh*
*Pittsburgh, Pennsylvania*

Few disorders pose a greater diagnostic or management challenge to the practitioner than the irritable bowel syndrome (IBS). This common disorder can affect patients of any age and exerts a major economic impact on medical care in the United States. Alteration of bowel frequency associated with abdominal cramps is the second most common cause of absenteeism in the United States. Symptoms related to intestinal dysmotility are the most common reason that patients seek medical evaluation for a gastrointestinal complaint and account for 40% of office visits to gastroenterologists. Previous synonyms for this syndrome (spastic colitis, mucous colitis, and nonulcerative colitis) should be abandoned, as they imply the presence of inflammation and may be confused with more serious forms of colitis.

**Symptoms.** IBS patients typically have a chronic and recurrent history of alternating diarrhea and constipation associated with abdominal pain. Pain in IBS is of variable location and severity and is improved by a bowel movement. Symptoms of colonic dysfunction include the passage of mucus, tenesmus, flatulence, and urgency. The frequent association of disordered upper intestinal motility and IBS accounts for the common finding of upper intestinal symptoms, such as nausea, borborygmi, early satiety, and bloating.

## DIAGNOSIS

**Differential Diagnosis.** Symptoms indistinguishable from those seen in patients with intestinal spasms are seen frequently in patients with more serious disorders, including adenocarcinoma, inflammatory bowel disease, diverticulitis, and intestinal infestations with parasites or bacteria. Diarrhea, bloating, and postprandial nausea are common symptoms in patients with a variety of other organic disorders, including peptic ulcer disease, malabsorption, and duodenal diverticulitis. Frequency, tenesmus, and urgency are symptoms seen most commonly in patients with proctocolitis and should not be attributed to irritable bowel syndrome until a thorough evaluation for this entity is negative. A large number of patients with previously diagnosed irritable bowel syndrome who in fact had diarrhea have been recently identified as having collagenous colitis. It is likely that there are many other entities within the large catchall diagnosis of irritable bowel syndrome.

The frequency of bowel movements alone should not be used to make the diagnosis of a motor disorder, unless they occur well beyond the broad range of normal, which is from three per day to one every 3 days. Any patient with a change in bowel habit, however, particularly if older than the age of 35 years, should be fully evaluated for a structural abnormality before the diagnosis of IBS can be made. Patients with extreme degrees of diarrhea associated with loss of greater than 250 ml per day should be evaluated for causes of chronic diarrhea, including causes of maldigestion or malabsorption. On the other hand, patients with chronic constipation with fewer than two bowel movements per week should be evaluated for causes of chronic severe constipation.

Upper intestinal symptoms in the absence of altered bowel habits or colonic symptoms suggest the presence of cholecystitis, peptic ulcer disease, or nonulcer dyspepsia.

**Importance of Psychologic Disturbances.** Intermittent alterations of bowel habit and abdominal cramping associated with extremes of stress are not an indication of motor disorder. Altered bowel habits are reported by 50% of healthy subjects when experiencing psychologic stress and therefore should be considered physiologic. The physician should address the cause of stress and assist the patient in its resolution or in strengthening the patient's coping mechanisms. Although variations in bowel frequency are common in otherwise healthy individuals, patients with IBS often show great concern over these apparently mild variations. Because of this, the role of psychosocial disturbances has been emphasized. Although no single psychologic disturbance can be generally applied to patients with functional bowel disorders, some abnormalities are found by formal psychologic interviews or personality testing in the majority of patients with IBS. More thoughtful studies have identified that the two most common problems are the patient's inability to cope with life's stresses and cancer phobia. IBS patients often seek medical care for other mild daily illnesses, including upper respiratory tract infections, headaches, musculoskeletal problems, and mild dermatologic abnormalities. An underlying fear of cancer occurs commonly. These subjects have weak social support systems: few close family members, limited friendships, and a poor self-esteem. They therefore seek physician's care not only for a diagnosis of their bowel problem but also in hopes of finding a compassionate ear and a caring, strong personality who can help them cope.

**Diagnostic Evaluation.** The diagnosis of irritable bowel syndrome can only be accepted in patients who have the following characteristics: (1) alternating bowel frequency, from diarrhea to constipation; (2) associated abdominal cramps and discomfort; and (3) absence of any structural or organic abnormalities. Key to the management of the IBS patient is the development of a thorough yet limited diagnostic evaluation that is tailored to the individual patient and based on his or her age, degree of disability, extent of prior history and evaluations, both real and perceived risk of colonic malignancy, and signs of organic disease. Certain examinations should be performed in every patient. A thorough metabolic and anatomic evaluation must be completed in every patient. The initial evaluation should include the discussion of the patient's social supports and psychologic stresses. A complete physical examination must be performed, including a thorough assessment of the abdomen and the rectum. Multiple checks for blood in the stool must be performed in every patient. The physical examination must also focus on the possibility of malabsorption, and a rectal examination must be performed to consider the possibility of rectal prolapse, anal sphincter incontinence, or Hirschsprung's syndrome. When the patient has classic symptoms, however, and normal physical examination findings, the concept of IBS should be introduced during the initial interview.

## MANAGEMENT

### Initial Approach

The initial approach to the IBS patient should be to develop a logical, yet limited evaluation during the first or second visit and refrain from expanding the evaluation because of resistance to treatments. The continued addition of tests after one has made a diagnosis of IBS only fuels the patient's concerns that there still may be an undiagnosed carcinoma.

The most important aspect of treatment is to be sympathetic to the patient's complaints and to reassure the patient that he or she has a syndrome with well-described physiologic disturbances, which can be documented if appropriately sophisticated measures are used. A brief discussion of the pathophysiology of the spastic colon may be helpful. Other disorders associated with severe pain but no structural abnormalities should be discussed with the patient, such as migraine headaches, low back pain syndromes, and muscle cramps. The patient should also be reassured that the physician is concerned with other symptoms and understands how uncomfortable they can become. The physician should avoid attempting to remove these symptoms or to belittle them. However, it is reasonable to encourage the patient to use relaxation exercises or other means of distraction to minimize the pain when it is present. Under rare circumstances, experts in pain management may also be helpful.

## Dietary Manipulations

Treatment of IBS should begin with the addition of fiber to the diet. IBS occurs rarely in societies in which there is a high fiber intake. Although soluble fiber is valuable for the management of hypercholesterolemia, whole-grain, insoluble fiber is most likely to benefit the patient with colonic motor disorder. Overall, the patient should strive to obtain 20 to 25 grams of raw fiber intake daily. The patient should be informed of the value of fiber not only in the management of abdominal cramps and spasms of colonic smooth muscle, but also in treating hypercholesterolemia and glucose intolerance and perhaps even in reducing the risk of colon cancer. Patients with IBS should also avoid fatty foods. Other dietary restrictions should be individualized. Patients often report that specific foods cause them distress. Although the physiologic mechanisms of such aversions are often difficult to explain, one or two simple food types can often be eliminated from the diet without producing nutritional deficiency. On the other hand, many patients severely restrict their diets without good cause, and this should be avoided.

## Pharmacotherapy

Every effort should be made to manage a patient with IBS without the use of pharmacotherapy; however, medications are sometimes necessary in resistant patients and refractory conditions. Other medications that may alter bowel habits should be eliminated. Irritant laxatives should be avoided.

Medical treatment of IBS rests primarily on the use of anticholinergic agents. These may be taken either on a continuous basis in more resistant patients or intermittently when the symptoms are sporadic. Dicyclomine (Bentyl), 10 mg orally up to four times per day, ½ hour prior to each meal and at bedtime, has been the standard of care. Anticholinergic therapy is often associated with side effects, including dry mouth, urinary retention, and blurred vision. Other anticholinergic agents have been developed and include hyoscyamine sulfate (Levsinex Timecaps). Intermittent anticholinergic therapy is valuable for the patient who has predictable symptoms in the presence of stresses or when eating specific foods.

Patients with diarrhea-predominant IBS may benefit from an opioid analogue or the calcium channel blocker verapamil (Calan). Verapamil must be used with caution because it is not approved for this indication by the U.S. Food and Drug Administration and may be associated with orthostatic hypertension and fluid retention. Phe-

nobarbital-containing solutions have been suggested but are of unproven benefit. Antianxiety and/or antidepressant therapy has no role in the management of most patients with IBS. In patients with obvious psychiatric disorders, however, these medications may be valuable.

Treatment of constipation-predominant IBS that does not respond to high fiber intake should begin with osmotic laxatives. Irritant laxatives should be avoided, not only because they may be habit forming but also because they may lead to damage of the colonic myenteric plexus. Rarely, repeated use of tap water enemas may be necessary.

# HEMORRHOIDS, ANAL FISSURE, AND ANORECTAL ABSCESS AND FISTULA

method of
RICHARD P. BILLINGHAM, M.D.
*University of Washington*
*Seattle, Washington*

## HEMORRHOIDS

Hemorrhoids are enlarged veins in the anal area, similar to varicose veins in the legs. *Internal* hemorrhoids are located *inside* the anal canal, above the dentate line, where the veins are covered with mucosa of the rectum; *external* hemorrhoids are located on the perianal skin. Although some authorities maintain that such structures represent "vascular cushions," contain arterioles, or contribute somehow to continence, such concepts are irrelevant from the standpoint of practical management. Humans are born with such submucosal rectal veins or other blood vessels, but these are only considered to be hemorrhoids when they become enlarged or otherwise symptomatic.

There are three areas where hemorrhoids usually occur: the right posterior, right anterior, and left lateral areas of the anus. People may be bothered *only* by internal hemorrhoids, *only* by external hemorrhoids, or by both. Symptomatic hemorrhoids may develop in response to chronic constipation and straining at stool, presumably owing to pulsion forces, or there may be a familial tendency. However, for the majority of people with such symptoms, no definite cause can be determined. Despite popular folklore, there is no evidence that the development of hemorrhoids is related to prolonged sitting, lifting of heavy objects, or other work-related activities, though these situations may exacerbate the symptoms of hemorrhoids that are already present.

It is important to question patients carefully regarding the specific symptoms that they may attribute to hemorrhoids, because most people are unaware of the possible existence of any other name for perianal pathologic changes. Inquiry should be made regarding *pain* (character, location, and association with bowel movements or other activity); *bleeding* (color, whether just with bowel movements or at other times, and whether noticed on the toilet paper, in the toilet bowl, on the outside of the stools, or mixed in with the stools); *protrusion* (if present, whether just with bowel movements or all the time, and, if associated with defecation, whether the swelling goes away spontaneously or manual reduction is required); and *itching* (called pruritis ani; rarely related to hemorrhoids), as well as the patient's *normal bowel pattern* and any recent alteration thereof.

*Internal hemorrhoids* may cause bleeding and/or prolapse, but are almost never associated with pain. Prolapse associated with bowel movements may resolve spontaneously or may require manual reduction in more severe cases. Bleeding is characteristically bright red and seen in the toilet bowl as well as on the toilet paper. *External hemorrhoids* are generally asymptomatic when small and may appear as skin tags; as they enlarge, they may cause some difficulty with cleaning after bowel movements. Thrombosis of one or more external hemorrhoids may occur suddenly and *is* associated with an acutely painful perianal nodule. Bleeding rarely occurs with such thrombosis unless the clot erodes through the perianal skin after a few days, in which case the resulting blood is usually dark red and may be seen on underclothes.

Examination of the patient with hemorrhoid symptoms should include external anal inspection, digital anorectal examination, anoscopy, and sigmoidoscopy. Other causes of similar symptoms must be ruled out, including neoplasms, which may cause increased straining; inflammatory bowel disease, which may cause bleeding; perianal tumors, which may be confused with external hemorrhoids; anal fissure, the most common cause of perianal pain; and anorectal abscesses, which are also painful and may occasionally be confused with thrombosed external hemorrhoids.

### Treatment

Treatment of hemorrhoids depends on the severity of symptoms. If these are mild or infrequent, bulk laxatives and/or topical hydrocorti-sone creams are often sufficient. The latter are most effectively applied with a finger cot inside the anus; suppositories are rarely of benefit.

### Office Procedures

*Thrombosed external hemorrhoids* are of sudden onset and are associated with varying degrees of pain. For patients in whom pain does not rapidly resolve, office *excision* of the involved hemorrhoid under local anesthesia is well tolerated and is associated with rapid resolution of pain. Local anesthetic agents containing epinephrine 1:100,000 are often helpful in achieving spontaneous hemostasis after such excision, as well as prolonging anesthesia. Sutures are rarely necessary, even with the excision of larger external hemorrhoids, as the wounds heal quite well without skin approximation, and there is less pain afterwards if no sutures are used. Following such treatment, sitz baths in warm water, 15 to 20 minutes at a time, three times daily, often give further symptomatic relief; medications for pain relief are occasionally helpful. *Incision* of the involved hemorrhoid, with an attempt at clot evacuation, is less than adequate therapy. It is often unsuccessful in relieving symptoms because of the multiloculated nature of the clots and leaves the hemorrhoid to continue to hurt for several days, as well as to remain to cause similar symptoms in the future.

For *internal hemorrhoids* that bleed but do not prolapse (first-degree internal hemorrhoids), injection sclerotherapy is usually both effective and painless. This is performed through an anoscope using an agent such as sodium tetradecyl sulfate (Sotradecol) for each of the friable internal hemorrhoids. Such injection should only be done above the dentate line, where there is generally no sensation to pain; three hemorrhoids can be done at one session, if necessary. For second-degree internal hemorrhoids (prolapsing, but with spontaneous reduction), rubber band ligation is usually helpful. This technique uses an applicator to place a tiny rubber band around the base of an internal hemorrhoid, devascularizing the prolapsing tissue and causing it to slough within 3 to 10 days. Care must be taken to place the band sufficiently above the dentate line to avoid pain. When the rubber band is properly placed, most people feel no discomfort. Following proper placement, approximately 15% of patients have a sensation of having to have a bowel movement, and 5 to 10% have a mild aching sensation, lasting in both cases for a day or two. Such treatments are usually best performed by ligating only one hemorrhoid at a time at three-week intervals. Complications include bleeding at the time of sloughing in 0.5 to 1% and thrombosis of adjacent external hemorrhoids in 1 to 2% of patients.

Rarely, life-threatening infections have been reported following rubber banding, without known precipitating factors. Such infections are usually heralded by the development of severe local pain and inability to urinate, occurring within 24 to 72 hours of the application of a band. Prompt, aggressive treatment of such problems may be lifesaving. Although such incidents have occurred, their incidence is less than 1 in 10,000; as such, rubber banding is safer than operative hemorrhoidectomy.

Recurrence of internal hemorrhoids may occur after rubber banding in 15 to 20% of patients within 5 years, but such patients can usually be treated again with rubber band ligation without the necessity of surgery.

Other methods of office treatment include cryotherapy, infrared photocoagulation, laser treatment, and electrical coagulation, but these techniques have not been demonstrated to have any advantage over the use of the rubber banding technique and are generally more expensive to the patient.

### Operative Measures

*Surgical hemorrhoidectomy* is reserved for those with third-degree (prolapsing, requiring manual reduction) and fourth-degree (prolapsing and irreducible) internal hemorrhoids and for those with both symptomatic internal hemorrhoids *and* symptomatic external hemorrhoids. Hemorrhoidectomy generally does not require an overnight hospital stay, and modern techniques have markedly decreased the discomfort, as well as other postoperative morbidity, commonly associated with this procedure. The procedure can be performed under local, regional, or general anesthesia. The recurrence rate following surgical hemorrhoidectomy is 1 to 2%.

Other therapies for hemorrhoids gain popularity from time to time, such as electrocautery, cryotherapy, laser therapy, and anal dilation. These techniques have not been shown to have the permanence offered by surgical hemorrhoidectomy, and claims of diminished pain, for example, have not been substantiated.

### ANAL FISSURE

An anal fissure is a crack, sometimes referred to as an ulcer, in the lining of the anus. This is associated with pain, particularly during and after bowel movements, as well as with a small amount of bleeding; usually, this is bright red and noted only on the toilet paper after bowel movements. A fissure may occur after a hard dry stool, after diarrhea, or with inflammatory bowel disease or other cause of local inflammation, or the specific event or cause may be undiscoverable. Most persistent fissures are associated with increased tone or spasm of the internal sphincter muscle; whether this is a cause or an effect of fissures is not known. More than 90% of anal fissures are located in the midline of the body—60% posteriorly and 30% anteriorly. Fissures *not* in the midline should raise suspicions about other systemic disease, such as inflammatory bowel disease and blood dyscrasias, though such conditions may equally likely not be found.

Many fissures may heal by themselves, often within a day or so; of those treated in the physician's office, about 50% heal with the combination of topical steroid cream, bulk laxatives, and sitz baths. Suppositories, foams, and topical pads containing witch hazel and other nostrums are generally ineffective. Topical cream is best applied by the patient, using a finger cot to place a small amount of cream directly into the anal canal and onto the painful area; the fenestrated applicators supplied with such preparations are, surprisingly, much less effective. In general, fissures that are going to heal by such conservative means do so within 1 month.

For those patients whose fissures remain symptomatic after a month of such treatment, outpatient surgery is quite effective and gives rapid relief. Excision of the fissure with suturing of the base is associated with a 90% success rate and moderate postoperative pain for several days. However, another procedure, "lateral internal sphincterotomy," divides the internal anal sphincter laterally in the anal canal, without removing the fissure. This procedure is effective in about 98% of cases, and most patients are able to return to normal activity the day after surgery, *without discomfort*. Because the internal anal sphincter is not under voluntary control and is not an important determinant of fecal continence, the procedure is rarely associated with transient incontinence or flatus and almost never with stool incontinence. Following such surgery, recurrence of anal fissure is extremely uncommon.

### PERIANAL ABSCESS AND FISTULA

*Abscesses* and *fistulas* of the perianal area are different phases of the same basic process—the abscess is the acute stage, and the fistula is the chronic aspect. The process almost always originates from an otherwise useless anal gland, of which there are 6 to 12 arranged radially around the anus. The opening of each gland is located in the base of one of the anal crypts at the dentate line; the body of each gland is thought to lie between the internal and external sphincters. When the neck or opening of a gland becomes occluded, whether by inflammation, inflammatory bowel disease, or unknown causes, the bacteria and secretions within the gland proliferate. This causes the body of the gland to swell and fester, producing pus. Symptoms at this stage include perianal *pain,* which is constant and increases over hours or days, is unaffected by bowel movements, and may be associated with fever or other evidence of systemic infection. Initially, pain can sometimes occur in the absence of perianal induration, erythema, or other physical findings. When an abscess is suspected in such instances, subsequent examination of the patient after a day or so is warranted.

As the process continues, the abscess either ruptures spontaneously, through the perianal skin, or is drained by a physician prior to the time of such rupture. This is usually accompanied by a dramatic improvement in symptoms.

Following rupture or spontaneous drainage, about 50% of all such abscesses rapidly resolve spontaneously, without sequelae; the other 50% go on to the stage of fistula. This is caused by the reopening of the original ostium and neck of the anal gland, and by the persistence of an external opening, at the site of abscess drainage. Symptoms of a fistula usually are limited to the drainage of small amounts of mucus or purulent material from time to time throughout the day, with rare small amounts of blood. Occasionally, the external opening of a fistula epithelializes and heals over, with the reaccumulation of pus and the return of abscess symptoms. This resolves either spontaneously or after repeated drainage.

Other causes of perianal inflammation and superficial abscess include hidradenitis suppurativa, pilondial cyst and abscess, inflammatory bowel disease (most commonly Crohn's disease), foreign bodies, and Bartholin's abscess.

### Treatment

Treatment of an *abscess* consists of incision and drainage. In most situations, this may be done in the office, under local anesthesia, but larger and more complex abscesses should be drained in the operating room. Antibiotics are generally neither necessary nor helpful in this setting; exceptions may include the diabetic patient, the presence of a prosthetic joint or heart valve, and extensive associated cellulitis. Drainage of the abscess is rapidly followed by resolution of associated signs and symptoms without further medications. Principles of such drainage include making the incision as close to the anal verge as possible (to reduce the length of any possible fistula) and removing an *ellipse* of skin, rather than making a small slit, to keep the skin opening from prematurely closing prior to the resolution of the abscess. Cultures of the abscess fluid universally show mixed aerobic and anaerobic bowel flora and are not helpful.

The practice of using gauze packing to "encourage drainage" is oxymoronic; it both is uncomfortable and actually discourages drainage and therefore the rapid resolution of the underlying process. It is unnecessary to "break up loculations" within the abscess cavity itself; if these even actually exist, they seem to manage themselves. Sitz baths in comfortably warm water, three times daily for 20 minutes each time, are helpful in encouraging rapid healing as well as in giving symptomatic relief.

Management of perianal *fistulas* is complex and requires a thorough knowledge of relevant anatomy and fistula types. A surgical approach is almost always required, unroofing the entire extent of the fistula tract, from external to internal opening; this requires division of the internal anal sphincter and usually a portion of the external anal sphincter. Following such unroofing, or *fistulotomy,* a careful search must be made for additional fistula tracts, and the granulation tissue in the bed of the fistula must be removed. Curettage is almost always sufficient for this purpose, rather than removal of the fistula tract itself, or *fistulectomy.* Following this, marsupialization of the resulting wound, tacking the edges down to the base of the fistula tract, is usually carried out. An alternative to fistulotomy, used when preservation of a maximal amount of sphincter muscle is critical, is the use of an *endorectal advancement flap* to cover the internal opening of a fistula.

Such procedures can almost always be done in an outpatient setting, with only a few days of moderate postoperative discomfort. Complete healing may take 6 to 12 weeks and does not interfere with normal function and lifestyle.

Some authors advocate fistulotomy, at the time of incision and drainage of an abscess, for those abscesses that must be treated in the operating room. With increased appreciation that office management is effective for the abscess itself, as detailed earlier, and with the consideration than only 50% of abscesses develop into fistulas, most specialists now advocate a delayed approach to fistula repair. The specific management of complex anorectal fistulas, such as horseshoe fistulas, suprasphincteric or extrasphincteric fistulas, or the role of setons, is beyond the scope of this discussion.

# GASTRITIS

method of
BARRY J. MARSHALL, M.D.
*University of Virginia Health Sciences Center*
*Charlottesville, Virginia*

## CLINICAL APPEARANCE

Gastritis is the name given to conditions that cause an inflammation of the gastric mucosa. The inside of the stomach is not generally accessible for examination by the primary care physician, so the diagnosis of gastritis may be suspected, inferred, or proved, depending on what investigations have been performed.

Initially, a patient with upper gastrointestinal symptoms may be suspected of having gastritis. In many countries the term "gastritis" is synonymous with the clinical syndrome of "nonulcer dyspepsia." The patient may complain of a burning or gnawing sensation in the epigastrium, perhaps relieved by food and/or antacids. Other components of the discomfort may include bloating sensations after meals, flatulence, belching, abdominal distention, and epigastric tenderness. In more severe cases, nausea and vomiting may occur. Usually symptoms arising in the stomach are affected in some way by eating, the pain is located above the umbilicus, and disturbance of bowel habit is uncommon.

The clinical syndrome of gastritis does not correlate well with endoscopic and histologic appearances of the gastric mucosa. Patients with severe symptoms may have normal mucosa, and patients with no symptoms may have severe erosive gastritis. It is important therefore to refer to a clinical impression of gastritis as "clinical gastritis" so that it is not confused with more well-defined types of gastritis.

## ENDOSCOPY

At endoscopy, the normal gastric mucosa is a pink color, like the palm of the hand. The endoscopic appearance of gastric mucosa when gastritis is present can vary along a continuum from normality to redness, widespread erosion, hemorrhage, and ulceration.

Gastritis affects the antrum more severely than the body of the stomach. Degrees of redness are common, especially in the antral mucosa. Slight changes may be called "mild gastritis" by some gastroenterologists, but are regarded as a normal variant by many endoscopists and are not reported. When the mucosa is very red, all gastroenterologists mention gastritis on the endoscopy report.

When small areas of the epithelium are eroded, brown spots attributable to the presence of changed blood on the mucosa can be seen. These spots may not be associated with a visible macroscopic lesion; depending on the number present, "mild erosive gastritis" may be reported. An erosion is defined as an interruption of the epithelial layer that does not extend deeper than the muscularis mucosae (about 1-mm deep). More extensive lesions are called ulcers. Severe erosive gastritis occurs when the mucosa is diffusely affected and both microscopic and visible erosions are present.

It should be emphasized that endoscopic identification of gastritis does not reflect the histologic status of the mucosa. For example, patients with extensive bleeding erosions resulting from nonsteroidal anti-inflammatory drug (NSAID) ingestion may have a completely normal histologic appearance in mucosa not actually affected by an erosion.

Endoscopically apparent gastritis, therefore, is the macroscopic lesion seen at endoscopy. It is affected by recently ingested or retained food, coloring agents (premedication mixtures at endoscopy may be colored pink), the microvasculature (congestion, vasodilation), the integrity of the overlying mucosa (erosion, ulceration), the presence of bile (edema, vasodilation), bleeding (new or altered blood), and, in some cases, by the presence of pus cells in the gastric mucus.

Thus, endoscopic identification of gastritis is the sum total of many factors that may affect, or appear to affect, the gastric mucosa. More accurate diagnosis of the endoscopic lesion requires histologic examination of a mucosal biopsy specimen.

## HISTOLOGY

Histologic evidence of gastritis is an infiltration of the gastric mucosa with neutrophils, lymphocytes, and plasma cells. This is the most common form of gastritis, and there are two types:

Type A gastritis is associated with pernicious anemia. It affects the parietal cells in the body of the stomach. It is uncommon and usually does not cause gastric symptoms because acid secretion is minimal or absent.

Type B gastritis is much more common. It affects the mucus-secreting epithelial cells that line the stomach. It is most severe in the antrum, where these cells are most plentiful. Type B gastritis is caused by chronic *Helicobacter pylori* infection.

Type B gastritis is referred to when the terms "acute," "active," "superficial," "chronic atrophic," and "nonspecific" are used by the pathologist. Other findings sometimes accompany Type B gastritis and may be sequelae of the disorder. Intestinal metaplasia is the replacement of the gastric mucus-secreting epithelial cells with intestinal-type (brush border and goblet) cells. The combination of chronic gastritis and intestinal metaplasia is associated with gastric carcinoma.

## SPECIFIC FORMS OF GASTRITIS

### Alcohol-Induced Gastritis

Acute gastritis, with or without erosions, may develop after the ingestion of any corrosive substance. Alcohol causes an acute erosive gastritis if it is consumed in excessive amounts, particularly as spirits. Occasionally, erosions and superficial ulcerations are also seen in the duodenum.

After the offending agent has been removed, the gastric mucosa heals rapidly. Symptoms and erosions therefore last no more than a few days after abstinence. Prolonged nausea or vomiting after 72 hours is more likely due to an underlying chronic gastritis, a peptic ulcer, or an associated metabolic disturbance. Alcohol in moderate amounts does not harm the gastric mucosa and is not implicated in the causation of chronic gastritis or peptic ulceration. Acute lesions due to alcohol do not lead to chronic gastritis or any kind of permanent mucosal defect.

Many alcoholics have chronic gastritis and peptic ulcer disease. It is now known that, in most cases, the chronic gastritis is caused by *H. pylori* infection (see later) so there is no need to invoke alcohol as a cause. *H. pylori* is more common in economically disadvantaged groups and, like other enteric infections, is more likely to be present in alcoholics. Conversely, alcoholics without *H. pylori* do not have chronic gastritis.

Hematemesis or coffee-ground vomitus is common after acute alcoholic binge drinking. Common causes are peptic ulcer disease, Mallory-Weiss tear, and erosive gastritis. It is important to ascertain whether the blood was present in the initial vomit or if it was only noted in subsequent vomiting episodes. In Mallory-Weiss syndrome, the initial vomit is normal and bright-red blood is seen in subsequent vomits. If acute erosive gastritis or peptic ulcer is present, frank blood or coffee ground vomit is likely to be present in the initial vomitus. More serious lesions, such as bleeding esophageal varices, should be considered in the appropriate clinical setting.

**Management.** Symptoms should resolve rapidly after alcohol ingestion has ceased. Pain should be treated with antacids and $H_2$ receptor antagonists. If bleeding is present, an endoscopy within 12 hours is necessary to identify the site of bleeding. Later endoscopy may not detect rapidly healing small mucosal tears or small acute erosions. Mucosal biopsy should always be performed to check for chronic gastritis due to *H. pylori*.

### Aspirin-Induced Gastritis

Aspirin and NSAIDs together may be the most common causes of erosive gastritis. These drugs inhibit prostaglandin synthesis and so impair the ability of the mucosa to secrete mucus and withstand acid or peptic attack. Although NSAIDs may also have a directly "corrosive" effect on the mucosa, even persons taking NSAIDs rectally are prone to gastric erosions.

Aspirin-induced erosions may occur anywhere in the stomach, rather than being localized to the antrum as erosions related to peptic ulcer disease are (see later). Histologically, NSAID erosions are associated with little inflammation, not more than would be expected from natural healing of any epithelial disruption. Apart from discontinuity of the epithelial layer and hemorrhage, there may be no histologic abnormality. Away from the actual erosion, the mucosa is relatively normal.

Nearly all persons receiving long-term NSAID therapy have some degree of erosive gastritis. Not all erosions cause symptoms and not all progress to form a chronic peptic ulcer. If another predisposing cause is present, however, NSAID ingestion may be additive and result in expression of peptic ulcer disease. For example, in persons with *H. pylori* who take NSAIDs, the ulcer risk is additive. Apart from *H. pylori*, NSAIDs are the only common cause of peptic ulcer.

**Therapy.** As for alcohol-induced erosive gastritis, erosions due to NSAID ingestion should ideally be treated by withdrawing the offending drug. If the NSAID can be ceased, the mucosa repairs itself in a few days. Peptic ulcers caused by NSAID require a month or so to heal, as do all ulcers.

Symptoms should be treated with antacids and $H_2$ receptor antagonists for 3 to 14 days. If symptoms persist, another cause of gastritis should be suspected, *H. pylori* and/or peptic ulcer disease.

In many patients, the NSAID cannot be stopped owing to a chronic rheumatic complaint. For example, rheumatoid arthritis is difficult to manage without the use of NSAIDs, all of which have ulcerogenic potential. There are several ways to approach this problem:

Misoprostol, a prostaglandin analogue, protects against NSAID-induced gastric lesions. Misoprostol should not be given to women of reproductive potential, and it may cause diarrhea, but can be given on a long-term basis to many patients, allowing them to continue receiving the NSAID. The dosage is 100 to 200 μg four times a day. Misoprostol has been shown to decrease the absorption of some NSAIDs.

$H_2$ receptor antagonists, sucralfate, or antacids given in ulcer-healing dosages may heal erosions and prevent the progression to frank peptic ulcer. These are drugs of choice in those who cannot take prostaglandins.

Because *H. pylori* and NSAIDs produce additive deleterious effects on the gastric mucosa, it may be possible to remove *H. pylori* and permit healing of symptomatic gastritis, erosions, or ulceration. If patients must continue taking an NSAID, one should check for the presence of *H. pylori* and treat *H. pylori*–associated gastritis if present (see later). Some patients improve clinically and are able to continue taking the NSAID.

## Helicobacter pylori Gastritis

*H. pylori* is the most common cause of gastritis. There are two clinical syndromes: the acute infection (hypochlorhydric gastritis) and the chronic infection (active chronic or Type B gastritis).

### Acute Hypochlorhydric Gastritis

Acute hypochlorhydric gastritis (AHG) should be suspected when gastritis symptoms appear in a previously well person, in whom there is no history of alcohol or aspirin ingestion. Three to 7 days after ingestion of the organism, the patient develops epigastric pain; feels bloated, anorectic, and nauseated; and may vomit very mucous clear fluid, which has reduced acidity (pH >4.0). This fluid also contains reduced amounts of urea because *H. pylori* urease enzyme destroys urea present in the gastric juice. Normal gastric juice contains 2 to 5 mM of urea, whereas the concentration is usually less than 1.0 mM if *H. pylori* is present.

Diagnosis is difficult if *H. pylori* has been suppressed with bismuth or antibacterial therapy. *H. pylori* may be detected at endoscopy, by examination of a gastric mucosal biopsy specimen with a rapid urease test, by histologic examination (Giemsa's stain of antral mucosa), or by a urea breath test (available in some centers).

In the United States, acute *H. pylori* infection is uncommon, but may be expected in children or young adults who are in intimate contact with another person (spouse, parent, or grandparent) who has *H. pylori*. Thus, new members of families with a history of dyspepsia or peptic ulcer disease are prone to be infected with *H. pylori* and develop the acute syndrome. (Acute hypochlorhydric gastritis is a well-known syndrome in gastroenterology research volunteers infected during acid secretion studies. In addition, the syndrome has been confirmed in experiments in which *H. pylori* was deliberately administered to healthy subjects.)

Symptoms usually subside in 3 to 5 days, after which time chronic gastritis is present in most persons. After the acute stage, acid secretion remains low and the patient may be asymptomatic for months, for years, or indefinitely. When acid secretion returns, dyspeptic symptoms may appear, owing to the action of acid on the inflamed gastric mucosa.

The acute syndrome is usually short lived and responds to simple measures such as a clear fluid diet, small snacks instead of regular meals, and administration of metoclopramide, antacids, and analgesics (avoid aspirin). Bismuth subsalicylate (Pepto-Bismol in the United States) or bismuth subcitrate (De-Nol)* is specific therapy for *H. pylori* gastritis and suppresses the infection.

### Chronic Gastritis

Chronic gastritis (Type B antral gastritis, ulcer-associated gastritis) is usually caused by *H. pylori* (>80%). It should be emphasized that most major "peptic" lesions in the stomach and duodenum occur in the region colonized by *H. pylori*—i.e., the distal lesser curve, the prepyloric antrum, the pyloric canal, and the first inch of the duodenal bulb. *H. pylori* lesions therefore affect the lower half of the stomach and display the full spectrum of clinical, endoscopic, and histologic findings of gastritis.

Chronic gastritis may be asymptomatic, with or without an endoscopic lesion. This is referred to as nonerosive chronic gastritis in some texts. Regardless of the endoscopic appearance, *H. pylori* gastritis is always associated with histologic changes called active chronic gastritis—i.e., infiltration of the mucosa with inflammatory cells. When pathologists call gastritis acute, they are usually referring to the presence of neutrophils in *H. pylori* gastritis. The changes are histologically acute, but not temporally acute. In some patients, they persist for many years.

Chronic *H. pylori* gastritis may lead to an endoscopically abnormal stomach, ranging from redness, through erosions, to ulcerations. One should remember that all ulcers must pass through the stage of redness and erosion and that most persons with chronic peptic ulcer disease have Type B gastritis, which remains even when the ulcer is healed.

Thus, patients with known or suspected peptic ulcer disease may have gastritis symptoms between episodes of frank ulceration. Typically, nausea is a prominent symptom in symptomatic patients who do not have a visible ulcer.

### Management

Symptomatic chronic gastritis due to *H. pylori* should be treated because it does not resolve spontaneously and may predispose the patient to peptic ulceration (20-fold risk) and, possibly, to gastric cancer. Before treatment, diagnosis must be confirmed.

Noninvasive methods of diagnosis include the urea breath test and serology. In the urea breath test, urea labeled with a carbon isotope is given orally. If *H. pylori* is present in the stomach, the urea is broken down by bacterial urease and the carbon isotope is quickly expired as $CO_2$ in the breath. Breath samples are read in a beta counter or a mass spectrometer. Serologic tests will be

---

* Not available in the United States.

TABLE 1. **Dose and Duration of Antibiotics Used in Combination with Bismuth**

| Drug | Dose | Times/Day | Start Day | Duration of Therapy (days) |
|---|---|---|---|---|
| Metronidazole | 250 mg | 4–6 | 4 | 10 |
| Tetracycline | 500 mg | 4 | 1 | 10–14 |
| Erythromycin | 250–500 mg | 4 | 1 | 10–14 |
| Amoxicillin | 500 mg | 4 | 1 | 10–14 |

*Note:* Triple therapy with bismuth, tetracycline, and metronidazole cures 80 to 90% of infections. If a metronidazole-resistant organism is present, replace the metronidazole with erythromycin. Amoxicillin has been associated with *Clostridium difficile* infection in 2% of patients.

available in the United States after 1990. They are sensitive screening tests for *H. pylori* antibody. Nearly all infected patients have high levels of IgG and IgA against the bacterium.

More accurate methods of *H. pylori* detection involve endoscopic biopsy of the stomach and testing of a mucosal biopsy specimen with a rapid urease test (fastest and cheapest), culture (most specific, but less sensitive), or histologic Giemsa's staining (most sensitive, but slow and expensive).

Therapy for *H. pylori* is presently imperfect. The organism is always sensitive to bismuth, so bismuth subsalicylate, 525 mg four times daily (Pepto-Bismol regular strength liquid, 30 ml or 2 tablets four times daily on an empty stomach) should be given. Bismuth suppresses *H. pylori* and probably heals any associated mucosal lesions. After bismuth therapy has been commenced, the results of most diagnostic tests (except serologic studies) are normal for 1 to 3 weeks. One should try to confirm the diagnosis of *H. pylori* before instituting therapy.

In patients who cannot take bismuth, suppression of *H. pylori* with amoxicillin (2 grams daily), erythromycin (2 grams daily), or tetracycline (2 grams daily) may be tried. Without bismuth, cure of infection is difficult.

Cure of *H. pylori* infection requires that an antibiotic be given concurrently with bismuth subsalicylate (Table 1). The best antibiotic is metronidazole (Flagyl) in a daily dosage of 20 mg per kg (1 to 1.5 grams per day), with a 70% cure rate if given from day 4 to day 10 of a 14-day course of bismuth subsalicylate. Other antibiotics are less successful in combination with bismuth. $H_2$ receptor antagonist therapy or other acid-reducing drugs (e.g., omeprazole) do not impair the efficacy of this therapy and may even enhance it. Addition of a third antibiotic may improve cure rates, but increases antibiotic side effects. Outside the United States, bismuth subcitrate (De-Nol) is used as an alternative to bismuth subsalicylate and gives about a 10% higher cure rate in combination with antibiotics. De-Nol is presently under evaluation in the United States.

## OTHER TYPES OF GASTRITIS

### Bile Reflux (Alkaline Reflux) Gastritis

In patients who have had previous gastric surgery, dyspeptic symptoms are common. They may complain of bilious vomiting, as well as the usual symptoms of gastritis. Endoscopically, the gastric mucosa may appear quite red. This change is probably a vascular effect, as histologic findings of inflammation are not present unless *H. pylori* infection is found. When other causes of gastritis are not present, the histologic examination may show a condition called "foveolar hyperplasia," which is associated with some edema and congestion.

Management principles are similar to those described earlier. First, one should exclude ingested agents as a cause and then exclude *H. pylori* infection (more than half of the patients have this and respond to appropriate therapy). Finally, some patients respond to surgical intervention with a Roux-en-Y bile diversion.

### Hypertrophic Gastritis

This is a rare cause of diarrhea and protein loss in which massive hypertrophy of the gastric mucosa occurs and albumin is lost from the gastric mucosa. The cause is unknown. Diagnosis is by endoscopy and biopsy. In children, *H. pylori* can also cause excessive protein loss from the gastric mucosa.

### FURTHER READING

The understanding of gastritis has advanced a great deal since *H. pylori* was recognized as the most common cause. Review articles on *H. pylori* have appeared (Dooley CP, and Cohen H: The clinical significance of *Campylobacter pylori*. Ann Intern Med *108*(1):70–79, 1988; Blaser MJ: Gastric *Campylobacter*-like organisms, gastritis, and peptic ulcer disease. Gastroenterology *93*(2):371–383, 1987; and Hendrix TR, and Yardley JH: *Campylobacter gastritis* and associated disorders. South Med J *81*(7):859–862, 1988).

# ACUTE AND CHRONIC VIRAL HEPATITIS

method of
GEOFFREY C. FARRELL, M.D.
*Westmead Hospital, University of Sydney*
*Sydney, Australia*

## ACUTE VIRAL HEPATITIS

Acute viral hepatitis refers to a clinicopathologic syndrome resulting from hepatocellular necrosis, which is characterized by malaise, anorexia, nausea, tender hepatomegaly, and high serum aminotransferase levels. Jaundice is a common but not invariable feature. The usual cause is one of the five hepatitis viruses, now termed A, B, C, D, and E. Other causes of the acute viral hepatitis syndrome include hepatic involvement with other infectious diseases (such as Q fever, infectious mononucleosis, and cytomegalovirus infection); however, hepatic drug reactions and hepatic infarction, such as occurs with venocclusive disease and ischemic hepatitis, can have similar features. These disorders are not considered further here. It is important to identify which hepatitis virus is the cause of the patient's acute illness because measures to prevent transmission of infection vary with the agent, as does the possibility that the infection will become chronic.

*Hepatitis A Virus (HAV)* is an enterically transmitted RNA virus, which is spread endemically or epidemically under conditions of poor sanitation and especially by contaminated food and water supplies. The virus is shed in stools for up to 2 weeks after the onset of jaundice. Recent infection is diagnosed by the presence of IgM anti-HAV antibodies. The presence of IgG anti-HAV reflects past infection and is present in 40% of the adult population in Western countries; most infections are acquired asymptomatically in childhood. There is no chronic carriage state for HAV infection.

*Hepatitis B virus (HBV)* is a DNA virus that consists of a surface lipoprotein coat, the hepatitis B surface antigen (HBsAg); several core proteins, including the hepatitis B core antigen (HBcAg) and the hepatitis B e antigen (HBeAg); and an incomplete double-stranded ring of DNA, the hepatitis B virus DNA (HBV-DNA). The presence of HBeAg and of HBV-DNA in peripheral blood indicates circulating virus particles. They therefore indicate both continuing HBV replication and infectivity of the patient. The development of antibodies to HBsAg (anti-HBs) confers complete protection against reinfection, even with a different serologic subtype of virus. This is the basis for the high efficacy of the genetically engineered and plasma-derived vaccines currently available for immunization against HBV (see under "Prevention"). HBV infection is acquired by parenteral inoculation with contaminated blood or other bodily secretions and by close physical and especially sexual contact. On a global scale, the most important mode of infection is vertical transmission—i.e., from mother to baby at the time of birth. HBV infection in the first 6 months of life leads to a chronic carrier state in 90% of infants compared with less than 10% of adults who are infected with HBV. This, together with other means of spread within families (which include sexual and to a lesser extent "horizontal" transmission), largely accounts for the endemicity of chronic HBV infection in some population groups. There are at least 250 million chronic HBV carriers worldwide, a substantial proportion of whom will die of complications of the disease, which include cirrhosis and hepatocellular carcinoma. Carrier rates vary from approximately 0.2% in some Western countries, through 5 to 10% in Southern Europe, to 15% in parts of Asia, the Pacific Islands, and subsaharan Africa.

*Hepatitis C virus (HCV)* is an RNA virus, which appears to be responsible for at least 90% of cases of parenterally transmitted non-A, non-B hepatitis. It may also account for 20 to 40% of sporadic acute viral hepatitis in the community, although first-generation tests for anti-HCV antibody are positive in only 60% cases of community-acquired non-A, non-B hepatitis. HCV is parenterally spread, usually by transfusion of blood or blood product or by contaminated needles, particularly in the context of intravenous drug abuse. Sexual transmission may occur to a limited extent, as the prevalence of anti-HCV in prostitutes and male homosexuals is about 5% compared with 1% in the general population.

*Hepatitis D virus (HDV)*, also often called the delta agent, is an incomplete RNA-containing particle that requires HBsAg to enter human hepatocytes. As a consequence of this unusual biologic dependence, HDV can only cause hepatitis when it is acquired as a coinfection with the HBV, or when a chronic carrier of HBV is superinfected with the agent. HDV infection is diagnosed by the presence of anti-HDV antibodies in peripheral blood. IgM anti-HDV antibodies are indicative of recent or continuing HDV infection.

*Hepatitis E virus (HEV)* is an incompletely characterized, enterically transmitted agent, which has been responsible for several epidemics of acute viral hepatitis in the Middle East and parts of Asia. These epidemics have been attributed to contamination of water supplies. HEV infection has not yet been described in North America or Western Europe.

The acute illnesses caused by the five hepatitis viruses are indistinguishable. In a particular patient, however, the existence of risk factors for infection may suggest that some agents are more likely than others. Complications of acute viral hepatitis differ with the etiologic agents, as considered later.

### General Management

There are no accepted treatments to shorten the course or alleviate the general symptoms of acute viral hepatitis. Putative hepatoprotective agents have not been demonstrated to be effective in shortening the duration of aminotransferasemia. On the other hand, corticosteroids almost certainly increase the risk of chronicity when administered to a patient with acute hepatitis B; they should be avoided in all patients with acute viral hepatitis, except in the rare circumstances indicated under "Complications." Patients are best managed at home unless domestic support is inadequate and the patient is too ill to prepare food and attend to personal needs. Patients with HAV infection should be subjected to simple enteric precautions, including confinement to a single room with separate eating utensils and bedding, careful disposal of excrement, and handwashing after physical contact. In patients with acute hepatitis B, C, or D, such precautions are illogical and can negatively affect the patient's morale. On the other hand, patients with acute hepatitis B, C, or D should be counseled about the increased risk of sexual transmission during the acute phase of infection with these viruses; about the need to avoid sharing potentially contaminated personal implements, such as toothbrushes, combs, and razors; and about the high infectivity of blood, serous discharges, and possibly saliva. Specific measures for preventing the transmission of viral hepatitis are discussed later.

It is not necessary to recommend strict bed rest for a patient with acute viral hepatitis, but it is sensible for individuals to rest from usual activities until well-being and appetite improve. As for any acutely ill person, it is important to prevent dehydration and to minimize the catabolic effects of starvation. Carbohydrate-rich foods and drinks are usually better tolerated. Avoidance of fat may decrease nausea, but is not otherwise essential. Alcohol should not be consumed during acute viral hepatitis but can be taken in modest amounts after normalization of serum aminotransferase levels occurs. In the presence of severe acute hepatitis, the metabolism of drugs and other foreign compounds, including theophylline, caffeine, phenytoin (Dilantin), warfarin (Coumadin), and oral hypoglycemic agents, may be impaired. This should be considered in patients taking medication. In some cases, monitoring of blood drug levels or reduction of dosage may be indicated temporarily. In general, avoidance of sedatives, hypnotics, and other drugs cleared by the liver is recommended, as metabolism may be impaired and the risk of side effects accentuated. However, hepatic pain can be alleviated by acetaminophen, maximal dose 3 grams per day; nausea or vomiting by metoclopramide (Reglan), 10 mg three times daily, or prochlorperazine (Compazine), 5 to 10 mg orally or 12.5 mg by intramuscular injection, two or three times daily; and pruritus by cholestyramine (Questran), 4 grams four times daily. Persistent vomiting, dehydration, bruising, clouding of consciousness, and the development of ascites all indicate severe hepatitis. In this setting, deterioration of hepatic function may occur and such patients should be admitted to the hospital for closer observation and supportive measures, such as the administration of intravenous fluids. Most patients with acute viral hepatitis begin to convalesce after 1 to 4 weeks, a phase which is marked by improvement in appetite and well-being. Patients should be encouraged to increase physical activity as soon as they feel capable and to return to work when serum biochemistry values are normal or almost normal.

### Complications

**Relapse.** This occurs in about 5% of cases, but is often milder than the initial attack. Relapse should respond to simple supportive therapy, and the patient usually makes a complete recovery.

**Prolonged Cholestasis.** Prolonged jaundice, often with intense pruritus, may occur after the initial illness with any of the hepatitis viruses, but seems to be particularly common after HAV infection. The serum biochemistry values reflect this "cholestatic syndrome" and can cause diagnostic confusion, particularly if the patient has this syndrome without a more obvious episode of acute viral hepatitis. Hepatitis virus serologic studies, ultrasonography of the biliary tract, and possibly liver biopsy or cholangiography may be required to confirm the diagnosis. Laparotomy is contraindicated in such circumstances, as hepatic decompensation may be precipitated. Symptoms may persist for up to 6 months, but pruritus should respond to cholestyramine. Corticosteroids used to be recommended for this complication, but I would only consider this for cholestasis after acute hepatitis A; a trial of prednisolone, 40 mg per day for 1 week, may hasten recovery in these circumstances.

**Fulminant Hepatitis.** This complication is defined by the development of hepatic failure, particularly characterized by encephalopathy, within 8 weeks of the onset of acute viral hepatitis. It occurs in about 0.2% of cases of HAV infection, in 0.5 to 1% of those with HBV or HCV infection, but in up to 20% of patients with HBV and HDV co-infection. In pregnant women, HEV infection commonly causes fulminant hepatitis, but other hepatitis viruses do not. In the elderly, the risk that acute viral hepatitis will run a fulminant course is probably increased, and the outcome of fulminant hepatitis is also less favorable in this group. The mortality of fulminant hepatitis varies from 50 to 90%, depending on the age of the patient and to a lesser extent on the etiology. If recovery does occur, it is associated with complete healing of the liver. The most important aspect of management is intensive supportive therapy. There is no longer enthusiasm for "hepatic support" by such devices as charcoal columns and filtration through dialysis filters to remove "middle-sized" molecules. As liver failure is a complex and uncommon problem, management is best carried out in a specialized facility with relevant experience and preferably in close proximity to a liver transplantation team. Early management should focus on close monitoring of the neurologic status and prompt correction of such complications as hypoxia, electrolyte imbalance, bacterial sepsis, and severe coagulation disorder if bleeding has occurred. Conservative measures for hepatic encephalopathy include lactose or lactulose enemas and oral neomycin. Should deterioration in consciousness occur, consideration must be given to inserting an intracranial pressure monitoring device. Early increases in intracranial pressure respond to intravenous mannitol, but refractoriness will eventually occur. It now seems likely that the outcome for patients with fulminant hepatic failure, when Grade 3 or 4 coma is present, is improved by liver transplantation. Because the availability of a suitable donor liver is the most difficult logistic problem to overcome, early consultation with or referral to a transplantation unit should now be considered for patients with fulminant hepatic failure.

**Subacute Hepatic Necrosis.** This term refers more precisely to the lesion of bridging hepatic necrosis, which may occur in some patients with severe viral hepatitis. It is associated with an increased risk of chronicity and of the development of cirrhosis. The patient may remain unwell for more than 8 weeks, with repeated vomiting, deepening jaundice, ascites, and a bleeding diathesis resulting from decreased synthesis of coagulation fac-

tors. Such patients should be carefully considered for hepatic transplantation.

**Posthepatitis Syndromes.** Prolonged fatigue after acute viral hepatitis is less common than is popularly imagined. As with other chronic fatigue syndromes, the basis for the symptoms is unclear. Strong reassurance about an eventual favorable outcome should be given if the serum biochemistry profile has returned to normal. Recovery from HBV infection is evidenced by loss of HBs antigenemia and the formation of anti-HBs. With HCV infection, even minor abnormalities of serum biochemistry values persisting for more than 6 months indicate the presence of chronic hepatitis and liver biopsy is indicated to assess the severity of the hepatic lesion.

**Aplastic Anemia.** Pure red blood cell hypoplasia is a rare and often fatal complication of acute viral hepatitis.

## CHRONIC VIRAL HEPATITIS

The propensity for chronicity means that HBV, HCV, and, to a lesser extent, HDV infections are common causes of chronic liver disease. In addition, chronic HBV and HCV infection both predispose to hepatocellular carcinoma. There is no chronic carrier state for HAV and HEV infections.

**Chronic Hepatitis B Virus Infection.** About 10% of adults and 90% of babies infected with the HBV fail to clear the virus. Lifelong HBV infection is associated with a 40% chance of dying of cirrhosis or hepatocellular carcinoma. A characteristic of HBV carriers is a specific immunoparesis, such that they are unable to clear the virus. However, the biologic state of HBV infection varies between patients and in each individual varies with time. The earlier years of chronic HBV infection tend to be characterized by continued viral replication as indicated by positive serum test results for HBeAg and HBV-DNA. Later, HBV-DNA and HBeAg disappear (seroconversion) from peripheral blood as hepatic replication of the virus ceases. Anti-HBe usually becomes positive at this time, but HBsAg tends to persist indefinitely. Serologic relapse (reappearance of HBV-DNA and HBeAg) can occur in some individuals. Another transition in chronic HBV infection appears to result from a mutation of the viral genome. It is associated with loss of HBeAg expression, but continued presence of HBV-DNA in plasma. These serologic changes correlate with the type (that is, the necroinflammatory activity) of associated liver disease. The majority of chronic HBV carriers have either no liver disease, so-called healthy carriers, or mild inflammatory lesions, such as chronic persistent hepatitis. Chronic active hepatitis (CAH) is present in about 5% to 25% of chronic HBV carriers, depending on the duration of viral carriage. This lesion is the forerunner of hepatic cirrhosis, and possibly hepatocellular carcinoma. Chronic active hepatitis B (CAH-B) is nearly always associated with detectable HBV-DNA in peripheral blood, even among the minority of patients who are HBeAg negative. Conversely, the arrest of hepatitis B viral replication by antiviral treatment is associated with HBeAg to anti-HBe seroconversion and transition of the liver disease from CAH to chronic persistent hepatitis. When loss of HBsAg is accomplished, it is associated with complete histologic resolution of hepatitis.

Although prolonged treatment with corticosteroids is effective in autoimmune CAH, it should not be used for CAH-B. In this disease, steroids may worsen the outcome. Their withdrawal is often associated with a flare of the disease, but controlled studies have shown that this does not increase the chance of HBeAg seroconversion. Acyclovir (Zovirax) is not effective and adenine arabinoside monophosphate is too toxic for use in chronic HBV infection. Interferon-alfa (IFN-α) has a place in treatment of CAH-B.* At present, use of IFN-α is probably best carried out by groups with experience in treating HBV infection. Appropriate selection of patients is the biggest difficulty. The best results are in patients who have been HBV carriers for less than 2 years, who have a serum alanine aminotransferase (ALT) level of more than 150 IU per liter, and whose serum HBV-DNA level is less than 200 fmol per liter. Females and those with histologic CAH rather than chronic persistent hepatitis may be more likely to respond. Lifelong carriers of HBV, including patients from ethnic groups in whom HBV carriage is endemic, are unlikely to respond to IFN. Patients who are anti-HDV positive or who exhibit immunosuppression produced by human immunodeficiency virus infection are unlikely to respond to IFN-α.

A complete response to IFN includes permanent loss of HBV-DNA, HBeAg to anti-HBe seroconversion, and loss of HBsAg, usually with formation of anti-HBs. Partial response to IFN is associated with permanent loss of HBV-DNA and HBeAg to anti-HBe seroconversion, but HBs antigenemia continues. Among patients with the more favorable characteristics listed above, a permanent response to IFN is obtained in 35 to 45%, and about one-third of these are complete responses. Among untreated patients with CAH-B, 10 to 15% may experience spontaneous HBeAg

to anti-HBe seroconversion within 1 to 2 years, but loss of HBsAg is rare. An important feature of the HBeAg seroconversion phenomenon is that it is preceded by biochemical and occasionally clinical features of acute hepatitis. Among patients with cirrhosis and impaired hepatocellular function, such a seroconversion illness can lead to the manifestations of liver failure and even death. Hence, advanced liver disease is a paradoxical contraindication to the use of IFN for chronic HBV infection.

The optimal dosage of IFN-α for CAH-B is 4.5 to 6 million U given by subcutaneous injection thrice weekly for 4 to 6 months. Higher dosages and more prolonged treatment do not appear to increase the chance of a successful outcome. On the other hand, IFN toxicity is dose dependent. The early side effects of IFN are virtually universal and include fever, rigors, muscle pain, headache, nausea, diarrhea, and fatigue. These influenza-like symptoms commence 2 to 4 hours after IFN injection and last 4 to 6 hours. They are partly ameliorated by acetaminophen. Treatment with IFN is possible, and in general is well tolerated by patients, because tachyphylaxis to these early IFN side effects develops after about 2 weeks of treatment. Persistent fatigue is the most common long-term side effect. More significant potential toxic effects include depression, leukopenia, thrombocytopenia, alopecia, neurotoxicity, nephrotoxicity, and hepatotoxicity. All these are uncommon with the dosages of IFN used to treat CAH-B, and most respond promptly to dosage reduction or drug withdrawal.

Table 1 summarizes possible approaches to treating chronic HBV infection according to different serologic patterns of the disease. In patients who are HBV-DNA and HBeAg positive but with serum ALT level less than 150 IU per liter, the chance of response to IFN-α is only about 20%. Some preliminary evidence indicates that this can be improved by giving patients a preceding course of prednisolone (60 mg for 2 weeks, then 40 mg for 2 weeks, and 20 mg for 2 weeks) followed by withdrawal of prednisolone in an attempt to facilitate enhancement of the immune response. IFN-α is commenced 2 weeks later. Such steroid priming does not improve the response rate to IFN in the HBV-DNA–positive, high–serum ALT group; I would only consider its use in low–ALT patients who have failed to respond to an initial course of IFN-α. In general, it seems unlikely that patients who fail to respond to one course of IFN-α would respond to a second course. Patients with CAH-B who are HBeAg negative but HBV-DNA positive may respond to IFN, although preliminary evidence suggests that they are also more likely to subsequently relapse after completion of IFN therapy.

---

*This use of interferon is not listed in the manufacturer's official directive.

TABLE 1. **Approaches to Treating Groups of Patients with Chronic Hepatitis B Virus Infection**

| | Serologic Tests | | ALT | | |
| Clinical Features | HBeAg | HBV-DNA | (IU/L) | Histology | Recommended Treatment |
|---|---|---|---|---|---|
| Symptoms (no liver failure*) | + | + | >150 | CAH + C<br>CAH<br>CPH | IFN |
| No symptoms | + | + | >150 | CAH + C<br>CAH | IFN |
| Liver failure | + | + | >150 | CAH + C | Avoid IFN, consider LT |
| N/R | + | + | <150 | CAH + C<br>CAH | IFN or prednisolone first,<br>then IFN |
| N/R | – | + | N/R | CAH + C<br>CAH | IFN |
| None of liver failure* | – | – | N/R | N/R | No treatment |
| Liver failure* | – | – | N/R | Cirrhosis | LT |

*Term used to include low serum albumin concentration, prolongation of prothrombin time, ascites, and hepatic encephalopathy.

*Abbreviations:* N/R = not relevant, CAH = chronic active hepatitis; CAH + C = chronic active hepatitis with cirrhosis; CPH = chronic persistent hepatitis; LT = liver transplantation.

There is no theoretical basis for treating patients with CAH-B who are HBV-DNA negative with IFN or with corticosteroids; the latter treatment has occasionally been advocated, but there are no literature reports of results and, in my view, it should be avoided. Because well over half of patients with chronic HBV infection and chronic liver disease are either unsuitable for or fail to respond to IFN treatment, progression to end-stage cirrhosis still occurs commonly. In this situation, and especially in HBV-DNA–negative subjects, liver transplantation should be considered. Although infection of the transplanted liver is inevitable, despite all attempts to eliminate residual virus before and at the time of transplantation, this may not necessarily be associated with poor graft function for several years.

**Chronic Hepatitis C Virus Infection.** Surveys with the new anti-HCV test indicate that chronic HCV infection may be present in 1% of the population, but the severity of associated liver disease remains to be determined. More than 40% of cases of parenterally transmitted acute hepatitis C and at least 15% of sporadically acquired cases are associated with chronicity. Among these patients, cirrhosis occurs in at least 25% after 10 years. Hepatitis C virus appears to be a major cause of hitherto "cryptogenic" cirrhosis. It is therefore reasonable to conclude that attempts to eliminate the virus are worthwhile, particularly in younger patients, in those with CAH-C (with or without cirrhosis), and in those with symptoms.

As for chronic HBV infection, corticosteroids should be avoided. IFN-α controls necroinflammatory activity of the disease in at least 50% of patients. The recommended initial treatment course is 3 million U subcutaneously thrice weekly for 6 months. Sustained remission of the disease (normal ALT level, histologic improvement) occurs in about half of those who respond to IFN-α—that is, about 25% of all patients treated. Unlike CAH-B, CAH-C usually responds rapidly to IFN and without a "seroconversion" type of illness. However, relapse of the disease on withdrawal of IFN is often associated with a transient episode of acute hepatitis, at least as indicated by serum ALT levels that greatly exceed pretreatment levels. The long-term management of patients who relapse after stopping IFN is unresolved. Patients who tolerated IFN well, and especially those with more severe histologic lesions, should probably be treated for a prolonged period, possibly indefinitely. Control of the disease is readily re-established after reintroduction of IFN. Because the dosage of IFN-α required to control CAH-C disease activity is less than for CAH-B, side effects are even less troublesome. However, long-term use of IFN may be associated with risks of autoimmune disease. The magnitude of this potential problem has not yet been ascertained, but vigilance is particularly required for autoimmune thyroid disease. It may be possible to maintain some patients with CAH-C with very low dosages of IFN. Conversely, "breakthrough" of control is seen in some patients and may require dosage escalation. Patients with end-stage liver disease due to chronic HCV infection appear to be suitable candidates for liver transplantation. The risk of infection of the grafted liver has not been reported at the time of writing.

**Chronic Hepatitis D Virus Infection.** Intravenous drug addicts and certain populations in Southern Europe are at greatest risk. Chronic HDV infection is associated with a poorer prognosis than uncomplicated chronic HBV infection, with more rapid progression to cirrhosis and death often occurring within 2 to 5 years. Treatment is unsatisfactory. Interferon-α has, at best, a marginal effect in slowing progression of disease. The dosage usually needs to be greater than for CAH-B, and improvement in serum ALT level (when obtained) is only maintained while IFN is administered continuously. In my view, this disease should not be treated with antiviral agents, except in a clinical trial setting. Liver transplantation is often the only option, but carries with it a 15 to 20% risk that infection of the transplanted liver with both HDV and HBV will cause death from fulminant hepatitis. The 1-year survival rate of patients with transplants for cirrhosis due to chronic HDV infection is about 50%.

### PREVENTION

Prevention remains the most important aspect of the management of viral hepatitis. Epidemics of enterically spread viral hepatitis (HAV and HEV) are preventable by provision of adequate sanitation and adherence to simple aspects of personal hygiene, particularly handwashing. A hepatitis A vaccine using attenuated live virus is being developed, but progress has been slow owing to the difficulties of culturing this agent. Eventually, immunization should be possible. Because HAV is a common infection, all batches of pooled immune serum globulin (ISG) contain high titers of IgG anti-HAV. Injection of ISG confers at least 70% protection against HAV. It should be administered to household contacts of a patient with acute hepatitis A and is also useful prophylaxis for those traveling to underdeveloped countries where HAV is common. ISG injection is unnecessary if an individual already has IgG anti-HAV antibodies. This includes 40% of the population in economically well-developed countries, many of whom do not have a history of acute viral hepatitis because most HAV infections are asymptomatic.

General measures to prevent infection with parenterally transmitted hepatitis viruses (B, C, and D) include prevention of post-transfusion hepatitis, sterilization of blood products, precautions to prevent accidental inoculation of health care workers, and public health and social measures in relation to such matters as intravenous drug abuse, use of acupuncture, and tattooing. Awareness and appropriate counseling about sexual transmission, particularly of HBV and HDV, are also pertinent. ISG does not provide passive immunoprophylaxis against HBV, HCV, or HDV. However, hepatitis B hyperimmune serum globulin (HBIG) is highly effective in preventing clinically significant infection with HBV. The indications for use of HBIG (the availability of which is scarce) are listed in Table 2. They can be summarized as any recent (within 48 hours) percutaneous inoculation of blood known to con-

TABLE 2. **Indications for Use of Hepatitis B Hyperimmune Serum Globulin**

Recent* exposure to acute hepatitis B
  Percutaneous
  Sexual
  Neonatal (mother during third trimester of pregnancy)

Recent* exposure to HBeAg (or HBV-DNA)–positive chronic HBV carrier
  Percutaneous
  Sexual
  Neonatal (HBsAg- and HBeAg-positive mother)

*Within 48 hours.
*Note:* In all these situations, hepatitis B vaccination should also be commenced.

tain HBV particles or sexual exposure to a patient who is both HBsAg and HBeAg positive. An indication for HBIG is an essential indication for hepatitis B vaccination.

Hepatitis B immunization is possible because the presence of anti-HBs in peripheral blood is protective against HBV infection. Pure preparations of HBsAg suitable for use as hepatitis B vaccines were initially prepared from the plasma of chronic HBV carriers. These plasma-derived vaccines have proved to be both highly protective and very safe. More recently, genetically engineered vaccines have become available and have been shown to be as effective as the plasma-derived products. Immunization of the entire population is the logical means to eliminate HBV infection in countries with HBV carrier rates of more than 5%. Such programs have begun in a few countries, commencing with the newborn and preschool children. Unfortunately, they are expensive and beyond the health budgets of most Third World countries. In regions with lower HBV carrier rates, such as North America and Western Europe, immunization of the whole population is not a cost-effective way of eliminating new HBV infections. A more appropriate strategy is to vaccinate all those in categories of special risk for HBV infection (Table 3). The responsibilities of individual physicians (as opposed to public health authorities) particularly include ensuring that at-risk contacts of patients with newly diagnosed acute or chronic HBV infection receive hepatitis B vaccination. Such at-risk contacts include newborns, sexual partners, and close family members, especially young children. It is worth noting that postexposure vaccination with hepatitis B vaccine is highly effective, even several weeks after contact, particularly sexual contact, which is associated with incubation times of up to 6 months. Hepatitis B vaccine should be injected into the deltoid (not the gluteal) muscle. Close adherence to the manufacturer's recommendations about storage is important. Doses are generally 5 µg for babies and small children and

TABLE 3. **Special Risk Categories for Hepatitis B Virus Infection**

| Group | Prevalence of HBV Markers (%) | HBV Carrier Rate (%) | Modes of Spread |
|---|---|---|---|
| Ethnic groups | | | |
|   Immigrants from endemic areas | 20–70 | 5–20 | Vertical, sexual, horizontal* |
|   Aboriginal populations—e.g., native Americans | 10–60 | 3–10 | |
| High-risk patients | | | |
|   Renal dialysis patients | 40–60 | 0–5 | Contaminated blood, blood |
|   Hemophiliacs | 75–95 | 5–10 |   products |
|   Thalassemia patients | 25–90 | 2–10 | |
| Sexually promiscuous | | | |
|   Male homosexuals | 60–80 | 5–8 | Sexual |
|   Heterosexuals—e.g., female prostitutes | 15–30 | 1–3 | |
| Intravenous drug addicts | 50–80 | 8–10 | Needle sharing |
| Health care workers† | | | |
|   Dentists | 15–30 | ?0.5–3 | Accidental inoculation of con- |
|   Surgeons | 20–30 | ?0.5–2 |   taminated blood |
|   Nurses in high-risk units | 10–50 | ?0.5–3 | |
| Laboratory technicians | 10–25 | ?0.5–1 | |
| Inmates of institutions | | | |
|   Mental retarded | 50–90 | 2–10 | Blood or saliva contamination, |
|   Prisoners | 25–60 | 1–5 |   intravenous drug abuse, sexual spread |

*Horizontal spread pertains to nonvertical, nonsexual transmission, usually within families. The mechanism of spread is unclear, but is likely to involve close physical contact. It is most prevalent among young children.
†These data are from older studies of highly selected groups.

10 µg for larger children and adults. After the first injection, the second is given at 1 month and the third at 6 months. Protective levels of anti-HBs are found in 70% of vaccine recipients after the second injection and in over 90% after the third injection. Of the remainder, a few have low levels of anti-HBs, which can be increased by further injections with vaccine, whereas about 4% of the population are unable to elaborate an immunologic response to the hepatitis B vaccine because of a genetic defect in antigen recognition. In patients at continued high risk for HBV infection, a modified regimen of hepatitis B vaccination—that is, injections at 0, 1, 2, and 12 months—may slightly accelerate the elaboration of protective antibodies. Titers of anti-HBs wane relatively quickly, with up to 30% of vaccine recipients losing detectable antibodies by 5 years. To date, immunization authorities have not made recommendations about the need for booster shots. Those concerned about loss of anti-HBs (which does not necessarily imply loss of protection against clinically important HBV infection) can be advised to have anti-HBs measured at 3 years, with booster injection given if titers are low, or simply to subject themselves to a booster injection.

For the reasons outlined earlier, protection against HBV infection also confers protection against HDV infection. Those at risk for HDV (intravenous drug addicts, families and sexual consorts of patients with HDV infection) should receive hepatitis B vaccination.

Post-transfusion hepatitis is now almost completely preventable. Introduction of HBV marker screening in the early 1970s eliminated most cases of post-transfusion hepatitis B. Unfortunately, it was then appreciated that 90% of cases of post-transfusion hepatitis were due to a viral agent (or agents) that was neither HAV nor HBV. This non-A, non-B form of post-transfusion hepatitis has now been shown to be due to HCV infection. Before identification of the HCV genome, the incidence of post-transfusion hepatitis in the United States had already been reduced from more than 10% 10 years ago to less than 5% in 1989. This improvement is due to the exclusion of paid donors, to the use of surrogate tests (ALT and anti-HBc), and to screening procedures for human immunodeficiency virus infection. Anti-HCV screening was licensed in the United States in May, 1990, and it is hoped that such screening will help eliminate transfusion of blood and blood products as a source of HCV infection. The nature of the HCV (which is rather similar to yellow fever virus) is such that, now that the genome has been identified, it should be possible to develop an HCV vaccine.

# THE MALABSORPTION SYNDROMES

method of
INGRAM M. ROBERTS, M.D.
*George Washington University School of Medicine*
*Washington, D.C.*

The evaluation of the patient with malabsorption should follow a clear sequence of screening and diagnostic testing that reveals the correct cause of the patient's condition. Often, the typical history and physical findings suggestive of malabsorption are not found. The clinician must suspect the presence of malabsorption and determine objectively whether evidence of malabsorption exists.

In addition to the loss of the highest dietary source of calories (fat contains 9 calories per gram in contrast to 4 calories per gram for carbohydrate and protein), deficiency of essential fatty acids, such as linoleic (18:2) and arachidonic (20:4) acids, may result from fat malabsorption. Essential fatty acids are the precursors of prostaglandins, thromboxanes, leukotrienes, and other biologically active compounds. Oral or intravenous supplementation with essential fatty acids has been successful in restoring serum essential fatty acid levels toward normal in some patients with malabsorption.

Selected patients with malabsorption may develop fat-soluble vitamin deficiency. In a similar situation to essential fatty acid deficiency, serum vitamin levels did not correlate well with the absolute degree of steatorrhea. Syndromes that may result include hypocoagulable state (vitamin K deficiency), osteomalacia (vitamin D deficiency), neurologic abnormalities (vitamin E deficiency), and night blindness (vitamin A deficiency) (Table 1).

As many different conditions can cause malabsorption, the precise diagnosis should be elucidated before the proper medical management can be instituted. In most disorders, fat, carbohydrate, and protein malabsorption occur concomitantly, and steatorrhea, the presence of excess fat in the stool, is the hallmark of malabsorption. However, enterokinase deficiency or protein-losing enteropathy may produce only protein malabsorption. Congenital lipase or colipase deficiency and abetalipoproteinemia may produce only fat malabsorption. Finally, disaccharidase deficiencies (lactase, sucrase-isomaltase, or trehalase) or transport abnormalities (glucose-galactose or fructose) may lead to malabsorption of carbohydrates alone.

## DIAGNOSTIC TESTS

The most extensively used test for malabsorption is the Sudan stain for fecal fat. The qualitative stool fat determination using the Sudan stain is 100% sensitive and 96% specific as a screening test for steatorrhea. Other tests lack the proper sensitivity and specificity for routine use.

Supported in part by Cystic Fibrosis Foundation Research Award G191 9–1 and by NIH/NIDDK FIRST Award #R29–DK38729–01.

The definitive test for the diagnosis of malabsorption is the 72-hour quantitative stool collection for fecal fat. There are several situations in which fecal fat excretion is increased under physiologic conditions: (1) when extremely high-fiber diets (100 grams per day of fiber) are consumed, (2) when dietary fat is ingested in a form such as whole peanuts, and (3) in the neonatal period when intraluminal levels of pancreatic lipase and bile salts are reduced. Excluding the above, the finding of a coefficient of fat absorption less than 93% confirms the presence of steatorrhea due to malabsorption.

When steatorrhea is demonstrated, one should determine whether malabsorption is caused by disease of the intestinal mucosa or by abnormalities of intraluminal digestion. To distinguish between these possibilities, the work-up follows a nomogram (Figure 1). An upper gastrointestinal series and small bowel follow-through (UGI/SBFT) may reveal anatomic abnormalities such as jejunal diverticuli, show the abnormal mucosal pattern (thickening of the folds, dilation, segmentation, etc.) found with many malabsorption syndromes, or demonstrate the "string sign" narrowing seen in Crohn's disease. Flat plate of the abdomen may show pancreatic calcifications, which are diagnostic of chronic pancreatitis.

The absorptive integrity of the intestinal mucosa can be determined by the D-xylose test. D-Xylose is a pentose sugar, which is absorbed from the small bowel via the same transport mechanism as for glucose and excreted unchanged in the urine. The usual dose is 25 grams administered orally after an overnight fast, and urine collection is for 5 hours. A normal urinary excretion should be greater than 5 grams. Measurement of the serum D-xylose level 1 hour after oral ingestion yields a higher sensitivity and specificity than the 5-hour urine collection. A normal serum level should be greater than 20 mg per dl. Low values for D-xylose are characteristic of diseases of the intestinal mucosa or bacterial overgrowth (due to ingestion of xylose by the bacteria), whereas normal values are compatible with pancreatic insufficiency.

The radioimmunoassay for serum trypsinogen is specific for the diagnosis of chronic pancreatitis, if the trypsinogen value is less than 10 ng per ml. Nonpancreatic causes of malabsorption almost always yield a normal serum trypsinogen level (10 to 75 ng per ml). If steatorrhea and a low serum trypsinogen level are found, the diagnosis of chronic pancreatitis is likely.

If the D-xylose test and UGI/SBFT results are abnormal, a small bowel biopsy should be performed for histologic diagnosis. Grasp forceps biopsies obtained from the distal duodenum via the endoscope may be

TABLE 1. **Clinical Syndromes Associated with Fat Malabsorption**

| Condition | Deficient Nutrient |
| --- | --- |
| Hyocoagulable state | Vitamin K |
| Night blindness | Vitamin A |
| Osteomalacia | Vitamin D |
| Neurologic abnormalities | Vitamin E |
| Dermatitis, hair loss, growth failure | Essential fatty acids |

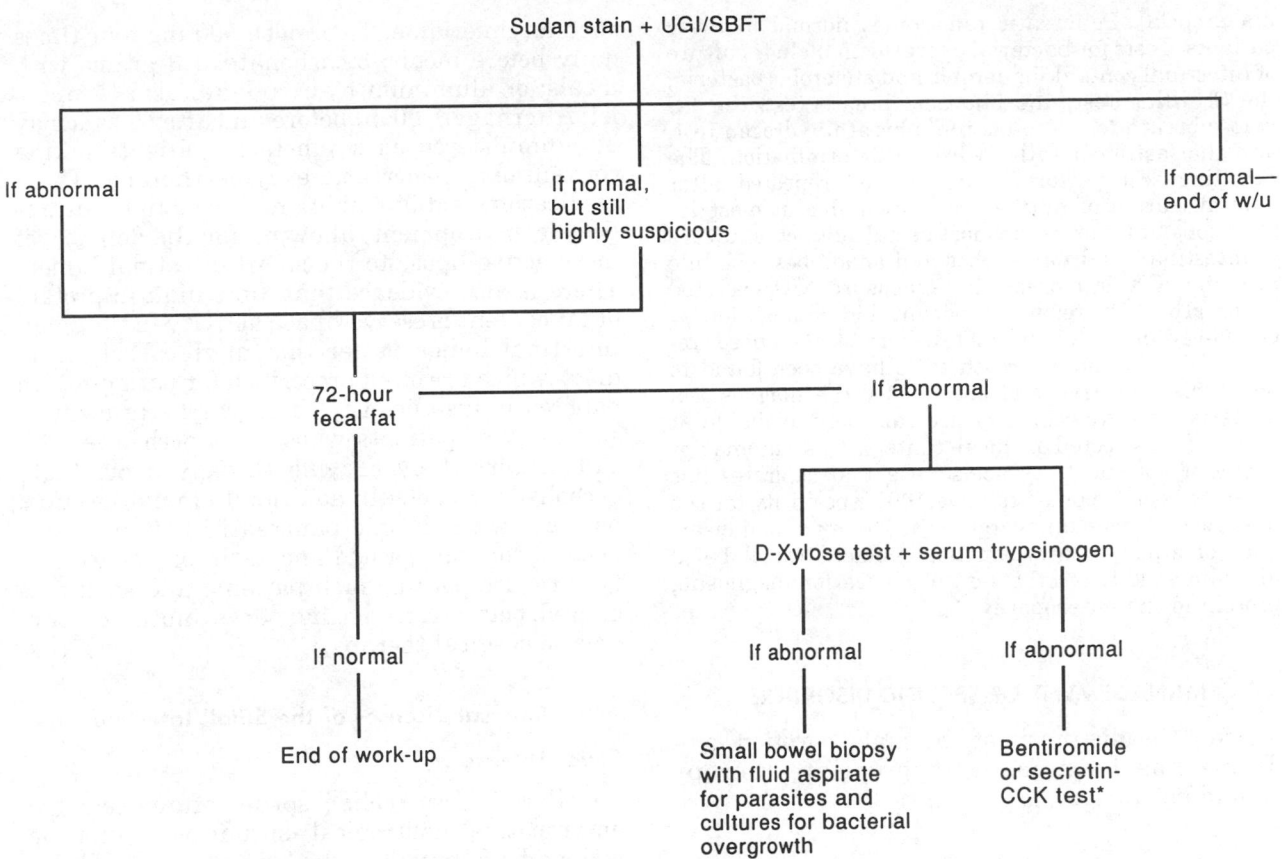

*If pancreatic calcifications present on abdominal x-ray, these tests are not necessary.

**Figure 1.** Decision tree for suspected malabsorption.

oriented properly for diagnostic interpretation like the larger biopsies obtained with a Quinton-Rubin tube. Small bowel biopsy is diagnostic in conditions such as Whipple's disease, abetalipoproteinemia, lymphoma, lymphangiectasia, parasitic infections, eosinophilic enteritis, amyloidosis, immunodeficiency syndromes, mastocytosis, and Crohn's disease. Although not diagnostic, the biopsy may suggest the diagnosis in celiac sprue, tropical sprue, bacterial overgrowth, and radiation enteritis. The small bowel biopsy is normal in conditions such as pancreatic insufficiency and postgastrectomy malabsorption that do not involve the intestinal mucosa.

A normal D-xylose test result and a low serum trypsinogen level are found in chronic pancreatitis. The finding of pancreatic calcifications on abdominal flat plate confirms the diagnosis, and further studies need not be performed. If calcifications are absent, the bentiromide test, a "tubeless" test of pancreatic function, or a direct pancreatic stimulation test with secretion or a combination of secretin and cholecystokinin (CCK) should be done. Bentiromide (Chymex) is *N*-benzoyl-L-tyrosyl-paminobenzoic acid. Pancreatic chymotrypsin cleaves this tripeptide in the intestinal lumen, producing para-aminobenzoic acid (PABA). PABA is absorbed by the intestine, conjugated in the liver, and excreted in the urine. The dosage is 500 mg

given orally, followed by a urine collection for 5 hours, as in the D-xylose test. Certain drugs (thiazides, chloramphenicol, sulfonamides, acetaminophen, phenacetin, sunscreens, and "caine" anesthetics) may lead to false-negative test results.

Pancreatic stimulation tests with pharmacologic doses of intravenous CCK and secretin or secretin alone are the most sensitive and specific methods for diagnosing chronic pancreatitis. Because these tests require small bowel intubation, collection of intestinal content, and detailed analysis of bicarbonate and enzymes (trypsin, lipase, or amylase), they have not achieved widespread popularity in the United States. Bicarbonate concentrations of less than 70 mEq per liter and secretion volume of less than 2 ml per kg of body weight per hour are considered abnormal.

Patients have malabsorption in association with disorders of intestinal motility (scleroderma, intestinal pseudo-obstruction, etc.), intestinal surgery, or anatomic abnormalities (small intestinal diverticuli). In these cases, the diagnosis of bacterial overgrowth should be considered. Patients with overgrowth (greater than $10^6$ organisms per ml of intestinal content) may have positive D-xylose test results after ingestion of the sugar by bacteria, and the small bowel biopsy is often nonspecifically abnormal (partially blunted villi, increased inflammatory cells in the lamina propria). Pancreatic function is normal in these patients. Tests for bacterial overgrowth include culture of intestinal content for aerobic and anaerobic bacteria, the Schilling test, the bile acid breath test, the [14]C xylose breath test, the lactulose breath hydrogen test, and the fasting breath hydrogen determination. The Schilling test performed before and repeated after administration of antibiotics is available at most institutions. It remains the most useful adjunct to culture of intestinal fluid for aerobes and anaerobes. The bile acid and [14]C xylose breath tests measure [14]$CO_2$ excreted in breath as a result of bacterial deconjugation of cholyl-glycine-1-[14]C and metabolism of [14]C xylose, respectively. Although breath tests have been found to be highly sensitive and specific for the diagnosis of bacterial overgrowth, they are routinely available at only a few selected medical centers. Gas chromatography of volatile fatty acids in jejunal aspirates has recently been reported to have 100% specificity for the presence of bacterial overgrowth. The intestinal clearance of alpha$_1$-antitrypsin has replaced radiolabeled albumin studies as the test of choice for diagnosing protein-losing enteropathy.

## MANAGEMENT OF SPECIFIC DISORDERS

After the diagnosis of the malabsorption syndrome has been made, appropriate therapy should be started.

### Abnormalities in Intraluminal Digestion

**Pancreatic Enzyme Replacement.** There is a tremendous amount of enzyme reserve in a healthy pancreas; patients with diseases of the pancreas do not develop steatorrhea until their lipase outputs drop to less than 10% of normal. In many patients, conventional enzyme replacement for pancreatic insufficiency reduces steatorrhea, but rarely completely eliminates fat malabsorption. All pancreatic enzymes are sensitive to acidic pH, but lipase is most labile, being irreversibly denatured at pH 4 or below. One should give approximately 30,000 U of lipase with each meal (this is 10% of the normal postprandial lipase output in health). The major advantage of enteric-coated preparations is that they do not dissolve until alkaline pH is reached. This presumably protects the enzymes during transit through the stomach. In Europe, some patients have been treated with enzyme preparations from fungi that have stability over a broader range (pH 2 to 8) than pancreatic enzymes. These preparations appear to have comparable efficacy with enteric-coated pancreatic enzymes, but are currently not available in the United States. In the future, other acid-stable lipases, such as lingual and gastric lipases, may be produced through recombinant DNA techniques, as both these genes have been cloned by investigators. In selected patients, $H_2$ blockers,

such as cimetidine (Tagamet), 300 mg four times daily before meals; bicarbonate, 1.3 grams with meals; or aluminum hydroxide antacid (Amphojel, Alternagel), 30 ml before and after meals may be administered as adjuncts in patients taking conventional pancreatic enzyme therapy. These medications aid in stabilizing lipase in the intragastric environment, allowing for the delivery of more active lipase to the small intestinal lumen. There is also evidence that diets high in protein or fat content preserve lipase activity in the small intestinal lumen better than high-carbohydrate diets, which are often prescribed for patients with pancreatic insufficiency. It might be prudent to suggest that patients whose steatorrhea is difficult to correct by enzyme therapy avoid high-carbohydrate diets. In addition to malabsorption, patients with chronic pancreatitis often experience abdominal pain. Pancreatic proteases may help reduce pain in such patients and should be offered before considering nerve blocks or pancreatic surgical therapy.

### Mucosal Diseases of the Small Intestine

#### Celiac Disease

Celiac disease (celiac sprue, gluten-sensitive enteropathy, nontropical sprue) was first described by Samuel Gee in 1888 who noticed that "if the patient be cured at all . . . the allowance of farinaceous food must be small." This observation went unnoticed until World War II, when Dicke noted that the illness could be alleviated by excluding wheat, rye, and barley from the diet (gluten is the water-insoluble protein fraction of wheat grain). It is interesting that during the Nazi occupation of Holland, celiac disease became a rare condition, as the Germans had successfully sequestered the Dutch grain. The mechanism by which gluten causes the disease is unknown. It is now understood that celiac disease is activated when the intestinal mucosa is exposed to alcohol-soluble wheat gliadins extracted from gluten. Gliadins are single polypeptide chains with $M_r$ from 30 to 75K. There is a homology between A-gliadin and the 54K early-region protein of human adenovirus Type 12. It has been speculated that the disease may result from immunologic cross-reactivity between the viral protein and the gliadin peptide. Haplotypes HLA-B8 and DW3 are found in 60 to 80% of patients with celiac disease, an increased association compared with that found in the general population. In addition, many patients with dermatitis herpetiformis have small bowel biopsy findings compatible with celiac disease.

The diagnosis of celiac disease is based on the finding of an abnormal small bowel biopsy specimen that improves toward normal histologic appearance when gluten is withdrawn from the diet. The disease most commonly involves the proximal small bowel, but can extend all the way to the ileum. The large majority of patients in the United States with "flat" (absent villi, elongated crypts) biopsy specimens have celiac disease. Complications of celiac disease include refractory sprue, collagenous sprue, and the development of malignancy (most commonly intestinal lymphoma).

**Treatment.** A gluten-free diet is the key to therapy for celiac disease (Table 2). The Celiac Society (45 Gifford Avenue, Jersey City, NJ 07304) can aid patients with newly diagnosed disease adjust to a gluten-free diet. Should a patient with celiac disease deteriorate clinically, noncompliance with the gluten-free diet should be suspected. If this is not the case, the development of refractory sprue, collagenous sprue, or lymphoma needs to be ruled out.

### Tropical Sprue

A disease of uncertain etiology, tropical sprue may cause a malabsorption syndrome in patients living in or visiting the Caribbean, India, or Southeast Asia. Nutritional deficiencies, selective overgrowth of aerobic bacteria that produce enterotoxins, or a transmissible infectious agent have all been theorized to cause tropical sprue. Hallmarks of the condition include steatorrhea, low serum folate and vitamin $B_{12}$ levels, megaloblastic anemia, and an abnormal D-xylose test result. Small bowel biopsy often shows a subtotal villous atrophy that does not improve after a gluten-free diet, distinguishing this disease from celiac sprue.

**Treatment.** Folate (5 mg per day), vitamin $B_{12}$ (100 µg per month), and antibiotics (tetracycline [Sumycin] 250 to 500 mg four times daily) are recommended for 6 months of treatment. Patients have been known to relapse on shorter treatment regimens.

### Whipple's Disease

This extremely rare disorder is a systemic illness, but frequently involves the small intestine

TABLE 2. **Gluten-Free Diet**

| Beverages | Milk, coffee, tea, carbonated drinks |
|---|---|
| Breads | Breads made from rice, corn, soybean, potato |
| Cereals | Cornflakes, rice cereals |
| Fats, meats, eggs, vegetables, fruits | No restrictions unless made with wheat flour or bread crumbs |
| Desserts | Gelatin, sherbet, tapioca, rice pudding, custard |
| Miscellaneous | Honey, sugar, corn syrup, nuts |

with the development of malabsorption. Lymphadenopathy, arthritis, and central nervous system involvement also commonly occur. The characteristic finding in the condition is the presence of large macrophages infiltrating the lamina propria of the small intestine that stain periodic acid–Schiff positive. Under the electron microscope, the macrophages appear to contain bacillary-like structures. Although most patients respond to antibiotic therapy, an infectious organism has not yet been isolated from these patients. The pathogenesis of the disease remains obscure.

**Treatment.** The usual initial therapy for Whipple's disease consists of parenteral antibiotics. Procaine penicillin, 1.2 million U, and streptomycin, 1 gram daily given for 2 weeks, are the drugs of choice for most patients with Whipple's disease. Trimethoprim-sulfamethoxazole double strength (Bactrim DS), given twice daily, is suggested as follow-up therapy for 1 year.

### Lactase Deficiency

This benign condition is quite common, occurring in about 70% of blacks, Asians, and Jews, and is due to low levels of intestinal brush border lactase. This results in an inability to digest lactose (the major sugar in milk products) to glucose and galactose. Osmotically active lactose remaining in the lumen of the bowel may cause diarrhea. Colonic bacteria produce hydrogen gas and lactic and acetic acids from the undigested lactose. This may result in a decreased stool pH. If a mucosal disease involves the brush border of the small intestine, secondary lactase deficiency may result. Often, a therapeutic dietary trial suggests the diagnosis, but the 25-gram lactose breath test is becoming a simple and sensitive way of making the diagnosis.

**Treatment.** Symptoms of lactose intolerance include bloating, cramps, diarrhea, and flatulence and can be relieved if the patient follows a low-lactose or lactose-free diet. Patients may add lactase (LactAid) pills (contain active lactase enzyme) to their milk products or they may purchase LactAid milk (with enzyme already added). Yogurt is well tolerated by lactose-intolerant patients, as it contains lactase supplied by the bacterial cultures.

## Impaired Lymphatic Delivery

### Abetalipoproteinemia

This is a rare inherited disorder (probably autosomally recessive) characterized by the absence of apo-B synthesis. The biochemical defect is an inability to transport absorbed triglyceride out of the enterocytes into the portal circulation with absent chylomicron and very-low-density lipoprotein formation. Clinically, the disease presents with fat malabsorption, progressive ataxic neurologic disease, acanthocytosis of red blood cells, congestive heart failure, and "atypical" retinitis pigmentosa. The disease is usually diagnosed in childhood, and small bowel biopsy reveals enterocytes swollen with accumulated lipid.

**Treatment.** Medium-chain triglycerides (MCT) and a low-fat diet are the mainstays of therapy. The prognosis is poor, with few patients surviving beyond the third decade.

### Intestinal Lymphangiectasia

This is a disorder of the lymphatic system characterized by asymmetrical lymphedema, hypoproteinemia (protein-losing enteropathy), and lymphocytopenia. Chylous ascites may also form in some of these patients. Gastrointestinal symptoms are often mild, but on occasion severe diarrhea may occur. The small bowel biopsy in these patients shows dilated lacteals in the lamina propria, which may distort the villi, and protein-losing enteropathy may be documented by an abnormal clearance of alpha$_1$-antitrypsin.

**Treatment.** Therapy consists of MCT and a low-fat diet (see later). Patients may have a localized intestinal lesion that may respond to surgical resection.

## Miscellaneous Conditions

### Short-Bowel Syndrome

See under "Dietary Therapies."

### Crohn's Disease (See Section 6, Article 7)

Crohn's disease is a transmural inflammatory process of unknown cause that may affect any part of the gastrointestinal tract. Commonly, the distal small bowel and proximal colon are involved. Malabsorption may result if enough surface area is inflamed or if the bile salt pool is depleted as a consequence of terminal ileal disease. Although sulfasalazine (Azulfidine) and corticosteroids are the mainstays of therapy for inflammatory complications of Crohn's disease, dietary therapies have a role in nutritional repletion (see under "Dietary Therapies").

### Giardiasis and Other Parasitic Infections

A common infection leading to diarrhea and occasionally to malabsorption is that with the parasite *Giardia lamblia*. This infection is usually spread through contaminated water. Often, stool samples are negative for the organism, but small intestinal aspirate and biopsy reveal the parasites between the villi. Patients who are IgA deficient are particularly susceptible to this infection. Coccidia, such as cryptosporidia, *Isospora belli,* and microsporidia, may produce watery diarrhea and malabsorption, primarily in immunocompromised patients (see under "AIDS and Malabsorption"). Other parasitic infections that less commonly cause malabsorption include ascariasis, strongyloidiasis, and capillariasis.

**Treatment.** Therapy for giardiasis usually consists of a course of quinacrine hydrochloride (Altabrine), 100 mg three times daily, or metronidazole (Flagyl), 250 mg four times daily given for 7 to 10 days. Therapies for coccidiosis have been largely unsuccessful; there are anecdotal reports of responses to treatment with spiramycin, 1 gram four times daily, and hyperimmune bovine colostrum (1:200,000 titer to cryptosporidia). Treatment of strongyloides infection or capillariasis usually consists of a course of an antihelminthic, such as thiabendazole (Mintezol), 25 mg per kg twice daily. Ascariasis responds to treatment with mebendazole (Vermox), 100 mg twice daily for 3 days.

### Bacterial Overgrowth

In health, the colon contains copious flora ($10^{11}$ per ml), which are mostly anerobic. The proximal gastrointestinal tract contains less than $10^5$ organisms per ml, with a transition zone of increasing bacteria in the ileum. In pathologic conditions (Table 3), bacteria may colonize areas of the small intestine, and several adverse consequences may develop. This may lead to malabsorption of vitamin B$_{12}$ (resulting from ingestion by the bacteria), steatorrhea (caused by deconjugation and precipitation of bile salts, leading to failure of micelle formation and poor fat absorption), and diarrhea (due to toxic bacterial metabolic products and unabsorbed fatty acids). The diagnosis is based on establishing increased bacteria on small intestinal aspirate and an abnormal result of a noninvasive test such as the stage II Schilling test, bile acid breath test, 80-gram glucose breath test, elevated fasting breath hydrogen determination, or $^{14}$C xylose breath test.

**Treatment.** Patients with bacterial overgrowth should undergo surgery if a discrete anatomic cause of overgrowth is the cause of the problem—e.g., jejunal diverticuli or postsurgical fistulas. In patients without obvious anatomic ab-

TABLE 3. **Causes of Bacterial Overgrowth**

| |
|---|
| Status postgastric surgery ("blind loop") |
| Small bowel diverticuli |
| Fistulas and stricture formation (often in Crohn's disease) |
| Radiation enteritis |
| Diabetic enteropathy |
| Pseudo-obstruction syndrome |
| Scleroderma |
| Idiopathic small intestinal motility disorders |

normalities, tetracycline, 250 mg; ampicillin, 250 mg; erythromycin, 250 mg; or metronidazole, 250 mg, is administered four times daily for 10 to 14 days. If patients have a clinical response, with less steatorrhea, etc., periodic courses of antibiotics may be used for relapses.

### Zollinger-Ellison Syndrome

Malabsorption and diarrhea in the Zollinger-Ellison syndrome is due to precipitation of bile salts and inactivation of pancreatic lipase by the large volumes of acidic gastric juice that are produced by the hypergastrinemia. If gastric acid secretion is successfully controlled, steatorrhea is corrected. In the past $H_2$ blockers, such as cimetidine, ranitidine (Zantac), famotidine (Pepcid), and nizatidine (Axid), were mainstays of therapy. Omeprazole (Losec), a parietal cell $H^+/K^+$ ATPase inhibitor, at a dosage of 60 to 100 mg per day, is the choice of therapy for Zollinger-Ellison syndrome.

### Eosinophilic Enteropathy

This disorder is characterized by inflammation throughout the wall of the bowel by eosinophils. Patients may have malabsorption, diarrhea, protein-losing enteropathy, iron deficiency anemia, abdominal pain, pleural effusions, and ascites. Peripheral eosinophilia may be seen, and biopsy of the stomach and small bowel may show the diagnostic infiltration with eosinophils. Corticosteroids, such as prednisone (Deltasone), 20 to 40 mg per day, are the usual treatment. In other countries, cromolyn sodium (Intal), 800 to 1200 mg per day orally, has been used as empiric therapy.

### Mastocytosis

Malabsorption is seen in addition to headache, tachycardia, pruritus, urticaria, and facial flushing in 10% of patients with this unusual syndrome. Intestinal biopsy reveals infiltration of the lamina propria with mature mast cells. It is thought that malabsorption in this condition is the result of injury to the enterocytes due to release of mast cell mediators in the lamina propria. As in the case of eosinophilic enteropathy, cromolyn sodium or cimetidine has been used to reduce the symptoms of diarrhea and abdominal pain. Steatorrhea, however, remains relatively unresponsive to these treatments.

### Postgastrectomy Malabsorption

Mild steatorrhea (7 to 10 grams of fat per day) after subtotal gastrectomy is more common after Billroth's II than Billroth's I anastomosis. It is thought to occur as a result of poor timing of the digestive process with rapid transit into the small bowel; fat emulsification is suboptimal, and preduodenal fat digestion may also be impaired. It has been suggested that pancreatic enzyme output is diluted owing to the rapid emptying into the intestine. Bacterial overgrowth in the afferent loop resulting from stasis may further exacerbate fat maldigestion.

**Treatment.** Six small feedings are given throughout the day, and liquid consumption during meals should be minimized. If bacterial overgrowth coexists, a course of antibiotics may be given. Empiric therapy with pancreatic enzyme preparations has helped in selected patients.

### Acquired Immune Deficiency Syndrome and Malabsorption

Diarrhea is a reported complication of AIDS in at least 50% of patients. One should always search for an infectious cause of malabsorption in these patients (see earlier), but, in the experience of most investigators, this work-up is often negative. Patients have frank steatorrhea with small bowel biopsies that are not clearly diagnostic of any known condition (partial villous atrophy, increased mononuclear cells in the lamina propria). Studies have demonstrated the presence of human immunodeficiency virus (HIV) antigens in enterocytes by immunocytochemical techniques. The malabsorption and secretory diarrhea present in these patients have therefore been attributed to infection with HIV itself. Antidiarrheal agents, such as diphenoxylate with atropine (Lomotil), two tablets up to four times daily, or loperamide (Imodium), up to 16 mg daily, and bulk-forming agents, such as psyllium (Metamucil), may be helpful in controlling symptoms. Anecdotal reports have shown responses in some patients treated empirically with somatostatin analogues.

### Vascular Disease of the Small Bowel

Chronic atherosclerosis of two or more of the major mesenteric vessels (celiac, superior mesenteric artery, and inferior mesenteric artery) may lead to sitophobia (fear of eating) as a result of abdominal pain, diarrhea, steatorrhea, and weight loss. This condition is often called "intestinal angina." Mesenteric arteriography reveals the stenosed vessels, and, if there are bypassable lesions, the patient may have a dramatic response to surgical treatment. In contrast, acute ischemia of the mesenteric circulation leads to severe abdominal pain often disproportionate to the patient's physical findings. Congestive heart failure, digitalis therapy, and evidence of peripheral vascular disease are often associated findings in such patients. Rarely, small bowel volvulus, incarcerated hernia, intussusception, or adhesions may compromise the blood supply. If suspicion is high enough, angiography should be pursued to establish the diagnosis, followed by surgery if necessary. Without rapid diagnosis, many of these patients undergo a fatal deterioration with transmural necrosis of the bowel.

Mesenteric venous disease is rarer than arterial insufficiency, but may cause similar symptoms in patients with abnormal coagulation syndromes (paroxysmal nocturnal hemoglobinuria, antithrombin III deficiency, cancer, etc.). Patients with inflammatory bowel disease may also be hypercoagulable and have mesenteric venous occlusion. Again, the diagnosis is difficult to make unless the physician is appropriately suspicious. Patients who survive surgery for mesenteric ischemia with necrosis often later have short-bowel syndrome (see under "Dietary Therapies").

## DIETARY THERAPIES

**Low-Fat Diet for Short Bowel and Intestinal Lymphangiectasia.** A reduced-fat diet (50 grams per day) may help decrease steatorrhea in patients with short bowel, intestinal lymphangiectasia, or abetalipoproteinemia. Foods that should be excluded from the diet to lower fat content are shown in Table 4. Medium-chain triglycerides may be added to the diet to add increased easily digestible calories (see later).

**Medium-Chain Triglycerides.** These triglycerides (composed of fatty acid chains from 6 to 12 carbons in length) are transported into enterocytes by simple diffusion and do not require lipase digestion for absorption. They are absorbed directly into the portal venous system without the need for re-esterification. The usual dosage is 15 ml (1 tablespoon, 115 calories) three times daily orally. MCTs serve as a good supplemental energy source, in addition to decreasing steatorrhea. Unfortunately, MCTs cannot completely replace the requirement for long-chain triglycerides, which still need to be given to prevent the development of essential fatty acid deficiency.

**Low-Oxalate Diet.** Patients with Crohn's disease may have development of calcium oxalate renal stones if they have ileal disease plus an intact colon. A low-oxalate diet, which excludes foods such as beets, carrots, greens, spinach, green pepper, yams, sweet potato, plums, berries, rhubarb, tea, cocoa, and chocolate, may diminish the incidence of kidney stones.

**Enteral Liquid Diets.** Certain selected patients with Crohn's disease, short-bowel syndrome, etc., may respond to enteral diets given either orally or with a nasoenteral feeding tube. In patients treated with tube feedings, No. 5–10 French silicone feeding tubes are often more comfortable than conventional No. 16–18 French Levin's nasogastric tubes. Liquid diets need to be initially diluted twofold to fivefold, with their concentration gradually increased to full strength over the first week of therapy. This helps in avoiding a hyperosmolar load and "dumping" syndrome. Therapy may be given during sleep using a constant infusion pump. Usually, preparations such as Ensure or Vivonex are utilized. Enteral alimentation may be compounded by pulmonary aspiration, dumping syndrome, or tube obstruction.

**Parenteral Alimentation for Severe Malabsorption.** Patients with short-bowel syndrome and inadequate absorptive surface (commonly less than 60 to 100 cm of jejunum) may require permanent total parenteral nutrition (TPN). An advantage of TPN is that solutions with 1800 mOsm per liter or greater can be infused, in the subclavian or jugular vein, as the solution is rapidly diluted by the high central blood flow. Data suggest that patients who absorb less than 60% of energy content by bomb calorimetry after a liquid test meal need TPN indefinitely. Many patients with short-bowel syndrome can learn to self-administer parenteral nutrition under sterile conditions at home with indwelling Broviac's or Hickman's catheters. Other patients with severe mucosal disorders, such as Crohn's disease, celiac sprue, etc., may also occasionally require inpatient parenteral nutrition until their disease process remits to a sufficient extent that oral feeding can

TABLE 4. **Low-Fat (50-gram) Diet**

| | |
|---|---|
| Beverages | Coffee, tea, skim milk, and carbonated beverages allowed<br>No whole milk products |
| Breads | White, rye, whole grain allowed<br>No pancakes, waffles, or doughnuts |
| Cereals | No granola or 100% bran<br>All others allowed |
| Fats | Exclude bacon<br>Margarine allowed |
| Soups | Only bouillon and fat-free broth allowed |
| Meat | 5 oz daily allowed: must be broiled, boiled, or baked |
| Cheese | Cottage cheese allowed |
| Eggs | 1 daily allowed, but no fried or creamed eggs |
| Vegetables | No creamed, scalloped, or fried vegetables allowed |
| Potatoes | Creamed, fried, and scalloped potatoes excluded<br>No egg noodles or potato chips allowed |
| Fruits | All allowed, except for avocado |
| Desserts and sweets | No pastries, pies, cake, ice cream, ice milk, chocolate, or coconut allowed |
| Miscellaneous | No cream sauces or gravies, no nuts, no olives, no buttered popcorn, no cocoa |

be reinstituted. A typical parenteral nutrition prescription is given in Table 5. Essential vitamins and trace elements are mixed in the solutions, along with the appropriate amounts of fat, glucose, and amino acids. Although parenteral hyperalimentation is at times lifesaving, several complications may ensue. The TPN catheter may become infected, leading to bacteremia or sepsis (the most common organism is *Staphylococcus epidermidis)*. Pneumothorax and subclavian or vena caval thrombosis may complicate catheter placement itself. Air embolism may develop if the intravenous infusion tubing is disconnected from the catheter by accident. Electrolyte imbalances, such as hypokalemia and hypophosphatemia, may occur, leading to cardiac arrhythmias and hemolytic anemia. Disturbances of glucose metabolism, such as hyperosmolar coma and dehydration attributable to the hypertonic sugar loads given in the parenteral nutrition formulas, may occur. Following urine specific gravity may help in the adjustment of infusion requirements. Abrupt discontinuance of parenteral nutrition results in hypoglycemia as a consequence of high endogenous insulin output; TPN should therefore be tapered slowly. Essential fatty acids and trace elements need to be given in TPN solutions to prevent deficiency states (see Table 5). Finally, the cost of TPN remains a difficult problem; $100 to $300 per day on either an inpatient or outpatient basis is a conservative estimate of the costs to the patient.

TABLE 5. **Typical Daily Requirements for Parenteral Nutrition**

| | |
|---|---|
| Calories (kcal/kg body weight) | 30–45 |
| Fat (% total calories) | 20–40 |
| Glucose (% total calories) | 50–60 |
| Amino acids (% total calories; g/kg) | 10–20; 1–4 |
| Water (L) | 2–4 |
| Vitamins | |
| D (IU) | 100 |
| E (mg) | 50 |
| A (IU) | 2500 |
| K (mg) | 1 |
| Water soluble (thiamine, folate, etc.) | 1 amp of MVI |
| Trace elements | |
| Cu (mg) | 1.6 |
| Cr (ug) | 2 |
| Se (ug) | 120 |
| Fe (mg) | 2 |
| Mn (mg) | 2 |
| Zn (mg) | 3 |
| Electrolytes (approximate mEq/day) | |
| K | 55–90 |
| Na | 100–200 |
| Ca | 25–30 |
| Mg | 20–30 |
| Cl | 120–250 |
| $HPO_4$ | 17–40 |
| $HCO_3$ | 22–40 |

*Abbreviations:* IU = International Units; MVI = multivitamins.

## Replacement in Common Vitamin and Mineral Deficiencies

VITAMIN B12. Vitamin B12 may be replaced in dosages of 100 μg intramuscularly every month. Vitamin $B_{12}$ deficiency is most commonly associated with conditions of the terminal ileum, such as Crohn's disease, ileal resection, or bacterial overgrowth.

FOLATE. Folic acid is usually given in a dosage of 1 mg daily orally in patients with malabsorption due to celiac disease or tropical sprue. Patients with bacterial overgrowth are often not folate deficient, as the bacterial produce copious amounts of folate derivatives.

IRON. Iron is absorbed in the proximal small bowel (duodenum and jejunum). Patients with severe proximal disease, such as celiac sprue, occasionally require intramuscular iron, but often patients with short-bowel syndrome require iron supplementation in their parenteral nutrition solutions.

# ACUTE PANCREATITIS

method of
JOAQUIN S. ALDRETE, M.D.
*The University of Alabama*
*Birmingham, Alabama*

"Acute pancreatitis" is a term that includes a wide spectrum of pathologic conditions involving the pancreas and the peripancreatic spaces. In some instances, the devastating effects of severe acute pancreatitis involve other organ systems, as in the respiratory or renal failure often seen in these patients. The morphologic changes observed in the pancreas vary from mild edema to total necrosis. Thus, the clinical course of acute pancreatitis can vary from a mild, self-limiting illness to a relentlessly lethal process. Therefore, the therapeutic approaches to acute pancreatitis are dictated by the variety of functional and morphologic changes.

The exact etiopathogenesis of acute pancreatitis remains elusive. Some etiologic factors, such as the presence of biliary lithiasis, alcohol abuse, and hyperlipoproteinemia, can be established in some patients. However, at the subcellular level, the exact mechanism by which these or any other possible etiologic factors cause the disease remains to be elucidated.

## CATEGORIZATION

Because the clinical manifestations, treatment, and outcome of patients with acute pancreatitis vary so much, some form of categorization is essential. The more relevant one, from the clinician's point of view, categorizes the cases into *mild acute pancreatitis*, characterized by interstitial edema and mild inflammation of the pancreas; *moderate acute pancreatitis*, character-

## TABLE 1. Acute Mild Pancreatitis

Morphologic changes: Edema of pancreatic cells, mild interstitial inflammation, no necrosis, minimal amount of fluid in the peripancreatic spaces

Symptoms: Mild epigastric pain, nausea, vomiting

Signs: Mild epigastric tenderness, no peritoneal irritation, no jaundice, mild tachycardia, no obvious hemodynamic changes

Diagnostic investigation: Amylase in serum and urine (elevated levels); ultrasound scan to assess biliary system

Treatment: Nothing orally, IV fluids, cholecystectomy if indicated

Expected evolution and prognosis: Rapid recovery in most cases, >90% survival rate

---

ized by diffuse inflammation with focal areas of necrosis in the pancreas; and *severe acute pancreatitis*, characterized by extensive necrosis of the pancreatic parenchyma extending into the peripancreatic spaces, often complicated by local or systemic sepsis, renal failure, respiratory failure, hemorrhage of the pancreas, and hemodynamic instability. Whether these categories of acute pancreatitis occur as sequential stages or independently of each other remains a matter of speculation (Tables 1, 2, and 3).

## DIAGNOSIS

### Symptoms and Signs

All patients with moderate to severe pain in the midabdomen should be suspected of having acute pancreatitis, and their serum amylase level should be measured. When it is elevated (usually >150 IU), the diagnosis of acute pancreatitis is highly probable. The findings on physical examination can vary from none or mild epigastric tenderness to prostration and shock.

## TABLE 2. Acute Moderate Pancreatitis

Morphologic changes: Severe diffuse edema, focal necrosis of the acinar epithelium with gross focal but minimal necrosis visible in the pancreas, small amount of fluid in the peripancreatic spaces

Symptoms: Moderate to severe epigastric pain, nausea, vomiting

Signs: Tachycardia, mild abdominal distention, mild peritoneal irritation, tachycardia, no other hemodynamic changes

Diagnostic investigation: Amylase in serum and urine (elevated levels); ultrasound scan to assess biliary system, CT scan to assess pancreas

Treatment: Nothing by mouth, IV fluids, antibiotics (?), cholecystectomy if indicated

Expected evolution and prognosis: Improvement in 3–5 days in 70% of patients; 30% progress to severe necrotizing pancreatitis

---

Obviously, the patients with severe forms of pancreatitis have the most noticeable physical findings. These patients can appear to be acutely ill and dehydrated; fever is not uncommon. Tachycardia may be present; hemodynamic instability is present in patients who have bleeding or systemic sepsis. The abdomen may be distended, with decreased or absent bowel sounds. Palpation may reveal a tender epigastric mass or just diffuse, generalized tenderness. True abdominal rigidity is uncommon.

### Laboratory Tests

The elevation of the serum amylase level is the main diagnostic clue to acute pancreatitis. The magnitude of this elevation is not in direct proportion to the severity of the disease; it simply indicates an increase in the production of the amylase enzyme by the pancreas, which is assumed to be caused by acute pancreatitis. Serum amylase measurements 24 hours after the onset of a mild attack of acute pancreatitis may reveal normal levels.

Amylase is normally cleared by the kidney at a rate of only about 3 ml per minute, and the amylase/creatinine clearance ratio is about 2.5%. In acute pancreatitis, the amylase cannot be totally reabsorbed by the renal tubule. Defective tubular reabsorption may exist, leading to an increase in urinary amylase excretion, amylase clearance, and the amylase/creatinine clearance ratio. These measurements are also

## TABLE 3. Acute Severe Pancreatitis

Morphologic changes: Severe inflammation of the pancreas with partial or total necrosis of the organ; necrosis usually extends to the peripancreatic spaces; hemorrhage throughout the pancreas (hemorrhagic pancreatitis) can occur in addition in 10–15% of cases

Symptoms and signs: Severe epigastric or diffuse abdominal pain, nausea, and vomiting; signs of peritoneal irritation may or may not be present; nausea and vomiting, mental confusion, abdominal distention; a mass may be palpable, and high fever can be present; tachycardia, hypotension, and shock can occur in some extreme cases associated with systemic sepsis

Diagnostic investigation: Amylase in serum and urine (elevated levels); electrolyte disturbances, reduced Ca, reduced K, and reduced Na, raised BUN and raised creatinine, reduced Hct. CT scan of the abdomen to assess extension of pancreatic necrosis

Treatment
  Nonoperative: Nothing orally, IV fluids and antibiotics, respiratory support and hemodialysis as needed, intensive care, parenteral nutrition

  Operation indicated:
    1. Signs of pancreatic abscess (air bubbles on CT scan)
    2. Uncertain diagnosis; extensive necrosis within or surrounding the pancreas
    3. Lack of improvement after 3 days of supportive treatment with signs of pancreatic necrosis on CT scan

---

*Abbreviations:* Ca = calcium; K = potassium; Na = sodium; BUN = blood urea nitrogen; Hct = hematocrit.

considered useful in diagnosing acute pancreatitis in questionable cases of hyperamylasemia.

## Plain Film Radiographs

Plain film radiographs of the chest are often (70%) abnormal in patients with severe pancreatitis. The most common findings are pleural effusions, left lower lobe consolidation, and widened mediastinum. Plain film radiographs of the abdomen are nonspecific for acute pancreatitis; however, fluid levels and dilation of the duodenum, gastric dilation, and generalized intestinal ileus are often found in patients with severe pancreatitis.

## Ultrasonography

Ultrasonography can detect both focal and generalized pancreatic enlargement, which may be associated with acute pancreatitis. Ultrasonography is also useful to detect pancreatic pseudocysts and the presence of biliary lithiasis.

## Computed Tomography

The image of the acutely inflamed pancreas, as assessed by computed tomography (CT), can vary from normal to greatly disrupted. CT also assesses the involvement of or damage to the peripancreatic spaces; however, it has been estimated that one-third of the patients with acute pancreatitis have a normal-appearing pancreas on CT. Pancreatic enlargement can be noted in two-thirds of the cases, diffuse enlargement in 55%, and focal enlargement in 45%. Blurring of the margins of the pancreatic gland, decreased CT density of the gland, and fluid collections in the peripancreatic spaces are almost always found in moderate or severe pancreatitis. More specifically, in severe necrotizing or hemorrhagic pancreatitis, the CT image of the pancreas is almost always abnormal. Because of the lack of uniformity in the terminology used, it has been difficult to establish firmly how the radiologic descriptions correlate with the different stages of the severe forms of acute pancreatitis, as observed at operation. Terms such as "phlegmon," "pancreatic pseudocyst," "pancreatic fluid collection," and "pancreatic abscess" have, unfortunately, been used indiscriminately by clinicians and radiologists alike, and fulfillment of the capabilities of the imaging procedures in acute pancreatitis has been curtailed by this lack of uniformity in terminology and description. As these imaging procedures are used more frequently, the terminology is becoming more uniform and relevant to the operative findings. The information obtained on CT scans is the most important basis for the decision-making process, indicating the appropriate and timely operative therapy of patients with severe acute pancreatitis.

## Endoscopic Retrograde Cholangiopancreatography

Endoscopic retrograde cholangiopancreatography (ERCP) can cause acute pancreatitis; therefore, most expert reviews state that ERCP is contraindicated in the acute phase of this disease. In a few cases of recurrent acute pancreatitis, ERCP can guide effective therapy, but it should be done only after the serum amylase level is normal and the patient has been completely free of symptoms for at least 15 days. These restrictions greatly limit its usefulness.

## TREATMENT

### General Principles

Although the majority of patients with mild to moderate pancreatitis require a short period of hospitalization without intensive care, patients with severe necrotizing pancreatitis cannot always be identified in the early stages of the disease. Therefore, patients with abdominal pain and hyperamylasemia should be admitted to the hospital.

There is no specific treatment for acute pancreatitis; the traditionally recommended therapeutic maneuvers are based on the principle that the requirements for pancreatic function should be kept at an absolute minimum as the first step in arresting whatever processes are producing the disease. Therefore, before taking specific therapeutic measures, it is essential to discuss a therapeutic concept for acute pancreatitis (Figure 1). This therapeutic concept involves two main areas: the general supportive therapy of the patient, and the operative treatment to correct specific complications or eliminate possible etiologic factors. The supportive measures include restoration and maintenance of the intravascular volume, correction of electrolyte disturbances, and

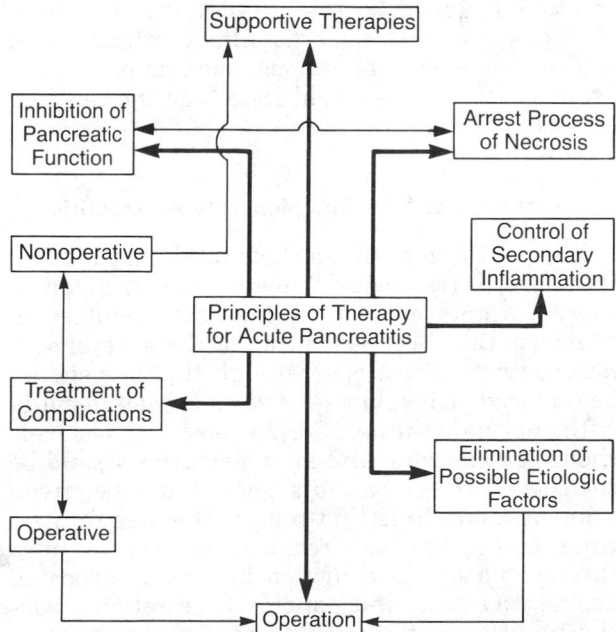

**Figure 1.** Therapeutic concept of acute pancreatitis.

adequate nutritional support, as well as support for failing systems or organs, including mechanical ventilation and hemodialysis when needed.

The general supportive and operative therapies should be complemented by efforts to inhibit pancreatic function, such as nasogastric intubation and administration of anticholinergics, glucagon, or cimetidine. However, none of these agents have proved effective in significantly inhibiting pancreatic secretion in humans. Other experimental approaches designed mainly to arrest the process of necrosis through inactivation of pancreatic enzymes by administering fresh-frozen plasma, aprotinin, or soybean trypsin inhibitor; inducing cytoprotection with prostaglandins; and decreasing the inflammatory response with corticosteroids do not affect the course of acute pancreatitis in humans. The recently available synthetic analogue somatostatin (octreotide acetate) appears to be the most promising method of inhibiting pancreatic secretion and function, but its clinical effectiveness has not yet been proved objectively.

Attempts to control secondary inflammation or to interrupt the pathogenesis mechanism, mostly comprising the administration of antibiotics, antacids, heparin, plasmin, low-molecular-weight dextran, and vasopressin, have also been made, but without impressive results.

The treatment of well-identified complications is the only specific therapeutic measure that can be applied to patients with acute pancreatitis; it can vary from correction of electrolyte and fluid imbalances to more invasive measures, such as ventilatory support and hemodialysis. Operative treatment should be reserved for the treatment of etiologic agents, such as biliary lithiasis, and well-identified complications, such as pancreatic pseudocysts, pancreatic abscess, and the removal of necrotic tissue.

### Treatment of Mild and Moderate Pancreatitis

Most of these patients show mild dehydration; therefore, intravenous fluids should be given to these patients as soon as they are admitted to the hospital. Because most of them receive a nasogastric tube, losses through the tube should be replaced on a volume-for-volume basis, usually with normal saline. Serum electrolyte levels should be checked, and all deficiencies should be corrected. These patients should not be given alimentation directly through the gastrointestinal tract; in fact, removal of gastric juice through nasogastric suction has been advocated as one way to inhibit pancreatic secretion. Sedatives and analgesics should be given as needed. There is no proof that prophylactic antibiotics

are useful for these types of pancreatitis; however, wide-spectrum antibiotics, such as cefoxitin, are often used on the empiric premise that they may prevent sepsis in the presence of mild pancreatic necrosis.

As previously noted, a synthetic analogue of somatostatin to inhibit pancreatic function appears promising. It is hoped that the results of trials with this new drug, currently under way, will confirm its effectiveness. As a general rule, the patient should not be given anything orally until the amylase level has returned to normal. Most patients with mild to moderate pancreatitis recover from the acute attack within 2 to 5 days; their improvement should be noticeable within 48 hours after admission to the hospital. If it is not, the possibility of a more severe form of the disease should be considered and evaluated with an abdominal CT scan. Once the amylase level returns to normal the nasogastric tube can be removed, and a liquid diet can be given and increased as tolerated to a soft diet. At this point, a decision should be made in regard to cholecystectomy in patients with biliary lithiasis. I recommend elective cholecystectomy during the same hospital admission, or no later than during the next 3 weeks.

### Nonoperative Management of Severe Acute Pancreatitis

Because of their more severe and persistent symptoms and signs, most patients with severe acute pancreatitis can be diagnosed at the time of admission or shortly thereafter. Such patients require close observation and intensive nursing care. Their pain is often severe and requires narcotic analgesics. They should be given a nasogastric tube and intravenous fluids to correct fluid and electrolyte imbalances. There is general agreement that prophylactic antibiotics should be given to these patients; cefoxitin and ampicillin are commonly selected. Because gastroduodenal stress ulcerations with bleeding are common complications, they should be prevented by the administration of one of the $H_2$ receptor antagonists.

Patients with severe pancreatitis may experience severe hemodynamic instability. In many cases, insertion of invasive monitoring devices, such as needles in a radial artery and Swan-Ganz catheters in the pulmonary artery, are justified. When oliguria occurs, a low dose of dopamine, 3 to 5 $\mu$g per kg per minute, should improve the patient's hemodynamics and, consequently, the renal output. Renal failure occurs frequently in patients with severe pancreatitis, is related to hypovolemia, and is usually prerenal. Acute tubular necrosis or cortical necrosis can occur; these conditions can best be prevented by maintaining adequate intravascular volume. When renal failure is established despite the use of diuretics (furosemide), hemodialysis should be promptly instituted. Metabolic complications such as hypoglycemia and hyperglycemia, as well as hypocalcemia, can develop in patients with severe pancreatitis. They should be recognized and treated.

Respiratory failure is common and is indistinguishable from other causes of adult respiratory distress syndrome; therefore, in patients who are seriously ill, serial measurements of arterial blood gases should be done. A falling $Po_2$ is always a worrisome sign; endotracheal intubation and mechanical ventilation should be promptly established when respiratory failure appears inevitable. Positive end-expiratory pressure is helpful to maintain adequate $Po_2$ in hypoxemic patients who require high fractional expiratory oxygen concentrations ($FI_{O_2}$ more than 50%). Some of these patients require prolonged respiratory support on a ventilator. When they improve, they should be weaned from the ventilator slowly, with close observation and guidance by improvements in $Po_2$, compliance, tidal volume, and vital capacity.

Once it is recognized that a patient has severe acute pancreatitis, a central line should be inserted and intravenous hyperalimentation begun. Such patients will probably not be able to eat for at least 3 weeks, and adequate nutritional support is essential.

The use of peritoneal lavage, with catheters such as those used for peritoneal dialysis, has been advocated by many authors as an effective method to treat or ameliorate the effects of severe acute pancreatitis. However, several prospective randomized studies have not documented the efficacy of peritoneal lavage in diminishing the mortality or morbidity of these patients. Furthermore, although the rationale for peritoneal lavage is that "toxins" freely floating in the peritoneal cavity are diluted or removed by this method, it is clear that pancreatic necrosis occurs primarily in the lesser sac and usually extends into the retroperitoneal space, rather than into the free peritoneal cavity. It appears unrealistic to think that lavaging the free peritoneum can reduce or eliminate necrosis located in a separate peritoneal compartment.

Needle aspiration done blindly or under radiologic guidance should be avoided in patients with suspected pancreatic necrosis, even if they have fluid. The problem is the thick necrotic tissue that does not drain even through large catheter tubes. In my experience, this procedure usually offers no diagnostic or therapeutic benefits and,

not uncommonly, contaminates an area of pancreatic necrosis that was previously uninfected.

### Operative Treatment of Severe Pancreatitis

It is essential to recognize that in patients with acute necrotizing pancreatitis and/or hemorrhagic pancreatitis, operative treatment can only be directed at the complications of the disease. It does not interrupt the pathogenesis of the necrotic or hemorrhagic process affecting the pancreas.

The decision on when to operate on a patient with severe pancreatitis remains difficult. Once the surgeon is convinced that there is extensive necrosis in the pancreas and peripancreatic tissues, based on the CT scan of the abdomen and the deteriorating clinical condition of the patient, serious consideration should be given to operating promptly to remove the necrotic tissue. Similar indications for surgery are applicable to "enlarging pancreatic pseudocysts" (>10 cm in diameter), which in the acute stage are actually fluid collections frequently associated with extensive necrosis in the pancreas and peripancreatic tissues. Nonspecific indications for operation, or operations to drain the gallbladder or place a tube gastrostomy or tube jejunostomy for feeding purposes, usually do not benefit the patient. Uncertainty about the diagnosis and the possibility of other abdominal catastrophes, such as infarcted bowel or perforated viscus, can also indicate the need for operation. Once the decision to operate has been made, a serious commitment is implied on the part of the surgeon to continue the intensive nonoperative treatment. There is also a strong possibility of repeated operations to remove and drain persistent necrotic tissue. The operation is done through a subcostal, often bilateral, incision. The free ascitic fluid is aspirated, the abdomen is carefully evaluated, and then the lesser sac is entered and the pancreas and its surroundings are examined. Then the necrotic tissue is carefully removed. This is best accomplished by "scooping out" the tissue, rather than by doing a formal pancreatectomy, which, in most cases, is nearly impossible because the anatomic margins have been destroyed by the necrotic process. Several closed system–type drains are left to irrigate and drain the area continuously. The continuous irrigation keeps the catheters open and removes the loose debris, but the thick residual necrotic tissue can be directly removed only at reoperation.

When infection appears in the necrotic tissue, a pancreatic and/or peripancreatic abscess develops. This abscess should also be treated by open drainage, packing, and removal of the necrotic tissue, sometimes leaving the lesser sac and pancreatic bed wide open into the open incision.

Extreme care should be taken to drain the complete area of necrosis and to avoid erosion or intrusion into one of the neighboring blood vessels. Often the process of necrosis obliterates most of the minor blood vessels in and around the pancreas; the entire lesser sac is packed with gauze rolls and left completely open. The dressings are changed under sterile conditions, preferably in the operating room, where the necrotic tissue can be débrided manually. The thickness of the necrotic material is the best confirmation that percutaneous drainage or needle aspiration is not totally effective in removing this thickened, often "sticky," necrotic tissue. In fact, two or three more operations are sometimes needed to complete its removal.

When the CT scan shows moderate pancreatic necrosis and fluid collections that measure 5 cm or less in diameter, aspiration or intervention is usually not needed. Follow-up CT scans eventually show spontaneous resolution of most of these "pseudocysts." However, when these fluid collections are more than 6 cm in diameter, they are often associated with extensive pancreatic necrosis that requires operation, as described earlier. Some patients with segmental pancreatic necrosis do not require operation during the acute phase, but their fluid collection becomes a pancreatic pseudocyst that usually measures 6 cm or more and often becomes symptomatic. Such patients should be treated by internal drainage of this well-established, noninfected cyst into a defunctionalized limb of jejunum (Roux-en-Y method).

# CHRONIC PANCREATITIS

method of
MICHAEL G. SARR, M.D., and
JON A. VAN HEERDEN, M.D.
*Mayo Clinic and Mayo Foundation*
*Rochester, Minnesota*

Chronic pancreatitis is a difficult management problem for physicians and surgeons alike. Not only does chronic progressive pancreatic injury affect both pancreatic endocrine and exocrine functions, but associated inflammatory and fibrotic changes within and around the pancreas may lead to biliary and duodenal obstruction, may cause structural damage in surrounding organs, and may induce a debilitating, chronic pain syndrome. Because no single treatment is appropriate in all patients and because many proposed medical and surgical therapies remain controversial, the spectrum of chronic pancreatitis presents as a diverse and fascinating disease process.

## ETIOLOGY

Throughout the world, the most common cause of chronic pancreatitis is chronic, persistent alcohol abuse. This effect of alcohol, although still poorly understood from the standpoint of pathogenesis, is well known to be a dose-related phenomenon. However, the detrimental effect of alcohol on the pancreas appears to vary in different individuals; some individuals may consume equal or greater daily amounts of alcohol and yet exhibit few, if any, pancreatic parenchymal changes. Other causes of chronic pancreatitis are much less common; these include a hereditary pancreatitis, an idiopathic form, and possibly forms of persistent pancreatic injury related to a partial anatomic, structural, or functional obstruction to the egress of pancreatic exocrine secretion into the duodenum. Whether the consequences of gallstone disease can lead to chronic pancreatitis is unclear. Although a direct causal relationship between gallstones and acute (gallstone) pancreatitis is undisputed, it is unclear whether the related, intermittent passage of gallstones through the ampulla into the duodenum, or chronic choledocholithiasis, can injure the ampulla and induce a chronic progressive pancreatic injury.

## SYMPTOMS

The clinical spectrum of chronic pancreatitis is quite diverse. In some patients, the disease process remains subclinical and asymptomatic. Progressive pancreatic destruction may eventually lead to pancreatic endocrine insufficiency and diabetes mellitus or to pancreatic exocrine insufficiency and maldigestion (steatorrhea). Pancreatic insufficiency usually occurs when pancreatic enzyme production has fallen to 10% or less of its capacity. Rarely, this exocrine insufficiency may give rise to vitamin $B_{12}$ malabsorption. Pain syndromes may manifest as repeated episodes of acute abdominal pain (chronic relapsing pancreatitis) or as the progressive development of a chronic debilitating pain syndrome with associated narcotic analgesic addiction. The pain usually has a boring epigastric quality that radiates to the back and prevents sleep and productive function in society. The patient with chronic pancreatitis may, at times, present with upper gastrointestinal hemorrhage from esophagogastric varices, which are secondary to splenic vein thrombosis (sinistral or left-sided portal hypertension). The common denominators in most of these varied presentations are the presence of destruction and inflammation within the pancreas superimposed on the setting of chronic alcoholism.

## DIAGNOSIS

The diagnosis is usually not difficult and should be highly suspect in most patients with these symptoms. Radiographic imaging techniques aid in confirming the clinical impression. Diffuse pancreatic calcifications seen on plain radiographs are relatively specific but are present in only approximately one-third of patients. Computed tomography (CT) or ultrasonography may reveal an enlarged gland with surrounding inflammatory changes, but, in the absence of calcification, this picture does not necessarily signify chronic pancreatitis. Endoscopic retrograde cholangiopancreatography (ERCP) provides one of the best objective means of confirming the diagnosis. Changes of primary and secondary pancreatic ductal irregularity, narrowing or saccular dilations ("chain-of-lakes" appearance), associated pseudocysts, and pancreatic ductal stones are pathognomonic, and virtually all patients harbor some form of these changes on ERCP. Pancreatic function tests, such as Lund's meal, the secretin stimulation test, or the bentiromide and pancreolauryl tests, can usually document the presence of pancreatic exocrine insufficiency in advanced cases. Demonstration of abnormalities of exocrine secretion in less-advanced cases is less reliable.

## TREATMENT

Management of the patient with chronic pancreatitis must assume a supportive role because the pancreatic damage is in large part irreversible. Discontinuation of all alcohol ingestion (in an attempt to prevent further glandular injury) and enrollment of the patient in some form of alcoholic rehabilitation program should be foremost. From a practical standpoint, treatment addresses the symptoms and complications that may arise.

### Endocrine and Exocrine Insufficiency

Generally, about 90% of the pancreatic parenchyma must be destroyed before pancreatic insufficiency is evident. Endocrine insufficiency manifests as diabetes mellitus and is treated as such with dietary modifications, oral hypoglycemics when possible, or, in a few selected patients, daily insulin administration. Insulin requirements are less than those in most spontaneous diabetics and, in contrast to genetic diabetes, these patients have no tendency toward ketoacidosis, are seldom resistant to insulin, and are often thin and malnourished. Exocrine insufficiency is best managed by oral pancreatic enzyme replacement with sufficient doses of Viokase, Pancrease, or Cotazym with each meal to improve the maldigestion and the associated malabsorption and steatorrhea.

### Pain

Pain remains the most difficult complication of chronic pancreatitis to treat effectively. All attempts at nonoperative management should be exhausted before surgical intervention is considered. The acute episodes of chronic relapsing pancreatitis are managed expectantly as for acute pancreatitis. However, when chronic pain becomes established, a multidisciplinary approach is necessary. Pancreatic pain can become debilitating and may be difficult or impossible to manage with non-narcotic analgesics. Nevertheless, every effort should be made to avoid use of narcotic analgesics. The introduction of narcotics sets the stage for a secondary drug dependency and addiction, which compounds the problem and makes it more difficult to differentiate visceral pain from narcotic withdrawal. Some investigators have provided evidence that oral pancreatic enzyme replacement therapy may ameliorate (not relieve) the pain of chronic pancreatitis in some patients by a still controversial feedback regulation of pancreatic exocrine function. Use of percutaneous celiac plexus block in an attempt to block afferent visceral pain fibers from the pancreas may provide transient relief (3 to 6 months) in a small percentage of patients and should be entertained. In some patients, the chronic pain syndrome is refractory to all the treatment modalities mentioned, and surgical therapy should be considered. Most investigators believe that the chronic pain from chronic pancreatitis eventually resolves; however, this resolution may take years and the physician must weigh the risks of operative intervention and its expected benefits and limitations against the quality of life of the patient and whether or not he or she can function satisfactorily.

When surgical therapy is necessary, the surgeon's principal concern should be the status of the pancreatic duct on ERCP (or on a good CT scan). If the pancreatic duct is dilated (>7 mm), a ductal drainage procedure is indicated. This usually entails opening the pancreatic duct for *its entire length* and anastomosing the "filleted" duct to a Roux-en-Y limb of jejunum—the so-called lateral pancreaticojejunostomy (Puestow's procedure). This is a safe procedure with little morbidity or mortality, and good results can be expected in about 80% of patients. This procedure relieves the associated pancreatic ductal hypertension (the possible cause of the pain), preserves pancreatic endocrine function, and allegedly preserves exocrine function by preventing further pancreatic parenchymal destruction. Attempts to promote better pancreatic ductal drainage by operative or endoscopic sphincterotomy or by distal pancreatectomy and distal pancreaticojejunostomy (Duval's procedure) alone are doomed to failure because of associated pancreatic ductal stones or multiple strictures.

When the pancreatic duct is not dilated (small duct or parenchymal disease), a formal pancreatic resection may be undertaken. Such ablative procedures should be avoided when possible because they sacrifice pancreatic endocrine and exocrine functions, are technically demanding, are accompanied by significant morbidity and mortality, and are far from uniformly successful. The preservation of endocrine or exocrine function is not as important in patients with overt pancreatic insufficiency but can be an important consideration in the poorly compliant alcoholic patient who may be rendered diabetic and dependent on parenteral insulin and oral pancreatic enzyme replacement postoperatively. Pancreatic resection should be directed at the major site of glandular involvement. This operation usually entails resection of the head of the gland (pancreaticoduodenectomy or Whipple's procedure), resection of the body and tail of the gland (distal or 80% subtotal pancreatectomy), or, in selected patients, resection of the entire pancreas (total pancreatectomy). These procedures carry a definite morbidity (approximately 20%) and mortality (1 to 4%), which must be acknowledged by both surgeon and patient. Such pancreatic resections give satisfactory long-term pain relief in 60 to 80% of patients. Previous attempts at autotransplanting the islets of Langerhans (islet cell autotransplantation) from the resected pancreas to the spleen or liver have generally proved to be unsuccessful.

Surgical pancreatic denervations, an extension of the percutaneous celiac plexus block, were designed as a more complete denervation of the pancreatic parenchyma by interrupting visceral afferent pain fibers. Many modifications have included transthoracic greater and lesser splanchnic neurotomies and transabdominal celiac and superior mesenteric ganglionectomies, but the long-term results in general have been disappointing. Recently, some interest has been generated by encouraging preliminary results with other forms of complete pancreatic denervation by autotransplanting the body and tail of the gland into the pelvis; however, the long-term success remains unknown.

### Inflammatory Complications

The progressive fibrosing reaction of chronic pancreatitis may cause a cicatrixing obstruction of either the proximal duodenum or the intrapancreatic portion of the common bile duct, which requires operative relief in the form of an enteric or biliary bypass. Pancreatic pseudocysts are not uncommon complications of chronic pancreatitis and, if symptomatic, are indications for operative intervention to provide enteric drainage and relief of symptoms. The peripancreatic inflammatory changes have been associated with visceral artery aneurysms (splenic or gastroduodenal arteries) that can rupture and bleed into the stomach or into the pancreatic duct (hemosuccus pancreaticus). Similarly, splenic vein thrombosis may occur and lead to left-sided or sinistral portal

hypertension, gastric varices, and intragastric hemorrhage necessitating curative splenectomy.

The best treatment of chronic pancreatitis is prevention. Chronic pancreatitis should be considered to be a medical disease until the patient proves to be a chronic medical failure or develops a serious complication; only then should surgical intervention be entertained.

# PEPTIC ULCER

method of
JAMES H. LEWIS, M.D.
*Georgetown University Medical Center*
*Washington, D.C.*

Over the past few years the increasingly wider array of therapeutic alternatives for the treatment and prevention of peptic ulcer disease (PUD) has made the selection of agents a more complicated process, demanding an increasing sophistication on the part of clinicians.

The pathogenesis of peptic ulcer disease (PUD) remains multifactorial, and it is still important that any therapeutic approach to ulcer healing address those factors that may be associated with an increased risk of PUD. These factors include continued smoking, the use of aspirin and other nonsteroidal anti-inflammatory drugs (NSAIDs), and certain underlying diseases (e.g., chronic lung disease, chronic renal failure, hyperparathyroidism). The relationship between PUD and environmental or emotional stress remains largely unproved, although most clinicians continue to recommend stress reduction techniques for selected patients. Similarly, diet therapy has never been shown to significantly alter the course of duodenal ulcer (DU) disease and has been relegated to a position of minor importance. The Inglefinger diet (three regular meals daily with avoidance of a bedtime snack or any foods or beverages that cause symptoms) remains the most sensible.

The natural history of PUD is one of recurrent exacerbations and remissions. Although the overall incidence of DU appears to be declining, the complication rate from ulcer disease has remained relatively constant, despite the introduction of the $H_2$ blockers and other new ulcer agents. Whether or not PUD ever eventually "burns itself out" after one or more decades (as has been suggested) is not known with any certainty. As a result, ulcer disease should be regarded as a chronic disorder and treated accordingly. Indeed, a growing emphasis is being placed on long-term ulcer maintenance therapy to prevent recurrences and subsequent complications, as will be discussed.

The role played by *Helicobacter pylori* (formerly *Campylobacter pylori*) in the pathogenesis of ulcer disease and its inherent tendency to relapse remains controversial. *H. pylori* is currently regarded as an important cause of nonerosive gastritis, which is found in most (but not all) patients with PUD, and which has been associated with many instances of ulcer relapse. However, since *H. pylori* is present in approximately 20% of asymptomatic individuals (nearly all of whom harbor unsuspected nonerosive gastritis), the relationship between the organism and dyspeptic symptoms has not been fully defined. Nor has the issue of whether to look for and/or treat *H. pylori* infection been settled, as will be discussed.

## TREATMENT

### Duodenal Ulcer

#### Short-Term Therapy

Several dozen pharmacologic agents have been developed for the treatment of DU. These drugs fall into five general categories: (1) acid-neutralizing agents, (2) antisecretory drugs, (3) mucosal protective compounds, (4) compounds with both antisecretory and mucosal protective properties and (5) agents aimed at the eradication of *H. pylori* (Table 1). No clinically important differences exist in the ability of any of the currently available agents to heal ulcers acutely or to relieve ulcer symptoms in the majority of patients. It is expected that 75 to 80% of DUs heal endoscopically at 4 weeks. Continuing therapy for an additional 2 or 4 weeks will increase healing to 90% or more. Even ulcers treated with placebos heal 25 to 60% of the time depending on geographic location.

Since healing and symptom relief are similar regardless of which agent is prescribed, the remaining factors that govern the rational choice of ulcer therapy must center on the issues of drug safety (adverse effects and drug interactions) and

TABLE 1. **Ulcer-Healing Drugs**

| Class | Examples |
| --- | --- |
| Acid neutralizing | Antacids |
| Antisecretory | |
|   H₂ receptor antagonists | Cimetidine, ranitidine, famotidine, nizatidine |
|   Proton pump inhibitors | Omeprazole* |
| Muscarinic receptor antagonists | |
|   Nonselective | Anticholinergics |
|   Selective | Pirenzepine* |
|   Gastrin antagonists | Proglumide* |
|   Tricyclic antidepressants | Trimipramine* |
|   Cell activation inhibitors | |
|     Calcium entry blockers | Verapamil,* nifedipine* |
| Mucosal protective | |
|   Sulfated disaccharides | Sucralfate |
|   Bismuth compounds | De-Nol,* Pepto-Bismol* |
|   Licorice derivatives | Carbenoxolone,* Caved-S* |
| Antisecretory-cytoprotective | |
|   Prostaglandins E₁, E₂ | Misoprostol,*† enprostil* |

*Not approved by the U.S. Food and Drug Administration for duodenal ulcer treatment.

†Approved for short-term prevention of NSAID-induced gastric ulcer.

patient acceptability (compliance and cost), as discussed later.

**Antacids.** Antacids are most commonly used by patients for the self-directed relief of heartburn and dyspepsia. A majority of chronic antacid users have been shown to have gastroesophageal reflux disease (GERD) rather than PUD. While antacids remain a time-honored therapy when prescribed for peptic ulcer disease, they are inconvenient because of a dosing schedule that generally calls for 30 to 60 ml of a liquid suspension to be taken 1 and 3 hours after meals and at bedtime. Even the use of lower acid-neutralizing capacity products or tablet antacid regimens requires dosing at least four times daily. Bowel dysfunction is common, with diarrhea resulting from magnesium-containing preparations and constipation from aluminum-containing products. Mineral and electrolyte disturbances, variable sodium content, the ability to interfere with the absorption of numerous drugs (including cimetidine, ranitidine, digoxin, ketoconazole, tetracycline, and isoniazid), and the fact that the cost of therapeutic amounts of many antacids can be more than for other classes of agents are several additional reasons why antacids are currently unattractive to many patients as well as physicians.

**H₂ Blockers.** These agents reduce acid secretion through competitive inhibition of the H₂ receptor on the parietal cell. Tens of millions of patients have been treated with cimetidine (Tagamet) and ranitidine (Zantac), and the safety and compliance profiles that have emerged for each drug are excellent. Short-term healing rates and symptom reduction are virtually identical for the two medications. The compounds are, however, structurally dissimilar, cimetidine having an imidazole ring and ranitidine a furan ring. This chemical difference probably accounts for many, if not all, of the important potential clinical differences that have become apparent between the two drugs. Famotidine (Pepcid) and nizatidine (Axid) are the two newest agents in this class. Both possess a thiazole ring structure. While clinical experience continues to be limited in comparison with that with cimetidine and ranitidine, the safety profiles of famotidine and nizatidine that have been seen to date are similar to that of ranitidine. However, neither agent appears to offer any advantages in terms of clinical efficacy, safety, or compliance as compared with ranitidine. In their usually prescribed doses, all three drugs are equipotent and are slightly more potent antisecretory agents than cimetidine.

Perhaps the most important distinction to be made among the H₂ blockers is the potential for cimetidine to inhibit the hepatic cytochrome P-450 mixed-function oxidase (MFO) system. The result of this dose-related MFO inhibition is a reduction in hepatic clearance, leading to an increased serum concentration of many drugs, including warfarin, theophylline, phenytoin, benzodiazepines, lidocaine, and propranolol. In some patients these increased blood levels may result in clinically evident toxicity: e.g., bleeding from warfarin; arrhythmias, diarrhea, and convulsions from theophylline; nystagmus, ataxia, and confusion from phenytoin; and so on. The true incidence of these drug interactions remains to be established, however. Nonetheless, when confronted by a potential cimetidine drug interaction, many clinicians elect to avoid the possibility entirely by using one of the newer $H_2$ blockers. Ranitidine, famotidine, and nizatidine have at most only one-tenth the affinity of cimetidine to inhibit the P-450 MFO system, and suspected instances of drug interactions are very rare (or have never been reported).

The antiandrogenic effects seen with cimetidine (impotence, gynecomastia, and breast tenderness) generally do not occur unless the drug is taken in large doses for long periods of time (e.g., in Zollinger-Ellison syndrome). Ranitidine is not antiandrogenic and has been used successfully in patients with these cimetidine-induced antiandrogenic effects. Both famotidine and nizatidine appear to be devoid of antiandrogenic side effects. Headaches are probably the most commonly reported side effect seen with ranitidine and famotidine. Mental confusion has been reported with all four drugs, but it anecdotally appears to be more common in cimetidine recipients, especially those with multiple organ failure in an intensive care unit setting.

None of the currently available $H_2$ blockers are intrinsically hepatotoxic, although mild hepatic dysfunction and rare instances of overt hepatitis have been reported for all four agents. The incidence and clinical severity of hepatitis appear similar for cimetidine and ranitidine. Instances of hepatitis were identified during clinical trials of both famotidine and nizatidine, and the true incidence of hepatic injury remains to be defined for these two newer $H_2$ blockers. There are no reports of hepatitis from the intravenous use of these drugs. The potential use of cimetidine in the prevention of hepatic injury from acute acetaminophen overdose remains theoretical and investigational. No instances of acetaminophen-induced liver injury have been reported in volunteers or patients receiving ranitidine or the newer $H_2$ blockers.

Each $H_2$ blocker is effective when used twice daily, and all have been approved for use as a single bedtime dose to control nocturnal acid and improve patient compliance. The move to bedtime dosing (800 mg cimetidine; 300 mg ranitidine; 40 mg famotidine; and 300 mg nizatidine) is based on studies suggesting that nocturnal acid secretion is most important in terms of ulcer pathogenesis. Taking these medications at bedtime leaves acid secretion intact during the waking hours, which is viewed by many as a more physiologic approach. Taking the $H_2$ blocker just after the evening meal may be an even more effective means of controlling acid and healing ulcers in smokers and in patients with large ulcers.

**Other Antisecretory Drugs.** *Anticholinergics* are not suited for primary therapy of peptic ulcer disease because of inferior healing rates and unwanted side effects. Their role is presently confined to that of adjunctive therapy in certain patients with the Zollinger-Ellison syndrome and other hypersecretory states that are poorly controlled with $H_2$ blockers. But even here, newer agents (e.g., omeprazole) are making this role obsolete.

*Tricyclic antidepressants* are not officially approved for use in peptic ulcer disease, but they have been successfully employed in ulcer patients requiring psychotropic drug therapy. Whether or not their effects are additive to those of $H_2$ blockers or other agents remains speculative. *Pirenzepine* is a drug with selective antimuscarinic and tricyclic antidepressant properties that is in use outside of the United States. Clinical experience has not demonstrated any advantages over $H_2$ blockers.

*Omeprazole*, a substituted benzimidazole, is a potent inhibitor of the $H^+/K^+$ ATPase (proton) pump of the parietal cell. It is currently indicated for treatment of Zollinger-Ellison syndrome (ZES) and other pathologic hypersecretory states, and for the short-term (4 to 8 weeks) treatment of severe reflux esophagitis that is resistant or nonresponsive to other therapy. In May 1990, the Gastrointestinal Drugs Advisory Committee of the U.S. Food and Drug Administration (FDA) made a recommendation that omeprazole also be approved for the short-term treatment of DU, including refractory ulcers, although studies in North America comparing cimetidine and ranitidine to omeprazole have not shown a consistently distinct clinical advantage over the $H_2$ blockers in terms of ulcer healing or pain relief at the 20 mg dose over a 4 to 8 week treatment period. Because of potential safety concerns (gastric carcinoid tumors developed in rats during long-term toxicity studies, presumably the result of achlorhydria-induced hypergastrinemia), omeprazole should be reserved for patients with resistant or refractory ulcer disease or GERD. Since the carcinogenic potential of omeprazole and its long-term safety profile in patients with non-ZES disorders have not been defined (a process that may yet require several additional years of study), it is not recommended for maintenance therapy for PUD.

**Mucosal Protective Drugs.** A number of agents that heal ulcers through mechanisms other than inhibition or neutralization of gastric acid have been termed "mucosal protective." *Sucralfate* (Carafate), the aluminum salt of sucrose octasulfate, is a coating agent that is thought to enhance mucosal defenses. It has been in use for nearly 20 years in various countries and has proved to be an excellent alternative therapy for short-term treatment of DUs. Although some patients have complained of slower initial pain relief compared with $H_2$ blockers, overall healing efficacy and symptom reduction at the end of 4- to 8-week trials are not significantly different from those of other agents.

Constipation is the most commonly reported side effect with sucralfate, the result of the high aluminum content of the compound. Since sucralfate is very poorly absorbed, no systemic side effects are expected. However, it may interfere with the absorption of other agents, such as tetracycline and phenytoin. Accordingly, it should not be given concomitantly with other drugs and should be taken at least 30 minutes prior to meals to avoid being bound to food. Although initially designed to be given as 1 gram four times daily, twice daily regimens may be equally effective but are not currently approved by the FDA.

**Antisecretory-Cytoprotective Agents.** Synthetic *prostaglandin* analogues of the $E_1$ and $E_2$ classes remain investigational for the acute treatment of DU in the United States. Although healing efficacy is similar to that of the $H_2$ blockers in some clinical trials, no clinical advantages over these or other agents have emerged, and concerns about safety (e.g., diarrhea and abdominal cramps in up to 39% of recipients and the potential abortofacient effects of misoprostol [Cytotec]) continue to delay FDA approval for use in PUD. However, misoprostol is approved for short-term prevention of NSAID-induced gastric (but not duodenal) ulcers, as will be discussed later.

### Combination Ulcer Therapy

Antacids are widely prescribed with $H_2$ blockers and other agents to help control ulcer symptoms, although they are usually unnecessary for this purpose. Only a few studies have examined the usefulness of two or more therapeutically active agents taken together to promote ulcer healing. In one well-controlled trial, no advantage was found for the combination of cimetidine plus sucralfate (both given four times a day) compared with either agent used alone. It is doubtful that any other combination would be of additional benefit. Combination therapy for bleeding ulcers or refractory ulcers has not been well studied.

### Follow-up of DU

In contrast to gastric ulcers, it is generally not necessary to document healing of a DU following short-term therapy. If ulcer symptoms remain well controlled throughout the course of treatment, most physicians do not repeat the endoscopy or upper gastrointestinal tract series, even though it is well known that there is a poor correlation between symptoms and the presence or absence of the ulcer after therapy with $H_2$ blockers. On the other hand, if the symptomatic response at the end of therapy is not satisfactory, or if an ulcer relapse is suspected, it may be useful to document healing (or nonhealing) to help determine the direction that future therapy or additional diagnostic evaluation should take.

### Prevention of DU

Endoscopic studies have consistently revealed that up to 80% of healed ulcers will relapse endoscopically within 1 year after therapy is withdrawn. This relapse rate is virtually the same regardless of whether healing is accomplished with antacids, $H_2$ blockers, sucralfate, omeprazole, pirenzepine, or other agents and no matter how long the acute therapy is extended prior to being discontinued. The one possible exception may be bismuth compounds, which may have been associated with significantly lower one-year relapse rates after acute healing than occur after treatment with $H_2$ blockers. This has been attributed to the eradication of *H. pylori* infection and resolution of the accompanying gastric (and possibly duodenal) inflammation. The possibility of reinfection remains high, however, and to date, no study has demonstrated a reduced relapse rate compared with $H_2$ blockers for bismuth-treated patients beyond 1 year after therapy is given.

Since most DUs remain in remission only during the time that active therapy is being administered, a number of long-term treatment approaches have been developed. The most commonly employed method utilizes an $H_2$ blocker (in half of the nocturnal dose used for short-term healing, e.g., cimetidine, 400 mg; ranitidine, 150 mg; famotidine, 20 mg; or nizatidine, 150 mg) given daily at bedtime. One-year DU relapse rates can be reduced from 80% to 20 or 30% using these agents. The relapse rate for patients on ranitidine is somewhat lower than that for cimetidine. The most likely explanation for this difference is that nocturnal acid inhibition is significantly greater with ranitidine 150 mg compared with cimetidine 400 mg h.s. Much less information and clinical experience is available for other agents. Maintenance therapy with sucralfate, 1 gram twice daily, is also effective and may soon receive FDA approval for this indication. Antacids given several times throughout the day have been shown to be as effective as other agents. However, they are not effective when given only at bedtime and are not recommended by this author for patients with a severe underlying ulcer diathesis, in whom ensuring compliance is essential.

Continuous daily maintenance therapy is not necessary or indicated for all patients with PUD. Those with either a first time, uncomplicated DU or no important relapse risk factors (Table 2) can usually be followed expectantly. If a symptomatic ulcer relapse occurs, these individuals are often treated with full-dose therapy for several weeks (intermittent therapy). Patients who develop frequent symptomatic relapses or who have a history of an ulcer-related complication such as hemorrhage or obstruction become candidates for continuous daily maintenance therapy with $H_2$ blockers (Figure 1). Recent studies indicate that continuous daily therapy is superior to an intermittent treatment approach.

A small number of patients will experience a "breakthrough" relapse while on maintenance therapy. These relapses tend to be clinically mild, relatively easy to reheal, and less likely to be associated with ulcer complications compared with relapses that develop in individuals not receiving preventive therapy.

### Long-Term Safety

Just how long maintenance therapy can or should be continued remains controversial. To date, the longest controlled maintenance trials conducted with $H_2$ blockers have lasted only 5 to 9 years. However, cumulative relapse rates suggest that an ulcer that remains healed during the first year of maintenance therapy will continue to do so during subsequent years. Few adverse side effects from long-term continuous

TABLE 2. **Predictors of Ulcer Relapse**

**Strongly Associated**

Cigarette smoking
Poor compliance with maintenance therapy
Incomplete healing after initial therapy
Acid hypersecretion
Continued use of nonsteroidal anti-inflammatory drugs
Prior ulcer complications (e.g., bleeding)
Presence of *H. pylori* infection

**Possibly Associated**

Family history of ulcer disease
Psychologic stress
Alcohol ingestion

administration of the $H_2$ blockers in maintenance doses have been observed or are expected. While some individuals have expressed concern that gastric cancer might develop from prolonged exposure to these agents, this complication remains more theoretical than practical, as it has not been borne out in experimental or clinical studies. In fact, the risk of not taking maintenance therapy or of stopping it prematurely appears to greatly outweigh any concerns about continuing the $H_2$ blockers indefinitely in high-risk patients. For example, use of daily ranitidine or cimetidine has been shown to significantly reduce the risk of recurrent ulcer bleeding over a period of several years in patients with a prior history of hemorrhage. It is this group, perhaps, that should be most strongly considered for maintenance treatment, the alternative being surgery following an ulcer bleed. The projected cost of daily maintenance therapy with $H_2$ blockers remains less than the cost of surgery for 15 to 30 years, based on current charges.

Indeed, for patients in whom chronic (perhaps several years and even possibly lifelong) maintenance therapy is recommended but is not acceptable for reasons such as cost, compliance, or the potential for long-term side effects, consideration can be given to a surgical means of ulcer prevention. Highly selective (proximal) vagotomy has been favored over more conventional operations (vagotomy and pyloroplasty or antrectomy) in some European centers. Although it has a lower perioperative and postoperative morbidity and mortality rate compared with more conventional operations, it also has a higher recurrence rate and currently is not being advocated by many U.S. surgeons. Nevertheless, its recurrence rate of 2 to 3% per year compares quite favorably with an annual relapse rate of 20 to 30% for medical therapy.

### Gastric Ulcer

#### Short-Term Therapy

The same drugs used in DU therapy are used to treat gastric ulcers (GU), but the healing rates are generally 10 to 25% lower than those observed for DU, reflecting, in part, differences in the pathophysiology of the two conditions. In European trials, omeprazole has been shown to have superior GU healing rates compared with $H_2$ blockers, but no clear healing advantages have been shown in several North American trials, and it is not currently indicated for this indication in the United States.

The risk of malignancy in a non–drug-related GU (approximately 1 to 3%) mandates that all GUs be followed endoscopically or radiographi-

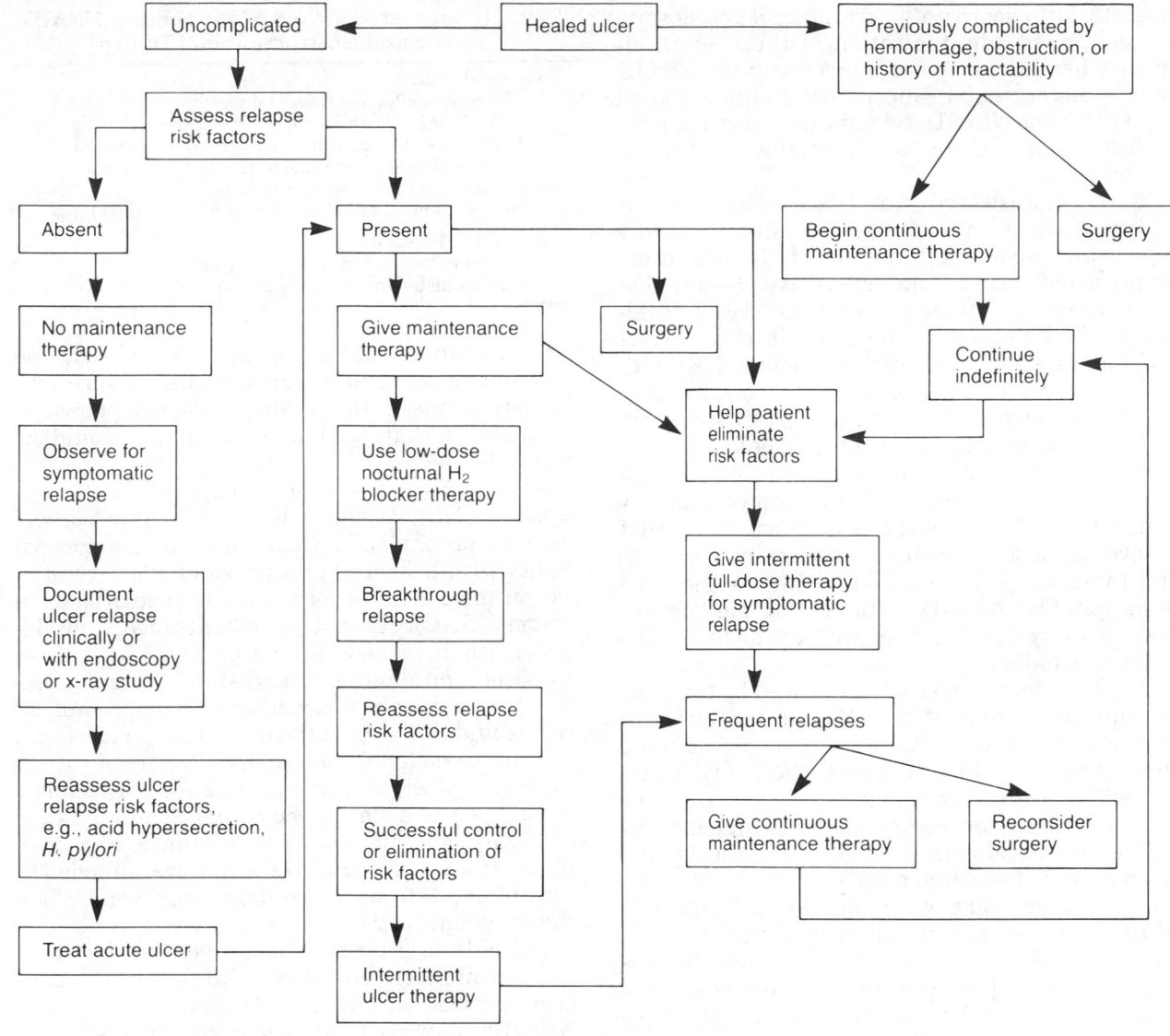

**Figure 1.** Prevention of peptic ulcer relapse.

cally until they heal completely, especially in older individuals. A combination of endoscopically directed biopsies and brushings for cytologic findings can accurately exclude malignancy in over 99% of cases and should be obtained early in all patients in whom the endoscopic or radiographic findings are equivocal or suspicious for gastric cancer.

Most benign GUs can be expected to heal after 6 to 8 weeks of therapy with an $H_2$ blocker. For large ulcers, up to 15 weeks may be required for healing, depending on their size. It should be remembered that even a malignant GU can partially heal on therapy. Therefore, any GU that does not heal completely on an intensive medical regimen after an appropriate length of time (e.g., 8 to 12 weeks for ulcer diameter <2.5 cm and 12 to 15 weeks for an ulcer >2.5 cm) should be seriously considered for surgery.

## NSAID-Related Gastroduodenal Injury

Approximately 20 per cent of chronic aspirin and other NSAID users develop either a GU or a DU (in a ratio of approximately 2:1), the majority of which are asymptomatic. The analgesic effects of aspirin and other NSAIDs may mask the pain of an ulcer and represent one possible reason for the poor correlation between NSAID injury and symptoms. These patients, however, remain at increased risk for ulcer-related complications such as hemorrhage and perforation with continued NSAID use. Healing of NSAID-related ulcers can be accomplished by using $H_2$ blockers, sucralfate, or misoprostol in standard doses, despite the continued administration of the NSAID, although healing rates are improved if the NSAID can be discontinued. Substituting enteric-coated aspirin for the NSAID did not allow gastric ulcers to heal in one study of cimetidine-treated patients.

Many unanswered questions remain about which course of action is best to minimize NSAID injury and about defining which NSAID users might benefit most from preventive therapy. Patients considered to be at increased risk of developing NSAID injury to the gastrointestinal tract include the elderly (especially women), those with a past history of an ulcer or ulcer complication, and those on comcomitant corticosteroids. Other possible risk factors are given in Table 3.

The actual risk of developing a serious NSAID-related ulcer complication is not known with any certainty. In England, it has been estimated that a severe reaction occurs in approximately 1 in 500 individuals. In the United States, the need to hospitalize NSAID patients for gastrointestinal toxicity has been estimated to be on the order of 1 to 5%.

The only agent currently approved by the FDA for the prevention of NSAID-induced ulcers is misoprostol. It is indicated, however, for only short-term (e.g., 3-month) protection of GUs at a dose of 100 to 200 μg four times daily with meals and at bedtime. Secretory diarrhea and abdominal cramps develop in up to 39% of patients, and relief of NSAID-related pain was not significantly different from that with placebo in controlled trials. The drug is contraindicated in pregnancy and in women of childbearing potential unless they are using effective contraception. Postmenopausal bleeding has been reported in some women.

Ranitidine in a dose of 150 mg b.i.d. has been shown to effectively prevent the development of DU in chronic NSAID users, but does not appear to prevent GU ( a finding completely opposite to misoprostol). The ability of the other ulcer-healing agents to prevent DU and GU among NSAID users has been less well studied, and no firm recommendations regarding their use can be made at this time. The combination of misopros-

### TABLE 3. Possible Risk Factors for the Development of NSAID-induced Gastroduodenal Injury

Prior GU or DU
Prior ulcer complication on or off NSAIDs
Concomitant corticosteroid therapy
Age >65 years
Female gender
High-dose NSAID therapy

### TABLE 4. Suggested Means of Preventing NSAID-associated Gastroduodenal Injury

**General Measures**
Use lowest effective NSAID dose
Take NSAIDs with meals
Substitute acetaminophen for other agents when
    possible (e.g., treatment of simple headache)
Switch to enteric-coated products
Switch to nonacetylated salicylates (e.g., salsalate)

**Specific Measures**
Coadminister misoprostol to prevent GU
Coadminister ranitidine to prevent DU

tol plus ranitidine has not been evaluated, and whether or not this regimen would ensure protection against both GU and DU is not known. It is doubtful that such a combination would be cost-effective.

As it does not appear to be cost-effective to treat all NSAID users in general, at present I reserve prophylactic treatment mainly for patients with a history of a previous ulcer complication (bleeding, perforations, or obstruction) in whom NSAIDS cannot be discontinued. Individuals with a history of an uncomplicated ulcer, those on concomitant corticosteroids, and those in whom a serious ulcer bleed or other complication could have devastating consequences can also be considered for prophylaxis (Table 4). If the prior ulcer was known to be gastric, misoprostol is the agent of choice (starting at a dose of 100 μg four times daily to minimize diarrhea). If, on the other hand, the ulcer was duodenal, ranitidine, 150 mg twice daily, is given. When the previous ulcer site is unknown, it is still reasonable to use ranitidine, given the fact that DUs outnumber GUs by several fold in the general population in the United States, and NSAIDS may reactivate a dormant or latent DU.

### Refractory Ulcers

Approximately 10% of DUs remain unhealed after 8 weeks of therapy with $H_2$ blockers in endoscopic trials. Noncompliance with the prescribed treatment regimen, cigarette smoking, the continued use of NSAIDs, and gastric acid hypersecretion are the most common reasons why ulcers fail to heal. Several early reports of "cimetidine-resistant" DUs that were subsequently responsive to ranitidine have appeared. However, in most instances the initial treatment period was only 4 to 6 weeks. This may have been too short a time to label an ulcer as truly "resistant," and it is equally as likely that continued treatment with cimetidine for an additional 2 to 4 weeks would have resulted in the same rate of healing as was accomplished by switching to ranitidine. Actual "resistance" to an active agent due to genetic or other factors is thought to be exceedingly rare.

If, however, an ulcer is judged to be refractory to a standard course of $H_2$ blocker therapy, treatment options include (1) continuing the same drug at the same or a higher dose, (2) adding a second agent such as sucralfate or an anticholinergic, or (3) switching to a completely different class of agent, e.g., omeprazole in a dose of 40 mg per day. In our unit many patients with refractory ulcers have been found to have idiopathic hypersecretion of acid. We have had very good success treating these patients with increased doses of $H_2$ blockers to keep the basal acid output below 10 mEq per hour. This can usually be accomplished by simply doubling the dose of ranitidine or other similarly potent $H_2$ blocker.

### Special Circumstances

**Ulcer Disease in Pregnancy.** Pregnancy is normally associated with a lower incidence of DU relapse and ulcer complications than is the nonpregnant state, although some patients may require treatment during gestation. Although no ulcer-healing drug is approved for use during pregnancy, antacids and sucralfate are probably safe, especially after the first trimester. The $H_2$ blockers may be used if the expected benefits are thought to outweigh the possible risks. These agents, however, are excreted in breast milk and are not recommended for nursing mothers.

**Ulcer Disease in Children.** The same drugs used in adults may be used to heal and maintain PUD in remission in children, recognizing that there is far less experience with these agents in the younger age groups.

### Treatment of *Helicobacter pylori* Infection

*H. pylori* continues to command our attention as an important factor in the pathogenesis and relapse of PUD. However, it remains controversial whether to look for or attempt to eradicate the organism. It is thought that with the future widespread availability of noninvasive diagnostic techniques such as the carbon-labeled urea breath test or newer serologic tests that are being developed, the indications for initial detection and the need for post-treatment follow-up may be met with less skepticism.

At present, treatment of *H. pylori* is best accomplished with the combination of a bismuth compound (e.g., Pepto-Bismol, two tablets or 30 ml four times daily on an empty stomach) for a total of 21 days plus one or preferably two antibiotics administered concomitantly for the final 10 to 14 days (e.g., amoxicillin, 250 to 500 mg three or four times daily, or tetracycline, 500 mg four times daily; with metronidazole, 250 to 500 mg three times daily). Approximately 80% of cases are treated effectively with this regimen, but relapse rates of *H. pylori* infection can be high, the possible result of reinfection from unsuspected family members who transmit the organism by fecal-oral or respiratory droplet routes.

Side effects of bismuth generally are only cosmetic (e.g., black stools and darkening of the tongue), but encephalopathy has been reported with prolonged use of certain bismuth salts. Antibiotics in this setting have been associated with the usual hypersensitivity reactions and *Clostridium difficile*–related colitis (even among those receiving metronidazole). Thus, the decision to treat *H. pylori* with these agents must take such risks into account. Since ulcers have been shown to heal quite well with $H_2$ blockers, despite the presence or persistence of *H. pylori* infection, treatment of *H. pylori* is not necessary if the therapeutic response to conventional ulcer therapy is satisfactory. However, if dyspeptic symptoms persist after treatment with $H_2$ blockers or if ulcer relapses are frequent when therapy is discontinued, the knowledge that *H. pylori* is present may provide for a reasonable treatment alternative.

Future ulcer-healing agents might well combine an antisecretory drug, such as an $H_2$ blocker, with a bismuth compound or even an antibiotic aimed at treating *H. pylori*. Whether we will ever have an agent that completely and permanently cures PUD after a single short-term course of therapy is certainly possible, but I consider it unlikely for the near future.

# TUMORS OF THE STOMACH

method of
FRANK L. LANZA, M.D.
*Baylor College of Medicine*
*Houston, Texas*

Adenocarcinoma is the most common gastric tumor. Because surgical resection offers the only real hope for cure, the most important aspect of treatment is early and accurate diagnosis. Most patients usually become symptomatic late in the course of their illness, resulting in 5-year surgical cure rates of only 5 to 10%. However, the increasing use of endoscopy, which has all but replaced radiography as the primary diagnostic tool for evaluation of upper gastrointestinal (GI) complaints, has led to more frequent early diagnoses of this disease. Japanese investigators have demonstrated that "early gastric cancer" limited to the mucosa and submucosa can be cured surgically in many patients. Benign gastric tumors are probably more frequent than generally thought, but are still less common than malignant tumors. They fall, generally, into two categories: mucosal lesions (polyps) or submucosal tumors, which are usually of mesenchymal origin. They are most often incidentally found by radiography or endoscopy and at surgery. Occasionally, they ulcerate and present as acute GI bleeding or occult anemia.

## TREATMENT

### Malignant Tumors

Ninety-five per cent of all malignant gastric neoplasms are adenocarcinoma. These patients have abdominal pain, nausea, vomiting, anorexia, weight loss, and anemia. It is extremely important that all patients with these symptoms undergo endoscopy. Biopsy should be performed for all gastric abnormalities, and, when there is a high suspicion of malignancy, washings and/or brushings should be obtained. All gastric ulcers, even those with benign histology, should undergo subsequent endoscopy after 6 to 8 weeks of therapy to assess healing. Unhealed ulcerations should be rechecked histologically. This method detects 98% of all gastric cancers. Duration of therapy should be individualized, but all gastric ulcers that fail to heal after an adequate course of therapy, usually 6 to 12 weeks, should be treated surgically. In Japan, with its high incidence of gastric cancer, mass endoscopic screening takes place, which leads to more early diagnosis; however, this is not feasible elsewhere. Patients with a higher risk of gastric cancer—i.e., those with pernicious anemia, a history of polyps or prior gastric resection, or a strong family history—should be endoscopically checked at least every 2 to 3 years.

The primary treatment of gastric cancer remains surgical, and all operable patients without evidence of distant metastases deserve surgical exploration for either cure or palliation. Preoperative computed tomographic scanning is extremely helpful in detecting both local and distant spread of disease. Subtotal radical gastrectomy or radical gastrectomy is the treatment of choice for potentially curable disease. The 5-year survival rate for patients thought to be curable at surgery is 20 to 25%, and "early gastric cancer" may have survival rates in the range of 90%. These rates again point out that early and accurate diagnosis is the most critical factor in the treatment of gastric cancer. Palliative surgery is indicated in patients with obstruction or anemia when curative resection is impossible. Patients with distant metastases may also undergo palliative surgery with elimination of these complications to improve quality of life.

The most commonly performed palliative procedure for bypass of obstruction is simple gastrojejunostomy; however, occasional subtotal distal gastrectomy may be indicated, especially when GI bleeding is a problem. Proximal gastric obstruction due to carcinoma of the cardia or the fundus can often be managed by endoscopic yttrium-aluminum-garnet (YAG) laser or large heater probe therapy, although palliative resection of the upper stomach is occasionally indicated.

Other gastric malignancies include lymphomas (4%) and various sarcomas (1%), the most common of which is leiomyosarcoma. The diagnostic considerations for these lesions are essentially the same as those for adenocarcinoma. These lesions, when confined to the stomach, are also treated surgically.

Chemotherapy is generally ineffective as primary treatment of gastric carcinoma. Combination chemotherapy has shown some promise as adjunct therapy to curative resection in increasing survival and delaying recurrence in treated patients. Radiation therapy is of no significant value in the treatment of gastric carcinoma and does not add to the efficacy of chemotherapy. Combination chemotherapy with or without radiation therapy is of considerable value in the treatment of malignant lymphoma of the stomach. This is used most often when gastric involvement is part of systemic disease, but may also be used when the disease is confined to the stomach, especially in patients with a high operative risk. Primary gastric lymphoma confined to the stomach is probably still best treated by surgical resection; however, cure can be accomplished in a significant number of patients with combination chemotherapy and/or radiotherapy.

### Benign Tumors

**Submucosal Tumors.** A great variety of pathologic entities present as benign submucosal gastric tumors, the majority of which are asymptomatic. The most common is leiomyoma, which is highly vascular in nature and may present with massive GI hemorrhage. Diagnosis is by endoscopic biopsy. Routine biopsy specimens usually reveal only normal overlying mucosa, however, newer techniques with large forceps and needles have markedly increased the diagnostic yield with these lesions. Other benign submucosal gastric tumors include other tumors of muscular origin (cellular leiomyoma, leiomyoblastoma); neurogenic tumors (neurolemmoma, neurofibroma); vascular tumors (glomus and lymphangiomas); and lipoma, fibroma, granular cell tumor, eosinophilic granuloma, and pseudolymphoma. These lesions are treated by surgical excision. Occasionally, if they are small (less than 2 cm) and on a well-defined stalk, they can be removed by endoscopic polypectomy. Small lesions in high-risk patients can also be followed endoscopically, especially when a benign histologic diagnosis has been made.

Ectopic pancreas is an extremely common submucosal lesion, characteristically found along the greater curvature of the prepyloric antrum and having a characteristic appearance, both on radiograph and endoscopy. It often has a dimple on its surface, which represents the orifice of its rudimentary secretory duct. Rarely, these lesions can produce symptoms of gastric outlet obstruction or pancreatitis. In these cases, they should be removed surgically. When asymptomatic, they do not need to be surgically excised. Biopsies should be obtained, and the lesions should be followed endoscopically or by X-ray for any change in size or appearance.

**Mucosal Lesions (Polyps).** There are two types of polyps, adenomatous and hyperplastic. Adenomatous polyps exhibit varying degrees of dysplasia and are categorized as tubular, tubulovillous, or villous adenomas. The incidence of carcinomatous change is far more common in the more atypical villous adenomas. The incidence of malignant change in villous adenomas greater than 2 cm in size is as high as 50%. Hyperplastic polyps are thought to be the result of reaction to chronic inflammation. The incidence of malignancy in hyperplastic lesions is extremely low, although the coexistence in the stomach of both hyperplastic and adenomatous polyps is not uncommon. All polypoid lesions in the stomach should undergo endoscopic biopsy. Large, atypical villous lesions should be surgically removed. Smaller polyps, especially those with well-defined stalks, can be removed endoscopically, and those showing invasive carcinoma require surgical exploration. Patients with large numbers of adenomatous polyps are often best treated by gastrectomy. Large hyperplastic polyps are extremely unusual. Often, they are mixed hyperplastic and adenomatous lesions and should be removed surgically. Smaller hyperplastic lesions, when they are few in number, can be endoscopically eliminated. Patients with large numbers of hyperplastic polyps can be followed by endoscopy and biopsy.

# TUMORS OF THE COLON AND RECTUM

method of
LEE E. SMITH, M.D.
*The George Washington University Medical
Center*
*Washington, D. C.*

## INCIDENCE AND EPIDEMIOLOGY

Colorectal cancer is the second most common visceral carcinoma after lung cancer. It is estimated that there will be 157,000 new cases in 1990, with 61,000 deaths. The disease affects members of both sexes approximately equally, but there has been a decreasing trend in women. Black and caucasian people in the United States are affected in equal numbers. It is predicted that 5 to 6% of the population will ultimately develop a colorectal cancer.

Genetics undoubtedly play a role in the development of this cancer. The frequency with which cancers are present throughout a family line is testimony to this fact. This genetic predisposition should guide relatives of affected individuals to seek careful surveillance for colorectal cancer.

Colorectal cancer is also a product of environment. Westernized industrial countries are far more likely to have people with this cancer as opposed to developing countries. For example, there are 3.4 cases per 100,000 in Nigeria as compared with 35.8 per 100,000 in Connecticut. Another means of exemplifying this propensity for development of colorectal cancer in Western countries is the observation that migrants to this country eventually develop colorectal cancer at rates similar to those of people already in the United States, even when they have come from an area of low incidence. For example, Japanese living in Japan have a low incidence of carcinoma of the colorectum; however, immigrants from Japan to Hawaii are a population that is prone to colorectal cancer.

Colorectal carcinoma is likely related to diet. Carcinogens may be associated with bile salts and animal fat. The action of the resident bacteria on these substances may create carcinogens as a byproduct. A low-fiber diet and a slow transit time might enhance exposure of the mucosa to such carcinogens.

## RISK FACTORS

Certain benign tumors of the colorectum are precursors of carcinoma. Tumors that are defined pathologically as tubular, tubulovillous, or villous are recognized as carcinoma formers. This is termed "the polyp to cancer sequence." This sequence may evolve over 5 to 10 years. The incidence of malignancy found within such polyps is based on the size of the tumor, the number of the tumors, and the amount of villous component making up the total tumor. Adenomas are found in about 2 to 15% of the population, and in 25% a second one is present. A carcinogenic diet is a direct inducement for development of polyps or cancer.

Familial polyposis syndromes are genetic disorders that lead to colorectal cancer. A specific gene is responsible for the development of familial polyposis. Patients carrying this genetic defect may develop polyps in their childhood or adolescence. It is a dominantly inherited disorder, and essentially half of the offspring will have polyposis. Gardner's syndrome is a variant of this disorder, and associated with the polyposis in Gardner's syndrome are certain benign tumors such as inclusion cysts, lipomas, osteomas, and desmoids. A serious new finding in 40% of patients with colonic polyposis syndromes is polyposis of the duodenum and stomach. Thus, annual upper gastrointestinal surveillance is needed in this subset. Half of the people who have this genetic disorder develop cancer by age 40 years. Thus, the total colon should be removed on diagnosis.

Inflammatory bowel disease contributes to cancer formation. Chronic ulcerative colitis in time can be expected to result in cancer. It is estimated that 35% of patients who have had the disease for 25 to 30 years will develop a cancer. Crohn's disease, on the other hand, may have some propensity to result in cancer, but not at that level.

Another genetic disorder is the familial cancer syndrome. These families have multiple types of cancer without polyposis. Other family trees demonstrate the formation of colorectal cancers in virtually every generation.

Those patients who have had an adenoma or a carcinoma have an increased risk of forming a second neoplastic growth. It is estimated that 3% of patients who have had one colorectal cancer will develop a metachronous colorectal cancer.

Colorectal cancers occur more frequently in the older age group. Even without a family history of cancer, growing old confers an additional risk on the population. It is clear that there is a dramatic increase in the incidence of colorectal cancer after age 50. Adenomas or villous tumors are the precursors that may be found in those 40 to 50 years of age; hence, surveillance should begin then.

## PREVENTION

A prudent diet may allow a patient to minimize the risk of colorectal cancer. As previously mentioned, a high-fiber, low-fat diet seems to be most appropriate for diminishing carcinogenesis. A new set of drugs entitled antioxidants are believed to minimize and perhaps cause regression of polyps of the colon. Substances such as selenium, a trace element, have been reported to be advantageous for colorectal neoplasm prevention in animal experiments. The administration of vitamins C and E, which are antioxidants, has also shown a modest improvement in the regression of polyps.

## SCREENING

The key to successful cure of a cancer is detection in its infancy and removal prior to metastasis within the body. As recommended by the American Cancer Society, three tests are used for screening: the digital examination, sigmoidoscopy, and occult blood testing of the stool. The digital examination and occult blood testing should be performed in patients starting at age 40 as part of an annual physical examination. Sigmoidoscopy should be performed for patients older than age 50 at three-year intervals. The flexible fiberoptic sigmoidoscope creates a new dimension for better examination of the distal colorectum.

Fecal occult blood testing showed promise in the past, but, practically speaking, it has not detected blood within the stool in many patients and it has not identified others who had a cancer that was not bleeding. Furthermore, there is a high false-positive rate owing to products that cause the guaiac reaction or ingested blood products. Unfortunately, there is not a cheap, easy to perform, specific test to substitute at this time.

## SYMPTOMS

The location of the tumor influences the type of symptoms that are encountered. The right side of the colon has liquid stool, which becomes more solid as it traverses the colon and ends as solid in the descending colon. In the right side of the colon, the patient often has minimal symptoms because there is not an element of obstruction with the liquid stool. On the other hand, cancer of the left side of the colon with solid stool manifests obstructive symptoms early. With rectal cancer, there may be tenesmus during defecation.

Blood in the stool is the most frequent complaint of patients with colorectal neoplasms. The most common cause of bleeding is hemorrhoids, but it is imperative that the physician not be misled and direct treatment at hemorrhoids and miss a proximal carcinoma. This is a scenario that is played out frequently. A change in bowel habits may be noted in later stages of tumor growth. This may take the form of constipation, diarrhea, or alternating diarrhea and constipation. A change in bowel habits in an elderly patient deserves a more careful look to see if there are lesions within the colon.

Abdominal pain, weight loss, fatigue, palpable mass, and frank bowel obstruction are rather late symptoms. The small tumors, which are the most curable, lie silent. Anemia may be the first finding in the patient with a colon cancer on the right side. Frank obstruction accounts for about 10% of the patients with colonic carcinoma. Sometimes pain in the right lower quadrant, suggestive of appendicitis, turns out to be a carcinoma of the colon on the right side at exploration.

### DIAGNOSIS

The diagnosis of colorectal cancer entails several examinations. Digital examination allows palpation of a rectal cancer at or below the 10-cm level. Sigmoidoscopy allows examination of the rectum and a portion of the sigmoid, and biopsies may be obtainable in this fashion. Historically, the sigmoidoscope has been rigid, but in the past decade flexible sigmoidoscopes were introduced. The rigid scope allows better evaluation of the size and fixation of the cancer and provides larger biopsy specimens. Colonoscopy is useful to identify a cancer at any level in the colon; also biopsies via the colonoscope are obtainable. Barium enema is not as good as colonoscopy for the detection of small neoplasms, but, when air contrast is added, it improves mucosal detail, which increases the chance of finding the carcinoma.

Colonoscopy should be part of the work-up because there is a 2 to 3% incidence of synchronous cancers and about a 40% chance of an adenoma's being present.

There is a search to identify specific tumor markers of colorectal cancer, but this has been relatively unsuccessful. The carcinoembryonic antigen (CEA) is a marker of extensive or metastatic cancer, but, unfortunately, it is produced in only about 80% of colon cancers.

### STAGING

In 1932, Cuthbert Dukes, a pathologist, described a classification of rectal cancer. The cancers were staged as A, B, or C lesions. The A lesion refers to growth into, but not through, the rectal wall. The B lesion penetrates the rectal or colonic wall. The C lesion has associated cancer in the lymph nodes. There have been many modifications of the Dukes' classification, especially with subsets of the B and C stages. Some people have added a D classification for distant metastasis. The TNM classification better defines the level of bowel wall invasion. T (for tumor) describes five levels of invasion into the wall. N (for nodes) is either positive or zero. M (metastasis) again is either present or not. With this information, prognosis can be predicted.

Ordinarily, there is an orderly progression of disease. Initially, there is local spread, which means circumferential growth around the wall and finally through the wall. Thereafter, lymph nodes become involved. Hematogenous spread allows tumor to metastasize, usually to the liver and the lung. A 5 to 10% metastasis rate is found in patients who undergo exploration of the abdomen for a colorectal cancer.

### TREATMENT

Benign polyps can be excised locally. Distal polyps can be removed via the sigmoidoscope, and those at a higher position can be removed through colonosocopy. Large sessile polyps may be removed piecemeal by snaring.

Patients believed to have curable cancer should be treated by colectomy. The amount of bowel removed is dependent on the colonic segment's vascular supply. The lymphatics tend to parallel the visible arteries and veins, and, by removing these, the involved lymphatics and nodes can be included in the specimen. Small lesions located low in the rectum and not overlying the vagina may be cured by local excision. Endorectal ultrasound has been an objective method for verifying the findings by sigmoidoscopy and digital examination. Abdominal perineal resection is necessary for low-lying cancers that impinge on the sphincter mechanism. When cancer occurs at that level, the sphincter mechanism must be removed en bloc to achieve cure. Because there is no sphincter mechanism remaining, a colostomy must be fashioned. In recent years, the blood replaced at surgery has been incriminated as interfering with the immune system.

Palliative surgery may be entertained for those who have local pain, bleeding, or obstruction. When these findings are encountered, removal of the primary lesion often alleviates those symptoms. When bone or nerve roots deep in the retroperitoneum or the pelvis are invaded, palliative surgery fails to provide pain relief. In recurrent cancer, an isolated cancer site should be resected, regardless of its location in the body.

Preoperative work-up includes a physical examination to palpate the tumors to help make decisions regarding the appropriate treatment. Complete staging is done by the pathologist after the specimen has been removed. Yet the ultrasound, especially the endorectal ultrasound and the computed tomography studies have allowed better determination of whether there is local, nodal, or distant metastasis prior to beginning the operation. Hence, the tumor can sometimes be staged preoperatively.

Radiation therapy has minimal use in the colorectum. However, in rectal cancer, there is a modest increase in survival shown in studies using radiation as preoperative or postoperative adjuvant therapy. Needless to say, radiation therapy has complications of its own and should not be undertaken lightly.

Chemotherapy as an adjuvant has not been particularly successful. 5-Fluororacil (5-FU) has been available for 30 years, and no great improvement in survival has been demonstrated. Long-term infusion, as opposed to intermittent peripheral injections, may produce some increase in survival time. Many drugs have been tried in the treatment of colorectal cancer, but until recently none have worked any better than 5-FU alone. Combination therapy may have an improved yield in survival. Recently, the combination of levamisole and 5-FU used after surgery in those patients who have nodal involvement has shown an increase in 5-year survival from 38% to 49%. This is a statistically significant improvement. Another exception is the combination of 5-FU, semustine (methyl CCNU), and vincristine (Oncovin), which improves disease-free survival and overall survival time in males.

Modification of the immune mechanism has been attempted as a treatment to allow the host better ability to attack the tumor cells. Interferon, interleukins, and monoclonal antibodies are being studied in research centers to effect change in the immune system.

### FOLLOW-UP

Of the patients who have had a colorectal cancer resected, half will be cured. Early detection of recurrences and institution of additional therapy give the patient the best chance for retreatment to achieve cure. The history and physical examination may reveal symptoms similar to those mentioned under "Diagnosis." The CEA, although not useful in screening, may be used as a marker for tumor escape. For example, if there is an elevation of the CEA level, which drops to normal after surgery, and later becomes elevated, a metastasis must be surmised and appropriate studies instituted.

Because of the propensity for those patients who have had a cancer or a polyp to subsequently have additional lesions, a surveillance program is advisable. Currently, colonoscopy is usually performed at 3-year intervals to look for metachronous neoplasms.

# INTESTINAL PARASITES

method of
FRANK J. BIA, M.D., M.P.H., and
MICHÉLE BARRY, M.D.
*Yale University*
*New Haven, Connecticut*

There is a broad range of intestinal parasitic infections caused by organisms that vary in size from invasive unicellular protozoa to large nematodes capable of causing mechanical obstruction. The significance of these parasitic infections, in both industrialized and developing countries, is expanding owing to increasing travel, tourism, and commerce. The era of allograft transplantation and potent immunosuppressive regimens for prevention of graft rejection has provided new opportunities for both enhancement and dissemination of these infections. The continuing epidemic of acquired immune deficiency syndrome (AIDS) has produced a group of chronically compromised hosts for whom intestinal parasitic infections threaten dissemination.

### EXPOSURE

The classic questions in the diagnosis of intestinal parasitic infection have been directed at obtaining a history of recent or remote travel, including the locations of prior military service. Many intestinal parasitic infections are long-lived, and they may disseminate if immunosuppression occurs. A history should consider factors such as previous blood transfusions, sexual preferences, and use of drugs associated with the sharing of intravenous needles—all are risk factors for acquisition of human immunodeficiency virus (HIV) infections. An additional question might be: "What medications are you taking?"—looking specifically for the use of immunosuppressive agents. Swimming in slow-moving fresh water poses a risk of schistosomiasis in some tropical countries. Farm animals, such as pigs, could transmit *Balantidium coli* infection. Dietary preferences for undercooked or raw foods may be the source for tapeworms, trichinosis, or anisakiasis. Children are increasingly exposed to day-care centers where infections with intestinal parasites such as *Cryptosporidium* are readily spread. Migrant workers and recent immigrants often carry evidence of their previous exposures to multiple parasitic infections.

### SYMPTOMS

Intestinal parasitic infection might present with a specific symptom complex. More often, they are either asymptomatic, nonspecific in their presentations, or associated with symptoms of concurrent parasitic or bacterial infections. Occasionally, a silent gastrointestinal infection is heralded by metastatic infection in visceral organs (amebic liver abscess) or brain (neurocysticercosis, trichinosis). Migration of an adult parasite or passage of an identifiable worm segment in stool (tapeworm proglottid) aids in diagnosis. Adult *Ascaris* can migrate through suture lines or be passed per mouth or rectum. *Anasakis, Trichuris,* and *Enterobius* adults are smaller than *Ascaris,* but can be readily identified when retrieved.

Upper gastrointestinal midepigastric discomfort suggests giardiasis or stronglyoidiasis, both of which may become chronic infections. Fever and blood in stools are not associated with these infections. Lower abdominal pain, fever, and passage of blood and mucus per rectum suggest dysentery caused by invasive bacterial or protozoal disease in the colon. Inflammatory bowel disease, such as ulcerative colitis or regional enteritis

TABLE 1. **Drug Therapy for Intestinal Protozoan Parasites**[1]

| Parasite | Drug | Adult Dose[2] | Pediatric Dose[2] | Availability |
|---|---|---|---|---|
| *Balantidium coli* | Tetracycline[3] or | As per *D. fragilis* | As per *D. fragilis* | |
| | Iodoquinol[3] or | As per *D. fragilis* | As per *D. fragilis* | Yodoxin (Glenwood, Inc.) |
| | Metronidazole | 750 mg tid × 5 days | 35–50 mg/kg/day in 3 divided doses × 5 days | Flagyl (Searle) |
| *Blastocystis hominis* | Iodoquinol or | As per *D. fragilis* | As per *D. fragilis* | |
| | Metronidazole | 750 mg tid × 10 days | 35–50 mg/kg/day in 3 divided doses × 10 days | Flagyl (Searle) |
| *Cryptosporidium* | Spiramycin[4] | 3 grams/day in divided doses for 2–4 wk | As per *E. histolytica* for 5 days | Rovamycine (Rhone-Poulenc/Montreal) (tablets) |
| | Octreotide | | 300–500 µg tid subcutaneously (controls diarrhea) | Sandostatin (Sandoz) (injection) |
| *Dientamoeba fragilis* | Iodoquinol or | 650 mg tid × 20 days or | 40 mg/kg/day in 3 divided doses × 20 days (max, 2 grams per day [use only for children over 8 yr of age]) | Yodoxin (Glenwood, Inc.) (tablets) |
| | Tetracycline or | 500 mg qid × 10 days or | 10 mg/kd qid × 10 days (max, 2 grams/day [use only for children over 8 yr of age]) | |
| | Paromomycin | 25–30 mg/kg/day in 3 doses × 7 days | 25–30 mg/kg/day in 3 doses × 7 days | Humatin (Parke-Davis) (tablets) |
| *Entamoeba histolytica* | See separate article on amebiasis | | | |
| *Giardia lamblia* | Quinacrine HCl or | 100 mg p.c. tid × 5 days | 2 mg/kg p.c. tid × 5 days (max. 300 mg/day) | Atabrine (Winthrop-Breon) (tablets) |
| | Metronidazole[3] | 250 mg tid × 5 days | 5 mg/kg tid × 5 days | Flagyl (Searle) (tablets) |
| | Furazolidone | 100 mg (tablet) qid × 7–10 days | 1.25 mg/kg qid × 7–10 days (suspension) | Furoxone (Norwich-Eaton) (tablets and suspension) |
| *Isospora belli* | Trimethoprim-sulfamethoxazole[3] (TMP-SMX) or | 160 mg TMP and 800 mg SMX qid × 10 days, then bid × 3 weeks; chronic suppression with 1 tablet daily may be necessary in immunocompromised patients | | Bactrim (Roche) Septra (Burroughs Wellcome) (tablets) |
| | Pyrimethamine | 50–75 mg daily for sulfonamide-sensitive patients | | Daraprim (Burroughs Wellcome) (tablets) |

[1]Adapted from previous editions of this text and The Medical Letter *32*:23–32, 1990.
[2]All recommended drugs given by mouth.
[3]Considered investigational for this indication by the FDA.
[4]Not approved in the United States. Permission to use this drug must be obtained from the FDA, telephone 301–443–4310. *Cryptosporidium* is self-limited in immunocompetent patients (see text).

exacerbated by traveler's diarrhea, could present similarly. If antibiotic treatment has already been initiated, antibiotic associated colitis, caused by *Clostridium difficile* toxin, is suspect.

The presence of gastrointestinal bleeding is a significant finding. When acute traveler's diarrhea is associated with passage of blood and mucus per rectum, invasive infections of the colon are suspect (amebic or bacterial dysentery). Upper gastrointestinal bleeding is less common, but has been noted with acute gastric anisakiasis acquired from raw or undercooked fish.

Any process that causes portal hypertension, such as chronic hepatic schistosomiasis, could present as a serious variceal bleed. Acute traveler's diarrhea is more likely to be both bacterial in origin and self-limited. Should more chronic symptoms occur, giardiasis, heavy *Blastocystis hominis* infection, or strongly-loidiasis must be considered. *Campylobacter* (now called *Helicobacter*) species can cause relapsing gastrointestinal infections. However, chronic infectious processes could be confused with a simple postinfectious irritable bowel syndrome or a serious nonpara-

TABLE 2. **Drug Therapy for Intestinal Helminths**[1]

| Parasite | Drug | Adult Dose[2] | Pediatric Dose[2] | Availability |
|---|---|---|---|---|
| *Anisakis* | Surgical removal | | | |
| *Ascaris lumbricoides* | Mebendazole or | 100 mg bid × 3 days | Same as adult dose (for children over 2 yr) | Vermox (Janssen) (tablets) |
| | Pyrantel pamoate or | 11 mg/kg single dose (max, 1 gram) | Same as adult dose (max, 1 gram) | Antiminth (Pfizer) (suspension) |
| | Piperazine citrate | 75 mg/kg/day × 2 days (max, 3.5 grams/day) | Same as adult dose (max, 3.5 grams/day) | Antepar (Burroughs Wellcome) (syrup) |
| *Enterobius vermicularis* (pinworm) | Pyrantel pamoate or | 11 mg/kg single dose; (max, 1 gram; repeat after 2 wk) | Same as adult dose (max, 1 gram) | |
| | Mebendazole | 100 mg single dose; repeat after 2 wk | Same as adult dose (for children over 2 yr) | |
| Hookworm: | | | | |
| *Necator americanus* and | Mebendazole or | As per *Ascaris* | As per *Ascaris* | |
| *Ancylostoma duodenale* | Pyrantel pamoate[3] | As per *Ascaris* daily for 3 days | As per *Ascaris* daily for 3 days | |
| Intestinal flukes: | | | | |
| *Fasciolopsis buski* | Praziquantel[3] or | 25 mg/kg tid for 1 day | Same as adult dose | Bitricide (Miles) (tablets) |
| | Niclosamide | As per *T. saginata* | As per *T. saginata* | Niclocide, Yomesan (Miles) (tablets) |
| *Heterophyes heterophyes* | Praziquantel | As per *F. buski* | As per *F. buski* | |
| *Metagonimus yokogawai* | Praziquantel | As per *F. buski* | As per *F. buski* | |
| Liver flukes: | | | | |
| *Clonorchis sinensis* *Opisthorchis viverini* | Praziquantel[3] | 25 mg/kg tid for 2 days | Same as adult dose | |
| *Fasciola hepatica* | Bithionol[3, 4] | 30 to 50 mg/kg on alternate days × 10 to 15 doses | Same as adult dose | Bitin (Parasitic Disease Service, Centers for Disease Control, Atlanta, GA) (tablets) |
| Schistosomiasis: | | | | |
| *Schistosoma mansoni* | Praziquantel or | 20 mg/kg bid for 1 day | Same as adult dose | Biltricide (Miles) (tablets) |
| | Oxamniquine | Caribbean & South American strains: 15 mg/kg single dose | 10 mg/kg bid | Vansil (Pfipharmecs) (tablets) |
| | | African strains: 15 mg/kg bid × 1 day East Africa; × 2 days Egypt and South Africa | Same as adult dose | |

sitic illness, such as tropical sprue, ulcerative colitis, or regional enteritis (Crohn's disease). Eosinophilia is a distinctly uncommon finding in association with infections with luminal intestinal parasites such as *Giardia lamblia* or *Cryptosporidium*. It is more commonly associated with migrating or invasive larvae (e.g., trichinosis, toxicariasis).

## TREATMENT

Currently recommended therapy for both intestinal protozoa and helminth infections is summarized in Tables 1 and 2.

**Anisakiasis.** Larvae of certain roundworms infecting marine animals can be acquired by humans from raw or undercooked fish of many species, causing acute gastric anisakiasis within hours. The motile larval roundworm is detected in the human stomach wall by upper endoscopy and must be removed via this procedure or surgical resection because no effective form of chemotherapy yet exists. A chronic intestinal form of the disease may occur following an acute intestinal syndrome and there is no effective drug for treating this disease. Freezing fish at $-10°$ C for a week kills most larvae.

**Amebiasis.** This infection is discussed in Section 2.

**Ascariasis.** These large adult roundworms usually live for less than 1 year in the small bowel. In cases of multiple infection with additional parasites, *Ascaris* should be treated first because some agents may cause these nematodes to migrate into the biliary pancreatic tree. Mebendazole (Vermox) and pyrantel pamoate (Antiminth)

TABLE 2. **Drug Therapy for Intestinal Helminths**[1] *Continued*

| Parasite | Drug | Adult Dose[2] | Pediatric Dose[2] | Availability |
|---|---|---|---|---|
| *Schistosoma japonicum* | Praziquantel | 20 mg/kg tid for 1 day | Same as adult dose | |
| *Schistoma mekongi* | Praziquantel | As per *S. japonicum* | As per *S. japonicum* | |
| *Schistosoma haemato-bium* | Praziquantel | As per *S. mansoni* | As per *S. mansoni* | |
| *Strongyloides stercoralis* | Thiabendazole | 25 mg/kg bid × 2 days (max, 3 grams/day)[5] | Same as adult dose | Mintezol (Merck, Sharp and Dohme) (tablets) |
| Tapeworms: | | | | |
| *Taenia saginata* | Niclosamide | Single dose of 4 tablets | 11–34 kg: single dose of | Niclocide, Yomesan |
| *Taenia solium* | or | (2 grams) chewed thor- | 2 tablets (1 gram); >34 | (Miles) (tablets) |
| *Diphyllobothrium latum and pacificum* | | oughly | kg: single dose of 3 tablets (1.5 grams) | |
| *Dipylidium caninum* | Praziquantel[3] | 10 to 20 mg/kg once | Same as adult dose | Biltricide (Miles) (tablets) |
| *Hymenolepis nana* | Praziquantel[3] or | 25 mg/kg once | Same as adult dose | |
| | Niclosamide | Single 2-gram dose (4 tablets) followed by 1 gram (2 tablets) daily × 6 days | 11–34 kg: single dose of 2 tablets (1 gram) × 1 day then 1 tablet (0.5 gram) daily × 6 days; >34 kg: single dose of 3 tablets (1.5 grams) × 1 day, then 2 tablets (1 gram) daily × 6 days | |
| *Trichostrongylus* sp. | Pyrantel pamoate | As per *Ascaris* | As per *Ascaris* | |
| | Thiabendazole | As per *Strongyloides* | As per *Strongyloides* | |
| *Trichuris trichiura* | Mebendazole | As per *Ascaris* | As per *Ascaris* | |

[1]Adapted from previous editions of this text and The Medical Letter *32*:23–32, 1990.

[2]All recommended drugs given by mouth.

[3]Considered investigational for this indication by the FDA.

[4]Limited data indicate that albendazole may be helpful and triclabendazole (Fasinex), a veterinary agent, may also be effective.

[5]For disseminated strongyloidiasis, thiabendazole should be continued for at least 5 days.

are well tolerated; the former may cause abdominal discomfort, diarrhea, and, rarely, leukopenia, agranulocytosis, or hypospermia. Pyrantel pamoate may cause some gastrointestinal disturbance, headache, rash, dizziness, or fever. Piperazine salts (many manufacturers) cure more than 90% of uncomplicated infections; occasionally gastrointestinal and central nervous system effects may occur (vertigo, difficulty in focusing, incoordination, and confusion). Epileptic patients could develop an exacerbation of seizures while taking piperazine salts.

During heavy *Ascaris* infection, intestinal obstruction or volvulus caused by a large mass of worms require piperazine therapy (150 mg per kg [75 mg/kg for 2 consecutive days], up to 3.5 grams maximum) via a nasogastric tube. Complete obstruction may require emergency surgery. Biliary and pancreatic disease are managed more conservatively with intravenous fluids, antispasmodics, and piperazine as outlined earlier; the worm may return to the duodenum. Endoscopic retrograde cholangiopancreatography (ERCP) and papillotomy could be required for helminth removal. After 2 weeks of conservative therapy, surgery may be required.

***Balantidum coli* Infection.** Infection with these large ciliated protozoa occurs mostly in developing countries and areas where there is close human contact with pigs and their excrement. As with amebiasis, the organisms may either live as commensuals or cause dysentery. Visceral invasion and intestinal perforation are rare. Tetracyclines and iodoquinol (Yodoxin) are effective therapy; metronidazole (Flagyl) has not been consistently effective.

***Blastocystis hominis* Infection.** Controversy exists regarding the status of this organism as a human pathogen. In small numbers, these parasites may cause asymptomatic infection. Treatment is indicated when otherwise unexplained diarrhea is associated with large numbers of organisms in stool. Therapy with a 3-week course of iodoquinol (Yodoxin) is effective, and metronidazole (Flagyl) for 10 days is a useful alternative. To avoid optic neuritis, the maximal dosage of 2 grams per day of iodoquinol should not be exceeded. This drug is contraindicated in patients with iodine intolerance or hepatic disease. It may also cause thyroid enlargement and interfere with thyroid function test results. Treating asymptomatic patients with *Blastocystis* is not indicated unless they are possible sources for transmission, such as food handlers.

**Cryptosporidosis.** The coccidia include three genera (*Isospora*, *Cryptosporidium*, and *Sarcocystis*), which may cause diarrhea and some abdominal discomfort. *Cryptosporidium* multiplies on the surface of epithelial cells in the intestine without invading tissue. Acute infection in normal hosts clears spontaneously within days to weeks. In U.S. day-care centers, prevalence ranges from 6 to 54%. *Cryptosporidium* infects as many as 7% of children in the developing world. Clinical infection may be mistaken for giardiasis or isosporiasis. Cysts are easily missed in stool samples; they are colorless in fresh iodine mounts, but stain with Kinyoun's acid fast technique.

In AIDS patients, *Cryptosporidia* infections persist, causing a chronic cholera-like diarrhea and producing a large volume of watery bowel movements daily. The resulting dehydration, wasting, and cachexia accelerate the demise of some AIDS patients. Immunocompromised patients can also develop cryptosporidial cholecystitis and cholangitis.

Therapy for cryptosporidiosis is not satisfactory. Resolution of infection is largely dependent on reversal of the immunocompromised state. Spiramycin (Rovamycine) is available from the manufacturer (Rhone-Poulenc Pharmaceuticals, Montreal, Canada 514–384–8220) after permission has been obtained from the Division of Anti-Infective Drug Products, U. S. Food and Drug Administration (301–443–4310). Somatostatin (Octreotide, Sandostatin)* is under investigation for control of the profuse diarrheal symptoms of the disease in AIDS patients.

**Dientamoeba fragilis Infections.** This organism is a noninvasive intestinal ameboflagellate related to *Trichomonas*. Prevalence rates for infection in North America range from 4 to 9%. Most infections are asymptomatic, but some are associated with abdominal discomfort and mild or explosive diarrhea. Iodoquinol (Yodoxin), tetracycline, or paromomycin (Humatin) is effective, as are the dosages of metronidazole (Flagyl) used to treat amebiasis.

**Enterobius vermicularis (Pinworm) Infection.** Infections are most common among children between the ages of 5 and 10, particularly in temperate climates and in overcrowded conditions. In women, worm migration may result in vaginitis, endometritis, or salpingitis. Several members of a household may require therapy to eliminate the organism from a family.

Pyrantel pamoate (Antiminth) as a single dose, repeated in 2 weeks, will cure most infections. Because mature worms are more susceptible to

drug therapy than are developing worms, the second dose is required to achieve 95% cure rates. Recurrent persistent infections may require multiple courses of therapy for all family members. Similar cure rates can be achieved with mebendazole (Vermox), but because of limited experience it is only used in children older than 2 years. Personal hygiene and laundering of bedclothes, sheets, and towels to kill ova are important control measures.

**Flukes.** The synthetic isoquinoline-pyrazine praziquantel (Biltricide) is effective against all liver, lung, and intestinal flukes,* but a role in the treatment of *Fasciola hepatica* infections is not certain. This drug alters calcium permeability, causing paralysis of worm musculature and death, but not for *F. hepatica*. Side effects are mild and transient, including headache, sedation, gastrointestinal upset, pruritis, rashes, and eosinophilia. Children tolerate the drug well. Bithionol (Bitin)† is an investigational alternative drug for *Fasciola* infections, but it is associated with vomiting, abdominal pain, diarrhea, urticaria, and photosensitivity.

**Giardia lamblia Infection.** This parasite is the most common intestinal protozoal pathogen in the United States and Europe and is ubiquitous in its distribution throughout the world. Transmission is largely via ingestion of cysts present in contaminated fresh water. Travelers on vacation may not develop symptoms until their return home. Hikers, campers, children in day-care centers, male homosexuals, and those with congenital IgA deficiency are at increased risk of acquiring symptomatic infection. Water-borne outbreaks have occurred in cities when filtration systems failed. Cysts are viable for months at cold temperatures. The malabsorptive acute diarrhea may progress to a more chronic pattern of gastrointestinal disturbances, which can last for years. Lactose intolerance, resulting from giardiasis, may require months to resolve after eradication of the parasite. Diagnosis usually is made by finding cysts or trophozoites in stool samples. Duodenal aspiration or biopsy of the small bowel may be necessary for diagnosis.

Quinacrine (Atabrine) is the most effective drug available in the United States, achieving cure rates of 95%. Alcohol intake is contraindicated owing to a disulfiram-like reaction. Children do not tolerate this agent as well as adults. Side effects include headache, diarrhea, nightmares, dizziness, and possibly toxic psychosis (1.5%). It should be avoided in those with a

---

*This use of Octreotide is not listed in the manufacturer's official directive.

*This use of praziquantel is not listed in the manufacturer's official directive.

†Can be obtained from the Centers for Disease Control 404–639–3670.

history of neuropsychiatric disorders. Fever and rash are described, but yellowing of the skin is generally not seen with the usual dosages used to treat giardiasis. Psoriasis and porphyria may be exacerbated by this drug. If giardiasis definitely requires treatment during pregnancy, quinacrine is likely the safest of the available agents, although therapy during pregnancy should be avoided when possible.

Metronidazole (Flagyl) achieves only slightly lower cure rates (85%) than quinacrine, and the drugs are considered about equally effective. Side effects include headache, gastrointestinal upset, a metallic after-taste, and a disulfiram-like reaction if taken with alcohol. It is mutagenic and carcinogenic in animals, and use is best avoided during pregnancy, particularly during the first trimester. Although short course therapy for giardiasis (2 grams per day for 3 days) may be effective, it is neither necessary nor recommended. If available, tinidazole (Fasigyn), another nitroimidazole, is effective as single-dose therapy (2 grams for adults; 30 to 35 mg per kg for children) and is better tolerated.*

Furazolidone (Furoxone) is an alternative therapy for giardiasis, which is slightly less effective than the above agents, but is available in liquid form for children. Adverse reactions include disulfiram-like reactions and hemolysis in glucose-6-phosphate dehydrogenase–deficient patients. Headache, nausea, vomiting, and allergic reactions, including pulmonary infiltrates, are described.

In patients with apparently chronic or persistent infections, congenital IgA deficiency and lactose intolerance secondary to giardiasis must be considered. Combined therapy for 10 days to 2 weeks with metronizadole and quinacrine could be attempted if giardiasis clearly persists after therapy with a single agent.

**Hookworms.** Regardless of the intensity of hookworm infection, treatment should include both antihelminthic agents and iron to correct anemia. For severe disease, parenteral iron and supplemental folate may also be required to reverse anemia. Mebendazole and pyrantel pamoate are both effective. These agents will also treat any accompanying *Ascaris* infection without inducing migration of this nematode.

*Isospora belli* is another human coccidial parasite. It develops within intestinal mucosal cells and, like *Cryptosporidium,* may cause acute watery diarrhea or result in a chronic syndrome in immunocompromised patients. In acute diarrhea, up to 50% of patients may have eosinophilia, which should suggest this diagnosis. Treatment

with the combination trimethoprim-sulfamethoxazole is useful and it should be continued for 3 weeks. Long-term suppression may be required for immunocompromised patients. Those who have become allergic to sulfonamides can be given pyrimethamine (Daraprim)* 50 to 75 mg daily, which can be used on a long-term basis for maintenance therapy. These patients require monitoring for development of leukopenia.

**Sarcocystosis.** This infection is another form of human coccidiosis caused by *Sarcocystis* species. These are ingested by humans as sporocysts present in the feces of an infected carnivore. Myositis may result from infection of human striated muscle and can be accompanied by fever and eosinophilia. Human enteric infections are generally mild with nonspecific symptoms, and diagnosis is made on finding the sporocysts in stool. Treatment of enteric infections is not satisfactory, and shedding of sporocysts may continue for up to 6 months.

**Schistosomiasis.** Praziquantel (Biltricide) is useful for all forms of schistosomiasis. Patients shedding ova harbor adult worms which can usually be eliminated, with a single day of therapy. Cure rates at 3 to 6 months are 63 to 100%, and schistosomiasis resistance to praziquantel is not observed. Praziquantel is well tolerated, but can cause malaise, dizziness, or drowsiness. Animal data dictate against use during pregnancy. Lactating women treated with praziquantel should not nurse on the day of treatment and for 3 days after the drug is given. Oxamniquine (Vansil), a semisynthetic hydroquinoline, is equally as effective for *S. mansoni* infections, but neuropsychiatric disturbances and seizures have been reported in some patients. Dizziness is the most common side effect.

***Strongyloides stercoralis* Infection.** This nematode has a life cycle which includes autoinfection of its human host, permitting chronic infections, which may last for decades. Mild eosinophilia and skin eruptions are clues to chronic infections. Under immunosuppressive regimens to prevent organ transplant rejection, hyperinfection and larval dissemination may occur in association with gram-negative bacteremias and meningitis. Larvae, not ova, are identified in stool samples, duodenal contents, small bowel biopsy specimens, or sputum. In light infections, serum antibody determinations may be useful in identifying patients who have resided in endemic areas, become infected, and are at risk should they receive immunosuppressive therapy.

For most uncomplicated infections, thiabenda-

---

*Not available in the United States.

*This use of Daraprim is not listed in the manufacturer's official directive.

zole (Mintezol) for 2 days is effective. For disseminated infections, often occurring in the compromised host, therapy for at least 5 days is required, until stools are free of larvae. If immunosuppression cannot be reversed and the nematode cannot be eradicated, monthly 2-day courses of thiabendazole have been suggested to prevent hyperinfection. Tablets must be chewed well. An oral suspension (Mintezol) is available. *Ascaris* may migrate during therapy if not first eliminated. Side effects of thiabendazole are mild and transient. Most common are dizziness and gastrointestinal syndromes. Erythema multiforme has occurred in children. Rarely cholestatic jaundice has occurred. When they become available, ivermectin* and albendazole* are two new alternatives with activity against *Strongyloides stercoralis*.

In patients from Southeast Asia and the Phillipines, in particular, intestinal capillariasis may be mistaken for strongyloidiasis. This infection is likely transmitted in raw or undercooked fish and may progress to malabsorption and a protein-losing enteropathy. Ova, larvae, or adult *Capillaria philippinensis* worms are found in stool. Thiabendazole therapy is unfortunately associated with relapses in about one-third of patients. Preferred treatment is mebendazole (Vermox), 200 mg orally twice daily for 20 days.

**Tapeworms.** For adult intestinal tapeworm infections, including *Diphyllobothrium latum* (fish), *Taenia saginata* (beef), *T. solim* (pork), and *Dipylidium caninum* (dog), a single dose of niclosamide (Niclocide) or praziquantel (Biltricide) is effective therapy. The dwarf tapeworm, *Hymenolepis nana,* should be treated with praziquantel, now actually the drug of choice for all tapeworm infections. Cure rates are close to 100%. If niclosamide is used as alternative therapy, drug tablets should be chewed well and swallowed with a small amount of water on an empty stomach. Meals on the day prior to therapy should be light, with only liquids on the evening prior to treatment. Purging is not necessary following therapy. Theoretically, *T. solium* proglottid disintegration and release of ova during therapy could cause autoinfection with risk of cysticercosis, so purging is recommended in treating this infection. Niclosamide may cause nausea and some abdominal discomfort. Paromomycin (Humatin)* (75 mg per kg,† to a maximal dose of 4 grams) is an alternative when the other two agents are unavailable, or during pregnancy, as it is not well absorbed. The cure rate is more than 90%, and the major side effect is diarrhea.

*Trichuris trichuria* (Whipworm) Infections. These are seen commonly in association with other nematode infections, such as hookworm and *Ascaris* infections. Adult worms reside in the cecum and upper colon. Appendicitis has resulted from heavy infections. Iron deficiency anemia has occurred in heavily infected children whose diarrhea and tenesmus may be severe enough to cause rectal prolapse. A 3-day course of mebendazole has an expected cure rate of 60 to 80%. Both *Ascaris* and hookworm infections are also treated with this regimen.

**Nonpathogenic Protozoa.** It is important to understand the problems that are associated with classifying "nonpathogens." At one time, *G. lamblia* was incorrectly considered such. Immunodeficient states, such as those associated with AIDS or prevention of transplant rejection, may alter the pathogenesis of any such infections. These "nonpathogenic" amebae and flagellates are usually not associated with symptoms of intestinal carriage by the normal host, nor do these organisms require therapy. If encountered, however, by inexperienced technicians, they could be confused with pathogenic organisms. These species include *Entamoeba coli, lodamoeba butschlii, Endolimax nana,* and *Chilomastix mesnili.* Their importance as a clinical finding for patients is that their presence serves as a useful indicator of fecal contamination of food and water supplies.

---

*Not available in the United States.

*This use of Humatin is not listed in the manufacturer's official directive.

†Exceeds dosage recommended by the manufacturer.

# Metabolic Disorders

## BERIBERI

method of
KAMALA KRISHNASWAMY, M.D.
*National Institute of Nutrition*
*Hyderabad, India*

The disease beriberi has been known for centuries. It was Takaki of Japan who described in detail the clinical syndrome of beriberi and related it to the introduction of polished rice in the diet. Eijkman later (1890–1897) described the experimental counterpart in fowls, which, when fed on polished rice, developed polyneuritic symptoms. Grijins cured the disease in fowls with rice polishings. It was Funk who isolated the material from rice polishings and coined the name "vitamin." Later, the crystalline form was obtained and the structure was clearly delineated. Beriberi (Singhalese for "I cannot" or "extreme weakness") is a disease of antiquity of rice-eating populations. The epidemiology of the disease is related to consumption of rice diet and alcohol.

### BIOCHEMISTRY AND FUNCTIONS

Thiamine, a water-soluble crystalline compound, is a pyrimidine-substituted thiazole with a pyrimidyl ring joined by a methylene bridge to a thiazole nucleus. The free vitamin is a base, and the principal coenzyme form is the pyrophosphate ester. It is readily absorbed in the small intestine by an active transport process that is probably carrier mediated. The free vitamin is present in plasma, and the coenzyme thiamine pyrophosphate (TPP) predominates in the cellular components. About 30 mg of thiamine are found in the body, of which 80% is pyrophosphates, 10% is triphosphate, and the rest is free thiamine/monophosphates. More than 50% of thiamine is found in skeletal muscles, and the rest is distributed in heart, liver, kidney, and nervous tissues, which contain mostly triphosphate. The multienzyme dehydrogenase complexes that effect decarboxylation conversion require TPP, and it is an important vitamin in the intermediary metabolism. TPP is the coenzyme for pyruvate dehydrogene, transketolase, and α-ketoglutarate dehydrogenase. Although much is known about the function of thiamine in metabolism, the basis for the manifestation of deficiency symptoms is largely unknown.

### FOOD SOURCES

Thiamine is found in most forms of life. Rich sources are lean meat, pork, beans, peas, nuts, whole-grain cereals, and organ meats like liver, heart, kidney, and brain. Thiamine, however, can be easily lost or destroyed before or during cooking. Twenty to 30% of the vitamin is lost during boiling, roasting, refining, dehydrating, and canning. An adequate intake will therefore depend on quality and quantity of foods consumed, cooking practices, and consumption of processed and stored food. Available evidence indicates that recommended dietary allowances are approximately 0.4 to 0.5 mg per 1000 calories. Thiamine requirement increases with increasing carbohydrate intake.

### THIAMINE DEFICIENCY SYNDROMES

Beriberi generally occurs in two distinct forms, wet and dry, in which the cardiovascular and nervous systems are affected, respectively. The wet cardiovascular beriberi can present as high-output or low-output failure and the dry beriberi as polyneuropathy, infantile beriberi, and Wernicke-Korsakoff's syndrome. The manifestations of deficiency appear to be related to the degree of deprivation, although for reasons unknown, the two forms rarely occur in the same patient. Severe deficiency often leads to encephalopathy and Korsakoff's psychosis, and less severe and perhaps chronic deficiency leads to beriberi heart disease and polyneuritis.

#### Occurrence

Classic beriberi as encountered in Asian rice-eating populations has disappeared to a great extent. The acute forms are rarely encountered, although the chronic entities are often seen, particularly in alcoholics. It can occur in populations with inadequate intakes of thiamine and faulty cooking practices, or it is associated with malabsorption and wasting diseases. There are several recent reports of its occurrence in Africa, particularly during lean seasons, in migrant workers. It can occur when energy requirement and expenditure go up considerably. Foods rich in thiaminases (raw fish) or antithiamine substances (fermented tea leaves) can precipitate thiamine deficiency. Being a heat labile and water soluble compound, thiamine can easily be denatured or lost if cooked at very high temperatures in excess water which is thrown away as waste water. Infants, adolescents, pregnant women, and the elderly can easily experience thiamine deficiency.

Recent reports indicate that beriberi can occur as a complication of total parenteral nutrition (TPN). Patients who are marginally nourished when they receive glucose intravenously without sufficient thiamine can develop fulminant forms of wet beriberi characterized by shock, cardiac failure, hyperlactic acidemia, and metabolic acidosis.

Primary or secondary thiamine deficiency that occurs in association with chronic diseases often takes a long time to develop, allowing metabolic adaptation to take place. The significance of subclinical thiamine status as assessed by biochemical parameters remains controversial. Further, the diagnosis of beriberi may be overlooked in cases of congestive heart failure and cardiomyopathy of unknown or undefined etiology and alcoholic cardiomyopathy. Thiamine deficiency is described in fulminant hepatic failures and in patients with chronic liver diseases.

There are several thiamine-responsive inborn errors of metabolism which include megaloblastic anemia of unknown mechanisms, lactic acidosis, and subacute necrotizing encephalomyelopathy (lack of thiamine triphosphate).

## CLINICAL PROFILE

The clinical signs and symptoms and the causes of the disease are extremely variable. The wet form occurs with physical exertion and high carbohydrate intake, whereas the dry, or polyneuritic, form occurs with relative inactivity and calorie restriction.

### Wet Beriberi

The most common high-output state manifests signs and symptoms of biventricular heart failure, the right side being affected more than the left, resulting in dyspnea, orthopnea, pulmonary rales, sinus tachycardia wide pulse pressure, and peripheral vasoconstriction with cold, cyanotic extremities and pedal edema. The low-output form is characterized by severe hypotension, lactic acidosis, and systemic vascular resistance. Peripheral edema is absent, and invariably the outcome is fatal. The acute form is termed "shoshin," or pernicious beriberi. The patient is severely dyspneic, complains of precordial pain, is restless with rapid but superficial respiration, has a weak pulse, as well as a systolic murmur and pistol shot sounds.

### Dry Beriberi

Dry beriberi involves the nervous system and presents with numbness of feet and heaviness of legs. Paresthesias develop in the hands and legs with sensation of pins and needles, tingling, and numbness, and tender calf muscles. Deep tendon reflexes may be exaggerated to begin with but disappear at later stages.

Glove-and-stocking type of anesthesia may be encountered, and muscle weakness occurs as foot- or wristdrop. Several factors appear to influence which areas are affected, such as the length of nerve fibers, amount of work done, and probably the blood supply. In advanced cases aphonia may be seen. Subclinical types with paresthesias and muscular pain are more often encountered.

### Infantile Beriberi

Infantile beriberi occurs in breast-fed infants between the second and fifth months. It is due to low thiamine content in breast milk. It may present in an acute cardiac form, often precipitated by infection. Death may occur within 24 to 48 hours. Aphonia is a characteristic feature. A chronic form may manifest itself as pseudomeningitis and convulsions with opisthotonus, edema, and head retraction. Infantile beriberi can also present as subacute necrotizing encephalomyelopathy (SNE). The relation of thiamine to SNE is not well established, and temporary remissions have been reported with thiamine supplementation.

## LABORATORY DIAGNOSIS

Urinary thiamine excretion correlates with dietary intake, and random urine samples can be collected and thiamine excretion related to creatinine excretion, particularly in community surveys involving a large population. Adults receiving adequate thiamine excrete more than 100 $\mu$g per 24 hours. The concentration of thiamine in blood may not be a sensitive index of thiamine nutriture; TPP concentration may be more sensitive. The best method now routinely employed to assess thiamine nutritional status is red cell transketolase activity and its in vitro stimulation by added TPP. Biochemical tests, such as the ratio of lactic to pyruvic acid after glucose load, have also been considered.

## TREATMENT

Severe manifestations of beriberi, such as cardiac failure or Wernicke's encephalopathy, can be treated by 10 to 20 mg of thiamine given intramuscularly several times daily. In infantile beriberi 2 to 5 mg of thiamine may lead to marked improvement within a few hours. In severe heart failure 20 to 25 mg of thiamine has been given intravenously. Oral administration of 5 to 10 mg two or three times a day will ensure maximum absorption of the vitamin for chronic or dry beriberi. Large doses of thiamine by the parenteral or oral route do not serve any additional purpose as the vitamin is not absorbed when taken by the external route and is excreted in urine when given by the parenteral route. Thiamine propyl disulfide has been observed to be better absorbed and retained with sustained response.

## TOXICITY

Thiamine is not toxic when administered by mouth. However, serious hypersensitivity reactions, particularly to large doses given by the parenteral route, are reported. Anaphylactic shock can occur with parenteral preparations. Megadoses of thiamine in the pharmacologic range must be regarded as potentially hazardous in humans.

## PREVENTION

Avoiding excessive milling and polishing of cereal grains can increase the thiamine intake from diets. Avoidance of faulty cooking practices and avoidance of consumption of excessive quantities of thiamine-poor refined foods, such as alcoholic drinks, carbonated beverages, and sugar, will improve thiamine status in general. Nutrition education and encouragement to follow a varied diet with sufficient thiamine-rich foods should be attempted in high-risk groups. Enrichment of flour and cereal grains has been tried. Parboiling of cereals and grains can preserve the vitamin. If subjects at risk can be identified, oral supplements may be regularly distributed. Thiamine fortification of alcoholic beverages has been suggested. However, the most desirable approach to meeting nutritional needs is using foods that are locally available and cheap and that improve dietary habits to provide a sufficient quantity of thiamine.

# DIABETES MELLITUS IN ADULTS

method of
DAVID M. NATHAN, M.D.
*Massachusetts General Hospital*
*Harvard Medical School*
*Boston, Massachusetts*

The estimated prevalences of 3.4% for diagnosed diabetes mellitus, 3.2% for undiagnosed diabetes, and 11.2% for impaired glucose tolerance (IGT) in persons 20 to 74 years old make disorders of glucose tolerance the most common diseases in the U.S. (Diabetes *36*:523–534, 1987). According to the National Diabetes Data Group (NDDG) criteria, the vast majority of the adult cases of diabetes are noninsulin dependent (Type II). Type II diabetes, in contrast to the etiologically distinct insulin-dependent (Type I) diabetes, is associated with older age and obesity and is secondary to a relative deficiency of insulin in combination with greater insulin requirements (insulin resistance). Table 1 describes the characteristics of Type I and Type II diabetes.

The extraordinary increase of Type II diabetes in the U.S., other industrialized nations, and recently "Westernized" populations is related to longevity and an increasingly sedentary lifestyle and its attendant obesity. The prevalence of diabetes in those 65- to 74-years old, the most rapidly growing segment of the U.S. population, approaches 20%.

While most patients with Type I diabetes diagnosed during childhood reach adulthood and a small but significant percentage of Type I patients develop their diabetes between ages 20 and 40, and, rarely, even later in life, the entire Type I population is less than 10% of the total adult diabetic population. Therefore, the treatment of diabetes in adults is predominantly the treatment of Type II diabetes.

## PATHOPHYSIOLOGY

In order to understand the treatment principles of diabetes, an appreciation of the pathophysiology of diabetes is important. Insulin acts by binding to specific cell surface receptors. Activation of the receptors involves one or more kinases that are part of the receptor. These kinases lead to the phosphorylation of other target proteins and the generation of putative second messengers. Ultimately, the expression of insulin activity in the cell involves the generation or activation of transport proteins (e.g., for glucose transport) or the activation of specific, generally anabolic enzymes such as glycogen synthetase.

In Type I diabetes, an absolute deficiency of insulin exists, secondary to the autoimmune destruction of insulin-producing pancreatic islet cells. In order to prevent catabolism, hyperglycemia with dehydration from osmotic diuresis, and ketoacidosis, patients are absolutely dependent on exogenous insulin. In Type II diabetes, patients generally require more insulin (i.e., they are insulin resistant secondary to obesity and other factors) and cannot synthesize enough to maintain normal metabolism. Type II diabetes is therefore characterized by a relative insulin deficiency. Although legitimate disagreement remains regarding the primary abnormality in Type II diabetes (abnormal insulin resistance or insulin secretory abnormalities), several studies have suggested that the earliest abnormality identifiable in impaired glucose tolerance may be insulin resistance. In order for diabetes with fasting hyperglycemia to develop, however, insulin secretory failure is necessary. Since patients with Type II diabetes continue to secrete some insulin (and may even have relatively high circulating insulin levels), they generally remain ketosis resistant and do not need exogenous insulin to sustain life. However, they may require insulin to normalize glucose metabolism.

A further advance in our understanding of the pathophysiology of Type II diabetes is that the abnormalities in insulin resistance and secretion are at least partially

TABLE 1. **Characteristics of Type I and Type II Diabetes**

|  | Type I | Type II |
| --- | --- | --- |
| Age at onset | Usually <20 | Usually >40 |
| Male:female ratio | 1:1 | 1:1 |
| Obesity | Rare | Common |
| Insulin requirement | Absolute | Variable |
| Ketosis | Common | Rare |
| Anti–islet cell antibodies | Positive | Negative |

reversible. Restoration of normal fasting blood glucose levels will reduce insulin resistance and improve insulin secretion. This improvement can be seen after diet therapy or sulfonylurea or insulin treatment. Thus, in Type II diabetes, improved glucose control begets improved glucose control.

## DIAGNOSIS AND SCREENING

Diagnosis of Type I diabetes is generally straightforward as patients usually present with symptoms of polyuria, polydipsia, fatigue, weight loss, and blurred vision concurrent with hyperglycemia. In the adult age population, however, the diagnosis of diabetes in a nonobese individual may be overlooked because presentation of Type I diabetes is unusual in this age group. Because the consequences of missing a diagnosis of Type I diabetes may be severe (i.e., development of ketoacidosis), physicians must be alert to the presentation of Type I diabetes in adults as well as children. Type I diabetes should be suspected in any thin, hyperglycemic patient. The presence of ketonuria in otherwise unstressed diabetic patients also strongly suggests Type I diabetes. Although anti-islet cell antibodies are relatively specific for Type I diabetes, they are not measurable in as many as 25% of the Type I population at the time of clinical presentation. In addition, the commercially available assays are not uniformly reliable. Therefore, measurement of anti-islet cell antibodies cannot be recommended at this time for general clinical use in the diagnosis of Type I diabetes.

The diagnosis of Type II diabetes is more problematic. The number of undiagnosed Type II diabetic patients equals the number of diagnosed Type II diabetic patients. Therefore, symptoms and usual blood and urine glucose testing during office visits and insurance exams may not be sufficient to diagnose as many as 50% of cases. The argument to perform 75-gram oral glucose tolerance tests (OGTT), which are necessary to detect the otherwise undiagnosed cases with any sensitivity, can only be supported if diagnosis of such cases will lead to an improvement in health status. Since no data exist to demonstrate improved outcome when asymptomatic patients are identified, there is no good argument for screening the adult population to detect asymptomatic patients with diabetes. Simply stated, since we cannot demonstrate any benefit in identifying asymptomatic patients, there is no reason to expend significant resources to identify them. In summary, the majority of Type II diabetic patients who can be helped will be identified by symptoms or by significantly elevated fasting blood glucose levels. Oral glucose tolerance tests are generally not necessary since the majority of symptomatic patients will have abnormal (greater than 140 mg per dl) fasting plasma glucose levels. The NDDG criteria are listed in Table 2.

The exception to the above is pregnant women who should have a 50-gram "screening" OGTT followed by a 100-gram "diagnostic" OGTT for those who screen positive during the 24th to 28th week of gestation (Table 3). The widely accepted argument in favor of screening for gestational diabetes (GDM) is that ap-

TABLE 2. **Diagnosis of Type II Diabetes in Nonpregnant Adults***

| |
|---|
| Typical symptoms with "unequivocal" elevation of plasma glucose |
| More than one fasting plasma glucose level ≥140 mg/dl |
| More than one 75-gram OGTT with 2-hr and other sample ≥200 mg/dl |

*From National Diabetes Data Group. Diabetes 28:1039–1057, 1979.

propriate treatment of GDM improves neonatal outcome.

Other measures of glycemia, such as hemoglobin $A_{1c}$ ($HbA_{1c}$), are generally considered to be too insensitive to use in the diagnosis of diabetes.

## TREATMENT

### Philosophy

In general, management of diabetes should promote health and well-being, including the absence of symptoms of hyper- and hypoglycemia; prevent the development of severe metabolic decompensation, such as diabetic ketoacidosis (DKA) and severe hypoglycemia; and treat or, if possible, prevent associated long-term complications. The level of blood glucose necessary to accomplish the goals above will vary from individual to individual, but in general, average blood glucose levels higher than 200 mg per dl ($HbA_{1c}$ greater than 9%) result in hyperglycemic symptoms and isolated levels less than 65 mg per dl can result in hypoglycemia. Whether intensive treatment regimens that aim for near-normal glycemia can prevent or alter the long-term complications is unknown. Therefore, enthusiasm for achieving normoglycemia, except in pregnancy, must be tempered by the primary goals of treatment. The major conflicts between primary therapeutic goals and the questionable need to achieve normoglycemia are the increased risk of hypoglycemia, increased expense, and the often unacceptable changes in lifestyle that accompany intensive therapy regimens. These burdens are

TABLE 3. **Screening and Diagnosis of Gestational Diabetes Mellitus***

| |
|---|
| 50-gm OGTT administered between weeks 24 and 28 of gestation in all nondiabetic pregnant women |
| If plasma glucose at 1 hr ≥140 mg/dl perform 100-gram OGTT after overnight fast |
| GDM criteria are *two or more* of<br>  fasting plasma glucose ≥105 mg/dl<br>  1-hr ≥190 mg/dl<br>  2-hr ≥165 mg/dl<br>  3-hr ≥145 mg/dl |

*From ADA Position Statement on Gestational Diabetes. Diabetes Care 9:430–431, 1986. Copyright 1986 by the American Diabetes Association. Reprinted with permission.

more common in treatment regimens for Type I than Type II diabetes.

Therefore, the choice of target blood glucose level and corresponding intensity of treatment must represent a careful balance between theoretical benefits and known risks/costs. The level of therapy selected by patient and physician in concert should depend on the patient's lifestyle, motivation, understanding of the risks and potential benefits, and interest in maintaining a given level of glycemia. Treatment regimens should be internally consistent. Intensive regimens require more frequent monitoring and greater attention to diet. Conversely, more simple regimens, with one injection per day, should not include monitoring four times a day; the information generated is usually superfluous.

### Monitoring by the Patient

Monitoring metabolic status is a major component of diabetes care and self-care. Type I diabetes is characterized by frequent and major fluctuations of blood glucose, with the potential risk of hypoglycemia and ketosis. Therefore, more frequent glucose monitoring, especially to prevent hypoglycemia and guide adjustment of insulin doses, is required. Urine glucose testing is insensitive to hypoglycemia and too inaccurate to be useful in this setting, and self-monitoring of blood glucose (SMBG) is recommended. The frequency of SMBG is dictated by individual patient factors. Patients who are treated more intensively with the aim of achieving glucose values close to the normal range, such as pregnant, Type I diabetic women, will require SMBG three to five times per day to adjust rapid-acting insulin doses. Other, less intensively treated patients may test themselves only once or twice a day in order to adjust their once or twice per day insulin injections. All Type I patients should, at a minimum, know how to perform SMBG to avoid hypoglycemia and to help guide sick-day care. Although urine glucose testing is not recommended, testing for urine ketones is important during sick days and when blood glucose values are consistently and unusually elevated for more than 24 to 48 hours. Careful attention to such monitoring can lead to early treatment and adjustment of regimens and prevent avoidable emergency room and hospital admissions for ketoacidosis and hypoglycemia.

Type II diabetes may be characterized by equally high blood glucose values as in Type I diabetes, but blood glucose profiles tend to be less chaotic, with fasting levels generally lower than the predictable postprandial glucose excursions.

Under usual unstressed conditions, Type II patients are ketosis resistant.

Since diet-treated Type II patients are not at risk for hypoglycemia, SMBG is not necessary. Insulin- and oral-agent–treated Type II patients, however, are at risk for hypoglycemia, so general recommendations for blood glucose monitoring as in Type I diabetes pertain. Since the blood glucose profile is relatively predictable in such patients and insulin regimens generally include only one injection per day, SMBG more than once a day is required only during periods when medications are being adjusted. No benefit to more frequent testing has been demonstrated. Urine ketone testing should be performed during sick days.

### Monitoring by the Physician

In addition to patient-performed monitoring, physicians must monitor some aspects of metabolic control. The unpredictable glucose profiles in Type I diabetes make sporadic office testing of blood glucose of little value. On the other hand, the stability of fasting glucose values in Type II diabetes suggests that examining fasting values every 3 months may suffice to determine average glucose control in stable Type II diabetes. Physicians can also validate accuracy of SMBG by comparing a concurrent laboratory and SMBG value during an office visit.

The availability of glycosylated hemoglobin assays ($HbA_1$, $HbA_{1c}$) allows physicians to measure objectively and accurately the average level of glucose control over the preceding 2 to 3 months. This measurement has been widely implemented and informs the physician (and patient) whether glycemic goals are being reached and changes in therapy have been effective. The frequency of testing must be individualized. Intensively treated Type I patients may be tested three to four times per year, while testing once or twice a year is appropriate in more stable Type II patients. Discrepancies between SMBG and $HbA_{1c}$ results suggest patient inaccuracy. More recently introduced measurements of glycated serum proteins (fructosamine assays) reflect only 2 to 3 weeks of glucose control and are less clinically useful than measurements of glycated hemoglobin. The relationship between $HbA_{1c}$ and mean blood glucose over the preceding 2 months is shown in Figure 1.

### Diet

Diet represents one of the key elements in diabetes therapy. Prescription of specific diets for diabetic patients is generally beyond the expertise of most physicians and is too time consuming

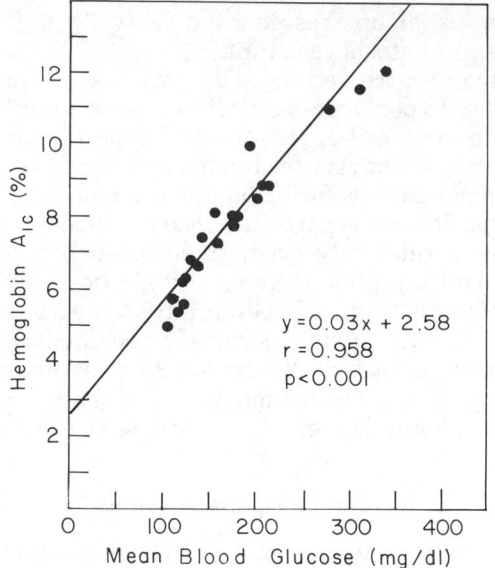

(Based on 200-300 HBGM Measurements)

**Figure 1.** Relationship between HbA$_{1c}$ and mean plasma glucose. Twenty-one subjects performed frequent (three to five times per day) self-monitoring of blood glucose (SMBG) for 8 weeks. At the end of the 8-week period, HbA$_{1c}$ was measured and compared with the mean of the blood glucose measurements. Each 1% change in HbA$_{1c}$ is approximately equivalent to a 33 mg per dl change in plasma glucose. HBGM = home blood glucose monitoring. (From Nathan DM, et al: Reprinted, by permission of the New England Journal of Medicine, *310*:341, 1984.)

for them to perform adequately in any case. Trained dietitians should be incorporated routinely into the care of patients with diabetes.

All patients with diabetes should be encouraged to follow a prudent low-fat diet as recommended by the American Heart Association and American Diabetes Association (Diabetes Care *10*:126–132, 1987). Beyond a prudent low-fat diet, principles of dietary therapy are different for Type I and Type II diabetes. The major dietary feature for obese Type II diabetes is caloric restriction. Caloric restriction with the goal of achieving ideal body weight can restore normoglycemia, as well as reduce blood pressure, lipids, and cardiovascular risk. Many insulin- and oral-agent–treated Type II diabetic patients will have a significant decrease in hypoglycemic medication requirements within hours to days of being placed on a hypocaloric diet, a fact that should be borne in mind when writing insulin or sulfonylurea orders for hospitalized patients who are likely to be on a lower calorie diet in the hospital.

Treatment with a balanced weight loss diet may be the most cost-effective therapy known. Unfortunately, less than 10% of obese diabetic patients succeed in maintaining weight loss over a 2-year period. Nevertheless, patients who fail

diet therapy should always be provided with another chance to succeed. In order to have any chance of success, realistic goals must be chosen and therapy individualized. In many cases, a modest weight reduction of 5 to 10 kg will result in a dramatic improvement in glycemia, even if the patient remains substantially above ideal body weight. Behavioral modification programs may be of use.

The fundamental features of Type I diabetic diets are the following: (1) to provide patients with a consistent diet, both in terms of timing and content; (2) to provide patients with a sense of the carbohydrate content of meals*; and (3) to educate patients on appropriate snacks to prevent hypoglycemia (e.g., with exercise) and how to treat hypoglycemia should it occur.

These fundamental features should be taught to all Type I diabetic patients and insulin-treated Type II patients. More sophisticated dietary manipulations and understanding, such as the use of glycemic indices, should be reserved for patients treated with more sophisticated, intensive regimens.

### Medication

**Type I Diabetes.** The treatment of Type I diabetes in adults is not very different from treatment of diabetic adolescents in that insulin is required, ketoacidosis is a risk, and monitoring to prevent hypoglycemia and adjust insulin doses is required. (Several recent monographs are available; see Nathan DM Med Clin North Am 72:1365–1378, 1988). There are, however, several pertinent differences in diabetes in this population, compared with younger patients, that have therapeutic implications. Although Type I diabetes in adults may be easier to manage since the travails and hormonal chaos that accompany childhood and puberty are not present, the increasing prevalence of asymptomatic hypoglycemia ("hypoglycemia unawareness"), cardiovascular disease, visual loss, renal failure, and hypertension that accompany diabetes of long duration make therapy problematic. Physicians must be alert for long-term complications and their effects on therapy.

In the absence of proof to demonstrate that blood glucose control more rigorous than the level necessary to ameliorate symptoms of hyperglycemia benefits patients, especially with regard to the prevention of complications, there is no firm rationale to support intensive therapies. More-

---

*Although a strict knowledge of carbohydrate exchanges is not absolutely required, they are of use in educating patients. Such knowledge facilitates matching of insulin requirements with insulin delivery.

TABLE 4. **Treatment of Type I Diabetes**

| | SMBG per day | Insulin Regimen | Diet | Exercise | Expected HbA$_{ic}$* (%) |
|---|---|---|---|---|---|
| Level of Therapy | | Injections/day (Type†) | | | |
| *Minimal* | 0–1 To prevent hypoglycemia and on sick days | 1 or 2 (I ± R) | 45–60% carbohydrates, limited sucrose <30 % fat <300 mg chol. protein 0.8 grams/kg Regular meals | Patient preference Snack to prevent hypoglycemia | 9.5–12 |
| *Average* | 1–3 (fasting and presupper or prebed) | 2 (I and R) | As in Minimal, plus exchange list | As in Minimal | 7.5–9.5 |
| *Intensive* | 4–7 (premeals & prebed; 3 a.m. once per week, postprandial as needed) | ≥3 injections (I or UL and R) or pump | More accurate carbohydrate exchange—use glycemic indices when appropriate | Adjust insulin and/or meals to prevent hypoglycemia | <7.5 |

*Nondiabetic range, 4.8–6.4%.

†Abbreviations: I = intermediate-acting (NPH or Lente); R = regular; UL = Ultralente.

over, although the putative benefits of tight control remain unproved, the risks (especially hypoglycemia) have been well documented. It is currently impossible to define the appropriate target for glucose control beyond the level that will ameliorate symptoms. Previous experience with different levels of therapy in Type I diabetes suggests that based on patient motivation and choice, one of three levels can be chosen. These, somewhat arbitrary, levels of therapy are shown in Table 4 along with the range of HbA$_{1c}$ that can be expected.

The only clinical setting in which intensive therapy with the goal of achieving near-normal glucose levels is currently supported by data is in the Type I diabetic woman who is planning pregnancy or who is pregnant. In this setting, the documented benefit to the neonate motivates implementation of intensive therapies.

**Type II Diabetes.** When diet therapy is not successful because of noncompliance and failure to lose weight or when, despite weight loss, glucose levels remain higher than acceptable, patient and physician must consider the use of medications. Because Type II diabetic patients do not usually run the risk of potentially life-threatening ketoacidosis, indications for starting insulin or oral agents are less pressing (and more debated) than in Type I diabetes. In considering therapy, the costs and risks must be balanced, as in Type I diabetes, against the as yet unproved benefit of lowering glucose levels beyond the level necessary to eliminate symptoms. Table 5 lists the indications, in order of importance, for starting drug therapy to control blood glucose levels in Type II diabetes.

**Sulfonylurea or Insulin.** If the physician and patient agree that medications are called for, the choice of medication, insulin or sulfonylurea, is the next step. The development of oral medications capable of enhancing glucose-stimulated insulin secretion provided a choice of therapy for Type II diabetic patients. The hypoglycemic potency of sulfonylureas, discovered during investigation of antibiotic sulfa drugs, is dependent on the ability of patients to secrete insulin. There is also an effect on insulin resistance. The arguments for and against insulin vs. sulfonylureas are noted in Table 6. The major problem with the sulfonylureas is that they are only variably effective and have primary failure rates of 10 to 25% and an additional secondary failure rate of 5 to 15% per year. Thus, by 5 years after the initiation of therapy, probably less than 50% of sulfonylurea-treated patients will continue to have acceptable glucose control. In addition to their limited efficacy, the safety of sulfonylureas has been called into question by the University Group Diabetes Program (UGDP). This multicenter, randomized study documented an increased risk for cardiovascular death in tolbutamide (Orinase)-treated patients compared with diet- or insulin-treated patients. Although the results of this study have been widely debated, an independent review group, The Biometric Society, con-

TABLE 5. **Indications for Beginning Drug Therapy in Type II Patients Who Fail Diet**

Presence of symptoms of hyperglycemia

Presence of ketones

Pregnant women (insulin)

Patients in whom dehydration poses a major threat, e.g., altered thirst mechanism

Certain cases of hyperlipidemia

TABLE 6. **Arguments Supporting Use of Insulin Versus Sulfonylureas in Treatment of "Diet Failure" Type II Diabetes**

| Insulin | Sulfonylureas |
| --- | --- |
| Insulin more effective than sulfonylureas—no maximum dose | Patients reluctant to use insulin |
| Insulin more physiologic | |
| UGDP* suggests that sulfonylureas are cardiotoxic | Insulin treatment results in hyperinsulinemia and may promote atherosclerosis |
| Hypoglycemia more severe with sulfonylureas | Hypoglycemia more common with insulin |

*University Group Diabetes Program.

firmed the validity of the major findings. For the reasons above, the author views sulfonylureas as second choice drugs, behind insulin, in the treatment of Type II diabetes.

A newer group of sulfonylureas, including glipizide (Glucotrol) and glyburide (Micronase, Diabeta), have been in use in Canada and Europe for 15 years and in the U.S. for more than 5 years. Although somewhat more potent and with fewer drug interactions than the first-generation sulfonylureas, the newer sulfonylureas are not substantively different. The cardiovascular risk associated with tolbutamide is assumed to be a class action effect. Patients who fail maximal doses of a first-generation sulfonylurea should not be expected to respond to a second-generation oral agent and should be changed to insulin.

Another group of oral agents, the biguanides, act through a poorly understood mechanism. Because of the risk of lactic acidosis associated with phenformin, none of the biguanides is currently approved for use in the U.S. The drug metformin, which has much less risk of lactic acidosis, is used in Europe and Canada, and is under active investigation in the U.S.

Insulin use in Type II diabetes is also debated. The major arguments against using insulin in Type II diabetes involve (1) the reluctance of some patients to accept insulin therapy—"the needle"; (2) the risks of hypoglycemia; and (3) the putative risk of aggravating hyperinsulinemia in these already hyperinsulinemic patients. In response to these arguments, the first objection cannot be tested unless physicians are less reluctant to suggest insulin to their patients. Second, hypoglycemia probably does not occur more frequently in insulin-treated patients compared with sulfonylurea-treated patients. Moreover, hypoglycemia with sulfonylurea drugs generally carries more morbidity and mortality. Finally, the evidence that hyperinsulinemia (endogenous) is a cardiovascular risk factor remains preliminary and is not a strong argument in favor of sulfonylurea therapy, especially with the UGDP data available.

Insulin therapy in Type II diabetes can be initiated with a single injection of an intermediate-acting insulin (NPH or Lente) in the morning. Since these patients are generally insulin resistant, they often require more than 50 units per day. If the morning dose exceeds 100 U without adequate control of afternoon or morning blood glucose levels, a second injection of intermediate-acting insulin at bedtime is recommended This dose, adjusted with the guidance of SMBG, should lower fasting glucose levels. When this is accomplished, the total insulin dose may begin to decrease. The risk of further weight gain, as the caloric drain of glycosuria is eliminated, must be borne in mind. Diet therapy remains important even after medications are begun. Other regimens, including the sole use of bedtime intermediate-acting insulin and the use of very long-acting Ultralente insulin, have been tried with varied success.

Although human insulin may be indicated in patients with a history of insulin allergy, antibody-mediated resistance, or interrupted use of insulin, it does not have documented clinical attributes, compared with insulin derived from animal species, to substantiate its use over the generally less expensive insulins prepared from beef or pig. In fact, the NPH formulation of human insulin tends to have a shorter duration and more rapid onset of action, which may be undesirable in some patients.

Finally, the use of "combination" therapy, insulin plus oral agents, has become popular recently. The majority of studies have demonstrated that the dose of insulin required to achieve similar metabolic control can be reduced if oral agents are added. However, if larger doses of insulin are used, the same results can be obtained. The generally acknowledged poorer compliance and increased adverse drug effects encountered when two drugs (instead of one) are used mitigate against this strategy.

The appropriate target glucose levels in Type II diabetes are as difficult to choose as in Type I diabetes. In the absence of a demonstrated benefit of lower glucose levels, the risk of hypoglycemia in the older population with a higher risk of underlying cardiovascular disease tempers enthusiasm for tight control. As in Type I diabetes, goals must be individualized.

### Exercise

Exercise is an important adjunct to diet therapy in weight loss regimens for obese Type II diabetic patients. In addition to promoting negative caloric balance and improving cardiovascular tone, insulin sensitivity is increased. Problems that can be encountered during exercise and that must be anticipated include (1) hypoglycemia in insulin- and oral-agent–treated patients; (2) the danger of foot trauma, diabetic foot ulcers, and Charcot joints in the presence of neuropathy and peripheral vascular disease; and (3) the danger of precipitating angina. Since diabetic patients have a higher prevalence of coronary artery disease, especially asymptomatic angina, than nondiabetic patients, an exercise tolerance test should be performed before any diabetic patient older than age 40 and with diabetes duration greater than 10 years initiates a new exercise program. In addition, diabetic patients should understand that absorption of insulin can be altered when injected into an exercising limb (e.g., increased rate of absorption from the arm with weight lifting) and that hypoglycemia can occur many hours after completion of exercise.

## MONITORING AND TREATING COMPLICATIONS

### DKA and Hyperosmolar Nonketotic Coma

The treatment of ketoacidosis in adults is not dissimilar to treatment in the adolescent population. Repletion of the large volume sodium and potassium deficits and insulin administration remain the hallmarks of treatment. The medical setting in which DKA is treated should provide the ability to monitor volume, acid-base status, and glucose levels on a frequent basis and perform cardiac monitoring. In most instances, this will be an intensive care unit. Although "low-dose" (i.e., 2 to 10 U per hour after a loading bolus) intravenous insulin infusion has become an increasingly popular means of treating DKA, any method that reliably repletes insulin is acceptable. The dangers of hypoglycemia and hypokalemia and the consequences of profound phosphate depletion are well documented.

Features of DKA in adults that are different from those in the pediatric population are the following: essentially no history of cerebral edema in adults; Type II diabetic patients who develop DKA often have extreme stress as a precipitant of the DKA, e.g., sepsis or myocardial infarction; and more care should be exercised in repleting patients with saline than in the pediatric population since the coincidence of significant coronary artery disease is high in the adult population.

Hyperosmolar hyperglycemic nonketotic coma develops in elderly Type II diabetics when blood glucose levels rise to extremely high levels (often because of added hyperglycemic stimuli such as infection, treatment with steroids, etc.), with resultant dehydration that is in turn exacerbated by limited access to free water because of abnormal thirst mechanism or other factors. Treatment is with repletion of volume and free water. Patients tend to be very sensitive to insulin and often do not require insulin after resolution of the acute event.

### Retinopathy, Nephropathy, and Neuropathy

Since all diabetic complications are duration dependent and generally require more than 10 years to develop, the vast majority of diabetic patients who develop complications will be adults. Moreover, patients with Type II diabetes have a risk for developing complications similar to that of Type I diabetic patients and, because of their large number, provide the majority of diabetic complications.

Retinopathy develops in more than 90% of all diabetic patients by 15 years of duration. Severe retinopathy, including macular edema and high-risk proliferative retinopathy, can affect vision. It is crucial to recognize such severe eye lesions since timely laser therapy can prevent loss of vision. Nonophthalmologists may miss as many as 70% of severe lesions during a nondilated or dilated ophthalmoscopic examination. Because of the severe consequences of missing such lesions, yearly examination with an ophthalmologist is recommended. Hypertension is the only other factor identified that may exacerbate retinopathy and should be treated aggressively.

Nephropathy leading to end-stage renal disease (ESRD) is the most serious of specific diabetic complications and may develop in 40% of Type I and 10% of Type II diabetic patients. The presence of microalbuminuria (25 to 40 mg of albumin per 24 hours) may presage renal failure by 10 to 15 years in both Type I and II diabetes. Since there is no proven intervention available at this stage in the evolution of diabetic nephropathy, routine measurement of microalbuminuria is not indicated. The development of nephropathy proceeds from microalbuminuria to gross proteinuria (greater than 500 mg per 24 hours) with accompanying hypertension, to nephrotic syndrome, and finally to declining glomerular filtration rate (GFR) with the ultimate development of ESRD. During this progression, assiduous attention to control of hypertension, with angiotensin-converting enzyme (ACE)–inhibitors providing certain theoretic advantages over other antihypertensives, can slow the rate of progression of nephropathy. Use of phosphate-binding antacids and low-protein diets may also play a role in slowing progression. Nephrologists should be consulted as GFR falls to less than 50% of normal.

Neuropathy occurs in one guise or another in most patients with diabetes. Usually, it is asymptomatic. Painful peripheral neuropathy can represent a severe problem, but it usually waxes and wanes and can be treated with non-narcotic analgesics, combinations of tricyclic antidepressants, and fluphenazine (Prolixin), carbamazepine (Tegretol), or phenytoin (Dilantin). No therapy is uniformly effective; narcotic analgesics should be avoided as much as possible since dependency is an all too frequent outcome.

The major severe consequence of peripheral neuropathy is foot trauma, which is poorly recognized or unrecognized by the patient, and, in conjunction with vasculopathy, can lead to penetrating foot ulcers, osteomyelitis, gangrene, and amputation. Patients must be instructed in appropriate foot care and, if they have extremities at risk because of the presence of peripheral sensory-motor neuropathy, should see a podiatrist on a regular basis. Foot examination should be part of the routine physical examination.

Autonomic neuropathy can present as impotence, gastroparesis, postural hypotension, resting sinus tachycardias, or, more rarely, diabetic diarrhea and incontinence. Impotence, which may develop in 50% of diabetic men, can be treated with penile injection therapy (papaverine) or with a variety of external or implantable devices. The implantable prostheses are generally safe and provide an acceptable sex life for the patient.

# DIABETES MELLITUS IN CHILDREN AND ADOLESCENTS*

method of
MICHAEL P. GOLDEN, M.D., and
DEBORAH L. GRAY, R.N., M.S.N.
*Indiana University Medical Center*
*Indianapolis, Indiana*

Diabetes mellitus in children is a relatively common disorder, with a prevalence rate of approximately 1 in

*Supported in part by the Indiana University Diabetes Research and Training Center, PHS P60-DK-20542.

800 children and adolescents in the United States. As such, it is regularly seen by pediatricians, and over 75% of general pediatricians in this country report caring for one or more (median, five) patients with diabetes. Peak incidence is in early adolescence, but congenital diabetes, while rare, has been reported and children of all ages can develop diabetes.

Diabetes presenting in childhood is almost always insulin-dependent diabetes mellitus (IDDM). Non–insulin-dependent diabetes mellitus (NIDDM) is unusual and is characterized by significant degrees of insulin resistance, usually associated with hyperinsulinemia. NIDDM accounts for 90% of diabetes in the United States but generally occurs during or after middle age in adults with some degree of obesity. Occasionally, adolescents with a very strong family history of obesity and diabetes, usually of African-American descent, present with early diagnosed NIDDM. Maturity onset diabetes of the young (MODY) is an inherited autosomal dominant condition, generally not associated with obesity, which manifests varying degrees of glucose intolerance. Patients may be asymptomatic and generally are not ketotic. However, they can develop complications and do require treatment.

Both NIDDM and MODY are unusual in the pediatric age range, and thus, the remainder of this discussion will focus on IDDM.

IDDM is characterized by progressive loss of pancreatic beta cells with concurrent loss of insulin secretory capacity. Clinically, there is absolute dependence on insulin, and signs and symptoms usually develop acutely. If untreated, patients will develop life-threatening ketoacidosis. The etiology of IDDM appears to be related to autoimmune phenomena. A variety of antibodies directed against the beta cell have been described as well as abnormalities in T cell functions relative to pancreatic beta cell antigens. The exact nature of the autoimmune disorder is not currently known, nor is the possible relationship between viral infections and the development of diabetes. Particularly in younger children, a variety of viral illnesses frequently seems to precede the acute development of symptoms of diabetes. However, it is more likely that these illnesses are an acute stress that precipitates symptoms rather than the cause of diabetes itself.

## CLINICAL PRESENTATION AND DIAGNOSIS

Once considered, the diagnosis of IDDM is usually not difficult. During the early course of the illness, typical symptoms are polyuria, polydipsia, and nocturia. Weight loss is variable. Most patients will feel well or, retrospectively, may complain of malaise. Diagnosis during this early phase is optimal, since a delay leads to progressively more dangerous symptoms that include increasing weight loss, malaise and lethargy with the onset of diabetic ketoacidosis (DKA), nausea, vomiting, dehydration, somnolence, and eventually coma. During DKA abdominal pain is common and can be confused with an acute surgical abdomen.

Laboratory diagnosis is generally unambiguous. A random blood glucose level over 200 mg per dl in association with typical symptoms is sufficient to make the diagnosis. A glucose tolerance test is rarely, if ever, indicated in children. Glycosuria is almost always detectable, although some patients may not be acidotic and urinary ketones may be absent.

## TREATMENT

### Diabetic Ketoacidosis

Diabetic ketoacidosis is a life-threatening condition for which the best treatment is prevention. However, when confronted with a patient with DKA, several basic principles should be observed. First, treatment requires an intensive care unit or equivalent with experienced pediatric staff and continuous monitoring of electrocardiogram (ECG) and blood pressure. There should be careful and frequent re-evaluation of both physical and laboratory status, and slow correction of metabolic abnormalities is preferable to rapid correction as long as there is continual improvement.

The most frequent causes of DKA are late diagnosis and the omission of insulin by patients; these account for more than 90% of admissions for DKA in our experience. Other causes include chronic poor control that is acutely decompensated by another illness. Gastroenteritis in young children can lead to development of mild ketoacidosis. Factors that do not induce DKA include overeating, menses, and stress.

On physical examination, it is important to evaluate the state of consciousness with careful documentation of baseline neurologic function. The state of hydration is necessary to determine the appropriate fluids. Kussmaul's respirations indicate metabolic acidosis. Reflexes are an indirect measure of potassium status. If abdominal pain is present, it is important to attempt to decide whether the pain is primary or secondary to DKA. Infections should be sought because they may contribute to insulin resistance and DKA.

Fluid and electrolyte management varies from center to center. For shock, we use a bolus of 350 ml per $M^2$ of normal saline over 20 to 30 minutes. If there are no signs of shock, begin treatment with normal saline without glucose until the blood glucose level is less than or equal to 300 mg per dl, then add in 5% dextrose normal saline. If the serum glucose concentration continues to decline, change to 10% dextrose. Dextrose is added to fluids before the serum glucose reaches 300 mg per dl if the insulin infusion rate is down to 0.05 U per kg per hour and the serum glucose level is falling at a rate greater than 100 mg per dl per hour.

Insulin is administered by continuous intravenous infusion using a controlled rate infusion system. Use a concentration of 0.1 U per ml in normal saline. An initial bolus of 0.05 to 0.1 U per kg of regular insulin may be administered. The lower dose is used with younger children. A bolus is not necessary if sufficient subcutaneous insulin has been given within the time frame of the insulin (4 hours for regular, 12 hours for Lente or NPH).

Begin the insulin infusion at 0.1 U per kg per hour (for children under 5 years start with 0.05 U per kg per hour). The goal of both insulin and glucose administration is to achieve a progressive decrease in blood glucose of 50 to 80 mg per dl per hour. Adjust the rate by 10 to 20% per hour to achieve it. Unless the patient is hypoglycemic, the insulin infusion should not be stopped as this will rapidly lead to metabolic decompensation. Except under unusual circumstances, the insulin infusion rate should not be decreased to less than 0.05 U per kg per hour. Insulin infusion should be continued until the patient is rehydrated, the serum glucose level is in the 150 to 250 mg per dl range, and the patient is able to eat.

Fluid replacement should be slow and careful. We calculate fluid maintenance as 1500 ml per $M^2$ per 24 hours plus replacement of dehydration. Patients with DKA are at least 10% dehydrated. Dehydration is corrected over 48 hours. For example, a 25-kg child (surface area 1 $M^2$) requires a maintenance rate of 1500 ml per 24 hour, or 66 ml per hour. For 10% dehydration, rehydration is 2500 ml divided by 48 hours, or 52 ml per hour. Total fluids are 112 ml per hour. Remember that marked hyperglycemia will lead to osmotic diuresis with excessive urinary loss. If urinary output exceeds the rehydration rate, the child will not improve. If this is occurring, urine output should be replaced ml for ml above the maintenance rate. One can measure urinary electrolytes to help select the replacement solution, or a solution of half-normal saline with 10 mEq per liter of potassium chloride can be used. Glucose should not be used in the urinary replacement fluids. Stop replacing urine when osmotic diuresis stops, usually when the glucose is less than or equal to 300 mg per dl.

Monitoring sodium (Na) level is important in assessing the degree of hydration and, potentially, in limiting the likelihood of development of cerebal edema. A declining Na level may indicate that excess free water is being administered, a probable risk factor for cerebral edema. In general, normal saline is used for the first 8 to 12 hours of treatment. After that, if the corrected serum Na level (corrected Na = measured Na + [serum glucose {mg per dl} − 100] × 0.016mEq) is not declining and is within the normal range, one can switch to half normal saline when dextrose is added to the fluids. Sodium needs to be corrected because of the artificial lowering of serum sodium related to the hyperosmolarity of hyperglycemia. If the calculated serum sodium is decreasing and reaching levels below normal, careful restriction of fluid administration rate is indicated.

Potassium administration should be started as soon as urination is established and hyperkalemia is excluded. If there is no urine production in the first 30 minutes, catheterization is indicated. Potassium should be started at 30 to 40 mEq per liter, and the dose should be adjusted in response to serum potassium and bicarbonate levels. Potassium requirements may exceed 40 mEq per liter. In general, potassium is administered as potassium chloride. If the serum chloride level is high or the phosphate is low, one can give half the potassium as chloride and half as phosphate. Carefully monitor potassium levels because a dramatic decrease in potassium can be expected with correction of acidosis.

Rapid administration of bicarbonate is used only for cardiac arrest or shock. With severe acidosis (pH less than 7.1), a slow infusion may be used, the total not exceeding 3 mEq per kg per 8 hours.

Frequent laboratory re-evaluation is important. An intravenous heparin lock or, if necessary, an arterial line should be placed. An arterial line is not mandatory and should be reserved for severe DKA or for DKA complicated by cardiac or pulmonary disease.

Initial laboratory evaluation should include an arterial or venous pH, glucose, electrolytes, blood urea nitrogen (BUN), creatinine, calcium, phosphorus, urinalysis, and others as needed. Serum glucose should be followed initially every hour and then every 2 hours, once a stable and declining pattern is established. Glucose levels can be monitored by glucose oxidase strips with meters for immediate results. Serum electrolytes are initially monitored every 2 hours. In general, the plasma bicarbonate level may be used to follow the degree of acidosis. Venous or arterial pH is also useful.

When the patient is able to resume caloric intake and is rehydrated, discontinue the insulin infusion immediately before beginning subcutaneous insulin. In a newly diagnosed patient, one can usually start with a mixed dose of regular and intermediate insulin in a dose of 0.5 U per kg per day. In a previously treated patient, the established dose may be appropriate.

The most dangerous complication of DKA, and the most common cause of death, is severe neurologic dysfunction related to cerebral edema. Typically, cerebral edema manifests itself clinically several hours to 24 hours after the start of treatment of a child who may begin to improve and then deteriorates neurologically. The onset can be abrupt or gradual. Signs include increasing confusion and deepening coma, fixed and dilated pupils or change in respiratory status, or other evidence of neurologic impairment. Neurologic checks should be performed frequently during initial treatment, and the patient should not be left unobserved for more than a brief period. If cerebral edema is suspected, mannitol (0.5 gram per kg) should be given immediately and appropriate neurologic or neurosurgical consultation obtained. Treatment at this stage is supportive and frequently not completely successful. Excessively rapid correction of dehydration with fluid overload has been implicated in the pathogenesis of cerebral edema.

## Long-Term Management

In pediatrics, diabetes is a relatively unique illness in that daily management is completely under the control of the patient and family. The physician and diabetes care team can best help by providing excellent education in diabetes management, recommending appropriate regimens, and by being available for long-term support, ongoing education, and introduction of new technology when appropriate. Education, addressed in more detail later, should include the complete family unit and should be based on appropriate education principles. It should take into account the normal variability in development of children and adolescents, and children should not be pushed too fast or too hard to assume responsibility for diabetes self-care procedures.

Therapeutic goals for metabolic control in diabetes are controversial and still evolving. There is consensus that all children should grow normally and be free of symptoms of hyperglycemia or significant hypoglycemia. It is as yet unclear to what degree blood glucose should be controlled in an attempt to minimize complications. At this time, our program uses the following assumptions. First, young children below the age of 5 or 6 are more susceptible than older children to developing hypoglycemia and may be more susceptible to development of permanent neurologic dysfunction related to even mild hypoglycemia. In particular, young children with diabetes are at risk for long-term learning disabilities. Therefore, our policy is to minimize even asymptomatic hypoglycemia below the age of 6 by attempting to maintain premeal blood glucose values in the range of 150 to 200 mg per dl.

In school-age children, good control is easier to attain, and we attempt to maintain premeal blood glucose levels between 80 and 150 mg per dl. Recent evidence suggests, however, that the risk for developing diabetes complications appears to be relatively unrelated to duration of IDDM before puberty, and we do not emphasize the need for excellent control in the prepubertal child.

At the time of puberty, however, the risk for developing complications does begin to become significant and is progressive with duration of diabetes postpuberty. Further, it seems that the level of metabolic control is related to the risk for developing complications. Therefore, one should attempt to achieve the best possible metabolic control. Ideally, we recommend attempting to achieve premeal blood glucose levels between 80 and 140 mg per dl whenever possible while minimizing the frequency of hypoglycemia. Health care providers should always bear in mind that it is almost impossible for patients with IDDM to achieve this narrow range much of the time and that one cannot insist upon excellent control at the cost of hypoglycemic seizures.

It is hoped that more definitive data will emerge from the Diabetes Control and Complication Trial (DCCT). This is a multicenter, long-term trial sponsored by the National Institutes of Health designed to evaluate the relationship between metabolic control and complications. The trial is approximately half-way complete, and its results should have a major bearing on the intensity with which diabetes is treated in the future.

### Experimental Treatment

Because IDDM is an autoimmune disease, a number of interventions involving immune suppression have been evaluated. Both cyclosporine and a combination of azothioprine and prednisone have been shown to decrease insulin requirements and to increase the frequency of complete remissions in the early phase of diabetes in some newly diagnosed patients. However, in all cases, the duration of the effect is limited, and once therapy is discontinued, diabetes rapidly recurs. In addition, there are ongoing concerns about side effects of any immunosuppressive regimen. At this time, immune suppression is experimental and should be implemented only as part of a randomized, blind therapeutic trial at a center where excellent immunologic monitoring is possible.

### Insulin Therapy

Optimal use of insulin requires knowledge of available insulin preparations and their pharmacologic properties, selection of an insulin regimen appropriate to the individual's needs, and consideration of other factors that affect insulin response and dosage requirements. Insulin is classified according to species (beef, pork, human), purity, strength, and duration of action (Table 1).

Most insulins now available in the U.S. are highly purified. Consequently, the incidence of local or systemic insulin allergy or lipoatrophy at the injection site has been greatly reduced. Nonetheless, both animal and human insulins may be immunogenic, with human being the least, perhaps the one clear advantage of its use over other species. In general, we prefer to use either biosynthetic or semisynthetic human insulins. Purified pork insulin seems to have an extended duration of action and may be helpful when insulin action is too short. Beef Ultralente has an extended duration of action and is used to provide a basal insulin level in patients using an intensified conventional therapeutic regimen (see later).

U–100 (100 U per ml) insulin concentration is used almost exclusively in children and adolescents with IDDM. The exception is very young children under the age of 4 or 5 years. Many of these children have very small insulin requirements and will benefit from the use of diluted insulin. We frequently use insulin diluted to U–10 concentration—i.e., 10 U of insulin per ml. This allows for smaller incremental dose changes (tenths of units). A disadvantage of using U–10 insulin is that a greater volume of insulin must be given. This can be modified by using a com-

TABLE 1. **Insulins by Relative Comparative Action Curves***

| Insulin | Onset (hr) | Peak (hr) | Usual Effective Duration (hr) | Usual Maximum Duration (hr) |
|---|---|---|---|---|
| *Animal* | | | | |
| Regular | 0.5–2.0 | 3–4 | 4–6 | 6–8 |
| NPH | 4–6 | 8–14 | 16–20 | 20–24 |
| Lente | 4–6 | 8–14 | 16–20 | 20–24 |
| Ultralente | 8–14 | Minimal | 24–36 | 24–36 |
| *Human* | | | | |
| Regular | 0.5–1.0 | 2–3 | 3–6 | 4–6 |
| NPH | 2–4 | 4–10 | 10–16 | 14–18 |
| Lente | 3–4 | 4–12 | 12–18 | 16–20 |
| Ultralente | 6–10 | ? | 18–20 | 20–30 |

*From *Physicians' Guide to Insulin-Dependent (Type I) Diabetes,* p 33, 1988. Reproduced with permission of the American Diabetes Association, Inc.

bination of U–10 with U–100. For example, 1.3 U can be given as 1 U of U–100 and .3 U of U–10 insulin. It is also important to point out that diluting insulin shortens its duration of action. Thus, it is preferable to use purified pork insulin rather than human insulin in this instance.

From a practical point of view, it is probably best to learn the properties of a few types of insulins. We use human regular and human Lente for most patients. In our experience, human NPH is absorbed more rapidly from the injection site, peaks sooner, and has a shorter duration of action than Lente. Patients using human NPH on standard insulin therapy seem more likely to experience early morning hyperglycemia than patients on human Lente or animal NPH formulations.

There are a number of ways in which insulin can be combined to moderate glucose excursions. Conventional insulin therapy, used for most children and adolescents, consists of regular insulin combined with Lente insulin given twice daily before breakfast and dinner. Most patients require a total daily dose between 0.6 U per kg to 1.0 U per kg per day, with some exceptions to be noted later. We initially place patients on a dose with 55% of their total insulin in the morning and 45% in the evening. The percentages of morning regular and Lente insulin are 45% and 55%, respectively. The evening insulin is divided equally. Thereafter, insulin is adjusted according to target goals and individual response (Table 2).

Other regimens can be used for specific problems. For patients with elevated prebreakfast (but normal 3 a.m.) glucoses, patients can take their combined insulin in the morning but take only regular insulin before dinner and Lente-NPH several hours later before bedtime. This delays the peak action of Lente-NPH to coincide with the early morning rise in blood glucose.

### TABLE 2. **Patient Instructions for Basal Insulin Adjustment**

1. Treatment goals for blood glucose:

| Glucose Reading | Acceptable Range |
|---|---|
| Before meals | 80–140 |
| Before bedtime | 100–140 |

2. Instructions:

   If your blood sugar level consistently exceeds these goals, increase the insulin listed below. Increase only one insulin at a time by 10%, and wait 3 days between changes. If your average blood sugar is below the treatment goal, decrease the appropriate insulin by 10%.

| Before Breakfast | Before Lunch | Before Supper | Before Bed |
|---|---|---|---|
| Evening NPH or Lente | Morning regular | Morning NPH or Lente regular | Evening |

More recently, we have found that Humulin Ultralente (Eli Lilly, Inc., Indianapolis, IN) is effective in eliminating the early morning rise in blood glucose when given before dinner. To increase flexibility of lifestyle while maintaining control, we use a multidose insulin regimen with three or four injections per day. Very-long-acting insulin (purified beef Ultralente) is combined with regular insulin before breakfast, and regular insulin is given alone prior to the remaining meals or snacks. With this regimen, meals and snacks can be delayed or missed altogether, although careful and frequent blood glucose monitoring is required. This regimen works particularly well for older adolescents and young adults who have widely varying schedules and can benefit from the greater flexibility. We recommend purified beef Ultralente because it is less immunogenic than beef-pork combinations. Human Ultralente does not lend itself to this type of regimen. Insulin is distributed as follows: Ultralente comprises about 40% of the total daily dose and the remaining 60% is divided equally among the three major meals. An evening snack requires approximately 4 to 6 U of regular insulin, depending on content and size. Adjustments of Ultralente are based on 3 a.m. and prebreakfast readings. Regular insulin is given according to a sliding scale designed to compensate for every 100 mg per dl of glucose above 100 up to 400. Our sliding scale increases in 10% increments up to a maximum of 50% above the starting scale.

Both puberty and insulin therapy in very young children present special problems. Insulin requirements usually remain fairly constant, between 0.6 to 1.0 U of insulin per kg per day, from about 2 years after diagnosis until puberty. During puberty, increased insulin requirements are associated with hormone-mediated insulin resistance, and many adolescents require between 1.1 to 1.4 U per kg per day from the onset of puberty until growth is complete. Thereafter, insulin requirements gradually return to prepubertal levels. Insulin resistance does not account solely for poor metabolic outcomes during adolescence.

Whereas insulin resistance characterizes adolescence, insulin sensitivity is an important factor in children under the age of 5. The combination of increased insulin sensitivity and the inability to recognize and communicate the symptoms of hypoglycemia places very young children at a significant risk for severe hypoglycemia. The incidence of severe hypoglycemia can be significantly reduced with frequent blood glucose monitoring and by maintaining premeal blood glucose levels between 150 to 200 mg per dl. Furthermore, most children under 5 require less than 0.7 U per kg per day. Increases above this level must be made gradually and accompanied by periodic 3 a.m. blood glucose screening.

### Diet Therapy

Diet is one of the cornerstones of therapy for IDDM. Management is directed toward normalizing plasma glucose levels, maintaining adequate nutrient intake to promote normal growth and development, promoting healthy eating habits, and minimizing the risk of long-term vascular complications. We follow the recommendations established by the American Diabetes Association with a slight modification in the percentage of carbohydrate and fat. Nutrients are distributed as 50 to 55% carbohydrate, 15 to 20% protein, and 30 to 35% fat. We teach a somewhat liberal attitude toward the use of sucrose, enabling families to incorporate favorite foods common to the pediatric population into the dietary plan. Families are taught to integrate food preferences, as with all other foods, into the dietary plan, based on the food exchange system.

During childhood and adolescence, caloric requirements will vary considerably and therefore must be individualized to reflect growth, activity, and food habits. A general guideline for establishing initial requirements follows:

| | |
|---|---|
| 0 to 12 years: | 1000 calories for the first year and 100 calories per year over 1 up to 12 |
| 12 to 15 years (female) | 1500 to 2000 calories and 100 calories per year over 12 up to 2400 |
| 12 to 15 years (male) | 2000 to 2500 calories and 200 calories per year over 12 up to 2800 |

Thereafter, calories are adjusted to maintain desirable body weight. Adolescent females, in particular, need to begin tapering caloric intake before the end of puberty to avoid excess weight gain.

While these guidelines are useful in approximating initial caloric needs, a thorough nutritional history by a dietitian well versed in diabetes care will provide a better method of determining nutritional requirements. Once requirements are established, calories are distributed over three meals and three snacks to moderate plasma glucose excursions.

Dietary management during sick days may pose a special problem. However, liquids containing sugar can be substituted and given at a rate of 50 grams of carbohydrate every 3 to 4 hours. When a child is not able to tolerate his or her usual diet, adjustments in insulin may need to be made accordingly.

## MONITORING METABOLIC CONTROL

Self-monitoring by patients of blood glucose levels at home is critical to management. Both patients and health care providers should use these home records for decisions about insulin therapy. When patients are not given appropriate education to understand their own blood glucose levels, they rapidly decrease the frequency with which they measure blood glucose. Optimally, blood glucose should be measured before each meal and before the bedtime snack. However, few children will test their blood during school. Therefore, decisions about the morning short-acting insulin are based on blood glucose measurements obtained occasionally at school or on weekends. When significant changes in the evening long-acting insulin dose are made, blood glucose levels should be monitored at 3 a.m. to ensure that nocturnal hypoglycemia is not occurring. For the same reason, an occasional 3 a.m. blood glucose in a patient who is well controlled is helpful. Many patients will not, cannot, or do not monitor themselves as often as recommended. It is important that they be encouraged to test at different times of the day and to accept what is offered. Urine glucose measurement is not necessary. Urine ketone measurement is helpful during periods of illness and significant hyperglycemia. Hypoglycemic reactions should be recorded. Occasional (two to three times per week) episodes of mild hypoglycemia are acceptable and probably are unavoidable with good control. Such episodes should not result in change in level of consciousness.

Glycosylated hemoglobin is a measure of integrated blood glucose control over the preceding 6 to 12 weeks. These tests are an objective means of documenting the previous mean blood glucose level. Glycosylated hemoglobin is a product of a nonenzymatic reaction between glucose and hemoglobin in which the higher the ambient concentration of glucose, the greater the percentage of hemoglobin glycosylated. Assays can measure either total glycosylated hemoglobin ($HbA_{1a} + {}_b + {}_c$) or the predominant glycosylated component which is hemoglobin $A_{1c}$. Assays may have different normative ranges, and it is important to interpret the results in view of the laboratory performing the test.

Few patients with IDDM of greater than 2 years' duration can maintain $HbA_1$ at or near the normal range. We consider that our patients are doing well if they are within 1.5% of the upper normal limit. Specifically, in our laboratory, the upper normal limit is 7.5%, and we consider 9% to be good control. An $HbA_1$ greater than 150% of the upper range of normal indicates poor control with the need for significant re-evaluation.

We obtain HbA$_1$ levels every 3 months and communicate these results to our patients and families.

## SPECIAL CIRCUMSTANCES

### Sports

Exercise has many well-known benefits, including increased cardiovascular fitness, an increased sense of well-being, maintenance of normal body weight, and in some instances, promotion of weight loss. For children and adolescents with diabetes, exercise offers the additional benefits of lowering blood glucose levels and increasing insulin sensitivity. However, these additional benefits also increase the likelihood of hypoglycemia. Thus, the effects of exercise must be counterbalanced with either a reduction in insulin or an increase in food intake.

Children's exercise generally takes the form of spontaneous bursts of activity. Consequently, families must be aware of a change in the quality and quantity of activity and be ready to compensate. For extra activity, we recommend an additional 100 to 150 calories for every hour of unplanned, uninterrupted vigorous play. Both simple and complex carbohydrates should be offered. Planned activity, such as an after school sports program, can be dealt with by a reduction in insulin or a combination of increased food intake and insulin reduction. A 10 to 15% decrease in insulin for every hour of continuous aerobic activity is generally sufficient. A reduction in insulin requires advance planning. For example, sports practice immediately after school requires a reduction in morning long-acting insulin. Patients should experiment by changing insulin regimens and food intake for activity and closely monitor their blood glucose before, during, and after participation in intensive exercise. The effects of exercise on insulin sensitivity may be prolonged (6 to 12 hours postexercise). Children who engage in unusually prolonged periods of activity are at increased risk for postexercise hypoglycemia during the night, and both increased food intake and decreased evening long-acting insulin can help avoid severe nocturnal hypoglycemia.

Contraindications to exercise are few. However, patients should be cautioned against exercise when the blood glucose level is excessively high or ketones are present in the urine. Exercise in the presence of a relative state of insulin deficiency stimulates gluconeogenic pathways, thereby elevating the plasma glucose level further. Once the blood glucose level falls below 300 mg per dl, exercise may be resumed.

### Sick Days

Insulin requirements may increase markedly during illness, including seemingly minor illness. Consequently, meticulous attention to blood glucose and ketone levels is very important in the presence of illness. Families should check blood glucose and ketone levels every 4 to 6 hours. In addition, families need to know how to respond to elevated blood glucose levels to avoid ketoacidosis. Table 3 gives algorithms to adjust insulin according to glucose level, ketones, and time of day during illness. Each patient needs individualized guidelines. It is important to note that these guidelines are calculated for patients on a coventional, twice daily regimen and on the basis of insulin dosage of 1 U per kg per day. Patients receiving less than 1 U per kg per day will require substantially less insulin. When vomiting or other GI symptoms preclude usual meals and snacks, less insulin must be used in order to avoid hypoglycemia. The presence of vomiting with elevated blood glucose and ketone levels requires that the patient be seen to rule out DKA. We absolutely recommend evaluation if vomiting persists more than 4 to 6 hours or if ketones are present with a blood glucose level above 250 mg per dl.

### Pregnancy and Birth Control

Birth control and prepregnancy planning are important. Risks of an unplanned pregnancy are substantial. The incidence of congenital anomalies among infants of women with poorly controlled diabetes is increased. Morever, background retinopathy or incipient nephropathy may progress without careful medical follow-up and tight metabolic control prior to and during pregnancy. Most adolescents respond honestly and openly to direct questions regarding sexuality and contraceptive use if such questions are stated nonjudgmentally and with an assurance of confidentiality.

Diabetes, in and of itself, is not a contraindication to using birth control pills. Birth control pills are often the only acceptable and reliable method of contracepton for adolescents, and the risks associated with their use must be weighed against the presence of other risk factors. When indicated, oral contraceptives with a low progesterone-estrogen formulation are generally best. Patients should receive screening for hypertension and lipid profiles prior to and during birth control use. Finally, young women must be informed about the importance of prepregnancy planning.

TABLE 3. **Insulin Adjustment for High Blood Sugar During Illness**

| | Blood Sugar 250 or Above with Ketones (Small, Moderate, Large) | Blood Sugar 300 or Above without Ketones |
|---|---|---|
| Breakfast | Take your usual dose of NPH or Lente insulin<br>Take your usual dose of REGULAR insulin *plus* 50% more REGULAR insulin | Take your usual dose of NPH or Lente insulin<br>Take your usual dose of REGULAR insulin *plus* 30% more REGULAR insulin |
| Lunch | Take ⅛ unit of REGULAR insulin per pound of your weight | Take ⅒ unit of REGULAR insulin per pound of your weight |
| Supper | Take your usual dose of NPH or Lente insulin<br>Take your usual dose of REGULAR insulin *plus* 50% more REGULAR insulin | Take your usual dose of NPH or Lente insulin<br>Take your usual dose of REGULAR insulin *plus* 30% more REGULAR insulin |
| Bedtime | Take ¹⁄₁₂ unit of REGULAR insulin per pound of your weight | Take ¹⁄₂₀ unit of REGULAR insulin per pound of your weight |
| *Remember:* | If the extra insulin brings your blood sugar to below normal, subtract 1–2 units from the amount suggested next time. | |

## DIABETES EDUCATION

Diabetes education is an integral component of treatment. Successful management of diabetes depends on the ability of the patient and his or her family to incorporate multiple facets of complex disease treatment into daily life. Thus, one of the primary goals of education is to teach families how to become effective self-managers.

We use a multidisciplinary approach to education, providing a series of organized learning experiences tailored to a family's particular needs. Content for each series is sequenced from the simple to the more complex, starting with basic survival skills and ending with algorithms for insulin adjustment.

Education of new-onset patients and their families begins with a 3- to 4-day hospitalization, during which education is focused solely on basic survival skills, that is, those skills necessary to survive outside the hospital. On the first day, families are introduced to members of the multidisciplinary team and are given basic explanations about diabetes and its treatment. We also use this time to assess the family's knowledge of diabetes, dispel myths, and begin to deal with anxieties and fears. Because injections represent perhaps the greatest fear, insulin administration is introduced to families on the first day in order to dissipate some of the anxiety. Blood glucose monitoring is also introduced. By focusing attention initially on mechanical skills, families may begin to regain a sense of control.

By the second day, concepts related to hypoglycemia and its treatment are discussed. Diabetes pathophysiology is taught in a little more detail, and insulin administration is reviewed, with families administering insulin under supervision. Dietary education is begun with a primary focus on basics with less emphasis on food types and more emphasis on consistency of meal timing and food amounts.

The third day deals with hyperglycemia, basic sick day management, over-the-counter medications, and follow-up care. Content from previous sessions is reviewed and reinforced. A determination by the diabetes team is made as to the family's readiness for the patient's discharge, and most patients are discharged at that time. Frequent contact by phone is maintained until their return visit for intensive outpatient education several weeks later.

Our outpatient education program lasts 3 full days and meets in groups of six families 1 to 2 months after diagnosis. This delay in more intensive education serves two purposes. First, it enables families to begin to incorporate diabetes management into their daily lives and determine what works and what doesn't. Second, families are more receptive to education once they have had an opportunity to dissipate some of the shock that may interfere with earlier learning.

The curriculum provides a more in-depth discussion of contents previously covered. In addition, we teach algorithms for daily dose adjustment, insulin and dietary management for sick days, and supplemental insulin coverage for hyperglycemia. Dietary education emphasizes flexibility in meal planning, including reading food labels, dealing with fast foods, and incorporating recipes to provide a wide range of food choices. Subsequently, nutritional needs are reviewed at 3- to 6- month intervals and modified as necessary to reflect changes in growth, activity, or food preferences.

The importance of exercise and strategies appropriate to compensate for exercise are taught. Home exercise programs are developed individually for use during inclement weather for younger children. Older adolescents are taught how to manage diabetes around school activities and jobs. Issues related to self-esteem, talking to friends, birth control, prepregnancy planning, and complications are also discussed. New technologies and a research update are included. Finally, as part of long-term management, education is reviewed and brought up-to-date as children develop and their concepts about diabetes and their abilities change.

## PSYCHOSOCIAL CONSIDERATIONS

Because of the complicated nature of diabetes management, psychologic and social health of the patient and family and the social milieu are particularly relevant to treatment. As with most chronic illnesses, the diagnosis of diabetes is traumatic. We treat this as a family crisis and encourage crisis psychotherapy for everyone.

It is important to evaluate the individual family and child to be able to appropriately guide them in assuming responsibility for the care of diabetes. There is no one age at which children assume specific tasks, such as insulin injection, self-monitoring of blood glucose, or decisions about insulin doses. Rather, parents should be encouraged to maintain an active interest in their child's diabetes care as long as the child wishes it. Even if the child wishes to assume an increasing responsibility, he or she should only very gradually take on new tasks and should demonstrate the ability to consistently perform them. A gradual transition is best, and it is clear that children whose families are actively involved with their diabetes care well into their mid- to late teenage years do best. At this later age, families may only be involved in self-adjustment decisions.

The effect of psychosocial dysfunction on metabolic control is of the most direct concern to physicians. Most dramatic are those children who consciously omit insulin in an effort to induce DKA, a common occurrence, particularly among preadolescents and adolescents. This pattern occurs more often in girls but is not limited to them. The first step in treatment is recognizing that recurrent DKA is not due to intrinsic lability but to sabotage of the diabetic regimen, specifically the omission of insulin by the patient and, less commonly, by families. To treat, first document that the patient does not develop DKA when under supervision. The patient is hospitalized, with the hospital staff administering all insulin and performing all blood glucose monitoring. Insulin should be kept away from the patient so that he or she is not able to surreptitiously administer extra insulin. Forthright discussion with the patient and family about the nature of the problem, followed by appropriate psychologic counseling and clarification that a responsible parent needs to administer the insulin, is imperative. If this is unsuccessful, legal avenues may need to be explored to ensure that the child is receiving adequate medical supervision either in or out of the home.

Finally, physicians should appreciate that diabetes, in and of itself, does not cause psychologic dysfunction and that the vast majority of children with diabetes do not develop any unusual psychologic or social dysfunction.

## MONITORING FOR RISK FACTORS AND ASSOCIATED ILLNESSES

Diabetes can lead to the risk of retinopathy and life-threatening cardiovascular and renal disease. Exemplary diabetes management includes regular monitoring for known risk factors (Table 4).

Cigarette smoking constitutes a major risk factor for macrovascular complications. Adolescents should be strongly counseled to either quit or not start.

Hypertension is a serious risk factor for nephropathy. Patients with blood pressures greater than the ninetieth percentile for age should be evaluated and usually treated. Consideration should be given to treating adolescent patients with blood pressures greater than 135/85. Angiotensin-converting enzyme (ACE) inhibitors are currently the agent of choice.

Cardiovascular disease is the leading cause of premature death in diabetic patients. Hyperlipidemia may occur in conjunction with diabetes. For all patients, dietary management is preferable, and a hypolipidemic diet is taught to all patients. Elevated lipids can also occur as a result of hyperglycemia. In such cases, blood sugar control should be maximally improved before considering other options. When hyperlipidemia is not responsive to dietary treatment and is not sec-

TABLE 4. **Monitoring Recommendations for Complications and Associated Diseases**

Each Visit
  Blood pressure
  Height (if growing)
  Weight

Annually
  Random urinary microalbumin level
  Random cholesterol
  T4, T3RU (TSH if positive antithyroid antibodies)
  Ophthalmologic examination (duration >5 yr)
  Smoking history

At initial visit only (unless clinically indicated)
  Antithyroid antibodies
  TSH

PRN
  Fasting total and high-density cholesterol and 16-hour fasting triglycerides (if random cholesterol >200 mg/dl); 24-hour urinary microalbumin level and creatinine clearance (if random urine microalbumin level is greater than 30 µg/mg/Cr).

ondary to high blood glucose, antihyperlipidemic agents are in order. Any excessive alcohol intake must be reduced or eliminated. The goal should be to keep total cholesterol under 200 mg per dl unless HDL levels are high.

A random first morning urine for microalbumin should be obtained yearly. If the result is greater than 30 μg per mg creatinine, a 24-hour microalbumin level and creatinine clearance should be obtained. If total daily urinary microalbumin is greater than 30 to 40 mg per day, increased effort should be made to tighten metabolic control, normalize blood pressure, and monitor renal function.

While development of retinopathy may be best delayed by optimal glucose control, early treatment of preproliferative or proliferative disease with photocoagulation is strikingly effective. All patients with diabetes of over 5 years' duration should have yearly ophthalmologic evaluations.

Patients with insulin-dependent diabetes mellitus are at increased risk for other autoimmune diseases, particularly hypothyroidism and adrenal failure. Thyroid function should be monitored yearly and hypoadrenalism considered when clinically indicated. Guidelines for thyroid evaluation arc presented in Table 4.

# HYPERURICEMIA AND GOUT

method of
CHRISTOPHER M. WISE, M.D.
*Bowman Gray School of Medicine*
*Winston-Salem, North Carolina*

Gout most commonly presents in middle-aged males as an acute mono- or oligoarthritis in the lower extremities, but it should also be considered in the differential diagnosis of any unexplained acute or chronic inflammatory arthritis. The documentation of monosodium urate crystals in synovial fluid or from tophaceous deposits remains the only means of making a definite diagnosis of gout. Most patients with gout have elevated levels of serum uric acid at some point in their clinical course, but normal levels may be seen during acute attacks. Asymptomatic hyperuricemia is common, particularly in ambulatory patients on diuretics or critically ill patients with fluid and electrolyte disturbances. Thus, arthrocentesis followed by evaluation of synovial fluid by polarized microscopy for needle-shaped, intracellular, negatively birefringent crystals is essential in any patient suspected of having acute gout, when this has not been previously documented. In the patient with a history of prior attacks of acute arthritis suggestive of gout, aspiration of an asymptomatic knee or first metatarsophalangeal joint may allow demonstration of crystals, and thus confirm a diagnosis, even between attacks. Even in clinical settings where gout is the leading diagnostic consideration, alternative diagnoses such as infection or pseudogout should be kept in mind, and every effort should be made to confirm a diagnosis, particularly when long-term hypouricemic therapy is being considered.

## TREATMENT OF ACUTE GOUT

Acute gouty arthritis is a self-limited process that will resolve spontaneously without therapy. However, several days to 3 to 4 weeks may be required for such resolution, and attacks are usually sufficiently disabling to warrant therapy. Since changes in serum uric acid levels may be associated with precipitating attacks, no attempt should be made to lower uric acid levels during this phase. Agents that can be effective in terminating acute gout include most of the nonsteroidal anti-inflammatory drugs, oral or intravenous colchicine, and intra-articular or systemic corticosteroids. An individualized approach, based on the patient's age and concomitant medical problems, should allow a safe, prompt resolution of the acute attack in all but a small minority of patients.

**Nonsteroidal Anti-inflammatory Drugs (NSAIDs).** Because of their proven efficacy and relatively low toxicity profile in the acute setting, drugs in this class have become the mainstay of therapy in most patients with acute gout. NSAIDs are ideal for ambulatory patients without concomitant medical illnesses. The major risks include gastric irritation and ulceration, impairment of renal function, fluid retention, and central nervous system toxicity, such as headache and confusion. Such toxicities are much more common in the elderly or patients with renal or hepatic insufficiency. Thus, these drugs should be used with caution, or alternative therapies sought, in these clinical settings. In general, NSAIDs are started at a high dose initially (e.g., indomethacin (Indocin) 50 mg three to four times daily), continued at this dose for 1 to 3 days until a substantial improvement is noted, and the dose is then gradually reduced to a lower maintenance level for 1 to 2 weeks, depending on response and tolerability. NSAIDs that have been found to be effective in the treatment of acute gout are listed in Table 1, along with suggested dosages.

Indomethacin is effective and well tolerated in most healthy, ambulatory patients, but it seems to carry a higher risk for gastrointestinal (GI), renal, or central nervous system (CNS) toxicities and should be used with caution in the elderly. Sulindac (Clinoril) has been shown in some studies to have less risk of renal toxicity. Most of the other drugs listed have similar profiles of efficacy and safety. Phenylbutazone (Butazolidin), not

TABLE 1. **Nonsteroidal Anti-inflammatory Drugs (NSAIDs) Useful in Acute Gout**

| Drug | Initial Dose | Maintenance Dose |
|---|---|---|
| Indomethacin (Indocin) | 50 mg tid–qid | 25 mg bid–tid |
| Sulindac (Clinoril) | 200 mg bid | 150–200 mg bid |
| Ibuprofen (Motrin) | 800 mg tid–qid | 400–600 mg tid–qid |
| Naproxen (Naprosyn) | 500 mg bid–tid | 250–375 mg bid–tid |
| Fenoprofen (Nalfon) | 600–800 mg qid | 200–600 mg tid |
| Piroxicam (Feldene) | 20 mg qd–bid | 20 mg qd |
| Ketoprofen (Orudis) | 50–75 mg tid | 50–75 mg bid |
| Tolmetin (Tolectin) | 400–600 mg tid | 200–400 mg bid–tid |
| Meclofenamate (Meclomen) | 100 mg tid–qid | 50 mg bid–tid |
| Diclofenac (Voltaren) | 75 mg tid | 50–75 mg bid |
| Flurbiprofen (Ansaid) | 100 mg tid | 100 mg bid |

listed in the table, is highly effective but seldom used in recent years because of its high toxicity profile. Salicylates, because of their potential for interfering with urate excretion (see later), are usually not used in gout.

**Oral Colchicine.** Originally given as an extract of the autumn saffron (*Colchicum autumnale*) in ancient times, oral colchicine has long been known as an effective therapy for acute gout. However, GI symptoms, including nausea, cramping, and diarrhea, are frequent when given in full therapeutic doses. Oral colchicine may be given for an acute attack in a dosage of 0.5 mg or 0.6 mg every 1 to 2 hours until GI side effects occur or until there is significant improvement. A maximum dosage of 6 mg (10 to 12 tablets) should not be exceeded in 24 hours. Because colchicine is excreted slowly, any further colchicine (by any route) should be avoided for 7 days when the above high dose regimen is used. A modification of the above regimen, which is reasonably effective and safe, is to give 0.6 mg three to four times daily for 1 to 2 days and then reduce to a twice-daily schedule for 1 to 2 weeks. Serious toxicities associated with colchicine include bone marrow failure, renal and hepatic injury, CNS dysfunction, neuropathy, and myopathy. These toxicities have been limited almost exclusively to cases where an inappropriately high cumulative dose was given acutely, or in the elderly, or in patients with renal or hepatic insufficiency.

**Intravenous Colchicine.** Intravenous colchicine will result in prompt resolution of an acute attack without the GI side effects frequently associated with oral administration. However, strict adherence to dosage guidelines is mandatory in order to avoid the rarely reported bone marrow toxicity that has been seen with overdosage. Because extravasation of colchicine can cause severe tissue necrosis, the drug should be diluted with at least 20 ml of normal saline and administered only through an adequately running intravenous line. An initial dose of 1 to 2 mg may be given, followed by 1-mg doses 6 and 12 hours later. No more than 4 mg should be given in a 24-hour period, and no further colchicine, in any form, should be given for 7 days. In patients with renal or hepatic insufficiency, a total dosage of 2 mg should not be exceeded, or alternative forms of therapy should be considered.

**Corticosteroids.** Given intra-articularly, orally, or intramuscularly, corticosteroids have been shown to be effective in acute gout. Intra-articular injections of depot corticosteroids (triamcinolone [Aristocort Forte], methylprednisolone [Depo-Medrol], etc.) are particularly useful in the patient with an attack in a single large joint. Oral prednisone (Deltasone) in a dosage of 30 mg per day and tapered over 5 to 7 days or a single dose of 40 units of intramuscular adrenocorticotropic hormone (ACTH) may be effective. However, because of concern over "rebound" flares, most practitioners have limited the use of systemic steroids to patients with contraindications to other agents or in resistant attacks.

## MANAGEMENT OF INTERCRITICAL GOUT

After resolution of the initial attack of gout, goals of management should be to prevent subsequent attacks, assess the patient's baseline serum uric acid levels and patterns of uric acid excretion, and determine the need for hypouricemic therapy. Although recurrences are common, up to 40% of patients may not have another attack within the next year. There is a general correlation between serum uric acid levels and frequency of subsequent attacks.

**Prophylaxis.** After the initial attack, a 1- to 12-month period of prophylactic therapy is usually indicated. Low doses of oral colchicine (0.6 mg once or twice daily) will prevent recurrences in 75 to 90% of patients and are well tolerated in most patients with normal renal and hepatic function. Small doses of NSAIDs (e.g., indomethacin 25 mg twice daily) are probably effective prophylactically, although these agents have not been as extensively studied in this setting. Patients with severe initial attacks, marked hyperuricemia, or tophaceous deposits should probably receive prophylactic therapy for 6 to 12 months after the last attack. Prophylactic therapy should also be continued for several months after the initiation of hypouricemic therapy, discussed below.

**Assessment.** Serum uric acid levels vary considerably depending on state of hydration, concomitant medications, and alcohol use. Measurements of serum levels during asymptomatic periods provide a more accurate assessment for chronic hyperuricemia. A 24-hour urine collection will allow classification of the hyperuricemic patient as an "overproducer" (i.e., over 700 mg uric acid excretion per day) or an "underexcretor" (i.e., less than 700 mg uric acid excretion per day, inappropriately low in the face of hyperuricemia). Such classification will help determine a more definitive approach to hypouricemic therapy, should this be indicated.

**Indications for Hypouricemic Therapy.** There is still some disagreement as to which patients with gout should be treated with agents to lower serum uric acid levels. Some patients will never have a second attack and will never have renal stones or renal damage. On the other hand, most patients have microscopic evidence of synovial urate deposition (microtophi) at the time of the first attack. General indications for the initiation of hypouricemic therapy are listed in Table 2. Patients with clinically evident tophaceous deposits are at high risk for joint damage, renal stones, and renal damage. Patients with marked uric acid overproduction (greater than 1000 mg per day), uric acid stones, or oxalate stones with hyperuricosuria are at increased risk for further stone formation and renal parenchymal damage. The patient with recurrent attacks despite prophylactic measures should be considered for hypouricemic therapy, although the decision in this setting can be based on the frequency and severity of attacks and the patient's level of compliance. In any case, a decision to initiate hypouricemic therapy usually implies a lifelong commitment, with an understanding of the cost and potential risks of the medications involved.

## MANAGEMENT OF HYPERURICEMIA

Uric acid levels can be lowered by the use of drugs that either decrease production or increase renal excretion of uric acid. A majority (70 to 80%) of patients with gout are underexcretors of uric acid (i.e., less than 700 mg of urinary uric acid per day). In such patients with normal renal function and no history of renal stones, uricosuric drugs can be used. Drugs that decrease uric acid production will be effective in both overproducers and underexcretors. Since uricosuric drugs tend to be less expensive and toxic, an initial trial of a uricosuric drug is usually indicated in underexcretors. The goal of therapy should be to lower serum uric acid levels well into the normal range, preferably below 7 mg per dl, in order to permit gradual reduction of tophaceous deposits. During the initiation of hypouricemic therapy, prophylaxis with colchicine or a low-dose NSAID for several months after the last attack of acute gouty arthritis is usually indicated.

**Allopurinol.** A potent inhibitor of the enzyme (xanthine oxidase) needed to convert hypoxanthine to uric acid, allopurinol is the only agent currently available that will decrease the synthesis of uric acid. Allopurinol (Zyloprim) is effective in lowering both serum and urine levels of uric acid in almost all patients. The dosage of allopurinol needed to normalize uric acid levels ranges from 100 to 600 mg per day, with the most commonly used dosage being 300 mg per day. Allopurinol should be started at 100 mg per day, and the dosage gradually increased over several weeks until normal serum uric acid levels are achieved. Dosage should be reduced in patients with renal insufficiency, usually to 200 mg per day when creatinine clearance (CrCl) is less than 60 ml per minute, to 100 mg for CrCl of less than 30 ml per minute, and 50 mg for CrCl of less than 10 ml per minute.

Drug interactions with allopurinol are well described and include potentiation of purine analogues (6-mercaptopurine (Durinethol), azathioprine (Imuran), interactions with anticoagulants, increased toxicity from cytotoxic drugs, and increased incidence of rashes with certain other drugs (ampicillin, thiazides). Thus, a careful review of concomitant medications is mandatory whenever allopurinol therapy is initiated.

Although allopurinol is relatively safe, rashes have been described in 3 to 10% of patients taking this agent. A more severe hypersensitivity reaction manifested by diffuse rash, fever, eosinophilia, renal, and hepatocellular injury has been

TABLE 2. **Indications for Hypouricemic Therapy in Gout**

Tophaceous gout
Destructive arthropathy attributable to gout
Marked overproduction (>1000 mg per day) of uric acid
History of nephrolithiasis (urate or other)
Frequent disabling attacks of acute gout (see text)
Patients without documented gout:
  Hyperuricemia associated with neoplasm, chemotherapy anticipated
  ?? "Asymptomatic" hyperuricemia with marked (>1000 mg per day) hyperuricosuria (see discussion under asymptomatic hyperuricemia)
  Hyperuricemia associated with heritable disorders of purine metabolism

described with an incidence as high as 1 in 250 patients treated and a mortality of 20 to 25%. Thus, allopurinol should be discontinued immediately in any patient with unexplained rash or fever.

**Uricosuric Drugs.** These agents increase urate excretion by interfering with tubular reabsorption of filtered urate. Uricosuric drugs should not be used in patients with a history of renal stones or those with increased urinary uric acid excretion and will be ineffective in patients with impaired renal function. Probenecid (Benemid) and sulfinpyrazone (Anturane) are uricosurics available in this country. Probenecid is more commonly prescribed. It should be started at 250 mg twice daily and increased at weekly intervals to a maximum of 3 grams per day and should be given in divided doses (three to four times daily). Sulfinpyrazone can be initiated at a dose of 50 mg twice daily and increased to a maximum of 400 to 800 mg per day in divided doses. Because of the potential for stone formation, high fluid intake should be encouraged, and occasionally, alkalinization of the urine with acetazolamide or bicarbonate may be necessary to prevent stone formation. Both drugs are otherwise relatively safe but can rarely cause GI side effects. In addition, uricosurics can interfere with excretion of several other medications. Thus, a careful review of concomitant medications is also mandatory when one of these agents is initiated.

## CLINICAL CONSIDERATIONS IN THE MANAGEMENT OF GOUT

**The Critically Ill Patient.** Acute attacks of gouty arthritis are frequent in hospitalized patients with major medical or surgical illness. Although usually seen in the patient with a previous diagnosis of gout, the initial attack may occur in such a setting. Treatment of acute gout in these patients is frequently compromised by an inability to take oral medications, unstable hemodynamic status, or tenuous renal or hepatic function. Intravenous colchicine may be given with care but probably should be limited to a single dose of 1 to 2 mg, and no further colchicine in any form should be given for 7 days. If a small number of joints are involved, intra-articular steroids may be the safest treatment in these patients. If joints are difficult to access by arthrocentesis or if multiple joints are involved, intramuscular ACTH may be preferable. No attempt should be made to initiate hypouricemic therapy in the critically ill patient.

**The Patient with Peptic Ulcer Disease.** In patients with recently active peptic ulcer disease, NSAIDs should be avoided. Although recent advances in cytoprotective therapy (i.e., misoprostil [Cytotec]) may allow the use of NSAIDs in patients with a history of peptic ulcer disease, this has not been adequately studied in this clinical setting. Oral or intravenous colchicine, intramuscular ACTH, or intra-articular steroids are preferable to NSAIDs for acute gout in patients with peptic ulcer disease.

**The Patient with Renal Insufficiency.** Patients with renal insufficiency are frequently hyperuricemic without clinically evident tophi, gouty arthritis, or renal stones, and such patients should not be treated with hypouricemic therapy. In acute gout, any of the usual therapies may be used, with certain limitations.

NSAIDs may cause worsening of renal function and should be used in reduced dosage if at all. Sulindac appears to have less nephrotoxic potential and may be preferable to other NSAIDs in this setting. Colchicine dosage in the acute setting should be reduced, and patients on chronic colchicine should be monitored for hematologic and neurotoxicity. Attempts to lower dosage or discontinue the drug should be considered earlier in these patients. Uricosuric drugs should not be used, and allopurinol dosage should be reduced in patients with renal insufficiency, as noted previously.

**Gout in the Elderly.** Recent literature suggests that gout may be under-recognized in the elderly and should be considered in the differential diagnosis of any unexplained arthritis, particularly in women who may present atypically. Therapy in elderly patients with gout should be undertaken cautiously, and dosages of most medications should be reduced to avoid potential toxicity. Many elderly patients have only a few mild attacks of gout and may never require hypouricemic therapy.

**Hyperuricemia in the Cancer Patient.** Patients with hyperuricemia associated with neoplasms are at increased risk for acute renal tubular precipitation of uric acid, particularly if chemotherapy is anticipated. Such patients should be treated prophylactically with allopurinol along with increased fluid intake. If there is a history of gout, low-dose oral colchicine should be considered to prevent the attack that can be seen with rapid changes in uric acid levels.

## SPECIAL AREAS OF INTEREST

**The Resistant Attack.** Although a vast majority of acute attacks can be controlled with colchicine or an NSAID, an occasional patient will respond poorly to initial therapy. Patients with resistant attacks should be carefully re-evaluated for alternative diagnoses, such as infectious arthritis, by repeat arthrocentesis and culture of synovial fluid. In the patient with an inadequate response to oral NSAID or colchicine, the addition of an intra-articular steroid or intramuscular ACTH may result in eventual control of the resistant attack.

**Coexistent Infection in Acute Gout.** Patients with underlying joint disease are at increased risk for joint infection, and coexistent infection should be considered in the patient with the severe or resistant attack. Although gout can cause fever and sometimes purulent-appearing synovial fluid, such patients should have synovial fluid cultures sent as part of their initial evaluation.

**Role of Diet and Alcohol.** Even the strictest purine-free diet will result in only modest reductions in serum uric acid, and such dietary restrictions are seldom helpful in management. However, weight reduction may be a very useful way to lower uric acid levels in some obese patients. Heavy alcohol consumption is frequently associated with hyperuricemia, and attacks may be precipitated by alcohol consumption, particularly in "binge" drinkers. All patients with gout should be counseled to reduce their alcohol consumption.

**Salicylates and Gout.** Salicylates affect renal tubular handling of urate, causing increased serum levels owing to decreased excretion at low doses and acting as a uricosuric at high (greater than 3 grams per day) doses. Because of these effects, salicylates should be avoided in patients with gout, and patients should be warned to avoid over-the-counter salicylate preparations.

**Asymptomatic Hyperuricemia.** Although there has been some concern over potential long-term renal damage in patients with persistent hyperuricemia, subsequent studies have shown that this is limited to patients with documented gout, tophi, or renal stones. Thus, truly asymptomatic hyperuricemia should not be treated. Exceptions to this include hyperuricemic cancer patients anticipating chemotherapy. In addition, asymptomatic patients who demonstrate marked overproduction of uric acid (greater than 1000 mg of urinary uric acid per day) appear to be at increased risk for renal stone formation and should be followed carefully.

**Allopurinol Hypersensitivity.** As discussed previously, the full-blown syndrome of allopurinol hypersensitivity carries such a high mortality that allopurinol should be avoided in any patient with a history of significant rash attributed to this drug. In such patients who require hypouricemic therapy, uricosuric drugs should be attempted, and weight reduction and avoidance of alcohol and salicylates should be re-emphasized. Successful regimens to desensitize patients with a prior history of rash from allopurinol have been published, but such regimens should be undertaken only under careful supervision.

**Associated Conditions.** The association of gout with hypertension, hyperlipidemia, renal disease, obesity, and alcohol overuse is well described. Patients with gout should be carefully evaluated for these treatable, and potentially morbid, conditions.

# HYPERLIPOPROTEINEMIA

method of
ERNST J. SCHAEFER, M.D.
*Tufts University School of Medicine*
*New England Medical Center*
*Boston, Massachusetts*

Elevated plasma or serum cholesterol and/or triglyceride levels are associated with increased levels of lipoproteins. Increased plasma low-density lipoprotein (LDL) cholesterol levels and decreased high-density lipoprotein (HDL) cholesterol levels are associated with the development of atherosclerosis, and severe hypertriglyceridemia with circulating chylomicrons in the fasting state is associated with recurrent pancreatitis.

## LIPOPROTEIN METABOLISM

Cholesterol is a sterol that is an important constituent of membranes and a precursor of various hormones as well as bile acids. The very properties that make this molecule important for membranes (i.e., its insolubility in aqueous media) also cause it to promote atherosclerosis in the artery wall when present in excess. About 70% of the cholesterol in the blood stream has one fatty acid attached to it (known as "cholesteryl ester"). Humans consume about 400 mg of cholesterol per day in the diet, and absorption from the intestine varies between 30 and 70% of the amount ingested. Triglyceride or triacylglycerol is a molecule composed of three fatty acids attached to a glycerol backbone. Humans consume about 20 to 150 grams of fat or triglyceride per day. Triglyceride is broken down into fatty acids in the intestine by lipases in the presence of bile acids. Fatty acid absorption in the intestine is very efficient (more than 90% of the amount ingested). Humans can synthesize both cholesterol and triglyceride.

Lipoproteins are round particles composed of cholesterol, triglyceride, phospholipid, and protein. Chylomicrons are very large, triglyceride-rich (90% by weight) particles made in the intestine in response to a fat-rich meal. On entry into the plasma, the chylomicron triglyceride content is rapidly depleted by lipoprotein lipase, an enzyme that is located on the surface of endothelial cells in the capillary bed. This enzyme, in the presence of a protein activator (apolipoprotein C-II) and albumin, removes fatty acids from the glycerol backbone of triglyceride. Fatty acids are stored as triglyceride in the fat cell. During the lipolytic process, chylomicron remnants are formed, which are taken up by the liver. In normal individuals, chylomicrons are not present in fasting plasma. When chylomicron catabolism is impaired, severe hypertriglyceridemia occurs, and such particles can be deposited in various tissues, including the liver and pancreas. Such deposition causes an enlarged, fatty liver and pancreatitis as a result of intracellular release of pancreatic lipase. Chylomicrons are not thought to be atherogenic particles because they contain very little cholesterol and are too large to be filtered into the arterial wall. However, accumulations of chylomicron remnants are probably atherogenic.

Very-low-density lipoproteins (VLDLs) are triglyceride-rich (60% by weight) lipoproteins that are made by the liver. VLDL is the major carrier of plasma triglyceride in normal individuals in the fasting state. After VLDL enters the plasma, its triglyceride content is rapidly depleted by lipolytic enzymes to form LDL. In certain instances, especially in the setting of hypertriglyceridemia, VLDL is removed from the plasma without being converted to LDL. In other instances, especially in the setting of hypercholesterolemia, LDL may be produced directly by the liver. There is debate as to whether VLDL particles are atherogenic. Patients with elevated triglyceride levels caused by increased VLDL often have decreased HDL levels, and this lipid pattern is often observed in patients with premature coronary heart disease (CHD). Small, cholesterol-rich VLDL particles are probably atherogenic.

LDL particles are cholesterol rich (60% by weight) and are the major carriers of plasma cholesterol in normal individuals. About 70% of LDL is removed from the blood stream by the liver, and about 70% of all LDL catabolism occurs via LDL receptor-mediated uptake. Dietary saturated fat (especially myristic and palmitic acids) and dietary cholesterol both downregulate LDL receptor activity, which results in increased plasma LDL cholesterol levels. LDL particles are known to be atherogenic and are deposited in the arterial wall.

HDL particles are protein rich (50% by weight). They are synthesized directly in both the liver and the intestine. In addition, HDL constituents are derived from components (proteins and lipids) shed from the surface of chylomicrons and VLDL during lipolysis. HDL has been shown to promote removal of free cholesterol from cholesterol-laden cells. The free cholesterol in HDL is rapidly esterified. It can then remain with the HDL particle or be transferred to other lipoproteins, such as chylomicron or VLDL remnants, by transfer proteins. HDL is catabolized mainly by the liver and appears to play a major role in reverse cholesterol transport. There is currently debate as to whether an HDL receptor exists. Moreover, the precise role of HDL in protecting against atherosclerosis remains to be defined.

## DIAGNOSIS OF LIPOPROTEIN DISORDERS

In 1985 a National Institutes of Health Consensus Conference panel concluded that elevated blood cholesterol levels (specifically, increased LDL cholesterol) were associated with premature CHD and that lowering LDL cholesterol levels was associated with a decreased risk of developing CHD. In addition, the panel concluded that the blood cholesterol levels of many Americans were undesirably high because of an excessive intake of dietary saturated fat and cholesterol. The panel recommended identification and treatment of individuals whose cholesterol levels were above the seventy-fifth percentile of normal. In 1987, the adult treatment panel of the National Cholesterol Education Program (NCEP), sponsored by the National Heart, Lung, and Blood Institute, released its guidelines for the diagnosis and treatment of elevated blood cholesterol levels in individuals older than 20 years of age; the guidelines focused on elevated LDL cholesterol.

Total plasma or serum cholesterol levels can be measured in the nonfasting state as well as in the fasting state. For screening programs, finger stick methodology is now available. A total cholesterol level below 200 mg per dl has been classified as desirable and should be rechecked in 5 years. A cholesterol level of 200 to 239 mg per dl is in the borderline category, and a level of 240 mg per dl or more is in the high-risk category. To proceed further with individuals in the borderline category, it is necessary to obtain information about the presence of CHD or CHD risk factors. CHD has been defined as prior myocardial infarction or angina. Other CHD risk factors include male sex, a family history of premature CHD (defined as myocardial infarction or sudden death in a parent or a sibling before age 55 years), cigarette smoking, hypertension, decreased HDL cholesterol level (below 35 mg per dl, confirmed by repeat measurement), diabetes mellitus, a history of cerebrovascular or peripheral vascular disease, and severe obesity (defined as 30 per cent or more above ideal body weight).

If the patient has a cholesterol level in the borderline category in the absence of CHD or two or more CHD risk factors, dietary information (see later) should be given to the patient and the cholesterol level should be rechecked in about 1 year. For the patient in the borderline cholesterol category with CHD or two or more CHD risk factors, or for the patient in the high-risk cholesterol category, a lipoprotein analysis is recommended. An alternative approach is to measure lipoprotein levels in all patients with cholesterol values of 200 mg per dl or greater. I prefer the latter approach because patients in the borderline category may be misclassified if their HDL cholesterol level is not measured. Alternatively, HDL cholesterol can be measured in the nonfasting state, but it may be 2 to 4 mg per dl lower than when measured in the fasting state.

To measure lipoprotein levels, the patient should be instructed to fast for at least 12 hours, except for water. Total cholesterol and triglyceride levels in plasma or serum are measured. Plasma levels are 3% lower than serum levels. HDL cholesterol is also measured in the supernatant fraction after the other lipoproteins have been precipitated. Ideally, laboratories should obtain coefficients of variation for these assays of 3% or less and should participate in a standardization program linked to the Centers for Disease Control Lipid Research Clinics program. To calculate the VLDL cholesterol level, the triglyceride level is divided by 5. The LDL cholesterol level is then calculated by subtracting the VLDL and HDL cholesterol levels from the total cholesterol level. This calculation is not valid if the triglyceride level is higher than 400 mg per dl. For an approximate measure of the LDL cholesterol level in patients with triglyceride levels higher than 400 mg per dl, the triglyceride level should be divided by 6 for levels up to 1000 mg per dl and by 8 for levels higher than 1000 mg per dl. Precise measurement of LDL cholesterol levels in these latter categories requires ultracentrifugation.

An LDL cholesterol level of less than 130 mg per dl has been classified as desirable, a level of 130 to 159 mg per dl as borderline, and a level of 160 mg per dl or more as high risk. An LDL cholesterol level of 160 mg per dl represents approximately the seventy-fifth percentile for middle-aged Americans. An LDL cholesterol level higher than 225 mg per dl is above the ninety-fifth percentile for all age and sex groups, and an HDL cholesterol level less than 27 mg per dl is below the fifth percentile for all age and sex groups. Triglyceride levels higher than 250 mg per dl, with VLDL cholesterol levels higher than 50 mg per dl, have been classified as elevated. A triglyceride level greater than 320 mg per dl is above the ninety-fifth percentile for all age and sex groups. Severe hypertriglyceridemia is characterized by triglyceride levels greater than 1000 mg per dl. In this latter category, chylomicrons are almost invariably present, as assessed by lipoprotein electrophoresis. It is important to confirm the presence of elevated levels by repeat determinations. Acute infections and myocardial infarction are known to affect plasma lipid levels, so patients should have these levels checked more than 6 weeks after such illnesses.

### Secondary Causes

Secondary causes of hypercholesterolemia should be ruled out before initiating dietary and drug therapy. Secondary causes of an elevated LDL cholesterol level include hypothyroidism, obstructive liver disease, and nephrotic syndrome. Rarer secondary causes include dysproteinemia and porphyria. Secondary causes of hypertriglyceridemia include excess alcohol intake, diabetes mellitus, renal insufficiency, use of beta-blocker medication, and estrogen therapy. Rarer causes include glycogen storage disease and lipodystrophy. Secondary causes of HDL deficiency include hypertriglyceridemia, diabetes mellitus, renal insufficiency, use of beta-blocker medication, male sex, obesity, and use of progestins and anabolic steroids.

## TREATMENT

### Hypercholesterolemia (Elevated LDL Level)

Hypercholesterolemia is defined as an elevated plasma cholesterol level (240 mg per dl or higher) in the setting of a normal triglyceride level. Rarely, patients in this category have markedly elevated HDL cholesterol levels but normal LDL cholesterol levels. These patients do not require therapy. Most hypercholesterolemic patients have elevated LDL cholesterol levels (160 mg per dl or higher, Type IIA hyperlipoproteinemia), as previously defined. The most common forms of these disorders have either an autosomal dominant or a polygenic mode of inheritance without xanthomas. Therefore it is worthwhile to screen family members. Some of these patients can be treated with dietary therapy alone, but many require medication in addition to diet. Before using medication, dietary therapy (see later) should be tried for at least 6 months. Drugs should be initiated in all patients who maintain an LDL cholesterol level higher than 190 mg per dl after dietary therapy, with the goal being to lower the LDL cholesterol level to less than 160 mg per dl. In addition, in patients with CHD or two or more CHD risk factors, drugs should be initiated after dietary treatment if the LDL cholesterol level remains higher than 160 mg per dl after dietary therapy, with the goal being to lower the LDL cholesterol level to less than 130 mg per dl. Patients should be encouraged to continue the dietary treatment even after receiving medication.

Anion exchange resins (see later) are currently the drugs of choice for the treatment of elevated LDL cholesterol levels. Patients who cannot tolerate these agents should be given niacin (see later). Both of these agents have been shown to reduce the incidence of CHD in prospective studies but are difficult for many patients to tolerate. A new medication, lovastatin, which inhibits hydroxymethylglutaryl coenzyme A (HMG CoA) reductase, the rate-limiting enzyme in cholesterol biosynthesis, is now available. This medication (see later) is extremely effective in lowering the LDL cholesterol level and is well tolerated by most patients. However, its long-term safety and efficacy in reducing the incidence of CHD have not yet been demonstrated. Current experience with the agent indicates excellent safety after at least 5 years of use. If its efficacy in reducing the incidence of CHD is established, this agent will become the drug of choice for reducing LDL levels. Lovastatin is currently the drug of choice in patients who are unable to tolerate either resins or niacin or who do not achieve an adequate LDL cholesterol reduction with these other agents. Probucol (see later) is another agent that is available for lowering cholesterol levels. This is a third line agent that is generally well tolerated. Probucol lowers LDL cholesterol levels modestly but also lowers HDL cholesterol levels significantly. Long-term efficacy data on reduction of the risk of CHD are not yet available for this agent. For this reason, I rarely use it. The combination of resins and niacin is extremely effective, as are the combinations of resin and lovastatin and of niacin and lovastatin. However, all these agents have side effects (see later) that require careful follow-up of the patient.

Occasionally, patients present with marked hypercholesterolemia (level often higher than 400 mg per dl, with LDL cholesterol levels well above the ninety-fifth percentile) and tendinous xanthomas. These patients are heterozygotes for classic familial hypercholesterolemia (autosomal dominant mode of inheritance) and often develop CHD before the age of 50 years. Homozygotes with this disorder are very rare, can develop CHD in their teens, and have been shown to have a variety of LDL receptor defects. Heterozygous patients almost invariably require treatment with medication in addition to diet. Moreover, they often require two medications used in combination. In children with this disorder (cholesterol levels higher than 300 mg per dl), I use low doses of resin. After puberty these patients are treated in the same manner as adult patients with elevated LDL cholesterol levels. Homozygotes with familial hypercholesterolemia generally require plasma exchange every 2 weeks. Some of these patients respond to medication but do not achieve adequate reductions in LDL cholesterol levels. Those patients who do respond should continue to receive medication in addition to plasma exchange.

### Hypercholesterolemia and Hypertriglyceridemia (Elevated VLDL and LDL Levels)

Combined elevations of plasma cholesterol levels (higher than 240 mg per dl) and triglyceride levels (higher than 250 mg per dl) are commonly observed. One form of this disorder, known as "familial combined hyperlipidemia," is an autosomal dominant disorder in which affected family members may have elevations of both plasma cholesterol and triglyceride levels (associated with VLDL cholesterol levels higher than 50 mg per dl and LDL cholesterol levels higher than 160 mg per dl, Type IIB hyperlipoproteinemia) or elevations of either one alone. These patients have overproduction of VLDL and LDL, and those with hypertriglyceridemia have some delayed VLDL clearance as well. Screening of family members is worthwhile. Some patients with this lipid pattern can be treated with dietary therapy alone (alcohol abstention, weight reduction, and an exercise program are also important). For patients who maintain an LDL cholesterol level higher than 190 mg per dl or for those whose LDL cholesterol level is higher than 160 mg per dl in the presence of CHD or two or more CHD risk factors after 6 months of dietary therapy, the drug of choice is niacin. For patients who are not candidates for this agent or who cannot tol-

erate it, the combination of resin and gemfibrozil can be used. Resins should not be used as the only agents in these patients because they elevate triglyceride levels. For patients who cannot tolerate the combination or obtain an inadequate response, lovastatin should be used. The combination of gemfibrozil and niacin can also be used.

Rarely, patients in this category may have dysbetalipoproteinemia or Type III hyperlipoproteinemia associated with a marked increase in cholesterol-rich VLDL of abnormal beta-migrating electrophoretic mobility. These patients may have palmar xanthomas (yellow creases in the palms) and tuberoeruptive xanthomas, especially on the elbows. This disorder is associated with genetic abnormalities in apolipoprotein E and with delayed clearance of chylomicron remnants and VLDL, as well as excess hepatic VLDL production. Diagnosis is not essential except for research purposes because the treatment is the same as that for other patients with combined elevations of cholesterol and triglyceride levels.

### Hypertriglyceridemia (Elevated VLDL Level)

Hypertriglyceridemia is defined as a triglyceride level higher than 250 mg per dl in the setting of a normal LDL cholesterol value (Type IV hyperlipoproteinemia). These patients often have decreased HDL cholesterol levels. Patients with elevated triglyceride levels may have familial hypertriglyceridemia, an autosomal dominant disorder. These patients have overproduction of hepatic triglyceride and may have defective VLDL catabolism as well. All patients with hypertriglyceridemia should be treated with dietary therapy. Emphasis should be placed on caloric restriction in overweight patients and abstinence from alcohol, as well as a regular program of exercise. An attempt should be made to switch patients who are on beta-blocker medication to other agents, such as calcium channel blockers, that do not raise triglyceride levels. The goal of therapy is to reduce triglyceride levels to less than 200 mg per dl and to raise the HDL cholesterol level to more than 40 mg per dl. Patients in this category are not covered by the new NCEP guidelines, and yet they are among the ones most commonly observed in any survey of patients with premature CHD. In one large recent primary prevention study (the Helsinki Heart Study), about 8% of the subjects had elevated VLDL cholesterol and normal LDL cholesterol levels. In this study, subjects in this category who received gemfibrozil had a lower incidence of CHD prospectively than subjects in this category who received a placebo. The question is whether such patients should be treated with medication if dietary therapy fails to normalize their triglyceride levels. Our practice is to treat such patients with medication if they have established CHD or a definite family history of CHD. The medication of choice is niacin. For patients who cannot tolerate this agent or who are not candidates for the drug, gemfibrozil should be used.

### Severe Hypertriglyceridemia

Severe hypertriglyceridemia is defined as a triglyceride level higher than 1000 mg per dl in plasma obtained from a patient after a 12- to 14-hour overnight fast. Patients can be subclassified further on the basis of lipoprotein electrophoresis into those who have both chylomicrons and excess VLDL present (Type V hyperlipoproteinemia) or those in whom only chylomicrons are present (Type I hyperlipoproteinemia). The former pattern is much more common, and these patients are often middle-aged, overweight individuals who commonly have concomitant adult-onset Type II diabetes mellitus and hyperuricemia. These patients have delayed clearance of triglyceride-rich lipoproteins of either intestinal or hepatic origin and increased hepatic production of VLDL. These patients may have arthritis, paresthesias, or dry eyes and mouth, as well as emotional lability. Family members of these patients often have moderate hypertriglyceridemia. Treatment with diet is very important (dietary fat should be restricted to less than 20% of calories), as is weight reduction via calorie restriction, abstinence from alcohol, and avoidance of estrogens, beta blockers, and thiazide diuretics. An exercise program is also recommended. In the diabetic patient, careful control of glucose levels is important. These patients are at high risk of developing recurrent pancreatitis and may present with eruptive xanthomas and lipemia retinalis. If dietary and other therapies are not effective in lowering the triglyceride levels to less than 500 mg per dl, the drug of choice is gemfibrozil. If additional triglyceride reduction is required or if patients cannot tolerate this agent, fish oil capsules should be used. In patients without diabetes, niacin can be used as well. Gemfibrozil is the single most effective triglyceride-lowering agent in this category of patient.

Occasionally, patients with severe hypertriglyceridemia are children or young adults and are not obese or diabetic. These rare patients often have chylomicrons as their major lipoprotein band on electrophoresis. They may have a deficiency of the enzyme lipoprotein lipase or of its activator protein (apolipoprotein C-II) and have a striking inability to catabolize chylomicrons. Treatment consists of dietary fat restriction to less than 20 grams per day. Niacin and gemfibrozil are generally not effective in these patients, but a trial of therapy is indicated. In my experience, fish oil capsules (see later) are effective in lowering triglyceride levels in some patients in this group.

### HDL Deficiency

HDL deficiency is defined as an HDL cholesterol level less than 35 mg per dl in the presence of normal VLDL and LDL cholesterol levels. Dietary therapy is recommended for these patients to optimize their LDL cholesterol levels. For overweight patients, caloric restriction is indicated. An exercise program is also important, as is cessation of smoking. Patients taking beta-blocker medication should be switched to lipid neutral medications if possible. For patients with established CHD with HDL deficiency that is still present despite attempts to use the previously described measures, niacin therapy can be used. In patients who cannot tolerate niacin or who do not obtain an adequate response, gemfibrozil should be used.

### Patients with Coronary Heart Disease

In such patients, efforts should be made to optimize levels of plasma lipids and lipoproteins. My goals in these patients, in addition to smoking cessation and control of hypertension, body weight, and glucose level, are to reduce LDL cholesterol levels to less than 130 mg per dl, to raise HDL cholesterol levels to more than 40 mg per dl, and to lower triglyceride levels to less than 200 mg per dl. In a recent 2-year study of hypercholesterolemic post–coronary artery bypass patients, use of the combination of niacin and colestipol was associated with marked reductions in LDL cholesterol levels, increases in HDL cholesterol values, and significantly less progression of angiographically documented coronary atherosclerosis compared with the placebo group. However, many CHD patients cannot tolerate these agents. I do not hesitate to use lovastatin in such patients because one can achieve similar LDL cholesterol reductions, along with modest decreases in triglyceride levels and increases in HDL cholesterol levels with this agent.

### Pregnant Women

Patients who become pregnant should immediately stop use of all lipid-lowering medications until after pregnancy and nursing are completed. Women who are attempting to conceive should also stop medication. Pregnant women who have severe hypertriglyceridemia and who have had pancreatitis should be treated with marked dietary fat restriction (less than 20 grams per day). If these measures are unsuccessful in reducing triglyceride values to less than 1000 mg per dl, fish oil capsules should be tried.

### Children

All children above the age of 2 years should be treated with diet if their LDL cholesterol levels are higher than 130 mg per dl. Children with LDL cholesterol levels higher than 225 mg per dl while eating an LDL-reducing diet are candidates for therapy with low doses of resin (see later). After puberty, adolescents should be treated in the same manner as adults.

### Diabetic Patients

Patients with Type I diabetes generally have normal lipid levels if their glucose levels are well controlled. In contrast, patients with Type II diabetes frequently have elevated triglyceride levels and decreased HDL cholesterol levels. Occasionally, these patients may have elevated LDL cholesterol values. Attempts should be made to optimize their lipid levels, as for CHD patients, because these patients are at high risk for developing clinically significant atherosclerosis. In addition to glucose control and modification of diet and lifestyle, gemfibrozil is useful for lowering triglyceride levels and raising HDL levels, and cholestyramine or lovastatin can be used to control LDL cholesterol levels.

### Dietary Management

Dietary therapy should be initiated in all patients with an LDL cholesterol level of 160 mg per dl or greater and in patients with levels of 130 mg per dl or greater if CHD or two or more CHD risk factors are present. Target levels for therapy in these two groups are identical to initiation levels. The current recommendation is to provide the patient initially with pamphlet information and counseling and then to determine if the patient has reached the target levels. Excellent pamphlets for patients can be obtained from the local American Heart Association affiliate or the NCEP Program (telephone 301–951–3260), which provide information about the NCEP Step 1 diet. The goal of this diet is to reduce dietary fat to less than 30% of calories, dietary saturated fat to less than 10% of calories, and dietary cholesterol to less than 300 mg per day. Such a diet has been recommended as prudent for the entire population by both the American Heart Association and the U.S. Surgeon General. Achieving optimal weight and exercising regularly are also recommended. These latter measures are often more effective in lowering triglyceride levels than cholesterol levels.

If the patient has not reached target levels within 3 months, referral to a trained registered dietitian is recommended for implementation of the Step 2 diet. This diet is designed to reduce dietary fat to less than 30% of calories, saturated fat to less than 7% of calories, and dietary cholesterol to less than 200 mg per day. In general, physicians should allow 6 months to determine whether target levels can be achieved with dietary therapy alone. Use of dietitians is encouraged, but the physician should also emphasize the importance of diet as the cornerstone of therapy. In our experience, this stepwise approach may be too cumbersome and lengthy for many patients to adhere to, and direct referral to a dietitian with implementation of the Step 2 diet is preferable. The same diet is used for all forms of hyperlipoproteinemia.

Some guidelines about the NCEP Step 2 diet follow. The use of fresh vegetables (as long as they are not prepared with saturated fat) and fruits is encouraged, as are cereals except for granola or "natural cereals" containing coconut oil. The use of skim milk, egg whites, and nonfat or low-fat yogurt products is encouraged, and the use of eggs, cheeses, and other dairy products such as butter, whole milk, cream, and ice cream is discouraged. Sherbet can be used. The oils that are lowest in saturated fat include rapeseed (canola), safflower, and sunflower oils. Soft margarine made from these oils should be used instead of butter. Foods containing palm or coconut oil should be avoided. Most breads are fine except for croissants and muffins. Fish is fine, as is turkey or chicken white meat without the skin. Lobster, crab, clams, and mussels are fine, but shrimp should be eaten only occasionally because of its high cholesterol content. Patients can occasionally eat lean beef (round) or extra lean ham. Spaghetti and macaroni are fine, but pizza, quiche, cookies, cakes, pies, chocolate, and french fries should be avoided unless they have been specially prepared.

Some authorities have recommended the use of a high-monounsaturated-fat diet instead of a high-polyunsaturated-fat diet or a high-carbohydrate, low-fat diet. It has been shown that monounsaturated fats are as effective in lowering LDL cholesterol levels as are polyunsaturated fats, compared with saturated fat, and have the advantage of not lowering HDL cholesterol levels. In addition, some studies suggest that polyunsaturated fats act as cocarcinogens when used in experimental animals in large amounts in the diet. Therefore the current recommendations are that polyunsaturated fat intake not exceed 10% of caloric intake and that no limitation be placed on monounsaturated fats. Studies suggest that a saturated fatty acid (stearic acid) found in beef and chocolate does not raise LDL cholesterol levels. It should be noted, however, that these food products contain more palmitic acid than stearic acid, and palmitic acid definitely raises LDL cholesterol levels. It should also be noted that a major source of monounsaturated fat in the U.S. diet is meat. The emphasis of the NCEP Step 1 and Step 2 diets on lowering dietary saturated fat and cholesterol intake is appropriate because these are the dietary constituents that raise LDL cholesterol levels in the blood stream. The NCEP Step 1 and Step 2 diets are lower in monounsaturated fat content than the current U.S. diet (about 15% of calories as saturated fat and monounsaturated fat and 6% of calories as polyunsaturated fat). In patients with severe hypertriglyceridemia, dietary fat should be restricted to less than 20% of calories.

## Drug Therapy

Drug therapy is indicated after at least a 6-month trial of diet in all patients with LDL cholesterol levels higher than 190 mg per dl, with the goal of reducing LDL cholesterol levels to less than 160 mg per dl. Drug therapy is also indicated after dietary therapy in patients with LDL cholesterol levels higher than 160 mg per dl if CHD or two or more CHD risk factors are present, with the goal of reducing the LDL cholesterol level to less than 130 mg per dl. Medications used for lipid reduction include anion exchange resins, niacin, fibric acid derivatives, HMG CoA reductase inhibitors, fish oil capsules, and probucol.

### Anion Exchange Resins

The resins bind bile acids in the intestine, which prevents their reabsorption and promotes their fecal excretion. This process causes conversion of more cholesterol to bile acids in the liver, depletion of the cholesterol content in hepatocytes, and up-regulation of liver LDL receptor activity. This process, in turn, leads to enhanced catabolism of plasma LDL resulting in reductions in plasma LDL cholesterol levels. The most common side effects are constipation, abdominal cramps, and distention. Less common effects include flatulence, nausea, vomiting, heartburn, and anorexia. These agents often increase plasma triglyceride levels and interfere with the absorption of digoxin, thyroxine, warfarin sodium (Coumadin), phenobarbital, phenylbutazone, beta

blockers, chlorothiazide, tetracycline, and potentially other agents. Therefore, such medications must be given either 1 hour before or 4 hours after the use of resins. Decreased levels of folate and of fat-soluble vitamins have been reported with chronic use of fairly high doses of resin. Therefore, annual measurements of the prothrombin time, as well as of folate, retinol, and alpha-tocopherol levels, are reasonable. Deficiencies of these nutrients are extremely rare in patients on resins.

Two different resins are available. Cholestyramine (Questran) comes in packets containing 4 grams of active compound, and colestipol (Colestid) comes in similar packets containing 5 grams of a different resin. Both agents have similar efficacy and side effects. Cholestyramine has an orange-like flavor and has extra filler, whereas colestipol is tasteless. Both agents also come in containers from which patients can scoop the powder. One packet is equal to one scoop, and the price of scoops is substantially less than the price of packets. Cholestyramine is also available as a bar (one bar is equal to one packet). The packets or scoops of powder must be mixed with water or juice and thoroughly stirred before use. Patients can try either resin formulation to see which they prefer. Some authorities recommend using resins in a dose of one or two packets orally four times per day. It has been shown that resin is equally effective if given in a comparable dose twice a day. I start by giving the patient one packet or scoop twice a day and increase the dose to two scoops twice a day. Many patients can tolerate this regimen and achieve LDL cholesterol reductions of 15 to 20%. If constipation develops, it can be treated with psyllium (Metamucil), 1 teaspoon orally twice daily, which may lower LDL cholesterol further. In a large prospective study (Lipid Research Clinics Study) in asymptomatic middle-aged men with elevated LDL cholesterol levels, the use of cholestyramine during a 7-year period resulted in a 12% reduction in LDL cholesterol levels in the drug group and a 19% lower rate of development of CHD compared with a placebo group. Subjects receiving the drug were supposed to use six packets per day, but the average subject used three and one-half; four and one-half packets per day were used in the placebo group. Clearly, long-term compliance is a problem with this agent. Those subjects in the study who actually took 24 grams per day of cholestyramine sustained a 35% reduction in LDL cholesterol levels. In my experience, using lower doses (16 grams per day of cholestyramine) markedly increases compliance. In children with marked hypercholesterolemia under the age of 5 years, I use one-half packet or scoop of resin twice daily; in children between the ages of 5 and 10 years, I use one scoop twice daily; and in older children and adults, I use two scoops of resin twice daily. In patients who develop vomiting, the drug should be discontinued immediately.

### Niacin

Niacin or nicotinic acid, when used in pharmacologic doses of 2 to 3 grams per day, decreases the production of VLDL and LDL and increases HDL cholesterol levels. Triglyceride levels are decreased by approximately 30% and LDL cholesterol levels by about 20%, and HDL cholesterol levels are increased by about 20%. In a large prospective study (the Coronary Drug Project), use of niacin in a dose of 3 grams per day in patients with previous myocardial infarction was associated with a 10% reduction in total cholesterol and a 20% reduction in prospective CHD incidence during a 5-year period compared with the placebo group. Fifteen years after initiation of the trial and 9 years after completion of the study and termination of medication, subjects who had been taking niacin had an 11 per cent lower mortality than those who had been taking a placebo. Responses are quite variable. Niacin is available as an over-the-counter medication in 50-, 100-, 250-, 500-, and 1000-mg tablets. The drug is started at a dose of 100 mg orally twice daily with meals and gradually increased during a 2-week period to 1 gram orally twice daily. Three times daily dosing may reduce adverse reactions. Doses of either 1 gram orally three times daily or 1.5 grams orally twice daily with meals can also be used. Some authorities use even higher doses, but the incidence of side effects increases markedly. I recommend using no more than 2 grams per day for most patients. Almost all patients have initial problems with flushing, but this effect decreases with time. Aspirin or nonsteroidal anti-inflammatory compounds decrease the flushing and may have to be used for the first month of therapy, or whenever niacin is stopped for even short periods. Long-acting or delayed-release niacin can also be used. The drug may also cause gastritis and should not be taken on an empty stomach, but after 1 month I switch the patient to regular niacin. There is evidence that long-acting niacin is less effective and is associated with more gastrointestinal side effects than regular niacin. Niacinamide has no lipid-lowering effect and cannot be used in place of niacin.

All patients receiving niacin should have baseline liver enzymes, glucose, and uric acid levels measured. These parameters need to be monitored in all patients initially every 6 weeks for the first 6 months, and then every 3 to 6 months.

Contraindications to niacin use include peptic ulcer, liver disease, and hyperuricemia (although the last problem can be treated with allopurinol). Niacin should not be used in diabetic patients unless they are taking insulin and one is prepared to increase the dose of insulin. There is a significant incidence of liver enzyme level elevation in patients taking niacin, and if these levels increase to greater than three times the normal mean, the drug should be discontinued. Other side effects include dry skin, dry eyes, postural hypotension, and, rarely, acanthosis nigricans.

### Fibric Acid Derivatives

The fibric acid derivatives gemfibrozil (Lopid) and clofibrate (Atromid-S) are extremely effective triglyceride-lowering agents and are generally well tolerated. These agents decrease VLDL synthesis and enhance VLDL degradation. Clofibrate is used less frequently than gemfibrozil because it is less effective in lowering triglyceride levels and because excess mortality was associated with its use compared with placebo in the World Health Organization Study. In this large prospective primary prevention study in middle-aged, hypercholesterolemic men, subjects taking clofibrate had 8% lower cholesterol levels and a 21% lower incidence of CHD during a 5-year period compared with the placebo group but had higher mortality. Clofibrate is known to promote lithogenic bile and to cause gallstones. In another study with clofibrate (the Coronary Drug Project), no increases in mortality were observed (even at the 15-year follow-up), but only a 6% reduction in cholesterol levels and a 10% decrease in prospective CHD incidence were observed during 5 years compared with the results achieved with a placebo. In contrast, in a recent large prospective primary prevention study in middle-aged, hypercholesterolemic men (the Helsinki Heart Study), the use of gemfibrozil at a dose of 600 mg orally twice daily was associated with a mean 9% lower total cholesterol level, a 35% lower triglyceride level, a 9% lower LDL cholesterol level, a 10% lower HDL cholesterol value, and a 34% lower incidence of CHD compared with the results achieved with a placebo. Gemfibrozil appears to be less lithogenic than clofibrate. No major adverse effects were noted with gemfibrozil in the Helsinki study.

Gemfibrozil is generally well tolerated. Occasional gastrointestinal side effects are noted, as are rare liver enzyme level elevations and changes in hematologic test results. Muscle cramps and increased creatine phosphokinase (CPK) levels are observed in about 1% of cases; therefore, CPK monitoring is warranted. Allergic skin reactions also occur rarely. The drug is contraindicated in patients with renal insufficiency or liver disease. It is available in 300-mg capsules and 600-mg tablets. The standard dose is 600 mg orally twice daily. The drug potentiates the action of Coumadin, so that patients taking both agents may have to have their Coumadin dose reduced by 50%. A new fibric acid derivative, fenofibrate, may soon be available in the United States. This agent is substantially more effective in lowering LDL cholesterol than either clofibrate or gemfibrozil and has been used in Europe for a long time. In patients with normal LDL cholesterol levels, gemfibrozil is the drug of choice for lowering triglyceride levels.

### Lovastatin

Lovastatin (Mevacor) inhibits HMG CoA reductase, the rate-limiting enzyme in cholesterol biosynthesis, which results in reduced intracellular cholesterol levels, up-regulation of LDL receptor activity, enhanced plasma clearance of LDL, and decreased LDL cholesterol levels in plasma. The drug may also decrease VLDL and LDL hepatic production. The drug is available in 20-mg tablets. The starting dose is 20 mg orally per day in the evening, and the maximal dose is 40 mg orally twice daily. Reductions of approximately 20% in LDL cholesterol are observed with 20 mg per day, 30% with 40 mg per day, and about 40% with 80 mg per day. Some patients obtain a maximal effect with a dose of 20 mg orally twice daily. The drug is generally well tolerated. There is about a 1% incidence of significant liver enzyme level elevation and a similar incidence of significant CPK level elevation and muscle cramping. Both of these side effects necessitate discontinuation of the drug. Other reported side effects include headaches, decreased sleep duration, insomnia, nausea, fatigue, gastrointestinal distress, weight gain, and rashes. Other HMG CoA reductase inhibitors will soon be available in the United States. One of these, pravastatin, does not cross the blood-brain barrier, so that the potential central nervous system side effects of lovastatin, such as headaches, decreased sleep, and insomnia, may be reduced.

It is recommended that patients taking lovastatin have their liver enzyme and CPK levels monitored at baseline and every 6 weeks for the first year, and every 3 to 6 months thereafter. Elevations in CPK levels, myalgia, and rhabdomyolysis have occasionally occurred in patients treated concurrently with niacin, gemfibrozil, or immunosuppressive agents. An annual eye examination is recommended to rule out the development of cataracts, although there is no evidence at present that this agent causes cataract formation in humans at the dose levels used. In contrast to other effective LDL-lowering agents (resins and niacin), lovastatin is generally well tolerated by most patients. If long-term safety is established and efficacy in CHD reduction is demonstrated, HMG CoA reductase inhibitors will become the drugs of choice for LDL reduction.

### Fish Oil Capsules

Fish oil capsules are effective triglyceride-lowering agents in patients with severe hypertriglyceridemia in whom sufficient triglyceride reduction has not been achieved with other agents. Fish oil capsules contain 1 gram of fish oil, which is almost entirely fat. These capsules contain as much saturated fat as they do omega-3 fatty acids. The capsules that we use are obtained from Bronson Pharmaceuticals (LaCanada, Calif.; 800–521–3322) and, based on our own analysis, contain the least saturated fat and the most omega-3 fatty acids of all commercially available capsules that we have tested. Moreover these capsules (SuperEPA) are much less expensive than some of the other heavily advertised products. The starting dose is three 1-gram capsules orally twice daily, which may have to be increased to five capsules twice daily. In some studies, 30 to 40 grams per day has been used. Ten capsules per day is a low dose compared with clinical trials. These capsules can be used in combination with any other lipid-lowering drug. They are generally well tolerated. They cause a modest increase in bleeding time and occasional gastrointestinal distress and may cause a fishy odor when the patient belches. Fish oil capsules may increase LDL cholesterol levels and may also increase glucose levels in diabetic subjects.

### Probucol

Probucol (Lorelco) is a potent antioxidant compound that is incorporated into both LDL and HDL particles. It enhances LDL clearance by non–receptor-mediated mechanisms and decreases HDL production. The drug is available in 250- and 500-mg tablets, and the dose is 500 mg orally twice daily. The drug lowers LDL cholesterol levels by about 10 to 15% and HDL cholesterol levels by about 20%. Some authorities recommend its use as a second- or third-line drug in the treatment of familial hypercholesterolemia. However, in my view, this drug cannot be recommended until its efficacy in CHD reduction has been documented because of its adverse effects on HDL cholesterol levels. Probucol is generally well tolerated but may cause diarrhea, flatulence, abdominal pain, and nausea and may prolong the QT interval on the electrocardiogram.

### Combination Therapy

The combination of resins and niacin is extremely effective in lowering LDL cholesterol and triglyceride levels and in raising HDL cholesterol levels. The combination of lovastatin with either resins or niacin is even more effective in lowering LDL cholesterol levels. However, the incidence of significant liver enzyme level elevation is quite high with the niacin-lovastatin combination. The combination of resins and gemfibrozil is effective in lowering triglyceride and LDL cholesterol levels and in raising HDL cholesterol levels. The combination of lovastatin and gemfibrozil is extremely effective in lowering triglyceride and LDL cholesterol levels and in raising HDL cholesterol levels, but the incidence of myositis and CPK elevation is about 7%. Therefore, patients taking this combination of drugs need to be carefully monitored.

# OBESITY

method of
BEATRICE S. KANDERS, Ed.D., M.P.H., R.D.,
R. ARMOUR FORSE, M.D., Ph.D., and
GEORGE L. BLACKBURN, M.D., Ph.D.
*Harvard Medical School*
*Boston, Massachusetts*

Obesity is a complex disease resulting in a condition of excess body fat which can contribute to important health and functional consequences. It is a cause of hypertension, diabetes, and lipid abnormalities. It also results in insulin resistance. This increased insulin resistance has been associated with a number of metabolic abnormalities, including hyperinsulinemia, hypertension, hypercholesterolemia, and hyperuricemia, now identified as syndrome X (Reaven's syndrome). Improvements in insulin resistance and the associated clinical outcomes are sensitive to 5 to 15% changes in body weight. Other co-morbidities of obesity include cardiomyopathy, respiratory failure, hypoventilation syndrome, gallbladder disease, and certain forms of cancer (Table 1). Indeed, recently, obesity was identified as a strong risk factor for coronary heart disease in middle-aged women—and even mild to moderate overweight was associated with a substantial elevation in coronary risk. The risk of mild obesity, once thought to be minimal, has recently been closely examined. New evidence suggests that even mild overweight will

increase the risk of heart disease particularly in individuals who smoke and have syndrome X.

The proportion of overweight adults in the United States has been steadily increasing in the past several decades, especially among women. Indeed, obesity is one of the most prevalent diet-related problems in the United States with the highest rates observed among the poor and minority groups. At present, about 34 million adults, or one in five Americans, ages 20 to 74, are obese, that is, 20% or more above the desirable level, and about 12 million individuals are severely overweight (40% or more above ideal body weight).

Given the complexity of the disease, obesity remains difficult to treat and long-term success rates remain poor. Its complex causes include genetic, environmental, psychologic, social, and metabolic components that interrelate. The American diet, which is high in fat and low in fiber, and the American lifestyle, which is largely sedentary, are strong contributors to the increasing prevalence of obesity in this country. As such, obesity has more recently been recognized as an important public health problem that has been highlighted in the Surgeon General's Report on Nutrition and Health (U.S. Department of Health and Human Services, 1988), and the Diet and Health Report of the National Research Council (Diet, Health and Chronic Diseases, National Research Council, Washington, D.C., 1988).

While no precise medical definition of obesity exists, the condition is one of excess body fat that adversely affects health. Insurance company tables suggest an "ideal" range of weight for given heights, derived from data on insured persons with the longest lifespans, yet these weight for height tables do not present an accurate estimate of excess body fat per se. A more useful calculation involves the determination of body mass index (BMI), body weight in kilograms divided by height in meters squared ($kg/m^2$). A simple nomogram (Table 2) has been developed for the rapid determination of BMI. The calculated BMI can then be used to classify the degree of severity of obesity (Table 3). In addition, the pattern of body fat distribution has important effects on the risk of disease. Patients with upper-body, or android, obesity (inferred from the waist to hip circumference ratio) sustain greater risk from obesity-related illness as compared with patients with lower body (femoral-gluteal), or gynoid, obesity.

Recent evidence demonstrated that as little as a 5 to 10% weight reduction that can be sustained for 3 to 5 years will ameliorate most obesity-related diseases and metabolic disorders involving insulin-sensitive glucose uptake ("insulin resistance"). Obesity can be an important contributor to 5 of the 10 major chronic illnesses; prevention and treatment can be factors in preventing primary disease and reducing risk. Thus, physicians must understand and actively begin to treat patients with obesity and weight gain.

State-of-the-art treatment of obesity is multidisciplinary and should include increasing physical activity; a healthy, nutrient-dense hypocaloric diet; and behavior modification leading to a permanent change in lifestyle. Treatment of obesity by conventional diet programs or by emphasizing weekly weight change without comprehensive therapy has yielded extremely poor results and is not recommended. Because obesity

TABLE 1. **Conditions Associated with Obesity**

| | |
|---|---|
| Diabetes mellitus | Hyperinsulinism |
| Hypertension | Polycystic ovary |
| Coronary heart disease | Hirsutism |
| Congestive heart failure | Acanthosis nigricans |
| Restrictive lung disease | Psychosocial incapacity |
| Sleep apnea | Certain cancers (e.g., colon, prostrate in men; endometrial, ovarian in women) |
| Degenerative arthritis | |
| Pickwickian syndrome | |
| Infertility | Hyperlipoproteinemia |
| | Gallbladder disease |

TABLE 2. **Medical Classification of Obesity Using Body Mass Index (BMI) for Men and Women***

| Grade of Obesity: | 1 | 2 | 3 | 4 | 5 | 6 |
|---|---|---|---|---|---|---|
| Definition: | Overweight | Obesity | Significant Obesity | Morbid Obesity | Super Obesity | Supermorbid Obesity |
| Height: | BMI 25 | 30 | 35 | 40 | 45 | 50 |
| 4' 10" | 120 | 144 | 167 | 191 | 215 | 239 |
| 4' 11" | 124 | 149 | 174 | 198 | 223 | 248 |
| 5' 0" | 128 | 153 | 179 | 205 | 230 | 256 |
| 5' 1" | 132 | 159 | 185 | 212 | 238 | 265 |
| 5' 2" | 137 | 164 | 191 | 219 | 246 | 273 |
| 5' 3" | 141 | 169 | 198 | 226 | 254 | 282 |
| 5' 4" | 146 | 175 | 204 | 233 | 262 | 291 |
| 5' 5" | 150 | 181 | 211 | 241 | 271 | 301 |
| 5' 6" | 155 | 186 | 217 | 248 | 279 | 310 |
| 5' 7" | 160 | 192 | 224 | 256 | 288 | 320 |
| 5' 8" | 164 | 197 | 230 | 263 | 296 | 329 |
| 5' 9" | 169 | 203 | 237 | 271 | 305 | 338 |
| 5' 10" | 174 | 209 | 244 | 279 | 313 | 348 |
| 5' 11" | 179 | 215 | 251 | 287 | 322 | 358 |
| 6' 0" | 185 | 222 | 259 | 295 | 332 | 369 |
| 6' 1" | 190 | 228 | 265 | 303 | 341 | 379 |
| 6' 2" | 195 | 233 | 272 | 311 | 350 | 389 |
| 6' 3" | 200 | 240 | 280 | 320 | 360 | 400 |
| 6' 4" | 206 | 247 | 288 | 329 | 370 | 411 |

*Adapted from Robert E. T. Stark, M.D., Phoenix, Arizona, 1987.

TABLE 3. **Medical Classification of Obesity Using Body Mass Index***

| Desirable Weight‡ (%) | Definition | Grade of Obesity | Excess Fat‡ (lb/kg) | BMI‡ (kg/m²) |
|---|---|---|---|---|
| *Men* | | | | |
| 225 | Supermorbid obesity | 6 | 173/79 | ≥50 |
| 200 | Super obesity | 5 | 139/63 | 45 |
| 180 | Morbid obesity | 4 | 111/50 | 40 |
| 160 | Medically significant obesity | 3 | 83/38 | 35 |
| 135 | Obesity | 2 | 48/22 | 30 |
| 110 | Overweight | 1 | 14/6 | 25 |
| 100 | Desirable weight | 0 | 0 | 22 |
| 70 | Medically significant starvation | −3 | −15/−7† | 15 |
| *Women* | | | | |
| 245 | Supermorbid obesity | 6 | 158/72 | ≥50 |
| 220 | Super obesity | 5 | 131/59 | 45 |
| 195 | Morbid obesity | 4 | 103/47 | 40 |
| 170 | Medically significant obesity | 3 | 76/34 | 35 |
| 145 | Obesity | 2 | 49/22 | 30 |
| 120 | Overweight | 1 | 22/10 | 25 |
| 100 | Desirable weight | 0 | 0 | 21 |
| 75 | Medically significant starvation | −3 | −20/−9† | 15 |

*Medical risk of obesity is further modified by concurrent illness(es), complicating organ dysfunction, body fat distribution, velocity of weight change, and age. Relative risk varies from 2–15-fold.

†Assuming 75% of weight loss in simple starvation is body fat.

‡% desirable weight = % desirable body weight − 154 pounds for Reference Man; 120 pounds for Reference Woman (1980 Recommended Dietary Allowance Table). Excess fat (pounds), assuming 90% of excess body weight is fat. BMI = Body Mass Index (weight/height²).

Developed by the Nutrition/Metabolism Laboratory, Cancer Research Institute, Boston, MA.

is a complex disease with a variety of etiologies, treatment strategies should be tailored to the physical and emotional needs of the individual. When considering treatment approaches, a comprehensive evaluation of an obese patient's background should be the first step toward identifying an appropriate treatment strategy.

## TREATMENT

### Comprehensive Weight-Control Program

A comprehensive, multidisciplinary approach to weight loss and long-term maintenance should include the following three components: (1) increased physical activity; (2) a hypocaloric diet followed by a balanced maintenance diet that is low in fat and high in fiber and emphasizes fruits and vegetables, whole grains, and lean meats; (3) behavior modification. Drug therapy in the form of an adjuvant to this multidisciplinary approach may also be indicated to treat depression or to control appetite. Patients with morbid obesity are candidates for surgical therapy. Although exercise and dietary restriction are central to the initial weight loss phase, long-term weight maintenance requires permanent lifestyle changes that necessitate increased physical activity and behavior change.

### Medical Treatment Program Overview

At the initial interview, attention should be given to the patient's rationale for seeking treatment and his or her expectations of the program. Physician involvement is essential in that the physician can best explain the program's rationale and requirements. It is especially important to establish a patient-physician partnership based on shared responsibility. Since many obese individuals suffer from obesity-related health problems, the physician can emphasize the health benefits as well as the potential improvement in the quality of life offered by long-term weight loss.

State-of-the-art medical treatment of obesity requires a team approach. This team should consist of a physician and dietitian specializing in weight control. Consulting psychologists and exercise physiologists can be brought in as needed. Due to the complex nature of the disease and the necessity of close medical supervision of these patients, only physicians experienced in the treatment of obesity (more than 50 cases per year) should offer treatment programs. Physicians not equipped to treat these patients can refer them to existing self-help programs, trained registered dietitians specializing in weight control, or other physicians with specialties in bariatric or nutritional medicine.

### Medical Evaluation

Often the physician's first encounter with an obese patient may result from a health complaint related to a weight gain. Typically, these patients will present with excess fatigue and low self-esteem as well as obesity-related medical problems. Hypertension, diabetes, high blood cholesterol, cardiovascular disease, sleep apnea, infertility, degenerative arthritis, and gallbladder disease are all associated with moderate to morbid obesity; overweight or a 20- to 40-pound weight gain also increases the patient's risk for certain types of cancer, neurologic disorders, and kidney diseases (see Table 1 for summary). When patients seek medical help for a weight-related disorder, physicians must explain that a simple prescription "or crash diet" will not resolve the problem and may compound it by aggravating other disorders due to the excess weight. Even if the obese patient has not yet experienced any additional problems, the physician should explain the potential risks and engage the patient in a thorough evaluation. Estimation of excess body fat from height/weight tables is accurate in only 40% of females and 80% of males. Determination of anthropometrics, body composition, and fat distribution is the key to a thorough assessment.

During the initial interview, the physician should emphasize the need for the patient to take responsibility for his or her treatment. Discussion of the patient's rationale for seeking therapy and his or her expectations of the program is also essential. While the patient is ultimately responsible for the success of the program, the physician must be involved as a sensitive, supportive partner. Obesity is generally misunderstood as an indication of personal slothfulness and gluttony rather than as a complex disease, and it is important for the medical professional to affirm his or her patient's self-esteem by relaying an understanding of the complex nature of this condition.

Medical screening should include not only a physical examination, body composition assessment, and routine biochemical and metabolic tests, but also psychologic testing, a fitness evaluation, and a nutritional history, including a description of previous dieting experiences. With the aid of a trained dietitian, patients should be instructed on keeping 3-day food diaries, in which they write down the type, amount, and time of consumption for all food eaten (include one weekend day). If possible, patients should also have a 20-year weight history questionnaire and 7-day activity diary mailed to them in advance with instructions to complete them prior to their visit. The physician will be able to use the weight history questionnaire to identify patterns of weight cycling and potential body weight set points and use the 3-day food diaries and activity records to identify unhealthy eating behavior and sedentary living. The process of record keeping helps patients begin to assume responsibility for their treatment. It also allows them to monitor their compliance and identify problems related to treatment.

At the first visit, the physician or dictitian should review with the patient the changes that will be required: lower fat consumption, increased physical activity, detailed planning, and modification in eating habits. Currently, Americans consume 37% of their total calories as fat, a level associated with many health problems regardless of body weight. Finally, food consumption trends indicate that more and more Americans are eating away from home, and these meals typically are high fat, low fiber, and not balanced. These are all habits that can be modified with the help of a trained dietitian without tremendous sacrifice on the part of the patient. Patients should be aware that these eating, exercise, and lifestyle changes are essential to successful weight loss and postobese weight maintenance.

Once the comprehensive medical evaluation has been completed, patients should be instructed to begin a nutrient balanced deficit diet. This low-fat diet provides 1200 to 1500 calories and a minimum of 2 liters of water or low-calorie beverages per day. A trained nutritionist or nurse can provide dietary instruction, sample menus, and low-fat recipes. Patients should also be told to begin a walking program, starting with a minimum of three to five 15-minute sessions each week. Less than 10% of the U.S. population exercises for 30 minutes at least three times per week, emphasizing the sedentary nature of people in this country. Detailed food and activity diaries, which record changes in mood as well, should be kept for the next week. These will then be used to evaluate the patient's commitment to serious medical treatment of obesity,

At the next visit (1 week later), the patient's commitment to undertaking comprehensive treatment program can be evaluated based on compliance with these recommendations. Patients who are unwilling to adhere to these initial strategies may not be appropriate for aggressive treatment and the cause of their reluctance should be discussed. Treatment is varied if personal or other problems exist that would inhibit a successful outcome. These patients may be better off waiting until they are physically and mentally capable of undergoing therapy. For those patients who are deemed appropriate and wish to continue with treatment, blood pressure and weight as well as mood changes, subjective feelings, and personal goals and objectives should be assessed. Target weight loss goals are to decrease obesity by one grade (see Table 3) or a 20- to 40-pound weight loss for the average obese individual.

At this point, the physician working with the patient should discuss the options for weight reduction, namely, dietary intervention, surgery (for morbidly obese patients), and pharmacotherapy. The prescription should be based on the amount of excess body weight, dieting history, physical and mental health status, and stated lifestyle preferences. The physician and patient work together to select the appropriate program.

### Dietary Intervention

All obese patients, regardless of the final choice of intervention, should start with a program of brisk walking, dietary intervention, and record keeping. Those planning to use surgery or drugs should continue with the initial prescription until the physician feels the patient is psychologically and physiologically ready to undertake further treatment.

Regardless of the calorie level prescribed, the active weight-loss phase should last from 12 to 16 weeks; few patients can successfully lose weight and maintain the same level of enthusiasm beyond 4 months. During this period of weight loss, patients on a low-calorie diet should lose 20 to 40 pounds (10 to 15% of their body weight), and patients on a very low-calorie diet should lose 30 to 60 pounds (15 to 20% of body weight). Patients should plan to come in weekly throughout active weight loss, as frequent contact with medical staff helps to support and motivate patients and assure safety. In addition, a nurse or physician should routinely monitor patients for adverse experiences, both related and unrelated to the diet.

**Low-Calorie Diets (LCDs).** Low-calorie diets are ideally suited for mildly overweight patients (BMI 25 to 30). The conventional American Diabetic Association exchange-list diets offer a varied diet that is easy to follow. The diets, based on "exchanges" of defined portions of food, are set up to provide from 800 to 1500 calories per day, although the calorie level should be individualized according to the initial weight and sex of the patient. Although it is possible to obtain adequate levels of all vitamins and minerals while on a low-calorie diet, supplementation with a multivitamin is recommended.

Patients should also be given the option of selecting meal replacements as part of their diet. For patients who live hectic, stressed lives, and for patients who have difficulty preparing and eating the appropriate amount of food, meal replacements and ready-to-serve, low-fat entrees offer nutritious and effective methods of portion control. Examples of meal replacements include Alba 77, Carnation Instant Breakfast, and Ultra Slim•Fast. Prepackaged (frozen or shelf stable) entrees or dinners that contain approximately 10 grams of fat or less for 300 calories can be used. Patients should, however, receive instruction on the proper use of meal replacements and supplementing prepackaged foods with additional foods by a nutritionist or other trained health professional.

**Very-Low-Calorie Diets (VLCDs).** Very-low-calorie diets are defined by an intake equal to or below 800 calories per day and are frequently referred to as semistarvation or supplemented fasting. Total starvation is no longer recommended for any obese patient as several deaths have been reported of patients on total fasts due to cardiac arrhythmias and excessive loss of lean body tissue. The modern VLCDs are designed to produce rapid weight loss while preserving lean body mass and are associated with only minor complications when administered by physicians trained in their use. As reported by the AMA Council on Scientific Affairs, because patients participating in these diets do incur some risk, VLCDs should be limited to persons who are a minimum of 50 pounds (more than 130% IBW) overweight. Patients should also undergo meticulous screening by a physician. In addition to the medical evaluation described above, these patients should receive an electrocardiogram, a chest roentgenogram, and a complete blood profile, including electrolytes, blood urea nitrogen, creatinine, fasting glucose, liver function tests, and calcium, phosphorus, and lipid panel. Patients should be free of any contraindications, such as pregnancy; very young or advanced age; recent myocardial infarction; cardiac conduction disorder; history of cerebrovascular, renal, or hepatic disease; cancer; or any significant psychiatric disturbance. Very-low-calorie diets must only be administered when the physician has received proper training and is experienced in their use, possible complications, and probable outcome.

Very-low-calorie diets should provide a minimum of 70 grams of protein per day and optimally 70 grams or more; this should supply 1.2 to 1.5 grams of protein per kilogram of ideal body weight and adjusted to restrict loss of lean body mass to less than 15% of weight loss. Carbohydrate, if provided at all, should be limited to no more than 100 grams per day. The VLCD can be either liquid or food based. The popular liquid-protein diets, such as Optifast, Medifast, and Health Management Resources (HMR), are administered as packets of milk- or egg-based protein powder that, when mixed with water, supply all necessary vitamins, minerals, and electrolytes as well as small amounts of carbohydrate and essential fatty acids. Very-low-calorie diets composed of poor quality protein, such as digested collagen, have been associated with a number of deaths and are not recommended. Morbidly obese patients should be instructed to supplement a liquid VLCD with one meal of lean meat, fish, or fowl (3 to 4 ounces) each day.

The alternative to liquid-protein VLCDs comes in the form of a protein-sparing modified fast (PSMF). This diet provides two or three servings of lean meat, fish, or fowl (3- to 4- ounce servings), which must be trimmed, cooked without fat, and weighed after cooking. No other food is allowed, although certain patients may be prescribed a small plain salad. Vitamin and mineral supplements are essential, and intake of 2 to 3 liters of fluids is recommended (Table 4). Special attention must be paid to supplementation of folic acid, potassium, calcium (Tums), and magnesium (milk of magnesia tablets). The consumption of three bouillon cubes is recommended to provide sodium chloride to counteract the natriuresis of early fasting.

The metabolic changes associated with both types of VLCD include loss of hunger and rapid rate of weight loss, which help motivate patients to remain in the program. During the weight-loss phase of the VLCD, patients must undergo weekly physical examinations and have their electrolyte levels and other laboratory values monitored biweekly or at the very least monthly. Blood pressure should also be carefully monitored to ensure that adequate sodium, potassium, and fluid supplementation does not lead to orthostatic hypotension. Other mild complications include headache, nausea, vomiting, diarrhea, constipation, amenorrhea, mild fatigue, hair loss, dry skin, and hypothermia. Abdominal pain represents a major concern, as the possibility of exacerbating gallstone attacks may arise.

Plasma uric acid levels generally increase during a VLCD, and patients with a prior history of gout are prone to develop symptoms, which can be alleviated with prescribed medication; no cases of gout have been documented in previously asymptomatic patients. Patients with adult-onset

TABLE 4. **Daily Composition of a Protein-Sparing Modified Fast (PSMF)**

1. 1.5 grams of high-quality protein per kg of ideal body weight
2. K-lyte, giving 25–50 mEq of potassium
3. One-a-day vitamin with minerals
4. Sodium chloride, 5 gm or more
5. Calcium carbonate (Tums), 4 tablets per day, providing 800 mg of calcium
6. Magnesium 400 mg
7. 2 liters or more of fluids

diabetes or significant hypertension should be weaned off oral hypoglycemic and diuretic agents at the onset of the diet. Other antihypertensive drugs, such as beta blockers and alpha agonists, may be continued but only with careful monitoring. The VLCD is not contraindicated for the Type I insulin-dependent diabetic; however, use of a VLCD requires close medical supervision by an experienced physician. We have successfully treated these patients as outpatients with a VLCD that is 800 kcal and contains 50% of these calories (100 grams) from carbohydrate. Patients will need to reduce their insulin by approximately 50%. Type II insulin-requiring diabetics should also be closely followed, as they will need to continue to reduce their insulin with weight loss and possibly discontinue its use.

Following the active weight loss phase of the VLCD, patients must be gradually refed over 4 to 6 weeks. This is a particularly high-risk period for cardiac arrhythmia, gallstone formation, and other morbidity. During refeed, vegetables, fruits, dairy products, and starches must be slowly reintroduced to the diet as the patient is weaned off the liquid supplement or lean meats. Liquid VLCD patients replace the supplement with lean meats. Low-fat, unprocessed foods are emphasized, and patients must undergo close monitoring.

**Exercise.** While on a low-calorie or a very-low-calorie diet, patients must increase their level of physical activity. Patients should always start with a walking program in which they start off with three sessions lasting 15 to 20 minutes each. Over the course of 12 weeks, patients are instructed to increase the duration (by 5-minute increments) and frequency of walking sessions until they have worked up to 200 minutes of purposeful exercise per week. Patients with orthopedic problems that limit weight-bearing activity should be instructed to swim and concentrate on upper body exercises that strengthen the upper torso. After the active weight-loss phase, because calorie levels will be increased by varying degrees, patients should set new weekly goals of 200 to 400 minutes of exercise per week. At this time, patients should begin to include physical activity that addresses the four areas of fitness: cardiovascular fitness, muscular strength (with emphasis on upper body conditioning), endurance training, and flexibility. Variety in the form of swimming, bicycling, weight training, or low-impact aerobics can be added to enhance compliance. The added bonus of improved well-being, self-esteem, and overall health that results from regular exercise should also be stressed when discussing the patient's physical activity.

**Behavior Modification.** Finally, without individual or group therapy, patients are unlikely to maintain weight loss achieved by the hypocaloric diet. Behavior modification is based on the concept that changing daily habits will promote long-term control of body weight. Self-monitoring is used to identify eating behaviors and moods that are associated with overeating or poor compliance, and patients are taught during the active weight-loss phase to recognize these adverse behaviors and to substitute healthier behaviors that promote compliance. Patients are also taught to reduce their exposure to food and to food cues (smells, locations, time of day, special event, etc.) and to reinforce their positive behaviors by rewarding them in ways that do not involve food. Finally, comprehensive programs provide cognitive restructuring to help the patients modify their attitudes and beliefs about their weight, body image, and self-esteem. Patients must be taught to think positively about themselves and their efforts to control their weight to encourage continued success. Contingency planning, problem solving, and visualization exercises are an important part of long-term treatment programs.

**Maintenance.** At the conclusion of the 12- to 16-week weight-loss phase, caloric level should be increased to maintain the new reduced body weight. The maintenance calorie level can vary considerably but is usually between 1300 to 2500 calories, depending on the weight, age, sex, and activity level of the patient. Each pound of weight loss will lower resting energy expenditure by about 10 kcals. Thus a 200- to 400-calorie reduction from prediet intake must occur to maintain a 20- to 40-pound weight loss. Because obesity is a chronic problem requiring lifelong diligence in preventing relapse, patients must enter a maintenance program or at least maintain regular contact with their physician. Maintenance contact should occur one to two times per month and should reinforce the patient's nutrition education, exercise goals, and behavior modification skills. Maintenance contact can be a phone call, individual visit, or group session led by a trained health professional. Patients who choose not to participate in a structured maintenance program are at great risk for weight regain and the associated health consequences.

### Surgical Intervention

Morbidly obese patients (100 pounds overweight) who fail at the more conservative dietary intervention become candidates for gastric restrictive surgery. Currently, surgical treatment has a mortality rate of less than 1%, a mortality rate that is lower than that expected for patients who otherwise remain morbidly obese. The operation produces rapid weight loss over 6 months, with a slower rate for the next 6 months, at which point the patient has lost one-third of his or her body weight, primarily as body fat.

When assessing morbidly obese patients as candidates for surgery, physicians should conduct a more detailed evaluation than that done for dietary intervention. Patients should generally be from 18 to 55 years of age, and their psychologic profile should be accurately assessed. Patients with prior surgical procedures for weight control, such as the jejunoileal bypass or failed gastric restrictive surgery, may also be considered for revisional surgery but only after a thorough examination of the cause of failure and of potential complications. Pulmonary function tests should be conducted as well as an analysis of blood gases, a repeat electrocardiogram, an abdominal ultrasound for cholelithiasis, and an upper endoscopy to check for gastrointestinal problems. Blood tests should include platelets and a coagulation profile to discount the presence of abnormal antithrombin III. Prior to surgery, the patient should undergo a 20- to 50-pound weight loss to decrease the pulmonary and vascular preload. In addition, the patient should have stopped smoking for at least 1 month before surgery.

The operations that are currently used include the gastric bypass and the vertical banded gastroplasty. Intestinal bypasses have been stopped because of the high incidence of complications, and the horizontal procedures because of the large number of failures. The surgical procedures basically provide a reversible mechanical obstruction to food by creating a small pouch with a limited outlet. This alteration causes early pouch filling while eating and hence early satiety.

The gastroplasty produces a small pouch by the application of four rows of vertically placed staples in the stomach. This pouch opens to empty into the rest of the stomach, and the opening is supported by a piece of mesh to prevent it from enlarging. The gastric bypass procedure also creates a small pouch, which is then attached to a segment of intestine. In this case, absorptive capacity is reduced. With the gastric bypass, the majority of the intestine is in circuit so that diarrhea and significant malabsorption are not major complications.

Patients who do have surgical therapy for their morbid obesity require careful and attentive follow-up to assure correct adaptation of eating behavior. A nutritionally balanced diet is vital to ensure that the patient does not suffer any degree of protein malnutrition nor any specific vitamin deficiencies. An exercise program is important for improved fitness, enhanced feeling of well-being, and long-term weight control. Like patients undergoing dietary intervention, these individuals must also enroll in a maintenance program to undertake lifelong lifestyle changes in eating and exercise behavior. Morbidly obese patients are at major risk for depression and low self-esteem and developing "new" eating disorders at any point during treatment emphasizing

TABLE 5. **Appetite-Suppressing Drugs**

| Generic and Proprietary Names | Common Trade Names | Dosage (mg) | Administration (mg) | Peak Blood Concentration (Hours after Oral Dose) | Half-Life in Blood (Hours) | % Excreted Unchanged in Acidic Urine |
|---|---|---|---|---|---|---|
| **Schedule IV\*** | | | | | | |
| Diethylpropion | Tenuate, propion | 25, 75 | 25 before meals (tid)* 75 in morning | 1–2 | 8–13 | 24 |
| Fenfluramine | Pondimin | 20 | 20–40 before meals | 1 | 20 | 20 |
| Mazindol | Sanorex, Mazanor | 1, 2 | 1 before meals 2 in morning | 2 | 13 | 22 |
| Phentermine | Ionamin | 15, 30 | 15 (tid) 30 in morning | | Free 7–8 | 75 |
| | Fastin | | | 1 | 20–24 | |
| **Schedule III†** | | | | | | |
| Phendimetrazine | Plegine, Obalan | 35 | 35 before meals | — | 4 | — |
| Benzphetamine | Didrex | 25, 50 | 25–50 before meals | 1–2 | 2 | — |
| **Schedule II** | | | | | | |
| Amphetamine | Dexedrine | 5, 10, 15 | 5–10 before meals (tid) | 1–2 | 5 | 55 |
| Methamphetamine | Desoxyn | 5, 10, 15 | 2.5 or 5 before meals (tid) 10 or 15 in morning | 1–2 | 13 | 45 |
| Phenmetrazine | Preludin | 25, 50, 75 | 25 (bid or tid) | — | — | 19 |

*tid = three times daily.

†The Federal Controlled Substances Act of 1970 places the prescription anorexiants into five schedule categories. Appetite suppressants in schedule II are most likely to be abused; those in schedule IV have little or no risk abuse.

−: Data not available.

the chronic nature of this disease. Every effort should be made to keep these patients in lifelong treatment programs. Gastric restrictive surgery is only one component of a comprehensive treatment plan for this chronic and complex disease.

### Pharmacologic Intervention

The pharmacologic effects of appetite-suppressant medications can be divided into three major categories. Most stimulate the central nervous system, but the extent will vary considerably. These drugs also affect the cardiovascular system by raising heart rate and blood pressure. Finally, metabolic effects also occur, such as a rise in the concentration of free fatty acids or glycerol.

In choosing an appetite suppressant the drug therapy must first be established as safe and effective (Table 5). The Food and Drug Administration has provided one of the largest reviews of effectiveness of these agents and concluded that, overall, patients treated with drugs lost an average of 0.25 kg (.56 pounds) per week more than did those in the placebo-treated group.

The safety of appetite-suppressant drugs has been the subject of considerable discussion. Amphetamine, methamphetamine, and phenmetrazine (schedule II) have been more frequently abused than other drugs. Thus, there is little or no indication for use of drugs in schedule II for the treatment of obesity. If appetite suppressants are to be used, they should be adjuncts in obesity treatment. Drugs in schedule IV obviously are preferred, but drugs in schedule III also have a low abuse potential. No drugs should be used in pregnant women or in obese children who are still growing.

Phenylpropanolamine (PPA) is one of the over-the-counter drugs available for weight control. A group of five clinical trial studies using PPA alone as compared with a placebo found that the drug-treated individuals lost an average of 0.24 kg per week more than the placebo-treated group—similar to the extra weight loss of 0.25 kg per week reported when prescription appetite-suppressing drugs and placebo are compared. An advisory panel to the FDA concluded that PPA is probably safe and effective, although at high doses (75 mg immediate release), some elevation in blood pressure occurs in some patients. The drug's abuse potential is also low. In patients with depression disorders, as defined by Diagnostic and Statistical Manual-III (DSM-III), antidepressant drugs that affect central nervous system uptake of serotonin (e.g., fluoxetine) have been associated with anorexia and weight loss. In patients with diagnosed DSM-III eating disorders and depression resulting in binge eating,

patients with significant weight gain or obesity are candidates for trial of this drug by qualified physicians.

### Long-Term Results

Among our moderately obese patients treated with a multidisciplinary VLCD, 25% are 40 pounds lighter, and 50% are 20 pounds lighter at 5-year follow-up. Two-year follow-up data available on moderately obese patients treated with low-calorie diets show that patients maintain an 11-pound weight loss, approximately a 5% reduction in body weight from program entry. Research from our lab and elsewhere reports that patients who lose 10 to 20% of their body weight and who can maintain at least one-third of this weight loss for 3 to 5 years will obtain significant health benefits. Given the significant risks incurred by excess body weight and the improved treatments for obesity that bring about appreciable health benefits, effective treatment of obesity is becoming a necessity and a reality.

# PELLAGRA

method of
STEPHEN R. NEWMARK, M.D.
*Diabetes Center of Excellence*
*Humana Sunrise Hospital*
*Las Vegas, Nevada*

## CLINICAL MANIFESTATIONS

Pellagra is the clinical symptom complex associated with niacin and tryptophan deficiency and characterized by the the three Ds: dermatitis, diarrhea, and dementia. The skin manifestations of pellagra are the most common manifestations of the syndrome and may be characterized by an erythematous reaction in sun-exposed areas, which is then followed by a deepening of the color to a dark reddish brown. Scaling may become prominent with subsequent vesicular and bullae formation. Skin creases may contain hyperkeratotic pigmented papules. The upper chest and neck areas are particularly vulnerable to these pellagrous dermatoses (Casal's necklace). Other manifestations include glossitis characterized by a bright red, smooth tongue along with other oral mucosal changes. Frequently, dermatitis will involve all the regions around body orifices with stomatitis, vulvovaginitis, and proctitis, as well as severe ulcerative scrotal lesions in males. Diarrhea is particularly common and may involve most of the gastrointestinal tract, which histologically shows inflammation and mucosal atrophy. Neurologic manifestations include peripheral motor and sensory neuropathy, loss of position and vibration sensation, and psychologic changes that may range from irritability to delirium and dementia.

## ETIOLOGY

Pellagra historically has occurred in population groups who use corn or maize as their staple food. In recent years, pellagra has been observed in alcoholic individuals, in patients receiving parenteral nutrition without adequate vitamin supplementation, and, rarely, in patients with carcinoid tumors or Hartnup's disease. Pellagra is caused by an inadequate intake of niacin or its amino acid precursor, tryptophan. Inadequate niacin synthesis results in decreased formation of nicotinamide acid mononucleotide and subsequently nicotinamide adenine dinucleotide (NAD) and nicotinamide adenine dinucleotide phosphate (NADP), which are important co-enzymes for many oxidation-reduction reactions. Recent evidence suggests that an amino acid imbalance created by excessive leucine ingestion may also precipitate pellagra in certain individuals by inhibiting nicotinamide acid mononucleotide synthesis. As 60 mg of tryptophan is converted to approximately 1 mg of niacin, any disease process, such as the carcinoid syndrome which diverts tryptophan to 5-hydroxytryptophan (serotonin) and Hartnup's disease in which there is a genetic disorder in the metabolism of tryptophan, could occasionally produce the manifestations of niacin deficiency or pellagra.

### PREVENTION AND TREATMENT

The Food and Agriculture Organization/World Health Organization Expert Group has recommended 6.6 niacin equivalents per 1000 kilocalories (one niacin equivalent = 1 mg niacin = 60 mg of tryptophan). The recommended daily allowance in the United States is 6 to 9 mg per day for infants, 11 to 18 mg per day for children, and 13 to 19 mg per day for adults. These recommendations can be met by the ingestion of a balanced diet which includes meats, fish, whole grain cereals, and legumes. Although milk and eggs do not contain high levels of niacin, they are rich in tryptophan. The average American diet provides 16 to 34 niacin equivalents per day.

The treatment of pellagra includes the oral administration of niacinamide, 300 to 500 mg per day in divided doses of 50 to 100 mg per dose along with appropriate fluid and electrolyte replacement. In cases of severe stomatitis or other oral lesions, 100 mg niacinamide may be given intramuscularly three times a day for the first 2 to 3 days. After the acute symptoms of pellagra have subsided, continued therapy with niacinamide, 50 mg orally three times a day, until all clinical symptoms have abated will be necessary. Young children usually will need only 50% of the above adult doses. As other vitamin deficiency states may coexist with niacin deficiency, it is usually prudent to provide supplementary vita-

mins along with a balanced diet. Usually the manifestations of pellagra will start improving within 2 to 3 days after initial therapy with marked improvement in 2 to 3 weeks.

# RICKETS AND OSTEOMALACIA

method of
SONIA BALSAN, M.D.
*Université René Descartes*
*Paris, France*

Rickets and osteomalacia are metabolic diseases resulting from defective mineralization of the skeletal matrix. The radiologic and histologic characteristics of rickets indicate that the growing plates are involved. Hence, rickets only occurs in children and adolescents before the end of puberty. Osteomalacia is a mineralization defect of the osteoid matrix of trabecular and cortical bones. This abnormality can be seen in both children and adults.

The clinical symptoms of rickets are well known and readily recognized in children. However, during the first trimester of life, the symptoms are mainly those of hypocalcemia (tremors, Bravais-jacksonian fits, convulsions, and laryngospasm). In contrast, osteomalacia is very difficult to diagnose clinically in adults, especially in the early stages, since its main symptoms are bone pain and muscular weakness, which are common features of a variety of pathologic conditions.

## BONE MINERALIZATION

Normal mineralization requires a normal matrix, which implies the presence of normally active cartilage and bone cells and optimum ambient calcium and phosphorus concentrations. The two main regulators of calcium and phosphorus homeostasis are parathyroid hormone (PTH) and the hormonal form of vitamin D—1,25-dihydroxyvitamin $D_3$, or calcitriol. The syntheses and biologic actions of these two hormones are closely interrelated.

### Parathyroid Hormone

Calcium is the major regulator of PTH synthesis and secretion. A decrease in circulating Ca concentration stimulates, and an increase inhibits, the secretion of PTH. The second potent regulator, which directly modulates parathyroid gland activity via a specific receptor on the gland itself, is the hormonal form of vitamin D, calcitriol.

PTH has a wide range of biologic actions, but its main action is the fine, minute-to-minute regulation of calcium concentration in the circulation and extracellular fluid. It does this by acting directly on the bone and kidney: In bone it promotes the liberation of Ca by stimulating resorption, and in kidney, it increases the tubular reabsorption of calcium, decreases that of phosphorus, and stimulates the activity of the enzyme 25-hydroxyvitamin D 1α-hydroxylase, which is responsible for the synthesis of calcitriol.

*Calcitriol*

Vitamin Ds—either cholecalciferol (vitamin D₃), the natural mammalian product synthesized in the skin by the action of ultraviolet light on epidermal 7-dehydrocholesterol, or ergocalciferol (vitamin D₂), an irradiated plant steroid used to fortify food or for pharmaceutical vitamin D and multivitamin preparations—have no biologic activity at physiologic doses. They must be hydroxylated to become active. The first hydroxylation takes place in the liver, to form 25(OH)D₃ (calcidiol). The second hydroxylation, to form 1,25(OH)₂D₃ (calcitriol), occurs mainly in the kidney. Several other tissues and types of cells can also convert 25(OH)D to 1,25(OH)₂D. However, the nearly undetectable levels of this metabolite in the plasma of anephric patients suggest that extrarenal sources of 1,25(OH)₂D contribute little to circulating calcitriol levels.

Many ionic or hormonal factors modulate the renal production of calcitriol. Previous deficiency of calcitriol, hypocalcemia, hypophosphatemia, hyperparathyroidism, growth hormone, cAMP, prostaglandins, sex hormones, prolactin, and calcitonin all stimulate calcitriol synthesis. In contrast, excess calcitriol, lack of or resistance to PTH, hypercalcemia, hyperphosphatemia, and acidosis decrease calcitriol production.

The mode of action of calcitriol is similar to that of steroid hormones. It is bound to a specific nuclear receptor, and there is a cascade of post-transcriptional events. Specific binding sites for calcitriol have been found in a variety of tissues and cells; the most important ones for calcium and phosphorus homeostasis are in the intestine, kidney, and bone. The main physiologic role of calcitriol is to enhance intestinal calcium and phosphorus absorption. In conjunction with PTH, it also mobilizes mineral from bone. Calcitriol has a short half-life in the circulation and is not stored in the body, in contrast to its precursors, calcidiol and vitamin D, which are stored in body fat and muscle. Because the vitamin Ds, calcidiol, and calcitriol are all fat-soluble, their intestinal absorption requires normal fat absorption, with intact biliary and pancreatic function and integrity of the intestinal mucosa.

There are many degradative pathways for the vitamin Ds, calcidiol, and calcitriol, including the formation of inactive sulfo- and glucuro- conjugates in the

TABLE 1. **Pathogenic Mechanisms of Rickets and Osteomalacia**

 I. Deficiency of Parent Vitamin D
   Dietary deprivation or lack of exposure to sunlight.
 II. Abnormalities of Vitamin Metabolism or Action
   II.1. Malabsorption of parent vitamin D
     a. Postgastrectomy
     b. Small bowel resection or bypass
     c. Fat malabsorption (celiac disease, mucoviscidosis, biliary obstruction, exocrine pancreas insufficiency)
   II.2. Impaired calcidiol formation
     a. Premature infants
     b. Severe hepatitis
   II.3. Increased catabolism of vitamin D, calcidiol, and calcitriol
     Enzyme induction by anticonvulsant drugs
   II.4. Increased loss of vitamin D, calcidiol, and calcitriol
     a. Nephrotic syndrome
     b. Chronic peritoneal dialysis
   II.5. Impaired 1-hydroxylation of calcidiol
     a. Inborn error: vitamin D dependency or pseudodeficiency rickets Type I
     b. Hypoparathyroidism and pseudohypoparathyroidism
     c. Chronic renal failure
     d. X-linked hypophosphatemia
     e. Ketaconazole treatment
   II.6. Impaired target-organ responsiveness to calcitriol
     a. Inborn error: Hereditary resistance to calcitriol (vitamin D dependency or pseudodeficiency rickets Type II)
     b. Chronic renal failure
 III. Isolated Calcium Deficiency
   Calcium-poor diets in children
 IV. Chronic Hypophosphatemia
   IV.1. X-linked and other forms of hereditary hypophosphatemia
   IV.2. Diseases and syndrome with phosphate diabetes (idiopathic de Toni-Debré-Fanconi syndrome, Wilson's disease, Lowe's syndrome, familial vitamin D–resistant rickets with hypercalciuria, cystinosis, multiple tubular dysfunction with aminoaciduria, calciuria, uricosuria, and phosphate diabetes)
 V. Chronic Metabolic Acidosis
 VI. Oncogenic Rickets and/or Osteomalacia
 VII. Iatrogenic: Mineralization Inhibitors
   VII.1. Aluminum (during antacid therapy or parenteral nutrition)
   VII.2. Bisphosphonates (disodium etidronate)
 VIII. Miscellaneous
   VIII.1. Hypophosphatasia
   VIII.2. Fibrogenesis imperfecta

liver. The enzymes responsible may be stimulated by substances such as phenobarbitals and phenytoin.

## GENERAL GUIDELINES

Rickets and osteomalacia may occur as complications in a variety of pathologic states, because normal extracellular calcium and phosphorus concentrations are important for correct mineralization, and because many tissues and factors are directly or indirectly involved in their homeostasis and in the metabolism of their main regulator, vitamin D (through the actions of its hormonal form, calcitriol). Hence, once a mineralization defect is diagnosed by physical examination, biochemical studies, and radiologic examination (bone biopsy is not necessary, especially for children), it is important to discriminate between simple nutritional rickets and secondary rickets or osteomalacia.

Knowledge of the pathologic mechanism(s) (Table 1) responsible for rickets or osteomalacia will help in selecting the appropriate drug, its dose, and administration route (Table 2). It should be stressed that the use of pharmacologic doses of any form of vitamin D (parent vitamin D, tachysterol, calcidiol, or calcitriol) requires regular biochemical monitoring at intervals not exceeding 1 to 2 weeks at the start of treatment and 2 months during long-term therapy. It should also be remembered that the first signal of vitamin D overdose, preceding any hypercalcemia, is hypercalciuria (24-hour urinary calcium excretion exceeding 0.75 mmol or 3 mg per kg body weight, or urinary calcium-to-creatinine ratio (mmol per mmol) greater than 0.30).

## PRIMARY VITAMIN D DEFICIENCY

### Risk Factors

The minimum daily vitamin D requirement for healthy individuals is estimated to be around 10 μg (400 units) for children and 2.5 μg for adults. Natural foodstuffs contain little vitamin D, but adequate exposure of the skin to sunlight can easily cover this need, since a few minutes exposure of a small area of skin to ultraviolet light increases the circulating level of 25(OH)D up to 60-fold 24 to 48 hours after exposure. However, skin pigmentation, seasonal variations, latitude, climatic conditions, air pollution, social or religious habits, or living conditions (institutionalized, bed-ridden patients) may prevent sufficient skin synthesis of vitamin D. Foodstuffs or milk are fortified with vitamin D in some countries, including the United States, to prevent vitamin D deficiency in the general population. Although this procedure has markedly reduced the number of individuals suffering from vitamin D deficiency, it has not totally eradicated this pathology: The poor and some food faddists do not have access to, or do not ingest, fortified foodstuffs.

More vitamin D is required during pregnancy. Therefore, a state of vitamin D depletion may develop when the interval between pregnancies is short, especially in women of socioeconomic groups at risk. Vitamin D and its metabolites cross the placenta, and the fetus possesses the machinery necessary for calcidiol and calcitriol synthesis. Nevertheless, newborns rapidly become depleted of vitamin D since they have no major fat stores and the half-life of calcitriol is short. In addition, breast milk does not contain sufficient vitamin D. Therefore, breast-fed babies, like those bottle-fed with nonfortified milk, are likely to become vitamin D deficient if they do not benefit from exposure to efficient sunlight or if they are not given prophylactic doses of vitamin D.

### Diagnosis

The two most reliable criteria of primary vitamin D deficiency are low circulating calcidiol (less than 6 ng per ml) and the rapid (within 1 to 2 weeks) normalization of the associated hypocalcemia or hypophosphatemia after small oral doses of parent vitamin D (see below). One of the first responses to this treatment is the increase in circulating calcitriol to high, or even very high, levels as early as 24 hours after beginning therapy. However, in contrast to circulating calcidiol, the levels of circulating calcitriol may be undetectable, low, normal, or above normal before treatment. The serum alkaline phosphatase activity and the plasma immunoreactive parathyroid hormone concentration (iPTH) are usually elevated. But these abnormalities also occur in a variety of secondary rickets or osteomalacia. The clinical and radiologic symptoms and the data from common laboratory tests may, as stated above, vary according to the age of the patient and the severity and duration of vitamin D deprivation.

## TREATMENT

The treatment of primary vitamin D deficiency does not require dihydrotachysterol or active derivatives of vitamin D (calcidiol or calcitriol). Parent vitamin D ($D_3$ or $D_2$) is the drug of choice.

TABLE 2. **Pharmaceutical Preparations of Vitamin D Sterols**

|  | Ergocalciferol | Dihydrotachysterol | Calcidiol | Calcitriol |
|---|---|---|---|---|
| Abbreviation | $D_2$ | DHT | 25(OH)D | 1,25(OH)$_2$D |
| Trade name | Calciferol, Drisdol | DHT, Hytakerol | Calderol | Rocaltrol |
| Dosage form | Capsules: 1250 μg (50,000 IU) | Tablets: 125, 200 and 400 μg | Capsules: 20 and 50 μg | Capsules: 0.25 and 0.50 μg |
| Normal serum levels | 0.5–18 ng/ml | — | 8 to 30 ng/ml | 27 to 80 pg/ml |
| Daily dosage in vitamin D deficiency | 5 μg | not required | not required | not required |
| Daily dosage range in resistant rickets* | 0.5–2 mg | 0.1–1 mg | 20–100 μg | 0.5–3 μg |

*Except in hereditary resistance to 1,25(OH)$_2$D that may require much higher doses.

A total dose of 5 mg (200,000 IU) of vitamin D, given either as a single dose or divided into weekly (50,000 IU per week for a month) or daily (2000 IU per day for 3 months) doses, is sufficient to restore even the most severe form of vitamin D lack, normalize the circulating level of calcidiol, and correct the usual biochemical parameters. The hypocalcemia or hypophosphatemia is usually corrected after 7 to 10 days; serum alkaline phosphatase activity increases in the days following the start of therapy, then slowly decreases to normal in about 1 month. Healing of x-ray rachitic lesions is indicated by the appearance of a calcification line (front) across the cartilage 2 to 3 weeks after the start of treatment. However, correction of long bone incurvature usually takes several months. Therefore, persistence of the lesions should not lead to repeated administration of vitamin D at pharmacologic doses. The clinical symptoms of muscular weakness and bone pain are alleviated by therapy in a matter of days.

In cases of primary vitamin D deficiency associated with hypocalcemia or severe osteopenia, calcium supplements must be given together with vitamin D treatment. Calcium should be infused intravenously when the serum calcium is below 2 mmol per liter (8 mg per dl); the dose should be 0.5 to 1 gram of elemental calcium per 1.73 $m^2$ in 500 ml isotonic saline per 12 hours, depending on the severity of the hypocalcemia. The amount of elemental calcium infused is then decreased progressively with careful biochemical monitoring. Oral calcium supplements (0.5 to 1 gram elemental calcium per day) may eventually be substituted for the calcium infusion. These supplements are continued until skeletal mineralization or the skeletal x-ray is normal (Table 3).

The prophylactic dose of parent vitamin D required in countries where foodstuffs and milk are not fortified is estimated to be 30 $\mu$g (1200 IU) per day for white caucasians and 50 $\mu$g (2000 IU) per day for heavily pigmented babies, or oral administration of 5 mg (200,000 IU) every 4 to 6 months. This treatment should be started as early as the first week of life, even in breast-fed babies, and continued until the age of 2 years. Thereafter, until the age of 5 years, children should be given the same daily dose for 6 months (or a single equivalent total dose) during the winter and spring.

Giving a single oral dose of 2.5 mg (100,000 IU) or a daily dose of 50 $\mu$g (2000 IU) of vitamin $D_2$ or $D_3$ to pregnant women, beginning at the seventh month of gestation, has been shown to prevent vitamin D depletion in the mother and neonatal hypocalcemia in the baby, especially when the last trimester of gestation corresponds to the less sunny winter months.

## SECONDARY RICKETS AND OSTEOMALACIA

The so-called vitamin D–resistant rickets and osteomalacia may occur in a child or adult for a variety of causes (see Table 1), despite the fact that they may have adequate exposure to sunlight, a diet fortified with vitamin D, or oral prophylactic doses of vitamin D. The basal calcidiol concentration in these patients is normal, but if it is found to be low (in countries where food is not fortified), simple vitamin D deficiency may be associated with other pathologic states without any direct inter-relationship between the two diseases. There is no rapid correction following *oral* administration of small doses of parent vitamin D. This situation defines in clinical terms

TABLE 3. **Pharmaceutical Preparations for Oral Calcium Supplementation**

| Preparation | Trade Name | % Elemental Calcium | Dosage Form | Amount Containing 1 Gm of Elemental Calcium | Comments |
|---|---|---|---|---|---|
| Calcium carbonate | Titralac | 40 | Suspension: 500 mg/5 ml | 12.5 ml | May cause constipation, flatulence |
| | | | | 6 tablets | |
| | | | Tablets: 420 mg | 4 tablets | |
| Calcium lactate | | 13 | Tablets: 325 mg; | 24 tablets | May be poorly absorbed by some people |
| | | | 650 mg | 12 tablets | |
| Calcium gluconate | | 9 | Tablets: 500 mg; | 17 tablets | Well tolerated |
| | | | 975 mg | 11 tablets | |
| Calcium glubionate | Neo-Calglucon | 7 | Syrup: 1.8 g/5 ml | 43.5 ml | Well tolerated |
| Calcium citrate | Citracal | 21 | Tablets: 950 mg | | |
| Dibasic calcium phosphate dihydrate | Dibasic Calcium Phosphate | 23 | Tablets: 486 mg | | |
| Tricalcium phosphate | Posture | 39 | Tablets: 300 mg | | |
| | | | 600 mg | | |

"resistance to vitamin D." However, progress in our understanding of vitamin D metabolism and mode of action has shown that many forms of secondary rickets and osteomalacia are not due to a true target organ resistance to the hormonal form of vitamin D, calcitriol. We have also learned that rickets and osteomalacia may occur even when serum levels of calcitriol are normal because of a calcium or phosphorus deficiency or because of the presence of substances inhibiting mineralization. In addition, there is usually not one, but several mechanisms, each contributing in varying degrees to the pathologic state of many diseases leading to secondary vitamin D–resistant rickets or osteomalacia.

The various forms of secondary vitamin D–resistant rickets and osteomalacia are presented according to their main pathogenic causes in order to simplify the treatment regimens.

### Malabsorption of Vitamin D

Vitamin D and its active derivatives are fat-soluble substances. Calcidiol undergoes entero-hepatic recycling after its synthesis in the liver. Hence, any situation leading to steatorrhea may result in both malabsorption of dietary vitamin D and depletion of calcidiol and vitamin $D_2$ and $D_3$ body stores. Small bowel resection or bypass may also result in parent vitamin D malabsorption, while calcium and magnesium malabsorption occurs in cases of steatorrhea. Hypomagnesemia may be responsible for decreased stimulation of PTH secretion.

Although the usual skeletal manifestations in these malabsorption syndromes is osteoporosis, as in celiac disease or cystic fibrosis, mild to severe symptoms of rickets and osteomalacia, associated with hypocalcemia and hypomagnesemia, may occur in some patients. Calcidiol levels are low in the serum of all these patients. Prevention or treatment is by monthly intramuscular injections of 2 to 2.5 mg (80,000 to 100,000 IU) of parent vitamin D. A daily magnesium supplement (350 to 750 mg of elemental magnesium) should be prescribed if hypomagnesemia is present. Magnesium oxide tablets contain 60% magnesium. Serum calcidiol, calcium and magnesium, and urinary calcium excretion must be regularly monitored to ensure optimizing therapy to each patient's needs.

### Impaired Calcidiol Formation

Very premature infants have a decreased capacity to transform vitamin D to calcidiol. Vitamin D deficiency in these babies can be prevented by daily doses of 100 µg (4000 IU) parent vitamin D until the infant reaches its term age. Thereafter, prophylactic therapy can be continued with fortified milk or, if the latter is not available, with the usual doses of parent vitamin D (see above).

Theoretically, liver diseases are indications for the use of calcidiol. However, measurements of serum calcidiol concentration show that the circulating level of calcidiol is not significantly depressed in these patients, except in the terminal stages of hepatic failure. Rickets and osteomalacia can be prevented in cases where cholestasis is associated with liver disease by parenteral vitamin D, as above, or daily oral doses of 20 µg calcidiol, as bile salts are necessary for normal fat, and hence vitamin D and calcidiol absorption.

### Increased Catabolism of Vitamin D and Its Active Metabolites

**Role of Anticonvulsant Drugs.** Rickets and osteomalacia with hypocalcemia, elevated serum alkaline phosphatase activity, and secondary hyperparathyroidism are all possible complications in patients on long-term anticonvulsant therapy. These drugs activate the hepatic microsomal enzymes involved in the catabolism of vitamin D and its active metabolites. Measurements of serum calcidiol have shown that the only patients on anticonvulsant medication who are prone to vitamin D deficiency are those treated with multiple drugs and on a diet not fortified with vitamin D, having little or no effective solar exposure. Although rare, this possible complication should be kept in mind since the aggravation of seizures by the secondary hypocalcemic state may indirectly lead to increased doses of anticonvulsant drug, provoking further aggravation of the symptoms of vitamin D deficiency.

The rickets and osteomalacia of patients on long-term anticonvulsant therapy may be treated with daily oral doses of 40 to 100 µg (1200 to 4000 IU) parent vitamin D or 20 µg calcidiol, with periodic assay of serum calcidiol and calcium concentration, and of 24-hour urinary calcium.

### Increased Loss of Vitamin D and Its Active Metabolites

Considerable wastage of vitamin D and its active metabolites, especially calcidiol, generally occurs in two pathologic conditions: nephrotic syndrome with normal glomerular function and marked proteinuria and during chronic peritoneal dialysis. Experimental studies have shown that, in nephrotic syndrome, this is due to urinary loss of the metabolites bound to specific vitamin D–binding protein. Losses of 2 to 22 µg calcidiol have been found in the dialysate of children on chronic peritoneal dialysis, and similar losses occur in adults.

Vitamin D deficiency, assessed in both situations by low circulating calcidiol, can be prevented or corrected in the nephrotic syndrome by daily supraphysiologic doses of parent vitamin D (1200 to 4000 IU) or 20 μg calcidiol. The serum ionized calcium or total calcium corrected for serum protein or albumin should be monitored in these patients because of the hypoproteinemia or hypoalbuminemia that occurs in these cases. The situation is more complex for patients on chronic peritoneal dialysis because of their terminal renal failure and, hence, their inability to synthesize calcitriol. The treatment of choice for these patients is daily doses of calcitriol, 0.25 to 1 μg, according to the presence or absence of overt signs of rickets or osteomalacia and of secondary hyperparathyroidism.

### Impaired 1-Hydroxylation, Vitamin D–Dependent Rickets, or Pseudodeficiency Rickets Type I

This inborn error of vitamin D metabolism is due to a renal 25(OH)D–1α-hydroxylase deficiency. Its inheritance is autosomal recessive. Symptoms are similar to those of severe nutritional rickets with hypocalcemia. Treatment with parent vitamin D at the doses usually active in simple vitamin D deficiency is followed by maintenance of normal serum calcidiol levels. However, in pseudodeficiency rickets Type I, this is not associated with the normalization of the biologic parameters and a marked increase in serum calcitriol. Serum calcitriol concentrations are found to be low or normal. Management of children with this disorder is easy but requires lifelong replacement therapy with calcitriol. The necessary daily doses are 1.5 to 2.5 μg for healing x-ray lesions. Thereafter, for replacement therapy, doses of 0.75 to 1 μg are usually sufficient. Before calcitriol or its synthetic analogue, 1α-hydroxyvitamin $D_3$, became available, these patients satisfactorily responded to pharmacologic doses of parent vitamin D (1 to 3 mg per day) or calcidiol (75 to 150 μg per day) during the active phase of the disease, followed by 5 mg (200,000 IU) of vitamin $D_2$ or $D_3$ once a week or 50 to 75 μg per day of calcidiol.

### Hypoparathyroidism and Pseudohypoparathyroidism

Reduced serum calcitriol in these disorders is due either to lack of PTH or to resistance to the renal action of the hormone. In hypoparathyroidism the activity of bone cells is decreased; little bone matrix is laid down and a mineralization defect is not common. The main problem is correction of the hypocalcemia. Since PTH is also responsible for the tubular reabsorption of calcium, its lack leads to a tendency to hypercalciuria as soon as serum calcium reaches 2 to 2.2 mmol per liter (8 to 8.8 mg per dl). Therefore, treatment with calcitriol (0.5 to 1 μg per day), plus oral calcium supplements (0.5 to 1 gram elemental calcium per day), should be used, with frequent laboratory monitoring to maintain serum calcium concentration in the low-normal range and to avoid hypercalciuria. Thiazide derivatives, which reduce urinary calcium output, have been successfully used with this treatment in adults.

In pseudohypoparathyroidism, resistance to the renal action of PTH (lack of cAMP stimulation and calcitriol synthesis) may be associated with the absence of or variable degrees of resistance to the bone effects of the hormone. A mineralizing deficiency is not exceptional in those patients with persistent skeletal sensitivity to PTH and may lead to deformities such as genu valgum. Patients with pseudohypoparathyroidism do not have exaggerated urinary calcium excretion. Their serum calcium, phosphorus, and immunoreactive PTH can be normalized, without inducing hypercalciuria, with daily doses of calcitriol and calcium supplement, using doses similar to those used in hypoparathyroidism.

Pharmacologic doses of parent vitamin D or calcidiol have been used to treat both hypo- and pseudohypoparathyroid patients. However, in cases of overdose, the toxic effects of these substances are long-lasting because of their extended half-lives (see Table 2). In addition, idiopathic hypoparathyroidism patients who are prone to chronic fungal infections and are treated with the antifungal drug, ketoconazole (Nizoral), may require increased parent vitamin D as the antifungal drug inhibits calcitriol synthesis.

### Chronic Renal Failure

Patients with chronic renal failure suffer from impaired calcitriol synthesis and resistance to the intestinal effects of this hormone. However, these abnormalities are usually associated with a variety of problems that all contribute, directly or indirectly, to the pathogeny of renal osteodystrophy. These factors include hypocalcemia, hyperphosphatemia, acidosis, and secondary hyperparathyroidism. The bone lesions vary but are mainly hyper-resorption with or without osteomalacia. Uremic bone disease may be prevented by the usual dietary restriction and correction of the acidosis, hypocalcemia, and hyperphosphatemia. Serum phosphorus should be maintained at 4 to 5 mg per dl (3.3 to 3.7 mmol per liter) in adults and less than 6 mg per dl (2 mmol per liter) in children. As aluminum is known to be toxic for the brain and bone, very high daily doses of calcium carbonate should be used (6 to 9 grams per day), rather than aluminum-containing antacids. This medication has the double advantage of chelating phosphorus in the intestine and providing a calcium supplement. As calcitriol is the hormonal form missing in severe uremia, it is the drug of choice in renal osteodystrophy. Initial doses of 0.25 to 0.5 µg per day should be modified in light of subsequent careful laboratory monitoring. Calcitriol or pharmacologic doses of any vitamin D preparation is proscribed for patients with aluminum intoxication because the inability of these patients to mineralize bone results in severe hypercalcemia.

## Impaired End-Organ Responsiveness to Calcitriol

**Hereditary Resistance to Calcitriol or Vitamin D–Dependent Rickets Type II.** This recently identified disorder is probably inherited as an autosomal recessive. There are several abnormalities at the calcitriol receptor and postreceptor levels. Rickets, osteomalacia, and current laboratory data are identical to those for simple vitamin D–deficient rickets. The circulating calcitriol levels are elevated and may reach nanogram levels during treatment with very high doses of vitamin D or calcidiol. Some patients also suffer from congenital alopecia. The bone lesions of some patients can be healed and the biologic parameters normalized with extremely high doses of parent vitamin D (up to 70 mg per day) or calcidiol (5 mg per day*). Patients have also been found to respond to large doses of calcitriol (17 µg per day). However, others remain resistant, and for these we have devised a therapeutic program with daily, then thrice weekly, parenteral administration of calcium (500 to 1000 mg elemental calcium infused in 500 ml isotonic solute over 12 hours via an intracaval catheter or arteriovenous fistula). This therapeutic model produces biopsy-proven healing of the osteomalacia in 3 months and normalization of blood biochemistry. Thereafter, infusions can be continued once a week. Others have used very high doses (up to 5 grams per day of elemental calcium) given daily. Spontaneous remissions have also been reported.

## Isolated Calcium Deficiency

Rickets and osteomalacia may develop in children receiving less than 200 mg of dietary cal-

cium per day. Elemental calcium, at 1 gram per day, corrects the hypocalcemia and elevated plasma PTH and alkaline phosphatase and heals the skeletal lesions.

## Chronic Hypophosphatemia

**Hereditary Hypophosphatemic Vitamin D–Resistant Rickets (VDRR).** This congenital disease is usually transmitted as an X-linked dominant trait, but the family history may be negative (sporadic form) and autosomal recessive or dominant transmissions have also been reported. The primary defect in all these forms is renal phosphate leakage (phosphate diabetes). Calcitriol synthesis is also disturbed, as is the activity of bone cells of the osteoblastic lineage. The basic therapy is phosphorus supplements (Table 4). The daily dose must be given in four to six divided doses as the administered phosphorus is rapidly excreted. The dosage varies from 0.75 gram in young infants to 3 to 4 grams in adults. Phosphorus supplementation is associated with a trend toward decreased serum calcium and, consequently, parathyroid gland overactivity. Hence, these patients must be given calcitriol in addition to phosphorus supplements. The daily initial dose of calcitriol is 0.5 to 1 µg, which is gradually increased, taking care to avoid hypercalciuria. If a liquid preparation of calcitriol is not commercially available, young children may be treated by dissolving the capsule in applesauce.

A liquid preparation of 1α-hydroxyvitamin $D_3$,* a synthetic analogue of calcitriol, is used in many countries, at doses twice that of calcitriol.

Treating patients with VDRR is not a rewarding task. Fasting serum phosphorus is not readily normalized except with phosphorus doses which are not well tolerated (gastritis, diarrhea) and calcitriol doses which are hypercalciuric and hypercalcemic. Therefore, no attempt should be made to normalize fasting serum phosphorus at all costs, but the concentration should be maintained as near as possible to 1 mmol per liter (3.1 mg per dl). Bone deformities may be corrected by medical therapy. If they persist, orthopedic surgery is not recommended until after growth has ceased. The disease usually becomes less active after puberty, and treatment of most patients can be stopped. The monitoring of these patients during therapy should include, in addition to serum calcium, phosphorus, and alkaline phosphatase and urinary excretion, serum iPTH (every 4 to 6 months) to avoid persistent secondary hyperparathyroidism. Interrupting oral phosphorus for 1 month usually restores any increased

---

*Exceeds dosage recommended by manufacturer.

*Not available in the United States.

TABLE 4. **Pharmaceutical Preparations for Oral Phosphate Supplementation**

| Trade Name | Amount Containing 1 Gm of Phosphorus | Comment |
| --- | --- | --- |
| Neutra-Phos | 4 capsules* | They may all induce gastritis, diarrhea,† |
| Neutra-Phos-K | 4 capsules | and secondary hyperparathyroidism |
| K-Phos Original | 9 tablets | |
| Fleet Phospho-Soda | 6.7 ml | |

*Each capsule is reconstituted with 75 ml of water, fruit juice, or cola. A powder concentrate is also available.
†Gastrointestinal tolerance to all preparations is enhanced if the drug is not taken on an empty stomach.

iPTH to normal. Treatment with oral phosphorus can then be restarted at a lower dose.

Although growth velocity during childhood is accelerated by calcidiol plus phosphate therapy, most affected boys reach short adult stature, whereas the majority of girls attain normal height. Parental stature has little or no influence on the final stature of males but is important for determining the adult height of girls.

Hypophosphatemic bone disease, a recently identified familial disorder, probably with autosomal dominant transmission, is also characterized by hypophosphatemia and bowing of the lower limbs, but the loss of adult stature is modest and the bone changes are more like metaphyseal chondrodysplasia than rickets. Treatment is essentially the same as that for VDRR.

**Disorders with Phosphate Diabetes.** A variety of metabolic disorders (see Table 1) may be responsible for multiple tubular dysfunction, including phosphate diabetes. One of the less complex is familial vitamin D–resistant rickets with hypercalciuria. There is generally no defect in calcitriol synthesis in any of these disorders, and the circulating concentration of this metabolite is adequately high with respect to the prevailing phosphatemia. Rickets and osteomalacia can be healed in these patients with normal renal function by giving divided daily oral phosphate at doses similar to those used for VDRR. Patients with any concomitant hypocalcemia may be given small doses of calcitriol (0.25 to 0.5 μg per day) with the phosphate therapy.

### Chronic Metabolic Acidosis

Acidosis affects normal mineralization and depletes the skeleton of its mineral resources via several mechanisms. It may occur in patients with chronic hyperchloremic tubular acidosis or following surgery in which a segment of bowel is placed in continuity with the urinary tract. The bone abnormality is usually osteoporosis in both groups of patients. However, rickets and osteomalacia can also occur. Alkali therapy alone corrects these bone lesions, but any hypocalcemia should be corrected with calcium supplements before beginning alkali treatment to guard against tetany.

### Oncogenic Rickets and/or Osteomalacia

Late-onset hypophosphatemic vitamin D–resistant rickets and osteomalacia have been described in association with a wide variety of benign soft-tissue or bone tumors. The skeletal lesions heal rapidly after resection of the tumor, but the tumor itself may not be easily detected in some patients. This syndrome, which occurs in previously healthy individuals, is characterized by a marked decrease in serum phosphorus (0.4 mmol per liter or less, 1.2 mg per dl) and severe muscular weakness. Treatment is phosphate supplements and calcitriol, as for VDRR. The tumors are thought to secrete a factor (or factors) that inhibits tubular reabsorption of phosphorus and acts as an antivitamin D.

### Iatrogenic Mineralization Defects

**Aluminum Overload.** Osteomalacia and aplastic bone disease may occur if aluminum accumulates along the bone tissue mineralization front and perturbs the osteoblasts' activity. This intoxication may come from aluminum-containing dialysis fluids, antacid drugs, milk formulas, casein hydrolysates used as a protein source for parenteral nutrition, or contaminated albumin used in plasma exchange therapy. The bone abnormalities may be associated with a relative PTH deficiency in renal patients. Serum aluminum concentration is not a reliable criterion of overload. Aluminum content in bone needle biopsy, if available, and the desferrioxamine infusion test, based on the ability of this drug to chelate and remove tissue aluminum, are the best methods of estimating aluminum stores. Treatment includes withdrawal of the aluminum source and intravenous infusion of desferrioxamine at doses of 1 to 2 grams per week for several months; the total treatment duration is adapted to the needs of each patient.

**Bisphosphonates.** There have been reports of a state associating x-ray lesions of rickets and hyperphosphatemia in therapeutic trials of etidronate (Didronel) in children with myositis ossificans. These complications are secondary to the inhibitory effects of this drug on cartilage and bone mineralization. This treatment is no longer used in children. New classes of phosphonates, with lower bone toxicities, are used successfully at present, or are being tested, especially on adults with Paget's disease of bone.

### Miscellaneous Disorders

Hypophosphatasia and fibrogenesis imperfecta are two rare inborn errors of metabolism. The former, an inherited disorder, is characterized by low circulating alkaline phosphatase activity. Defective mineralization leads to x-ray pictures resembling rickets, presumably as a result of the deficient activity of this enzyme in bone and cartilage. The primary defect in fibrogenesis imperfecta is in the bone organic matrix. There is no specific therapy for either disorder. Correct diagnosis is important because treatment with vitamin D is not only useless, but it may lead to severe hypercalcemia and hypercalciuria.

# SCURVY AND VITAMIN C DEFICIENCY

method of
JOHN H. CRANDON, M.D.
*Tufts University Medical School*
*Boston, Massachusetts*

### INCIDENCE

During the past 30 years, scurvy has virtually vanished from the American scene. Coincidentally, requests for blood ascorbic acid levels, the sine qua non for a positive diagnosis of subclinical ascorbic acid deficiency, have become so infrequent that even the larger hospitals now send these blood samples to special laboratories for analysis.

During this period, nevertheless, there has been a marked proliferation of studies, both experimental and statistical, relating to the possibly beneficial actions of ascorbic acid, particularly in megadoses, for diseases ranging from cancer to colds. Many of the conclusions drawn from these studies must remain hypothetical because ethics committees and a litigious society have reduced human experimental studies to zero.

### CLINICAL FINDINGS

The clinical diagnosis of scurvy is made on the basis of the dietary history, petechiae or hyperkeratotic plugs in the hair follicles, scattered ecchymoses, bleeding gums (if teeth are present), hemarthroses, lassitude, postural hypotension, and a markedly limited ability to perform strenuous work. A tourniquet test for petechiae is of no value. In infants there may be tenderness over the tibiae, bony epiphyses, or costo-chondral junctions, with a characteristic x-ray picture in these areas.

The fundamental finding seen by the pathologist (generally in wound biopsy specimens) is lack of intercellular "cement substance," or collagen, between proliferating fibroblasts in the soft tissues and between endothelial cells in the small blood vessel walls. A diagnosis of scurvy on the basis of perifollicular petechiae alone is incorrect in at least one-third of the cases.

When blood determinations, wound biopsy specimens, or gum biopsy specimens are not available, a therapeutic test with oral or parenteral ascorbic acid in doses of 500 mg per day in adults and 100 to 200 mg per day in children for 10 days should be performed. It should be borne in mind that petechial hemorrhages of the extremities from whatever cause may show some improvement with bed rest alone.

### ACTION

Ascorbic acid is a strong reducing agent that is easily destroyed by alkalis. Aside from its vital role in the formation of intercellular substance, ascorbic acid facilitates the absorption of heme iron and enhances the action of the immune system and leukocytes; the action of catecholamine, norepinephrine, and dopamine; and the biosynthesis of carnitine. It participates in the conversion of folic acid to folinic acid, in the metabolism of tyrosine, and in the oxidation-reduction of sulfhydryl groups. It also protects against certain toxic substances, such as the heavy metals (e.g., cadmium).

An exciting discovery was the action of ascorbic acid in preventing the formation in the stomach of cancerogenic nitrosamines produced by the ingestion of nitrate-rich foods (foods to which nitrate had been added as a preservative). Coincidental with the advent of better vitamin C nutrition, there has been, in the opinion of most surgeons, a considerable decline in the incidence of gastric carcinoma. Improved control of peptic ulcer disease could also be a factor in this decline.

TABLE 1. **Ascorbic Acid Required to Maintain Adequate Blood Levels**

| Condition | Daily Dose (mg) |
|---|---|
| Tuberculosis | 100–200 |
| Burns (severe) | 200–500 |
| Ulcerative colitis | 200–400 |
| Urinary infection | 200–300 |
| Wounds (granulating) | 100–200 |
| Postoperative benign course | 100 |
| Diarrhea (severe) | 200 |
| Hyperthyroidism | 200 |
| Pregnancy or lactation | 100 |

*Deficient Blood Ascorbic Levels*
Plasma: less than 0.2 mg/dl*
Buffy coat: less than 4 mg per 100 grams†

*Roe and Kuether method.
†Butler and Cushman method.

In the treatment of cancer, ascorbic acid has been found to be of no value.

## REQUIREMENT

The recommended daily allowance of ascorbic acid for the average adult is 60 mg, for pregnant women 80 mg, and for infants 35 mg. With disease or increased metabolism, stress, trauma (particularly severe burns), or extensive inflammatory processes, the requirement is much higher. With surgery, the blood ascorbic acid level generally falls, and among heavy smokers it is usually below average. The minimal amounts of the vitamin necessary on a surgical ward to maintain adequate blood levels in adults with various diseases and surgeries are shown in Table 1.

In recent years, megadoses of vitamin C (1000 to 3000 mg per day) have been recommended by some people for a variety of reasons ranging from promoting good health to preventing cancer and colds. Ascorbic acid is relatively inexpensive and can serve as a good placebo. However, it has now been established that overdoses cause oxaluria, with production of renal stones, and may cause iron poisoning from too much absorption of heme iron. Megadoses in pregnant women may produce a rebound phenomenon in the newborn infant. Large doses may interfere with Clinitest and Testape determinations in the urine and Hemoccult tests of the feces.

It is noteworthy that most pharmaceutical firms have reduced the amount of ascorbic acid in their multivitamin tablets from 500 to 600 mg to 100 to 200 mg. In addition, ascorbic acid is added to some canned foods and bottled drinks as a preservative and to some drugs as a buffer (parenteral Achromycin, Tofranil).

# VITAMIN K DEFICIENCY

method of
WILLIAM D. HAIRE, M.D.
*University of Nebraska College of Medicine*
*Omaha, Nebraska*

Vitamin K is a term applied to a group of fat soluble vitamins derived from 2-methyl–1,4-naphthoquinone that are required for hepatic synthesis of the plasma coagulation Factors II (prothrombin), VII, IX, and X and the naturally occurring anticoagulant proteins protein C and protein S. Under normal circumstances, the liver produces inactive forms of these coagulation factors that are then acted upon by a vitamin K–dependent carboxylase, converting some of their glutamic acid residues to gamma-carboxyglutamic acid residues. This change allows the molecules to become fully functional coagulation factors. In the absence or antagonism of vitamin K, the production of these nonfunctional molecules continues but they are not converted to their active forms.

Vitamin K is present in a wide range of plant and animal tissues, with the highest concentrations in green leafy vegetables. Vitamin K is also produced by microorganisms comprising the normal human intestinal flora. The vitamin K used in humans can come from either of these two sources. Once in the intestinal tract, vitamin K requires an intact lipid absorption mechanism to enter the circulation. Under normal circumstances, the daily adult requirement of this vitamin is probably less than 100 μg. Because the body stores of vitamin K are limited, a deficiency can occur in as little as a few weeks on a diet deficient in this vitamin. If broad-spectrum antibiotics are given simultaneously (limiting production of vitamin K by the gut flora), deficiency can occur more rapidly.

## CAUSES

Any process that limits oral intake, impairs lipid absorption, or limits production by intestinal microorganisms can cause absolute vitamin K deficiency. The restricted oral intake inherent with the newborn state and the postoperative period and the reliance on total parenteral nutrition are clinical examples of the first category. Biliary obstruction, either intra- or extrahepatic, and malabsorptive syndromes such as celiac disease or cystic fibrosis belong to the second category. Broad-spectrum antibiotic use, especially in the face of limited oral intake, can cause vitamin K deficiency via the third mechanism. Coumarin derivatives are competitive inhibitors of vitamin K and prevent vitamin K from acting as an enzyme cofactor. The presence of these compounds, either given therapeutically or ingested surreptitiously, can lead to all the manifestations of vitamin K deficiency in the absence of dietary deficiency. The newer cephalosporins with a methyl-thiatetrazole side chain (such as cefamandole, moxalactam, and cefoperazone) can act to limit vitamin K production by intestinal flora and may also act as inhibitors of vitamin K activity at the hepatocyte level.

## CLINICAL AND LABORATORY MANIFESTATIONS

The only known clinical manifestation of vitamin K deficiency is a hemorrhagic diathesis due to deficiencies in functional forms of coagulation Factors II, VII, IX and X. The hemorrhagic complications may be as mild as ecchymosis or as severe as fatal intracranial or retroperitoneal bleeding. The deficiency may be detected prior to any hemorrhagic manifestations by abnormal coagulation studies—generally a prolongation of the prothrombin and partial thromboplastin times. Because the vitamin K–dependent coagulation factors are involved in both the intrinsic and extrinsic pathways of coagulation, a deficiency of this vitamin will result in a prolongation of both the prothrombin time and partial thromboplastin times. If one of these studies is abnormal and the other is normal, the diagnosis of vitamin K deficiency should be questioned. Since the coagulation defect that occurs in the absence of vitamin K is due to a deficiency of coagulation factors, the abnormal prothrombin and partial thromboplastin times can be corrected by simply mixing the patient's plasma with normal plasma. The diagnosis can be suspected in the appropriate clinical setting by a prolongation of the prothrombin and partial thromboplastin times that corrects after mixing with normal plasma. Rarely, assays of the vitamin K–dependent coagulation factors are helpful in establishing the diagnosis. The diagnosis can be confirmed if administration of vitamin K totally corrects these studies.

## TREATMENT

Therapy is generally directed at replacement of vitamin K and/or the vitamin K–dependent coagulation factors along with treatment of the underlying disease that predisposed the patient to the deficiency. The type of treatment chosen depends on the severity of the clinical situation. Asymptomatic patients with mild abnormalities of coagulation studies and an intact lipid absorptive mechanism can often be treated with an oral vitamin K analogue.

Patients with active hemorrhage or marked abnormalities of coagulation studies should receive parenteral therapy, usually with vitamin $K_1$ (AquaMEPHYTON or Konakion). In patients with a severe coagulopathy, intramuscular administration of these and other medications can cause local hematoma formation and is contraindicated. The subcutaneous route can be used, but the absorption of the drug may be erratic, especially in patients with cutaneous vasoconstriction. The use of slow intravenous infusion of vitamin $K_1$ offers the advantages of rapid and reliable delivery of the drug to the liver and can restore hemostatic levels of coagulation factors within 12 to 24 hours. This route of administration is rarely associated with hypotension that can be fatal and should be used only when the clinical situation warrants this type of risk. Generally, intravenous therapy is indicated only if the patient is actively bleeding at a rate or in a location that jeopardizes either life or organ function. Patients with marked abnormalities of coagulation tests (prothrombin times of over 30 seconds) are at high enough risk of severe bleeding that parenteral therapy is warranted. In this situation, the subcutaneous route of administration is preferred to the intravenous route unless the patient has cutaneous vasoconstriction. The dose of parenteral vitamin $K_1$ varies with the size of the patient: 0.5 to 1.0 mg is generally adequate for newborns, 2 to 3 mg is given to children, and 5 to 10 mg is the dose for adults.

Even after the intravenous administration of vitamin K, the liver requires several hours to synthesize active coagulation factors. In the face of overt hemorrhage requiring immediate correction of the deficiency in coagulation factors, transfusion of fresh-frozen plasma is indicated. A reasonable dose of plasma is 10 to 15 ml per kg. Because of the potential for hepatitis transmission and thrombotic complications, prothrombin complex concentrates (Konyne-HT, Proplex) should not be used in this setting. Repeating the coagulation studies immediately after transfusion or 12 to 24 hours after vitamin K replacement is imperative to confirm the adequacy of treatment.

In clinical situations posing high risk of vitamin K deficiency, this disorder can often be prevented. In patients without restriction of oral intake, this can be accomplished with 5 mg of a water-soluble vitamin K derivative, such as Synkayvite, two to four times weekly. In patients receiving total parenteral nutrition, this can be done with 1 to 2 mg of AquaMEPHYTON or Konakion, two to three times weekly.

# OSTEOPOROSIS

method of
URIEL S. BARZEL, M.D.
*Albert Einstein College of Medicine and*
*Montefiore Medical Center*
*Bronx, New York*

Osteoporosis is a condition, present primarily among the aged, in which there is a propensity to fracture bones spontaneously or as a result of minimal trauma. In this condition, there is too little bone tissue to provide adequate skeletal support for the physical stresses of normal daily life and for commonly encountered minor accidents. Osteoporosis is not clinically apparent until the patient presents with a fracture, since there is no unique medical or biologic marker that would identify it. There are some nonspecific radiologic findings associated with this condition, and some patients may be suspected of having osteoporosis as the result of incidental observations made in radiologic procedures.

## CLINICAL MANIFESTATIONS

Wrist fracture (Colles' fracture) is the most common presenting condition of osteoporosis, followed in frequency by collapse-fractures of spinal vertebrae and by hip fractures. In extreme cases, patients may sustain rib fractures as a result of leaning against a hard surface such as the side of a bathtub. Osteoporotic hip fractures are associated with 25 to 50% 1-year mortality.

## NATURAL HISTORY

The natural history of osteoporosis is one of recurrent, unexpected, discrete occurrences of fractures, interspersed with periods of months or years of freedom from clinical symptoms. Bone in osteoporosis is completely normal, both histologically and biochemically. Osteoporotic fractures heal normally; there is formation of callus and the development of union of the broken bones within a few weeks. Fractures in the dorsal spine may result in round back deformity, especially if there are anterior collapses of upper thoracic vertebrae. Fractures in the lower thoracic and lumbar spine result, eventually, in the rib cage coming to rest on the iliac crest, a condition identified by the patient as the total loss of the waistline. All of these cause a marked reduction in height; osteoporotic patients have been known to lose 6 to 10 inches as a result of multiple fractures. The round back deformity and the loss of vertebral height bring about a bulging of the abdominal muscles and the development of chronic constipation because of inability to develop intra-abdominal pressure for adequate evacuation.

## ETIOLOGY

A major contributory factor to osteoporosis is the *failure to achieve maximum skeletal density at peak development* in early adulthood. To some extent this may be genetic or familial, and to some extent it may be the result of inadequate calcium intake during the formative years (Table 1).

Superimposed on this failure to achieve maximal density is an imbalance in bone turnover in both men and women throughout adult life, with bone resorption quantitatively exceeding bone formation, which results in a slow and inexorable loss of bone. There are multiple potential contributory factors to this imbalance: *inadequate calcium intake* throughout adult life and *calcium malabsorption,* which is frequently present in the elderly, may be two such factors. Experimental *inactivity* in volunteers and complete bed rest in orthopedic or neurologic cases cause negative calcium balance and osteopenia, suggesting that inactivity may play an etiologic role in osteoporosis. Recent studies imply an *abnormal parathyroid response* to hypocalcemia in this condition, and some investigators propose that an *abnormality of vitamin D metabolism* may be a contributory factor in osteoporosis. *High protein intake, obligatory urinary calcium loss* as a result of high sodium intake, and *renal tubular calcium leak* have all been described in osteoporosis and may also play a contributory role in its development.

In women, there is an acceleration and exaggeration of the imbalance between formation and resorption of bone as a result of the *cessation of gonadal function* as seen at the time of *menopause,* whether natural or artificial (e.g., bilateral oophorectomy). Because women reach at maturity a smaller skeletal mass than men and because men do not normally lose gonadal function, women are much more commonly afflicted by this disease.

## ACHIEVEMENT OF SKELETAL INTEGRITY

The achievement of maximal skeletal development requires an adequate intake of vitamin D and calcium and physical exercise. Vitamin D may be endogenously synthesized through the exposure of the skin to the ultraviolet rays of the sun for a few minutes a day. Vitamin D is available exogenously in cod liver oil, in deep sea fish, and, in the United States, in milk that is fortified with vitamin D. It is also widely available in *therapeutic* vitamin capsules. In the teenager and the adult, the amount of vitamin D required is 200 to 400 U per day. Because ingestion of excess vitamin D may result in vitamin D toxicity—hypercalciuria and hypercalcemia—megadoses of this vitamin should be discouraged, except in cases of fat malabsorption and of hypoparathyroidism. The recommended amount of dietary calcium is 800 to 1000 mg daily (and twice as much in the teenager). Both vitamin D and calcium can be obtained in adequate amounts from the ingestion of three to four glasses of milk daily. Calcium is also easily available in multiple over-the-counter products, generally as calcium carbonate, and can be taken as a supplement if the amount of milk ingested is less than recommended. Maintenance of adequate muscle strength, by the performance of calisthenics for 30 to 60 minutes three times weekly, is also useful. Excessive exercise may induce amenorrhea and is, therefore, counterproductive because the cessation of estrogen production in this situation results in a negative calcium balance and decreased skeletal mass.

## MAINTENANCE OF SKELETAL INTEGRITY AND PREVENTION OF OSTEOPOROSIS

Maintenance of the skeletal integrity, once maximal development has been achieved, requires continuation of adequate intake of calcium and vitamin D and maintenance of an exercise program. Furthermore, it is recommended that cigarette smoking and excessive alcohol consumption be avoided because these are associated

TABLE 1. **Factors Associated with Osteoporosis**

Female sex
Menopause
Fair skin
Low calcium intake
Low body weight
Smoking
Alcoholism
Diabetes mellitus
Anorexia nervosa
Pernicious anemia
Inactivity
Excessive activity with secondary amenorrhea

with osteoporosis as well as with other disabilities.

A most important measure in the prevention of osteoporosis in females is cyclic hormone therapy at the time of menopause. Epidemiologic studies, performed in postmenopausal white women, reveal that estrogen ingestion reduces the risk of osteoporotic fractures in half. Similar studies reveal that the protective effect of estrogen is independent of so called risk factors such as lean body weight or smoking. Thus, if there is no contraindication for hormone therapy, this therapy should be offered to *all menopausal women,* since rapid bone loss is a universal phenomenon that occurs in all women when estrogen production ceases. To be effective in preventing the rapid loss of bone, estrogen replacement therapy should be started immediately after bilateral oophorectomy or as soon as possible following, and no later than 5 years after, the onset of natural menopause. Once started, estrogen therapy should be continued for at least 5 or 6 years. The optimal treatment regimen that is recommended today is cycling therapy with estrogen and progesterone. The minimum effective oral estrogen dose is 25 μg ethinyl estradiol (Estinyl) or 0.625 mg conjugated estrogen (Premarin) (0.300 mg conjugated estrogen if coupled with high calcium intake) and medroxyprogesterone (Provera, Amen, Curretab), 10 mg per day for the last 10 days of cycle. Transcutaneous and subcutaneous implantation may become alternative routes of estrogen administration.

In special situations, appropriate medical intervention and treatment will help prevent the development of osteoporosis. These include certain endocrine conditions, such as acromegaly, hyperadrenocorticism, and thyrotoxicosis, as well as excess thyroid hormone replacement, gastrectomy, and liver disease. To the extent possible, endocrine disease should be under optimal control. If patients are given pharmacologic doses of corticosteroids as a long-term therapy, some element of protection of the skeleton can be achieved by the coadministration of pharmacologic doses (50,000 to 100,000 U per week) of vitamin D (Calciferol) and an adequate calcium intake. Patients receiving thyroxine replacement should be given this hormone in amounts that would maintain normal serum thyroxine and serum thyroid stimulating hormone (TSH) levels. Suppression of the serum TSH level below the normal range should be avoided (except in cases of thyroid cancer in which this is the therapeutic goal). In postgastrectomy states, osteomalacia may develop unless adequate vitamin D is chronically given to overcome a degree of malabsorption that is present in this condition.

## THERAPY FOR ESTABLISHED OSTEOPOROSIS

When presented with a case of apparent osteoporosis and a fracture, we treat the actual fracture and at the same time review the differential diagnosis (Table 2) and initiate a treatment regimen for whatever underlying condition may be responsible for the development of osteoporosis.

Colles' fracture is treated by casting. Spinal collapse is treated with complete bed rest until the acute pain has substantially diminished (72 hours to 2 weeks), followed by gradual mobilization, first to an inclined chair and later to full upright position and re-ambulation. Pain treatment should avoid narcotics, if possible, because of their tendency to produce constipation. A corset may be used for a few weeks to give the spine some support during the period of recovery. Hip fracture requires surgical pinning or hip replacement, followed by aggressive physiotherapy.

Beyond the repair of the acute fracture, the anatomic goal of medical therapy in established osteoporosis is to increase the amount of bone tissue. The prescription of adequate vitamin intake, adequate calcium ingestion (which in the postmenopausal woman rises to 1500 mg per day), and exercise remains true in women who have established osteoporosis but will not, per se, improve their bone mineral status.

Rapid bone loss had ceased, in most cases, a long while earlier. Because estrogens slow down bone turnover, they alone are also unlikely to have a beneficial effect if started at this stage in the natural history of the disease. Furthermore, estrogens' side effects are unacceptable to most elderly women with established osteoporosis. For example, in a 1-year study in which 70-year-old normal women were given estrogen-gestagen, 44% left the study before its conclusion, two-thirds of them due to "menstrual troubles." In another study, 13% of women with established osteoporosis who were given estrogen therapy required hysterectomy or dilatation and curettage. Thus there is no room for estrogens in the management of established osteoporosis.

A large number of pharmacologic agents have been under investigation for their possible positive effect on skeletal metabolism (Table 3). In

TABLE 2. **Differential Diagnosis of Osteoporosis**

Osteomalacia
Acromegaly
Hyperthyroidism
Hyperparathyroidism
Hyperadrenocorticism
Multiple myeloma
Prolonged heparin therapy
Lipid storage disease
Liver disease
Chronic anemia

TABLE 3. **Treatments in Established Osteoporosis**

**Generally Accepted or Approved**
High calcium diet
Alkaline calcium supplements
  Calcium carbonate
  Calcium citrate malate
  Calcium citrate*
Adequate vitamin D intake
Exercise
Calcitonin

**Investigational**
Sodium fluoride (enteric coated)
anabolic agents—methandrostenolone
Low-dose parathyroid hormone
Vitamin D metabolite
  1α-Hydroxyvitamin D
  1,25-Dihydroxyvitamin D (calcitriol)
  24,25-Dihydroxyvitamin D
Hydrochlorothiazide
Low sodium intake
ADFR, or "coherence therapy"
  *Activate*: phosphorus, $T_3$—3 days
  *Depress*: etidronate—2 wk
  *Free*: 8 to 10 wk
  *Repeat*

*Preferred preparation in hypochlorhydria.

reviewing the literature dealing with the treatment regimens of this condition, and with osteoporosis in general, a few caveats must be kept in mind: (1) Much of the information presently available on osteoporosis is the result of cross-sectional studies in which people born in different years are compared. Clearly, such comparisons may not always be justifiable. Comparisons of maximal skeletal development of subjects born in 1910, for instance, with those born in 1945 may be totally invalid because standards of diet and health were markedly different during the times these two cohorts of patients grew up and reached maturity. (2) Many ongoing studies of osteoporosis use currently available methods of bone densitometry and quantitation of bone mineral at different bone sites as their end points of efficacy of interventional regimens. These provide clearly valuable information about bone at these specific, measurable sites, but must be viewed critically until proved to have a significant correlation with fracture rates. With these caveats in place, one can now examine osteoporosis therapy.

*Calcitonin,* an injectable hormone with significant effect in Paget's disease, has been approved by the FDA for treatment of osteoporosis. Available data show that, administered at a dose of 50 to 100 IU subcutaneously or intramuscularly daily or every other day, salmon calcitonin does have a salutary effect on bone density, but the studies are too short and contain too few subjects to prove that calcitonin treatment prevents osteoporotic fractures. *Sodium fluoride* has been the subject of intense investigations for over 10 years. There are epidemiologic data to suggest that, within narrow limits, lifelong exposure to low-level fluoride results in better skeletal resistance to the development of osteoporosis. When used therapeutically, in doses of 35 to 70 mg per day, fluoride effectively increases bone density in only 60% of osteoporotic subjects, the resultant bone is not histologically normal, and, most importantly, fracture prevention has not been demonstrated unequivocally. Furthermore, fluoride therapy is associated with a high rate of gastric and joint complications (a lesser rate of these complications is reported for enteric-coated tablets). *Anabolic agents* (e.g., stanozolol [Winstrol], 2 to 6 mg daily, 3 weeks out of 4) have a positive effect on bone economy but are unacceptable to most female patients because of the associated masculinizing side effects and because of their negative effects on lipid metabolism. A theory that very-low-dose *parathyroid hormone* administered parenterally may result in an improved skeletal density and strength is under investigation. The possibility that *vitamin D* metabolism is faulty in osteoporotic subjects fuels a number of studies of various metabolites of the vitamin. The jury is still out on vitamin D metabolite treatment, as it is on parathyroid hormone injection therapy. There is epidemiologic evidence that subjects who have been taking *thiazide diuretics* for over 10 years have a lesser rate of osteoporotic fractures. The use of these preparations in subjects with hypercalciuria is clearly justified, but it is not known whether thiazide therapy or a low sodium diet will lead to a positive skeletal balance.

A new approach to the problem of osteoporosis is to be found in the recent development of *ADFR* (activate, depress, free, repeat), also called *coherence therapy* (see Table 3). This treatment method is designed to exploit the physiologic sequential coupling of bone resorption and bone formation in bone turnover. Bone turnover and remodeling can be visualized as beginning with osteoclastic resorption, which is later followed by osteoblastic deposition of bone in the same anatomic locations. ADFR aims to stimulate coherent bone resorption (A = activate) and then stop it prematurely (D = depress). Thereafter, bone formation will proceed normally (F = free), and eventually the cycle will be repeated (R = repeat). The success of this method hinges on the fact that while bone resorption would be interrupted pharmacologically, bone formation would be allowed to proceed, physiologically, unhampered. By interrupting the resorptive phase and not the formative phase, one would achieve excess formation relative to resorption and a reversal of the previously negative bone balance.

"Activation" can be achieved by ingestion of phosphorus (Neutra-Phos), 2.0 grams daily. This lowers serum calcium and generally causes an increase in parathyroid hormone secretion, which stimulates bone resorptive activity. Triiodothyronine ($T_3$) has also been used for the same end. This phase is continued for only a few days. "Depression" is achieved by the use of the diphosphonate etidronate (Didronel).* This orally administered agent arrests osteoclastic activity and has been used extensively, for a number of years, to suppress osteoclastic bone resorption in Paget's disease. It is administered in the ADFR sequence at a dose of 400 mg daily for a period of 2 weeks. Thereafter, patients are provided with adequate calcium and vitamin D but are otherwise "free"—not treated. The treatment cycle is repeated every 10 to 12 weeks. Histologic examinations of bone are reported to find no abnormality after 150 weeks of ADFR therapy and do demonstrate a reduction in the depth of resorption cavities. Furthermore, preliminary data show that over 2 years there is continuous increase in bone density in all sites examined, *as well as* a reduction in fracture activity. Of special interest is the fact that some investigators report equally good results with this cycling therapy without the A ("activation") leg of the protocol. If confirmed to be effective, this therapeutic approach may prove to provide a safe and simple long-term management opportunity in established osteoporosis.

---

*This use of Didronel is not listed in the manufacturer's official directive.

# PAGET'S DISEASE OF BONE

method of
WILL G. RYAN, M.D.
*Rush–Presbyterian–St. Luke's Medical Center*
*Chicago, Illinois*

Paget's disease of bone is a disorder that usually manifests itself in middle or old age, although because it is very slowly progressive it likely begins at a young age, possibly in childhood. It is estimated that from about 1% of the United States population in their forties to as many as 10% in their eighties will have some evidence of the disease, although less than 10 to 20% of these individuals will ever become symptomatic as a result.

The skeleton is normally remodeled at a rate of about 1% per year under the control of the osteoclasts (the cells that break down bone) and osteoblasts (the cells that build up bone). In Paget's disease in the areas of the skeleton involved, the osteoclasts are excessively numerous and active, resulting in initial excessive lytic activity. There is some evidence that this process may be induced by a virus, but this is not established. Nucleocapsids that react to antibodies to measles or respiratory syncytial viruses are often seen in pagetic osteoclasts but are seen in osteoclasts of certain other bone diseases as well. By some as yet poorly understood coupling process, the osteoblasts in the area are stimulated to be numerous and active as well and attempt to repair that bone that has been lysed by the osteoclasts, resulting in a markedly increased bone turnover rate in the areas involved with consequent increased blood flow. This abnormally rapid turnover results in normally lamellar bone being replaced by embryonic or "woven" bone that is structurally inferior. In some phases of the disease, the radiographs will have primarily a lytic appearance but most of the time a mixed lytic and blastic appearance will be seen. The advancing wall of disease activity tends to progress at a rate of about 1 cm per year. As the disease progresses, varying degrees of deformity of the bones involved will appear.

The disease appears somewhat randomly distributed throughout the skeleton, with predominance in the axial and weight-bearing skeleton and with usual sparing of the extreme distal extremities; it is rare to see it in the phalanges. The disease may range from a single small bone being detected incidentally on a bone scan to one of virtually every bone in the skeleton being involved and producing marked skeletal deformities. *The manifestations of the disease are largely related to its strategic location in the skeleton.* Large areas of the pelvis or calvaria may be involved and yet produce little or no symptoms. However, if the pelvic disease progresses to involve the acetabulum, it tends to cause degenerative disease of the hip joint with attendant mild to marked disability, which may require replacement with a mechanical device for continued function. The same is often true if the head of the femur is involved. Calvarial skull disease may cause some enlargement of the skull and on occasion may be associated with headaches. Basilar skull disease tends to cause mild to marked deafness if the area around the cochlea or other parts of the auditory mechanism are involved. Involvement of other cranial nerves occurs but is much less common. Extensive basilar skull disease results in platybasia and if severe may on occasion produce hydrocephalus by mechanical interference with the flow of cerebrospinal fluid. Involvement of facial bones sometimes results in grotesque facial deformity. Long-bone involvement, particularly of the lower extremities, usually results in considerable bowing and easy fracture. Long-bone involvement tends to occur near one end (epiphysis) or the other and progress toward the middle (metaphysis). If the disease manifests in the distal femur or proximal tibia, a process similar to that previously described for the hip may occur at the knee and result in similar disability. Upper extremity involvement may produce deformity but usually not significant disability, presumably because of lack of weight bearing. Finally, involvement of one or multiple vertebrae may cause sufficient neural compression (or on occasion a vascular "steal" syndrome) to result in paraparesis or plegia. Patients with extensive disease and with already compromised myocardial function may develop congestive heart failure because of increased blood flow through pagetic bone. Osteogenic sarcoma is the most dreaded complication of Paget's disease but fortunately occurs in less than 1% of patients.

## DIAGNOSIS

Paget's disease is characterized by having at least five useful objective parameters of the disease process. The serum alkaline phosphatase reflecting increased osteoblastic activity is the most useful of these for assessing the disease. In these days of routine chemistry panels performed on patients' sera, Paget's disease, like hyperparathyroidism and other diseases, is being diagnosed more frequently in the asymptomatic state. In this situation, it must be distinguished from possible hepatic disease, although with the latter several of the serum enzymes are usually increased. Although bone alkaline phosphatase is more heat sensitive than that of liver and isoenzyme determinations are available, they tend not to be very reliable clinically, particularly at levels only slightly increased over normal. In this situation, a bone scan is the most reliable and sensitive means of making the diagnosis. Efforts are underway, however, for increasing the specificity of the alkaline phosphatase determination.

Because the collagen-rich matrix of bone that is digested by the osteoclast has a high (approximately 20%) concentration of hydroxyproline, urinary hydroxyproline determinations are another means of assessing disease activity. However, they are relatively expensive (about $100) and inconvenient (24-hour urines) and they are not as useful under routine clinical conditions. Because osteoclastic and osteoblastic activities are so tightly coupled in this disorder, the serum alkaline phosphatase, although not representing the primary disease process, is satisfactory for assessing disease activity, and my impression is that it is somewhat more sensitive than urinary hydroxyproline. Patients with small amounts of disease may have normal serum alkaline phosphatase and urinary hydroxyproline. This small amount of disease may be detectable only by bone scan. We detected such in a 25-year-old woman who was the daughter of one of my patients with a strong family history (mother and four of eight siblings) during a study using bone scanning of the offspring.

Less expensive (except for total body survey) than bone scanning is roentgenography of involved areas, and its images are also usually sufficiently characteristic for diagnosis. Computed tomography (CT) and magnetic resonance imaging (MRI) may also be useful on occasion, particularly when occult sarcoma is suspected, but are unnecessary as a routine. For usual diagnosis, bone biopsy is rarely if ever indicated but may be mandatory when osteosarcoma or other malignant degeneration is suspected. Serum osteocalcin (bone GLA protein) is not nearly as precise for monitoring disease activity as is serum alkaline phosphatase.

In the initial phases of therapy (with calcitonin or bisphosphonates), obtaining a serum alkaline phosphatase at about monthly intervals is sufficient to determine response in most cases. In later stages of monitoring treatment, the determinations may be extended to 3- to 12-month intervals depending on the response obtained.

## TREATMENT

Many patients with Paget's disease have only mild symptoms of bone pain or arthritis and can be treated with simple analgesics or the nonsteroidal anti-inflammatory agents. Prior to the late 1960s, there were no specific effective antipagetic (antiresorptive) agents; now there are several, which fall into three general classes—calcitonins, bisphosphonates (formerly called diphosphonates), and plicamycin (formerly called mithramycin; the name was changed to avoid confusion with mitomycin). The point at which to begin antiresorptive therapy is somewhat problematic at this time, particularly with the asymptomatic patients. It is estimated that 80% of patients are elderly and asymptomatic. In my opinion, if the disease is in a location likely to produce complications at a later time (such as near but not yet involving the acetabulum or cochlea), early antiresorptive therapy is indicated, whereas if the disease involves the wing of the ilium or a small amount of calvarium, such treatment is probably not needed. It is also important, particularly in treating back pain, to determine if the site of the disease is likely to be causing the patient's symptoms. However, with the development of new, more potent and safe agents (the newer bisphosphonates) over the next several years, it is likely that physicians will be treating virtually all patients to prevent progression or possibly cure the disease before it has a chance to produce significant disability.

### Calcitonins

Two forms of calcitonin are available in the United States—synthetic human (Cibacalcin) and synthetic salmon (Calcimar). Eel calcitonin* is also being used in other parts of the world. Salmon is the most potent of the calcitonins, which presumably has something to do with the fish's habit of migrating from fresh (very low calcium concentration) to sea water (very high calcium concentration). Whether or not human calcitonin serves a physiologic function is still being debated, mostly as to whether or not it may have a role in the prevention of osteoporosis. At pharmacologic doses the calcitonins have a potent osteoclast inhibitory activity, and this property makes them effective in the treatment of Paget's disease. At present, they are likely the safest agents to use for long-term treatment. Unfortu-

---

*Not available in the United States.

nately, they tend to be the least effective, are the most expensive ($8 to $10 per day at full starting dose), and have to be given by subcutaneous injection. Nasal spray delivery is currently under development and may be available in the U.S. by the time this book is published. Generally, a 50 to 75% reduction in the serum alkaline phosphatase is seen within the first few months of initiating therapy, but there is often loss of effectiveness over time. If the serum alkaline phosphatase is increasing in the face of continued therapy, there is likely no good reason to continue it. The cause of loss of effectiveness is sometimes related to excessive antibody production as a result of injection of a foreign substance but mostly occurs for unknown reasons. A number of patients have a sustained response for the duration of therapy, exceeding 10 years in some individuals. Resistance to human calcitonin likely occurs less frequently than to salmon, but there are no controlled clinical trials to my knowledge in this regard. I have seen some patients respond to the human form after failing to respond to salmon calcitonin, but in others I have not seen such response.

Human calcitonin (Cibacalcin) is packaged as a dry powder (0.5 mg) in conjunction with a syringe filled with diluent and does not require refrigeration. The usual starting dose is 0.5 mg daily, but this may be reduced to three times a week or less if the patient has a good sustained response. Skin testing for possible allergenicity does not appear to be indicated, but the usual precautions for injecting a foreign protein are suggested.

Salmon calcitonin (Calcimar) is packaged as 2-ml vials containing 200 IU per ml. It should be refrigerated or at least kept cool for the short periods when refrigeration might not be possible. The usual starting dose is 100 IU per day (0.5 ml), but this may later be reduced to as little as 50 IU three times a week. Because a foreign peptide is being injected, it is advisable to skin test the patient for possible allergenicity using the directions in the package insert. Severe anaphylactoid reactions are unusual but do occur sometimes after institution of therapy, although I am not aware of any resulting in death. Use of insulin syringes with needles is a convenient mode of administration.

Both calcitonins have associated side effects, the most troublesome of which is nausea, occurring in up to 10% of patients. This may be minimized by having patients take their dose at bedtime. Flushing also occurs, usually more so with human than with salmon calcitonin, but is not often troublesome enough to discontinue therapy. Local skin reactions are usually minor, and other side effects are infrequent.

## Bisphosphonates

Bisphosphonates (formerly called diphosphonates) are compounds structurally related to pyrophosphate but are resistant to destruction by pyrophosphatase. They have a great avidity for the actively metabolizing areas of the skeleton, and it is this type of compound, with radioactive technetium attached, that is used currently in performing bone scans. Bone scanning is the most sensitive means of detecting the activity of Paget's disease and assessing its distribution throughout the skeleton. Also because of the markedly increased metabolic activity in the areas involved, these compounds are highly concentrated in such areas when administered to the patient with active Paget's disease. Although it is not known with certainty, it is likely that the high concentration in these areas results in the compounds being ingested by the pagetic osteoclasts, resulting in toxicity to them and thus accounting for the therapeutic effect.

Etidronate (Didronel) has been available for general therapeutic use in Paget's disease in the U.S. for over a decade; it is the only one of these compounds currently available here. However, it is likely that aminopropylidene diphosphonate (APD, Pamidronate) will be available by the time or shortly after this text is published, and several other agents are under investigation in the "therapeutic pipeline." Although Didronel is an effective agent in the treatment of Paget's disease, it has the side effect of inhibiting crystallization of hydroxyapatite, the major mineral component of bone. Thus, if used at high dose or for prolonged periods of time, it tends to cause clinically significant osteomalacia resulting sometimes in increased bone pain and/or susceptibility to easy fracture. Compounded by the already structurally inferior pagetic bone, this may result in very adverse consequences, and I tend to avoid its use in patients with disease in weight-bearing long bones (femur and/or tibia). I have seen a few patients in whom the drug was used inappropriately (at high dose or for prolonged periods) and in whom this has occurred. One of these patients had fractured his tibia several times with only weight-bearing stress. In fact, this compound was first and is still used for inhibition of extraskeletal calcification.

The newer therapeutic bisphosphonates are characterized by increased antiresorptive effect and by lessened or virtual abolishment of the inhibition of crystallization of hydroxyapatite, and unless unexpected consequences occur it is likely that they will replace Didronel for use in Paget's disease.

When used appropriately, Didronel is a very effective agent in the therapy of most patients with Paget's disease. It has the advantage over other agents of being active orally and less expensive ($1 to $2 per day). The recommended dosage is 5 mg per kg per day, and it is available in 200- and 400-mg tablets. Because it is poorly and variably absorbed, it should be taken with water on an empty stomach once daily. The patient should be advised not to eat or drink (particularly milk or milk products) other than water for 2 hours before and after taking it to prevent interference with absorption. The usual dosage for a normal weight adult is 400 mg per day, and because of the variable absorption fine tuning of the dose is irrelevant. To avoid significant production of osteomalacia, it *should not be given for longer than 6 months without interruption.* The usual and recommended approach is to give the drug for 6 months at a time. The serum alkaline phosphatase is usually lowered by 50 to 75%, although some patients may reach normal levels that may persist for variable periods of time. If the patient is showing signs of relapse as indicated by an increasing serum alkaline phosphatase or has had an inadequate initial response, the *course may be repeated after 3 to 6 months off therapy* and many patients have been managed in this manner for several years. Some patients have a prolonged (over 2 years) response after a single course. In those not having an adequate response to the usual dosage, higher-dose therapy is likely not advisable because of the attendant previously discussed side effects. In such patients, combination therapy with a calcitonin may be effective. Because calcitonins tend to inhibit osteoclast activity, they likely tend to inhibit ingestion of the bisphosphonate by the osteoclast. Therefore, when combination therapy is used, bisphosphonate should probably be used first or when the patient is in a state of relapse off calcitonin.

### Plicamycin

Plicamycin (Mithracin) is a cytotoxic antibiotic originally used in cancer chemotherapy. It binds to DNA and interferes with DNA-directed RNA synthesis. Why it has particularly osteoclast toxicity is unknown, but it must have such activity because it is useful in therapy in any form of life-threatening hypercalcemia.

Although plicamycin is the most potent agent against Paget's disease generally available in the U.S. (although not officially FDA approved for this indication) at this time, because of its toxicity it should be used primarily in patients who have failed to respond to other therapies or in whom a rapid response is required, such as patients with neural compression syndromes. Also because of

its toxicity (hepatic, renal, platelet), it should be used only by physicians thoroughly familiar with the principles of chemotherapy. It generally is given as 7- to 10-day courses infused intravenously at a dosage of 15 to 25 $\mu$g per kg body weight per day with careful daily monitoring for excessive toxicity. Physicians contemplating its use may receive detailed information from me by calling (312–942–6163) or writing.* It may also be given by bolus injection for outpatient therapy. Another major side effect is nausea, and although my colleagues and I have seen no cumulative toxic effect, the nausea (sometimes anticipatory) may limit prolonged use. It can, however, be a valuable therapy when used in patients with appropriately severe problems resistant to other therapies.

### General Comments

Obviously, orthopedic or neurosurgical intervention is appropriate in certain situations (hip replacement, etc.), and pagetic bone usually heals well. If there is time, suppression of disease activity with calcitonin prior to surgery is likely of value. I tend to avoid use of Didronel for 1 to 2 months perioperatively. Unless neural compression syndromes require urgent intervention, a trial of medical therapy is indicated and often gratifying, particularly in those with extensive vertebral disease. Other investigators have indicated that antiresorptive agents may be useful in therapy of nonunion fractures of pagetic bone, and although I have had no experience with this type of treatment, it seems worth consideration.

---

*Rush–Presbyterian–St. Luke's Medical Center, 1653 W. Congress Pkwy., Chicago, IL 60612.

# TOTAL PARENTERAL NUTRITION IN ADULTS

method of
ROBERT J. ELSEN, M.D., and
BRUCE R. BISTRIAN, M.D., Ph.D.
*New England Deaconess Hospital*
*Boston, Massachusetts*

Malnutrition is a frequent complication in the hospitalized patient that can greatly influence morbidity and mortality. Particularly for the stressed, malnourished patient, nutritional intervention can provide significant therapeutic benefit. There are two primary methods of involuntary feeding: enteral and parenteral. Enteral feeding is the method of choice except in those instances in which the gut cannot (i.e., obstruction) or should not (i.e., severe pancreatitis) be used and total parenteral nutrition (TPN) must be employed. The role of parenteral nutrition has evolved since its first use in 1968. There is a clear consensus based on clinical trials in regard to certain indications for its use, but for most patients, its use is still based largely on clinical grounds. Other important aspects of TPN delivery include the route of administration, the components of the solution, and additives that allow the specific tailoring of the solution to patient needs. The first and most critical step in evaluating a patient for TPN is a complete nutritional assessment.

## NUTRITIONAL ASSESSMENT

A fundamental and essential part of the nutritional assessment is to simply look at the patient. Cachexia, resulting from prolonged semistarvation, and significant dehydration are fairly obvious and reliable physical findings. The loss of fat and lean tissue alone does represent some risk, but this risk is increased dramatically when metabolic stress is superimposed (Table 1). The history is also easily obtained and can provide very valuable information. Particular attention should be paid to dietary intake history; drug usage; alcohol use; gastrointestinal disturbances, such as vomiting and diarrhea; and recent weight loss, most importantly the amount of weight lost and over how long a period. Weight loss of greater than 10% body weight in the last 6 months can be considered significant because it is at this level that effects on patient outcome can be reliably forecast. Greater amounts of weight loss over shorter periods are proportionately more pathologic, with greater than 20% weight loss in less than 3 months reflecting severe protein-calorie malnutrition (PCM). The physical examination, again, is focused on the patient's general appearance. Temporal wasting, thin extremities, and marked reduction in weight are

### TABLE 1. **Nutritional Assessment**

**History**

Recent food intake to establish degree and duration of semistarvation

Medications that affect dietary intake, intestinal loss, or intermediary metabolism

Gastrointestinal disturbances (anorexia, nausea, vomiting, diarrhea)

Recent unintentional weight loss (greater than 10%, 15%, 20%)

**Physical Examination**

General appearance

Height-weight (1959 build and blood pressure standards)

Presence of edema

Muscle and subcutaneous fat wasting

**Ancillary Studies**

Anthropometrics (triceps skin fold, upper arm muscle circumference—greater or less than fifth percentile)

Creatinine-height index (less than 75% standard)

Serum albumin (less than 3.5 grams/dl, less than 2.5 grams/dl)

White blood cell count and differential

Temperature

all signs of adult cachexia or the marasmic form of PCM, which is the most commonly encountered form of malnutrition in patients admitted to the hospital. The second factor in the pathophysiology of hospital PCM is the metabolic response to the stress of injury, inflammation, or infection that is stereotypical in type but varies in degree and duration. Although metabolic stress, by causing anorexia and increasing energy expenditure, leads to semistarvation, the greater impact on the need for nutritional support is the poor tolerance for metabolic stress in the semistarved, and particularly in the semistarved marasmic, individual. Nutritional assessment then requires knowledge of three variables: the amount of lean tissue loss, duration and degree of semistarvation, and presence and degree of metabolic stress.

Along with the history and physical examination, certain measurements and laboratory tests are essential and others helpful for a complete nutritional assessment. Triceps skin fold and mid–upper arm circumference estimate fat and muscle protein stores, the latter of principal value when fluid retention (cardiac, hepatic, renal disease) invalidates weight-height and per cent weight loss. Although serum albumin has traditionally been considered to reflect protein status, it does this poorly. However, it is a superb indicator of the stress response to trauma, infection, or surgery, although somewhat slow to normalize after stress remits, given its half-life of 18 to 20 days. In certain special situations such as liver disease with ascites or the nephrotic syndrome, hypoalbuminemia may not reflect stress, but the presence of fever, leukocytosis, or a left-shifted white blood cell count can be employed for this purpose. Although serum transferrin and prealbumin have shorter half-lives than that of albumin, the use of secretory proteins as short-term indicators of protein nutritional status is limited. Thus, the simple assessment of lean tissue loss by weight-height, per cent weight loss, and upper arm anthropometry; the presence of semistarvation for longer than 7 to 10 days; and the presence of metabolic stress as reflected by serum albumin, fever, leukocytosis, and number of bands enable the clinician to estimate whether nutritional intervention would be beneficial.

## INDICATIONS FOR TPN

Stressed patients should not undergo semistarvation for periods longer than 7 to 10 days, and for much shorter periods if severely malnourished (greater than 15% weight loss, less than 85% weight-height, arm muscle circumference less than the fifth percentile) or if severely stressed (major trauma, severe burns, head injury, severe sepsis). The decision of whether to refeed the severely malnourished patient who is not stressed is a relatively uncommon problem because, in many instances, the disease process may not be amenable to therapy (e.g., cancer, chronic obstructive pulmonary disease) or will be managed by long-term enteral feeding (e.g., strokes) in chronic care institutions or at home. General indications for TPN include some combination of PCM, semistarvation, and stress along with a nonfunctional gastrointestinal tract (Table 2). Patients fitting these criteria would include those with

TABLE 2. **Common Indications for TPN**

**General**

Semistarvation >7–10 days plus moderate stress
Severe stress (major burns, multiple trauma, head injury, severe sepsis)
Semistarvation >3 days, moderate malnutrition, moderate stress
Severe cachexia

**Specific**

*Small Bowel Disease*
Small bowel obstruction
Inflammatory bowel disease
Extensive small bowel resection
Radiation enteritis
Intestinal fistulas

*Preoperative Patients for Thoracoabdominal Surgery*
Hypoalbuminemia
Weight loss >15%

*Cancer Patients*
Malnourished and facing:
  Surgery
  Chemotherapy
  Radiation
  Bone marrow transplantation

*Pancreatitis*
Prolonged period of bowel rest

*Bone Marrow Transplantation*
Prolonged period of stress and semistarvation

*Acute Renal Failure*

*Acute Hepatic Failure*

*Thoracic Duct Fistula*

small bowel disease, including small bowel obstruction, inflammatory bowel disease, extensive small bowel resection, or radiation enteritis; hepatic disease (hepatitis, hepatic failure); pancreatitis; acute renal failure; or long bone fracture, to name a few specific disorders. Parenteral nutrition, as a course lasting at least 7 to 10 days, is also presumed to be beneficial in preoperative patients scheduled to undergo major thoracoabdominal surgery with significant weight loss, particularly if greater than 15%, as well as with any evidence of stress (albumin less than 3 grams per dl). Preoperative TPN appears to decrease operative mortality and postoperative complications and also improves wound healing. Postoperative TPN, although of benefit, is much less effective than preoperative feeding in reducing morbidity. In cancer patients undergoing chemotherapy, the routine provision of nutritional support without regard to nutritional status has not been beneficial. However, if the patient is already malnourished and needs nutritional support through a period of therapy that will render the gastrointestinal tract nonfunctional, such as surgery, radiation, or chemotherapy, nutritional support should be given under the same general rules as for patients without cancer. There is no known benefit of nutritional support in the terminally ill cancer patient, although, on a case-by-case basis, the therapy may occasionally be valuable. Pancreatitis is an indication for parenteral nutrition only if the patient is to be at bowel rest for an extended period. Often in such cases, tube feeding into the jejunum placed endoscopically or at surgery will work as well or better.

It must be remembered that enteral nutrition is always the preferred route of administration and parenteral nutrition is indicated only if the gut cannot be used. With enteral feedings, there is improved gastrointestinal mucosal integrity leading to decreased bacterial translocation across the bowel wall as well as better glucose homeostasis, presumably producing fewer septic complications. If parenteral nutrition does need to be initiated, enteral feedings should be started as soon as the gut is functional. A transitional feeding period should then follow, in which parenteral nutrition is gradually decreased as enteral feedings are advanced until they provide the patient's full needs.

## ADMINISTRATION

### Access

Once a patient is determined to be an appropriate candidate for parenteral nutrition, the route of administration must be chosen. The two options are peripheral parenteral nutrition and total parenteral nutrition (TPN). Nutritional solutions given through a peripheral vein alone generally cannot provide full nutritional needs within volume constraints for many patients, since the tolerated osmolality is usually under 700 mOsm per liter. To minimize the risk of phlebitis, 1000 U of heparin and 5 mg of hydrocortisone per liter can be added to the solution. Peripheral nutrition can best be used as a source of supplemental protein and calories as well as certain micronutrients that may require repletion (magnesium, calcium, zinc, phosphorus, iron) in patients with suboptimal oral intake or tube feedings.

To provide full calories and protein parenterally, central access is required. TPN solutions have high osmolalities (1000 to 1900 mOsm per liter) and cannot be tolerated in peripheral veins. Infraclavicular subclavian vein cathererization is the preferred approach for TPN administration. If the patient has distorted anatomy secondary to surgery, irradiation, or trauma, internal jugular catheterization is used. Subclavian central lines tend to be more comfortable for the patient, and the catheter site has a tendency to remain cleaner. If long-term TPN is planned, a tunneled venous access catheter or venous access disk is preferred. With any central line, as few lumens as possible should be used to minimize the risk of catheter sepsis.

Meticulous catheter care is essential, since catheter sepsis can be a major complication of TPN delivery. Routine catheter care should include dressing changes two to three times per week by an experienced nurse. The indications for changing central venous lines over a guide-wire are controversial, but the protocol used at our institution has been associated with an acceptable infection rate of less than 3% while preserving most catheter sites. This protocol uses the technique of changing a catheter over a guidewire, which poses less risk to the patient than recatheterization and has not been associated with serious infectious morbidity (Table 3). In addition to the criteria listed, any catheter should be removed, cultured, and re-sited if there is a catheter infection due to *Staphylococcus aureus* or any fungal species, suppuration at the insertion site, or life-threatening sepsis of unknown origin. An often unrecognized but potentially hazardous complication of central line insertion is cardiac arrhythmias induced by overinsertion of the guidewire. Atrial or ventricular arrhythmias can occur frequently with guidewire insertion, although serious arrhythmias are rare. This problem can be avoided by kinking the wire at a point 2 to 3 cm longer than the catheter so that the wire will be advanced only as far as needed. With these techniques in central venous catheter care and insertion, the potential for risks and complications can be significantly reduced.

### Formula

To prescribe a TPN formula, the protein and calorie needs of the patient must be determined. The Harris-Benedict equation can be used to calculate basal energy expenditure (BEE):

Men:  $\text{BEE} = 66.47 + 13.75 \,(\text{weight}) + 5.0 \,(\text{height}) - 6.76 \,(\text{age})$

Women:  $\text{BEE} = 65.51 + 9.56 \,(\text{weight}) + 1.85 \,(\text{height}) - 4.68 \,(\text{age})$

Maintenance energy needs are approximately 1.2 times the BEE. Energy needs are increased with the stress of sepsis, trauma, or burns, with an estimated increase of 1.3 to 1.5 times the BEE, but can be as high as 2 times the BEE with severe burns. These estimates are generally seen in the young who are not severely malnourished. In many hospitals, parenteral feeding is principally employed in critical care units, where the recipients are often elderly and have less lean tissue. A simpler estimate of their energy needs can be estimated at 25 to 30 kcal per kg per day. Given that the goal of feeding in most stressed patients is meeting rather than exceeding energy needs, providing 30 kcal per kg for the elderly stressed patient and 40 kcal per kg for the young is usually sufficient for the short term of 3 weeks that most TPN is provided. The patient's actual weight is used to calculate caloric needs unless the patient is morbidly obese, when the ideal body weight is appropriate. Although this will not meet actual energy expenditure, TPN glucose calories are less well tolerated in the obese. Another method to calculate caloric needs is the portable indirect calorimeter to measure oxygen consumption and $CO_2$ production, which can then be used to calculate energy requirement. This method is especially useful in the ventilated patient who is difficult to wean from ventilation. Overfeeding, and thus increased $CO_2$ production, can then be avoided. The severely marasmic patient can also sometimes benefit from actual measurement, because estimates of energy expenditure are least accurate in this group.

Protein needs are somewhat easier to calculate, since almost all stressed patients need 1.5 to 2.0 grams of protein per kg of ideal body weight per day. In the nonstressed, protein-depleted patient, this will aid in repleting lean tissue, while in the stressed, critically ill patient, it will maintain the increased protein synthetic rates characteristic of the injury response. A 24-hour urinary urea nitrogen (UUN) measurement, which is possible in all hospital clinical laboratories, can be used to estimate nitrogen balance:

Nitrogen balance = protein intake (grams) /6.25 − (24-hour UUN [grams] + 4)

TABLE 3. **Guidelines for Defining Catheter Sepsis**

| CTC | CBC | PBC | Interpretation | Response |
|-----|-----|-----|----------------|----------|
| − | − | − | No catheter infection-sepsis | Continue TPN, change wire in 1 wk if fever persists |
| − | − | + | Sepsis (not catheter related) | |
| − | + | + | Sepsis (? catheter seeding) | Repeat catheter change over wire with culture and remove catheter, reinsert at different site if repeat CTC or CBC is positive |
| + | − | − | Catheter infection | |
| − | + | − | Catheter infection | |
| + | + | − | Catheter infection | |
| + | − | + | Catheter-related sepsis | Remove catheter with cultures and reinsert at different site |
| + | + | + | Catheter-related sepsis | |

CTC = Catheter tip culture; CBC = catheter blood culture; PBC = peripheral blood culture.

Each gram of nitrogen is equivalent to 30 grams of lean tissue. For most stressed patients, nitrogen balance (i.e., no gain or loss) is achieved with 1.5 to 2.0 grams of protein per kg per day, although the severely catabolic patient may be in negative nitrogen balance in the acute phase. Increasing protein intake beyond 2.0 grams per kg is not of benefit in these patients, although matching energy intake to measured energy expenditure may be of value. With protein and calorie needs determined, a formula can be made using the three fuel sources of TPN: carbohydrates, lipids, and amino acids.

## Carbohydrates

Carbohydrates are the major fuel source in TPN. Although the caloric density of glucose is 4 kcal per kg, in the hydrated form used in TPN it is 3.4 kcal per kg. Glucose has unique advantages, owing to its protein-sparing effects and also as an essential fuel source for red blood cells, the brain, and the renal medulla. In ischemic or injured tissue, anaerobic glycolysis allows the generation of adenosine triphosphate from glucose metabolism in the absence of oxygen. The major complication of glucose administration is alteration in glucose homeostasis as a result of the insulin resistance of illness and systemic rather than portal venous glucose administration. This often leads to hyperglycemia and is a factor in accelerated lipogenesis in the liver. Overfeeding with glucose can lead to a high respiratory quotient ($Vco_2/Vo_2$) and difficulty in weaning the patient, with $CO_2$ retention from mechanical ventilation. Glucose overfeeding also exacerbates hepatic lipogenesis, which when severe can produce hyperbilirubinemia, although hepatic enzyme elevations are much more common.

The endogenous production of glucose ranges between 1 and 2 mg per kg per minute, or 100 to 200 grams of dextrose in a 70-kg man per day. By providing this amount of glucose intravenously to the unstressed individual, endogenous production is near totally suppressed. Metabolic stress limits the suppressive effects of exogenous glucose on endogenous glucose production, and thus total glucose flux is additive. Therefore, when initiating TPN, it is best to give no more than 2 mg per kg per minute, or 200 grams per day, in the event there may be underlying glucose intolerance, especially in the presence of metabolic stress. If this formula is tolerated, glucose can be gradually advanced to 4 mg per kg per minute, where optimal glucose oxidation and protein sparing occur. A rate of glucose infusion more rapid than 4 mg per kg per minute can increase total glucose oxidation but also leads to a significant rise in the respiratory quotient and lipid deposition in the liver. Obviously, known diabetic patients should receive relatively lower amounts of glucose, initially at about 1 to 1.5 mg per kg per minute and at full feeding, about 2 mg per kg per minute. To provide sufficient calories to meet energy requirements without increasing glucose infusion rate, the second fuel source, lipid, can be used.

## Lipids

Presently available lipid emulsions are composed of polyunsaturated long chain triglycerides from soybean oil or a mixture of safflower and soybean oils. Their caloric density is 9 kcal per gram, and they provide essential fatty acids. Lipids also have the beneficial effect of protein sparing, equivalent to dextrose at levels above the basal energy expenditure, but do not have the adverse effect of increasing the respiratory quotient. If lipids are not needed as a source of calories but are to be given only as a source of essential fatty acids, daily lipid infusion is unnecessary. The daily requirement for essential fatty acids is provided by 5 to 10 grams of a standard lipid emulsion. This is most easily given as an infusion of 500 ml of a 10% fat emulsion per week. If lipids are needed daily as a caloric source, there are two methods of infusion—either as a separate infusion or as part of a mixed fuel system with dextrose and amino acids.

The route of administration is an important consideration in lipid delivery because if done improperly, it can adversely affect the function of the reticuloendothelial system. When long chain triglycerides comprise greater than 50% of total caloric intake, there is a risk of decreased reticuloendothelial system function, particularly when lipids are provided over the standard 10- to 12-hour intermittent infusion period. With a mixed fuel system, the rate of lipid infusion is much more controlled because lipids are given over 24 hours with dextrose and amino acids. Another advantage of this mixed fuel system is the better metabolic utilization of the fat, as well as a reduced likelihood of dramatically altering eicosanoid metabolism, which can adversely affect pulmonary function in the critically ill. The past concern over bacterial growth in lipid emulsions has not been realized. A mixed fuel solution given over 24 hours does not preferentially support bacterial growth over that found with standard amino acid and dextrose solution. A mixed fuel system is, therefore, the preferred method of lipid delivery, with amounts restricted to less than 30 to 40% of the total daily calories. The only disadvantages to 3-in-1 solutions are the incompatibility with in-line filtering and certain admixtures such as albumin and hydrochloric acid and less tolerance to high concentrations of multivalent cations and anions (calcium, magnesium, zinc, iron, phosphate).

### Amino Acids

Protein in TPN is in the form of amino acids, and stock solutions provide both essential and nonessential amino acids. One gram of amino acids has a caloric density of 4 kcal. Standard amino acid solutions are sufficient for most patients, but there are certain patients who benefit from a solution with a high percentage of branched chain amino acids (BCAAs.) Leucine, isoleucine, and valine are the three BCAAs and are unique because they are oxidized in skeletal muscle and adipose tissue, increase hepatic protein synthesis, and reduce post-injury catabolism. The two clinical conditions in which BCAAs seem to afford clinical advantage are hepatic encephalopathy and uremia. If encephalopathy is mild or blood urea nitrogen (BUN) is less than 100 mg per dl without signs or symptoms of uremia, protein restricted to 70 grams of a conventional amino acid solution is sufficient. However, in patients with severe encephalopathy, BCAA-enriched solutions can decrease symptoms and improve nitrogen balance at any given level of intake between 40 and 70 grams daily. Similarly, with significant uremia, BCAA-enriched mixtures over this range of intake can help to slow the rise of BUN by improving nitrogen balance. BCAA-enriched solutions have not yet been shown to be of clinical benefit in other conditions (sepsis, trauma, cancer) and are far more expensive than standard amino acid solutions.

### Electrolytes and Minerals

Because for many patients TPN is the only source of intake, close attention must be paid to electrolyte and mineral requirements. These requirements obviously vary among patients, but generally, most patients' needs can be met by the intakes summarized in Table 4. There are a number of clinical situations in which these requirements need to be modified. Sodium should be restricted in volume-overloaded states and in sodium-retaining states such as renal failure and cirrhosis to no more than 40 mEq above initially measured nonurinary losses. Potassium should likewise be restricted in renal failure as well as in the more common acquired renal tubular dysfunction. Magnesium excretion is significantly decreased by renal failure, particularly if oliguric

TABLE 4. **Electrolytes and Minerals in TPN***

| Ion or Element | Requirement |
|---|---|
| Sodium | 60–150 mEq |
| Potassium | 30–160 mEq |
| Magnesium | 8–12 mEq |
| Calcium | 10–12 mEq |
| Phosphorus | 26–40 mmol |
| Zinc | 3 mg |
| Copper | 1.2 mg |
| Chromium | 12 μg |
| Manganese | 0.3 mg |
| Selenium | 60 μg |
| Iodine | 50–12 μg |
| Iron | 1–5 mg |

*24-hr recommendations.

or anuric, and excretion is often increased in renal tubular dysfunction (cisplatin, amphotericin). Phosphorus excretion is decreased with renal failure but is increased substantially by therapeutic corticosteroids. Hypophosphatemia should be especially avoided in patients with cardiorespiratory illnesses, because it can decrease cardiac and diaphragmatic contractility. Serum levels of total calcium are often misleading secondary to hypoalbuminemia or hyperlipidemia. In questionable cases, an ionized calcium determination is more reliable. Maintenance iron needs are usually met by 2 mg per day, but more iron can be added for iron deficiency anemia, although 15 mg per day should be an upper limit provided by this route. Zinc losses can be significant with elevated intestinal fluid output through ostomies or diarrhea, and these patients will need up to 10 mg per day. Selenium deficiency is rare, and its occurrence is essentially eliminated by provision of the amounts found in the commercial trace element solution. Chromium, manganese, and iodine needs are not usually altered by clinical states, and sufficient amounts are also provided in the trace element solution. Copper may need to be restricted in patients with biliary obstruction.

### Vitamins

The AMA-FDA intravenous vitamin requirements for adults are listed in Table 5 and are commercially available in these amounts. Vitamin K is given separately as 10 mg subcutaneously or in the TPN solution each week. Some vitamins are fairly labile and should not be stored in TPN solution over 36 hours. This property becomes important in home TPN patients who receive a large supply of solution at once. In this situation, the patient should add the multivitamin source to the TPN solution on the day of use.

TABLE 5. **Intravenous Vitamin Requirements in TPN***

| Ascorbic acid | 100.0 mg |
|---|---|
| Retinol | 1.0 mg (3300 U) |
| Ergocalciferol | 5.0 μg (200 U) |
| Thiamine | 3.0 mg |
| Riboflavin | 3.6 mg |
| Pyridoxine | 4.0 mg |
| Niacinamide | 40.0 mg |
| Dexpanthenol | 15.0 mg |
| Tocopherol | 10.0 mg (10 U) |
| Biotin | 60.0 μg |
| Folic acid | 400.0 μg |
| Cyanocobalamin | 5.0 μg |
| Phytonadione | 5.0 mg weekly |

*24-hr requirements per FDA/AMA 1979.

## TPN and Diabetes Mellitus

Control of blood glucose in the diabetic patient receiving TPN can be difficult. Severe stress or infection can make insulin resistance a serious problem in the known diabetic patient and can also expose glucose intolerance in the previously undiagnosed diabetic, as glucose provided through a central vein stimulates more insulin than a similar amount of glucose fed enterally. Maintenance of reasonable blood glucose control is essential in TPN delivery in order to limit the risk of infection. It has been found that in vitro, a glucose concentration greater than 200 mg per dl has adverse effects on leukocyte phagocytic function, and in vivo, poor glucose control dramatically increases the incidence of systemic infection. Because many patients on TPN already have depressed immune function, further depression could adversely affect patient outcome, nullifying the immunoenhancement of nutritional repletion and thus the benefits of feeding.

As discussed earlier, all patients being started on TPN should initially receive no more than 2 mg dextrose per kg per day or 200 grams per day for the 70-kg individual. In the insulin-dependent diabetic patient, insulin is added to the TPN solution on the first day in the same proportion to usual insulin intake as amount of calories in the TPN is to the usual calorie intake. Because up to one-half of the insulin binds to the TPN container and tubing, insulin provided in this manner is almost invariably an underestimate, which limits the risk of hypoglycemia. For example, if the patient normally takes a daily total of 40 U of insulin for 2000 kcal, for a TPN solution of 1000 kcal, one-half of 40 U, or 20 U, is added. Capillary blood glucose concentrations are checked every 6 to 8 hours, and a sliding scale for subcutaneous insulin is used. On the second day, two-thirds to all of the total amount of insulin given through the sliding scale, depending on the level of control, is added to the TPN.

This process continues until serial capillary glucose levels are under 200 mg per dl. In the non–insulin-dependent diabetic patient or the patient who develops glucose intolerance, a similar strategy can be used. On the first day of TPN, no insulin is added but a sliding scale is written. If any insulin from the sliding scale is given, two-thirds to all of the total amount is added to the TPN solution. Insulin on subsequent days is then adjusted as described earlier for the insulin-dependent diabetic. Once adequate blood glucose control is obtained, which for the diabetic receiving TPN is blood glucose values below 200 mg per dl, dextrose can be increased, using the same glucose/insulin ratio. It is important to remember the detrimental effects of severe hyperglycemia on immune function, and good glucose control should not be sacrificed simply to supply adequate calories.

## TPN and Critical Care

Patients requiring TPN are often critically ill and have a number of metabolic disturbances. TPN solution, in addition to providing protein and calories, can be specifically tailored to treat many of these disorders. Acid-base disturbances are common in the intensive care unit (ICU) patient. Metabolic alkalosis is a frequent complication, related to corticosteroid or diuretic use or to nasogastric suction. Mild alkalosis of the chloride-responsive type can be treated with chloride replacement using sodium or potassium chloride. More significant alkalosis may require the addition of hydrochloric acid to the TPN solution in amounts of 50 to 150 mEq per day. Generally, enough HCl is added to neutralize one-half of the calculated base excess per day. For metabolic acidosis, usually associated with acquired renal tubular dysfunction, acetate is added, which can be metabolized by the Krebs cycle to carbon dioxide and water. Sodium bicarbonate must never be used in TPN solution, owing to incompatibility. In stable conditions, replacement should be gradual, administering one-half of the calculated base deficit in the first 24 hours. The acid-base status of the patient can be followed by arterial blood gases, but venous gases are adequate in most cases except in circulatory collapse. Venous pH is 0.03 to 0.04 lower than arterial pH. Excess volume is frequently a problem in the ICU patient, and often the patient can tolerate only 1 liter of TPN solution. In this setting, maximally concentrated solutions with 70 grams of protein are preferred, which can be given as a 7% amino acids and 21% dextrose solution ($A_7D_{21}$). The mixture will usually fall below caloric needs but protein intake will be adequate, which is considered to be of more importance in the severely stressed patient. Hypocalcemia is often seen in the critical care setting, and the serum calcium concentration is most effectively raised and maintained by a constant infusion of calcium, not by boluses. Hypoalbuminemia is another common problem in the critically ill, and albumin can be added to the TPN solution when levels are very low (less than 2 grams per dl). There is no good evidence to support albumin supplementation at higher serum albumin levels. The ICU patient, as well as the less severely ill patient, can often benefit from a number of other additives that can be placed in TPN solution.

### Other Additives

Central vein thrombosis can be a frequent complication of intravenous catheters. By adding heparin to the TPN solution in sufficient amounts, this problem can usually be avoided. The continuous infusion of heparin at 6000 U per day in the TPN solution significantly reduces the incidence of thrombosis without increasing the risk of bleeding in most patients. Greater amounts (up to 10,000 U per day) may be given when the patient is at greater risk of thrombosis as evidenced by a partial thromboplastin time more than 3 seconds shorter than control. Lesser amounts (less than 3000 U per day) can be used if there is somewhat greater concern about bleeding (i.e, platelet count 50,000 to 100,000). Heparin should generally not be provided if the patient has a heparin sensitivity, is anticoagulated either therapeutically or due to disease, or has a platelet count less than 50,000.

Because of volume constraints, it is often advantageous to add compatible medications to the TPN solution. This practice also decreases the number of intravenous catheters required for drug delivery as well as minimizing the expense of drug administration. Commonly used medications compatible with TPN solutions are cimetidine, corticosteroids, and metoclopramide. Aminophylline is also compatible but should be added only when a stable dose has been established. Care must be taken to ensure the compatibility of a drug with specific TPN solutions, especially when a mixed fuel system is used.

### Cycled TPN

In the long-term TPN patient, cyclic feeding at night is often used for greater patient mobility during the day, which for the home TPN patient fosters the development of a more normal lifestyle. Patients on cycled TPN must be able to tolerate infusion rates of 200 to 300 ml per hour for 10 to 12 hours. During the last 1 to 2 hours of administration, the rate is decreased by one-half to avoid problems with hyperinsulinemia and rebound hypoglycemia induced by the concentrated dextrose solution. Besides the convenience, cycled TPN also decreases the duration of hyperinsulinemia and of the accentuated hepatic lipogenesis and improves hepatic function. Cycled TPN is not recommended for insulin-dependent diabetics, owing to difficulties in management of glucose homeostasis. However, home TPN should not be denied on this basis, since a combination of infusion insulin plus subcutaneous insulin during the off-cycle can provide reasonable control in the stable patient. To avoid complications of venous thrombosis in home TPN, low-dose warfarin therapy (1 to 2 mg orally so as not to prolong prothrombin time) should be considered. The patient receiving home TPN needs to be properly trained, and home monitoring requires a visiting nurse.

### Team Approach

TPN is an important therapeutic modality for the stressed and semistarved patient, but improper administration can be harmful and provision to poorly selected patients is wasteful of an expensive resource. Many patients requiring TPN have organ disease causing dysfunction of multiple organs, a heightened risk of infection and potential adverse drug effects and interactions, and underlying protein-calorie malnutrition (PCM), which require the participation of more than one type of health care worker. A nutrition support team consisting of a physician, nurse, pharmacist, and dietitian seems to address best the total care of the patient.

# PARENTERAL FLUID THERAPY IN INFANTS AND CHILDREN

method of
WILLIAM A. PRIMACK, M.D.
*Fallon Clinic*
*University of Massachusetts Medical School*
*Worcester, Massachusetts*

Fluid and electrolyte therapy consists of three components: (1) *maintenance therapy* replaces the daily *normal expenditure* of fluids and electrolytes; (2) *deficit therapy* replaces *pre-existing abnormal losses* of fluid, electrolytes, or both; and (3) *replacement therapy* replaces *ongoing abnormal losses* such as those caused by nasogastric drainage or persistent diarrhea. Fluid therapy may be given orally, but it is given parenterally if the infant or child is unable to meet his or her needs by the oral route.

Dehydration from gastroenteritis is the most common clinical situation where fluid therapy is required in infants and children. Since the 1930s, parenteral (i.e., intravenous) fluid therapy has been the standard route of rehydration. Recently, following the lead of health care workers in the Third World, the need in the Western World for parenteral fluid therapy in the treatment of gastroenteritis has been lessened by the use of oral rehydration solutions (ORSs) and glucose and electrolyte oral maintenance solutions.

## MAINTENANCE FLUID AND ELECTROLYTE THERAPY

Maintenance therapy replaces normal metabolic losses from respiration, urine, sweat, and stool. This therapy should allow fluid and electrolyte homeostasis with minimal renal compensation and provide sufficient calories to prevent protein catabolism and ketosis. Parenteral maintenance therapy should meet all the daily needs of an adequately hydrated child with normal renal function who is temporarily unable to ingest oral fluids and who has no excessive ongoing water or electrolyte losses. An example is the preoperative or postoperative patient who is allowed no oral hydration.

In the infant, about two-thirds of *insensible water losses* are from the skin and one-third are from the lungs. These losses are evaporative and account for about 50% of daily maintenance water requirements in the infant and about 30 to 35% of daily needs in the older child. *Urinary losses* account for the remainder of maintenance fluid needs, except in infants, in whom stool water averages 10 to 20 ml per kg per day. Because daily physiologic insensible water losses are proportional to caloric expenditure, correlating the maintenance water requirement with the caloric expenditure gives a convenient estimate of fluid needs that is reliable for most infants and children. The hospitalized child requires approximately 120 ml of water for every 100 kcal metabolized. Because water of oxidation and pre-formed water provide about 17 ml and 3 ml per 100 kcal metabolized, respectively, approximately 100 ml of water is required for each 100 kcal metabolized. A formula to estimate caloric expenditure based on body weight is given in Table 1. Thus,

a hospitalized 16-kg child should receive about 1300 kcal or about 1300 ml of water per day (1000 ml for the first 10 kg plus $50 \times 6 = 300$ ml for the remaining 6 kg). Similarly, a 38-kg child requires about 1860 kcal or 1860 ml of water daily (1000 ml for the first 10 kg, plus $50 \times 10 = 500$ ml for the next 10 kg, plus $20 \times 18 = 360$ ml for the remainder).

Insensible losses are increased by about 12% for each degree of body temperature above 38° C. An increased respiratory rate or a high ambient temperature also increases insensible fluid losses, which are decreased if the child is in a mist tent or is breathing humidified air via an endotracheal tube.

Water loss from the kidneys depends on the solute load that must be excreted. The clinician may assume that the average child who requires fluid therapy is not receiving an excessive dietary solute load, so that the estimated renal solute load can be assumed to be 10 to 40 mOsm per 100 kcal. Unless the child has significant renal abnormalities, a urinary concentration range of 150 to 600 mOsm (specific gravity 1.005 to 1.020) can be achieved. Thus, an average renal solute load of 30 mOsm per kcal can be excreted in as little as 50 ml of urine (urine osmolarity = 600 mOsm) or as much as 200 ml (urine osmolarity = 150 mOsm). Most infants and children can easily excrete their renal solute load in approximately 70 ml of water per 100 kcal.

Average daily urinary electrolyte losses are approximately 2 to 3 mEq of sodium and 1 to 2 mEq of potassium per kg of body weight. Chloride is the principal inorganic anion in urine. Water lost from the lungs is electrolyte free. Daily electrolyte losses in sweat are about 0.5 mEq per kg each of sodium and potassium. Electrolyte losses in stool are minimal in the absence of diarrhea. Thus, replacement should approximate 2 to 3 mEq of sodium and 2 mEq of potassium per 100 kcal metabolized (or per 100 ml of fluid required). A solution containing 20 to 30 mEq per liter of sodium chloride (NaCl) and 20 mEq per liter of potassium chloride (KCl) given at a rate calculated from Table 1 will meet the maintenance fluid requirements of the average hospitalized infant or child. Glucose is added to the intravenous solution to provide sufficient calories (about 20% of basal caloric needs) to prevent protein catabolism and the osmotic diuresis of starvation ketosis.

The euvolemic child with normal renal function should excrete 1 to 3 ml per kg of urine per hour. Urine output of less than 0.8 ml per kg per hour suggests oliguria. The anuric patient should receive replacement only for insensible losses, or approximately one-third of the fluid recommended in Table 1, with 0.5 to 1.0 mEq of sodium

TABLE 1. **Estimate of Maintenance Fluid Requirements**

| Body Weight (kg) | Maintenance Fluids (ml/day) |
|---|---|
| 4–10 | 100 ml/kg |
| 11–20 | 1000 ml + 50 ml/kg over 10 kg |
| 21–80 | 1500 ml + 20 ml/kg over 20 kg |

TABLE 2. **Estimate of the Degree of Isotonic Dehydration by Physical Signs**

| Physical Sign | Symptoms of Dehydration for Degree Shown* | | | |
| | < 5% | 5–10% | 10–15% | >15% |
|---|---|---|---|---|
| Turgor | Normal | Decreased | Tenting | Poor |
| Mucous membranes | Moist | Dry | Very dry | Parched |
| Eyeballs | Normal | Soft | Sunken | Very sunken |
| Fontanelle | Flat | Soft | Sunken | Very sunken |
| CNS | Consolable | Irritable | Lethargic | Comatose |
| Pulse | Normal | Orthostatic | Increased | Thready |
| BP | Normal | Normal | Orthostatic | Shock |

*Hypotonic dehydration: physical signs accentuated; hypertonic dehydration: physical signs diminished, with "woody" turgor.
*Abbreviations:* CNS = central nervous system; BP = blood pressure.

per kg daily and no potassium. An anuric child should lose about 0.5% of body weight daily, or overhydration may occur.

## DEFICIT THERAPY

Dehydration is caused by an acute loss of body fluids and electrolytes, with a resulting deficit of total body water and variable deficits of electrolytes. In infants and children, the most common causes of dehydration are gastrointestinal losses from diarrhea or vomiting. Less common causes include the osmotic diuresis of diabetic ketoacidosis or dehydration from vigorous activity in a warm environment.

The most accurate estimation of dehydration is the direct measurement of body weight loss. Often an accurate pre-illness weight is not available, and the clinician is forced to use subjective physical signs to estimate the degree of dehydration (Table 2). Estimates of the degree of dehydration assume that the observed changes are not caused by malnutrition or chronic illness. In infants and small children, estimates are usually no more accurate than 5% of body weight. *Mild or 5% dehydration* occurs with a history compatible with fluid and electrolyte loss, but with relatively few physical signs, except possibly thirst and dry mucous membranes. *Moderate or 10% dehydration* occurs when there are clear physical signs of fluid loss, such as loss of subcutaneous tissue turgor ("tenting") or a sunken fontanelle, but no signs of circulatory or central nervous system compromise. *Severe or 15% de-*

*hydration* indicates more dramatic physical signs with impending circulatory compromise, and the patient may be near shock. In older children and young adults, similar clinical findings are used to estimate dehydration. In these children, states of mild, moderate, and severe dehydration are estimated as 3, 6, and 9% of body weight loss, respectively.

Classification of dehydration depends on the quantity of electrolytes lost relative to water losses. Most fluids lost have sodium concentrations ranging from 30 to 70 mEq per liter, with the notable exception of the situation in cholera, in which the sodium concentration of stool is nearly isotonic with plasma (Table 3). *Isotonic dehydration* (sodium level 130 to 150 mEq per liter) indicates that the loss of free water and electrolytes is proportional to normal physiologic concentrations.

*Hypertonic dehydration* (sodium level greater than 150 mEq per liter) occurs when too little free water is given. The classic example is replacement of the relatively low sodium losses of rotavirus diarrhea with a relatively high-sodium solution such as boiled skim milk (see Table 4). The high sodium concentration protects the extracellular space at the expense of the intracellular space. Consequently, the child often has few classic physical signs of dehydration, and the clinician tends to underestimate the degree of volume deficit (see Table 2). Hypertonicity causes the formation of intracellular osmotically active substances (idiogenic osmole) that protect intracellular volume from the high extracellular os-

TABLE 3. **Electrolyte Content of Common Body Fluids**

| Electrolyte | Electrolyte Content (mEq/Liter) of Diarrheal Fluid | | | Electrolyte Content (mEq/Liter) of Body Fluid | | |
| | Cholera | Rotavirus Infection | ETEC Infection | Gastric Fluid | Sweat | Ileal Fluid |
|---|---|---|---|---|---|---|
| Sodium | 88 | 37 | 53 | 60 | 45 | 129 |
| Potassium | 30 | 38 | 37 | 10 | 5 | 11 |
| Chloride | 86 | 22 | 24 | 84 | 58 | 116 |
| Bicarbonate | 32 | 6 | 18 | 0 | 0 | 29 |

*Abbreviation:* ETEC = enterotoxic *Escherichia coli.*

TABLE 4. **Electrolyte Content of ORS, Maintenance, and Commonly Used Oral Fluids**

| Solution | Sodium (mEq/Liter) | Potassium (mEq/Liter) | Chloride (mEq/Liter) | Base (mEq/Liter) | CHO (Grams/ Liter) | Type of CHO | Storage Form* |
|---|---|---|---|---|---|---|---|
| *Rehydration Solutions* | | | | | | | |
| WHO ORS | 90 | 20 | 80 | 30 | 20 | Glucose | Powder |
| Rehydralyte | 75 | 20 | 65 | 30 | 25 | Glucose | Liquid |
| *Maintenance Electrolyte Solutions* | | | | | | | |
| Infalyte | 50 | 20 | 40 | 30 | 20 | Glucose | Powder |
| Lytren | 50 | 25 | 45 | 30 | 20 | Glucose | Powder |
| Pedialyte | 45 | 20 | 35 | 30 | 25 | Glucose | Liquid |
| Resol | 50 | 20 | 50 | 34 | 20 | Glucose | Liquid |
| *Clear Fluids* | | | | | | | |
| Gatorade | 21 | 17 | 17 | 6 | 61 | Glucose | Liquid |
| Kool-Aid | 0–5† | 0.1 | 0 | † | 88 | Sucrose | Powder |
| Soda | 0–8† | 1–12† | ?? | 0 | 80–120† | ‡ | Liquid |
| Apple juice | 0.4 | 26 | ?? | 0 | 119 | Fructose | Liquid |
| Chicken soup | 105 | 2 | 100 | 0 | 32 | ?? | Liquid |
| Cherry Jell-O | 25 | 0.25 | 10 | † | 166 | Sucrose | Powder |
| *Milk and Infant Formula* | | | | | | | |
| Skim milk | 23 | 47 | 29 | 0 | 50 | Lactose | Liquid |
| Formula | 8–12† | 18–28† | 12–18† | 0 | 67 | Lactose | Liquid |

*All values represent powders diluted according to directions.
†Range for commonly used brands.
‡High-fructose syrup, sucrose, or both.
*Abbreviations:* WHO = World Health Organization; CHO = carbohydrate.

molarity. If hypertonicity is corrected too rapidly, the cells swell as water is osmotically drawn in before the idiogenic osmole can leave. In the brain, the swelling can cause cerebral edema, seizures, intracerebral bleeding, or all three.

*Hypotonic dehydration* (sodium level less than 130 mEq per liter) occurs when solute is lost in excess of water, causing the serum sodium level to fall. It may be seen in children with dehydration in whom free water is replaced in excess of solute, especially when sodium-containing losses persist. An example is an infant with several days of moderately severe diarrhea who is receiving replacement solely with low-sodium–containing solutions such as soda or diluted infant formula (Table 4). Because sodium is the principal extracellular cation, hypotonic dehydration indicates a disproportionate loss of electrolytes and fluid from the extracellular space, with consequent exaggerated physical signs of dehydration (see Table 2).

*Hyponatremia* can occur in many clinical settings other than hypotonic dehydration. As Table 5 shows, the child with hypotonic dehydration should have evidence of weight loss and clinical findings of dehydration. The urinary sodium level should be low (<10 mEq per liter) and the urine osmolarity high. Similar urinary findings are observed with congestive heart failure and nephrosis, but the patient shows weight gain and edema. Hyponatremia can also occur when free water is received in excess of solute, such as with

water intoxication. The urine sodium level is low and the urine is hyposmotic to plasma. An inability to concentrate the urine, as may be seen with renal insufficiency or obstructive uropathy, produces a high urine sodium level (greater than 50 mEq per liter) and an isotonic or mildly hypotonic urine. Similar findings associated with hyperkalemia suggest adrenal insufficiency. Inappropriate release of antidiuretic hormone (SIADH) produces hyponatremia from excessive renal reabsorption of free water, resulting in urine with a high sodium level and an osmolarity inappropriately high for the hypotonic serum. High serum concentrations of osmotically active materials can cause an artificially low serum sodium level (pseudohyponatremia). Examples include marked hyperglycemia, severe hyperlip-

TABLE 5. **Hyponatremia**

| Clinical Condition | Weight | Urine Sodium (mEq/Liter) | Urine Osmolarity (mOsm/ kg H2O) |
|---|---|---|---|
| Hypotonic dehydration | Decreased | <10 | >500 |
| CHF or nephrosis | Increased | <10 | >500 |
| Water intoxication | Increased | <10 | <200 |
| Chronic renal insufficiency | No change | >50 | <300 |
| Adrenal insufficiency | Decreased | >50 | <300 |
| SIADH | Increased | >50 | >500 |

*Abbreviations:* CHF = congestive heart failure; SIADH = syndrome of inappropriate release of antidiuretic hormone.

idemia, and high serum concentrations of mannitol or radiocontrast materials.

## ONGOING LOSSES

Replacement of ongoing losses is essential to successful fluid therapy. Common examples are persistent diarrhea and nasogastric drainage. The volume of these losses can be accurately measured and the electrolyte content measured or estimated (see Table 3), so that accurate replacement can be planned. Diarrheal losses in infants are accurately estimated by weighing dirty diapers and subtracting the weight of the empty diaper.

## TREATMENT PRINCIPLES

Most mild and moderate dehydration can be safely and effectively treated by the use of ORS, to be discussed later. If the oral route is unavailable, the intravenous route is the only parenteral route usually required. In extreme situations, isotonic fluids can be administered to infants or young children by intraosseous infusion. An 18-gauge Jamshidi bone marrow needle or a Cook intraosseous needle is placed thorugh the medial surface of the anterior tibia 2 to 3 cm below the tibial tubercle.

**Fluid Resuscitation.** If dehydration is moderate or severe, immediate expansion of the extracellular space is begun to preserve cardiovascular function and renal perfusion. An infusion of 0.9% NaCl (normal saline) with 5% dextrose or Ringer's lactate solution with 5% dextrose at a rate of 10 to 20 ml per kg per hour for 1 to 2 hours usually provides adequate fluid resuscitation while awaiting the results of initial laboratory tests and planning further therapy. Plasma or albumin infusions are rarely required.

**Rate of Fluid Infusion and Treatment Duration.** Fluid repair usually takes about 24 hours. One-half of the deficit is replaced in the first 8 hours and the remainder over the next 14 to 16 hours. In hypertonic dehydration, treatment is usually planned over 48 hours. Maintenance fluid requirements are added to the deficit fluids. Replacement of all losses, including restoration of full nutrition, usually takes several days.

**Body Fluid Spaces.** Knowledge of the body fluid spaces and their principal constituents aids in the prescription of fluid and electrolyte therapy. The *total body water* of an infant is about 70% of body weight, decreasing to the adult value of 60% by 1 year of age. Of the total body water, approximately two-thirds is in the *intracellular fluid* (ICF), where potassium is the major cation and proteins and energy-containing phosphate compounds are the major anions. The remaining one-third of body water is in the *extracellular fluid* (ECF), which includes the interstitial space and the intravascular space. The major cation of the ECF is sodium at a concentration of about 140 mEq per liter, and the major anion is chloride at a concentration of 100 mEq per liter. The potassium concentration in the ECF is only 5 mEq per liter.

In the typical clinical situation, acute weight loss from dehydration is nearly all from the total body water space. Approximately one-half of the loss is from the ECF and one-half from the ICF. Consequently, if electrolyte loss is isosmotic to fluid loss (isotonic dehydration), each liter (kilogram) of acute body weight loss suggests an approximate deficit of sodium of $140 \times 0.50 = 70$ mEq and of potassium of $150 \times 0.50 = 75$ mEq. The more rapid the onset of dehydration, the greater the relative deficit of the ECF.

**Potassium.** Potassium losses vary, depending on the source of the electrolyte deficit, with relatively high losses caused by gastric or intestinal drainage (see Table 3). Extracellular (serum) potassium values are only an approximate reflection of intracellular potassium values and may be misleading. For example, metabolic acidosis raises the serum potassium level as hydrogen ions displace potassium ions within the cell. Some of the displaced potassium is rapidly excreted, so that the child with acidosis may have a normal, or even elevated, serum potassium level but a large potassium deficit. There are no clinical signs of potassium loss, unless it is extreme, with muscle weakness or electrocardiographic changes (usually the potassium level less than 2 mEq per liter).

Potassium replacement should be gradual, as the total intracellular store of potassium is much greater than the extracellular store, and potassium should never be added to an intravenous solution until urine output is assured to avoid the arrhythmias associated with severe hyperkalemia. In most clinical situations potassium replacement of 20 to 30 mEq per liter of intravenous fluid is adequate because total replacement of potassium losses may take several days. A potassium concentration more than 40 mEq per liter should never be exceeded in parenteral fluids without administration into a central line, where a great deal of mixing can occur. High potassium concentrations should be given only in a patient care setting where adequate monitoring is available. Potassium is usually added as KCl or occasionally as potassium phosphate.

**Hyponatremia.** Treatment of hyponatremia depends on the etiology. If it is caused by water intoxication, it resolves spontaneously when the excess water is withheld. Mineralocorticoids are required in adrenal insufficiency. Water restriction is essential to treat SIADH successfully.

In hypotonic dehydration, solute (NaCl) must be replaced (see Case 2, later). The quantity of NaCl necessary to replace a solute deficit is calculated as

$$(\text{Na desired} - \text{Na measured}) \times \%\text{TBW} \times \text{body weight}$$

where %TBW is percentage of total body water. Because about one-half of the solute losses are intracellular potassium, only about one-half of the amount of the calculated sodium deficit is placed in the fluid prescription.

If hyponatremia is severe (sodium level less than 120 mEq per liter) and the patient has symptoms such as seizures, hypertonic (3 or 5%) saline can be infused at a maximal rate of 5 mEq per kg per hour (10 ml per kg per hour) until symptoms remit. Rapid repair of severe hyponatremia is controversial and should be done only if absolutely required.

**Hypernatremia.** Correction of hypernatremia must proceed slowly to minimize the risk of cerebral edema, seizures, or both. Most authorities recommend replacement of the total deficit over 48 hours or more and believe that *the serum sodium level should decrease by no more than 10 to 12 mEq per liter per day.* Hypertonicity represents a greater deficit of free water compared with solute. The water deficit equals the normal water volume minus the measured water volume, as shown:

$$\text{Deficit} = \frac{\%\text{TBW} \times \text{body weight (kg)} \times \text{measured osmolarity}}{\text{normal plasma osmolarity}} - \%\text{TBW} \times \text{body weight}$$

If the measured serum osmolarity value is not available, substituting two times the serum sodium value gives a usable estimation. This formula is used in Case 3. Hypotonic solutions must be given carefully to prevent a too rapid fall of the serum osmolarity. Hypocalcemia and hyperglycemia are frequent complications of hypernatremic dehydration. Severe hypernatremia (sodium level greater than 180 mEq per liter) may require peritoneal dialysis.

**Acid-Base Disturbances.** The poor tissue perfusion in severe dehydration or the loss of bicarbonate ($HCO_3$)-rich fluids, such as in profuse diarrhea, may result in a *metabolic acidosis.* Unless the acidosis is severe, adequate rehydration with re-establishment of tissue and renal perfusion usually causes rapid resolution of the acidosis without requiring exogenous base therapy. If the

acidosis is severe (serum $HCO_3$ level less than 10 to 12 mEq per liter) or a large anion gap is present, the initial resuscitation fluid can contain up to 40 to 60 mEq per liter of sodium bicarbonate ($NaHCO_3$). This should be mixed into a hypotonic solution such as 0.45% (half-normal) saline with 5% dextrose. Routine intravenous infusion of hypertonic solutions should be avoided, as should rapid infusion of undiluted $NaHCO_3$, which may result in a paradoxical intracellular acidosis in the central nervous system.

*Metabolic alkalosis* can be caused by loss of hydrogen ions in gastic juice, as with frequent vomiting or nasogastric suction. The classic example in infants is the persistent vomiting of pyloric stenosis (Case 4). Chloride losses are also high, usually resulting in a hypochloremic metabolic alkalosis, often associated with hypokalemia. Replacement with chloride-containing solutions such as NaCl and KCl is necessary because administration of HCl or $NH_4Cl$ is impractical.

**Re-Evaluation of the Treatment Plan.** In the acute setting, the patient should be frequently re-examined, and repeated measurements of body weight, serum electrolytes, or both (e.g., every 8 to 12 hours) may be required. The fluid prescription can then be revised appropriately. This is especially true when large ongoing losses occur.

## EXAMPLES OF TREATMENT PLANS

The patient in the first three cases is a 10-kg infant with a temperature of 37° C and without abnormal ongoing losses. All laboratory results are given in Table 6. From Table 1, the infant's maintenance fluid requirements would be 1000 ml per day or about 40 ml per hour. Electrolyte requirements would be about 25 mEq of NaCl and about 20 mEq of KCl daily.

This infant develops gastroenteritis and rapidly becomes 10% dehydrated. This indicates that the fluid deficit is about 1 liter ($0.1 \times 10$ kg). The infant's initial fluid resuscitation requires 0.9% saline with 5% dextrose at a rate of 100 ml per hour for the first 1 or 2 hours (10 ml per kg per hour). Because the degree of dehydration is a rough estimate, the resuscitation fluids are not usually included in the calculation of the fluid prescription.

TABLE 6. **Case Examples**

| Case No. (Dehydration Type) | Weight (kg) | mEq/Liter | | | |
|---|---|---|---|---|---|
| | | *Na* | *K* | *Cl* | *CO₂* |
| 1 (isotonic) | 10 | 140 | 4.5 | 108 | 18 |
| 2 (hypotonic) | 10 | 125 | 4.5 | 93 | 18 |
| 3 (hypertonic) | 10 | 163 | 5.0 | 128 | 19 |
| 4 (pyloric stenosis) | 4.2 | 128 | 3.4 | 75 | 34 |

**Case 1: Isotonic Dehydration.** Because the total estimated deficit of 1 liter is approximately evenly divided between the ECF and the ICF, the sodium and potassium deficits are 70 and 75 mEq, respectively. These are added to the maintenance requirements of 25 and 20 mEq each. Thus, 2 liters of solution containing a total of 95 mEq each of sodium and potassium is required (given as 50 mEq per liter of NaCl and 30 mEq per liter of KCl). Because one-half of the deficit is to be replaced in the first 8 hours, the initial rate of infusion would be 500 ml per 8 hours + maintenance (40 ml per hour), or about 100 ml per hour, and the remainder would be infused at a rate of 500 ml per 16 hours + 40 ml per hour, or about 70 ml per hour.

**Case 2: Hypotonic Dehydration.** The sodium and potassium deficits from dehydration and the rate of fluid administration are the same as in Case 1. The formula to replace the additional sodium deficit is

$$(\text{Na desired} - \text{Na measured}) \times \%\text{TBW}$$
$$\times \text{ body weight}$$
$$\text{or}$$
$$135 - 125 \times 0.6 \times 10 \text{ kg} = 60 \text{ mEq}$$

Thus, using the calculations from Case 1, a total of 160 mEq of sodium and 60 mEq of potassium is mixed into 2 liters of water (80 mEq per liter of NaCl and 30 mEq per liter of KCl) administered at the same rate as in Case 1.

**Case 3: Hypertonic Dehydration.** Correction should be planned over 48 hours once initial fluid resuscitation is complete. The formula to calculate the water deficit is:

$$\text{Deficit} =$$

$$\frac{\%\text{TBW} \times \text{body wt (kg)} \times \text{measured osmolarity}}{\text{normal plasma osmolarity}}$$

$$- \%\text{TBW} \times \text{body wt}$$
$$\text{or}$$
$$= \frac{0.6 \times 10 \text{ kg} \times 326}{280}$$
$$- 0.6 \times 10 \text{ kg} = 6.98 - 6 = 980 \text{ ml}$$

The maintenance requirements for 48 hours are 2000 ml of water, 50 mEq of sodium, and 40 mEq of potassium. The deficit of water is 1000 ml from the dehydration and 980 ml from the hypernatremia. Even though the serum sodium level is elevated, sodium must be added to the rehydration solution, as in the other examples, because there is a total body deficit of sodium associated with the dehydration, and too rapid correction of hypernatremia must be avoided. The hyperton-

icity results from an excess loss of free water relative to sodium. Thus, 75 mEq of sodium and 70 mEq of potassium are added to the maintenance electrolyte requirement, giving a total of 125 mEq of sodium and 110 mEq of potassium in 3980 ml (about 35 mEq per liter of NaCl and 30 mEq per liter of KCl) to be administered over 48 hours: The volume deficit should be replaced in the first 12 hours.

**Case 4: Pyloric Stenosis.** A 6-week-old infant who weighed 4.2 kg 3 days before becoming ill has had projectile vomiting of all fluids for 30 hours. The weight is 3.7 kg (12% dehydration), and there is an "olive" mass in the right upper abdomen. Laboratory results (see Table 6) show a hypochloremic metabolic alkalosis with hyponatremia.

Therapy must repair the dehydration because volume contraction causes the proximal tubule of the kidney to reabsorb excess $HCO_3$, aggravating the metabolic alkalosis. Normal saline rather than Ringer's lactate must be used as the initial resuscitation fluid. The infant's deficit from dehydration is $0.12 \times 0.7 \times 4 \text{ kg} = 336 \text{ ml}$ of water and $(0.34 \text{ liter} \times 70 \text{ mEq per liter}) = 24$ mEq of sodium. The sodium deficit is $(135 - 128 \text{ mEq}) \times 0.7 \times 4 \text{ kg} = 20 \text{ mEq}$. The potassium deficit is often large and takes several days to replace. The infant's maintenance needs are 400 ml of water and 10 and 8 mEq of sodium and potassium, respectively. Thus, a total of 54 mEq of sodium in about 740 ml of water is required (about 75 mEq of NaCl and 40 mEq of KCl per liter) and should be administered at a rate of 46 ml per hour for the first 8 hours and 23 ml per hour for the rest of the day. Any ongoing losses from nasogastric suction must also be replaced (see Table 3).

## ORAL REHYDRATION THERAPY

The observation that the coupled transport of sodium and glucose in the small intestine persists despite infectious gastroenteritis has led to the development of glucose and electrolyte solutions for the oral treatment of patients with dehydration. Glucose facilitates the absorption of sodium. Water is absorbed osmotically after sodium absorption. Potassium is transported passively by solvent drag with absorbed water. Properly formulated glucose and electrolyte ORS provide a net positive absorption of electrolytes and water despite persisting diarrhea. A glucose concentration of 2% (111 mmol) allows maximal sodium absorption. Much higher concentrations of glucose may not be fully absorbed from the intestine, and the osmotic effect of the remaining glucose may cause excess water to be lost in the stool.

Experience has shown success with ORS in all

forms of mild and moderate dehydration both in the Third World and the West. ORS use allows rapid rehydration, with a complication rate similar to that of parenteral rehydration, at a much lower cost. The principal contraindications to ORS use are altered consciousness or seizure activity, severe hypotension or shock, persistent vomiting (as in pyloric stenosis), or absent bowel sounds. In these situations, parenteral rehydration therapy should be used until the patient stabilizes, at which time ORS may be added or substituted. Because continuing losses from the stool are often somewhat higher in patients receiving ORS than when the gut is put "to rest" (the child is receiving no oral feeding) during parenteral rehydration, the volumes recommended for rehydration with ORS are larger than those recommended for parenteral rehydration. The child's thirst and appetite assist in determining the rate, volume, and type of fluid administration with ORS.

The prototype ORS is the World Health Organization (WHO) solution (Table 7). This solution has been used successfully for more than 20 years in the treatment of cholera. It can be mixed by adding the ingredients in Table 6 to 1 liter (1.05 quarts) of clean water. Recent work has shown that glucose can be replaced by sucrose or rice powder, both of which are less expensive and easier to store. $HCO_3$ can be replaced by citrate, which is much more stable in solution. The ingredients should be provided in premixed packets or solutions to avoid iatrogenic errors in mixing.

In developed countries, the organisms causing gastroenteritis result in a stool sodium concentration that is much lower than that typically seen in cholera (see Table 3). Consequently, rehydration solutions developed for the West are lower in sodium content than is the WHO solution (see Table 7). Oral rehydration solutions have higher sodium concentrations than do oral maintenance electrolyte solutions. Oral maintenance solutions are formulated to prevent dehydration when an infant or child has mild gastroenteritis or another acute illness limiting the intake of food or milk (see Table 7).

Clear fluids, such as fruit juices or soda, which are often recommended in the United States for mild gastroenteritis maintenance, are not as effective as the oral maintenance electrolyte solution. Clear fluids are low in sodium, and fructose

is often the most prevalent carbohydrate, because high-fructose corn syrup has replaced sucrose as the major sweetener in many soda pops and juice drinks (see Table 7). Fructose is an ineffective substitute substrate for the glucose-sodium transporter in the small intestine. Also, if clear fluids are used alone for oral rehydration, or if they are used alone for prolonged periods as oral maintenance solutions, their low sodium content may cause hyponatremia. Clear fluids are good sources of additional fluids and calories once the recommended volumes of ORS or oral maintenance solutions have been ingested.

## TREATMENT PLAN USING ORAL REHYDRATION SOLUTIONS

Clinical assessment of the degree and type of dehydration is identical to that given before parenteral therapy (see Table 2). The rehydration phase generally should last for 3 to 6 hours, with the estimated deficit being replaced with ORS. For example, replacement of 50 ml per kg over 4 hours should be planned for mild dehydration, and 100 ml per kg over 6 hours should be planned for moderately severe dehydration. If the child has hypertonic dehydration, oral rehydration should be planned over 12 to 24 hours. If the infant or child continues to vomit, as is common with rotavirus infections, small amounts (less than 30 ml) of ORS administered frequently are usually tolerated.

*After rehydration is complete, ORS should not be used as the only fluid intake,* because the high sodium content may lead to hypernatremia. ORS can be replaced with a maintenance electrolyte solution, or ORS can be ingested with extra free water in the form of breast milk in nursing infants, or as plain water, fruit juices, or other low-sodium clear liquids. The ratio of ORS to clear fluids should be approximately 1:1. Refeeding should begin as soon as the rehydration phase is complete. Breast-feeding should continue ad libitum. Generally, solids such as a BRAT diet (*B*anana, *R*ice, *A*pple sauce, *T*oast) or other carbohydrate-rich, low-lactose foods such as boiled potatoes are well tolerated. Refeeding may cause an increase in stool volume, which the infant or child usually tolerates well by increasing the appetite for fluids.

The timing of the reintroduction of lactose-containing formulas is controversial. The usual practice in the United States has been to delay the reintroduction of milk-based formula for several days, because some experienced pediatricians have observed recurrence of dehydrating diarrhea with early reintroduction of such for-

TABLE 7. **WHO ORS Formula**

| To 1 liter of water add | Substitutions |
|---|---|
| ½ tsp NaCl | |
| ½ tsp NaHCO₃ | ½ tsp sodium citrate |
| ¼ tsp KCl | |
| 2 tbsp glucose | 4 tbsp sucrose |

mulas. However, breast milk, which is rich in lactose, is well tolerated. Nevertheless, delay in reintroducing milk-based formulas is probably still prudent. Infants can temporarily use a casein hydrolysate or other non–lactose-containing formula. The older infant or child should be able to tolerate the normal diet for several days before the use of cow milk.

# The Endocrine System

## ACROMEGALY

method of
SHLOMO MELMED, M.D.
*Cedars-Sinai Medical Center–UCLA School of
Medicine*
*Los Angeles, California*

The anterior pituitary consists of at least five separate differentiated cell types secreting their specific trophic hormones, including growth hormone (GH), prolactin (PRL), thyroid stimulating hormone (TSH), luteinizing hormone (LH), follicle stimulating hormone (FSH), and the ACTH-related pro-opiomelanocortin peptides. Functional hypersecretory pituitary adenomas may arise from any of these cells. GH-secreting tumors causing acromegaly account for about one-third of the functional pituitary adenomas. Gigantism occurs when these tumors present prior to epiphyseal closure.

The hypothalamus controls the secretion of GH by two regulatory hormones: growth hormone–releasing hormone (GHRH), which stimulates growth hormone secretion; and somatostatin (SRIF), which inhibits the secretion of GH. GH is secreted from the pituitary and stimulates peripheral hepatic and extrahepatic synthesis of insulin-like growth factor I (IGF-I), which in turn stimulates bone chondrocytes, skeletal growth, and replication of epithelial cells. GH also has direct anti-insulin actions and affects carbohydrate and fat metabolism. In treating acromegaly, the concern, in addition to suppressing GH levels, is also with lowering IGF-I levels that contribute to many of the somatic changes seen in acromegaly.

Over 95% of patients with acromegaly harbor pituitary tumors, expressing either GH alone, or GH with PRL (Table 1). The remaining patients have extrapituitary causes of acromegaly as a result of ectopic tumor production of GHRH, or very rarely ectopic GH. Tumors elaborating GHRH include bronchial and abdominal carcinoids; and rarely tumors of other endocrine organs, including the pancreas and adrenal glands.

### DIAGNOSIS

Acromegaly is diagnosed by failure to suppress GH levels to less than 2 $\mu$g per liter within 2 hours after an oral glucose load. Elevated IGF-I levels are invariably present. Diagnosis of pituitary adenoma is made by magnetic resonance imaging or computed tomography scanning of the pituitary gland. Diagnosis of extrapituitary acromegaly is made by measuring ele-

**TABLE 1. Causes of Acromegaly**

| Excess GH Secretion by Tumor | Estimated Relative Frequency (%) |
|---|---|
| Pituitary | 95 |
| Abdomen or chest | <1 |
| **Excess GHRH Secretion by Tumor** | |
| Carcinoid | 5 |
| Other abdominal | <1 |

vated levels of circulating GHRH and by confirming the presence of a thoracic or intra-abdominal mass.

### TREATMENT

Besides the physical disfigurement of acromegaly and the local pressure effects of the tumor, the effects of elevated GH and IGF-I levels contribute to a significantly increased morbidity and mortality. The deleterious effects of hypersomatotrophism include diabetes mellitus, hypertension, ischemic heart disease, hypercalcemia, renal dysfunction, arthritis, and nerve entrapments. Increased prevalence of benign and malignant neoplasms, including skin tags, lipomas, colon polyps, and colon carcinoma further emphasizes the importance of attaining a sustained suppression of GH secretion in these patients.

The criteria to be fulfilled in order to effectively treat the patient with acromegaly are outlined in Table 2. Firstly, unrestrained GH secretion should be abolished and the tumor mass itself should be ablated or reduced. The latter is particularly important, owing to the critical location of the pituitary leading to local pressure effects including visual field defects, cranial nerve palsies, cavernous sinus invasion, internal hydrocephalus, and invasion of the temporal or frontal lobes. Therapy should correct any visual or neu-

**TABLE 2. Criteria for Effective Management of GH-Secreting Anterior Pituitary Adenomas**

1. Suppression of autonomous growth hormone secretion
2. Ablation or reduction of pituitary tumor mass
3. Correction of visual and neurologic defects
4. Preservation of pituitary trophic hormone function, especially adrenal, thyroid, and gonadal axes
5. Prevention of biochemical or local recurrence

rologic dysfunction caused by the tumor. Successful treatment should also preserve residual pituitary trophic hormone function and prevent the development of pituitary failure. Effective therapy should also prevent recurrence of the tumor and hypersecretion of GH. These criteria have unfortunately not satisfactorily been fulfilled with available surgical, radiation, or medical modes of management of somatotroph adenomas (Table 3).

### Surgical Management

Trans-sphenoidal resection of the somatotroph adenoma invariably results in a brisk fall in circulating GH levels, improvement in well-being, and amelioration of symptoms including excessive perspiration and soft tissue swelling. Unfortunately, the results of most surgical series are difficult to interpret because the criteria for cure are usually reported as a percentage fall in GH levels. Alternatively, random GH levels less than 10 or 5 μg per liter, respectively, are reported. Naturally, these criteria are inadequate to define a true "cure" of the disorder. About 60% of patients have GH levels less than 5 μg per liter after surgery. The success of surgery is highly dependent on the skill of the neurosurgeon and the expertise of the center. Larger tumors (greater than 5 mm), local invasiveness, and higher preoperative GH levels (greater than 50 μg per liter) portend a less favorable surgical outcome.

Side effects of surgery include new pituitary failure, diabetes insipidus, CSF leaks, and meningitis. These complications are seen in 5 to 15% of patients undergoing trans-sphenoidal surgery. Long-term biochemical and/or clinical recurrence rates are difficult to assess from the literature. It would appear, however, that recurrence rates are low in those patients who are initially truly cured as defined by strict biochemical criteria.

### Radiation Therapy

Two modes of irradiation of GH secreting tumors are employed. Conventional external irradiation (4000 to 6000 rad) is administered over 6 weeks. GH levels fall slowly, often taking up to 10 years to normalize. The tumor mass invariably shrinks. Unfortunately, about 50% of patients will develop some degree of hypopituitarism within 10 years and require replacement of adrenal, thyroid, and/or sex steroids. Furthermore, cranial nerve damage, visual defects, cerebral radionecrosis, and personality disturbances are serious side effects. Proton beam irradiation causes a more rapid reduction in GH levels but is associated with a higher incidence of cranial nerve damage and should therefore be reserved for intrasellar tumors only.

### Medical Therapy

**Bromocriptine.** Bromocriptine (Parlodel), a dopamine agonist, effectively normalizes GH levels in about 20% of patients. The drug, given at a dose of up to 20 mg daily, will also shrink about 10% of tumors. Despite the failure to suppress GH in the majority of patients, clinical benefit is almost invariably noted, with most patients reporting a subjective feeling of improvement. Side effects of bromocriptine include transient nausea and abdominal discomfort and hypotension. Uncommon side effects include Raynaud's phenomenon, nasal stuffiness, and depression.

**Octreotide Acetate.** Because somatostatin suppresses GH secretion, it seemed a natural candidate peptide for treatment of acromegaly. GH secretion in acromegaly is indeed suppressed by intravenous somatostatin infusions. However, the rapid half-life of somatostatin results in an immediate rebound hypersecretion of GH, precluding the use of native somatostatin for the treatment of acromegalic patients. In contrast, octreotide acetate (Sandostatin), an octapeptide synthetic somatostatin analogue, suppresses elevated GH levels to normal for 8 to 10 hours after subcutaneous injection. The drug is relatively resistant to peripheral degradation and has a circulating half-life of about 2 hours. Unlike native somatostatin, it does not cause significant insulin suppression. When acromegalic patients are treated with a 50-μg single injection of octreotide, 95% exhibit lower GH levels, with GH levels in two-thirds of patients falling to less than 2 μg per dl. Long-term subcutaneous injection (100 to 300 μg every 8 hours), or continuous subcutaneous infusion of octreotide, normalizes GH and IGF-I levels in up to 80% of patients.

Octreotide also shrinks pituitary tumors in up to half of patients with acromegaly. These patients experience remarkable improvement in their symptomatology. Arthralgias, soft tissue swelling, facial coarsening, paresthesias, and

TABLE 3. **Acromegaly: Management Options**

**Surgical Ablation of Excess GH or GHRH Source**
Trans-sphenoidal pituitary adenomectomy
Extrapituitary tumor resection

**Irradiation of Source of Excess GH Secretion**
Conventional external x-ray therapy
Proton beam

**Functional Suppression of Excess GH or GHRH Secretion**
Bromocriptine
Octreotide acetate

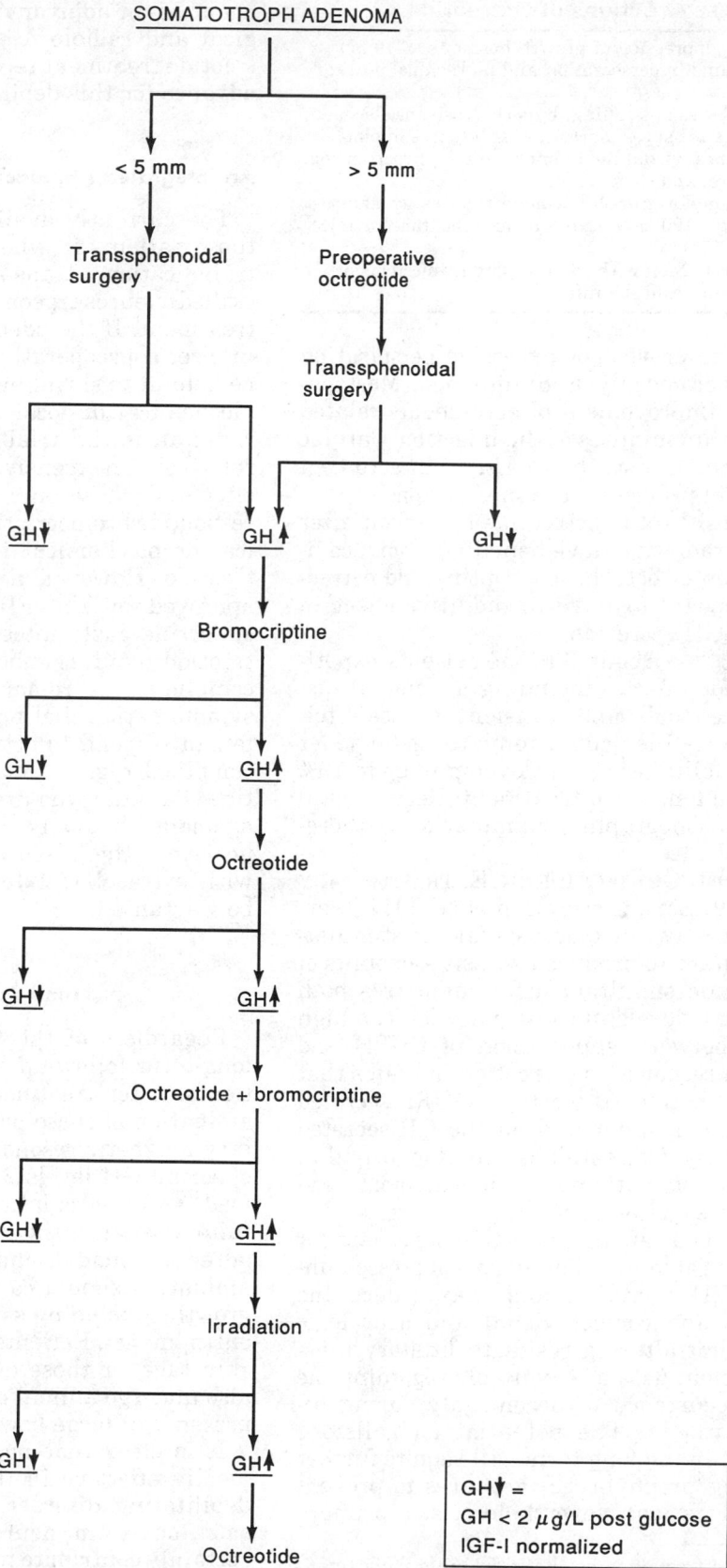

**Figure 1.** Management of acromegaly.

TABLE 4. **Actions of Octreotide**

1. Long-acting suppression of growth hormone (8–10 hr) with no rebound hypersecretion and no residual pituitary damage
2. Improves soft tissue swelling, hyperhidrosis, headaches, menstrual disturbances, paresthesias, glucose intolerance, impotence, visual field abnormalities, hypertension, cardiac failure, and sleep apnea
3. Optimal dosage for growth hormone suppression and tumor shrinkage: 100–500 µg q 8 hr as subcutaneous injection
4. Maximal effects seen with more frequent injections or continuous subcutaneous infusion

tiredness all improve. The excessive perspiration peculiar to acromegaly is diminished. Most patients report improvement of acromegaly-related headache within minutes of the injection. Cardiac failure and renal disturbances seen in acromegaly are also improved by the medication.

Patients resistant to octreotide treatment after surgery or irradiation have benefited from a combined regimen of both bromocriptine and octreotide that appears to have an additive effect in suppressing GH secretion.

SIDE EFFECTS. About 30% of patients experience mild side effects, including abdominal discomfort, loose stools, and transient glucose intolerance. Because the drug attenuates gallbladder motility, cholelithiasis may develop in up to 10% of patients on long-term treatment. Regular gallbladder ultrasonographic examination is therefore recommended.

EFFICACY OF OCTREOTIDE IN EXTRAPITUITARY ACROMEGALY. Ectopic secretion of GHRH by carcinoid tumor may cause acromegaly by stimulating the pituitary to produce excessive amounts of GH. Octreotide simultaneously suppresses both GHRH and GH levels in these patients. The high correlation between suppression of GHRH and GH levels in response to octreotide indicates that the drug acts both on the ectopic GHRH secreted by the carcinoid tumor and on the GH secreted by the pituitary. Octreotide is therefore useful in management of patients with carcinoid and chronic hypersomatotrophism.

Octreotide is a safe and effective treatment for acromegaly (Table 4).* The drug suppresses unrestrained GH secretion and may reduce the tumor mass and correct visual and neurologic defects without altering residual pituitary function. Insufficient data are available regarding the long-term recurrence of acromegaly during octreotide treatment. The potential for gallstone development in the long term will require further studies using prophylactic measures to prevent gallstone formation. Nevertheless, as a primary

---

*This use of octreotide is not listed in the manufacturer's official directive.

agent or an adjuvant to currently available surgical and radiologic therapeutic modalities, octreotide treatment represents a major therapeutic advance for this debilitating disease.

### An Integrated Approach to Management (Figure 1)

The currently available data indicate that in those patients in whom there is no medical contraindication, trans-sphenoidal surgery by a skilled neurosurgeon is the preferred primary treatment. If the adenoma is greater than 5 mm in size, a preoperative course of octreotide may be helpful in shrinking the tumor mass. Residual biochemical or local disease after surgery warrants an initial trial of bromocriptine, which is relatively inexpensive and has few major side effects. Because only about 20% of patients will respond to bromocriptine, most patients with clinical or biochemical recurrence will require octreotide. However, at present the medication is approved by the FDA only for carcinoid and endocrine gastrointestinal tumors. Although octreotide requires subcutaneous injection, patient compliance is remarkably high, owing to the symptomatic relief provided. Some patients who fail to respond to octreotide may benefit from a combined regimen of octreotide with bromocriptine. Patients who are resistant to medical management should be referred for irradiation. If, however, the disease recurrence is associated with extrasellar extension, repeat surgery may be warranted.

### Long-Term Follow-up

Regardless of the treatment mode employed, long-term follow-up is imperative for these patients. After treatment, long-term follow-up examination of these patients should include pituitary magnetic resonance imaging, measurement of serum GH levels 2 hours after an oral glucose load, and a circulating IGF-I level. Anterior pituitary reserve should also be tested, including adrenal, gonadal, and thyroid axes. Physical examination should carefully note new soft tissue growths, including skin tags, lipomas, and nerve entrapments. Patients harboring more than three skin tags, or those over 50 years of age, should also undergo annual colonoscopy to search for the presence of large bowel polyps.

It is clear that no single mode of therapy is ideally effective in the therapy of this chronic, debilitating disorder. Development of new and safe long-term neuropeptide preparations will certainly contribute to successful biochemical and clinical management.

# ADRENOCORTICAL INSUFFICIENCY

method of
JAMIE DANANBERG, M.D., and
ROGER J. GREKIN, M.D.
*University of Michigan and*
*Veterans Administration Medical Center*
*Ann Arbor, Michigan*

The causes of adrenocortical insufficiency are diverse and include immunologic, infectious, hemorrhagic, malignant, and drug-induced etiologies. The proportion of cases due to these processes has changed over time, with infectious etiologies becoming significantly less frequent. As a result, immunologic causes make up the preponderance of cases. The evolution of diseases caused by human immunodeficiency virus (HIV) infection may broaden the spectrum further. In that adrenal disease can affect any of the classes of steroid hormones produced in the cortex, and the presentation can vary from acute to chronic, several syndromes can also be distinguished. The mainstay of therapy is prompt replacement of glucocorticoids, vigorous fluid rehydration, and diagnosis and treatment of any coexisting precipitant illnesses. The definitive diagnosis of this disorder rests on selected tests of the hypothalamic-pituitary-adrenal (HPA) axis; however, treatment of acute symptoms should never be delayed pending results of these investigations.

## PATHOPHYSIOLOGY

### Primary Adrenal Insufficiency

Adrenal insufficiency can be separated into classes based on the level of the HPA axis affected. Primary adrenal insufficiency (Addison's disease) specifies adrenal dysfunction, whereas secondary insufficiency defines those diseases affecting pituitary or hypothalamic function. Primary adrenocortical insufficiency is due to the inability of zona glomerulosa or fasciculata cells to secrete mineralocorticoids or glucocorticoids, respectively, in amounts sufficient to meet bodily requirements (Table 1). In both cases, there must be loss of greater than 90% of the normal secretory capacity of the adrenal cortex in order for signs and symptoms to develop under basal conditions. Approximately 80% of the cases appear to be due to autoimmune phenomena. Of these cases, women outnumber men by about 3:1, a variety of age groups are affected, and antiadrenal antibodies are detected approximately 60% of the time. This syndrome is frequently associated with autoimmune polyglandular disease as well as vitiligo and pernicious anemia. In patients who have prior evidence of autoimmune endocrine disease, the appearance of antiadrenal or antisteroidal cell antibodies is highly predictive of adrenal failure. Despite a reduction in the overall frequency of infectious causes of adrenal failure, tubercular and fungal etiologies remain important considerations in the differential diagnosis. Coccidioidomycosis, blastomycosis, and candidiasis have all been described as causing adrenal insufficiency. Most patients with acquired immune deficiency

TABLE 1. **Causes of Primary Adrenocortical Insufficiency**

Idiopathic-autoimmune
Infectious
  Tuberculosis, coccidioidomycosis, blastomycosis, histoplasmosis, candidiasis, HIV
Vascular
  Hemorrhage, infarction
Infiltration
  Metastases, lymphoma, amyloidosis, sarcoidosis, hemochromatosis
Iatrogenic
  Irradiation, surgical excision
Drugs
  Metyrapone, aminoglutethimide, mitotane
Hereditary
  Congenital adrenal hyperplasia-hypoplasia, familial glucocorticoid deficiency

syndrome (AIDS) have normal adrenal function, although there have been occasional reports of HIV-induced Addison's disease. Nevertheless, the predisposition to tuberculosis, to fungal and Epstein-Barr viral infections, and to lymphomatous infiltrative diseases in AIDS puts these patients at risk for adrenal insufficiency. Malignant replacement of the adrenal glands, by metastatic or primary disease, is the third most likely cause of primary adrenal failure. Up to one-third of patients with bilateral adrenal metastases will have suppressed adrenal function as assessed by cosyntropin stimulation testing. Tumors that metastasize to the adrenal glands include carcinoma of lung, breast, gastrointestinal tract, and prostate.

Among the rarer etiologies of primary adrenal insufficiency are hemorrhage, infarction, late onset enzymatic deficiencies, and iatrogenic causes. Adrenal hemorrhage occurs most commonly in adults during anticoagulation with warfarin (Coumadin) and in association with other causes of thrombocytopenia, including that induced by heparin. Intra-adrenal bleeding has also been shown to occur in association with bacterial sepsis, classically associated with meningococcemia (Waterhouse-Friderichsen syndrome) or *Pseudomonas* septicemia, and can lead to rapid deterioration with frequent mortality. Adrenal infarction has been described, although glandular insufficiency on this basis is uncommon. Various drugs can depress adrenal function, including ketoconazole (Nizoral), aminoglutethimide (Cytadren), and metyrapone (Metopirone), which block various steroid biosynthetic enzymes. o,p'-DDD (mitotane [Lysodren]), a chemotherapeutic agent used to treat adrenal carcinoma, blocks mitochondrial enzymes and is toxic to adrenal cortical tissue.

The spectrum of congenital adrenal disease has been shown to include deficiencies of the majority of enzymes in the steroid biosynthetic pathway. The nature of the clinical syndrome relates to the specific enzyme involved and the degree of activity loss. Deficiency of 21-, 18-, 17α-, and 11β-hydroxylase; 3β-hydroxysteroid dehydrogenase; and desmolase may all cause partial or complete adrenal insufficiency as part of the syndrome of congenital adrenal hyperplasia.

## Secondary Adrenal Insufficiency

The loss of glucocorticoid secretion can also be due to loss of pituitary adrenocorticotropic (ACTH) or corticotropin releasing (CRH) hormones (Table 2). Therefore, the scope of diseases that can precipitate adrenal failure is a set of those diseases that will reduce normal hypothalamic-pituitary (HP) function. The most common suppressant of pituitary secretion of ACTH is exogenous glucocorticoids. Even low doses of potent glucocorticoids such as dexamethasone (Decadron) can suppress normal HP responsiveness for months. Reduction of exogenous glucocorticoids can therefore lead to relative adrenocortical insufficiency. Any of the other diverse diseases or treatments affecting the pituitary or hypothalamus, including adenoma, malignancy, infection, infiltrative disease, infarction, surgery, and radiation therapy, can lead to a secondary decrease in adrenal function.

## CLINICAL PRESENTATION

The precise presentation of patients with adrenocortical failure generally relates to the rate at which loss of adrenal steroids developed and the presence of any coexisting illnesses or precipitants. The majority of patients will present with chronic symptoms of glucocorticoid deficiency. Adrenal hemorrhage will frequently be manifested on an emergent basis. Severe congenital forms are generally diagnosed in the first week of life, whereas nonclassic enzyme deficiencies will be seen at various times in later life.

### Primary Chronic Adrenal Insufficiency

The most common signs and symptoms of Addison's disease are also the most nonspecific. Virtually all patients complain of weakness and fatigue, initially with generalized aching. Weight loss and anorexia are also invariably present. Hyperpigmentation, hypotension, nausea, and vomiting are also usually noted. The presence of these features, particularly hyperpigmentation as it occurs in the palmar creases, nail beds, buccal mucosa, tongue, periareolar area, or navel, should vastly increase clinical suspicion for the disease. The deposit of pigment can often predate many other sequelae of the syndrome. Other objective findings may

TABLE 2. **Causes of Secondary Adrenocortical Insufficiency**

Tumor
  Adenoma, craniopharyngioma, meningioma, glioma
Vascular
  Ischemic necrosis, aneurysm, cavernous sinus thrombosis
Infectious
  Tuberculosis, syphilis, meningitis, fungal
Infiltrative
  Hemochromatosis, sarcoidosis, amyloidosis, lipid storage
    disease, granulomatosis
Iatrogenic
  Surgical, irradiation, glucocorticoids
Empty sella syndrome
Nutritional
  Starvation, obesity, anorexia nervosa
Idiopathic

include hyperkalemia and fever. Lymphocytosis and eosinophilia have also been noted in a number of patients. Hypoglycemia, although reported, is a rare finding at presentation in chronic deficiency states. In a smaller number of cases, patients may also note a history of salt craving.

### Addisonian Crisis

This can be life threatening and often presents as such. In most cases, the patients will be either those with known Addison's disease or those with undiagnosed, chronic, borderline adrenal dysfunction who develop an intercurrent illness. In addition to the findings noted in the preceding section, patients will present with profound volume contraction if not frank shock, nausea and vomiting, abdominal pain, and lethargy and confusion, along with findings of hyperpyrexia, hyponatremia, azotemia, and renal failure.

A separate consideration must be made of acute adrenal hemorrhage. In this condition, the hallmark manifestations of hyperpigmentation, early weakness, and electrolyte abnormalities are usually absent. In contrast, fever, shock, nausea, and vomiting in conjunction with severe abdominal or flank pain are expected, particularly when they occur in a patient with significant illness. This composite of findings can be confused with an acute surgical abdomen.

### Secondary Chronic Adrenal Insufficiency

The features of adrenal failure secondary to hypothalamic-pituitary disorders are similar to those of primary disease. These patients will frequently present with a history of chronic glucocorticoid insufficiency, either undiagnosed or previously treated with exogenous steroids and precipitated by an intercurrent illness. Two important features that differentiate secondary from primary adrenal insufficiency are the lack of skin pigmentation and the absence of signs and symptoms related to mineralocorticoid deficiency. These are explained by the absence of ACTH, pro-opiomelanocortin (POMC), melanocyte-stimulating hormone (MSH), and β-lipotropin (β-LPH) in inducing pigment formation and by normal renin-controlled aldosterone secretion, respectively. Cortisol is important in normal water metabolism, and therefore water excretion may be impaired. In these instances, however, hyponatremia is not accompanied by hyperkalemia, acidosis, or azotemia. In addition to the features of adrenal dysfunction, many patients will display signs and symptoms related to the pituitary disease (mass effect, loss of other pituitary hormones) or may have evidence of chronic exogenous glucocorticoid use. Patients with pituitary tumors frequently have evidence of gonadotropin or thyrotropin deficiency, as these tend to be more sensitive to mass effect than is ACTH.

## DIAGNOSIS

The use of ancillary testing in the diagnosis of adrenocortical insufficiency serves as confirmation of clinical suspicion and is required to establish the diagnosis. The fundamental impairment in this group of disorders is insufficient amounts of plasma cortisol under a given circumstance.

Functional assessment of the adrenal gland is accomplished with the synthetic ACTH cosyntropin (Cortrosyn). After a baseline cortisol level is determined, cosyntropin, 0.25 mg, is rapidly injected intravenously. Two additional samples are drawn at 30 and 60 minutes following injection, or a single sample taken at 45 minutes is acceptable. It is expected that plasma cortisol will increase to values greater then 20 $\mu$g per dl. If basal cortisol levels are particularly low (less than 5 $\mu$g per dl), this result may not be achieved and the specificity of the test diminishes. If there is a question of primary versus secondary disease, a plasma ACTH sample should also be drawn with the baseline sample. An abnormal cosyntropin stimulation test with elevated basal ACTH levels is diagnostic for primary adrenal insufficiency, whereas suppressed levels of ACTH would suggest a secondary etiology. A normal cosyntropin stimulation rules out dysfunctional adrenal glands but does not exclude the possibility that pituitary function is impaired. Evaluation of hypothalamic and pituitary function must be performed if moderate but subnormal responses to cosyntropin occur. An alternative, albeit less informative, screening test is the measurement of an 8 a.m. cortisol sample. In patients who are not acutely ill and who have plasma cortisol values in the upper normal range (approximately 20 to 25 $\mu$g per dl), the likelihood of adrenal insufficiency is low.

These tests are functional in nature and will not determine the etiology of the disorder. Adjunct tests of importance may include computed tomography of the abdomen and/or pituitary; magnetic resonance imaging of the pituitary; tuberculin skin testing; measurement of antiadrenal antibodies, electrolytes, glucose, calcium, and phosphate; and thyroid function tests, depending on the clinical history. In addition, appropriate diagnostic studies will be required to determine the nature of underlying precipitant diseases.

A final point regards the diagnosis of acute adrenal insufficiency. As discussed in the next section, these individuals can be investigated and treated simultaneously. Treatment should not be delayed pending laboratory results.

## TREATMENT

### Acute Adrenal Crisis

The primary therapy of acute adrenal crisis is administration of intravenous glucocorticoids in doses that approximate maximal stress adrenal output. Intravenous saline and glucose should be given rapidly, and other electrolyte and acid-base disturbances should be corrected. Treatment of underlying precipitant diseases, if present, should be undertaken. Patients should be given a water-soluble preparation of cortisol, specifically hydrocortisone sodium succinate (Solu-Cortef), 100 mg intravenously immediately and every 6 hours. If the patient is critically ill, this dose should be continued until improvement is noted; otherwise, the dose can be tapered to 50 mg every 6 hours on day 2, and tapered gradually thereafter. Doses of hydrocortisone at this level have sufficient mineralocorticoid activity to make mineralocorticoid replacement unnecessary. Once the total daily dose is less then 50 mg, a mineralocorticoid may be necessary in the treatment of primary adrenal failure. The importance of volume replacement should also be emphasized. Aggressive administration of intravenous saline is critical to a successful outcome.

It is often necessary to combine treatment and diagnosis on an emergent basis when adrenal insufficiency is suspected in an acutely ill patient. In these cases, a blood sample should be obtained for the simultaneous measurement of ACTH and cortisol. Following this, replacement cortisol can be immediately started as recommended earlier. If the results of these assays are equivocal in making the diagnosis of adrenal insufficiency, a cosyntropin stimulation test may be performed at a later date when the patient is less critically ill.

### Chronic Adrenal Insufficiency

In those patients with documented disease, lifetime therapy is required. In these patients, the drug of choice is typically hydrocortisone, 20 to 30 mg daily given orally in divided doses. Generally, patients will take 15 mg in the morning and 10 mg in the evening or, alternatively, 10 mg in the morning, 10 mg in the afternoon, and 5 mg in the evening. Patients with primary adrenal failure will usually, although not always, need a maintenance mineralocorticoid as well and should be given fludrocortisone acetate (Florinef), 0.05 to 0.2 mg daily. These patients should closely monitor their weight, blood pressure, and general health status on a routine basis. All patients should be instructed to increase their hydrocortisone dose immediately in the event of a stressful illness, which for most purposes can be determined by the presence of fever. The general rule is to double the hydrocortisone dose at each time interval. Gastrointestinal disorders that cause vomiting and prevent ingestion of medication usually require hospitalization and parenteral therapy. Patients with chronic adrenal insufficiency should be instructed to carry an emergency identification card or bracelet as well. Follow-up should consist of yearly office visits. Physical examination must look for evidence of iatrogenic Cushing's syndrome, suggesting overreplacement; and for skin pigmentation, which would indicate underreplacement (in primary disease). Recumbent and upright blood pressure and serum electrolytes should also be checked.

## HYPOALDOSTERONISM

The isolated loss of adrenal mineralocorticoid secretion can occur in the face of low, normal, or high plasma renin activity (PRA). The differentiation of these is important in selecting treatment modalities for the condition. Hyporeninemic hypoaldosteronism occurs in patients with renal impairment and presents as hyperkalemia with an associated hyperchloremic metabolic acidosis. The exact cause of the defect in renin release is unknown. The disorder is associated with diabetes mellitus and interstitial nephritis. The treatment can be twofold. Frequently, improved diabetic control can restore normokalemia and make the need for additional therapy unnecessary. Occasionally, patients will need to be treated with small doses of fludrocortisone acetate to restore potassium balance. For patients with hypertension or edema, furosemide is preferable therapy. Removal of aldosterone secreting tumors can lead to a transient hyporeninemic state, which may require temporary doses of mineralocorticoid until normal renin secretion resumes. Preoperative treatment of patients with spironolactone usually prevents this problem.

Patients with hypoaldosteronism and normal or increased PRA have been shown to have isolated zona glomerulosa destruction with subsequent mineralocorticoid deficit. The setting for this is in critically ill patients, often those who have had periods of hypotension. If hypotension or hyperkalemia is present, treatment with fludrocortisone should be instituted.

# CUSHING'S SYNDROME

method of
THEMISTOCLES C. KAMILARIS, M.D., PH.D., and GEORGE P. CHROUSOS, M.D.
*National Institutes of Health*
*Bethesda, Maryland*

Cushing's syndrome results from prolonged exposure to high levels of glucocorticoid hormones. The cause can be exogenous, owing to administration of glucocorticoids or ACTH; or endogenous, as a result of increased secretion of ACTH or cortisol. Endogenous Cushing's syndrome can be classified as ACTH-dependent, which accounts for about 80% of endogenous cases; and ACTH independent, which accounts for the remaining 20%. ACTH-dependent pituitary Cushing's syndrome (Cushing's disease), which accounts for about 80% of adult and 35% of childhood cases, most commonly occurs

during the third and fourth decades of life and is more common in females than males. It is most often caused by ACTH-secreting pituitary microadenomas (90%) or macroadenomas (10%). Rarely, diffuse corticotroph hyperplasia is found in association with ACTH hypersecretion. Recently, the identification and characterization of corticotropin releasing hormone (CRH) has led to an increasing number of reports of ectopic CRH production by tumors, as a possible rare cause of pituitary ACTH Cushing's syndrome.

ACTH-dependent Cushing's syndrome due to ectopic ACTH production accounts for about 20% of ACTH-dependent cases and is most often associated with small cell carcinoma of the lung, thymoma, pancreatic islet cell tumor, lung or thymic carcinoid, medullary carcinoma of the thyroid, and pheochromocytoma. It more commonly occurs in males than females and is usually seen during the fourth to sixth decade of life.

ACTH-independent Cushing's syndrome, which accounts for about 20% of adult cases and 65% of cases in children under 7, is usually the result of a benign cortisol secreting adrenal adenoma or an adrenocortical carcinoma. The frequency of adrenocortical tumors as a cause of Cushing's syndrome is greater in females in every age group. A rare form of Cushing's syndrome, micronodular adrenal disease, is caused by multiple, small, bilateral, autonomous adrenocortical cortisol secreting adenomas. It is mainly a disorder of children and adolescents and is presumed to be of autoimmune nature.

Depressed or alcoholic patients often have mild hypercortisolism. The hypercortisolism disappears with resolution of depression or discontinuation of alcohol. This condition is referred to as a "pseudo-Cushing's state."

## DIAGNOSTIC EVALUATION

Cushing's syndrome has a highly variable presentation. There is no feature that occurs in all cases. Common clinical features include obesity (predominantly truncal), acne, hirsutism, facial rounding (moon facies), plethora, easy bruising, purple skin striae, menstrual abnormalities (oligoamenorrhea), muscle weakness, emotional disturbances, hypertension, edema, carbohydrate intolerance, and osteopenia. Patients may present with only a few or many of these features, depending to some extent on the severity and duration of the disorder. In addition to the history and clinical evaluation, biochemical and imaging evaluation is necessary to establish the diagnosis and determine the cause.

The first step is to establish the presence of hypercorisolism (Table 1). Urinary free cortisol is the best single laboratory test for this purpose. There are virtually no false-negative results, and, with the exception of patients with depression and alcoholism or the rare syndrome of primary glucocorticoid resistance, there are few false-positives. In pediatric patients, correction per body surface area is necessary for evaluation of hypercortisolism. Urinary 24-hour 17-hydroxysteroid excretion, corrected per gram of urinary creatinine excretion, is also useful and can be used when assays for urinary free cortisol are not available.

TABLE 1. **Evaluation of Hypercortisolism**

**Diagnosis**

Single-dose dexamethasone suppression test (screening)
Urinary free cortisol or 17-hydroxysteroid excretion (per gram creatinine)

**Differential Diagnosis**

*Feedback Regulation of the Hypothalamic-Pituitary-Adrenal Axis*
Basal plasma ACTH and CRH
Standard dexamethasone suppression test
Metyrapone stimulation test
CRH stimulation test
Measurement of other hormones or metabolites if multiple endocrine neoplasia or ectopic ACTH secretion is suspected (i.e., plasma calcitonin, gastrin, urinary 5-HIAA, catecholamines, POMC derivatives, etc.)

*Localization-Imaging Studies*
Bilateral inferior petrosal sinus sampling combined with CRH stimulation*
Pituitary MRI-CT
Adrenal MRI-CT
Chest and abdominal MRI-CT if ectopic ACTH secretion is suspected
Iodocholesterol scan to examine bilateral or unilateral adrenal uptake or to localize functional adrenal tissue

*Abbreviations:* ACTH = adrenocorticotropic hormone; CRH = corticotropin releasing hormone; 5-HIAA = 5-hydroxyindoleacetic acid; POMC = pro-opiomelacortin.

*In centers with experience, it appears that the differential diagnosis can be made on the basis of the combined test alone.

Isolated plasma ACTH and cortisol determinations are of limited value because both hormones are secreted episodically and their secretion is influenced by physical or emotional stress. Serial measurements, however, can be of assistance, since a high 24-hour mean total plasma cortisol value with loss of circadian variation suggests the diagnosis of Cushing's syndrome. The overnight 1-mg dexamethasone (Decadron) suppression test may also be employed as a screening test when a clinician suspects hypercortisolism. It is simple (plasma cortisol determination at 8:00 a.m. following the administration of 1 mg dexamethasone orally at 11:00 p.m.) and has a low incidence of falsely normal suppression. If the urinary free cortisol excretion is above normal or the plasma cortisol fails to suppress to 5 μg per dl or less after dexamethasone, the diagnosis of hypercortisolism is likely.

Once hypercortisolism has been confirmed, testing should be undertaken to determine the specific etiology of the syndrome (Table 1). This entails using tests that examine the integrity of the feedback regulation of the hypothalamic-pituitary-adrenal axis, such as the low-dose–high-dose standard dexamethasone suppression test, the metyrapone (Metopirone) stimulation test, the corticotropin releasing hormone (CRH) stimulation test, and localization-imaging studies. In the standard dexamethasone suppression (low dose, 0.5 mg orally every 6 hours for 2 days; high dose, 2 mg orally every 6 hours for 2 days), urinary free cortisol and 17-hydroxysteroid excretion should normally suppress to less than 80% or less than 50%, respectively, of the baseline values during the low-dose dexamethasone administration. Failure to suppress to these levels confirms the diagnosis of hypercortisolism. Failure to suppress significantly during the high-dose dexamethasone test points towards the diagnosis of ectopic ACTH syndrome or primary adrenocortical disease. Metyrapone (750 mg orally every 4 hours for six doses) stimulation is also useful in this regard. Eighty per cent of patients with Cushing's disease respond with an approximate doubling of their urinary 17-hydroxysteroid excretion. Most patients with the ectopic ACTH syndrome fail to respond in this manner.

Recently, the ovine CRH (oCRH) stimulation test has been introduced into clinical practice. This test appears to be equivalent to the standard dexamethasone suppression test in distinguishing between Cushing's disease and the ectopic ACTH syndrome. Patients with Cushing's disease usually show a normal or exaggerated ACTH and cortisol response to intravenous bolus oCRH administration (1 μg per kg body weight), whereas patients with ectopic ACTH secretion and non–ACTH-dependent causes of hypercortisolism fail to respond to this test. The diagnostic accuracy of the oCRH and the dexamethasone suppression tests are similar—about 85%. Our diagnostic power, however, is enhanced when both tests are employed. Negative results from both tests exclude the diagnosis of Cushing's disease with an accuracy greater than 98%.

The differential diagnosis between mild Cushing's syndrome and the hypercortisolism of depression can be a problem. It should be kept in mind that the natural histories of the two conditions are different. Depression is usually a self-limited condition, and resolution of the clinical picture of hypercortisolism is associated with improvement in the degree of depression. Patients with Cushing's syndrome, on the other hand, experience slow progression of their disease and the deterioration of their clinical status makes the diagnosis clear.

When the results of the evaluation for Cushing's syndrome are inconclusive, periodic hypersecretion of cortisol should be suspected. Long-term monitoring (1 to 2 months) with weekly urine collections for the measurement of free cortisol or 17-hydroxysteroid excretion will usually clarify this situation.

Rarely, a patient with factitious Cushing's syndrome is encountered. These individuals usually have Cushing's syndrome with low levels of urinary free cortisol excretion because synthetic glucocorticoids, such as prednisone, prednisolone, or dexamethasone, are the most frequently abused agents. Specific plasma or urine assays for these steroids are usually necessary to confirm the diagnosis.

Once the diagnosis of hypercortisolism and its likely etiology are established, specific imaging techniques are required to help confirm the diagnosis and to guide therapy. Magnetic resonance imaging (MRI) and high-resolution computer-assisted tomographic (CT) scanning have been used for identifying pituitary adenomas. In spite of the remarkable advances in imaging technology, however, abnormal pituitary CT and MRI scans are found in less than 10% of patients with pituitary corticotropinomas. The use of gadolinium enhancement with MRI improves the sensitivity of this procedure significantly. Thus, this technique detects up to 40% of pituitary ACTH secreting adenomas. If there is failure to demonstrate a pituitary abnormality by CT or gadolinium-enhanced MRI, bilateral simultaneous petrosal sinus sampling for measurement of ACTH concentrations is one of the most specific and accurate tests available both to unequivocally establish the presence of an ACTH secreting hypophyseal tumor and to provide lateralization information. The latter is often useful to the neurosurgeon when attempting to resect very small (2 to 3 mm) microadenomas. A plasma ACTH concentration gradient between the petrosal sinus and a peripheral vein greater than or equal to 1.6 verifies a pituitary source of ACTH. The utility of the test is enhanced if CRH is administered during the procedure. Stimulation with CRH results in a dramatic outpouring of ACTH, principally from the side of the microadenoma. The absence of or a reduced response contralaterally indicates glucocorticoid-induced suppression of the normal pituitary corticotrophs in the presence of a functional microadenoma. Imaging studies of the adrenal glands in Cushing's disease would be expected to demonstrate mild, bilateral enlargement. Approximately 10 to 15% of patients with Cushing's disease, however, demonstrate unilateral or bilateral nodules. This entity is then called "macronodular adrenal hyperplasia." When the appearance of nodules is asymmetrical, it may be confused with unilateral cortisol secreting adenoma, especially in the older patients with Cushing's disease and in patients with "atypical" or equivocal biochemical tests.

Enlargement of both adrenals and the infrequent presence of adrenocortical macronodules are also expected in the ectopic ACTH syndrome. If the patient's evaluation suggests the diagnosis of ectopic ACTH secretion, the primary tumor should be sought. Over 50% of these tumors are within the thorax (oat cell carcinomas, bronchial carcinoids, thymomas), and chest radiograms, lung tomograms, and thoracic CT scans will often localize the lesion. Once a tumor has been detected, ACTH production can be verified by percutaneous needle aspiration. Other ACTH secreting tumors are found in the pancreas, the thyroid gland, and the adrenal medulla. In 20% to 30% of patients with the ectopic ACTH syndrome, the tumor cannot be identified anatomically. A bronchial or thymic carcinoid is usually discovered as the source of ACTH after a 1- to 2-year period has elapsed. The presence of an occult medullary thyroid carcinoma producing ACTH can be suggested by elevated calcitonin levels.

Most adrenocortical carcinomas are large when patients present with Cushing's syndrome. These tumors can be palpable and are usually visible on ultrasonography, CT, or MRI. Benign adenomas are usually small (less than 5 cm in diameter), and the majority can be demonstrated with these techniques and/or a radiolabeled iodocholesterol scan. The latter is useful in differentiating adrenocortical carcinomas from adenomas or ACTH-dependent macronodules. Carcinomas fail to be imaged with this technique, whereas benign adenomas and ACTH-dependent macronodules concentrate iodocholesterol and, hence, produce an image. A major contribution of MRI is its ability to differentiate between benign and malignant hyperfunctioning adrenocortical masses. The latter are bright on the second time of relaxation ($T_2$). Contrary to previous reports, it appears that primary micronodular adrenal disease can be often diagnosed by CT and/or MRI scans of the adrenals.

## TREATMENT

Therapy is indicated in all patients with clinical signs and laboratory confirmation of Cushing's syndrome. The treatment of choice depends upon the specific cause of the hypercortisolism, which must be established unequivocally (Table 2). Optimal treatment is the correction of hypercortisolism without permanent dependence on hormone replacement.

### Cushing's Disease

Most cases of Cushing's syndrome are caused by ACTH secreting pituitary adenomas. These

TABLE 2. **Therapy of Cushing's Syndrome**

**Cushing's Disease (Pituitary)**

Trans-sphenoidal microadenomectomy or hemipituitectomy
Pituitary x-radiation
Adrenolytic mitotane (low dose) ⎫
Steroid synthesis inhibitors      ⎪
　Aminoglutethimide              ⎬ Alone or in combination
　Metyrapone*                    ⎪
　Trilostane                     ⎪
　Ketoconazole†                  ⎭
Bilateral adrenalectomy

**Ectopic ACTH Secretion Syndrome**

Removal of primary tumor and solitary accessible metastases
Adrenolytic mitotane (low dose) ⎫
Steroid synthesis inhibitors      ⎪
　Aminoglutethimide              ⎬ Alone or in combination
　Metyrapone*                    ⎪
　Trilostane                     ⎪
　Ketoconazole†                  ⎭
Glucocorticoid antagonist RU 486
Bilateral adrenalectomy
Palliative x-radiation
Somatostatin analogue SMS 201-995

**Adrenal Cushing's Syndrome**

*Benign Adenomas or Micronodular Adrenal Disease*
Unilateral or bilateral-adrenalectomy

*Adrenocortical Carcinomas*
Surgery
Adrenolytic mitotane (high dose)
Steroid synthesis inhibitors
　Aminoglutethimide
　Metyrapone*
　Trilostane
　Ketoconazole†
Glucocorticoid antagonist RU 486‡
Chemotherapy for solid tumors
Palliative radiotherapy for bone metastases

*This use of metyrapone is not listed in the manufacturer's official directive.

†This use of ketoconazole is not listed in the manufacturer's official directive.

‡Not available in the United States.

are usually benign and small (90% are less than 10 mm in diameter) and cause no sellar enlargement. Currently, four therapeutic modalities are available for the treatment of these tumors: trans-sphenoidal adenomectomy, pituitary irradiation with concomitant therapy with the adrenolytic agent mitotane (*o,p'*-DDD [Lysodren]), therapy with mitotane or steroidogenic enzyme inhibitors (aminoglutethimide [Cytadren], metyrapone, ketoconazole [Nizoral]*), and bilateral adrenalectomy.

Trans-sphenoidal adenomectomy is the treatment of choice for most cases of Cushing's syndrome caused by pituitary microadenomas. If preoperatively the presence of a pituitary microadenoma can be demonstrated by imaging techniques or inferior petrosal sinus sampling, trans-sphenoidal selective resection of the adenoma is indicated. If the microadenoma is not detected by radiographic techniques but typical diagnostic criteria for Cushing's disease exist and inferior petrosal sinus sampling has lateralized the microadenoma, 90% of patients can be cured by ipsilateral hemihypophysectomy, even though in some of the patients the adenomas may not be identified at surgery. We recommend hemihypophysectomy on the side of the ACTH gradient when adenomas cannot be found, although adenomas close to the pituitary stalk or embedded into the wall of the cavernous sinus are probably not resected by this procedure. Successful surgery leads to cure of hypercortisolism with no need for permanent glucocorticoid replacement. The overall success rate of the operation exceeds 80 to 90% in the best series, with considerable variability. A small percentage of patients (approximately 5%) suffer recurrences. The currently employed diagnostic methods appear to be improving the results. The success rate of transsphenoidal operation is considerably lower (60%) in patients with recurrent Cushing's disease after a previously successful operation, or in patients with previously failed trans-sphenoidal operations, invasive macroadenomas, or "atypical" diagnostic criteria for Cushing's disease. Transient diabetes insipidus may occur during the early weeks following surgery. Permanent diabetes insipidus and cerebrospinal fluid rhinorrhea are uncommon complications but may occur more frequently in patients with repeated trans-sphenoidal surgery. The mortality rate is probably less than 1%, lower than that of bilateral adrenalectomy (approximately 4%). Treatment failures are most common in patients with pituitary macroadenomas. A CRH stimulation test has been used in the postoperative evaluation of patients cured of Cushing's disease by selective microadenomectomy. At the early postoperative period, these patients are hypocortisolemic with subnormal ACTH responses to CRH, presumably on the basis of suppression of the pituitary gland and/or hypothalamic CRH neurons, as a result of long-standing hypercortisolism. Normal cortisol levels and a normal response to CRH in this period may identify a subgroup of patients at risk for suboptimal resection and recurrence of the disease.

Pituitary x-irradiation is a reasonable alternative form of treatment following failure of trans-sphenoidal surgery or as the first line of treatment in patients judged unsuitable for surgery. The most widely used dosage of pituitary irradiation is 4500 to 5000 rad total. High-voltage, conventional x-radiation is given in 180- to 200-rad fractions over a period of 6 weeks. This treatment cures only 10 to 15%, but markedly improves another 25 to 30% of untreated adult patients (better responses in adults under 40 years of age) and about 80% of children younger than 18 years. Biochemical and clinical amelioration occurs with preservation of pituitary and adrenal function but is delayed by several months (6 to 18 months). Heavy particle beam irradiation and Bragg peak proton irradiation therapy appear to be equally effective to conventional irradiation; however, the prevalence of postirradiation panhypopituitarism is higher with the former techniques. The side effects, as well as the efficacy of therapy, may be related to the dosage of radiation administered. Progressive anterior hypopituitarism, including growth hormone deficiency, hypothyroidism, and hypogonadism, occurs in 30 to 40% of patients. Radiation-induced atrophy of the brain may also be seen with high dosages. These complications may occur several years after radiotherapy. Usually, concomitantly with and following pituitary radiation, drug therapy (mitotane) is given at low doses, ranging from 1 to 4 grams per day. Combined pituitary radiation and mitotane improves the success rate of either modality given alone.

Drug therapy alone is rarely used to treat Cushing's disease except temporarily, prior to definitive treatment. Mitotane (Lysodren) is the only available pharmacologic agent that both inhibits biosynthesis of corticosteroids (inhibits 11-beta hydroxylase and cholesterol side chain cleavage enzymes) and destroys adrenocortical cells secreting cortisol, thus producing a long-lasting effect. Therapy with mitotane alone can be successful in 30 to 40% of patients with Cushing's disease. Addition of aminoglutethimide, up to 1 gram a day orally in four divided doses, or

---

*This use of ketoconazole is not listed in the manufacturer's official directive.

metyrapone,* up to 1 gram a day† in four divided doses, can improve the success rate. During treatment, the urinary free cortisol excretion should be monitored and the dose of mitotane titrated to maintain urinary free cortisol excretion in the normal range. If adrenal insufficiency is suspected, oral hydrocortisone should be added. Although mitotane is a selective inhibitor of the *reticularis* and *fasciculata* zones of the adrenal cortex, it may on occasion affect the *zona glomerulosa*, leading to hypoaldosteronism that requires replacement with oral fludrocortisone (Florinef), 50 to 300 μg per day. Because mitotane induces liver mono-oxygenases (cytochrome P-450 enzymes) that metabolize steroids and other drugs, an adequate dose of hydrocortisone and fludrocortisone may be higher than expected. Measuring urinary 17-hydroxysteroid excretion does not provide a reliable index of adrenal suppression by the drug, since an early fall in the urinary excretion of this metabolite occurs independently of the effect of the drug on cortisol secretion. This phenomenon is a result of mitotane-induced enhancement of liver 6-hydroxylase activity that results in side tracking cortisol metabolism to 6-alpha-hydroxylated and related metabolites that are not detected by the Porter-Silber reaction, which detects 17-hydroxycorticosteroids. Side effects with mitotane therapy include anorexia, nausea, vomiting, diarrhea, skin reactions, hyperlipoproteinemia, hepatotoxicity and neurologic manifestations (primarily somnolence), lethargy, dizziness, and muscle weakness. All of the side effects described can be reversed by reducing the dose of the drug or by discontinuing therapy.

Adrenal enzyme inhibitors—aminoglutethimide, metyrapone, trilostane, and ketoconazole‡—have been used alone or in combination with mitotane or each other to control some of the symptoms and metabolic abnormalities associated with the hypercortisolemia in Cushing's disease and the ectopic ACTH syndrome. Combinations are recommended because they most frequently alleviate "breakthroughs" that occur when the drugs are used alone. In addition, one can employ moderate doses with less side effects.

Aminoglutethimide (Cytadren) acts in the first step of steroid biosynthesis, where it blocks the conversion of cholesterol to delta-5-pregnenolone in the adrenal cortex. As a result, the synthesis of cortisol, aldosterone, and androgens is inhibited. The drug has been used both in adults and in children in doses of 0.5 to 2 grams daily. Aminoglutethimide alone is only transiently effective, since the inhibitory effect of the drug on cortisol synthesis is overcome by increasing plasma concentrations of ACTH. Aminoglutethimide has gastrointestinal (anorexia, nausea, vomiting) and neurologic (lethargy, sedation, blurred vision) side effects and can cause hypothyroidism in 5% of patients. A skin rash is frequently observed during the first 10 days of therapy, which usually subsides despite continuation of treatment.

Metyrapone (Metopirone), an 11-beta hydroxylase inhibitor, blocks the final step of cortisol biosynthesis by preventing the conversion of 11-deoxycortisol to cortisol. Treatment with metyrapone alone (250 mg twice daily to 1 gram divided four times daily) or in combination with mitotane or aminoglutethimide can result in biochemical and clinical remission in patients with Cushing's disease. Metyrapone causes hypertension and hypokalemic alkalosis, a result of blockade of 11-hydroxylase and accumulation of 11-deoxycorticosterone. It also produces gastrointestinal irritation, nausea, vomiting, and allergic rash, and may worsen hirsutism. Combination of metyrapone and aminoglutethimide should lead to increased therapeutic effectiveness with decreased individual drug doses and fewer side effects.

Trilostane (Modrastane), which until recently was an investigational drug, inhibits the conversion of pregnenolone to progesterone, another critical step in cortisol biosynthesis. Trilostane at doses of 200 to 1000 mg daily* has similar side effects to those observed with aminoglutethimide.

Ketoconazole,† an antifungal agent, is a recent addition to our armamentarium of cortisol synthesis inhibitors. The drug can be given at 600 to 1200 mg a day‡ in three or more divided doses. Amelioration of clinical and metabolic manifestations of hypercortisolism has been seen within 4 to 6 weeks of treatment. The drug is well tolerated but has some hepatoxicity, primarily of the hepatocellular type. Ketoconazole can also cause nausea, vomiting, abdominal pain, and pruritus in 1 to 3% of patients. Etomidate, an imidazole containing anesthetic agent, has also been found to inhibit cortisol secretion in a manner similar to that of ketoconazole. At the present time, etomidate has not been used for treatment of patients with Cushing's syndrome in the United States.

The indications for adrenal surgery for Cushing's disease have been altered radically by the

---

*This use of metyrapone is not listed in the manufacturer's official directive.
†Exceeds dosage recommended by the manufacturer.
‡This use of ketoconazole is not listed in the manufacturer's official directive.

---

*Exceeds dosage recommended by the manufacturer.
†This use of ketoconazole is not lised in the manufacturer's offical directive.
‡Exceeds dosage recommended by the manufacturer.

success and low morbidity of trans-sphenoidal surgery. Bilateral total adrenalectomy could be considered for adults who have failed selective pituitary adenomectomy or hypophysectomy and in whom ectopic ACTH secretion has been unequivocally ruled out. When performed properly, it leads to cure of hypercortisolism. The major disadvantages of bilateral adrenalectomy are that the individual after surgery is committed to lifelong daily cortisol and fludrocortisone replacements; that it fails to attack the cause underlying the hypersecretion of ACTH; and that relapses, although uncommon, can occur as a result of growth of adrenal rest tissue or an adrenal remnant. In addition, perioperative mortality is approximately four times higher than that of transsphenoidal surgery, although it can be minimized by careful perioperative preparation. Nelson's syndrome (large pituitary macroadenomas secreting great amounts of ACTH and β-lipotropin resulting in skin hyperpigmentation) may occur in approximately 10 to 15% of patients with Cushing's disease treated with bilateral adrenalectomy. Clinically apparent Nelson's syndrome may occur months or years after bilateral adrenalectomy. These ACTH secreting macroadenomas may be locally invasive and extend above the diaphragma sellae, causing visual field defects. Rarely, they can metastasize locally in the brain and distant hepatic metastatic nodules have been reported. Treatment for such ACTH secreting macroadenomas is usually difficult and includes trans-sphenoidal surgery (if not too large) followed by 5000 rad of conventional pituitary x-radiation.

## The Ectopic ACTH Syndrome

Treatment of the ectopic ACTH syndrome is directed, if possible, at the primary tumor. If the tumor is totally excised, hypercortisolism will be cured. Tumors secreting ACTH, however, are often occult or disseminated at the time of diagnosis, and other therapeutic options must be employed. Therapy, other than primary tumor excision, is directed toward the adrenal glands and at the glucocorticoid receptor level. The use of the adrenolytic mitotane and steroidogenic enzyme inhibitors, such as aminoglutethimide, metyrapone, and ketoconazole, is the first line of defense to control hypercortisolism and ameliorate the clinical manifestations of the syndrome. However, the very high ACTH levels usually present in the ectopic ACTH syndrome may overcome rapidly the suppressive effect of these drugs. The glucocorticoid receptor antagonist RU 486*

*Not available in the United States.

has been used recently to treat the hypercortisolism of patients with ectopic Cushing's syndrome. It is relatively well tolerated and nontoxic at doses ranging between 10 and 20 mg per kg per day. However, because cortisol production fluctuates in many patients with the ectopic ACTH syndrome, treatment of these patients with a fixed dose of RU 486 introduces the risk of adrenal insufficiency. RU 486 is still an investigational drug, and its use is limited to investigational protocols. Recently, another drug, the long-acting somatostatin analogue SMS 201–995 (octreotide acetate; [Sandostatin]), has been used successfully in the treatment of patients with the ectopic ACTH Cushing's syndrome and probably could be valuable for the long-term medical management of such patients. SMS 201–995 may reduce ACTH secretion by occasional tumors, but has no effect on tumor growth. The usual dose is 100 μg three times per day, subcutaneously. Bilateral adrenalectomy is indicated in a patient with Cushing's syndrome caused by ectopic ACTH production when the patient is severely ill, the primary tumor is disseminated or not found, or when medical therapy fails or is poorly tolerated. Preparation of the patients for bilateral adrenalectomy with cortisol synthesis inhibitors or RU 486 is recommended.

## Adrenocortical Tumors

Surgical resection is the treatment of choice for all primary adrenocortical tumors. Unilateral total adrenalectomy is recommended for the autonomous benign cortisol secreting adrenal adenomas. Bilateral adrenalectomy is recommended for patients with micronodular adrenal disease. Complete resection of the tumor is the treatment of choice for adrenal carcinoma. If complete resection cannot be achieved, however, as much of the tumor as possible should be removed. Solitary local recurrences or metastases of adrenocortical carcinoma should also be removed surgically, if possible. Adrenal carcinomas causing Cushing's syndrome are highly malignant neoplasms. Long-term remissions, however, have been reported following complete resection of adrenocortical carcinoma and long-term remissions have followed surgical resection of hepatic, pulmonary, or cerebral metastases. Once it is known that the patient does not have surgically curable disease, therapy with the adrenolytic agent mitotane is usually initiated. Mitotane given at maximally tolerated oral doses (up to 16 grams per day) has been the only drug that has some effectiveness in patients with metastatic adrenocortical carcinoma. Tumor regression or arrest of growth has been observed in as many as one-third of the patients, while the agent ameliorates the endocrine syndrome in approximately two-thirds of these patients. Mean survival time, however, does not appear to be altered, although there are occasional patients with unresectable carcinomas who achieve long-term survival. The side effects of mitotane are found to be dose dependent and have been previously mentioned. Starting with low doses of mitotane (250 to 500 mg four times a day) and gradually advancing to therapeutic levels (12 to 16 grams daily), one can minimize to some degree the side effects. Before initiation of therapy, a tumor mass should be defined, which can be followed objectively by radiologic procedures (usually CT scan or MRI) for monitoring therapeutic efficacy. Patients taking mitotane may develop hypocortisolism and hypoaldosteronism, and hydrocortisone or fludrocortisone should be added as needed. Occasionally, for the correction of hypercortisolism, steroid synthesis inhibitors (aminoglutethimide, metyrapone, ketoconazole) or the glucocorticoid antagonist RU 486 is required. Radiation therapy is occasionally helpful for palliation of metastases.

### Postoperative Steroid Replacement

Following a successful trans-sphenoidal operation in Cushing's disease or removal of an autonomous ACTH or cortisol secreting tumor, a period of adrenal insufficiency ensues, during which glucocorticoids must be replaced. This abnormality of the hypothalamic-pituitary-adrenal axis can last as long as 1 year. Intraoperatively, and during the first 2 postoperative days, 100 mg per $M^2$ per day of hydrocortisone or its equivalent is given intravenously. Once the patient has recovered from the surgical procedure, oral replacement doses of hydrocortisone, 20 to 30 mg (12 to 15 mg per $M^2$) per day, are initiated. Patients who are cured often complain of weakness and lack of energy at these doses, a sign of successful surgery. The replacement dose of hydrocortisone is maintained for 1 month and then tapered. Tapering starts by doubling the daily dose and giving it on alternate days for 2 months. Then the patient is tested with a short ACTH stimulation test (Cortrosyn, 250 µg intravenously, with cortisol measured at 60 minutes). If the response to this test is normal (plasma cortisol above 18 µg per dl), an attempt is made to discontinue hydrocortisone therapy. If the result is subnormal, the therapy is continued for another 2 months and the test repeated. The majority of patients can discontinue glucocorticoid replacement within 10 to 12 months postoperatively. During this period, patients should be given extra glucocorticoids during stress. During minor stress

(nausea, vomiting, fever above 100° F), they should double the daily dose until the illness is resolved. During major stress (surgery), they should be given 300 mg of parenteral hydrocortisone daily, beginning 1 day before surgery and tapered to normal replacement as rapidly as recovery allows. All patients should wear medical alert badges indicating that they are receiving glucocorticoid replacement and be prepared to use an emergency kit.

### Exogenous Cushing's Syndrome

This is most commonly seen in patients with renal, autoimmune, hematologic, and neoplastic conditions that require chronic pharmacologic glucocorticoid therapy. Exposure to glucocorticoids for periods of time sufficient to produce symptoms and signs as those found in endogenous Cushing's syndrome can be expected to also produce hypothalamic-pituitary-adrenal axis suppression that may require up to 1 year to recover. Therefore, every effort should be made to minimize the period during which steroids are given daily. Once the disease process has been controlled, the daily dose should be doubled and administered on alternate days. An alternate schedule of administration is crucial in children, in whom daily administration stunts growth. Many glucocorticoid-responsive diseases are now successfully controlled in this manner, whereas signs and symptoms as those of Cushing's syndrome are diminished. Patients should be given extra glucocorticoids during stress like postoperative cured patients with Cushing's syndrome.

# DIABETES INSIPIDUS

method of
MARYA GENDZIELEWSKI, M.D., and
ARNOLD M. MOSES, M.D.
*SUNY Health Science Center and Veterans
    Administration Medical Center*
*Syracuse, New York*

Central or neurogenic diabetes insipidus occurs when there is deficiency of arginine vasopressin (AVP) release in response to osmotic stimuli in the physiologic range. The causative lesion may be at any locus within the hypothalamic neurohypophyseal tract. However, lesions confined to the posterior pituitary usually cause only transient symptoms because AVP can be released in adequate quantities from the pituitary stalk. Deficiency of AVP results in an excessive excretion of dilute urine. This causes a small increment in plasma osmolality, which stimulates thirst and the intake of sufficient water to dilute plasma solutes to a normal osmolality. In the presence of thyroid or adrenocortical insufficiency, polyuria becomes evident only after initiation of appropriate replacement therapy. Occasionally diabetes insipidus occurs in association with impaired thirst sensation.

Central diabetes insipidus may be caused by a variety of lesions that disrupt hypothalamic function. Most commonly, these lesions are head trauma, primary brain tumors pre- or postoperatively, and metastatic malignancy, most often from the breast. Sarcoidosis and histiocytosis X are less common causes. The incidence of idiopathic diabetes insipidus has decreased with the availability of more sophisticated diagnostic techniques.

Nephrogenic diabetes insipidus is a form of hypotonic polyuria characterized by the inability of renal tubules to respond to endogenous or exogenous AVP. Although a congenital form exists that most severely affects males, this disorder is usually seen as an acquired defect. Causes include many chronic renal diseases, electrolyte abnormalities (hypokalemia and hypercalcemia), and nephrotoxic drugs (most commonly lithium). Specific interventions against the underlying disease may help to ameliorate the polyuria. However, in some cases nonhormonal or hormonal therapy may be necessary.

The diagnosis of diabetes insipidus can generally be made without measurement of AVP levels in blood or urine and without saline infusion studies. The diagnosis can almost always be established when urine osmolality is low in association with an elevated plasma osmolality. If these random values do not differentiate between diabetes insipidus and overhydration, repeat measurements made after a short period (1 or 2 hours) of controlled water restriction usually allow a distinction to be made. An impaired antidiuretic response to injected vasopressin (Pitressin) or desmopressin (DDAVP) usually distinguishes nephrogenic from central diabetes insipidus.

As long as patients with diabetes insipidus are conscious, retain normal thirst, and have enough fluid to drink, they seldom allow themselves to become more than mildly dehydrated. Severe dehydration with markedly elevated serum sodium concentrations may occur when diabetes insipidus is associated with thirst center failure or with inability to take sufficient water because of unconsciousness, infancy, or unavailability of fluid for other reasons. Occasionally, bladder emptying may not keep pace with urine flow, resulting in bladder distention, hydronephrosis, and renal insufficiency.

## HORMONAL TREATMENT

Diabetes insipidus is treated hormonally with synthetic peptides (vasopressin or desmopressin). Arginine vasopressin is the natural hormone of humans, whereas desmopressin is a synthetic analogue with a prolonged action. Unlike vasopressin, desmopressin is minimally vasoactive and can thus be used without fear of precipitating angina or of causing abdominal cramping and headaches. Some characteristics of these preparations are listed in Tables 1 and 2.

Aqueous AVP is used primarily in the initial management of unconscious patients with diabetes insipidus following head trauma or neurosurgical procedures. Its short duration of action allows recognition of the recovery of neurohypophyseal function and helps prevent the development of water intoxication in patients receiving intravenous fluids. As with all forms of vasopressin, it is safest to administer subsequent doses when polyuria reappears.

For most patients with diabetes insipidus, the treatment of choice is intranasal administration of desmopressin (100 μg per ml). Two delivery systems are available: a nasal tube, which the patient uses to blow measured amounts (.05 to .2 ml) of desmopressin into the nose, and a compression pump system which can deliver only 0.1 ml. Table 2 gives the duration of action of the nasal preparation when 10, 15, and 20 μg of the drug (0.1 to 0.2 ml) are instilled. The duration of action and lack of side effects of desmopressin have largely eliminated the use of lypressin. The nasal absorption of desmopressin may be decreased in the presence of conditions that alter the absorptive capacity of the upper respiratory mucosa. In such circumstances, and in the unconscious or uncooperative patient with diabetes insipidus, desmopressin should be given by injection. The mean duration of action of desmopressin injected in amounts ranging from 0.5 to 4.0 μg is listed in Table 2. The major clinical effect of increasing the dose of either the intranasal or the injectable form of DDAVP is to increase the duration of antidiuresis rather than its magnitude. Occasional patients with lithium-induced nephrogenic diabetic insipidus and some female patients with congenital nephrogenic diabetes insipidus may obtain substantial clinical improvement from the injection of large amounts (6 to 8 μg) of desmopressin.

Previously, diabetes insipidus was often treated with vasopressin (Pitressin) tannate in oil. However, this preparation is no longer being manufactured.

## NONHORMONAL TREATMENT

Patients with diabetes insipidus who have some residual releasable AVP may respond to oral treatment with several nonhormonal agents. These agents are occasionally used despite the safety and efficacy of desmopressin. Chlorpropamide (Diabinese) stimulates AVP release from the neurohypophysis and potentiates the action of submaximal amounts of AVP on the renal tubule. Oral doses of 200 to 500 mg taken once

TABLE 1. **Characteristics of Vasopressin Preparations Used in the Treatment of Patients with Neurogenic Diabetes Insipidus**

| Generic Description | Trade Name | Concentration | ml/Ampule or Bottle | Manufacturer |
|---|---|---|---|---|
| Arginine vasopressin | Pitressin synthetic | 20 U/ml | 0.5 and 1.0 | Parke-Davis |
| Desmopressin | DDAVP injection | 4 μg/ml | 1.0 | Rorer |
| Desmopression | Stimate* | 4 μg/ml | 10.0 | Armour |
| Desmopressin | DDAVP intranasal | 100 μg/ml | 2.5 and 5.0† | Rorer |
| Lypressin | Diapid | 50 U/ml (185 μg/ml) | 8.0 | Sandoz |
| Vasopressin tannate in oil‡ | Pitressin tannate in oil | 5 U/ml | 1.0 | Parke-Davis |

*Marketed for the treatment of von Willebrand's disease.
†The nasal tube form contains 2.5 ml, and the metered dose form contains 5.0 ml.
‡Must be shaken vigorously and warmed in water or hand to suspend powder in peanut oil. The manufacturer discontinued production of this product early in 1990.

daily are usually sufficient for an antidiuretic effect. The response starts within several hours of administration and usually lasts for 24 hours. Hypoglycemia may occur, but usually can be avoided by adherence to a regular schedule of meals. Clofibrate (Atromid) is capable of stimulating the release of residual AVP and in doses of 500 mg four times a day often results in a prompt and sustained antidiuresis. Clofibrate has been associated with the development of "flu-like" symptoms and myalgias and must be used with caution in patients with a history of peptic ulcer disease and in patients on oral anticoagulants. In some patients, combined treatment with chlorpropamide and clofibrate results in restoration of normal water balance. Carbamazepine (Tegretol) frequently produces antidiuresis in patients with diabetes insipidus by stimulation of AVP release. Doses of 400 to 600 mg daily are effective, but the drug is not widely used because of toxic side effects. Patients with nephrogenic diabetes insipidus may have substantial improvement of polyuria by inducing a sodium-depleted state by restricting sodium intake and administration of a diuretic such as 50 mg per day of

hydrochlorothiazide. This should not be attempted in patients whose nephrogenic diabetes insipidus is due to lithium.

## GENERAL PRINCIPLES OF FLUID BALANCE

**The Alert Conscious Patient.** When antidiuretic therapy is initiated in the alert conscious patient with diabetes insipidus, excessive drinking must be consciously prevented for at least several days. Because some patients have diabetes insipidus combined with a form of primary polydipsia, they must constantly be alerted against excessive drinking, which would result in water intoxication with an SIADH-like (inappropriate antidiuretic hormone) syndrome. Thirst may be perceived with a normal or low plasma sodium concentration because of a dry mouth, which can occur with mouth breathing, anticholinergic drugs, beta-adrenergic blockers, or cigarette smoking. In some patients, education about water intake must constantly be reinforced with emphasis about drinking only when thirsty. For instance, difficulty ensues when patients drink fluids such as beer when they are not thirsty.

TABLE 2. **Mean Time That Urine Remains Hypertonic to Plasma After Administration of Vasopressin to Adult Patients with Neurogenic Diabetes Insipidus**

| Generic Description | Route of Administration | Amount Administered | Mean Duration of Action (hr)* |
|---|---|---|---|
| Arginine vasopressin | Subcutaneous, Intramuscular | 5 U (12.5 μg) | 4 |
| Desmopressin | † | 0.5 μg | 8 |
| Desmopressin | † | 1.0 μg | 12 |
| Desmopressin | † | 2.0 μg | 16 |
| Desmopressin | † | 4.0 μg | 20 |
| Desmopressin | Intranasal | 10 μg (0.1 ml) | 12 |
| Desmopressin | Intranasal | 15 μg (0.15) | 16 |
| Desmopressin | Intranasal | 20 μg (0.2 ml) | 20 |
| Lypressin | Intranasal | 2 sprays in each nostril (about 10 U) | 5 |
| Vasopressin tannate in oil | Intramuscular | 5 U | 48–72 |

*These durations are variable from patient to patient but are quite consistent in individual patients.
†Subcutaneous, intramuscular, or intravenous.
*Note:* Onset of antidiuretic actions of all the above (except vasopressin tannate in oil) is about 30–45 min. Onset of action of vasopressin tannate in oil is 2–4 hr).

**The Alert Conscious Patient with Adipsia.** This type of patient presents a very difficult management problem. The patient and his or her family must closely and continuously monitor intake and output of fluids, body weight, vital signs, and plasma sodium concentrations. This type of patient must always relate his or her fluid intake to urine output plus fluid losses in perspiration and via the gastrointestinal tract. He or she may fail to experience thirst despite the development of hypovolemic shock with a serum sodium concentration of up to 180 to 200 mEq per liter.

**The Confused, Obtunded, or Unconscious Patient.** These patients, who are usually seen postoperatively or after head trauma, are monitored in the same way as the alert conscious patient with adipsia. The volume and osmolality of 4- or 8-hour urine collections should be closely monitored and fluid losses replaced with intravenous fluids to match urinary losses plus insensible (and other) fluid losses. The patient's serum sodium concentration should be determined at least daily, along with body weight, vital signs, blood urea nitrogen (BUN), uric acid, and creatinine concentrations. Normal saline in the presence of hypernatremia is required only to help restore pulse and blood pressure to normal in hypovolemic patients. Otherwise, patients with hypernatremia should be treated with dextrose in water (see later) while appropriate hormonal therapy is instituted and maintained.

## SPECIAL PROBLEMS OF FLUID BALANCE

**Preparation for Diagnostic Tests or Treatment.** Special care must be taken when patients with treated diabetes insipidus are subjected to certain "standard protocols" associated with many diagnostic and therapeutic procedures. These protocols require the patient either to be fluid restricted, like when being prepared for intravenous pyelography, or to be hydrated, as after the administration of contrast media or for chemotherapy. Tests that require patients to have no oral fluids should not be performed without adequate intravenous hydration matched to their urine output. Intravenous fluids should be started from the time the patient is no longer able to take oral fluids and may be discontinued when oral fluids are again allowed. In contrast, patients receiving antidiuretic therapy for diabetes insipidus should not be made to "force fluids" beyond the amounts determined by thirst or to have hydration orders at rates not related to urinary output. If high urine flow rates are desired, the patient's antidiuretic therapy should be discontinued so that polyuria results. Oral or intravenous fluids can then be given to match the large urine volumes. Sometimes it may be appropriate (in order to obtain more precise timing of a diuresis) to continue antidiuretic therapy and administer intravenous furosemide. The monitoring of serum sodium levels will greatly assist in determining the status of fluid balance in these situations.

**The Hypernatremic Patient.** Hypernatremia in patients with diabetes insipidus is usually associated with normal total body sodium. The hypernatremia is due to loss of free water by way of the kidneys, but losses from the skin and lungs can aggravate the problem. The hypernatremia may cause neurologic symptoms such as restlessness, irritability, lethargy, muscle twitching, and spasticity, which may culminate in coma, seizures, and death. Neurologic sequelae, particularly in children, are not uncommon.

Postoperative hypernatremia should be prevented by the early recognition of diabetes insipidus before and during, as well as after, surgery and by discouraging the use of osmotic diuretics during surgery. Patients should be changed to oral fluids as soon as possible, and the adequacy of the patient's thirst mechanism to control fluid intake appropriately should be evaluated. Diabetes insipidus that occurs in the postoperative or head trauma patient may be variable (biphasic or triphasic), and frequently the diabetes insipidus is transient. Therefore, hormonal treatment should occasionally be withheld to determine if the diabetes insipidus recurs. There may be amelioration of symptoms after several months and, rarely, after 6 months.

The goals of treating hypernatremia in patients with diabetes insipidus are the restoration of normal plasma volume and tonicity. If there are circulatory disturbances due to hypovolemia, isotonic sodium chloride should be given until systemic hemodynamics are stabilized. Subsequently, the hypernatremia should be treated with 5% dextrose in water. The water deficit in these patients can be calculated on the basis of the serum sodium concentration and on the assumption that 60% of body weight is water. For example, if the usual weight is 75 kg, the patient would normally have $75 \text{ kg} \times 0.6 = 45$ liters of total body water. If serum sodium is 154 mEq per liter, the patient has a 10% deficit of water

$$\frac{(154 - 140)}{140}$$

and needs 4.5 liters of water to correct his or her deficit. Obviously, continuing losses of water must also be replaced. Despite inaccuracies, this approach provides an approximate value that can be used in planning therapy. Most authors feel that the hypernatremia should be corrected slowly over 48 to 72 hours, and not at a rate greater than 2 mOsm per kg per hour. More rapid correction can be associated with the development of seizures, apparently owing to cerebral edema.

Treatment of hypernatremia due to water loss must also address associated electrolyte abnormalities and underlying medical and surgical conditions. A special example of this would be the patient with coexisting diabetes insipidus and diabetes mellitus. When marked hyperglycemia exists, the "corrected" serum sodium value should be used when calculating the water deficit. Slightly low or normal serum sodium concentrations in the presence of extremely high serum glucose concentrations often result, when corrected, in hypernatremic values. The "corrected" serum sodium concentration can easily be calculated by increasing the serum sodium concentration by 1.5 mEq per liter for every 100 mg per dl increment in the serum glucose concentration above 100 mg per dl. For example, in a patient with a sodium level of 138 mEq per liter and glucose of 700 mg per dl, the "corrected" serum sodium concentration would be $138 + (1.5 \times 6)$ or 147 mEq per liter. Water can be given by mouth if the patient is conscious and able to drink. Water should never be given by nasogastric tube to a comatose patient unless a cuffed endotracheal tube is in place.

**The Hyponatremic Patient.** Hyponatremia is closely correlated with the degree of water overload. The magnitude of the excessive body water can be calculated by use of the same approach as described earlier under *hypernatremia*. Occasionally, hyponatremia is aggravated by large losses of sodium in the urine, probably related to increased levels of atrial natriuretic peptide (ANP), inhibition of aldosterone, and an increased glomerular filtration rate. Urine sodium concentrations should occasionally be obtained to determine if it is in the usual range (20 to 40 mEq per liter), high (around 100 mEq per liter), or very high (around 180 mEq per liter). The treatment of such natriuresis in the water-overloaded patient can only be partially corrected with saline infusions, since the natriuresis continues until the hypervolemic state is corrected. In the overhydrated hyponatremic patient, urine should be measured every 4 to 8 hours for volume and osmolality, and fluid replacement should be ordered *in relation to urine volume*. It is inappropriate to write for a fixed amount of fluid replacement, and an NPO order should never be written. If the patient is being under-replaced with fluids to correct for previous over-replacement, plasma sodium concentration should be checked frequently. The complaint of thirst in a water-restricted patient should never be ignored. Insensible fluid losses of about 600 ml per day should be considered when ordering fluid replacement. The direct cause of the hyponatremia in patients with treated diabetes insipidus is over-replacement with fluids. The hyponatremia is only indirectly related to the antidiuretic hormone used in treatment. Therefore, it is usually much less disruptive of long-term management to adjust fluid intake than to discontinue hormonal therapy and allow the patient to "break through." In severe situations, however, interruption of hormonal therapy may be justified under a closely monitored situation. When the patient has symptomatic hyponatremia, several hundred milliliters of 3 or 5% saline may be given intravenously, perhaps together with intravenous furosemide. Even in the presence of vasopressin, furosemide (Lasix) causes the excretion of a slightly hypotonic or an isotonic urine. Thyroid or adrenal insufficiency may cause or aggravate the hyponatremia in these patients and should be treated.

The symptoms of hyponatremia depend on the acuteness of the condition. Rapid lowering of serum sodium concentration to below 125 mEq per liter may cause nausea, emesis, muscular twitching, convulsions, and coma. The mortality rate may be as high as 50%. When plasma sodium is lowered slowly to the same level, patients usually have fewer symptoms.

Hyponatremia should be corrected slowly, which is generally considered to mean correction of one-third of the abnormality in sodium concentration per day for 3 days. The frequently fatal condition of central pontine myelinolysis may be caused by the overly rapid correction of hyponatremia.

# GOITER

method of
GILBERT H. DANIELS, M.D.
*Massachusetts General Hospital*
*Boston, Massachusetts*

The term *goiter* refers to any enlargement of the thyroid gland. When a goiter is palpated, the clinician must ask several important questions: (1) Is the goiter due to one or more nodules or is the thyroid diffusely enlarged? (2) Are there symptoms related to the goiter? (3) Is a malignancy likely? (4) Is the thyroid function normal? The answers to these questions help determine what kind of goiter is present and how it should be treated.

In iodine-deficient areas of the world, goiter is very common. With iodine deficiency, thyroid hormone output falls and serum thyroid stimulating hormone (TSH) is elevated. Although TSH-induced diffuse goiter might be predicted, multinodular goiters are the rule.

Multiple cell populations are present within these goiters, with variable rates of proliferation and variable ability to concentrate iodine. Rapidly proliferating cells give rise to nodular areas that may be either "hot" or "cold" on radioisotope scanning. The elevated serum TSH concentration accelerates cell proliferation and facilitates nodule development. In the United States, nodular goiters presumably develop in similar fashion, from cell populations with variable proliferative rates. Whereas iodine deficiency–induced TSH elevation is not present in the United States, the prevalence of nodular goiter is not as high as in iodine deficiency areas.

In the United States, diffuse goiter is usually due to autoimmune thyroid disease: Hashimoto's thyroiditis, postpartum thyroiditis, silent thyroiditis, or Graves' disease. If marked thyroid tenderness is present, subacute thyroiditis is likely. Drugs that inhibit thyroid hormone release (e.g., lithium or iodides) or thyroid hormone synthesis (e.g., propylthiouracil [PTU] or methimazole [Tapazole]) can produce a diffuse goiter or lead to growth of a Hashimoto's gland. Thyroid cancer uncommonly presents as a diffuse or asymmetrical goiter.

## CLINICAL DIAGNOSIS

When multiple thyroid nodules are palpated, the likely diagnosis is multinodular goiter. Careful measurement of individual nodules and the neck circumference provides important baseline information. The firm lobes of Hashimoto's thyroiditis are often misinterpreted as nodules. An easily palpable pyramidal lobe favors the diagnosis of Hashimoto's thyroiditis.

When the thyroid is diffusely tender, subacute thyroiditis is most likely, although Hashimoto's thyroiditis is occasionally painful. A painful nodule suggests that hemorrhage into or infarction of an adenoma has occurred. Although neck pain is a rare presentation of thyroid cancer, any unusually prolonged thyroid pain should be viewed with suspicion.

Large goiters may cause obstructive symptoms such as dyspnea (due to tracheal narrowing) and dysphagia (due to esophageal compression). Difficulty in swallowing saliva is a common complaint, but is usually due to globus, rather than the goiter itself. Hoarseness may be secondary to involvement of the recurrent laryngeal nerve leading to vocal cord palsy and requires appropriate laryngoscopic evaluation.

Cancer is not common in patients with multinodular goiter, but previous head or neck irradiation increases the likelihood of a malignancy. Rapidly growing thyroid nodules or goiters, especially in older patients, are of concern.

Thyroid function tests are mandatory, with the measurement of serum TSH by ultrasensitive assay being most important. In the United States, patients with nodular goiters have normal or low serum TSH concentrations. Patients with undetectable serum TSH concentrations are either hyperthyroid (elevated serum $T_4$, free $T_4$, or $T_3$) or borderline hyperthyroid (normal serum $T_4$, free $T_4$, and $T_3$). A low or undetectable serum TSH concentration implies thyroid autonomy and a patient at risk for developing spontaneous or iodine-induced hyperthyroidism (e.g., after radiocontrast dye exposure). Thyroid hormone therapy is contraindicated in patients with thyroid autonomy, as hyperthyroidism often results from such therapy.

A "nodular goiter" with an elevated serum TSH concentration is most likely Hashimoto's thyroiditis. If a thyroid scan (or ultrasound) is obtained in such patients, the presumed nodules are found to correspond to the thyroid lobes. The finding of high-titer antithyroid antibodies supports the diagnosis of Hashimoto's thyroiditis, even with a normal serum TSH. Rapid growth of the thyroid in a patient with known or presumed Hashimoto's thyroiditis suggests a thyroid lymphoma.

When a nodular goiter contains a dominant or clinically suspicious (e.g., firm, fixed, rapidly growing) nodule a thyroid scan should be obtained. If the nodule is "cold," a needle biopsy should be performed. Small multinodular goiters rarely require scans. Although a thyroid ultrasound examination may be useful in following the size of selected nodules, it is usually unnecessary and is rarely helpful in following the goiter itself.

A chest x-ray or CT scan is necessary to look for substernal extension of large or low lying goiters and in patients with tracheal deviation. If the trachea appears narrowed on chest x-ray or if shortness of breath is present, a flow-volume loop should be obtained to judge the severity of tracheal obstruction.

## THERAPY

Does the goiter need to be treated? The questions asked in the first paragraph are helpful in answering this question. Large, symptomatic goiters causing hoarseness, shortness of breath, or esophageal compression should be excised. Although suppressive therapy is often attempted in such patients, large multinodular goiters are often fibrotic and hemorrhagic and rarely shrink significantly. Surgery should also be offered to patients with huge, cosmetically disfiguring multinodular goiters, even when asymptomatic. Substernal goiters are difficult to follow clinically and are best treated surgically. Substernal goiter excision can generally be accomplished through a neck incision and rarely requires splitting of the sternum. Dominant cold nodules or clinically suspicious cold nodules should be biopsied and a surgical decision based on the biopsy findings. Patients with prior head or neck irradiation and multinodular goiters may require surgery or biopsy of suspicious nodules.

Patients with toxic nodular goiters are best treated with radioactive iodine ($^{131}$I) therapy, generally after pretreatment with antithyroid drugs (methimazole [Tapazole] or propylthiouracil [PTU]). Thyroid function will return to normal even when the size of the thyroid gland does not change. If patients with known autonomous multinodular goiters require intravenous contrast material or iodine containing drugs (such as amiodarone [Cordarone]), prophylactic antithyroid drug therapy (to prevent hyperthyroidism) should be considered.

The majority of nodular goiters are small to medium sized and are asymptomatic. These can be suppressed with L-thyroxine (Synthroid or Levothroid), provided that a pretreatment (ultrasensitive) serum TSH measurement is within normal limits. The object of such therapy is to inhibit TSH release and shrink the thyroid (minority) or to prevent further growth (majority). L-Thyroxine should be prescribed in graded doses to lower the serum TSH to low or, less commonly, undetectable values. This is a reasonable approach in younger patients. In the elderly or in those with heart disease, such therapy is often unnecessary or potentially hazardous. L-Thyroxine is commonly prescribed after total or subtotal goiter surgery and for irradiated patients with nodular goiter who do not seem to require surgery.

A follow-up examination 3 months after the initial goiter assessment will ensure that rapid growth is not taking place. Although the sudden increase in size of a individual nodule is commonly due to fluid formation or hemorrhage, a needle aspiration should be performed to confirm this. Should a nodule or goiter actually grow under observation or on suppressive therapy, surgery is indicated. Stable goiters can be followed at 6-month and eventually yearly intervals. Thyroid function (including serum $T_4$, free $T_4$, $T_3[RIA]$,* and TSH) should be measured yearly to be sure that subtle thyrotoxicosis is not developing and that thyroid hormone therapy is not excessive.

---

*$T_3(RIA)$ = serum triiodothyronine measured by radioimmunoassay.

# HYPERPARATHYROIDISM AND HYPOPARATHYROIDISM

method of
SOLOMON POSEN, M.D.
*University of Sydney*
*Sydney, Australia*

## PHYSIOLOGY OF PARATHYROID HORMONE

Parathyroid hormone (PTH) is secreted by the parathyroid glands and is delivered, via the blood stream, to various target tissues, particularly the kidneys and the skeleton. In the kidneys, PTH enhances the synthesis of cyclic adenosine monophosphate (AMP), the reabsorption of calcium from the tubules, and the synthesis of 1,25-dihydroxyvitamin D. In addition, PTH diminishes the tubular reabsorption of phosphate. In bone, PTH stimulates osteoblastic activity with an increase in bone formation and an increase in the synthesis of alkaline phosphatase and osteocalcin. Osteoclasts, which are also stimulated by PTH (possibly indirectly), release bone mineral into the circulation. As a result, hyperparathyroid individuals have high serum calcium concentrations, while serum inorganic phosphate concentrations are low. In hypoparathyroid states, the situation is reversed—serum calcium concentrations are low, while serum inorganic phosphate concentrations are high.

The effects of PTH on urine calcium are complex. Whereas the enhanced tubular reabsorption of calcium reduces urinary calcium, a high serum calcium concentration has the opposite effect. It raises the filtered load with an increase in urinary calcium. The second of these effects predominates, so that the majority of patients with hyperparathyroidism have high urinary calcium values.

## PRIMARY HYPERPARATHYROIDISM

This condition, which usually affects only one of the four glands, is characterized by adenoma formation or hyperplasia of PTH secreting cells with hypersecretion of the hormone. As the name suggests, the cause of primary hyperparathyroidism is unknown. In a few patients it follows neck irradiation or long-term lithium carbonate consumption, but in the vast majority of patients (most of whom are middle aged or elderly women) no underlying mechanism is discernible. In about 5% of patients, other glands such as the pituitary are also involved ("multiple endocrine neoplasia"). Parathyroid carcinoma is extremely rare and accounts for less than 0.5% of cases of primary hyperparathyroidism.

It is now realized that far from being a rare disorder, primary hyperparathyroidism is at least as common as hyperthyroidism. The old modes of presentation ("stones, bones, and abdominal groans") have become uncommon, and most of the patients are now discovered during the diagnostic work-up for apparently unrelated disorders. Patients with such diverse conditions as ischemic heart disease, gallbladder disease, depression, or nonspecific pain syndromes are increasingly found to have high serum calcium concentrations, and further investigations show that they have primary hyperparathyroidism.

### Diagnosis

A patient who is found to be hypercalcemic may have one of several disorders. These include sarcoidosis, the milk-alkali syndrome, hyperthyroidism, and immobilization, but for practical purposes these rare causes can usually be diagnosed by the clinical scenario (immobilization), a few simple questions (calcium consumption, vitamin D consumption), and physical examination (lymphadenopathy or pulmonary signs). Ninety-five per cent of hypercalcemic patients suffer from just two conditions—primary hyperparathyroidism or various malignancies. In general, hypercalcemia of malignancy occurs in patients who look ill and whose malignant conditions are overt rather than occult. Moreover, hypercalcemia of malignancy is highly unlikely in a patient whose serum calcium was elevated more than 6 months previously.

The diagnosis of primary hyperparathyroidism should be suspected in every patient with serum calcium elevation. Serum inorganic phosphate is usually low or in the low-normal range, whereas urine calcium is high or in the high-normal range (see Physiology of Parathyroid Hormone). Serum alkaline phosphatase activites and serum $1,25(OH)_2$-vitamin D concentrations are not consistently abnormal and are therefore not useful as diagnostic tests.

PTH assays are now widely available, and in good laboratories these assays are generally reliable. An elevated serum PTH concentration in the presence of hypercalcemia is virtually diagnostic of hyperparathyroidism, so that additional tests such as serum ionized calcium and urinary cyclic AMP measurements are not usually required. There is a positive correlation between the severity of hypercalcemia and the serum PTH concentration; therefore, patients with gross hypercalcemia and unimpressive serum PTH elevation should be suspected of suffering from conditions other than hyperparathyroidism.

A large number of imaging procedures such as ultrasonography, subtraction isotope scanning, and CT scanning have been used in attempts to localize the lesions preoperatively. None of these techniques are satisfactory. An experienced surgeon can localize 95% of abnormal parathyroid glands at the first operation, and there is no imaging procedure with an equivalent yield. Moreover, preoperative imaging techniques frequently display large lesions (which do not require imaging) while failing to display glands that measure less than 1 cm in diameter. The estimation of PTH in blood obtained from the venous drainage system has also proved disappointing.

### Treatment

The major problem of hyperparathyroidism relates not to the diagnosis (which is usually easy) or the preoperative localization (which is gener-

ally unhelpful) but to treatment. There is no satisfactory medical therapy for primary hyperparathyroidism. Ethinyl estradiol (Estinyl) (30 $\mu$g per day) lowers serum calcium in hyperparathyroidism, but elderly women unable or unwilling to undergo surgery are frequently unsuitable for estrogen therapy. The options are therefore either no treatment or neck exploration. Obviously, a 50-year-old patient with a serum calcium concentration of 3.5 mmol per liter (14 mg per dl) and symptoms and signs of dehydration requires surgery. The situation is less clear in a 75-year-old woman who feels well, who is being treated for symptomless hypertension, and whose serum calcium is 2.9 mmol per liter (11.6 mg per dl). There are at present (1990) no data to indicate that life expectancy or the quality of life will be improved by parathyroidectomy in such a patient. In general, the younger the patient, the more severe the symptoms, and the higher the serum calcium concentration, the greater the need for surgery. The presence of renal calculi is also taken as an indication for neck exploration, even though existing stones will not go away after a successful parathyroidectomy and no guarantee can be given to a patient that he or she will stop forming further stones. Hypertension is neither an indication for nor a contraindication to parathyroidectomy, which lowers blood pressure only temporarily.

There is some controversy as to whether hyperparathyroidism does or does not cause pancreatitis. Although even in patients with documented hyperparathyroidism pancreatitis is frequently due to other causes such as gallstones or alcoholism, it is generally thought that the history of pancreatitis in a patient with hyperparathyroidism constitutes an indication for neck exploration.

Bone mineral measurements generally give low results in hyperparathyroidism, especially in peripheral bones such as the forearm, though this finding does not seem to be associated with an increase in the prevalence of fractures. Longitudinal studies show a slight initial improvement in forearm mineral content after parathyroidectomy, but this improvement is not continued after 2 years.

The greatest problem relates to patients with chronic pain and chronic fatigue syndromes who are investigated for organic pathology and who are found to have the biochemical features of hyperparathyroidism. Such patients have frequently seen many physicians, and there is a strong temptation to "do something." There are anecdotes of individuals who lost their symptoms after parathyroidectomy (possibly owing to the cyclical nature of some depressive syndromes), whereas others experience no improvement and actually feel worse in spite of normalization of serum calcium. There is at present no way of predicting which nonspecific symptoms will improve and which will persist after parathyroidectomy.

If nonoperative treatment is decided upon, the patients should be told to avoid dehydration, calcium containing medications, and thiazide diuretics. They should carry a note in their wallet indicating that they suffer from primary hyperparathyroidism. Their serum calcium and serum creatinine concentrations are checked at 6-month intervals, and bone mineral measurements are made every 2 years. Deterioration in one of these parameters may lead to a decision to treat the patients surgically rather than conservatively.

Surgical treatment should be carried out only in specialized units with experience in thyroid and parathyroid operations. In essence, the operation consists of the identification of all parathyroid glands and the removal of macroscopically abnormal tissue. Postoperative tetany is rare, but when it occurs the patients may require magnesium as well as calcium (see Hypoparathyroidism—Treatment).

## SECONDARY HYPERPARATHYROIDISM

This condition is said to be present when parathyroid hyperplasia and hypersecretion are due to some identifiable cause. The most common of these is chronic renal failure, though the mechanism whereby renal failure causes hyperparathyroidism is still the subject of much speculation. It has been claimed that PTH has deleterious effects on a variety of tissues (myocardium, peripheral nerves, hemopoietic cells) and that it is *the* or at least *a* uremic toxin.

Patients with hyperparathyroidism secondary to renal failure have increased osteoblastic and osteoclastic activity in skeletal tissue. However, the renal responses to PTH are defective in these patients, who do not become hypophosphatemic and whose serum calcium concentration either remains in the normal range or is only mildly elevated in relation to the degree of PTH elevation.

Patients with hyperparathyroidism secondary to renal failure, whether at the predialysis stage or after renal transplantation, require intervention if hypercalcemia is considered a threat to residual renal function. Parathyroidectomy may also be required for patients with skeletal pain attributable to hyperparathyroidism or with ectopic calcification not amenable to treatment with phosphate binders. Parathyroidectomy for secondary hyperparathyroidism involves the removal of all parathyroid tissue except for a rem-

nant considered by the surgeon as equivalent to all four glands in a normal individual.

## HYPERCALCEMIC CRISIS

Patients with severe hypercalcemia due to hyperparathyroidism or other causes (including malignancies) may present in a diabetes insipidus–like state with polyuria, dehydration, and drowsiness. This syndrome requires urgent treatment, sometimes before the cause of hypercalcemia can be established. Rehydration can usually be accomplished with 3 to 4 liters of normal saline per 24 hours with careful monitoring of the jugular venous pressure, if necessary, with a central venous line. Intravenous furosemide (Lasix) in doses of 40 mg every 6 hours increases the urinary excretion of calcium but may also cause or aggravate dehydration and hypokalemia. Agents available for the medium-term treatment of hypercalcemia include salmon calcitonin (Calcimar) at a dose of 100 U given subcutaneously four times daily. Calcitonin in these doses frequently causes nausea. Moreover, the hypercalcemic state generally becomes resistant to calcitonin within a few days, so that this agent is useful for only short periods of time. Corticosteroids in high doses (e.g., 200 mg hydrocortisone per day) reduce serum calcium in some malignancies and in sarcoidosis and may potentiate the effect of calcitonin. However, hyperparathyroidism and a number of tumors do not respond to prednisone or other corticosteroids. The best medium-term agent currently available for the treatment of hypercalcemia is aminohydroxypropylidene* diphosphonate (APD—30 mg given intravenously in saline over 3 hours). A single infusion lowers serum calcium within 48 hours, while normalization of serum calcium is usually achieved within 5 to 6 days. APD is well tolerated, and its effect lasts long enough (several weeks) for the patients to be investigated and appropriately treated. If APD is not available, mithramycin (plicamycin [Mithracin]) may be used but this material has a large number of side effects. The usual dose is 1.5 mg given intravenously in 5% dextrose over 4 hours, taking care to avoid extravasation into the surrounding tissues. Mithramycin administration may have to be repeated the next day, but its toxic effects on platelets, clotting factors, kidney function, and liver function should be checked before second or third doses are given.

## HYPOPARATHYROIDISM

### Causes

Hypoparathyroidism occurs when biologically active PTH is circulating in inadequate amounts

---

*Not available in the United States.

or when the response of the target tissues is impaired. In the majority of cases, the parathyroid glands have been accidentally or deliberately removed during surgical procedures on the neck. In patients who suffer from nonsurgical or "idiopathic" hypoparathyroidism, the glands are believed to have been destroyed by "autoimmune" processes. In some of these patients, there are demonstrable abnormalities affecting B cell and T cell lymphocyte function with or without failure of other endocrine organs such as the adrenals or the gonads. Transient parathyroid insufficiency occurs in premature infants who may also be hypoglycemic and hyperbilirubinemic. Hypoparathyroidism may be due to PTH resistance associated with receptor or postreceptor abnormalities ("pseudohypoparathyroidism"). Patients with these syndromes do not respond normally to endogenous or exogenous PTH. Magnesium deficiency, which may complicate acute postoperative situations (see Treatment), results in both inadequate PTH release and inadequate target tissue responses. Isolated patients have been described with hypoparathyroidism due to the secretion of an abnormal hormone.

### Clinical Presentation

Hypocalcemia leads to "leaky" membrane systems, particularly in the central and peripheral nervous systems. Depolarization occurs more readily than in normal individuals resulting in tetany, epileptic seizures, or both. In long-standing hypocalcemia there is paradoxically an accumulation of intracellular calcium, particularly in the brain and the ocular lens. Hypoparathyroidism should be suspected in patients presenting with carpopedal spasms, in patients with unexplained fits and/or dementia, and in patients who develop cataracts before the age of 55.

### Investigations

The major biochemical change associated with hypoparathyroidism is hypocalcemia in the presence of normal plasma protein concentrations. In hypoproteinemic states, serum calcium concentrations may be low because some 40% of blood calcium is protein bound. Patients with this type of "hypocalcemia" require attention to plasma proteins rather than to hypoparathyroidism, which may not be present. The majority of patients are hyperphosphatemic (see Physiology of Parathyroid Hormone) and have no detectable immunoreactive PTH. Infusions of human PTH cause a massive increase in plasma and urinary cyclic AMP concentrations. In pseudohypoparathyroidism, serum PTH values are high and the responses to infused PTH are blunted.

Additional investigations include the measurement of plasma magnesium (see Causes) and CT scans of the brain, which may show cerebral calcification. Slit lamp examination of the lens may show characteristic lenticular opacities. Many patients with surgical hypoparathyroidism also suffer from hypothyroidism and/or paralysis of a vocal cord.

### Treatment

Patients with symptoms and/or biochemical features of hypoparathyroidism require treatment. Calcium supplements by themselves are usually insufficient for patients whose serum calcium values are below 2 mmol per liter (8.0 mg per dl). Such patients require pharmacologic doses of ergocalciferol (vitamin D, calciferol) (1 mg per day) or calcitriol (Rocaltrol) (1 μg per day). The therapeutic doses of these substances are close to the intoxicating doses and should be individualized for each patient. It is also advisable to prescribe calcium supplements (1 gram of elemental calcium per day) for hypoparathyroid patients so as to prevent wide fluctuations in calcium consumption. Treatment generally has to be given on a permanent basis. For patients who appear to be "resistant" to conventional doses of ergocalciferol or who become vitamin D intoxicated, serum 25-hydroxy vitamin D measurements are available to monitor compliance and to predict hypercalcemic episodes.

Serum calcium should be maintained in the low-normal range. Measurements are made monthly for the first 3 to 6 months after the commencement of vitamin D therapy or more frequently if the patients report symptoms of hypercalcemia (especially polyuria). Once a plateau has been reached, serum calcium measurements are required only two or three times per year.

Vitamin D and calcium supplements should be discontinued at once if a patient is found to be hypercalcemic. Withdrawal of medication and recommencement at a lower dose once serum calcium has fallen to 2.1 mmol per liter (8.4 mg per dl) are generally all that is required. The obtunded, dehydrated patient requires to be admitted to hospital and to be treated according to the principles set out under Hypercalcemic Crisis.

Patients who develop acute hypoparathyroidism after thyroidectomy or parathyroidectomy may be hypomagnesemic as well as hypocalcemic. Treatment of such individuals is also complicated by the fact that they may be unable to take oral medications. Intravenous calcium chloride (10% in 10 ml given intravenously over 10 minutes) usually controls carpopedal spasms, at least temporarily. Care should be taken to avoid extravasation into the perivascular area, as calcium chloride may cause tissue necrosis. The acute intravenous injection of calcium chloride is followed by a slower infusion. Three ampules of 10% calcium chloride (approximately 800 mg elemental calcium) are added to 1 liter of normal saline, which is given intravenously over 24 hours. Although this may not be sufficient to make the patient normocalcemic, it usually prevents tetany.

If patients in this situation have documented hypomagnesemia (or are liable to be chronically magnesium depleted as in malabsorption or chronic alcoholism), they should be given intravenous magnesium also. Magnesium sulfate is available in ampules as a 50% solution, each milliliter containing 2 mmol of magnesium). Ten milliliters of this material is added to 1 liter of normal saline, which is then given intravenously over 24 hours in a separate line from the one carrying calcium chloride. Serum calcium and serum magnesium concentrations should be checked at least once a day in such patients.

If 72 hours after thyroidectomy a patient is still hypocalcemic, it is likely that he or she will require vitamin D therapy. In this situation, calcitriol is preferable to ergocalciferol and the initial dose may have to be higher than 1 μg per day. Long-term oral magnesium supplements are rarely required.

## NORMOCALCEMIC TETANY

Some patients develop carpopedal spasms in the absence of any major biochemical changes. These patients display the classic posture of the hand (adducted thumb, flexed metacarpophalangeal joints, and extended interphalangeal joints) either spontaneously or after the application of a tourniquet (Trousseau's sign). They may also have a positive Chvostek's sign (contraction of facial muscles when branches of the facial nerve are percussed). This syndrome is often attributed to hyperventilation, and the patients are advised to breathe into a paper bag during attacks. Neither the pathogenesis nor the treatment of this condition has been subjected to critical analysis. The attacks of tetany tend to be episodic, and the patients (most of whom are young women) should be given a good prognosis. Remissions may last for many years.

# HYPOPITUITARISM

method of
BARRY SHERMAN, M.D., and
ANN JOHANSON, M.D.
*Genentech, Inc.*
*South San Francisco, California*

The anterior lobe of the pituitary secretes at least six hormones: growth hormone (GH), adrenal corticotropin (ACTH), thyroid stimulating hormone (TSH), follicle stimulating hormone (FSH), luteinizing hormone (LH), and prolactin (PRL). ACTH is synthesized as part of a peptide of substantially greater molecular weight—pro-opiomelanocortin. Another portion of this same precursor peptide is beta endorphin, an endogenous opiate. The existence and exact nature of the hormone responsible for regulating skin pigmentation are at present in doubt. The hypothalamus regulates the release of these hormones from the pituitary through secretion of both stimulatory and inhibitory factors. The concentration of circulating hormones from the target glands (such as thyroid, adrenal, or gonad) exerts a negative feedback control on secretion of its corresponding tropic hormone. High concentrations of thyroid hormones or of cortisol, for example, diminish pituitary TSH and ACTH secretion, respectively. These effects are mediated at the level of the hypothalamus, the pituitary, or both. For prolactin, a hypothalamic inhibiting factor predominates, whereas for growth hormone both a releasing hormone and a release inhibiting hormone (somatostatin) have been demonstrated.

Pituitary hormone deficiency may involve one or more hormones. Panhypopituitarism is a relatively rare occurrence. The causes of hypopituitarism are listed in Table 1. Pituitary adenomas, craniopharyngiomas, and idiopathic hypopituitarism of childhood are by far the most common causes. A pituitary tumor may be recognized because of excess hormone production, hormone deficiencies, or mechanical consequences such as headache and visual field abnormalities. In

TABLE 1. **Causes of Hypopituitarism**

| Classification | Causes |
| --- | --- |
| Neoplasms | Primary intrasellar tumors<br>Craniopharyngioma<br>Metastatic carcinoma<br>Histiocytosis |
| Granulomas infection | Sarcoidosis<br>Fungal diseases<br>Tuberculosis<br>Syphilis (gumma)<br>Pyogenic infections<br>Meningitis (sequela) |
| Vascular | Infarction—intrapartum or postpartum<br>Ischemic vascular disease<br>Aneurysm of internal carotid artery |
| Idiopathic | Hypopituitarism of childhood<br>Isolated hormone deficiency |
| Surgical trauma | Hypophysectomy or stalk section |

some patients, especially those with pituitary tumors, there may be progressive loss of pituitary function. The pituitary hormones usually become deficient in the following order: (1) GH, (2) LH and FSH, (3) ACTH, and (4) TSH; in adults, the first clinical manifestation may be related to disturbed gonadotropin secretion. Prolactin deficiency is very unusual. Because of these considerations, periodic reassessment of pituitary function is important. The initiation of hormone replacement usually commits the patient to lifelong therapy. For that reason, a diagnosis of pituitary hormone deficiency should be carefully documented, using appropriate testing procedures.

Patients with hypopituitarism should be instructed to register with the Medic Alert Foundation, P. O. Box 10099, Turlock, CA 95380, and to obtain an identification tag that lists their hormone treatment.

## GROWTH HORMONE DEFICIENCY

In the adult patient, few symptoms directly referable to growth hormone deficiency are recognized. Insulin-requiring diabetics may have a dramatic increase in insulin sensitivity with a decrease in requirement for insulin therapy. The availability of growth hormone produced by recommended DNA methods has increased interest in the study of GH deficiency in adults and the potential benefits of GH replacement. Growth hormone–deficient children will have greatly retarded growth with the history of normal birth weight. This type of dwarfism is characterized by normal body proportions and may be associated with other endocrine deficiencies.

For more than 30 years, the diagnosis of growth hormone deficiency was based on the analysis of serum GH concentrations following two or more pharmacologic stimuli of pituitary growth hormone secretion. Because of the limited amount of pituitary-derived GH, the criteria were established so that only the most severely growth hormone–deficient children would receive GH treatment. Gradually, improved pituitary collection and extraction strategies resulted in some increase in the availability of GH for treatment, so that the criteria for treatment were somewhat relaxed. Whereas originally GH concentrations after stimulation of less that 5 ng per ml defined the GH deficient state, later values up to 7 or 10 ng per ml were consistent with GH deficiency. Children with levels in the higher range were determined to have partial GH deficiency. One disadvantage of pharmacologic tests for the diagnosis of GH insufficiency is that some children who respond normally to one or more tests may in fact have significant abnormalities of GH release demonstrated under normal physiologic circumstances. Growth failure due to severe GH deficiency is a universally accepted therapeutic indication for GH. Treatment of partial GH defi-

ciency is also standard practice. However, the evaluation and diagnosis of short children who may have milder forms of GH deficiency or some abnormality in GH action remain uncertain.

Human growth hormone produced by recombinant DNA methods was first tested in 1981 and became generally available in 1985. The greater availability of GH has permitted optimization of treatment for GH-deficient children. When the GH supply was limited, the usual dosage was 0.05 mg per kg three times per week. Recent studies suggest that a dosage of 0.3 mg per kg per week divided into daily subcutaneous injections of 0.04 to 0.05 mg per kg per day is associated with an improved growth response.

In children with multiple pituitary hormone deficiencies, treatment with other hormones requires careful attention. Adequate thyroid hormone is necessary for optimal growth. Excessive glucocorticoid hormone therapy can reduce the response to growth hormone. Sex hormone replacement speeds epiphyseal closure and should be delayed consistent with the patient's emotional and social needs. Optimal, early growth hormone replacement therapy will permit age appropriate initiation of sexual development.

## GONADOTROPIN DEFICIENCY

Gonadotropin deficiency results in loss of libido in both men and women, impotence in men, and amenorrhea. In women, this secondary estrogen deficiency causes atrophy of breast tissue and vaginal epithelium and development of fine wrinkles around the eyes and mouth. In men, the testes may become smaller and softer, and the rate of beard growth is often reduced. Preadolescent gonadotropin deficiency results in failure to develop secondary sex characteristics.

A functional form of gonadotropin deficiency that results in amenorrhea and infertility occurs in patients with hyperprolactinemia. Lowering the prolactin concentration to normal, either surgically or medically, results in resumption of menstrual cycles and return of fertility in premenopausal women.

Another functional form of gonadotropin deficiency occurs in patients with eating disorders such as anorexia nervosa and bulemia and with weight loss associated with extreme exercise. More common in women, these situations are reversible when weight is regained.

Treatment of gonadotropin deficiency is possible by administration of the synthetic releasing hormone (GnRH). However, the pulsatile administration of GnRH shown to be effective in restoration of gonadal function in an investigational setting is not a practical approach to treatment.

Administration of human LH or FSH by injection could also result in stimulation of ovarian and testicular function, but these materials are not available for clinical use.

In men, androgen replacement is carried out using the parenteral preparations testosterone enanthate (Delatestryl) or testosterone cypionate (Depo-Testosterone). These are more effective in maintaining secondary sex characteristics than are oral preparations such as fluoxymesterone. In adults, the usual dosage is 200 mg intramuscularly every 3 to 4 weeks. The serum testosterone concentration can be measured before the next dose to adjust the dosing interval to maintain the serum testosterone level in the normal range. The dose can be reduced in older men to reduce the likelihood of prostatic hyperplasia and obstructive uropathy.

There are other considerations in the initiation of treatment in adolescents. Sex hormone therapy results in epiphyseal closure. Ideally, treatment of androgen deficiency should be delayed to provide an opportunity for maximal linear growth, and when started is begun in a lower dosage, 25 to 50 mg monthly with 25 to 50 mg increments every 6 months. This consideration often has to be balanced against the needs of the patient for normal adolescent changes.

In the adolescent male, it is often difficult to distinguish physiologic delayed puberty from permanent hypothalamic-pituitary gonadotropin deficiency. Normal puberty may follow a 4- to 6-month trial of androgen replacement in some patients with physiologic delay. Such a therapeutic trial should be followed by a reassessment of pituitary-gonadal function. In these circumstances, some physicians prefer to use human chorionic gonadotropin (hCG), 2000 IU three times a week, to stimulate Leydig cell testosterone production. This is usually effective but is expensive and requires frequent injections.

Side effects of androgen replacement include the development of acne and transient gynecomastia in adolescents. Adults may be troubled by mild fluid retention.

The treatment of the infertility that accompanies pituitary dysfunction in men is unsatisfactory. This has been attempted in a variety of ways with hCG, purified LH, and FSH or GnRH. Research with each of these methods continues, but none has yet been shown to be consistently effective.

Gonadotropin deficiency in women is treated by cyclical replacement of both estrogen and progesterone. This is done conveniently with a combination oral contraceptive containing 20 to 50 µg of ethinyl estradiol. An alternative approach is 20- to 50-µg tablets of ethinyl estradiol or 0.625-mg tablets of conjugated estrogens (Premarin) for 25 days, with 5 to 10 mg of medroxyprogesterone (Provera) for the last 7 to 10 days of the cycle. These programs provide for cyclical sloughing of the endometrium and avoid the potential consequences of persistent estrogen stimulation.

Induction of fertility in women with LH and FSH deficiency can be accomplished by administration of gonadotropins. Ovulation induction is carried out with human menopausal gonadotropin (hMG [Pergonal]). This material is recovered from the urine of menopausal women and is rich in both LH and FSH. Each ampule contains 75 IU of FSH and 75 IU of LH. Induction of ovulation requires the qualitative, quantitative, and temporal replication of the events of the normal ovulatory cycle, resulting in follicular maturation ovulation and corpus luteum function. Follicular maturation is promoted by daily administration of 1 or more ampules of hMG for 9 to 12 days. Serum and/or urinary estrogen concentrations are measured daily to assess the adequacy of follicular maturation and to judge the appropriate timing of a single dose of hCG, 5000 or 10,000 U. The bolus of hCG mimics the midcycle LH surge and causes follicular rupture and ovulation.

The success rate of ovulation induction is approximately 35%. This treatment is complex and expensive, and should be done only by physicians experienced in the use of these drugs and with adequate laboratory support. Complications include ovarian enlargement, multiple pregnancies, and the hyperstimulation syndrome characterized by abdominal pain, nausea, vomiting, ruptured ovarian cysts, and ascites.

## ACTH DEFICIENCY

Loss of ACTH secretory capacity usually results in decreased stamina, exhaustion, hypopigmentation, and loss of axillary and pubic hair. In general, symptoms referable to mineralocorticoid deficiency such as postural hypotension and vascular collapse are not prominent in the absence of unusual stress.

Most adult patients do well on a program of cortisone acetate, 25 mg orally in the morning and 12.5 mg in the late afternoon. An alternative is hydrocortisone, 10 mg in the morning, 10 mg at noon, and 5 mg in the late afternoon. Individual dose adjustment is necessary, depending upon the patient's response. Some will experience an increase in appetite and weight gain, even on standard doses. Laboratory tests are not helpful in determining the precise replacement dose for an individual patient.

Children who need cortisone replacement should be dosed on a weight basis (25 mg per $M^2$

per day or less). The smallest dose needed to prevent symptoms should be used in order to permit adequate growth. Even a 5 mg per day excess can seriously impair normal growth.

Postural hypotension and hyponatremia, although uncommon, will occur in some patients with hypopituitarism and indicate the need for mineralocorticoid replacement. Fludrocortisone acetate (Florinef) is used in a dose as small as 0.05 mg on alternate days and rarely more than 0.1 mg daily. If ankle edema or hypertension develops, the dose should be reduced.

Patients taking glucocorticoid replacement should receive special instructions. They should register with and obtain an appropriate identification tag from the Medic Alert Foundation. During intercurrent illnesses or gastroenteritis, they should double their usual steroid dose. They should have available a parenteral dose of glucocorticoid hormone in a prefilled syringe, either 4 mg of dexamethasone phosphate or 100 mg of hydrocortisone sodium succinate (Solu-Cortef). Children should have 25 mg administered intramuscularly. The patient and family member should be instructed on how to use the syringe in the event of an acute catastrophic illness or when nausea and vomiting preclude oral medications.

Patients with pituitary disease require special hormone treatment before and during surgery. One routine is to give cortisone acetate, 100 mg intramuscularly, on the morning of surgery. During surgery, hydrocortisone sodium succinate (Solu-Cortef) is given intravenously in a dosage of 10 mg per hour. Another 100-mg dose of cortisone acetate is given intramuscularly after surgery and is continued in a dosage of 100 mg twice daily during the immediate postoperative period. Thereafter, the dose can be reduced commensurate with the clinical course. Children should be dosed commensurate with weight, so that a 20-kg child should receive one-quarter of the above doses.

Patients with hypopituitarism and ACTH deficiency can develop the syndrome of acute adrenal insufficiency just as patients with primary adrenal disease. Treatment is as for acute primary adrenal insufficiency, including immediate intravenous administration of hydrocortisone sodium succinate (Solu-Cortef), 100 mg, and intravenous saline.

### THYROID DEFICIENCY

The entire spectrum of symptoms and signs of thyroid deficiency can be observed in hypopituitarism and is indistinguishable from, though often milder than, primary hypothyroidism. The same therapeutic considerations apply as in the treatment of primary hypothyroidism.

L-Thyroxine (Synthroid) is the standard therapy for hypothyrodism. The usual dosage is 0.05 to 0.2 mg in a single daily dose. Treatment can usually be started with a 0.05- or 0.10-mg dose. Similar doses are used in children. Desiccated thyroid hormone is a suitable alternative, but triiodothyronine or combinations of thyroxine and triiodothyronine have no place in the management of hypothyroidism.

The adequacy of therapy is assessed by the patient's clinical response and by measurement of the serum thyroxine concentration in patients taking L-thyroxine.

It is prudent to begin treatment with low doses of thyroxine (0.025 or 0.05 mg daily) in the elderly; in patients with ischemic heart disease; and in those with long-standing severe hypothyroidism. That dose is doubled at 3- to 4-week intervals, depending on the patient's response and the serum thyroxine concentration.

Most patients with secondary hypothyroidism will have other pituitary hormone deficits, including that of ACTH. Unless patients have had prior testing to document adequate adrenal reserve, treatment with replacement doses of glucocorticoid hormone should be started when thyroid hormone treatment is begun.

# HYPERPROLACTINEMIA

method of
NICHOLAS P. CHRISTY, M.D.
*Columbia University College of Physicians and Surgeons*
*New York, New York*

Hyperprolactinemia is persistent, chronic elevation of the plasma prolactin concentration; it is fairly common in the population at large and is the most prevalent neuroendocrine disorder. Prolactinoma, that is, prolactin-secreting tumor of the pituitary gland, an important cause of hyperprolactinemia, is the most frequent hormone-producing tumor of the human adenohypophysis, occurring in as many as 10%, and in some studies up to 25%, of random autopsies.

Hyperprolactinemia is observed as a result of or in association with various clinical conditions. Those diverse circumstances dictate the diagnostic plans and procedures and determine the need for and nature of the treatment. The consensus of endocrinologists is that most patients with hyperprolactinemia require treatment under most circumstances. If the decision is made to withhold treatment, continuous, careful monitoring is necessary. Certain categories of patients, to be discussed, do not need treatment of the hyperprolactinemia per se, although they may require correction of the associated disorder. Proper therapy or a rational decision to withhold it demands precise diagnosis.

## CLINICAL PRESENTATION

Many patients with hyperprolactinemia have no symptoms or signs ascribable to a raised plasma prolactin concentration. This is true of most patients who have drug-induced or drug-related hyperprolactinemia, which usually abates when the drug is stopped. Examples are some agents that block dopamine agonist receptors or reduce dopamine synthesis in various parts of the brain. Specific drugs include neuroleptics such as chlorpromazine, perphenazine, haloperidol, metoclopramide, and sulpiride; antidepressants such as imipramine and amitryptiline; and antihypertensives such as reserpine and methyldopa. Opiates, verapamil, and intravenous cimetidine may induce hyperprolactinemia, as may administered estrogens, but not in the small doses found in contraceptive agents. Asymptomatic hyperprolactinemia is observed in hypothyroidism, correction of which slowly brings down the raised plasma prolactin concentration. The same is true in patients with chronic renal failure, wherein the mechanism is completely unknown. Especially high values are seen with renal hemodialysis. Successful renal transplantation and correction of the zinc deficiency of renal failure restore the serum prolactin concentration to normal.

In some other conditions associated with hyperprolactinemia, the laboratory abnormality may have clinical significance. Abnormally high prolactin concentrations are sometimes observed in women with syndromes of hyperandrogenicity, such as polycystic ovary (Stein-Leventhal) syndrome. It is now known that hyperprolactinemia may stimulate the adrenal cortex to secrete excessive quantities of dehydroepiandrosterone sulfate. In isolated galactorrhea (i.e., galactorrhea without oligo- or amenorrhea), where one would expect to find hyperprolactinemia, the situation is complex. The incidence of this type of galactorrhea in hyperprolactinemic women is variably reported as 30 to 80%, whereas, conversely, galactorrhea can occur with normal serum prolactin concentrations in many women, more than 85% in one series.

The hyperprolactinemia of Addison's disease and that associated with the presumably neurogenic injuries to the chest wall are of no known clinical significance.

Hyperprolactinemia is most often observed in the setting of gonadal dysfunction: amenorrhea or infertility in women, loss of libido or impotence in men. Reduced sexual activity is a frequent finding in both sexes, as are headache and other signs of hypothalamic or pituitary tumor, including visual disturbances and visual field defects. This group of patients most often has prolactinoma. In these patients, hyperprolactinemia induces hypoestrogenism, probably through inhibition by the excessive prolactin of hypothalamic gonadotropin-releasing hormone, although the mechanism is still debated.

## DIAGNOSIS

Symptomatic hyperprolactinemia is closely associated with prolactinoma. Even under ideal conditions, diagnosis is imperfect in some cases and treatment may have to be either protracted or repeated. Close, continuous follow-up with laboratory and radiologic monitoring is required.

Because prolactin is secreted episodically, with a sharp rise during sleep, and because the plasma prolactin concentration is labile in the face of multiple stimuli, sustained hyperprolactinemia can be documented only by repeated measurements (on 3 different days) under basal, trauma-free conditions. The best time for this determination is in the morning, 2 hours after waking. The upper limit of normal serum (plasma) prolactin concentration is 18 to 20 ng per ml. The importance of a large, experienced, and busy laboratory for the measurement of prolactin concentration resides in two characteristics of the prolactin radioimmunoassay: Prolactin is fairly easily damaged by prolonged storage, which may result in loss of immunoactivity and cause falsely high readings on plasma specimens; and an altered molecular form of either the standards or the circulating prolactin ("big" or "big-big" prolactin) may result in serial dilutions that yield curves wherein the standard and the specimen (unknown) are not parallel, which produces errors in assays done at high versus low dilutions. Small laboratories that perform only occasional prolactin assays cannot be expected to circumvent all these difficulties, so that their results are not reliable.

The many patients who have obvious symptoms or signs of disease of the sellar region or who, in the setting of gonadal insufficiency, are prime candidates for a diagnosis of prolactinoma or pseudoprolactinoma require careful radiographic study of the pituitary fossa and contiguous structures. Large supra- and intrasellar tumors and pseudoprolactinomas (large hypothalamic, pituitary, or parapituitary tumors) can sometimes be visualized by plain skull films taken in the sagittal and coronal planes. Nevertheless, the best results are now obtained with computed tomography (CT) scanning or magnetic resonance imaging (MRI). These are particularly useful in distinguishing hypothalamic from pituitary tumors. Provocative (chlorpromazine, thyrotropin-releasing hormone) stimulation and inhibition tests are not discriminatory because both the hypothalamus and the pituitary contain dopamine agonist receptors. Such pharmacologic tests do not enable a differential diagnosis between a diencephalic and a pituitary etiology of prolactin hypersecretion. The most accurate technique for the definition of the pituitary anatomy now available is the high-resolution CT scan (with or without contrast medium enhancement), with 1.5-mm sections through the substance of the pituitary gland.

MRI can demonstrate prolactinomas. The pituitary fossa is often slightly enlarged by the tumor.

As to the relative advantages of CT scanning and MRI, it has been found that CT is superior in about 10% of studies, MRI is better in 10%, and the results are equivalent in 80%. MRI may yet show better resolution of the sellar region. It has the advantages that there is no need for contrast medium and there is no exposure to radiation. A potential disadvantage is that MRI often fails to demonstrate lateral spread or extension of tumor into the cavernous sinuses. More observations with MRI are needed to establish its relative or absolute value.

One more detail must be added concerning plasma prolactin concentrations in prolactinoma. Roughly speaking, the larger the tumor, the higher the prolactin concentration. In several clinics, it has now been established that concentrations of 200 to 250 ng per ml may have any cause; concentrations above 250 ng per ml indicate a prolactinoma; and concentrations higher than 300 ng per ml always indicate a prolactinoma.

The cause of hyperprolactinemia can usually be accurately identified by the history, the clinical picture, or both. The patients who have the most important clinical indications for treatment, namely, those with prolactinoma, require intense radiologic examination. Even in the best hands, some prolactinomas, especially small ones (1 to 2 mm in diameter), will be missed; some workers suggest that the portion escaping detection may be up to 30%. Nevertheless, as CT and MRI techniques improve and become more widely used, we may expect that the number of cases of "idiopathic," "undefined," or "functional" hyperprolactinemia will grow progressively smaller.

## TREATMENT

Most patients with hyperprolactinemia should be treated at large medical centers with extensive laboratory facilities, experienced endocrinologists, and neurosurgeons who have had wide experience with trans-sphenoidal pituitary adenomectomy.

Once pregnancy, postpartum lactation, hypothyroidism, primary adrenocortical insufficiency, polycystic ovary syndrome, and drugs have been excluded, the diagnosis of prolactinoma is established by CT scan or MRI. Then, as will be seen, there are several therapeutic choices, including some that entail combining two or more treatment modalities. Several considerations enter into the best choice of therapy for the individual patient.

A few general statements can be made. If a microadenoma is suspected but cannot be rigorously proved, there is a reasonable option not to treat. In the face of a proven hypothalamic tumor or prolactinoma of the pituitary, one is obliged to treat if only because the tumor mass itself is a threat to life or to normal neuroendocrine function. In the presence of prolactinoma associated with infertility, treatment is mandatory if fertility is desired. Galactorrhea with a normal menstrual cycle and hyperprolactinemia need not be treated unless the inappropriate lactation is so voluminous as to constitute a major nuisance. Treatment of hyperprolactinemia with the aim of preventing or ameliorating the osteopenia associated with hypoestrinism and for the possible prevention of coronary artery disease in women

will be discussed under "Hyperprolactinemia of Unknown Cause."

### Pituitary Microadenoma

Microadenoma, defined as a tumor with radiographic (CT) dimensions less than 10 mm in diameter, is the most common assignable cause of hyperprolactinemia when no other etiology can be identified. The first step is to rule out drug-induced hyperprolactinemia; the second is to eliminate medical conditions (alcoholism and liver disease) and neurologic disorders (epileptic seizures, electroconvulsive therapy; rarely, empty sella). Then the question of whether and how to treat rests on associated symptoms and signs, the specific needs or wishes of the patient, and knowledge of the natural history of hyperprolactinemia. This has been studied in three groups of patients with pituitary tumors, mostly microadenomas. Over 3 to 20 years of observation, most patients with demonstrated microadenoma have shown little or no progression of growth of the pituitary tumor. Criteria for treatment are thus other than the tumor considered simply as an intrasellar mass lesion (e.g., infertility).

In a group of 41 hyperprolactinemic patients without evidence of pituitary tumor (by definition, idiopathic hyperprolactinemia) followed for as long as 12 years, more than 80% had either no change or a fall in serum prolactin concentration; in more than one-third, it fell to the normal range; more than one-half of the patients demonstrated a decrease to less than 50% of the control level. In general, the higher the initial prolactin concentration, the smaller was its fall. Pituitary tumor developed in only 1 of these 41 patients.

For hyperprolactinemic patients who are asymptomatic, a good case can be made to withhold treatment and to observe over time. Observation includes prolactin measurements about every 6 months and CT scanning of the sellar region every 2 to 4 years. Given the likelihood that a number (up to 30%) of small (<1 to 3 mm in diameter) microadenomas will be missed by CT scan, the clinician should assume that a few patients will develop significant pituitary tumor. The data show that the number of patients will be small and the rate of progression slow.

#### Symptomatic Pituitary Microadenoma

The decision to treat a microadenoma is based on symptoms of disturbance in or near the sella and the status of gonadal function. The natural history of treatment by observation only has been discussed. Apart from theoretical considerations, other factors entering into the decision are the infrequency and slow rate of progression of microadenomas, the high rate of recurrence of treated tumors over the long term, and, if pharmacotherapy is used, the need for indefinite treatment because hyperprolactinemia recurs when the therapeutic agent is stopped. The major indication for treatment is the need to restore relatively normal pituitary function to achieve normal gonadal activity, including normal menses, ovulation, and fertility in women; and to improve libido, sperm count, and potency in men. There are five therapeutic options: surgery, bromocriptine, radiotherapy to the sellar region, various combinations of these three therapies, and observation alone.

**Surgery: Trans-sphenoidal Adenomectomy.** This procedure is most often the treatment of choice in the United States because endocrinologists and surgeons here have had the widest experience with it. It should be emphasized that the data presented here are based on results obtained by experienced neurosurgeons. It should also be added that the procedure used is an adaptation of the one revived at the turn of the twentieth century by Harvey Cushing; by the mid-1920s, Cushing had reduced the mortality rate to 5.6%, a figure now decreased to less than 1% in most centers. The effectiveness of this treatment is variable. In the British experience, the initial cure rate (substantial reduction of the prolactin concentration or its restoration to or near normal) is 80 to 85% and mortality is 0.27%, with major morbidity occurring in 0.4% and cerebrospinal rhinorrhea fluid being observed in 1 to 2%. The rate of recurrence of hyperprolactinemia is 20 to 50%; relapse occurs within 1 to 2 years, a few becoming evident at 2 to 5 years. Most often, the recurrent tumor cannot be seen by CT scan. The inference is either that residual tumor fragments have grown back or that there is a stimulatory hypothalamic influence, new or recurrent. Other large series have reported a long-term recurrence rate of 50%; lower rates (of 0 to 30%) have been described. Most workers hold that these rates, like all others, will continue to increase over the years of postoperative follow-up.

In patients who show an initial cure, there is a high rate of return of normal ovulatory menses and of achievement of pregnancy. The treatment of prolactinomas, microadenomas, or macroadenomas is further discussed under "Pregnancy." Surgical treatment involving craniotomy (never used for microadenoma) is far more hazardous than the trans-sphenoidal approach.

**Pharmacotherapy: Bromocriptine.** The use of the ergot derivative bromocriptine (Parlodel) started in 1970, chiefly in Europe and the United Kingdom. There, most endocrinologists regard this drug and its congeners as the treatment of choice.

Bromocriptine is a dopamine receptor agonist. Dopamine is the natural hypothalamic hypophysiotropic hormone that exerts the principal tonic inhibitory influence on pituitary prolactin secretion; that is, it is a prolactin-inhibiting factor or hormone (PIF, PIH). Untoward effects of bromocriptine are nausea, vomiting, and orthostatic hypotension; psychic effects (rarely, psychosis) are uncommon, but they may persist and become more or less troublesome in about 10% of patients. These disadvantages can be minimized by very gradual attainment of the therapeutic dose and by careful follow-up. A practical regimen is this: A dose of 1.25 mg (orally) is given with a bedtime feeding; after a week without side effects, this dose is moved to the time of the evening meal; after another week or so, another 1.25-mg dose is added with another meal. Thereafter, the dose is gradually increased to 2.5 mg two to three times a day until the serum prolactin concentration has fallen into the normal range. This usually occurs within days to a few weeks (some favorable effect on the prolactin concentration is seen within hours) and at a total dose of 7.5 mg a day, which after some weeks can sometimes be given as a single dose. Patients develop tolerance to the side effects of the drug within days to weeks. Only occasionally are larger doses, up to 30 mg per day, required. Long-term therapy is safe; untoward effects of clinical significance are not seen even after years of treatment (see also under "Pregnancy").

Bromocriptine therapy is rapid and effective. At the usual dose, 7.5 mg per day, the general experience has been that microadenomas shrink—by as much as three-quarters of their volume—in 50 to 100% of cases. Menses return in 85% of treated women, and documented ovulation is restored in 60 to 100%. Coexistent deficiencies of pituitary function tend to improve to or toward normal; an exception is failure of serum testosterone concentrations to rise in about one-half of the treated men. After continuous treatment for 2 years or more, it is sometimes possible to reduce the bromocriptine dose if the serum prolactin concentration has fallen and the tumor has shrunk. Prolactin concentrations rise when bromocriptine is stopped, but after prolonged drug therapy, that rise may be delayed until many months after cessation of the drug.

Bromocriptine therapy is only rarely curative. When the drug is stopped, the tumor or the hyperprolactinemia or both recrudesce. Treatment therefore must be continued indefinitely. Symptoms and signs of the pituitary adenoma as a tumor mass are relieved as the tumor shrinks. As indicated, there is a very high rate of restoration of gonadal function, especially among women, and a number of hyperprolactinemic men with hypogonadism and depression respond to bromocriptine with improvement in emotional state, libido, potency, and sperm count, whether or not there is an accompanying rise in the serum testosterone concentration.

Disadvantages of long-term treatment with bromocriptine are these: The drug is expensive; no one knows how long treatment must be continued; and, in theory, there may be untoward effects—so far not identified—of therapy over many years.

**Radiation Therapy.** This modality is never used as primary treatment for microadenoma. If used adjunctively, the dosage is 4500 rad to the sellar region, delivered through three portals at a rate of 200 rad per day. The serum prolactin concentration falls to normal in fewer than 25% of patients, even over many years. The fall, if it occurs, is exceedingly slow, like that of growth hormone in radiation-treated acromegaly. There is also a substantial risk of hypopituitarism after 20 years or more: hypogonadism in more than one-half of the patients, hypoadrenalism in about one-third, and thyroid deficiency in 15 to 20%. Therapeutic results and unwanted sequelae are about the same with alpha-particles or proton beam therapy as with conventional radiotherapy.

**Combination Therapy.** Various combinations have been used to treat microadenoma. Second surgical procedures after tumor recurrence with initial surgical cure carry a much higher rate of untoward effects and sequelae. Bromocriptine is safe and effective if re-treatment is needed several years after trans-sphenoidal resection. Some workers have advocated initial treatment with bromocriptine, followed by surgery. The drawback with this sequence is that the planes of dissection between the adenoma and the contiguous normal pituitary tissue may be partly or completely obliterated, which renders surgery more difficult. Surgery followed by radiotherapy (or the reverse) is more likely to effect a permanent cure, but the incidence of hypopituitarism is higher and the patient is exposed to the risks of both procedures. The most useful combination appears to be prepregnancy radiation followed by bromocriptine (see under "Pregnancy"). To date, there are not enough reported statistics on the results of combination therapies to establish a clear preference. Treatment has to be individualized.

**Observation Only.** "Expectant" treatment is usually safe. Microadenomas progress in very few cases (well under 4%). With alert monitoring (prolactin measurements, CT scans every 6 months to 2 or more years) and following patients for signs of tumor enlargement (headache, vision and visual field changes), recurrences can be anticipated or treated promptly. The larger the original tumor, the less likely is expectant therapy to be a reasonable alternative.

### Pituitary Macroadenoma

By definition, macroadenomas are tumors with a diameter of greater than 10 mm (by CT scan). They are far less common than microadenomas. They seem to be more frequent in men than in women, perhaps because they are discovered later. Without the obvious clinical sign of amenorrhea as a marker, the clinical presentation is slower and more gradual; furthermore, male patients are reluctant to complain of reduced frequency of shaving, loss of libido, or impotence. The plasma prolactin concentration correlates only roughly with the tumor size. Values range from 300 to higher than 1000 ng per ml. With these large tumors, the tumor viewed as a mass is often the primary factor in governing treatment, not the hyperprolactinemia and its consequences (e.g., infertility).

**Trans-sphenoidal Adenomectomy.** Cure (normal prolactin concentration) is achieved in only 10 to 40% of patients; results are far less favorable than those for microadenomas. The larger the tumor, the lower the success rate. In some series, the rate of recurrence has been 20 to 80% over several years; some workers believe that this rate will approach 100% after enough time has passed. The mortality is 0.9%, with a major morbidity of 14%, which includes a 10% incidence of diabetes insipidus, sometimes transitory and sometimes permanent. Repeat trans-sphenoidal operation is far more hazardous than a first or primary procedure, as is any approach that requires craniotomy. Secondary treatment is usually done with bromocriptine.

**Bromocriptine.** The tumor shrinks by one-half or more in about 70% of the treated patients; some shrinkage occurs in the remaining 30%. The prolactin concentration always falls but does not correlate with the tumor size before or during treatment. The rate of shrinkage is rapid; reduction occurs within 1 to 2 weeks and almost always by 6 to 12 weeks. There are no indices that enable prediction of the amount or rate of reduction. A good plan is to treat during a period of many months. Even with signs of chiasmal compression, clinical improvement occurs in more than 90% of patients, so that such signs do not necessarily imply a surgical emergency. This method tends to be the treatment of choice in the United Kingdom; in the United States, most clinics favor trans-sphenoidal surgery as primary therapy.

**Combination Therapy.** For macroadenomas, many, perhaps most, patients require the addition of radiotherapy or trans-sphenoidal resection to the bromocriptine regimen. Not enough patients have been systematically followed to enable a clear statement as to the optimal order of therapeutic methods.

**Observation Only.** Because of the size of the tumor mass, this method is not appropriate for macroprolactinomas.

### Pseudoprolactinomas

These hypothalamic or pituitary tumors, which induce hyperprolactinemia by their pressure effects on the infundibulum or the pituitary stalk, can sometimes be effectively treated with bromocriptine. Usually the treatment of choice is trans-sphenoidal resection (if the tumor is not too large and does not extend too far outside the pituitary fossa) or radiotherapy. It is probably true that many of these tumors are what endocrinologists used to call "chromophobe" or "null cell" adenomas; many of them are now known to be prolactinomas.

### Pregnancy

Probably the best method of treating microadenomas and some macroadenomas in women who desire pregnancy is by initial radiation, followed by bromocriptine therapy (the latter to achieve a more rapid fall in the serum prolactin concentration). Once several ovulatory cycles (three or more) are achieved, conception may be tried. If the attempt is successful, the patient is closely monitored. If in the course of the normal pituitary swelling during gestation there is apparent tumor recurrence, bromocriptine can be safely reinstituted. So far, there is no evidence of bromocriptine teratogenicity; the frequency of congenital anomalies in the fetus is no higher than that in the population of pregnant women at large. The question of whether breast-feeding should be permitted has not yet been settled (compare the stimulatory influence of suckling on pituitary secretion of prolactin).

Bromocriptine treatment has been successfully carried out in more than 3000 pregnant women. In a few patients, trans-sphenoidal surgery—where strongly indicated—has been done with perfect safety during gestation.

### Hyperprolactinemia of Unknown Cause

As indicated earlier, many of these patients do not need treatment. It is not possible to predict with certainty to which patients this statement applies. Still, it is certain that only a tiny minority of microadenomas, even those that can be demonstrated, progress to macroadenomas and

that this evolution is slow. Arguments in favor of treating these patients include restoration of fertility (if desired), restoration of normal estrogen levels (in premenopausal women), restoration of libido and potency (in men), and prevention of possible pituitary tumor (theoretical).

Arguments against treatment include lack of evidence that "idiopathic" hyperprolactinemia is harmful, the observation that in some patients the hyperprolactinemia disappears spontaneously, the possibility that prolonged bromocriptine treatment may induce untoward effects not yet recognized, the high cost of the drug, and the apparent need for indefinite treatment.

# HYPOTHYROIDISM

method of
CHARLES P. BARSANO, M.D., PH.D.
*North Chicago VA Medical Center and the
University of Health Sciences/The Chicago
Medical School
North Chicago, Illinois*

### OBJECTIVES OF THERAPY

In the broadest sense, hypothyroidism is a cellular thyroid hormone deficiency state. If the cellular deficiency of thyroid hormone has been of sufficient degree and duration, the characteristic symptoms and signs of "clinical" hypothyroidism are evident by history and physical examination. "Subclinical" hypothyroidism implies a state in which a cellular thyroid hormone deficiency has not yet generated clinically evident features of hypothyroidism. The logical objective of therapy therefore should be to relieve hypothyroidism of either sort when its existence is clear and unlikely to be transient.

### ESTABLISHING A BASIS FOR TREATING HYPOTHYROIDISM

Several key questions are important to address prior to the institution of thyroid hormone replacement:

1. Do the symptoms, signs, and laboratory findings represent true hypothyroidism? The symptoms and signs of hypothyroidism are notoriously nonspecific. Reductions of serum thyroxine ($T_4$) and, to a much lesser extent, elevations in serum thyroid stimulating hormone (TSH) can occur in clinical situations other than hypothyroidism.

2. Is the hypothyroidism remediable without thyroid hormone replacement? Thyroid hormone replacement is not always the appropriate therapy for hypothyroidism. Drug-induced hypothyroidism—e.g. from propylthiouracil, methimazole or lithium—is usually best managed by a dosage reduction or discontinuation of the responsible medication.

3. Is the hypothyroidism transient? Transient periods of clinical or serologic hypothyroidism can occur in

subacute thyroiditis, in "silent" thyroiditis, and after discontinuation of chronic suppressive thyroxine therapy. In most cases the hypothyroidism is mild and requires no therapy.

4. Should adjunctive therapy precede or accompany the institution of thyroid hormone replacement? Hypothyroid patients with angina pectoris may require antianginal drugs or even coronary bypass grafting prior to thyroid hormone replacement. Patients with secondary hypothyroidism or severe primary hypothyroidism may require concurrent corticosteroid coverage.

## PREPARATIONS

Synthetic L-thyroxine is the drug of choice for the treatment of hypothyroidism. Near-physiologic proportions of serum $T_4$ and triiodothyronine ($T_3$) are achieved with little if any fluctuation in the serum levels of either hormone after once-daily administration. Desiccated thyroid USP, thyroglobulin, and combinations of $T_4$ and $T_3$ (liotrix) result in postingestion peaks in the serum $T_3$ that, in a few patients, may be associated with palpitations or other symptoms of hyperthyroidism. These preparations also complicate the monitoring of therapy. The serum $T_3$ concentrations may be considerably supraphysiologic in the presence of normal serum $T_4$ concentrations for several hours after dosing yet be well within the normal range at other times of the day. Thus the metabolic status of the patient may be neither uniform nor accurately represented by the serum $T_4$ or TSH concentrations.

## TREATMENT

### Initiation of Therapy

Several factors are particularly important to consider with regard to when and how to initiate thyroxine replacement therapy.

### Severity of Hypothyroidism

In the mildly hypothyroid patient unlikely to have significant coronary artery disease (e.g., a premenopausal woman), thyroxine replacement can often be started at a full replacement dosage—0.100 to 0.125 mg daily (Table 1). I gener-

TABLE 1. **Initiation and Advancement of Thyroxine (Levothyroxine) Dosage**

| Severity of Hypothyroidism | Initial Daily Dosage (mg)* | Monthly Increment in Daily Dosage (mg)* |
|---|---|---|
| Mild | 0.050–0.125 | 0.050 |
| Moderate | 0.050 | 0.025–0.050 |
| Severe† | 0.025 | 0.025 |

*In the presence of significant coronary artery disease, known or suspected, medical and surgical antianginal therapy should be considered prior to the institution of thyroxine replacement. The above dosages may also require reduction by ~50%.

†Myxedema coma is a special situation that requires high-dose thyroxine therapy and concurrent supportive measures.

ally provide a prescription for 0.100-mg or 0.125-mg tablets with the instructions to take one-half tablet daily for 1 or 2 weeks before advancing to one tablet daily. In my experience, this practice helps to minimize the occasional complaint of palpitations early after the initiation of replacement therapy.

In moderate hypothyroidism, therapy can be initiated with 0.050 mg daily and, if well tolerated, increased by the same amount 1 month later. Further adjustments in dosage are determined on the basis of the history, examination, and hormone levels as discussed later.

In the severely hypothyroid patient without significant coronary artery disease and without the neurologic features of myxedema coma, thyroxine therapy should begin with 0.025 mg daily. If well tolerated, the daily dosage can be increased by 0.025 mg at monthly intervals. Therapy in each case must be individualized, but it is often best to initiate treatment of the severely hypothyroid patient on an inpatient basis with particular vigilance for the unmasking of cardiac ischemia or hypoadrenalism.

In the presence of well-controlled angina or suspected myocardial ischemia, the initial thyroxine doses and increments of dose advancement recommended in Table 1 may need to be reduced by approximately 50%. Careful, frequent clinical evaluations are very important for assessing the need and efficacy of the antianginal regimen.

### Coronary Artery Disease

It has long been recognized that thyroid hormone replacement can unmask latent myocardial ischemia, exacerbate pre-existing angina, and even precipitate myocardial infarction. There are also reports of thyroid hormone replacement relieving pre-existing angina. In practice, however, the possibility of exacerbating cardiac ischemia must take precedence over the possibility of ameliorating ischemia. In recent years, it has been shown that the hypothyroid patient with severe angina can undergo coronary catheterization, angiography, and bypass grafting with little risk beyond that of the same procedures in euthyroid patients. Indeed, the risks attending initiation of hormone replacement before bypass grafting appear to be greater than the risks of bypass surgery in the untreated hypothyroid patient. In this light, coronary bypass surgery should be considered as a very early, if not the first, step in the treatment of the hypothyroid patient with pre-existing angina or angina appearing in the course of thyroid hormone replacement therapy. Postoperative initiation of thyroid hormone replacement, and its advancement to complete euthyroidism, is usually well tolerated.

It is also noteworthy that hypothyroid patients are as highly sensitive to the effects of cardiac drugs as they are to medications in general. Because of the slower drug metabolism or clearance in hypothyroidism, exaggerated drug effects are often observed with standard doses of many medications. More pronounced or frequent hypotension and bradycardia may result from ordinary doses of nitrates and beta blockers, respectively. Lower initial doses of digoxin should be considered to avoid digitalis toxicity.

Until the relevant risk factors are better defined, cautious advancement of thyroxine dosage should also attend the treatment of hypothyroid patients with cardiac arrhythmias. As demonstrated in a recent study, the number of "benign" atrial (but not ventricular) premature beats per 24 hours is likely to increase after hormonal restitution of euthyroidism. Additional studies of the effects of thyroid hormone replacement on specific cardiac arrhythmias would be of much interest and value.

### The Perioperative Period

The potential complications of surgery in the severely hypothyroid patient are numerous and include perioperative respiratory problems, exaggerated effects of anesthetics and sedatives, and precipitation of myxedema coma, hypothermia, hypotension, congestive heart failure, adynamic ileus, and imbalances of fluids and electrolytes. The risks of such complications are expectedly less, and in fact not always demonstrable, in mildly to moderately hypothyroid patients. Current opinion is that surgery in mild to moderate hypothyroidism, although not risk-free compared with surgery in the euthyroid patient, is decidedly safer than was previously believed. When balanced against the risks of unmasking latent coronary artery disease during the perioperative period and the risk/benefit ratio of delaying surgery to accommodate at least partial hormone replacement, there will be occasions when surgery in the moderately hypothyroid patient should be performed without delay and without a token attempt to treat the hypothyroidism preoperatively.

It is important to recognize that although normal serum levels of thyroid hormones can be restored very rapidly if desired, the restoration of the euthyroid state is a process typically requiring months of therapy. Moreover, there is reasonable doubt that a few days of preoperative thyroxine replacement would provide the moderately hypothyroid patient with any benefit commensurate with the risks of initiating therapy and delaying surgery.

It is impossible to formulate rigid recommendations regarding urgent surgery in the severely hypothyroid patient. If symptomatic myocardial ischemia is present, it is probably best to proceed without institution of thyroxine replacement. When coronary artery disease is not a major factor in a severely hypothyroid patient, some investigators recommend starting 0.025 mg of thyroxine daily and delaying surgery for at least 48 hours if possible. If urgent surgery is required in a patient with myxedema coma, it would seem prudent to begin specific therapy for myxedema coma immediately. In view of the substantial mortality of myxedema coma under the best of circumstances, the potentially serious risk from delaying surgery for a few days may at times be less than the risk of proceeding without delay. Because of the impaired adrenocortical stress response in severely hypothyroid individuals, these patients, regardless of mental status, should receive perioperative glucocorticoid coverage in stress doses—e.g., 100 mg of hydrocortisone every 8 hours.

Elective surgery in mild or subclinical hypothyroidism can usually be performed without delay and without preoperative initiation of thyroxine replacement. In moderate or severe hypothyroidism, however, elective surgery should be delayed until euthyroidism is restored.

### Maintenance and Monitoring of Therapy

Estimates of the average daily replacement dosage of thyroxine have declined over the years to a present consensus of approximately 0.110 mg to 0.130 mg per day (approximately 1.6 $\mu$g per kg per day). These estimates should not be regarded as end points in the titration of thyroxine dosage, since many well-managed patients require a greater than average dosage while many others require a less than average dosage. Rather, the average daily thyroxine replacement dosage serves as a useful guideline. I would reevaluate the adequacy or appropriateness of therapy in any individual purported to be well managed on a daily thyroxine dosage considerably greater or less than the average daily replacement dosage—e.g., >0.175 mg or <0.075 mg daily.

A conventional and generally effective strategy for thyroxine replacement in primary hypothyroidism is the titration of thyroxine to the lowest dosage required to maintain clinical euthyroidism, a nonelevated serum TSH, and a normal or slightly elevated serum $T_4$ or free $T_4$ index (Table 2). Serum $T_3$ levels are almost always normal and need not be monitored. The serum $T_4/T_3$ ratio in patients receiving thyroxine replacement is

TABLE 2. **Conventional Criteria for the Titration of Thyroxine (Levothyroxine) Dosage**

| Parameter | End Point* |
|---|---|
| History and examination | No signs or symptoms of hypo- or hyperthyroidism |
| Serum TSH† | Nonelevated |
| Serum $T_4$ (or free $T_4$ index) | Normal to slightly elevated |

*The lowest daily dosage of thyroxine required to meet the above conditions in patients with primary hypothyroidism is considered optimal.

†Determined by either conventional thyroid stimulating hormone by radioimmunoassay (TSH-RIA) or high-sensitivity TSH assays.

generally higher than the ratio observed in normal individuals.

In the first year of replacement therapy, the serum $T_4$, $T_3$, and TSH concentrations do not always remain the same on a constant daily dosage of thyroxine. In the early months of therapy, the serum $T_4$ and $T_3$ levels may fully normalize as the serum TSH decreases. In the ensuing weeks or months, the serum $T_4$ and $T_3$ may begin to fall while the serum TSH begins to increase without any change in thyroxine dosage. It is probable that with the gradual amelioration of hypothyroidism, the turnover of thyroid hormone is restored to the more rapid, euthyroid rate. Thus, lower serum thyroid hormone levels are maintained at a fixed input of hormone. Surveillance should not be reduced as soon as clinical and serologic euthyroidism is first achieved. Rather, adequacy of therapy should be re-evaluated every 2 to 3 months during the first year of therapy. After the first year, or when it is clear that the patient's clinical status and serum $T_4$ and TSH concentrations are both appropriate and stable, the patient can be evaluated on an annual basis.

### Recent Considerations in the Monitoring of Replacement Therapy

Conventional monitoring of thyroxine replacement therapy employing clinical assessment, serum $T_4$, and serum TSH by radioimmunoassay (TSH-RIA) is not as sensitive for the detection of thyroxine overmedication as it is for the detection of undermedication. Gross overmedication is usually clinically evident by the symptoms and signs of hyperthyroidism. The symptomatology of mild hyperthyroidism, however, is often equivocal or too nonspecific to use for modifying ongoing hormone replacement. It remains controversial if an elevated serum $T_4$ concentration necessarily represents excess thyroxine dosage. Patients with slightly elevated serum $T_4$ levels are usually euthyroid clinically. Because their corresponding

serum $T_3$ levels are typically lower than those of normal or hyperthyroid individuals with equivalent serum $T_4$ levels, slight elevations of the serum $T_4$ need not imply an excess of net thyroid hormone activity. Likewise, undetectable serum TSH levels by conventional radioimmunoassay do not imply an excessive dosage of thyroxine.

The new generation of high-sensitivity TSH assays (HS-TSH) may provide a means for reliable detection or exclusion of thyroxine overmedication. In contrast to the conventional TSH-RIA, the HS-TSH assays can separate normal serum TSH concentrations (approximately 0.3 to 5 µU per ml) from the suppressed serum TSH concentrations consistent with, but not necessarily diagnostic of, hyperthyroidism (less than 0.1 µU per ml).

In recent years, much attention has been focussed on the potential adverse effects of "subclinical" hyperthyroidism—i.e., a postulated degree of hormone excess sufficient to impair tissue function but inadequate to generate concurrent symptoms or signs of hyperthyroidism. At present, many studies document abnormalities of systolic time intervals, bone mineral density, or serum markers of hepatic "tissue thyrotoxicosis" in serologically defined states of "subclinical" hyperthyroidism. The implication that "subclinical" hyperthyroidism sustained for years would eventuate in clinical disease is speculative but reasonable and deserving of serious consideration.

Thyroxine-replaced patients with "subclinical" hyperthyroidism are asymptomatic by definition. However, there is no unanimity on which laboratory parameters indicate the presence of "subclinical" hyperthyroidism. Although there are insufficient data at this time to equate with certainty a fully suppressed or undetectable HS-TSH (less than approximately 0.1 µU per ml) with "subclinical" hyperthyroidism, by force of logic "subclinical" hyperthyroidism must be much less likely in the presence of an incompletely suppressed HS-TSH (greater than 0.1 µU per ml) than in the presence of a fully suppressed HS-TSH level. Accordingly, it has been my practice to modify the conventional strategy for thyroxine replacement in primary hypothyroidism such as to maintain a nonelevated, incompletely suppressed HS-TSH in a clinically euthyroid patient (Table 3). The serum $T_4$ and $T_3$ concentrations are not employed as end points of therapy but do fall within the normal reference intervals. Although not necessary in the decision-making process of this strategy, the serum $T_4$ is useful for gauging the extent of over- or undermedication when the HS-TSH is fully suppressed or elevated, respectively.

TABLE 3. **Modified Criteria for the Titration of Thyroxine Dosage**

| Parameter | End Point* |
|---|---|
| History and examination | No signs or symptoms of hypo- or hyperthyroidism |
| Serum HS-TSH† | Nonelevated but not fully suppressed‡ |
| Serum T$_4$ (or free T$_4$ index) | Normal to slightly elevated |

*The lowest daily dosage of thyroxine required to meet the above conditions in patients with primary hypothyroidism is considered optimal.

†Determined in a high-sensitivity thyroid stimulating hormone (TSH) assay—i.e., an assay whose sensitivity is ≤0.1 μU/ml.

‡"Fully suppressed" is defined as a serum TSH concentration equal to or less than that exhibited by known thyrotoxic patients in the same assay, typically ≤0.1 μU/ml.

## Special Clinical Situations

### Secondary (Pituitary) Hypothyroidism

Thyroid hormone replacement in secondary hypothyroidism is governed by the same general principles recommended in primary hypothyroidism, with two important exceptions. In the event of concurrent hypoadrenalism, traditional wisdom has been to initiate glucocorticoid replacement at or before institution of thyroid hormone replacement. In principle, the initiation of thyroxine replacement constitutes a metabolic "stress" capable of precipitating an "adrenal crisis" in untreated hypoadrenalism.

The second important exception is that in secondary hypothyroidism serum TSH is not a valid criterion for assessing the adequacy of thyroid hormone replacement. In secondary hypothyroidism, thyroxine dosage is based upon the restoration of euthyroidism by clinical parameters in conjunction with a normal serum T$_4$ concentration.

### Myxedema Coma

Severe hypothyroidism accompanied by a marked depression of the sensorium—myxedema coma—is a medical emergency requiring prompt therapy. In contrast to severe hypothyroidism without sensorial changes, myxedema coma is best treated by the intravenous administration of 0.250 mg to 0.500 mg of thyroxine followed by intravenous administration of 0.100 mg of thyroxine on a daily basis. No less important are various supportive measures, best provided in an intensive care unit. Occasionally these patients require mechanical ventilation. Administration of intravenous fluids must be judicious because of the deficient free water clearance in severe hypothyroidism. Hypothermia is best treated by passive warming to prevent excessive peripheral vasodilatation and hypotension. Glucocorticoid

coverage, 100 mg hydrocortisone every 8 hours, is also recommended because of the impaired adrenocortical stress response observed in severe hypothyroidism. Even with prompt and intensive treatment, mortality in myxedema coma is high.

### Hypothyroidism in Pregnancy

Hypothyroidism in the pregnant woman is a potentially serious problem that, if untreated, is associated with an increased risk of spontaneous abortion. Of importance to the clinician, the marked increase in serum thyroxine binding globulin (TBG) in normal pregnancy predictably raises the serum T$_4$ concentration above the normal reference interval by up to approximately 50%. The free T$_4$ index generally corrects well for this binding aberration and remains within its established norms. The diagnostic and therapeutic implications of augmented TBG levels in pregnancy are (1) that primary hypothyroidism is not excluded by a serum T$_4$ concentration within the normal reference interval; and (2) that appropriate thyroxine replacement should ordinarily achieve a serum T$_4$ concentration at or above the normal reference interval—e.g., 12 to 16 μg per dl. The interpretation of serum TSH and the general management of hypothyroidism in the pregnant patient are otherwise the same as in the nonpregnant individual.

# HYPERTHYROIDISM

method of
JOHN T. NICOLOFF, M.D.
*USC School of Medicine*
*Los Angeles, California*

Hyperthyroidism and thyrotoxicosis are synonymous terms used to describe the signs and symptoms produced in patients who are chronically exposed to excessive levels of thyroid hormone. Emphasis should be placed on the chronicity of this process, since it requires many weeks and even months to develop or recover from hyperthyroidism. This is not only because of the long biologic half-life that thyroid hormones possess in the circulation but also because of their prolonged effects on target tissues. As a result of these characteristics, the therapeutic management of hyperthyroidism is a somewhat lengthy process falling into three distinct phases. The first consists of an *acute medical management phase* in which the physician initiates a variety of supportive measures designed to assist the patient in tolerating the thyrotoxicosis until antithyroid therapy has an opportunity to mitigate the underlying hyperthyroid condition. The second relates to *establishing a specific diagnosis and antithyroid therapy program*, while the final phase concerns the *achievement of a permanent euthyroid state and a long-term follow-up plan.*

Throughout this treatment program, certain temporal milestones should be kept in mind. Within 2 or 3 days of starting therapy, the patient's general nutritional, medical, and psychiatric status should be stabilized; by 2 weeks, there should be evidence of substantial biochemical and clinical improvement; by 4 to 10 weeks, a near-euthyroid status should be achieved; and by 6 months, a permanent stable state of eumetabolism, or the strategy for accomplishing it, should be apparent. To meet these goals, the physician and patient must work closely together as a team. The failure to do so, in this author's experience, is the most common cause for lack of therapeutic success.

## PHASE I. ACUTE MEDICAL MANAGEMENT OF HYPERTHYROIDISM

With all of the therapeutic tools available for treatment of hyperthyroidism, it is surprising that none of them directly reverse the action of thyroid hormones at the peripheral tissue level. Thus, until antithyroid therapy produces a sustained normalization in circulating thyroid hormone levels, medical management must be directed at providing supportive care to ameliorate the effects of hyperthyroidism. In order to accomplish this task, the physician must have an understanding of the major metabolic demands placed on the thyrotoxic patient.

Increased thermogenesis and an exaggerated response to beta-adrenergic stimuli represent the two most important metabolic challenges facing the hyperthyroid patient. In response to this endogenously generated thermogenic load, the cardiovascular system shunts blood to the skin for purposes of dissipating heat. This increased shunting results in a greater return of blood to the heart, producing a high-output state characteristic of hyperthyroidism. This condition is physiologically similar to the high-output state normally observed in exercising euthyroid subjects. Therefore, the cardiovascular system in thyrotoxic patients is chronically overburdened, not only to meet increased tissue oxygen requirements but also to assist in losing excess body heat. The exaggerated beta-adrenergic responses often cause patients to experience an increased sense of nervousness and anxiety, rapid heart action, and tremor. To counter these effects, supportive care should be directed toward four general areas: (1) educating patients as to the character of the underlying disease condition, (2) improving nutrition to compensate for the hypermetabolic state, (3) reducing cardiovascular demands, and (4) employing beta-blocking drugs.

**Patient Education.** It is important to counsel patients that hyperthyroidism characteristically produces emotional instability and that they should not be unduly worried if they are having problems in this regard. Often after raising this subject, patients, as well as their spouses or family members, will spontaneously bring forward a multiplicity of concerns regarding their emotional stability. Explaining in lay terms the mechanism by which this emotional lability is produced, indicating that the condition is reversible and that there are medications available to help in its management, will have a beneficial effect on easing such concerns. It is also prudent to advise patients not to make any critical personal decisions until their illness is well controlled for several months. The physician should then outline the general goals of their treatment program. It is also helpful to provide appropriate reading material, since the patient's attention span and ability to retain information may be impaired.

**Nutritional Therapy.** Most hyperthyroid patients lose weight despite increased dietary intake. If the patient reports a poor appetite, this may be a sign of a poor prognosis, as well as a possible harbinger of an intercurrent illness and/or thyroid storm. More commonly, however, patients are simply "too nervous" to eat and with adequate beta blockade, rest, and reassurance, they will usually reverse this pattern to a more appropriate hyperphagic state that will allow them to stabilize or possibly restore some of the lost weight. If anorexia persists despite the institution of these measures, careful evaluation for some intercurrent illness and consideration of hospitalization may be indicated until the nutritional status improves.

**Reduction in Cardiovascular Workload.** Some modest reduction in physical demands is usually advisable for most patients. When dealing with younger patients who are otherwise healthy, one may advise avoiding extremes of physical exertion such as competitive sports. In the elderly or in those patients with possible underlying heart disease, a more cautious approach should be taken. This might include reduction in working hours, use of frequent rest periods, and avoidance of exposure to high environmental temperatures. For those demonstrating signs of heart failure, bed rest, a calm supportive environment, reduction in dietary salt intake, and judicious use of diuretics serve as the cornerstone of therapy. Usually these patients are also digitalized; however, the inotropic benefits of digitalization are usually not striking in hyperthyroid patients. Digitalization is effective, however, for controlling heart rate in cases of atrial fibrillation and/or flutter, which is seen in approximately 15% of patients with hyperthyroidism. Reduction in the ventricular response rate to the range of 90 to 120 serves as an appropriate end point while the patient is in a hypermetabolic state. Attempts to slow the heart rate further are not desirable and may be associated with precipitation of heart failure. Serum digoxin levels may require monitoring, since drug clearance is accelerated with hyperthyroidism and will slow as the patient is brought into an eumetabolic state.

**Beta-Adrenergic Blocking Drugs.** Beta-adrenergic blocking drugs have proved to be very useful agents for controlling a wide variety of hyperadrenergic manifestations associated with hyperthyroidism. Such common features as tremor, diaphoresis, palpitations, and anxiety dramatically improve with their use. For the ambulatory patients who are attempting to pursue an active life, beta-adrenergic drugs are particularly valuable in allowing them to perform in a more normal manner. It should also be stated that reduction in emotional and physical demands placed on the patient will also produce similar beneficial results. Thus, the physician should discuss with the patient the need to achieve an appropriate balance between the use of beta-blocking drugs and reducing physical and emotional environmental stress.

There are certain instances in which beta-blocking drugs have benefits in hyperthyroidism that would not be predicted on the basis of their adrenergic blocking effects. These conditions include reduction in hypercalcemia, prevention of hypokalemic periodic paralysis, and reversal of acute hallucinatory psychosis. In all of these instances, beta-blocking drugs will promptly and dramatically improve the aberrant function if it is secondary to thyrotoxicosis. Propranolol (Inderal) also inhibits thyroxine ($T_4$) to triiodothyronine ($T_3$) conversion by peripheral tissue deiodinase systems and thereby decreases serum $T_3$ levels. This effect is, however, not mediated through its beta-blocking action, but by its membrane stabilizing effects.

The dose of beta-blocking drug required varies considerably from patient to patient. For propranolol, the most widely employed beta-blocking drug, the oral dose may vary from 10 to 80 mg administered three or four times daily. The reasons for this large variation in dose requirement probably relates to variability in bioavailability and therapeutic end point employed. Nadolol (Corgard), metoprolol (Lopressor), and atenolol (Tenormin) have also been used with apparent therapeutic success. These other beta-blocking drugs have the purported advantages of being longer acting, cardioselective, or not passing through the blood-brain barrier. The contraindications for employment of beta-blocking therapy are relative but rarely absolute. In patients with coexisting bronchospasm, bradycardiac conduction disorders, and congestive heart failure, beta-

blocking drugs should not be employed or used with caution. Because these drugs reduce vascular shunting, they may be beneficial in reducing cardiac workload in patients with high-output heart failure. However, in such cases, they should not be used as the initial form of therapy until the congestive failure is brought into better control by bed rest and diuresis. When used orally and starting at low doses, adverse effects are rarely seen. In contrast, life-threatening difficulties may be encountered with their intravenous use, particularly in severely ill patients whose cardiovascular status is unstable.

## PHASE II. DIAGNOSIS AND CHOOSING THE ANTITHYROID THERAPY PROGRAM

**Diagnosis.** Before one initiates an antithyroid therapy program, it is essential to establish the underlying cause of the hyperthyroidism because the therapeutic approaches differ depending upon etiology. Graves' disease, which compromises the majority of cases, is usually not a difficult diagnosis to establish, owing to its characteristic clinical features and laboratory findings. The remaining 5 to 15% of cases result mostly from toxic nodular goiter or thyroiditis. These latter entities should be entertained, if the typical clinical picture for Graves' disease is not present. More troublesome is the identification of rarer forms of hyperthyroidism, such as factitious, thyroid stimulating hormone (TSH) secreting tumors, and ectopic hormone secretion. Critical assessment of atypical clinical presentations and the employment of the new sensitive serum TSH methods appear to provide the best means for recognizing these unusual etiologies. Because Graves' disease constitutes the most common cause of hyperthyroidism, the greatest emphasis will be placed on its therapeutic management.

**Choice of Antithyroid Therapy Program for Graves' Disease.** There are three antithyroid therapy programs available to the clinician for treatment of Graves' disease: (1) thioamide drugs, (2) radioiodine, and (3) surgery. All three methods control hyperthyroidism by impairing hormone secretion—the first by chemical blockade, and the latter two by ablation of the thyroid gland itself. However, none of the three significantly alter the underlying autoimmune disorder producing Graves' disease. The choice of therapy should, therefore, be a pragmatic one balancing the therapeutic benefits against potential adverse side effects for each form of therapy. Based on this line of reasoning, radioiodine therapy has deservedly gained the reputation as the most effective therapy for treatment of hyperthyroid Graves' disease, while thioamide and surgical therapy have been relegated to a secondary role to be employed in certain selected instances. It is our present view that *radioiodine ablative therapy should be considered the treatment of choice for hyperthyroid Graves' disease.*

The reasons why radioiodine therapy has gained this pre-eminent position in the management of hyperthyroid Graves' disease are multiple and deserve emphasis. They include (1) *simplicity*—its administration is the ultimate of simplicity in that the patient merely drinks a tasteless radioactive solution; (2) *safety*—during the more than 35 years of its use in more than a million patients, no adverse side effects have been observed; (3) *cost*—overall, this is the least expensive form of therapy; (4) *definitiveness*—relapse following radioablation is rare; and (5) *effectiveness*—once radioablation has been achieved, thyroxine replacement therapy provides a dependable means of maintaining a euthyroid status.

The apparent advantage of thioamide therapy is that a remission in Graves' disease may be achieved during the course of antithyroid drug treatment that is sustained following cessation of drug therapy. However, long-term remissions probably do not occur in any more than 25 to 35% of cases. Follow-up studies of such apparently remitted cases often reveal concurrent chronic thyroiditis that eventually will produce thyroid failure or, alternatively, persistent subclinical hyperthyroidism, as shown by suppressed serum-sensitive TSH values. Despite this rather negative view of long-term antithyroid drug therapy, there is a defined subgroup of patients who may benefit from a trial of antithyroid drugs. Even if a complete remission is achieved, however, such patients must be carefully monitored for the remainder of their lives for possible relapse or spontaneous thyroid failure.

The use of subtotal thyroidectomy as a form of primary treatment for hyperthyroid Graves' disease has limited indications. This is principally due to the fact that radioiodine treatment has proved to be a much easier, simpler, and safer form of ablative therapy.

## GENERAL GUIDELINES FOR THERAPY IN HYPERTHYROID GRAVES' DISEASE

Our current recommendations regarding an antithyroid treatment program are as follows: (1) *Radioiodine therapy* is the primary form of treatment for all nonpregnant patients over the age of 20 years. (2) *Thioamide therapy* may be given as a long-term trial in selected patients who are likely to undergo spontaneous remission. These drugs are also indicated for control of hyperthy-

roidism during the course of pregnancy and in young patients until they reach an age at which they can assume personal responsibility for management of their [131]I-induced hypothyroidism. (3) *Subtotal thyroidectomy* is indicated in pregnant patients during the second trimester if thioamide drugs are ineffective or when a concurrent neoplastic nodule is discovered in a Graves' disease gland. Subtotal thyroidectomy may also be employed as a secondary choice in those patients who refuse radioiodine therapy.

### Radioiodine Therapy for Graves' Disease

The primary goal of radioiodine therapy for Graves' disease is ablation of the thyroid gland. It is important that the primary physician and nuclear medicine consultant fully inform the patient as to the potential side effects and consequences of [131]I therapy. The physician should be fully satisfied that the patient understands the consequences of this form of therapy and is willing to assume the basic responsibility for long-term follow-up.

**Dosage.** Recommended dosages of [131]I may vary considerably depending on the nuclear medicine unit administering the radioiodine. Smaller dosages have been employed in an attempt to avoid the induction of hypothyroidism, whereas larger doses have been favored by those wanting to achieve rapid and certain control of the hyperthyroidism while accepting the fact that primary hypothyroidism will be produced. We favor the latter approach of using the larger [131]I doses because it is evident that all patients will eventually become hypothyroid after radioiodine therapy regardless of size of the original dose employed. The only difference is that with the larger dose this occurs more rapidly. We currently recommend a dose of 15 mCi as the initial treatment. This large dose will achieve ablation in about 90% of patients by 6 months. If ablation is not achieved and thyrotoxicosis persists, a repeat dose ranging between 15 to 29 mCi is recommended.

**Response.** During the first 2 weeks following radioiodine therapy, there is usually little chemical or clinical evidence of change in the hyperthyroid state. Thereafter, there is typically a rapid drop in serum thyroid hormone indices that achieves a nadir somewhere between 6 and 12 weeks after therapy. The thyroid gland size usually diminishes in parallel with the falling serum thyroid hormone indices. A fall in these two parameters, in association with an increase in serum TSH levels, serves as a harbinger of successful ablation and the need to initiate thyroid hormone replacement therapy. When thyroid glandular size does not decline as serum hormone indices fall, this indicates that a relapse may occur in 2 or 3 months after recovery from the acute radiation effects. This latter pattern is more common when lower doses of radioiodine are employed.

**Pretreatment Before Radioiodine Therapy.** In patients with severe hyperthyroidism and/or very large thyroid glands, it may be advisable to pretreat the patient with thioamide drugs to control the hyperthyroidism prior to radioiodine therapy. Such thioamide therapy should be discontinued 2 or 3 days prior to the scheduled radioiodine so that it will not interfere with the retention of the radioiodine in the thyroid gland. This withdrawal period from thioamide therapy should be no longer than 3 days, since the hyperthyroidism may rapidly reoccur. Such pretreatment has the additional advantage of bringing the patient more rapidly to a euthyroid state than would occur if radioiodine were used alone.

In the mild or moderate forms of hyperthyroidism, pretreatment with beta blockade to control the hyperadrenergic symptoms of hyperthyroidism is often helpful. This pretreatment has the advantage of requiring no delay in the administration of radioiodine therapy as well as being a simpler and more straightforward treatment approach.

**Side Effects.** Permanent hypothyroidism is the principal side effect of radioiodine therapy. It should be emphasized to the patients before they receive the radioiodine therapy that they are deliberately being made hypothyroid and that their thyroid status will subsequently depend on exogenous thyroxine replacement therapy. It should also be stressed that it is the patient's primary responsibility for taking the replacement therapy.

Patients frequently voice fears that radioiodine therapy may induce cancers, such as leukemia, or cause an increased incidence of birth defects. Although such concerns are understandable, they have proved to be unfounded. Although the patient should be told that radiation can do harm to the body, they should also be informed that most of it is directed at the thyroid gland where tissue destruction is desired. Outside the thyroid gland, the radiation dose to the body is only at modest levels comparable with what would be received from a standard diagnostic study such as with a gastrointestinal x-ray series. One can also emphasize the precision of radioiodine therapy by the fact that the parathyroid glands, immediately adjacent to the thyroid gland, are not functionally impaired by the radioiodine therapy.

**Radioiodine Therapy in Young Patients.** We have previously emphasized that the age limitation on administration of radioiodine primarily relates to the maturity of the patients in accepting the management responsibilities for their hypothyroidism. An additional consideration is that radiation therapy, especially in young patients, is associated with an increased frequency of subsequent nodularity in the radiated thyroid remnant. Such nodularity could cause concern regarding the possibility of the induction of a malignant growth that might eventually require thyroid surgery. When one employs the higher radioiodine dosages as recommended, near-total thyroid ablation will result, which will virtually abolish this problem.

### Thioamide Drug Therapy

The two most widely employed thioamide drugs are methimazole (Tapazole) and propylthiouracil (PTU). Both of these drugs act by inhibiting the synthesis of thyroid hormones by the thyroid gland. The potency of methimazole is at least 10 times greater than that of PTU on a milligram-for-milligram basis. PTU, but not methimazole, will also inhibit the peripheral tissue conversion of thyroxine ($T_4$) to triiodothyronine ($T_3$), which is a useful characteristic in the management of severely thyrotoxic patients. However, methimazole is preferred over PTU for outpatient therapy because of its longer duration of action, which makes compliance a less critical issue. *The greatest problem with the use of thioamide drugs is the necessity for excellent compliance. Failure of patient compliance is the most common cause for treatment failures with thioamide drugs.*

**Dosage Schedule.** The recommended starting dosage of methimazole is 20 mg (two tablets) twice daily or alternatively 300 to 400 mg of PTU in two to three divided doses daily. Dosages greater than 60 mg of methimazole or its equivalent in PTU are not recommended, even in severely hyperthyroid patients, since these higher dosages are associated with a greater frequency of adverse side effects and afford only a minimal increase in thyroid blocking action.

**Assessment of Therapeutic Response.** Regardless of the severity of elevations in serum thyroid hormone indices observed, if the patient adheres to the therapeutic schedule, chemical euthyroidism will be achieved in 4 to 8 weeks following the initiation of thioamide therapy. Therefore, normal serum free thyroxine levels will be achieved in 4 to 8 weeks regardless of the magnitude of elevation in the original serum $T_4$ values. Serum $T_4$ concentrations should be assessed during the first 2 weeks after starting therapy to confirm that serum $T_4$ levels are declining in the expected fashion. If they are not, it can be assumed that the patient is not fully complying with the medication regimen. It cannot be emphasized enough that even a brief period of noncompliance will result in a rapid relapse in hyperthyroidism.

After the restoration of normal serum thyroid hormone indices, the thioamide dose should be reduced. In the case of methimazole, this is accomplished by reducing the frequency of administration to a single morning dose. Often this daily methimazole dose can be as low as 5 mg. Some clinicians will also add oral thyroxine to the regimen in the dosage range of 100 µg daily to prevent hypothyroidism induced by overtreatment. However, this is usually not necessary.

**Adverse Side Effects.** All patients should be carefully instructed regarding adverse effects produced by thioamide drugs. Although most of these side effects will rapidly remit following cessation of drug therapy, some of them may be severe and potentially fatal. Mild gastric irritation is a common problem of thioamide drug therapy that can be largely overcome by administering the drug with meals. In approximately 3 to 5% of patients, an urticarial skin eruption may develop several weeks after starting therapy. If is mild, it can usually be managed with antihistaminic drugs without stopping thioamide therapy. If severe, medication should be switched to the alternative thioamide drug preparation.

Less common side effects include cholestatic *jaundice*, arthralgias, drug fever, and neuritis, which usually regress on discontinuance of therapy. These complications are potentially serious, making an alternative therapy, such as radioiodine, indicated.

The most dangerous adverse effect is agranulocytosis, which fortunately occurs in less than 0.1% of cases. This complication usually occurs during the first few months of therapy and appears, to some degree, to be related to the size of the dose. There is no prognostic benefit of performing routine white cell counts, since differential white cell counts may be entirely normal immediately before the onset of agranulocytosis. The only safeguard is to warn all patients that with the onset of a sore throat or fever they should immediately stop their thioamide medication and have their blood cell count determined. If agranulocytosis does occur, patients should be placed in reverse isolation and given broad-spectrum antibiotic coverage. A detectable monocyte count, even in the absence of granulocytes, is a good prognostic sign that recovery will occur. A fatal outcome occurs in about 10% of patients experiencing this complication.

**Long-Term Thioamide Therapy.** There is a subset of hyperthyroid Graves' disease patients who may be candidates for long-term thioamide therapy with the hope of obtaining a remission in their Graves' hyperthyroidism. Such patients should meet most of the following criteria: (1) recent onset, (2) small thyroid gland, (3) negative family history for autoimmune thyroid disease, (4) absence of concurrent chronic thyroiditis, (5) high motivation to follow through on therapy, and (6) female gender.

**Assessment of Remission.** Probably the simplest gauge for determining whether a remission has occurred during the course of thioamide therapy is reduction of the thyroid gland size. Regression to a normal or near-normal gland size while on thioamide therapy indicates that a remission has likely taken place and that consideration should be given to withdrawing antithyroid drug therapy. An arbitrary therapy trial period ranging between 6 and 18 months may also be employed. Approximately 80% of those who are going to achieve remission will do so by 6 months.

There have been a number of methods proposed for verifying whether a remission has occurred. The simplest method is to measure serum thyroid hormone indices just prior to and 2 weeks following the withdrawal from antithyroid drug therapy. If thyroid indices rapidly increase, particularly serum $T_3$ levels, the patient is likely to experience a relapse. If thyroid indices remain essentially unaltered, a remission may have occurred. However, the patient should be carefully monitored over the next several months for evidence of biochemical and clinical relapse. If this is observed, reinstitution of the thioamide therapy for purposes of achieving an eventual remission or alternatively selection of an ablative form of treatment, such as radioiodine, is indicated.

### Thyroidectomy

The main indication for thyroidectomy is the patient with an exceptionally large goiter that may require multiple radiotherapy doses or when there is a question that there may be concurrent neoplastic growth contained within the thyroid gland. Infrequently, pregnant thyrotoxic patients who are poorly managed with thioamide therapy may also require thyroidectomy in the second trimester.

**Preoperative Preparation.** All patients undergoing elective thyroidectomy should first receive a course of thioamide therapy to render them chemically and clinically euthyroid. After achieving this goal, exogenous iodine (5 drops of saturated solution of potassium iodine twice daily) is then added to the thioamide treatment regimen for 5 to 10 days to reduce vascularity and fragility of the thyroid gland, thereby facilitating its surgical removal.

**Risks.** The complications from subtotal thyroid-ectomy vary considerably, depending upon the skill of the surgeon and the extent to which the thyroid gland is removed. In the properly prepared patient, the mortality risk should be essentially that of anesthesia. The complication of recurrent laryngeal palsy or permanent hypoparathyroidism should be a rare occurrence for the skilled thyroid surgeon, being about 1%. Recurrence of hyperthyroidism may vary from 2 to 18%, depending on the degree to which the thyroid gland was surgically removed.

## TREATMENT OF TOXIC NODULAR GOITER

Most cases of toxic nodular goiter result from a superimposition of a thyrotoxic state in a patient with a long-standing nontoxic nodular goiter. Less commonly, a single hyperfunctioning benign adenoma in an otherwise normal thyroid gland is the cause. Often the cases of toxic multinodular goiter are seen in patients who are elderly and who are born and raised in iodine-deficient regions of the world. When such patients move to an area where dietary iodine is sufficient, as in the United States, the gradual onset of hyperthyroidism will take place within 4 to 5 years. When such patients are exposed to massive levels of iodine, such as are contained in radi-opaque dyes, povidone-iodine (Betadine), and saturated solution of potassium iodide, hyperthyroidism will be precipitated within a few weeks following exposure (Jod-Basedow effect). The clinical presentation of hyperthyroidism in these patients is often subtle, owing to the mildness of the hyperthyroidism and the apathetic presentation often seen in the elderly. Thyrocardiac disease is also a common finding because of the higher frequency of underlying heart disease present in such a patient population.

Thioamide drug therapy is effective in either form of toxic nodular goiter, but it may take somewhat longer for the achievement of a biochemical and clinical euthyroid state than is seen in Graves' disease. Although thioamide drugs are useful in ameliorating the thyrotoxicosis, long-term control of the hyperthyroidism requires ablative treatment.

Radioactive iodine and surgery comprise useful techniques for carrying out ablative therapy in cases of toxic nodular goiter. Where a single toxic adenoma is present, a partial or total thyroid lobectomy is the treatment of choice if the patient is a good surgical risk. In toxic multinodular goiter, [131]I therapy probably provides the most convenient and safe form of ablative treatment. Larger doses of radioiodine are usually required than for Graves' disease glands, since these glands usually do not concentrate radioiodine as efficiently as the Graves' disease glands and are intrinsically more resistant to radiation effects. It is advisable to give a dose of 29 mCi to these patients as the initial dose. Despite using this large dose, more than one therapy dose is frequently required. Even if the hyperthyroidism is controlled, usually gland size is minimally affected. Thus, the goal of the iodine therapy is control of the hyperthyroidism rather than achieving ablation of the thyroid gland as in Graves' disease. Surgery is a reasonable alternative approach for the patient with toxic multinodular goiter who is a good operative risk. This is especially true for patients with large goiters that are causing local obstructive complications.

## OTHER FORMS OF HYPERTHYROIDISM

Care must be taken to identify those forms of hyperthyroidism that will spontaneously resolve, such as subacute (de Quervain's) and lymphocytic (silent, painless, postpartum) forms of thyroiditis, which at times may be confused with hyperthyroidism caused by Graves' disease or nodular goiter. If thyroiditis is suspected on a clinical basis, appropriate laboratory testing should be performed and, in particular, radioiodine uptake test should be performed, which is uniformly suppressed in such patients. Because the hyperthyroidism is transient, it can be conservatively managed with beta-blocking agents until it remits. If there is associated pain and tenderness of the thyroid gland, glucocorticoid therapy (prednisone, 20 mg twice daily) is effective in rapidly relieving symptomatology. The failure to achieve rapid relief should raise the question as to the accuracy of the diagnosis of subacute thyroiditis. Following the hyperthyroid phase of the disease, which usually lasts for 4 to 6 weeks, a period of transient hypothyroidism may occur that may require temporary intervention with thyroxine therapy.

Hyperthyroidism due to surreptitious ingestion of thyroid hormone is a very rare occurrence that can be diagnosed by the combination of a suppressed radioiodine uptake and inappropriately low serum thyroglobulin levels. In all other forms of hyperthyroidism, serum thyroglobulin levels are elevated. Hyperthyroidism caused by TSH secreting pituitary adenomas, decidual tumors, and thyroid hormone secreting struma ovarii is equally rare. Surgical excision of the neoplasia is usually indicated in such cases. Somatostatin analogue may also be quite effective in controlling TSH secreting pituitary adenomas.

## SPECIAL SITUATIONS IN THE MANAGEMENT OF HYPERTHYROIDISM

### Thyroid Storm or Crisis

This syndrome represents a potentially fatal complication of severe hyperthyroidism that usually occurs in patients who have more severe forms of thyrotoxicosis. Key clinical manifestations of the pending thyroid storm include *accentuated signs and symptoms of hyperthyroidism; fever*, which responds poorly to conventional therapy; *and altered mental status*, ranging from disorientation to psychosis, delirium, stupor, and coma. In most cases, there is an identifiable precipitating event such as infection, trauma, psychiatric disturbance, or surgical stress. These stressful events place an increasing burden on the cardiovascular system, which if not treated appropriately may eventually lead to cardiovascular collapse and death. Younger patients generally have a more rapid and severe course than do elderly patients, who usually have a slower evolving apathetic presentation. The key to therapeutic success is the early recognition of the onset of this syndrome and the institution of general supportive measures that will assist the cardiovascular system in dealing with this crisis until the underlying hyperthyroid condition can be ameliorated. These measures include the liberal use of intravenous glucose containing fluids to ensure adequate hydration and a cooling mattress if body temperature is elevated. The use of intramuscular chlorpromazine (Thorazine) doses ranging between 50 and 100 mg every 8 to 12 hours and/or codeine, 30 to 60 mg, may be very helpful in preventing a shivering response so that cooling measures can be maximally effective. Propranolol (Inderal) can be given either orally, as outlined earlier, or by intravenous infusion, starting with 1 mg every 5 minutes until the heart rate is reduced to the range of 90 to 120 beats per minute, followed by a sustaining dose of 5 to 10 mg per hour therafter. Propranolol therapy is particularly important in those patients in whom an excessive adrenergic response is suspected. Beta blockade is considerably less effective when the febrile event is due to an infectious process. When heart failure is present, diuretic and digitalis therapy should be employed prior to the institution of propranolol. Efforts should also be initiated to bring the hyperthyroid state rapidly under control by the use of combination therapy employing PTU (100 mg every 8 hours), intravenous sodium iodide (0.5 grams daily), and glucocorticoids (20 mg prednisone every 8 hours). This combined therapeutic regimen will result in a rapid fall in serum thyroid hormone indices, including a reduction in serum $T_3$ levels to the normal range within 24 to 48 hours. In cases in which patients cannot take oral PTU, methimazole can be formulated into an 80-mg rectal suppository. If this is not feasible, iodide and glucocorticoid therapy can be given alone until the patient's status has improved enough to allow oral PTU therapy to be initiated. Another alternative is the use of the gallbladder dye iopanoic acid (Telepaque), 0.5 gm daily, which provides the therapeutic benefits of iodine blocking action and also inhibits peripheral conversion of $T_4$ to $T_3$.

### Treatment of Hyperthyroidism in Pregnancy

Thioamide drugs constitute the treatment of choice for the thyrotoxic pregnant patient. Either PTU or methimazole may be employed. Some clinicians prefer PTU because it does not as readily cross the placenta as methimazole. If compliance is a problem, however, methimazole would appear to be the preferred agent. Past concerns that methimazole may cause a scalp disorder called cutis aplasia appear not to have been substantiated and therefore should not serve as a contraindication to the use of methimazole. The addition of oral thyroid hormone to the thioamide therapy is not recommended, since it does not protect the fetus against the possibility of developing a goiter and/or hypothyroidism owing to the fact that thyroid hormones do not easily cross the placenta. Maintenance thioamide therapy should be reduced to the minimal amount necessary to control hyperthyroidism as soon as the patient's condition has clinically abated. Thioamide therapy is generally easier to manage in pregnancy because the underlying autoimmune disease partially remits. The goal of therapy is to use the minimal dose of thioamide medication necessary to maintain the mother in a near-euthyroid state, gaining appropriate weight and generally maintaining good health. The physician should avoid overtreating because hypothyroidism is not conducive to a normal gestation. If the hyperthyroidism is detected early in the course of pregnancy and managed appropriately, the incidence of prematurity and other obstetric problems should be no greater than is found in the nonhyperthyroid state.

Radioiodine should not be employed for either diagnostic or therapeutic purposes in pregnancy, since it rapidly passes across the placenta and can be concentrated in the fetal thyroid. However, if a therapeutic dose of radioiodine is inadvertently administered early in pregnancy, it is highly unlikely that the fetal thyroid will suffer, since the thyroid gland is not capable of concentrating iodine until the twelfth week. Stable iodine preparations, such as saturated solution of potassium iodide (SSKI), Lugol's solution, or Betadine, should never be used during pregnancy because they will often induce a goiter in the fetus. The only exception would be their brief use preoperatively if surgical thyroidectomy were required during the second trimester because of inability to control the hyperthyroidism with thioamide drugs.

The newborn should be carefully observed for signs of thyrotoxicosis if the mother has a history of thyrotoxic Graves' disease. In either case, thyroid stimulating immunoglobulins (TSI) are actively transported across the placenta in the later portions of gestation and may result in neonatal hyperthyroidism. Significant neonatal hyperthyroidism probably occurs in only 10% of cases. Those mothers having the highest titers of TSI in their serum are most likely to have infants who will suffer from transient hyperthyroidism during the neonatal period. The neonatal hyperthyroidism, if it does occur, can be treated with thioamide and beta-adrenergic blocking drugs. Neonatal hyperthyroidism is a self-limited disease that will disappear in 3 or 4 months as the maternal immunoglobulin levels disappear. However, exacerbation of the maternal hyperthyroidism often occurs 2 to 4 months post partum, resulting from a rebound in the immunosuppressive state of pregnancy.

### Preparation of the Hyperthyroid Patient for Emergency Surgery

The physician may be faced with the problem of preparing a hyperthyroid patient for emergency nonthyroidal surgery. This can be rapidly accomplished by the use of propranolol intravenously in a manner similar to that outlined for thyroid storm; namely, 1-mg infusions of propranolol should be administered every 5 minutes until the heart rate is controlled in the range between 90 and 120 beats per minute. Usually, three to seven doses are required to achieve this end point. This is followed by a constant infusion of propranolol ranging between 5 and 10 mg per hour. Anticholinergic drugs, such as atropine or scopolamine, should be withheld. During the course of anesthetic induction, throughout surgery, and during the acute postoperative period, the patient's heart rate, temperature, and ECG pattern should be carefully monitored. With the stress of intubation, surgery, and extubation, increases in circulating catecholamines may result in a rapid increase in heart rate, which should be countered by the increasing infusion of propranolol. If the heart rate falls below 80 beats

per minute, atropine or scopolamine should be given to counter vagal influence.

Hyperthyroid patients tolerate surgery remarkably well when adequate beta blockade is employed. Further, the thyroid "storm" picture, frequently induced by surgical stress, is prevented by adequate propranolol therapy. Therefore, if there are clear indications for an emergency surgical procedure, the physician should not hesitate to proceed once adequate beta blockade has been established.

# THYROID CANCER

method of
BLAKE CADY, M.D.
*New England Deaconess Hospital*
*Boston, Massachusetts*

Cancer of the thyroid is an uncommon disease that provokes considerable interest and controversy in its management because of the frequency of thyroid nodules and the often puzzling clinical evaluation of patients in terms of the need for surgery or other therapy. There is enormous variability in the outcome of cancers in the old and the young, which adds to the confusion and uncertainty about how to manage this disease. There are 11,000 cases of thyroid cancer in the United States per year but only 1100 deaths. Therefore, this is a relatively uncommon cancer and deaths are very uncommon, representing only 10% of cases, compared with other visceral organ cancers. Thyroid cancer is predominant in women (more than 70% of cases), particularly in the younger age groups. One of the confusing aspects of thyroid cancer is the frequency of occult, microscopic foci of papillary carcinoma seen in thyroid glands removed for benign problems. The incidence of these occult papillary carcinomas in microscopic foci may be as high as 30% in routine autopsies in some parts of the world and is at least 10% in autopsies in this country. The frequency is related, in part, to the number of sections of the thyroid gland inspected.

The known etiologic factors of thyroid carcinoma include radiation in childhood, which has been shown to be associated with an increased frequency of thyroid nodules and thyroid cancers many years later. This susceptibility to radiation occurs only in the developing thyroid glands of infants and children, however, and is reported in patients after radiation treatments of the thymus, adenoids, and skin in the years before 1950. Few patients with radiation-associated thyroid cancer are seen currently because of the complete cessation of childhood irradiation after the 1950s. Although family histories are common in benign thyroid disorders, only a few family clusters of differentiated thyroid carcinoma have been reported. In contrast, 20% of medullary carcinomas of the thyroid occur in familial clusters, particularly in association with multiple endocrine neoplasia syndromes.

There is a relationship between environmental and dietary iodine levels and the frequency and type of differentiated thyroid carcinoma. Iodine-deficient areas have a higher incidence of cancers by a factor of about three; these cancers are more commonly follicular carcinomas.

## PATHOLOGY

The most frequently used pathologic classification of thyroid carcinoma is seen in Table 1.

Any cancer with papillary features is classified as papillary carcinoma, whether it is pure papillary, mixed papillary and follicular, or predominantly follicular with only minor papillary elements. All cancers with papillary features behave in a biologically similar fashion. In contrast, pure follicular adenocarcinomas have a distinct biologic behavior, with few if any lymph node metastases and more common distant metastases, particularly to the lungs. Follicular carcinomas must be separated into low-grade, encapsulated lesions with minimal tumor capsular invasion by cancer cells and lesions marked by significant tumor capsular invasion by malignant cells and with blood vessel invasion. These latter tumors have a more aggressive behavior and a high incidence of metastatic disease. Hürthle's cell carcinomas are considered to be a separate entity by some investigators, but we view them as a variant of follicular adenocarcinoma, with biologic behavior similar to that of other follicular carcinomas. Medullary thyroid carcinoma is not a cancer of the thyroid cells but arises within the thyroid gland from parafollicular cells that produce calcitonin. Eighty per cent of medullary carcinomas are sporadic, with a unifocal origin in one thyroid lobe. The other 20% are associated with familial syndromes and are characterized by multifocal origin throughout in the thyroid gland. Calcitonin produced by the parafollicular C cells is easily detectable in the serum and can be used as an accurate tumor marker. With few exceptions, the calcitonin level is elevated in cases of either familial or sporadic medullary carcinoma, and is particularly useful in screening familial endocrine syndrome persons without apparent clinical disease so that an early curative operation can be performed.

Undifferentiated thyroid carcinomas consist of anaplastic varieties with spindle and giant cells but also include some small cell types; they are extremely aggressive, lethal, and rapidly growing cancers. Fortunately, they have occurred with far less frequency in recent years and now make up only 2 or 3% of all cancers, in contrast to more than 20% in the 1930s and 1940s. In some parts of the world, they are still common. Thyroid lymphoma is relatively uncommon, but it is necessary both to recognize it and to separate it from generalized lymphomas that involve the thyroid gland. Thyroid lymphoma frequently arises in the background of Hashimoto's lymphoid thyroiditis, and this must be recognized in the differential diagnosis of thyroid masses in Hashimoto's thyroiditis. Rare cases of squamous cell carcinoma of the thyroid must be separated from squamous cell carcinomas of the larynx that grow into the thyroid gland and present as a thyroid mass.

## RISK GROUP ASSESSMENT

Although the pathologic features of thyroid carcinoma are important, the age of the patient with differentiated thyroid carcinoma is the most important prognostic feature. No other human cancer has such a wide disparity of outcome on the basis of age. For many years, the excellent prognosis in the young and the modest prognosis in the old have been recognized, but in recent years this age separation has been more carefully analyzed and quantified. In differentiated thyroid cancer of childhood and in adults up to the age of 40 years in men and 50 years in women, less than 1 or 2% of patients die of this disease. Children and young to middle-aged adults make up two-thirds of these cases. In contrast, men over age 40 years and women over age 50 years have a recurrence rate of at least 25% and a death rate of more than 20%.

The reasons for this great separation in outcome based on age are obscure. However, age is such a strong determinant of the prognosis that it supersedes the effects of size, extent, pathologic type, type of surgery, use of radioactive iodine, and all other clinical and therapeutic features of the disease.

In attempts to make the risk group assessment of cases more inclusive, clinical scoring systems have been developed. They indicate that in addition to age, the size and invasiveness of the differentiated cancers in the older age group should be taken into account to produce a more inclusive low-risk group that includes almost 90% of all patients. In this more inclusive low-risk group, the cancer mortality rate is less than 2% and the recurrence rate is less than 5%. In the residual high-risk group, which makes up about 10% of patients, the mortality rate is close to 50%. Simple clinical criteria can be used to separate patients into low-risk and high-risk groups for help in assessing therapeutic options and outcomes. The definition of low-risk and high-risk patients is given in Table 2.

## CLINICAL ASSESSMENT OF PATIENTS

Thyroid cancer patients usually present with either thyroid nodules or lymph node metastases in the neck. Rarely is a distant metastasis from thyroid carcinoma the presenting complaint in the absence of a thyroid mass. Assessment of the likelihood of cancer in the patient with a thyroid nodule hinges on its size; a history of recent growth; firmness, hardness, or fixation

TABLE 1. **Classification of Thyroid Cancers**

1. Differentiated (from follicular epithelium):
   represents more than 95% of cases
   Papillary; mixed papillary and follicular
   Follicular (Hürthle's cell)
2. Undifferentiated (from follicular epithelium)
   Anaplastic, spindle and giant cell, small cell
3. Medullary (from parafollicular C cells)
4. Lymphoma
5. Other rare forms
   Squamous, sarcoma, teratoma
6. Metastatic
   Renal, lung, melanoma, breast

TABLE 2. **Differentiated Thyroid Carcinoma: Inclusive Risk Group Definition**

**Low Risk (90% of All Patients)**
1. Men 40 years or younger and women 50 years or younger
   A. All papillary cancers, regardless of local extent
   B. All follicular cancers with minor tumor capsular invasion
   C. Without distant metastases

2. Men >40 years and women >50 years
   A. Cancers less than 5 cm in diameter
   B. Follicular cancers with minor tumor capsular invasion
   C. Papillary cancers confined within the thyroid gland capsule

**High Risk (10% of All Patients)**
1. Men 40 years or younger and women 50 years or younger
   A. Follicular cancers with major tumor capsular invasion
   B. With distant metastases

2. Men >40 years and women >50 years
   A. Cancers greater than 5 cm in diameter
   B. Follicular cancers with major tumor capsular invasion
   C. Papillary cancers extending outside the thyroid gland capsule
   D. With distant metastases

of the nodule; and symptoms suggestive of invasion of surrounding tissue, such as hoarseness from vocal chord paralysis, dysphagia from compression of the esophagus, or stridor from compression of the trachea. In young patients, 25% present with an enlarged lymph node in the neck, sometimes without a palpable mass in the thyroid gland itself. Older patients usually present with a thyroid nodule.

Physical examination is essential and should be performed in detail from both in front of and behind the patient. A careful evaluation of all the cervical lymph nodes is necessary, as well as evaluation of the thyroid gland itself.

Because thyroid cancer is an anatomic rather than a functional disease, measurements of thyroid function are of little help in assessing the risk of thyroid carcinoma in a particular nodule.

Anatomic studies of the thyroid gland, such as ultrasonography, radioactive thyroid scans, or computed tomography scans, may be helpful but are not diagnostic. Nodules that show increased activity may also harbor thyroid carcinoma. Thus, radioactive iodine scans of the thyroid gland should not be used as the sole basis for decisions about the surgical approach. Similarly, ultrasonic examination of thyroid nodules that reveals cystic lesions does not rule out the cystic presentation of a papillary carcinoma, which is not uncommon. Thus, the laboratory evaluation of thyroid nodules offers little specificity and should be viewed with caution.

*Needle Biopsy*

In contrast, thyroid needle aspiration of palpable thyroid masses or cervical lymph nodes is an extremely valuable technique. Although a specific diagnosis of cancer frequently cannot be made by thyroid needle cytology or biopsy, the essential discrimination be-

tween thyroid nodules that need to be removed surgically and those that can be observed can be made. Thyroid needle aspiration cytology showing a microfollicular pattern of cells consistent with either a benign or a malignant follicular neoplasm should lead to surgical removal. The thyroid needle aspiration may give a definitive diagnosis of papillary, anaplastic, or medullary carcinoma. Needle aspiration cytology or biopsy of the thyroid is usually not accurate enough to discriminate between Hashimoto's thyroiditis and lymphoma of the thyroid. Thus, an argument can be made for thyroid nodule needle aspiration cytology or biopsy as the first diagnostic procedure after the history and physical examination. Once thyroid needle aspiration cytology has revealed cells consistent with adenomatous goiter and the nodule does not require removal because of its size or symptoms, functional tests can be performed to assess that aspect of thyroid physiology, and scans can be obtained to confirm the diagnosis of multinodular gland or act as a baseline for the follow-up of such patients. The separation of follicular thyroid lesions into benign or malignant categories by aspiration cytology is not possible at the present time; indeed, accurate discrimination between an adenomatous nodule in a multinodular gland and a follicular adenocarcinoma cannot be made. Therefore, any thyroid aspiration cytology that reveals a microfollicular pattern should lead to surgical removal. If there is any uncertainty about the interpretation of the thyroid needle cytology, it can be repeated, if necessary, before settling on a course of management.

Studies that have compared core cutting needle biopsy with fine needle aspiration cytology of the thyroid indicate that both techniques are highly accurate and equivalent. Fine needle aspiration has fewer complications, such as bleeding, and is easier and more acceptable to patients. Thus, at present, most thyroid needle biopsies should be aspiration cytology examinations. Use of a No. 18 or No. 19 needle for the aspiration cytology is recommended because more thyroid tissue can be obtained and even clumps of cells can be produced as a microbiopsy for examination by the pathologist.

Thyroid needle aspiration cytology is a laboratory test and, like all tests, needs to be put into a clinical context. If the patient has a mass that is so large that it should be removed anyway, there is little purpose in performing thyroid needle biopsy. If the nodule has clinical characteristics of cancer, it should be operated on regardless of the thyroid needle cytology findings. Although thyroid needle cytology can be extremely helpful in separating patients into those who require surgery and those who do not, it may not supply a specific diagnosis and must be placed in the clinical context.

## TREATMENT

### Operative Approach

Thyroid surgery is extremely safe and uncomplicated in experienced hands. The rate of recurrent laryngeal nerve injury should be less than 1%, and hypoparathyroidism should not occur unless a bilateral thyroid operation is undertaken, in which case its incidence postoperatively should be less than 1% to justify bilateral thyroid surgery. Death after thyroid surgery is extraordinarily rare. The average patient can walk the night of surgery, have food by mouth the next day, and leave the hospital within 3 days, if not earlier. Thus, the simplicity, ease, safety, and lack of complications after thyroid surgery should be appreciated to place the role of thyroid surgery in the management of thyroid nodules in context. Seventy-five per cent of patients operated on for thyroid disease today are explored for the possibility of cancer. Roughly one-third of patients with solitary thyroid nodules or predominant thyroid nodules in a multinodular gland undergoing aspiration cytology do not need surgery. The incidence of carcinoma ranges between 25 and 50% in patients undergoing thyroid surgery for nodules. Benign follicular adenomas should also be removed because they apparently progress and later lead to follicular adenocarcinoma. Thus, the large majority of patients operated on have pathology that should be removed. The widespread use of thyroid needle aspiration cytology has perhaps doubled the incidence of carcinoma in surgical specimens by the elimination of small, innocuous nodules, but it is better to err on the side of surgical removal of ambiguous thyroid nodules.

The surgical approach to the thyroid gland is made through a low collar incision, which heals rapidly with a thin scar and minimal disfigurement. The median diameter of thyroid cancers operated on in recent years has decreased to less than 2 cm in diameter; thus patients can be easily handled with a thyroid lobectomy, either total or subtotal, as the initial operative step. Once the pathologist has examined the specimen and made the diagnosis, benign lesions need no further surgery; cancers sometimes need additional tissue removal. Most cancers in young patients at extremely low risk of death from disease are adequately treated by a unilateral thyroid operation. The opposite thyroid lobe should be examined at surgery because multicentric cancers sometimes occur in the opposite thyroid lobe in patients with papillary thyroid carcinoma; those abnormal lobes should also be removed. Lymph node metastases in papillary carcinoma are common. When encountered in the area of the thyroid bed they can be removed by a "node-picking" operation. If lymph node metastases were palpable before surgery, the thyroid incision can be extended to perform a modified neck dissection, preserving the spinal accessory nerve and usually the sternocleidomastoid muscle and the jugular vein.

In patients with a significant risk of recurrence and death, the thyroid operation needs to be more extensive for ease in the use of radioactive iodine. This mandates a total lobectomy on the side of the primary thyroid cancer and a subtotal thyroid gland removal on the opposite side. On occasion, total thyroidectomy may be required for multifocal thyroid carcinoma, but this does not increase curability and is associated with significant increases in complications.

For patients with medullary carcinoma of the thyroid, total thyroidectomy should be performed because, at the time of surgery, the complete family history is usually not known; the patient may be the index case of a familial cluster and may have multicentric cancer. If thorough documentation of a medullary carcinoma is available before surgery, so that its sporadic nature is completely confirmed, total thyroidectomy is not required. In medullary carcinomas, ipsilateral neck dissection should be performed in a more traditional fashion, including the sacrifice of the jugular vein, sternocleidomastoid muscle, and all the lymph nodes from the superior mediastinum and lateral and upper neck, with sparing of the spinal accessory nerve. Submandibular dissections are not required. Node metastases are common and imply a poor prognosis in patients with medullary carcinoma, although the typical disease course is indolent and may extend over many years.

Patients with anaplastic thyroid carcinoma can seldom have a complete removal of the tumor because it usually invades the surrounding tissues widely and is large. The major therapeutic goal in surgery of anaplastic carcinoma is to achieve a satisfactory airway by unroofing the trachea and, if necessary, performing a tracheostomy. In thyroid lymphoma the tumor should be completely removed if possible because the prognosis is excellent if the lymphoma is confined to the thyroid gland. Frequently, complete removal is impossible because of the large size of the tumor and the extensive involvement of surrounding tissues.

### Follow-up of Thyroid Cancer Patients

Postoperative management of thyroid carcinoma remains controversial. In low-risk patients, because the prognosis is so good, radioactive iodine therapy cannot add to the control of disease. In patients with high-risk, differentiated thyroid carcinoma, radioactive iodine should be routinely used postoperatively, first to ablate any normal thyroid gland and later diagnostically to seek out the presence of metastases. Metastases can be treated with therapeutic radioactive iodine if they concentrate the tracer dose, which unfortuntely occurs in a minority of cases.

Although thyroid hormone administration postoperatively to suppress thyroid-stimulating hormone is routine, there is some doubt about whether it makes a difference in the long-term prognosis. Standard therapy today includes thyroid hormone administration, but for young patients with a small carcinoma and a hemithyroidectomy with a 100% chance of cure, thyroid hormone administration postoperatively should be optional if patients are euthyroid.

The use of thyroglobulin as a tumor marker postoperatively is effective only in the presence of a total thyroid ablation and thus is not widely applicable. It has little use in young patients, who have almost no risk of recurrence or death, but it can be used in high-risk patients for follow-up. Unfortunately, treatment of metastatic disease is uniformly unsuccessful in older patients. Chest x-ray films should be taken if symptoms are present or pulmonary metastases are suspected. Thyroid function tests should be performed occasionally to analyze the success of thyroid-stimulating hormone suppression if thyroid hormone is administered. Routine bone scans, radioactive iodine scans, and other tests in the low-risk group are probably of little value. They may be used in the high-risk group for follow-up when metastases are suspected.

Lymphoma of the thyroid is curable with the use of multidrug chemotherapy and radiotherapy after surgery. Multidisciplinary management of anaplastic carcinomas should include both chemotherapy and radiotherapy, but unfortunately, cures are essentially unprecedented.

# PHEOCHROMOCYTOMA

method of
WILLIAM MUIR MANGER, M.D., PH.D.
*New York University and Columbia Medical
    Centers*
*New York, New York*

There is no more important and treacherous cause of hypertension to recognize than pheochromocytoma, since, if left untreated, it will almost invariably prove to be fatal. This tumor has been justifiably described as a pharmacologic bomb, since the sudden secretion of catecholamines from a pheochromocytoma often causes a rapid (explosive) and dramatic appearance of clinical manifestations. Mortality and morbidity result mainly from complications of severe hypertension and/or excess circulating catecholamines (e.g., cerebrovascular and cardiovascular accidents, cardiomyopathy, cardiac decompensation, arrhythmias); only about 10% of tumors are malignant.

The clinical expressions of pheochromocytoma are so variable that it can mimic a large variety of diseases. The secret for clinicians is to maintain a high index of suspicion when dealing with hypertension, whether sustained or paroxysmal. With the diagnostic modalities available today, the diagnosis of pheochromocytoma should rarely be missed.

## ORIGIN

Pheochromocytomas arise from chromaffin cells of the adrenal medullae (90% of tumors; more often in the right) and the organ of Zuckerkandl, and from chromaffin cells associated with sympathetic nerves and plexuses in extra-adrenal sites in the abdomen (including the urinary bladder), chest (less than 2% of tumors), and neck (less than 0.1% of tumors); very rarely tumors arise at the base of the skull, in the heart, or in the spermatic cord. Multiple and extra-adrenal tumors are more common in children (35% of cases) than in adults (8%). About 10% of pheochromocytoma cases are familial, and at least 70% of these familial tumors are bilateral.

## INCIDENCE

It is estimated that fewer than 0.05% of Americans with sustained diastolic hypertension have pheochromocytoma as the cause of their hypertension; however, in estimating this tumor's prevalence, it must be remembered that roughly 45% of patients with pheochromocytoma have only paroxysmal hypertension.

Pheochromocytoma may occur at any age but is most common in the fourth and fifth decades, with a slight predilection for women. In children, about two-thirds of these tumors occur in boys, suggesting an endocrine influence on pheochromocytoma development prior to puberty.

## BIOSYNTHESIS AND CATABOLISM

The catecholamines occurring in humans (dopamine, norepinephine, and epinephrine) are synthesized by a series of enzymatic reactions in the following sequence: tyrosine $\rightarrow$ dopa $\rightarrow$ dopamine $\rightarrow$ norepinephrine $\rightarrow$ epinephrine. A major portion of the catecholamines is conjugated, but some dopamine is catabolized to homovanillic acid (HVA), whereas some epinephrine and norepinephrine is converted to the metanephrines and vanillylmandelic acid (VMA). Catecholamine biosynthesis occurs in chromaffin cells and in parts of the brain, but only norepinephrine and dopamine are synthesized in postganglionic nerves. Epinephrine and norepinephrine can increase metabolism, augment the rate and force of myocardial contraction, and cause intense vasoconstriction. Dopamine can cause vasodilatation in the splanchnic and renal beds and can augment myocardial contraction; it also has a diuretic and natriuretic action. Some chromaffin cells in the adrenal medulla and certain cells in the brain are capable of converting norepinephrine to epinephrine through the action of the enzyme phenylethanolamine-N-methyltransferase (PNMT). Plasma dopamine accounts for about 13% of free catecholamine, whereas epinephrine and norepinephrine account for roughly 14% and 73%, respectively. Only small amounts of free epinephrine and norepinephrine are excreted in the urine; the relatively larger amount of urinary free dopamine results from conversion of dopa to dopamine in the kidney. Catecholamines are mainly eliminated in the urine as their metabolites (metanephrines, VMA, HVA) and conjugates.

Catecholamines, synthesized and secreted by pheochromocytomas, account for the physiologic and pharmacologic effects caused by these tumors. Catecholamines exert their cardiovascular and metabolic effects by stimulating specific protein cellular receptors (adrenoceptors). Why some tumors cause paroxysmal hypertension whereas others cause sustained hypertension is unclear. Most tumors secrete both epinephrine and norepinephrine; however, norepinephrine is usually the predominant amine. Some secrete only norepinephrine or, rarely, only epinephrine. Very rarely, dopamine and even dopa may be secreted.

## PATHOPHYSIOLOGY

The average pheochromocytoma is 5 cm in diameter and 70% weigh 70 grams or less, but they may be microscopic or weigh 4000 grams. Most tumors are very vascular, although occasionally they are relatively avascular or cystic, and rarely they contain calcium. Usually they are encapsulated and benign. Roughly 10% are malignant, as evidenced by metastases or invasion of adjacent structures. Because cells of benign and malignant pheochromocytoma may appear identical, it is impossible to determine malignancy from histologic examination; however, recent experience indicates that determination of DNA patterns in pheochromocytoma cells by flow cytometry is highly reliable in differentiating malignant from benign tumors. Although malignancy is more common in tumors containing dopamine than in those containing only epinephrine and/or norepinephrine, the presence of dopamine or its precursor does not establish malignancy. Extra-adrenal pheochromocytomas are more often malignant than tumors arising in the adrenal.

Severity of symptoms depends primarily on the amount of catecholamines liberated into the circulation and whether the liberation is sustained or episodic. There is no good correlation between the size of the tumor and clinical or laboratory manifestations; small tumors often have a more rapid turnover of catecholamines and secrete more catecholamines into the circulation than large tumors. Secretion from pheochromocytomas (none of which have any nervous innervation) seems to occur mainly by passive diffusion from tumor cells; however, some tumors appear to secrete catecholamines simultaneously with other contents of catecholamine storage vesicles (e.g., dopamine beta-hydroxylase and chromogranin A) by an active exocytotic process.

Some pheochromocytomas may contain serotonin, vasoactive intestinal polypeptide (VIP), opioids (enkephalins and beta-endorphin), alpha-melanocyte stimulating hormone ($\alpha$-MSH), adrenocorticotropic hormone (ACTH), serotonin, calcitonin, somatostatin, and others; secretion of these substances into the circulation may play a role in the symptomatology of some patients with pheochromocytoma.

## CLINICAL PRESENTATION

Manifestations of pheochromocytoma are often diverse and numerous, suggesting a variety of diagnostic possibilities. Of great diagnostic importance is the occurrence of hypertension, since attacks with symptoms suggesting excess circulating catecholamines in the absence of sustained or paroxysmal hypertension almost rule out the presence of pheochromocytoma. An exception is the rare case of familial pheochromocytoma in which hypertension is not infrequently absent and plasma and urinary concentrations of catecholamines and their metabolites may be normal or only slightly elevated.

About 75% of patients have one or more symptomatic attacks weekly; some experience one or more attacks daily, whereas others have attacks only once every few months. Attacks may be precipitated by pressure in the region of the tumor, postural changes, exertion, anxiety, trauma, pain, micturition or bladder distention, ingestion of certain foods or beverages containing tyramine (certain cheeses, beer or wine) or synephrine (citrus fruit), administration of certain drugs (histamine, glucagon, tyramine, phenothiazines, naloxone [Narcan], metoclopramide [Reglan], ACTH), arteriography in the region of the tumor, intubation, anesthesia, operative manipulation, or child birth.

Manifestations mainly represent the effects of hypercatecholaminemia and hypertension. Patients may complain of headaches; excess sweating; palpitations; tachycardia or sometimes bradycardia; anxiety; tremulousness; chest or abdominal pain; nausea; vomiting; weakness; weight loss; dyspnea; warmth; visual disturbances; faintness; constipation; arm paresthesias; grand mal seizures; and, in pheochromocytoma of the urinary bladder, painless hematuria, frequency, nocturia, and tenesmus. The physician may observe hypertension with or without wide BP fluctuations, paroxysmal hypertension, orthostatic hypotension in the hypertensive patient, and rarely hypertension alternating with hypotension; a paradoxic blood pressure response to antihypertensive drugs may be noted. Pallor may be pronounced (rarely flushing appears), and patients often become frightened. Hypertensive retinopathy occurs in some patients with sustained hypertension, and occasionally there is a slight fever. Children may display atypical manifestations; polydipsia, polyuria, and convulsive seizures are not uncommon, and puffy, red or cyanotic hands may appear.

Headache, the most common symptom, usually occurs during a paroxysm of hypertension and is usually severe, but some patients have only mild headaches. Sweating, generalized and sometimes drenching, and palpitations (with tachycardia or reflex bradycardia) occur frequently. Patients often experience severe acute anxiety but do not exhibit chronic anxiety unless they also have a neurosis. Weight loss is common, but some patients with only paroxysmal hypertension do not lose weight. Severe constipation occurs in a few individuals with persistent hypertension; however, secretion of VIP or serotonin from a pheochromocytoma (or a coexisting medullary thyroid carcinoma) can cause severe diarrhea.

Orthostatic hypotension in the untreated hypertensive, resistance to antihypertensive therapy or paradoxic BP increases following administration of certain antihypertensives (e.g., beta blockers, guanethidine, ganglionic blockers), or marked pressor responses to any of the conditions (mentioned earlier) that may precipitate attacks should suggest the diagnosis of pheochromocytoma. Attacks may subside or worsen during pregnancy.

## ASSOCIATED PATHOLOGIC ENTITIES

Coexistence of familial pheochromocytomas with neoplasms and/or hyperplasia of the thyroid (Sipple's syndrome) and parathyroid glands characterizes multiple endocrine neoplasia (MEN) Type 2. (In MEN Type 2, medullary thyroid carcinoma and pheochromocytoma coexist in about one-fourth of cases.) The combination of pheochromocytoma, medullary thyroid carcinoma, mucosal neuromas, thickened corneal nerves, alimentary tract ganglioneuromatosis, and frequently a marfanoid habitus constitutes another entity: MEN Type 3 (thyroid carcinoma occurs in about 80% of cases, whereas pheochromocytoma coexists in 30%). Hyperparathyroidism occurs in 50% of patients with MEN Type 2 but rarely complicates MEN Type 3. Secretion of calcitonin, serotonin, or prostaglandin by thyroid carcinomas may cause diarrhea. Patients with pheochromocytomas should be screened for evidence of medullary thyroid carcinoma or premalignant thyroid C cell hyperplasia as well as for hyperparathyroidism; screening should be performed after pheochromocytoma removal, since some pheochromocytomas may themselves cause hypercalcitonemia and/or hypercalcemia. Secretion of ACTH-like substances from thyroid carcinomas or from pheochromocytomas causes Cushing's syndrome in rare cases.

Neurofibromatosis (von Recklinghausen's disease), often with café au lait spots, afflicts about 5% of patients with pheochromocytoma; hence, screening patients with hypertension and neurofibromatosis for pheochromocytoma is indicated. Rarely, pheochromocytoma coexists with von Hippel–Lindau disease (retinal angiomatosis and cerebellar angiomatosis) or with acromegaly.

Pheochromocytomas and associated lesions of the thyroid and neurocutaneous tissues have common embryonic origins, which strongly suggests these entities may arise from maldevelopment of the neural crest.

## DIAGNOSIS

Many conditions exist whose manifestations may suggest pheochromocytoma, some of which can yield increased urinary catecholamines and their metabolites. Most of these conditions can be excluded on clinical grounds.

Consumption of certain illegal drugs (cocaine, phencyclidine, lysergic acid diethylamide) and some prescription (amphetamines, monoamine oxidase inhibitors) and over-the-counter drugs (decongestants and anorectics containing phenylpropanolamine) may cause hypertensive crises and symptoms mimicking pheochromocytoma. Factitious production of symptoms (pseudopheochromocytoma) by an emotionally disturbed person having access to drugs should always be considered in the differential diagnosis.

Hemorrhagic necrosis of a pheochromocytoma is a rare but serious complication that may present as an acute abdomen or cardiovascular catastrophe. Without prompt stabilizing treatment and tumor extirpation, the patient will almost certainly die.

Because 95% of patients with pheochromocytoma complain of headaches or sweating or palpitations or any combination of these, a detailed history and physical examination are essential in deciding who should be screened.

All symptomatic patients with sustained or paroxysmal hypertension should be screened for pheochromocytoma unless the cause of their hypertension is known. Even asymptomatic patients with hypertension should be screened if they have abnormal laboratory or electrocardiographic findings that may be caused by increased circulating catecholamines, or if they have radiologic evidence suggesting pheochromocytoma or if they have diseases known to coexist with pheochromocytoma. Screening pregnant patients with hypertension of uncertain cause is indicated because pregnancy and childbirth in the presence of an unsuspected pheochromocytoma carry high risks of maternal and fetal mortality.

Screening usually consists of quantitating 24-hour urinary metanephrines or plasma catecholamines; assay of urinary catecholamines and VMA is less reliable.

### Laboratory and ECG Abnormalities

Hyperglycemia, hypermetabolism, and increased plasma free fatty acids can result from elevated circulating catecholamines. Hypovolemia afflicts the majority of patients, particularly those with sustained hypertension. Polycythemia (due to erythropoietin secretion by some pheochromocytomas) occasionally occurs. Cushing's syndrome, rarely observed with sporadic or familial pheochromocytoma, may result from elaboration of an ACTH-like substance by the pheochromocytoma or an associated thyroid carcinoma.

A wide variety of electrocardiographic (ECG) changes include arrhythmias and abnormalities consistent with myocardial ischemia, damage, or strain. The transient appearance of ECG changes during a paroxysm of hypertension and symptoms suggesting pheochromocytoma supports the diagnosis, especially in the absence of other causes. Permanent ECG changes may result from hypertension, coronary atherosclerosis, myocardial infarction, and catecholamine myocarditis or cardiomyopathy.

### Specific Biochemical Tests

Plasma and urinary catecholamines and their metabolites are invariably elevated in patients with sustained hypertension due to pheochromocytoma. However, in some patients urinary catecholamines and their metabolites do not rise substantially while the BP remains relatively normal. To establish the diagnosis in these individuals, one must either obtain blood during a spontaneous or provoked hypertensive period or collect urine shortly following a hypertensive episode.

Occasionally individuals with essential hypertension or blood pressure hyperlability have borderline or modest elevations of plasma (500 to 2000 pg per ml) or urinary catecholamines and their metabolites. The clonidine suppression test is exceptionally reliable in differentiating neurogenic from pheochromocytic hypertension. Clonidine suppresses the sympathetic nervous system, reducing plasma norepinephrine concentrations (by 50% and to normal levels) in patients with neurogenic hypertension but not in those with pheochromocytoma.

Measurement of total metanephrines (metanephrine plus normetanephrine) in a 24-hour urine collection is a highly reliable screening test because more than 95% of patients with pheochromocytoma have elevated levels.

Table 1 gives the upper limits (these vary somewhat among laboratories) of normal concentrations for catecholamine and metabolites, as well as substances that can interfere with these determinations. Very few drugs can lower urinary catecholamines or their metabolites to normal in pheochromocytoma cases; however, radiopaque contrast media containing methylglucamine (meglumine) can cause false-negative metanephrine assays. Increased excretion of catecholamines and their metabolites may occur with other neural crest tumors, adrenal medullary hyperplasia, intracranial lesions, autonomic hyper-reflexia, use of some illicit drugs, carcinoid, hypoglycemia, acrodynia, acute porphyria, tetanus, lead poisoning, Guillain-Barré syndrome, clonidine withdrawal, factitious hypertension, and conditions causing severe hypotension or stress (e.g., shock, heart failure, myocardial infarction, anoxia, acidosis, some anesthetics, CNS stimulation, and strenuous physical activity).

Occasionally, a provocative test with glucagon or histamine (combined with quantitation of plasma catecholamines) can prove to be indispensable in detecting a paroxysmally secreting pheochromocytoma. A provocative test is contraindicated in hypertensives (with BPs greater than or equal to 170/100 mmHg) and in patients with conditions (e.g., cerebrovascular or cardiovascular disease) that might deteriorate with a sudden BP elevation; a hypertensive response can be avoided by administering 10 mg of nifedipine (Procardia) sublingually shortly before the test or administering prazosin (Minipress) for several days before testing. Provocative tests are safe in patients who do not have contraindications or premedication if performed correctly and with precautions to counteract hypertensive crises, arrhythmias, and hypotension.

## PREOPERATIVE LOCALIZATION OF PHEOCHROMOCYTOMA

If a relatively large amount of plasma or urinary epinephrine (or its metabolite, metanephrine) is detected, it is likely that the pheochromocytoma is in the adrenal area; however, other tests can establish the location.

Computed tomography (CT) can identify about 95% of pheochromocytomas; it is extremely accurate in revealing lesions 1 cm or larger in the adrenals or 2 cm or larger in extra-adrenal abdominal locations. CT scan is usually initially performed without contrast; if this shows no tumor, the scan should be repeated with intravenous and oral contrast for optimal interpretation. CT is superior to and safer than angiography (now rarely indicated). It should prove to be valuable in identifying pheochromocytomas in the thorax and neck, but experience is limited.

Isotope scanning with [$^{131}$I]-metaiodobenzylguanidine ($^{131}$I-MIBG) constitutes a fairly sensitive and specific technique for localizing pheochromocytomas, since $^{131}$I-MIBG usually concentrates in these tumors. Nevertheless, such scanning misses up to 15% of all pheochromocytomas and up to 50% if these tumors are malignant.

Magnetic resonance imaging (MRI) provides an especially valuable modality for determining the presence of a pheochromocytoma. Although MRI does not afford the resolution of CT, a particular pattern of high-signal intensity appears to be characteristic for pheochromocytoma and is almost never seen in other adrenal tumors except primary or metastatic malignancy.

If there is any hematuria or a suggestion that hypertensive attacks occur with micturition or bladder distention, cystoscopy should be performed under alpha-adrenergic blockade.

If all preoperative attempts to localize a pheochromocytoma fail, sampling blood from various levels of the vena cava may localize abdominal, thoracic, and cervical tumors.

## PREOPERATIVE MANAGEMENT

Successful management of pheochromocytoma requires expertise and teamwork. Surgical removal, the only curative procedure, should be performed expeditiously in all patients for whom surgery is not contraindicated. Medullary thyroid carcinoma and hyperparathyroidism must be excluded, especially in patients with familial pheochromocytoma (and their relatives), although diagnosis and treatment of these conditions should wait until after pheochromocytoma removal.

Before surgery, the presence and degree of bilateral renal function should be established in case the surgeon considers sacrificing a kidney during tumor removal.

A hypertensive crisis, malignant hypertension, or acute abdominal or cardiovascular complications may require immediate medical and/or surgical therapy. Acute hypertensive crises occurring spontaneously or induced by angiography or provocative tests or resulting from anesthesia or operation can usually be controlled by a rapid intravenous bolus of phentolamine (Regitine), 3 to 5 mg; if this elicits no response within a minute

TABLE 1. **Effects of Drugs and Other Interfering Substances on Concentrations of Plasma and Urinary Cathecholamines and Their Metabolites***

| | | Effects | |
|---|---|---|---|
| **Urine Concentrations** | | *Increased Apparent Value* | *Decreased Apparent Value* |
| *Adult upper limit of normal (mg/24 hr)* | | | |
| Catecholamines | | *Catecholamines* | Fenfluramine |
|   Epinephrine | 0.02 | *Drugs containing catecholamines* | *Methenamine mandelate (Mandelamine)*† |
|   Norepinephrine | 0.08 | Isoproterenol† | Bromocriptine |
|   Total | 0.10 | *Levodopa* | Some antihypertensives that suppress adrenergic activity |
|   Dopamine | 0.20 | *Methyldopa*† | |
| | | *Labetalol*† | |
| | | Erythromycin† | |
| | | Phenothiazines | |
| | | Tricyclic antidepressants | |
| | | Other fluorescent substances† (e.g., quinine, quinidine, bile, B complex vitamins) | |
| | | *Rapid clonidine withdrawal* | |
| | | Ethanol | |
| | | *Ether* | |
| Metanephrines | | *Catecholamines* | *Meglumine* (x-ray contrast media) |
|   Metanephrine | 0.4 | *Drugs containing catecholamines* | Fenfluramine |
|   Normetanephrine | 0.9 | *Labetalol*† | Bromocriptine |
|   Total | 1.3 | *Monamine oxidase inhibitors* | Some antihypertensives that suppress adrenergic activity |
| | | *Phenothiazines*† | |
| | | Benzodiazepines | |
| | | Tricyclic antidepressants | |
| | | *Rapid clonidine withdrawal* | |
| | | Methyldopa† | |
| | | Ethanol | |
| | | *Ether* | |
| Vanillylmandelic acid | 6.5 | Catecholamines | *Clofibrate* |
| | | Drugs containing catecholamines | *Disulfiram* |
| | | *Glycerol guaiacolate*† | *Ethanol* |
| | | *Levodopa* | *Monoamine oxidase inhibitors* |
| | | *Labetalol*† | Methyldopa |
| | | *Nalidixic acid*† | Fenfluramine |
| | | Methocarbamol *(Robaxin)*† | Phenothiazines |
| | | *Rapid clonidine withdrawal* | Tricyclic antidepressants |
| | | *Ether* | Some antihypertensives |
| | | | Bromocriptine |
| **Plasma Concentrations** | | *Catecholamines* | Fenfluramine |
| *Adult upper limit of normal (pg/ml)*‡ | | *Drugs containing catecholamines* | Bromocriptine |
|   Epinephrine | 275 | *Rapid clonidine withdrawal* | Some antihypertensives that suppress adrenergic activity |
|   Norepinephrine | 500 | Isoproterenol | |
|   Dopamine | 120 | *Labetalol*† | |
| | | *Levodopa* | |
| | | Methyldopa | |
| | | *Ether* | |

*Many drugs interfere with fluorometric, colorimetric, and less specific assays, making them unreliable; with most specific assays (e.g., spectrophotometric, radioenzymatic, and high-pressure liquid chromatography), only *italicized* drugs may falsely indicate the presence or absence of pheochromocytoma. *Vasodilators (e.g., minoxidil, hydralazine) or hypoglycemic drugs may cause marked elevations of catecholamine and their metabolites.*

†Probably spurious interference.

‡Radioenzymatic assay.

or two, an additional 5 mg can be given and repeated as needed. Because effects of phentolamine boluses are transient, it may be necessary to control repeated hypertensive crises (especially during surgery) with infusions of phentolamine or preferably sodium nitroprusside (Nitropress), usually 100 mg of either drug in 500 ml of 5% dextrose solution, at a rate sufficient to maintain a relatively normal BP. (With impaired renal function or prolonged nitroprusside infusion, thiocyanate levels should be monitored; concentrations over 10 mg per dl can cause thiocyanate toxicity and psychosis.)

If immediate operation is indicated, significantly contracted blood volume requires correction with whole blood or appropriate fluids during the day before surgery in order to minimize postoperative hypotension. However, normalization of BP with alpha-adrenergic blocking drugs for 1 to 2 weeks preoperatively will usually correct a blood volume deficit and avoid risks of blood transfusion.

Abdominal palpation and diagnostic procedures that entail any trauma or stress should be performed with caution and with drugs available to treat potential hypertensive crises, arrhythmias, and hypotension. Morphine and phenothiazines should be avoided, since they may precipitate hypertensive crises or hypotension. Bilateral adrenalectomy mandates steroid replacement before surgery.

Preoperative alpha-adrenergic blockade with phenoxybenzamine (Dibenzyline), 10 to 20 mg twice daily, or prazosin (Minipress), starting with 1 mg and increasing to 1 or 2 mg two to three times daily for a week or more and continued to the time of surgery, usually prevents hypertensive crises and serious clinical manifestations, reverses hypovolemia, and promotes smooth induction of anesthesia and a relatively stable BP during surgery.

Complete blockade (evidenced by marked orthostatic hypotension) should be avoided, since this prevents the surgeon from (1) using BP increases with palpation during laparotomy as a guide to tumor location; and (2) immediately recognizing, by persistence of hypertension after tumor removal, presence of additional tumor(s).

Beta-adrenergic blockade is indicated for hazardous arrhythmias or tachycardia or angina, if there are no contraindications; however, *beta blockers should not be used without first creating alpha-adrenergic blockade, since beta blockade alone can markedly increase BP*. Ventricular arrhythmias should be treated with lidocaine (Xylocaine). Labetalol (Normodyne), an alpha- and beta-adrenergic blocker, may control BP in some patients with pheochromocytoma, yet it can occasionally cause hypertensive crises.

## OPERATIVE AND POSTOPERATIVE MANAGEMENT

Preoperative medication with diazepam (Valium) or meperidine (Demerol) will allay anxiety that could trigger catecholamine release. Fentanyl (Innovar) and droperidol (Inapsine) should not be used because they may cause tumor secretion of catecholamines. Atropine should be avoided, since it can cause severe tachycardia in the presence of excess circulating catecholamines.

The anesthesiologist must begin monitoring arterial BP, central venous pressure, and ECG and administer muscle relaxants before endotracheal intubation. During intubation and surgery, prompt control of hypertensive crises with phentolamine and/or nitroprusside and of arrhythmias with intravenous propranolol (Inderal) or esmolol (Brevibloc) and/or lidocaine is critical. Intraoperative correction of blood volume deficits is also essential. Isoflurane is the most popular anesthetic, although enflurane and holothane are suitable agents.

Intra-abdominal pheochromocytomas should be removed through an anterior transperitoneal incision to facilitate removal of multiple and extra-adrenal tumors. Operative mortality is 3.3% or less in medical centers with wide experience in treating pheochromocytoma.

Although controversial, bilateral adrenalectomy has been recommended in patients with MEN Type 2 or 3 syndromes because of the high probability that both adrenals harbor or will eventually develop pheochromocytomas. If cholelithiasis, intra-abdominal neurofibromatosis, or vascular abnormalities are encountered, they may require additional surgery.

Pheochromocytomas of the neck, chest, and urinary bladder require special surgical techniques; otherwise, management is similar to that described earlier. However, existence of multiple pheochromocytomas must always be excluded. Pheochromocytomas discovered during pregnancy are usually removed and the pregnancy continued if possible. If pregnancy is carried to term, cesarean section and tumor extirpation at delivery are advisable to avoid the stress of labor and vaginal delivery.

Close postoperative monitoring must continue until the patient's condition stabilizes. Hemorrhage at operative sites or a blood volume deficit can cause hypotension. Hypertension may result from fluid overload, pain, urinary retention, hypoxia, hypercarbia, or residual pheochromocytoma. Inadvertent ligation of a renal artery (resulting in kidney ischemia and hyper-reninemia) can cause hypertension but not until a few days or weeks after surgery.

Hypoglycemia with CNS manifestations, including coma, can occur within two hours after tumor removal; although this is a transient phenomenon, prompt infusion of a dextrose solution is mandatory. Starting an infusion of 5% dextrose and water immediately following tumor removal and continuing it for 24 hours will prevent hypoglycemia and its potentially serious consequences.

About 75% of patients become normotensive after successful tumor removal; the cause of persistent hypertension in the remainder is unclear. Five-year survival for patients with benign tumors is 95%, whereas it varies from 36% to 50% when tumors are malignant.

To determine whether patients remain free of

tumor, 24-hour urine metanephrines are measured every 6 to 12 months for 5 years.

## CHRONIC MEDICAL MANAGEMENT

When pheochromocytomas cannot be totally removed, the surgeon should resect as much as possible to minimize functioning tissue. Radiotherapy has sometimes proved highly effective, especially with bone metastases. Irradiation with large doses of [131]I-MIBG has occasionally reduced tumor size, catecholamine secretion, and symptomatology; however, long-term results have been so disappointing that this therapeutic modality has been discontinued. Combination chemotherapy (cyclophosphamide [Cytoxan], vincristine [Oncovin], and dacarbazine [DTIC-Dome]) should be considered if malignant pheochromocytomas are causing signs and/or symptoms from metastases. A complete or partial response (i.e., reduced tumor mass, catecholamine secretion, and symptoms) may occur in over 50% of patients for up to 2 years.

Prolonged treatment with alpha- and beta-adrenergic blockade can effectively control BP and symptoms for many years. Metyrosine (Demser) can be especially valuable in prolonged treatment of malignant pheochromocytoma, since it can markedly decrease catecholamine synthesis and reduce or abolish manifestations of excess circulating catecholamines.

Patients may occasionally survive for 2 or 3 decades after partial tumor removal and adequate control of BP and symptoms.

# THYROIDITIS

method of
ALAN M. McGREGOR, M.D.
*King's College School of Medicine*
*London, England*

The infiltration of the thyroid gland by inflammatory cells seen in thyroiditis results from a spectrum of both infective and inflammatory conditions. The disease process may be thyroid specific or part of a multisystem process. Depending on the etiology of the condition, the disease may be acute and self-limiting or chronic and progressive and altered thyroid function may result. The spectrum of diseases leading to thyroiditis are listed in Table 1.

## ACUTE SUPPURATIVE THYROIDITIS

This extremely rare condition is most commonly due to a gram-positive bacterial infection. Immunocompromised individuals are at an in-

TABLE 1. **Classification of Thyroiditis**

| |
|---|
| **Acute** |
| Suppurative |
| de Quervain's (subacute) |
| **Chronic** |
| Autoimmune |
|   Hashimoto's (lymphocytic) |
|   Fibrous |
|   Juvenile |
|   Atrophic |
|   Focal |
|   Painless |
| Riedel's (invasive fibrous) |
| Suppurative |
| Nonsuppurative |

creased risk. A short nonspecific prodrome is followed by intense pain in the thyroid radiating towards the ears and associated with difficulty in swallowing. The thyroid is extremely tender, so that neck movements are painful, and is usually enlarged and warm with erythema of the overlying skin. The patient is febrile, and there may be localized lymphadenopathy. Laboratory tests reveal a leukocytosis, and blood cultures may be valuable in identifying the organism. Recurrent attacks should lead to the exclusion of possible local fistulas. Appropriate parenteral antibiotic therapy is required, and occasionally surgical drainage may be necessary if an abscess forms and may also contribute to the identification of the organism.

## DE QUERVAIN'S (SUBACUTE) THYROIDITIS

Although it is assumed that this is a virally induced disease, there are little convincing supportive data for this assumption. There is considerable geographic and seasonal variation in the frequency with which the disease is reported. A prodromal viremic illness generally precedes the development of thyroiditis by a few weeks. Pain in the thyroid may develop relatively acutely and be associated with thyroid tenderness and dysphagia. The gland is enlarged and tender to palpation. The severity of the illness is variable, but the symptoms and signs are never as marked as those described in acute suppurative thyroiditis. In more severe disease, there may be systemic symptoms including fever and malaise and, not uncommonly, the initial presentation may be with clinical hyperthyroidism. Laboratory evaluation at this stage demonstrates a high erythrocyte sedimentation rate. A leukocytosis may be present. Biochemical evidence of hyperthyroidism and the demonstration on a thyroidal radioactive iodine uptake scan of no uptake of isotope into the thyroid are almost diagnostic of the condition in this situation. Most commonly, all that is required in managing the condition is providing the patient with a clear explanation of the disease and reassurance, since the natural history of the disease will be to remit spontaneously. Importantly, however, prior to complete recovery, there may be a period of transient hypothyroidism that follows the hyperthyroid phase and, again, the patient should be made aware of this and the possible clinical impact of symptoms of hypothyroidism. During the acute phase of the illness if there is severe discomfort in the thyroid and systemic symptoms and signs, simple anti-inflammatory agents such as aspirin in its coated form (Ecotrin), 600 mg every 6 to 8 hours, can be used until the symptoms subside, which usually occurs within 2 weeks of the acute onset of the condition. In patients with more severe disease, the problem can be rapidly controlled by steroids, and prednisone (Deltasone) given as 30 to 40 mg daily in an enteric coated form* and then rapidly reduced over the succeeding 2 weeks may be necessary. The transient hyperthyroidism occasionally associated with the disease does not usually require treatment, but use of a beta blocker such as propranolol (Inderal) taken at a dosage of 40 mg every 8 hours for 1 to 2 weeks should resolve the problem. It is important to be aware of the fact that in a small percentage of patients following the acute episode of hyperthyroidism, persistent hypothyroidism may result and therefore follow-up is important and replacement therapy with thyroxine may be required in this subgroup.

## AUTOIMMUNE THYROIDITIS

The term autoimmune thyroid disease defines a group of conditions that are characterized by the presence of circulating thyroid autoantibodies and immunologically competent cells that through their interaction with autoantigenic determinants on thyroid cells, are capable of inducing thyroid destruction and therefore dysfunction. The diseases that fall into this group include, in particular, Hashimoto's (goitrous) thyroiditis and atrophic thyroiditis (primary myxedema). The painless variety is considered separately. The fibrous, juvenile, and focal forms of the disease probably represent variants of the two major groups of Hashimoto's and atrophic thyroiditis. The mechanisms leading to thyroiditis remain to be completely characterized, but it seems increasingly likely that antibodies and T cells directed against the autoantigen thyroid peroxidase may have a key role in the destruction

of thyroid cells in these autoimmune diseases and, in addition, in the atrophic variant, that a proportion of patients may develop disease in response to antibodies directed against the thyroid stimulating hormone (TSH) receptor that bind to the receptor and block its function. Whatever the etiology, the presentation of these diseases is characteristic and common to the group. In the majority of patients, thyroid function remains normal and most patients are therefore asymptomatic. In this situation, they may be alerted to the possibility of the disease by the recognition by themselves or their families or family physician of a goiter; by a strong family history of autoimmune thyroid disease; or by a strong family or personal history of other organ-specific autoimmune diseases such as insulin-dependent diabetes mellitus, Graves' disease, pernicious anemia, vitiligo, and myasthenia gravis. Thyroid enlargement is uncommon, since the atrophic variant is the more common subgroup. The majority of patients presenting with this condition are female and usually in the fourth or fifth decade of life. In patients presenting asymptomatically, with a goiter, or because of hypothyroidism, the diagnosis of autoimmune thyroiditis is confirmed by the demonstration of high levels of autoantibodies to the thyroid peroxidase as well as (in a smaller percentage of patients) to thyroglobulin. In the presence of antibodies, there is really no indication to investigate further the etiology of the condition by scan or biopsy of the thyroid gland. Assessment of thyroid function is best performed by measurement of basal TSH and a measure of the free thyroxine level. There is no specific treatment against the autoimmune process, and therefore when treatment of thyroid failure is required, this should be done using thyroid hormone replacement. The indications for treating hypothyroidism are treating symptoms or when, despite biochemical evidence of hypothyroidism, a patient who is clinically asymptomatic is concerned about the appearance or local effects of an enlarged goiter. In patients with subclinical hypothyroidism who have minimal evidence biochemically of thyroid failure but who also demonstrate autoantibodies in their sera, there is an increasing and progressive risk of development of overt clinical hypothyroidism with time, and they should therefore be followed at regular intervals. Treatment of the hypothyroidism, besides ensuring symptomatic improvement, may also have a role to play in protecting against the development of coronary artery disease and certainly in reducing hypercholesterolemia, though this area is still surrounded by considerable controversy. The aim of treatment with thyroxine is clearly to relieve symptoms and, historically, the adequacy of the replacement

*The enteric coated form of prednisone is not available in the United States.

of thyroxine has been monitored by the serum TSH level. In commencing treatment with thyroxine, the severity and the duration of hypothyroidism and the age of the patient are important considerations, since in those with severe long-standing disease who are elderly, rapid replacement of thyroxine is contraindicated because, at the very least, a too rapid replacement may induce insomnia, weight loss, and palpitation and, at the very worst, may precipitate frank myocardial infarction. In the latter group of individuals, particularly if prior to treatment they have a history or ECG evidence of ischemic heart disease, they should be commenced on 0.025 mg daily of thyroxine (synthroid), which should be increased every 4 to 6 weeks by a further 0.025 mg daily until a satisfactory replacement dose is achieved and the patients are asymptomatic. In the remainder of patients presenting with this condition, commencement on thyroxine at a dosage of 0.05 mg daily with an increase at monthly intervals to a maintenance dosage of between 0.1 and 0.15 mg daily of thyroxine as determined by serial serum TSH measurements is all that may be required. Different patients will clearly have different requirements and, importantly too, one needs to bear in mind the recent recognition that over-replacement with thyroxine may in fact contribute to the development of osteoporosis. Once thyroxine replacement has been established, the treatment usually needs to be maintained for life, although in very rare instances patients have been reported to develop hyperthyroidism following an initial episode of hypothyroidism and this needs to be borne in mind. In patients in whom thyroxine is prescribed for reduction in goiter size, smaller doses of thyroxine may suffice than the normal maintenance levels of 0.1 to 0.15 mg daily. Where thyroxine fails to reduce goiter size sufficiently and the patient remains concerned about the goiter, surgery is the only means of resolving the problem.

## PAINLESS THYROIDITIS

Painless thyroiditis has been increasingly recognized over the past decade or so and has been referred to variously as silent, painless, or post-partum thyroiditis. The condition is usually subacute in its clinical presentation and therefore requires differentiation from subacute, de Quervain's thyroiditis. Unlike the latter, there is strong evidence that painless thyroiditis is autoimmune rather than viral in origin, with clear evidence of positive family histories, autoimmune-type HLA associations, high titers of persisting autoantibodies, goiter formation, lymphocytic infiltration in the goiter, frequent recurrences of the condition, and a much higher incidence of progression to permanent hypothyroidism. Clinically, the disease is characterized by the development of clinical and biochemical evidence of hyperthyroidism that is self-limiting, having often developed acutely in an individual in whom the thyroid gland, though enlarged, is painless and demonstrates a low iodine uptake on radioactive iodine scan. If the thyroid is biopsied as stated, the characteristic infiltration is lymphocytic rather than the giant cell and granulomatous changes seen in de Quervain's thyroiditis. The disease can be contrasted with hyperthyroid Graves' disease because of the absence of ophthalmopathy and the low rather than high thyroidal radioactive iodine uptake seen in the hyperthyroid phase. As in the de Quervain variant, the hyperthyroid phase may be followed by a hypothyroid phase that is far more commonly persistent, often after several episodes of recurrence. Treatment of the condition, provided it is recognized, is usually unnecessary and reassurance of the patient is all that is required. During the hyperthyroid phase, should the patient be symptomatic, beta-adrenergic blockers may be used to control the symptoms. Occasionally the succeeding hypothyroid phase may be severe enough to require thyroxine replacement, though this is very much the exception rather than the rule. In these individuals, because of the risk of further recurrence or of permanent hypothyroidism, regular follow-up is indicated.

## RIEDEL'S (INVASIVE FIBROUS) THYROIDITIS

This exceedingly rare condition is of uncertain etiology. It may be associated with fibrosis outside of the thyroid gland and has been reported to occur in conjunction with retroperitoneal and mediastinal fibrosis, fibrosing cholangitis, and pseudotumors of the orbit. The thyroid gland in this condition may be involved wholly or in part by a dense invasive fibrosis that extends out of the capsule to involve surrounding tissues without any evidence of cellular infiltration in the gland. Presentation is usually with an enlarged thyroid that is frequently associated with symptoms of tracheal or esophageal compression. The gland is nontender but exceedingly firm to palpation, and there may or may not be evidence of fibrosis at sites outside of the thyroid. Thyroid failure may occur if the disease is extensive. The diagnosis is confirmed by biopsy, and treatment is directed at replacing thyroid hormone where needed and relieving pressure symptoms by thyroid surgery, though because of the invasiveness of the fibrotic process, surgery may be very difficult.

## CHRONIC SUPPURATIVE AND NONSUPPURATIVE THYROIDITIS

Rarely, chronic infective processes such as tuberculosis and fungal infections may lead to thyroiditis. The history is of a longer presentation of enlargement of the thyroid with diagnosis being made by thyroid scan and biopsy. Nonsuppurative conditions such as sarcoidosis and amyloidosis may also involve the thyroid leading to chronic thyroiditis and, again, the diagnosis is made by biopsy of the gland. In the latter situation, thyroid failure may result if there is extensive involvement of the gland and thyroxine replacement may therefore be required.

# The Urogenital Tract

## BACTERIAL INFECTIONS OF THE URINARY TRACT IN MALES

method of
JOHN N. KRIEGER, M.D.
*University of Washington School of Medicine*
*Seattle, Washington*

Urinary tract infections include a variety of clinical conditions whose common denominator is invasion of the organs and tissues extending from the renal cortex to the urethral meatus. Infection may occur predominantly at a single site, such as the bladder (cystitis), prostate (prostatitis), or kidney (pyelonephritis). It is also possible for an infection to be restricted to the urine. The entire urinary tract is at risk for invasion by bacteria when any of its parts has become infected.

The key issue for therapy is to distinguish uncomplicated (medical) infections from complicated (surgical) infections of the urinary tract. An uncomplicated infection occurs in the absence of underlying structural or neurologic disorders of the urinary tract. These infections usually respond well to antimicrobial therapy. In contrast, complicated infections occur when the urinary tract has been repeatedly invaded by bacteria, leaving residual inflammation, or, in cases accompanied by obstruction, stones, or neurologic conditions that interfere with urinary drainage. Antimicrobial therapy alone is markedly less effective in complicated urinary tract infections. An important differential point is that patients with complicated infections tend to have persistence of bacteria within the urinary tract in the face of antimicrobial agents to which the bacteria appear to be sensitive in laboratory tests. Often, it is necessary to correct an underlying obstructive lesion or voiding problem to clear the infection. The goal of therapy for any patient with a urinary tract infection should be total elimination of the infecting organism from the urinary tract.

### NATURAL HISTORY

In infancy, the incidence of symptomatic urinary tract infections is higher in males than in females. Recently, this has been related to circumcision status. It appears that bacteria can adhere to the prepuce of uncircumcised male children and gain access to the urinary tract. After the neonatal period, symptomatic infections in male children and adults are distinctly uncommon until middle age. This is in marked contrast to the situation in females, who experience an increasing incidence of both symptomatic and asymptomatic infections with a marked increase following initiation of sexual activity in young adulthood and a continued gradual rise with age. Asymptomatic bacteriuria is also distinctly unusual in males compared with females.

Well-documented bacterial urinary tract infections in male children mandate thorough urologic investigation. This is because of the high prevalence of structural abnormalities of the genitourinary tract in such patients. Often, the bacterial urinary tract infection is the key diagnostic presentation for major abnormalities of the urinary tract. For example, vesicoureteral reflux of urine, posterior urethral valves, and other major structural abnormalities may present initially with a bacterial urinary tract infection. Early diagnosis and appropriate therapy offer the best chance for preservation of maximal renal function. Such abnormalities remain a major cause of renal failure in children, and morbidity may be minimized by appropriate evaluation and therapy. My choice for evaluation of a male child with a urinary tract infection includes an intravenous pyelogram and a voiding cystourethrogram. These studies allow assessment of both upper and lower urinary tract structure and function. An alternative, which is particularly satisfactory in neonates and young children, is to evaluate the upper urinary tract with renal ultrasonography and to evaluate the lower urinary tract with nuclear medicine cystography.

In young men, there are few well-done studies of the natural history of bacterial urinary tract infections. In patients without obvious neurologic or structural abnormalities, sexual intercourse, particularly among homosexual men or heterosexual men who practice insertive anal intercourse, may be a risk factor. The overall contribution of these practices to bacterial urinary tract infections in adult men is uncertain. Standard urologic teaching is to carry out a thorough evaluation for structural abnormalities in such patients, including radiographic studies and cystourethroscopy. However, my belief is that an excretory urogram with a postvoiding film and a uroflow study are adequate to screen for structural abnormalities in this population. I reserve cystoscopy for those patients determined to be at risk for significant abnormalities on the basis of these screening studies. The other major risk factors for urinary tract infections in men are instrumentation of the urinary tract and bacterial prostatitis.

### DIAGNOSIS AND LOCALIZATION

Because accurate diagnosis is a prerequisite for appropriate therapy, I obtain culture and sensitivity testing on urine specimens from any male with symptoms or signs suggesting urinary infection. In patients who do not have obstructive lesions, stasis, stones, or foreign bodies, recurrent and persistent urinary tract infections are often related to bacterial prostatitis. Segmented localization cultures can be used to differentiate cystitis and urethritis from bacterial prostatitis. This procedure should be carried out at a time when the patient does not have bacteriuria. After cleaning the glans with sterile water, the initial 5 to 10 ml of urine is collected in a sterile container. Next, a midstream specimen is obtained. The patient is asked to stop voiding and prostatic fluid is obtained by digital rectal examination. The next 5 to 10 ml is collected as the postmassage urine specimen. Culture and sensitivity testing are then carried out. It is critical to make certain that the laboratory is aware of the purpose of these studies so that they will evaluate small numbers of uropathogens.

Diagnosis of bacterial prostatitis can be made if the postmassage urine specimen or expressed prostatic secretion contains a 10-fold or greater increase in the concentration of the uropathogen compared with that in the first-void urine specimen. In patients with well-documented bacterial prostatitis, the causative organism is identical to that causing recurrent episodes of bacteriuria.

## BASIC PRINCIPLES IN THERAPY

There are three keys to successful therapy. First, one should eliminate or control predisposing factors. For example, removal of catheters, obstructive lesions, stones, or strictures or improved drainage of the lower urinary tract may be successful in eliminating the focus of infection. Second, one should eradicate the infection as soon as possible to prevent colonization of the prostate and other structures. Third, one should ensure that the infection has been eliminated by obtaining cultures during or immediately after therapy and at follow-up at 1 to 2 months following therapy.

### Uncomplicated Infections

Uncomplicated infections generally present with symptoms of bacterial cystitis, with a combination of urinary frequency, urgency, dysuria, nocturia, suprapubic discomfort, low-back pain, and hematuria. Systemic symptoms of fever, chills, and rigor are absent. Urine culture confirms the diagnosis, with *Escherichia coli* being the most common pathogen. Uncomplicated infections introduced by a single or short course of indwelling ureteral catheterization generally respond promptly to a short course of antimicrobial therapy. The infection may persist and become difficult to eradicate if the prostate becomes colonized or if the patient has a stone or structural abnormality of the urinary tract. Thus, an effort

should be made to eliminate predisposing factors while routine therapy is guided by in vitro susceptibility tests. I generally prefer oral therapy with one of the agents listed in Table 1. The duration of therapy should be at least 2 weeks.

For patients with persistent infections, longer courses of therapy are indicated. Often, I have used 3 to 4 months of therapy in this situation. In elderly patients or those in nursing homes, continuous therapy may be necessary to suppress bacteriuria, even though eradication of infecting organisms may prove impossible. Thus, for patients with recurrent or complicated infections, I recommend an attempt to eradicate the focus of infection following thorough evaluation of the urinary tract. The therapy is usually with the same drugs listed in Table 1, although duration is for 3 months. For patients with persistent or frequently relapsing infections, I consider long-term therapy (months or years) using low dosages of antimicrobial drugs for prophylaxis or suppression with periodic monitoring by culture to be sure that the agent continues to be effective.

### Complicated Infections

Patients with systemic signs or those with a history of structural or neurologic abnormalities merit thorough anatomic investigation of the urinary tract. It is important to do this early in the course of therapy because antimicrobial therapy alone may fail to cure the infection and urosepsis may develop unless there is specific management of the underlying problem. The initial choice for evaluation of these patients is an excretory urography with postvoiding film and/or renal ultrasonography, depending on the patient's overall medical status and level of renal function. If an abscess in the retroperitoneal space or the prostate is suspected, computed tomographic scanning has proved superior to the other modalities for diagnosis.

Acute and chronic bacterial prostatitis may

TABLE 1. **Oral Antimicrobial Agents Prescribed for Urinary Tract Infections in Adult Males**

| Antibiotic | Recommended Oral Dosage |
|---|---|
| Nitrofurantoin macrocrystals (Macrodantin) | 50 mg 4 times daily |
| Trimethoprim-sulfamethoxazole (Septra, Bactrim) | Two tablets (80 mg trimethoprim, 400 mg sulfamethoxazole) or one double-strength tablet (160 mg trimethoprim, 800 mg sulfamethoxazole) twice daily |
| Cephalexin (Keflex) | 250–500 mg 4 times daily |
| Cephradine (Velosef) | 250–500 mg 4 times daily |
| Norfloxacin (Noroxin) | 400 mg twice daily |
| Ciprofloxacin (Cipro) | 500 mg twice daily |

also present with systemic signs and symptoms. Acute bacterial prostatitis is usually manifest with a sudden onset of chills, fever, and low-back and perineal pain, as well as difficulty in urination. On rectal examination, the prostate is tense and exquisitely tender. Excessive palpation may induce septicemia. I usually hospitalize patients and treat them with 5 to 14 days of parenteral antimicrobial therapy. Most often, my initial choice is the combination of a beta-lactam drug and an aminoglycoside until the results of antimicrobial sensitivity testing are available. Following parenteral therapy, the patient is managed with continued antimicrobial therapy for at least 4 weeks. Patients with acute bacterial prostatitis usually respond well to a variety of antimicrobial agents that penetrate an acutely inflamed prostate. Many of these agents are not effective in chronic bacterial prostatitis.

In contrast to acute bacterial prostatitis, chronic bacterial prostatitis is often insidious in onset. Patients usually have recurrent urinary tract infections and sometimes recurrent episodes of acute prostatitis. Between symptomatic intervals, the patients may be totally asymptomatic. Diagnosis depends on the localization cultures described earlier. Treatment must be prolonged, as diffusion of antimicrobial agents into the prostate is poor. My initial choice is usually trimethroprim-sulfamethoxazole (Septra, Bactrim). Alternative drugs include the newer quinolones, norfloxacin, and ciprofloxacin. Carbenicillin indanyl sodium (Geocillin) is also approved for this indication, but has not been particularly effective in my hands. It is important that one not confuse bacterial prostatitis with other prostatitis syndromes. Nonbacterial "prostatitis" syndromes are much more common than bacterial prostatitis, and antimicrobial therapy does not prove particularly effective.

## OTHER CONSIDERATIONS

Patients with long-term urinary catheters or other devices and chronic asymptomatic bacterial colonization should not be treated. It is not possible to permanently sterilize the urine. Furthermore, resistant organisms will likely emerge, making subsequent therapy difficult. I prefer to treat such patients if they develop acute symptoms or prior to genitourinary tract instrumentation.

Prophylaxis for genitourinary tract instrumentation in patients who are uninfected has been the subject of considerable controversy. In my opinion, patients who do not have other indications for prophylaxis (prosthetic or valvular heart disease, for example) and who have sterile urine cultures do not require prophylactic therapy. In contrast, patients with indwelling catheters, or active urinary tract infections, who require genitourinary tract instrumentation should receive therapy with appropriate parenteral agents to prevent bacteremia and other complications.

# BACTERIAL INFECTIONS OF THE URINARY TRACT IN WOMEN

method of
ABDOLLAH IRAVANI, M.D.
*University of Florida College of Medicine*
*Gainesville, Florida*

Urinary tract infections (UTIs) are highly prevalent in women of childbearing age. It is estimated that 6 to 8% of young women develop UTIs each year, compared with only 2 to 3% of female infants and prepubertal girls. Bacteria responsible for these infections originate from the normal constituents of fecal flora that contaminate the urogenital area and adhere to and colonize the periurethral mucosa. Because of both a variety of host factors and bacterial pathogenicity, bacteria ascend the urethra and invade the urinary tract. The most common urinary tract pathogens in women are *Escherichia coli* and *Staphylococcus saprophyticus*. The other organisms, in order of decreasing incidence, are strains of *Proteus, Klebsiella,* and *Enterobacter* species. Infections may be limited to the lower tract (cystitis) or also involve the upper tract (pyelonephritis). More than 95% of young women with UTIs have simple uncomplicated infections with anatomically normal urinary tracts; nevertheless, the recurrence rate is high. Urinary tract infections carry a great risk of renal damage and scarring when they are complicated by underlying anatomic or functional abnormalities, such as obstructions, calculi, and neurogenic bladder; during pregnancy; or in systemic diseases, such as diabetes mellitus, systemic lupus erythematosus, and sickle cell disorders.

## CLINICAL SYMPTOMS

Clinical presentations of UTI are not consistent. Presence of dysuria and frequency with suprapubic pain and tenderness is a good indicator of UTI. Patients

TABLE 1. **Urinary Pathogens in Women**

| Common | *Escherichia coli* |
| | *S. saprophyticus* |
| Uncommon | *Proteus mirabilis* |
| | *Klebsiella pneumoniae* |
| | *Enterobacter* spp. |
| Rare | *Pseudomonas* spp. |
| | Enterococcus |
| | *Citrobacter* spp. |
| | *Acinetobacter* spp. |

may be asymptomatic or have dysuria symptoms with negative urine cultures, known as dysuria syndrome. Dysuria syndrome may be due to other causes and infections of the lower urogenital area with *Chlamydia trachomatis*, genital *Mycoplasma* infection, genital herpes, and *Candida* vaginitis.

## DIAGNOSIS

Diagnosis of UTI is based on the presence of clinical symptoms, pyuria, and more than $10^5$ colony-forming units (cfu) of a bacterium per ml of a clean catch midstream urine specimen. Presence of one bacterium per high-power field (hpf) ($100\times$) of microscopic examination of an unspun urine specimen correlates with greater than $10^5$ cfu of a bacterium per ml of urine. Semiquantitative urine culture devices such as dipslide (Culturia), roll tube (Bactercult), and small culture plate (Testuria) are practical office devices that have facilitated the diagnosis of UTIs.

Pyuria (white blood cell [WBC] >1 per hpf of unspun urine) supports diagnosis of UTI, but documentation of UTI cannot be based on the presence of pyuria alone. Pyuria is noted in 50 to 60% of women with UTIs. Pyuria may also occur without bacterial infection or may be due to contamination of urine with vaginal secretions.

A variety of tests such as those for nitrate (Griess' test), glucose oxidase, tetrasolum reduction, leukocyte esterase, and catalase are good only for screening purposes. It is unsound medical practice to treat a patient for UTI without performing a urine culture for a definite diagnosis.

## MANAGEMENT

### Duration of Therapy and Selection of Antimicrobial Agents

The duration of antimicrobial therapy can range from single-dose to short-term (3 to 10 days) therapy for cystitis and uncomplicated UTIs to long-term (longer than 10 days) courses for severe infections, pyelonephritis, and infections accompanied by underlying urologic abnormalities.

Antimicrobial agents that attain a high urinary concentration in active form generally result in a rapid and effective therapeutic response,

provided the urinary photogene is susceptible. Other selection criteria for drugs include (1) little or no systemic toxic effect, (2) minimal emergence of fecal bacterial resistance, (3) low incidence of *Candida* vaginitis, (4) low cost, and (5) convenient administration. The following antimicrobial agents generally have these characteristics.

**Sulfonamides.** Sulfonamides are synthetic bacteriostatic agents. They prevent the incorporation of para-aminobenzoic acid (PABA) into folic acid, which is necessary for purine and DNA synthesis in the bacteria. Of the common urinary pathogens, 70 to 75% are susceptible to these agents. Commonly used oral sulfonamides are sulfisoxazole (Gantrisin), 0.5 to 1 gram every 6 hours, or sulfamethoxazole (Gantanol), 0.5 to 1 gram every 12 hours. Sulfonamides are low in cost. Common side effects are headaches, rashes, and nausea.

**Trimethoprim.** Trimethoprim (Proloprim, Trimpex) is a synthetic bacteriostatic agent. It blocks a step in microbial folate metabolism that immediately follows the reaction inhibited by sulfonamide. Trimethoprim is absorbed well from gastrointestinal (GI) tract and is secreted in high concentration as active form in the urine. Trimethoprim, 100 mg twice daily or 200 mg once daily orally, is an effective agent against more than 95% of common urinary tract pathogens. *Pseudomonas* species and enterococci are resistant to this drug. Because trimethoprim is secreted in high concentrations in the vagina, it is suitable for use in prophylaxis of recurrent UTIs. Trimethoprim is tolerated well by more than 90% of patients. The common adverse reactions encountered are maculopapular rash and nausea.

**Trimethoprim-Sulfamethoxazole.** Because of the synergistic antibacterial action of trimethoprim and sulfonamides, a fixed combination of trimethoprim, 80 mg, and sulfamethoxazole, 400 mg (Bactrim, Septra, or double-strength tablets) is available. This combination is active against more than 90% of common urinary tract pathogens. The combination is less frequently associated with emergence of bacterial resistance than either of its components. Adverse reactions commonly noted are the same as those known to occur with sulfonamides and trimethoprim when used separately. Severe rashes, including erythema multiforme, and Stevens-Johnson syndrome have been reported with the use of sulfonamides and the combination.

**Aminopenicillins.** Aminopenicillins are beta-lactam antibiotics. Their antibacterial action is in inhibiting bacterial cell wall synthesis. Ampicillin (Totacillin, Polycillin, Omnipen), 250 to 500 mg every 6 hours; amoxicillin (Amoxil, Polymox, Wymox), 250 to 500 mg every 8 hours, and bacampicillin (Spectrobid), 400 mg every 12 hours, are the commonly used aminopenicillins.

TABLE 2. **Single-Dose Therapy of Urinary Tract Infections in Women**

| Antimicrobial Agent | Dosage |
|---|---|
| Trimethoprim-sulfamethoxazole (Bactrim, Septra) | 3 double-strength tablets (160 mg trimethoprim, 800 mg sulfamethoxazole each) orally |
| Amoxicillin (Amoxil, Polymox, Wymox) | 3 grams orally |
| Cephalexin (Keflex) | 3 grams orally |
| Ceftriaxone (Rocephin) | 0.5–1 gram intramuscularly |
| Cefuroxime axetil (Ceftin) | 1 gram orally |

TABLE 3. **Antimicrobial Agents Used in the Treatment of Urinary Tract Infections in Women**

| Agents | Dosage | Daily Dosing | Comments |
|---|---|---|---|
| Sulfonamides | | | |
| Sulfisoxazole | 0.5–1 gram | 4 | Bacterial resistance on the rise; frequent side |
| Sulfamethoxazole | 0.5–1 gram | 2 | effects; low cost |
| Trimethoprim-sulfamethoxazole | 160 mg trimethoprim, 800 mg sulfamethoxazole | 2 | Highly active against common urinary tract pathogens; frequent adverse effects, most commonly rash and headache |
| Trimethoprim | 100 mg | 2 | Highly active against common urinary tract |
| | 200 mg | 1 | pathogens; good for prophylaxis |
| Amoxicillin | 250–500 mg | 3 | Bacterial resistance on the rise; well tolerated; high incidence of *Candida* vaginitis |
| Amoxicillin-clavulanate | 250 mg amoxicillin, 125 mg clavulanate | 3 | Active against most common urinary tract pathogens that are resistant to amoxicillin; high incidence of GI side effects and *Candida* vaginitis |
| Nitrofurantoin | 50–100 mg | 4 | Effective treatment for cystitis; high incidence of nausea and vomiting; good for prophylaxis |
| Cephalosporins | | | |
| Cephalexin | 250–500 mg | 4 | Active against most common urinary tract pathogens; high cost; occasional GI symptoms; high incidence of *Candida* vaginitis |
| Cefadroxil | 250–500 mg | 2 | |
| Cefaclor | 250–500 mg | 3 | |
| Cefuroxime axetil | 125–250 mg | 2 | |
| Cefixime | 400 mg | 1 | |
| New quinolones | | | |
| Ciprofloxacin | 250–500 mg | 2 | Highly active against most urinary tract pathogens; occasional CNS and GI adverse reactions; high cost |
| Norfloxacin | 400 mg | 2 | |

They have similar activity against the urinary tract pathogens. Bacampicillin is a prodrug and is not active against bacteria in vitro but is converted to ampicillin in the intestinal wall. Amoxicillin and bacampicillin are preferable to ampicillin because of less frequent dosing and better patient tolerance. More than 35% of the common urinary tract pathogens of UTIs treated on an outpatient basis are resistant to these agents. The most common mechanism of bacterial resistance is inactivation by beta-lactamases. A fixed combination of amoxicillin, 250 mg, and the beta-lactamase inhibitor potassium clavulanate, 125 mg (Augmentin) has become available. This combination is effective against most bacteria resistant to amoxicillin. An approach to therapy of UTI is to initiate with the combination until the results of bacterial susceptibility testing become available. Aminopenicillins must, of course, be avoided in patients with histories of allergy to penicillins. Common adverse reactions include nausea, vomiting, diarrhea, and rashes. *Candida* vaginitis is a common side effect, occurring in 10 to 16% of patients.

**Cephalosporins.** Cephalosporins are beta-lactam antibiotics related to penicillins. Like penicillins, they are bactericidal by inhibiting bacterial cell wall synthesis. Numerous cephalosporins have been developed, each with distinct and unique pharmacologic, pharmacokinetic, and antibacterial properties. Cephalosporins are active in vitro against a wide variety of gram-positive and gram-negative microorganisms. First-generation cephalosporins (cephalexin [Keflex], cephalothin [Keflin] and cephadroxil [Duracef, Ultracef]) are more active against gram-positive microorganisms. However, bacterial resistance is increasing and approximately 25% of *E. coli* of outpatients with UTIs are resistant to these agents. Cephalexin (Keflex) 250 to 500 mg every 6 to 8 hours, or cefadroxil (Duracef or Ultracef), 500 mg every 8 to 12 hours, is used for treatment of UTIs.

Second-generation cephalosporins (cefuroxime axetil [Ceftin], cefaclor [Ceclor], cefuroxime [Zinacef], and cefamandole [Mandol]) have more antibacterial activity than their predecessors. They are active against both gram-positive and gram-negative microorganisms. Enterococci and *Pseudomonas* species are usually resistant to first- and second-generation cephalosporins. Cefaclor (Ceclor), 250 to 500 mg every 8 hours, and cefuroxime-axetil (Ceftin), 125 or 250 mg twice daily, are effective in treatment of UTIs.

Third-generation cephalosporins (cefixime [Suprax], ceftriaxone [Rocephin], and ceftazidime [Fortaz]) are highly active against a broad spectrum of gram-negative bacilli, including *Pseudomonas* species (ceftazidime). They are less active against gram-positive cocci, including *S. saprophyticus*. Ceftriaxone (Rocephin) is a parenteral cephalosporin with long half-life, allowing once or twice daily dosing. In patients with nausea and vomiting, a single dose of ceftriaxone, 500 to 1000 mg intramuscularly or intravenously, may help to alleviate the symptoms and subsequent oral antibiotic therapy can be better tolerated. Cefixime (Suprax), the only orally active third-generation cepholosporin, is beta-lactam–stable and has a long plasma half-life, permitting once-daily dosing. Cefixime has broad antibacterial activity similar to that of ceftriaxone. Cefixime, 400 mg once a day, is effective in treatment of UTIs.

Untoward effects of cephalosporins in general include nausea, vomiting, diarrhea, bleeding diathesis, positive direct Coombs' test result and cross-sensitivity reaction in 10 to 20% of individuals with allergy to penicillins. Cephalosporins may produce overgrowth of *Clostridium difficile* in the bowel and cause pseudomembranous colitis. *Candida* vaginitis is a common side effect and occurs in 6 to 16% of the patients.

**Nalidixic Acid.** Nalidixic acid (Neg Gram) has bactericidal activity by selective inhibition of bacterial DNA synthesis. Nalidixic acid is active against common gram-negative urinary tract pathogens. *Pseudomonas* species and *S. saprophyticus* are resistant to this drug. The presence of *S. saprophyticus* should be ruled out by microscopic examination of the urine before nalidixic acid is prescribed. Cinoxacin (Cinobac) is a derivative of nalidixic acid with a longer plasma half-life and otherwise similar antibacterial spectrum. Nalidixic acid is used as 1 gram every 6 hours orally and cinoxacin as 250 to 500 mg twice daily orally. Common side effects of these agents include visual and sensory neural disturbances, photosensitivities, dizziness, headaches, nausea, and rashes.

**New Quinolones.** New fluoroquinolones are derivatives of nalidixic acid with highly increased activity against bacterial DNA-gyrase. DNA-gyrase is essential for bacterial DNA replication and repair.

The commercially available new fluoroquinolones are ciprofloxacin (Cipro) and norfloxacin (Noroxin). These agents have broad antibacterial activity against Enterobacteriaceae, *Pseudomonas* species, and *Staphylococcus* species, including *S. saprophyticus*. They are also active against enterococci, although some quite resistant strains have been reported.

New fluoroquinolones are absorbed well and rapidly after oral administration and attain high serum, tissue, and urine concentrations in active form. Calcium and magnesium compounds interfere with intestinal absorption of new quinolones. Fluoroquinolones interfere with and decrease caffeine and theophylline (Theo-Dur) metabolism. Simultaneous administration of new fluoroquinolones and theophylline may result in high serum theophylline levels and severe toxicity. Ciprofloxacin, 250 to 500 mg twice daily, and norfloxacin, 400 mg twice daily, are highly effective in therapy of UTIs in women. They are not recommended in children and pregnant or lactating women. Ciprofloxacin is available in parenteral forms for intravenous administration in more serious infections. New fluoroquinolones are generally safe and are tolerated well by a majority of patients. The common adverse reactions include nausea, vomiting, abdominal pain, dizziness, nervousness, headaches, insomnia, anxiety, rashes, myalgia, arthralgia, photosensitivity with bullous skin lesions, and, rarely, generalized seizures.

**Nitrofurantoin.** Nitrofurantoin (Macrodantin) is an antibacterial agent that acts by interference with several bacterial enzymes. Nitrofurantoin is absorbed well from the small intestine and is rapidly excreted in the urine without development of significant blood levels. Nitrofurantoin is active against most common urinary tract pathogens, including enterococci and *S. saprophyticus*. *Proteus* species and *Pseudomonas* species are resistant to this agent. Nitrofurantoin rarely causes emergence of bacterial resistance or disturbs bowel bacterial flora. Nitrofurantoin macromolecule (Macrodantin), at oral dosages of 50 to 100 mg every 6 hours, should be taken after meals to decrease incidence of nausea and vomiting.

Common adverse reactions are nausea, vomiting, rashes, and anorexia. Other reactions are chronic active hepatitis, chronic allergic pneumonitis, anemia, and lupus-like syndrome. The drug is contraindicated in patients with glucose-6-phosphate dehydrogenase deficiency. *Candida* vaginitis is rare. Nitrofurantoin is a good agent for prophylaxis in recurrent UTIs, prescribed at 50 to 100 mg once daily at bedtime.

**Aminoglycosides.** Gentamicin (Garamycin) and tobramycin (Nebcin) are parenteral antibiotics and have broad antibacterial activity against gram-positive and gram-negative organisms, including *Pseudomonas* species. They are useful at 60 to 80 mg intravenously or intramuscularly every 8 hours in patients with severe infections or in those patients with multiple drug allergies to other antibiotics. Aminoglycosides are well known for their ototoxicity and nephrotoxicity. In patients with decreased renal function, dosing intervals should be extended according to the degree of renal function. Serum levels may have to be monitored 2 to 3 days after starting therapy.

**Erythromycin.** Erythromycin is not recommended in the treatment of UTIs because of the hepatobiliary route of excretion.

**Tetracyclines.** Tetracyclines are not recommended in the treatment of UTIs because of their low urinary excretion and high bacterial resistance.

## Simple Uncomplicated Infections

The majority of UTIs (>95%) in women are simple and uncomplicated. Simple uncomplicated infections are differentiated from complicated infections by their good response to a short course of antibiotic treatment. In patients with uncomplicated infections, symptoms are usually relieved and urine becomes sterile within 2 days of therapy. Persistence of symptoms and bacteriuria may be due to a variety of conditions, such as bacterial resistance, urinary calculi, obstructive uropathy, or the patient's poor compliance in taking her medication. On the other hand, resolution of symptoms alone is not a reliable indicator of therapeutic success and elimination of the urinary tract pathogen, especially in complicated UTIs; therefore, it is suggested that urine cultures be repeated at 1 week and 1 month after therapy.

The length of antibiotic treatment of UTI is a controversial issue. Factors to be considered are recent history of UTI, presence of fever (temperature >38° C), costovertebral angle tenderness, vomiting, dehydration, duration of symptoms, and the degree of pyuria. Patients with a few days of symptoms of lower tract infections and mild pyuria (WBC 1 to 5 per hpf) usually respond well to a single dose or 3 to 5 days of therapy, and those with longer duration of symptoms and heavy pyuria (WBC 10 to 20 per hpf) require a 7- to 10-day or longer course of therapy. Antimicrobial therapy should be started with the finding of bacteriuria on urinalysis rather than be delayed for the results of urine culture and susceptibility testing.

## Acute Pyelonephritis

Acute pyelonephritis is a bacterial infection of the renal parenchyma. It is distinct from and more serious than lower tract infections. The symptoms may vary from flank pain, fever (temperature >38.5° C), chills, vomiting, and dysuria to no symptoms at all. Approximately 30% of women with only symptoms of cystitis may have covert pyelonephritis. Depending on the severity of the clinical findings and the general condition of the patient, antimicrobial agents may be administered orally or parenterally. Each of the following antimicrobial agents may be given intravenously for 3 to 5 days or until the patient can tolerate an oral antimicrobial agent: ceftriaxone, 0.5 to 1 gram every 12 to 24 hours; ampicillin, 1 gram every 6 hours; trimethoprim-sulfamethoxazole (Bactrim, Septra), 160 mg of trimethoprim and 800 mg of sulfamethoxazole every 12 hours with large volume of fluid; cefazolin (Ancef, Kefzol); or cefamandole (Mandol), 1 gram every 6 hours. Therapy with an oral antimicrobial agent should be continued for a total of 10 to 14 days, according to the bacterial susceptibility testing results.

A sonogram of the urinary tract or an intravenous pyelogram is suggested within 1 month after therapy.

## Recurrent Urinary Tract Infections

Recurrent UTIs are a costly, inconvenient, and annoying problem in women. A recurrent infection occurs in 40% of women within 3 months and in 75 to 80% within 2 years after an episode of UTI. More than 90% of recurrences are reinfections caused by a different bacterium from that producing the initial infection.

Each episode of recurrent infection is treated with an appropriate antibacterial agent for 3 to 10 days. Personal hygienic precautions alone are not effective in preventing these infections, whereas long-term, low-dose antimicrobial therapy has proved effective. Prophylactic therapy is indicated when recurrences occur at frequent, closely spaced intervals. After the active infection is cleared, a low dose of an antimicrobial agent is prescribed to be taken at bedtime for 3 to 9 months. The antimicrobial agents commonly used for prophylaxis include trimethoprim, 100 mg; trimethoprim-sulfamethoxazole, 80 mg of trimethoprim and 400 mg of sulfamethoxazole; nitrofurantoin, 100 mg; cinoxacin, 250 mg; and cephalexin, 250 mg. A complete blood cell count (CBC) and liver profile tests (aminotransferase enzyme levels) are indicated every 3 months to evaluate the safety of the drug being used. Sulfonamides and aminopenicillins cause rapid emergence of bacterial resistance in fecal flora and are not recommended for prophylactic therapy.

A renal sonogram or an intravenous pyelogram is suggested for patients with more than four recurrences in a 12-month period.

## Asymptomatic Urinary Tract Infections

Asymptomatic UTIs may occur in patients with either anatomically normal or abnormal urinary tracts. Treatment of these infections is controversial. Asymptomatic UTIs, detected on a medical screening, are usually treated with a short course of an antimicrobial agent, after which the patient is observed for recurrent infections. Asymptomatic UTIs are of great significance and should be treated in patients with ureteral reflux, obstructive uropathies, or primary parenchymal renal disease and during pregnancy.

### Urinary Tract Infections in Pregnancy

Urinary tract infections can be a serious problem in pregnancy. Pregnant women are more susceptible to UTIs than are nonpregnant women, largely as a result of hormonal and physiologic changes. During pregnancy, hydroureter and vesicoureteral reflux may develop and facilitate pyelonephritis and renal scarring. The incidence of symptomatic UTI in pregnant women is reported to be as high as 15%, whereas the incidence of asymptomatic UTI is 4 to 6% (similar to that in nonpregnant women). Acute pyelonephritis is a common sequela of untreated asymptomatic bacteriuria. Recommended antimicrobial agents include aminopenicillins, cephalosporins, nitrofurantoin, and sulfonamides. A 7- to 10-day course of therapy usually eradicates the infection. Sulfonamides should not be used during the third trimester because they may cause kernicterus in the neonate. Periodic screening for asymptomatic bacteriuria is required during pregnancy.

### Complicated Urinary Tract Infections

The incidence of significant underlying urologic anomalies is less than 5% in young women with UTIs. *Pseudomonas* species, enterococci, and Enterobacteriaceae other than *E. coli* commonly cause complicated infections. Urinary tract pathogens are usually resistant to most antimicrobial agents. Management of these infections requires both antimicrobial therapy and surgical intervention to resolve the urinary retention. Consequent renal damage and scarring depend on the nature and the degree of the obstruction and the time lapse between the onset of infection and the establishment of antimicrobial therapy and adequate drainage. In complicated infections, bacteriuria may often persist or frequent relapses may occur at short intervals, necessitating extensive long-term antimicrobial therapy.

# URINARY TRACT INFECTIONS IN FEMALE CHILDREN

method of
BRUCE BROECKER, M.D.
*Emory University School of Medicine*
*Atlanta, Georgia*

Urinary tract infections (UTIs) are a common cause of morbidity and an occasional cause of mortality in children. Five to 6% of girls have at least one bacterial urinary tract infection during childhood, and many have multiple recurrences. Pediatric UTIs occur predominantly in girls (female/male ratio of 30:1), except during the first 30 days of life, when males predominate by a ratio of 10:1. During the past 30 years, the treatment of UTIs has become highly successful as a result of the many effective antibacterials that concentrate in the urine, but the pathophysiology of individual susceptibility and the natural history continue to be less well understood, despite intense research efforts.

Urinary tract infections may be classified in ways that are useful in selecting therapy and further diagnostic evaluation. One such classification divides UTIs into (1) neonatal infections, (2) uncomplicated cystitis, (3) recurrent cystitis, and (4) acute pyelonephritis. It should be recognized that this classification is clinical and does not limit the infection to a specific location in the urinary tract. It should also be recognized that the patient's symptoms in infections in each of these categories may be caused by nonbacterial infections (from *Chlamydia* and *Candida* species and adenoviruses) as well as by noninfectious conditions.

Methods of anatomically localizing bacteria have been exhaustively studied in an effort to tailor therapy more objectively. As yet, those methods that are noninvasive (antibody-coated bacteria, C-reactive protein, capsular antigen, and lactate dehydrogenase isoenzyme determinations) are unreliable. The most reliable techniques (bladder washout and ureteral catheterization) are invasive, requiring general anesthesia, and, therefore, are not generally employed.

The most common organism responsible for bacterial UTIs continues to be *Escherichia coli,* followed by enterococci, *Pseudomonas, Klebsiella*, and *Proteus* species.

## TREATMENT AND EVALUATION

### Neonatal Urinary Tract Infections

Neonatal UTIs occur predominantly in males, with an incidence of approximately 1.5% and 0.15% in males and females, respectively. Recent data suggest a role of the foreskin as a predisposing factor in these infections, with uncircumcised neonates being more susceptible than their circumcised counterparts. The most common organism is *E. coli,* accounting for 80% of the infections. These are serious infections and must be treated promptly and aggressively. Recommended treatment is with ampicillin and an aminoglycoside (gentamicin, tobramycin, or amikacin) (Table 1) until an organism is identified and sensitivity test results are available. Peak and trough aminoglycoside levels should be obtained regularly to monitor and adjust dosage. Treatment should be continued for 10 to 14 days, at which time a urinalysis should reveal acellular urine. A urine culture should be repeated 5 to 7 days after completion of therapy. The incidence of anatomic abnormalities in these children is significant (30 to 50%), with vesicoureteral reflux being the most common. All infected neonates should be evalu-

TABLE 1. **Treatment of Urinary Tract Infections in Female Children**

| Type of Therapy | Dosage/ kg/Day | Daily Dosing |
|---|---|---|
| Parenteral | | |
| Ampicillin | 100 mg | 4 |
| Amoxicillin | 50 mg | 3 |
| Cefazolin (Ancef) | 50 mg | 4 |
| Cefamandole (Mandol) | 100 mg | 4 |
| Gentamicin (Garamycin) | 5–7 mg | 3 |
| Tobramycin (Nebcin) | 5 mg | 3 |
| Amikacin (Amikin) | 15 mg | 3 |
| Oral | | |
| Ampicillin | 100 mg | 4 |
| Amoxicillin | 40 mg | 3 |
| Cephradine (Velosef) | 25 mg | 4 |
| Erythromycin | 30 mg | 4 |
| Nitrofurantoin (Furadantin) | 5–7 mg | 4 |
| TMP-SMX* (Bactrim, Septra) | 0.5–1 ml | 2 |
| Prophylactic | | |
| Nitrofurantoin | 3 mg | 1 |
| TMP-SMX | 0.5 ml | 1 |

*TMP/SMX = 8 mg of trimethoprim and 40 mg of sulfamethoxazole per ml.

ated radiographically (Table 2). A renal ultrasonogram should be done early in the course of a neonatal infection to rule out obstruction. The timing of delayed evaluation is not critical, but generally it is carried out between 2 and 4 weeks after the completion of treatment. It is desirable, however, for the child to take oral antibiotics until the evaluation is completed.

Radiographic evaluation should include a voiding cystourethrogram (VCUG) and a renal nuclear scan or an intravenous urogram (if the VCUG demonstrates vesicoureteral reflux). The urogram or nuclear scan is preferred in infants with demonstrable reflux because of its better delineation of subtle degrees of reflux nephropathy. It has been recommended that the neonate with UTI who is febrile and has normal radiographic studies should have a follow-up ultrasonogram at age 2 years, because the evolution of renal scarring may take this long to appear on imaging studies.

## Uncomplicated Cystitis

Uncomplicated cystitis denotes a bacterial infection of the bladder occurring for the first time in an anatomically normal urinary tract. This infection is overwhelmingly found in females, generally with irritative voiding symptoms and without fever. Radiographic evaluation is indicated in all children who present with clinical symptoms of uncomplicated cystitis and have a culture-proven bacterial infection. The particular imaging studies may, however, be tailored to the patient's age. It is my practice to evaluate older children (older than 5 years) with the first afe-

brile infection with ultrasonography alone. If that study is normal, no further imaging studies are done. A child with an abnormal study is evaluated with additional studies as dictated by the abnormal findings. In younger children (younger than 5 years) or in any child with febrile or recurrent infections, a VCUG is done in addition to the ultrasonographic examination. The ultrasonographic examination of a child with a UTI should include views of both the kidneys and the bladder.

Treatment of uncomplicated cystitis is extremely effective. The following antibiotics are all useful: sulfisoxazole (Gantrisin), ampicillin, amoxicillin, erythromycin, cefradine (Velosef), trimethoprim-sulfamethoxazole (TMP-SMX) (Bactrim, Septra), trimethoprim, and nitrofurantoin (Furadantin) (see Table 1). The appropriate length of treatment has been the subject of a number of articles during recent years. The standard treatment course of 10 to 14 days has been challenged by courses lasting 7, 5, 3, and 1 day(s). Advocates of the shortest regimen point to advantages of decreased cost, decreased toxicity, greater compliance, and comparable success rates, whereas advocates of the longer courses argue that there is a greater recurrence rate with abbreviated treatment. For uncomplicated cystitis, I favor a 3- to 5-day course of one of the above antibiotics, most commonly TMP-SMX or nitrofurantoin.

## Recurrent Cystitis

Recurrent cystitis denotes a repetitive UTI and is a particularly prevalent feature of UTIs in children. Up to 75% of children with a UTI develop one or more recurrent infections. A recurrent infection is defined as a second new infection and is to be distinguished from bacterial persistence, which means failure of eradication of the original organism. This differentiation is

TABLE 2. **Evaluation of Female Child with Urinary Tract Infection**

**Neonate**
During therapy (early): renal/bladder ultrasonogram*
After resolution of UTI (delayed): VCUG*
**Uncomplicated Cystitis**
Older than 5 years of age: renal/bladder ultrasonogram
Younger than 5 years of age: VCUG, renal ultrasonogram (IVP)
**Recurrent Cystitis**
VCUG, renal ultrasonogram (IVP)
**Acute Pyelonephritis**
As per neonatal UTI

*Further studies (IVP, renal scan, computed tomographic scan) may be indicated by abnormalities discovered on the above studies.
*Abbreviations:* UTI = urinary tract infection; VCUG = voiding cystourethrogram; IVP = intravenous pyelogram.

usually readily done with the urine culture and sensitivity test. Even when infections are closely spaced, recurrent infection is the rule. Bacterial persistence generally occurs only with bacterial resistance (wrong antibiotics), treatment noncompliance, or anatomic abnormalities. Nitrofurantoin and TMP-SMX are the most useful antibiotics in treating this category, with a dosage modification for prophylactic use (see Table 1). In those children in whom the recurrent infections are closely spaced (several days to a week), it is my belief that the infections have altered the normal bladder defense mechanisms, rendering the child susceptible to an early recurrence. I have found a prophylactic dose of TMP-SMX or nitrofurantoin for 4 to 6 weeks immediately following the therapeutic course useful in interrupting this process. In the child whose recurrences are most widely spaced (weeks to months), I use the finding of three infections in 6 months or four infections in 1 year as indication for prophylactic therapy lasting 3 to 6 months. Infections occurring at less frequent intervals are treated individually with a 3- to 5-day therapeutic course of one of the standard antibiotics mentioned earlier.

### Acute Pyelonephritis

This category consists of those children with an acute febrile UTI associated with leukocytosis and flank pain. It is a serious upper UTI that needs prompt and effective treatment to prevent renal damage. These children should have an ultrasonogram of the kidneys and the bladder early during treatment to rule out obstructive anomalies of the urinary tract. Further imaging studies are postponed until after resolution of the infection. Parenteral antibiotics with ampicillin and aminoglycoside are indicated as initial therapy until results of culture and sensitivity studies are available. Parenteral therapy should continue until the patient has been afebrile for 24 hours and the urinalysis reveals absence of pyuria or bacteriuria. Oral antibiotics are continued for a total of 14 days.

# CHILDHOOD ENURESIS

method of
MARK PUCZYNSKI, M.D.

*Allegheny General Hospital*
*Pittsburgh, Pennsylvania*

Enuresis is defined as the involuntary discharge of urine occurring in children beyond the expected age of bladder control. Wetting during the night is termed nocturnal enuresis, whereas daytime wetting constitutes diurnal enuresis. A person with both types present is said to have mixed enuresis.

Most children are approximately 4 years of age before they have achieved a degree of bladder control, but are often 5 to 6 years of age before they can withhold urination associated with bladder distention. The term "enuresis" describes wetting in girls older than 5 years of age and is reserved for boys at least 6 years of age. Ten to 15% of 5-year-olds, 7% of 10-year-olds, and 2% of 15-year-olds experience at least one episode of enuresis a month.

Primary enuresis describes the situation in which the child has never achieved dryness. Secondary enuresis is reserved for children who have achieved a period of dryness of at least 3 to 6 months. Twenty-five per cent of children who have achieved bladder control experience self-limited bed-wetting, which may only appear during times of infection or stress. Fifteen to 20% of children with nocturnal enuresis also experience daytime wetting, a frequency that decreases after 5 years of age.

## ETIOLOGY

Males are affected more frequently than females at a ratio of 1.5:1. Genetic influences are a determinant and, in 70% of families with an enuretic child, symptoms occurred in more than one family member. This symptom is also seen more frequently in children of lower socioeconomic status and in larger families.

Primary enuresis may be the result of a maturational delay in the acquisition of normal bladder control. Recent studies in children with nocturnal enuresis failed to demonstrate any abnormal bladder activity, inadequate bladder capacity, urethral sphincter dysfunction, or the presence of a sleep arousal disorder. Children with nocturnal enuresis appear to have a high urinary output that results from a lack of an increase in antidiuretic hormone secretion at night. It is not clear why these children do not arouse when their bladder is full. Secondary enuresis may be the result of stress and be accompanied by other somatic symptoms. Enuresis has been associated with urinary tract infections, diabetes mellitus, renal tubal disease, diabetes insipidus, psychogenic water drinking, and disorders that affect bladder innervation.

The evaluation of children with enuresis must begin with a thorough history and physical examination. History should include information about the family, a behavior profile of the child, the type and duration of the enuresis, a description of the urine stream, the presence of urgency, the frequency of voiding, prior episodes of urinary tract infection, and the existence of other illnesses. The physical examination should include documentation of growth variables, vital signs, and a thorough neurologic and genitourinary examination. The neurologic examination should include examination of the lower back for abnormal growths of hair, lipomas, dimples, and angiomas, which may be suggestive of an occult spinal dysraphism. An evaluation of the lower extremities should include a motor and sensory examination, assessment of peripheral reflexes, documentation of anal sphincter tone, and observation of the urine stream. A urinalysis and culture should be included in the initial evaluation.

The child with nocturnal enuresis, normal history and physical examination findings, normal urinalysis and culture, and a family history of enuresis has uncomplicated enuresis and generally requires no further work-up. Children with positive urine culture, history of a prior urinary tract infection, encopresis, voiding dysfunction, and an abnormal genitourinary and/or neurologic examination have complicated enuresis. In these instances, further evaluation with a renal or bladder ultrasound and voiding cystogram (with spine films) is warranted. Abnormalities discovered on these tests indicate the need for further urodynamic and neurosurgical evaluation.

## TREATMENT

The treatment of the underlying cause of complicated enuresis, such as a urinary tract infection, may result in immediate resolution of the symptom. In cases of uncomplicated enuresis, spontaneous resolution generally occurs at a rate of 12 to 15% of cases per year. Reassurance and the elimination of blame and punishment may be all that is needed. When uncomplicated enuresis creates undue stress for a child, further intervention is warranted. Management of nocturnal enuresis is generally behavioral (wetness alarm) or medical and directed at the central nervous system, the bladder, or the kidney. Other interventions, such as withholding of fluid, bladder retention training exercises, and random awakening, have met with some success. Conditioning therapy involves the use of an alarm system that is triggered during the process of voiding. Alarm systems have a long-term success rate of 65 to 70%, but an initial relapse occurs in 30% of patients. A more favorable outcome is to be expected when retreatment occurs. Newer alarm systems (Wet-Stop, Nytone) avoid some of the complications associated with the pad and buzzer systems, such as "buzzer ulcers." Devices that vibrate rather than ring are useful for deaf children or in situations in which it is important not to disturb other family members.

Pharmacologic agents have been used to treat enuresis, but their therapeutic value must be weighed against their toxic effects. A tricyclic antidepressant, imipramine (Tofranil), has a long-term success rate reported to be 25%. However, a high relapse rate occurs after discontinuation of the drug. It exerts peripheral anticholinergic and antispasmodic effects, which may explain its efficacy in the treatment of enuresis. Imipramine should be reserved for children 6 years of age or older, with a starting dose of 25 mg for a 6- to 8-year-old child and 50 to 75 mg for a 6- to 8-year-old child and 50 to 75 mg in older children. Medication should be given 1 hour before bedtime. The optimal duration of treatment is unknown, although it has been suggested to maintain treatment for 3 to 6 months, followed by a gradual reduction in dosage. To accurately assess the effectiveness of therapy, children should be treated at least 2 weeks before considering adjustment of the dosage. Possible side effects of imipramine in children treated for enuresis include anxiety, sleep disturbances, lethargy, and mild gastrointestinal disorders. Overdoses can lead to potentially fatal toxicity, with arrhythmias, respiratory depression, and convulsions. Oxybutynin (Ditropan), an anticholinergic drug, may be beneficial to patients who have enuresis associated with uninhibited bladder contractions, but it is of little benefit in those who exclusively experience nocturnal enuresis. The experience with this drug in the treatment of nocturnal enuresis is limited.

Desmopressin (1-desamino-8-D arginine vasopressin, DDAVP), an analogue of vasopressin, administered intranasally at 10 to 40 µg at bedtime, is effective in the treatment of nocturnal enuresis with no serious side effects reported to date. Fifty to 70% of children with nocturnal enuresis achieve dryness, but experience a high relapse rate if treatment is suddenly discontinued. Weaning from the medication requires a minimum of 3 months. Allergic rhinitis or an upper respiratory tract infection may interfere with absorption and effectiveness of this drug.

Psychotherapy may be of value in treating emotional problems that may coexist in the child and/or the family, but is not the treatment of choice. If undue stress is present within the family environment, counseling should be considered as part of the overall management of the child with enuresis.

# URINARY INCONTINENCE

method of
RICHARD W. DEMMLER, M.D.
*Baylor College of Medicine*
*Houston, Texas*

Normal micturition occurs when intravesicular pressure exceeds intraurethral pressure. Urinary incontinence occurs when this balance is disrupted. For treatment, urinary incontinence can be divided into four categories: detrusor instability, stress, overflow, and functional incontinence. Of these, detrusor instability is by far the most common, accounting for as much as 70% of all incontinence.

To appropriately treat this condition, the physician must keep in mind the mechanism of bladder innervation. The relaxation or filling component is under sympathetic control. The detrusor contains predominantly beta-sympathetic receptors, which when stimulated result in increased vesicular volumes without increased pressures. The distal third (including the internal sphincter) contains predominantly alpha receptors, whose stimulation results in increased intraurethral pressure. Parasympathetic stimulation results in contraction of the detrusor and relaxation of the internal sphincter.

## DETRUSOR INSTABILITY

Detrusor instability is also termed unstable bladder, spastic bladder, or uninhibited bladder. It is caused by decreased cortical inhibition as a result of lesions in the anteromedial frontal lobe, such as intracranial tumors, aneurysms of the anterior cerebral artery, penetrating brain injuries, or lobotomy. Cerebrovascular accidents, Parkinson's disease, Alzheimer's dementia, and multiple sclerosis have also been associated with incontinence because of their effect on micturition centers in the central nervous system. Detrusor instability may also be precipitated by states of bladder hyperexcitability, as in cases of infection, inflammation, fecal impaction, genitourinary or rectal neoplasias, uterine prolapse, prostatic hypertrophy, Valsalva's maneuvers, coughing, or surgical manipulation.

Detrusor instability typically presents as voiding frequent small amounts immediately after the initial urge to micturate. A simple office procedure can be used for diagnosing detrusor instability. The procedure requires a sterile catheter and a 50-ml catheter tip syringe.

1. After completely voiding, the patient should be placed in a recumbent position with a fracture pan or urinal placed to collect any overflow. A No. 12 or 14 French catheter is inserted and the residual volume recorded.

2. The syringe is attached to the catheter and held 15 cm above the symphysis pubis.

3. The bladder is filled at 50-ml increments, until the patient reports feelings of bladder pressure.

4. After the appreciation of bladder filling, the bladder is filled using 25-ml increments until there is involuntary bladder contraction or the patient reports an inability to hold more fluid. Detrusor instability is associated with volumes of less than 300 ml of instilled volume.

Treatment of detrusor instability attempts to increase bladder volume without increasing pressures. Oxybutynin (Ditropan) is a parasympathetic antagonist, which is the most effective agent with the least side effects when administered initially at 2.5 mg twice daily and titrated up to 5 mg three times a day. Imipramine (Tof-

ranil) is theoretically the best drug for this disorder, as it blocks detrusor contractions and has alpha-sympathomimetic properties, which increase the intraurethral pressure. However, agitation in the elderly population limits the usefulness of this agent. Calcium channel blockers have met with considerable success, but, owing to the attendant reduction in blood pressure, considerable caution must be used.

## STRESS INCONTINENCE

Stress incontinence results from mechanical and structural changes of the internal sphincter. It is most commonly seen in multiparas or women who have had a hysterectomy. This incontinence results when micturition occurs at lower intravesicular pressures. In elderly women, however, detrusor instability is commonly co-existent with stress incontinence and must be appropriately managed.

Initial treatment of stress urinary incontinence should always be medical and is aimed at increasing the intraurethral pressure. Kegel's exercises are preferred, if the patient is capable. Intravaginal or orally administered estrogen improve the urethrovesicular angle by increasing the support of the vaginal subcutaneous tissue. Alpha-adrenergic agonists, such as phenylpropanolamine or pseudoephedrine, increase the intraurethral pressure. Imipramine may also be considered for increasing intraurethral pressure. Surgical intervention should be considered only after failure of these therapies and if the patient desires further treatment. An anterior repair, the Marshall-Marchetti-Krantz procedure, is the recommended surgical intervention.

## OVERFLOW INCONTINENCE

Overflow incontinence occurs in two pathologic states, neurogenic bladder and outlet obstruction. In these states, the intravesicular pressures exceed the intraurethral pressures only at high volumes. Diagnosis is made when the postvoiding residual is greater than 100 ml of urine. Obviously, a rectal examination is instructive in delineating possible causes.

If overflow incontinence is due to outlet obstruction, therapy is directed by the physical findings. Removal of a fecal impaction results in immediate resolution of the urinary incontinence. Urethral dilation is required for urethral stricture. Prostatic hypertrophy would be treated with transurethral resection or radical prostatectomy, depending on the needs of the patient. An atonic or neurogenic bladder should be treated by intermittent catheterization, which minimizes the risk of infection.

## FUNCTIONAL INCONTINENCE

Functional incontinence is a result of a person's inability to get to toileting facilities in an appropriate time and fashion. Both physical and medicinal restraints, which are frequently used, result in incontinence. In addition, patients with strokes, Parkinson's disease, or impaired vision may be unable to navigate through environmental hazards. Physicians must remain ever mindful of their ability to precipitate urinary incontinence. In many cases, treatment of underlying illnesses or choosing aids that improve mobility resolves the problem.

## DIAPERS AND INDWELLING FOLEY'S CATHETERS

Only if the earlier mentioned therapeutic maneuvers do not adequately treat the condition should one consider using diapers. Yet more often than not diapers are used primarily. There are occasional instances when indwelling Foley's catheters can be used, but they are few and far between. In general, the use of either of these entities should be discouraged until all therapeutic avenues have been addressed.

# EPIDIDYMITIS

method of
PETER T. NIEH, M.D.
*Lahey Clinic Medical Center*
*Burlington, Massachusetts*

Inflammation of the epididymis is characterized by scrotal pain and by enlargement and induration of the posterior-lying epididymis, with eventual scrotal edema, testicular involvement, and hydrocele formation. Epididymitis usually is caused by infection of the urinary tract but may be associated with trauma, tuberculosis, or even syphilis or gonorrhea. Reflux of sterile urine down the vas deferens after prostatectomy may produce a chemical epididymitis. Men with bladder cancer receiving intravesical bacille Calmette-Guérin for immunotherapy may develop tuberculous-like granulomas of the epididymis.

In males younger than age 35 years, chlamydia is the common pathogen, usually presenting with expressible urethral discharge. In older men, the typical coliform bacteria predominate, often associated with distal urinary tract obstruction. Tuberculosis should be considered in the older patient with sterile pyuria and nodularity of the vas deferens.

In prepubertal boys, the rare instances of epididymitis are usually caused by bacteria, and careful evaluation for congenital urinary anomalies, such as vesicoureteral reflux or ectopic ureter, should be undertaken. In adolescents and young adults, acute epididymitis must be differentiated from testicular torsion, which is a surgical emergency. Radionuclide scan or Doppler ultrasonography may be useful in this situation.

Urinalysis may reveal pyuria and sometimes bacteriuria. A smear of any urethral discharge should be made and stained for *Neisseria gonorrhoeae*. A urine culture should be obtained before any antibiotic therapy is instituted. If tuberculosis is suspected, a sample for acid-fast bacilli should also be submitted.

## TREATMENT

### Immobilization

In mild cases, scrotal support is adequate. However, in more severe cases, the testis may need to be elevated on several soft folded towels or even strapped to the pubic symphysis by using cloth tape after the scrotum is shaved.

Strict bed rest for the first 24 to 48 hours minimizes further irritation and pain. The patient should be permitted to leave the bed only to use the bathroom.

### Analgesia

Application of an ice pack limits edema and provides appreciable relief. Codeine with acetaminophen or aspirin, combined with nonsteroidal anti-inflammatory drugs such as ibuprofen, usually suffices to control pain. In particularly severe cases, a local anesthetic block provides further relief and permits better examination of the enlarged scrotal contents. Local anesthesia is performed after appropriate preparation of the skin with iodine, by using 10 ml of 0.5% lidocaine (Xylocaine) or bupivacaine (Marcaine) injected carefully through a 21-gauge needle into the spermatic cord at the level of the pubic tubercle.

### Broad-Spectrum Antibiotics

The therapy for gonorrhea is described elsewhere. For the patient younger than age 35 years with nongonococcal epididymitis, chlamydia is most effectively treated with tetracycline, 500 mg orally every 6 hours for 10 days, or doxycycline, 100 mg orally twice daily for 10 days. If bacteria are seen on urinalysis, either ciprofloxacin (Cipro), 250 mg, or trimethoprim-sulfamethoxazole (Septra or Bactrim), one tablet orally twice daily for 10 days, is advisable. If the patient appears to be in a toxic condition with a high fever and leukocytosis, use of a third-generation cephalosporin or parenteral aminoglycoside is preferable.

## Surgery

Aspiration of an acute hydrocele under local anesthesia allows a more careful examination of the underlying structures and often permits more rapid resolution of scrotal discomfort. If there is any doubt whether epididymitis or testicular torsion is the problem, early surgical exploration is recommended. If a area of fluctuance develops, which suggests abscess formation, surgical drainage or excision may be necessary. If pain and fever persist in an older man, an epididymo-orchiectomy must be considered. If a mass persists after treatment, the possibility of an underlying testicular tumor should be considered, and ultrasonography and inguinal exploration may be required.

## COMPLICATIONS

Most patients with acute epididymitis respond to proper treatment with relatively rapid resolution of pain, although induration may take several weeks to resolve completely. In some instances, chronic epididymitis may persist, with recurrent episodes of scrotal pain and induration. In these patients, fibrosis and ductal obstruction are usually present, with resultant sterility if involvement is bilateral. In patients who are immunocompromised, epididymitis may progress to produce Fournier's gangrene, a necrotizing, synergistic infection of the scrotal wall. This condition requires radical excision of all infected tissue and epididymo-orchiectomy in selected patients.

# GLOMERULAR DISORDERS

method of
GERALD C. GROGGEL, M.D.
*College of Medicine, University of Vermont,
Burlington, Vermont*

Glomerular disorders may result from a variety of pathologic processes, the primary one being immunologic. The principal clinical manifestations of glomerular disorders are hematuria, proteinuria, hypertension, edema, and reduction of the glomerular filtration rate.

Glomerular disorders can be divided into four major clinical syndromes: acute glomerulonephritis, rapidly progressive glomerulonephritis (RPGN), the nephrotic syndrome, and asymptomatic urinary abnormalities (proteinuria and hematuria). They can also be divided into primary disorders, in which only the kidney is involved in the disease process and all clinical manifestations arise from alterations in glomerular structure or function, and secondary or systemic disorders, in which the kidney is part of a disorder affecting multiple organs, such as diabetes mellitus.

## ACUTE GLOMERULONEPHRITIS

Most patients with acute glomerulonephritis have had a recent infection of the pharynx or skin with a group A beta-hemolytic *Streptococcus*. Acute glomerulonephritis similar to poststreptococcal glomerulonephritis may occur after many bacterial, viral, or parasitic infections. Certain systemic diseases such as systemic lupus erythematosus, infective endocarditis, and vasculitis may also cause acute glomerulonephritis.

### Poststreptococcal Glomerulonephritis

This form of acute glomerulonephritis is secondary to an infection with certain strains of group A beta-hemolytic *Streptococcus*. The hallmark of this disorder is depression of the levels of the third and fourth components of complement. These levels return to normal after 6 to 8 weeks. If the component levels remain persistently low, another diagnosis should be sought. Treatment of the streptococcal infection does not prevent the occurrence of glomerulonephritis, but it may suppress the development of streptococcal antibodies. Treatment of the infection is recommended with a 10-day course of either penicillin or erythromycin. Treatment with antibiotics probably does not affect the course of acute glomerulonephritis. Thus only conservative management is used to treat the symptoms of the glomerulonephritis, including the management of hypertension and edema. There is no evidence that corticosteroid therapy is of value in acute glomerulonephritis. An occasional patient with acute poststreptococcal glomerulonephritis presents with crescentic glomerulonephritis and rapid loss of renal function. In these instances, it is appropriate to treat the patient with RPGN just as any other patient with this condition would be treated (see the section on RPGN). The prognosis for this disorder is in general very good.

### Infectious Glomerulonephritis

Glomerulonephritis may be associated with subacute bacterial endocarditis, infected ventriculoatrial shunts, or visceral abscesses. In each situation, the primary purpose of therapy should be to eradicate the infection as rapidly as possible. The glomerulonephritis usually resolves with appropriate antibiotic or surgical treatment of the underlying process.

In the rare patient who develops diffuse crescentic glomerulonephritis with rapid loss of renal function, the use of high-dose steroid therapy may be considered. However, the benefits of steroid therapy need to be weighed against the detrimental and potentially life-threatening effects of such therapy on the course of the underlying infection. I consider the administration of high-dose steroids only if the infection has been adequately treated. In that case, the physician could consider using intravenous methylprednisolone, 15 to 30 mg per kg, given over several hours every other day for three doses, followed by a short course of oral prednisone, 60 mg per day, for 4 weeks.

### Systemic Lupus Erythematosus

The therapeutic approaches to the management of lupus nephritis are controversial. All patients with active lupus have some form of renal involvement, but only those with significant glomerular involvement require treatment. When there is no evidence of clinical renal disease, the physician can assume that the patient does not have significant glomerulonephritis. But if the patient has proteinuria, hematuria, an active urinary sediment, or an elevated serum creatinine level, treatment should be considered. Before treatment is instituted in this setting, it is appropriate to perform a renal biopsy to classify the patient according to the microscopic appearance of the kidney. The major forms of lupus nephritis, according to the World Health Organization's classification, are minimal, mesangial, focal proliferative, diffuse proliferative, and membranous glomerulonephritis.

#### Minimal and Mesangial Lupus Nephritis

Minimal lupus nephritis is characterized by rare mesangial immune deposits in otherwise normal-appearing glomeruli. In mesangial nephritis there are more mesangial deposits, and these are associated with mild mesangial expansion and proliferation. Usually these patients have normal renal function and minimal proteinuria. The goal of therapy is to control the extrarenal manifestations of the lupus. No specific therapy is required for this form of glomerular disease. If the serum creatinine level rises or heavy proteinuria develops, the clinician should suspect the development of a more severe form of lupus nephritis.

#### Focal and Diffuse Proliferative Lupus Nephritis

Focal lupus nephritis is characterized by focal and segmental glomerular lesions that are often associated with necrosis and intercapillary thrombi. The immune deposits are extensive, involving both the mesangium and the glomerular capillary wall, primarily in a subendothelial location. Diffuse proliferative lupus nephritis involves almost all the glomeruli and is characterized by extensive glomerular hypercellularity, necrosis, capillary wall thickening, and fibrinoid changes. Crescent formation may be present in both of these diseases. In diffuse proliferative lupus nephritis, immune deposits may be found in the mesangium, the subendothelium, and even the subepithelial space. These patients typically have heavy proteinuria, an active urinary sediment, frequent hypertension, and a reduced glomerular filtration rate.

Present evidence indicates that steroid therapy alone is probably not effective. These patients also require some form of cytotoxic therapy. They can be initially treated with high-dose oral prednisone, 60 to 80 mg per day, with tapering after 1 month of therapy. After the prednisone has been tapered, they should be treated with either cyclophosphamide or azathioprine. Regimens that have proved to be successful in treating lupus nephritis include cyclophosphamide, 1 to 3 mg per kg per day; azathioprine, 1 to 3 mg per kg per day; a combination of cyclophosphamide, 1 mg per kg per day, and azathioprine, 1 mg per kg per day; or cyclophosphamide, 500 to 1000 mg per $M^2$ of body surface intravenously. There is some preliminary evidence that the intravenous form of cyclophosphamide is associated with fewer adverse reactions than the other regimens and may provide better preservation of renal function.

Thus, presently I recommend treating proliferative lupus nephritis with intravenous cyclophosphamide, beginning with a dose of 500 mg per $M^2$ of body surface. This is given in 250 ml of normal saline and is followed by a minimum of 1 liter of normal saline. The white blood cell count is followed carefully, with a goal of reaching a nadir of approximately 2000 to 3000 cells per $mm^3$. If this dose is tolerated, it is increased the next month to 750 mg per $M^2$ and again to a maximal dose of 1000 mg per $M^2$. This dose is given monthly for a total of 6 months.

It should be emphasized that extensive scarring seen on renal biopsy, particularly with interstitial fibrosis and tubular atrophy, suggests that the lupus nephritis is less amenable to therapy. In this situation, the risks of continuing immunosuppressive therapy probably do not outweigh the potential benefits.

#### Membranous Lupus Nephritis

In this form of lupus nephritis there is diffuse capillary wall thickening, with immune deposits located in the subepithelial space. In contrast to idiopathic membranous nephropathy, there can also be mild mesangial changes with mesangial immune deposits. The clinical course of this form of lupus nephritis is usually more indolent than that of the proliferative forms. Although there are no controlled therapeutic trials of this form of lupus nephritis, I would recommend treating these patients just as patients with idiopathic membranous nephropathy are treated. They should receive 120 mg of prednisone orally every other day for 8 weeks, with the dose tapered over a 4-week period. These patients may require lower doses of prednisone to control their extrarenal lupus.

### Necrotizing Vasculitis

Systemic necrotizing vasculitis is a heterogeneous disorder in which blood vessels of various sizes in many different organs may be involved with inflammatory necrotizing lesions. Polyarteritis nodosa, hypersensitivity vasculitis, and Wegener's granulomatosis may all involve the kidney.

As initial therapy, it is appropriate to treat these patients with a combination of high-dose prednisone, 60 to 80 mg per day, and oral cyclophosphamide, 1 to 3 mg per kg per day. The prednisone can be tapered over 1 to 3 months. The cyclophosphamide is continued for at least 3 months or until the disease becomes quiescent.

For Wegener's granulomatosis, therapy consists of cyclophosphamide, 1 to 3 mg per kg per day, and prednisone, 40 to 60 mg a day. After 1 year of therapy, the cyclophosphamide can be slowly discontinued. In all forms of vasculitis, it is important that treatment be initiated early to maximize the preservation of renal function.

### Henoch-Schönlein Purpura

Henoch-Schönlein purpura is a syndrome consisting of dermal, articular, abdominal, and renal manifestations. It is a leukoclastic vasculitis with deposits of IgA in both the skin and the kidney. The glomerulonephritis can vary in severity from mild to severe. In general, this is a benign, self-limited disease, with less than 10% of patients progressing to renal failure. Treatment does not appear to alter the course of the renal disease. An occasional patient may have crescentic glomerulonephritis on renal biopsy. These patients should be treated just as other patients with crescentic glomerulonephritis are treated, as described in the next section.

## RAPIDLY PROGRESSIVE (CRESCENTIC) GLOMERULONEPHRITIS

RPGN is a form of glomerulonephritis associated with progressive renal insufficiency that develops over weeks to months. The morphologic hallmark of this disorder is extensive glomerular crescent formation. If it remains untreated, end-stage renal disease always develops. Thus early diagnosis and treatment are essential.

Any type of acute glomerulonephritis can result in crescentic glomerulonephritis. The term "idiopathic rapidly progressive glomerulonephritis" is reserved for patients who do not have evidence of another type of glomerulonephritis and do not have evidence of a systemic disease. In the presence of pulmonary involvement, this disorder is called Goodpasture's syndrome. This disorder has been divided into three types. Type I is characterized by linear deposits of IgG along the glomerular capillary membrane and is associated with circulating antiglomerular basement membrane antibodies. Approximately 20% of the patients have this form. Type II is characterized by granular immune deposits of IgG and complement. Approximately 40% of the patients have this form. Type III is characterized by no glomerular immune deposits on immunofluorescence. Approximately 40% of the patients have this form. There are few studies of the treatment for this disorder, and none of them have been well controlled.

The initial treatment for the antiglomerular basement membrane antibody–mediated disease should be plasma exchange (plasmapheresis) combined with oral prednisone, 60 mg per day, and cyclophosphamide, 1 to 3 mg per kg per day. Plasmapheresis should consist of 2- to 4-liter exchanges daily for the first 2 to 5 days. The frequency of plasmapheresis can then be gradually reduced over 2 to 4 weeks until the serum antiglomerular antibody level decreases and a good clinical response is obtained. The cyclophosphamide can be discontinued after 2 to 3 months, and then the prednisone can be slowly tapered. These patients are monitored by following serum levels of antiglomerular basement membrane antibody. This therapy is most effective in nonoliguric patients with an initial serum creatinine level of less than 6 to 7 mg per dl. Patients who have oliguria and severe renal failure should be treated conservatively with dialysis and transplantation. Plasmapheresis should not be instituted without simultaneous immune suppression because there is often a clinical relapse caused by a rebound in circulating antibody levels after the plasmapheresis is stopped.

The treatment of patients with Type II RPGN or granular immune deposits is pulse methylprednisolone. Methylprednisolone, 30 mg per kg per day, is given intravenously over 30 minutes three times on alternate days, followed by oral prednisone, 1 mg per kg per day, tapered over several months. In contrast to the situation in

Type I RPGN, the benefit of treatment has been seen even in patients who are oliguric and receiving dialysis, but the best results occur in patients treated early. There is no evidence that plasmapheresis is superior to pulse steroids in Type II RPGN. If there is evidence of an underlying vasculitis based on clinical features and focal necrotizing glomerular lesions, a cytotoxic agent should be added, usually cyclophosphamide, in a dose of 1 to 3 mg per kg per day for 3 to 6 months.

The treatment of Type III RPGN or no immune deposits disease is identical to the treatment of Type II. Again, if there is evidence of an underlying vasculitis, patients should be treated with cytotoxic therapy, usually cyclophosphamide, as noted earlier. Although there have been anecdotal reports of the use of anticoagulants (heparin, warfarin) and antithrombotics (dipyridamole) in this disorder, the risk of life-threatening complications clearly outweighs any potential benefit.

### Goodpasture's Syndrome

Goodpasture's syndrome is an antiglomerular basement membrane antibody–mediated disease with systemic involvement manifested primarily by pulmonary hemorrhage. The therapeutic approach to these patients is similar to that used for patients with idiopathic antiglomerular basement membrane antibody–mediated disease. The pulmonary manifestations should respond to plasmapheresis in the vast majority of patients. In patients with advanced renal disease, that is, with a serum creatinine level greater than 7 mg per dl and/or oliguria, the response of the renal disease to plasmapheresis will probably be poor. In these patients, the renal disease should be treated conservatively with dialysis and transplantation. Patients who are to undergo transplantation should have low or undetectable serum antibody levels for at least 3 to 6 months to minimize the risk of disease recurrence in the transplanted kidney.

### IDIOPATHIC IgA NEPHROPATHY

IgA nephropathy is one of the most frequent forms of glomerulonephritis. Its clinical features are variable. Many patients have recurrent episodes of gross (macroscopic) hematuria, particularly after virus-like syndromes. On examination of the renal biopsy specimen, the hallmark of this disorder is deposits of IgA in the mesangium by immunofluorescence. A subset of patients with IgA nephropathy may have the nephrotic syndrome. Patients with heavy proteinuria, hypertension, and abnormal renal function at the time of presentation probably have a worse prognosis. Approximately 20 to 25% of patients with IgA nephropathy develop end-stage renal disease during a period of 20 years. Henoch-Schönlein purpura is the systemic form of this disease.

Presently, the treatment for IgA nephropathy is entirely supportive. There is no evidence that any therapeutic measures are effective in this disorder. Therapies that have been tried include corticosteroids, cytotoxic agents, antibiotics, and phenytoin.

### ASYMPTOMATIC PROTEINURIA

Patients with low-grade proteinuria (less than 1 gram per 24 hours) and a normal urinary sediment are said to have asymptomatic proteinuria. The vast majority of these patients have postural proteinuria, which occurs only when they are in the upright position. This can be documented by collecting a split 24-hour urine sample consisting of the urine produced both while the patient is recumbent and while the patient is upright. If protein appears only in urine collected in the upright posture, the patient can be identified as having postural proteinuria. These patients can be reassured that the prognosis is good, and they do not need further evaluation or treatment. If the proteinuria is not postural, these patients should be followed closely. If they develop evidence of severe proteinuria (more than 2 grams per 24 hours), an abnormal urinary sediment, or loss of renal function, they should undergo a renal biopsy. Based on the biopsy findings, specific therapy can then be instituted.

### NEPHROTIC SYNDROME

The nephrotic syndrome is a clinical syndrome manifested by heavy proteinuria (usually more than 3.5 grams per day per 1.72 $M^2$ body surface area), hypoalbuminemia, hyperlipidemia, lipiduria, and edema. The hallmark of this syndrome is hypoalbuminemia. This, rather than the degree of proteinuria, defines the syndrome.

There are many causes of the nephrotic syndrome, idiopathic as well as systemic. In children the vast majority have the idiopathic form, whereas in adults approximately one-third are associated with a systemic disease, drug, or toxin. The most common systemic diseases causing the nephrotic syndrome are diabetes mellitus, systemic lupus erythematosus, amyloidosis, drugs, and neoplasms. Diabetic nephropathy is always accompanied by other manifestations of microangiopathy, particularly retinopathy. There is no known specific therapy for the renal disease.

Rigorous control of blood pressure and blood glucose level may delay the development of end-stage renal failure. There are some anecdotal reports that converting enzyme inhibitors are effective in reducing the proteinuria in this disorder and possibly in slowing the progression to end-stage renal disease. Further studies are needed before the therapeutic benefits of converting enzyme inhibition are established.

Amyloidosis may be primary or associated with a variety of systemic diseases. If the underlying disease can be identified, it should be treated if possible. Unfortunately, no specific therapy is of proven benefit. In patients with familial Mediterranean fever, colchicine diminishes the frequency of attacks and prevents the development of amyloidosis. Many drugs have been associated with the nephrotic syndrome, including the nonsteroidal anti-inflammatory agents, gold, captopril, and penicillamine. The nephrotic syndrome usually resolves when the offending agent is discontinued. Many neoplasms have also been associated with the nephrotic syndrome. If the neoplasm can be effectively treated, the nephrotic syndrome usually remits.

## Causes of the Idiopathic Nephrotic Syndrome

### Minimal Change Disease

This disease accounts for 85 to 90% of children with the nephrotic syndrome and 15 to 20% of adults. Generally the urinary sediment is benign, blood pressure is normal, and there is little tendency toward loss of renal function. Thus the indications for treatment are primarily symptomatic.

These patients, both adults and children, should be treated initially with oral prednisone, 2 mg per kg (up to 80 mg per day), given as a single daily dose for 4 weeks, and then on an alternate-day basis for an additional 4 weeks. As soon as the nephrotic syndrome completely remits (urinary protein level less than 200 mg per day), one should switch to alternate-day steroid therapy. Prednisone should then be slowly tapered over the remainder of the 8-week treatment period. If alternate-day treatment is used as initial therapy, it usually takes longer to induce a remission.

With this approach, more than 90% of patients achieve a remission. However, 60% of these patients have subsequent relapses. For patients with infrequent relapses (one or two per year), repeating the initial therapy is usually effective. Patients who have frequent relapses may benefit from either oral cyclophosphamide, 1 to 2 mg per kg per day, or chlorambucil, 0.15 mg per kg given for 6 to 8 weeks, plus prednisone.

Patients who relapse as the prednisone is being tapered or immediately after it is discontinued are considered to be steroid dependent. In these patients the benefits of long-term, low-dose steroid therapy are probably outweighed by the side effects. Therefore, treatment with cyclophosphamide or chlorambucil to induce a long-lasting remission would be appropriate. These patients may require slightly higher doses of chlorambucil (0.15 to 0.2 mg per kg per day). All adult patients should have a renal biopsy before being treated. For children, who are usually assumed to have minimal change disease and are treated without a renal biopsy, it is appropriate to perform a renal biopsy before instituting cyclophosphamide or chlorambucil therapy.

There are significant side effects associated with both of these alkylating agents, and they should be used with caution. The white blood cell count, hematocrit, and platelet count need to be measured weekly. If signs of bone marrow toxicity develop, the dose of the alkylating agent should be reduced or discontinued. To avoid gonadal dysfunction, the patient should be treated with cyclophosphamide for 6 weeks or less, and the total cumulative dose of chlorambucil should be kept below 7 mg per kg. A urinalysis should be performed at regular intervals to detect hemorrhagic cystitis from the cyclophosphamide. The use of these agents has also been associated with a high risk of malignancies, particularly leukemia and lymphoma, in later life. Given the natural history of this disease and the risk of side effects with the use of alkylating agents, the majority of patients should not be so treated. These drugs should be reserved for the patient who frequently relapses and is debilitated from both the consequences of the nephrotic syndrome and the long-term side effects of steroid therapy.

### Mesangial Proliferative Glomerulonephritis

Mesangial proliferative glomerulonephritis is characterized by increased cellularity in the mesangial region in a patient without systemic illness. There are usually immune deposits of IgM in the mesangium. Treatment of mesangial proliferative glomerulonephritis is similar to that of minimal change disease. The drug of choice is prednisone. Patients should be treated to the point of remission or for up to 8 weeks. With this treatment, approximately 50% of the patients can be expected to achieve a complete remission of the nephrotic syndrome. However, the majority of patients relapse as soon as the steroid dose is tapered or discontinued. If prednisone is ineffective or if the patient is steroid dependent and the nephrotic syndrome is significant, cyclophosphamide can be used at a dose of 1 to 2 mg per kg per day for 8 weeks. Adding prednisone to the cyclophosphamide does not improve the outcome. The cyclophosphamide does not need to be tapered. Some of these patients develop focal glomerulosclerosis.

### Focal Segmental Glomerulosclerosis

Focal glomerulosclerosis accounts for approximately 10 to 15% of the adults with idiopathic nephrotic syndrome. The majority of these patients have progressive renal failure and hypertension and develop end-stage disease after 5 years. Patients who achieve a partial remission of the nephrotic syndrome tend to have a better prognosis than those with persistent, heavy proteinuria. There have been no controlled clinical trials, but certain patients have had a remission of proteinuria associated with steroid therapy. Patients who respond to therapy appear to have a better prognosis than nonresponders or patients who have not been treated. Thus, if there are no contraindications to steroid therapy and renal function is well preserved, I recommend a trial of corticosteroids. Patients should be treated with 100 to 120 mg of prednisone on alternate days until a complete remission occurs or for a maximum of 8 weeks. The prednisone can then be tapered over the next 4 weeks. Although there is no proven benefit at this time, the risks and side effects from a short course of alternate-day prednisone therapy are low and the potential benefits may be great. If there are contraindications to steroid therapy or the patient has advanced renal failure, conservative management with control of blood pressure is indicated. There is no evidence that alkylating agents are of benefit. Recent preliminary work suggests that cyclosporine may be effective in inducing a remission, but patients appear to have relapses as soon as the drug is discontinued. Thus, at this time, cyclosporine cannot be recommended for these patients. In patients who respond to steroids but who have frequent relapses or are steroid dependent, a prolonged remission in proteinuria may be induced with the use of cyclophosphamide, 1 to 2 mg per kg per day, or chlorambucil, 0.1 to 0.2 mg per kg per day, in addition to the prednisone for an 8-week course. But this therapy should be reserved for patients with significant side effects from the nephrotic syndrome and the steroid treatment. Patients with focal sclerosis who have non-nephrotic proteinuria should be treated conservatively because they generally do not progress to end-stage renal disease.

### Membranous Nephropathy

Idiopathic membranous nephropathy is the most frequent cause of the nephrotic syndrome in adults, accounting for about 50% of these cases. The outcome is highly variable. Spontaneous remission can occur. The treatment of membranous nephropathy remains highly controversial. However, a number of well-done prospective studies have demonstrated the benefits of therapy in slowing the progression of the renal disease.

Initial treatment of membranous nephropathy is 120 mg of prednisone orally given on alternate days for 8 weeks. The drug is then tapered and discontinued over the next 4 to 8 weeks. The patient who relapses later should be treated in a similar manner. This treatment has been shown to preserve renal function and slow the progression to end-stage renal disease. These benefits have been achieved even without remission of the proteinuria. A second form of treatment that has been shown to be effective is methylprednisolone, 1 gram intravenously for 3 days, followed by oral prednisone, 0.5 mg per kg per day for a month, alternated with chlorambucil, 0.2 mg per kg per day for a month, for a total of 6 months. The dose of chlorambucil is reduced if the white blood cell count falls below 5000 per mm³. This therapy has also been shown to be beneficial in preserving renal function.

Recently it has been shown that cyclophosphamide in a dose of 1.5 mg per kg per day for 12 to 24 months slows the progression to end-stage renal disease. This treatment is particularly effective in patients with serum creatinine levels higher than 1.8 mg per dl. In patients with membranous nephropathy and non-nephrotic, asymptomatic proteinuria (< 2 grams protein per 24 hours), the prognosis is good and treatment is not recommended.

### Membranoproliferative Glomerulonephritis

Membranoproliferative glomerulonephritis is an uncommon cause of the idiopathic nephrotic syndrome, accounting for less than 5% of adults with this syndrome. These patients usually present with the nephrotic syndrome or with acute glomerulonephritis manifested by hematuria and low-grade proteinuria. Many patients have a decreased serum complement level at some stage of their disease. Most patients with membranoproliferative glomerulonephritis progress to end-stage renal disease. Occasional spontaneous remission may occur. There are two histologic subtypes of membranoproliferative glomerulonephritis. Type I is characterized by prominent C3 deposits along the glomerular capillary and in the mesangium, and by electron-dense deposits in subendothelial and mesangial locations. In Type II membranoproliferative glomerulonephritis (intramembranous deposit disease), C3 deposits are present in the capillary walls and mesangium, but immunoglobulin is absent. The glomerular basement membrane is usually thickened with electron-dense deposits. I recommend treating patients with both Type I and Type II membranoproliferative glomerulonephritis with dipyridamole, 75 mg three times per day, and aspirin, 325 mg three times per day. In Type I membranoproliferative glomerulonephritis, this regimen has been shown to delay the progression to end-stage renal disease.

A number of other therapeutic regimens have been tried in patients with membranoproliferative glomerulonephritis. Particularly in children, uncontrolled trials of alternate-day prednisone have been shown to be of benefit in slowing the progression of the renal disease. But until controlled trials show a benefit of this form of therapy, I cannot recommend it. The combination of cyclophosphamide, dipyridamole, and warfarin (Coumadin) has been shown to be ineffective in the treatment of membranoproliferative glomerulonephritis.

## GENERAL MANAGEMENT OF GLOMERULAR DISEASE

In addition to the treatment of the underlying disorder, management of patients with glomerular disease, particularly the nephrotic syndrome, includes therapy directed at relief of symptoms, correction of deficiencies resulting from urinary losses, and preservation of renal function.

### Edema

Edema may occur in patients with glomerular diseases for various reasons. First, hypoalbuminemia resulting from the nephrotic syndrome reduces plasma oncotic pressure, leading to a disturbance in Starling forces in the peripheral capillary. Intravascular fluid is redistributed into the interstitial compartment, producing edema. The decreased intravascular volume then leads to increased resorption of sodium chloride and water by the kidney. Second, avid sodium chloride resorption can be found in the absence of hypoalbuminemia in glomerular disorders marked by intense glomerular inflammation. Third, a decrease in the glomerular filtration rate may limit urinary sodium chloride and water excretion, which leads to intravascular volume expansion. The consequences of the fluid retention in addition to edema can include hypertension and pulmonary congestion. Patients with mild to moderate edema do not need treatment except for moderate salt restriction (dietary sodium limit of 2 grams per day). Ony severe symptomatic edema should be treated. Diuretics can be used to treat this condition. Hydrochlorothiazide, be-

ginning at a dose of 25 mg per day, can be used in patients with a glomerular filtration rate exceeding 50 ml per minute. For patients with more compromised renal function, the loop diuretics furosemide or ethacrynic acid should be used in doses of 40 to 160 mg per day. If the hydrochlorothiazide or loop diuretics alone are not effective, a potassium-sparing agent such as amiloride, spironolactone, or triamterene can be added. These agents must be used with great caution in patients with compromised renal function because the risk of hyperkalemia is considerable. These patients must be monitored carefully for overdiuresis and the development of volume depletion. The goal of therapy should not be the eradication of edema but the control of the symptoms of edema. All of these patients have edema to some extent at all times.

### Hypertension

Hypertension associated with glomerular disorders may be secondary to volume expansion or excessive systemic vasoconstriction. Clearly sustained hypertension accelerates the progression and irreversible loss of renal function, whatever the underlying disorder. Thus hypertension must be aggressively treated in these patients because it is an important factor in the progression of the renal disease. Generally a diuretic should be the initial therapy. The thiazide diuretics can be used in patients with serum creatinine levels less than 2.5 mg per dl. In those with serum creatinine levels higher than 2.5 mg per dl, the loop diuretics should be used. If the blood pressure is not controlled with a diuretic alone, a second agent, either a converting enzyme inhibitor, captopril and enalapril, or a beta blocker such as propranolol should be used. Captopril should be instituted at a dose of 25 mg twice per day and increased to a total of 150 mg per day. Enalapril should be initiated at a dose of 5 mg once per day and increased to a total dose of 20 or 30 mg per day. Propranolol should be started at a dose of 40 mg twice per day and increased to a total dose of 160 to 240 mg per day. Other agents that can be used include a calcium channel blocker such as nifedipine or diltiazem. For resistant hypertension, minoxidil can be effective, beginning at a dose of 2.5 to 5 mg per day and increasing to 20 to 30 mg per day.

A few words of caution about the use of drugs in patients with glomerular disease must be kept in mind. Because many drugs circulate bound to albumin, the hypoalbuminemia present in these patients may lead to high levels of free drug and increased toxicity. Certain agents, particularly the sulfonamide diuretics, can cause acute interstitial nephritis and lead to deterioration of renal function. Certain agents, such as the beta blockers nadolol and atenolol, are excreted primarily by the kidney, and their dosage needs to be adjusted for the level of renal function. The angiotensin-converting enzyme inhibitor captopril has been associated with the development of membranous nephropathy in a small number of patients. Doses greater than 150 mg per day should not be used in patients with impaired renal function or in those with systemic lupus erythematosus.

### Thrombosis

Patients with the nephrotic syndrome have an increased prevalence of thromboembolic disease, which may be related in part to loss of inhibitors of coagulation, particularly antithrombin III, and to increased platelet aggregation. Renal vein thrombosis is particularly common in patients with the nephrotic syndrome secondary to membranous nephropathy. Pulmonary emboli can complicate renal vein thrombosis. Patients who present with evidence of either pulmonary emboli or an acute worsening of proteinuria or renal function that cannot be explained by other means should undergo venography. Patients with documented renal vein thrombosis or thromboembolic events need to be treated with oral anticoagulants. This therapy should be continued for as long as they remain nephrotic and hypoalbuminemic. There is no evidence that prophylactic anticoagulation is of benefit.

### Hyperlipidemia

One of the hallmarks of the nephrotic syndrome is hyperlipidemia, manifested primarily by elevation of the serum cholesterol level but also, in patients who are severely nephrotic, by elevation of serum triglyceride levels as well. The etiology of the hyperlipidemia is multifactorial in these patients. Clearly, patients with persistent, long-term proteinuria and long-term elevations of serum lipid levels are at risk for premature atherosclerosis. Until recently there has been no safe, effective treatment for this disorder. Now, however, the fibric acid congener gemfibrozil has been found to be safe and effective at a dose of 600 mg twice per day. A combination of gemfibrozil plus the bile acid–binding resin colestipol, at a dose of 10 grams twice per day, was particularly effective in these patients. Unfortunately, many patients are unable to tolerate the gastrointestinal side effects of the bile acid–binding resins. Recent studies also suggest that the new lipid-lowering agents, the hydroxymethylglu-

taryl coenzyme A reductase inhibitors, particularly lovastatin (Mevacor), may also be effective in this disorder. Lovastatin can be administered in a dose of 10 to 40 mg twice daily.

### Nutritional Therapy

In patients with the nephrotic syndrome, deficiencies of a variety of plasma proteins may occur. Significant hypogammaglobulinemia may be present and may be associated with increased susceptibility to infections. Hyperimmune gamma globulin may be beneficial in patients with recurrent infections. The loss of vitamin D–binding globulin may lead to vitamin D deficiency, hypocalcemia, and bone disease. These patients may require therapy with oral vitamin D preparations. There may be urinary losses of trace metals such as iron, zinc, and copper.

The optimal dietary intake for patients with the nephrotic syndrome and renal insufficiency remains to be established. There is some clinical evidence that moderate dietary protein restriction may retard the progression of renal disease in patients with chronic renal failure. There is also evidence that moderate protein restriction, rather than increased protein intake, may be more effective in maintaining serum albumin levels in patients with the nephrotic syndrome. However, the long-term safety and efficacy of protein-restricted diets in patients with heavy proteinuria, diabetes, and systemic diseases have not been demonstrated. In selected patients, moderate protein restriction may be appropriate. Initial therapy should include dietary counseling and a diet containing 0.7 to 0.8 gram per kg of protein per day. These patients need to be monitored closely for maintenance of body weight and serum albumin concentrations. Frequent visits with a nutritionist are probably required to ensure dietary compliance.

# PYELONEPHRITIS

method of
STEVEN M. OPAL, M.D.
*Brown University*
*Providence, Rhode Island*

Pyelonephritis is defined as acute or chronic inflammation of the kidney resulting from the presence of microorganisms within the renal pelvis and interstitium. The disease generally presents as a clinically apparent, toxic illness with symptoms referrable to the urinary tract. However, it is important to note that infection of the upper urinary tract may occur in the absence of localizing symptoms. This condition is referred to as subclinical pyelonephritis and is observed primarily in children or the elderly. Pyelonephritis is the most common recognized source of bacteremia in hospitalized patients with gram-negative sepsis, and urinary tract infections remain the most common cause of nosocomially acquired infection. Although the optimal therapy for pyelonephritis is yet to be defined, general guidelines for this clinical entity have been developed. The recent introduction of various new antimicrobial agents has improved and widened the therapeutic options available to clinicians who treat pyelonephritis.

## ACUTE PYELONEPHRITIS

The diagnosis of acute pyelonephritis is based on clinical findings of urinary frequency, dysuria, pyuria, and bacteriuria accompanied by fever, flank pain, and systemic toxicity. Despite the development of various techniques to localize infection in the upper urinary tract (antibody-coated bacteria, ureteral catheterization, Fairley's bladder washout, and imaging techniques), no method is sufficiently safe and reliable to be used routinely.

Pyelonephritis generally occurs as a result of ascending urinary tract infection from the urethra and urinary bladder. Infection of the kidney via the hematogenous route occurs infrequently ($< 5\%$ of cases) after disseminated infection with invasive microbial pathogens such as *Staphylococcus aureus*, *Candida* species, and *Salmonella* species. The Enterobacteriaceae and *Enterococcus faecalis* account for more than 95% of the microorganisms causing pyelonephritis. Infection of the upper urinary tract is abetted by functional or mechanical obstruction of urinary flow and vesicoureteral reflux. Urinary calculi may contribute to pyelonephritis by producing urinary obstruction. Certain organisms (*Proteus* species, some *Klebsiella* species, *Staphylococcus saprophyticus*) may promote urolithiasis by producing urease, which alkalinizes the urine by releasing ammonia. The change in urinary pH results in precipitation of magnesium-ammonium-phosphate (struvite) stones. These stones may encase viable bacteria, which results in recalcitrant urinary tract infections.

Acute pyelonephritis is generally caused by a single strain of bacteria. Polymicrobial urinary tract infections are uncommon and should prompt a search for enterovesical fistulas or other structural abnormalities of the urinary tract. Polymicrobial infection is occasionally associated with urinary tract instrumentation or urolithiasis.

A Gram's stain of urine provides a rapid and reliable technique for diagnosis of pyelonephritis. The finding of one or more organism per oil immersion field on Gram's stain of uncentrifuged urine indicates at least $10^5$ organisms per ml. Gram's stain also distinguishes gram-negative bacilli from gram-positive cocci (enterococci or staphylococci), which permits an early guide to empiric therapy. Urine culture and susceptibility studies, when available, can be used to direct antimicrobial therapy. Blood cultures are generally warranted in patients with acute pyelonephritis. White blood cell casts in the urinary sediment are specific for renal medullary infection and are often found in urinary tract infections that are complicated by obstruction or papillary necrosis. Pyelonephritis in the absence of significant bacteriuria may occur under the following circumstances: pyelonephritis with complete urinary obstruction, prior antimicrobial therapy, or suppurative complications (intrarenal or perinephric abscess).

### Treatment

The toxic-appearing patient with acute pyelonephritis should be hospitalized for intravenous antimicrobial therapy. A rapid assessment of fluid and electrolyte status should be conducted, in addition to a review of potential complicating factors such as recent use of urinary tract instrumentation, prior antimicrobial therapy, pregnancy, diabetes mellitus, prior urinary tract infections, or functional or mechanical abnormalities of urinary flow. Intravenous fluids are indicated to promote an adequate urinary output and to treat volume depletion, which may develop secondary to fever and loss of urinary concentrating ability. After urine and blood cultures have been obtained and urinalysis and Gram's stain have been reviewed, empiric therapy is warranted based on an assessment of the most likely pathogen.

Uncomplicated pyelonephritis may be treated with a variety of acceptable antimicrobial regimens. Parenteral ampicillin, cefazolin (Ancef), or trimethoprim-sulfamethoxazole (Septra, Bactrim) are acceptable empiric agents. Combination therapy with aminoglycosides in addition to beta-lactam drugs is generally reserved for severely ill patients with presumed gram-negative sepsis, or for nosocomially acquired infections in which resistant gram-negative bacilli (*Pseudomonas, Providencia*) are more likely to occur. Antimicrobial therapy should be modified once the susceptibility pattern of the offending pathogen is known. Directed therapy should make use of the simplest and least expensive effective agent.

A number of second- and third-generation cephalosporins and newer antimicrobial agents such as aztreonam (Azactam), imipenem (Primaxin), and beta-lactamase inhibitor combinations such as ticarcillin plus clavulanic acid (Timentin) are well suited for treatment of acute pyelonephritis. These agents have the advantage of being active against a wide variety of resistant gram-negative bacilli (including *Pseudomonas* species) while avoiding the potential nephrotoxicity associated with aminoglycoside antibiotics. They are particularly useful in treating nosocomially acquired pyelonephritis. The fluoroquinolones norfloxacin (Noroxin) and ciprofloxacin (Cipro) have an excellent spectrum of activity and pharmacokinetic properties for use in the treatment of urinary tract infections. Intravenous preparations of fluoroquinolones will soon be available and will provide a useful alternative for the treatment of acute pyelonephritis. Enterococcal urinary tract infections are successfully treated with ampicillin alone unless the patient is septic, which indicates the need for the addition of an aminoglycoside. *S. saprophyticus* is susceptible to trimethoprim-sulfamethoxazole, ampicillin, or vancomycin.

Intravenous therapy should continue until 48 hours after the patient becomes afebrile. At that time, the patient may be switched to an effective oral antimicrobial agent for a total duration of therapy of at least 2 weeks. Therapy should continue for a total of 4 to 6 weeks in patients who have frequent relapsing infections or complicated structural abnormalities of the urinary tract. Most patients are rendered afebrile within 72 hours of initiation of appropriate antimicrobial therapy. Lack of clinical response by this time should prompt an investigation to rule out local suppurative complications (intrarenal or perinephric abscess, papillary necrosis) or urinary obstruction. Computed tomography and renal ultrasonography are useful in providing diagnostic information as well as a means of directing therapeutic percutaneous drainage if an abscess is identified.

A follow-up urine culture 1 week after completion of therapy should be obtained in patients with documented pyelonephritis. Evidence of relapsing infection should be treated with a prolonged course (4 to 6 weeks) of an appropriate antimicrobial agent. Frequent relapsing infections in women and any urinary tract infection in men should prompt urologic evaluation to exclude potentially correctable structural abnormalities.

### CHRONIC PYELONEPHRITIS

Chronic pyelonephritis connotes chronic interstitial nephritis with scarring associated with recurrent urinary tract infections. This entity is seen almost exclusively in patients who have structural abnormalities of the genitourinary tract with evidence of recurrent infection since childhood. Recurrent urinary tract infections in adults without structural anomalies of the genitourinary tract rarely, if ever, result in chronic renal insufficiency. Chronic pyelonephritis is associated with small contracted kidneys that have uneven scarring and thinning of the renal cortex. The clinical presentation is one of chronic renal insufficiency associated with hypertension, urinary concentrating defects, metabolic acidosis, hyperkalemia, and renal salt wasting.

### Treatment

The optimal therapy of chronic pyelonephritis is prevention of its occurrence before irreversible loss of renal function occurs. Prevention is accomplished by careful evaluation and treatment of patients with structural abnormalities of the urinary tract. Urinary tract infections in children, in males, in women with recurrent relapsing infections, and in patients with abnormal renal function deserve a urologic investigation to exclude potentially correctable obstructive lesions.

Prolonged suppressive antimicrobial therapy may occasionally be useful in patients with recurrent urinary tract infections associated with renal scarring. A 6- to 12-week course of an oral antimicrobial agent such as trimethoprim-sulfamethoxazole, trimethoprim alone, a fluoroquinolone, or urinary acidification with methenamine mandelate (Mandelamine) is often effective.

Complete sterilization of the urine in patients with multiple genitourinary tract abnormalities is often impossible. It is recommended that patients be treated during acute symptomatic infections with a 10- to 14-day course of antimicrobial agents in an attempt to alleviate symptoms and prevent systemic infection. Continuous antimicrobial suppression is ill advised in such patients because this treatment creates selection pressures favoring the development of an antibiotic-resistant bacterial population.

# GENITOURINARY TRAUMA

method of
SAMUEL R. WATKINS, JR., M.D., and
MICHAEL O. KOCH, M.D.
*Vanderbilt University Medical Center*
*Nashville, Tennessee*

Injuries to the genitourinary tract account for about 10% of traumatic injuries seen in emergency departments. Early diagnosis is essential to prevent complications. Initial assessment is directed toward control of life-threatening injuries. After this has been accomplished, a thorough and systematic approach to the evaluation of genitourinary injuries should be undertaken. A thorough history of the mechanism of injury and the physical examination can provide much insight into the patient's clinical situation as it pertains to the genitourinary system. For example, pelvic fractures due to blunt pelvic trauma are often associated with bladder and urethral injuries, whereas rapid deceleration may be associated with renal injuries. Generally, the roentgenologic evaluation proceeds in a caudad to cephalad direction (i.e., urethrogram, cystogram, intravenous pyelogram, and computed tomographic [CT] scan). The history and physical examination may suggest which of these are not required.

## RENAL INJURIES

The kidney is the most commonly injured organ in the genitourinary system. The kidneys are well protected owing to their location high in the retroperitoneal space, which is protected and guarded by the overlying ribs and thick muscle. They are surrounded by perirenal fat, Gerota's fascia, and the renal capsule, which resists rupture. These structures tend to limit renal hemorrhage via a tamponade effect. The kidneys are protected posteriorly by the psoas and quadratus lumborum muscles and anteriorly by the abdominal viscera. Another major factor offering some protection is the mobility of the kidney. The kidney can move one to three vertebral levels while remaining fixed to the renal vein, the renal artery, and the ureter.

Renal injuries are most commonly classified according to the mechanism of injury: blunt or penetrating. Blunt trauma accounts for 80 to 90% of renal injuries, whereas penetrating trauma accounts for the remaining 10 to 20%. Blunt renal injuries may be due to deceleration mechanisms or to a crush effect, the most common cause being motor vehicle accidents. Other causes of blunt renal trauma include sports injuries, falls, and assaults. Gunshot and stab wounds are the principal causes of penetrating renal trauma.

Hematuria is the major indication of renal injury. However, up to a third of patients with renal injury from blunt trauma may not have hematuria, and unfortunately there is only a poor correlation between the amount of hematuria and the degree of renal injury. Thus, in patients with a history compatible with renal injury or signs and symptoms suggestive of a renal injury, investigation is warranted. The signs and symptoms suggestive of renal injury include flank pain or ecchymosis, gross or microscopic hematuria, hypotension, fracture of the lower ribs, or flank mass.

Following initial assessment, examination, and resuscitation, patients with suspected renal injuries should be evaluated radiographically. The principal radiographic study utilized in staging a suspected renal injury is the intravenous urogram with nephrotomograms. The majority of patients can be assessed accurately with the intravenous urogram without the need for more sophisticated and expensive studies. There are four major classifications or stages of renal injuries: (1) renal contusions, which involve ecchymosis or subcapsular hematomas associated with an intact renal capsule and collecting system; (2) minor renal cortical lacerations of the kidney, which do not involve the medulla or collecting system; (3) major renal lacerations, which extend into the medulla or collecting system or the fractured kidney with multiple devitalized areas of renal parenchyma; and (4) renal pedicle injuries, involving lacerations, avulsions, or thrombosis of the renal artery or vein.

In renal contusions, intravenous urography demonstrates delayed function with compression of the collecting system from renal parenchymal swelling. The renal outline is smooth and intact, and there is no extravasation of contrast. Subcapsular hematomas generally appear as a flattened portion of the renal cortex because the renal cortex is compressed by the hematoma under the renal capsule. Similar findings are noted with minor renal lacerations, with the additional finding of a disruption of the renal cortical outline, usually best seen on tomography. Major renal lacerations are usually readily apparent on intravenous urography and manifest severe disruption of the renal cortical outline, extravasation of contrast, and poor function. Renal pedicle injuries result in complete nonvisualization of the kidney on intravenous urography. When the results of the intravenous urogram are abnormal or nondiagnostic, further evaluation is warranted. The most common and widely applicable test is contrast-enhanced CT. This has generally supplanted arteriography in the evaluation of renal trauma, except if there is complete nonvisualization of the kidney on urography. Patients in this setting would be likely to have a renal pedicle injury, which would be delineated most precisely with an arteriogram. The advantages of CT include its noninvasiveness, its ability to identify associated injuries in other organs, and its ability to accurately assess the extent of renal injury.

### Management

Minor renal injuries from blunt trauma account for 85% of cases and would include renal contusions, subcapsular hematomas, and minor renal lacerations. Hematuria and perirenal bleeding generally stop with bed rest and hydration. Patients with gross hematuria are admitted to the hospital for bed rest and observation, serial blood counts, and serial determinations of vital signs. These patients usually have no long-term sequelae from their renal injury. Patients with more severe renal injuries may require surgical exploration. Indications for operation include persistent retroperitoneal bleeding, extensive urinary extravasation, evidence of nonviable renal parenchyma, and renal pedicle injuries. These patients are usually unstable, require multiple transfusions, or have an expanding flank mass. When surgery is performed, renal trauma should be explored through a midline incision. This allows examination and assessment of other intraperitoneal injuries and early control of the renal vasculature. This is accomplished through an incision in the retroperitoneum over the aorta, just medial to the inferior mesenteric vein. This allows quick and accurate control of the renal vessels. Following vascular control, the colon is reflected medially and the hematoma surrounding the kidney is opened. After débridement of devitalized renal parenchyma, an assessment is made of the repairability of the injury. If possible, the kidney is repaired and the area is drained appropriately. Management of traumatic renal artery occlusions is controversial. Renal ischemia time before complete loss of renal function is only 60 minutes, thus, even with aggressive surgical management, renal salvage is unusual. Absolute indications for repair of renal pedicle injuries include bilateral renal artery lesions, injuries in solitary kidneys, and partial injuries. Renal pedicle avulsions generally present with expanding hematomas and require emergency nephrectomy.

Eighty per cent of penetrating renal injuries have associated intra-abdominal injuries. Penetrating renal injuries should generally be surgically explored. The degree of damage from injuries due to gunshot wounds is dependent on the mass and velocity of the bullet. High-velocity bullet wounds are associated with more significant soft tissue destruction owing to the blast effect. This requires more extensive débridement intraoperatively. Stab wounds to the kidneys generally have their entrance points in the lower thorax, the flank area, or the upper abdomen. Stab wounds to the flank can be managed non-operatively if the patient is stable and CT has demonstrated only minor renal injury. Hemorrhagic shock may or may not be present, depending on the location and severity of the injury. Stab wounds to the anterior abdomen have a high incidence of associated intra-abdominal injuries, whereas the incidence of associated injuries with flank or posterior stab wounds is much less.

The long-term complications of renal trauma from any cause include arteriovenous fistula, hy-dronephrosis, hypertension, and renal atrophy. Arteriovenous fistulas are seen mainly with penetrating renal injuries. Hydronephrosis and hypertension are caused by scarring and fibrosis around the kidney. The hypertension in this setting is mediated by renin that results from renal ischemia. To detect these late complications, intravenous urography should be performed 3 to 6 months following the renal injury.

## URETERAL INJURIES

The ureter is extremely well protected and is thus not commonly injured. Ureteral injury may thus be classified according to the type of injury sustained. These include avulsions, lacerations, crush injuries, ligations, devascularizations, and burns. A high index of suspicion must be maintained, as ureteral injuries can be easily overlooked. This can occur with external trauma as well as iatrogenic injuries. If unrecognized, urinary extravasation and possible fistula formation or functional loss of the kidney can occur. Ureteral trauma is most commonly surgical in origin, related to gynecologic, general, or urologic surgery. Blunt trauma is a rare cause of ureteral injury, but disruption of the ureter from the renal pelvis can be seen following hyperextension injuries. This is most common in children, as they have more pliable spinal columns. With penetrating injuries, the most common site of ureteral involvement is the midureter. Penetrating injuries are also frequently associated with other internal injuries that require treatment. Diagnosis of a ureteral injury is made by excretory urography if possible. Findings vary and include hydronephrosis, extravasation, and nonvisualization of the ureter. If the ureter is not visualized and the clinical situation warrants, a retrograde ureterogram is indicated.

### Management

Treatment of ureteral injuries is dependent on the site, the severity, and the cause of the injury. Partial lacerations of the ureter are best treated with placement of an internal ureteral stent and suture repair of the laceration. If the laceration is complete, the site of the injury becomes critical. Those injuries in the distal third of the ureter are managed with débridement and ureteroneocystostomy. Those injuries in the more proximal portions of the ureter are managed with ureteroureterostomy. Ureteral injuries in seriously ill patients may be treated on a temporary basis with percutaneous drainage of the kidney until the patient is stabilized.

## BLADDER INJURIES

Blunt trauma is the most common cause of injury to the bladder. This is most often due to motor vehicle accidents but can result from falls, crush injuries to the pelvis, and blows to the abdomen. Penetrating trauma is less frequently associated with bladder injury. In the setting of blunt trauma, pelvic fracture accompanies bladder rupture in 80% of cases. Moreover, about 15% of all pelvic fractures are associated with bladder or urethral injuries.

When the bladder is full, a direct blow to the lower abdomen may result in rupture of the bladder. This generally occurs at the dome of the bladder, leading to intraperitoneal extravasation of urine. If the diagnosis is delayed or the urine is infected, the presentation may be that of peritonitis, azotemia, and acidosis. The majority of bladder ruptures due to pelvic fractures are extraperitoneal. Some of these ruptures are felt to be secondary to laceration of the bladder wall by bone fragments. Bladder injury should thus be suspected in patients with pelvic fracture, lower abdominal trauma, hematuria, or an inability to void.

Abdominal plain films may reveal a pelvic fracture, and intravenous urography usually establishes whether renal or ureteral injuries are present. A normal bladder contour on intravenous urography does *not* exclude a bladder rupture. Twenty per cent of bladder ruptures are missed on intravenous urography. Cystography is the procedure of choice to evaluate for a bladder injury. The bladder is filled with 300 ml of contrast material, and a plain film of the abdomen is obtained. A second film is obtained after the bladder is drained of the contrast. With intraperitoneal rupture of the bladder, free contrast material is seen within the abdominal cavity, highlighting bowel loops. In extraperitoneal rupture, areas of contrast localization outside the bladder are seen usually in a feathery appearance, as contrast extends through the pelvic connective tissues. This is often seen only on the postdrainage film and is thus the rationale for the routine use of both the filling and postdrainage films in cystography in the trauma setting.

### Management

Penetrating injuries must be surgically explored to repair the bladder injury and to assess for associated intraperitoneal injuries. Patients with intraperitoneal bladder ruptures are treated with a transperitoneal approach consisting of closure of the bladder rupture in multiple layers. A large suprapubic tube is used for bladder drainage and the area is drained. Patients with iso-

lated extraperitoneal bladder rupture can be treated surgically or nonoperatively with catheter drainage for 10 days. The nonoperative approach is dependent on prompt diagnosis, the absence of associated injuries that require exploration, and sterile urine.

## URETHRAL INJURIES IN MALES

Urethral injuries are generally divided into those that involve the anterior urethra and those that involve the posterior urethra. The anterior urethra consists of the bulbous and pendulous portions of the urethra, whereas the posterior urethra consists of the prostatic and membranous portions.

### Anterior Urethral Injuries

The anterior urethra is that portion of the urethra that is distal to the urogenital diaphragm. The most common cause of an anterior urethral injury is a fall with a straddle-type perineal injury, such as falling from a height, straddling a fence, or falling onto a crossbar or a ladder. Bleeding from the urethra, difficulty in voiding, and pain and swelling of the perineum or penis are usually seen. The perineum is tender, and a mass (hematoma) may be found.

Localization of the site of injury is done with a retrograde urethrogram. Catheterization prior to the urethrogram should be avoided to prevent conversion of a partial disruption to complete disruption. If there is no extravasation, the diagnosis of urethral contusion can be made. This may be treated with catheterization or observation if the patient is able to void and the urine is clear. A partial rupture can be treated with a urethral catheter for 1 to 2 weeks or can be treated with a suprapubic cystostomy tube for urinary drainage until the injury heals. Complete rupture of the anterior urethra is best managed by exploration, débridement, and sutured repair of the disruption.

### Posterior Urethral Injuries

Injuries to the posterior urethra most often result from blunt trauma and pelvic fractures. Ninety per cent of posterior urethral disruptions are associated with pelvic fractures; 10% of pelvic fractures are associated with urethral injuries. The urethra is torn off just proximal to or at the urogenital diaphragm, and the prostate is displaced superiorly by the pelvic hematoma. Patients generally have blood at the urethral meatus and urinary retention. Findings of a pelvic fracture with inability to void or blood at the urethral meatus mandate radiographic evaluation of the urethra. Catheterization of the urethra in this setting is contraindicated. A retrograde urethrogram should be performed. With a complete tear, extravasation is noted into the perivesicular space or the perineum. Incomplete tears of the prostatomembranous urethra reveal some extravasation of contrast, but continuity of the urethra into the bladder. This distinction may be difficult to make if a cystogram or an intravenous urogram has been previously performed. If there is no extravasation of contrast and the urethra is intact, a catheter should be inserted followed by cystography. Frequently, a catheter may have previously been placed prior to the patient's presentation. If the catheter is not draining well and/or the suspicion of a urethral injury is high, a retrograde urethrogram should be performed around the indwelling catheter.

**Management.** The treatment of complete posterior urethral injuries is controversial. Some authors prefer placement of a suprapubic tube followed by delayed urethral reconstruction in 3 to 6 months. The support for this treatment regimen is based on a possibility of decreased incidence of impotence, less likelihood of infection of the pelvic hematoma, and the relative ease of placement of a suprapubic tube in a patient who often has sustained other significant injuries and is critically ill.

A second method of treatment involves manipulation of the urethra and bladder into continuity with realignment of the urethra. A catheter is placed through the urethra and into the bladder to maintain this realignment and a suprapubic tube is placed as well. This treatment is dependent on the patient's being stable with no immediate life-threatening injuries. Either form of treatment results in impotence rates of approximately 25% and incontinence rates of 2%. Long-term strictures and voiding dysfunction may be problems.

### GENITALIA INJURIES IN MALES

Serious injuries of the penis are unusual owing to its relative mobility. Injuries of the penis include fracture of the corporal bodies, traumatic amputation, avulsion of the penile skin, strangulation injuries, and penetrating trauma. Diagnosis of these injuries is usually apparent from the history and physical examination. Fracture of the penis refers to rupture of the tunica albuginea surrounding the corpora cavernosa. This most often occurs during sexual intercourse and should be treated with surgical exploration and repair of the rupture. Penetrating trauma, most often from gunshot wounds, should be treated

with surgical exploration and débridement and closure of any defects. Urethral injuries must be ruled out with urethrography. Penile amputation is a rare injury that is often self-induced. Repair with microsurgical techniques is sometimes possible. Minor injuries such as contusions are treated conservatively. Avulsion of the penile skin is most often from injuries involving farm or industrial machinery. Skin distal to the injury should be removed to within 2 to 3 mm of the coronal sulcus and skin grafting to the penile shaft performed. Failure to remove the skin distal to the avulsion results in lymphedema of the distal portion of the penis.

Injuries to the scrotum and testes can be caused by blunt trauma, penetrating trauma, or avulsion-type injuries. Avulsion of the scrotal skin, like that found in penile avulsion, is most often due to accidents involving farm or industrial machinery. Immediate treatment includes broad-spectrum antibiotics and tetanus prophylaxis, followed by immediate surgical débridement and repair. This is best accomplished by coverage with remaining scrotal skin if possible. If the avulsion injury is complete, the testicles should be placed in subcutaneous thigh pouches with plans for later reconstruction of the scrotum utilizing a skin graft or thigh flap.

Trauma to the testicle generally results from blunt injury. Patients present with large scrotal hematomas, pain, nausea, and vomiting. The hematoma around the testicle may make delineation of the testicle difficult. Ultrasonography of the testicle usually determines if tunica of the testicle is intact. If there is rupture of the testicle, treatment is open surgical repair consisting of débridement, closure of the defect in the tunica albuginea, and drainage. With an aggressive surgical approach, the risk of testicular loss is reduced to less than 5% and morbidity is dramatically reduced.

# BENIGN PROSTATIC HYPERTROPHY

method of
JERRY G. BLAIVAS, M.D.
*Columbia-Presbyterian Medical Center*
*New York, New York*

Benign prostatic hypertrophy (BPH) is probably the most ubiquitous affliction of old age. Approximately 50% of men develop BPH by the age of 60 and by age 80 the incidence is almost 80%. The symptoms are either obstructive or irritative in nature. Obstructive symptoms include difficulty initiating the urinary stream (hesitancy), a weak or intermittent stream, a feeling of incomplete bladder emptying, postvoid dribbling of urine, and, finally, acute urinary retention. Irritative symptoms include urinary frequency, urgency, urge incontinence, and nocturia.

Historically, all of the symptoms of prostatism have been attributed to simple mechanical obstruction of the prostatic urethra by the hyperplastic prostate gland. However, the pathophysiology and differential diagnosis actually involve additional factors that may coexist with BPH or may be the sole cause of the symptoms (Table 1).

## PATHOPHYSIOLOGY AND DIFFERENTIAL DIAGNOSIS

**Prostatic Obstruction.** The most overt effect of BPH is mechanical obstruction of the prostatic urethra by the hypertrophied prostate gland. Available data suggest that approximately 70% of patients with clinical prostatism fulfill urodynamic criteria for obstruction.

**Involuntary Detrusor Contractions.** Approximately two-thirds of patients with prostatism have involuntary contractions of the bladder, which cause urinary frequency, urgency, and urge incontinence. Involuntary detrusor contractions may also cause obstructive symptoms by the following mechanism: The bladder contracts involuntarily, and this is perceived by the patient as an urge to void. He rushes to the bathroom, but by the time he gets there the contraction has abated and when he tries to void he has difficulty starting because of the small volume in his bladder. The patient complains of hesitancy and weak stream, which are misinterpreted by the physician as being due to prostatic obstruction.

The etiology of involuntary detrusor contractions is either neurologic (detrusor hyper-reflexia), idiopathic, or associated with obstruction. The proper term for the latter two conditions is "detrusor instability."

**Impaired Detrusor Contractility.** Recent data suggest that as many as 15 to 25% of patients with clinical BPH actually have weak or poorly sustained bladder contractions as the proximate cause of their symptoms. Impaired detrusor contractility results in a weak stream and a feeling of incomplete bladder emptying.

Paradoxically, many of these patients also complain of urinary frequency and urgency.

**Sensory Abnormalities of the Bladder.** In some patients with prostatism, the symptoms are due to sensory abnormalities of the bladder wall. Sensory abnormalities include hypersensitivity and hyposensitivity. Hypersensitivity (sensory urgency) causes urinary frequency, urgency, and bladder and urethral pain. Hyposensitivity can lead to overdistention and urinary retention.

**Adrenergic Activity.** The sympathetic nervous system plays an important role in the pathogenesis of symptoms in patients with clinical prostatism. Alpha-adrenergic overactivity contributes to vesical neck and prostatic urethral obstruction, and alpha-adrenergic hypoactivity may result in urinary incontinence.

## DIAGNOSIS

Because BPH is so common in older men, it follows that most men with clinical prostatism do in fact have prostatic obstruction and in most the diagnosis seems quite straightforward. The work-up begins with a thorough history and physical examination. Particular note should be made of neurologic conditions such as stroke, multiple sclerosis, and Parkinson's disease, because in patients with these conditions the symptoms of prostatism are often due to the underlying neurologic condition and are not improved by prostatectomy. A list of medications that might affect micturition is seen in Table 2. The size, configuration, and consistency of the prostate should be assessed by rectal examination. Palpable nodules or areas of "hardness" should be considered to be prostate cancer until proved otherwise by biopsy. Abnormalities of perianal sensation, anal sphincter tone and control, and the bulbocavernosus reflex suggest lower motor neuron neurologic lesions.

Although it has been suggested that the diagnosis of prostatic obstruction can be confirmed by measurement of urine flow rate, this is actually not the case because the flow curve that results from a weak bladder contraction is indistinguishable from that of prostatic obstruction. The only technique for distinguishing

TABLE 1. **Benign Prostatic Hypertrophy (BPH)**

| Symptom | Pathophysiology | Etiology |
|---|---|---|
| Frequency<br>Urgency<br>Urge incontinence | Sensory urgency | BPH<br>Urinary tract infection<br>Bladder stone<br>Carcinoma of bladder<br>Carcinoma of prostate<br>Interstitial cystitis |
| | Involuntary detrusor contractions | Idiopathic: detrusor instability<br>BPH<br>Neurogenic: detrusor hyper-reflexia (stroke, multiple sclerosis, Parkinson's disease) |
| Hesitancy<br>Weak stream retention<br>Postvoid dribble | Urethral obstruction | BPH<br>Carcinoma of prostate<br>Vesical neck obstruction<br>Urethral stricture |
| | Weak bladder contraction | Neurogenic (diabetes, lower motor neuron lesions)<br>BPH, myogenic |
| | Involuntary detrusor contractions | |

TABLE 2. **Medications That Affect Micturition**

Anticholinergics
    Propantheline (Pro-Banthine)
    Oxybutynin (Ditropan)
    Flavoxate (Urispas)
    Hyoscyamine (Cysto-Spaz)
Cholinergic agonists
    Bethanechol (Urecholine)
Adrenergic agonists
    Ephedrine
Adrenergic blockers
    Phenoxybenzamine (Dibenzyline)
    Prazosin (Minipress)
    Clonidine (Catapres)
    Terazocin (Hytrin)
Tricyclic antidepressants
    Imipramine (Tofranil)

these two entities is measuring detrusor pressure and urine flow simultaneously (by multichannel and video urodynamic studies). A diminished urine flow in the presence of a detrusor contraction of adequate duration and magnitude confirms the diagnosis of urethral obstruction.

At the present time, the role of urodynamic studies in evaluating patients with prostatism has not been well defined. However, in equivocal conditions, sophisticated pressure and flow and video urodynamic studies are necessary to confirm the proper diagnosis. Specific indications for the routine application of sophisticated urodynamic studies include (1) prostatism in men younger than one would expect for BPH; (2) men with equivocal urine flow criteria for obstruction; (3) men who remain symptomatic after seemingly appropriate treatment; (4) men with neurologic disorders, particularly stroke, Parkinson's disease, multiple sclerosis, and spinal cord injury; and (5) men with excessive bladder capacity (greater than 800 ml).

The role of intravenous pyelography (IVP) in patients with prostatism is also controversial unless there are specific indications, such as microscopic hematuria or abnormal urinary cytologic findings. In patients with symptomatic BPH who have elected to undergo surgical treatment, IVP is unnecessary. However, in those who do not elect surgery, IVP is an important diagnostic modality. The argument against routine IVP is that it is so often normal. However, a normal IVP in a patient with symptomatic prostatism reconfirms the elective nature of treatment and ensures that it is safe to defer prostatectomy indefinitely. An IVP that shows significant hydronephrosis with "hockey sticking" of the ureters may provide sufficient evidence that prostatectomy is indicated for medical reasons.

It is generally agreed that cystourethroscopy is necessary prior to prostatectomy, but whether it is performed separately as part of the routine evaluation or whether it is performed at the same time as the surgery remains the option of the surgeon. I believe that the diagnosis of BPH is a clinical one based on symptoms, the age of the patient, and the size and consistency of the prostate gland and that the diagnosis of prostatic obstruction is a urodynamic one based on the relationship between destrusor pressure and urine flow. Cystoscopy aids in neither diagnosis, but provides impor-

tant information about (1) the feasibility of performing transurethral versus open prostatic surgery, (2) unsuspected urethral stricture, (3) unsuspected bladder tumor, (4) bladder stones, and (5) bladder diverticuli. Accordingly, separate diagnostic cystoscopy is only necessary when, in the opinion of the urologist, it is important to know about these entities prior to prostatectomy or when there is a specific indication such as hematuria or abnormal urinary cytologic findings. Finally, because cystoscopy may precipitate urinary retention or infection, it should not be undertaken unless one is prepared to deal with the consequences of these complications.

## TREATMENT

In the vast majority of patients, treatment of symptoms of BPH is entirely elective. There is no convincing evidence that delaying prostatectomy in patients with prostatic obstruction has any significant deleterious effect on the patient's health unless there are signs of obstruction to the kidneys. Nevertheless, when complications arise from prostatic obstruction, treatment is more strongly indicated. These include elevated blood urea nitrogen and creatinine levels, hydronephrosis, acute urinary retention, recurrent urinary tract infection, and bladder stones.

Although prostatectomy remains the mainstay of treatment, there has recently been a surge of interest in less invasive forms of therapy, such as drugs, prosthetics, behavior modification, and balloon dilation of the prostatic urethra.

### Surgery

The main goal of surgical treatment is to relieve bladder outlet obstruction; none of the operations for benign disease removes the entire prostate. There are two generic surgical techniques commonly in use for BPH: open surgery and transurethral surgery.

Transurethral surgery is performed with a specialized cystoscope (resectoscope). In transurethral resection of the prostate (TURP), the resectoscope is introduced through the urethra and the prostate gland is cut into small pieces with an electrocautery loop. The prostatic chips are periodically removed from the bladder by irrigation. Bleeding is controlled by cautery. In prostatotomy or transurethral incision of the prostate, single or multiple incisions are made through the substance of the prostate. The main advantage of prostatotomy is that it can be performed in about 20 minutes, thus greatly reducing operative morbidity. In selected patients it can even be performed with local anesthesia.

Ideally, transurethral surgery should be performed under regional anesthesia (spinal or epidural) because of the lower morbidity and particularly because of the potential for early diagnosis and treatment of the TURP syndrome (see later). Postoperatively, a Foley's catheter is left in place for 2 or 3 days. Because of the lower morbidity of transurethral surgery, more than 90% of the operations for BPH are performed by this technique.

Open surgery is performed through a lower abdominal incision. The retropubic space is entered, and the prostate is approached either directly through an incision in the prostatic capsule (retropubic prostatectomy) or by an incision in the bladder (suprapubic prostatectomy). The prostate gland is enucleated and hemostasis secured with absorbable sutures. Either transurethral or suprapubic catheters are left in place for 5 to 7 days.

### Complications of Surgery

MORTALITY. The surgical mortality after prostatectomy is in the range of 1 to 2%. It is slightly higher after open procedures and higher still in those with severe cardiopulmonary disease or bleeding disorders and in those older than the age of 85 years.

HEMORRHAGE. Some degree of blood loss occurs in all surgical procedures on the prostate, and in some instances hemorrhage can be life-threatening. The magnitude of the blood loss depends on a number of factors, including the duration of the operation (usually, the longer the operation, the greater the blood loss), the skill of the surgeon, the size of the prostate, and the presence of preexisting risk factors, such as preoperative use of anticoagulants.

Delayed bleeding occurs in 5 to 10% of patients 1 to 2 weeks postoperatively. In most instances, the bleeding is self-limited and characterized only by the passage of gross hematuria. Sometimes, the patient passes clots or develops clot retention requiring catheter drainage and irrigation of the clots. Delayed bleeding is often precipitated by heavy physical exercise or straining at stool. For this reason, it is advised that the patient refrain from excessive physical activity for at least 1 month postoperatively and that he take stool softeners and cathartics to prevent straining during defecation.

TRANSURETHRAL PROSTATECTOMY SYNDROME. The TURP syndrome is a unique complication of transurethral prostatectomy. This potentially life-threatening condition is due to intraoperative absorption of large volumes of irrigating fluid by the venous sinuses of the prostate. Because the irrigating fluid is hypotonic, both hypervolemia and hyponatremia ensue. Early findings include restlessness, irritability, and a rise in central venous pressure, which progresses to nausea, vomiting, bradycardia, hypertension, mental con-

fusion, congestive heart failure, seizures, and coma. The most effective treatment is immediate recognition of the condition during surgery, the prompt administration of diuretics, and termination of the procedure as soon as possible. Although the TURP syndrome is more common when resection time is long (very large prostate gland or excessive bleeding), it may be encountered for no apparent reason.

ACUTE URINARY RETENTION. Occasionally, patients are unable to void after removal of the catheter. This may be due to either urethral obstruction or impaired detrusor contractility. Most commonly, obstruction is due to retained prostatic chips or blood clots, but occasionally is caused by residual prostatic obstruction. Immediate management consists of reinsertion of a urethral catheter to check the residual urine volume and to exclude clot retention. If the patient fails a second voiding trial, an indwelling catheter is left for 2 to 4 weeks. If subsequent voiding trials are unsuccessful, cystoscopy and pressure and flow urodynamic studies are necessary for diagnosis. Persistent prostatic obstruction may necessitate repetition of transurethral resection.

Urinary retention due to impaired detrusor contractility is usually refractory to prostatectomy, unless there is concomitant obstruction (which is usually not the case). Ideally, these patients should be diagnosed accurately and surgery avoided. The only effective treatment is intermittent self-catheterization.

URINARY TRACT INFECTION. In patients who have not undergone previous instrumentation, symptomatic urinary tract infection after prostatectomy is uncommon, and urosepsis is rare, although bacteriuria is seen in the majority of patients.

URINARY INCONTINENCE. Persistent urinary incontinence is uncommon after prostatectomy, but many patients have transient frequency, urgency, and urge incontinence or sphincteric incontinence for several days or weeks after surgery. Persistent incontinence is due to either involuntary detrusor contractions or damage to the sphincter mechanism.

URETHRAL STRICTURE AND VESICAL NECK CONTRACTURE. Strictures may occur at any location in the urethra after prostatectomy, but are most common at the vesical neck, the bulbomembranous urethra, or the urethral meatus. These complications are seen in about 10% of patients. In many instances, they are asymptomatic, but, when therapy is indicated, optical urethrotomy is the treatment of choice. Extreme caution must be exercised when the stricture is at the bulbomembranous junction, lest urinary incontinence ensue.

SEXUAL DYSFUNCTION. The majority of patients develop retrograde ejaculation after prostatectomy, but erections and orgasm remain unchanged. Retrograde ejaculation causes no medical damage; the seminal contents are simply mixed with urine in the bladder. Obviously, infertility is the rule, although sperm for artificial insemination may be recovered from centrifuged urine.

### Nonsurgical Treatment

**Pharmacologic Treatment.** Pharmacologic treatment has received widespread attention in the lay press, but there have been few well-controlled studies to document their efficacy. Treatment has generally been in the form of alpha-adrenergic blockers such as phenoxybenzamine (Dibenzyline) or prazosin (Minipress). Because of reports of carcinogenesis in mice, phenoxybenzamine is not recommended for long-term use. Prazosin has been used in dosages ranging from 1 to 3 mg three times a day.

**Behavior Modification.** Behavior modification using micturition diaries and gradual prolongation of the intervoiding interval may be effective in treating the irritative symptoms of BPH, but has no role to play in treating outlet obstruction.

**Balloon Dilation of the Prostatic Urethra.** This has also received widespread publicity in the lay press, but its overall efficacy remains to be determined.

**Prosthetics.** Several prosthetic devices have been developed that are inserted transurethrally into the prostatic urethra for the purpose of relieving prostatic obstruction. At the present time, these are also experimental forms of treatment.

# PROSTATITIS

method of
RODNEY U. ANDERSON, M.D.
*Stanford University School of Medicine*
*Stanford, California*

The medical diagnosis of prostatitis includes a constellation of clinical findings, few of which demonstrate an offending pathogenic microorganism and many of which show little evidence of gland inflammation. The clinician is confronted with unsophisticated diagnostic tools and questionable therapeutic efficacy, leaving him or her to offer only symptomatic treatment and supportive consolation.

In spite of this pessimistic assessment of a common disorder in the male, there are specific diagnostic and management decisions that need to be made. The fundamental questions include: Are bacteria involved? Is there significant inflammation occurring within the prostate tissue? If the answer is no to both of these questions, one is dealing with a syndrome that has been variously labeled prostatosis, prostatodynia, pelvic myalgia, or pelviperineal pain. The multiple descriptions affirm our lack of knowledge concerning etiology, much less treatment.

Histologic findings of prostatitis, then, may be classified as bacterial or nonbacterial and should be accurately diagnosed to facilitate appropriate management and counseling of the patient.

## BACTERIAL PROSTATITIS

### Acute Bacterial Prostatitis

This unusual problem may occur in both younger and older men and is typically characterized by fever, chills, perineal and suprapubic discomfort, dysuria, and inhibited urinary voiding. The urine examination reveals pus cells and bacterial rods. Digital examination of the prostate is painful, and the gland is swollen and boggy in texture; it may occasionally harbor an abscess. The gland should never be massaged in this condition, however, for fear of disseminating bacteria into the blood stream and inciting fulminant gram-negative sepsis. If there is enough swelling to inhibit urine flow to any significant degree, particularly in the elderly male, I advocate placing a temporary small-bore suprapubic catheter for drainage after injection of a first dose of an empiric broad-spectrum parenteral antibiotic such as ampicillin plus aminoglycoside. I usually hospitalize these patients pending outcome of peripheral white blood cell count, blood cultures, identification of the pathogen to switch to oral antibiotics, and clinical response to treatment.

It is important to treat acute prostatitis aggressively and for enough days to ensure elimination of the bacteria from the gland. Drugs that may be taken orally and reach adequate bactericidal concentrations in the prostatic tissue include trimethoprim-sulfamethoxazole (Septra, Bactrim), carbenicillin indanyl sodium (Geocillin), norfloxacin (Noroxin), and ciprofloxacin (Cipro). No one knows the precise period of time one should continue oral antibiotic agents following acute prostatitis, but most clinicians agree that 4 weeks is adequate. After completing treatment, and when the patient is asymptomatic, it is good practice to confirm that no chronic bacterial colonization of the prostate has occurred by performing a lower urinary tract localization study (see later).

### Chronic Bacterial Prostatitis

The hallmark of this diagnosis is recurrent urinary tract infection, usually with the same organism. These men are typically asymptomatic and the urine clear between episodes; the acute relapses are less impressive than the classic acute prostatitis. In older men, the bacteriuria may even be asymptomatic. A recent report from Paris suggests that approximately 8 to 10% of human immunodeficiency virus–infected men have bacterial prostatitis; many of these cases also have an associated prostatic abscess diagnosed by ultrasound.

One approach to prove colonization of the prostate by pathogenic bacteria consists of utilizing nitrofurantoin (Macrodantin) as a urinary tract–sterilizing antimicrobial agent and then performing segmented urine cultures with prostate massage. Collecting and culturing urine and expressed prostatic secretion (EPS) requires diligence on the part of the treating physician and attention to detail by the clinical laboratory. The first specimen obtained is the urethral washout using the patient's first 5 to 10 ml of voided urine. The foreskin should be retracted to prevent skin flora contamination. The second specimen is midstream urine (30 to 50 ml), and I tell the patient to always retain a little urine in reserve for a final urethral washout specimen following prostate massage. The third specimen is the prostatic fluid obtained by patiently massaging from lateral to midline in each lobe of the gland and expressing a drop or two of fluid down the urethra with compression of the bulbar urethra. I use a sterile test tube to collect these precious drops of fluid. The patient then collects a fourth specimen as a final urethral washout of 5 to 10 ml. Each of these specimens is cultured and colony counts of identified bacteria obtained. The laboratory personnel must be willing and able to report absolute colony counts, even when less than 1000 colony-forming units per ml. I advocate streaking at least 0.1 ml on the agar plate to accommodate the lower counts. If the culture shows a difference of 10-fold in growth of the same organism between the urethral washout specimen and the postmassage specimen or EPS, the prostate is considered the source of infection. The organism must be identical to the positive urine culture obtained prior to sterilizing the urine.

Cytologic analysis should simultaneously be performed to establish the presence of inflammation within the urethra, the bladder, or the prostate. A drop of sediment stain, such as Sternheimer-Malbin, helps differentiate leukocytes from lecithin granules or spermatids. I prefer to quantify the count in a hemacytometer as white blood cells per mm$^3$ (normal up to 1000 in EPS), but most urologists accept greater than 10 per high-power field as indicative of inflammation. Oval fat bodies (macrophages) in the prostatic fluid also suggest chronic inflammation. More than 15 leukocytes per high-power field in the urethral washout and more than 5 in the midstream urine are considered indicative of inflammation. This analysis of the leukocyte pattern, along with assessment of bacterial identification and colony count, should allow the clinician to determine if chronic bacterial prostatis exists.

Therapeutic management of chronic bacterial prostatitis poses a challenge. Diffusion of drug into the prostatic tissue is limited, and only those agents mentioned earlier qualify for the job. Erythromycin (E-Mycin) and clindamycin (Cleocin) also penetrate well, but are seldom the drugs of choice. If one uses the criteria of cure to include symptom free and bacteria free for a minimum of 6 months following completion of oral therapy, the success rate is often on the order of only 30 to 40%. Recently, ciprofloxacin has been reported to yield cure rates in the range of 75% at 3 months' follow-up. The mean duration of treatment averaged approximately 2 months. Other, more aggressive, treatment regimens include parenteral therapy with aminoglycosides for 7 to 10 days, direct injection of antibiotics into the gland tissue through ultrasound guidance, and extensive removal of prostate tissue through transurethral resection or even total prostatectomy. The transurethral resection may be specifically indicated if there exist multiple calculi within the gland acting as infection stones. When specific therapy fails to eradicate the offending organism, one is left with using chronic prophylaxis of bacteriuria using low-dose oral antibiotics. My preference is 50 mg of nitrofurantoin (Macrodantin) or trimethoprim-sulfamethoxazole (Septra, Bactrim), 80 mg of trimethoprim and 40 mg of sulfamethoxazole, taken each night if the organism is sensitive to these.

## NONBACTERIAL PROSTATITIS

The diagnosis of nonbacterial prostatitis implies objective evidence of prostatic inflammation, but no documentation of a microorganism as inciting agent. The patient has symptoms, but no laboratory evidence of a causative microorganism—a frustrating dilemma. It is true that some virulent pathogens fail to grow on routine culture media. Considerable effort has been given, for example, to document that *Chlamydia trachomatis* is an offending organism in these cases. This is a gram-negative bacterium with only intracellular growth. This organism, as well as *Ureaplasma urealyticum,* may be found as urethral commensals, adding confusion to the localization. Similarly, a large proportion of patients with inflamed prostates and no bacteria have a history of sexually transmitted diseases. Although no prostatic fluid antibodies to either organism can be found in these patients, they do have elevated IgA and IgG levels that may represent some yet unproved inflammatory agent or autoimmune phenomenon to a preceding infection. Prostatic fluid antibodies to either organism have not been documented. In a recent study of 50 consecutive males diagnosed with nonbacterial prostatitis, only one had a positive finding of *Chlamydia* in EPS, and, although 44 out of 50 had inflammation on transperineal biopsy, none had *Chlamydia* cultured from the tissue. Nevertheless, other clinicians have been able to demonstrate 8 to 10% of symptomatic males with *Chlamydia* localized to the prostate and clear the organism and symptoms with 3 to 4 weeks of trimethoprim-sulfa or tetracycline (Sumycin). In any case, it is probably prudent to look for significant colonization of possible pathogens only when the patient has been completely off all antimicrobial agents for at least 30 days. Until further evidence to the contrary, a clinical trial of 2 weeks of tetracycline, doxycycline (Vibramycin), or erythromycin is warranted.

It has been suggested that refluxing urine is an inflammatory agent, causing formation of calculi and perpetuation of the irritated prostate. Outflow obstruction in the form of external sphincter spasm or urethral stricture as well as internal sphincter dyssynergia may play a role. Because of this, I establish a working diagnosis of nonbacterial prostatitis with at least two documented localizations of inflammation without bacteria, and then study patients with complex urodynamic and selected endoscopic examinations. In some patients, a transrectal ultrasound examination of the prostate and seminal vesicles is warranted. There are criteria being developed to describe the ultrasound appearance of chronic prostatitis, and a transrectal biopsy will confirm the inflammatory process in the stromal tissue. I continue to look for dilated seminal vesicles as a cause of discomfort as well.

If the presence of urinary outflow obstruction is established—usually a form of internal sphincter dyssynergia—I initiate a trial of alpha-adrenergic blocking agents. I urge patients to use hot sitz baths (100° F) and occasionally use agents such as diazepam (Valium) or tricyclic antidepressants in the obviously stressed and anxious patient. I urge avoidance of common substances known to irritate the membranes of the genitourinary tract: tobacco, caffeine, chocolate, alcohol, spices, etc. At the same time, I recommend moderation in sexual ejaculation—neither too often nor too seldom.

Adding to the confusion about etiology in this malady is a report that in rats spontaneous nonbacterial prostatitis seems to be genetically predetermined, age related, and influenced by hormones; estrogen worsens the condition and testosterone is helpful. Human studies are needed to clarify any hormonal aspects in man.

## PROSTATODYNIA OR PELVIPERINEAL PAIN SYNDROME

This wastebasket medical diagnosis is an admission of failure in medical science. Patients are lumped into this category when they have pain in or near the prostate and no shred of evidence of either microorganisms or inflammatory condition. The patient describes, usually in excruciating detail, aching, pulling, coldness, itching, orchalgia, subpubic and suprapubic discomfort, rectal discomfort, dysuria, postejaculatory pain, urethral burning, and any combination of the above. These individuals often have high stress and anxiety levels with a propensity to somatic awareness. In my experience, many of these pelviperineal pain conditions occur as a result of lifestyle: long-distance running, long-distance driving or airflight, weight lifting, biking, etc. It is also coincidental how many of these individuals have a history of back injury or complaints of chronic low-back aching. In a few convincing instances I perform magnetic resonance imaging of the lumbosacral nerve roots to seek a cause of their problem. If there is also good evidence of urinary dysfunction, I proceed with urodynamic testing.

One disease process that may be uncovered in pelviperineal pain and associated urge and frequency complaints is interstitial cystitis; although a rare entity in males, it should be kept in mind when dealing with a complaint of painful prostate. Of course, prostate cancer and bladder carcinoma-in-situ, as well as anal and rectal problems, need to be ruled out.

There is a tendency for the physician to judge patients with no abnormal findings as having a psychosomatic disorder. Accordingly, the best treatment may be psychotherapy, but given by a wise and caring physician who has assured himself or herself and the patient that no serious medical illness exists. Otherwise, the patient gives up on the doctor in frustration and begins the process all over again with some other practitioner—often in another city.

# ACUTE RENAL FAILURE
method of
JOHN T. HARRINGTON, M.D.
*Tufts University School of Medicine*
*Newton-Wellesley Hospital*
*Newton, Massachusetts*

Acute renal failure (ARF) is the origin of clinical nephrology. In 1941 Bywaters and Beall reported their experience with patients with ARF from crush injuries after the bombing of London. A few years later in the Netherlands, Kolff used the artificial kidney for the first time on a patient with uremia from malignant hypertension. Kolff made eight artificial kidneys during World War II; after the war, three were dispatched abroad—one to London, one to New York, and one to Montreal. Merrill's group at the Brigham Hospital in Boston built its own machine, using Kolff's blueprints, and, according to Kolff, "probably did more for the further propagation of dialysis than any other group." ARF was the major indication for the early use of the artificial kidney. Chronic hemodialysis did not become feasible until the early 1960s, after the invention of the Quinton-Scribner shunt.

In the 45 years since the end of World War II, an enormous amount has been learned about ARF at the cellular, nephronal, whole-kidney, and whole-body levels. Nevertheless, survival of ARF patients still hovers about 50%, a figure not dissimilar to that seen in the first decade after the end of World War II. Thus, ARF remains a challenging clinical entity. The fact that a patient can survive for a prolonged period with total loss of a vital organ system and then recover virtually complete function highlights the unique aspect of ARF.

Acute renal failure remains a generic term, encompassing a variety of clinical situations. I restrict the use of this term to patients in whom renal function deteriorates over a period of 2 weeks or less. At a macroscopic level, ARF, like Gaul, can be divided into three parts: prerenal azotemia, postrenal azotemia, and intrinsic renal failure. It is important to rule out both prerenal and postrenal azotemia before deciding that intrinsic renal failure is present. The reason for this is obvious: Rapid correction of prerenal azotemia (e.g., dehydration) or relief of postrenal azotemia (e.g., benign prostatic hypertrophy with obstruction) can rapidly return renal function to normal. In both of these circumstances, the kidney is intrinsically normal, at least during the early phases. Historically, ARF was almost always associated with oliguria (<400 ml per day). The last decade has demonstrated that intrinsic renal failure caused by acute tubular necrosis (see later) is associated with urinary output of approximately 1000 ml per day in at least 20 to 30% of cases.

*Prerenal azotemia* is caused by inadequate renal perfusion. Inadequate renal perfusion results either from salt and water depletion (e.g., severe diarrhea or "third space" accumulations from acute pancreatitis) or from volume overload (e.g., congestive heart failure, where renal function deteriorates because of the impaired cardiac output). In either case, prerenal azotemia is manifested by a reduction in urinary output, a benign urinary sediment, excretion of concentrated urine (specific gravity > 1.015 to 1.020), and urinary sodium excretion of less than 5 to 10 mEq per liter (in the absence of diuretic administration).

Given that prerenal azotemia can be caused by either volume depletion or volume overload, determination of the volume status of the ARF patient is essential. This determination requires careful attention to the patient's immediate history, accurate knowledge of fluid intake and ouput, analysis of daily weight (still all too often lacking in hospitalized patients in the United States), and a careful physical examination.

Physical examination of a patient in whom one is attempting to determine the intravascular volume should stress (1) measurement of orthostatic blood pressure and pulse; (2) skin turgor, particularly over the anterior thigh, where the presence of "tenting" is an excellent sign of intravascular volume depletion even in elderly patients; and (3) a careful search for edema, either pretibially or in the sacral region. All too often, I see "dehydrated" patients (a diagnosis erroneously made on the basis of a dry tongue—simply a function of mouth breathing) who have 4 + pitting sacral edema—edema that has been missed by attending physicians and house staff alike. The presence of edema establishes the fact that total body sodium overload exists. Although in unusual circumstances edema can be present with a decrease in effective intravascular volume, statistically it is much more likely to be accompanied by increased intravascular volume. If doubt remains regarding the status of the intravascular volume after the history and physical examination, a recent chest x-ray film may be helpful; findings consistent with congestive heart failure establish the presence of volume excess. Finally, invasive hemodynamic measurements, using either a central venous pressure line or a Swan-Ganz line, can be made. Volume challenges, if used in the patient with prerenal azotemia who is thought to be volume depleted, should consist of 250 ml isotonic saline or lactated Ringer's solution (no difference between these two replacement solutions has ever been shown), given over 15 minutes, with repeated clinical observations or hemodynamic measurements made. In patients with severe third space accumulations (e.g., acute pancreatitis), 10 liters or more may be required in extreme circumstances before intravascular volume, blood pressure, and renal perfusion are restored.

*Postrenal failure,* defined as obstruction to urine flow, is seen most typically in elderly men with prostatic hypertrophy. The presence of total anuria or alternating swings between high and low urinary output strongly suggests the possibility of obstruction and the need for appropriate urologic investigation. Abdominal percussion and palpation, rectal examination, and an estimate of postvoid residual urine (by Foley's catheter or by ultrasonography) should be done in all oliguric patients. A pelvic examination is mandatory in any woman with oliguria or ARF to eliminate the possibility of bilateral ureteral obstruction secondary to widespread pelvic cancer. Detection of obstructive uropathy was once difficult, frequently requiring cystoscopy and retrograde catheterization; the advent of ultrasonography has virtually eliminated their use. Renal ultrasound provides not only evidence regarding the possibility of obstruction, but also information on postvoid residual urine and renal size (see later).

Recalling that the kidney has only four main structures (i.e., glomeruli, blood vessels, renal tubules, and interstitium) is helpful in focusing on the precise cause of *intrinsic renal failure*. Globally, ARF may be caused by acute glomerulonephritis, renovascular disease, acute tubular necrosis (ATN), or acute interstitial nephritis (AIN). In patients with *hospital-acquired ARF,* the vast majority of instances are caused either by prerenal azotemia or by ATN. In patients who *enter* the hospital with ARF, the likelihood of finding entities other than ATN is considerably higher, and more attention must be paid to the differential diagnosis in these patients.

## DIAGNOSIS

My approach to the differential diagnosis of intrinsic renal failure relies heavily on a recent history; a careful physical examination establishing the patient's volume status; measurement of urine specific gravity (or osmolality) and urinary sodium level (the latter only in the patient who is not receiving furosemide, a rare finding in today's hospitalized oliguric patient); and, most importantly, a careful examination of the spun urinary sediment. A plethora of urinary diagnostic indices has been promulgated during the last 2 decades. In my experience, they rarely add anything beyond what can be obtained by the methods just noted. As mentioned earlier, the patient with prerenal azotemia has a benign urinary sediment, concentrated urine, and a low urinary sodium concentration. The patient with postrenal azotemia has a benign urinary sediment and, occasionally, red blood cells (caused by previous urologic investigation or the disease causing the obstruction); urine specific gravity and urinary sodium concentration are not helpful in making the diagnosis of postrenal azotemia.

In the patient with ARF caused by intrinsic renal disease, urinary sediment examination by the experienced clinician-uroscopist is particularly helpful. Classically, one finds proteinuria, hematuria, and red blood cell casts in the patient with acute glomerulonephritis; white blood cells, perhaps eosinophils, and, rarely, white blood cell casts in the patient with AIN; and renal tubular cells, muddy brown pigmented casts, and occasionally renal tubular cell casts in the patient with ATN. In my experience, diagnostic urinary sediment abnormalities are found in more than 95% of patients with acute glomerulonephritis, in a comparable percentage in patients with AIN, and in approximately 75 to 85% of patients with ATN. Jaundiced patients have a urinary sediment typical of that seen in patients with ATN, with the obvious addition of bilirubinuria.

Urine specific gravity is elevated and urinary sodium excretion is decreased in patients with acute glomerulonephritis (of any sort), whereas in ATN, urine specific gravity is usually in the 1.010 to 1.012 range and urinary sodium concentration is more than 30 to 40 mEq per liter. Urine specific gravity and sodium concentration are not helpful in the diagnosis of AIN. The remainder of this discussion focuses on the patient with ATN because that is the likely cause of ARF in hospitalized patients. Renal biopsy may be required in instances where there is little clinical evidence of ATN, in helping to distinguish cortical necrosis from ATN, and in diagnosing suspected acute glomerulonephritis or AIN.

## ACUTE TUBULAR NECROSIS

### Epidemiology, Risk Factors, and Prognosis

Two recent, major reports have defined the epidemiology of hospital-acquired ARF, its risk factors, and its prognosis. ARF, variably defined by a rise in the serum creatinine concentration, occurred in 2 to 5% of hospitalized patients in these studies. In one study, 80% of the episodes of hospital-acquired renal insufficiency were caused by decreased renal perfusion, postoperative renal insufficiency, radiographic contrast media, or aminoglycoside administration. In the second study, volume depletion, aminoglycoside use, congestive heart failure, radiographic contrast media, and septic shock were the major risk factors identified. Poor prognostic factors include the presence of oliguria (nonoliguric patients seem to have both less severe ATN and a lower likelihood of dying), urinary sediment abnormalities, and severe renal insufficiency. The adverse effect of volume depletion was increased in diabetics; the risk of aminoglycoside use increased with increasing age. In one study, an increase in the serum creatinine level of 3 mg per dl or more was associated with a mortality rate of 64%! In most instances, however, patients did not die of renal failure per se but rather of the diseases that precipitated it.

### Prevention

Knowledge of the limited number of risk factors associated with hospital-acquired ARF should provide the clinician with all the ammunition needed to reduce its incidence dramatically. To prevent ARF, attention should be directed at avoiding nephrotoxic aminoglycoside antibiotics, avoiding radiocontrast media, and moderating the use of diuretics to prevent too rapid diuresis, particularly in a diabetic patient. All clinicians have the tools to monitor their own patients efficiently and cheaply. The requirements are simple: (1) *mandatory* daily weight determinations in all patients admitted to medical and surgical units; (2) avoidance of nephrotoxic agents when possible; (3) measurements of peak and trough serum levels of aminoglycosides at appropriate intervals, coupled with measurement of the serum creatinine concentration every other day; and (4) infection surveillance and control programs. In this regard, careful attention must be directed especially at the use of Foley's catheters and indwelling arterial and venous lines.

### Treatment

Treatment of ARF encompasses both conservative (nondialytic) therapy and various dialytic modalities. At present, treatment of established ATN is primarily supportive in that no demonstrated, effective method of hastening recovery from ATN exists. A number of innovative treatment protocols, including the intravenous administration of adenosine triphosphate–magnesium chloride, are being examined experimentally, but information on their use in clinical ARF is scanty. High-dose furosemide (200 to 400 mg intravenously) and mannitol (12.5 to 25 grams intravenously) have been shown to convert early oliguric renal insufficiency into nonoliguric renal failure. No effect on overall mortality rates has been demonstrated, however.

### Conservative Therapy

Conservative therapy of the oliguric patient, based on principles established in the 1950s, is still applicable to ARF patients as we enter the 1990s. The physician must be attuned to abnormalities in all organ systems, not simply to those of the kidneys. Normal volume status must be maintained. Fluid (water) should be administered only to replace urinary output and nonrenal losses, and to provide an additional 400 to 500 ml per day. If the serum sodium level falls below 130 mEq per liter, more rigid water restriction must be used; the input may need to be reduced to as little as 400 ml per day. Sodium should be given to the oliguric patient only to the extent that it is lost by nonrenal routes or to replace third space losses. The oliguric patient should have a sodium chloride intake of 2 grams per day or less orally and no sodium chloride in intravenous fluids. The administration of 0.5 N sodium chloride to the edematous, oliguric patient, inexplicably still a common practice in U.S. hospitals, results only in further edema and more profound hyponatremia. Potassium administration should be forbidden in the oliguric patient unless hypokalemia and potassium depletion from a nonrenal route are present. The daily diet should consist of an adequate protein intake (40 to 60 grams) and large amounts of carbohydrates (at least 100 grams). In fact, the introduction of a low-sodium, low-potassium diet that contained adequate protein, coupled with 100 grams of glucose, resulted in a decline in the mortality of ARF from approximately 90% in the 1940s to its current level of approximately 50% even by the early 1950s. Although these conservative maneuvers are in a sense old-fashioned, they remain the bedrock of modern treatment of the patient with ARF.

### Dietary Treatment

Dietary treatment has been a major area of investigation in ARF in the past 20 years. No one dietary prescription can be given to all patients with ARF, but some general guidelines can be provided for patients with ARF of varying severity. First, in the patient with mild ARF who is in mild negative nitrogen balance, a diet that includes 20 to 30 grams per day of high-biologic value protein or its equivalent as essential amino acids is indicated (along with sodium and potassium restriction, as just noted). At least 100 grams of carbohydrate per day should be given; increased calories should be supplied if renal failure lasts for more than 5 to 7 days. In patients with moderately severe ARF (e.g., secondary to sepsis), intravenous nutritional support is often required. One should give sufficient calories to maintain the nitrogen balance (clinically estimated by a stable weight in the edema-free patient); carbohydrates should compose 60 to 70% of the total calories, with the remaining calories being given as a 20% fat emulsion. Essential amino acids given intravenously may be required; a variety of commercial preparations are available. Concentrated dextrose is the major caloric source in most of these feeding solutions, along with 10 to 20% fat emulsions. In the severely catabolic patient (e.g., the patient with ARF after trauma and rhabdomyolysis), 3000 calories per day or more is required. From 20 to 30 grams per day of essential amino acids may be needed, along with large amounts of glucose and 10 to 20% fat emulsions.

In the patient who cannot be fed, parenteral nutrition is required. Hypertonic nutrient solutions must be infused centrally through a subclavian vein catheter. Knowledge of a number of technical details is required to provide total parenteral nutrition safely; the clinician is referred to specialized textbooks on ARF for such details. Finally, it should be pointed out that although maintenance of nitrogen balance is a reasonable goal of therapy, it has not been demonstrated that advances in nutritional therapy have improved survival rates in ARF patients.

Conservative management of the patient with ARF must also focus on prevention of infection, prevention and treatment of gastrointestinal bleeding, and maintenance of normal cardiac and pulmonary functions. Foley's catheters should not be used unless urologically indicated; urine volumes can be obtained by intermittent bladder catheterization, with less risk of infection in the oliguric patient. Although not proved effective in reducing uremic gastrointestinal bleeding, my approach is to use aluminum hydroxide (antacids) and an $H_2$ receptor antagonist (e.g., cimetidine, 300 mg orally twice daily). In patients in whom bleeding continues, particularly those in whom any surgical procedure is required, administration of desmopressin (1-desamino-8-D-arginine vasopressin, DDAVP), 0.3 μg per kg over 20 minutes intravenously, or intranasally at 3.0 μg per kg; cryoprecipitate, 7 to 10 bags; or conjugated estrogens, 0.6 mg per kg per day for 4 to 5 days, helps to correct the platelet dysfunction that causes the bleeding in these patients. I prefer to use DDAVP. Adequate dialysis (daily in the bleeding patient with a prolonged bleeding time) is the initial treatment of choice in uremic bleeding.

Finally, *any drug* that is being given to a patient with renal failure should be carefully scrutinized both for its absolute necessity and for the appropriateness of its dosage and of the intervals between doses. A number of tables are available to guide the clinician on the dosage and time intervals of the most commonly used drugs. These tables also provide information on the dialysis of drugs, either by hemodialysis or by peritoneal dialysis.

### Dialytic Therapy

Dialysis is required in patients with ARF for the same indications as in chronic renal failure. Absolute indications include volume overload, severe acidosis, hyperkalemia, and gross manifestations of uremia, such as seizures or pericarditis. Dialysis may be required daily to keep the blood urea nitrogen level below 100 mg per dl and the serum creatinine level below 10 mg per dl. Three techniques of dialytic therapy are currently available: hemodialysis, peritoneal dialysis, and continuous arteriovenous hemofiltration (CAVH). Peritoneal dialysis, although still an excellent therapeutic modality, is not used as often as in the past, having been superseded by hemodialysis, with its greater ease, convenience, and rapidity. Peritoneal dialysis suffers from the problem of slow clearance and frequently cannot be used in patients who have undergone major abdominal surgical procedures. Because of the ability to dialyze hemodynamically unstable patients and to use small amounts of anticoagulants (without causing clotting in the external device), as well as the ease of insertion of double-lumen dialysis catheters, hemodialysis is now relied on heavily for management of ARF patients.

I do not wait for the absolute indications for hemodialysis noted earlier. My approach is to use hemodialysis on a prophylactic basis, starting before the major uremic complications appear. Dialysis should be done for 4 hours per treatment for a minimum of three times per week until the onset of the postoliguric phase and stability or a decline in blood urea nitrogen and serum creatinine levels are observed. Bicarbonate, not acetate, should be used as the source of alkali in dialysis in ARF patients. In my experience, subclavian venous access provides a better alternative than femoral vein catheterization because the subclavian route allows the patient to move about, thereby reducing the likelihood of deep venous thrombosis and other complications of strict bed rest.

The last decade has seen the introduction of several nondialytic techniques for the treatment of ARF, including CAVH and slow continuous arteriovenous ultrafiltration (SCUF). Both techniques, which are essentially the same, consist of continuous removal of a large volume of uremic ultrafiltrate via a dialyzer. When the ultrafiltrate removed is replaced by a nearly equal volume of an appropriate electrolyte solution, the technique is considered CAVH; when the fluid is not replaced, it is considered SCUF. Proponents of CAVH argue that it is particularly useful in ARF patients who cannot be peritoneally dialyzed or in those who are hemodynamically unstable and therefore not suitable for acute hemodialysis. The hemofiltration device, in essence a high-flux dialyzer, operates without the use of a blood pump, requiring the patient's systolic blood pressure to be higher than 70 mmHg. Blood flow rates of approximately 100 ml per minute can be obtained by cannulation of the femoral artery, with return of blood to any peripheral vein. Large amounts of fluid can be removed by ultrafiltration with these devices; 10 liters or more per day of ultrafiltrate is not unusual. It is thus obvious that unless the patient is grossly volume overloaded, physiologic solutions must be infused to match the fluid lost. In contrast to hemodialysis, which removes fluids and waste products by ultrafiltration and diffusion, convective forces account for removal of uremic molecules in CAVH. Many complications of hemodialysis, peritoneal dialysis, and CAVH exist. Accordingly, these techniques should be used only by a nephrologist who has experience with them.

# CHRONIC RENAL FAILURE

method of
SAULO KLAHR, M.D.
*Washington University School of Medicine*
*St. Louis, Missouri*

Chronic renal disease is the irreversible loss of renal function and may result from a variety of insults. It may be caused by systemic disease, such as diabetes, collagen vascular disorders, or hypertension, or it may result from diseases intrinsic to the kidney, such as glomerulonephritis or polycystic kidney disease (Table 1). The hallmark of chronic renal disease is a decrease in glomerular filtration rate (GFR). Patients with slight to moderate decrements in GFR may be completely asymptomatic, whereas patients with markedly reduced GFR values and end-stage renal insufficiency may require renal replacement therapy (dialysis, transplantation) for survival.

TABLE 1. **Causes of Chronic Renal Disease**

Primary renal diseases: immunologically mediated, drugs, toxins, etc.
Hypertensive nephrosclerosis
Renal diseases due to systemic diseases: diabetes mellitus, collagen vascular disorders, etc.
Inherited or congenital conditions: polycystic kidney disease, renal dysgenesis
Urologic diseases: obstructive uropathy
Rarely, acute renal failure may be irreversible, resulting in end-stage renal disease

As GFR falls, solutes that are excreted by the kidney mainly by filtration (urea, creatinine) accumulate in body fluids, and their concentration in plasma rises. Indeed, the plasma levels of urea and creatinine provide a crude estimate of the decrease in GFR. However, it should be remembered that serum levels of both of these substances may be misleading because such levels may be affected by events other than changes in GFR. For example, serum creatinine levels are highly dependent on total muscle mass, and blood urea nitrogen concentrations can be altered by changes in protein intake and/or protein metabolism. The decline in GFR can be assessed more accurately by serial measurements of creatinine clearance, although at later stages of renal insufficiency the creatinine clearance tends to overestimate the true GFR values.

As GFR decreases below 25% of normal (about 30 ml per minute), other solutes that are filtered and either secreted or reabsorbed by the renal tubules also accumulate in body fluids. These include phosphate, sulfate, uric acid, magnesium, and hydrogen. Finally, a number of other substances are increased in body fluids when renal insufficiency is far advanced. These include guanidines, organic acids, phenols, and certain peptides. Some of these solutes may achieve concentrations that are "toxic" and could contribute to the symptoms and signs of advanced chronic renal insufficiency (uremia).

As renal function deteriorates, the ability of the patient to adjust to changes in dietary intake of sodium, potassium, and water is markedly restricted. Although the excretion of solutes and water per nephron increases as renal function decreases, the fewer the number of functional nephrons, the narrower is the range of solute and water excretion achievable by the composite nephron population. Thus, the upper limit of excretion ("ceiling") for many solutes and water is less in patients with renal insufficiency than in normal subjects, and for sodium and water there is also a restriction of the minimal amount ("floor") that can be excreted. Thus, as renal disease progresses, there is decreased flexibility in response to changes in the intake of sodium, other solutes, and water. Therefore, the volume and composition of the extracellular fluid may change as renal function decreases, particularly when dietary intake is not modified.

Patients with GFR values between 50 and 80% of normal are usually asymptomatic. These patients can perform their daily activities and tolerate stress without difficulties. The presence of renal disease in such patients can be detected by accurate measurements of creatinine clearance and are suspected by their inability to concentrate the urine or by the presence of proteinuria. Although patients with GFR values between 25 and 50% of normal may be asymptomatic, they may not tolerate undue stress very well. Patients with GFR values below 25% of normal are usually symptomatic. Symptoms may include gastrointestinal manifestations such as nausea and vomiting, dyspnea on exertion, bone pain, articular pain, and peripheral edema. Anemia is usually present in these patients, and electrolyte abnormalities, such as hyperphosphatemia, hypocalcemia, and moderate metabolic acidosis, may be seen. Patients with GFR values less than 5% of normal are usually markedly symptomatic and have manifestations that reflect the involvement of several organ systems, including neurologic, cardiovascular, pulmonary, and gastrointestinal manifestations.

## CONSERVATIVE MANAGEMENT

The conservative management of patients with chronic renal failure (CRF) includes measures intended to prevent or correct the metabolic derangements of renal failure and efforts to preserve remaining renal function so as to postpone or delay the need for dialytic therapy. In these patients, it is particularly important to identify potentially reversible causes that may contribute to the decline in renal function. The reversible causes of worsening renal function in patients with chronic renal disease are summarized in Table 2. Circumstances that decrease renal perfusion may result in rapid deterioration of renal function. Such events include the development of congestive heart failure; changes in extracellular fluid volume, particularly volume contraction due to salt and water restriction or aggressive administration of diuretics; the development of pericar-

TABLE 2. **Potentially Reversible Causes of Rapid Decrease in Renal Function in Patients with Chronic Renal Disease**

Decreased renal blood flow
  Congestive heart failure
  Volume depletion
  Pericardial effusion with tamponade
  Hypotension—excessive antihypertensive medication
Uncontrolled hypertension
Worsening of metabolic abnormalities, including
  Metabolic acidosis
  Hypercalcemia, hyperuricemia, hyperphosphatemia
  Hyperkalemia or hypokalemia
Infection
  Renal
  Extrarenal
Urinary tract obstruction
Drugs and nephrotoxic agents
  Radiographic dyes
  Diuretics—volume depletion
  Certain antibiotics—aminoglycosides
  Nonsteroidal anti-inflammatory agents
  Acute renal failure of any cause, including renal arterial thrombosis and renal vein thrombosis
Pregnancy

ditis with pericardial effusion and tamponade; and the development of hypotension due to excessive administration of antihypertensive drugs.

Other causes of rapid deterioration of renal function in patients with chronic renal disease include uncontrolled hypertension, metabolic abnormalities, infection, obstructive uropathy, and the administration of nephrotoxic agents or drugs.

**Decreased Renal Blood Flow.** *Congestive heart failure* may decrease renal function owing to a fall in renal blood flow and a rise in venous pressure. Congestive heart failure is treated in the standard fashion with diuretics and digitalis. However, certain precautions are necessary in the patient with CRF. First, the dosage of digitalis must be adjusted, on the basis of the levels of creatinine clearance in patients with CRF. Second, potassium-sparing diuretics should be avoided because hyperkalemia may result from the decrease in renal function. Third, the diuretic response to commonly used drugs such as loop diuretics may be decreased in patients with CRF owing to a lesser number of functional nephrons, and consequently larger doses of the diuretics may be necessary to achieve a diuretic effect in the presence of fluid retention and volume expansion.

*Volume depletion* resulting in decreased renal perfusion is a common cause of rapid renal function deterioration in patients with CRF. This usually results from too stringent dietary salt restriction and/or administration of diuretics. Ideally, patients with CRF should be allowed a salt intake between 4 and 8 grams of sodium chloride (68 to 136 mEq of Na per day) until late in the course of their disease, unless blood pressure control is difficult. In general, the presence of trace pedal edema should be tolerated.

Other causes of decreased renal blood flow include pericardial effusion and hypotension, resulting from excessive levels of antihypertensive agents.

**Hypertension.** Approximately 80 to 90% of patients with far-advanced renal insufficiency are hypertensive. Significant evidence has accumulated to indicate that hypertension may accelerate the progression of renal disease. Consequently, blood pressure should be adequately controlled in patients with CRF. It should be remembered that, when diuretics are used to control blood pressure, the response to these agents may be reduced in patients with renal failure, and the risk of inducing volume contraction severe enough to result in a deterioration of renal function should be kept in mind. Evidence also exists that thiazide diuretics tend to decrease GFR. Thus, loop diuretics such as furosemide are preferred. Other agents should be employed to control blood pressure, especially when no evidence of increased extracellular fluid volume is apparent. Antihypertensive agents that do not decrease renal blood flow are preferred. Agents such as beta blockers, hydralyzine, alpha-methyldopa, clonidine, and prazosin have been utilized. Recently, many groups have begun to treat hypertension in patients with renal disease with inhibitors of the angiotensin I converting enzyme such as captopril and enalapril. The rationale for the use of these agents relates to their potential effect in decreasing intraglomerular pressures in addition to decreasing systemic blood pressures. Their potential beneficial effects on slowing the progression of renal disease may relate also to events other than adequate blood pressure control. Calcium channel blockers are also being utilized with increasing frequency. The goals of blood pressure control should be blood pressure of 130/80 mmHg or less. In cases resistant to therapy, minoxidil (Loniten), 5 to 30 mg daily, can be used. It should be remembered, however, that, in the elderly patient with CRF, aggressive antihypertensive therapy may result in postural hypotension, which in turn may decrease renal perfusion, aggravate the degree of renal insufficiency, and result in decreases in cerebral blood flow.

**Metabolic Abnormalities.** Several metabolic abnormalities, including metabolic acidosis, changes in calcium and uric acid concentration, hyperkalemia, and hypokalemia, may decrease renal function by affecting GFR either directly or indirectly. Severe *metabolic acidosis* tends to decrease blood pressure owing to a decrease in cardiac output and decreased responsiveness of vascular smooth muscle to the vasoconstrictive effects of norepinephrine. Consequently, correction of metabolic acidosis may improve renal perfusion that is a consequence of vasoconstriction. *Hypercalcemia* may reduce GFR and its correction may result in reversal of the decrement in GFR.

**Infection.** Infections, both renal and extrarenal, may decrease renal function and should be excluded when a sudden deterioration in GFR occurs in patients with a known course of decline in renal function.

**Urinary Tract Obstruction.** Urinary tract obstruction, of course, can occur in patients with already established parenchymal renal failure and may accelerate the degree of renal functional impairment. Noninvasive methods, such as ultrasonography, should be utilized to investigate the presence of urinary tract obstruction.

**Drugs and Nephrotoxic Agents.** In addition, the use of certain drugs and the performance of some diagnostic procedures that may decrease renal function in the patient with established CRF should be avoided, unless they are essential to treatment or diagnosis. For example, the injection of *radiographic contrast materials* into patients with chronic renal disease decreases GFR. Although in many of these patients the decrease in GFR is reversible, in others the injection of dye results in a permanent decrement in GFR. Hence, careful consideration should be given to the need for radiographic studies requiring contrast material in patients with CRF. If the studies are absolutely necessary, adequate hydration must be maintained in these patients to avoid renal failure or a reduction in GFR. Mannitol may also be given to prevent this event. The use of certain nephrotoxic drugs such as aminoglycosides or agents such as nonsteroidal anti-inflammatory agents that inhibit renal prostaglandin production, which is usually increased in patients with chronic renal disease, perhaps as a potential compensatory mechanism to maintain GFR, may result in marked decreases in GFR.

**Pregnancy.** Pregnancy may aggravate the rate of progression of certain renal diseases and careful monitoring of these patients in association with an obstetrician is mandatory.

In addition to identifying and treating or preventing these reversible causes of renal deterioration, one can use other therapeutic modalities designed to ameliorate or treat extrarenal complications of renal failure.

### Protein Restriction and Caloric Intake

It has been known for years that dietary protein restriction ameliorates the symptoms and signs of uremia in patients with relatively far advanced renal insufficiency. The beneficial effect is thought to be due to a reduction in the generation of nitrogenous waste products resulting from protein metabolism. There is also suggestive but not conclusive evidence that a low-protein diet, 0.6 to 0.7 gram of protein daily per kg of body weight, may reduce the progression of renal disease, particularly in patients whose GFR values are less than 30 ml per minute, or approximately 25% of normal. However, an effect of reduced protein intake on the progression of renal disease has not been established unequivocally, and a multicenter study designed to examine this question in a prospective manner is under way. Adequate caloric intake, between 35 and 40 calories per kg, should be provided to avoid endogenous protein catabolism and allow adequate utilization of exogenous protein. Patients ingesting a protein-restricted diet should be followed carefully for signs of malnutrition, which include a decrease in serum albumin levels, a fall in the levels of transferrin, a decrease in body weight,

and a decrease in anthropometric measures such as biceps circumference, skin fold thickness, etc. Decreases in serum cholesterol levels, particularly below 150 mg per dl, also suggest malnutrition in patients with chronic renal disease who are ingesting protein-restricted diets.

### Sodium Intake

There is usually no need for marked restrictions in salt intake in the garden variety patient with renal insufficiency. Because the range for salt excretion narrows as renal disease progresses, limitations in dietary salt intake may be necessary. However, because the floor for sodium excretion is raised in patients with chronic renal disease, such patients should not be prescribed diets markedly restricted in sodium. Such patients should be warned also not to ingest an amount of sodium chloride in excess of 6 to 8 grams per day.

### Potassium Intake

Potassium intake has to be restricted to less than 40 mEq per day when GFR falls below 20% of normal. More severe restrictions may be necessary later in the course of the disease, particularly if patients are catabolic. Foods rich in potassium should be avoided. Correction of metabolic acidosis decreases serum potassium levels by shifting this cation from the extracellular to the intracellular space. Occasionally, cation exchange resins are required to control hyperkalemia. Sodium polystyrene sulfonate (Kayexalate) taken orally removes about 1 mEq of $K^+$ per gram of resin administered. Because the resin is constipating, it should be given with poorly absorbed agents such as sorbitol.

### Phosphate and Calcium Intake

With progressive renal insufficiency, particularly when GFR levels fall below 25% of normal, phosphate retention occurs because of the inability of the kidney to further decrease phosphate reabsorption and maintain phosphate balance. Hyperphosphatemia results in a reciprocal fall in serum calcium levels. As a consequence of decreased synthesis of $1,25\text{-}(OH)_2D_3$ by the kidney, there is a fall in the absorption of calcium from the gastrointestinal tract. The hypocalcemia and decrease in the circulating levels of $1,25\text{-}(OH)_2D_3$ result in increased parathyroid hormone secretion and a state of secondary hyperparathyroidism. This occurs almost universally in patients with CRF unless phosphate restriction is initiated early in the course of renal insufficiency.

Also, hyperphosphatemia and increased phosphaturia per nephron may contribute to the progression of renal disease. Consequently, phosphorus intake should be restricted to 900 mg per day or less when GFR is less than 50% of normal. As GFR falls further, more strict phosphate restriction becomes necessary (Table 3). However, at a certain level of GFR (usually 25% of normal), phosphate restriction alone cannot maintain serum levels of phosphorus within the normal range. At this time, the administration of phosphate binders becomes necessary to forestall the development of hyperphosphatemia (see Table 3). Although aluminum-containing gels such as aluminum hydroxide gel (Amphogel) and basic aluminum carbonate gel (Basalgel), 15 to 30 ml or 1 to 3 capsules, given with meals have been used as effective phosphate binders, it has become evident that some of these preparations may cause aluminum toxicity when administered for long periods. Some of the consequences of elevated tissue aluminum levels in patients with chronic renal disease include the development of osteomalacia and sometimes an encephalopathy. Consequently, other phosphate-binding agents have been utilized. Of particular benefit has been the use of calcium carbonate, 1 to 2 grams given orally with meals (see Table 3). However, sometimes larger doses of calcium carbonate may be required to control phosphate. This may result in hypercalcemia with a potential for extraskeletal calcification. It should be remembered that calcium carbonate should not be administered unless the serum phosphate has been reduced to less than 7 mg per dl and the calcium phosphate product is less than 65 to avoid the possibility of metastatic calcification. Therefore, particularly in very hyperphosphatemic patients, the initial approach may consist of administering aluminum-binding gels. When the serum phosphate levels are decreased below 7 mg per dl, some of the aluminum gels can be replaced, at least

partially, by the administration of calcium carbonate. It should also be remembered that, in patients with reductions in both protein and phosphorus intake, the amount of calcium ingested is below the amount required to maintain calcium balance. It is, therefore, imperative to administer calcium supplements (500 to 1500 mg per day) to patients ingesting diets restricted in protein and phosphate (see Table 3). In patients undergoing dialysis in whom the serum levels of $1,25\text{-}(OH)_2D_3$ are markedly decreased, administration of $1,25\text{-}(OH)_2D_3$ may be necessary to control hyperparathyroidism. It must be remembered that calcium carbonate as a phosphorus-binding agent should be given with meals. By contrast, when calcium carbonate is given as a calcium supplement, it should be taken on an empty stomach.

### Magnesium Intake

As renal function decreases, magnesium tends to accumulate in body fluids. Although magnesium balance is maintained until late in the course of renal insufficiency owing to an increase in magnesium excretion per nephron, the administration of extra magnesium may result in marked hypermagnesemia in patients with CRF. Consequently, administration of preparations (enemas) or drugs (milk of magnesia) containing magnesium should be avoided, particularly in patients with GFR values below 40% of normal.

### Metabolic Acidosis

Metabolic acidosis may contribute to the decrement in renal function and also aggravate some of the symptoms and signs of uremia. Consequently, treatment of acidosis is recommended, particularly when serum bicarbonate level falls below 16 mEq per liter. The administration of oral sodium bicarbonate tablets (650 mg) three times a day is recommended. However, it should

TABLE 3. **Recommended Treatment Schedules for Abnormal Calcium, Phosphorus, and Vitamin D Metabolism of Chronic Renal Failure***

| Stage of Chronic Renal Failure | Calcium Supplement (mg) | Dietary Phosphorus Restriction | Vitamin D Supplement |
|---|---|---|---|
| Early | 500–1000 | 900 mg or less | |
| Moderate | 1000–1200† | 700–900 mg, plus mealtime Ca++ carbonate | |
| Advanced | 1200–1500† | 700–900 mg, plus 1200 mg of Ca++ carbonate with meals | |
| Dialysis | 1200–1800† | Same as advanced, but higher dosages of phosphate binder may be required | $1,25 = (OH)_2D_3$ 0.25–1 μg/day |

*Adapted with permission from Hruska, K: Requirements for calcium, phosphorus, and vitamin D. *In* Mitch, WE, and Klahr, S (eds): Nutrition and the Kidney. Boston, Little, Brown, 1987, p. 113.

†Apart from any calcium carbonate used as a phosphorus binder. Calcium supplements should be taken when the stomach is empty.

be remembered that the administration of extra sodium in the form of sodium bicarbonate may pose problems in some patients with a tendency to retain salt. Consequently dietary sodium may have to be reduced to allow for the extra sodium being administered in the diet in the form of sodium bicarbonate. It also may be necessary to utilize a diuretic, but it should be emphasized that the response to diuretics may be decreased, particularly in patients with moderately to severely advanced renal insufficiency. Although protein restriction decreases the generation of hydrogen and hence ameliorates metabolic acidosis in some patients, it may not be sufficient to maintain serum bicarbonate levels above 18 mEq per liter. In these patients, sodium bicarbonate administration may be required. Metabolic acidosis should be corrected because it contributes to bone disease; may cause symptoms, such as dyspnea and malaise; may impair cardiac performance; and may aggravate other uremic symptoms.

### Anemia of Chronic Renal Disease

Severe anemia develops almost universally in patients with end-stage renal disease. Anemia is primarily due to the inability of the diseased kidney to produce adequate amounts of erythropoietin. Although modest reductions in the half-life of red blood cells and the potential presence of inhibitors of erythropoiesis in the serum of uremic patients may contribute to the anemia, the effect could not be great because there is a rapid response of practically all patients undergoing hemodialysis to the administration of human recombinant erythropoietin (epoetin alfa [Epogen]). A number of patients require periodic blood transfusions during hemodialysis to keep their hematocrits from falling much below 20 to 25%. With the advent of recombinant human erythropoietin, the need for transfusions may be greatly diminished in patients with end-stage renal disease. In a recent multicenter clinical trial involving more than 300 hemodialysis patients, the baseline hematocrit of 22% increased to 35% within 12 weeks in 97.4% of the patients treated with erythropoietin. Red blood cell transfusions were eliminated in all patients within 2 months of therapy. The median maintenance dosage of recombinant human erythropoietin used was 75 units per kg three times per week. The range was from 12.5 to 525 units per kg. In 68 patients who had iron overload, there was a 39% reduction in serum ferritin levels after 6 months of therapy. The small minority of patients who did not respond to therapy had complicating causes, which included myelofibrosis, osteitis fibrosa, osteomye-litis, and acute or chronic blood loss. Adverse effects of therapy include myalgias in 5% of patients, iron deficiency in 43%, increased blood pressure in 45%, and seizures in 5.4%. The creatinine, potassium, and phosphate levels increased slightly, but significantly. The platelet count increased slightly, but there was no increase in clotting episodes of the vascular access.

Administration of recombinant human erythropoietin is also effective in correcting the anemia in patients with renal insufficiency who are not as yet receiving dialysis therapy. The drug has been given either intravenously three times a week or subcutaneously three times a week for 4 to 8 months with no marked untoward effects and with a correction of the hematocrit from the mid-20% to the mid-30% range. However, the experience with untoward effects of erythropoietin administration in patients with renal insufficiency not yet undergoing dialysis therapy is small compared with that obtained in patients receiving dialysis. Additional information is required in a greater number of patients to establish the safety of administration of the drug in patients prior to dialysis and to determine whether correction of the anemia accelerates the progression of renal disease in patients who still have sufficient residual renal function to preclude the need for dialysis.

### Drug Administration

A decrease in renal function, as occurs in patients with CRF, imposes restrictions on the dosage and frequency of administration of certain drugs, particularly those whose metabolism is greatly dependent on renal excretion. Drug interactions may be modified in patients with uremia. Binding to albumin may also be affected owing to the accumulation of organic acids in uremic serum. This may result in greater concentrations of free drug. Tables are available regarding dosage and frequency of administration of drugs in patients with different degrees of renal insufficiency.

In summary, the aims of conservative therapy (Table 4) in patients with chronic renal failure are to treat any reversible forms of renal failure; prevent or treat extrarenal complications of renal failure; and formulate a plan for treatment (dialysis, transplantation) when conservative therapy can no longer control the clinical or biochemical manifestations of uremia. This requires careful management of the patient by a skilled nephrologist or internist and also significant participation and input from dietitians, social workers, and nurses.

TABLE 4. **Treatment of Chronic Renal Disease**

| Glomerular Filtration Rate* | Management |
|---|---|
| Between 20% and 80% of normal | Prevent hyperparathyroidism ($PO_4$ restriction, Ca supplementation) |
| | Control blood pressure |
| | Adjust dosage of drugs |
| Between 5% and 20% of normal | All of the above. Limited ranges for sodium, potassium, and water excretion. Treat acidosis |
| | Protein restriction usually necessary to control increased $PO_4$, increased K, and acidosis |
| Less than 5% of normal | All of the above. Plans for chronic dialysis or transplantation. Placement of vascular access |

*At all stages of GFR, search for reversible causes that may accelerate renal insufficiency. Avoid use of contrast material or nephrotoxic drugs if possible. Watch for evidence of malnutrition if protein intake is reduced.

## DIALYSIS

Dialysis usually is defined as the process of separating crystalloids (such as sodium or potassium) from colloids (such as albumin), utilizing the differences in their rates of diffusion through a semipermeable membrane. Crystalloids pass through the membrane readily, whereas colloids do not. Although extensively modified, the process of removing particles from a solution on the basis of permeability characteristics is the fundamental mechanism for the treatment of patients with end-stage renal disease. Dialysis of uremic patients is predicted on the assumption that toxic substances accumulate in the body during the course of progressive renal failure. Currently, levels of more than 50 compounds have been found to be elevated in the blood of uremic patients. Some of these substances have known harmful effects. Excessive sodium and water retention, for example, may lead to edema and hypertension. High levels of serum potassium may cause cardiac arrhythmias. These substances readily diffuse from the patient's blood through a semipermeable membrane to the artificially prepared solution on the other side. Other readily dialyzable substances (urea, creatinine) that routinely can be shown to be elevated in severe renal failure probably do not cause uremic symptoms. During dialysis, some essential nontoxic substances are also removed, and hence the diet must be supplemented with such substances to prevent a depletion state. For example, folic acid, a relatively low-molecular-weight, water-soluble vitamin is dialyzable and, without adequate oral supplementation, folic acid depletion and subsequently megaloblastic anemia may occur.

There are two major forms of dialysis currently available in the treatment of patients with terminal renal failure, hemodialysis and peritoneal dialysis. Approximately 130,000 patients are undergoing dialysis, both hemodialysis and peritoneal dialysis in the United States.

### Hemodialysis

Hemodialysis involves the passage of a patient's blood continuously through a dialyzer (artificial kidney) at the rate of 200 to 300 ml per minute. In the dialyzer, the blood of the patient is separated by a semipermeable membrane from an artificial solution (dialysate) whose ionic composition resembles plasma. Some of the substances in the blood diffuse across the semipermeable membrane and are removed by the circulating dialysate. The partially cleansed blood returns to the patient's circulation, and the dialysate is discarded. During a typical 4-hour hemodialysis, 48 to 72 liters of blood flow through the dialyzer. Thus, hemodialysis is a rapid and efficient (for low-molecular-weight solutes) method to remove potential uremic toxins. The rate of removal of a specific substance depends on the characteristics of the semipermeable membrane, the differences in concentration gradient between blood and the dialysate, and the physical properties of the solute being removed. Hemodialysis requires access to the circulatory system via Quinton-Scribner shunt, arteriovenous fistula, vascular graft, or vascular catheter. The treatment is performed in a hospital-based or free-standing dialysis center (in-center hemodialysis) or at home after several weeks of training of the patient and an assistant (home hemodialysis).

### Peritoneal Dialysis

The physiologic principles of peritoneal dialysis are similar to those of hemodialysis. Instead of an artificial membrane, however, the lining of the peritoneum serves as a semipermeable barrier to solute. The dialysate is instilled within the peritoneal cavity and allowed to equilibrate with the solute circulating through the peritoneal vessels. Because the osmolality of the dialysate exceeds that of the plasma of the uremic patient, water leaves the peritoneal circulation and enters the peritoneal cavity. Thus, with peritoneal dialysis, ultrafiltration is achieved because of the hyperosmolality of the dialysate fluid, whereas with hemodialysis ultrafiltration is the result of transmembrane hydrostatic pressure differences.

Peritoneal dialysis also differs from hemodialysis in the permeability characteristics of the membrane. The clearance rates of low-molecular-weight solutes across the peritoneal membrane are less than with hemodialysis. In contrast, the removal of middle-molecular-weight substances is significantly greater with peritoneal dialysis. The procedure requires the insertion of a catheter into the abdominal cavity and repeated instillation of free dialysate. Each time the dialysate is drained by gravity, toxins, electrolytes, and fluid are removed. The dialysate is then replaced with fresh dialysate. Several options for treatment by peritoneal dialysis are available. Intermittent peritoneal dialysis requires frequent exchanges of dialysate usually in twice-weekly sessions lasting 10 to 12 hours. Intermittent peritoneal dialysis can be performed in center or at home. Since 1979, home intermittent peritoneal dialysis has been gradually replaced by continuous ambulatory peritoneal dialysis (CAPD) as the preferred home treatment. For CAPD, the patient generally performs five exchanges with prolonged dwell times of the dialysate on a daily basis. Continuous cycling peritoneal dialysis (CCPD) is also a home treatment. This modified CAPD technique utilizes several exchanges every night with one long dwell time during the day. Peritoneal dialysis is frequently used in patients who prefer the independence of self-care or for those who have difficulty with vascular access or hemodialysis therapy because of cardiovascular problems.

## TRANSPLANTATION

In renal transplantation, the donor kidney is placed in the iliac fossa. Its renal artery is anastomosed to either the hypogastric or the iliac artery and its distal ureter is anastomosed to the patient's bladder. An adequate function of the renal transplant changes dramatically the internal milieu of the uremic patient. Renal excretory and nonexcretory function is normalized to a large extent. By contrast, dialysis can only partially correct the former, and has no direct effects on the latter defect. Most patients receiving a renal transplant require long-term immunosuppressive therapy to prevent rejection. The effects of these drugs, usually steroids and cytotoxic agents, such as azathioprine or cytoxan, are complex. The untoward effects and complications of these drugs are beyond the scope of this chapter. The kidney to be transplanted may be from a living donor, usually a blood relative, or from a cadaveric donor. Whereas transplantation from a living related donor can be scheduled and may be done as an initial or early therapy, transplan-

tation from a cadaveric donor usually requires a prolonged waiting time, averaging 1 year or longer. The survival of the transplanted kidney (allograft or graft) is influenced by a variety of factors, such as pretransplant blood transfusions, duration of warm and cold ischemia of the transplant kidney during harvesting of the organ, pulsatile perfusion times, percentage of reactive antibodies, HLA matching, patient demographic data, and immunosuppressive therapy. The latter has changed in most cases after the introduction of cyclosporine (Sandimmune) therapy which became widely available toward the end of 1983. Long-term use of cyclosporine may result in nephrotoxicity and damage to the kidney as a direct consequence of this drug. Approximately 8500 to 9000 transplants were performed in the United States in each of the last 3 years.

It should be pointed out that dialysis and transplantation are not mutually exclusive therapeutic modalities in patients with end-stage renal disease. In many instances, renal transplantation is performed at an optimal time after a patient has been undergoing dialysis for a certain period. In addition, patients who reject their transplanted kidney may be maintained on dialysis subsequently or until a second renal transplant is performed. Thus, the treatment modalities available to the patient with end-stage renal disease should be considered complementary.

End-stage renal disease has a drastic impact on the life of the affected patient and his or her family. Changes in lifestyle, economic constraints, and sentiments of self-pity all contribute to psychosocial problems in patients with end-stage renal disease. Patients and relatives should be made clearly aware of the therapeutic options available, and appropriate support should be provided to the patient and the family. The integrated teamwork of the physician, the social worker, the dietitian, and the nurse is required to ameliorate the negative impact of end-stage renal disease on the daily life of the patient and the family.

# MALIGNANT TUMORS OF THE GENITOURINARY SYSTEM

method of
WILLIAM L. NABORS, M.D., and
E. DAVID CRAWFORD, M.D.
*University of Colorado*
*Denver, Colorado*

## ADRENAL TUMORS

Adrenocortical carcinomas are rare and represent less than 0.2% of all cancers. The majority are functional and produce virilization, Cushing's syndrome, or feminization. The combination of virilization and Cushing's syndrome is most common. Functional tumors are found most often in women, reflecting the relative ease of detection of functional tumors in females.

Incidental adrenal adenomas are being found more and more often as a consequence of increased use of abdominal computed tomographic (CT) scans and ultrasound. Differentiation of these benign adenomas from nonfunctioning adrenal carcinomas is important. Generally, adrenocortical carcinomas are greater than 6 cm in diameter at presentation. Smaller lesions are evaluated using CT scan, magnetic resonance imaging (MRI), and biochemical assessment. Close follow-up is mandatory in those who do not undergo surgical resection. Needle biopsy is not reliable for diagnosis.

The treatment of malignant lesions is by surgical removal. Prolonged remissions have been reported following resection of metastases. At present, there is not an effective chemotherapeutic agent, or combination of agents, for the treatment of metastatic adrenocortical carcinoma. Mitotane (o,'-DDD) produces the highest percentage of responders, although most relapse. The drug is associated with potentially serious side effects; almost 100% have significant gastrointestinal toxicity (anorexia, nausea and vomiting, and diarrhea), and approximately 40% have central nervous system (CNS) toxicity (lethargy, sedation, and vertigo).

Pheochromocytomas can be found anywhere that chromaffin cells are present, and the vast majority occur in the adrenal medulla. Ten per cent are extra-adrenal, and 10% are malignant. Surgical removal remains the only effective treatment. Scanning with $^{131}$I-MIBG improves preoperative localization. Preoperative treatment with phenoxybenzamine (Dibenzyline), an alpha-adrenergic blocker, helps to control the associated symptoms and hypertension and, over a 2-week period, allows restoration of a normal plasma volume. Propranolol (Inderal), a beta-adrenergic blocker, is added if tachycardia develops and should not be started prior to adequate alpha blockade. Adequate preoperative preparation prevents or decreases the hypertensive episodes associated with anesthetic induction and manipulation during surgery.

## RENAL TUMORS

Renal cell carcinoma accounts for approximately 3% of all adult malignancies and 85% of primary renal tumors. Urothelial tumors account for approximately 10%. The remainder are squamous cell carcinomas, sarcomas, and Wilms' tumors in children.

With improvement in the newer-generation CT scanners, CT has become the primary method of diagnosis and staging of renal cell carcinomas, although intravenous pyelography (IVP), ultrasonography, and arteriography continue to have a role. If the renal vein cannot be clearly visualized and deemed free of thrombus by CT scan, venacavography or MRI is obtained to rule out renal vein and/or vena caval involvement.

Treatment is by surgical removal. A radical nephrectomy should be performed if possible. By definition, this procedure involves removal of Gerota's fascia and its contents, including the ipsilateral adrenal gland. Patients with a tumor in a solitary kidney or with bilateral synchronous tumors require individualized treatment. Extension of the tumor into the renal vein and/or vena cava is not uncommon and occurs in up to 15% of cases. Surgical removal, although technically more difficult, can produce cure rates approximately equal to those achieved with tumors confined to the kidney.

Renal cell carcinoma is resistant to both chemotherapy and radiotherapy. Patients with an apparent solitary metastasis can benefit from resection of the primary tumor and metastasis.

The use of radiation therapy is mainly palliative. Palliation of bone pain requires high doses, up to 5000 cGy, and generally the remission is of short duration. Chemotherapy for metastatic renal cell carcinoma generally is not successful. Most single-agent chemotherapy regimens produce little or no results. Vinblastine (0.2 to 0.3 mg per kg per week) produces responses of 15 to 30%, and combination therapy adds little except an increase in toxicity.

Hormonal therapy has been used since the 1940s. Progesterones (medroxyprogesterone [Depo-Provera] 10 mg intramuscularly weekly) generally are used. Responses, when present, are of a short duration; however, the lack of significant side effects prompts its continued use. Androgens and antiestrogens also have been used.

Immunotherapy offers the most exciting possibility for treatment of metastatic renal cell carcinoma. Various interferons have been evaluated, of which interferon alpha is the most effective. Responses up to about 25% have been reported. Adoptive therapy using lymphokine-activated cells and interleukin-2* has produced the greatest response rates, usually in patients who have undergone prior nephrectomy.

---

*Investigational drug in the United States.

## UROTHELIAL TUMORS: UPPER URINARY TRACTS AND BLADDER

The renal pelvis, ureters, bladder, and prostatic urethra all share the same transitional epithelium. A tumor may present at any point or at multiple points along this tract. The vast majority of the tumors are transitional cell carcinomas, followed in frequency by squamous cell carcinoma and adenocarcinoma. Most present with hematuria, either gross or microscopic.

**Upper Urinary Tracts.** An upper urinary tract tumor is demonstrated as a filling defect or nonvisualization during IVP. Retrograde ureteropyelography frequently is utilized to further evaluate the etiology of the filling defect or nonvisualization.

Urine cytologic specimens can be obtained at the same time retrograde ureteropyelography is performed. Cytology is helpful in establishing the diagnosis but is hampered by a high false-negative rate, particularly in lower-grade carcinomas. Flow cytometry may improve the ability to diagnose these lesions correctly, particularly those of low grade. The use of brush biopsy and direct visualization using a rigid or flexible ureteropyeloscope may aid in diagnosis, but must be weighed against the possible complications of bleeding, infection, and perforation.

Traditionally, management has consisted of radical nephroureterectomy, which, by definition, includes removal of Gerota's fascia and its contents, along with the ipsilateral ureter with a cuff of bladder. The ipsilateral ureter is removed in its entirety because the incidence of tumor recurrence in the ipsilateral ureter approaches 30%. Two to 4% of patients diagnosed with a transitional cell tumor of the upper urinary tract develop a tumor on the contralateral side, and up to 30% develop a bladder tumor. For this reason, long-term follow-up is mandatory. We generally follow our patients with cystoscopy and urine cytology at 3-month intervals for 2 years, then at six-month intervals for 1 year, and then yearly if there is no recurrence.

More conservative renal-sparing surgical procedures generally are reserved for patients with a solitary kidney or with synchronous bilateral lesions. Low-grade tumors in the distal ureter can be managed conservatively with distal resection and reimplantation of the ureter into the bladder using a psoas hitch with or without a Boari's bladder flap to bridge the gap. Segmental resection with ureteroureterostomy or transureteroureterostomy can be performed for low-grade tumors in the mid and upper ureter in selected patients. Fulguration, laser coagulation, or resection of low-grade lesions is possible, but still should be considered experimental. Various chemotherapeutic agents can be instilled directly into the renal pelvis and ureter, again in carefully selected patients. Treatment of metastatic disease is as for metastatic bladder cancer.

**Bladder Cancer.** All patients with unexplained hematuria, microscopic or gross, should undergo an intravenous urogram followed by cystoscopy. Cystoscopy, followed by transurethral resection, remains the first-line treatment. As for upper tract tumors, cytology is not reliable for the diagnosis of low-grade tumors. Random bladder biopsies also are obtained routinely, as coexisting field change abnormalities may be present.

Treatment is dependent on cell type, stage, and grade. The majority of bladder tumors are transitional cell carcinomas and, of these, 85% are superficial (not invading the muscle). Up to 70% of these patients have one or more tumor recurrences, and 15% of these become invasive. By definition, carcinoma in situ is confined to the mucosa. However, it is frequently found in conjunction with a papillary tumor and is associated with a high risk of subsequent muscle invasion.

Patients with superficial tumors generally are followed with cystoscopy and cytology every 3 months for 2 years, then every 6 months for 1 year, and then yearly. Should a recurrence be documented, the schedule for close follow-up is repeated. A neodymium: yttrium-aluminum-garnet (YAG) laser can be used to control the primary tumor and, in theory, would not be associated with recurrence from cancer cell implantation. However, laser treatment does not allow for tissue examination for staging purposes.

Intravesical chemotherapy or immunotherapy is used to prevent or decrease the rate of recurrence. Intravesical therapy allows direct contact of the agent with the bladder mucosa with little or no systemic absorption. The agents most commonly used in the United States are thiotepa (triethylenethiophosphoramide), doxorubicin (Adriamycin), mitomycin-C (Mutamycin), and bacille Calmette-Guérin (BCG). Thiotepa is given in either 30- or 60-mg weekly instillations for 6 to 8 weeks, followed by monthly treatments for up to 2 years. A white blood cell count should be checked prior to each administration, as systemic absorption can occur, leading to myelosuppression. Doxorubicin produces approximately the same response rate as thiotepa in the treatment of superficial tumors, and it has been shown to be an effective treatment of carcinoma in situ. A chemical cystitis frequently occurs and can result in a contracted bladder. Mitomycin-C (Mutamycin) is given most commonly as 20 to 40 mg weekly for 8 weeks,* followed by monthly main-

---

*Exceeds dosage recommended by the manufacturer.

tenance therapy. This agent is more effective than thiotepa or doxorubicin. Toxicity is minimal. Chemical cystitis or a contact dermatitis on the hands or genitalia can be present. Mitomycin-C also is effective in carcinoma in situ. BCG may be somewhat more effective than mitomycin-C; it too is effective in the treatment of carcinoma in situ. The mechanism of action of BCG remains unknown, and the most effective strain and the optimal dosage also have not been determined. BCG is substantially less expensive than mitomycin-C but is associated with more toxicity. Irritative symptoms are frequent and may progress to severe cystitis, and influenza-like symptoms and polyarthralgias may develop. Systemic infections with BCG have occurred and require treatment with antituberculous drugs. Conversion to a positive purified protein derivative skin test and/or a granulomatous reaction in the bladder wall has been associated with a higher tumor response rate.

In the United States, invasive (into muscle) transitional cell carcinoma generally is managed by radical cystectomy, with radiation therapy reserved for those who are not candidates for or who refuse radical surgery. British urologists advocate radiation therapy with salvage cystectomy for those who do not respond or relapse. Several trials of concomitant radiation therapy and chemotherapy are in progress and include misonidozole,* 5-fluouracil, cisplatin, and methotrexate (Mexate); cisplatin (Platinol); and vinblastine (Velban) followed by radiation plus cisplatin.

The neodymium:YAG laser is not an effective treatment of tumors with deep muscle penetration. Partial cystectomy is possible in only a limited number of patients because these tumors tend to be multiple. The tumor must be solitary, well away from the trigone, and without any concomitant mucosal atypia on random bladder biopsies. Preoperative radiation therapy provides no therapeutic benefit.

Radical cystectomy, by definition, involves the removal of the bladder, prostate, and seminal vesicles in men and the bladder, urethra, uterus, ovaries, fallopian tubes, and anterior vaginal wall in women. A bilateral pelvic lymph node dissection is performed prior to cystectomy in all patients, except those who have received prior high-dose radiation therapy. Some patients with only a few microscopic nodal metastases may be cured by a meticulous dissection. If there is tumor involvement in the trigone or the prostatic urethra or when carcinoma in situ is present, the male urethra is removed en bloc at the time of cystectomy.

Potency-sparing radical cystectomy is now possible and followed the demonstration of the anatomic relationship of the branches of the pelvic plexus by Walsh and Donker in 1982. An ileal conduit is the most common form of urinary diversion following radical cystectomy. Numerous methods of creating a continent reservoir are now available and appear to offer a better quality of life.

Metastatic transitional cell carcinoma of the bladder has been shown to be responsive to various chemotherapeutic agents. The most active single agents are cisplatin (Platinol) and methotrexate (Mexate). The combination of methotrexate, vinblastine, Adriamycin, and cisplatin (MVAC) produces a complete response in 20 to 35% of patients; and those patients achieving a complete response have been shown to enjoy a survival advantage. The regimen can be very toxic. Nausea and vomiting, mucositis, and myelosuppression are common, requiring dosage modification or delay in therapy. As mentioned, trials of adjuvant and neoadjuvant MVAC are in progress.

## PROSTATE CANCER

In the United States, carcinoma of the prostate has the highest incidence of any cancer found in men. The estimated incidence in 1989 is 21% (lung cancer estimate is 20%), and it will be responsible for approximately 11% of the reported cancer deaths. However, the true incidence is unknown because many men harbor occult tumors. A higher incidence and decreased 5-year survival tend to occur in black men.

**Diagnosis.** Digital rectal examination continues to be the "gold standard" for screening patients at risk for prostate cancer. The use of transrectal ultrasonography for screening remains controversial, although it is useful in staging and for directed needle biopsy. Diagnosis generally is made in the United States by histologic examination of a core-needle biopsy, although cytologic examination of fine-needle aspirates is accurate and is used much more frequently in Europe.

**Treatment.** The treatment of prostatic carcinoma is dependent on the stage of tumor at presentation. The age and health of the patient also determine how aggressive the treatment can be.

STAGE A. Cancer is found in approximately 10% of all patients who undergo a transurethral resection of the prostate (TURP) for presumed benign disease. The preoperative rectal examination reveals no induration suggesting carcinoma. Stage A1 is defined as either three or fewer positive chips or less than 5% of the total

---

*Investigational drug in the United States.

volume and is histologically well differentiated. This stage was thought to be clinically insignificant. However, tumors in up to 16% of patients have been found to progress by 8 years. Stage A2 represents greater tumor volume or any grade other than well differentiated. Stage A2 tumors tend to behave more like stage C tumors and have lymph node metastases in up to 23% of patients at the time of diagnosis.

Traditionally, patients with stage A1 tumors have been followed conservatively. Now that we know that up to 16% of these tumors will progress by 8 years, urologists tend to be more aggressive in the younger, healthier patients. The treatment for selected stage A1 and all stage A2 tumors is as for stage B tumors.

STAGE B. Stage B tumors are detectable by digital rectal examination and are confined within the capsule. B1 tumors are less than 1.5 to 2 cm in diameter; B2 tumors are of greater volume. The incidence of positive nodes at the time of staging lymphadenectomy increases with the stage and grade of tumor.

Radical prostatectomy remains the most effective treatment of locally confined carcinoma. A nerve-sparing radical prostatectomy can now be performed, allowing the patient to remain potent postoperatively. A further benefit of the nerve-sparing technique is a decrease in the postsurgical incontinence rate. Should impotence or incontinence result, effective treatment is available.

Radiation therapy can produce long-term survival as well. However, at 60 months, there is a significant increase in treatment failure. Abnormal biopsy findings after radiation therapy are now considered treatment failure and occur in up to 30% of patients treated. If the disease remains locally confined and the patient is a surgical candidate, salvage prostatectomy should be considered. Both radical prostatectomy and radiation therapy usually are reserved for men with a greater than 10-year life expectancy.

STAGE C. Stage C tumors have extended outside the capsule of the prostate gland, but with no evidence of distant metastases. Because of the local extension, these patients are not considered candidates for cure by radical prostatectomy or radiation therapy. Further, at least 50% of these patients will have positive lymph nodes at the time of staging lymphadenectomy. It is our policy to offer these patients radiation therapy in the hope of delaying progression. Early hormonal manipulation also is a treatment option.

STAGE D. Stage D tumors represent distant metastases. Stage D0 tumors are clinically localized and the bone scan is normal; however, the serum prostatic acid phosphatase level remains persistently elevated. It is our policy not to explore surgically patients with a persistently ele-

vated acid phosphatase level, as the vast majority have occult metastases and early progression.

Stage D1 tumors represent local lymph node involvement. Distant nodal (outside the pelvis), bone, or visceral metastases is denoted by stage D2. Chemotherapy, whether single-agent or combination therapy, produces little significant benefit at present. Since the early 1940s, treatment of advanced prostate cancer has centered around hormonal manipulation. In the United States, this was generally achieved by orchiectomy or by the administration of estrogens, principally diethylstilbestrol (DES), 3 mg per day. Sixty to 80% of patients respond. DES at 3 mg per day will produce anorchid levels of testosterone, but is associated with many well-known toxicities, including thrombosis, phlebitis, pulmonary emboli, and myocardial infarction. Lower dosages of DES may not produce anorchid levels of testosterone.

Luteinizing hormone–releasing hormone (LHRH) agonists (leuprolide [Lupron, depot Lupron] and goseralin [Zoladex]) have been approved for use in the United States. With administration of an LHRH agonist, there is an initial stimulatory phase with a rise in the levels of luteinizing hormone and, subsequently, testosterone. Clinically, this may cause an increase in bone pain and/or bladder outlet obstruction. Increases in serum creatinine can occur, as can spinal cord compression. This can be blocked by prior administration of a number of agents, including cyproterone acetate and nonsteroidal antiandrogens.

Flutamide (Eulexin) is a synthetic nonsteroidal antiandrogen recently approved for use in the United States. Anandron (Nilutamide),* also is a nonsteroidal antiandrogen and currently is undergoing clinical testing.

Total androgen ablation (control of the androgens of both testicular and adrenal origin) was first attempted in the early 1940s. In a recent multicenter trial in the United States, the combination of leuprolide plus flutamide versus leuprolide plus placebo was compared. Median progression-free survival (16.5 months versus 13.9 months) and median length of survival (35.6 months versus 28.3 months) were superior in the leuprolide plus flutamide combination arm. Patients with minimal disease experienced a much greater benefit, although the number of patients in these groups was small. We believe that, if an LHRH agonist is chosen to treat prostate cancer, flutamide should be added to the regimen.

## TESTICULAR CANCER

Testicular cancer is the most common cancer in young men, although it represents only ap-

---

*Investigational drug in the United States.

proximately 1% of all male malignancies. The tumor generally presents as a painless mass, although a dull, aching pain may be present. Acute pain may mimic the symptoms of epididymitis. A delay in diagnosis is common.

Testicular ultrasound is helpful and can detect even small tumors. If there is any doubt as to the diagnosis, an inguinal exploration should be undertaken, as it allows early control of the vascular and lymphatic channels. Transcrotal orchiectomy may precipitate scrotal or inguinal lymph node involvement. Normally, the lymphatic drainage from the testes follows the spermatic veins. On the right, the testicular vein drains into the vena cava below the level of the renal vein. Lymphatic involvement primarily involves the precaval, interaortocaval, and preaortic nodes. On the left side, the spermatic vein drains into the renal vein. Lymphatic involvement from this side primarily involves the left para-aortic and preaortic nodes.

Staging is completed using CT of the abdomen, chest x-ray, and serum alpha-fetoprotein (AFP) and serum human chorionic gonadotropin-beta (hCG-beta) determinations. Though a variety of histologic types may be present, for treatment purposes, they are typed as either seminomatous or nonseminomatous tumors. Staging for both groups is as follows:

Stage A—Confined to testes
Stage B1—Minimal retroperitoneal metastases
Stage B2—More than five positive nodes or any node greater than 2 cm
Stage B3—Palpable abdominal mass secondary to retroperitoneal metastases
Stage C—Supradiaphragmatic or extranodal metastases

Elevation of AFP level indicates a nonseminomatous tumor (NSGCT), even in a patient whose primary is interpreted as pure seminoma, and should be managed as such. Pure seminoma can produce elevation of hCG-beta. It is important to remember that not all NSGCT produce serum markers and that some may lose the ability to produce these markers, though still be viable tumors.

**Seminoma.** Pure seminoma represents greater than 40% of all tumors and is the most common histologic type. Patients with stage A or low Stage B1 and B2 seminoma are treated with radiation therapy. Supradiaphragmatic radiation is no longer used, as it has little effect on recurrence in this area. Chemotherapy, if needed, would be difficult to administer because of compromised bone marrow function. Survival rates of greater than 95% and approaching 100% are reported for Stages A, B1, and B2 tumors.

Higher-volume disease (Stages B3 and C) does not respond well to radiation therapy, and chemotherapy regimens are utilized. Seminomas are exquisitely sensitive to chemotherapy.

The management of any residual tumor after chemotherapy is controversial. Retroperitoneal lymphadenectomy (RPLND) is difficult owing to dense fibrous scarring: pathologically, the vast majority are scar tissue only with no tumor present. The benefit of postchemotherapy irradiation has not been fully delineated. Close observation appears to be best at present.

**Nonseminomatous Tumors.** There are a number of different histologic types. Pure embryonal carcinoma is sensitive to chemotherapy. Pure choriocarcinoma traditionally is associated with a poor prognosis. For patients with low-stage disease (A, B1, and B2), RPLND remains the primary treatment. Adjuvant chemotherapy for those with positive nodes remains controversial. Less than 50% of those with low-volume Stage B tumors have a recurrence of their tumor, usually in the lungs. With close follow-up, virtually all that progress can be cured with appropriate chemotherapy. Adjuvant chemotherapy reduces the recurrence rate to less than 5%. With microscopic involvement only, a nerve-sparing RPLND can be performed. This allows preservation of the sympathetic nerves on one or both sides, thus preserving ejaculation. Erection is not affected by RPLND.

Several centers are recommending that patients with clinical Stage A tumors and no local invasion be observed. Extremely close follow-up is mandatory. Currently, we present both options to patients, but strongly recommend RPLND.

For higher-stage disease, the optimal results are obtained with initial chemotherapy. Several regimens are in use; all are cisplatin based. The combination of cisplatin, vinblastine, and bleomycin (Blenoxane) was introduced in 1974 at Indiana. Newer regimens substitute vincristine (Oncovin) or etoposide (VP-16-213, VePesid) for vinblastine and produce the same or better cure rates with less toxicity. Maintenance therapy is not necessary.

The end point for chemotherapy is the normalization of the tumor markers. RPLND surgery should not be performed if the marker levels remain elevated. Salvage chemotherapy using ifosfamide (Ifex) and cisplatin is given for those with persistent tumor.

Persistent masses after completion of chemotherapy and normalization of serum markers are surgically removed. Forty per cent of these patients are found to have mature teratomas, 40% have fibrosis, and 20% are found to harbor carcinoma. Those with residual carcinoma are given salvage chemotherapy. Patients with a complete response to the initial chemotherapy do not derive any benefit from RPLND and are simply followed closely for recurrence. We follow our patients monthly for 2 years, every 2 months for the third year, and then every 6 months.

## PENILE CARCINOMA

Carcinoma of the penis is rarely seen in the United States, with an incidence of approximately 1 per 100,000. Most of these are squamous cell carcinomas. Circumcision early in life is protective; later circumcision is not. Poor hygiene is associated with an increased incidence. Venereal disease may have an association as well, and sexual partners have been reported to have an increased incidence of carcinoma of the cervix.

The primary lesion generally involves the glands or the prepuce. Diagnosis is obtained by an incisional biopsy. If carcinoma is limited to the prepuce, in carefully selected patients, circumcision can be curative. In the United States, most urologists use the staging system by Jackson:

Stage I—Tumor confined to the glans or the prepuce
Stage II—Invasion into the shaft or corpora of the penis
Stage III—Inguinal metastases, but operable
Stage IV—Local extension, inoperable nodes, or distant metastases

Partial penectomy for distal lesions, with a 2-cm proximal margin, produces good local control. Total penectomy with a perineal urethrostomy is necessary for more proximal lesions.

Management of the regional lymph nodes remains controversial. Inguinal nodes are clinically palpable in up to 60% of all patients. A high false-positive rate is present, as up to 50% of palpable lymphadenopathy is due to secondary infection and inflammation. Up to 20% of patients with clinically negative nodes have metastatic disease present. Lymphangiography and CT are of no help in differentiating between benign and malignant nodes.

It is our policy to treat the patients with broad-spectrum antibiotics for 4 weeks after management of the primary tumor. No resolution of palpable adenopathy is an indication for ilioinguinal lymphadenectomy. Extensive lesions of the base of the penis and/or involvement of the corpora cavernosa is also an indication for lymphadenectomy, as is the development of inguinal adenopathy in a patient without prior adenopathy. Skinny-needle aspiration may allow pathologic confirmation of positive nodes. Ilioinguinal node dissection can be associated with significant morbidity, including skin flap necrosis, leg and/or scrotal edema, infection, and delayed healing.

Radiation therapy can produce good local control in early-stage lesions and also can produce good palliative effects in patients with advanced disease. Chemotherapy for metastatic disease is in evolution; and, at this time, the results are dismal. Methotrexate, bleomycin (Blenoxane), and cisplatin are the more effective single agents. Patients should be placed into multicenter clinical trials to aid in the development of appropriate drug combinations.

# URETHRAL STRICTURE IN THE MALE

method of
JAMES M. PIERCE, Jr., M.D.
*Wayne State University*
*Detroit, Michigan*

Urethral stricture disease in the male is due to a number of causes. In the United States, the classic cause of urethral stricture was postinflammatory disease in the anterior urethra. This was most commonly a long-term sequela of gonorrheal urethritis. The incidence of this cause is much diminished because of the advent of adequate antibiotic therapy for the gonococcus. The major causes of urethral stricture in the United States today are traumatic. *External* trauma, such as straddle injury to the bulbous urethra, can occur. These are individuals who fall on the perineal body, such as straddling a fence or a bar, and compress the perineum up against the arch of the ischial rami and pubis and cause damage to the bulbous urethra. The other type of external trauma is pelvic crushing injury with dismemberment, either partial or complete, of the urethra just distal to the apex of the prostate and at the level of the urogenital diaphragm. The other type of trauma is *iatrogenic* following urethral catheterization with development of urethritis or due to traumatic damage to the wall of the urethra, such as by transurethral-type operative procedures or operative damage during surgery on contiguous organs. The final cause of urethral stricture is *congenital*. Meatal stenosis may fall into this category.

## DIAGNOSIS

The magnitude of the obstruction produced by a stricture is best determined by a urethral flow study. This is done with the patient having a full bladder of at least 200 ml in the adult, and the patient is instructed to void without straining. A maximal flow of less than 12 ml per second may indicate a situation in which treatment has to be considered. The anatomic location and extent of the stricture is best determined by urethrogram. A retrograde urethrogram, injecting radiocontrast material through the urethral meatus, demonstrates the distal extent of the stricture, but may not adequately demonstrate the length or proximal limits of the stricture. The latter are best demonstrated by a voiding urethrogram. This shows the proximal extent of the stricture. These studies are obtained for baseline data. Strictures that are just at the urethral meatus can sometimes be handled by self-dilation of the meatus with an obturator, such as the plastic cover of hypodermic needles. If this does not work, the patient may require an urethral meatotomy.

## MANAGEMENT

Endoscopy should be performed for all strictures of the anterior urethra, except for meatal stenosis, because the first symptom of carcinoma of the urethra is usually obstruction. The stricture is best handled initially with urethral dilation. This can be done with filiforms and followers. If only a filiform or a small No. 6 follower can pass through the stricture, it is left in place for 24 hours and then the stricture is dilated further.

The more difficult strictures can be handled endoscopically with a direct vision internal urethrotomy in which, under endoscopic control, a knife blade in the endoscope can be used to cut the strictured area anteriorly in the midline from a point in normal tissue just proximal to the stricture to a point just distal to the stricture. A catheter is often left in place for several days and then removed.

If the stricture then recurs, a flow study and then the internal urethrotomy should be repeated. At the second internal urethrotomy, it is best to have the patient self-catheterize himself twice a day for 30 days so that the cut edges do not grow together and the cut urethra will heal with a wide-caliber lumen. This is all that is necessary in many patients.

### Formal Urethroplasties

In those strictures that fail to resolve with urethral dilation and internal urethrotomy as described earlier, one has to consider a formal urethroplasty. In those patients who have a post-infectious stricture with infection of tissues, a two-stage procedure is often best. In these individuals, the infected area of the urethra with the stricture is excised and covered with a 12/1000-inch split-thickness skin graft. This is especially important in areas of the penile urethra where, if one excises the stricture and brings the skin on each side to the midline, there is not enough skin for a second-stage procedure. By putting the split-thickness skin in this area, the normal skin is brought down to the edges of the graft, and

this allows enough loose skin to roll a tube of urethra as a second stage and close the skin over it without tension.

In strictures due to either iatrogenic trauma or trauma from external injury, such as straddle injury with a bulbous stricture, the strictured area is usually relatively short, about 1 cm or 1.5 cm in length. This can be excised and the ends of the normal urethra anastomosed. If a long area of urethra has to be excised, one can consider a free defatted full-thickness skin tube. The best skin for this is the foreskin if the patient is uncircumcised. Otherwise, distal penile shaft skin can be used. The skin is made into a tube around a catheter and the ends sutured to the urethra. The catheter is usually left in place for 2 to 3 weeks and then removed.

Straddle injuries, which usually occur in the bulbous urethra, can also be treated with patch grafts from scrotal or perineal skin in which the blood supply is kept intact to the subcutaneous tissue, and then this is rolled into a partial or complete tube and patched onto the area of urethral incision or excision. One has to be careful to maintain the blood supply in this type of graft.

In some individuals in their 60s and older, a permanent perineal urethrostomy proximal to the stricture may be the best solution.

### Prostatomembranous Urethral Stricture (Posterior Urethra)

This is an entirely different group of problems. Most of these are secondary to a crushing pelvic injury in which the urethra just a few millimeters distal to the apex of the prostatic urethra is partially or completely dismembered from the membranous urethra. This occurs just above or in the area of the so-called urogenital diaphragm. Initially, this injury can be treated in one of two ways. The safest way is to put a cystostomy tube into the bladder and leave the patient alone. Then after 3 or 4 months when the damaged tissue and hematoma resolve, one can decide what to do. Most of these patients require operative excision of the "strictured" area and end-to-end anastomosis of the bulbous urethra to the apex of the prostatic urethra. The second way to treat these initially at the time of injury is to try establishment of continuity of the urethra. Unfortunately, these people have a lot of other injuries in their pelvis. There is a big hematoma, and sometimes one can do more damage than if a simple cystostomy was done with repair later on. The damage may be to the man's erectile function. Permanent impotence can occur in approximately 50% of patients who have had severe traumas and in about 20% of those who have had less serious injuries. Some of those who are impotent initially after the injury regain their potency later.

Establishment of urethral continuity is not always feasible. I recommend that the surgeon only occasionally seeing this injury perform a suprapubic cystostomy. Then a formal urethroplasty can be done if necessary in 3 to 4 months. These should be done by individuals with experience in this difficult area.

The procedure of choice in doing the urethroplasty is to use a transperineal approach, excise the scar, and anastomose the end of the bulbous urethra to the apex of the prostatic urethra. On some occasions, one has to remove some of the inferior portion of the pubic arch. This is done in my hands with a mallet and osteotome, for it may be necessary to expose the proximal portion of the prostatic urethra adequately. In my experience, this has to be done in only 10% of the cases. Again, the frequency is determined by the severity of the crushing injury. Total pubectomy—i.e., excising the entire pubis—is no longer necessary. A catheter is usually left in place for about 3 weeks and then removed. These people have to be followed practically forever because of the possibility of restricturing. This can usually be handled by internal urethrotomy on one or two occasions at the most. The patients can best be followed by a urine flow study intermittently. If the vesical neck itself has not been injured, the patient is continent. If there has been a concomitant lesion of the vesical neck, incontinence may result.

In my experience, the most common cause of incompetence of the vesical neck in these pelvic crushing injuries is due to putting a Foley's catheter on tension and leaving it on tension for a number of days. This causes ischemia and then fibrosis of the vesical neck and therefore makes it incompetent. These can be tricky injuries and sometimes require a lot of experience in deciding exactly what needs to be done. They can be complex, and thus the surgeon must be experienced in this area.

# RENAL CALCULI

method of
G. FORREST QUIMBY, M.D., and
MANI MENON, M.D.
*University of Massachusetts Medical Center*
*Worcester, Massachusetts*

Urolithiasis has afflicted humans since antiquity and is commonly acknowledged to be a significant medical problem. The annual frequency of hospitalization for urinary stone disease in the United States in 1978 was approximately 1 in 1000. However, the actual incidence of this disease is clearly higher because not all patients with renal lithiasis require hospitalization. The age at which patients are evaluated for renal lithiasis is usually between 30 and 60 years, with the majority of patients reporting onset of clinical symptoms in the second decade of life. In North America, calcium stones account for approximately 80% of the total incidence of urolithiasis and are primarily composed of calcium oxalate and calcium phosphate, 73% of the time occurring in mixtures. The remaining stones are composed of magnesium ammonium phosphate (struvite), uric acid, and cystine. When considering only calcium stones, males predominate over females by a ratio of 3:1. Long-term follow-up of patients reveals a surprisingly high recurrence rate; estimates for the recurrence of renal calculi range from 9 to 73%, with 50% of patients having a recurrence in 10 years.

The risk factors for the development of renal calculi can be divided into two sets. The first of these may be considered intrinsic factors or a genetic predisposition to stone formation. This is best seen in conditions such as renal tubular acidosis and cystinuria, which are well-defined inherited traits. Other intrinsic factors include poorly defined polygenic defects that increase the predisposition to stone formation in certain ethnic, racial, and familial groups. The second group of risk factors are termed extrinsic or environmental. These include geography, climatic and seasonal factors, water intake, diet, and occupation. Surveys in the United States have identified geographic "stone belts" of urolithiasis in the Northwest, the Southeast, and the Southwest. The peak incidence of stone disease in the United States occurs in the hot summer months of July, August, and September. Other risk factors for renal calculi that are well defined include low water intake, a high–animal protein diet, and a sedentary lifestyle.

## DIAGNOSIS

*Medical History*

A personal and family history should be obtained for all patients. Particular attention should be paid to eliciting a history of inflammatory bowel disease, recurrent urinary tract infections, prolonged periods of immobilization, gout, or familial occurrence of certain inherited renal diseases, such as renal tubular acidosis or cystinuria. A complete list of all medications and vitamins taken should be obtained. Acetazolamide (Diamox), often taken in the treatment of glaucoma, has been implicated as a possible cause of calcium stones. Ascorbic acid taken in megadoses of greater than 5 grams per day may increase urinary excretion of oxalate and contribute to the formation of calcium oxalate stones. Further, any drug that decreases the urinary pH may contribute to the formation of uric acid stones. Finally, in patients with a history of stone disease, information concerning previous diagnostic evaluation, methods of previous treatment, and details of previous stone composition should be obtained.

## Symptoms

It is generally accepted that renal stones are initially formed in the proximal urinary tract and pass progressively into the renal calyces, the renal pelvis, and the ureter. Although it has been thought that most small caliceal and renal pelvic stones are asymptomatic, recent evidence suggests that they can cause dull loin pain. Stones become symptomatic on passage into the ureter. The ureter has anatomic narrowing at three sites. Beyond the narrowing of the ureteropelvic junction, the ureter assumes a diameter of about 10 mm (30 French), until the level at which the ureter crosses over the iliac vessels. At this point, the diameter of the ureter narrows to about 4 mm (12 French). The final site of ureteral narrowing exists at the level of the ureterovesical junction, where a diameter of 1 to 5 mm is reached. It is at this site that most ureteral stones become lodged.

The patient with "renal colic" has an acute onset of excruciating pain, occurring in waves, with no association with a particular activity. The sufferer is seldom pain free between spasms, owing to an element of fixed flank pain that is due to renal capsular distention. In contradistinction to patients with acute peritonitis, individuals with renal colic writhe about and are unable to find comfort in any position. The location of the pain and its radiation depends on the site of impaction of the stone. Proximal ureteral stones usually present with pain localized to the flank, with radiation to the lateral flank and abdominal area. As the stone passes into the distal ureter, the pain becomes intermittent and sharp, corresponding to ureteral peristalsis. In men, the pain frequently radiates along the inguinal canal into the groin and the corresponding testicle and into the medial aspect of the thigh. In women, the pain radiates to the labia. Finally, after a calculus reaches the ureterovesical junction, symptoms of vesical irritation are frequently noted. Associated symptoms include nausea and vomiting and abdominal distention resulting from reflex ileus.

## Findings on Physical Examination

A thorough physical examination is an essential part of the initial evaluation of the patient who may have a urinary calculus. Diaphoresis, tachycardia, and tachypnea are frequent signs. Hypertension attributable to the excruciating pain may also be present. Fever is not usually present unless infection is associated with obstruction. Examination of the back usually reveals costovertebral angle tenderness. The abdomen should be examined carefully to rule out other causes of abdominal pain. Abdominal distention, hypoactive bowel sounds, and radiographic evidence of ileus are not unusual.

## Laboratory Findings

Urinalysis in the patient with urinary lithiasis frequently reveals microscopic hematuria. Indeed, the presence of significant microscopic hematuria (10 to 20 red blood cells per high-power field) in a patient with abdominal pain should warrant a complete investigation for renal stones. Moderate pyuria occurs even in the absence of urinary tract infection. The presence of crystals in the urine should also be recorded, because they often occur in the acute phase of urinary lithiasis and may provide a diagnosis of the type of stone disease present. The presence of "benzene ring" crystals is diagnostic of cystinuria. Urinary pH may help in the diagnosis. Typically, patients with uric acid stones have acidic urine, whereas alkaline urine is often found when struvite stones are present.

In a patient with suspected ureteral calculus, a plain roentgenogram of the abdomen often is diagnostic. Approximately 90% of urinary calculi are radiopaque. Stones composed of calcium phosphate are the most radiopaque, followed by calcium oxalate, struvite, and cystine stones in decreasing order. Uric acid stones are considered radiolucent. However, a stone must be about 2 mm in its widest diameter and radiopaque to be visualized. A lower ureteral stone often looks like the root of a tooth. This sign helps to distinguish it from a phlebolith. Nonvisualization of the stone on a plain film in the presence of a suggestive clinical history mandates the performance of excretory urography. If nonvisualization of the kidney is present 15 minutes after injection of the contrast medium, delayed films need to be obtained at 1 hour, 4 hours, and 24 hours. Oblique films are important both for distinguishing ureteral calculi from phleboliths and for visualizing small calculi impacted at the ureterovesical junction in a postvoiding film. The role of newer imaging techniques in the diagnosis of renal calculi is limited. Computed tomography (CT) is often useful in the presence of a radiolucent filling defect for differentiating between ureteral calculi (which are densely opaque on a nonenhanced CT scan) and other causes, such as malignancy. Ultrasonography or retrograde pyelography may be needed in patients allergic to contrast media.

## TREATMENT

### Initial Management

Most patients with urinary lithiasis require prompt therapy for pain relief. The intramuscular injection of meperidine (Demerol), 50 to 100 mg, is usually adequate. Fluid management should be aggressive, with the goal of maintaining a urinary output of 3 to 4 liters per day. More than 90% of patients with ureteral calculi can be managed on an ambulatory basis. The indications for hospitalization are listed in Table 1. In the presence of fever associated with leukocytosis or bacteriuria, prompt administration of intrave-

TABLE 1. **Indications for Hospital Admission**

Stone in a solitary kidney
Stone in a patient with fever and leukocytosis or bacteriuria
Stone greater than 6 mm in diameter
Stones and associated azotemia
Excessive nausea and vomiting negating adequate oral hydration
Symptoms too severe for ambulatory management

nous antibiotics should occur. Ordinarily, the majority of calculi less than 5 mm in width pass spontaneously within 4 weeks of the onset of symptoms. These patients should simply be observed and followed up on an outpatient basis. Calculi greater than 6 mm have less than a 50% chance of spontaneous passage and usually need intervention. The presence of obstruction for longer than 4 to 6 weeks can result in irreversible renal damage. For this reason, we recommend intervention for all stones, regardless of size, if obstruction is present after 4 weeks and the stone is not moving down the ureter. Finally, during outpatient follow-up or inpatient treatment, several studies should be initiated.

### Metabolic Diagnosis

Following acute treatment, stone recovery is of immediate importance, and all patients should be instructed to strain their urine. Stone analysis is a necessary step and aids the clinician in tailoring further therapy. If a stone cannot be recovered, a urine nitroprusside test should be performed to detect cystine. If this is positive, a 24-hour urine specimen should be evaluated for total cystine content. The evaluation of all patients with a single stone episode should also include intravenous urography, urinalysis, urine culture, a complete blood count, and an SMA-18. The cause of calcium oxalate stone disease is multifactorial. In patients with calcium urolithiasis, less than 5% have a well-defined pathologic condition, such as renal tubular acidosis, primary hyperparathyroidism, sarcoidosis, or inflammatory bowel disease. The other causes of calcium stones include hypercalciuria resulting from either excessive absorption of calcium (absorptive hypercalciuria) or renal loss of calcium (renal hypercalciuria). Hyperuricosuria, hyperoxaluria, hypocitraturia, and hypomagnesiuria also play a role.

In the caucasian male patient who has formed his first calcium oxalate stone, if hypercalcemia, renal tubular acidosis, sarcoidosis, and iatrogenic causes are ruled out and if the intravenous urogram is normal, no further metabolic work-up is necessary. The patient is informed of the importance of hydration, instructed to decrease his meat intake to less than 8 oz per day, and advised to increase the amount of fiber and bran in his diet.

The remaining patients are submitted to a more detailed ambulatory metabolic evaluation for stone disease similar to that of Pak and associates. In brief, the test protocol consists of two 24-hour urine collections, the first with patients on their customary diet 4 weeks after discontinuing drugs known to affect metabolism of calcium, oxalate, or uric acid. Following the first specimen, patients are placed on a calcium- and oxalate-restricted diet (400 mg of calcium; 100 mEq of sodium) for 1 week and then a second 24-hour urine collection is obtained. Both 24-hour urine specimens are analyzed for calcium, uric acid, magnesium, oxalate, citrate, creatinine, and pH. The relative supersaturation of calcium oxalate, calcium phosphate, and uric acid are calculated. If necessary, urine samples can be sent to a commercial laboratory for these measurements. In patients with severe stone disease, on completion of the second 24-hour collection, a calcium load test is performed with 1 gram of calcium glubionate after a 12-hour fast. Preload and postload urine samples are collected and evaluated for calcium, creatinine, and pH. This protocol allows the differentiation of absorptive hypercalciuria from renal hypercalciuria and provides data on the presence or absence of hyperuricosuria, hyperoxaluria, hypocitraturia, and hypomagnesiuria. In patients in whom no urine pH is less than 5.5, an ammonium chloride test is performed to diagnose incomplete distal renal tubular acidosis.

### Stone-Specific Medical Therapy

All patients with calcium stone disease are instructed to drink enough fluids to maintain a urinary output of greater than 3000 ml per day. Because there are critical periods of supersaturation of the urine, maximal intake of fluids should occur within 3 hours after meals, during periods of strenuous physical activity, at bedtime, and once in the middle of the night. Because of conflicting data and poor patient compliance, we do not recommend dietary calcium and oxalate restriction. Rather, patients are instructed to limit their daily intake of meat to less than 8 oz per day and to increase their consumption of dietary fibers, especially bran. If excessive calcium intake is present, it is moderated.

Patients with absorptive hypercalciuria are adequately treated with phosphates. Our first choice is treatment with neutral phosphates (K-Phos Neutral). The minimal effective doses of phosphate in men and women are 1500 mg and 1250 mg respectively, administered in three divided doses daily. However, adequate therapy should be titrated to produce a 24-hour urinary phosphorus level between 1900 and 2000 mg. Phosphate therapy is ideally indicated in patients with hypophosphatemic hypercalciuria. Phosphates are contraindicated in patients with struvite stones and in patients with a glomerular filtration rate (GFR) less than 30 ml per minute, and they are not tolerated in patients with malabsorption. Diarrhea is the most frequently noted side effect. Sodium cellulose phosphate, a nonabsorbable ion exchange resin with an affinity for divalent cations, is an expensive alternative. Dosage is 5 grams two or three times daily; however, magnesium supplementation and oxalate restriction must also be implemented.

The mainstay of treatment for patients with either renal hypercalciuria or unclassified hypercalciuria is thiazide diuretics. Hydrochlorothiazide, 50 mg twice daily, is usually adequate. In most individuals, potassium supplementation need not be given routinely; however, individuals receiving digitalis therapy are an exception. Thiazides may precipitate an acute attack of gout in patients with hyperuricemia. They are not the agent of choice in patients with absorptive hypercalciuria because they may result in soft tissue calcification.

On the basis of the metabolic work-up, specific therapy for calcium stone disease can be "fine tuned." Allopurinol (Zyloprim), 100 mg 3 times daily, is a useful addition in the patient with hyperuricosuric calcium oxalate urolithiasis. Potassium citrate (Urocit-K or Polycitra), 20 mEq three times daily, can be added in patients with hypocitraturia. Magnesium hydroxide, 400 to 500 mg per day, is used in patients with low urinary magnesium levels or gastrointestinal malabsorption.

Uric acid stones are the most easily dissolved. Adequate alkalinization of the urine to a pH of 6.5 to 7 is necessary. Potassium citrate at dosages listed earlier is usually effective. Sodium bicarbonate, 650 to 1000 mg every 6 to 8 hours, can also be used. Adequate hydration to produce urinary outputs of 2500 to 3000 ml per day is necessary. The urinary pH should be monitored regularly with a pH indicator tape to avoid excessive or insufficient alkalinization. Urinary uric acid excretion is lowered by limiting dietary meat intake to less than 8 oz per day. Allopurinol in dosages listed earlier is added for the treatment of frank hyperuricemia.

Cystine stones require more aggressive therapy. To produce adequate cystine stone dissolution, the urine pH must be maintained at greater than 7. This can be accomplished with potassium citrate, but at very high dosages. However, when urine pH is increased above 7, there is increased risk for the formation of calcium stones. Fluid therapy, with urinary outputs greater than 2500 ml per day, is also mandatory. With failure of conservative therapy, treatment with D-penicillamine (Cupimine), may be instituted. The dosage utilized is titrated to that amount required to reduce urinary cystine concentration to below its solubility limit (< 250 mg per liter). The occurrence of side effects may be minimized by starting with a low dosage of 150 mg 3 times a day. Maintaining adequate hydration, and alkalinization therapy may help to decrease the dosage necessary to achieve cystine solubility. D-Penicillamine produces serious side effects, including agranulocytosis, thrombocytopenia, and the nephrotic syndrome, and often must be stopped. A newer agent, alpha-mercaptopropionylglycine,* has an action similar to that of penicillamine and has fewer side effects. However, clinical experience with this drug is limited.

Struvite stones are associated with chronic urinary tract infections, typically infections with urea-splitting organisms. They occur twice as often in women as in men. In general, surgical removal of struvite stones is the procedure of choice.

### Interventional Treatment

Indications for interventional treatment in patients with renal calculi correspond to indications for admission (see Table 1), with the exception that patients admitted for intravenous hydration secondary to intractable vomiting do not necessarily need intervention. In addition, stones that cannot be dissolved, infected struvite stones, and stones in the presence of 4 weeks of obstruction with no stone progression are also treated with interventional therapy. The choice of approach to remove a given stone depends on its size, location, and composition, as well as the clinical status of the patient. Today's urologist has a variety of powerful techniques at his or her disposal, including percutaneous chemolysis, endourologic stone extraction, open surgery, and extracorporeal shock wave lithotripsy (ESWL). With the continuing improvement of these techniques, the open surgical removal of stones is rare.

In addition to the systemic chemolysis used in the treatment of cystine and uric acid stones, and as an adjunct to the surgical treatment of struvite calculi, percutaneous chemolysis is often employed. In struvite stones, hemiacidrin (Renacidin) is employed as an irrigating solution in those patients that retain stone fragments after interventional therapy. The significant complications, including death, that plagued the initial use of this agent have been resolved with the development of established guidelines for therapy. The chemolysis of uric acid calculi can be accomplished rapidly through the percutaneous irrigation of tromethamine (tris [hydroxymethyl] aminomethane, THAM). This agent can also be used to dissolve cystine stones, although with much slower results.

---

*Not available in the United States.

Extracorporeal shock wave lithotripsy is the treatment of choice for most renal stones. ESWL involves the electric generation of shock waves in a water medium, which are then focused onto the target stone. ESWL is greater than 90% effective in fragmenting renal calculi. It is limited to stones less than 2.5 cm in size. Stones composed of calcium oxalate monohydrate and cystine are often difficult to pulverize owing to their hardness. ESWL is contraindicated in the presence of any condition that prevents stone fragment passage. Because ESWL is only 30 to 50% effective in the treatment of ureteral calculi, proximal ureteral stones are often manipulated into the renal pelvis where they are subsequently disintegrated using ESWL.

Endourologic stone extraction is particularly useful in treating ureteral calculi. For stones in the distal to mid ureter, a transurethral approach is used. Cystoscopy is performed, and the intramural ureter is dilated, utilizing an angioplastic balloon catheter. On dilation, the rigid ureteropyeloscope is advanced to visualize the calculus, and the stone is engaged in a stone basket that is passed through the scope. If the stone is small enough, it is then removed under direct vision as the scope is withdrawn. Larger stones must be disintegrated prior to removal. A variety of probes that pass through the ureteropyeloscope may be used. Ultrasonic lithotripsy has the ad-vantage of safety, in that it does not damage the ureteral wall. However, stone disintegration is often slow and tedious. Electrohydraulic lithotripsy is faster, and harder stones can be fragmented with this method. Its major disadvantage is a much greater risk of ureteral injury. With the recent commercial availability of the flexible ureteropyeloscope, and the development of a laser fiber that can pass through its smaller instrument channel, laser disintegration through a flexible scope may be the wave of the future. After stone extraction, a double-J stent is passed to prevent ureteral occlusion secondary to edema.

Stones impacted in the proximal ureter, large renal stones, and stones associated with congenital anomalies such as a caliceal diverticulum are most easily approached percutaneously. In percutaneous lithotripsy, a nephrostomy tract is created through the parenchyma of the kidney and adequately dilated to accommodate the nephroscope. Stones are then removed utilizing the methods described earlier.

In the recent past, open surgical removal of calculi was performed with regularity. As the indications for open surgery have narrowed with the advent of the less invasive techniques mentioned earlier, open stone surgery is now reserved for stones in the presence of coexisting ureteral or renal pathologic changes.

# The Sexually Transmitted Diseases

## CHANCROID

method of
ELIZABETH F. SHERERTZ, M.D.

*Bowman Gray School of Medicine of Wake Forest
    University
Winston-Salem, North Carolina*

The incidence of chancroid has continued to rise in the United States, with a 10-fold increase in rate per 100,000 population in the past decade. There have been many regional outbreaks, often associated with prostitutes. Chancroid, caused by gram-negative *Haemophilus ducreyi*, presents acutely as tender genital ulcer(s), regional lymphadenopathy, and tender buboes, which may suppurate and lead to abscesses. Stained smears of ulcer exudate or bubo aspirate may demonstrate a "school of fish" pattern, but are subject to experience in interpretation and possible contamination.

Laboratory confirmation of chancroid has improved since culture media have been developed that are more reliable for isolation of *H. ducreyi*. Either an enriched chocolate agar or a heart infusion agar with fetal bovine serum, both with added vancomycin, can be used with $CO_2$ (or candle jar) incubation at 33° C with good recovery of *H. ducreyi*. Many laboratories are now using such a culture medium, and sensitivity testing also becomes increasingly important as antibiotic resistance occurs.

Examination, culture, and serologic testing for other concomitant sexually transmitted diseases should be done. Prompt recognition and treatment to heal the genital ulcers are important because such ulcerations can allow easier transmission of human immunodeficiency virus (HIV) infection. Sexual partners should also be identified and treated with a regimen effective for the index case.

### TREATMENT

Plasmid-mediated antibiotic resistance has been an emerging problem with chancroid in the past decade. This has occurred with tetracycline in particular and is seen in the United States as well as other endemic countries. Despite the increasing resistance patterns, there have been improved treatment options, as summarized in Table 1. Erythromycin, orally 500 mg four times daily, and ceftriaxone (Rocephin), 250 mg intramuscularly in a single dose, are options currently recommended by the Centers for Disease Control. Source of infection (contact with prostitute, during foreign travel, with immigrant) may help dictate choice of therapy. HIV-infected patients may be more difficult to clear of their chancroid infection.

Aspiration of suppurative buboes is recom-

TABLE 1. **Chancroid Treatment**

|  | Antibiotic | Route | Dosage | Duration |
|---|---|---|---|---|
| Recommended | Erythromycin | PO | 500 mg qid | 7–10 days |
|  | Ceftriaxone (Rocephin) | IM | 250-mg injection | Single dose |
| Alternatives | Trimethoprim-sulfamethoxazole (double strength) (Bactrim DS, Septra DS) | PO | 1 double-strength tablet (160 mg trimethoprim, 800 mg sulfamethoxazole) bid | 7 days |
|  | Amoxicillin–clavulanic acid (Augmentin) | PO | 1 tablet (500 mg amoxicillin, 125 mg clavulanic acid) tid | 7 days |
|  | Ciprofloxacin (Cipro) | PO | 1000 mg *or* 500 mg bid | Single dose 3 days |
|  | Norfloxacin (Noroxin) | PO | 800 mg | Single dose |
|  | Enoxacin* | PO | 400 mg q 12 hr | Three doses over 36 hr |
|  | Spectinomycin (Trobicin) | IM | 2000 mg | Single dose |

*Investigational drug in the United States.

mended, preferably through normal skin. Topical therapy with saline compresses is helpful for the ulcerations. Patient follow-up is essential, because treatment failure can occur. Evidence of other sexually transmitted diseases should also be sought in follow-up. Abstinence from sexual activity should be encouraged until lesions are healed. Patients should be educated about condom use.

# GONORRHEA

method of
CRAIG E. SMITH, M.D., and
C. KENNETH McALLISTER, M.D.
*Brooke Army Medical Center*
*Fort Sam Houston, Texas*

Since the discovery of penicillinase-producing *Neisseria gonorrhoeae* (PPNG) in 1976, the antibiotic susceptibility of *N. gonorrhoeae* has changed, with the emergence of resistance not only to the penicillins but also to the tetracyclines, spectinomycin (Trobicin), and second-generation cephalosporins, such as cefoxitin (Mefoxin). Resistance mechanisms may be either chromosomally (CMRNG) or plasmid mediated. Continuous surveillance of local susceptibility patterns is imperative because resistant clinical isolates may be "imported" and become epidemic at any time. Cultures should be obtained from every patient so that susceptibility testing may be done. Recommendations for treatment are based on the prevalence of resistant strains. In areas with a low prevalence of PPNG (<1% of isolates) or CMRNG (<5% of isolates), regimens using penicillins should be as efficacious as those with third-generation cephalosporins, e.g., ceftriaxone (Rocephin). In areas where resistant strains are endemic, susceptibility testing should be performed on each isolate to ensure optimal antibiotic selection.

The susceptibility of *N. gonorrhoeae,* including strains resistant to penicillins and tetracyclines, to third-generation cephalosporins, e.g., ceftriaxone (Rocephin), remains exquisite with a usual minimal inhibitory concentration of less than 0.008 µg per ml. To date, no clinically significant strains have been reported to be resistant to ceftriaxone (Rocephin). Single-dose therapy of gonorrhea with ceftriaxone (Rocephin) may be efficacious in treating concurrent chancroid caused by *Haemophilus ducreyi*, but not against concurrent established syphilis. Ceftriaxone (Rocephin) appears to be effective against incubating syphilis; however, spectinomycin and quinolones are not.

Concurrent infection with *Chlamydia trachomatis* occurs in up to 45% of heterosexual patients with gonorrhea. Presumptive antichlamydial therapy is therefore recommended for all patients with gonorrhea. No single antimicrobial agent has been shown to be uniformly effective for both gonorrhea and chlamydial infections when given as a single dose.

All patients with gonorrhea should also be offered testing and counseling for human immunodeficiency virus (HIV) infection. No change in drug regimens for the treatment of gonorrhea is necessary in the presence of concurrent HIV infection.

The diagnosis of gonorrhea is based on appropriate clinical syndromes with a positive Gram's stain or culture. No specific serologic test is available. Reinfection is also common because no protective immunity develops, even with recurrent infection. Although clinical trials have been attempted, no effective vaccine has been developed.

## UNCOMPLICATED MUCOSAL INFECTION

Cure rates of essentially 100% may be achieved with single-dose therapy, which eliminates problems with compliance. Although urethral gonorrhea is usually symptomatic, cervical, rectal, and pharyngeal infections are frequently asymptomatic. Ceftriaxone (Rocephin) in a single dose reliably treats gonorrhea at all anatomic sites (Table 1). Failures are common when treating pharyngeal infections with spectinomycin (Trobicin) and cefoxitin (Mefoxin). Many authorities prefer using a lower dose of ceftriaxone (125 mg intramuscularly once) because it is less expensive and needs a smaller volume for administration (0.5 ml). However, a higher dosage is recommended because it may delay the emergence of ceftriaxone-resistant strains and is required to treat pharyngeal infections, which may be asymptomatic. Approximately 20% of individuals with gonococcal infection have a second sexually transmitted disease, such as syphilis. Syphilis serologic tests should be routinely performed in all patients with gonorrhea.

Sexual partners of patients with gonorrhea should be examined, cultured, and treated presumptively for gonorrhea.

## PREGNANCY

Because gonorrhea infection in females is commonly asymptomatic, all patients should be cultured for *N. gonorrhoeae* at their first prenatal visit. High-risk patients should be recultured during their third trimester to prevent neonatal infection. Pharyngeal infection is more prevalent during pregnancy and may not respond to spectinomycin (Trobicin). If chlamydial diagnostic studies are not available, pregnant patients should receive treatment with erythromycin for concurrent chlamydial infection. Quinolones and tetracyclines are contraindicated during pregnancy owing to potential adverse effects on the fetus.

TABLE 1. **Therapy for Adult Gonorrhea Syndromes**

| Syndrome | First Choice | Alternative Regimens |
|---|---|---|
| **Mucosal infection**† | | |
| Urethral | Ceftriaxone, 250 mg IM once | Spectinomycin, 2 grams IM once |
| Cervical | | Ciprofloxacin, 500 mg PO once |
| Rectal | | Norfloxacin, 800 mg PO once |
| Pharyngeal | Ceftriaxone, 250 mg IM once | Ciprofloxacin, 500 mg PO once |
| **Pregnancy**‡ | Ceftriaxone, 250 mg IM once | Spectinomycin, 2 grams IM once |
| **Conjunctivitis (adults)** | Ceftriaxone, 1 gram IM once, with buffered saline irrigation | Ceftriaxone, 250 mg IM for 3–5 days, with buffered saline irrigation |
| **Complicated infections** | | |
| Bacteremia§ | Ceftriaxone, 1 gram IM or IV daily for 7 days | Cefotaxime or ceftizoxime, 1 gram IV q 8 hr for 7 days<br>Spectinomycin, 2 grams IM q 12 hr for 7 days |
| Meningitis | Ceftriaxone, 2 grams IV daily for 10–14 days | |
| Endocarditis | Ceftriaxone, 2 grams IV daily for 4 weeks | |
| **Pelvic inflammatory disease** | | |
| Hospitalized | Cefoxitin, 2 grams IV q 6 hr<br>*or*<br>Cefotetan, 2 grams IV q 12 hr for 48 hr after clinical improvement<br>*plus*<br>Doxycycline, 100 mg IV q 12 hr until clinically improved, then 100 mg PO bid to complete a 10–14 day total course | Clindamycin, 900 mg IV q 8 hr<br>*plus*<br>Gentamicin, 2 mg/kg IV or IM loading and 1.5 mg/kg q 8 hr maintenance dose for 48 hr after clinical improvement<br>*followed by*<br>Doxycycline, 100 mg PO twice daily to complete a 10–14 day total course |
| Ambulatory | Cefoxitin, 2 grams IM once, with probenecid, 1 gram PO<br>*or*<br>Ceftriaxone, 250 mg IM once, with probenecid, 1 gram PO<br>*plus*<br>Doxycycline, 100 mg PO bid for 10–14 days | |

*All patients with gonorrhea should either be tested for concurrent chlamydial infection or treated presumptively. Tetracycline, 500 mg orally 4 times per day or doxycycline, 100 mg orally twice daily for 7 days, may be used.

†In nonendemic PPNG areas, ampicillin, 3.5 grams, or amoxicillin, 3 grams orally, with probenecid, 1 gram orally.

‡Quinolones, e.g. ciprofloxacin, and tetracyclines are contraindicated in pregnancy because of potential adverse effects on the fetus. Simultaneous chlamydial infections should be treated with erythromycin, 500 mg orally 4 times per day for 7 days.

§Bacteremia with penicillin-sensitive *N. gonorrhoeae* may be treated with ampicillin, 1 gram q 6 hr. When compliance is not a problem, patients may complete a 7-day course of oral antibiotics with cefuroxime axetil, 500 mg twice daily; ciprofloxacin, 500 mg twice daily; or amoxicillin–potassium clavulanate (500 mg amoxicillin, 125 mg potassium clavulanate), 3 times per day.

## COMPLICATED INFECTIONS

Complicated infections are a result of bacteremia and include disseminated gonococcal infection (DGI), endocarditis, and meningitis. Patients with DGI may have minimal symptoms or present with the "dermatitis-arthritis" syndrome. Disseminated gonococcal infection is the most common cause of infectious arthritis in young adults. Therapy for DGI should initially be administered parenterally on an inpatient basis. If compliance is not a problem, 24 to 48 hours after symptoms resolve, patients may be switched to an oral regimen to complete their 10-day course of antibiotics. A single diagnostic arthrocentesis may be useful, but irrigation of affected joints with antibiotic solutions and/or open drainage is not indicated.

Endocarditis and meningitis are rare complications of gonococcal infection. Susceptibility testing should be done in all cases to ensure in vitro susceptibility. Patients with endocarditis, meningitis, or recurrent DGI should be evaluated for terminal complement deficiencies.

## EPIDIDYMITIS

Acute epididymitis in young heterosexual adults (younger than 35 years old) is primarily due to *C. trachomatis* or *N. gonorrhoeae*. Antibiotic therapy is the same as for mucosal infections, including the antichlamydial therapy. Epididymitis in older males is more commonly secondary to gram-negative rods such as *Escherichia coli* or *Pseudomonas aeruginosa*.

## CONJUNCTIVITIS

Gonococcal conjunctivitis in adults is an acute, purulent infection usually caused by autoinoculation from a genital source. Careful ophthalmologic assessment is necessary to rule out progression to corneal ulceration. Parenteral antibiotics are the primary therapy with adjunctive buffered saline irrigations. Topical antibiotics offer no additional benefit to parenteral antibiotics. Concurrent chlamydial infection may occur, necessitating longer therapy and closer follow-up.

## PELVIC INFLAMMATORY DISEASE

Pelvic inflammatory disease (PID) is a term that encompasses endometritis, salpingitis, tubo-ovarian abscess, and peritonitis secondary to polymicrobial infection with a mixture of *N. gonorrhoeae* (40 to 95% of cases), *C. trachomatis,* and endogenous vaginal facultative and anaerobic bacteria, including genital mycoplasma. Diagnosis is based on clinical presentation with fever, chills, bilateral back pain, adnexal tenderness, and mucopurulent cervicitis. The diagnosis may be confirmed by laparoscopy with intraperitoneal cultures. If laparoscopy is not available, antibiotic selection should be empiric and broad spectrum to include all potential pathogens. With the exception of positive gonococcal or chlamydial cultures, routine endocervical cultures may be misleading and should not be used to guide antibiotic selection.

Ideally, all patients with possible PID should be hospitalized for initial treatment with parenteral antibiotics. Patients with certain associated conditions—i.e., pregnancy, adolescence, severe symptoms, and possibility of other surgical diagnosis (appendicitis or ectopic pregnancy)—should always be admitted. Patients may be switched to an oral regimen 48 hours after their symptoms resolve and complete a total 10- to 14-day course of antibiotics. If ambulatory treatment is attempted, close follow-up within 72 hours is imperative to ensure adequate therapy. Appropriate therapy of PID is important to avoid fallopian tube obstruction, which may lead to infertility or ectopic pregnancy. Intrauterine devices (IUDs) are a risk factor for the development of PID. IUDs should be removed after antibiotic therapy has been initiated, and the patient counseled regarding other forms of contraception.

## PEDIATRIC INFECTIONS

Infants born to mothers with untreated gonorrhea are at high risk for developing DGI or ophthalmia neonatorum. All such infants should be carefully examined and observed for signs of infection—e.g., septic joints or meningitis. Disseminated infection should be treated with cefotaxime (Claforan), 25 to 50 mg per kg intravenously every 8 to 12 hours for 10 to 14 days. If the isolate is penicillin sensitive, aqueous penicillin G, 75,000 to 100,000 U per kg per day intravenously in three or four doses for 7 to 10 days, is given.

Ophthalmia neonatorum secondary to *N. gonorrhoeae* is contagious and may lead to blindness if not treated. Infants should receive parenteral therapy with ceftriaxone (Rocephin), 50 mg per kg (up to 125 mg) intramuscularly once, or cefotaxime (Claforan), 25 mg per kg intravenously every 8 to 12 hours for 7 days, and buffered saline irrigation to clear the exudate. Topical therapy is not adequate to treat ophthalmia neonatorum. The mother should also be tested for simultaneous chlamydial infection. Ceftriaxone (Rocephin) should be used cautiously in hyperbilirubinemic or premature infants.

Gonococcal ophthalmia neonatorum may be prevented by prophylaxis of all newborn infants within 1 hour of birth with silver nitrate (1%) aqueous solution, erythromycin (Ilotycin) 0.5% ophthalmic ointment, or tetracycline (Achromycin) 1% ophthalmic ointment. However, the best method for preventing neonatal gonococcal or chlamydial infection is screening and treating of pregnant women. Bacitracin ointment should not be used.

Gonococcal infections in children older than 1 year of age are essentially all associated with sexual abuse. Evaluation should also rule out other sexually transmitted diseases, such as *Chlamydia* infection, syphilis, and HIV infection. Uncomplicated mucosal infection in children less than 45 kg may be treated with ceftriaxone (Rocephin), 125 mg intramuscularly once; spectinomycin (Trobicin), 40 mg per kg once; or amoxicillin, 50 mg per kg orally once, with probenecid, 25 mg per kg (maximum 1 gram) orally. Complicated infections require ceftriaxone (Rocephin), 50 to 100 mg per kg (maximum 2 grams), or cefotaxime (Claforan), 50 to 200 mg per kg in divided doses intravenously daily for 7 to 10 days. Chlamydial therapy for children younger than 8 years old should be erythromycin, 12.5 mg per kg orally four times per day for 14 days, or for those older than 8 years old, doxycycline (Vibramycin), 100 mg two times per day for 7 days.

## PREVENTION AND FOLLOW-UP

The use of barrier forms of contraception—e.g., condoms and spermicidal agents, such as nonoxynol 9—may reduce but not prevent transmission of gonorrhea. Nonpharmacologic practices, such as urinating, washing, or douching after intercourse, also fail to prevent infection.

"Test of cure" cultures are no longer recommended for patients with uncomplicated infection treated with intramuscular ceftriaxone (Rocephin). However, all patients treated with alternative therapies should be recultured 3 to 7 days after completion of treatment. Persistent symptoms may be secondary to inadequate treatment of concurrent chlamydial infection, resistant strain of *N. gonorrhoeae*, or, most commonly, reinfection.

# NONGONOCOCCAL URETHRITIS

method of
MICHAEL F. REIN, M.D.
*The University of Virginia Health Sciences*
*Center*
*Charlottesville, Virginia*

Nongonococcal urethritis (NGU) is diagnosed when urethral inflammation is detected and gonococcal infection has been ruled out. In men, the diagnosis is initially based on a Gram's stain smear of urethral discharge that shows the presence of polymorphonuclear neutrophils (PMNs) but no gram-negative diplococci consistent with *Neisseria gonorrhoeae*. Although some texts use 5 PMNs, per X1000 oil immersion field as the criterion for urethritis, a smaller number of PMNs are seen in 16 to 50% of cases and should be regarded as indicating disease, especially if the patient has recently urinated. Diagnosis in women is more difficult because the symptoms of NGU mimic those of bacterial cystitis. NGU should be suspected in women whose dysuria and pyuria are associated with negative routine bacterial cultures of urine or in whom symptoms frequently recur following sexual contact. NGU in men and women may be asymptomatic.

*Chlamydia trachomatis* causes 30 to 50% of the cases of NGU. *Ureaplasma urealyticum*, formerly known as the T-strain mycoplasma, has been isolated from about 80% of men with chlamydia-negative NGU. The causes of the remaining 20% of cases are less well defined and include *Trichomonas vaginalis*, herpes simplex virus, other mycoplasmas, and a variety of other bacteria and viruses. Clinical etiologic differentiation is impossible, and NGU is usually treated as a syndrome.

## TREATMENT

Initial treatment of men and nonpregnant women consists of doxycycline (Doryx, Vibramycin, Vibra-Tabs), 100 mg orally twice daily for 7 days. Minocycline (Minocin) in equivalent dosages has no advantage over doxycycline, and its propensity to produce dizziness makes it a less desirable alternative. Tetracycline, 500 mg orally, four times daily, can be substituted, but this medication must be taken 1 hour before or 2 hours after meals, and the additional dosing and complexity reduces compliance. There is no advantage to extending any regimen for more than 7 days.

Pregnant women or patients intolerant of tetracyclines can be treated with erythromycin base (E-Mycin, Ery-Tab, ERYC), 500 mg, or erythromycin ethylsuccinate (E.E.S.), 800 mg, orally four times daily for 7 days. If either regimen produces intolerable gastrointestinal symptoms, one may cut the dosages in half, but extend therapy to a total of 14 days.

If the NGU is *known* to be chlamydial, patients may be treated with sulfisoxazole (Gantrisin), 500 mg orally four times daily for 10 days. Equivalent dosages of other sulfonamides can be used, but trimethoprim-sulfamethoxazole (Septra, Bactrim) has no advantage over sulfonamides alone.

Sexual partners of index cases should be treated with equivalent regimens on the basis of their high risk of infection (epidemiologic treatment).

**Management of Recurrences.** The pattern of recurrence can serve as a guide to subsequent management. Patients noting complete resolution of symptoms only to have them return days to weeks after re-exposure to a sexual partner are likely experiencing reinfection and may be retreated with the initial regimen. Efforts to ensure that sexual partners are treated should then be redoubled.

Patients whose symptoms persist after initial treatment with a tetracycline must be re-evaluated. The disappearance of PMN from the urethra suggests an adequate response to initial therapy, and such patients should be followed to ensure that symptoms indeed eventually resolve. Patients with objective evidence of persistent urethral inflammation (PMN) must be regarded as being infected with a tetracycline-resistant etiologic agent. Two well-characterized organisms are *T. vaginalis* and tetracycline-resistant *U. urealyticum*. Patients with persistent urethritis may thus be empirically treated with metronidazole (Flagyl, Protostat, Metric 21), 2 grams orally as a single dose, and erythromycin, to which these ureaplasmas remain sensitive, in the dosages listed earlier. Patients whose urethritis still fails to resolve should be given a thorough microbiologic and urologic evaluation.

Least well understood are those patients whose urethritis initially responds to treatment, but then recurs in the absence of re-exposure. Such patients are not likely to be infected either with *C. trachomatis* or *U. urealyticum*. Treatment of these patients remains somewhat controversial, but some are cured by extending regimens of doxycycline or erythromycin to 3 to 6 weeks.

Some patients who repeatedly relapse and in whom urologic work-up is unrevealing (e.g., absence of stricture or prostatitis) may need chronic suppressive therapy with a low dose of tetracycline (e.g., 500 mg orally once daily).

# GRANULOMA INGUINALE
## (Donovanosis)

method of
NANCY ANDERSON WILMS, M.D.
*Loma Linda University*
*Loma Linda, California*

Granuloma inguinale is a rare, slowly progressive, anogenital infection caused by an intracellular gram-negative bacillus, *Calymmatobacterium granulomatis*, which is serologically related to *Klebsiella*.

The incubation period ranges from several days to several months. The lesions begin as firm papules or vesiculopapules and later erode to a painless ulcer. Four variants in morphology include

1. Ulcerative or ulcerogranulomatous form, with a granulomatous ulcer, which is nonindurated and hemorrhagic.
2. Hypertrophic or verrucous form, which has an irregular surface and is drier than the ulcerative form, with a granulomatous base.
3. Necrotive form, which leads to destructive, exudative lesions.
4. Sclerotic or cicatricial form, which presents as a band-like scar of the genitalia.

*C. granulomatis* is demonstrated by Wright's or Giemsa's stain of biopsy or crushed samples of granulation tissue taken from the periphery of a lesion. The gram-negative bacilli are seen as intracytoplasmic inclusions of mononuclear cells. Histopathologic changes show nonspecific pseudoepitheliomatous changes, plasma cells and lymphocytes, and pathognomonic mononuclear cells with intracytoplasmic cysts filled with darkly staining bodies. The condition is generally classified as a veneral disease, although nonsexual transmission has been reported in epidemiologic studies.

### TREATMENT

No standardized approach to treatment exists. The treatment of choice is tetracycline, 2 grams daily (500 mg four times a day) for 14 to 21 days or until lesions are healed. If tetracycline fails, streptomycin should be used, 0.5 to 1 gram intramuscularly twice daily for 10 to 14 days. Alternative techniques include chloramphenicol, 500 mg four times a day for 10 to 14 days; gentamicin, 40 mg twice daily intramuscularly for 10 to 21 days; and co-trimoxazole (trimethoprim 160 mg, sulfamethoxazole 800 mg), 2 tablets (or one double-strength tablet) twice daily for 10 to 15 days. In pregnant women, erythromycin, 500 mg every 6 hours, is useful treatment. Good hygiene facilitates healing and should be encouraged.

# LYMPHOGRANULOMA VENEREUM

method of
NANCY ANDERSON WILMS, M.D.
*Loma Linda University*
*Loma Linda, California*

Lymphogranuloma venereum (LGV) is an uncommon, systemic, sexually transmitted disease caused by the L1, L2, and L3 serotypes of *Chlamydia trachomatis*. The incubation period seems highly variable and ranges from several days to several weeks. Infection is recognized more frequently in men than in women.

The infection starts as a small, tender vesicle of the genitalia or the perineum that rapidly ulcerates, becomes painful, and then disappears. The inguinal lymph nodes become enlarged then progress to buboes with multiple areas of suppuration and drainage. Multiple draining sinuses are seen in the groin and vulvar area. If the rectum is involved, there is associated painful proctocolitis and rectal strictures. Lymphogranuloma venereum is often accompanied by malaise, fever, myalgia, and arthralgia.

Diagnosis is made by complement fixation titers, of which 1:64 is considered diagnostic. *C. trachomatis* may be identified by rapid diagnostic testing employing either an enzyme-linked immunosorbent assay or a direct fluorescent antibody method. Cultures of the organisms are technically difficult, and the Frei test is no longer available.

### TREATMENT

The recommended treatment is tetracycline hydrochloride, 500 mg four times a day for 3 to 4 weeks or until all symptoms and signs have resolved. If lymphadenopathy fails to respond within 10 to 14 days or if a relapse occurs, an alternative antimicrobial should be used. Alternative regimens include 2- to 6-week courses of either sulfamethoxazole, 1 gram four times a day, or erythromycin, 500 mg four times a day. The latter is the preferred treatment for pregnant women.

Fluctuant lymph nodes should be aspirated with a large-bore needle and syringe to prevent tissue breakdown and the formation of chronic draining sinuses. If strictures of the vagina or rectum occur, periodic dilation at 2-week intervals may be necessary. Refractory cases may need surgical intervention.

# SYPHILIS*

method of
ROBERT C. NOBLE, M.D.
*University of Kentucky Medical Center*
*Lexington, Kentucky*

Syphilis is a chronic disease caused by the spirochete *Treponema pallidum,* which is highly sensitive to penicillin G. The disease is characterized by several distinct stages, and, as the disease progresses, the difficulty in treating it increases. Both the diagnosis and the treatment of syphilis rely heavily on the understanding of the serologic tests for syphilis, as the definitive tests (dark-field examination and direct fluorescent antibody test on tissues) are not readily available to most physicians.

Syphilis serologic tests are of two types. Treponemal tests are more specific and rely on antigens from *T. pallidum.* The two most common tests are the fluorescent treponemal antibody absorption (FTA-ABS) or one of the microhemagglutination (MHA-TP) tests. The treponemal antibody tests are not quantitated—that is, results are reported as either positive or negative; they do not correlate with disease activity. When test results become positive, they are generally positive for life. The treponemal antibody tests should not be used as an initial screening test, but rather as a confirmation of a positive nontreponemal test result.

The nontreponemal serologic tests rely on antigens that cross-react with *T. pallidum.* These tests include the Venereal Disease Research Laboratory (VDRL) and the rapid plasma reagin (RPR) tests. The nontreponemal tests are quantitated and reported as a positive titer. A fourfold change in the titer is significant and reflects a two-tube rise or fall in titer. Examples of this are a rise in titer from 1:8 to 1:32 or a fall in titer from 1:16 to 1:4. The VDRL and the RPR tests are equally useful, but only one test from one laboratory should be used to compare rises or falls in titers. The RPR titers are often slightly higher than the VDRL titers. The nontreponemal antibody titers correlate with activity of disease. Titers rise with infection and fall with treatment.

Early in primary syphilis, the serologic test results may be negative (thus the usefulness of the dark-field examination). The serologic tests are almost always positive in secondary and tertiary syphilis. Neurosyphilis cannot be accurately diagnosed from any single test. The cerebrospinal fluid (CSF) should be examined for cell count, protein, and VDRL. When neurosyphilis is present, the CSF leukocyte count is generally greater than 5 white blood cells (WBC) per mm³. The VDRL is the standard test for CSF. When the CSF VDRL is positive, it is considered diagnostic of neurosyphilis. However, it may be negative when neurosyphilis is present and cannot be used to rule out neurosyphilis. When used in CSF, the FTA-ABS has false-positive results, but when this test is negative, it provides evidence that neurosyphilis is not present.

## TREATMENT

Penicillin is the drug of choice for the treatment of syphilis. This is particularly true for patients with neurosyphilis, congenital syphilis, and syphilis during pregnancy because other drugs are less well studied in these conditions. If there is a question of penicillin allergy, penicillin skin tests and penicillin desensitization should be considered.

The Jarisch-Herxheimer reaction is thought to be due to the release of antigens from dead spirochetes following antibiotic therapy. The reaction usually consists of fever, headache, myalgia, and intensification of skin lesions. The Jarisch-Herxheimer reaction more commonly follows therapy of patients with primary or secondary syphilis. It is usually self-limited, but may be treated with antipyretics. Pregnant patients should be warned that this reaction may precipitate early labor.

Persons who are exposed to a patient with early syphilis should be examined and tested serologically. If the exposure took place within 90 days, the person may be seronegative even if he or she is infected and should be treated. Patients with any sexually transmitted disease should be serologically tested for syphilis as well. The current regimen recommended for gonorrhea (ceftriaxone [Rocephin] and doxycycline [Vibramycin]) is probably effective against incubating syphilis. If another nonpenicillin regimen for gonorrhea is used, the patient should have a subsequent serologic test for syphilis in 3 months.

Early syphilis means primary and secondary syphilis and early latent syphilis of less than 1 year's duration. The treatment of early syphilis is benzathine penicillin G, 2.4 million U intramuscularly in one dose. The alternative regimen for nonpregnant patients who are allergic to penicillin is doxycycline, 100 mg orally twice daily for 2 weeks, or tetracycline, 500 mg orally four times daily for 2 weeks.

If follow-up or compliance cannot be ensured, the patient should have skin testing for penicillin allergy, and desensitization to penicillin should be considered. Erythromycin, 500 mg orally four times daily for 2 weeks, can be used in a compliant patient who will return for follow-up. Ceftriaxone, 250 mg intramuscularly once a day for 10 days, may be considered in patients whose penicillin allergy is of a delayed type.

Follow-up of treated patients should be performed at 3 months and 6 months, and a nontreponemal serologic test should be performed. A

---

*This article is based on the syphilis treatment schedule found in Centers for Disease Control: 1989 sexually transmitted treatment guidelines. MMWR *38*(S-8):5–13, 1989.

favorable result would be a fourfold decline in titer by 3 months with primary or secondary syphilis. In patients with early latent syphilis, a fourfold decline should be present by 6 months. If these declines have not occurred or if signs and symptoms persist in the absence of reinfection, patients should have a CSF examination and be retreated.

Patients who are infected with human immunodeficiency virus (HIV) should have follow-up and serologic testing at 1, 2, 3, 6, 9, and 12 months. Any HIV-positive patient with a fourfold increase in titer in the absence of reinfection should have a CSF examination and should be treated as if the patient had neurosyphilis. All patients with syphilis should be counseled concerning the risks of HIV and be encouraged to be tested for HIV.

Patients with early syphilis may develop CSF abnormalities, but, when treated appropriately, few develop neurologic syphilis. Therefore, lumbar punctures are not routinely advised for patients with early syphilis, even if they are infected with HIV.

The treatment of patients with late latent syphilis or syphilis of more than 1 year's duration, gummas, and cardiovascular syphilis is different from the treatment of early or early latent syphilis. All patients with syphilis of more than 1 year's duration should have a CSF examination. Although in older individuals, the yield from a lumbar puncture is low, a lumbar puncture should be performed in patients with neurologic signs or symptoms; patients with treatment failures; those who have a serum nontreponemal antibody titer of 1:32 or greater; patients with other evidence of active syphilis, such as aortitis, iritis, and gumma; those who have HIV infection; and patients who will be treated with a nonpenicillin therapy. If the CSF results are suggestive of neurosyphilis or if the patient has cardiovascular syphilis, treatment should include an antibiotic regimen that is effective for neurosyphilis. For syphilis of greater than 1 year's duration, one should use benzathine penicillin G, 2.4 million U intramuscularly weekly for 3 consecutive weeks to a total of 7.2 million U. For penicillin-allergic nonpregnant patients, one should first exclude neurosyphilis with a lumbar puncture, and then give doxycycline, 100 mg orally twice daily for 4 weeks, or, tetracycline, 500 mg orally four times daily for 4 weeks.

Quantitative nontreponemal serologic tests should be repeated at 6 months and 12 months. If titers increase fourfold, if an initially high titer (≥1:32) fails to decrease, or if the patient has signs or symptoms attributable to syphilis, the patient should be evaluated for neurosyphilis and retreated appropriately.

Central nervous system disease may occur during any stage of syphilis. If the patient has evidence of neurologic involvement, such as optic or auditory symptoms and cranial nerve palsies, the patient should have an examination of the CSF.

The recommended regimen for the treatment of neurosyphilis is aqueous crystalline penicillin G, 12 to 24 million U per day given as 2 to 4 million U every 4 hours intravenously for 10 to 14 days.

Outpatient therapy of neurosyphilis is procaine penicillin, 2 to 4 million U intramuscularly daily, plus probenecid, 500 mg orally four times a day for 10 to 14 days; followed by benzathine penicillin G, 2.4 million U intramuscularly weekly for 3 consecutive weeks. Patients who cannot tolerate penicillin should be skin tested and desensitized, if necessary, or managed in consultation with an expert.

If initial CSF pleocytosis was present, the CSF examination is repeated, every 6 months until the cell count is normal. If the cell count has not decreased by 6 months, or is not normal by 2 years, retreatment should be strongly considered.

Pregnant women should be screened for syphilis early in pregnancy. Any pregnant woman who is seropositive for syphilis should be considered infected, unless she has already been treated and the follow-up serologic tests show an appropriate response. In areas where syphilis is prevalent and in high-risk patients, the serologic test for syphilis should be repeated in the third trimester and again at delivery.

Pregnant women should be treated with a penicillin regimen appropriate for the woman's stage of syphilis. Tetracycline and doxycycline are contraindicated in pregnancy. Erythromycin should not be used because of a high failure rate in curing fetal infections. Pregnant women who are allergic to penicillin should be skin tested to confirm this. If they are allergic to penicillin, they should be desensitized to penicillin.

If the therapy precipitates a Jarisch-Herxheimer reaction, women in the second half of pregnancy are at risk for premature labor and/or fetal distress. If they note any change in fetal movements or have any contractions following therapy, they should seek medical attention. Stillbirth is a rare complication of treatment, but treatment is necessary to prevent fetal damage. Treatment of pregnant women should not be delayed because of these concerns. The patients should be followed monthly after treatment. The antibody response is the same as for nonpregnant patients.

Untreated congenital syphilis has devastating consequences. Until the serologic status of the mother is known, an infant should not be released from the hospital.

Infants should be evaluated for syphilis if they are born to seropositive (nontreponemal test confirmed by a treponemal test) women in the following categories: those who have untreated syphilis; were treated for syphilis less than 1 month before delivery; were treated for syphilis during pregnancy with a nonpenicillin regimen; did not have the expected decrease in nontreponemal antibody titers after treatment for syphilis; do not have a well-documented history of treatment for syphilis; or were treated, but had insufficient serologic follow-up during pregnancy to assess disease activity.

The infant should have a thorough physical examination for evidence of congenital syphilis; a nontreponemal antibody titer; a lumbar puncture to examine CSF for cells, protein, and VDRL; roentgenograms of the long bones; and if possible, an FTA-ABS test on the purified 19S-IgM fraction of serum (e.g., separation by Isolab columns).

Infants should be treated if there is any evidence of active disease by physical or radiographic examinations, a reactive VDRL in the CSF, an abnormal CSF finding regardless of the CSF serology (WBC >5 per mm$^3$ or protein >50 mg per dl), quantitative nontreponemal titers that are fourfold (or greater) higher than their mother's, or a positive FTA-ABS 19S-IgM antibody, if performed.

Even if the evaluation findings are normal, infants should be treated if their mothers have untreated syphilis or evidence of relapse or reinfection after treatment. Those infants who are suspected of having syphilis, but who are not fully evaluated, should be assumed to be infected and should be treated.

Treatment is 100,000 to 150,000 U per kg of aqueous crystalline penicillin G daily (given as 50,000 U per kg intravenously every 8 to 12 hours) or 50,000 U per kg of procaine penicillin daily (given once intramuscularly) for 10 to 14 days. If more than 1 day of therapy is missed, the entire course should be restarted. All symptomatic neonates should also have an ophthalmologic examination.

Infants who, after evaluation, do not meet the criteria for therapy are at low risk for congenital syphilis. If their mothers were treated with erythromycin during pregnancy or if close follow-up cannot be assured, they should be treated with benzathine penicillin G, 50,000 U per kg intramuscularly as a one-time dose.

Seropositive untreated infants must be followed at 1, 2, 3, 6, and 12 months of age. In the absence of infection, nontreponemal antibody titers should be decreasing by 3 months of age and should have disappeared by 6 months of age. If the titers are found to be stable or increasing, the child should be re-evaluated and fully treated. Additionally, in the absence of infection, treponemal antibodies may be present for up to 1 year. If they are present beyond 1 year, the infant should be treated for congenital syphilis.

Infants who have been treated should be observed for falling nontreponemal titers. By 6 months of age, the titers should have disappeared. Treponemal test results generally remain positive for life. Those infants with CSF pleocytosis should have CSF examinations repeated every 6 months until the cell count is normal. If the CSF cell count is abnormal after 2 years or if a downward trend is not present at each CSF examination, the infant should be retreated. The CSF VDRL should be rechecked at 6 months; if it is still reactive, the infant should be retreated.

Children who are not in the newborn period who have syphilis should have a CSF examination to rule out congenital syphilis. If the child has CSF or congenital syphilis, the child should be given 200,000 to 300,000 U per kg per day of aqueous crystalline penicillin G (administered as 50,000 U per kg every 4 to 6 hours) for 10 to 14 days. Older children with acquired syphilis and a normal CSF examination result should be treated with benzathine penicillin G, 50,000 U per kg intramuscularly, up to the adult dose of 2.4 million U intramuscularly. Children with a history of penicillin allergy should be skin tested and, if necessary, desensitized. Follow-up for these children is as described earlier.

Syphilis in HIV-infected patients presents special problems. One should encourage all sexually active patients with syphilis to be tested for HIV. Patients with HIV infection who have neurologic symptoms may have neurosyphilis as well. Some HIV-positive patients who have early syphilis may have negative serologic results. If clinical signs or symptoms suggest syphilis, dark-field examinations, biopsies, and staining of lesion materials by direct fluorescent antibody staining should be performed. When an infant is found to have congenital syphilis, the mother should be encouraged to be tested for HIV infection.

For HIV-infected patients, several things should be taken into account for their syphilis treatment. Penicillin regimens should be used whenever possible for all stages of syphilis in HIV-infected patients. In HIV patients who give a history of penicillin allergy, it is not known how well the penicillin skin tests predict the immediate reactions to penicillin G. Desensitization to penicillin may be attempted.

No change in therapy for early syphilis is recommended for patients co-infected with HIV. However, some authorities advise a CSF examination and/or treatment with a regimen appropriate for neurosyphilis for all patients co-infected with syphilis and HIV, regardless of the clinical stage of syphilis. As with all cases of syphilis, follow-up is necessary to ensure the adequacy of treatment.

Patients with HIV infection who are treated for syphilis should be followed clinically and with quantitative nontreponemal serologic tests (VDRL or RPR) at 1, 2, 3, 6, 9, and 12 months after treatment. Patients with early syphilis whose titers increase or fail to decrease fourfold within 6 months should have a CSF examination and be retreated. In such patients, CSF abnormalities could be due to HIV-related infection and/or neurosyphilis.

# Diseases of Allergy

## ANAPHYLAXIS AND SERUM SICKNESS

method of
RENEE LANTNER, M.D.
*Loyola University Medical Center*
*Maywood, Illinois,*

MARK BALLOW, M.D.
*State University of New York at Buffalo and*
*The Children's Hospital of Buffalo*
*Buffalo, New York,*

and

RICHARD D. deSHAZO, M.D.
*University of South Alabama School of Medicine*
*Mobile, Alabama*

### EPIDEMIOLOGY

Anaphylaxis is a potentially life-threatening symptom complex resulting from the sudden release of mast cell– or basophil-derived mediators into the circulatory system. Anaphylaxis is a major medical problem because 1 in every 2700 hospitalized patients experiences drug-induced anaphylaxis and between 400 and 800 patients die each year from allergic reactions to beta-lactam antibiotics alone. Serum sickness results in a different symptom complex whereby immune complexes activate the complement system, resulting in localized inflammatory tissue damage. Serum sickness reactions are much less common than they were several decades ago, when animal-derived antitoxins were used for passive immunizations.

### ANAPHYLAXIS

#### Pathophysiology

Classic anaphylaxis results from the bridging of IgE molecules on the surface of mast cells or basophils by an antigen-causing mediator release (Figure 1). Mediators released from mast cells and basophils include histamine, arachidonic acid metabolites (leukotrienes and prostaglandins), platelet-activating factor, and chemotactic factors, which contribute to smooth muscle contraction, increased vascular permeability, secretion of mucus, and inflammatory responses characteristic of anaphylaxis.

Anaphylactoid reactions are reactions that mimic the symptoms of classic anaphylaxis but are produced by non–IgE-mediated mechanisms, such as direct mast cell degranulation, modulation of arachidonic acid metabolism, or activation of the complement cascade by immune complexes. Anaphylatoxins derived from complement component fragments (e.g., C3a, C5a) cause increased vascular permeability, smooth muscle contractility, and inflammatory cell mobilization, as well as release of additional mediators from mast cells. The distinction between anaphylaxis and anaphylactoid reactions has little clinical meaning because the symptom complex and the treatment are the same for each.

### Etiology

**IgE-Mediated Reactions (Anaphylaxis).** Hundreds of agents are known to cause anaphylaxis. Some examples of these are shown in Table 1. Recent additions include anaphylaxis associated with murine monoclonal antibodies used for diagnostic purposes or in transplantation rejection therapy, reactions to chymopapain used for chemonucleolysis, anaphylaxis to the venom of the imported fire ant (a growing problem in the southern United States), reactions occurring during dialysis to ethylene oxide gas used in the sterilization of dialysis tubing, and anaphylaxis to natural rubber, which is found in latex surgical gloves, balloons, and ileostomy bags. IgE-mediated hypersensitivity to many of these agents can be demonstrated in vivo by immediate-type skin testing or in vitro by the radioallergosorbent test.

**Non–IgE-Mediated Reactions (Anaphylactoid).** A similarly diverse group of agents has been associated with anaphylactoid reactions. Included in Table 2 are agents that cause the same symptom complex as that of anaphylaxis but are mediated by non-immunologic mechanisms. Anaphylactoid reactions to iodinated contrast media have been studied extensively. These agents not only cause direct release of mediators from mast cells and basophils but also activate the complement and coagulation systems. Nonsteroidal anti-inflammatory agents and bisulfite preservatives may cause acute anaphylactoid reactions in individu-

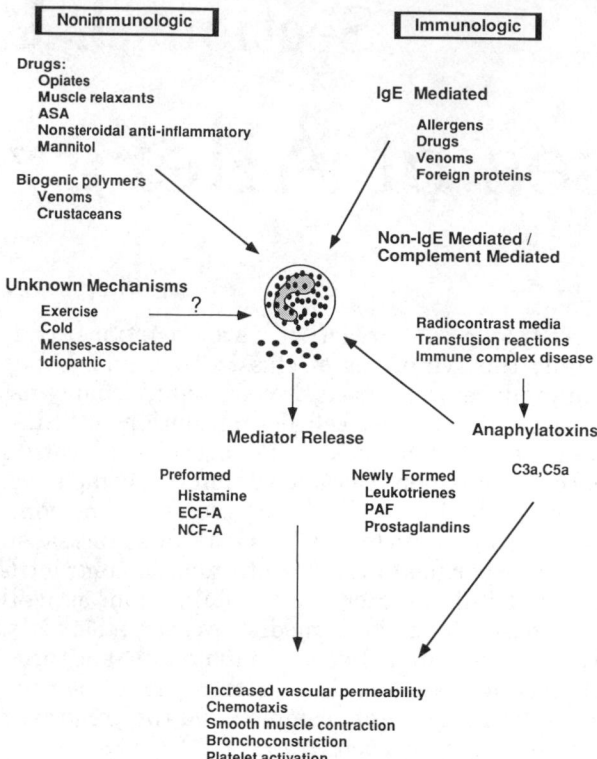

**Figure 1.** Diagram of anaphylactic and anaphylactoid mechanisms. ASA = acetylsalicylic acid; ECF-A = eosinophilic chemotactic factor of anaphylaxis; NCF-A = neutrophil chemotactic factor of anaphylaxis; PAF = platelet-activating factor.

als with no previous history of asthma or, more commonly, bronchospasm in a subpopulaton of patients with chronic asthma.

**Reactions with Unknown Pathogenesis.** Exercise-induced anaphylaxis occurs with prolonged, strenuous exercise, frequently in conditioned run-

TABLE 1. **Classes and Examples of Agents That Cause Anaphylaxis**

Hormones: adrenocorticotropic hormone, insulin, hydrocortisone, estradiol, synthetic luteinizing hormone–releasing hormone, parathormone

Animal or human proteins: horse serum (snake antivenin, antilymphocyte globulin), seminal fluid, Factor VIII, protamine sulfate, monoclonal antibodies, human serum albumin

Enzymes: chymotrypsin, chymopapain, streptokinase, asparaginase

Venoms: fire ants, wasps, yellow jackets, snakes

Animal danders: cat, horse, dog, and others

Foods: eggs, milk, shellfish, nuts, and others

Drugs: penicillin, cephalosporin, and others

Polysaccharides: dextran, iron dextran

Miscellaneous: ethylene oxide gas on dialysis tubing, hydatid cyst rupture, natural rubber (latex)

TABLE 2. **Representative Agents That Cause Anaphylactoid Reactions**

Nonsteroidal anti-inflammatory agents: acetylsalicylic acid, indomethacin, ibuprofen, and others

Diagnostic agents: iodinated contrast media*

Muscle relaxants:† d-tubocurarine, succinylcholine

Preservatives: bisulfites, metabisulfites

Opiates: codeine, morphine, and others

Mannitol

Blood products: intravenous gamma globulin, blood, plasma, cryoprecipitate

*Incidence of repeat reactions decreased to <5% by pretreatment with prednisone, 50 mg PO, at 6-hr intervals for three doses, with the last dose 1 hr before the procedure, plus diphenhydramine, 50 mg PO or IM, and ephedrine, 25 mg PO, 1 hr before administration (the latter not to be used in the presence of cardiac disease).
†Some of these reactions may be IgE-mediated.

ners, and is usually preceded by a short prodrome of generalized pruritus. In some cases, exercise-induced anaphylaxis occurs only after the ingestion of certain foods, such as shellfish or celery. Recently, a group of women who experienced attacks of anaphylaxis associated with menses were successfully treated with a luteinizing hormone–releasing hormone analogue and/or oophorectomy, implying a role for sex hormones in the pathogenesis of this condition. The mechanism of cold urticaria, which can lead to severe hypotension with total body exposure, is not totally understood; however, cryoglobulins may be involved, causing mast cell mediator release. A syndrome of repeated episodes of anaphylaxis for which no cause can be determined despite extensive evaluation is idiopathic anaphylaxis.

### Clinical Manifestations

The signs and symptoms of anaphylaxis reflect the effects of the released mediators on target organs, involving either a single organ, such as the skin, or multiple organ systems in more severe cases (Table 3). These reactions usually occur within seconds to minutes after exposure to the responsible agent but may be delayed for hours with some agents, especially foods. Anaphylactic reactions are commonly preceded by a short prodrome of nasal, eye, and genital itching or burning and then by urticaria and angioedema. In cases of massive mediator release, laryngospasm, bronchospasm, hypotension, arrhythmias, syncope, diarrhea, and uterine cramping may ensue. Some patients experience recurrence of symptoms up to 8 hours after the initial reaction. These recurrences termed "biphasic anaphylactic reactions," may be caused by partial therapy of the initial reaction or may constitute a secondary response similar to the late-phase response in asthma. Persistent anaphylaxis is a form of anaphylaxis that may last for 5 to 32 hours and occurs in up to 28% of patients.

### Differential Diagnosis

Vasovagal reactions that occur under stress— for example, during dental surgery—must be distinguished from anaphylactic reactions. In vasovagal reactions (compared with anaphylaxis), the pulse is slow rather than rapid, the blood pressure is normal or elevated rather than decreased, and the skin is cool rather than warm from vasodilation. Patients with systemic mastocytosis have recurrent episodes of flushing, tachycardia, pruritus, headache, abdominal pain, diarrhea, or syncope. Pseudoanaphylactic reactions have been described after intramuscular injection of procaine penicillin and are thought to be caused by the release of free procaine. Symptoms include visual hallucinations, unusual tastes, fright, combativeness, twitching, and seizures. Factitious anaphylaxis is defined as repeated, self-induced episodes of anaphylaxis. Patients with hereditary angioedema have episodes of laryngeal edema and painless, nonpruritic swelling of the extremities, frequently associated with abdominal pain and often occurring after trauma, such as dental surgery. Globus hystericus should be considered when the major complaint is a chronic "lump in the throat" and no anatomic abnormalities are found.

### Treatment

The treatment of anaphylaxis depends on the severity of the reaction. The use of aqueous epinephrine is key because it inhibits mediator release, restores vasomotor tone, and relaxes bronchial smooth muscle. The early use of antihistamines blocks histamine effects such as car-

#### TABLE 3. Signs of Anaphylaxis

| Organ System | Signs and Symptoms |
|---|---|
| General | Sense of impending doom, malaise, weakness, dizziness, syncope |
| Cutaneous | Erythema, urticaria, angioedema, pruritus, warmth |
| Respiratory | Sneezing, rhinorrhea, nasal congestion, dysphagia, laryngospasm, bronchospasm, stridor, dyspnea, tachypnea, wheezing, cyanosis |
| Cardiovascular | Tachycardia, hypotension, arrhythmias, faintness, palpitations |
| Gastrointestinal | Vomiting, diarrhea, abdominal cramps, tenesmus, nausea |
| Genitourinary | Uterine contractions, bladder urgency |

#### TABLE 4. Treatment of Anaphylaxis

1. Establish secure airway with oropharyngeal or endotracheal tube or, if necessary, by cricothyroidotomy. Administer oxygen if appropriate.

2. Inject aqueous epinephrine 1:1000, 0.01 ml/kg, up to 0.3 ml SC; repeat every 15–20 min as needed.

3. If anaphylaxis followed an injection, apply tourniquet proximal to injection site, removing briefly every 10–15 min, and give additional epinephrine 1:1000, 0.01 ml/kg, up to 0.2 ml, into injection site.

4. Give diphenhydramine, 1–2 mg/kg, up to 50 mg IV or IM; repeat every 4–6 hr as needed for urticaria and angioedema.

5. Monitor vital signs frequently.

6. Place patient in recumbent position and elevate legs.

7. If patient is hypotensive, begin IV infusion with isotonic crystalloid or colloid solutions, using large-bore catheter.

8. If hypotension persists, consider slow administration of IV epinephrine 1:10,000, 0.1 ml/kg, up to 10 ml (1 mg), over 5–10 min; this may be administered as a continuous infusion of 0.5–5 μg/min (0.1–1 μg/kg/min in children).

9. If preceding regimen fails, administer dopamine, 2–50 μg/kg/min, titrating to blood pressure.

10. For resistant hypotension caused by beta blockade, glucagon, 1–5 mg IV over 1 min, may be beneficial; because of short-term effects, a continuous infusion, 1–5 mg/hr, may be required. Side effects may include nausea, vomiting, and hypoglycemia. Bronchospasm may not be affected.

11. For bronchospasm, infuse aminophylline, 6 mg/kg IV over 20 min, followed by a continous drip of 0.5–0.8 mg/kg/hr (base on pre-existing plasma theophylline level, if applicable) and administer inhaled beta adrenergics (metaproterenol, albuterol, terbutaline) every 1–2 hr as needed.

12. Corticosteroids should be administered to prevent late-phase reactions as hydrocortisone, 250–500 mg IV every 4–6 hr (4–8 mg/kg for children); or methylprednisolone, 40–120 mg IV every 4–6 hr (1 mg/kg/dose for children); or prednisone, 30–40 mg PO every 12 hr (1–2 mg/kg/day for children) if less severe. Taper doses appropriately, if necessary.

13. For resistant or prolonged anaphylaxis, cimetidine, 300 mg IV or IM, may be beneficial in some cases.

diac arrhythmias and peripheral vasodilation. Establishing an airway, as in any critical situation, is imperative. A step-by-step approach to the management of anaphylaxis is outlined in Table 4. If the agent causing anaphylaxis has been injected into an extremity, continued absorption of the agent can be decreased by the use of tourniquets and the local injection of epinephrine. If the patient is cyanotic, oxygen should be administered. If bronchospasm is present, administration of an inhaled beta agonist or intravenous aminophylline should be added, keeping in mind that aminophylline may cause hypotension if infused too rapidly. If the patient is hypotensive, rapid infusion of intravenous fluid is indicated. If peripheral administration of epinephrine is unsuccessful, cautious intravenous administration of epinephrine, preferably with cardiac monitoring, should be considered. If hypotension persists, the use of vasopressors and the monitoring of pulmonary wedge pressure should be undertaken. Individuals who experience anaphylaxis while taking beta-adrenergic blockers are at risk for severe reactions that may be difficult to reverse. These individuals require much larger volumes of fluid replacement and vasopressor drug treatment than does the usual patient with anaphylaxis. Glucagon may reverse the hypotension in these patients. However, effects may be short-lived (less than 30 minutes unless a continuous infusion is used), and side effects include hypoglycemia with prolonged use resulting from depletion of glycogen stores, nausea, and vomiting, which can be hazardous in a patient with altered consciousness. Further studies are required to determine optimal dose regimens. Besides beta-adrenergic blocking drugs, pre-existing asthma and cardiac disease increase the risk of severe anaphylaxis, with significant morbidity and mortality. The administration of corticosteroids does not help in the early stages but may prevent late or prolonged reactions and should be given in all severe cases of anaphylaxis. All patients should be observed for several hours after anaphylaxis has resolved because symptoms may recur up to 8 hours later in 20% of the patients.

## SERUM SICKNESS

Serum sickness develops when antigen-antibody complexes form in the presence of slight antigen excess, are of critical size, and are present in sufficient amounts to be deposited in the blood vessels of various tissues. Symptoms are not present when the inciting antigen is first introduced. The appearance of host antibody 1 to 2 weeks later results in immune complex formation. These immune complexes lodge in the vascular walls, where complement activation occurs. Activated complement components, particularly C3a and C5a anaphylatoxins, increase vascular permeability and are chemotactic to neutrophils, which cause tissue damage by releasing proteolytic enzymes. As the immune response continues and antibody excess develops, these larger complexes are taken up by the mononuclear phagocytic system, and symptoms eventually resolve.

The causative antigens may be exogenous, from infecting organisms or drugs, or endogenous (organ specific or nonspecific), from damaged tissues. Drugs are the most common cause of these reactions and include heterologous sera (antilymphocyte globulin, antivenins), antibiotics (penicillin, sulfonamides), nonsteroidal anti-inflammatory

TABLE 5. **Features of Serum Sickness**

| Signs and Symptoms | Frequency (%) |
| --- | --- |
| Fever, malaise | 100 |
| Cutaneous eruptions (urticarial, morbilliform) | 90–95 |
| Arthralgia | 50–77 |
| Generalized vasculitis | Rare |
| Peripheral neuritis | Rare |
| Glomerulonephritis | Rare |
| Guillain-Barré syndrome | Rare |

drugs (phenylbutazone, naproxen), hydantoins, and thiazides. Serum sickness can also occur in association with infections such as hepatitis B, rickettsial disease, and subacute bacterial endocarditis.

Patients with serum sickness experience fever, urticarial or morbilliform eruptions, lymphadenopathy, arthralgia or arthritis, and vasculitis with palpable purpuric lesions on the skin of the extremities (Table 5). Patients may also have a purpuric or erythematous band at the junctions of plantar and palmar skin. In severe cases, neuritis, glomerulonephritis, and hypertension may occur and, rarely, a Guillain-Barré–type picture is seen. The diagnosis of serum sickness is made on the basis of the typical symptom complex, although certain laboratory findings are helpful. Total hemolytic complement ($CH_{50}$) and the specific complement components C3 and C4 may be decreased, suggesting complement consumption. The erythrocyte sedimentation rate may be elevated. Circulating immune complexes are often detected by C1q binding or Raji cell assay, as well as by immunofluorescence of skin or kidney biopsy specimens.

If the agent causing serum sickness can be identified, exposure to it should be stopped and subsequently avoided. Most commonly, symptoms resolve within 2 to 3 weeks after exposure to the causative agents ceases, and recovery is generally complete. If exposure is chronic, a syndrome of systemic vasculitis may result.

During the acute phase of serum sickness, the patient should be treated with antihistamines such as hydroxyzine (Atarax, Vistaril), 25 to 50 mg at bedtime or every 4 to 6 hours if needed. If arthralgia or arthritis is present, nonsteroidal anti-inflammatory agents may be helpful. More commonly, prednisone, 1 to 2 mg per kg per day (maximum, 60 mg), is administered as two divided doses for 5 to 7 days, followed by a single daily dose for several days. This dosage is then tapered over an additional 7 to 10 days. In severe cases, prednisone may be required for longer periods.

# ASTHMA IN THE ADOLESCENT AND ADULT

method of
JOHN M. WEILER, M.D., and
KAREN KELLEY MAVES, M.D.*
*University of Iowa*
*Iowa City, Iowa*

Asthma remains difficult to define. The American Thoracic Society (ATS) has struggled for years to define asthma to encompass all of the variants and yet to exclude diseases which clearly are not asthma. For the purposes of this discussion we adopt the ATS definition of 1982: "Asthma is. . . a syndrome whose primary characteristic is: (1) reversible (2) airway obstruction."

Reversibility is important because it distinguishes asthma from chronic nonreversible lung obstruction (COPD). In general, an improvement of 15 to 20% in the forced expiratory volume in 1 second ($FEV_1$) after treatment is sufficient to document reversibility. In addition, a spontaneous improvement of 15 to 20% in $FEV_1$ may be taken as evidence for reversibility.

Airway obstruction may be manifested by symptoms of wheeze, cough, shortness of breath, chest tightness, or even burning in the chest. Airway obstruction may be documented objectively by a decrease in $FEV_1$ after exercise, hyperventilation, or spontaneously, particularly if that decrease can be reversed by the administration of a pharmacologic agent. Furthermore, a decrease in $FEV_1$ after inhalation of antigen to which the patient is sensitive may be used to confirm allergic (extrinsic) asthma. However, a decrease in $FEV_1$ after pharmacologic treatment (e.g., inhalation of histamine or methacholine) does not by itself diagnose asthma.

Asthma is common and may afflict as much as 10 to 15% of the population at some time in their lives. Past reports from the National Institutes of Health estimate the prevalence of asthma in adults at 7%, but this estimate may be low when one includes all of the asthma variants. For example, asthma is often missed in adolescents who manifest the symptoms only after exercise in cold weather. This diagnosis may also be missed in adults who never exercise because they always feel out of shape, with tightness and burning in the lungs when they do exercise. It is more likely that asthma occurs in about 12% of adults.

## PATHOGENESIS

Patients challenged to breathe allergen to which they are sensitive may have a dual response. Within minutes (early response) there is a drop in flow rates (e.g., $FEV_1$, mid expiratory flow rate [MEFR], and peak expiratory flow rate [PEFR]) which return toward the baseline within 1 hour. This is followed 3 to 4 hours later (late response) by a more prolonged decrease in flow rates which may even persist for days. The late response is thought to play a predominant role in chronic allergic asthma because of the presence of

*Recipient of an NIH Immunology Training grant.

inflammatory cells such as mast cells, neutrophils, and eosinophils.

An assortment of mechanisms appear to be important in the pathogenesis of asthma. Mast cell degranulation and eosinophil degranulation cause release of a vast number of important chemical mediators of inflammation (e.g., leukotrienes, prostaglandins, histamine, eosinophil chemotactic factors, eosinophil granule major basic protein, and platelet activating factor). In addition to these cells, neutrophils and lymphocytes also are found in bronchoalveolar lavage fluid from patients with asthma. The cholinergic nervous system and neuropeptides have recently been studied for an important role in asthma. Asthma should properly be viewed as a heterogeneous clinical syndrome; thus it is likely that all of these mechanisms combine in a variety of ways to produce clinical asthma.

## DIAGNOSTIC CATEGORIES

Allergic (extrinsic) asthma is often differentiated from nonallergic (intrinsic) asthma. The following diagnostic groups might be used:

Allergic
  Triggered by mold, pollen, dust mite, and/or dander
  Allergic bronchopulmonary aspergillosis (ABPA)
Nonallergic
  No specific trigger
  Chemical induced
  Exercise induced
  Drug induced
  Postinfectious
  Associated with sinus infection

Another way to classify asthma might be by the frequency of airway obstruction:

Perennial symptoms
  Allergic (e.g., dust, mold, dander)
  Nonallergic
    No specific trigger
    Chemical exposure
    Occupational exposure
Seasonal symptoms
  Allergic (e.g., pollens)
  Nonallergic
    Occupational exposure
Acute intermittent symptoms
  Allergic (e.g., foods, animals, molds)
  Nonallergic
    Exercise induced
    Drug induced
"Variant" Asthma
  Cough

These categories demonstrate the many faces of asthma, some easily recognizable (e.g., exercise-induced asthma) and others which are often hidden diagnoses (e.g., cough variant asthma). It is important to remember the old adage that all that wheezes is not asthma and asthma does not always cause wheezing. The astute physician recognizes the many patterns by which asthma presents and is able to fit the diagnosis to the patient.

However, even with a long and cumbersome definition, some presentations defy diagnosis and remain for the clinician to resolve. For example, do any of the following patients with reversible airway obstruction have asthma?

1. Wheezing and obstruction that occur only after upper respiratory infections caused by specific agents.

2. Wheezing and obstruction that are provoked only by polluted air.

3. Wheezing and obstruction only during the height of the ragweed season in a patient with severe allergic rhinitis after high pollen exposure.

## ASSESSMENT OF THE PATIENT WITH ASTHMA

A full history must be obtained. First, it is important to determine whether the patient is presenting with an acute attack, continuing chronic symptoms, or a flare in chronic asthma. The following historical details are crucial:

1. Previous occasions when the patient sought treatment for asthma, including childhood episodes.

2. Medications taken in the past to control symptoms of asthma, including prescription and nonprescription drugs.

3. The nature of the symptoms at present.

4. Recent and past exposure history (e.g., to pets, dust, mold, irritants).

5. Occupation and hobby history (including exposure to isocyanates and other chemicals known to cause asthma).

6. Seasonal variation in symptoms.

7. The role of exercise, cold air, and hyperventilation in causing symptoms.

8. Medicines, foods, and additives that cause symptoms (e.g., penicillin, aspirin, peanuts, metabisulfites).

9. Presence of other allergic disease (e.g., rhinitis).

10. Presence of symptoms suggesting sinus infection.

A thorough history will often uncover details about the nature of the syndrome which will help in its control. For example, a veterinary student who is allergic to animals may be best advised to change his or her field of study. A body shop painter who has developed asthma after exposure to the chemicals in automobile paint might seek employment where there will not be continued exposure to these chemicals.

The physical examination has traditionally emphasized chest auscultation and this remains important. However, treatment of asthmatic patients also requires access to simple office spirometry. Patients may present with moderate or even severe asthma and have findings on physical examination which will trick the physician into thinking that the patient is doing well. Patients during the recovery phase from an asthmatic attack may become asymptomatic and have a normal chest examination and yet have significant impairment on pulmonary function testing. At a minimum, the clinician must have a machine that will record $FEV_1$ and FVC (forced vital capacity). It is ideal to have a machine that will also determine flow rates (e.g., $FEF_{25-75}$, PEFR) and present a flow loop. However, occasionally a patient who has both a normal physical examination and normal pulmonary function tests will complain of symptoms at hours when the clinic is not open. These patients should not be dismissed as being healthy without obtaining flow rates at times when the symptoms occur. A mini-Wright peak flow meter is ideal for these patients, who can be taught how to use the meter and to record flow rates at the appropriate times. We often have patients obtain twice daily flow rates (upon arising and at bedtime). In athletes, the mini-Wright peak flow meter may document the presence of exercise-induced asthma in the sports-specific setting (described later).

The remainder of the physical examination should focus on the nose, sinuses, pharynx, and heart to evaluate the patient for the presence of rhinitis, polyps, sinus disease, and cardiac asthma. In the patient with acute respiratory difficulty, the clinician should seek clues to the severity of the attack such as intercostal retractions, upright posture, sweating, and tachycardia.

All newly diagnosed asthma patients should receive a complete blood count with differential to document the presence of eosinophils, a sputum examination for eosinophils, and skin testing for sensitivity to common aeroallergens (molds, weed pollens, grass pollens). In general, a chest x-ray should also be obtained. A plain x-ray sinus series or coronal sinus computed tomography (CT) films should be obtained on patients in whom sinus disease is suspected. In a patient with a pulmonary infiltrate on chest x-ray, the diagnosis of allergic bronchopulmonary aspergillosis (ABPA) should be entertained. This diagnosis can be made when the patient is found to have a positive immediate intradermal skin test to aspergillus, increased total IgE, precipitating antibodies to aspergillus in plasma, peripheral blood eosinophilia, and central bronchiectasis. This diagnosis is important because it indicates the need for prolonged steroid therapy.

In the initial evaluation of the mild asthmatic patient ($FEV_1$ greater than 80% predicted), it is occasionally helpful to determine that the patient with airway obstruction responds to the inhalation of methacholine (Provocholine) or histamine. Exquisite sensitivity to either of these agents tends to support strongly the diagnosis of asthma. However, frequently in cases where the diagnosis of asthma is in some doubt, the methacholine or histamine bronchial provocation test is also equivocal.

## TREATMENT

The physician must work energetically to teach the patient about asthma so that the patient can actively participate in treatment. The patient should be encouraged to keep a symptom diary to determine when therapy is needed and the effectiveness of that therapy. A mini-Wright peak flow meter can often be used by the patient at home to document objectively the course of the asthma.

### Inhaled Medications

**Metered-Dose Inhaler (MDI).** No inhaled medication can be effective unless it is properly administered. Each patient should be taught the correct method of using the inhaler and the technique should be reviewed frequently. The technique we use is to hold the MDI just at the entrance to the open mouth. The patient is advised to exhale normally, a tidal breath (not an exaggerated breath), and then to begin slowly to inhale. As the patient begins to hear the air being inspired around the inhaler, the patient compresses the canister and continues to inhale at a constant speed to completely fill the lungs. The patient then holds his breath for 10 seconds before exhaling. This constitutes one puff (one inspiration or one dose).

Patients who have difficulty with the mechanics of this technique may benefit from the use of a spacer. We use either the Aerochamber or the InspirEase. Spacers may also be useful in patients who develop oral candidiasis from inhaled steroids. Accessory devices are available for patients with arthritis or other hand deformities. Rotahaler breath-triggered devices are now available; Rotacaps containing albuterol (Ventolin, Proventil) in powdered form are inserted into a Rotahaler which separates the capsule. When the patient breathes, the powdered medication is inhaled into the lungs. The Rotahaler does not require patients to coordinate pushing a canister with breathing.

**Inhaled Beta$_2$ Adrenergic Agonists.** Inhaled beta$_2$ adrenergic agonists are often the first-line therapy for asthmatic patients. Most of the standard drugs used in the United States, including metaproterenol (Alupent, Metaprel), albuterol (Proventil, Ventolin), terbutaline (Brethaire), pirbuterol (Maxair), and bitolterol (Tornalate), are strongly beta$_2$ receptor selective. Stimulation of beta$_2$ receptors, located in the airways, is thought to increase cyclic-AMP production in airway smooth muscle and mast cells. This in turn causes airway dilation and inhibits further mast cell degranulation, thereby reducing asthma symptoms. Side effects of these medications include palpitations and tremor which may result from stimulation of cardiac (beta$_1$) and peripheral skeletal muscle (beta$_2$) receptors.

Inhaled beta$_2$ adrenergic agonists have rapid onset with duration of action, which is about 4 to 6 hours. The usual dose is two inhalations. We prescribe beta$_2$ adrenergic agonists to be taken by MDI on an as needed basis or a regular schedule. For regular use, the patient is typically told to inhale one breath of albuterol every 4 hours while awake (e.g., at about 8:00 a.m., 12 noon, 4:00 p.m., and 8:00 p.m.). Then about 20 minutes later the patient inhales an additional breath of albuterol (e.g., at about 8:20 a.m., 12:20 p.m., 4:20 p.m., and 8:20 p.m.). We recommend a 10- to 20-minute separation between inhalations of beta$_2$ adrenergic agonist because this appears to be considerably more efficacious than if the two inhalations are taken in rapid succession. If additional inhalations are needed between dosing intervals, the patient is told to take only one inhalation. Generally the dosage is established so that the patient should take no more than 12 inhalations per day. If more beta$_2$ adrenergic agonist is needed, the patient is told to contact the physician. Occasionally, a patient who is having an increase in asthmatic symptoms may require MDI therapy every 1 to 2 hours, and in those cases, a physician must evaluate the severity of the symptoms. Patients who have asthma attacks brought on by cold air or exercise exposure may use an inhaled beta$_2$ adrenergic agonist 5 to 15 minutes prior to exposure and again after symptoms develop.

**Inhaled Steroids.** We often prescribe inhaled steroids to be taken with regular doses of inhaled beta$_2$ adrenergic agonists in the treatment of chronic asthma. With the recognition of the role that inflammation may play in asthma, inhaled steroids may soon overtake theophylline in the early therapy of asthma. Inhaled steroids can also be viewed as "steroid-sparing" agents for patients who are dependent on oral steroids, occasionally allowing oral steroids to be discontinued. However, it is important to emphasize that chronic daily steroids must be tapered slowly when inhaled steroids are begun to prevent serious consequences of steroid withdrawal.

The inhaled steroid preparations approved in the United States include beclomethasone dipropionate (Vanceril, Beclovent), triamcinolone acetonide (Azmacort), and flunisolide (AeroBid). Generally, the most common side effects of inhaled steroids are oral candidiasis and hoarseness. Candidiasis can sometimes be prevented by using a spacer device and by rinsing the mouth with saline after use of the inhaler. Few systemic side effects have been observed after the use of topical steroids when administered at recommended dosages. However, higher doses of inhaled steroids, particularly in combination with oral steroids, may cause adrenal suppression and possibly bone demineralization.

Inhaled steroids are anti-inflammatory agents. They have no bronchodilator activity, and thus, the patient must be told not to expect a quick response to these medications. Inhaled steroids cannot be used on an as needed (prn) basis, taken only on the days when the patient is particularly symptomatic. Instead, the patient should find a stable dose that will control symptoms and then not vary the dose except during seasons when symptoms would not otherwise occur. Furthermore, inhaled steroids are not adequate therapy for severe acute asthma attacks.

The recommended dosage for beclomethasone and triamcinolone is two puffs (84 μg and 200 μg, respectively) three to four times a day, usually after beta$_2$ adrenergic agonist therapy. In theory, the beta$_2$ adrenergic agonist opens the airway to allow maximum distribution of the inhaled steroid. Therefore, when inhaled steroid is added to albuterol therapy, we tell the patient to take the beclomethasone after the albuterol (e.g., after 8:20, 12:20, 4:20, and 8:20). The flunisolide dose is two puffs (500 μg) twice daily. These doses may be increased if needed to control symptoms in patients who are severely affected.

**Cromolyn Sodium.** Cromolyn sodium (Intal) is available in either MDI canisters or liquid form (for use in a nebulizer). Cromolyn has long been thought to stabilize mast cell membranes and inhibit degranulation and release of mast cell mediators such as histamine and leukotrienes. Cromolyn has no bronchodilator activity. This drug is more frequently useful in children but may also be used in adults. It is only used prophylactically and has no value in the treatment of acute asthma. Patients initiated on cromolyn therapy should be monitored for effectiveness in decreasing frequency of attacks, severity of cough, and sputum production for about 6 weeks. If no effect is seen, cromolyn should be discontinued. Occasionally, cromolyn may serve as a steroid-sparing agent and may have efficacy equal to theophylline. Cromolyn is very effective in preventing exercise-induced bronchospasm but again cannot be used to treat symptoms once they occur after exercise.

The typical cromolyn dosage is two sprays (1.6 mg) every 6 hours. The cromolyn dose necessary to prevent exercise-induced asthma must be determined by the patient. Typically as many as five inhalations must be administered 15 to 20 minutes before exercise or before exposure to a known trigger. Frequently, when lower doses are used, the medicine is ineffective in preventing exercise-induced symptoms. A repeat dose may be used if the exposure is prolonged.

The most frequent side effects of cromolyn are mucosal irritation and dryness of the throat and trachea and cough or bronchospasm caused by inhalation of the powder. When cromolyn is administered by MDI, it may also cause unpleasant aftertaste. Nevertheless, cromolyn is one of the safest medications available and is extremely well tolerated by most patients. Its use is limited primarily because it is not always effective in controlling symptoms.

**Anticholinergics.** Ipratropium bromide (Atrovent) is a quaternary ammonium compound, structurally similar to atropine, which exerts bronchodilator activity by antagonizing cholinergic release from the vagus nerve. Anticholinergics seem to be most effective in patients who have chronic airway obstruction and should be considered for use only in asthmatics who have an element of irreversible lung disease. Ipratropium bromide is rarely of value in patients with "pure" asthma and is not approved by the Food and Drug Administration for treating asthma.

The typical initial dosage of ipratropium is two inspirations (36 μg) every 6 hours. Anticholinergic systemic side effects are rare because ipratropium is not readily absorbed. The most common adverse reactions are cough and dry mouth.

**Nebulizer Therapy.** Motor-driven mist nebulizers may be used to administer beta$_2$ adrenergic agonists, cromolyn, or atropine. However, recent studies in adults demonstrate that nebulized medication is no more efficacious than is medicine administered by MDI, particularly when the MDI device is used with a spacer and when larger doses of the MDI medication are taken. The nebulizer is less convenient and much more expensive than MDI medications and should be reserved for emergency room treatment of acute asthmatic exacerbations and for home use by children and the elderly. Patients should be told that MDIs are more convenient and less expensive forms of the same medication with efficacy comparable to that of nebulized medication.

### Oral Medications

**Theophylline.** Theophylline, a methylxanthine, in one form or another, has been used as a bronchodilator for over 50 years. The oldest form is aminophylline, which is 85% theophylline. In recent years, anhydrous theophylline preparations have become more popular, particularly when administered in a sustained-release form because of the increased dosing interval, resulting in greater compliance and less variation in the peak and trough blood levels.

Theophylline is a bronchodilator that acts to inhibit phosphodiesterase which converts 3'5'-cyclic-AMP to 5'-cyclic-AMP. Theophylline also:

1. Improves contractility and decreases fatigability of the diaphragm.
2. Stimulates medullary respiratory centers.
3. Has a diuretic effect.
4. Causes inotropic and chronotropic effects on the heart.
5. Relaxes vascular smooth muscle.
6. Increases ciliary action.

In addition, xanthines may cause transient hyperglycemia and increased secretion of gastric acid. Nevertheless, the primary mechanism by which these drugs improve asthma remains unknown.

Theophylline used to be the mainstay of the

treatment of asthma, but in recent years, its popularity has begun to wane. The history of theophylline is instructive. Early in its use, blood levels were not available, and it was necessary to use the drug cautiously. With the advent of blood levels, it was possible to control the dosage to prevent serious adverse reactions, such as seizures, by keeping the plasma level below 22 μg per ml. However, even with the availability of drug levels, it became apparent that unacceptable side effects (gastrointestinal side effects, tremor, nervousness, and palpitations) occur in as many as one-third of patients who take theophylline and often continue as long as the drug is taken. Finally, it has become clear in recent years that asthma is an inflammatory process, and theophylline is not an anti-inflammatory drug. Consequently, theophylline is falling in popularity and being replaced by other more efficacious medications, particularly medications that have anti-inflammatory activity (e.g., inhaled topical steroids). Currently, we favor the use of theophylline in selected patients who do not have adverse reactions to the drug. For example, sustained release theophylline may be particularly efficacious for patients with nocturnal asthma.

Close monitoring of serum theophylline levels is necessary because of variability in absorption of the various oral theophylline preparations (Table 1), as well as individual patient variability in the rate of hepatic metabolism. The desired therapeutic range is 8 to 20 μg per ml to minimize side effects. However, if the patient is having few asthma symptoms and has a blood level at the lower end of the range, it is not necessary to raise the dosage just to increase the blood level.

The oral starting dose is usually 200 mg every 12 hours, which can then be increased based on patient tolerance and blood levels. The mainte-

nance dose should be reduced in patients with congestive heart failure, liver disease, or advanced age. Patients taking cimetidine (Tagamet) or erythromycin also require dosage reduction. Higher than standard doses are required in smokers. However, blood levels must be monitored closely in these patients and should not exceed 20 μg per ml. Signs of toxicity occur as the serum levels increase and include nausea, vomiting, diarrhea, nervousness, headache, and insomnia. High levels, greater than 40 μg per ml, are associated with encephalopathy, seizures, and cardiac arrhythmia. Seizures are fatal in about half of the cases. Typical parenteral loading and maintenance doses are 5 to 7 mg per kg for aminophylline and 4 to 6 mg per kg for theophylline in 5% dextrose. Usual maintenance doses of aminophylline for nonsmokers, smokers, the elderly, and those with heart or liver failure are 0.5 to 0.7, 0.9, 0.4, and 0.2 to 0.3 mg per kg per hour, respectively. Routine maintenance doses of theophylline in 5% dextrose for nonsmokers, smokers, the elderly, and those with heart or liver failure are 0.4 to 0.6, 0.75, 0.3, and 0.2 mg per kg per hour, respectively.

**Oral Steroid Therapy.** Corticosteroids decrease bronchial inflammation and are the most powerful agents available for treatment of asthma. They are also associated with myriad side effects, such as osteoporosis, cataracts, weight gain and fat redistribution, glucose intolerance, hypertension, and immunosuppression.

Steroid side effects are minimal when they are used infrequently for short courses as treatment for acute asthma exacerbations. Typically, we "burst" the dose of prednisone (Deltasone), a short-acting steroid; we give the average patient 60 mg of prednisone each day in the morning for 7 days. Occasionally, we give the patient a longer course (10 to 14 days), and depending on the patient's tolerance of steroid bursts, we may taper the dose. However, tapering is not always necessary when the drug is given for only 7 days. Occasionally, when the patient does not respond initially to prednisone, we give the drug in divided doses (15 mg every 6 hours). Rarely, patients may require frequent steroid bursts. When frequent bursts of prednisone are required, it is mandatory to look for causes for the asthma flares such as allergic bronchopulmonary aspergillosis and recalcitrant sinus infection. It may also be necessary to administer a daily oral steroid dose. In those cases we frequently attempt to wean the patient from the steroids (e.g., at least once a year) and attempt to administer the steroids on an every-other-day basis if possible. Ideally, maintenance prednisone should be administered at a dose of 10 to 30 mg every other day as a single dose in the morning in such patients in

TABLE 1. **Slow Release Theophylline Compounds**

| Brand Name | Available Doses (mg) | |
| | *Capsules* | *Tablets* |
| --- | --- | --- |
| Constant-T | | 200, 300 |
| Elixophyllin SR | 125, 250 | |
| Quibron-T/SR | | 300 |
| Slo-bid Gyrocaps | 50, 100, 200, 300 | |
| Slo-Phyllin Gyrocaps | 60, 125, 250 | |
| Sustaire | | 100, 300 |
| Theobid Duracaps | 130, 260 | |
| Theo-Dur Sprinkle | 50, 75, 125, 200 | |
| Theovent LA | 125, 250 | |
| Theo-24* | 100, 200, 300 | |
| Theo-Dur | | 100, 200, 300, 450 |
| Theolair-SR | | 200, 250, 300, 500 |
| Uniphyl* | | 200, 400 |

*Once-a-day preparations.

order to minimize adrenal suppression and other side effects. However, it must be remembered that steroid-induced osteoporosis is not alleviated by every-other-day steroid administration. When switching from oral daily to every-other-day steroids, we recommend a slow tapering of the everyday dose. One regimen we advocate involves decreasing the daily dose by 1 mg and increasing the alternate-day dose by 2 mg. Thus, the patient would take the following daily doses of prednisone: 10, 9, 12, 8, 14, 7, 16, etc. At the end of 3 weeks, the patient would be taking 30 mg of prednisone every other day. It is critical to pattern the doses of steroid to the individual patient.

Patients with asthmatic symptoms severe enough to require hospitalization always deserve rapid initiation of steroid therapy. Often steroids are administered by an intravenous route to hospitalized asthmatics, although there is no definite evidence that this is superior to steroids delivered orally. Typically, the intravenous dose of methylprednisolone (Solu-Medrol) is 60 mg every 6 hours.

Steroids are occasionally used to aid in the diagnosis of asthma; a lack of improvement in airway obstruction after an adequate trial of oral steroid tends to make the diagnosis of asthma doubtful. Physicians should not be reluctant to use steroids in patients with significant flares of asthma. A short course of steroids administered early in a flare can be lifesaving, can limit or even obviate the need for hospitalization, and can prevent the return of serious symptoms.

**Oral Adrenergic Agents.** Terbutaline (Brethine), metaproterenol, and albuterol are available for oral administration. Oral preparations are easier to use than MDIs in the elderly and the very young; however, a much higher dose of medication is delivered by the oral route, which may be associated with unwarranted systemic side effects. Consequently, we rarely use these formulations in our practice. They should be reserved only for patients unable to use MDIs. The recent spate of new MDI devices (such as spacers, triggers, and breath-activated devices) have made MDIs available to virtually all patients.

## Parenteral Medications

**Parenteral Sympathomimetics.** Epinephrine administered subcutaneously (0.3 to 0.5 ml of a 1:1000 dilution) is still considered to be useful to treat acute exacerbations of asthma. Epinephrine may be re-administered every 30 minutes for a total of three doses. Relative contraindications are severe hypertension or a pulse greater than 140 beats per minute.

Terbutaline is more specific for beta$_2$ receptors but should not be used initially to treat an acute attack because the onset of action is delayed by 30 to 60 minutes. A typical dose would be 0.25 mg administered subcutaneously. This may be repeated, but a total dose of 0.5 mg should not be exceeded in a 4-hour period.

Patients who require epinephrine or terbutaline in the emergency room or clinic should not be sent home until more intensive therapy (e.g., with Sus-Phrine, regular beta$_2$ adrenergic agonist, inhaled steroid, theophylline, and/or oral steroid) is instituted and follow-up is arranged. Furthermore, it is important to inform the patient that he should return if the disease flares.

## Miscellaneous Therapies

**Oxygen.** During severe asthma attacks, ventilation-perfusion defects occur which may cause marked hypoxia as well as respiratory alkalosis resulting from hyperventilation. Oxygen should be administered in the case of hypoxia and the patient monitored in the hospital. Arterial blood gases should be repeated to detect carbon dioxide retention, which indicates impending respiratory failure.

**Immunotherapy and Avoidance Therapy.** Immunotherapy remains controversial in the treatment of asthma. One well-controlled series of experiments has been performed in patients with cat allergy to demonstrate the potential effectiveness of immunotherapy in decreasing bronchial hyperresponsiveness. Nevertheless, the efficacy of immunotherapy using commercially available materials to treat clinical asthma is not universally accepted. In any case, the decision to initiate immunotherapy should be made by an allergist who will take into consideration whether the patient has had full medical therapy and whether the immunotherapy agent is likely to work. Immunotherapy using pollens (e.g., ragweed and grass) is reasonable in a patient highly sensitive to these pollens because these seasons are reasonably long. Immunotherapy with commercially available mold extracts and dust remains unproven. We do not advocate immunotherapy with tree pollen because the seasons for each pollen are too short (5 to 7 days) to make this therapy practical. We do not advocate immunotherapy for allergies to animals and prefer to recommend avoidance.

No therapy is as effective as avoidance in the patient who is highly sensitive to allergen. The patient who is very sensitive to ragweed will suffer a flare in asthma if he insists on working in fields of ragweed. A farmer who is ragweed sensitive should either hire help to harvest the fields during the ragweed season or use elaborate protective gear to prevent exposure. The body-shop worker who has isocyanate-induced asthma must avoid exposure to the agent in any form so that asthma can be avoided or controlled. The importance of avoidance in these situations cannot be overemphasized.

## MILD TO MODERATE ASTHMA: GENERAL GUIDELINES

We recommend the regular administration of inhaled beta$_2$ adrenergic agonist (albuterol) for patients with mild perennial asthma. Alternatively, the patient may be treated with theophylline (if it is tolerated by the patient and felt to be efficacious) or cromolyn as first-line drugs. We recommend inhaled beta$_2$ adrenergic agonists for patients with mild asthma which occurs only on an intermittent basis. The patient with a known trigger (e.g., animals, exercise, or pollen exposure) is advised to take preventive inhalations of the beta$_2$ adrenergic agonist or cromolyn prior to exposure. Beta$_2$ adrenergic agonists are often very effective in these situations in patients with mild asthma. We may prescribe inhaled steroids for patients with chronic symptoms of asthma, depending on whether the patient has evidence of inflammation in the airways.

If the patient's symptoms are not easily controlled by administration of a single medication, we will add a second medication. Thus, the patient receiving only inhaled albuterol may have theophylline added, and the patient receiving only theophylline may have inhaled albuterol added; alternatively, cromolyn may be added. Furthermore, as the severity of the symptoms increases, we are more pressed to add inhaled steroids to treat pulmonary inflammatory disease.

It is extremely important for patients with either chronic perennial or acute intermittent asthma to be followed closely. On these follow-up visits we ask about and grade asthma symptoms to determine efficacy of therapy. We ask about cough, wheeze, shortness of breath, chest tightness, and sleep disturbance. We also obtain office spirometry at each visit. In selected cases we might also ask the patient to obtain flow rates at home in the mornings and evenings.

## MODERATE TO SEVERE CHRONIC ASTHMA: GENERAL GUIDELINES

As the severity of asthma increases, we are inclined to add more medications and to be even more certain that important triggers have not been missed. Pharmacotherapy should include inhaled beta$_2$ adrenergic agonist, inhaled topical steroid, theophylline, if tolerated and shown to be efficacious, and cromolyn, if efficacious. As the frequency of flares increases, we may also add oral steroids. In these cases, it is again vital to determine that no important trigger has been overlooked. For example, the patient whose steroid-dependent asthma is caused by his pet cat must be warned to avoid exposure to the cat.

Severe asthma that requires chronic mid- to high-dose steroids presents a difficult challenge to the physician. These patients should be referred to a specialist so that alternative therapies can be considered. Methotrexate, troleandomycin (TAO), and gold (Myochrysone, Solganal) therapy are all experimental but must be considered for patients with intractable asthma who require moderately high doses of steroids. These patients are at risk for the side effects of continuing steroid administration as well as the risk of continued asthma.

## TREATMENT OF ACUTE ASTHMA

An acute flare in asthma presents special problems that require rapid recognition and institution of therapy. First, it is important to have a full and comprehensive history. If the patient has not been treated previously, this will require taking an extensive history and physical examination. The physician must look for specific triggers which would explain this flare in asthma; recent respiratory infection, animal exposure, or ingestion of specific food may explain the flare in asthma. It is especially important to determine whether the patient has been receiving and taking medications to treat asthma in order to determine which additional medications are needed to treat the flare. The treatment of an acute flare in a patient who is diligent about taking medications will vary considerably from the treatment of a patient who has not been seen previously by a physician for asthma or who has been seen and treated but who has not taken the medicines prescribed.

On physical examination, the physician must seek clues to the severity of the acute respiratory difficulty. Office spirometry is frequently more valuable than blood gases and should be obtained. The FEV$_1$ may be severely depressed before there is a decrease in PO$_2$, so a reliance on blood gases may give a false sense of security. The blood gas will demonstrate respiratory alkalosis early in an asthma flare (PO$_2$ nearly normal, PCO$_2$ less than 30, pH greater than 7.45). As the patient tires, the blood gas normalizes (PCO$_2$ = 40, pH = 7.40). The blood gas only becomes abnormal (PCO$_2$ greater than 40, pH less than 7.4) late in the course of an acute flare, whereas the FEV$_1$ is depressed early when treatment may avert more serious respiratory difficulty.

Treatment should be initiated prior to the completion of the assessment. Initial therapy might include subcutaneous epinephrine (0.3 ml of 1:1000) and inhaled beta$_2$ adrenergic agonist (albuterol) administered by MDI or nebulized. Steroids should be started early; give 60 mg of prednisone, by an oral route if possible. Oxygen and intravenous fluids should also be administered depending on the seriousness of the flare. There is no role for cromolyn or inhaled steroids in the treatment of an acute flare of asthma. These medications may be started but should not be expected to alleviate the flare in asthma. Similarly, we rarely initiate theophylline therapy in patients having an acute flare because recent studies suggest that theophylline has no role in the emergency treatment of flares.

Admission to the hospital is determined by the severity of the flare and response to therapy. Patients who require oxygen and intravenous therapy obviously need admission. Patients with a risk for respiratory collapse also need admission because they will need to be intubated if they become too fatigued. A variety of schemes exist to evaluate the need for hospitalization. The decision to hospitalize the patient with acute asthma primarily rests upon the response to treatment. Patients who are sent home without hospitalization require initiation of intensive therapy and must be scheduled for follow-up. It is also important for the patient to be told to return to the emergency room or clinic if the disease should flare up again before the scheduled appointment.

## EXERCISE-INDUCED ASTHMA

Exercise has long been known to be a trigger for asthma in susceptible individuals. Indeed, most studies show that about 90% of patients with chronic asthma have increased airway obstruction after exercise. Another group of healthy individuals will experience asthma symptoms only after exercise. These individuals may think that they are out of shape and that, if they were in better shape, they might not suffer chest symptoms such as tightness, coughing, and burning.

The treatment for exercise-induced asthma depends on whether the patient has chronic asthma or has only acute attacks brought on by exercise. Chronic asthma should be treated as described above. In general, as the chronic symptoms decrease so will the exercise-induced symptoms, and the patient will be better able to tolerate exercise. Pure exercise-induced asthma should be treated with inhalers. Many patients find that a single breath of beta$_2$ adrenergic agonist (albuterol) taken 5 to 15 minutes before exercise will prevent symptoms. A repeat inhalation may be taken just prior to the beginning of exercise and then 2 to 4 hours later, depending on the sport. Cromolyn sodium is particularly effective in the prevention of exercise-induced asthma symptoms. The MDI form of cromolyn should generally be used, and it may require five or more breaths in order to prevent the symptoms of exercise-induced asthma. In more severe cases, theophylline, administered chronically to produce therapeutic blood levels, has been used to prevent exercise-induced asthma. Rarely, chronic inhaled steroids can be used, but this should be reserved for patients with chronic asthma.

Physicians should be aware that some sports are more likely to produce asthma than others. The following list grades exercise from most to least likely to cause asthma: free running, treadmill, cycling, downhill skiing, swimming, walking. Furthermore, it is wise to suggest that individuals who are prone to exercise-induced asthma avoid breathing cold air. When walking in cold air, the patient should use a scarf wrapped over the mouth to help pre-warm the air; masks are effective but unpopular because they imply contagious illness. Recent studies suggest that pre-exercise warm-ups, if performed properly, can decrease the symptoms of exercise-induced asthma. For example, a football player may run across the field ten times with a minute rest between runs prior to practice or a game, and this can result in lessening or abolition of bronchospasm after the subsequent exercise. Exercise-induced asthma can generally be treated easily and can result in a much higher quality of life for the patient.

## CONCLUSION

Asthma is common and usually responds well to therapy. However, asthma may also be fatal, and the frequency of deaths from asthma appears to be on the rise in recent years. Consequently, it is important for the physician to recognize asthma and to initiate treatment promptly.

# ASTHMA IN CHILDREN

method of
NANCY P. CUMMINGS, M.D.
*Stanford University Hospital*
*Menlo Park, California*

Asthma is a common disorder affecting millions of children. It appears to be increasing in Western countries, with an incidence of approximately 5% in 1974 and 8% in 1980. Black persons are more commonly affected than caucasians, with an incidence of 9% compared with 6%. Asthma is the leading cause of morbidity in childhood, with an estimated 2.8 million restricted activity days per year attributed to asthma in 1983. Asthma and wheezing were the tenth most frequent causes of visits to the pediatrician's office in 1980–1981, accounting for 2.2 million visits. Most children with asthma have the first episode by their third birthday. Ninety per cent improve during adolescence. However, mild persistent wheezing is relatively common, and it is estimated that only 20% of those with childhood asthma become totally asymptomatic in adult life. Children who have persistent symptoms at age 14 and abnormalities in spirometric measurements often have persistent and severe symptoms in young adulthood.

The spectrum of the disorder ranges from a very mild, intermittent course to severe, life-threatening disease. Until recently, mortality caused by asthma had been stable or declining slowly. However, during the past 5 years, it has been increasing in a number of Western countries, including the United States. The reasons for this increase are not yet clear. However, considerations have included increased prevalence, increased severity of the disease, drug toxicity, and management deficiencies such as inadequate long-term treatment, discontinuity of medical care, poor patient compliance, and inadequate monitoring of lung function, especially between acute exacerbations.

The key feature of asthma is airway hyper-reactivity, an exaggerated bronchoconstrictor response to a variety of stimuli. Airway hyper-responsiveness is associated with inflammation of the airways. Postmortem lungs show marked inflammation of the airways with infiltration of inflammatory cells (particularly eosinophils), disruption of airway epithelium, and plugging of the airway lumen by viscous mucus. Mast cells have been assumed to play a role in the pathogenesis of asthma, with mast cell–released mediators such as histamine, prostaglandins, and leukotrienes causing bronchial smooth muscle contraction, microvascular leakage, and airway mucous secretion and acting as chemotactic agents for other inflammatory cells. Eosinophilic infiltration, a characteristic feature of asthmatic airways, differentiates asthma from other inflammatory conditions of the airways. Eosinophils release a variety of mediators including leukotriene $C_4$, platelet-activating factor, major basic protein, and eosinophilic cationic protein. These mediators are toxic to airway epithelium, and this epithelial damage may be a critical feature of airway hyper-responsiveness. In addition, the cholinergic and adrenergic autonomic nervous systems are involved in control of the airways. Recently, neuropeptides such as vasoactive intestinal peptide and substance P have been identified as having effects on airway function.

When a child presents with asthma or symptoms suggestive of asthma, a careful history and physical examination should precede therapy. Important points in the history include the precipitants of symptoms, the duration of symptoms, and current and past medications. If symptoms or attacks have occurred, the details of, as well as the response to, therapy are important. Usually the diagnosis is easy, especially when the asthma is severe. The diagnosis may be more difficult when the asthma is mild or if it presents in an atypical manner. Children who present six to eight times each winter with a diagnosis of "bronchitis" are unusual unless they have an underlying immunodeficiency disorder or chest problem. The common diagnosis is asthma. Chronic cough without wheezing or shortness of breath has been well described as a primary manifestation of asthma. In children who can perform the spirometry test, the most appropriate evidence is the demonstration of reversible obstructive airways disease. In older children in whom baseline pulmonary functions are normal and asthma is suspected, a provocative challenge either with exercise or by inhalation of methacholine or histamine may be needed to make the diagnosis of asthma apparent. Methacholine challenge has been safely performed in children as young as 2 years of age by experienced investigators. A therapeutic trial of oral or inhaled bronchodilators may also be diagnostic for asthma.

## TREATMENT

There are four basic approaches to the outpatient management of the child with asthma: (1) identifying the precipitants of the asthma and manipulating the environment to control the child's exposure to them; (2) controlling bronchospasm and the inflammatory component of asthma with medication; (3) altering the immune response to environmental allergens with immunotherapy; and (4) educating the patient and family to improve their ability to manage this chronic illness adequately.

The goals of asthma therapy are to obtain maximum control of symptoms with a minimal number of the safest medications. Ideally, children should be able to participate in normal daily activities and sports with few or no restrictions. School absenteeism should be minimized. Decreasing the number of acute episodes of wheezing that require emergency treatment and reducing the number and frequency of hospitalizations are desirable. Normal growth and development should occur. Ideally, there should be complete relief of airway obstruction and normalization of pulmonary function. The patient and family should be able to understand, accept, and manage the asthma within the context of the family's lifestyle.

### Identifying Precipitants of Asthma and Instituting Environmental Controls

Asthmatic children have a higher prevalence of allergies than the normal population. Approximately one-half of the children with asthma demonstrate allergen skin test reactivity compared with approximately 20% of nonasthmatics.

Pollens and molds, house dust, dust mites, and animal danders may all induce wheezing in asthmatic children. Allergen-induced asthma generally occurs within minutes after exposure to an allergen, peaks 10 to 15 minutes later, and lasts for 1 to 2 hours. Symptoms develop rapidly and are readily apparent. In some children, often those with severe asthma, a late asthmatic response may occur 2 to 4 hours after allergen exposure, peaking 5 to 12 hours later, and lasting for 1 to several days. Both immediate and late responses are precipitated by exposure to various allergens to which the patient has antigen-specific IgE, as demonstrated by skin test or in vitro measures of specific IgE. Dust mites, animal danders, pollens, and molds may be associated with both early and late asthmatic reactions. Avoidance of allergens can lead to a decrease in IgE–mediated reactions and may also decrease nonspecific airway hyper-reactivity. Avoidance of dust and dust mites requires special attention to the child's bedroom. Pillows, mattresses, and box springs should be encased in plastic covers and wiped weekly. Bedding should be washed weekly in hot water. Furniture and wall hangings should be limited. Bare floors are preferred, and if carpeting is present, a low pile is best. Carpeting should be vacuumed several times a week. Room air vents should be closed and covered with cheesecloth. Closets should contain only the current season's clothes. The bedroom should be dusted frequently. Animal allergens that may precipitate both early and late asthmatic reactions should be removed from the home. Allergy to air-borne fungi is an especially difficult problem, and a search for possible mold growth should be made in the home. Use of a dehumidifier may be considered to keep the general area as dry as possible.

Nonallergic precipitants of asthma include inhaled irritants, both particulate and gaseous. The most important of these irritants is cigarette smoke. Maternal cigarette smoking correlates most closely with the frequency and severity of acute asthmatic attacks in the child. Both parents, however, should be encouraged to stop smoking, and smoking should be prohibited in the home of an asthmatic child. Asthmatic teenagers should be strongly discouraged from smoking. Other pulmonary irritants include sulfur dioxide, nitrogen dioxide, and ozone; thus, smog exposure should also be avoided if possible. Irritants from wood-burning stoves, fireplaces, assorted oil-based heaters, and various chemicals (e.g., formaldehyde, cleaning products) may also cause bronchoconstriction.

Air purification systems may be useful for both allergen- and irritant-induced symptoms. Room units can be purchased for the bedroom (see *Consumer Reports,* January 1985). Central air purification systems can also be purchased; however, they are often expensive (between $500 and $1,000). A Humidist (Honeywell) can be installed in homes with central air conditioning and heating systems as an aid in controlling indoor humidity. Relative humidity of 40 to 50% is ideal because higher humidity (70 to 80% relative humidity) encourages the presence of dust mites and molds.

A major precipitant of asthma in children is viral respiratory infection, especially in young children. Viral infections can also increase nonspecific airway hyper-reactivity, which may persist for weeks after resolution of the viral infection. Major pathogens implicated in triggering asthma in children include *Mycoplasma,* parainfluenza virus, rhinovirus, respiratory syncytial virus, adenovirus, and influenza virus. Except for the use of erythromycin for *Mycoplasma* infections and possibly ribavirin (Virazole) for respiratory syncytial virus, no effective treatment is available once the infection begins. Consideration can be given to removing children from high-exposure environments such as day care centers. Careful handwashing should be emphasized for all persons who care for children.

Exercise, hyperventilation, and cold air trigger bronchospasm, possibly by shared mechanisms of heat and/or water loss from the bronchial mucosa. At least 90% of asthmatic children have exercise-induced bronchospasm. Despite this, most asthmatic children should be encouraged to exercise, with appropriate pharmacologic pre-treatment beforehand. Swimming tends to cause the least bronchoconstriction and long periods of running the most bronchoconstriction.

Emotions can occasionally be involved in triggering asthma. However, parents should be assured that asthma is not a psychosomatic disease.

Asthma may also be aggravated by changes in weather, such as an increase in relative humidity or a sudden change in barometric pressure. Smog, storms, and air turbulence may contribute to an asthmatic episode. The reasons for these changes are largely unknown.

### Pharmacotherapy

The major drugs employed for the treatment of asthma are (1) adrenergic or sympathomimetic drugs, (2) theophylline, (3) sodium cromoglycate (cromolyn), and (4) corticosteroids. Other less often used medications include atropine and its derivatives, antihistamines, antibiotics, anti-inflammatory medications, and antimetabolites.

**Adrenergic or Sympathomimetic Drugs.** A major advance in recent years has been the development of adrenergic compounds, which are predominantly beta$_2$ agonists that produce more prolonged bronchodilation and fewer cardiovascular side effects than previously available medications. In the early part of this century, both ephedrine and epinephrine, nonselective adrenergic agents, were used. With the identification of the beta$_1$ and beta$_2$ receptors, more specific beta$_2$ agonists were developed for wide use. The beta$_2$ receptor is the primary adrenergic receptor that stimulates relaxation of bronchial smooth muscle. The most widely used beta$_2$ agonists include metaproterenol (Alupent and Metaprel), terbutaline (Brethine, Bricanyl), albuterol (Ventolin, Proventil), and bitolterol (Tornalate). These medications are available in liquid preparations, tablet form, metered-dose inhalers (MDI), and liquid solutions for inhalation. The usual doses of these agents are shown in Table 1.

These drugs are generally well tolerated, although increased heart rate, tremor, and irritability can occur. Side effects often decrease with time. Liquid and tablet preparations are rapidly absorbed from the gastrointestinal tract and often produce more hyperactivity and tremor than inhalants. Inhaled forms of medications are particularly useful, with rapid onset of action and minimal side effects. Their use is limited primarily by the child's ability to coordinate activation of a MDI or to use a nebulizer.

**Theophylline.** Theophylline has been used as a bronchodilator since the 1940s. It is probably the most commonly prescribed drug for asthma in this country. The mechanism of action remains unclear. Although it was previously assumed that it acted as a phosphodiesterase inhibitor, it now appears that other mechanisms are responsible for theophylline's action. Theophylline effectively prevents symptoms of asthma but has a low therapeutic index. Serum levels thought to produce the maximal bronchodilating effect are between 10 and 20 $\mu$g per ml, although some children have relief of symptoms and improved pulmonary function with lower doses. Many children have difficulty tolerating theophylline. Side effects include irritability, restlessness, nightmares, decreased attention span, sleepwalking, misbehavior, enuresis, and poor school performance. Adverse effects can be noted with doses that produce serum levels within or below the therapeutic range.

There is significant intersubject variation in theophylline metabolism, and individualizing therapy is critical. Generally, if a child is initially given a low dose of theophylline and is gradually increased to therapeutic doses based on body weight (Table 2), side effects can be avoided or decreased. For young children, theophylline capsules may be used that are opened and the contents sprinkled in food. Most young children must take the drug three times a day. In older children and adolescents, a new longer-acting theophylline preparation that maintains blood levels for 24 hours may be beneficial when asthma has

TABLE 1. **Dosing Guidelines for Adrenergic Drugs**

| Drug | Subcutaneous Administration | Oral Administration | Aerosol Administration | Metered-Dose Inhaler |
|---|---|---|---|---|
| Epinephrine | 0.01 ml/kg up to 0.30 ml (1:1000 solution) | — | — | — |
| Isoetharine | — | — | 0.02 ml/kg/dose up to 0.05 ml diluted with 1.5–2 ml normal saline (1% solution) | Two inhalations q 2–3 hr (340 $\mu$g/inhalation) |
| Metaproterenol | — | 0.3–0.6 mg/kg/dose 4 times/day (10- and 20-mg tablets; 10 mg/5 ml syrup) | 0.01 ml/kg/dose up to 0.30 ml diluted with 1.5–2 ml normal saline (5% solution) or 1-unit dose (0.6% solution) | Two inhalations q 4 hr (65 $\mu$g/inhalation) |
| Albuterol | — | 0.1–0.15 mg/kg/dose 3–4 times/day (2- and 4-mg tablets; 2 mg/5 ml syrup) | 0.01–0.03 ml/kg/dose up to 0.5 ml diluted with 1.5–2 ml normal saline (0.5% solution) | Two inhalations q 4 hr (90 $\mu$g/inhalation) |
| Terbutaline* | 0.01 ml/kg up to 0.30 ml (1% solution) | 0.075–0.10 mg/kg 3–4 times/day (2.5- and 5.0-mg tablets) | 0.1 mg/kg diluted up to 2 ml with normal saline (marketed for subcutaneous use) | Two inhalations q 4 hr (200 $\mu$g/inhalation) |
| Bitolterol* | — | — | — | Two inhalations q 6 hr (370 $\mu$g/inhalation) |

*This use of terbutaline and bitolterol in children less than 12 years of age is not listed in the manufacturer's official directive.

TABLE 2. **Dosing Guidelines
for Oral Theophylline***

| Age | Total Daily Dose (mg/kg/24 hr) |
|---|---|
| 6–51 wk | $(0.30) \times$ (age in weeks) + 8 |
| 1–9 yr | 24 |
| 9–12 yr | 20 |
| 12–16 yr | 18 |
| More than 16 yr | 13 (or 900 mg/day, whichever is less) |

*Data From Weinberger M, Hendeles L, and Ahrens R: Clinical pharmacology of drugs used for asthma. Pediatr Clin North Am *28*:47–75, 1981.

significant diurnal variation and nocturnal exacerbations.

Theophylline levels should be determined and should be a guide for therapy. Peak (2 to 4 hours after a dose) and trough (before the preceding dose) levels have been recommended; however, long-acting theophylline preparations may be variable in their peak and trough times.

**Cromolyn.** Cromolyn has been thought to inhibit IgE–dependent release of mediators from human lung mast cells. However, recent evidence has shown this property to be surprisingly weak. Cromolyn may inhibit secretory properties of other inflammatory cells, thereby modulating mechanisms that contribute to the inflammatory component of asthma. Cromolyn has minimal side effects and appears to be as effective as theophylline in the first line treatment of asthma. It is especially useful in children who tolerate theophylline and beta-adrenergic agents poorly. It must be used prophylactically, and most children require it at least three times a day. As the asthma improves over months of routine use, many children can be adequately maintained with lower doses of cromolyn.

Cromolyn is available for administration in three forms. The oldest is a 20-mg capsule using lactose as a carrier, which is opened using a Spinhaler device. Because lactose is present inside the capsule and can be swallowed, gastrointestinal symptoms can occur in the lactose-intolerant patient. Cromolyn available as an MDI is generally chosen by older children and adolescents. A solution containing 20 mg per ml of cromolyn solution in 2-ml ampules is available for use with nebulizers.

**Atropine and Ipratropium Bromide (Atrovent).** Atropine has been used in the treatment of asthma for almost 2 centuries. It inhibits bronchoconstriction by its action as an anticholinergic agent. Atropine is rarely used in children. The pharmacist can prepare it by dissolving atropine tablets, 0.6 mg in normal saline (without preservatives) to a concentration of 1 mg per ml and sterile filtered. From 1 to 2 ml (0.05 mg per kg, maximum 2 mg) of this solution may be placed in a nebulizer and used either alone as a bronchodilator or with a beta-adrenergic drug or cromolyn. Atropine solution may also be used; however, it is more expensive. Atropine can be absorbed into the systemic circulation and is associated with anticholinergic side effects such as dry mouth, blurred vision, and altered heart rate.

Ipratropium bromide is a quaternary isopropyl derivative of atropine. It is poorly absorbed and has few systemic side effects. It has only recently been approved for use in the United States and can be used only with adults. However, a number of studies have shown its efficacy in childhood asthma. It is active as a bronchodilator, with a peak onset at 10 minutes and a duration of 4 to 6 hours. When it is used in combination with an inhaled beta agonist, prolonged bronchodilation occurs. The dose is generally two inhalations three or four times a day. Atropine and ipratropium bromide are drugs of choice in patients who have asthma induced by beta-blocking agents.

**Corticosteroids.** Corticosteroids are very effective drugs in the treatment of both acute and chronic asthma. They do not produce immediate bronchodilation but instead act at many sites to help reverse the pathologic process of asthma. Some of the actions of corticosteroids include enhancement of the beta-adrenergic response to relieve bronchospasm, reversal of mucosal edema, decrease in vascular permeability by vasoconstriction, inhibition of the release of leukotrienes, reduction of mucous secretion, and interference with chemotaxis (this action may be caused by leukotriene $B_4$). Corticosteroids also produce an eosinopenic effect, which may help prevent the cytotoxic effects of major basic protein and other inflammatory mediators released from the eosinophil. Corticosteroids have no direct effect on immediate hypersensitivity. They block the late asthmatic reaction and the increased airway hyper-reactivity observed after the late asthmatic reaction.

Toxicity of corticosteroids is related primarily to the duration rather than to the dose and includes a cushingoid appearance, growth suppression, striae and purpura, cataracts, osteoporosis, and muscle weakness. Because of their side effects, corticosteroids have traditionally been reserved for highly intractable disease in children who respond poorly to other medications. However, early intervention with corticosteroids in children who become unresponsive to bronchodilators may, with minimal risk, abort a severe impending asthma attack and prevent hospitalization. A dose of 2 mg per kg per day to a maximum of 60 to 80 mg in two divided doses may be administered for 4 to 7 days and discontinued abruptly or tapered. Although it would be ideal to target intervention with corticosteroids at patients who will not improve spontaneously, it is difficult to distinguish those in whom spontaneous resolution will not occur.

Aerosolized corticosteroids have been of considerable value in the management of patients with moderate to severe asthma. These preparations allow effective control of symptoms and improve pulmonary function in the majority of patients, with minimal risk of the systemic side effects associated with long-term oral steroid therapy. Preparations available for use by inhalation include beclomethasone (Beclovent, Vanceril), flunisolide (AeroBid), and triamcinolone (Azmacort). Therapy with aerosolized steroids is generally initiated after asthma is under maximal control with aggressive bronchodilator therapy and, if necessary, a short course of oral steroids. A starting dose for beclomethasone is generally 84 $\mu$g four times a day. A twice-a-day schedule may be equally effective. In patients who respond poorly to conventional doses of inhaled corticosteroids, the use of high-dose inhaled beclomethasone (up to 1600 $\mu$g per day) may improve asthma control and reduce systemic steroid requirements. Serious systemic side effects such as iatrogenic Cushing's syndrome and growth suppression have not yet been noted with the usual doses of inhaled corticosteroids. Abnormal pituitary and adrenal function has been reported with high-dose therapy. All patients should rinse their mouths after using these agents to avoid both nonspecific throat irritation and the development of oral candidiasis. Oral candidiasis may also be prevented by using spacer devices.

**Other Medications.** Antihistamines carry a warning that they should not be used in asthma patients. However, a number of studies have shown that not only are they safe in patients with severe asthma, they may have a bronchodilator effect. Newer antihistamines and antihistamines available in Europe have been shown to give dose-dependent protection against histamine-induced bronchoconstriction.

Antibiotics have not been shown to be beneficial in the treatment of asthma. However, an exception is the presence of sinusitis, which should be aggressively treated in patients with asthma because it has been demonstrated that treatment of sinusitis may improve the asthma. Erythromycin is often necessary to treat *Mycoplasma* infections that may precipitate an episode of wheezing. Erythromycin and troleandomycin (TAO) are two antibiotics that are steroid sparing. TAO has been well studied, and when used with methylprednisolone but not prednisone, it decreases the clearance of methylprednisolone, allowing the steroid dose to be decreased. These drugs also reduce the clearance of theophylline. Thus, the theophylline dose should be decreased at least 25 to 33% when initiating therapy with erythromycin or TAO. TAO has been associated with significant liver abnormalities, which can necessitate discontinuation of the drug.

Expectorants have not been demonstrated to benefit the child with asthma. Their use cannot be recommended.

Medications for anxiety and sedation are generally contraindicated in patients with asthma.

In a small number of adult patients, pulmonary functions have been shown to improve after ingestion of nonsteroidal anti-inflammatory agents such as aspirin. However, a larger number of asthmatic patients may develop bronchoconstriction after taking aspirin, so it is recommended that aspirin not be given to asthmatic children. Aspirin allergy is rare in childhood asthma and more common in adult-onset asthma.

Gold salt preparations have been used for the management of asthma in Japan. Although their mode of action is uncertain, they are thought to be effective through their anti-inflammatory mechanisms.

Methotrexate has been used in severe steroid-dependent asthma in adults. Use of this antimetabolite has allowed a decrease in the daily dose of steroids.

**Use of Aerosols.** Therapeutic aerosols used in the treatment of asthma include MDIs, dry powder inhalers, and nebulizer solutions. Beta agonists, cromolyn, ipratropium bromide, and inhaled corticosteroids are available in aerosol form for the management of patients with asthma. MDIs are compact and portable and are ideal for children older than 6 to 7 years of age. Approximately 10% of the drug reaches the airways, even with perfect inhalation technique. Because many studies have shown that these medications are improperly used, proper inhalation technique should be reviewed at each visit to the physician. MDIs should be shaken well before inhalation. The head is tilted back to straighten the airway. Children should be instructed to breathe out fully (but not forcibly). The MDI is held between the index finger and thumb, and the mouthpiece is placed just outside a wide-open mouth and directed toward the back of the throat. Inhalation should be slow and even, and the canister should simultaneously be firmly pressed. Deposition of aerosol particles in the lung can be enhanced by low inspiratory flow rates and breath holding for 10 seconds after inhalation. A second dose may be given immediately.

To increase the efficiency of the MDI, various extension tubes (spacer devices) can be placed between the MDI and the mouth. Activation of the MDI releases the aerosol into the spacer, from which the patient slowly inhales. Inhal-Aid, InspirEase, and the Monahan aerochamber have all been useful for children who are unable to use an MDI properly. Spacers do not confer any advantage in children who use an MDI correctly.

Several beta agonists, cromolyn, and pharmacist-made atropine solutions are available as solutions that can be delivered by nebulization with either a face mask or mouthpiece. They are delivered by using a compressor (Pulmo-Aide, De-Vilbiss, Somerset, Pa. 15501) or powered by wall oxygen. Many types of nebulizers are available. The main advantage of the nebulizer is that little patient coordination is required, and it can be used in crying and dyspneic children and in those too young to coordinate an MDI. The addition of intermittent positive pressure breathing does not improve the efficacy of nebulized solutions.

### Approaches to Treatment

**Mild Asthma.** More than one-half of children with asthma have mild asthma that occurs infrequently. Often their symptoms are precipitated only by viral respiratory infections, and they may be completely symptom free, with normal or near-normal pulmonary functions, between episodes. This group includes patients who have primarily exercise-induced bronchospasm, who present only with cough, and who have fewer than two or three mild non–life-threatening acute asthmatic episodes a year. These children generally require only intermittent medications and rarely need corticosteroids.

Exercise-induced bronchospasm is best managed with either an inhaled beta-adrenergic bronchodilator or cromolyn before exercise. Albuterol has the longest duration of effect and is generally considered to be the beta agonist of choice. Cromolyn, either one capsule by Spinhaler or two inhalations of an MDI, also effectively blocks exercise-induced bronchospasm. In children in whom a beta agonist and cromolyn only partially block exercise-induced bronchospasm, the combination of albuterol followed by cromolyn is recommended. An adequate warm-up period also improves children's response to exercise.

Mild acute exacerbations of asthma can generally be treated with inhaled beta-adrenergic agents. These can be given by MDI, two inhalations every 4 to 6 hours, or as solution delivered by nebulization. An oral agent, either theophylline or an oral beta agonist, may also be beneficial. The doses given in Table 1 are provided only as guidelines. Treatment usually begins with a smaller dose and, if needed and tolerated, is increased to a larger dose. Therapy should be continued for 5 to 7 days after the child is asymptomatic and then discontinued.

**Moderate Asthma.** Approximately 20% of asthmatic children have moderate asthma. They have frequent acute exacerbations that significantly affect their ability to function normally at their age level. Generally, these children have acute symptoms at least every 4 to 6 weeks (if not properly managed). Pulmonary functions may remain abnormal until proper control is achieved. These children generally require continuous use of medications. The initial medication may include either an inhaled or oral beta agonist, inhaled cromolyn, theophylline, or a combination. Because of the importance of inflammation in asthma, the second drug added to a beta agonist is often cromolyn, which decreases the inflammatory response, decreases bronchial hyper-reactivity, and inhibits both immediate IgE-mediated bronchoconstriction and the late asthmatic response. Occasionally, a short course of steroid therapy is required for acute exacerbations of asthma. If there is a seasonal pattern to the asthma, there may be times when less intensive therapy is adequate to control symptoms.

**Severe Asthma.** From 1 to 5% of asthmatic children have daily symptoms, limitation of physical activity and exercise, abnormal pulmonary functions at initial evaluation, and evidence of chronic hyperinflation on physical examination. These patients require aggressive management to control their disease, including an inhaled beta agonist, cromolyn, and theophylline. If this therapy proves to be inadequate, corticosteroids are indicated. Inhaled corticosteroids should be initiated after a course of oral steroids to maximize pulmonary functions. In children who continue to experience difficulty, even with optimal doses of inhaled bronchodilators and inhaled anti-inflammatory agents such as cromolyn and/or corticosteroids, and who require large doses of oral corticosteroids to treat acute episodes, consideration should be given to alternate-day corticosteroid therapy. The use of alternate-day corticosteroids often provides optimal control of the asthma and may result in the use of lower total doses of corticosteroids. Control of the asthma should be achieved with larger doses of prednisone initially, then tapering to 20 to 40 mg every other day, using the minimal dose that controls symptoms. If the child remains well for 6 to 8 weeks, the dose should be slowly tapered.

**Severe Acute Asthma (Status Asthmaticus).** Treatment of severe acute asthma ideally requires an understanding of the child's history, the treatment given before presentation, and the duration and symptoms of the present episode. This information should be elicited as briefly as possible while preparations for the child's care are undertaken. Once treatment has begun, the remainder of the child's history can be obtained.

The physical examination should also be brief and should be directed at assessing the severity of the respiratory distress and detecting the complications of the attack. Signs associated with severe obstruction include intercostal and suprasternal retractions, sternocleidomastoid contractions, pulsus paradoxus greater than 20 mmHg, cyanosis, agitation or lethargy, and poor air movement with a quiet chest. With a few exceptions, there is no clear benefit to obtaining various laboratory or radiologic tests. Complete blood tests are frequently ordered, but because of various medications the child may be taking, they seldom provide useful information. Electrolyte evaluations are useful if dehydration is suspected. Chest x-ray examinations are rarely necessary unless the presence of pneumothorax or pneumonia is considered likely. Arterial blood gas levels should be obtained if there is any question as to how the child is responding and certainly if the development of ventilatory failure is suspected. A theophylline level may be useful, especially to assess compliance or to rule out toxicity. However, care should be taken if long-acting oral theophyllines have been administered because the peak level can vary from patient to patient.

Oxygen should be administered but may be discontinued as the patient's condition improves. Administration of adrenergic drugs by aerosol has been shown to be as effective as administration of injected epinephrine or terbutaline. Effective bronchodilation is achieved with a much smaller inhaled than parenteral dose, and side effects are reduced. The onset and duration of action are similar. Nebulizers should be powered by wall oxygen in the emergency room and, if available, in the office, although compressors may be used. Older children may use nebulized solutions through a T tube, and infants may sit on their mothers' laps with a mask attached to the nebulizer. Doses for nebulized beta agonists are listed in Table 1. Nebulized treatments can be repeated every 20 minutes as long as the heart rate remains less than 80% of the predicted maximum. If there is no satisfactory response after two or three treatments, or sooner if the patient's condition deteriorates, hospitalization and observation are probably necessary. Alternatively, treatment may begin with aqueous epinephrine (0.01 ml per kg subcutaneously) or terbutaline (0.01 ml per kg subcutaneously). If there is a good response, epinephrine crystalline suspension (Sus-Phrine, 0.005 ml per kg subcutaneously) may provide longer clinical effects; however, tachycardia and tremor are significant. Intravenous theophylline does not appear to add

significantly to the bronchodilator effects of inhaled beta-adrenergic agents and should be administered cautiously if a long-acting theophylline preparation is present.

The decision to hospitalize should be made if there is severe obstruction with little response to the medications just mentioned, if improvement is not complete within 3 to 4 hours after therapy, or if an infant has symptoms with less than a complete response. Most children with an attack that has recurred within 48 hours should be hospitalized. Careful observation is the most important goal of hospitalization, and vital signs should be recorded frequently every 30 minutes to 1 hour for the first 8 hours of hospitalization. The basic laboratory studies include a chest x-ray film, arterial blood gas analysis, and peak expiratory flow measurements. A complete blood count is generally done; however, it may reveal information that is difficult to interpret. Urinalysis may demonstrate the presence of ketones and elevated specific gravity. Treatment consists of aerosolized beta agonists given every 30 minutes to 1 hour, with decreasing frequency as the child improves. Aminophylline can be administered as a bolus dose of 7 mg per kg if theophylline has not previously been given, followed by a constant infusion of 1.2 mg per kg per hour. Corticosteroids should be administered to all patients who are already using oral or inhaled corticosteroids. Corticosteroids appear to decrease the subsequent need for hospitalization. However, studies have not confirmed whether children who receive corticosteroids actually improve faster than those who are not given corticosteroids. Most hospitalized children should receive either hydrocortisone, 5 to 7 mg per kg bolus, followed by approximately 15 mg per kg per day,* or methylprednisolone, 1 to 2 mg per kg bolus, followed by 1 to 2 mg per kg every 4 to 6 hours.

Whether the patient is discharged from the hospital or the office, a treatment plan for the next 10 to 14 days should be carefully considered and reviewed with the patient and parents. Oral theophylline is begun at a dose extrapolated from the intravenous requirement (24-hour aminophylline dose × 0.85 divided by the dosing interval of the oral preparation). Inhaled adrenergic agonists are continued using an MDI or nebulizer. An outpatient return visit should be scheduled for less than 1 week.

### Immunotherapy

Although there is no absolutely convincing evidence from controlled double-blind studies

---

*Usual dose is 4 mg per kg, then 2 to 10 mg per kg per day, but dose varies with disease.

that immunotherapy is effective for children with allergic asthma, there is strongly suggestive published evidence and respectable anecdotal evidence that immunotherapy may be helpful. Experimental evidence shows that airway hyperreactivity to inhaled allergens is reduced after high-dose appropriate immunotherapy. Immunotherapy is indicated for children who have a history of allergen-induced asthma and who demonstrate IgE-mediated sensitivity to the suspected allergen by properly performed epicutaneous prick skin tests or in vitro measures of specific IgE. Immunotherapy is not indicated if there is an adequate response to environmental control and appropriate pharmacotherapy without side effects. It is important to determine the appropriate allergens to be used in patients with allergic asthma. These should include unavoidable allergens such as pollens, house dust mites, and possibly certain molds, especially *Alternaria,* which is prevalent in many parts of the United States. There is no place for immunotherapy with bacterial vaccines, tobacco, histamine, or food allergens. It is essential that reliable and potent extracts be used for both diagnosis and therapy, and that the administration of allergen extracts be started with appropriately low doses and increased progressively during a period of weeks and months at a rate that the patient can tolerate without risk of systemic anaphylactic reactions. Injections should always be administered in the office under the guidance of a physician. The child should be observed carefully for 20 minutes after each injection.

### Education

To many patients and families, asthma remains a mystery. They are angry that they have the problem, confused about what triggers asthma, and frustrated in their attempts to deal with it. The goal of an educational program is to acknowledge these issues and to convince the family that they are able, with help and support, to control the problem. The physician's attitude in this regard is critical. There is no substitute for spending enough time with the child and family to deal with these issues.

Excellent materials can be obtained from the Asthma and Allergy Foundation of America (1717 Massachusetts Ave. N.W., Suite 305, Washington, D.C., 20036, 202–265–0265); and the American Lung Association (1740 Broadway, New York, N.Y., 10019, 212–315–8700). A number of self-management programs (Air Power, Open Air, Air Wise, Living with Asthma, Family Asthma Program) have been developed and are frequently sponsored by local chapters of the Asthma and Allergy Foundation and the American Lung Association. Most asthma self-management programs deal with the following four principles: (1) asthma is a common disease, and having asthma is annoying but not disgraceful; (2) people with asthma can lead full and active lives; (3) it is much easier to prevent than to treat an asthmatic attack; and (4) people do not become addicted to asthma medications.

Armed with knowledge from the physician, and perhaps self-management programs, the patient and family can deal more easily with the stress that accompanies an acute episode of asthma, as well as the stress associated with chronic disease.

# ALLERGIC RHINITIS DUE TO AEROALLERGENS

method of
MICHAEL J. SCHUMACHER, M.B.B.S.
*University of Arizona Health Sciences Center*
*Tucson, Arizona*

Allergic rhinitis is the most common chronic disease of the respiratory tract, affecting nearly 30% of the population in North America. Its symptoms are usually trivial or limited in incidence to a short, airborne-pollen season each year. However, allergic rhinitis can cause significant morbidity in patients who are sensitive to perennially prevalent allergens, while other patients may have seasonal symptoms that are so distressing that normal daily activities become impossible. Allergic rhinitis is frequently accompanied by allergic conjunctivitis, postnasal discharge, vocal hoarseness, fatigue, cough, and bronchial hyper-responsiveness. Subacute or chronic sinusitis may also be more common in patients with allergic nasal disease. Treatment of sinusitis may be useful in improving the course of coexisting severe asthma, but it is not known whether topical drug treatment of allergic rhinitis is similarly beneficial for asthmatics. There is no conclusive evidence that immunotherapy of allergic rhinitis in childhood is able to prevent the subsequent onset of asthma. Although highly recurrent otitis media is common in young children with allergic rhinitis, and allergen challenge of the upper airways can provoke eustachian tube dysfunction, it is not known whether effective treatment of allergic rhinitis can reduce the incidence of otitis media in young children.

## DIAGNOSIS

Allergic rhinitis requires differentiation from nonallergic nasal conditions including vasomotor rhinitis, rhinitis medicamentosa, bacterial rhinosinusitis, rhinosinusitis with aspirin sensitivity, and nonallergic rhinitis with eosinophilia. Distinguishing allergic rhinitis from these nonallergic conditions is usually a simple matter, particularly if the physician takes a thorough history to show that the symptoms vary seasonally or are provoked by aeroallergens recognized by the patient. Moderate to severe itching of the upper airways or the conjunctivae is virtually diagnostic of allergy. Examination of the cytology of nasal scrapings may be helpful in distinguishing bacterial rhinosinusitis from eosinophilic rhinitis: neutrophilic (as distinct from eosinophilic) purulent secretions may indicate the need for sinus radiographs.

The main indications for skin testing are when extensive allergen avoidance or immunotherapy is contemplated or when the diagnosis remains unclear after an exhaustive history and careful physical examination. Selection of allergens for skin testing or radioallergosorbent testing (RAST) to identify IgE-mediated reactivity to specific allergens is not necessary for most patients with allergic rhinitis that is easily controlled by occasional doses of antihistamines or decongestants. Moreover, these tests are *never* a substitute for a thorough history and evaluation of the patient's allergenic environment, because it is common for positive skin tests or RAST results to be falsely positive or irrelevant. Serum levels of total IgE are usually not helpful unless they are elevated in a patient who has a strong history of allergy but entirely negative skin tests or RAST determinations, suggesting the presence of allergy to an allergen not included in the testing procedures. An undetectable level of IgE may help to rule out a diagnosis of allergic rhinitis in older children or adults whose history of allergy is not diagnostic.

When the history is not strongly suggestive of inhalant allergy, radiographs of the paranasal sinuses may be necessary to exclude subacute chronic sinusitis, because postnasal discharge may not be evident and transillumination may be negative in some patients with sinus disease. Failure of allergic rhinitis to respond to aggressive antihistamine decongestant therapy should also prompt exclusion of coexisting sinus disease. Fiberoptic nasopharyngoscopy and coronal computer-assisted tomography may also be necessary in selected patients.

## TREATMENT

### Allergen Avoidance

The simplest treatment of allergic rhinitis is to avoid the offending allergen. In most patients, complete avoidance of allergens significant in provoking the symptoms is rarely, if ever, possible because of sensitivity to ubiquitous aeroallergens.

Nevertheless, avoidance of potent aeroallergens, such as cat allergens, may reduce the need for medication to control symptoms from unavoidable allergens such as pollen or mold. House dust mites may cause nasal allergy in coastal cities or humid environments, and if symptoms cannot be controlled with occasional doses of antihistamines, it may be necessary to reduce exposure to mite allergens by use of allergen-proof encasings for the mattress and pillow, removal of carpeting from the bedroom, or use of acaricides. Blankets should be washed in hot water (greater than 56°C) on a regular basis. Feather pillows or down comforters should be replaced by synthetic materials. Disposable filters in the air intake of the furnace should be changed regularly and, in the case of severe house dust allergy, should be replaced with a high efficiency filter, e.g., the Newtron Electrostatic Air Cleaner. Heavy exposure to pollen can often be avoided: for example, when a patient allergic to grass pollen is obliged to mow the lawn, he should wear a pollen mask (3M Company). Seasonal exposure to high concentrations of mold spores is inevitable, particularly in rural areas where cultivation liberates soil molds into the atmosphere. Patients allergic to molds may benefit from an air purifier with an HEPA-type filter in the bedroom.

In most patients, additional measures as illustrated in Figure 1 are needed because environmental control provides only partial relief of symptoms.

### Pharmacologic Therapy

Patients with allergic rhinitis often come for treatment when self-medication with over-the-

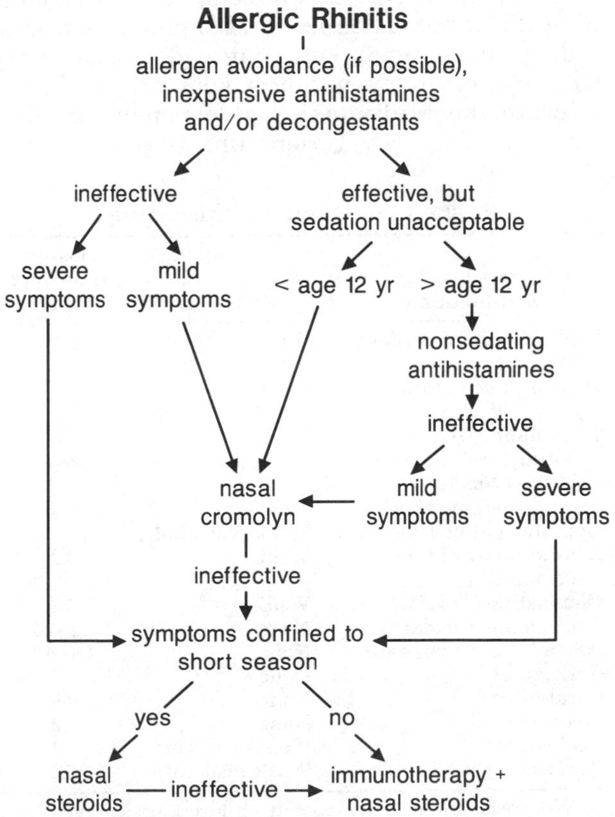

**Allergic Rhinitis**

**Figure 1.** Decision tree for the management of allergic rhinitis.

counter antihistamine-decongestant combinations, usually chlorpheniramine and pseudoephedrine, has become ineffective or causes excessive sedation. $H_1$ antihistamines, usually effective in controlling hypersecretion, sneezing, and itching, are often less effective for nasal congestion. Patients who have predominant nasal congestion without much increase in secretions may respond well to decongestant therapy alone. It is possible that the commonly observed loss of effectiveness of antihistamines may be caused by the development of subsensitivity to the antihistamine, a problem that has been documented with chlorpheniramine. However, there is insufficient evidence to support the claim that switching from one class of antihistamines to another has merit that transcends the placebo effect of a new medication.

Most of the antihistamines available in the U.S. are highly sedating. Their other main adverse effect, prolongation of voluntary reaction times, is not related to the degree of sedation, making it difficult to assess the safety of driving or operating hazardous equipment from subjective side effects. Antihistamines with reduced sedative side effects, such as clemastine (Tavist) and azatadine (Optimine, Trinalin), and newer antihistamines with no significant central nervous system (CNS) side effects, such as terfenadine (Seldane), astemizole (Hismanal), and loratadine (Clarityne), may provide satisfactory therapy for many patients who are unable to tolerate the traditional, less expensive antihistamines (Table 1). Terfenadine is probably less effective than most antihistamines in the currently recommended dose (60 mg twice daily). Astemizole and loratadine differ from most antihistamines in their very long biologic half-lives and have been reported to inhibit skin test responses to allergens for several weeks.

Inadequate response to antihistamine therapy may be a result of mediators other than histamine that are not antagonized by the drug. When drugs effective in antagonizing nonhistamine mediators of rhinitis become available, they may prove to be useful in combination with antihistamines. Antihistamines that also have activity against leukotrienes and other mediators, e.g., mequitazine* and azelastine,* are showing promise of efficacy for rhinitis in trials. Cetirizine* is an antihistamine that also reduces prostaglandin production and late inflammatory responses to allergen. Ketotifen* (Zaditen) has the additional effects of antagonizing platelet-activating factor (a mast cell mediator) and inhibiting mediator release from mast cells, but it is not yet clear whether these additional pharmacologic effects confer a significant therapeutic advantage in the management of allergic rhinitis. Guaphenesin and anticholinergic drugs are frequently added to antihistamine-decongestant combinations, but proof of efficacy in good double-blind control studies of these formulations is lacking.

When antihistamine-decongestant therapy fails, topical therapy with nasal sprays may be indicated. Aside from burning or irritation experienced by some patients, 4% cromolyn nasal spray (Nasalcrom) is effective when used at least four times a day. Nasal sprays containing topical corticosteroids, such as beclomethasone (Beconase, Vancenase) or flunisolide (Nasalide), are more effective than cromolyn and usually need only be used two to three times per day. Aqueous steroid formulations are tolerated better than the metered-dose aerosol steroids. In the first week of topical steroid or cromolyn therapy, it may be necessary to decongest the nose with a long-acting drug such as oxymetazoline (Afrin) sprayed into the nose two to three times a day, because swelling of the nasal turbinates may prevent adequate penetration of the nasal spray into the nasal cavity. More prolonged daily use of this drug will lead to rhinitis medicamentosa. The nose should also be cleared of excess secretions prior to using nasal sprays to aid their penetration into the mucosa. Very rarely, symptoms of allergic rhinitis may be so severe that systemic steroid therapy may be required for a 4-day period. In this situation, prednisone in doses of 1 mg per kg per day, up to a maximum

TABLE 1. **Selected Antihistamines**

| Antihistamine | Sedation | Dosing Intervals (hr) |
|---|---|---|
| Diphenhydramine (Benadryl) | Strong | 6–8 |
| Hydroxyzine (Atarax, Vistaril) | Strong | 12 |
| Triprolidine (Actifed) | Moderate | 6 |
| Chlorpheniramine (CTM, Chlor-Trimeton) | Moderate | 8–12 |
| Tripelennamine (PBZ) | Moderate | 6–8 |
| Cyproheptadine (Periactin) | Weak, variable | 8 |
| Azatadine (Optimine, Trinalin)* | Weak | 12 |
| Clemastine (Tavist) | Weak | 12 |
| Terfenadine (Seldane)* | None | 12–24 |
| Astemizole (Hismanal)* | None | 24–48 |
| Cetirizine† | None | |
| Loratadine† | None | 48 |
| Mequitazine† | None | 12 |
| Azelastine† | Weak-moderate | 12 |
| Ketotifen† | Weak-moderate | 12 |

*Not recommended for use in children under age 12, in U.S.

†Not currently available in U.S.

*Investigational drugs in the United States.

of 50 mg per day, could be used. Injectable corticosteroids, particularly the intramuscular depot formulations, are not recommended because their effects are prolonged and unpredictable, and the side effects of systemic corticosteroid therapy are unacceptable in a relatively benign, chronic disease.

### Immunotherapy

Immunotherapy by injection with allergen extracts may be necessary to control symptoms in patients who are inadequately controlled by medications. For example, full compliance with directions for the regular use of nasal sprays is likely to be achieved in only a small minority of patients, since it is known that compliance with therapy for life-threatening diseases such as asthma is often poor. Immunotherapy of allergic rhinitis with ragweed, grass, and birch pollen has been shown to be effective in reducing symptom-medication scores in double-blind controlled trials. Accordingly, appropriately administered immunotherapy can be expected to reduce needs for medication in most patients.

Patients with allergic rhinitis should not be started on immunotherapy unless they have had symptoms for more than 12 months, because it is not possible to establish seasonal relationships between allergen exposure and symptoms for shorter periods. Moreover, IgE antibody production may be predominantly confined to the target organ soon after the onset of disease. IgE antibodies may not be produced in amounts large enough to achieve serum levels above the lower limits of sensitivity of the RAST test or in amounts large enough to sensitize cutaneous mast cells in distant sites. Thus, skin testing early in the onset of allergic rhinitis may be negative or may be limited to one or two allergens, whereas the local IgE response may encompass a larger number of allergens. Similarly, skin testing and immunotherapy should never be started in patients who have recently moved from a botanically different environment because at least 1 year is required for the establishment of a significantly vigorous IgE antibody response to be reflected in positive skin tests.

Life-threatening or fatal anaphylactic reactions to allergen immunotherapy may occur. Therefore, it should be used only in patients in whom vigorous drug therapy and allergen avoidance has been tried unsuccessfully. The injections must be given only in an office fully equipped for emergency resuscitation from systemic anaphylaxis, including oxygen, epinephrine, and supplies for intravenous infusion and endotracheal intubation. Observation for 30 minutes after each injection is also essential.

Allergen injections usually lead to improvement inside 12 months, but progressive improvement may continue over the following 2 to 3 years. Injections should not be discontinued before a total period of 4 years in a patient who is responding satisfactorily because of the possibility of early relapse. Discontinuance of treatment after 5 years followed by a period of observation is recommended because further improvement beyond this period is unlikely, and improvement may be maintained for several years without restarting the injections. Some patients may deteriorate after stopping the injections. In these patients, the development of new sensitivities may require another course of immunotherapy with a reformulated allergen extract mixture.

## SPECIAL CONSIDERATIONS IN THE MANAGEMENT OF ALLERGIC RHINITIS

Allergic rhinitis in children presents special problems. In young children, antihistamines may cause excitation and hyperactivity instead of sedation. This age group is particularly difficult to treat with nasal sprays because of their intolerance of vehicles used in the spray formulations, whereas older children do not like using a nasal spray in the school environment. The nonsedating antihistamines are not recommended for children under age 12 (Table 1). Therefore, it may be necessary to rely on traditional oral medications and allergen avoidance or to recommend immunotherapy more readily in children.

Allergic rhinitis may also be difficult to treat during pregnancy. Very few of the currently available antihistamines have been proved to be safe through many years of use in the pregnant patient and few have been proved to be not teratogenic in animals. Thus, antihistamine therapy in pregnancy should be limited to tripelennamine (PBZ) and decongestant therapy to pseudoephedrine. Corticosteroids have also been shown to be safe in pregnancy, and therefore topical beclomethasone may be used in patients resistant to tripelennamine and pseudoephedrine. Systemic anaphylaxis with hypoxia or hypotension can be expected to have adverse consequences for the fetus, and therefore, risks of systemic reactions to allergen immunotherapy should be reduced to an absolute minimum. To this end, immunotherapy should not be started during pregnancy, and if pregnancy starts while the patient is currently receiving allergen injections, the dose should be reduced by at least 50% and maintained without any dose increases until after delivery.

Cardiovascular diseases may present additional risks in the use of immunotherapy for allergic rhinitis. Beta adrenergic–blocking drugs may increase the risk of systemic anaphylaxis after an allergen injection, requiring a choice between the use of the beta blocker or immunotherapy. The mortality from anaphylaxis is considerably higher in individuals over 40 years of age, requiring additional caution in the use of immunotherapy in patients in this age group. The presence of ischemic heart disease or cerebral vascular disease is a contraindication in the use of immunotherapy for allergic rhinitis because of the risk of myocardial infarction or stroke during hypotension or hypoxia during an anaphylactic complication from an immunotherapy injection. Fortunately, the decreasing severity of allergic rhinitis in middle and old age generally makes immunotherapy less necessary.

# ALLERGIC REACTIONS TO DRUGS

method of
MACY I. LEVINE, M.D.
*University of Pittsburgh School of Medicine*
*Pittsburgh, Pennsylvania*

Allergic reactions to drugs may be classified according to the Gell and Coombs scheme as Types I, II, III, and IV, or according to the major clinical manifestations.

Type I, or anaphylactic, hypersensitivity is mediated by IgE antibodies that attach to the surface of mast cells and basophils in the skin, respiratory and gastrointestinal tracts, and blood. Clinical manifestations of the antigen-antibody reaction include urticaria, angioedema, bronchospasm, hypotension, nausea, vomiting, diarrhea, and even death. Many drugs may induce this type of reaction, including antibiotics, many foreign proteins used in treatment, allergen extracts, and a host of drugs that are relatively simple chemical compounds. A number of chemicals used in medicine, such as radiocontrast media, produce anaphylactic-like reactions by a nonimmunologic mechanism.

Type II, or cytotoxic, hypersensitivity is due to an IgG or IgM antibody, but the antigen is on the surface of a tissue cell, such as one of the blood cells. The antigen-antibody interaction results in agglutination or lysis of cells, producing various cytopenias, hemolytic anemia, Hashimoto's thyroiditis, or Goodpasture's syndrome.

Type III hypersensitivity, or immune-complex disease, results from circulating or soluble antigen-antibody complexes, which appear responsible for classic serum sickness, some drug reactions, necrotizing angiitides, and connective tissue diseases.

Type IV, or cell-mediated immunity, is also known as delayed hypersensitivity and is manifested by contact dermatitis from various simple chemical compounds.

## DIAGNOSIS

The diagnosis of drug allergy may be very obvious, but usually it is very difficult to determine whether a specific drug, or any drug, was responsible for the clinical problem. To some extent this is because the hospitalized adult patient receives an average of ten drugs during his confinement, and the adult outpatient takes an average of two medications regularly. Furthermore, few tests are available for the positive identification of an allergic reaction to a drug. Sometimes the reaction is due to a metabolite of the drug rather than the drug itself.

Thus, the diagnosis is based on the presence of signs and symptoms known to occur from reactions to a specific drug, provided the reaction developed in the appropriate time following administration of the drug. Besides the clinical picture, other considerations include the history of previous exposure to the same or other drugs, the specific drugs to which the patient was exposed in the previous month, the propensity of specific drugs to cause the reaction under investigation, the response to withdrawal of the drug, and the results of any available immunologic tests.

## IMMUNOLOGIC TESTING

Since Type I hypersensitivity is due to IgE antibodies, tests that identify the presence of these antibodies may be helpful. These include scratch, prick, intradermal, or in vitro (e.g., RAST) tests, which determine whether IgE antibody is present or not.

However, a positive test may be confirmatory of a specific sensitivity or may only suggest that the specific drug is responsible for the reaction. Tests with drugs that are proteins are most useful, while tests with simple chemical compounds, if negative, may not rule out the role of that substance in causing the reaction. Other types of tests are undergoing investigation at present and may become available to the clinician in the near future.

In Type II hypersensitivity, the laboratory is necessary to determine the nature of the disease, but specific tests are not available to establish the role of drugs in the etiology. In some medical centers, tests may be available to identify drug-related platelet antibodies in cases of drug-induced thrombocytopenia or antidrug antibodies in drug-related hemolytic anemia. The disappearance of the condition following withdrawal of the drug usually establishes the diagnosis.

Type III hypersensitivity may be associated with IgE antibodies in addition to soluble antigen-antibody complexes. Appropriate tests for IgE antibodies or IgG and IgM hemagglutinating antibodies may be helpful in diagnosis. Tests for drug-induced immune complexes are not available so far for clinical use.

In allergic contact dermatitis due to drugs, a form of Type IV hypersensitivity, the proper test is the patch test with the appropriate concentration of the suspected chemical compound. A local inflammatory response at 48 hours may confirm the identity of the causative agent. Testing should not be performed while the dermatitis is active because of a risk of aggravating the rash.

## PREVENTION

The incidence of drug reactions may be minimized by observing the following precautions:

1. The patient must be questioned carefully regarding previous reactions to drugs. He must avoid any drug to which he has reacted in the past.

2. All drugs must be used with proper indication, preferably by mouth rather than by injection when appropriate.

3. If the patient has had an adverse reaction to a specific drug, use an unrelated drug that may be effective when possible.

4. When patients use any medication, they must read labels carefully, particularly when buying something over the counter.

5. The use of topical antibiotics, antihistamines, and local anesthetics should be avoided or minimized because of their potential for sensitization.

6. Drugs must be used with caution and discrimination during pregnancy.

7. Drugs that commonly cause allergic reactions, such as penicillin and its relatives, should be given by mouth rather than by injection in order to minimize the frequency of reactions. When the patient has a history of a previous allergic reaction to penicillin and has an illness for which penicillin or other beta lactam drug is required, skin testing with penicillin compounds is helpful in determining the degree of risk and the method for administration of the beta lactam drug.

Skin testing is performed using benzyl penicilloyl polylysine (Pre-Pen) and benzylpenicillin, 6000 units per ml, using the scratch or prick technique. If these tests are negative, the same tests are performed by the intradermal route. Negative results indicate that the patient has a minimal risk of an acute anaphylactic reaction from administration of a beta lactam drug. One cannot predict or prevent a later development of urticaria or other adverse reaction. Should the patient develop a positive skin test with either of the penicillin products, the patient is considered to be at significant risk of further allergic reaction. In that case, further consideration should be made for an alternative antibiotic. If a beta lactam drug is of sufficient indication to warrant some risk, the patient will be given the penicillin or related drug by "desensitization." Penicillin would then be given in a dosage of 0.1 unit subcutaneously, doubling the dose every 15 to 20 minutes until the desired therapeutic dose is reached.

8. Before administration of any drug, the patient should be advised about possible side effects or allergic reactions. The doctor must keep careful records of the drug history of every patient and the name and dosage of every drug prescribed.

## TREATMENT

The treatment of any reaction to a drug involves discontinuation of that drug plus symptomatic therapy.

Acute anaphylactic reactions require immediate treatment with aqueous epinephrine, 1:1000, 0.3 ml subcutaneously. This may be repeated every 10 to 20 minutes for two or three injections if there is no response. An $H_1$ antihistamine, such as diphenhydramine (Benadryl), 50 mg, should be given orally or intramuscularly. This, or other antihistamine, may be continued every 4 hours by mouth until the reaction has subsided. If the cause of the reaction was an injection or an insect sting, a tourniquet should be applied on the extremity proximal to the injection site in order to slow absorption of the allergen. The tourniquet must be released every 15 or 20 minutes. The patient should be placed in the recumbent position when hypotension is present. Intravenous aminophylline and inhaled bronchodilators should be administered for bronchospasm. The airway must be kept open and oxygen administered if the patient is having trouble breathing. Shock may be controlled by subcutaneous epinephrine or by its slow intravenous administration, 0.5 ml of the 1:1000 solution in 5 to 10 ml isotonic saline solution. Other vasopressor drugs may be substituted for epinephrine. If the reaction persists, adrenal corticosteroid therapy should be initiated and hospitalization arranged.

When the patient has urticaria or other rashes, antihistamines by mouth in addition to topical calamine lotion, cool baking soda or starch paste, and cold compresses may relieve the discomfort.

Antihistamines, bronchodilators, and other symptomatic measures, given orally, may be all that is required in less severe cases.

Contact dermatitis usually responds to topical steroids and oral antihistamines. Systemic steroids should be reserved for very severe or persistent cases. Prednisone (Deltasone) is the steroid of choice and should be initiated in a dose of 30 to 60 mg a day and should be decreased gradually over a period of 1 or 2 weeks.

Management of the patient who becomes allergic to insulin involves skin testing with various types of insulin in order to confirm the diagnosis and help find a type of insulin that the patient will tolerate. Single peak pork insulin is preferable to beef insulin, and highly purified or synthetic insulin may be tolerated. If no satisfactory insulin preparation can be found, the patient may require insulin desensitization in a fashion similar to penicillin desensitization.

# ALLERGIC REACTIONS TO INSECT STINGS

method of
JAMES R. WARPINSKI, M.D.,
MARK A. HUFTEL, M.D., and
WILLIAM W. BUSSE, M.D.
*University of Wisconsin Medical School*
*Madison, Wisconsin*

Allergic reactions to insect stings have a wide spectrum of severity. While most stings produce minor self-limited reactions, severe reactions also occur and cause an estimated 40 to 50 deaths per year in the United States. Most severe sting reactions are caused by insects of the Hymenoptera order, including the honey bee, yellow jacket, yellow hornet, white-faced hornet, wasp, and imported fire ant. During severe reactions, hypotension, anaphylaxis, or respiratory compromise may be profound and refractory to treatment, especially in individuals receiving beta-blocker therapy. Using purified venom from individual insects, Hymenoptera sensitivity can now be effectively diagnosed and treated in susceptible patients. Because of the rapidity of anaphylaxis to Hymenoptera venom, all individuals at risk for systemic reactions should carry epinephrine for self-treatment and be considered for immunotherapy.

## CLINICAL FEATURES

Stinging insect allergy affects individuals of all ages without regard to personal or family history of atopy and occurs in up to 3% of the general population. Reactions to stinging insects range from mild local irritation to fatal anaphylaxis. Local reactions are characteristic of most Hymenoptera stings. With most stings there is a circumscribed area of pain, warmth, and induration up to 1 cm in size. This is a normal response and relates to the pharmacologic action of venom substances. In some individuals, however, a large local reaction develops characterized by extensive swelling at the sting site, which peaks 48 to 72 hours later, and can last up to 1 week. If the stinger is retained, it should be flicked or scraped off, not pulled out; squeezing the stinger will discharge more venom into the area and host.

Occasionally, a sting site may become infected. For those circumstances, treatment would be similar to that used for other local infections. While large local reactions may be IgE-mediated, subsequent stings do not tend to result in systemic reactions so venom skin testing and immunotherapy are not indicated.

Systemic reactions to insect stings range from isolated cutaneous reactions (urticaria or angioedema) to fatal anaphylaxis. The pathologic features of Hymenoptera fatalities are indistinguishable from fatal anaphylaxis from other causes, e.g., penicillin or food induced. Respiratory tract obstruction is the major cause of death in more than two-thirds of such cases, while vascular involvement, anaphylactic shock, and neurologic reactions are responsible for the remaining fatalities. Myocardial ischemia, and even infarction, can complicate anaphylactic reactions to Hymenoptera and severely complicate treatment. Although most systemic reactions occur in children and adolescents, mortality is greatest in adults, particularly those with pre-existing cardiac disease and those receiving beta-blocker therapy.

Idiosyncratic reactions to Hymenoptera stings include vasculitis, nephritis, serum sickness, and neurologic conditions such as Guillain-Barré syndrome and cerebritis. These reactions are generally thought not to be IgE-mediated and do not warrant venom immunotherapy. Toxic reactions are caused by multiple stings with systemic absorption of large concentrations of venom. Because venom contains chemicals with actions similar to mast cell mediators, toxic reactions can have symptoms similar to those in anaphylaxis.

## DIAGNOSIS

The diagnosis of stinging insect hypersensitivity is based on the clinical history and the demonstration of venom-specific IgE. It is critical to document the circumstances surrounding the sting, concurrent medical problems and therapy, and signs of anaphylaxis such as hypotension, laryngeal edema, urticaria, and bronchospasm. Individuals who experience a severe systemic reaction to a Hymenoptera sting should undergo venom skin testing after an interval of at least 2 to 4 weeks. Skin testing is preferred over RAST or other *in vitro* tests as it is more sensitive and specific, although in selected cases, RAST may be used for diagnostic purposes. Allergy skin testing consists of initial prick tests followed by intradermal injections of dilute solutions of venom up to a maximum concentration of 1 µg/per ml. Testing is *not* indicated in instances of large local reactions or non–IgE-mediated reactions.

## TREATMENT

The treatment of local and large local reactions includes ice to the affected area, elevation if the entire limb is involved, and oral antihistamines such as diphenhydramine (Benadryl) 25 to 50 mg every 4 hours. Short courses of prednisone, 10 mg three times daily for 5 to 7 days, have been used for the more severe and extensive cases.

Since most fatalities from Hymenoptera stings occur within 30 to 60 minutes of the sting, all individuals at risk of a repeated systemic reaction to a Hymenoptera sting should be instructed in self-treatment with injectable epinephrine (Epi-Pen and Epi-Pen Jr., Center Laboratories, Port Washington, NY; Ana-kit, Hollister-Stier, Spokane, WA) before discharge from the emergency room or doctor's office. The Epi-Pen is preferred by us because of its ease of administration. If an Ana-kit is prescribed, the patient should be required to demonstrate proper self-injection technique. For emergency self-treatment to be effective, patients must carry the epinephrine

714

whenever at risk of Hymenoptera sting. Self-treatment with epinephrine should be administered at the first sign of a severe systemic reaction, such as throat swelling or respiratory difficulty, or immediately post-sting in those patients with a history of a preceding severe anaphylactic reaction. Repeat episodes of anaphylaxis tend to be similar to the initial episode. If a patient experienced hypotension on one occasion, this is likely to be the recurring symptom complex. Medical evaluation and treatment should then be promptly obtained in view of the potential for prolonged anaphylaxis.

Prompt treatment of systemic reactions is mandated because most fatal reactions occur quickly after the sting. The emergency management of anaphylaxis includes airway management, volume expansion, blood pressure support, and aminophylline for bronchospasm and is discussed in the section on anaphylaxis. Epinephrine 1:1000, 0.3 to 0.5 ml subcutaneously, should be promptly administered for a systemic reaction and repeated as necessary. Adjunctive therapy includes parenteral antihistamines, such as diphenhydramine 50 to 100 mg (1 to 2 mg per kg). Corticosteroids (prednisone 30 mg) may be given acutely, primarily to prevent the late allergic response to the sting and enhance efficacy of other therapy. With hypotension, vigorous fluid replacement is mandatory. Concomitant use of beta-blocker therapy may necessitate particularly vigorous therapy. Prophylactic treatment of stinging insect allergy involves avoidance and venom-specific immunotherapy. Measures designed to minimize the likelihood of repeat Hymenoptera stings include avoidance of perfumes and brightly colored clothing in addition to exercising caution (wearing of shoes) when outdoors during summer and fall.

Over the past decade venom-specific immunotherapy has been shown to be both safe and effective in preventing severe systemic reactions to stinging insects. Untreated individuals are at about a 60% risk of repeated systemic reaction to a subsequent Hymenoptera sting. However, with venom-specific immunotherapy, the risk for anaphylaxis is reduced to less than 5%. Furthermore, in those having a reaction *while* on immunotherapy, the intensity of the reaction is likely reduced.

Venom immunotherapy is indicated for those individuals with a history of a systemic reaction to a Hymenoptera sting in whom venom-specific IgE can be demonstrated. In contrast to adults, children less than 16 years old with only cutaneous symptoms do not require venom immunotherapy. Venom immunotherapy is administered through a series of weekly or twice weekly injections until a maintenance dose of 100 µg of each venom is reached. The interval between injections is then lengthened to 4 to 6 weeks. Recent evidence suggests that 5 years of venom immunotherapy *may* be sufficient to impart lasting protection.

The imported fire ant is now found in 13 southern states where it is a major cause of insect sting allergy. The imported fire ant is distinctive in that its sting is characterized by almost immediate pain, itching, and burning. Within 4 to 8 hours, clear vesicles develop with surrounding erythema, and by 24 hours, a characteristic sterile pustule is seen. Skin testing and immunotherapy for individuals at risk of severe systemic reactions to fire ants can be performed with whole body extract.

# Diseases of the Skin

## ACNE VULGARIS AND ROSACEA

method of
ALAN R. SHALITA, M.D.
*SUNY–Health Science Center at Brooklyn*
*Brooklyn, New York*

Acne vulgaris is the most common skin disease. It affects approximately 80% of the teenage and young adult population and, contrary to popular belief, may persist well into the third and fourth decades of life. Acne is a disease of the pilosebaceous follicle with a multifactorial cause. The pathogenesis includes an androgen-dependent increase in sebum production, proliferation of the follicular microflora (principally *Propionibacterium acnes*), alterations in follicular keratinization, and inflammation. This results in the clinical lesions of acne, namely, open comedones (blackheads), closed comedones (whiteheads), papules, pustules, and nodulocystic lesions. Current therapy is directed toward prevention and suppression of these lesions by affecting one or more of the pathogenic factors. Treatment is remarkably effective in most patients.

### TREATMENT

#### Topical Therapy

Many patients may be successfully treated with topical therapy alone. For comedonal and mild inflammatory acne, therapy is initiated with tretinoin (Retin-A) cream, 0.025%, or 0.01% tretinoin gel applied daily. The patient should be advised that an initial erythema and exfoliation may occur, that an exacerbation of inflammatory lesions is possible during the first month of therapy, and that an increased sensitivity to sunburn is likely. For the latter condition it is advisable to limit sun exposure and to recommend a suitable (SPF 15 or higher) sunscreen.

Patients who demonstrate little or no response and who have exhibited little or no erythema or desquamation may be placed on higher concentrations of the drug, either the 0.05% or 0.1% cream or 0.025% gel. A few patients may require the 0.05% liquid, the most irritating form of the drug, before achieving a satisfactory therapeutic response. Significant therapeutic improvement does not usually occur before 4 to 6 weeks, and 12 weeks are usually required for optimal therapeutic benefit. Topical tretinoin appears to exert its effect on the keratinizing epithelium of the follicle.

For the more inflammatory forms of acne, the addition of a benzoyl peroxide gel (Desquam-X, Persa Gel, PanOxyl) is frequently beneficial. Benzoyl peroxide is a potent antibacterial agent that significantly reduces the intrafollicular population of *P. acnes*. Therapy is usually initiated with the 5% gel applied daily, although some patients may achieve a satisfactory response to the 2.5% concentration. Refractory cases and patients with considerable involvement of the back and chest may require the 10% concentration. Although little erythema usually occurs, there may be considerable desquamation. In addition, a small percentage of the population may exhibit contact allergy to benzoyl peroxide.

Topical antibiotic solutions, such as those containing erythromycin (T-Stat, Staticin, ATS, Ery-Derm, Erycette) and clindamycin (Cleocin-T), are useful alternatives to benzoyl peroxide in the treatment of inflammatory acne. They offer the advantage of being essentially nonsensitizing but may result in the overgrowth of resistant organisms. Erythromycin solution or gel 1.5 to 2.0% and clindamycin solution or gel 1.0% appear to be equal in therapeutic value.

Our preferred method of topical treatment is the sequential use of topical tretinoin and a topical antibacterial, one applied in the morning and the other at night. The effects of the two drugs appear to be additive. Some patients, however, will not tolerate the "dryness" produced by this regimen. One may then try therapy with each drug on alternate days. Eventually, most patients will accommodate to these local side effects and will be able to use both drugs on the same day.

The combination of benzoyl peroxide and a topical antibiotic produces better results than when either agent is used alone. A stabilized formulation of erythromycin, 3%, and benzoyl peroxide, 5% (Benzamycin), is very effective and may be used in the sequential regimen with tretinoin. For those patients easily irritated by hydroalcoholic gels or solutions, meclocycline cream (Meclan) or erythromycin ointment (Aknemycin) may be used satisfactorily.

Preparations containing various combinations of sulfur, resorcin, and salicylic acid, particularly in tinted lotions and creams, may be useful when used judiciously. They accelerate the resolution of inflammatory lesions while providing cover. In addition, cleansers containing salicylic acid may be useful, particularly in patients who do not tolerate topical tretinoin. Salicylic acid has mild comedolytic properties (SalAc wash).

### Systemic Therapy

Broad-spectrum antibiotics are valuable in the treatment of inflammatory acne. They are generally reserved for patients with moderate to severe inflammatory acne and have achieved a remarkable record of safety in long-term use. Therapy is usually initiated with 500 to 1000 mg of tetracycline hydrochloride or erythromycin. The dose is decreased at appropriate intervals according to the therapeutic response. Minocycline (Minocin), 50 mg up to four times daily, is useful in those patients who appear to be refractory to the aforementioned agents. An alternative is larger doses of tetracycline, up to 3000 mg daily.

Recent evidence suggests that many women with inflammatory acne may have elevated androgens, either of adrenal or ovarian origin. In these patients, treatment with oral contraceptives, low-dose dexamethasone (Decadron)*, or a combination of the two may be quite beneficial. Spironolactone (Aldactone),† 50 to 200 mg per day, may also be effective.

Patients with severe, recalcitrant, nodulocystic acne who have failed to respond to the treatment regimens outlined may achieve remarkable improvement with isotretinoin (Accutane). Isotretinoin is administered in a dose of 0.5 to 1.0 mg per kg daily. Patients with severe involvement of the back and chest may require as much as 2 mg per kg daily. The course of treatment is from 4 to 5 months, and improvement is variable during this time period. Some patients may not achieve maximum improvement until after they have completed the course of treatment. Relapses are rare, and remissions lasting as long as 6 years have been reported. In any case, it is advisable to wait at least 3 to 4 months before retreating the refractory patient.

---

*This use of dexamethasone is not listed in the manufacturer's official directive.

†This use of spironolactone is not listed in the manufacturer's official directive.

Isotretinoin therapy is accompanied by numerous side effects. Most noteworthy is the fact that the drug is teratogenic in humans. Women of child-bearing age, therefore, should have pregnancy tests before initiation of therapy, practice strict contraception during treatment, and be constantly reminded of the teratogenic effects of the drug. It appears safe for conception to occur 1 month after discontinuing treatment. The drug is not mutagenic and has no effect on the ability to conceive and no apparent effects on spermatozoa. Most additional side effects relate to the fact that the drug causes a pronounced reduction in sebum production. Thus there is dryness of the skin, marked chapping of the lips, and cheilitis; dryness of the mucosa, which can lead to epistaxis and conjunctivitis; and some pruritus. All of these can be alleviated by the use of emollients. Although a variety of laboratory abnormalities may occur, the most significant is triglyceride elevation. For this reason it is recommended that baseline fasting triglycerides be obtained before treatment and every 2 weeks thereafter until a plateau has been reached. Dietary modification, prohibition of alcohol, and dose reduction will usually reduce these triglyceride elevations. If not, it is recommended that patients whose triglyceride levels rise above 750 mg per dl discontinue the drug. Bone pain, muscle aches, headache, and fatigue have been reported with some frequency. Most are relieved with simple analgesics. Pseudotumor cerebri has also been reported and appears to occur with increased frequency in patients taking isotretinoin and a tetracycline concomitantly. Therefore, the use of these two drugs together appears contraindicated. Finally, there are rare reports of decreased night vision and bony exostoses of the vertebrae. The latter appear to be asymptomatic. Given this side effect profile, it is evident that the drug should be limited to the most severe forms of the disease or to those patients who have proved to be totally refractory to conventional forms of acne treatment.

Systemic glucocorticoids are rarely required in the management of acne, except as noted in the low-dose treatment of women with increased androgen secretion. Larger doses (30 to 40 mg daily) may be used for brief periods of time in patients who develop flares of their disease during the course of isotretinoin treatment. Local injections of glucocorticoids such as triamcinolone acetonide (Kenalog) (2.5 to 5.0 mg per ml) are useful for the treatment of individual nodulocystic lesions and for the exuberant granulation tissue that may develop during treatment with isotretinoin. The use of a 1-ml syringe with a 30-gauge needle provides excellent control of the amount of material injected. No more than 0.5 mg should be injected in any one site. Triamcinolone hexacetamide (Aristospan Intralesional), 5 mg per ml, is longer lasting but may produce more atrophy and should be limited to lesions of the chest and back. It is also useful for the treatment of hypertrophic scars.

The physical removal of comedones with a comedo extractor is frequently beneficial. Incision and drainage of inflammatory lesions rarely accomplishes more than intralesional steroids.

## ROSACEA

Rosacea is a not uncommon disease of the skin that usually occurs from the fourth decade of life onward. It may be preceded by seborrheic dermatitis and appears to be more common in fair-skinned individuals of Celtic background. It is characterized by facial erythema, particularly of the perinasal area. More pronounced involvement may include the glabella, perioral areas, and the chin. As the disease progresses, telangiectasia, papules and pustules, and granulomatous tissue may form. The disease appears to be aggravated by all factors that increase blood flow to the head and neck, such as strenuous exercise, hot foods, increased temperature, hypertension, alcohol ingestion, and emotional stress.

## THERAPY

Most patients with rosacea will respond to combined therapy with oral tetracycline and topical anti-inflammatory measures. Tetracycline therapy is initiated at 1000 mg daily and reduced at monthly intervals to a maintenance dose of 250 mg daily. Many patients will achieve enough of a response to discontinue tetracycline for varying periods of time, but most will relapse at one time or another. Topical therapy should consist of the judicial use of hydrocortisone alone or in combination with 3% precipitated sulfur or 10% sodium sulfacetamide. Fluorinated steroid preparations are contraindicated since they will produce rebound telangiectasia. Even hydrocortisone (1 to 2.5%) should be limited to twice daily applications for brief periods of time to control the symptoms. Topical antibiotic therapy is occasionally beneficial, but many patients with rosacea do not tolerate the hydroalcoholic vehicles. For these patients, erythromycin ointment (Aknemycin) or meclocycline cream (Meclan) may be tried, although neither has been subjected to rigorous clinical evaluation for this purpose. Topical metronidazole gel (Metrogel) has recently been approved for this indication and may be highly effective, particularly in the pustular forms of the disease. It is applied twice daily and is well tolerated.

Isotretinoin has been reported to be particularly effective in patients with the more severe papulopustular and granulomatous forms of the disease. Reports conflict as to whether or not this drug has any effect on the telangiectasia. A dose of 0.5 mg per kg has been reported to be effective for this disease.

Telangiectasia may be treated by gentle electrodesiccation using an epilating needle with the lowest current available. Exuberant tissue, such as that found in rhinophyma, may be removed by electrosurgery, dermabrasion, or laser treatment.

Some patients with rosacea may develop ophthalmologic complications. Blepharitis is common and frequently is accompanied by conjunctivitis. Keratitis is less common but, left untreated, may result in visual impairment. All respond to oral tetracycline therapy. The addition of sodium sulfacetamide ophthalmic ointment is frequently of benefit. Refractory patients should be referred to an ophthalmologist.

# HAIR DISORDERS

method of
DAVID A. WHITING, M.D.
*Baylor Hair Research and Treatment Center*
*Dallas, Texas*

An essential element in the diagnosis and management of alopecia is the time needed to listen to the patient's history and anxieties. An explanation of the hair growth cycle is often helpful: Hairs go through continuous cycles of growth and rest. The resting, or telogen, hair is eventually displaced by the new growing, or anagen, hair below. It is assumed, for convenience, that the average number of scalp hairs equals 100,000, comprising 90% anagen and 10% telogen hairs. If the average duration of the anagen phase is 1000 days and the telogen phase 100 days, then a daily loss of up to 100 hairs is normal. The average growth rate of the large, visible, or terminal scalp hairs is 0.35 mm per day, or 1 inch every 2 1/2 months. Hair cycles and growth rate are affected by genetic factors, age, sex, race, and season, resulting in wide variations of normal. In the human scalp, growth cycles in individual hairs are not synchronized to ensure an even hair coverage.

The investigation of alopecia starts with a careful examination of scalp hair, noting the pattern of hair loss, and the length of affected hairs. The scalp itself, facial and body hair, and skin, nails, and teeth should also be checked. Simple pull tests in different areas of the scalp will indicate whether hairs detach too easily and whether they break off or come out by the roots. Easily detachable hairs with depigmented, clubbed roots indicate telogen hairs, and more adherent hairs with pigmented roots and long, white, root sheaths

TABLE 1. **Common Causes of Alopecia**

| | |
|---|---|
| Androgenetic alopecia | 68.8% |
| Diffuse alopecia | 11.3% |
| Alopecia areata | 9.9% |
| Cicatricial alopecia | 4.9% |
| Trichotillomania | 1.3% |
| Trauma, traction | 1.1% |
| Other (infections and infestations, hair shaft abnormalities, hereditary and congenital) | 2.7% |
| | 100.0% |

indicate anagen hairs. Light microscopy is an easy office procedure to identify hair roots, fiber diameter, and most structural abnormalities of the hair shaft. Potassium hydroxide preparations of affected hair fragments can demonstrate fungal infections, which can be typed by fungal culture. Scalp biopsies are indicated for diagnostic purposes in all cases of cicatricial and unexplained noncicatricial alopecia. The new technique of horizontal sectioning of scalp biopsies supplements the diagnostic capability of vertical sectioning and has some value in the prediction of future hair regrowth. Laboratory tests should depend on clinical indications, but a basic work-up in the unexplained case should include a complete blood count, routine chemistry studies, serum iron, urinalysis, tests of thyroid function, and a serologic test for syphilis. Tests of androgenic function are indicated in female pattern alopecia if acne, hirsutism, menstrual disorders, deepening of the voice, and/or severe male type of alopecia with both temporal recession and vertical baldness are present.

The common causes of alopecia are listed in Table 1.

## ANDROGENETIC ALOPECIA

Androgenetic alopecia affects both sexes and is of dominant inheritance. Scalp hairs on the vertex in these patients are unduly susceptible to the action of androgens and become progressively miniaturized. The hair is lost predominantly on the crown with relative sparing of the back and sides of the scalp. In a young patient the complaint of increased hair loss often precedes the appearance of alopecia. Telogen hairs are often more easily detached from the vertex than from the occipitoparietal areas.

In males, the onset may be any time after puberty and is not infrequent by the age of 17 years. The sequence of hair loss usually starts with a typical M pattern of bitemporal recession, followed by vertical loss. The amount of progression through frontal and vertical loss is variable, is influenced by genetic factors, and is often intermittent rather than continuous. Male-pattern androgenetic alopecia is graded according to severity from Types I through VII on the Hamilton-Norwood scale (Table 2). It affects 50% of males aged 50 years.

In females, androgenetic alopecia may commence at any age after puberty but is not often clinically apparent in women below 25 years of age. The incidence figures lag behind those of males by approximately one decade. The hair loss usually appears over the frontovertical region as a widened part line. Later, hair is lost more diffusely over the frontal and vertical regions, but an intact frontal hairline is preserved, without the bitemporal recession seen in males. Female-pattern androgenetic alopecia is graded as mild, moderate, or severe on the Ludwig scale and causes diffuse vertical thinning but not complete baldness.

### Treatment

No treatment is required for Types I and II male-pattern androgenetic alopecia, nor is it helpful for Type III with bitemporal recession only. Topical 2% minoxidil (Rogaine) applied twice daily for a minimum of 1 year is indicated in Type III male-pattern androgenetic alopecia with midfrontal recession and/or vertical hair loss, and in Types IV and V. The first observed effect from minoxidil is often a reduced rate of hair loss, usually after 6 to 8 weeks of treatment. Visible regrowth of hair, to be expected in approximately one-third of cases, may occur mostly on the vertex but rarely in the temples, after 3 to 9 months of treatment. The increasing hair growth rate may slow down and plateau after one year or continue to improve slowly over several years. Patients who respond best to this treatment are usually aged below 40 years, have a history of hair loss for less than 10 years, and have a bald area less than 10 cm in diameter. There is some evidence to suggest that minoxidil will stop further hair loss in 90% of cases of male-pattern alopecia, and it should therefore be used for its preventive effects in young patients with early hair loss. If positive results are noted after 1 year of treatment, minoxidil should be continued twice daily indefinitely. No adverse systemic effects have been demonstrated, but local irritation may occur in a few cases. Present indications

TABLE 2. **Hamilton-Norwood Classification of Male-Pattern Androgenetic Alopecia**

| | |
|---|---|
| Type I: | Full hair (e.g., normal prepubertal hair) |
| Type II: | Mild bitemporal recession (e.g., normal postpubertal hair) |
| Type III: | Deep bitemporal recession, possible midfrontal recession, possible vertical thinning |
| Type IV: | Increased frontotemporal recession, marked vertical thinning |
| Type V: | Marked frontotemporal and vertical thinning, becoming confluent |
| Type VI: | Large areas of frontotemporal and vertical alopecia, indefinite band of sparse hair in between |
| Type VII: | Complete confluence of frontotemporal and vertical areas of alopecia |

TABLE 3. **Causes of Diffuse Alopecia**

| | |
|---|---|
| Telogen effluvium | Nutritional |
| Anagen effluvium | Malabsorption |
| Drugs | Renal failure |
| Other chemicals | Hepatic failure |
| Thyroid disorder | Systemic disease |
| Iron deficiency | Miscellaneous |

TABLE 4. **Causes of Telogen Effluvium**

| | |
|---|---|
| Childbirth | Crash diets |
| Febrile illnesses | Traction |
| Surgical operations | Severe emotional stress |
| Chronic systemic disease | Physiologic in newborn |
| Drugs: Antithyroid, anticoagulants, sodium valproate, beta blockers | |

are that minoxidil has similar effects in female-pattern androgenetic alopecia, at least in mild and moderate cases.

If androgenetic alopecia is associated with undisputed evidence of androgenic overactivity, then the source of the androgen excess must be identified and treated appropriately. Topical antiandrogens have not as yet been shown to produce consistent regrowth of hair in androgenetic alopecia. Estrogen-dominant oral contraceptives currently obtainable in the USA, such as ethynodiol diacetate with ethinyl estrodiol (Demulen), are similarly disappointing. Oral spironolactone (Aldactone)* in doses of 75 to 200 mg daily is antiandrogenic and may be beneficial in some cases. Dexamethasone in doses of 0.125 to 0.5 mg daily can be used to suppress adrenal overactivity. The side effects of and contraindications to systemic antiandrogens should be reviewed before initiating treatment.

If medical treatment fails or is not desired, the remaining alternatives are surgery with hair transplants, scalp reductions or transposition of hair-bearing flaps, creative hairstyling, or hairpieces.

## DIFFUSE ALOPECIA

Diffuse alopecia is deceptive, since 40 to 50% of scalp hairs have to be lost before it becomes visible. Hairs can easily be detached from the back and sides of the scalp, as well as from the crown. The main causes are listed in Table 3.

### Telogen Effluvium

Telogen effluvium is a diffuse loss of normal club hairs from normal resting follicles. It is usually due to a premature interruption of growth in many anagen hairs, which then cycle through catagen into a telogen phase, so that the proportion of telogen hairs rises to 25 to 50%. When the resting phase ends 2 to 4 months later, new anagen hairs displace the club hairs, which loosen and fall out abruptly in large numbers from all over the scalp. A useful diagnostic marker of telogen effluvium in females is the presence of bitemporal recession, which is usually

less prominent in female pattern androgenetic alopecia. Causes are listed in Table 4.

### Treatment

If a definite cause in the recent past can be identified and if necessary eliminated, an explanation of the mechanism involved and reassurances about impending regrowth should suffice. Follow-up is necessary, since a disappointing number of patients progress to a chronic form of telogen effluvium. Minoxidil (Rogaine) applied twice daily may stimulate more anagen cycles in these patients and should be continued until the rate of hair loss returns to normal and hair regrowth is visible.

### Anagen Effluvium

Anagen effluvium is characterized by the diffuse loss of anagen hairs from growing follicles. Arrested cell division in the hair bulb matrix leads to progressive narrowing of the hair shaft or to failure of hair formation. The weakened hairs easily fracture and their proximal ends are tapered (pencil pointing). The alopecia is severe and easily diagnosed, since some 90% of scalp hairs are normally in anagen. Anagen alopecia occurs within a few weeks, and if the inhibitory influence is removed, hairs will regrow promptly. Causes are listed in Table 5.

### Treatment

The treatment of anagen effluvium lies in identifying the cause and treating or removing it, if possible.

### Drugs and Chemicals

Alopecia due to drugs and chemicals is usually diffuse and confined to the scalp. Drug-related

TABLE 5. **Causes of Anagen Effluvium**

| | |
|---|---|
| Cytostatic drugs | X-ray therapy |
| Endocrine diseases | Alopecia areata |
| Cicatricial alopecia | Trauma and pressure |
| Severe protein calorie malnutrition: kwashiorkor, marasmus | |
| Other toxic drugs: Retinoids, triparanol, thallium, thiourea, arsenic, gold, bismuth, borax, levodopa, colchicine | |

---

*This use of spironolactone is not listed in the manufacturer's official directive.

alopecia may be due to telogen or anagen effluvium or may be of a nonspecific dystrophic variety. In general, the only reliable way to confirm the diagnosis is to stop the suspected drug for a sufficient time to verify improvement and, later, if desirable and feasible, to rechallenge with the same drug, unless the drug is well known to cause alopecia. Fortunately, most of the alopecia caused by drugs is reversible. Many drugs can cause alopecia, including androgens, anticancer drugs, anticoagulants, anticonvulsants, antithyroid drugs, beta blockers, cholesterol reducers, gold, histamine $H_2$ receptor blockers, lithium, nonsteroidal anti-inflammatory drugs, oral contraceptives, retinoids and retinol, and tricyclic antidepressants.

### Treatment

The treatment lies in identifying and eliminating the cause, if possible.

### Other Causes of Diffuse Alopecia

Thyroid disorders, iron deficiency, nutritional deficiencies, malabsorption, renal failure, syphilis, collagen vascular diseases, carcinomatosis, and other miscellaneous underlying causes of alopecia require appropriate investigation and treatment.

### Alopecia Areata

Alopecia areata can occur at any age and affects both sexes equally. An onset in early childhood is likely in the 10% of cases associated with atopy, in which a high incidence of alopecia totalis is present (75% in Japan). An onset in middle age is usual in the 5% of cases associated with organ-specific autoimmune diseases, which have a 10% incidence of alopecia totalis. The age of onset varies in the remaining 85% of cases not associated with any particular disease, which have a 6% incidence of alopecia totalis. Alopecia areata is characterized by the development of one or more circumscribed patches of hair loss associated with smooth, atrophic skin. Exclamation point hairs may be present in the active borders of the lesions. The disease may remain limited to a few patches or may progress to widespread mosaic forms, to horizontal or vertical wave forms of ophiasis, or to alopecia totalis or universalis. In doubtful cases, scalp biopsies may be diagnostic.

### Treatment

Alopecia areata has an unpredictable course not easily altered by treatment. Localized patches

TABLE 6. **Causes of Cicatricial Alopecia**

| | |
|---|---|
| Hereditary and Congenital: | Aplasia cutis, epidermal nevi, epidermolysis bullosa |
| Infections: | |
| Bacterial: | Acne keloidalis, dissecting cellulitis, folliculitis, syphilis |
| Fungal: | Favus, kerion, mycetoma |
| Protozoal: | Leishmaniasis |
| Viral: | Herpes zoster, varicella |
| Physical Injuries: | Burns, mechanical trauma, radiodermatitis |
| Neoplasms: | Angiosarcoma, basal cell epithelioma, cylindroma, lymphoma, melanoma, metastatic tumors, squamous cell carcinoma |
| Dermatoses: | Cicatricial pemphigoid, dermatomyositis, folliculitis decalvans, lichen planopilaris, lupus erythematosus, neurotic excoriations, pseudopelade, scleroderma |

in adults and older children are best treated with intralesional corticosteroid injections such as triamcinolone acetonide (Kenalog) 5 to 10 mg per ml. High-potency topical corticosteroids such as fluocinonide gel 0.05% (Lidex gel) are preferred for young children and for widespread disease. The use of systemic steroids in alopecia areata is controversial, but prednisone 20 to 40 mg daily for 1 to 2 months can reverse rapid deterioration in widespread cases, although subsequent relapses are common. Minoxidil (Rogaine) has been tried with some success in alopecia areata, especially in cases with less than 75% hair loss. It should be continued until full regrowth occurs. Contact dermatitis can stimulate regrowth of hair and can be induced by short contact therapy for ½ to 1 hour daily with 0.25 to 1% anthralin (Drithocreme*), a therapy suitable for children.

### CICATRICIAL ALOPECIA

Common causes of cicatricial alopecia are listed in Table 6. The scarring may be subtle or obvious. Always check the scalp for other changes such as folliculitis, follicular plugging, absent follicular orifices, scaling, telangiectasia, and broken hairs. Look for associated lesions elsewhere on the skin and mucous membranes, including the mouth, ears, and nails, which may be useful in confirming the diagnosis of diseases such as lichen planus and lupus erythematosus. If disease activity is present, a specific diagnosis may be possible. In burned-out cases, the end result of scarring with permanent destruction of hair follicles may look much the same regardless of the cause. All cases of suspected cicatricial alopecia warrant a scalp biopsy, and special stains and/or immunofluorescence may be required.

---

*This use of anthralin is not listed in the manufacturer's official directive.

### Treatment

The treatment depends on the cause. Surgical treatment by excision, with scalp reduction or hair transplantation, may be suitable for nevoid lesions, tumors, and old scars. Infections can be treated appropriately. Folliculitis decalvans may respond to long-term antibiotics, such as tetracycline, erythromycin, or to trimethoprim/sulfamethoxazole (Bactrim, Septra), or to topical retinoic acid (Retin A*). Lichen planopilaris, lupus erythematosus, and pseudopelade can be treated with topical, intralesional, or oral corticosteroids and/or antimalarials.†

## TRICHOTILLOMANIA

Trichotillomania is an abnormal compulsion to pull out hair and is more common in females. It can lead to large areas of alopecia which vary from a symmetric to a predominantly unilateral location. The scalp is usually unaffected and is neither atrophic and smooth nor inflamed and scaly. The hairs are broken off at different lengths.

### Treatment

In children, underlying emotional problems are often identifiable and susceptible to problem solving. Adults usually require psychiatric treatment.

## TRACTION AND TRAUMA

Hair loss can result from many forms of physical and chemical trauma associated with overzealous hairstyling, from prolonged pressure on the scalp in motionless patients, from head rolling and habit tics, and from excoriations in pruritic dermatoses. The underlying cause requires identification and treatment.

## INFECTIONS AND INFESTATIONS

### Tinea Capitis

Tinea capitis causes patchy alopecia, especially in children. In the United States today it is usually due to *Trichophyton tonsurans*. This endothrix infection weakens the hairs, which snap off flush with the skin surface, giving rise to characteristic black dots. A kerion should always be suspected in prepubertal children with persistent, boggy abscesses on the scalp resistant to antibiotics and associated with hair loss. The treatment of choice for tinea capitis or kerion is prolonged oral griseofulvin therapy.

### Pediculosis Capitis

Head lice cause severe pruritus, and the resultant excoriations can cause alopecia. The most effective treatment is 1% permethrin creme rinse (Nix).

# CANCER OF THE SKIN

method of
RAMON L. SANCHEZ, M.D.
*University of Texas Medical Branch at Galveston*
*Galveston, Texas*

The skin is the organ most often involved by cancer, its incidence directly related to the age of the patient, skin color, and sun exposure, i.e., most instances of cancer of the skin are in elderly patients with fair skin who live in southern states.

Fortunately, the majority of skin cancers have a very low potential for dissemination and metastases, albeit they may show quite aggressive local growth with invasion of adjacent structures. When planning the treatment of skin cancer, prior consideration should be given to the type of tumor, location, and modifying circumstances.

### TYPE OF TUMOR

The majority of skin cancers are basal cell carcinomas, squamous cell carcinomas, or melanomas.

Basal cell carcinomas are the most common type of skin cancer, often seen in sun-exposed skin, although they may occur also in sun-protected skin. An early basal cell carcinoma appears clinically as a pearly-gray papule with associated telangiectasia. Tumors that have been present for some time often are ulcerated. For practical purposes, basal cell carcinomas never metastasize, although they often show local aggressive behavior.

Squamous cell carcinomas of the skin are seen almost exclusively in the sun-exposed skin of head and neck, anterior chest, and dorsum of hands and forearms. They usually are seen in association with actinic keratosis, which precedes the development of cancer. They present as hyperkeratotic papules or as ulcers with elevated, infiltrated borders. Squamous cell carcinomas may arise also in the setting of old burn scars (Marjolin's ulcer) or of chronic inflammatory processes such as an osteomyelitis drainage sinus. Squamous cell carcinomas may arise also in mucosae such as the lips or glans penis. The latter are associated sometimes with previous papilloma virus infections, i.e., condyloma.

Melanomas occur in any given location. Most mela-

---

*This use of retinoic acid is not listed in the manufacturer's official directive.

†This use of antimalarials is not listed in the manufacturer's official directive.

nomas arise de novo, although as many as one-fourth may arise in pre-existing nevi. Giant congenital nevi (over 18 cm in diameter) are often associated with development of melanoma, and the risk of malignant transformation increases with age. Melanomas are usually pigmented, although nodular melanomas may be totally devoid of pigment (amelanotic melanoma). Other lesions that may be pigmented and, therefore, resemble melanoma are seborrheic keratosis and basal cell carcinomas.

## LOCATION

Location of the tumor to be treated should be taken into consideration prior to surgery for several reasons. One is the possible involvement of adjacent structures by the tumor, such as the eyelids or the superficial temporal artery, which may lead to complications at the time of surgery or afterwards (such as ectropion or hemorrhage). The second reason is the different behavior of squamous cell carcinomas depending on the location of the tumor. While squamous cell carcinomas arising in sun-damaged skin in general have a very low metastatic potential (about 0.5% will metastasize), those tumors that arise on the lip, temple, dorsum of the hands, and ears have been associated with increased metastatic rates that approach 10 to 20% and, therefore, should be treated more aggressively than tumors in other locations. The increased metastatic potential is also true for squamous cell carcinomas arising in mucosae (lips, glans penis), burn scars, and chronically damaged skin (osteomyelitis sinus). It is therefore very important to understand the clinical setting of a given tumor before attempting therapy.

The third reason to consider location is the cosmetic results. Curettage and electrodesiccation often will result in flat discrete scars, and they are therefore preferred for small tumors on the face amenable to such treatment.

## MODIFYING CIRCUMSTANCES

Modifying circumstances are the size of the tumor, the time elapsed since first noticed by the patient, and consideration of primary vs. recurrent lesions. In general, with larger tumors and longer history, the treatment should be more aggressive. Recurrent lesions should always be treated by excision with control of the margins rather than by curettage. A specific type of basal cell carcinoma is the morphea-like or fibrosing basal cell carcinoma in which the tumor presents clinically as a flat, indurated, and depressed plaque, instead of the typical nodular or ulcerated presentation. In these cases, the tumor nests are encased in fibrous tissue and, therefore, are not amenable to be treated by curettage and electrodesiccation but by excision.

## BIOPSY

Skin biopsies are obtained sometimes as a step prior to the definitive surgical treatment of skin tumors. Among the reasons to obtain a skin biopsy are the need of a histologic diagnosis when the clinical diag-

nosis of malignancy is not certain. In large tumors or in tumors that infiltrate adjacent structures, a skin biopsy is obtained as part of the presurgical evaluation and preparation. The three methods commonly used to obtain skin biopsies are shave, punch, and ellipse.

Shave biopsy is a simple technique that can be performed quickly, yet it yields enough tissue for histologic diagnosis and does not require sutures. After the area to be biopsied has been cleaned with alcohol and a bactericidal soap, 1% lidocaine (Xylocaine) and epinephrine is injected to anesthetize the biopsy site. The shave biopsy can be performed with a razor blade or with a scalpel blade (we use #15 scalpel blades). The advantage of the razor blade is that it can be curved by holding it between the thumb and the middle finger, thereby assuring the depth of penetration. A shave biopsy should be deep enough to ensure that invasion of the dermis by the tumor can be histologically evaluated. Once the sample has been obtained, bleeding is stopped by applying 30 to 50% aluminum chloride in 50% isopropyl alcohol or Monsel's solution (ferric subsulfate in aqueous solution) with a cotton swab under pressure.

Shave biopsies are contraindicated in pigmented lesions that are suspicious for melanoma. If the tumor is a melanoma, the shave biopsy probably would be more shallow than the tumor, therefore preventing the histologic evaluation of its thickness and depth of penetration.

Punch biopsies and incisional biopsies have the advantage of being deep, and therefore, they are the only modality to be used in pigmented lesions. An incisional biopsy will provide more tissue for examination than a punch biopsy, so it is usually the modality of choice in large pigmented lesions that require previous diagnosis.

## TREATMENT OF NONMELANOMA SKIN CANCERS

### Curettage and Electrodesiccation

This technique is used for treatment of primary basal cell carcinomas and squamous cell carcinomas of the skin. It is not used for recurrent lesions or for morpheaform basal cell carcinomas. If the tumor is located on the nasolabial fold or near the inner canthus of the eye, only small superficial lesions should be treated in this fashion, as the possibility of recurrence is less likely to occur with excisions with histologically controlled free margins. In other settings, properly performed curettage and electrodesiccation yields results that are comparable to other modalities of treatment.

**Method.** After the area to be treated has been cleaned and anesthetized, a shave biopsy is obtained for histologic diagnosis (if there is not a previous biopsy). Thereafter, the tumor is scooped out with a curette of proper size. The tumor is usually soft and comes off easily until normal dermis is encountered, when no more tissue is obtained.

The base of the lesion and the borders are then electrodesiccated until the complete surface has been treated in this fashion. The whole procedure is then repeated once more.

### Excision

The skin area is prepared as before, by washing with an antiseptic such as 4% chlorhexidine (Hibiclens) detergent. It is a good idea to mark the excision to be performed with gentian violet or a felt-tip pen. In general, the elliptical fusiform excision should have a length-to-width ratio of 3-4:1 and the angles should be of about 30 degrees. The excision should be parallel to the skin wrinkle lines whenever possible.

The area is then anesthesized with 1% lidocaine, with or without epinephrine, and covered with a sterile fenestrated drape. It is better to wait for 5 to 10 minutes before starting the incision to allow time for the epinephrine to have maximum effect in decreasing the bleeding.

The incision is performed with a scalpel with a #15 disposable blade. The skin is held tight between the thumb and index finger. The blade is kept perpendicular to the skin surface while incising through the full thickness of the skin and some of the upper subcutaneous tissue. The depth of the incision will depend on the size of the tumor, but it should be deep enough to ensure an adequate amount of normal tissue under the tumor. Likewise, the lateral margins should appear clear to the naked eye. Once the incision is made, the specimen is removed by dissecting the deep plane with curved, dissecting blunt-end scissors or with a scalpel.

If the excision is large and the borders close only after applying considerable lateral pressure, undermining the borders is usually recommended. The undermining is done, as a rule, in the upper subcutaneous fat except on the scalp, where the undermining is done under the galea aponeurotica. Undermining is performed with either a scalpel or scissors. The next steps are hemostasis and closure of the wound.

The specimen should be placed in 10% formaldehyde and sent to a pathology laboratory conveniently documented. If the margins of excision are going to be examined by frozen section, the specimen should arrive at the laboratory "fresh." Examination of the margins, either on frozen or on permanent section, is a priority in skin cancer treatment in order to minimize recurrences. In general, the margins are better examined histologically with transverse sections perpendicular to the long axis of the incision. Unfortunately, to be absolutely sure that the margins are free, serial sections of the whole specimen are needed, which is possible only in small specimens. In large specimens, a combination of transverse sections and sections parallel to the lateral margins is used to ensure adequate examination of the entire margin. If the histologic examination discloses positive margins, re-excision is mandatory.

### Mohs' Micrographic Surgery

This form of surgery evolved from the original "chemosurgery" devised by Dr. Frederick Mohs using a chemical fixative consisting of a paste of zinc chloride. At present, the fixative has been eliminated, but the basic principles of the method still remain. Mohs' micrographic surgery (MMS) is indicated in recurrent lesions or in primary carcinomas of large size or in those located in important anatomic sites such as the inner canthi of the eyes, the nasolabial groove, or the digits. The method consists in summary of the following: (1) after local anesthesia, the bulk of the tumor is eliminated by curettage; (2) a section of tissue including skin around the tumor as well as underlying soft tissue is removed with a scalpel; (3) the specimen is then placed flat on a tray and its orientation is maintained identical to its position in the patient and a map of the specimen is drawn; (4) the tissue is then divided into segments with its margins color coded for identification in the histologic sections and the segments are drawn on the map; (5) frozen sections parallel to the external surface of the specimen are obtained from all the segments; (6) new specimens are obtained from the area containing tumor. The histologic examination of the sections and the correlation within the map allow the exact location of the residual tumor to be determined. A map is redrawn as above and frozen sections are examined. The procedure is repeated until the tumor has been completely removed. The wound heals by second intention, or reconstructive surgery is performed.

Tumors treated by MMS have the lowest rate of recurrence, when compared with other methods. However, it is not a surgical method available in the office of a general practitioner, as it requires a setting that includes laboratory and adequate surgical facilities. Training in MMS is necessary in order to perform the method.

## OTHER FORMS OF TREATMENT

### Cryosurgery

The tumor is destroyed by cold. Usually, liquid nitrogen, which lowers the temperature of the tissue to under $-25°$ C and probably to as low as $-40°$ C, is used. The most convenient method of applying the liquid nitrogen is to use a cryospray gun, which allows precise application. The method is extensively used for benign and premalignant lesions such as warts, seborrheic keratosis, and actinic keratosis. It is also indicated for small primary basal cell carcinomas, squamous cell carcinomas, and Bowen's disease. The area to be treated is sprayed with liquid nitrogen for 5 to 10 seconds. Malignant tumors may require longer exposure (up to 30 seconds). In small lesions, local anesthetic is not necessary. The patient has a burning sensation, and the pain is variable depending on the location. The periungual area is notoriously painful. The frozen tissue is allowed to thaw, and the treatment is repeated once or twice. Blister formation is quite common and expected after cryotherapy. Postoperative care includes cleaning with hydrogen peroxide.

### Laser

Lasers can be used for destruction or excision of tumors. In general, the advantage of using lasers is that they produce instant hemostasis, the beam sterilizes as it cuts, and there is minimal postoperative pain. The main disadvantages are slow healing and increased incidence of hypertrophic scars or keloids. The two lasers most commonly used for the treatment of skin tumors are the carbon dioxide laser and the argon laser. The $CO_2$ laser emits light in the infrared range, which is not visible. The energy is uniformly absorbed and there is low penetrance (0.1 to 0.2 mm). The argon laser operates in the visible light range, and the energy is selectively absorbed by melanin, hemoglobin, and bilirubin. Because of this, it is particularly useful in the treatment of vascular and pigmented lesions.

Retinoids including tretinoin* (topical) (Retin-A), isotretinoin* (Accutane), and etretinate* (Tegison) (oral) have been advocated for treatment of preneoplastic and frankly neoplastic conditions, including actinic keratosis, dysplastic nevi, keratoacanthoma, basal cell carcinoma, and inoperable squamous cell carcinoma. For both basal and squamous cell cancers, the dosages of etretinate and isotretinoin recommended have been very high—3 to 5 mg per kg per day† compared with the usual dosage of 1 mg per kg per day used for treatment of psoriasis or acne. The reported results have been mixed, with apparent regression and control but not complete cure.

---

*This use of tretinoin, isotretinoin, and etretinate is not listed in the manufacturer's official directive.
†Exceeds dosage recommendations by the manufacturer.

## TREATMENT OF MELANOMA

### Biopsy

Incisional biopsies are indicated for diagnosis and histologic grading of large pigmented lesions. The biopsy does not increase the risk of dissemination or local recurrence of melanoma. An incisional biopsy should be elliptical, should go through the thickest area of the tumor, and should be deep enough to contain full-thickness tumor.

Excisional biopsy including the whole lesion and 1 to 2 mm of the lateral margin is the procedure of choice for diagnosis of small pigmented lesions. If it proves histologically to be a melanoma, additional surgery can be performed at a later date.

### Surgery

Surgical treatment is the most effective treatment for early stages of melanoma. Although the recommended margins have been changing throughout the years, in general, a wide excision is curative in more than 90% of patients with a thin melanoma of less than 0.76 mm thickness. For melanomas of intermediate thickness (between 0.76 and 3 mm), a margin of 1 to 2 cm around the lesion is recommended, whereas for lesions 3 mm or more in thickness, a margin of 2 to 3 cm should be excised around the tumor. Prophylactic lymphadenectomy appears to be beneficial in melanomas of intermediate thickness, but it is not clearly indicated in patients with thick melanomas. Metastatic melanoma is also best treated by surgery, which may include radical lymph node dissection when there is lymph node metastasis.

## OTHER TREATMENTS

Other modalities of treatment have been used in melanoma, particularly for metastatic disease, including radiation therapy, chemotherapy with DTIC (dacarbazine) (response rate of 15 to 20%), nitrosoureas, the vinca alkaloids vincristine (Oncovin) and vinblastine (Velban), and cisplatin (Platinol). Other agents used alone or in conjunction with chemotherapy in the treatment of melanoma are the interferons and interleukin-2. In all of them, the probability of response ranges between 10 to 25%, and they are often associated with considerable toxicity.

# PAPULOSQUAMOUS ERUPTIONS

method of
DAVID C. GORSULOWSKY, M.D.
*Veterans Administration Medical Center and
University of California
San Francisco, California*

and

MATTHEW H. KANZLER, M.D.
*Santa Clara Valley Medical Center and Stanford
University School of Medicine
Stanford, California*

Papulosquamous eruptions are those that are palpable and scaly. They may or may not appear to be inflammatory in nature. This section will cover the common papulosquamous eruptions encountered in clinical practice. The clinical appearance of each condition will be described, followed by a synopsis of treatment goals and modalities.

## SEBORRHEIC DERMATITIS

Seborrheic dermatitis is one of the most common papulosquamous eruptions. Although it may occur at any age, it is most common during infancy or after the second decade of life. Although excessive sebum production was originally thought to be the cause, this is probably not the main factor necessary for the development of seborrheic dermatitis. Hormonal influences may play a role in this disorder, however, and anxiety may be an indirectly related factor in exacerbation. Recently, the yeast *Pityrosporum orbiculare* has been shown to play an etiologic role in some, but not all cases.

This eruption is characterized by mild to moderate erythema with overlying fine white to yellow scaling. Occasionally, scaling may be present without underlying inflammation. It is for this reason that patients often complain of "dry skin" in the areas involved. Seborrheic dermatitis most often affects the nasolabial folds, eyelids, eyebrows, scalp, and outer ear areas. Other areas of involvement include the sternal, axillary, and groin areas. Pruritus of mild to moderate degree is often a chief complaint.

It is of note that seborrheic dermatitis, especially when severe, may be a presenting sign of acquired immunodeficiency syndrome (AIDS). In these cases, the dermatitis may be very extensive and resistant to therapy.

### Therapy

The goal of therapy in seborrheic dermatitis is to control the underlying inflammation and to remove scales. For mild to moderate facial involvement, very mild topical corticosteroid therapy may be effective. The choice of corticosteroid is important and generally should not exceed the potency of 1% hydrocortisone. Occasionally, compounding 2% precipitated sulfur with 1% hydrocortisone will manage cases resistant to hydrocortisone alone.

For longer term therapy, especially with scalp involvement, shampoo regimens will be of help. Shampoos containing selenium sulfide (Selsun), zinc pyrithione (Head & Shoulders 1%, Sebulon 2%), salicylic acid, tar, or detergents are indicated. Generally, these are over-the-counter preparations. The patient should be instructed to shampoo three to five times weekly; the shampoo should be applied and left in place for 5 to 10 minutes before rinsing. A conditioner may be used after the medicated shampoo, since these preparations tend to dry the hair. The most cosmetically elegant preparations available at this time include T/Gel, DHS Zinc, DHS Tar, and Ionil T Plus shampoos. Mineral oil or products containing salicylic acid, such as Baker's P & S solution or Meted shampoo, may be necessary for areas with thicker scaling.

Recently, topical ketoconazole cream (2%) (Nizoral) has been shown to be very effective in some patients with seborrheic dermatitis. This is probably due to this drug's activity against *Pityrosporum orbiculare*. The advantage of topical ketoconazole is its lack of potential atrophogenic properties. Such properties may be associated with long-term corticosteroid therapy.

Whichever therapy is chosen, patients should be made aware that this may be a recurrent condition and that clearing with therapy is not a "cure." Topical emollients are of no benefit, since this condition is not merely dry skin.

## PSORIASIS

Psoriasis, which affects 1 to 3% of the population, is characterized by a chronic course with periods of remission and exacerbation. Psoriasis appears to be inherited in some cases and has been found to be associated with certain antigens of the histocompatibility locus. Its onset may be at any age.

Environmental and iatrogenic factors play a role in psoriasis as well. Infection and trauma have been associated with onset and exacerbation. Psoriasis may appear in areas of local trauma, the so-called Koebner phenomenon. Upper respiratory infections often precede psoriasis of the guttate or papular form. Medications, including lithium and beta-adrenergic blockers, as well as some nonsteroidal anti-inflammatory drugs, may exacerbate psoriasis. Anxiety plays a role in exacerbation as well. The patient must recognize that this is a multifactorial condition.

Characteristic lesions consist of well-demarcated erythematous plaques with overlying silvery-white to gray scales. These plaques often involve extensor surfaces such as elbow and knee areas. However, they may involve the skin of the scalp, trunk, intertriginous areas, or virtually any location. Nail findings associated with psoriasis include pitting, oil spot discoloration, splinter hemorrhages, distal onycholysis, and subungual debris. Another feature that may be helpful in making a diagnosis is the presence of psoriatic arthritis. Fifteen to 25% of patients may exhibit this seronegative condition, many of whom have clinical features identical with rheumatoid arthritis.

Several variants of psoriasis exist. Generalized erythroderma may be associated with an acute flare and may be accompanied by fever or other systemic signs, often mimicking sepsis. Guttate psoriasis is characterized by 0.5 to 1.0 cm papules and, as mentioned above, may follow an upper respiratory infection. Pustular psoriasis consists of numerous small, sterile pustules overlying erythematous plaques. These pustules may be localized to the palms and soles (palmoplantar pustulosis) or may be generalized.

The overall clinical appearance and history of the patient are important in establishing the diagnosis of psoriasis. Other conditions, including atopic dermatitis, may resemble psoriasis. It is important to differentiate these conditions, however, since treatments such as systemic corticosteroids, which may improve atopic dermatitis, may cause a severe flare of psoriasis.

## Therapy

The mainstay of outpatient therapy for psoriasis is topical corticosteroid preparations. Table 1 lists some of these medications, arranged by potency, as determined by the McKenzie-Stoughton scale. In general, the more occlusive bases, such as those found in the ointments, provide increased potency. The lesser occlusive bases, such as creams and lotions, afford less potency. Most corticosteroid preparations may be applied once or twice daily with good results. For more resistant lesions, occlusion by Saran Wrap or other dressing may be added after application of the corticosteroid. However, since this may increase the atrophogenic properties of the preparation, occlusion should be used for only a few days. Patients should be monitored closely for development of side-effects, including folliculitis, skin atrophy, telangiectasia, and striae. Even hypothalamic-pituitary-adrenal axis suppression

**TABLE 1. Currently Available Topical Corticosteroids (Partial List)**

| Brand Name | Generic Name |
|---|---|
| *Group I* | |
| Diprolene cream and ointment 0.05% in optimized vehicle | Betamethasone dipropionate |
| Temovate cream and ointment 0.05% | Clobetasol propionate |
| *Group II* | |
| Cyclocort ointment 0.1% | Amcinonide |
| Lidex cream and ointment 0.05% | Fluocinonide |
| Topicort cream 0.25% | Desoximetasone |
| *Group III* | |
| Diprosone cream 0.05% | Betamethasone dipropionate |
| Valisone ointment 0.1% | Betamethasone valerate |
| *Group IV* | |
| Aristocort ointment 0.1% | Triamcinolone acetonide |
| Kenalog ointment 0.1% | Triamcinolone acetonide |
| Synalar ointment 0.025% | Fluocinolone acetonide |
| *Group V* | |
| Locoid cream 0.1% | Hydrocortisone butyrate |
| Synalar cream 0.025% | Fluocinolone acetonide |
| Westcort cream 0.2% | Hydrocortisone valerate |
| *Group VI* | |
| Synalar solution 0.01% | Fluocinolone acetonide |
| Tridesilon cream 0.05% | Desonide |
| *Group VII* | |
| Topicals with hydrocortisone | |

Adapted from Cornell RC: Topical steroids. *In* Lowe NJ (ed): Practical Psoriasis Therapy. Chicago, Year Book Medical Publishers, Inc., 1986.

may occur with the highest potency corticosteroids.

The choice of a particular corticosteroid preparation depends on several factors, including the site of treatment, patient preference, resistance to therapy, and cost. In addition, if a patient is sensitive to preservatives, the choice of an ointment base may be appropriate, since they usually contain fewer of such chemicals. The superpotent corticosteroid preparations listed in group I in Table 1 are indicated only for treatment of resistant lesions in thick-skinned areas. Treatment beyond 2 weeks is generally not recommended. In intertriginous areas, penetration and absorption are increased, and therefore, creams and lotions with lower potency should be chosen. Lesions in hair-bearing areas respond well to the lotions.

Other preparations may be of help in specific cases. These include keratolytic agents such as salicylic acid (2 to 20%), urea (2 to 40%), and lactic acid (6 to 12%). These are helpful in thick scaly lesions, especially in hyperkeratotic lesions of the palms and soles. Two commonly available preparations are Keralyt Gel, which is 6% salicylic acid, and the newer Lac-Hydrin lotion, which is 12% ammonium lactate.

Preparations containing tar are probably the oldest form of therapy for psoriasis. Crude coal tar (1 to 5%) may be used to treat large, thick psoriatic plaques and is often reserved for hospitalized patients because of its messy effect. Less irritating and more cosmetically acceptable are other tar-related preparations, including liquor carbonis detergens (LCD) and ichthammol. These preparations may be used in concentrations of 1 to 10% in an emollient base and should be applied once daily to psoriatic lesions. Over-the-counter preparations such as Estar and Psorigel include tar in a cosmetically elegant base. The main advantage of tar-based preparations is that they may be used for long-term therapy and actually may induce remissions that are more long-lasting than those induced by corticosteroid preparations.

Another topical tar-related preparation is anthralin. It has been used for about 80 years in various forms. Commercially available anthralin preparations include Drithocreme (0.1 to 1%) and Anthra-Derm ointment (0.1 to 1%). Recently, short contact therapy with anthralin has been shown to be as effective as treatment lasting several hours. Specifically, the anthralin preparation is applied in a concentration of 0.1 to 3.0% for 10 to 30 minutes, and then washed off. The main disadvantages of anthralin are that irritation of normal skin may occur, and staining of normal skin and environmental objects is almost unavoidable. Therefore, the preparations should be applied specifically to the psoriatic lesions, taking care to avoid normal skin.

A more cumbersome, but very effective, form of therapy is phototherapy. For patients with extensive involvement with psoriatic plaques, acute and long-term management with ultraviolet B and ultraviolet A therapy may be the most effective and most appropriate choice of treatment. When combined with psoralen (PUVA therapy), ultraviolet A may be very effective. However, the practitioner must be very familiar with dosing of the light, frequency of treatments, and side effects such as pruritus, erythema, and blistering. Long-term side effects of PUVA therapy include cataract formation and increased incidence of skin cancer.

For patients who are unresponsive to the above therapies, other systemic agents may be indicated. However, these potent medications should be prescribed only by those physicians familiar with their use. Methotrexate is a well-established therapy for psoriasis and may be used long term if the patient is monitored appropriately. The dosage ranges from 5 to 25 mg once weekly. Patients must be monitored very carefully for hepatic dysfunction, and liver biopsies are necessary. Etretinate (Tegison) may be used at a dosage of 0.5 to 1.0 mg per kg per day alone or in combination with other therapies and is especially effective in the treatment of generalized erythrodermic or pustular psoriasis. Other agents such as cyclosporine (Sandimmune) and hydroxyurea (Hydrea) may also be of help but should be used only in patients who are unresponsive to more conventional therapy.

No matter which form of therapy is chosen, other important adjuncts include liberal use of emollient preparations, avoidance of hot water and other irritants, and avoidance of scratching, which may produce the Koebner phenomenon. An understanding physician is of utmost importance, since the chronic course of psoriasis may be difficult and frustrating to all involved.

## LICHEN PLANUS

Lichen planus is an eruption consisting of violaceous polygonal papules of the flexor surfaces, genitalia, and mucous membranes. Idiopathic in nature, the lesions frequently resolve within 1 to 2 years. Pruritus may be intractable.

Helpful in making the diagnosis, when present, are fine, white lace-like discolorations overlying some papules. These are referred to as Wickham's striae and may be especially evident in the lesions of the mucous membranes.

### Therapy

Topical or intralesional corticosteroids are of some help in treating localized lesions of lichen planus. Topical retinoic acid gel (e.g., Retin-A) has been shown recently to be effective, especially in oral lesions. For extensive or eruptive forms of the condition, phototherapy may also be helpful. Antipruritic lotions or antihistamine preparations may be necessary to relieve severe pruritus.

## PITYRIASIS ROSEA

Pityriasis rosea is an idiopathic pruritic eruption that occasionally follows an upper respiratory or other viral infection by 1 to 4 weeks. Patients may relate that a single lesion signaled the onset. This lesion is called the herald patch. Lesions usually are oval, pink to erythematous, accompanied by a circinate fine white scale, and in a "fir tree" distribution on the trunk. When the axilla is involved, the diagnosis is usually certain. The clinical presentation may mimic that of secondary syphilis.

### Therapy

The most important factor in treating the patient is reassurance that the condition is not contagious and is temporal. Mild topical corticosteroid preparations may be of help if pruritus is present. One such preparation includes hydrocortisone and a topical anesthetic and is sold under the brand name of Pramosone. A 1% or 2.5% lotion preparation of this agent is often helpful. Emollients are also important in reducing the pruritus. Natural sunlight has been shown to decrease the duration of this disorder. It is helpful to explain to patients that the condition will resolve within 6 to 12 weeks.

### SYPHILIS

Secondary syphilis may closely mimic the lesions of pityriasis rosea, as described above. Therefore, in the clinical setting of oval to round erythematous plaques with overlying fine scaling, serologic testing is necessary. The therapeutic approach should follow guidelines included in the section on syphilis elsewhere in this publication.

### PITYRIASIS RUBRA PILARIS

This condition is characterized by large salmon-colored to erythematous plaques with fine adherent scale. There are patches of uninvolved skin located within these plaques, "islands of sparing," which are fairly typical of this condition. Marked hyperkeratosis of the palms and soles and severe scalp involvement are common in pityriasis rubra pilaris.

#### Therapy

Topical corticosteroids may be of some help. However, systemic therapy with methotrexate or etretinate may be necessary. Long-term therapy is usually indicated.

### MYCOSIS FUNGOIDES

This cutaneous T cell lymphoma may present as a papulosquamous eruption during its early patch or plaque stages. Large or small erythematous to violaceous plaques may exhibit a fine adherent scale and may be located anywhere on the body. Some dermatologists consider parapsoriasis to be a precursor of mycosis fungoides. Parapsoriasis is characterized by large, oval plaques of the trunk. Biopsy is necessary to differentiate the premalignant and malignant conditions.

#### Therapy

Parapsoriasis may be treated with topical corticosteroid preparations or phototherapy. Mycosis fungoides, if involving only the skin, may be treated by phototherapy (PUVA), topical nitrogen mustard, or electron beam therapy. However, when there is systemic involvement, as in Sézary's syndrome, systemic chemotherapy is indicated.

# CONNECTIVE TISSUE DISORDERS: LUPUS ERYTHEMATOSUS, DERMATOMYOSITIS, AND SCLERODERMA

method of
JAY H. WARRICK, M.D., and
M. BASHAR KAHALEH, M.D.
*Medical University of South Carolina*
*Charleston, South Carolina*

### SYSTEMIC LUPUS ERYTHEMATOSUS

Appropriate therapy of systemic lupus erythematosus (SLE) depends on the clinical activity of disease as well as the systems involved. Therapy for nonvisceral involvement (constitutional, cutaneous, and joint manifestations) is generally less aggressive and employs less toxic agents than that for visceral involvement (hematologic, renal, and central nervous system manifestations).

#### Nonvisceral Manifestations of SLE

Constitutional symptoms such as malaise, fever, anorexia, and weight loss are common manifestations of SLE. They may occur independently or in combination with more serious visceral disease. In the latter case, treatment of the visceral disease often results in resolution of the constitutional symptoms. In the absence of visceral involvement, only conservative therapy is indicated. Attention to measures such as adequate rest and nutrition is most important. If fever is present, a complete physical examination is indicated to rule out evidence of infection. Acetaminophen, not aspirin, should be given for fever, as aspirin has been associated with transaminase elevation in lupus patients. In the rare instance of severe constitutional symptoms with failure to thrive, systemic steroid therapy (prednisone 20 to 40 mg daily) is justified.

**Skin Manifestations.** Abnormalities of the skin, hair, and mucous membranes are prevalent manifestations of SLE. The spectrum of skin involvement ranges from the classic butterfly "blush," a nonspecific maculopapular rash resembling a drug eruption, to subacute lesions and discoid lesions.

Treatment of the skin lesions should first include avoidance of sun exposure. Adequate clothing and sunscreens with a solar protection factor of 15 or higher should be used even for brief anticipated sun exposure. In the summer months, patients should develop the habit of applying sunscreen on a daily basis, whether or not sun exposure is anticipated.

Topical corticosteroids comprise the most effective arsenal against the skin manifestations of lupus. It is generally preferable to use the least potent preparation effective for a particular patient. One per cent hydrocortisone applied twice daily is mild in potency, safe, and often effective for poikiloderma as well as for early discoid lesions. Moderate potency preparations, such as 0.1% triamcinolone (Kenalog), are usually necessary for established discoid lesions. Potent fluorinated steroids such as fluocinonide 0.05% (Lidex) or flucinolone acetonide (Synalar) may be necessary for thick discoid lesions. Intralesional steroid injections may be effective but should be done by an experienced physician. Systemic corticosteroids are effective but should be reserved for only the most refractory skin disease.

For skin disease poorly controlled with topical preparations alone, hydroxychloroquine (Plaquenil) 200 mg orally twice daily is usually effective. It may take 8 to 12 weeks of therapy, however, before its benefits are seen. Ophthalmologic side effects limit its use in doses higher than 400 mg per day. Retinal toxicity may occur at conventional doses; therefore, patients should have a baseline ophthalmologic exam prior to starting therapy and at 6-month intervals thereafter.

**Joint Manifestations.** Arthralgia occurs commonly, usually without objective findings of synovitis on physical exam. Both large and small joints may be involved, and the pattern may or may not be symmetric. Arthralgia usually is effectively controlled with nonsteroidal anti-inflammatory drugs (NSAIDs) such as ibuprofen (Motrin) 800 mg three times daily, piroxicam (Feldene) 20 mg once a day, sulindac (Clinoril) 150 to 200 mg twice daily, or diclofenac (Voltaren) 50 to 75 mg twice daily.

Occasionally, arthralgia may be accompanied by frank synovitis, with joint tenderness, warmth, swelling, and effusion. NSAIDs are again the drugs of choice. For arthralgia and/or synovitis that persists despite NSAIDs, hydroxychloroquine (Plaquenil) 200 mg orally twice daily is often effective. As with its use in skin disease, 8 to 12 weeks may elapse before an effect is seen.

The patient should have an ophthalmologic exam every 6 months to screen for retinopathy.

For painful synovitis refractory to the above, low dose prednisone is appropriate. A dose of 15 to 20 mg daily may be given until the synovitis is controlled, then tapered to the lowest maintenance dose possible (preferably no greater than 7.5 mg daily). Low-dose prednisone may be used as a therapeutic "bridge" for several weeks after beginning hydroxychloroquine, then tapered.

### Visceral Manifestations of SLE

**Hematologic Manifestations.** Hemolytic anemia in SLE results most frequently from the production of erythrocyte autoantibodies of the "warm type" (IgG, IgA, or IgM binding to erythrocytes at 37° C). These antibody-coated RBCs are then phagocytized by reticuloendothelial cells of the liver and/or spleen. Clinical manifestations of hemolytic anemia include depressed hematocrit, positive Coombs' test, elevated lactate dehydrogenase, elevated indirect bilirubin, elevated reticulocyte count, depressed haptoglobin, and the presence of free hemoglobin in the plasma.

Patients with significant hemolysis should be started on 60 mg of prednisone per day in divided doses until the hemolysis is controlled, at which time the prednisone may be tapered by 5 mg per day per week. If no response to prednisone is seen within a 2- to 3-week period, or if the patient requires a prednisone maintenance dose of greater than or equal to 15 mg per day, splenectomy is indicated. Danazol (Danocrine)*, an androgenic steroid, may be a useful adjunct to splenectomy if hemolysis continues postoperatively. The effective dose is 200 mg orally three or four times daily. For life-threatening fulminant hemolysis, "pulse" steroid therapy (1 gram of intravenous methylprednisolone daily for 3 days) and plasmapheresis may be helpful.

Immune thrombocytopenia may occur in SLE by a similar mechanism. Platelet autoantibodies (usually IgG) coat circulating platelets, resulting in their removal by the reticuloendothelial system. Antiplatelet antibodies may be present in the serum, and a bone marrow examination reveals normal to increased numbers of megakaryocytes. The initial treatment strategy is the same as that for immune hemolysis; however, danazol can be quite effective as initial therapy in thrombocytopenia. If splenectomy is necessary and the platelet count is inadequate for surgery, intravenous immune globulin (Sandoglobulin) in the dose of 400 mg per kg per day for 5 days is

---

*This use of danazol is not listed in the manufacturer's directive.

usually successful in temporarily raising the platelet count. It is not unusual for splenectomy to be unsuccessful in SLE because the liver is often the primary organ of platelet sequestration. In this event, danazol may sustain the platelet count adequately. Another option is slow intravenous infusion of vinca alkaloids, which are taken up by platelets and subsequently inactivate reticuloendothelial cells after phagocytosis. Vinblastine* (Velban) 0.1 mg per kg or vincristine* (Oncovin) 0.02 mg per kg dissolved in 1 liter of normal saline infused intravenously over 6 to 8 hours is an effective regimen. Infusions may be repeated every 5 to 10 days as required. Once a normal platelet count is obtained, intervals between infusions may be slowly increased. Side effects of these infusions include neutropenia, epigastric discomfort, alopecia, fever, phlebitis, and peripheral neuropathy.

**Nephritis.** Lupus nephritis is clinically manifested by proteinuria, hematuria, and decreasing creatinine clearance. Serology often reveals hypocomplementemia and a high antinative DNA titer. Lupus may result in membranous glomerulonephritis with nephrotic range proteinuria, usually without hematuria, which progresses to end-stage renal disease infrequently, and thus rarely requires aggressive therapy. Focal or diffuse proliferative glomerulonephritis may occur, which may rapidly progress to severe renal insufficiency if not treated. Distinction of these forms can be readily made by renal biopsy.

For treatment of proliferative glomerulonephritis, high-dose prednisone (60 mg per day in divided doses), plus monthly pulse intravenous cyclophosphamide (Cytoxan)† in the dose of 0.5 to 1 gram‡ per m², is indicated for 6 months. The patient should be re-evaluated at this time; if renal function has stabilized, prednisone may be tapered and the cyclophosphamide dosing interval increased to every 3 months for 1 year. If there is rapid deterioration of renal function on initial presentation, pulse intravenous methylprednisolone (Solumedrol) in a dose of 1 gram daily for 3 days is indicated, followed by oral prednisone and intravenous cyclophosphamide as above.

Side effects of cyclophosphamide include nausea, vomiting, leukopenia, hemorrhagic cystitis, and development of hematologic malignancy. A complete blood count and urinalysis should be obtained prior to each dose.

**Central Nervous System (CNS) Manifestations.** Seizures and psychosis are common CNS manifestations of SLE. Standard antiepileptic therapy is usually sufficient to suppress seizures. For mild psychiatric manifestations, an antipsychotic such as haloperidol (Haldol) 1 to 4 mg orally or intramuscularly every 12 hours may be used. For florid psychosis, diffuse cerebritis, or transverse myelitis, corticosteroids are usually necessary. It is best to begin with high-dose prednisone (60 mg daily in divided doses) and taper slowly after resolution of the symptoms. Rapid improvement is often seen after pulse steroid therapy (methylprednisolone 1 gram intravenously daily for 3 days). For symptoms unresponsive to steroids, an intravenous dose of cyclophosphamide* (Cytoxan) in a dose of 1 gram† per m² may be effective. Since lupus cerebritis is a diagnosis of exclusion, lumbar puncture and computed tomography of the head are usually indicated to rule out other treatable organic causes of epilepsy or psychosis.

**Vasculitis.** Deposition of immune complexes in blood vessel walls may lead to inflammatory cell infiltration and activation of complement resulting in vasculitis. Symptoms and signs of vasculitis include fever, malaise, purpura, ulcerative skin lesions, abdominal pain, and mononeuritis multiplex. Diagnosis can often be made by sural nerve biopsy if nerve conduction velocities are abnormal. Mesenteric angiography may show tapering of medium-size vessels with pseudoaneurysm formation. Therapy consists of immunosuppression with high-dose prednisone (60 mg per day in divided doses) in combination with monthly pulse intravenous cyclophosphamide (Cytoxan) until the vasculitis is controlled.

**Pregnancy.** Women with SLE who become pregnant should be followed closely by both an obstetrician and a rheumatologist for disease flares. Systemic symptoms should be treated with the lowest corticosteroid dose possible (usually 10 to 20 mg of prednisone per day). The presence of anticardiolipin antibody or lupus anticoagulant in the serum is associated with a higher incidence of spontaneous abortions as well as thrombotic events and should be treated with prednisone until serum titers fall to normal. Low-dose aspirin (325 mg daily) may be effective in reducing the incidence of thrombosis.

If previous obstetric history includes flares in the peripartum period, 10 to 20 mg of prednisone daily starting 1 week before the estimated date of confinement may be used. If the patient's disease remains inactive, prednisone may be tapered 1 to 2 weeks after delivery.

---

*This use of vinblastine or vincristine is not listed in the manufacturer's official directive.

†This use of cyclophosphamide is not listed in the manufacturer's official directive.

‡Exceeds dosage recommended by the manufacturer.

---

*This use of cyclophosphamide is not listed in the manufacturer's official directive.

†Exceeds dosage recommended by the manufacturer.

## DERMATOMYOSITIS

Dermatomyositis is an autoimmune disease characterized by inflammation of the skin and muscles. Patients typically complain of progressive proximal muscle weakness. An erythematous rash over the extensor surfaces of the extremities may be present. Gottron's papules, scaly hyperpigmented plaques over the knuckles of the fingers, are characteristic. A violaceous "heliotrope" rash over the eyelids is often seen. Serum muscle enzyme levels (creatine phosphokinase and aldolase) are almost always elevated. Electromyography and muscle biopsy are essential tools to confirm the diagnosis.

### Treatment

Skin manifestations of the disease are generally benign and usually regress with treatment of the muscle disease. High-dose corticosteroids are appropriate initial therapy. Prednisone 60 mg daily in divided doses (1 to 2 mg per kg per day in children) is an adequate starting dose. A response is usually seen within 4 to 6 weeks, after which the steroids may be slowly tapered. If no response is seen within 4 to 6 weeks or the muscle disease progresses despite treatment, addition of an immunosuppressive agent is indicated. Azathioprine (Imuran)* at a dose of 2 mg per kg per day or methotrexate (Rheumatrex)† at a dose of 15 to 25 mg orally per week is an effective second-line agent. Both have steroid-sparing effects and often allow tapering of prednisone to an acceptable maintenance level (less than 15 mg per day). Regular monthly complete blood counts should be done to screen for cytopenias, which are side effects of both drugs. Methotrexate also has the potential for hepatotoxicity and pneumonitis. For muscle disease refractory to the previously described therapy, cyclophosphamide (Cytoxan) 1 to 2 mg per kg orally per day may be effective. Careful follow-up for cytopenias and hemorrhagic cystitis is mandatory.

Other manifestations of this disease include dysphagia, aspiration, and pulmonary fibrosis. It is important to ensure that the patient's gag reflex is intact so as to prevent aspiration of food. Often, placement of an enteral feeding tube is necessary in cases of severe esophageal involvement. Shortness of breath may occur secondary to respiratory muscle fatigue with resulting hypercapnia. Intubation and mechanical ventilation may be necessary. Bedside spirometry to measure daily forced vital capacities is an excellent way of monitoring respiratory muscle function. Interstitial pulmonary inflammation with resultant fibrosis may occur. This may or may not respond to immunosuppressive therapy.

Muscle rest is important in the inflammatory stages of the disease. Passive range of motion exercises are beneficial in maintaining joint mobility. More intensive physical therapy to actively rebuild muscle mass is indicated when the disease is in remission.

## SCLERODERMA

Scleroderma (systemic sclerosis) is a multisystem vascular and microvascular disorder of unknown etiology characterized by abnormal production of connective tissue and subsequent fibrosis of the skin and viscera. Though thickened, tightened, or hidebound skin is the hallmark of the disease, its cardiopulmonary, renal, and gastrointestinal manifestations produce significant morbidity and mortality.

### Dermatologic Manifestations

Raynaud's phenomenon is usually present prior to the onset of skin changes. Vasospasm may be severe, resulting in digital infarcts which may become secondarily infected. Patients should be instructed to wear warm clothing, including gloves, in the winter months, as Raynaud's phenomenon is precipitated by low temperatures. Calcium-channel blockade is often effective in reducing the severity of Raynaud's phenomenon. Nifedipine (Procardia) 10 to 30 mg orally every 8 hours or diltiazem (Cardizem) 30 to 90 mg orally every 6 hours is effective. Both of these drugs are available now in "extended release" forms. The dose is often limited by systemic hypotension. Nitroglycerine ointment (Nitrobid) can be helpful in treating digital infarcts when applied topically two to three times daily at the base of the affected digits.

Skin tightening usually begins distally and progresses proximally. Moisturizing lotions are useful to condition the skin and minimize pruritus. Physical therapy is essential to maintain mobility of joints covered with hidebound skin. To date there is no proven effective therapy to reverse sclerodermatous skin changes. However, D-penicillamine* has been suggested to be beneficial in reducing the rate of disease progression. Initial doses of 250 mg orally per day are recommended, with gradual increase in the dose every 1 to 3 months to a maximum dose of 1000

---

*This use of azathioprine is not listed in the manufacturer's official directive.

†This use of methotrexate is not listed in the manufacturer's official directive.

---

*This use of D-penicillamine is not listed in the manufacturer's official directive.

mg per day. The reported incidence of side effects varies from 10 to 98% and includes skin rash, dyspepsia, taste disturbance, nephropathy, and bone marrow suppression. Interferon gamma and photopheresis are currently under investigation with initial results that are encouraging.

### Gastrointestinal (GI) Manifestations

The esophagus is the major GI target organ. Distal esophageal dysmotility results in an incompetent lower esophageal sphincter and gastroesophageal reflux. This often produces chronic distal esophagitis, stricture formation, and dysphagia. All patients with esophageal abnormalities should elevate the head of the bed with 6-inch blocks to minimize nocturnal reflux. Antacids and/or $H_2$ blockers provide symptomatic relief. For radiographic or endoscopically proven ulcerative esophagitis unresponsive to $H_2$ blockers, omeprazole (Losec) 20 mg daily for 6 to 8 weeks usually allows healing. If dysphagia develops, a barium esophagram or esophagoscopy should be performed to rule out presence of a stricture. If a stricture is seen, malignancy should be excluded by biopsy.

Small bowel involvement can result in intestinal tract hypomotility and a functional "blind loop" syndrome in which chronic bacterial overgrowth results in diarrhea. This syndrome usually responds to cyclic intermittent antibiotic therapy. In patients with severe gastrointestinal hypomotility, intermittent ileus, and malnutrition, home hyperalimentation is the only effective supportive therapy.

### Pulmonary Manifestations

Inflammatory lung disease commonly complicates scleroderma. Dyspnea, cough, rales, restrictive pulmonary function tests, and decreased diffusion capacity are characteristic. These patients should optimally be evaluated with bronchoalveolar lavage (BAL) or gallium scan. If alveolitis is demonstrated, a 6-month course of cyclophosphamide (Cytoxan) 1 to 2 mg per kg orally per day, or 1 gram per $m^2$ intravenously per month may be given. Pulmonary function tests, BAL, and/or gallium scanning should be repeated at 6 months to assess response to therapy.

In patients with pulmonary hypertension, vasodilators such as hydralazine (Apresoline), isoproterenol, prazosin hydrochloride (Minipress), nifedipine (Procardia), diltiazem (Cardizem), or verapamil (Isoptin) may be of benefit. Objective response to therapy is determined most accurately by echocardiography, or better yet, by right heart catheterization with concomitant vasodilator administration.

### Cardiac Manifestations

Cardiac involvement in scleroderma is subtle and presents as restrictive cardiomyopathy with a high incidence of arrhythmia with atrioventricular conduction disturbances. Therapy consists of inotropic drugs, afterload reduction, calcium-channel blockers, and appropriate antiarrhythmic agents. Diuretics should be used with caution because of their potential to produce hypovolemic renal failure.

### Renal Manifestations

Scleroderma renal crisis is an unpredictable, rapidly progressive syndrome of hypertension and renal failure seen in approximately 10% of patients. Hypertension is often the initial manifestation of the renal disease. All scleroderma patients, especially those with rapidly progressing skin involvement or truncal skin involvement, should have weekly blood pressure checks. Any scleroderma patient with new onset hypertension should immediately begin treatment with an angiotensin-converting enzyme inhibitor. Captopril (Capoten) in a starting dose of 6.25 mg orally every 6 hours should be titrated upward to control hypertension. Other agents such as hydralazine (Apresoline), clonidine (Catapres), prazosin (Minipress), minoxidil (Loniten), and nitroprusside (Nipride) have been effective alone or in combination in controlling this process.

Renal failure may progress despite therapy necessitating dialysis. Rarely, patients may recover renal function during dialysis. Successful renal transplantation has been reported. In patients with mild renal disease, it is important to maintain renal perfusion by avoiding volume depletion, diuretics, and overtreatment of hypertension. Drugs that lead to selective renal vasoconstriction such as nonsteroidal anti-inflammatory agents should be used with extreme caution in this setting.

# CUTANEOUS VASCULITIS

method of
JEFFREY P. CALLEN, M.D.
*University of Louisville*
*Louisville, Kentucky*

Vasculitis is an inflammatory reaction characterized by a variety of presumed immunologically mediated phenomena that result in vessel wall invasion and damage. Cutaneous vasculitis refers to this phenomenon's occurring within the vessels of the skin. In some cases the inflammatory reaction may only be manifested as cutaneous disease, while in other instances the disease may affect multiple internal organs. The most common type of cutaneous vasculitis involves an inflammatory reaction characterized by neutrophilic destruction of the small vessels, usually the postcapillary venules, and is termed leukocytoclastic vasculitis (LCV). Although other inflammatory vasculitides can affect the skin, this discussion will be limited to the evaluation and treatment of LCV.

Leukocytoclastic vasculitis is characterized clinically by a variety of manifestations, including palpable purpura, urticaria-like lesions, livedo reticularis, necrosis of the skin, ulceration, nodular lesions, or fixed erythematous plaques. The most commonly observed findings are palpable purpura or urticarial lesions. The diagnosis is confirmed by histopathologic evaluation of the skin, in which the typical changes consist of polymorphonuclear leukocyte invasion of the vessel wall, fibrinoid necrosis of the vessel wall, a breakdown of the leukocytes with nuclear dust present (leukocytoclasis), and extravasation of erythrocytes. These findings are not static, and thus, timing of the biopsy may be critical in order to adequately demonstrate the classic changes. Although the skin may be the only organ system involved clinically, this disorder is felt to be representative of an immune complex disorder and, thus, should truly be considered a systemic disease process. The most frequently observed organ systems to be involved other than the skin are the joints, the kidneys, the gastrointestinal tract, and the nervous system. Significant involvement within these systems must be dealt with via a different approach from that outlined within this section.

## EVALUATION

Before instituting therapy for the patient with vasculitis of the skin, it is necessary to thoroughly evaluate for a possible causative factor (Table 1) and for the presence of recognizable systemic manifestations. The evaluation begins with a careful and thorough history and physical examination. This will aid in identifying a potentially removable or treatable etiologic factor and/or the presence of systemic disease symptoms. The laboratory evaluation should be extensive for similar reasons and includes a complete blood count, a serum multiphasic analysis, a urinalysis, a chest x-ray, and tests evaluating potential immunologic associations such as total hemolytic complement, antinuclear antibody, anti-Ro (SS-A) antibody, hepatitis B surface antigen, cryoglobulins, serum protein electrophoresis, and rheumatoid factor. Immunofluorescence microscopy is probably not essential except in rare instances, such as when one suspects Henoch-Schönlein purpura (HSP), which is due to IgA immune complexes. HSP is a tetrad manifested as palpable purpura with arthritis, nephritis, and gastrointestinal involvement. Recently, the identification of patients with cutaneous vasculitis in the setting of Ro positive Sjögren's syndrome has been associated with the potential for serious central nervous system involvement; thus, the identification of these patients is necessary to adequately predict prognosis.

Vasculitis is not a static process, and although there

TABLE 1. **Common Etiologic Factors and Associated Diseases of Leukocytoclastic Vasculitis**

*Infectious agents include:*
  Streptococcal infections (often precede Henoch-Schönlein purpura)
  Hepatitis B infection (associated with polyarteritis more often than with LCV)

*Drugs of ingestants include:*
  Antibiotics
  Thiazides
  Anticonvulsants
  Food dyes

*Collagen vascular diseases:*
  Lupus erythematosus
    Systemic LE (associated with a poor prognosis)
    Subacute cutaneous LE (associated with the presence of Ro antibody)
    Sjögren's syndrome (Ro positive associated with CNS disease)
    Rheumatoid arthritis

*Abnormal proteins:*
  Cryoglobulinemia
  Macroglobulinemia
  Hyperglobulinemic purpura

*Neoplasia (rare):*
  Hairy cell leukemia
  Lymphoma
  Solid tumors

*Miscellaneous:*
  Complement component deficiency (usually $C_2$)
  Inflammatory bowel disease
  Serous otitis media

is no demonstrable systemic involvement on the initial evaluation, the patient with continued disease should be periodically re-evaluated. This re-evaluation need not be as extensive as the initial testing. It is not clear how often re-evaluation is necessary, but my general rule is to monitor patients on an approximately annual basis.

## TREATMENT

The treatment of cutaneous vasculitis first includes the removal of any identified potential etiologic agent. Next, one must consider treatable diseases, for example, streptococcal infection. Evaluation of the nature of the patient's problem should then be undertaken, and the following questions should be considered prior to the selection and initiation of any proposed therapeutic agent: (1) Is the vasculitis self-limited in this patient? and (2) Does the patient have or is the patient likely to develop serious systemic disease? Only those patients with the potential for continued disease should be treated, and those with serious systemic involvement should be treated with more aggressive agents.

In general, the agents used to treat cutaneous vasculitis nonspecifically inhibit inflammation and thus do not result in more than a suppression of the disease manifestations. Most of the reports regarding therapy of LCV involve small open trials or anecdotal information gained from individual cases. There are many agents that have been reported to be effective, such as nonsteroidal anti-inflammatory drugs (NSAIDs), dapsone, antihistamines, antimalarials, and sulfa drugs, which in my experience are effective only in a minority of the patients treated. In contrast, corticosteroids, immunosuppressive agents, and colchicine seem to appropriately control the disease in a majority of the patients in whom they are used.

Patients with urticaria-like lesions may be effectively treated with antihistamines or occasionally with NSAIDs such as ibuprofen or indomethacin. When using oral antihistaminic agents, it is often necessary to elevate the dosage to soporific levels in order to control the process. Furthermore, agents that have effects on both the $H_1$ and $H_2$ receptors may be more effective. In those patients who do not respond to antihistamines, oral indomethacin (Indocin) 25 to 50 mg four times per day may be attempted. Another option is to use the sustained-release formula (Indocin-SR) twice daily. When these measures are not effective, colchicine may be tried (see later). Often, the disease is not totally controlled, and in these patients oral corticosteroids are effective but may also be toxic. Careful and thorough discussion of the benefits and toxicity of corticosteroid therapy should precede the initiation of this therapy.

For patients with primarily cutaneous disease, I have found that oral colchicine 0.6 mg twice daily is effective in two-thirds to three-fourths of the patients treated. The onset of benefit with the use of colchicine is rapid, usually occurring within the first 4 to 7 days, but almost always within the first 2 weeks of therapy. Toxicity with colchicine is minimal, but the acute toxicity is usually manifested by gastrointestinal symptomatology. Since colchicine is potentially teratogenic, it should not be given to women unless adequate birth control measures are practiced. The long-term potential toxicities include anemia, thrombocytopenia, hepatic dysfunction, and renal dysfunction. Thus, periodic evaluation of the complete blood count and serum multiphasic analysis are required during chronic therapy with colchicine. In addition to the beneficial effects on the skin, colchicine may also result in improvement in arthritis, but it has little effect on any of the other systemic manifestations.

Patients with severe systemic disease should be treated more aggressively with corticosteroids and/or an immunosuppressive agent. Frequently, the doses of corticosteroids necessary to control the disease result in iatrogenic Cushing's syndrome, and thus the use of either azathioprine or cyclophosphamide can result in a steroid-sparing effect. Only rarely is it necessary to treat the patient with "pure" cutaneous vasculitis with an immunosuppressive agent. However, in a recent trial, we have used azathioprine (Imuran) 150 mg per day to successfully treat five of six patients with recalcitrant cutaneous LCV. In addition, intravenous pulse therapy with methylprednisolone may give rapid clearing of disease manifestations, which can then be continued to be suppressed with an immunosuppressive agent. Finally, plasmapheresis and leukapheresis may be used in patients with demonstrable circulating immune complexes and recalcitrant disease.

# DISEASES OF THE NAILS

method of
RICHARD K. SCHER, M.D.
*Columbia University–Presbyterian Medical
   Center
New York, New York*

It is estimated that about 10% of dermatologic patient visits are for nail problems. The nail protects the underlying digit, scratches, aids fine touch, and provides an important cosmetic aspect to those who are so inclined. In addition, it serves occasionally both as an offensive and defensive weapon.

Fifty per cent of all nail disorders are due to fungal infection. Other problems include psoriasis, lichen planus, a wide range of miscellaneous onychodystrophies, as well as benign and malignant tumors. In addition, the nail unit may be the first sign of a systemic disease in a patient without other manifestations. Therefore, a knowledge of nail pathology can provide the physician with a quick diagnosis and thereby render his patient's care more effective. The discussion that follows will provide the physician with an approach to the treatment of nail disorders.

The comprehension of the anatomy of the nail unit is mandatory for one seeking to treat the patient with nail dystrophy. The nail unit is composed of the following structures: the nail matrix, the nail bed, the hyponychium, the nail plate, and the surrounding proximal and lateral nail folds. Some authorities also include the distal phalanx as part of this overall structure. The nail matrix—analogous to the hair matrix—lies beneath the proximal nail fold. It is the site wherein the nail plate is manufactured, and therefore injury to the nail matrix will subsequently appear in the nail plate several weeks to several months hence. The nail matrix extends proximally about 5 mm beneath the proximal nail fold and extends distally to include the lunula, or half-moon. The lunula represents the distal portion of the nail matrix. Where the lunula ends the nail matrix ends and the nail bed begins. The nail bed anatomically is composed of longitudinal grooves and ridges consisting of an epithelium and a dermal connective tissue. These longitudinal grooves and ridges explain the mechanism of formation of the splinter hemorrhage. If there is a small bleeding focus beneath the nail plate in the area of the nail bed, the blood becomes trapped in that confined site and gives the clinical appearance of a splinter. Other structures located in the nail bed are the glomera. These arteriovenous bodies occasionally enlarge into tumors, which cause considerable pain and discomfort. The nail matrix and bed do not possess subcutaneous tissue as does skin, but rather their undersurface rests on the underlying phalanx periosteum. The nail bed extends distally to approximately the point at which the overlying nail plate begins to separate. It is in this area that the hyponychium begins. The hyponychium is a small structure that is histologically distinct and is important in that fungus microorganisms in distal subungual onychomycosis enter at this site. The hyponychium extends distally and ends at the distal groove, the site at which the normal epidermis of the digit begins. There is no keratohyaline layer in the nail matrix and the nail bed, but it reappears at the site of the hyponychium. The proximal nail fold, which overlies the nail matrix, is a modified extension of the digit and is an actual fold of skin containing both epidermis and dermis. It is continuous with the similarly structured lateral nail fold on each side, and these folds of skin form three-quarters of the boundary of the nail plate; collectively they are referred to as the perionychium. The proximal nail groove has a roof and a floor. The roof is the undersurface of the proximal nail fold, and the floor is the nail matrix. Fitting securely into this groove is the nail plate itself. That portion of the plate at this site is referred to as the nail root, which is thinner, softer, and less tightly adherent to the underlying tissue than the more distal plate. The horny end product of the proximal nail fold is the cuticle and beneath the undersurface of the cuticle often can be seen the horny structure known as the eponychium.

## ONYCHOMYCOSIS

Onychomycosis may be defined as infection of one or more of the components of the nail by fungal organisms. The clinical appearance of onychomycosis caused by any one species in general is indistinguishable from that caused by any other species. However, it may be stated that there are some clinical clues that might allow the clinician to surmise that an organism of one species or another is probably not responsible for a particular variety of onychomycosis. Fungal infection of the nails may be classified into four clinical varieties: (1) distal subungual onychomycosis; (2) white superficial onychomycosis; (3) proximal subungual onychomycosis; and (4) Candida onychomycosis.

### Distal Subungual Onychomycosis

In distal subungual onychomycosis the primary involvement is the distal nail bed and hyponychium with secondary involvement of the inferior surface of the nail plate. This is the most common variety and has its onset from the entrance of the fungal microorganisms in the area of the hyponychium, which then begin to migrate proximally. Only later in the course of the disorder will it involve the proximal nail unit. The resultant effect is dermatitis and increased thickness of the cornified layer of the nail bed and hyponychium, which results in subungual hyperkeratosis and onycholysis or uplifting of the nail plate. As a rule, subungual hyperkeratosis may be regarded as the most reliable sign of onychomycosis. Actual destruction of the nail plate may take place secondary to its invasion. In the toenails trauma plays a significant role in the development of onychomycosis. This is particularly true in the first and second toes, depending upon which toe is longer in each individual. Often, after the instigating factor of trauma is eliminated, the onychomycosis may resolve spontaneously.

The most common etiologic organism in distal subungual onychomycosis is *Trichophyton rubrum*. Other species may also be causative but to a much lesser degree. Treatment of onychomycosis should not be instituted until the diagnosis is confirmed. This is done by means of mycologic studies, which include potassium hydroxide wet mounts, cultures, and, if necessary, a biopsy of the involved nail unit. For a KOH wet mount, one uses 10% potassium hydroxide in aqueous solution. This is applied to the glass slide after scrapings from the cornified layer of the nail bed are placed upon it. It is the subungual debris that contains the largest numbers of fungal microorganisms, and it is that site which should be used for investigative studies. Looking at the nail plate may prove futile because it often is not involved until late in the course of the disease. The slide should be warmed slightly and time allowed for digestion of the nonfungal material by the potassium hydroxide. If the KOH is dissolved in dimethylsulfoxide, a more rapid and easier diagnosis can be made. If the diagnosis of onychomycosis is confirmed by a KOH wet mount, it is still necessary to perform a culture. This is obviously because the wet mount in many situations cannot distinguish between different causative organisms requiring different therapy. The same material is used for culture on appropriate fungus-growing medium such as Sabouraud's and is examined in from 10 to 14 days to identify the causative organism. It is known that as much as 30% of mycologic studies for fungal organisms may be negative even in the presence of onychomycosis. Therefore, at least three specimens with wet mounts and cultures are recommended. If these studies still fail to produce the organism, one should consider performing a nail biopsy. A punch biopsy in the area of the pathology will often provide a confirmatory diagnosis of onychomycosis. In the event that the disorder is not onychomycosis, the biopsy will provide a correct diagnosis and therefore enable the clinician to begin proper treatment. All nail biopsies with the intent of establishing a diagnosis of onychomycosis should be stained with periodic acid–Schiff stain. The latter is done because often the numbers of microorganisms are few and they may be easily overlooked by routine hematoxylineosin stain. In the event that the biopsy confirms the diagnosis of onychomycosis, it is advisable to reattempt culture. This is true because the therapy may differ should one be dealing with a dermatophyte, Candida, or saprophyte infection.

### White Superficial Onychomycosis

In white superficial onychomycosis there is noted clinically multiple well-marginated opaque white islands on the surface of the nail plate. This is most common in toenails; it is an example of true leukonychia. These individual islands may coalesce and eventually involve the entire nail surface, which may then become rough, soft, and crumbly. Further on in the development of this disorder a yellowish discoloration may appear, but inflammatory reaction is almost always minimal. In this variety it is the superficial surface of the nail plate that is invaded by the fungal microorganism. There is no particular predilection for either the distal or the proximal portion of the nail unit. The most frequently implicated organism in this variety is *Trichophyton mentagrophytes*. The diagnosis in this type is determined in a fashion similar to that for distal subungual onychomycosis. There is a slight difference here, however, in that the fungal specimens for potassium hydroxide wet mounts and cultures are taken from the surface of the nail plate, which is the site of entrance of the attacking organisms. In contradistinction to distal subungual onychomycosis as well as proximal subungual onychomycosis, the organisms in this type invade the nail plate early and the cornified layer of the nail bed and hyponychium later.

### Proximal Subungual Onychomycosis

In proximal subungual onychomycosis the point of entry is in the region of the proximal nail fold. The organisms enter at the proximal groove and migrate proximally before proceeding in an acral direction. Many authorities believe that since this variety is infrequent, a preceding episode of trauma is necessary for it to occur.

Clinically there is subungual hyperkeratosis, onycholysis, leukonychia, and destruction of the proximal nail plate. Here the distal portion of the nail unit remains normal until late in the course of the disease. The etiologic organism that predominates is *Trichophyton rubrum*. The diagnosis of proximal subungual onychomycosis is arrived at in a fashion similar to that for the other onychomycoses. If a biopsy must be performed to make a diagnosis in this variety, however, caution must be exercised. Since the pathology is in the nail matrix area, surgery could result in a permanent nail dystrophy. Recently this type of onychomycosis has been reported with increasing frequency in patients with acquired immune deficiency syndrome (AIDS).

### Candida Onychomycosis

The common clinical manifestation of Candida onychomycosis is most often seen as a paronychia. Distal primary onycholysis may also be seen. Direct invasion of the nail plate by Candida organisms is a rare occurrence except in the immunocompromised individual. In this case, it will appear as the so-called Candida granuloma or chronic mucocutaneous candidiasis. Invasion of the nail plate in other individuals is a secondary phenomenon. Clinically what is seen are opaque nails with longitudinal white strands, transverse depressions (Beau's lines), and swelling of the proximal and lateral nail folds. The latter produces so-called pseudoclubbing when Lovibond's angle is less than 180 degrees. Diagnosis is made by the usual mycologic studies, except here the specimen must be obtained from material in the area of the proximal nail fold for paronychiae or from the distal nail bed and hyponychium in the case of onycholysis. The necessity of a biopsy in candidiasis is infrequent, since large numbers of organisms are usually present.

### Treatment

Treatment of onychomycosis of the nails may be subdivided according to the etiologic organism, namely, dermatophyte, Candida, or saprophyte.

**Dermatophyte Therapy.** Topical treatment for dermatophyte infections includes miconazole nitrate cream or lotion (Monistat-Derm), 1% clotrimazole cream or lotion (Lotrimin, Mycelex), haloprogin cream or lotion (Halotex), 1% econazole nitrate cream (Spectazole), ciclopirox olamine cream (Loprox), ketoconazole cream (Nizoral), and naftifine cream (Naftin). Although topical agents may provide some benefit, their effectiveness is generally not great. They may be applied to the involved area with a soft toothbrush, gently massaging in twice daily after the abnormal nail plate and debris have been removed. Systemic therapy, on the other hand, is the cornerstone of treatment. It should be stated, however, that even adequate oral treatment may produce only a limited cure. In those patients in whom a cure is obtained the recurrence rate is very high, 25% for fingernails and 75% for toenails. In addition, therapy is prolonged, requiring at least 6 to 18 months, depending on whether fingernails and/or toenails are treated. Therefore, the patient should be made aware, prior to onset of therapy, of the realities of this regimen. Oral griseofulvin is the treatment of choice. The treating physician should be certain there are no contraindications to its use such as allergy or hematologic abnormalities. The preferable form is the microsized Grisactin, Fulvicin U/F, or Grifulvin V, 500 mg once or twice daily. There is an elixir of griseofulvin available for children at appropriately reduced dosage schedules. The ultramicrosized form, Gris-PEG or Fulvicin P/G, may also be used. A minimum of 125 mg three times daily is usually required. It has been shown that nail avulsion in combination with oral therapy considerably improves both the cure rate and the recurrence rate. This may be done either surgically or chemically. The latter method uses 40% urea or 50% potassium iodide ointment under an occlusive dressing. This approach is preferable for patients in whom surgical treatment is not recommended. Ketoconazole (Nizoral) also is highly effective. It produces a greater percentage of cures and a lower percentage of recurrences. However, it must be used cautiously because of its adverse effects on the liver as well as its antiandrogen potential. It is FDA approved, however, only for chronic mucocutaneous candidiasis and resistant moccasin-type pedal dermatophytosis. The indications for ketoconazole are griseofulvin resistance, griseofulvin intolerance, and griseofulvin drug interaction. The treatment of white superficial onychomycosis consists simply of scraping the fungal organisms from the surface of the nail plate. In those cases in which white superficial onychomycosis has become more advanced and simple therapy is not adequate, systemic and topical antifungal agents may have to be used. Treatment of Candida onychomycosis includes the same topical preparations of miconazole, clotrimazole, haloprogin, econazole, ciclopirox olamine, and ketoconazole. In addition, amphotericin B (Fungizone), nystatin (Mycostatin), and sulfacetamide (Sulamyd 30%) have also been employed with some success. Mycolog II and lotrisone cream are also of value in this situation. Systemic treatment for Candida infection includes nystatin (Mycostatin), oral tablets 500,000 units four times a day for 2 weeks. The effectiveness of this drug is in its elimination of the causative organism from the gastrointestinal tract despite its lack of absorption. Many Candida paronychias are mixed infections with bacteria such as Pseudomonas. In these situations a combination of tetracycline with nystatin may be useful. However, it should be stressed again that prior to instituting any form of systemic therapy, proper microbiologic studies should be performed. Ketoconazole is also effective for Candida onychomycosis in a dosage of 200 mg daily. It is essential that patients with Candida onychomycosis keep their hands dry, as moisture is a significant factor in the proliferation of this organism. In addition, all patients should be checked for the possible presence of diabetes mellitus, and females should be investigated for the possibility of associated Candida vaginitis. X-ray therapy has been employed in the past for the acute exacerbation of Candida paronychia, and intralesional corticosteroids are also used. These modalities are better left to the specialist in dermatology. Finally, for intractable, recurrent Candida paronychia, surgical resection of the proximal nail fold (marsupialization) may be employed. Onychomycosis of the nails caused by saprophytes (Scopulariopsis and Aspergillus are the most common) is best treated by nail avulsion in combination with topical therapy such as miconazole, haloprogin, clotrimazole, econazole, and ciclopirox olamine. All patients on systemic antifungal therapy must have regular laboratory evaluations to monitor possible adverse effects from the medications.

## PSORIASIS

The diagnosis of psoriasis of the nails is not difficult in the patient who has significant cutaneous involvement. However, it is known that 1 to 5% of patients have normal skin with only psoriatic nail involvement. Since the prevalence of psoriasis in the United States is about 2 or 3% in nonpsoriatic families and as high as 35% in psoriatic families, it is important to be familiar with the clinical features of psoriasis of the nails. Psoriatic nail changes are dependent upon the site of the disease. When there is psoriasis of the nail matrix, the characteristic change is pitting. Since pitting occurs on the surface of the nail plate, it indicates that the proximal nail matrix is affected. Other nail changes seen are transverse depressions, crumbling of the nail plate, and leukonychia with rough or smooth surface. When the primary area of involvement is the nail bed or the hyponychium, there is noted distal onycholysis, discoloration of the nail bed (the "oil drop" sign), subungual hyperkeratosis, and the frequent finding of splinter hemorrhage. The splinter hemorrhage occurs because of the anatomic configuration of the nail bed and the characteristic histology of psoriasis. There are increased numbers as well as greater tortuosity of the dermal blood vessels within the dermal papillae that lie beneath the thinned suprapapillary plate. This finding correlates well with the Auspitz sign seen in psoriasis of the skin. The brownish discoloration is believed to be due to an accumulation of glycoprotein within the nail bed and is a unique change of psoriatic nails found virtually nowhere else. The etiology of psoriasis is, of course, unknown but trauma plays a particular role. This effect of trauma corresponds to the Koebner phenomenon noted in the skin. In order to confirm with certainty the diagnosis of psoriatic nails that are atypical it may be necessary to perform a nail biopsy after obtaining negative mycologic studies (KOH and culture) on three separate occasions.

### Treatment

Once the diagnosis of psoriasis of the nails has been confirmed therapy consists mainly of some form of corticosteroid. High-potency corticosteroids under occlusion are of some benefit, although the positive effect may be limited. Such preparations as 0.05% diflorasone diacetate ointment (Florone), 0.5% triamcinolone acetonide ointment (Aristocort), 0.2% fluocinolone acetonide cream (Synalar), betamethasone (Diprosone or Diprolene), and clobetasol (Temovate) are among the most effective. These latter three drugs should be used for a maximum period of 2 weeks, avoided in those below age 12, and without occlusion. However, the mainstay of treatment for psoriatic nails is intralesional corticosteroids. Using triamcinolone acetonide suspension (Kenalog-10) injected into the area of the proximal nail fold once a month for three or four injections with a concentration of 2.5 mg per ml is most effective. Other therapeutic modalities that have been used for psoriatic nails include x-ray, PUVA, 1% fluorouracil (Fluoroplex), and more recently the systemic aromatic retinoid etretinate (Tegison). Unfortunately, however, the treatment of psoriasis even when successful is fraught with frequent recurrences. This fact must be made clear to the patient prior to beginning therapy. Another problem associated with intralesional steroid injection is the considerable discomfort associated with it. It is preferable for these specialized modalities to be administered by a qualified dermatologist. The nail changes of psoriasis are frequently associated with psoriatic arthritis. It has been estimated that over 80% of patients with psoriatic arthritis have some form of nail dystrophy. This is particularly true in the characteristic distal interphalangeal joint psoriatic arthritis. Other forms of psoriatic arthritis associated with nail changes include asymmetric oligoarthritis, serum negative polyarthritis, arthritis mutilans, and spondylitic arthritis.

## LICHEN PLANUS

As with psoriasis, lichen planus of the nails may be readily recognized when there are characteristic cutaneous and/or mucous membrane lesions. However, less than 5% of the time there may be lichen planus nail changes without concomitant changes elsewhere. It is important in lichen planus of the nails to confirm the diagnosis as early as possible. Treatment should be started quickly because lichen planus of the nails may be very destructive, resulting in permanent damage with irreversible scarring, including total destruction of the nail unit.

The clinical picture of lichen planus of the nails depends on the site of the pathology. When the matrix is involved, there are noted longitudinal grooves and ridges of the nail plate (onychorrhexis), thinning of the nail plate (hapalonychia), and pterygium formation. When the nail bed is involved, there is shedding of the nail plate (onycholysis, onychomadesis), atrophy of the nail bed (onychatrophy), subungual hyperkeratosis (onychauxis), and subungual hyperpigmentation. The characteristic pterygium of lichen planus develops because of a permanent destruction of the nail matrix, resulting in a direct attachment of the cornified layer of the underlying surface of the proximal nail fold to the cornified layer of the nail bed. Since there is no intervening nail plate, these structures grow out together, forming the characteristic winglike appearance of the pterygium. This is an irreversible change. Pterygium formation is virtually pathognomonic of lichen planus, occurring additionally only in patients with peripheral vascular disease such as scleroderma or secondary to trauma. The etiology of lichen planus is unknown, although it has been reported to occur associated with such drugs as thiazides, phenothiazines, and benzodiazepines. The diagnosis of lichen planus of the nails can be made only by performing a nail biopsy after appropriate mycologic studies have eliminated the possibility of a fungus infection.

### Treatment

Successful treatment to date for lichen planus of the nails is best achieved with corticosteroid therapy. Although intralesional steroids may be of benefit and arrest the rapid progression of this disorder, there are times when systemic corticosteroids may be required. If there is no medical contraindication to this latter therapy, dosages of 20 to 40 mg daily of prednisone have been administered. Alternate day therapy should be established as quickly as possible so as to minimize the probability of steroid side effects. The positives and negatives of this form of treatment in patients with lichen planus of the nails must be discussed in great detail with the patient prior to starting treatment.

## DISCOLORATION AND NEOPLASMS OF THE TOENAILS

Perhaps the most frequent cause of nail discoloration is the subungual hematoma. This will result in a brown to black appearance of the involved nail unit. The cause is usually trauma, but the presence of blood must be proved. If it is not, the possibility of overlooking a melanoma of the nail unit exists. The proof of subungual hematoma is generally determined either by histologic confirmation or in some instances by being able to wash away the blood that is trapped beneath the nail plate. So-called tennis toe or sportsman's toe, for example, is a frequent producer of subungual hemorrhage of the big toenail. Jogger's toe, which has recently been on the increase, will often cause a subungual hematoma of toes four and five. Likewise, the second and third toes seem to be most frequently involved in soccer players. However, depending on the type of shoe and foot structure, there may be considerable crossover as to which toes are involved in these various athletic activities.

A longitudinal pigmented band in a nail requires a biopsy to rule out the presence of a malignancy. The examining physician must be alert to the fact that the presence of such a streak of melanin in the nail plate results from a pigment source in the nail matrix. It is at this latter site from which the biopsy must be taken.

The periungual and subungual wart or verruca vulgaris also occurs in the nail unit. This disorder may be difficult to treat and may require surgical intervention, cryotherapy, or the application of appropriate keratolytic agents. A persistent or intractable periungual or subungual verrucous lesion may require a biopsy to rule out the possibility of a verrucous squamous cell carcinoma.

A nail with an erythematous focus that does not blanch totally with pressure and is associated with pain probably represents a glomus tumor. These lesions require surgical excision because of the persistence of discomfort. When they are large enough, erosion of the underlying bone is possible. X-ray of these lesions should always be performed.

## INGROWN TOENAILS

Ingrown toenails may be caused by an overcurvature of the nail plate, hypertrophy of the lateral nail folds, or the perforation of the nail fold epithelium by a spicule of nail plate. These changes may be precipitated by external pressure, internal pressure, or systemic disease. External pressures include improper foot care from poorly fitted shoes, poor stance or gait, digestive disturbances, and faulty trimming of the nails. Internal pressures due to subungual tumors, abnormally formed phalanges, certain inflammatory processes, and various arthropathies are etiologic as well. Systemic diseases that may contribute to ingrown toenails include obesity, abnormal metabolism (e.g., thyroid disorders), and geriatric changes, as well as cardiac and renal disease (e.g., edema). The therapy of ingrown toenails consists first of attempting to correct the etiologic agents mentioned above. In addition to this, there is generally some form of surgical therapy required in order to restore the toe to its normal state. If the ingrown toenail is caused by a spicule of nail penetrating the epithelium, it must be removed. If the problem is overcurvature of the nail plate, nail avulsion or a partial destruction of the nail matrix in both corners to provide a narrower nail plate may be required. This destruction may be performed by the use of phenol, surgical excision, or electrofulguration and curettage. In the event that hypertrophy of the lateral nail fold is causative, resection of this portion of the nail unit must be done. Simpler procedures may be attempted at first, but in the event they are unsuccessful, the more definitive techniques discussed above are required.

## NAIL SIGNS OF SYSTEMIC DISEASE

The nail unit is susceptible to change in the presence of systemic disease, as are the skin, hair, and mucous membranes. There are times when the nail changes may precede the symptoms of systemic illness. Therefore, it is important for the clinical dermatologist to be able to recognize them. Connective tissue disorders (scleroderma, dermatomyositis, lupus erythematosus) may present with telangiectasia of the proximal nail fold or periungual erythema. In association with Raynaud's phenomenon, these findings suggest medical evaluation for these conditions. The yellow nail syndrome presents as a yellowish discoloration of the nails associated with slow nail growth.

It may be associated with bronchiectasis, chronic bronchitis, and lymphatic abnormalities with edema. White nails (leukonychia) have been reported in patients with low serum albumin associated with liver disease as well as renal disease when the proximal half of the nail bed is white and the distal half is red or brown. Systemic malignancies may reveal themselves in nail changes. For example, the severe subungual and periungual hyperkeratosis with destruction of the nail plate and associated sterile pustules resembling pustular psoriasis known as paraneoplastic acrokeratosis of Bazex is associated with respiratory carcinoma. Clubbing of the digits may be accompanied by bronchogenic carcinoma, heart disease, thyroid disease, or ulcerative colitis. Finally, koilonychia (spoon nails)—when there is a concave appearance to the nail plate—may be present in patients with iron deficiency anemia. Abnormal peripheral vascular syndromes may also present these findings.

## NEW DEVELOPMENTS

The recent increase in patients with acquired immune deficiency syndrome (AIDS) has produced a variety of different nail manifestations. Yellow discoloration of the nail plate in AIDS patients has been reported. A severe form of candidiasis of the nail unit is being seen which has required higher dosages of ketoconazole for longer periods of time. Unusual forms of dermatophyte onychomycosis have also been noted. A severe proximal white onychomycosis caused by *Trichophyton rubrum* occurs which requires increased levels of systemic antifungal agents for extended lengths of time. Other nail changes of a bizarre nature in AIDS patients include an extensive and destructive form of psoriasis. Large recalcitrant verrucae vulgaris (warts) occurring peri- and subungually develop. Therefore, in patients presenting clinically with unusual nail manifestations, the possibility of HIV infection must be entertained.

New drugs being assessed for onychomycosis are itraconazole,* a second-generation ketoconazole currently being used in Europe with great success. Topical nail lacquers containing allyl amines, ciclopirox, and pyrithiones are also promising for nonsystemic treatment of onychomycosis. Finally, topical minoxidil (Rogaine)† is being tested as a growth-enhancing agent and may have a future role in the therapy of brittle nails and even possibly for difficult mycotic infections.

---

*Not available in the United States.

†This use of minoxidil is not listed in the manufacturer's official directive.

# KELOIDS

method of
ROSS RUDOLPH, M.D.
*Scripps Clinic and Research Foundation*
*La Jolla, California*

Patients may complain of "keloids" when they may have either widespread scars, hypertrophic scars, or true keloids, and the physician must be able to distinguish between these deformities. A widespread scar is flat or even depressed, and the proper treatment is surgery. Both hypertrophic scars and keloids have red, raised itchy masses of collagenous scar tissue. Hypertrophic scars lie within the original wound margin, whereas true keloids extend beyond the original wound in a crab-like fashion.

True keloids are almost always secondary to trauma which may be quite mild. There is a racial and age predisposition, with darker pigmented patients, especially blacks, more prone to keloids. The young are more likely to develop keloids than the old. Certain locations on the body are prone to keloids, specifically the anterior chest, deltoid region of the shoulder, most of the trunk, and the face and neck, with the curious exception of the eyelids.

## PREVENTION

Keloid formation should be guarded against by careful patient and site selection. Particularly in blacks, a history should be taken both of the patient and of the family relative to keloid experience. If a patient appears to be keloid prone, surgery should be avoided if possible, especially in age groups and locations where keloids are more likely. If skin lesions must be removed, intradermal shaving rather than a full-thickness excision may make keloids less likely, particularly if the deep dermis is not violated. At all costs, avoid crossing joint lines at a right angle. Prophylactic injection of triamcinolone acetonide (Kenalog) may be useful (see under Treatment).

## TREATMENT

True keloids have a distressing tendency to recur, particularly after surgical excision, and they may recur worse than the original lesion. Hypertrophic scars are less likely to have recurrence and almost never worsen. Surgery for true keloids is often a last resort unless there is the situation of a large keloid and a relatively small stalk, particularly on the ear lobe region.

Triamcinolone (Kenalog) injection is the mainstay of treatment. This long-acting depot glucocorticoid decreases collagen synthesis and increases collagen breakdown. The triamcinolone is usually diluted with lidocaine (Xylocaine) for pain relief, although injection is nevertheless painful. Injection must be into the lesion, which is difficult with the first injection and easier subsequently. The concentration of triamcinolone selected for keloid treatment is generally 20 to 40 mg per ml. Ideally, a tuberculin syringe is used to allow maximum pressure, using a 27-gauge needle firmly applied; a Luer-lock is particularly useful. Injection should be avoided outside the lesion as it can lead to subcutaneous atrophy or depigmentation, particularly in blacks. Injections into the keloid are repeated 3 to 4 weeks apart until atrophy has been achieved, which usually requires three or four injections. Some physicians suggest prior freezing of the lesion surface with liquid nitrogen for topical anesthesia. Triamcinolone injections may be used prophylactically after trauma in keloid-prone areas.

Pressure has been shown to help in prevention and treatment of keloids. Custom-fitted Jobst garments can be used to apply constant pressure. For the earlobe keloid, a small clip simulating an earring is available. Regrettably, treatment with pressure both of keloids and hypertrophic scars must be constant and meticulously followed, and patients often resist the use of pressure garments.

Surgery for keloids must be judicious, owing to the risk of recurrence and worsening. Almost always, surgical maneuvers that increase the length of the scar (such as Z-plasties and W-plasties) should be avoided. Surgical excision of keloids is most useful with the small-stalked lesion. Careful, meticulous technique is essential using small sutures close to the wound edges; the sutures are removed as soon as the wound is healed. Simultaneous injection with triamcinolone 5 to 20 mg per ml is used at surgery. Follow-up should be for 12 to 24 months. Repeat injections of triamcinolone are used if there is a recurrence of itching or lumpiness; patients should be informed to return immediately if these symptoms develop. Earlobe lesions are particularly amenable to excision and triamcinolone treatment; trunk keloids may respond less well.

### Other Treatments

Carbon dioxide or Nd:YAG lasers have been used to excise recalcitrant keloids, with the wounds being left open to close secondarily. There may be a specific laser effect on fibroblasts that explains the beneficial effect of the laser (which is still relatively experimental). Other experimental treatments include the use of beta amino propionitrile (BAPN); systemic treatments proved somewhat toxic and current experimentation involves topical BAPN. Other chemotherapeutic agents have been used with mixed results, including antimalignant chemotherapeutic agents such as methotrexate*, nitrogen mustard*, and thiotepa*.

---

*This use of these drugs is not listed in the manufacturer's official directive.

# VERRUCA VULGARIS
## (Warts)

method of
### J. CORWIN VANCE, M.D.
*University of Minnesota*
*Minneapolis, Minnesota*

Warts are epithelial growths caused by the human papilloma virus (HPV). They were recognized as contagious during Greek and Roman times. Folk cures are as old, with the concept of transferring them to other individuals or objects being frequent. The cures recorded by Mark Twain in Tom Sawyer are good examples. One of my acquaintances "purchases" warts from children, giving them money which they are not to spend until the warts are transferred to her. Applications of various substances have been tried, such as "milkweed" sap, potatoes, tree sap, and fat pork. Some currently used methods undoubtedly were discovered by employing such empiric remedies.

### TRANSMISSION

HPV is species specific, so study is difficult. It can withstand exposure so that transmission on various surfaces is possible. It remains viable in liquid nitrogen, and therefore, aliquots of the liquid should be used rather than dipping a swab into a reservoir which could be contaminated. Heating does inactivate the virus. Maceration and abrasions facilitate HPV infection, and spread of warts in scratches produced by shaving is a common observation, such as in the presence of "kissing" warts at adjacent areas of skin.

### MALIGNANT POTENTIAL

Although they are generally considered little more than bothersome skin bumps, they have recently been recognized to be associated with precancerous as well as frankly cancerous growths of the anogenital and other areas. The most common invasive cancer associated with HPV is carcinoma of the cervix.

### VIRUS TYPES

More than 50 types of HPV have been identified using sophisticated DNA hybridization techniques, and each has distinguishing clinical and histologic findings. Type 1, for instance, infects the highly keratinized skin of the sole or palm but rarely invades the thinner, less keratinized skin of the genital areas where Types 6, 11, 16, and 18 predominate. Certain types are particularly associated with malignant degeneration.

## IMMUNE RESPONSE

There is an immune response to warts, but it is difficult to measure. Lymphocyte-mediated immunity is felt to be the predominant defense, but antibody-mediated and localized skin immune functions may also be active. Plantar and common warts become dark and hard before spontaneously resolving, while flat warts become red and itchy. "Infection" of warts has been felt to indicate the development of immunity.

Children commonly develop warts, but after a period of months to years, the warts spontaneously regress and those individuals resist reinfection. The duration of immunity and its HPV type specifically are not known. Adults are less likely to have a spontaneous regression. It is possible that by treating children we abort their immune response and therefore make them more susceptible to wart infections as adults. That may be partially responsible for our current increase in warts in adults. It may therefore be best not to treat children, unless there are good emotional or physical reasons to do so.

Immune deficiency results in particularly widespread and troublesome wart infections, whether the deficiency is caused by an inherited immune defect, a malignancy such as a lymphoma or leukemia, a disease process such as sarcoidosis or lupus erythematosus, or artifically induced such as during chemotherapy, by corticosteroid administration, or for organ transplantation.

## GENERAL PRINCIPLES OF TREATMENT

There are no easy cures. Home treatments such as salicylic acid will be effective only if applied conscientiously and for a period of about 12 weeks. Conservative, nonscarring methods must be attempted before using more aggressive methods. Detailed, printed instructions should be given to the patient together with good oral teaching.

### Locally Destructive Chemicals

Salicylic acid is one of the first recorded treatments for warts, and it remains one of the best (Table 1). It is available in a collodion base (Compound W), with lactic acid (DuoFilm), and is incorporated into moleskin pads at a 40% concentration (Mediplast) as well as in karaya gum patches (TransVerSal). Soaking to enhance penetration of the acid and paring down the hyperkeratosis enhances the cure. Contamination of the surrounding skin causes irritation, and there is often discomfort before the wart is cured. The reappearance of normal skin lines usually heralds the cure. Acids should never be applied to facial, genital, or perianal skin because of irritation.

Trichloroacetic acid (TCA) and bichloroacetic acid (BCA) are particularly useful for treatment

### TABLE 1. Treatments for Warts

*Locally destructive chemicals*
  Salicylic acid (in films, plasters, and pads)
  Lactic acid
  Trichloroacetic acid (TCA)
  Bichloroacetic acid (BCA)
  Nitric acid
  Glacial acetic acid

*Surgically destructive methods*
  Excision
  Electrocautery
  Electrodesiccation
  Curettage
  Blunt dissection
  Laser vaporization or coagulation

*Blister-producing methods*
  Liquid nitrogen cryotherapy
  Carbon dioxide cryotherapy
  Nitrous oxide cryotherapy
  Cantharidin

*Cellular inhibition*
  Podophyllin and podophyllotoxin
  5-Fluorouracil
  Bleomycin
  Colchicine
  Interferon local injections
  Radiation

*Altering the cutaneous environment*
  Retinoids
  Formalin
  Gluteraldehyde
  Aluminum chloride
  Heat therapy

*Immune stimulation*
  Dinitrochlorobenzene (DNCB)
  Interferon systemic injections
  Vaccination, autologous or intralesional

*Miscellaneous*
  Hypnosis
  Tape occlusion

of anogenital warts, but they must be carefully applied by the physician weekly. They are also effective in treating common and plantar warts but are painful, so anesthesia is required. The strong acids such as nitric and glacial acetic acid are useful only when applied by experts aware of the risks.

### Surgical Methods

Surgical intervention is often demanded by patients seeking a quick and easy cure. It should be reserved for resistant cases that have failed conservative therapy because of potential scarring, pain, and a recurrence rate ranging from 10 to 30%. Recurrences are due to inapparent HPV present in the surrounding skin. All methods require anesthesia. During excision, care must be taken not to contaminate the scalpel with HPV since it will implant new warts along the incision. Curettage of warts is effective in keratinized areas. Application of TCA or silver nitrate or use of electrocautery or electrodesiccation at the curetted site assists in hemostasis and destroys the contaminating virus. Blunt dissection is particularly effective in removing isolated plantar warts.

The carbon dioxide laser has improved wart treatment by being more precise and causing less damage to surrounding tissues, producing less edema, pain, and scarring. The rate of cure approximates other surgical modalities. However, it has the added problem of producing a smoke plume that contains intact viral particles. Care must be taken to evacuate the smoke safely. It is expensive but is excellent for treating resistant warts, particularly if combined with methods to prevent recurrences, such as localized interferon injections.

### Blistering Modalities

Liquid nitrogen cryotherapy is one of the best all-around modalities. A proper blister removes all of the infected cells while sparing the dermis, thereby minimizing scarring. It may be applied by a swab, which is inexpensive, or by a spray apparatus, which is quicker. A 1 mm rim of frozen (white) skin should surround the wart and be held for 10 to 30 seconds, depending on the thickness of the skin, and repeated once. Record the time of the freeze so that it may be increased if inadequate blistering occurs. Pare down hyperkeratotic skin before freezing, and avoid freezing underlying bone, cartilage, or nerves. A flare occurs on thawing, and an often painful blister forms in a few hours. The blister falls off in about 2 weeks, and the area is retreated, an average of four treatments being necessary.

Cantharidin (Cantharone) produces a chemical blister that is less predictable but is particularly useful in children and in periungual warts.

### Cellular Inhibition

Podophyllin is the best initial treatment for genital and perianal warts, being easy to apply, nonpainful, inexpensive, and nonscarring. It is toxic if absorbed, so it must be used sparingly and never on pregnant women. Multiple treatments are necessary. Be careful to avoid normal skin, and apply a powder to dry it and prevent spread. Perianal treatment may be painful. It must be washed off after 4 hours.

A purified, less toxic and more reliable podophyllin formulation has been developed in Europe, where it is used as a home treatment.

5-Fluorouracil (Efudex)* cream can be applied to multiple flat warts and can be used in combination with laser or other destructive methods to prevent recurrences.

Bleomycin is diluted to 1 unit per ml and injected into recalcitrant warts, particularly periungual. If multiple warts are treated, anesthesia, such as a nerve block, is recommended because of pain. Long-term safety is unknown.

Alfa-2b interferon (Intron-A) is given intralesionally into anogenital warts, giving a course of nine injections over 3 weeks, injecting up to 5 million units per treatment (1 million units per lesion). A flu-like syndrome occurs but is well tolerated, responds to acetaminophen, and tachyphylaxis occurs. It is particularly useful in prevention of recurrences after ablative treatment such as laser or cautery. It is being tested as a systemic treatment, and delayed-release formulations are under development. It has antiviral, antiproliferative, and immune stimulatory effects.

Topical colchicine* is useful for periurethral warts where scarring is not tolerated.

Radiation is rarely used because of potential side effects, but it is effective in localized plantar or periungual warts.

### Altering the Cutaneous Environment

Retinoic acid† (Retin-A) cream can be applied to flat warts or used as an adjuvant to other therapies in resistant plantar warts.

Formalin, 20% in an ointment, or gluteraldehyde 10% solution applied daily and occluded is effective in plantar warts. The skin becomes dark brown and very dry, with painful fissures occurring in thin skin areas, and sensitization can occur.

Aluminum chloride to reduce sweating and heat therapy are unproved methods often used in combination with others.

### Immune Stimulation

Stimulation of a local immune response with dinitrochlorobenzene (DNCB) can be helpful in clearing widespread warts. DNCB is a powerful sensitizer, and extreme caution must be used.

Vaccinations are unapproved and potentially dangerous. Systemic interferon injections are potentially useful but unproved.

---

*This use of 5-FU is not listed in the manufacturer's official directive.

*This use of colchicine is not listed in the manufacturer's official directive.

†This use of retinoic acid is not listed in the manufacturer's official directive.

### Miscellaneous

There is a distinct placebo response in wart treatments, with about a 20% cure. Hypnosis and tape occlusion probably use this effect.

# NEVI AND MELANOMAS

method of
RICHARD G. BENNETT, M.D.
*University of Southern California School of Medicine*
*Los Angeles, California*

A mole is one of the most common skin lesions that cause a patient to seek the opinion of a physician. Although the majority of moles, also known as nevocytic nevi or, less specifically, nevi, are benign, occasional evolution into melanomas can occur. If the physician can detect early a nevus that has become malignant and if an adequate excision is performed, the patient's life will be saved.

Nevocytic nevi are divided into two groups: congenital nevocytic nevi and acquired nevocytic nevi. Congenital nevocytic nevi are present at the time of birth, and acquired nevocytic nevi arise after about 1 or 2 years of age.

## CONGENITAL NEVOCYTIC NEVI

Congenital nevocytic nevi (CNN) are pigmented lesions that present in about 1% of all live births. Although they may be flat, many are papular and hairy. On the basis of size, CNN can be divided into small (less than 1.5 cm in diameter), medium (1.5 to 19.9 cm in diameter), and large (greater than 20 cm in diameter). The large CNN that occur on the buttocks and lower trunk have been termed "bathing trunk nevi." In general, CNN tend to be larger than acquired nevocytic nevi. Histopathologically, the nevus cells in CNN lie at various depths in the skin, from the superficial dermis into fat. Nevus cells in CNN are also found clustered around hair follicles and other skin appendages.

### Prognosis

The evolution of a CNN into a melanoma partially depends on its size. A large CNN is probably more likely to evolve into a melanoma than a small CNN, although exact figures are lacking. When careful follow-up of several large CNN is done, the incidence of malignant degeneration is about 12%.

### Treatment

Excision of CNN is done for two reasons: either to improve the patient's appearance or to preclude malignant degeneration. Each case should be weighed individually. Since only a minority of large CNN undergo malignant degeneration and even very small CNN have become malignant, no rules apply. Certainly the risk of malignant degeneration should outweigh the risk of excision. For small CNN, we usually recommend simple excision and closure. For very large CNN, excision is also recommended followed by skin grafting or other appropriate closure techniques. For medium-size lesions, the decision to excise is complicated by the fact that a significant scar will ensue and the chance of malignant degeneration is probably minimal.

Excision of CNN is predicated upon complete removal of all nevus cells. Because nevus cells in CNN may be quite deep, complete excision will also necessarily be deep. Dermabrasion has been suggested in lieu of excision for removal of CNN. However, careful studies have shown that dermabrasion usually leaves significant numbers of deep nevus cells. Therefore, at best, dermabrasion can only be considered a cosmetic procedure for CNN.

## ACQUIRED NEVOCYTIC NEVI

Acquired nevocytic nevi (ANN) occur usually after 1 or 2 years of age and are uniformly present in all individuals. The ANN is commonly referred to as a mole. Usually, there are about 15 to 40 ANN per adult. ANN are usually much smaller than CNN, and ANN have a life span of their own. Usually, an ANN appears in childhood, may at first be flat with pigment, then becomes papular with pigment in young adulthood. It then persists without pigment and eventually involutes in old age. The very young and very old are almost devoid of ANN. (It is interesting to note in comparison that most CNN are relatively stable in terms of size and pigmentation.) The clinical appearance of ANN is thought to correspond to the location of the nevus cells within the skin. The initial flat pigmented lesion (known as a junctional nevus) has nevus cells in nests along the dermal-epidermal junction. The papular pigmented lesion (known as a compound nevus) has nevus cell nests both along the dermal-epidermal junction and also deeper within the dermis. The papular nonpigmented lesion (known as an intradermal nevus) has nevus cells in nests in the upper dermis only.

### Prognosis

Most ANN remain benign, and transformation into melanoma is rare.

## Special Problems

Occasionally, ANN will contain a hair follicle or several hair follicles. Infection may occur if these follicles become occluded, and the ANN will become red and tender. It is thought that this occlusion occurs because the growth of nevus cells may constrict the follicular opening. Bleeding may also occur into an ANN, especially after trauma. These problems need to be carefully assessed and the infected or hemorrhagic ANN distinguished from malignant transformation of an ANN. Pregnancy can cause an ANN to darken and may be associated with the development of melanomas. Any suspicious pigmented lesions developing during pregnancy should be biopsied.

## Treatment

Not all ANN require treatment. Removal is recommended for those lesions that enlarge, change color, or bleed. Removal is also frequently done on those lesions irritated by clothing or cosmetically objectionable. Treatment of ANN is by excision, either incomplete (shave) excision or complete excision. When complete excision is done, the nevus cells are completely removed and the resultant wound sutured; complete excision usually leads to noticeable scarring, especially on the trunk. Incomplete excision is done to minimize scarring. To preclude a depressed scar from an incomplete (shave) excision, a small portion of the ANN is left above the skin surface during the shave, and this small amount of nevus tissue is lightly electrodesiccated. It should be stressed to the patient that subtotal removal of ANN frequently results in slow regrowth and repigmentation.

The excised ANN, whether complete or incomplete, should be sent for histopathologic examination. Occasionally, a lesion that appears completely benign is found, on histopathologic examination, to be malignant.

## Variants of ANN

The halo nevus is an ANN with a ring of surrounding hypopigmented skin. It is thought that the hypopigmented skin is due to immunologic destruction of melanocytes and nevus cells. Halo nevi usually occur sporadically but may be seen in association with melanoma.

The blue nevus is another ANN variant that appears very dark blue owing to the pigment being at a deeper level in the dermis than in common ANN. This depth of brown pigment results in a dark blue appearance because of differential light scattering and absorption.

The Spitz nevus, also mistakenly called a ju-venile melanoma, occurs as a pink papule, usually on the face of a child. The nevus cells are spindle shaped and may be deep.

The dysplastic nevocytic nevus (DNN) is a special variety of ANN that has been recently described. The DNN usually is larger than the ANN, is more irregularly pigmented, and arises later in life (Table 1). The importance of recognizing a DNN is that this lesion may be more likely to progress to a melanoma than is an ANN. When multiple, DNN may be markers of a familial predisposition to melanoma development. This familial predisposition has been termed the dysplastic nevus syndrome or the familial atypical mole melanoma (FAMM) syndrome.

Dysplastic nevocytic nevi should be watched for any signs of growth or increased pigmentation. Photodocumentation is suggested. Excisional biopsies on suspicious lesions should be done. Biopsies should be evaluated carefully by a trained dermatopathologist. Patients with DNN who especially need careful re-evaluation at intervals are those who have multiple dysplastic nevi and a family history of melanoma. In those patients with multiple DNN who do develop a melanoma, the melanoma frequently arises de novo rather than from a pre-existing DNN. Patients with multiple DNN should be re-evaluated at 1-year intervals.

## MELANOMA

Melanomas are the most common deadly tumor arising in the skin. The current incidence of melanoma is 1 in 250 people. This incidence has been increasing yearly, and it is estimated that by the year 2000 it will be 1 in 150 people. Although melanomas are seen with increasing frequency, it is unknown whether this is because of earlier detection than in previous times.

TABLE 1. **Comparison of Acquired Nevocytic Nevi (ANN) with Dysplastic Nevocytic Nevi (DNN)**

|  | ANN | DNN |
|---|---|---|
| Size | ≤5 mm | >5 mm |
| Appearance | Regular macular, papular | Pebbled or irregular papular |
| Pigmentation | Evenly distributed, tan or brown | Uneven and may be variegated, red/blue/brown |
| Surface | Regular | Irregular |
| Border | Regular, sharply defined | Irregular, indistinct |
| Age at appearance | Childhood, puberty, rarely after age 40 | Young adulthood until after age 40 |
| Location | Sun-exposed areas | Sun-exposed and sun-protected areas |

## Types of Melanomas

Cutaneous melanomas are not a homogeneous tumor type but are divided into four main types:

Lentigo maligna melanoma (LMM) arises on sun-damaged skin, usually the face. Atypical melanocytes are elongated and usually extend down the external root sheath of hair follicles. LMM evolves slowly over many years and often does not metastasize, even when deep.

Superficial spreading melanoma (SSM) arises anywhere on the body surface, spreads laterally within the epidermis, and appears as a lesion with an irregular border, irregular surface, and irregular pigmentation. The atypical melanocytes will, at a certain point, invade in-depth, and the melanoma then may have a nodular appearance with surrounding macular hyperpigmentation.

Nodular melanoma (NM) is a papular or nodular lesion with little or no surrounding macular pigmentation. Almost from the beginning, the atypical melanocytes in an NM are quite deep in the dermis. Usually, the prognosis is poor.

Acral lentiginous melanoma (ALM) is a flat, pigmented lesion of the finger or toe, often involving the nail bed. When involving the nail bed, the proximal nail fold is frequently pigmented (Hutchinson's melanotic whitlow). An ALM is often unrecognized early and may have a poor prognosis unless adequately treated.

All these melanoma types have different clinical appearances, different growth rates, and different prognoses. About 20% of SSM or NM arise from pre-existing acquired nevocytic nevi or congenital nevocytic nevi.

## Recognition

The clinical appearance of melanoma is best remembered by the mnemonic ABCD—asymmetry, border, color, and diameter. The melanoma surface is frequently asymmetric, as is the distribution of pigmentation. The border is irregular, often indented. The color is nonuniform with shades of brown, black, gray, or red. The diameter of a melanoma is usually greater than 6 mm.

## Prognosis

The most reliable prognostic indicator in nonmetastatic (Stage I) melanoma is tumor thickness. The thickness of each melanoma is assessed histopathologically by both Clark's level of thickness and Breslow's measured thickness. Both types of assessment (Clark's and Breslow's) are not uniform from one pathologist to the next; nonetheless, the deeper the tumor penetration, the worse the prognosis. Breslow's intervals of thickness (measured from the top of the granular cell layer to the deepest portion of the tumor) are as follows: less than .76 mm, .76 to 1.50 mm, 1.51 to 2.25 mm, 2.26 to 3.00 mm, and greater than 3 mm. Clark's levels of thickness are as follows: intraepidermal (Level I); into papillary dermis (Level II); to reticular dermis (Level III); into reticular dermis (Level IV); and below dermis (Level V). Melanomas with an excellent prognosis include Clark Level II lesions with a measured Breslow thickness of less than .76 mm. However, metastases may occur from even these superficial tumors.

## Treatment

Treatment is by excisional surgery. For small superficial lesions less than .76 mm, a 5- to 10-mm margin of normal tissue, including underlying fat, is now considered sufficient. For lesions thicker than .76 mm, the amount of normal tissue required is unknown. Certainly local recurrence is rare with SSM and NM so that very large margins of 5 cm are now considered unnecessary and needlessly mutilative. For large lesions where an excisional biopsy cannot be done easily, incisional biopsy may be necessary. It is now thought that incisional biopsy of a melanoma does not increase the likelihood of metastasis.

Recurrent melanomas or melanomas in cosmetically important areas, such as the nose or ear, are best treated by conservative excision with careful assessment of all margins. This ideal type of excision is provided best by Mohs micrographic surgery so that the maximal amount of normal tissue will be saved. LMM is also best treated by Mohs micrographic surgery, as this particular melanoma is more likely to recur locally.

For very thin (less than .76 mm), Level II tumors and very thick tumors (Level V), the type of therapy chosen has little influence on the prognosis. For lesions in between, the method of treatment has an unknown influence on the prognosis.

# PREMALIGNANT LESIONS

method of
JULIO HERNANDEZ, M.D.
*New Orleans, Louisiana*

The term premalignant implies that under various circumstances a lesion has a propensity to become a malignancy. The importance of recognizing and treating these lesions is that a lot of morbidity can be prevented. These lesions are the first warnings given by our body that there might be a problem later. The conditions discussed here are generally slow-growing. Malignant degeneration is insidious in onset. Patients and family members become accustomed to the presence of the slow-growing changes or other abnormalities and often do not seek medical examination until overt changes or other signs or symptoms occur.

Fortunately, with few exceptions, the precancerous stages are slow to develop into malignancy, and most of these conditions have a low rate of conversion to a malignant state. The incidence of premalignant lesions, especially those associated with sun exposure, is increasing.

## DIAGNOSTIC CONSIDERATIONS

To diagnose a premalignant lesion of the skin, good lighting is essential. Also, a high degree of suspicion will help to identify them. Traditionally, only sun-exposed areas were examined for the presence of premalignant lesions on the skin. However, non–sun-exposed areas can also harbor premalignant skin lesions. In particular, some of the melanoma precursors have been discovered in non–sun-exposed areas. Therefore, it is important to examine the whole body surface if one is to find an early indication of a malignancy.

Biopsy techniques are tailored to the specific features and distribution of lesions. Shave biopsies of the skin can be performed for a majority of lesions if enough dermis is obtained to allow the diagnosis of a lesion. However, the goal in dealing with premalignant conditions is to establish a definite diagnosis. If there is a doubt about the depth of the lesion, a punch biopsy would be preferred since one would want to provide enough material for pathology exam. If the lesion is small enough, biopsy in toto is recommended, as this will avoid the need for a secondary treatment whether the pathology is benign or premalignant. For premalignant lesions, a full-thickness biopsy is indicated so that if the lesion is found to be melanoma, proper therapeutic decision can be made based on the thickness and level of the lesion.

## PRIMARY LESIONS

### Actinic Keratosis

These scaling, erythematous or hyperpigmented plaques are found on sun-exposed areas and are the most common premalignant conditions. They often cause concern because of their cosmetic disfigurement. Their malignant potential is low; therefore, treatment should provide excellent cosmetic results. Because these lesions are superficial, I prefer to remove them under local anesthesia by thin, tangential shave excision, with the scalpel or razor blade slicing through the papillary dermis. A few millimeters of margin of epidermis surrounding the treatment site is then lightly electrodesiccated at a low power setting so that slow blanching (without bubbling or charring) of the surface is seen. In general, therapy should be individualized, depending on the number and extent of the lesions, the condition of the surrounding skin, the ana-

tomic subsite, and the general condition of the patient. Since some of the therapeutic modalities cause discomfort and temporary unsightliness, it is well to consider whether the patient has any impending socially important events or has the ability to care for himself or herself.

After assessing the lesion and these variables, it is best to outline a therapeutic plan that includes the sequential and judicious use of a combination of the available therapeutic techniques. It is advisable to tell the patient that, although therapy may cure all apparent lesions, new lesions caused by prior sun damage may be expected to continue to appear for a while. No matter which mode of therapy is chosen, all patients should be instructed to limit further sun exposure and are advised strongly to use a sunscreen whenever they go outside, regardless of the season. In addition to the previously discussed therapy, other choices for definite therapy include cryotherapy with liquid nitrogen, topical 5-fluorouracil (Efudex) therapy, curettage and electrodesiccation, surgical excision, chemocautery with various acids, and dermabrasion.

### Treatment

**Cryotherapy.** Cryotherapy is a method frequently used because of its effectiveness, ease of application, and availability. It is also fairly noninvasive, and it does not require anesthesia because usually the pain is only mild yet tolerable. However, this will vary greatly according to the patient's pain tolerance. Liquid nitrogen is effective in treating individual lesions, with treatment of as many lesions as the patient can tolerate in one sitting as the goal. It can be applied with either a commercially available spray device or a cotton tip applicator. The goal is to apply the liquid nitrogen directly to the center of the lesion until frosting occurs. The length of time the cryogen is applied is learned only with experience. Thinner lesions in an old patient with atrophic surrounding skin require less time than the thicker lesions on a younger patient. I personally use applicator sticks in an attempt to keep the lesions frosted for about 5 to 10 seconds and then wait for a comparable or slightly longer thaw time before repeating the process. The freeze time and number of freeze-thaw cycles depend on the thickness of the lesion and its response, upon visual inspection, to the cryogen. The keratosis and surrounding areas usually become erythematous and edematous within minutes, and the effects persist for 24 to 48 hours. A blister or hemorrhagic bulla may develop. The blister splits the skin at the dermal/epidermal junction and, if troublesome, may be punctured with a sterile needle and deflated. Otherwise, a necrotic crust forms within days and sloughs off within a week or two, depending on the thickness of the lesion. I recommend local care with hydrogen peroxide and polysporin ointment, two to three times daily until healing occurs. Complications of this therapy are usually related to excess freezing of the skin which might lead to scar formation. Also hypopigmentation can be seen and, in darker skinned patients, high risk of hyperpigmentation. In addition, if the therapy is too superficial, recurrence of the lesions will be seen. The main drawback that I have found is that patients complain of more discomfort (especially males) than is mentioned in the literature.

**5-Fluorouracil.** Multiple actinic keratosis involving major portions of the head and neck, trunk, and upper extremities can be treated with topical 5-fluorouracil (5-FU). The 5% cream is usually applied twice daily. Treatment should be continued for 3 to 4 weeks on the face and neck and for 4 to 6 weeks on the scalp, trunk, and upper extremities. Patients must be cautioned that several days after treatment begins and long before it is complete, the skin will become inflamed and will have a burning pain. For these reasons, I discourage 5-FU therapy. Once my patients have undergone one such treatment, they rarely choose it again. Therapy with 5-FU is terminated when most of the lesions that were initially inflamed become eroded and exudative. Lesions on the scalp, trunk, and upper extremities usually need 2 weeks of pretreatment and/or concomitant therapy with tretinoin (Retin-A) 0.025 or 0.05% cream for removal or softening of thick scales. Combination treatment with 5-FU and Retin-A should be administered only by physicians who have had extensive experience with both agents, since retinoid dermatitis or a very severe contact dermatitis can develop if therapy is managed improperly. After treatment, any residual lesions must be biopsied so that squamous cell carcinoma can be ruled out. Be forewarned that topical therapy with 5-FU may provide superficial but ultimately inadequate therapy for other forms of cutaneous tumors, such as basal cell carcinoma and squamous cell carcinoma, which will recur later as more biologically active lesions.

Another acceptable treatment for actinic keratosis is superficial curettage. As previously mentioned bleeding after shave excision or curettage occurs, but it is rarely a problem and can be controlled by pressure or by application of a chemical such as 35% aluminum chloride. Any lesion that recurs after treatment or one that initially has a thick surface scale should be considered for total excision, if feasible.

Three surgical procedures that effectively remove multiple actinic keratosis are the trichloroacetic acid (TCA) peel, the phenol peel, and facial dermabrasion. These are considerably more effective than topical 5-FU and should be used when numerous lesions are present or in patients who have a poor response to 5-FU (or no compliance with that treatment). A procedure used extensively in my practice, mainly on the head and neck, is peeling with 35% TCA. Higher concentrations of TCA can be used but are much more likely to cause scarring and therefore are not recommended. Actually, unless very experienced in the use of TCA, one shouldn't even have a bottle of TCA with a concentration higher than 35% in one's office.

The TCA peel can be enhanced by pretreatment with Jessner's solution or with the use of the newer alphahydroxy acid such as 50 to 70% lactic acid or glycolic acid. After these surgical procedures, the skin is rejuvenated. In addition to providing marked therapeutic effects, these treatments provide excellent cosmetic improvement. The main drawback of using TCA is a transient burning sensation, which might last 15 to 20 minutes, that patients might experience. The patient is instructed to wash off the area with soap and water after 4 hours and start applying hydrogen peroxide and polysporin ointment two to three times a day, the day after the procedure. After about 4 or 5 days the area will peel off and new skin will develop. The skin will have a pink appearance, and it might take up to 3 months before it gets its normal color back. This is due to destruction of melanocytes in the area, and the patient has to be forewarned of the need for strict use of sunscreens in this area until the skin color returns. Failure to do so might lead to permanent pigment changes. In addition, postinflammatory hyperpigmentation could be a problem in darker skinned people.

In addition, phenol solution using Baker's formula can be used for actinic keratosis. This is a more invasive procedure, and depending on the amount of skin to be treated, toxicity with phenol can occur. Anybody using phenol should be well trained in its complications, which include cardiac toxicity. If used in extensive areas of the skin, the patient should be monitored. Also, an assessment of the hepatic and renal status should be done prior to surgery. I personally do not use phenol for actinic keratosis and reserve it exclusively for the treatment of those patients with extensive actinic keratoses and severe solar elastosis in whom I want to achieve the goal of facial rejuvenation. An alternative, although more invasive, method of therapy is superficial dermabrasion of the face. In the hands of a trained physician, dermabrasion offers a great therapeutic advantage and is a fast and easy method. In this modality the skin is planed into the papillary dermis with subsequent regeneration of a keratosis-free epidermis and papillary dermis. This procedure not only treats the actinic damage but gives the face a rejuvenated appearance and adds a degree of prophylaxis against the development of new keratosis. Dermabrasions require more skill than any of the other previously mentioned treatments and should be used only by physicians trained in this procedure.

**Retin-A Therapy.** Tretinoin (Retin-A) has become fashionable for the treatment of aging skin, since it was first shown to aid in the rejuvenation of collagen in animal models a number of years ago. Clinical studies are very encouraging, and there are a few ongoing studies at present to further define therapy. Retin-A appears to reverse actinic damage to collagen (which may cause a reversal of some wrinkles), to shrink and eradicate minute actinic keratoses, and to abort the development of new lesions. The most important use of tretinoin will be for the reversal of the actinic damage, thereby decreasing, it is hoped, the incidence of skin cancer development. Side effects of Retin-A are minor and include irritation, redness, and increased phototoxicity during its use. A retinoid dermatitis has been described and should be promptly recognized and treated. The physician using this treatment modality should be aware of all the possible side effects and how to control them. All patients using Retin-A should be encouraged to use a moisturizing sunscreen in the daytime and avoid excessive sun exposure. Scaling and dryness might be noted by some patients within 1 to 2 weeks of initiating therapy and appears to decrease with continued use of the medication. Some patients will experience a severe reaction, and the treatment may have to be discontinued and then restarted at a lower dosage or lower frequency once symptoms have resolved. Patients should be started on the 0.025% cream, and the gel base or liquid should be avoided as it is more drying than the cream base. Starting with the higher concentrations will increase the chance of a significant side effect's developing. Patients should be instructed also to watch for any blemishes that do not fade within 3 to 4 weeks. Some early skin cancers have developed during Retin-A therapy. This is not to say that Retin-A induces skin cancer, but it may accelerate the development of already existent skin cancers. Appropriate therapy should be instituted if this happens. Finally, the patient should be warned that this is a non–FDA approved treatment, although it is used extensively in this country and there is sufficient clinical and laboratory evidence already in existence to warrant its use in the treatment of actinic keratoses and sun-induced damage. Dermatologists have over 15 years of experience using Retin-A therapy.

## Leukoplakia

This condition may be seen on the vermilion border of the lips and the mucous membranes of the oral, anal, and genital regions. The white hyperkeratotic changes of leukoplakia on the lips can be best defined clinically by grasping the lip at the angles of the mouth and placing it under stretch pressure. Not all leukoplakia is premalignant. When leukoplakia occurs in a sun-exposed area, it is more likely to be premalignant, and multiple selected biopsies are in order. I perform biopsy of the most suspicious areas, using a 2- or 3-mm punch, followed by primary closure with silk suture, which is more comfortable than the stiff monofilament suture materials. Leukoplakia in the lips most commonly results from chronic sun exposure, irritation from smoking, or chronic biting of the lip. Ill-fitting dentures, poor oral hygiene, excessive use of tobacco, and sharp or chipped teeth may create intraoral changes of leukoplakia.

When lesions occur within the oral cavity but have a reddish hue, they may be known as erythroleukoplakia. They have a much higher rate of degeneration to malignancy. Such lesions should be excised in toto.

**Treatment.** Definite treatment consists of infiltration of the affected area with local anesthesia, followed by cautery using a flat, spatula-shaped electrode capable of evenly distributing the destructive force. The affected area and some normal-appearing adjacent tissue are cauterized until a white hue is obtained. A curette is used to loosen the treated tissue. Repeat cautery may be necessary to eliminate a deeper, more stubborn area. An antibiotic ointment, such as polymixin B or bacitracin (Polysporin) should be applied three to four times a day to keep the surgical site soft (avoid cross formation). Re-epithelialization generally is complete between 7 and 15 days, postoperative pain is mild, and the healing is usually complete, without any visible scar formation. Initial evaluation and follow-up examination are performed at least on a semiannual basis and should include examination of the regional lymph nodes in the cervical chain and those that are palpable, while performing an intraoral bimanual examination using a gloved hand.

Laser surgery accomplishes the same result as electrodesiccation cautery. In severe cases of leukoplakic changes involving a major portion of the lower lip, and occasionally part of the upper lip, vermilionectomy and resurfacing of the lip using an advancement flap from the labium mucosa is a satisfactory procedure. It may leave some deformity of the lower lip. If the disease is localized, a wedge resection might be preferred.

Leukoplakia on the genital or anal area requires special consideration. It is absolutely imperative to rule out malignant degeneration before any surgical or medical treatment is initiated. Multiple selected biopsy sites may be used to establish the diagnosis.

When leukoplakia occurs on the vulva or perianal area, there is no satisfactory and reliable medical treatment. Therefore, planed excisional therapy, if location and size of the lesions are amenable, is the preferred method. Consideration of anatomic function and structure is part of the surface planing. Often, the leukoplakic areas are small in relation to overall pathologic areas, and hence, specific excisions may be accomplished.

Other treatment modalities for leukoplakia include the use of trichloroacidic acid, phenol, and liquid nitrogen.

### Lentigo Maligna (Melanotic Freckle of Hutchinson)

These are hyperpigmented and often irregularly colored macular (flat) lesions, commonly found on sun-exposed areas of the elderly. Some people consider them a form of actinic keratosis. The malar or lateral cheek areas are most commonly involved. They begin initially as small, brownish macules which can in time, usually years, enlarge peripherally and may become as large as a silver dollar or larger.

The significance of these lesions is primarily in regard to malignant degeneration. Because degeneration of these lesions leads to malignant melanoma, I prefer to treat them early. Punch biopsy shows dysplastic melanocytes along the basement membrane. Once the dysplastic or malignant changes penetrate the basement membrane, they should be considered melanoma and treated as such.

Focal areas of increased pigmentation, papule or nodule development, or variegated color changes should be sampled for biopsy to determine whether they are malignant or premalignant.

**Treatment.** Because the abnormal melanocytes may extend deep into the hair follicles, complete excision is indicated. Curettage and cautery, liquid nitrogen, and chemical peel using full-strength phenol have been recommended but do not adequately treat the deeper portions of the lesions and usually result in a disfiguring, hypopigmented scar. Dermabrasion, when carried below the hair follicles, cures the lesion but produces permanent scarring. Radiation therapy is not recommended.

Complete surgical excision with serial microscopic evaluation of the tissue is the treatment of choice. The lesion may be so large that it requires several surgical sessions of simple excision for complete removal. In more complex lesions, resurfacing with skin flaps is superior to grafting.

### Bowen's Disease

This condition is a particular type of squamous cell carcinoma in situ and usually presents on sun-exposed areas as a well-defined, erythematous, scaling flake. It is often mistaken for an actinic keratosis; however, its malignant potential is considerably greater. When found in areas not normally exposed to sunlight, it may result from earlier exposure to arsenic ingestion and may be associated with internal malignancy. Therefore, such patients deserve a clinical workup for occult malignancy, most particularly of the gastrointestinal tract and pulmonary system. Lesions on sun-exposed areas are statistically less likely to be a sign of internal malignancy. Nevertheless, reports over the years have raised significant questions as to whether or not Bowen's disease is a precursor or indicator of internal malignancy.

Essentially all lesions of Bowen's disease are slow growing and small. The average size of presentation is about ½ to 2 cm in diameter. They tend to be annular or circular, flat, slightly scaly, and slightly pinkish or erythematous. The extremities are the most common site. When nodularity or erosion is present, biopsy should encompass these areas.

**Treatment.** Complete excision of the lesions of Bowen's disease is imperative, and these specimens should be sent for serial section to determine definitely tumor-free borders. Most lesions are small and can be closed by using primary closure. Margins must be adequate to encompass areas of involvement that are not clinically perceptible. Other methods of treatment include cautery and curettage, radiation therapy, chemotherapy using 5-FU, and cryotherapy with liquid nitrogen. A disadvantage of these methods is that they do not provide a surgical specimen for microscopic evaluation.

### Queyrat's Erythroplasia

This is a unique disease occurring on the glans penis or foreskin. It is equivalent to Bowen's disease occurring elsewhere. Because of the glabrous type of skin, with the epidermis and dermis much thinner than that of the extremities, the possibility of developing into squamous cell carcinoma with regional lymph node metastasis is more likely.

**Treatment.** Diagnosis is the key to treatment. A

punch biopsy is invaluable before definite surgery. When the lesion is clinically definable, surgical excision with adequate margins is an effective cure. On uncircumcised males, circumcision is advised.

For extensive lesions of Queyrat's erythroplasia, particularly where considerable foreskin is involved in an uncircumcised male, Mohs' chemosurgery may be the treatment of choice. Because of the serious nature of this condition, I do not use topical chemotherapy with 5-FU, cryotherapy with liquid nitrogen, or cautery and curettage, as has been recommended by some.

## Keratoacanthoma

Keratoacanthomas are pseudomalignant tumors. They exhibit a characteristic clinical morphology and course and a tendency for spontaneous resolution. The typical solitary keratoacanthoma appears initially as a firm, red, round papule, which grows rapidly over a period of 4 to 6 weeks to attain its final size of 1 to 2 cm. In its fully developed form, it is a skin-colored, dome-shaped lesion, which has been likened to a volcano having smooth slopes and a central keratin-filled crater. There is a tendency for these lesions to resolve spontaneously over a period varying from 6 months to many years. Despite this spontaneous resolution, keratoacanthomas can be destructive as they evolve leaving disfiguring atrophic scars. Rapidly growing lesions, attaining the size of 2 cm or greater, are referred to as giant keratoacanthomas and can also be aggressive and destructive. The significance of these lesions, despite their rapid onset, is their histologic similarity to squamous cell carcinoma.

**Treatment.** A punch biopsy of keratoacanthoma lesions may be very misleading. A microscopic appearance of portions of lesions may so resemble squamous cell carcinoma that the pathologist cannot make a definite diagnosis under the light microscope. Therefore, unless the lesion is excessively large, complete excision is the preferred method of treatment. A wedge biopsy on selected lesions may be a preferred method of diagnosis prior to complete excision. The wedge biopsy should contain a portion of the center and should extend peripherally to apparently normal skin.

Rarely, multiple keratoacanthomas may occur as a consequence of either a hereditary condition or an immunosuppressed state or in conjunction with Torres's syndrome. In cases of multiple keratoacanthomas, selected lesions may be excised, and after several lesions have been evaluated to rule out squamous cell carcinoma, those remaining may be treated through several options. These include cryosurgery with liquid nitrogen, intralesional infiltration of full-strength 5-FU, or intralesional triamcinolone (Kenalog) 20 to 40 mg per ml. Other reported treatment methods for multiple keratoacanthomas are oral methotrexate, and a compounded 3.5% ointment of bleomycin. Multiple keratoacanthomas of the eruptive type are resistant to most forms of therapy.

## Arsenical Keratoses

These are keratotic lesions that tend to involve the epidermis and the outer keratin layers and may occur in the palms, soles, or anywhere on the body. Histologically, they are similar to actinic keratoses.

Usually, the source of arsenic is unknown to the patient. It may have been ingested or inhaled. In certain types of mining and smelting, particularly of copper, gold, or bauxite, the smeltering will perfuse the air with arsenic fumes for several miles around. For years, arsenic was contained in pesticides and other farm products, and over many years, well water became contaminated with detectable levels of arsenic. Persons using such water were subject to development of arsenical keratoses. Tobacco products may contain detectable levels of arsenic. Certain famous brand name cigars and pipe tobaccos have been measured by reliable laboratories and found to contain from 15 to 29 ppm of arsenic.

**Treatment.** Palmar and plantar arsenical keratoses rarely develop into malignancy, but lesions on other areas of the skin or mucous membrane margins are likely to become malignant. Therefore, treatment for arsenical keratoses should be equivalent to that for actinic keratosis except when they occur on the palms and soles.

Palmar and plantar arsenical keratoses can be treated by simple curettage, electrosurgery, cryotherapy, or the use of keratolytic topical agents. Treatment with 5-FU is not very effective, possibly because of thickness of the epidermis. Patients with arsenical keratosis are at a slightly increased risk for visceral carcinoma, and this should be kept in mind when evaluating these patients.

## Tar Keratoses

This unusual condition is seen in persons with a long history of exposure to coal, pitch, tar, or their by-products. Treatment may be simple, using electrodesiccation, cryosurgery, or shave excision and light dermabrasion. Preventive measures include avoidance of exposure to tar, pitch, soot, crude paraffin, asphalt, and related by-products. Sunscreens are helpful to decrease photoactivation of tar products. Occupational changes may be most practical.

## Giant Condyloma of Buschke and Löwenstein

Genital warts that have persisted for a long time in the normal or immunosuppressed host can undergo malignant degeneration into a verrucous carcinoma.

Infection with certain papilloma viruses appears to be closely correlated with the development of cervical carcinoma in infected women; female sexual partners of males with genital condyloma should be examined closely. Conditions analogous to the giant condyloma of Buschke and Löwenstein, epithelioma cuniculatum of the hands and feet and oral florid papillomatosis, are rare disorders that are also locally destructive.

Primary treatment with cryosurgery, 6-hour applications of podophyllin resin in the nonpregnant patient, or conservative local electrofulguration can be used on primary lesions. Nonresponsive disease should be biopsied to rule out malignant degeneration. However, electrofulguration should be used by properly trained physicians in a facility with adequate ventilation. Recent studies suggest that potentially infectious viral DNA from the papilloma virus is found in the smoky plume of vaporized condylomas.

Radiation therapy is absolutely contraindicated in the treatment of these lesions because it enhances their ability to metastasize.

## Oral Florid Papillomatosis

These lesions resemble leukoplakia of the oral mucosa and are usually found on the lower lips. The tendency to malignant degeneration is much less than that of actinic keratosis.

**Treatment.** After biopsy to establish diagnosis, conservative treatment, such as special topical or intralesional steroids, may merit a trial. Vermilionectomy may be definitive. Pipe smoking, chewing tobacco, and snuff are possible causative agents. Radiation therapy is contraindicated.

## Epithelioma Cuniculatum

This unusual condition involves the inner digital and plantar surfaces. Lesions may be quite large and difficult to cure because the most satisfactory treatment is complete surgical excision.

**Treatment.** Acceptable modes of therapy for small lesions detected early include electrodestruction, using curettage and electrodesiccation, and cryotherapy. Radiation therapy should be avoided.

## Congenital Melanocytic Nevi

Congenital pigmented nevi may be precursors of melanoma. The precise frequency of malignant degeneration is unknown but appears to increase dramatically with larger lesions (more than 10 cm; for example, giant hairy nevus, bathing trunk nevus), and appears to be almost negligible in small lesions.

**Treatment.** Removal of the small lesions by surgical excision is generally easy to accomplish and can eliminate the small but definite risk of malignant degeneration. The larger lesions, which have a higher incidence of malignant degeneration, are more difficult to remove, but a greater effort should be made to remove them. Treatment of giant congenital melanocytic nevi can consist of staged excisions, excision and grafting, or excision and the insertion of tissue expanders that allow additional normal skin to be used for reconstruction, or any combination thereof. Recently, dermabrasion has been recommended for large lesions. When used during the first 8 weeks of life, this method is effective in permanently removing pigmentation and destroys most of the melanocytes before they migrate to the deeper portions of the dermis. The procedure must be performed by a dermatologic surgeon who is well trained in the technique of dermabrasion.

## Dysplastic Nevi

Nevi with asymmetric configuration, irregular borders, multiple colors ranging from tan through dark brown to black, and frequently a diameter greater than 1 cm may be dysplastic, Dysplastic nevi are often hereditary but can occur sporadically, especially in individuals with a history of sun exposure resulting in a severe burn. These lesions also appear to arise in users of tanning salons who give a history of burning in the tanning salon. Mounting evidence suggests that dysplastic nevi are the histogenic precursors of malignant melanoma. Even if a particular dysplastic nevus does not itself become malignant, the patient still has a 7- to 70-fold increased risk of developing melanoma in some other area of the body. About 90% of dysplastic nevi occur on the trunk, but they can also appear in some protected areas such as the female breast, the scalp, or the buttocks. The latter three areas are diagnostically important, since common acquired nevi are less common in these locations. For the most part, dysplastic nevi proper appear only after puberty, although rudimentary nevi have been identified in individuals as young as 5 years old. If the syndrome has not developed by age 25, it most likely will not do so. A complete examination of the skin, scalp, and mouth of the patient is important. Also, it is important to examine the eyes since ocular nevi and melanoma are a possibility. Attention should be paid to any moles in which the dimensions, pigment, or border has changed. Symptoms such as bleeding or burning could be a sign that the mole is in the process of transformation.

On the microscopic level, dysplastic nevi are characterized by variable atypical melanocytes, a lentiginous epidermal pattern, fibrosis of the upper dermis, and a nevocytic component. Occasionally, the qualities are not always sufficient for a definite diagnosis, and it is essential for an experienced dermatopathologist to confirm any clinical diagnosis.

The dysplastic nevus syndrome, also known as the atypical mole syndrome (or B-K mole syndrome) was described in two families with familial melanoma. This syndrome can also be sporatic. Individuals with the sporadic condition, Type A, have no family history of either the syndrome or melanoma. The familial condition consists of several types. A patient who has dysplastic nevus syndrome and a family history of the syndrome is designated as having Type B. In Type C, in addition to the syndrome, the patient has a personal history of melanoma but a family history of neither the syndrome nor melanoma. Type D consists of two forms: Type D-1 patients have one family member with the syndrome and melanoma, whereas D-2 patients have two or more relatives with the syndrome and melanoma. It is estimated that dysplastic nevi may be found in 30 to 50% of sporadic, nonfamilial melanoma patients. Sporadic dysplastic nevus syndrome (Type A), which occurs in 5 to 10% of the general population, raises one's chances of developing melanoma by 5- to 7-fold, even if there is just one dysplastic nevus.

**Treatment.** Treatment of dysplastic moles is simple: local excision. Any suspicious lesion should be excised with a margin of 2 to 5 mm of normal tissue. Photographic documentation every 6 months is helpful, and family members should be screened for the condition.

### Organoid Nevus (Jadassohn's Sebaceous Nevus)

This congenital tumor can develop into a basal cell carcinoma, apocrine carcinoma, adnexal carcinoma, or squamous cell carcinoma. Because malignant degeneration usually occurs in adulthood, it is advisable to excise these lesions during adolescence. Superficial cautery and curettage do not destroy the deeper portions of this tumor and, in addition, produce an alopecic scar.

**Treatment.** The pathologic nature of these lesions implies involvement of the appendages to mid and deep dermis; hence, superficial curettage and electrodesiccation, cryosurgery, and chemo-exfoliation (peel) are not indicated. Most chemosurgery may be the preferred treatment once a malignant lesion has been detected.

### Chronic Conditions

Malignant degeneration in chronic irritant conditions is well known. It is often associated with chronic discharge or pruritus. These conditions include, but are not limited to, thermal burn scars, radiation dermatitis, cutaneous ulcers, ill-fitting appliances (e.g., dentures), cheilitis, lichen sclerosus et atrophicus, lichen planus, and lupus vulgaris. The practitioner must be aware that these conditions predispose to malignant degeneration. Periodic follow-up is indicated, and any suspicious change should prompt a skin biopsy.

### Large Plaque Parapsoriasis

This chronic, dermatitic, inflammatory eruption may progress into frank fungoides. Treatment can include potent topical corticosteroids, photochemotherapy, and systemic chemotherapy. Extracorporeal photophoresis may eventually play a role in the treatment of this disorder.

## PREMALIGNANT MARKERS FOR INTERNAL MALIGNANCY

### Leser-Trélat Sign

The sudden onset of a large number of seborrheic keraratoses with or without inflammation is often a marker for underlying gastrointestinal malignancy. Individual skin lesions can be treated accordingly, but the goal of therapy is to identify the hidden malignancy.

### Erythema Gyratum Repens

This is a woody-appearing polycyclic and annular scaling eruption which is a marker for internal malignancy. The treatment is to identify the underlying disease.

### Acrochordons (Skin Tags)

These are fleshy, pedunculated papules, usually found about the neck and in the axilla, that increase in number with age and increasing weight. Recently an association with colonic polyposis has been noted, but the veracity of this observation is questionable.

## Cowden's Disease

This rare and unusual complex cutaneous disorder is characterized by multiple hamartomas and by coexistence of multiple ectodermal, mesodermal, and endodermal neoplasias that tend to develop after the third decade. Abnormalities may occur in any or all of the internal organs or glands, most notably the breast. Fibrocystic disease may be an early manifestation, followed by carcinoma. Neural tumors are known to develop and result in mental and neurologic changes. This disease is named after its originally presenting patient. Multiple diagnostic regimens are required, with surgical therapy directed toward individual lesions and organ systems. There is no known medical therapy for this rare, unusual, and slowly devastating disease.

## Bowenoid Papulosis

This relatively new condition occurs on the skin and mucous membrane tissue on the genital area. Lesions are small and usually multiple and generally involve the shaft and glans of the penis but may also involve the foreskin. Although the etiology is not specifically defined, Bowenoid papulosis is believed to be caused by the human papilloma virus, perhaps Type 16. Although the micropathology is fairly distinctive, there is sufficient similarity to condyloma acuminatum to consider Bowenoid papulosis a variant. There has been recent concern in the literature that this disorder is a precursor to invasive carcinoma.

Bowenoid papulosis usually is nonresponsive to podophyllin therapy but is amenable to electrodesiccation, which is the preferred method of treatment. In cases in which large clusters of such lesions exist on the foreskin, it may be amenable to circumcision as a form of surgical removal. Cryotherapy is recommended by some physicians, but I have found it thoroughly unacceptable to the patient and its therapeutic effectiveness may be questionable in such instances. More recently, good results have been obtained with laser surgery using the $CO_2$ machine.

# BACTERIAL DISEASES OF THE SKIN
method of
JAMES E. RASMUSSEN, M.D.
*The University of Michigan Medical Center*
*Ann Arbor, Michigan*

## IMPETIGO

This is the most common bacterial infection of the skin. It frequently occurs in children or young adults and is often seen in warmer climates and during the summer months. Local trauma such as cuts, abrasions, and insect bites frequently represents the portal of entry. In the past, impetigo was clinically divided into two groups—bullous and nonbullous—based upon morphology as well as etiology. Coagulase-positive *Staphylococcus aureus* was invariably the cause of bullous impetigo, whereas nonbullous impetigo (crusted) was usually caused by group A beta-hemolytic streptococci, often mixed with *S. aureus*. Recently, however, numerous reports from around the world suggest that coagulase-positive *S. aureus* has become the dominant organism in all types of impetigo and is frequently found as the only organism in crusted impetigo. This has significance in therapy, since the staphylococci are invariably penicillin resistant and, depending upon the region of the country, are often resistant to methicillin and erythromycin.

### Treatment

Patients with mild to moderate amounts of impetigo can be treated either topically or systemically. A recently introduced topical agent—2% mupirocin (Bactroban)—has proved to be very effective in the topical treatment of impetigo. Numerous studies attest that it is better than any other available topical antibiotic and as good as some antibiotics (erythromycin) even against staphylococci.

Erythromycin, 250 mg orally every 6 hours for 7 to 10 days, is still an excellent choice for treatment, provided that you know the cultural sensitivities of the commonly occurring staphylococci in your community. If erythromycin resistance is a problem, dicloxacillin (Dynapen), 250 mg orally every 6 hours for 7 to 10 days, or ciprofloxacin (Cipro),* 250 mg orally every 6 hours for 7 to 10 days, is an excellent antistaphylococcal drug.

### ECTHYMA

Ecthyma is a slightly deeper cutaneous infection than is impetigo. It is usually caused by a mixture of staphylococci and streptococci and appears as a yellow, crusted area surrounded by a moderate zone of erythema and induration. It is usually located on the extremities and should be treated systemically with antibiotics directed against the staphylococci (erythromycin, dicloxacillin, ciprofloxacin). These are often more resistant to therapy than impetigo.

Ecthyma due to staphylococci and streptococci

---

*This use of Cipro for children is not listed in the manufacturer's official directive.

should be clearly differentiated from ecthyma gangrenosum, which is a much more serious infection usually occurring in debilitated patients with severe metabolic or malignant disorders such as leukemias and lymphomas. Ecthyma gangrenosum is usually caused by gram-negative bacteria such as *Pseudomonas aeruginosa* and is often accompanied by septicemia. Consequently, these patients should always be managed in a hospital setting with appropriate cultures and sensitivities. Antibiotics should be given parenterally, with the choice depending upon a thorough knowledge of the resistance patterns of the causative organism.

## CELLULITIS

Cellulitis represents infection of the dermis and subcutaneous tissues usually caused by group A beta-hemolytic streptococci. In its most common manifestation, it is called erysipelas. This usually occurs on the face or legs as an erythematous, sharply defined, indurated lesion that is often accompanied by fever and chills. Children under 4 years of age can develop a darker facial cellulitis often of a violet color that is secondary to *Haemophilus influenzae* infection. This is invariably accompanied by sepsis and needs to be treated in a hospital setting.

With the widespread availability of organ transplantation and the accompanied use of long-term immunosuppression in these patients as well as others with a variety of medical conditions, the etiology of cellulitis has changed appreciably in the past 15 years. In these immunosuppressed individuals, a wide variety of bacteria, fungi, and viruses must be considered as potential causes of cellulitis. Patients with AIDS may also present with cellulitis secondary to an unusual organism. Appropriate cultures must be taken in these settings. These may be obtained by injecting sterile saline solution (without preservatives) into the advancing edge and then aspirating. It may also be necessary to biopsy areas of cellulitis in immunosuppressed patients (for microscopic examination and cultures) if they do not respond rapidly to antibacterial therapy.

### Treatment

In a nonimmunosuppressed individual with streptococcal cellulitis, penicillin is the drug of choice. Penicillin VK, 250 to 500 mg orally every 6 hours for 7 to 10 days, is adequate in patients who are not septic. Intravenous penicillin G, 200,000 to 250,000 U every 6 hours, is often necessary for patients with severe systemic symptoms. Erythromycin, 250 to 500 mg orally every 6 hours for 7 to 10 days, is also appropriate provided that the patient can be managed as an outpatient.

## ATYPICAL MYCOBACTERIAL INFECTIONS OF THE SKIN (SWIMMING POOL GRANULOMA, FISH TANK GRANULOMA, BURULI ULCERS)

A wide variety of atypical mycobacterial organisms *(Mycobacterium marinum [balnei], kansasii, fortuitum,* and *ulcerans [buruli])* can produce ulcers, abscesses, or granulomas usually on a previously traumatized area of the body. They are notoriously resistant to treatment.

### Treatment

1. Obtain generous biopsy specimens (usually a deep skin biopsy is necessary) for culture and sensitivity. Request cultures for fungi, bacteria, and acid-fast organisms from the same specimen, since reliable differentiation from other types of bacterial infection of the skin is usually not possible on clinical examination.

2. If the lesions are small and few, surgical excision should be followed by chemotherapy. If they are large or multiple, surgery is usually not indicated except in the case of Buruli ulcers. Isoniazid (INH), para-aminosalicylic acid (PAS), and streptomycin are not usually helpful unless combined with rifampin (Rifadin), 10 to 20 mg per kg in a single dose but not more than 600 mg per day, or ethambutol (Myambutol), 15 mg per kg per day. Minocycline (Minocin), 100 mg twice daily to four times a day, is sometimes effective.

## STREPTOCOCCAL PERIANAL CELLULITIS

This is a recently described entity occurring primarily in children. The affected area is usually the intertriginous perianal skin, but a similar process has also been reported from an infection of the foreskin. The organism is a group A beta-hemolytic streptococcus that is usually, but not invariably, resistant to penicillin. Infected patients usually complain of tenderness, a mildly purulent exudate, and fissures. The infection responds promptly to treatment with erythromycin orally in doses of 20 to 30 mg per kg per day given in equal-divided doses every 6 hours for 7 to 10 days.

# VIRAL DISEASES OF THE SKIN

method of
BRENT G. PETTY, M.D.
*The Johns Hopkins University School of*
 *Medicine*
*Baltimore, Maryland*

This chapter deals with the treatment of viral infections that are usually limited to the skin (Table 1). Drug therapy specific for viral inhibition is available for treatment of the herpesviruses, but to date, no specific antiviral chemotherapy has been found for the other viral diseases discussed.

## HERPES SIMPLEX VIRUS TYPE 1

### Clinical Manifestations

**Orolabial Herpes.** Painful ulcerative pharyngitis and stomatitis caused by herpes simplex virus type 1 (HSV-1) are usually seen in children and resolve within 2 weeks without complications. When the disease is severe and extensive, however, the patient may become dehydrated because of inability to maintain adequate fluid intake.

The most common manifestation of HSV-1 infection is herpes labialis, the typical cold sore. It usually emerges at the vermilion border of the lip, frequently recurring in the same location in association with an illness or exposure to sunlight, after surgery, or after other physiologic stress. Herpes labialis is usually self-limited and is problematic primarily because of pain and cosmetic concerns.

**Cutaneous Herpes.** A patch of vesicular lesions with surrounding erythema, the appearance typical of herpetic lesions, may develop anywhere on the skin. Like herpes labialis, the eruption may recur in the same location. These lesions are usually less extensive than the dermatomal dis-

TABLE 1. **Viral Infections of the Skin**

| Herpesviruses |
| --- |
| Herpes simplex virus type 1 |
| Orolabial |
| Cutaneous |
| Whitlow |
| Herpes simplex virus type 2 |
| Genital herpes |
| Herpetic proctitis |
| Varicella-zoster virus |
| Localized |
| Disseminated |
| |
| Poxviruses |
| Molluscum contagiosum |
| Orf (ecthyma contagiosum) |
| Milker's nodules |
| |
| Papillomavirus |
| Warts |

tribution of herpes zoster (see later). Although cutaneous herpes is generally self-limited, in some patients it causes extensive erythema multiforme as a nonspecific response, often extending well beyond the area where the cutaneous viral infection was localized.

**Herpetic Whitlow.** The term "whitlow" refers to an infection localized to a finger tip after direct inoculation of virus through a break in the skin. It is usually seen in dentists or medical personnel or occurs as a result of self-inoculation by a patient with herpes elsewhere. Although the majority of cases are caused by HSV-1, many are caused by herpes simplex virus type 2 (HSV-2). Pain and swelling associated with vesicular lesions, pustular lesions, or both are typical at presentation.

### Diagnosis

The diagnosis of HSV-1 infection is largely clinical, and treatment is often initiated on the basis of clinical suspicion alone. Additional diagnostic aids are Tzanck's smear, viral culture, and antigen detection methods. Tzanck's smear is a toluidine blue stain of the material scraped from the base of a punctured, fresh vesicle. The presence of multinucleated giant cells supports the diagnosis of herpetic infection. Viral culture is perhaps the most specific and reliable method for confirming the presence of infectious virus, but it requires 2 to 3 days for the characteristic cytopathic effect to appear. The time needed to confirm the diagnosis can be shortened to 16 hours by detecting HSV antigens from cultured specimens, using monoclonal antibodies or biotinylated DNA probes. The monoclonal antibodies have the slight advantage of providing type-specific identification (either HSV-1 or HSV-2), whereas the biotinylated DNA probes react with both serotypes.

Serologic assays are available to identify individuals who were previously infected with HSV and who, by presumption, still have latent viral infection in ganglia. Identifying such individuals from among those who are to undergo organ transplantation is important in the prophylaxis of reactivated disease.

### Treatment

The development of the nucleoside analogue acyclovir allows specific treatment for HSV infections. This substantial step forward was part of the reason for awarding the 1988 Nobel Prize in Medicine and Physiology to Dr. Gertrude Elion, the developer of acyclovir. Acyclovir selectively inhibits viral replication because the virus contains an enzyme (thymidine kinase) that converts acyclovir to its active form (acyclovir triphosphate) in infected cells; uninfected human cells do not have this enzyme and so cannot produce the active triphosphate in a significant amount. This property allows acyclovir to act as a "magic bullet," affecting virus-infected cells and having no effect on uninfected cells.

Acyclovir is marketed in topical, oral, and intravenous formulations, with increasing degrees of efficacy, respectively. Topical therapy is no more or only slightly more beneficial clinically than placebo; the oral formulation is so well tolerated that, in my opinion, the topical preparation is not worth the mess and inconvenience. For either primary or recurrent HSV-1 infections, oral acyclovir, 200 mg five times per day for 5 days, is recommended. This dose is effective for orolabial or cutaneous disease and herpetic whitlow. When orolabial herpes is severe or is associated with herpes esophagitis, thereby preventing oral therapy, or if the patient is immunosuppressed, intravenous acyclovir, 5 mg per kg every 8 hours, should be administered. Because acyclovir is eliminated primarily by the kidneys, the dosage, whether given orally or intravenously, should be reduced in patients with renal insufficiency.

Inasmuch as herpes tends to be a recurrent disease, often with known precipitating factors (e.g., ultraviolet light exposure or surgery for trigeminal neuralgia), smaller doses of acyclovir have been found to decrease the incidence of recurrences. Doses of 200 mg of oral acyclovir twice daily* may provide protection from recurrent disease. This prophylactic therapy can be given continuously in patients who have severe recurrent disease or who are prone to develop serious complications with recurrences, such as erythema multiforme. On the other hand, many patients fare well if they simply take the prophylactic therapy in anticipation of an exposure likely to initiate a recurrence, such as extended exposure to sunlight. In patients with serologic evidence of past infection who are to undergo bone marrow, renal, or cardiac transplantation, intravenous acyclovir, 5 mg per kg every 8 hours, is highly effective in preventing the morbidity of recurrent herpes infection in such immunocompromised hosts.

## HERPES SIMPLEX VIRUS TYPE 2

### Clinical Manifestations

**Genital Herpes.** Genital herpes presents as multiple bilateral lesions on the external genitalia.

*This dose may be lower than that recommended by the manufacturer.

The lesions may be vesicular, pustular, or ulcerative. With time the lesions crust over and heal. In women there may be associated vaginal and cervical involvement. The symptoms include pain, dysuria, and vaginal and urethral discharge. Although some cases of genital herpes are caused by HSV-1, the majority are caused by HSV-2. The painful lesions usually remit spontaneously, but there is a propensity for recurrence, particularly with HSV-2, and, less frequently, with HSV-1.

**Herpetic Proctitis.** Pain, discharge, tenesmus, and ulcerative rectal lesions on proctoscopy are the hallmarks of rectal herpes infection. Like genital herpes, this condition is more often caused by HSV-2 than by HSV-1. It has become increasingly recognized in homosexual men and in heterosexual women who practice anal receptive intercourse.

### Diagnosis

The diagnostic considerations for HSV-2 were mentioned in the discussion of HSV-1.

### Treatment

Again, acyclovir provides specific antiviral treatment. Given in doses of 200 mg orally five times a day for 5 days, acyclovir causes initial or recurrent episodes of HSV-2 infection to remit more quickly than the resolution observed in patients treated with placebo. An alternative regimen of 800 mg twice daily for 5 days* may be equally effective, but it has been studied far less extensively. Because recurrence remains a major problem, prophylaxis with low-dose oral acyclovir is indicated in patients who have frequent and/or extensive recurrences. Doses as low as 200 mg orally twice daily have been shown to have a significant effect in reducing the frequency of the painful, debilitating episodes in predisposed patients. If 200 mg twice daily proves to be inadequate to reduce the incidence of recurrence, the dose can be increased to 200 mg three times daily or 400 mg twice daily. A single oral dose of 800 mg of acyclovir also appears to be superior to placebo in preventing recurrences, but it has not been compared with the lower-dose regimens.

## VARICELLA-ZOSTER VIRUS

### Clinical Manifestations

Varicella (chickenpox), usually contracted in childhood, invariably leads to latent viral infection of dorsal root ganglia. Reactivation of latent

*This dosage regimen is not listed by the manufacturer.

virus, with migration along sensory nerves to the skin, leads to the syndrome known as herpes zoster. Clinically, there may be a brief (3- to 5-day) period of pain, hyperesthesia, or both, in a dermatomal distribution before the eruption of typical grouped vesicles with surrounding erythema in a patchy distribution along the dermatome. Generally, herpes zoster is a self-limited disease with spontaneous remission. Nevertheless, there may be occasions, most commonly in immunosuppressed patients, when the involvement extends beyond single or contiguous dermatomes and affects distant dermatomes, visceral organs, or both, particularly the lungs and liver. Such "disseminated zoster" constitutes a serious disease. Even in the absence of dissemination, about 30% of patients have persistent pain after resolution of the cutaneous lesions, a condition known as postherpetic neuralgia. Postherpetic neuralgia increases in incidence with increasing age.

### Diagnosis

Herpes zoster is commonly a clinical diagnosis, based on the characteristic combination of clusters of vesicular lesions with surrounding erythema associated with pain in a dermatomal distribution. Tzanck's smear should be positive, just as with HSV, and viral culture can confirm the diagnosis but is rarely used outside of rigorous clinical trials or epidemiologic investigations.

### Treatment

Acyclovir has activity against varicella-zoster virus. Given orally or intravenously, it significantly reduces the duration of viral shedding, new lesion formation, and acute pain. Nevertheless, because the majority of immunocompetent patients with herpes zoster experience a self-limited illness, it is not clear whether acyclovir should be used, except when the disease affects the ophthalmic branch of the trigeminal nerve, thereby threatening the eye. In spite of its antiviral effect, acyclovir has been disappointing in preventing postherpetic neuralgia, either alone or in combination with corticosteroids. If oral acyclovir is used to treat herpes zoster,* it should be used as early as possible in the illness, and because varicella-zoster virus is less sensitive to acyclovir than is HSV, larger doses must be used, namely, 800 mg five times a day for 5 to 7 days.† Prodrugs of acyclovir and sustained-release preparations of oral acyclovir have been under investigation, but none have yet been marketed.

*This use is not listed by the manufacturer.
†This dosage regimen is not listed by the manufacturer.

TABLE 2. **Acyclovir Treatment of Herpesvirus Infections**

| Infection | Treatment | Prophylaxis |
|---|---|---|
| HSV-1 | 200 mg PO 5 times a day* | 200 mg PO bid† |
| HSV-2 | 200 mg PO 5 times a day* | 200–400 mg PO bid |
| Herpes zoster | | |
| Localized disease in slightly immunosuppressed patients | 800 mg PO 5 times a day‡ | |
| Localized disease in severely immunosupppressed patients | 10 mg/kg IV q 8 hr‡ | |
| Disseminated disease | 10 mg/kg IV q 8 hr‡ | |

*For extensive disease, when oral therapy is not possible, or in immunosuppressed patients, 5 mg/kg IV q 8 hr is recommended.
†May be lower than manufacturer's recommended dose.
‡May exceed manufacturer's recommended dose.

Because immunosuppressed patients are at special risk to develop disseminated disease, oral therapy must be monitored carefully to detect the earliest evidence of dissemination; alternatively, intravenous acyclovir, 10 mg per kg every 8 hours,* should be given instead of oral therapy. If dissemination occurs, even in an immunocompetent patient, intravenous acyclovir treatment with this dose should be started promptly and continued for 7 to 10 days, or longer if there is no positive clinical response. Human leukocyte interferon-alpha appears to be just as effective as intravenous acyclovir but has more adverse side effects, such as fever and nausea.

The treatment recommendations for herpesvirus infections are summarized in Table 2.

### POXVIRUSES

#### Clinical Manifestations

**Molluscum Contagiosum.** This illness is characterized by small, papular lesions with a central depression. It occurs primarily in children, in whom the lesions are located on the face, trunk, and limbs. In adults, the lesions most commonly occur in the genital and inner thigh areas, probably related to sexual contact. In both children and adults, the lesions are present without systemic symptoms. Molluscum contagiosum is usually a self-limited illness, requiring no treatment. The lesions clear in 6 months to 3 years after their appearance.

**Orf.** Also known as ecthyma contagiosum, orf

*May exceed manufacturer's recommended dose.

is an endemic viral illness among sheep and is transmitted to humans by contact with the animals' secretions by those responsible for handling them (e.g., sheepherders, veterinarians). The virus causes the development of nodules on exposed areas, which are self-limited but may become secondarily infected; this is the main concern in this disease.

**Milker's Nodules.** This poxviral illness is spread from infected cattle to handlers and causes a self-limited nodular eruption that lasts for 4 to 6 weeks. No therapy is recommended.

### Treatment

If treatment for molluscum contagiosum is contemplated because of the extent of the lesions, one can consider removal with a curette or liquid nitrogen, use of a keratolytic agent such as Duofilm (combination salicylic acid and lactic acid), or stimulation of a local inflammatory reaction in the dermis by puncturing the lesions and applying iodine. Orf nodules may be resected if they are extensive or necrotic. Secondary infections can be treated if they develop.

## PAPILLOMAVIRUS

### Clinical Manifestations

**Warts.** Warts are caused by over 40 different types of human papillomavirus. Each type is largely specific for warts erupting at a particular body site. Warts are generally spread by direct contact, including self-inoculation, but may also be spread by fomites, particularly with plantar warts, which can be acquired through contact with shower floors. Although they may be persistent or long-standing, most warts spontaneously regress. Venereal warts (condylomata acuminata) may be especially extensive, persistent, and resistant to treatment.

### Treatment

Removal by electrodesiccation, curettage, or blistering agents such as liquid nitrogen or cantharidin has been used. Keratolytic agents, such as salicylic acid paint, and formalin soaks have been used particularly for plantar warts. A 25 to 50% podophyllin solution is used, with or without surgical excision or liquid nitrogen application, in the treatment of genital warts. Intralesional interferon injections have been successful in the treatment of some patients with vulvar warts.

# PARASITIC DISEASES OF THE SKIN

method of
PHILIP D. SHENEFELT, M.D.
*University of South Florida*
*Tampa, Florida*

### SCABIES

Scabies is a skin infestation by the mite *Sarcoptes scabiei*. The mite lives and breeds in the stratum corneum. Usually the human host does not notice the initial exposure infestation until several weeks have passed. Sensitization to the mite or its scybala (fecal droppings) then results in intense pruritus, accentuated at night. Reinfestation will result in pruritus, within a day or two. Because of the asymptomatic initial phase of infestation, close contacts of a scabies patient should be treated even if not symptomatic. Because the mite lives in miniature tunnels in the stratum corneum called burrows, treatment kills the mite but does not remove the sensitizing material from the burrow. Thus, a successfully treated patient may continue to experience pruritus for a couple of weeks after treatment. The patient will stop itching only after the burrow and its contents are shed as the natural skin turnover occurs.

The distribution of scabies on the body typically involves the finger-webs, wrists, ankles, elbows, axillae, and waistline; it is seen under the breasts and on the nipples in women; and also involves the umbilicus, genitalia, and buttocks. Typically, lesions are small red papules, often excoriated. Secondary impetiginization may supervene. Uncommonly, nodules may appear on the genitalia, groin, or axilla. Vesicles can occur, especially in children. A pathognomonic lesion, the burrow, can sometimes be identified as a tiny line on a finger-web or lateral finger. The tiny black dot at the end of the burrow locates the mite. Lesions do not ordinarily occur above the neck except in infants and toddlers. If the reaction to scabies has been partially suppressed by topical or systemic corticosteroids, scabies incognito may occur and be difficult to recognize. At the other extreme, a mentally retarded or debilitated or immunocompromised patient may have thick crusted areas and thousands of mites, even burrowing into the fingernails. This condition is known as Norwegian scabies.

A presumptive diagnosis of scabies can be made from the preceding clinical presentation. To confirm the diagnosis, one should locate new excoriated papules or burrows. Using a No. 15 scalpel blade dipped in mineral oil, one should then scrape several of these lesions down almost to the point of pinpoint bleeding and transfer the scrapings to a drop of mineral oil on a clean glass slide. After placing a coverslip over the specimen, one then examines the slide under a microscope using the $10\times$ or $40\times$ objective. Finding the mite, its eggs, or its scybala (droppings) clinches the diagnosis.

### Treatment

Treatment of scabies is generally quite effective. To prevent reinfestation, asymptomatic close contacts should be treated simultaneously. Bedsheets and all clothing worn in the past 3 days should be laundered in hot soapy water or dry cleaned. The mite will not survive off the body for more than 3 days, so noncleanable items can be set aside for at least 3 days before being used again.

Lindane 1% (Kwell, Gamene) lotion is applied from the neck down and left on overnight for 8 to 12 hours. Reapplication after 5 days is often advisable. Lindane should usually be avoided in infants, pregnant women, and epileptics, owing to its neurotoxicity. If used on infants and toddlers, lindane should be applied to the head and scalp also. Following lindane treatment, many individuals experience a mild dry irritant dermatitis. Use of emollients will help to alleviate this side effect.

Crotamiton 10% (Eurax) lotion is applied daily from the neck down for 5 days. It is antipruritic but is usually less successful as a scabicide than lindane. If the eruption is pruritic but the diagnosis of scabies is highly questionable, crotamiton can be used to help relieve the pruritus.

Permethrin 5% (Elimite) cream is applied from the neck down and left on overnight for 8 to 12 hours. One treatment is adequate. For infants and toddlers, permethrin should be applied to the head and scalp also. Permethrin is much less toxic than lindane for young children.

Precipitated sulfur 6% in petrolatum is applied daily for 3 consecutive days without removal or bathing during the 3-day time interval. Treatment of infants and toddlers should include the face and scalp. This agent is preferred for infants, toddlers, and pregnant women, owing to its minimal toxicity. It also is indicated if lindane treatment has failed.

Symptomatic treatment for pruritus and scabies dermatitis consists of topical corticosteroid creams and oral antihistamines. Secondary impetigo may be treated with topical mupirocin 2% (Bactroban) ointment three times daily or appropriate oral antibiotics. Scabies nodules may require intralesional corticosteroid injections to obtain resolution.

## PEDICULOSIS

Human lice are of two types. *Phthirus pubis,* the pubic louse or crab louse, is squat and slow moving. It prefers the pubic hair but can be found on body and axillary hair, eyebrows, eyelashes, and occasionally the occipital scalp. *Pediculus humanus* var. *capitus,* the head louse, and var. *corporis,* the body louse, are elongate and fast moving. The head louse prefers the scalp, whereas the body louse hides in seams in clothing. The eggs or nits of the pubic and head louse are cemented to the bases of hairs, while those of the body louse are laid on clothing. Nits remain viable for up to a month. They hatch and evolve into adults within 2 or 3 weeks. Lice live for about a month, requiring blood meals to survive. Without blood meals, they die within a few days. Spread occurs from one person to another by close contact or sharing a bed or clothing. The louse bite results in a red macule with a central hemorrhagic center. The bite is typically pruritic.

### Pediculosis Pubis

Crab lice are identified by their characteristic shape and slow movement. They are difficult to see unless one looks closely. The nits also can be seen attached to the bases of hairs. In addition to the pubic hair, the body hair, axillary hair, eyebrows, eyelashes, and occipital scalp should also be examined. Pruritus and excoriations are common, and secondary impetiginization may supervene. Scattered bite sites may be seen on the skin near hairs.

**Treatment.** Lindane (Kwell, Gamene) shampoo should be applied to the affected areas for 5 to 10 minutes, then showered off. A fine-toothed nit comb may be used to remove nits by combing the hairs. The treatment may be repeated once in 5 to 7 days. Eyelash infestations may be treated with careful mechanical removal of nits and lice using a fine forceps. Alternately, petrolatum may be applied in a thick layer twice a day for a week. Clothing and bedding should be laundered in hot soapy water and mechanically dried for at least 20 minutes. Close contacts should be treated if infested.

### Pediculosis Capitis

Head lice move quickly, so one must be alert for sudden movement when parting the hair. The nits are easier to find. The areas of heaviest nit involvement typically are at the occipital scalp. Nits are attached at the bases of hairs. Scalp hair grows at about 1 cm a month, so distance of old nits from the scalp gives an estimate of the length of infestation. Pruritus with excoriations is usually present. Secondary impetiginization may occur. Because head lice are highly contagious in children, all closely associated children should be treated.

**Treatment.** Malathion (Prioderm) is an effective pediculocide and ovacide. It is applied to the moistened scalp, allowing it to dry. In 8 to 12 hours, it is shampooed out. A fine-toothed metal nit comb should be used subsequently to remove the nits.

Permethrin (Nix) is also effective as a single-dose treatment. It is applied after shampooing and toweling dry. After 10 minutes, it is rinsed out with water. A nit comb is used to remove nits.

Pyrethrin piperonyl butoxide liquid (Rid) is applied to dry hair and then shampooed out after 10 minutes. Because it is less effective as an ovacide, treatment should be repeated once in a week. Nits should be removed using a nit comb.

Lindane (Kwell, Gamene) shampoo has poor ovacidal activity. It is applied in contact with the scalp and hair for 4 minutes, then removed by shampooing. Nit combing must be thorough. Repeat treatments may be necessary.

### Pediculosis Corporis

Body lice are most commonly found on vagabonds or in wartime. Because the louse lives in the seams of clothing, it is not often observed on the skin. Typical feeding sites are on the trunk and buttocks. The resulting red papules are often extensively excoriated. Secondary impetiginization is common. Nits and lice should be sought in the seams of clothing for diagnosis.

**Treatment.** Laundering or dry cleaning the clothes and bedding kills the lice and nits. Sealing the clothing and bedding airtight in plastic bags for a month will also kill the lice and nits. The skin should be cleaned with soap and water. Pruritus may be treated with topical corticosteroid creams and oral antihistamines. Impetiginized areas may be treated with mupirocin (Bactroban) ointment three times daily or with appropriate oral antibiotics.

## CUTANEOUS LARVA MIGRANS

Cutaneous larva migrans, or creeping eruption, occurs when the larvae of the cat and dog hookworm *Ancyclostoma braziliense* penetrate skin in contact with the ground. Animal droppings containing the ova are deposited on the soil. Within a day or two, the rhabditiform larvae hatch. In a few days they mature into the filiform larvae, which can penetrate the skin directly or through clothing in contact with the ground. Freezing kills the organisms, so they are more prevalent in the South. The infestation usually occurs in warm, moist, sandy areas such as the beach, playgrounds, sandboxes, and under houses. Sunbathers, children, gardeners, plumbers, and electricians risk exposure. Within a few hours of contact, an erythematous papule appears at the site of skin penetration. Within a day or two, pruritic erythematous serpiginous tracks develop. The larvae are accidental intruders and usually die within a few weeks, although some may persist for up to a year with cycles of remission and exacerbation.

### Treatment

Small numbers of lesions can be treated with ethyl chloride or liquid nitrogen freezing. Larger numbers can be treated topically with thiabendazole (Mintezol), 500 mg per 5 ml suspension applied three times a day until the lesions have resolved. Oral thiabendazole (Mintezol), 10 mg per lb per day in two divided doses up to a maximum of 1.5 grams per day for patients over 150 lb, may be given for 2 consecutive days after weighing the benefits with the potential adverse reactions.

Patients should be instructed in preventive measures. Minimizing contact with the ground, covering sandboxes when not in use, and draping the ground with plastic prior to performing work in areas frequented by domestic animals help to prevent further exposure.

# FUNGAL DISEASES OF THE SKIN

method of
CHARLES CAMISA, M.D.
*Cleveland Clinic Foundation*
*Cleveland, Ohio*

In most cases, the diagnosis of superficial fungal infections is suspected clinically and confirmed by examining scales, nail debris, or hair in 10% potassium hydroxide (KOH), gently heated, under a microscope. Fungal cultures may be performed instead of the KOH test for dermatophytoses and candidiasis, or in the case of a negative or equivocal KOH test. The Wood's light is most valuable for confirming the diagnosis of either tinea versicolor or erythrasma.

### TOPICAL ANTIFUNGAL PREPARATIONS

Many patients have already tried tolnaftate (Tinactin, Aftate) or compound undecylenic acid (Desenex, Cruex) twice daily for 4 weeks before coming to the office. These over-the-counter antifungals are not as effective as prescription drugs or miconazole (Micatin), a broad-spectrum azole with activity against yeast and fungi.

There are many other prescription azole creams and lotions available. They act by inhibiting production of ergosterol, a basic component of the cell membrane. At higher concentrations, they may directly damage the cell membrane and disrupt mitochondrial function, thus causing cell death. The clinician should become familiar with a few different azole preparations, their local irritant potential, patient preferences, and relative costs. All of the azoles are highly effective, clearing up to 90% of skin infections. The older azoles such as clotrimazole (Lotrimin, Mycelex) and miconazole (Monistat-Derm) are less expensive and must be applied twice daily. The newer ones are approved for once-daily application, which may improve compliance—e.g., ketoconazole (Nizoral); oxiconazole (Oxistat); and sulconazole (Exelderm). There are currently two other prescription classes of antifungals that are unrelated to azoles: ciclopirox olamine (Loprox), a substituted pyridone; and naftifine (Naftin), an allylamine. Both are fungicidal. Although their advantages are slight, Naftin may have a quicker onset of action and Loprox may penetrate the hard keratin of nails better.

## SYSTEMIC ANTIFUNGAL DRUGS

There are only two oral medications in use for the treatment of superficial fungal infections: griseofulvin (Grisactin, Gris-Peg, others) and ketoconazole (Nizoral).

### Griseofulvin

Griseofulvin was introduced in 1959. It is most active against growing dermatophyte species. The drug binds to intracellular microtubules, inhibiting mitosis and accounting for its fungistatic effect. It is important to note that *yeast infections, including Candida and Pityrosporum, do not respond to griseofulvin.* Gastrointestinal absorption of griseofulvin is variable and incomplete but may be enhanced by taking the drug with a fatty meal and by prescribing formulations with "ultramicrosize" particles suspended in polyethylene glycol (Gris-Peg, Fulvicin P/G, Grisactin Ultra). The 250-mg tablet of the ultramicrosize is roughly equivalent to 500 mg of microsize griseofulvin. The usual adult dosage is 500 mg of microsize or 330 mg of ultramicrosize griseofulvin daily; higher doses are required in some cases. There is a liquid form of microsize griseofulvin available for children (Grifulvin V, 125 mg per 5 ml). The recommended dosage for children is

approximately 5 mg per lb body weight per day. For children weighing 30 to 50 lb, order 5 to 10 ml daily; if over 50 lb, order 10 to 20 ml daily.

Griseofulvin is a remarkably safe medication. Laboratory abnormalities and serious adverse reactions are rarely seen, and no deaths have been directly attributed to the drug. Griseofulvin can precipitate attacks of acute intermittent porphyria and is therefore contraindicated in the hepatic porphyrias. Minor side effects include headache, gastrointestinal symptoms, urticaria, and photosensitivity. Headache has been the single most important cause of discontinuation of griseofulvin in my practice; however, the majority of patients can overcome this problem without treatment, with standard analgesics, or by lowering the dose of griseofulvin and gradually increasing it. Griseofulvin can be given with caution to patients with pre-existing photosensitivity diseases such as lupus erythematosus.

There are three drug interactions with griseofulvin that are well established (alcohol, warfarin, phenobarbital) (Table 1). The package insert warns of a possible cross-reaction between griseofulvin and penicillin, since griseofulvin is derived from *Penicillium* fungi. However, in my experience, this has not been a problem, and I *do* prescribe griseofulvin for penicillin-allergic patients.

### Ketoconazole

Ketoconazole (Nizoral) was introduced in 1979. It is an azole derivative with a broad spectrum of action that includes the dermatophytes, *Candida* and *Pityrosporum* species, and many of the deep fungi. Its mode of action is disruption of the plasma cell membrane by inhibition of ergosterol synthesis. Gastrointestinal absorption is best on an empty stomach and is diminished by antacids and histamine$_2$ blockers. If the latter medicines are also required, they should be taken at least 2 hours before ketoconazole. The usual adult dosage is 200 to 400 mg as a single dose in the morning.

Ketoconazole is generally a safe and well-tolerated medication. The most common side effects are gastrointestinal symptoms. Anaphylactic reactions may occur rarely. Inhibition of steroid hormone biosynthesis occurs at doses of ketoconazole that are much higher than clinically relevant for superficial fungal infections.

The most serious potential adverse effect of ketoconazole is hepatotoxicity. Asymptomatic elevations of liver enzymes have been reported in up to 11% of patients with various fungal diseases during treatment. Symptomatic toxic hepatitis resembling viral hepatitis may occur in 1 in

TABLE 1. **Comparison of Systemic Antifungal Agents**

| | Griseofulvin | Ketoconazole |
|---|---|---|
| Generic name | Griseofulvin | Ketoconazole |
| Trade names | Grifulvin V | Nizoral |
| | Grisactin | |
| | Fulvicin P/G | |
| | Gris-Peg | |
| | Grisactin Ultra | |
| Mechanism | Fungistatic | Fungistatic |
| Indication | Dermatophytosis | Candidiasis |
| | | Tinea versicolor |
| | | Dermatophytosis |
| Minor toxicity | Headache | Gastrointestinal |
| | Gastrointestinal | Pruritus |
| Major toxicity | None | Hepatitis |
| Drug interactions | Alcohol—flushing tachycardia | Warfarin—more anticoagulation |
| | Warfarin—less anticoagulation | Rifampin—decreases blood levels of ketoconazole |
| | Phenobarbital—decreases activity of griseofulvin | Isoniazid—less absorption of ketoconazole |
| | | Phenytoin—alteration of metabolism of both keto- conazole and phenytoin |
| | | Cyclosporine—blood levels of ketoconazole increased |
| Safety monitor- ing | None for 8 wk or less | None for 2 wk or less |
| | CBC, creatinine, and aspartate amino- transferase (AST, SGOT) q 3 mo | Baseline liver function tests, repeated at 2 wks, monthly for 3 mo, then q 3 mo |

15,000 patients treated with ketoconazole. Several deaths resulting from hepatic necrosis have been reported. The reaction is presumed to be idiosyncratic. The majority of patients were female, over 40 years of age, with onychomycosis that required prolonged therapy. Periodic monitoring of liver function tests is essential if ketoconazole is to be administered safely for periods of more than 2 weeks. *For chronic dermatophytosis, ketoconazole is indicated only if the patient has failed to respond to or is intolerant of griseofulvin.* Ketoconazole should be stopped if progressive elevations or greater than three times normal values of transaminases are observed, or if the patient develops symptoms of jaundice, dark urine, pale stools, malaise, anorexia, nausea, or vomiting.

Pertinent drug interactions may occur with warfarin (Coumadin), rifampin, isoniazid, phenytoin (Dilantin), and cyclosporine (Sandimmune). Ketoconazole increases the blood level of cyclosporine, which in turn increases the risk of renal toxicity. Concomitant administration of ketoconazole and cyclosporine requires close monitoring of cyclosporine levels.

## DERMATOPHYTOSES

Invasion of a living host's skin, hair, or nails by dermatophytes, fungi belonging to the genera *Trichophyton, Microsporum,* or *Epidermophyton,* is called a dermatophytosis. The various clinical presentations are referred to as *tineas,* according to the anatomic site of involvement.

### Tinea Pedis

As many as 70% of the general population suffer from tinea pedis, a dermatophytosis of the toe-web spaces and soles. Limited and early involvement should be treated with one of the azole creams (Table 2) for at least 4 weeks. Wet, macerated toe-web spaces may be treated with Castellani paint to promote drying. Fissures and breaks in the skin caused by tinea pedis may later be the portal of entry for bacterial cellulitis, particularly in diabetics and immunosuppressed patients. The relapse rate is high even in normal hosts. For chronic cases, I recommend sprinkling of the inside of shoes overnight with tolnaftate powder and once-daily application of tolnaftate or miconazole to prevent recurrence.

### Tinea Manum

Dermatophyte infections of the palm are seen less commonly. Involvement of one palm may occur with bilateral sole involvement (the "one hand, two foot syndrome"). The clinical appearance often mimics that of psoriasis or eczema, but a positive potassium hydroxide (KOH) test and culture of *T. rubrum* confirm the diagnosis. Topical treatment with Whitfield's ointment at bedtime thins the horny layer and prepares the skin for a morning application of ketoconazole (Nizoral), econazole, oxiconazole, or sulconazole for 4 to 6 weeks. Failure to respond or relapse is an indication for an additional 6-week course of griseofulvin (1000 mg daily microsize or 500 mg daily ultramicrosize).

### Tinea Cruris

Infection of the groin, perineum, and perirectal area is referred to as tinea cruris. If there is exudation, compressing the area once or twice

TABLE 2. **Topical Antifungal Agents**

| Generic Name | Trade Names | OTC | R$_X$ | Dermatophyte | *Candida* | Tinea Versicolor |
|---|---|---|---|---|---|---|
| Tolnaftate | Aftate Tinactin | X | | X | | X |
| Undecylenic acid | Cruex Desenex | X | | X | | |
| Whitfield's ointment (6% benzoic acid, 3% salicylic acid) | USP | X | | X | | |
| Castellani paint (Carbol fuchsin solution) | | X | | X | X | |
| Gentian violet 1% | USP | X | | | X | |
| Selenium sulfide 2.5% | Exsel Selsun | | X | | | X |
| Haloprogin | Halotex | | X | X | X | |
| Nystatin | Mycostatin Nilstat | | X | | X | |
| Naftifine | Naftin | | X | X | | |
| Ciclopirox | Loprox | | X | X | X | X |
| **Azoles** | | | | | | |
| Clotrimazole | Lotrimin | X | X | X | X | X |
| | Mycelex | | X | X | X | X |
| Miconazole | Monistat-Derm | | X | X | X | X |
| | Micatin | X | | X | X | X |
| Econazole | Spectazole | | X | X | X | X |
| Ketoconazole | Nizoral | | X | X | X | X |
| Oxiconazole | Oxistat | | X | X | X | X |
| Sulconazole | Exelderm | | X | X | X | X |

daily with a dilute solution of aluminum acetate (Burow's solution 1:40, Bluboro, Domeboro) will help dry it, followed by the application of an azole cream for 4 to 6 weeks. Systemic therapy is usually not necessary.

### Tinea Capitis

Fungal infections of the scalp may present as light scaling resembling seborrheic dermatitis, bald patches with black dots resembling alopecia areata, or kerion formation that mimics an abscess or furuncle. A fungal culture is most valuable in tinea capitis. Hairs must be plucked close to the scalp to include the roots within or near the edge of the involved area and cultured on dermatophyte test medium (DTM) or Mycosel, a selective agar containing cycloheximide and chloramphenicol, or submitted to a mycology laboratory for identification. Dermatophytes will turn the DTM red within 2 weeks and can be interpreted in the office. I do rely on the culture for confirmation of diagnosis because the KOH test of hair is difficult to interpret. The overwhelming majority of tinea capitis in the U.S. is caused by the nonfluorescent *T. tonsurans*. Therefore, Wood's light examination of the scalp hairs is of little value.

Tinea capitis must be treated systemically in order to effect a cure. The treatment of choice is griseofulvin for 6 to 8 weeks. Because most of the patients are children, I use Grifulvin V, a minimum of 5 mg per pound body weight per day. In adults, 1000 mg of microsize or 500 mg of ultramicrosize tablets daily may be substituted.

The inflammation of a kerion may cause permanent damage to the hair follicles and hair loss. If the diagnosis can be confirmed and pyoderma has been ruled out, a brief tapering course (1 to 2 weeks) of methylprednisolone (Medrol Dosepak) or prednisone (40 mg, 35 mg, . . . 5 mg, 0) may be beneficial.

While waiting for the culture to grow, I will treat the child with daily 2.5% selenium sulfide shampoo (Selsun, Exsel) because it is sporicidal and prevents contagion to other children. However, griseofulvin must be given in order to cure the infection.

### Tinea Corporis

Dermatophyte infections of the trunk, extremities, and face (tinea faciale) may have the typical reddish scaly active border with central clearing ("ringworm"). They respond promptly to any of the prescription antifungal creams or miconazole applied for 4 weeks. Certain individuals acquire extensive tinea corporis infections that make widespread and thorough topical applications impractical. These patients may be genetically predisposed, have diabetes or iatrogenic immunosuppression (e.g., organ transplant recipients), or have AIDS. I treat such patients concomitantly with an azole cream and griseofulvin for 6 weeks.

### Tinea Unguium

Dermatophyte infections of the nail apparatus may involve the nail plate superficially, the distal subungual skin, or the most proximal matrix. The first infection is curable by scraping the white surface and applying an antifungal solution. In general, the other nail infections require systemic therapy to achieve cure. An occasional early proximal subungual infection may be cured by the diligent application of ciclopirox (Loprox) or econazole solution twice daily under and around the nail plate for several months.

Because tinea unguium of the toenails would require 6 to 12 months of systemic therapy, I usually discourage such treatment and treat only coexisting tinea pedis as described earlier. Moreover, the cure rate with either griseofulvin or ketoconazole is only about 20%.

Fingernail infections are worth treating with griseofulvin. I start with ultramicrosize 500 mg daily and notch the nailplate at the most proximal extent of disease. I see the patient in followup every 2 months. If the disease extends proximal to the notch, during treatment, I increase the dose by 250 mg daily. It may take 6 to 9 months to effect cure. Because of the long commitment to therapy, I recommend confirmation of diagnosis with a positive KOH test or culture. It is best to obtain subungual debris for testing from the most proximal location possible.

## CANDIDIASIS

*Candida albicans* is a ubiquitous yeast that constitutes part of the normal flora of the oral, gastrointestinal, and vaginal mucous membranes. The organism causes opportunistic infections in the face of altered immunity states, diabetes mellitus, antibiotic therapy, pregnancy, oral contraceptives, and extremes of age. The diagnosis can be confirmed by visualizing pseudohyphae and/or budding yeast forms under a KOH preparation or by culture.

### Intertriginous Candidiasis

Moisture in skinfold areas such as the axillae and groin predisposes an individual to candidal overgrowth, particularly in infants, obese adults, and diabetics. The appearance is usually redder and wetter than a dermatophytosis, and there may be characteristic satellite pustules at the periphery. Keeping these areas as dry as possible, weight reduction, and better glucose control in diabetics are beneficial. Wet compresses with Burow's solution 1:40 twice daily followed by the application of nystatin (Mycostatin) or miconazole (Monistat-Derm) for 2 weeks will clear most infections. An alternative treatment is the application of 1% gentian violet to involved areas.

### Oral Candidiasis

The classic presentation of acute pseudomembranous candidiasis or thrush consists of white curd-like matter that can be wiped away to expose a raw red base. In infants, I favor removing the yeast and applying 1% gentian violet. Asking adults who wear dentures to remove them at night may help. Corticosteroid inhalers for asthma such as beclomethazone (Vanceril) predispose patients to candidiasis.

In most adults, I treat with either clotrimazole (Mycelex) troches five times daily for 2 weeks or nystatin pastilles four per day for 2 weeks. When candidiasis affects the corners of the mouth, it is referred to as angular cheilitis or perlèche. The patient may have an ill fitting denture. I treat it with either nystatin ointment or econazole cream twice per day until clear.

### Genital Candidiasis

Vaginal candidiasis is treated with anticandidal vaginal suppositories: clotrimazole (Gyne-Lotrimin), 500 mg once, or miconazole (Monistat 3), 200 mg for 3 nights. If there is also vulvar candidiasis, it could be treated with a topical cream, but I would consider treating with ketoconazole, 200 mg daily for 10 to 14 days.

### Paronychia

Inflammation and swelling of the nail fold skin has many predisposing factors: wet work, irritants, detergents, solvents, eczema. *Candida* may be cultured from the skin or under the nail. This is usually a mixed infection with bacteria.

Patients should be asked to avoid immersion of bare hands and contact with solvents by wearing heavy duty vinyl gloves (Allerderm) for wet work. A drying solution of 3% thymol in chloroform or 95% ethanol may be applied twice daily. A topical antifungal solution such as haloprogin (Halotex), clotrimazole, or ciclopirox (Loprox) may be used instead or concomitantly. Oral ketoconazole is reserved for recalcitrant cases, 200 mg daily for 2 weeks.

## PITYROSPORUM INFECTIONS

*Pityrosporum orbiculare,* also called *Malassezia furfur,* is a yeast that comprises the normal flora of hair follicles. Under certain conditions the yeast becomes a pathogen, causing at least two patterns of skin disease.

### Tinea (Pityriasis) Versicolor

This common infection can be recognized by its typical truncal distribution, although the neck and arms may also be affected. The KOH preparation demonstrates short fat hyphae and piles of spores ("spaghetti and meatballs"). Wood's light examination reveals a greenish yellow fluorescence in infected areas. I treat tinea versicolor with selenium sulfide shampoo applied as a lotion from the neck to the waist and arms, left on for at least 15 minutes, daily for a week, followed by a shower and shampoo. I warn that there is a high relapse rate, particularly in warm humid climates. Although many of the topical antifungal creams would be effective, they are practical only for very limited disease that is visible and accessible to the patient. Oral ketoconazole is also very effective for tinea versicolor, but I reserve it for recalcitrant cases, noncompliant patients, and those who are immunosuppressed or physically disabled and otherwise unable to apply the lotion and take showers regularly. A dose of 400 mg daily for 5 days gives a very high cure rate.

### Pityrosporum Folliculitis

This presents as an acneiform eruption of the trunk and scalp that itches, unlike common acne. *Pityrosporum* cannot be cultured routinely. The KOH and Wood's light tests are usually not helpful. A skin biopsy of a lesion, however, shows numerous budding yeast forms in the follicular infundibulum. I usually treat *Pityrosporum* folliculitis with ketoconazole cream twice daily. If that is ineffective, I give the tablets: 200 to 400 mg daily for 2 weeks.

## ERYTHRASMA

Erythrasma is actually a bacterial disease caused by *Corynebacterium minutissimum,* but it is included in this article because it is a common, superficial infection that clinically mimics a fungal infection. It presents as reddish brown patches in the axillae, genitocrural folds, and toe-web spaces. I suspect erythrasma whenever an expected positive KOH test turns out to be consistently negative. The Wood's light shined on the involved areas reveals a brilliant orange or coral red fluorescence that confirms the diagnosis of erythrasma. It responds nicely to a 2-week course of either tetracycline (1 gram daily) or erythromycin (1 gram daily). An alternative approach would be the twice-daily application of erythromycin cream (Akne-mycin) for 3 weeks. Relapses may occur after successful treatment.

# DISEASES OF THE MOUTH

method of
ROBERT A. BURNS, D.D.S., M.S.
*Medical College of Ohio*
*Toledo, Ohio*

Gingivitis, periodontal disease, and dental caries are the most common local diseases of the oral cavity. However, appropriate preventive measures have substantially reduced the prevalence of these disorders, the most important of which includes supplemental intake of oral fluorides, especially in children and geriatric patients who suffer from varying degrees of xerostomia and salivary gland atrophy. Prevention of the formation of dental plaque also significantly protects against the development of dental caries as well as the development of gingivitis and periodontal disease. The daily use of dental floss and proper toothbrushing techniques will prevent the oral bacterial and mycotic flora from colonizing on the tooth surfaces and the gingival sulcus, and this in turn prevents dental plaque from organizing.

## LESIONS OF THE LIPS

### Mucocele (Mucus Retention Phenomenon)

The etiology of this condition is related to mechanical trauma to the minor salivary gland excretory duct, resulting in its severance, with extravasation of mucus into the surrounding connective tissue stroma. A granulation tissue response ensues, walling off the mucus and giving the lesion a pseudocyst-like quality.

Clinically, these lesions develop an elevated, smooth surface swelling with a bluish hue, frequently located in the lower labial mucosa midway between the midline and commissural angle. The size may fluctuate depending on the degree of mucin production. A viscous material is found if aspiration is attempted.

Treatment of choice is surgical excision with removal of the associated minor salivary glands in order to prevent recurrence. Aspiration provides no lasting clinical benefit.

## Chapped or Cracked Lips

This condition is usually factitial in origin due to alternate wetting and drying resulting in inflammation and secondary infection. Clinically, the surface of the vermilion is rough, peeling, and ulcerated with crusting. The normal vertical fissuring may be lost. Treatment is accomplished by application of an anti-inflammatory agent in a petrolatum or adhesive base that interrupts the irritating factor and promotes healing. Betamethasone valerate (Valisone) ointment 0.1% applied to the lips after each meal and at bedtime is recommended. For maintenance, the frequent application of petrolatum-based products—e.g., Chapstick or cocoa butter—should be used.

## Actinic Cheilitis (Solar Cheilosis)

This condition results from prolonged exposure to sunlight and results in irreversible degenerative changes in the vermilion border of the lips, especially the everted lower lip. The normal, red translucent vermilion border with regular, vertical fissuring of a smooth surface is replaced by a keratinized, flat surface that may exhibit periodic ulceration. If exposure to the UV light is allowed to continue, the degenerative changes may progress to a malignancy. This lesion is therefore considered to be premalignant.

Sunscreens with a high skin protection factor should be used constantly and the patient followed at close periodic intervals. If suspicious areas develop, a complete lip shave or cheiloplasty should be performed, with serial sections of the lip specimen evaluated microscopically for malignant transformation.

## Angular Cheilitis-Cheilosis

This condition refers to painful, fissured, erosive lesions in the corners of the mouth and is caused by a mixed infection of the following microorganisms: *Candida albicans*, staphylococci, and streptococci. The lesions are formed more frequently in children and geriatric patients. Predisposing factors include local habits of lip sucking, drooling, a decrease in the intermaxillary vertical dimension, nutritional deficiencies (vitamin B), and an extension of oral infections. Clinically, the commissures appear wrinkled, red, fissured, cracked, or crusted. Because this is usually a mixed infection, an effective therapeutic agent is a preparation of multiple ingredients containing nystatin–neomycin sulfate–gramicidin–triamcinolone acetonide (Mycolog). Apply to the affected area after each meal and at bedtime.

## Cheilitis Glandularis

This is an edematous condition of the lower lip, which becomes enlarged, firm, and finally everted. The labial salivary glands become enlarged, while the orifices of the secretory ducts become inflamed and dilated. A viscid secretion may seep from these openings. The condition may be caused by exposure to sun, wind, and dust, as well as the use of tobacco.

There is no definitive treatment, although some authorities consider this lesion to be premalignant. Studies have shown epidermoid carcinoma of the lips to be associated with cheilitis glandularis in 18 to 35% of the reported cases. Surgical stripping of the lip is recommended, since in most cases this has been shown to eliminate the disease while providing acceptable esthetic results.

## Secondary or Recurrent Herpes Labialis

Secondary herpes represents the reactivation of latent virus. There are usually prodromal symptoms of tingling, burning, or pain at the site in which clusters of fragile, short-lived vesicles appear that rupture within hours and then crust. Treatment should be initiated as early as possible in the prodromal stage. Acyclovir (Zovirax) topical ointment 5% applied to the affected area every 2 hours is recommended. Systemic acyclovir capsules may be considered when frequent recurrent herpetic episodes interfere with daily function and nutrition. If recurrence on the lips is precipitated by exposure to sunlight, the lesion may be prevented by the application to the area of a sunscreen with a high skin protection factor (greater than 15). The amino acid lysine (Enisyl), 600 mg daily, may also be suppressive for recurrent episodes.

## Squamous Cell Carcinoma of the Lip

Most frequently seen on the vermilion border of the lower lip on one side of the midline, squamous cell carcinoma of the lip usually appears as a nonhealing ulcer with a raised, rolled, and indurated margin that may be fixed to the underlying tissues. Pipe smoking and UV light are important in causing lower lip cancer. Lip carcinomas account for 25 to 30% of all oral cancers. Metastasis to regional lymph nodes is uncommon, and prognosis is excellent (85% 5-year survival) if detected and treated early. Surgical excision with 1 cm clear margins is the treatment of choice. Radiation therapy may be equally effective.

## TONGUE LESIONS

### Hairy Leukoplakia

Hairy leukoplakia is an unusual white lesion, often folded or corrugated, that occurs along the lateral margins of the tongue. The lesion may extend onto the dorsal surface of the tongue and rarely onto the buccal mucosa and floor of the mouth. Evidence has suggested this represents an opportunistic infection related to the Epstein-Barr virus (EBV) and associated with the subsequent development of the clinical and laboratory features of the acquired immune deficiency syndrome (AIDS) in up to 80% of the cases. There is no specific treatment for hairy leukoplakia, although it is critical for this diagnosis to be confirmed subsequent to its clinical identification.

### Hairy Tongue

In this condition, the dorsal surface of the tongue is covered by yellowish white to brownish black "hairs" that represent hypertrophied filiform papillae with retardation of the normal rate of desquamation. The etiology is unknown but is often seen in association with broad-spectrum antibiotics, smokers, the use of oxygenating mouthrinses, and radiation therapy. A form of chronic hyperplastic candidiasis should also be ruled out. The condition is self-limiting, and the tongue will return to normal following physical débridement and proper oral hygiene.

### Geographic Tongue

Geographic tongue is an inflammatory condition of unknown etiology that is seen in 2% of the U.S. population and is characterized by the presence of small, round, circinate patches of dekeratinization and desquamation of filiform papillae. These areas appear as depressed reddish lesions with elevated margins of yellowish white. Characteristically, this pattern of distribution changes over a period of days to weeks, appearing to move across the dorsal surface of the tongue. It is often seen in association with a fissured tongue. The condition may persist for years. This condition is usually asymptomatic and requires no treatment. If symptoms occur, a topical steroid preparation may be helpful. Assure the patient of the benign nature to relieve anxiety.

### Fissured Tongue

This congenital anomaly may be an isolated finding or associated with Down's, Melkersson-Rosenthal, or Sjögren's syndromes. The tongue is deeply fissured, predisposing the patient to food trapping, inflammation, and infection. Good oral hygiene, including brushing the tongue with a soft toothbrush and a mild hydrogen peroxide oral rinse after meals and at bedtime, is the only treatment required.

### Macroglossia

Enlargement of the tongue may be due to a variety of conditions, including neoplasms, developmental anomalies such as hemangioma and lymphangioma, and metabolic derangements such as amyloidosis. Infection, angioedema, and superior vena cava syndrome may also produce tongue enlargement.

### Median Rhomboid Glossitis

Median rhomboid glossitis is characterized by an irregularly shaped, smooth red patch located on the mid-dorsum of the tongue. This condition may be developmental or perhaps related to chronic low-grade candidiasis. It is usually asymptomatic, but if symptoms are present an antifungal agent may be tried. If symptoms persist, surgical excision is indicated.

## GINGIVAL AND PERIODONTAL LESIONS

### Gingivitis and Periodontitis

These diseases are the most common inflammatory reactions of the mouth and involve the supporting structures of the teeth. Periodontitis, if untreated, may cause extensive bone resorption and eventual tooth loss and infection (pyorrhea). These patients should be referred to a dentist for removal of plaque and calculus.

### Primary Herpetic Gingivostomatitis

This primary disease is usually found in children and those adults not previously exposed to herpes simplex virus (HSV). The prodromal symptoms will usually manifest as an intense gingivitis accompanied by fever, malaise, headache, and cervical lymphadenopathy. Within 24 to 36 hours, vesicular eruptions will appear on any mucosal surface. These rupture within hours and form shallow, painful ulcers. This is a transmissible infection with either HSV type 1 or type 2. This systemic infection runs its course in about 10 days to 2 weeks. The virus then migrates to the trigeminal ganglion to reside in a latent form. Acyclovir (Zovirax), 200 mg orally five times a day for 10 days, is the suggested initial therapy to relieve and decrease the duration of symptoms. Topical anesthetics such as lidocaine HCl (Xylocaine) viscous 2% as an oral rinse (one tablespoon before each meal and expectorate) help to relieve local symptoms. Supportive therapy includes forced fluids, protein, and vitamin and mineral food supplements.

## Gingival Hyperplasia

Localized gingival hyperplasia is usually the result of local factors—i.e., periodontal pockets, plaque, calculus deposits, and faulty dental restorations. Generalized gingival hyperplasia is seen frequently in association with puberty and pregnancy as a result of hormonal influences. A hereditary type of gingival fibromatosis produces a generalized overgrowth of the gingiva, usually involving both arches, and appears at the time of eruption of the permanent incisors. This is an autosomal dominant trait and requires surgical removal. This condition must be differentiated from a similar overgrowth that occurs in individuals on phenytoin (Dilantin) therapy, which also requires surgical management and maintenance of excellent oral hygiene procedures to retard recurrent growth.

Rarely, gingival enlargement may seem in the terminal stages of leukemia and in certain types of bleeding dyscrasias—i.e., thrombocytopenia and polycythemia.

## Pyogenic Granuloma

This lesion represents exuberant overgrowth of granulation tissue in response to local irritating factors; the interdental papilla area is a common location. It appears as a soft, reddish, lobulated mass that bleeds very easily. Pyogenic granuloma is frequently seen in pregnant females at about the third month of pregnancy. It is often called a "pregnancy tumor." The overgrowth tends to recur if not adequately excised.

## Acute Necrotizing Ulcerative Gingivitis (Trench Mouth, Vincent's Infection)

This is a sudden, intense, generalized, inflammatory condition of the gingiva that is characterized by ulceration and necrosis of the interdental papilla. This condition is caused by a mixed fusiform-spirochete infection and may be associated with fever and cervical lymphadenopathy. A typical fetid odor usually develops. This disease is often confused with primary herpetic gingivostomatitis and is precipitated by stress, fatigue, and poor oral hygiene. Treatment consists of antibiotics (penicillin, tetracycline) coupled with local débridement, hydrogen peroxide–saline rinses, and supportive therapy.

## Chronic Desquamative Gingivitis

This is an unusual inflammatory reaction of the attached gingiva. It presents as diffuse erythema of attached gingiva associated with vesiculation, erosion, and desquamation. Its etiology is obscure and is more often seen in postmenopausal women. This form of gingivitis is often a reaction to various stimuli—i.e., plaque-control toothpastes. It may be a manifestation of disorders such as bullous pemphigoid, cicatricial pemphigoid, or pemphigus vulgaris.

A biopsy specimen for histologic and direct immunofluorescent examination should be obtained. The inflammatory reaction can sometimes be suppressed by the application of a topical steroid such as dexamethasone (Decadron) elixir, 0.5 mg per 5 ml as an oral rinse three times a day.

# VESICULOULCERATIVE CONDITIONS

## Recurrent Aphthous Stomatitis

This condition is characterized by minor aphthae (canker sores), which are small, shallow, painful ulcerations covered by a gray membrane surrounded by a narrow erythematous halo and are less than 1 cm in size. They occur on nonkeratinized (movable) oral mucosa. Major aphthae may also be present and are large, painful ulcers greater than 1 cm that penetrate deep into muscle and heal with scarring. The ulcers may be present for weeks or months at a time. Herpetiform ulcers are crops of small, shallow, painful ulcers that occur on any mucosal surface and resemble recurrent intraoral herpes simplex.

An altered immune response is postulated as the predisposing factor. Decreased tissue integrity may result from deficiencies of iron, vitamin $B_{12}$, and folic acid. Patients should be screened for diabetes mellitus and inflammatory bowel diseases. Precipitating factors include stress, trauma, allergies, and endocrine alterations as well as acidic foods, nuts, and juices. Inspect the oral cavity to rule out sources of trauma. Treatment includes topical antibiotics of tetracycline (Achromycin-V) oral suspension, 125 mg per 5 ml; rinse with two teaspoons for 2 minutes and swallow every 6 hours for 7 days. This treatment is contraindicated in pregnant women and children under 8 years of age. Topical triamcinolone (Kenalog) in Orabase applied every 4 hours may suppress local symptoms. For diffuse lesions, use dexamethasone (Decadron) elixir as an oral rinse for 2 minutes four times a day. Do not swallow. Nutritional supplements may be indicated. Oral conditions may result from topical steroid and antibiotic therapy. In severe cases, systemic prednisone, 40 mg daily, may be necessary to suppress an episode; however, remission is only temporary. Azathioprine (Imuran) may be prescribed concomitantly with prednisone for managing very severe conditions of aphthae. Complications with systemic candidiasis should be considered.

### Erosive Lichen Planus

Erosive lichen planus is postulated to be an autoimmune disorder that is possibly initiated by a variety of factors, including emotional stress, debility, hypersensitivity to drugs, bacterial or viral infections, or a genetic predisposition. Characteristic lesions are painful, eroded areas ranging in size from a few millimeters to several centimeters surrounded by typical radiating, white striations. The lesions are commonly found on the buccal mucosa, gingiva, and tongue. The nonerosive form tends to be more common. There is often an association with diabetes mellitus and hypertension. Chronic, erosive lesions should be biopsied to rule out premalignant changes. Systemic and local relief is achieved with anti-inflammatory and immunosuppressant agents. Topical steroids, such as fluocinonide (Lidex) gel .05% applied to the infected area four times daily, are useful for localized lesions. Dexamethasone (Decadron) elixir as an oral rinse (one teaspoon four times a day and expectorate) is good for diffuse lesions. For very severe cases, one can use prednisone tablets, 10 mg four times a day for 2 weeks and taper as indicated by clinical response. A maintenance dose may be necessary to keep the erosions suppressed. The treatment of or the prevention of a secondary fungal infection needs to be considered.

Injectable steroids—dexamethasone phosphate injectable, 1 ampule (4 mg per ml)—may be used by injecting 0.5 to 1 ml around margins of the ulcer with a 25-gauge needle twice a week until the ulcer heals.

### Pemphigus-Pemphigoid

These are relatively uncommon oral lesions. They should be considered whenever a patient gives a history of blister-like lesions and chronic, persistent oral ulcerations. The oral symptoms commonly precede the onset of skin lesions. Diagnosis is based on the history and on histologic and immunofluorescent characteristics of a biopsy specimen of a primary oral lesion. Either refer the patient to a dermatologist or treat as indicated in the section on very severe lichen planus.

### Erythema Multiforme

Oral lesions of erythema multiforme develop as erythematous macules and papules. They may form vesicles and bullae, which rupture quickly, resulting in shallow, painful erosions. There is a cyclic and repetitive pattern to the disease, and the labial mucosa is typically involved. Drugs (particularly sulfonamides) and infections (herpes simplex and *Mycoplasma*) are common precipitating factors. However, in 50% of the cases the etiology remains unknown.

Treatment includes topical steroid ointment as well as frequent mouthwashes with Cepacol diluted 1:4 with water several times daily. Secondary infection should be treated with oral antibiotics. For severe lesions, systemic prednisone, 40 to 60 mg daily for 3 weeks, is most effective. Differentiation from pemphigus vulgaris and bullous pemphigoid may be difficult. Biopsy differentiation and recognition of precipitating factors may be helpful diagnostic clues.

## WHITE LESIONS OF THE ORAL MUCOSA

### Hyperkeratosis

Hyperkeratosis refers to a benign, white, plaque-like thickening of a localized area of the oral mucosa. It is usually caused by chronic irritation, such as that commonly seen on the buccal mucosa at the occlusal line, so-called linea alba. It may also be caused by lip or cheek biting and by ill-fitting dentures. These lesions do not rub off and require a biopsy to rule out any evidence of dysplasia.

### Nicotine Stomatitis

This is a benign condition that involves the palate and is directly related to smoking, particularly pipe smoking. Chemical and thermic factors are significant. Clinically, there are small (1 to 5 mm) papules with red dots in the center. These represent mucous duct ostia. Later in the course of the disease, the palate assumes a diffuse grayish white, wrinkled appearance. Cessation of smoking leads to gradual resolution. This condition is not considered precancerous.

### Nonerosive Lichen Planus

The oral condition may occur in association with the typical skin lesions in about 40% of the cases. The majority of oral lesions, however, do not tend to be seen with skin lesions. There is a great variation in clinical appearance, with papular, reticular, plaque-like, white lesions with a bilateral distribution seen especially on the buccal mucosa. The typical lesion presents as a delicate, white, lace-like pattern (Wickham's striae) and may resemble leukoplakia. Biopsy is usually not necessary to establish a diagnosis. Drug-induced lichen planus–like reactions can occur and should be excluded. Drugs that may cause this reaction in the oral mucosa include gold; thiazide diuretics; antimalarial agents; and, rarely, phenothiazine, methyldopa (Aldomet), penicillamine (Cuprimine), and lithium.

The nonerosive form is usually asymptomatic and only requires recognition. If the lesions become painful, use the prescribed treatment as indicated for erosive lichen planus.

## Candidiasis

Candidiasis of the oral mucosa presents as soft, white, slightly elevated plaques that can usually be wiped away leaving an erythematous area. It may also appear as generalized erythematous, atrophic areas especially in the hard palate in association with ill-fitting maxillary dentures. If there is questionable clinical diagnosis, a cytology smear or culture for *Candida albicans* is advisable.

*Candida albicans* is a yeast-like fungus. It is an opportunistic organism that tends to proliferate with the use of antibiotics, corticosteroids, and cytotoxic drugs. Conditions contributing to this disease include xerostomia, diabetes mellitus, pregnancy, poor oral hygiene, prosthodontic appliances, and suppression of the immune system or radiation therapy. If oral candidiasis occurs in an otherwise healthy young male, AIDS should be suspected. The presence of oral candidiasis in patients with AIDS-related complex indicates probable esophageal involvement.

Treatment consists of nystatin (Mycostatin) oral suspension, 100,000 U per ml, using one teaspoon as a rinse for 2 minutes and swallow. Medication should be continued for 48 hours after disappearance of clinical signs to prevent recurrence. Clotrimazole (Mycelex) troches, 10 mg, one troche dissolved in the mouth five times a day, are also very effective. If there is association with an ill-fitting denture, nystatin ointment can be applied to the inside of the denture base daily. When topical therapy is ineffective, ketoconazole (Nizoral) is an effective, well-tolerated, systemic drug for mucocutaneous candidiasis. Liver function tests should be conducted monthly if the drug is prescribed for an extended period.

## Other Conditions

Pachyonychia congenita and dyskeratosis congenita are rare syndromes that may present with white, keratotic plaques affecting the oral mucosa and gastrointestinal tract. Other cutaneous signs include thickened nails, keratoderma of the palms and soles, and a scalloped tongue. Oral lesions may become malignant and should be removed surgically if they become irritated or ulcerated.

Darier's disease (keratosis follicularis) may present with small, flat, coalescing papules that give the buccal or palatal mucosa a whitish "cobblestone" appearance. This disorder is seen in association with widespread keratotic follicular papules on the skin. It has a distinctive histopathologic presentation and is inherited in an autosomal dominant manner.

## NEOPLASIA

### Premalignant Lesions

Leukoplakia is a nonspecific, white keratotic, plaque-like lesion found primarily in those people who abuse all forms of tobacco, but especially smokers. These lesions are not associated with any other specific disease entity. Those lesions found on the lateral border of the tongue, floor of the mouth, and retromolar trigone area should always be viewed with great suspicion because they frequently are premalignant or carcinomatous. In various studies, the percentage of cases of clinical leukoplakia that had premalignant or malignant microscopic features present at the time of initial biopsy varied between 14 and 23%. Early detection of malignancy is extremely important, since patients with Stage I lesions have a 5-year survival rate of 90%.

Erythroplakia or a "speckled leukoplakia" is a much more sinister finding. These red lesions have a much higher risk for premalignant and malignant transformation. In some studies, as many as 65% of all red lesions of the oral mucosa have premalignant or malignant changes at the time of biopsy. Therefore, all white lesions and red lesions of the oral mucosa should be histologically examined; an exception to this is when an infection or other obvious entity is recognized.

### Squamous Cell Carcinoma

In the United States, oral cancer accounts for approximately 4 to 5% of all cancers, with over 30,000 cases reported annually. Of this number, squamous cell carcinoma accounts for 92% of the malignant lesions diagnosed in the mouth. It may present as a white keratotic lesion, erythroplasia, or chronic ulcer; have a verrucal, exophytic, or endophytic appearance; or present as a combination of all the above. The most important etiologic factors are smoking, alcohol abuse, and poor oral hygiene. The typical patient is usually male, in the fifth or sixth decade. Most cases are already Stage II or III at the time of diagnosis. The lesions invade locally and tend to metastasize to regional lymph nodes. Treatment consists of local excision with radical neck dissection, and radiation therapy, usually in combination.

In addition to squamous cell carcinomas, which account for the vast majority of oral carcinomas, adenocarcinomas may arise from minor salivary glands. Treatment of adenocarcinomas is surgical. One per cent of oral malignancies are metastatic from the breasts, lungs, kidneys, thyroid, prostate, and occasionally other sites. Melanomas are rare malignant tumors of the oral mucosa and have a marked tendency for metastases. Other unusual oral tumors include lymphoma, fibrosarcoma, rhabdomyosarcoma, liposarcoma, neurofibrosarcoma, angiosarcoma, and Kaposi's sarcoma. Kaposi's sarcoma involving the oral mucosa is seen more commonly in patients with AIDS. These oral lesions may present as macular or papular red to bluish red lesions involving all areas of the oral mucosa.

### Benign and Reactive Lesions

Irritation fibroma is a well-circumscribed, elevated, fibrous proliferation and is one of the most common lesions in the oral cavity. It is not a true tumor because it lacks potential for unlimited growth. The buccal mucosa and commissure of the lips are the most common locations. The patient usually gives a history of biting or sucking his or her cheek. Treatment is simple excision.

Papilloma is a localized benign neoplastic growth of the surface epithelium. It has a papillary or wart-like appearance and arises from a stalk or a sessile base. It is not precancerous, and simple excision is the treatment of choice. Multiple lesions of a similar nature may indicate condyloma acuminatum, a highly contagious virus infection of genital origin.

Torus palatinus is regarded as a developmental disturbance, resulting in an overgrowth of bone in the midline of the hard palate. It assumes various sizes and may undergo a delayed growth spurt. It is benign and usually requires no treatment unless it interferes with mastication or the placement of a maxillary prosthesis. A similar condition also occurs in the lower jaw—bilateral mandibular tori—usually found on the lingual aspect of the mandible.

Pleomorphic adenoma is a benign minor salivary gland tumor most commonly found in the hard and soft palate. It appears as a smooth, firm, well-circumscribed mass lateral to the midline.

Any swelling in this area should be considered a salivary gland tumor until proved otherwise by incisional biopsy.

Aspirin burn is related to placing an aspirin tablet against the mucosa with the intention of getting relief from a toothache. The caustic action produces painful, discrete white areas as a result of coagulation necrosis of the tissue. This white film can be wiped off, leaving a painful erythematous area.

Traumatic ulcer has the clinical characteristics to suggest carcinoma. It is an ulcer with firm, elevated margins and can occur in areas where carcinoma is commonly found. Traumatic ulcers heal within 10 to 14 days. If the lesion does not heal within this time, biopsy is mandatory.

Melanocytic nevi of all types may be seen in the oral cavity. They are not common and are rarely malignant. All types may be encountered, including lentigines; blue nevi; and junctional, compound, and dermal nevi. Excision is the best treatment if there is asymmetry, unusual enlargement, or color variability.

## OTHER CONDITIONS OF THE ORAL CAVITY

### Mucositis

This is a condition that occurs in postmenopausal women. It is frequently compounded by *Candida* infection. Drugs may frequently be associated with sore mouth. Phenytoin (Dilantin) can cause gingival hyperplasia. Mouth ulcers result from cytotoxic drugs, and antibiotics can cause black hairy tongue or overgrowth of *Candida*. Lichen planus stomatitis can be induced by a variety of medications, including gold and penicillamine therapy.

### Xerostomia

Causes of dry mouth include emotional stress and drugs such as anticholinergics and hypertensives. In addition, xerostomia may be idiopathic or may be a symptom of an autoimmune disorder of salivary glands. Other factors include age and radiation therapy of the head and neck. Underlying systemic disorders should be investigated, including Sjögren's syndrome, scleroderma, rheumatoid arthritis, lupus erythematosus, sarcoidosis, and malignancies.

Symptomatic relief may be obtained by frequent sips of water or saliva substitute (Xerolube, Scherer Laboratories). Because dental caries commonly occurs in patients with xerostomia, good oral hygiene and dental referral are necessary.

### Contact Stomatitis

The oral mucous membranes are less susceptible to allergic sensitization than is the skin. Symptoms such as burning, soreness, or loss of taste may be more prominent than physical findings. Sharply limited forms of contact stomatitis may be secondary to denture stomatitis in which the erythema is sharply localized to the denture site. Strong mouthwashes not uncommonly cause oral irritation.

A wide variety of contact allergens, including dentifrices, mouthwashes, and oral medications, must be suspected as etiologic factors. Routine patch testing is occasionally helpful. Cheilitis may be treated with cool tap water compresses and the application of a topical fluorinated steroid gel together with protective ointments. Gargling with 5 ml of diphenhydramine (Benadryl) may give symptomatic relief. Triamcinolone in a dental paste (Kenalog in Orabase) also may be applied three to four times daily. In the meantime, the patient should eliminate all commercial dentifrices and mouthwashes as well as chewing gum, candy, and lozenges.

### Burning Tongue Syndrome

In the majority of cases, it is difficult to find a cause for burning or painful tongue. Xerostomia, candidiasis, referred muscle pain, other chronic infections, dental disease, reflux of gastric acid, medications, blood dyscrasias, nutritional deficiencies, allergies, psychogenic or idiopathic factors, and factitial habits all need to be considered. On the basis of history, physical evaluation, and specific laboratory studies, rule out all possible etiologies. Minimal blood studies include CBC and differential, glucose, iron, folic acid, and vitamin $B_{12}$.

For symptomatic relief, diphenhydramine (Benadryl) elixir is useful as a topical rinse (one teaspoon for 2 minutes and swallow before each meal). When burning tongue is considered to be idiopathic, tricyclic antidepressants in low doses provide analgesia and sedation in reducing or eliminating the symptoms after several weeks. The recommended regimen is amitriptyline (Elavil) tablets, 25 mg, one tablet at bedtime for 1 week, then two tablets at bedtime and maintained at that dosage. The dosage should be adjusted according to the individual response of the patient.

# STASIS DERMATITIS AND STASIS ULCERS

method of
JESS R. YOUNG, M.D.
*Cleveland Clinic Foundation*
*Cleveland, Ohio*

Stasis dermatitis and stasis ulcerations are frequent complications of chronic venous insufficiency. Five hundred thousand Americans have or have had venous stasis ulcers. There is an estimated loss of 2 million work days annually in the United States. These complications account for 10% of all admissions to general hospitals.

## ETIOLOGY

Rarely do varicose veins, even severe varicosities, result in significant venous insufficiency. Insufficiency usually results from previous deep venous thrombosis. During the healing process of the thrombosis, even if patency is restored, the venous walls become thickened and distorted and the valves are often incompetent. This results in a high venous pressure, which in turn upsets the normal capillary fluid exchange. As a result, excessive fluid and red blood cells are lost to the extracellular spaces and there is poor nutrition of the surrounding tissue. The stasis ulcer itself is often associated with an incompetent perforating vein leading into the area of the ulcer.

The stasis changes of edema and dermatitis are often aggravated by scratching, overtreatment, or sensitization to the many preparations applied to the leg before the patient seeks professional help.

## CLINICAL FEATURES

Following deep venous thrombosis, prominent superficial veins may appear. Rarely are these incompetent. Edema is often the first sign of venous insufficiency. It will first be noted at the end of the day, disappearing overnight, but will slowly become more persistent if untreated. The next evidence of venous insufficiency is usually pigmentation. This results from rupture of tiny venules and capillaries caused by excessive venous pressure and subsequent extravasation of hemoglobin into the tissues. In some patients stasis dermatitis will develop with erythema, weeping, scaling, and pruritus. A few patients with stasis dermatitis will develop a generalized eczematous eruption as a sensitization or autoallergic (id) reaction.

In some patients an indurated, tender, subcutaneous cellulitis will develop on the medial aspect of the leg just proximal to the medial malleolus. This sterile, indurated cellulitis may spread up and down the calf on the medial side and occasionally may involve the posterior and lateral aspects of the lower leg. This condition has also been termed *liposclerosis*. It is often mistaken for thrombophlebitis or bacterial cellulitis.

Venous stasis ulcerations usually occur in the vicinity of the malleoli, especially the medial malleolus.

Less commonly, they may occur on the posterior and lateral aspect of the calf. Brown pigmentation is usually present in the surrounding skin, and the leg is often edematous. The base of the ulcer is usually moist with extensive granulation tissue, and is often secondarily infected. The ulcer may vary greatly in size, at times extending around the whole circumference of the calf. Pain is not a prominent feature of these ulcerations. If pain is present, it is usually relieved by elevation of the limb. Once healed, a tendency exists for recurrence in the same area if good elastic support is not used.

## TREATMENT

Many different treatments of venous stasis dermatitis and ulcerations have been proposed. The multitude of approaches attests to the fact that no one outstanding method exists for treating venous insufficiency. The choice of treatment is somewhat dependent on the type and extent of the dermatitis, the size of the ulceration, the presence of arterial insufficiency, and the severity of secondary infection. For this reason, treatment of the various aspects of venous insufficiency will be considered separately.

### Acute Stasis Dermatitis

Occlusive dressings must be avoided in treating acute dermatitis because they result in further maceration of tissues. Treatment should include bed rest to reduce the edema and the use of wet compresses that are changed every 2 to 4 hours. If the weeping discharge does not appear to be infected, the compression dressing may consist of isotonic saline solution 0.9% or aluminum acetate (Burow's solution) 0.5%. If the discharge appears to be infected, acetic acid 1% or boric acid solution 3% or ethanol-iodine complex (Wescodyne) solution 3% may be used. Between compresses, a drying anti-inflammatory steroid spray, topical anti-inflammatory steroid, or steroid-antibiotic cream may be employed to help clear the dermatitis. Ointments should be avoided in acute dermatitis because they can aggravate any maceration. If there is evidence of secondary infection with cellulitis or bacteremia, a culture should be taken and appropriate antibiotic therapy should be initiated.

### Subacute Or Chronic Stasis Dermatitis

When the acute phase of the dermatitis has subsided and the patient once again becomes ambulatory, recurrence of edema must be prevented. If this is not done, acute dermatitis often will return. The use of a modified Unna's paste boot (Dome-Paste) is most effective in this situation. The boot consists of flesh-colored rolled bandages impregnated with a paste of zinc oxide, calamine, glycerin, and gelatin. Its use permits the patient to return to work and to continue usual activities and eliminates the need for extensive bed rest or hospitalization. Directions for applying the paste boot are well illustrated on the package. The boot is usually changed at weekly intervals unless excessive drainage necessitates changing more frequently. If excessive discomfort occurs at home, the patient should be instructed to cut off the dressing and to return to the physician's office for further evaluation.

Even though Unna's boot is effective, problems are associated with it, including a long learning curve for correctly applying the cast, maceration of the skin when drainage is excessive, and inability to observe or bathe the leg while the cast is on. We have recently been favorably impressed by an alternative to Unna's boot. This is a compression dressing program, consisting of an absorbent dressing, which is held in place by a lightweight compression liner stocking (Jobst UlcerCARE program). During the day, when the patient is active, this compression liner stocking is covered by a heavy support stocking. The dressing is changed at bedtime. It appears to be simple, easy to learn, effective, and also gives the patient an opportunity to be an active participant in his or her own care.

Areas of chronic, thickened, lichenified dermatitis may require more potent topical steroid preparations, e.g., betamethasone valerate (Valisone), halcinonide (Halog), and triamcinolone acetonide (Kenalog). A discrete nodular lesion secondary to persistent scratching may require intralesional injections of triamcinolone acetonide, 5 mg per ml.

### Indurated Stasis Cellulitis

Usually no bacterial infection is present in chronic stasis cellulitis, and the inflammation does not respond to antibiotics. Best results are achieved by bed rest for 1 to 3 weeks with the leg elevated and applications of heat to the area. Warm, wet dressings are probably more effective than dry heat. The healing process may be expedited at times by giving nonsteroidal anti-inflammatory agents. When the patient can tolerate an elastic stocking, this should be worn with a one-quarter inch thick foam rubber pad placed over the indurated area. Wearing this pad may be discontinued once inflammation is no longer noticeable.

In a very few patients, cellulitis appears to resist all forms of treatment. If no improvement is noted after 6 to 8 weeks of treatment, excision of the indurated subcutaneous tissue and necrotic fat with skin grafting should be considered. The patient must continue to wear a heavy elastic support stocking after the operation.

## Stasis Ulcers

The general principles outlined for subacute or chronic stasis dermatitis apply to the management of a stasis ulcer. The ulcer and surrounding skin should be cleaned and gently débrided. When secondary infection or excessive drainage is present, Unna's boot should not be applied. Bed rest and compresses should be continued until the infection and drainage subside. Topical antibiotic creams or sprays may be used between compresses. If cellulitis, lymphangitis, or septicemia is present, systemic antibiotic therapy is indicated. The choice of antibiotics would depend on culture and sensitivity reports.

When secondary infection has cleared sufficiently and the drainage has diminished, Unna's paste boot may be applied. Alternatively, the newer compression dressing program mentioned previously may be used.

Topical enzymes have been advocated to expedite the débridement of leg ulcers. We have not been impressed that these agents offer any advantages over the more conservative measures outlined earlier, and the patient may become sensitized to the enzymes if they are used long enough.

Dextran polymer beads (Debrisan or DuoDerm beads) are also available for cleaning infected, draining ulcers. The beads are highly hydrophilic and absorb fluid until saturated. They are expensive, however, and usually equally good results may be obtained by the measures outlined previously.

In the past few years, new dressings have been developed that do more than just cover the wound and keep it clean. These occlusive or semiocclusive dressings vary in the degree of débridement, cleaning, and wound granulation that speed the healing process. Some examples are Opsite, Tagaderm, Bioclusive, Vigalon, and DuoDerm. Most of these dressings, except DuoDerm and Vigalon, transport water, and all except DuoDerm will transport oxygen. All of these dressings absorb bacteria, except Vigalon, and only DuoDerm is not transparent. All except Vigalon are self-adhesive to the skin. Exacerbation of infection and cellulitis may occur if these dressings are used on an infected ulcer. They are best used when all infection is cleared and good granulation tissue exists and re-epithelialization is sought. Some clinical trials have indicated that ulcer healing is equally effective with the older elastic compression dressings.

If the stasis ulcer does not appear to be developing granulation tissue at a satisfactory rate with the above measures, the growth can be stimulated by the use of benzoyl peroxide (Benoxyl), an oxidizing agent widely used in the treatment of acne vulgaris. The 10% lotion is applied by cutting terry cloth to the exact size and shape of the ulcer. The cloth is moistened with isotonic saline solution, covered on one side only with benzoyl peroxide lotion (10%), and applied lotion side down to the ulcer. The normal skin margins are protected with petroleum jelly, and the padded ulcer is then occluded with plastic film. The dressing is changed every 8 to 12 hours. If excessive granulation tissue occurs, it may be cauterized with silver nitrate applicators.

Large ulcers, small ulcers that fail to respond to these conservative measures, or persistently recurring ulcers should be referred for split thickness skin grafting or pinch grafting.

## Autoeczematization

If the patient with venous insufficiency develops a generalized eczematous eruption secondary to an id (autoallergic) reaction, this can usually be controlled by topical corticosteroids and oral antihistamines such as cyproheptadine (Periactin), 4 mg four times daily, or diphenhydramine (Benadryl), 50 mg four times daily. In patients with severe autoeczematization, systemic corticosteroids, orally or intravenously, may be necessary.

## Chronic Venous Insufficiency

Once the dermatitis has subsided and the ulcerations have healed, treatment of the leg with chronic venous insufficiency must continue. It must be stressed to the patient that continuous measures are necessary to prevent future recurrences of complications. He or she should be placed in a good elastic support stocking before arising and should remove it when ready to retire at night. Patients with very large legs or those with severe edema or recurrent ulcerations should obtain individually measured Jobst pressure gradient stockings. Patients with mild to moderate venous insufficiency can usually do well with an "off-the-shelf" elastic stocking, such as the Jobst Vairox, or Sigvaris support stocking. Unless the patient has impressive thigh edema, a below-knee stocking usually suffices. If thigh edema is a problem, a leotard elastic support is usually easier to wear and more effective than the thigh-high elastic stocking.

The patient should be advised to use a lubricating cream or lotion at bedtime to keep the skin of the legs from becoming excessively dry. Exercise of the leg should be encouraged, but the patient should be instructed to avoid prolonged standing or sitting with the legs hanging down.

# PRESSURE ULCERS

method of
RICHARD M. ALLMAN, M.D.
*University of Alabama at Birmingham*
*Birmingham, Alabama*

Pressure ulcers may present as nonblanchable erythema, soft tissue loss, blisters, or eschar over bony prominences. Synonymous terms include pressure sores, decubitus ulcers, and bedsores. The term pressure ulcer reflects the primary pathophysiologic factor responsible for these lesions. Shearing forces, friction, and moisture are contributing factors to skin breakdown and may decrease the amount of pressure required for the development of a pressure ulcer. Pressure ulcer severity is reflected, in part, by the stage of the lesion. Stage 1 lesions are manifested by nonblanchable erythema of intact skin. Stage 2 ulcers involve only the epidermis and/or dermis. Stage 3 ulcers extend into subcutaneous tissues and frequently are associated with undermining. Stage 4 lesions extend through deep fascia into muscle and/or bone.

## PREVENTION

Identification of persons at risk is the first step in a rational approach to pressure ulcer prevention. Immobility is generally required for the development of pressure ulcers, but other factors may increase risk. In the acute care hospital, hypoalbuminemia, fecal incontinence, and fractures may help identify particularly high-risk immobile patients. Chair- and bedbound patients in nursing homes with impaired nutritional intake or stroke are also vulnerable. Patients with spinal cord injury, functionally impaired older patients, and persons with skin breakdown are all predisposed to the development of pressure ulcers. Prevention in such patients includes attention to the general condition of the patient, including maintenance of adequate nutrition, evaluation and treatment of incontinence, and rehabilitative measures designed to improve mobility. The use of multidisciplinary teams has been shown to be able to reduce the incidence of pressure ulcers by more than 50%.

Repositioning to relieve pressure on the sites most prone to pressure-induced cutaneous injury involves turning the patient alternately from the 30 degree left side-lying position, the supine, and the 30 degree right side-lying positions. The patient should never be repositioned at a 90 degree angle to the support surface causing direct pressure over the greater trochanter and lateral malleolus. Prolonged sitting and excessive elevation of a chair- or bedbound person's upper torso also should be avoided. The frequency of repositioning required will depend on the risk status of the patient and the support surface. High-risk patients should be placed on a pressure reducing support surface (e.g., the Geo-Matt foam mattress or the Sof-Care air mattress). Replacement foam mattresses (e.g., the DeCube mattress) with pressure reducing capabilities are also appropriate support surfaces for high-risk patients. Convoluted foam mattresses (2-inch "egg-crate" mattresses) do not lower pressures sufficiently under bony prominences for high-risk patients. Although not popular in the acute care hospital because of their weight and the possibility of leakage, water mattresses may be helpful for the prevention of pressure ulcers in some patients. Pressure reducing cushions and chairs should be available for chairbound persons. More expensive air-fluidized beds and low air-loss beds should generally be used for treatment rather than prevention (see Treatment).

Patients should be repositioned on a regular schedule in conjunction with the use of an antipressure device and careful monitoring of all bony prominences every 2 to 4 hours. If blanchable or nonblanchable erythema (a Stage 1 pressure ulcer) occurs, more frequent repositioning is required or a different antipressure device may be indicated. Despite the best efforts of all members of the health care team, all pressure ulcers may *not* be preventable.

## ASSESSMENT

Evaluation of patients with pressure ulcers should include assessment of nutritional status, continence, and underlying medical problems contributing to immobility. Pressure ulcers need to be distinguished from ulcers due to vascular disease, inflammatory disorders, primary dermatologic conditions, and malignancy. Assessment of lesions should include documentation of location, size, number, and stage. Clinical evidence of infection should also be noted: necrotic tissue, purulent drainage, odor, and/or surrounding cellulitis. Palpation and probing with a clean cotton swab are required to assess the extent of undermining of deeper lesions. Fistulograms or computed tomography may be required to define the extent of some complicated lesions. A nonhealing ulcer, an elevated leukocyte count, an increased erythrocyte sedimentation rate, and an abnormal bone radiograph or bone scan may suggest the presence of underlying osteomyelitis, but histologic examination and culture of a bone biopsy specimen are required to confirm the diagnosis. On the other hand, the use of routine swab cultures is not helpful because all pressure ulcers are colonized. Although gram-negative rods and anaerobic organisms account for most isolates from patients with pressure ulcer–associated bacteremia, nearly a third of isolates are gram-positive organisms such as *Staphylococcus aureus,* enterococci and other streptococci.

## TREATMENT

### Systemic Measures

Adequate nutrition and correction of nutritional deficiencies are critically important for patients with pressure ulcers. Protein intake is one of the most important predictors of ulcer outcome. Vitamin C, 500 mg orally twice daily, may improve pressure ulcer outcome. Zinc sulfate, 220 mg orally three times per day, may be helpful for recalcitrant ulcers.

Systemic antibiotics are indicated only for ulcers complicated by cellulitis, osteomyelitis, bacteremia, or sepsis. Because transient bacteremia occurs in as many as 50% of patients undergoing débridement of necrotic lesions, bacterial endocarditis prophylaxis may be indicated for persons with cardiac valvular lesions. Aggressive surgical débridement is required along with appropriate antibiotic treatment for sepsis, but the in-hospital mortality of pressure ulcer–associated sepsis approaches 50% or greater despite such therapy. An aminoglycoside and clindamycin (Cleocin) are appropriate initial empiric antibiotics for presumed sepsis.

### Local Wound Care

Relief of pressure at the site of the ulcer, lowering wound bacterial counts by removing all necrotic tissue, and providing a moist, clean environment in which wound healing may occur are the major components of pressure ulcer treatment. The preventive measures described previously are generally sufficient for the treatment of Stage 1 pressure ulcers. Although colonized with bacteria, Stage 2 ulcers are generally not infected clinically. If necrotic tissue is present, careful débridement accompanied by the use of wet-to-dry dressings two to three times per day is usually sufficient to lower the bacterial count and leave a clean wound base. Enzymatic débridement agents (e.g., collagenase) also may facilitate the removal of necrotic tissue, but wet-to-dry dressings and the enzymatic agents should not be used once the ulcer is clean. The healing of a clean Stage 2 ulcer is improved by the use of an occlusive dressing such as Opsite, Tegaderm, or Duoderm. Such dressings may be left in place for 2 to 3 days and facilitate epidermal migration by keeping the wound surface moist. The occlusive dressings have not been shown to improve outcome for patients with deeper or infected pressure ulcers.

In contrast to Stage 1 and 2 lesions, which may heal in a few weeks without scarring, Stage 3 and 4 lesions may require weeks to months to heal and often become chronic. Lesions totally covered by eschar require surgical débridement accompanied by the use of wet-to-dry gauze dressings moistened by normal saline. Enzymatic débridement agents may be of help. Hydrophilic agents (e.g., dextranomer [Debrisan]) may be used for suppurative wounds, but dressing changes three to four times per day are generally sufficient even for draining ulcers.

Topical antiseptics may be used for short periods to assist in lowering bacterial counts, but agents such as povidone-iodine, acetic acid, Dakin's solution, and hydrogen peroxide have all been shown to be toxic to fibroblasts and may impair wound healing. Their use should be limited to a fixed period of time (1 to 2 weeks), and they should be discontinued when the ulcer base is clean. In contrast to antiseptics, topical antibiotics, such as silver sulfadiazine (Silvadene) and gentamicin, may facilitate healing of clinically infected ulcers. The use of topical antibiotics also should be limited to fixed periods of time to avoid selection of resistant organisms, systemic toxicity, or sensitization to the antibiotic. Once the base of a Stage 3 or 4 ulcer is clean and demonstrates granulation tissue, the ulcer should be kept moist at all times by covering it with gauze dressings saturated in normal saline. Moist dressings should be kept off of surrounding intact skin. Stage 4 ulcers may be complicated by underlying osteomyelitis. Surgical removal of infected bone may be required in such cases in addition to systemic antibiotics.

Pressure-induced cutaneous injury may be manifested by the presence of a blister over a bony prominence. Until such lesions are unroofed, it is difficult to determine their stage, but they are generally at least Stage 3 ulcers. In general, the blisters should not be unroofed unless there is evidence of cellulitis or purulent drainage. If the lesions need to be unroofed, they are treated the same as other Stage 3 and 4 lesions.

### Specialty Beds

In most patients, a foam or air mattress is an adequate antipressure device for treatment as well as prevention of pressure ulcers. Such devices have a one-time cost of about $50. In contrast, air-fluidized and low air-loss beds generally cost $40 to $100 per day to use. Air-fluidized beds (e.g., Clinitron) have been shown to improve pressure ulcer outcome among hospitalized patients, particularly those with large ulcers. Patients for whom conventional measures fail and those who have multiple ulcers, so that repositioning off the ulcers is difficult, may benefit from the use of the beds. However, large Stage 3 or 4 ulcers frequently do not heal despite prolonged therapy with the air-fluidized beds. A realistic treatment goal may be to avoid deterioration of the wound in some patients.

Low air-loss beds are made with multiple fabric

cushions attached to a regular hospital-type frame (e.g., Flexicare, Kin-Air, Mediscus). These beds are able to lower pressures under bony prominences as well as air-fluidized beds, but clinical trials comparing the devices have not been conducted. Low air-loss beds may be raised or lowered, and the head and foot of the bed may be adjusted to permit the head to be elevated and transfers to be made more easily than from the air-fluidized beds. For these reasons, and their somewhat lower cost, low air-loss beds are more popular than air-fluidized beds.

### Surgical and Future Treatments

Clean Stage 3 or 4 lesions are frequently managed by the use of myocutaneous flaps among patients with spinal cord injuries. Before surgery, the ulcers need to be treated using the strategies outlined earlier until the wound base is clean and covered with granulation tissue. Ulcers with more than $10^5$ organisms per gram of tissue do not have acceptable surgical outcomes. After appropriate preparation of the ulcer, postoperative recovery generally involves a 1- to 2-week hospital stay on an air-fluidized bed with a gradual increase in weight-bearing time on the flap. Such procedures result in rapid closure of the lesions but are associated with recurrences in many patients. Older patients who are otherwise acceptable operative candidates should be considered for such treatments. Although various growth factors, topical agents, wound margin exposure to electrical stimulation, and the use of synthetic materials may prove to be beneficial in the future, the best approach to pressure ulcers will remain prevention.

# ATOPIC DERMATITIS

method of
JEROME B. KOPSTEIN, M.D.
*Windsor, Ontario, Canada*

Atopic dermatitis may be defined as a chronic cutaneous disease occurring primarily but not exclusively in individuals from families in which asthma and hay fever are prevalent. The clinical appearance and location of skin involvement are fairly characteristic. Certain fungal, bacterial, and viral infections are particularly common in these patients.

## RECOGNITION

Atopic dermatitis occurs in all racial groups, but Caucasians and Orientals are most frequently affected. The disease appears to have an unusually high prevalence in Asians emigrating to temperate areas of North America. Approximately 90% of cases appear to occur by the age of 2 years. Approximately 70% of patients have family members with atopic diseases. Adult-onset atopic dermatitis occurs rarely. Most of the new cases seen in adults are recurrences of childhood atopic dermatitis that may not be recalled. Itching is a paramount symptom. The classic presentation is in an infant with an eczematous eruption on the cheeks, anterior aspect of the legs, and dorsa of the arms. An associated diaper dermatitis is not infrequent. Scalp involvement also occurs and must be distinguished from the yellowish, greasy scales seen in seborrheic dermatitis. Nummular, or coin-like, patches, especially on extensor surfaces, may occur. These patches frequently form crusts, and a seropurulent discharge from their surfaces may occur. This variety also occurs in adults and is not always atopic in origin.

The Dennie-Morgan atopic fold is a pleat of skin around the eyes that may be an early cutaneous marker of atopic dermatitis. In black skin, the eczema tends to be more papular and may leave areas of hyper- or hypopigmentation on clearing. The infantile phase of the disease may subside or progress to the childhood variety, in which flexural eczematous patches appear, especially in the antecubital and popliteal areas. Infraorbital darkening with facial pallor also is frequently seen in children and adults with the disease. Excoriation and rubbing may lead to thickening or lichenification of the skin. The adult variety is similar, with additional involvement around the eyes and neck, although this may also be seen in the childhood variety. Accentuation of the palmar lines, with or without ichthyosis, frequently coexists with atopic dermatitis. The ichthyosis is of the dominant type (ichthyosis vulgaris).

Juvenile plantar dermatitis is a dry, scaly form of eczema that is almost always atopic in origin. It may be the only manifestation of the disease. This condition is especially prevalent in older children and teenagers, particularly males. Keratosis pilaris often coexists with atopic dermatitis and is characterized by large numbers of keratotic papules on the upper arms, the anterior thighs, and occasionally the face. Pityriasis alba is a disorder that is also likely atopic in origin and is characterized by whitish, scaly patches, especially on the face and arms. It may persist for long periods, often into the twenties or even the thirties. Chronic hand eczema, especially in young adult women, is often seen, and a history of atopic disease is frequently obtained in this group. Primary household irritants are etiologically important in these patients. Similarly, much industrial contact dermatitis of the primary irritant variety occurs in atopic individuals, which accounts for its frequent intractability.

## PRECIPITATING FACTORS

It is well known that atopic dermatitis is seasonal, with worsening especially at seasonal changes. Most atopics appear to do better during the warmer months in temperate climates if excessive humidity and high temperatures are avoided. Some appear to do better during the winter. Atopic skin appears to cope with sudden temperature changes poorly, and flare-ups may occur with prolonged exposure to cold, windy weather. Emotional factors may be operative in older children and adults and may be associated with exacerbations of the disease. The role of diet is controversial, but many believe that in infancy some foods do play a role in flare-ups of the disease (see later).

## COMPLICATIONS

Atopic patients appear to have diminished T cell numbers and functions, as well as defects in chemotaxis. IgE levels are often but not always increased. These abnormalities may account for the unusual susceptibility of these patients to herpes simplex and molluscum contagiosum infections. These infections may be quite widespread in the case of herpes simplex, causing serious, widespread inoculation lesions within the patches of eczema. This is known as Kaposi's varicelliform eruption. Systemic or oral acyclovir (Zovirax) may be required in these patients if they have severe, widespread involvement. Fungal infections with dermatophyte pathogens also appear to have an increased frequency and are responsive to oral ketoconazole (Nizoral) or griseofulvin or topical miconazole (Micatin) or clotrimazole (Lotrimin). Atopic patients are also highly susceptible to cutaneous infection with coagulase-positive staphylococci. Boils, carbuncles, folliculitis, and impetigo are seen with high frequency in patients with atopic dermatitis. However, colonization of lesions with these organisms without obvious infection is extremely frequent and may be important in causing persistence of the lesions. Scabies may coexist in patients with atopic dermatitis and may produce a clinical picture that may be unrecognizable. Nevertheless, a careful search with a hand lens may reveal burrows around the wrists, axillary folds, breasts, or penis. Scrapings suspended in mineral oil may reveal the acari under low-power microscopy. The use of lindane in coexistent scabies and widespread atopic dermatitis may result in potentially toxic levels of the drug. Careful monitoring of such patients is required, as convulsions may occur, especially in young children. If there is any doubt about the use of lindane, physicians are advised to apply 6% sulfur in petrolatum twice daily for 3 days as an alternative therapy.

## NATURAL HISTORY AND PROGNOSIS

Atopic dermatitis tends to decrease with age, with fewer relapses during adult life. In perhaps 60 to 70% of infants and children with atopic dermatitis, the disease resolves before adulthood. However, recurrences in the form of adult hand eczema or industrial dermatitis are frequently seen after earlier remissions. It is best not to prognosticate to parents about the future in childhood atopic dermatitis. Furthermore, at least one-third of infant and childhood patients will develop bronchial asthma, and another one-third will develop hay fever.

### MANAGEMENT

There seems little doubt that infantile atopic dermatitis may be aggravated by certain foods, especially cow milk, eggs, and wheat products. It is probably better to avoid these foods when they appear to be a factor. Prolonged, restrictive diets with little or no rationale may interfere with nutrition and should not be prescribed. Anaphylactic reactions to peanuts, chocolate, and eggs are relatively rare but can be fatal. Allergy to penicillin is also more frequent in atopic individuals. Tomatoes and citrus products may produce a characteristic circumoral erythema in some of these patients. The use of a straw when ingesting liquids may be helpful in young children in whom this occurs. Wool, dust, feathers, cats, dogs, horses, and guinea pigs should be avoided. Atopic infants and children should not be allowed to play directly on household carpets, whether these are wool or synthetics. Cotton garments and socks should be worn, if possible, although smooth synthetic fabrics may be tolerated. The use of regular alkaline soap is contraindicated. Cleansing can be achieved with Cetaphil Lotion, Aveenobar, Lowila Cake, and numerous other soapless cleansers. In my opinion, bleaches, fabric softeners, and antistatic pads should be avoided in washing clothing. Double rinsing may sometimes be required to rid the clothing completely of detergents.

Topical corticosteroids are the single most important modality in the management of this disease. Most importantly in children, the least potent steroid that is effective should be used. One per cent hydrocortisone cream or ointment may be quite effective, especially in children, and there is little, if any, absorption. If it is ineffective, desonide cream (Tridesilon) or ointment and 0.2% hydrocortisone valerate (Westcort) are slightly more potent alternatives. Sometimes a diluted form of a more potent steroid may be useful. In this regard, 15 grams of 0.1% triamcinolone acetonide cream diluted to 120 or 240 grams with one of the commercial cream or ointment bases, is often effective and is quite economical. The high-potency topical steroids such as betamethasone dipropionate (Diprosone) and valerate (Valisone) or clobetasol propionate (Temovate) may have a place in localized, intractable atopic dermatitis. Widespread use for prolonged periods should be avoided because of the risk of absorption and adrenal suppression. There is also evidence that in childhood, widespread use of intermediate or strong topical steroids may delay or reduce the adolescent growth spurt. On the scalp, the alcohol–propylene glycol steroid lotions may burn and may not be tolerated. There are several light steroid creams and lotions available for use in this location. Nothing stronger than 1% hydrocortisone should be used in intertriginous sites or on the face because of the risk of atrophy and striae formation. Ichthyosis frequently coexists

with atopic dermatitis. Emollients such as petrolatum, Eucerin, Nivea, or Aquaphor should be
applied after a bath. Urea 5 to 20% ointments
often are used in ichthyosis but may burn if
applied to hot, wet skin. Similarly, lactic acid
and some of the newer hydroxy acid creams may
be useful in ichthyosis. Burning and stinging
may also be occasional problems here as well.
Tar preparations are rarely indicated in the modern management of this disease, although they
are occasionally helpful in nummular eczema.

Bath oils may be helpful in either the bath or
the shower. If applied to the entire skin in the
shower, they should be partially rinsed off. These
oils should be unscented. Lubath and Aveeno
Oilated are two bath oils that are often used.
Natural sunlight or professionally supervised
shortwave ultraviolet light therapy may be helpful in some cases of atopic dermatitis. Home sun
lamps and tanning facilities are best avoided.

Systemic corticosteroids may be indicated for
severe flare-ups that cannot be controlled by
topical therapy alone. They should be withdrawn
as soon as possible after clearing occurs. Their
use in children is difficult to justify unless an
emergency situation exists. Hospitalization may
provide great benefit in cases where the disease
has become intractable. Here intensive nursing
care with ultraviolet light, baths, and supervised
administration of ointments and oral sedation
results in rapid resolution in many cases.

Antihistamines such as hydroxyzine (Atarax)
or diphenhydramine (Benadryl) may be useful for
their sedative and antipruritic properties. The
newer nonsedative antihistamines have no antipruritic or sedative properties and are not indicated in atopic dermatitis. As previously indicated, staphylococcal infection or colonization
often occurs in these patients. Erythromycin and
cloxacillin (Tegopen) or its derivatives may be
used for frank infections. In addition, in some
cases of recalcitrant atopic dermatitis, empiric
use for 7 to 10 days may result in clearing of the
disease, presumably because of removal of staphylococcal colonization.

# FIXED ERYTHEMAS

method of
ROBERT G. CARNEY, Jr., M.D.
*University of Illinois College of Medicine*
*Urbana–Champaign, Illinois*

The fixed erythemas are a group of immune dermatoses, so named because with one exception the eruptions are more prolonged than urticarial reactions. The

potential list of causes is large and varied, but the
lesions are generally erythematous and annular.

## ERYTHEMA MULTIFORME

This is by far the most common of the fixed
erythemas. It may occur at any age, although
children are more commonly afflicted with the
more severe forms. It occurs about three times
more frequently in males.

The eruption of erythema multiforme is usually
symmetrical and may consist of erythematous
macules, urticarial plaques, or even nodules. The
most common and characteristic presentation is
"target" or "iris" lesions, which enlarge centrifugally and may show concentric rings. More severe forms have central vesicle or bulla formation, often with hemorrhage.

Erythema multiforme may affect both skin and
mucous membranes. The oral and other mucosae
are often severely affected in the major form,
called Stevens-Johnson syndrome. In this form,
bullous erythema multiforme can cause permanent damage and even death.

The reaction pattern of erythema multiforme
may be induced by a wide variety of agents. Most
common are recurrent infection with herpes simplex viruses and the *Mycoplasma* organisms.
Many drugs, notably the penicillins and sulfonamides; other infections; malignancies; pregnancy; collagen vascular diseases; sarcoidosis;
and ingestants can also be causative. The inducing agent should be diligently sought for elimination or treatment, but unfortunately cannot be
found in at least one-half of the patients.

### Treatment

Mild eruptions should be treated symptomatically. Cool compresses, oatmeal baths, calamine
lotion, and the like are helpful. If vesicles are
present, saline or Burow's 1:40 compresses may
be applied for 20 minutes several times daily.
Pruritis may be treated with oral antihistamines,
with astemizole (Hismanal) and terfenadine (Seldane) potentially useful for the easily sedated.

More severe reactions with bullae and mucous
membrane involvement may require parenteral
fluids and medications if the patient is unable to
eat or drink. Erosive oral lesions may be treated
with hydrogen peroxide 3% in combination with
Chloraseptic, diphenhydramine (Benadryl) elixir,
and/or viscous lidocaine 2% locally. Other mucosae should be lubricated liberally with antibiotic ointment, which should also prevent secondary infection. Severe ocular lesions should
lead to early ophthalmologic consultation.

The use of systemic corticosteroids, such as

intravenous hydrocortisone, 100 mg every 8 hours, or oral prednisone, 60 to 80 mg daily in divided doses, remains controversial. Parenteral steroids usually result in symptomatic relief, but probably do not alter the course of the disease. The steroids normally can be tapered over 2 to 4 weeks.

When recurrent erythema multiforme is caused by herpes simplex, prophylaxis with oral acyclovir (Zovirax), 200 mg three times daily (or in children, twice daily), is often very useful. Cimetidine, 200 mg every 8 hours, has been reported to be helpful in patients who do not respond to acyclovir.

## ERYTHEMA NODOSUM

Erythema nodosum is characterized by the sudden onset of tender, erythematous nodules on the anterior shins and, less often, thighs, arms, or elsewhere. One to six lesions are present, usually several centimeters in diameter.

Etiologic factors include drugs (especially oral contraceptives, estrogens, and sulfonamides), infections (streptococcal, acid-fast, viral, and fungal), sarcoidosis, and occasionally malignancy. Although the cause cannot be found in 30 to 50% of patients, the variants—erythema induratum (caused by tuberculosis) and erythema nodosum leprosum—serve as reminders that the cause should be diligently sought.

### Treatment

Erythema nodosum is generally a self-limited disease of 3 to 6 weeks' duration, unless the cause cannot be eliminated quickly. Bed rest, leg elevation, analgesic and anti-inflammatory agents, and mild sedation are usually all that are necessary. Bed rest and leg elevation are often contrary to the lifestyle of active students and others, but failure of the physician to stress these simple measures may prolong greatly both patient discomfort and course of disease.

In severe cases, intralesional triamcinolone (Kenalog), 2.5 mg per ml (2 ml Kenalog 40 mixed with 30 ml sterile saline), or oral prednisone, 40 to 60 mg daily in divided doses, tapered over 2 to 3 weeks, is most helpful.

### FIGURATE ERYTHEMAS

The figurate erythemas include a variety of annular and polycyclic eruptions which usually last for weeks to months. The most common condition, in widening endemic areas, is the once-rare *erythema chronicum migrans*. Historically it was seen occasionally as a mainly solitary, expanding red ring on exposed skin, usually following rickettsial or viral inoculation from a tick bite. It is now recognized as the marker for infection by the tick-borne spirochete *Borrelia burgdorferi*, the cause of Lyme disease (see article on Lyme disease).

Also not rare is *erythema annulare centrifugum*, usually one or several slowly enlarging, asymptomatic annular or polycyclic rings. Treatment is unnecessary, but causes include medication and ingestant reactions as well as infections, such as tuberculosis, ascariasis, candidiasis, Epstein-Barr virus, and streptococcal disease, so work-up is important. The same is true of the rare *erythema gyratum repens*, characterized by polycyclic waves of erythema over much of the body. About 85% of patients have an internal malignancy. Finally, *erythema marginatum*, with its narrow-bordered migratory rings, is a marker of rheumatic fever.

### Treatment

In all the figurate erythemas, treatment takes a back seat to the search for etiologic factors. Lesions are more a temporary cosmetic nuisance than they are symptomatic or harmful.

# BULLOUS DISEASES*

method of
KIM B. YANCEY, M.D., and
NOUHA DOMLOGE-HULTSCH, M.D.
*Uniformed Services University of the Health
Sciences*
*Bethesda, Maryland*

Bullous skin diseases are currently considered to be autoimmune diseases, and hence their management largely attempts to suppress the immunologic and inflammatory aspects of these reactions.

## PEMPHIGUS VULGARIS

Pemphigus vulgaris (PV) is a blistering skin disease seen predominantly in adults. This disorder is characterized by acantholysis—a process in which epidermal cells lose their cohesiveness resulting in intraepithelial blister formation. Clinically, patients with PV typically demon-

*This work was suported by USUHS Protocols G48403 and 208400 as well as NIH Grant AR 37446. The opinions or assertions contained herein are the private ones of the authors and are not to be construed as official or reflecting the views of the Department of Defense or The Uniformed Services University of the Health Sciences.

strate oral mucosal blisters and erosions as well as flaccid blisters on either normal or erythematous skin. These blisters rupture easily, resulting in denuded lesions that tend to enlarge peripherally and crust. Lesions in patients with PV usually predominate on the scalp, face, oral mucosa, neck, and flexural areas; selected cases demonstrate extensive sites of involvement. Of these sites, oral mucosal involvement is seen in approximately 90% of PV patients at some time during the course of their disease; in 50 to 70% of patients, PV originates in the mouth. In PV, blistered skin typically heals without scar formation. Postinflammatory hyper- or hypopigmentation at sites of healed lesions is common and usually resolves over several months. Patients with active PV (as well as several other skin diseases) often demonstrate a positive Nikolsky's sign—a finding whereby lateral manual pressure to perilesional skin elicits separation of a sheet of epidermal cells from its underlying base. This finding exemplifies how these patients are prone to develop widespread cutaneous denudation.

Biopsy specimens of early lesional skin from patients with PV show acantholytic blister formation within the portion of the epidermis just above the basal keratinocyte cell layer (i.e., suprabasal acantholysis). Lesional skin may also contain focal collections of eosinophils and/or neutrophils. Direct immunofluorescence microscopy of normal appearing, perilesional skin from patients with PV demonstrates deposits of IgG with or without C3 on the surface of epidermal cells. Almost all patients with active disease show evidence of IgG autoantibodies directed against epithelial cell surface antigens when their sera are studied by indirect immunofluorescence microscopy. These autoantibodies are felt to be directly responsible for lesion formation in this disease. Moreover, their titer roughly correlates with disease activity.

PV is a potentially life-threatening skin disease. Prior to the availability of systemic glucocorticosteroids, the incidence of mortality associated with this disease ranged from 60 to 90%. Current estimates suggest a mortality incidence of approximately 10%. This improved prognosis likely relates to the availability of systemic glucocorticosteroids and other immunosuppressive agents, better diagnostic capabilities, earlier institution of therapy, and more favorable management of various complications of treatment. Interestingly, current common causes of mortality in patients with PV usually directly relate to complications of therapy with systemic glucocorticosteroids. Bad prognostic factors in these patients include advanced age, extensive involvement, and a history of treatment with high doses of systemic glucocorticosteroids with or without

other immunosuppressive agents. It should be kept in mind that the severity of disease varies among patients and that in an individual patient the course of disease is unpredictable. Whereas some patients have extensive disease refractory to treatment, others may achieve remission or demonstrate moderate involvement characterized by periods of activity and remission.

### Treatment

The goal of treatment in patients with PV is to bring the eruption under control as well as lessen its severity and (if possible) its duration utilizing the minimal amount of medication. Response to treatment is determined by quantitating numbers of new lesions as well as the healing time of existing erosions. Systemic glucocorticosteroids are the mainstay of treatment. Most patients respond to prednisone in dosages of 60 to 80 mg per day in single morning or divided doses. If new lesions continue to develop after 5 to 7 days of treatment, the dosage of prednisone should be increased to approximately 2 mg per kg daily in divided doses orally. Once PV is controlled, the patient's prednisone regimen should be consolidated to a single morning dose then tapered to approximately 40 to 60 mg per day. Patients whose acute disease has been controlled usually tolerate rather rapid tapering of daily morning prednisone to the level noted earlier (i.e., 40 to 60 mg per day) and can then be converted to an alternate-day regimen. Likewise, alternate-day prednisone therapy should be tapered as tolerated. As is true for most inflammatory and immunologic disorders, one should not attempt to control acute PV or a flare of disease by either initiating, or increasing doses of, alternate-day prednisone. Such problems are best managed by increased doses of daily prednisone in either single morning or divided dose schedules.

To lessen complications of high maintenance doses of systemic glucocorticosteroids in PV patients, adjunctive therapy with a cytotoxic immunosuppressive such as azathioprine (Imuran)* or cyclophosphamide (Cytoxan)† is often initiated. However, it should be noted that these agents require several weeks (i.e., 3 to 6 weeks) to exert their effects and hence are not the first choice for control of acute flares of disease. Moreover, to lessen immunosuppression, these agents are often withheld until a patient's acute disease has been controlled and the daily prednisone dose

---

*This use of azathioprine is not listed in the manufacturer's official directive.

†This use of cyclophosphamide is not listed in the manufacturer's official directive.

has been tapered to 40 to 60 mg. Patients treated with a combination of prednisone and one of these cytotoxic immunosuppressives may be able to gradually taper and discontinue the former, relying solely on the cytotoxic agent for control of PV. In selected patients, it may be possible to gradually reduce the dose of the cytotoxic agent and eventually discontinue all therapy. Specific considerations regarding these cytotoxic agents include the following: Cyclophosphamide is typically administered to PV patients in dosages of 1 to 2 mg per kg per day. Although this agent is an excellent immunosuppressive with acknowledged efficacy in PV, it is associated with a number of significant adverse side effects such as bone marrow suppression, hair loss, hemorrhagic cystitis, urinary bladder fibrosis, sterility, teratogenicity, and some risk for development of secondary malignancies. This profile of side effects (particularly concerns related to azospermia, anovulation, sterility, and teratogenicity) suggests that cyclophosphamide may be a more suitable adjunctive agent in older PV patients. All patients treated with cyclophosphamide must receive regular clinical and laboratory evaluations. Azathioprine is also acknowledged for its effectiveness in controlling PV; the usual dosage is approximately 1 to 2 mg per kg per day. Side effects associated with azathioprine include bone marrow suppression, hepatotoxicity, teratogenicity, and some risk for development of secondary malignancies. As is true for cyclophosphamide, PV patients receiving azathioprine require regular clinical and laboratory evaluations.

A number of other agents have been successfully employed in patients with PV. These alternate therapies include methotrexate, parenteral gold, dapsone, and etretinate (Tegison)*. Each of these agents has specific limitations and adverse side effects that warrant careful and experienced management. A number of studies have also demonstrated that plasmapheresis has utility as an adjunctive technique to manage acute, refractory PV. However, such cases must be treated concomitantly with systemic glucocorticosteroids (with or without cytotoxic agents) to avoid a rebound in circulating autoantibody levels after plasmapheresis has been completed. Patients with severe disease may benefit from hospitalization and direct supportive care.

Local therapy of specific lesions includes saline or tap water wet dressings for 10 to 15 minutes every 6 to 8 hours for removal of crusts and cleaning. Bacteriologic cultures of lesions and systemic antibiotics (when indicated) are also important aspects of wound care. PV patients with involvement limited to their oral mucosa may benefit from local therapy with topical triamcinolone acetonide in an adherent base (e.g., Kenalog in Orabase). A soft diet (with or without premeal topical analgesia with viscous lidocaine) may also be useful in PV patients with oral mucosal involvement. It should be noted that it is not uncommon for lesions to have longer healing times in patients on high maintenance doses of systemic glucocorticosteroids.

## PEMPHIGUS FOLIACEUS

Pemphigus foliaceus (PF) is a variant form of pemphigus characterized by superficial sites of acantholytic blister formation. Clinically, PF patients rarely demonstrate intact flaccid blisters; instead, these patients typically exhibit superficial erosions and sites of erythema, scaling, and crust formation. Mucous membrane involvement in PF is rare. Mild cases of PF may resemble seborrheic dermatitis, whereas severe cases may produce an exfoliative dermatitis. A blistering skin disease endemic to south central Brazil known as fogo selvagem is clinically, histologically, and immunopathologically indistinguishable from PF. The major distinguishing histologic feature of PF is acantholytic blister formation superficially within the epidermis, usually just beneath the stratum corneum. Patients with PF have immunopathologic findings in common with PV patients (see earlier discussion).

### Treatment

In general, PF is a far less severe blistering skin disease than PV. Mild to moderate involvement can sometimes be successfully managed with mid- to high-potency topical glucocorticosteroids two to four times each day. Selected patients with local involvement may also benefit from intradermal injection of triamcinolone acetonide (2 to 10 mg per ml infiltrated around the edge of active lesions). More severe cases of PF require treatment with systemic glucocorticosteroids to bring disease under control. Prednisone in dosages of 40 to 60 mg per day in single morning or divided daily doses is usually effective in such patients. General considerations about the use of these agents, alternative therapies, and local wound care in patients with PF are the same as those outlined for individuals with PV.

## BULLOUS PEMPHIGOID

Bullous pemphigoid (BP) is a subepidermal blistering skin disease usually seen in elderly

---

*This use of methotrexate, gold, dapsone, and etretinate is not listed in the manufacturer's official directive.

patients. Clinically, lesions are characterized as tense blisters situated on inflamed or normal appearing skin. As lesions evolve, blisters rupture and are replaced by crusted erosions. Lesions predominate in flexural areas; 10 to 25% of BP patients demonstrate oral mucosal involvement.

Biopsy specimens of early lesional skin demonstrate subepidermal blister formation and a granulocyte-rich leukocytic infiltrate. Direct immunofluorescence microscopy of normal appearing, perilesional skin from BP patients demonstrates linear deposits of C3 with or without IgG in the epidermal basement membrane. The sera of approximately 70% of these patients contain circulating IgG autoantibodies that bind the epidermal basement membrane of normal human skin in indirect immunofluorescence microscopy. These autoantibodies are felt to deposit in the epidermal basement membrane, activate complement, and produce an inflammatory reaction that culminates in blister formation. Although useful diagnostically, there is no strict correlation between the titer of these autoantibodies and disease activity in BP patients.

### Treatment

In general, BP is a more benign blistering skin disease than PV; however, it may persist for months to years with periods of exacerbation and remission. Although the mortality rate in BP is low even in the absence of treatment, deaths may occur in elderly or debilitated patients. The mainstay of treatment for patients with BP is systemic glucocorticosteroids. Most patients respond to prednisone in dosages of 40 to 60 mg per day. Once BP is controlled, prednisone should be tapered and converted to an alternate-day regimen as described for management of patients with PV. In severe cases, patients requiring high maintenance doses of systemic glucocorticosteroids or individuals intolerant of the latter, treatment with a cytotoxic immunosuppressive may be warranted. Azathioprine or cyclophosphamide (both at dosages of 1 mg per kg per day) is an appropriate choice for such cases. The various adverse side effects of these agents have been previously listed, as well as the fact that they require several weeks to exert their maximal effect. Patients with local or minimal disease can sometimes be managed with mid- to high-potency topical glucocorticosteroids applied three to four times per day. Recommendations for care of blistered sites and erosions are the same as those suggested for patients with PV.

## DERMATITIS HERPETIFORMIS

Dermatitis herpetiformis (DH) is an intensely pruritic, chronic, papulovesicular skin disease that typically presents in early to mid-adulthood. Lesions are usually symmetrically distributed over extensor surfaces such as elbows, knees, buttocks, back, and scalp. The primary lesion in DH may consist of a papule, papulovesicle, or urticarial plaque. However, because pruritus is a prominent feature of this disease, patients may only manifest excoriations and/or crusted papules. Almost all DH patients have an associated, usually asymptomatic, gluten-sensitive enteropathy, and more than 90% express the HLA-B8, DRw3, and DQw2 haplotypes.

Biopsy specimens of early lesional skin from patients with DH reveal neutrophil-rich leukocytic infiltrates within dermal papillae. As lesions progress, edema, microvesicles, and fibrin deposits appear within dermal papillae and eventuate in subepidermal bullae. Interestingly, direct immunofluorescence microscopic examination of normal appearing, perilesional skin from patients with DH reveals granular deposits of IgA (a sine qua non for the diagnosis of this disease) and complement components within dermal papillae and along the epidermal basement membrane. Circulating IgA autoantibodies directed against normal epidermal basement membrane are not demonstrable in patients with DH. Deposits of IgA within the epidermal basement membrane of these patients are unaffected by control of disease with medication but may diminish or disappear in individuals maintained for long periods on a strict gluten-free diet.

### Treatment

The mainstay of treatment for patients with DH is dapsone.* DH patients usually respond promptly to this agent, reporting decreased pruritus and new lesion formation within 24 to 48 hours. Discontinuation of dapsone in these patients leads to recurrence of disease in a similar amount of time. In addition, it should be noted that dapsone has no effect on the gastrointestinal manifestations of this disease. All candidates for treatment with dapsone require careful pretreatment clinical and laboratory evaluations as well as close follow-up to ensure that complications are avoided, recognized, and controlled (see later).

The usual initial adult dosage of dapsone for patients with DH is 50 to 100 mg per day orally. Some patients require higher maintenance doses, though most can be controlled on less than 200 mg of dapsone per day orally. A single daily dose of dapsone is adequate for most DH patients. Patients should be treated with the lowest pos-

---

*This use of dapsone is not listed in the manufacturer's official directive.

sible maintenance dose of dapsone. In this regard, some minimal degree of disease activity is acceptable because much higher doses of dapsone may be required to completely suppress all lesions. Moreover, because DH is characterized by periods of varying severity, patients should be intermittently given lower doses of dapsone to assess their status. As stated earlier, DH is a chronic disorder that essentially always requires some form of therapy. A gluten-free diet can lessen dapsone requirements of DH patients and, if maintained carefully for sufficient time, may alleviate the necessity of dapsone completely. However, this diet must rigidly exclude gluten for as long as 6 to 12 months (or longer) to be of benefit. Careful counselling by a trained dietitian is critical for patients who want to adhere to this diet.

Hemolysis and methemoglobinemia are pharmacologic effects of dapsone. Patients treated with more than 50 mg per day of dapsone will experience hemolysis, have their hemoglobin level reduced, and develop some degree of reticulocytosis in response to treatment. Patients of Mediterranean, Asian, or black ancestry should have pretreatment determinations of glucose-6-phosphate dehydrogenase (G6PD) levels because major hemolytic events are prone to occur in patients deficient in this enzyme following oxidative stress (such as occurs with dapsone administration). Additional pretreatment evaluations include a complete hemogram, serum chemistry profile, and urinalysis. After initiation of treatment, complete hemograms should be obtained weekly for the first month, every 2 weeks for the next 2 months, and every 3 to 4 months thereafter. It should be noted that increased amounts of hemolysis may develop secondary to subsequent increases in dapsone doses. Most patients tolerate a reduced hemoglobin level as well as the appearance of methemoglobinemia; however, patients with cardiopulmonary disease are more susceptible to these effects, which reduce the oxygen carrying capacity of blood. In rare instances, dapsone induces granulocytopenia or agranulocytosis; these idiosyncratic reactions are more common during the early phase of treatment. Because dapsone is metabolized in the liver and excreted by the kidneys, it is important to monitor serum chemistry and urinalysis profiles periodically. Other less common adverse effects of dapsone include toxic hepatitis, cholestatic jaundice, peripheral neuropathy, psychosis, and drug eruptions.

## LINEAR IgA DERMATOSIS

Linear IgA dermatosis (or linear IgA disease) was formerly considered a variant of DH but is now regarded as a separate entity. Clinically, patients with linear IgA dermatosis demonstrate pruritic papulovesicular and/or urticarial lesions in an extensor distribution. Selected patients with this disorder exhibit oral mucosal involvement. Histologically, these patients develop subepidermal vesiculobullous lesions that may be indistinguishable from those seen in patients with DH or other subepidermal blistering skin diseases. Direct immunofluorescence microscopic examination of normal appearing, perilesional skin of these patients reveals linear deposits of IgA within their epidermal basement membrane. Selected patients with linear IgA dermatosis possess circulating IgA autoantibodies against normal epidermal basement membrane. However, patients with linear IgA dermatosis do not have an associated enteropathy or an increased incidence of the HLA-B8, DRw3, and DQw2 haplotypes.

### Treatment

Patients with linear IgA dermatosis respond promptly to dapsone in single daily doses between 50 and 200 mg orally. These patients require the same pretreatment and follow-up evaluations described for DH patients receiving dapsone. Because these patients do not have an associated enteropathy, there is no rationale for their treatment with a gluten-free diet.

# CONTACT DERMATITIS

method of
JOSEPH F. FOWLER, JR., M.D.
*The University of Louisville School of Medicine*
*Louisville, Kentucky*

Dermatitis is a type of inflammation of the skin that may result from endogenous or exogenous factors, or both. Contact dermatitis is a subtype resulting in a clinical cutaneous reaction pattern caused by interaction with exogenous environmental factors. The term eczema is synonymous with dermatitis, although in practice it is often used to imply an acute, severe form of dermatitis as opposed to a chronic, low-grade process. Contact dermatitis is further split into irritant contact dermatitis and allergic contact dermatitis. The more common, irritant contact dermatitis, is caused by a direct, toxic effect of an environmental agent on the skin. The immune system is not involved in the development of this type of dermatitis. Detergents, solvents, acids, and alkalis are all capable of causing a direct irritant contact dermatitis. A dose-response curve is operative for irritant contact dermatitis. For instance, a much diluted solvent or detergent may not cause skin irritation, whereas a more concentrated agent or more prolonged exposure would break down the skin's natural barriers and result in irritant dermatitis. Conversely, allergic contact dermatitis is caused by an immunologic hypersensitivity to an allergen applied to the skin. Therefore, the immune system, specifically cell-mediated immunity, must be intact for development of allergic contact dermatitis. Virtually any chemical or agent can cause allergic contact dermatitis. Poison ivy or oak *(Rhus)* is by far the most common cause in North America. Other common contact allergens include nickel, rubber compounds, preservatives, and fragrances.

Clinically, acute contact dermatitis presents with weeping, vesicular lesions with edema, crusting, and possible secondary infection. Chronic contact dermatitis usually presents with scaling, lichenified plaques, and excoriations. Both types of dermatitis are often very pruritic. The eruption shows sharp borders with angular corners and geometric outlines that suggest that an external contact occurred. Although history may identify the precipitating factor or factors, the only reliable method of diagnosing allergic contact dermatitis is by patch testing. Irritant contact dermatitis is a clinical diagnosis without definitive testing currently available.

## SKIN PROTECTION

As in many diseases, contact dermatitis is best "treated" by prevention. Once an allergen or irritant is identified, avoidance of skin contact with that material is essential. Sometimes this can be rather easily done by removing the offending agent from the home or workplace. For instance, an individual sensitive to a chemical preservative present in a skin care product can simply avoid contact with that chemical by checking the labels of products to be used. When the allergen is ubiquitous, such as formaldehyde, or when an individual is sensitive to items in the work environment, substitution of other products may not be possible. Protective gloves and clothing can be very beneficial in some instances but require continuous vigilance on the part of the affected individual. Barrier creams are of minimal benefit. For poison ivy, however, several compounds that may block the absorption of the allergen, urushiol, have shown promise and may be available soon. In the workplace, highly allergenic chemicals ideally should be present only in closed manufacturing processes where the employee's contact with the material is minimal.

Hyposensitization, or immunotherapy, as is used for pollen and food allergies, holds great theoretical interest but has failed to be beneficial for allergic contact dermatitis. Animal testing can be used to predict the likelihood of sensitization to new compounds. Pre-employment testing for prospective workers is controversial and not usually practiced.

## TREATMENT

### Acute Contact Dermatitis

Acute poison ivy dermatitis is the most common example of an acute allergic contact dermatitis. Systemic corticosteroid therapy is of great benefit and should be considered in all but mild cases of acute allergic contact dermatitis. For adults, prednisone, 40 to 60 mg per day, in two or three divided doses is the treatment of choice. Generally, this dosage should be tapered gradually, resulting in a total treatment time of 10 to 14 days. An easily remembered dosage schedule is prednisone, 10 mg four times daily for 3 days, three times daily for 3 days, two times daily for 3 days, then once daily for 3 days. Further tapering is not necessary, and steroid side effects, although possible, are very rare with this length of treatment. Tapering the treatment too soon often results in a rebound of the initial dermatitis. In cases of localized acute contact dermatitis, or in patients in whom even a short course of systemic steroids is contraindicated, a potent topical corticosteroid cream is used. Betamethasone dipropionate (Diprosone, Maxivate) or fluocinonide (Lidex) or one of many other similar brands are useful on open skin areas. Fluorinated steroids such as these, however, should not be used on the face or intertriginous areas except for periods of less than 1 to 2 weeks. Cream bases, which may provide some drying effect, are preferable to ointments, which may trap moisture.

To further enhance the drying of acute, weepy lesions, moist compresses that have a soothing effect and remove crust and debris are helpful. A clean, absorbent cloth is moistened with an astringent, such as aluminum sulfate and calcium acetate (Domeboro), or even plain tap water, and applied for 20 to 30 minutes several times a day. Alternatively, bathing in oatmeal baths (Aveeno) is useful when large body areas are involved.

Itching is often severe in acute contact dermatitis and is usually best treated by steroids rather than antihistamines. However, antihistamines initially may have an added effect and also may induce drowsiness, which may be beneficial to the patient. Hydroxyzine (Atarax), 10 to 25 mg, or diphenhydramine (Benadryl), 25 to 50 mg, two to four times daily as needed and tolerated, may be useful.

### Chronic Contact Dermatitis

In contrast to the treatment of acute contact dermatitis, systemic steroids should be used cautiously in the treatment of chronic contact dermatitis because the condition may require months or even years of therapy. The first line of treatment beyond prevention and avoidance is the use of emollients to decrease itching and reduce dryness and scaling. Lotions containing alpha-hydroxy acids, such as glycolic acid (Aqua Glycolic Lotion) or lactic acid (Lacticare), are available over the counter and are especially useful for thick, scaly plaques. Low- to medium-strength topical steroids, such as hydrocortisone valerate (Westcort), aclometasone (Aclovate), or desonide (Tridesilon), are useful. Some ointments, however, are greasy and the patient's acceptance of them must be considered when prescribing these products. Intralesional injection of triamcinolone acetonide (Kenalog), 4 to 10 mg per ml, is useful in occasional thick plaques, but caution must be exercised because of potential for atrophy. Antihistamines are of some benefit in minimizing itching, but intolerance may develop, thus limiting their effectiveness. In selected cases, Kenalog, 40 mg to 60 mg intramuscularly, which has a beneficial effect of 3- to 6-week duration, may be used without serious risk of adverse effects, but should only be employed when other more conservative measures have failed.

Rare cases of persistent severe allergic contact dermatitis may be treated with immunosuppressive agents, such as azathioprine (Imuran), or with psoralen (Oxsoralen) and ultraviolet light (PUVA). Because of the risks, costs, and commitment from the patient and physician involved, these therapies are utilized only in the most desperate cases.

# SKIN DISEASES OF PREGNANCY

method of
CHÉRIE M. DITRE, M.D., and
KEVIN D. COOPER, M.D.

*School of Medicine, University of Michigan*
*Medical Center*
*Ann Arbor, Michigan*

### SPECIFIC DERMATOSES IN PREGNANCY

#### Herpes Gestationis (HG)

Herpes gestationis, also known as bullous pemphigoid of pregnancy, is a rare recurrent vesiculobullous disease occurring in 1 in 50,000 to 60,000 pregnancies. The onset is frequently in the second trimester, but the range is generally from 9 weeks' gestation to 6 days post partum. The disease is felt to be one of exacerbations and remissions. Remission can occur within 2 weeks to 3 months post partum. Spontaneous clearing during the last 6 to 8 weeks of gestation has been

observed, but the disease is exacerbated at delivery in 75 to 80% of patients. The reoccurrence in subsequent pregnancies tends to be earlier and with more serious manifestations. So far, only four cases have been reported in blacks, which may be due to the decreased frequency of the HLA-DR4 haplotype in the black population and the finding that this haplotype is higher in the HG population. The disease begins with a prodrome of malaise, fever, nausea, headache, hot and cold sensations, burning, and pruritus. The cutaneous lesions begin as urticarial papules and erythematous polycyclic wheals. Approximately 4 weeks later, tense bullae develop. The lesions start at the umbilicus in 87% of cases and move peripherally to include the thighs, palms, and soles and may become generalized but spare the face and oral mucosa. When the bullae rupture, a hemorrhagic or brown yellow crust may remain. Uncomplicated healing without scar formation is the rule, but postinflammatory hyperpigmentation can be seen. Histologically, there is epidermal and upper dermal edema with a superficial and deep dense perivascular lymphocytic and eosinophilic infiltrate. As the edema increases, there can be found eosinophilic spongiosis, necrosis of basal cells at the dermal papillae, and subepidermal bullae. In all cases of HG, direct immunofluorescent (DIF) examination of lesional, perilesional, and normal skin reveals a band-like deposition of C3 at the lamina lucida of the basement membrane zone (BMZ) with line deposition of IgG at the lamina lucida occurring in 30 to 40% of HG patients. The complement deposition may last months to years after the disease has resolved. Indirect immunofluorescent (IIF) studies demonstrate the presence of circulating HG factor in 85 to 100% of cases, which is an IgG that fixes complement, crosses the placenta, and can be found in cord serum and can bind to the BMZ of the amnion and chorion but not to the placental syncytiotrophoblast. A pregnancy factor different from HG factor but able to fix complement on the syncytiotrophoblast has been proposed by Ortonne. His group suggests that HG factor may be induced by BMZ antigen of extravillous cytotrophoblasts. These factors may be responsible for the skin lesions in the newborn. The HG factor appears in low agglutination titers and therefore is undetectable by routine immunoelectron microscopy. Therefore, complement IIF is used and allows patients' HG factor to activate normal serum C3 to bind to the substrate along the BMZ. The HG titer does not reflect disease activity. Laboratory findings may show a leukocytosis with prominent eosinophilia in up to 50% of cases.

The pathophysiology of HG is not yet known, but hormonal modulation may play a significant role as suggested by recurrence of the disease in subsequent pregnancies, menstruation, or oral contraceptive usage. Maternal prognosis is excellent, whereas infant prognosis is debated. Perhaps the advent of steroids has decreased the frequency of premature labor, and the average gestation is now 39 weeks with minimal fetal risk.

The incidence of small for gestational age infants may be increased, but stillbirths are not. When the patient is in the bullous stage of the disease, treatment consists of prednisone, 40 mg per day, which is then tapered slowly; the dose is increased immediately post partum to prevent a flare.

Plasmapheresis has been used successfully during and after gestation. Further, newborn cutaneous disease is transient, resolving over days to week's and long-term sequelae are not known, but so far no increase in autoimmune disease has been seen. The clinical, histopathologic, and immunologic features of HG and bullous pemphigoid (BP) are somewhat similar, and one group of investigators has suggested renaming HG pemphigoid gestationis. Nevertheless, there are dissimilarities that allow one to differentiate between the two. First, HG occurs in young pregnant females for a short period of time, has an increased frequency of umbilical predilection, and is exacerbated by hormonal influences such as pregnancy or oral contraceptives. Second, histopathology of HG shows isolated necrotic basal keratinocytes not found in BP. Furthermore, immunologically there is an increased frequency of HLA-B8, -DR-3, and -DR4 antigen and anti-HLA antibodies, whereas there is normal HLA antigen in BP. HG factor can more effectively fix complement than BP antibody. IgG is more readily detected in 70% of patients with BP, as compared with 30 to 40% in HG. There is one case report by Holmes describing an evolution of HG into BP.

## Pruritic Urticarial Papules and Plaques of Pregnancy (PUPPP)

Originally described by Lawley in 1979, PUPPP is now considered a distinct and specific dermatosis of pregnancy. Retrospective studies have helped to differentiate it from Bourne's toxemic rash of pregnancy and Nurse's prurigo of pregnancy. PUPPP is felt to be more common than HG, but figures are lacking. PUPPP is seen in 71 to 76% of primigravidas and therefore is felt to be a disease of first pregnancies. According to Yancey's study, there was no tendency toward recurrence in subsequent pregnancies or with oral contraceptives. However, Holmes and col-

leagues state that though recurrence is rare, it is also less severe. About 90% of patients report erythematous papules and urticarial plaques with 48% having urticated abdominal striae and disease presenting in the abdomen. There is severe pruritus in 88% but minimal excoriations, which occur after the thirty-fourth week of gestation. Generally the lesions are less than 2 mm and bullae are not seen. The disease is usually confined to the abdomen but can generalize. Lack of facial involvement was felt to be a consistent feature, but Alcalay now disputes this. Carruthers believes that facial involvement is a Koebner or isomorphic phenomenon. The histologic appearance consists of early epidermal and upper dermal edema with a superficial and mid-dermal perivascular lymphocytic infiltrate with prominent eosinophilia in 24%. Vesicular spongiosis and papillary dermal edema can be found and lead to subepidermal vesicle formation. DIF was negative in 76%, with few weakly positive granular C3 at the dermal-epidermal junction. There are no laboratory abnormalities. The reoccurrence of urticaria during lactation suggests hormonal modulation. The treatment is topical steroids to control the pruritus. Difficult cases may require prednisone, 40 mg per day. There have been no fetal or maternal complications, though there is one report of a newborn with erythema neonatorum in a mother with PUPPP. Congenital abnormality is not seen. Hormonal evaluations show no difference from controls in beta-hCG–estradiol, estriol, and cortisol levels.

**Relationship Between PUPPP and HG.** HG begins in the second trimester and remits after 34 weeks' gestation, at the time PUPPP is felt to begin. HG flares post partum, when PUPPP resolves. HG shows complement deposition at the BMZ of lesional skin; such deposition is not seen in PUPPP. Immunogenetic studies show increased HLA-B8 and -DR3 with HG but not with PUPPP.

## Prurigo Gravidarum (PG)

Also known as intrahepatic cholestasis of pregnancy, PG is generally seen in the last trimester and is characterized by generalized pruritus but without primary skin or liver disease. The incidence of PG has been reported as 0.02 to 2.4%. Excoriations are common and may be the only overt manifestation. In more severe cases, clinical jaundice is found with laboratory evidence of cholestasis and a positive liver biopsy for centrizonal patchy dilatation of bile canaliculi and accumulation of bile pigment with layered mitochondria in parenchymal cells; this is a distinct entity from the acute fatty liver of pregnancy. The pruritus, jaundice, and laboratory abnormalities all resolve post partum and may recur in subsequent pregnancies or on oral contraceptives. Laboratory abnormalities include possible increased alkaline phosphatase above normal pregnancy levels from the placental unit; slight increase in gamma-glutamyl transpeptidase; bilirubinemia below 5 with a normal to modest increase in aspartate aminotransferase, prothrombin time, and lactate dehydrogenase; and a 10 to 100× increase in serum bile acids with an abnormal lipoprotein X in the serum. Natural and synthetic estrogens have been shown to produce cholestatic effects by interfering with normal diffusion of fluid across the canalicular membrane of the hepatocyte. The mechanism is felt to be inhibition of hepatic glucuronyl transferase by progesterones and therefore decreased clearance of estrogen from blood leading to bilirubin-impaired conjugation and excretion and decreased storage. It also has been suggested that there is an alternate bile acid synthesis pathway producing pruritogenic cholesterol metabolites. In any event, the level of serum bilirubin does not correlate with the degree of pruritus or the incidence of complications as previously thought.

### Impetigo Herpetiformis (IH)

In 1872, von Hebra described IH as a rare and serious variant of pustular psoriasis precipitated by and recurring with pregnancy. Because all of von Hebra's five patients were pregnant females, this disease was felt to be a dermatosis of pregnancy. Since that time, other authors have noted this condition in men and nonpregnant females and in patients with hypoparathyroidism and hypocalcemia, and therefore its classification as a specific dermatosis of pregnancy is in doubt. Nevertheless, it is generally seen in the third trimester but may present as early as the third month and in patients with a history of psoriasis. So far, only 100 cases have been reported. The cutaneous lesions consist of irregular erythematous patches beginning in intertriginous areas— e.g., axillae, nape of neck, groin, inframammary folds, gluteal crease—that then extend centrifugally, sparing the face, hands, and feet. Hundreds of superficial, sterile, pinhead-sized pustules develop at the periphery of the erythematous patch and can be arranged in groups or rings. As the pustules break down centrally, impetiginization results, with activity at the margin. Advancing vegetating verrucous plaques may also develop in moist flexural areas. Pruritus is not a major problem. There can be painful mucous membrane involvement of oral mucosa, esophagus, and tongue and respiratory tract; subungual pustules may cause onycholysis. The cutaneous eruptions are accompanied by malaise, fever, delirium, diarrhea, vomiting, and tetany secondary to decreased calcium and dehydration. As many as 25% of patients have serious complications of hyperthermia or renal or cardiac failure secondary to the enormous loss of albumin and calcium. It is important to note that increased temperature, leukocytosis with lymphopenia, increased uric acid, hypoalbuminemia, and hypocalcemia can be seen in both IH and pustular psoriasis.

Histologically, IH is identified by the spongiform pustule of Kogoj, which is a large collection of neutrophils within a focus of spongiotic epidermis. Also seen are parakeratosis, elongated rete ridges, and migration of mononuclear cells from dermal capillaries into epidermis. DIF and IIF are negative. This picture can also be seen in Reiter's disease (keratoderma blenorrhagica), Hallopeau's acrodermatitis continua, and von Zumbusch's gene. In pustular psoriasis, the differential diagnosis would also include autoimmune progesterone dermatitis of Bierman and when impetiginized may resemble HG, subcorneal pustular dermatosis, infectious impetigo, and DH.

The pathophysiology of IH is unknown but may be an outbreak of pustular psoriasis in a latent psoriatic patient triggered by the hormonal milieu of pregnancy.

Treatment consists of prednisone, 15 to 30 mg per day, with antibiotics for any secondary infection. Hypocalcemia should be corrected and fluid balance maintained. If prednisone is used, placental estrogen decrease and urine or serum *estriol cannot be used to monitor fetal well-being*. Therefore, oxytocin challenge with measurement of the lecithin/sphingomyelin ratio should be used as a monitor. Prior to steroids, abortion, stillbirth, and neonatal death were frequent. Now maternal mortality is rare, but stillbirth and placental insufficiency may occur and fetal monitoring is advised. The disease remits post partum but may recur in subsequent pregnancies.

*Autoimmune progesterone dermatitis of pregnancy* is the name describing the lesion in a single report by Bierman in 1973 of an East Indian woman who in two successive pregnancies developed an acneiform eruption on her extremities and buttocks associated with arthritis and a positive intradermal skin test to progesterone. Both pregnancies were spontaneously aborted. This entity is distinct from that *not* associated with pregnancy in which 7 to 10 days prior to menses a pruritic, vesiculobullous or urticarial eruption develops on the trunk or extremities and can be seen with synthetic progesterone use. In Bierman's patient, her cutaneous eruption of follicular and perifollicular comedones and papules began on the fingers, arms, and legs and spread to her buttocks. The pustules became firm, turbid, and tender, and an associated arthritis of the wrists, knees, and metacarpophalangeal joints ensued. She was challenged later with oral contraceptives, and the dermatitis and arthritis recurred.

On laboratory evaluation, serum IgG and IgM were increasing and an abscess was caused at the intradermal injection site of progesterone but not with estrogen.

Histologically, the lesion showed an acanthotic epidermis with focal spongiosis and exocytosis of lymphocytes and histiocytes. A predominance of eosinophils was seen throughout the dermis, and the subcutaneous tissue contained a lobular panniculitis with abscess formation. DIF and IIF were negative. The pathophysiology is felt to be hypersensitivity to endogenous progesterone.

### Linear IgM Dermatosis of Pregnancy

Alcalay and colleagues have reported a case of a woman in her third trimester having an intensely pruritic, red, 2 to 4 mm dome-shaped follicular papular eruption occurring symmetrically on her forearms, abdomen, thighs, and legs with a few pustules. The histopathology showed irregular acanthosis of epidermis and mid-dermal perifollicular fibrosis with perivascular infiltrate of lymphocytes and neutrophils. There was no evidence of folliculitis. DIF of perilesional skin revealed dense linear IgM along the dermal-epidermal junction. IIF was negative. The patient delivered at 40 weeks, and 6 weeks post partum the eruption disappeared. Repeat DIF examinations were negative near the original biopsy sites. Allergic contact dermatitis was excluded by patch tests. Alcalay and associates feel that the occurrence of the disease in the third trimester with resolution post partum entitles this entity to be ranked with specific dermatoses of pregnancy.

# PRURITUS ANI AND VULVAE

method of
REES B. REES, M.D.
*University of California School of Medicine*
*San Francisco, California*

In pruritus ani and vulvae, itching of the anogenital area—chiefly nocturnal—occurs. Skin changes may be absent on overt examination, or excoriations, inflammation, and even lichenification may be seen. Rare malignancies, such as Bowen's disease or extramammary Paget's disease may be present, with skin changes so inapparent that biopsy may be necessary. If lichenification is present, scraping the lesion may

yield scales that show dermatophyte or yeast infection when examined microscopically in sodium or potassium hydroxide 15%.

### GENERAL CONSIDERATIONS

Usually no obvious cause of the condition exists but may be lichen simplex chronicus; intertrigo; seborrheic dermatitis; inverse psoriasis; general uncleanliness; or contact dermatitis from soaps, bubble baths, colognes, douches, contraceptives, and irritating secretions. Diarrhea, leaky anal sphincter, leukorrhea, or trichomoniasis also may be present.

In women, pruritus ani by itself is rare, but up to 10% of gynecologic patients may have pruritus vulvae. When all possible causes have been ruled out, the words "idiopathic" or "essential pruritus" may be used. Deep gluteal clefts, moisture, friction, chafing, or sitting or standing too long may be at fault.

Proctoscopic examination is usually not helpful. Erythrasma is seen with a Wood's light as a coral red fluorescence. It is cured by topical and oral erythromycin.

### TREATMENT

The anogenital area should be cleaned with plain water after each trip to the lavatory. Moistened toilet paper or paper towels will suffice, although the ideal cleaning method is use of a douche or a bidet. Diabetes should be ruled out and treated if present. Stool examinations are rarely conclusive. Spicy food should be curtailed.

Topically, 1% hydrocortisone ointment is useful and safe. Creams contain suspending agents and preservatives, which may themselves cause pruritus. Rule out oral medications that might be contributory. Potent topical corticosteroids may lead to pseudoatrophy and striae formation. Painting the involved areas with a tightly wound cotton-tipped applicator dipped in Castellani's solution or 1% aqueous gentian violet may be helpful if applied sparingly. This should only be applied in the office (repeated use may be irritating) but may give instant relief. Sitz baths with a quarter cup each of baking soda and starch may be used if subacute inflammation is present.

# URTICARIA

method of
ROBERT P. WARIN, M.D.
*Department of Dermatology, Bristol Royal*
  *Infirmary*
*Bristol, England*

### ANTIHISTAMINES USED FOR URTICARIA

#### H₁ Antagonists

$H_1$ antagonists were introduced about 1946 and until the 1980s their use was limited by side effects, particularly drowsiness. In 1982 terfenadine (Seldane; Triludan in UK, Teldane in many other countries) and a few years later astemizole (Hismanal) became available and sedative side effects are no greater than those experienced with a placebo tablet. Terfenadine is now the drug of choice unless it is thought that a mild sedative side effect is of value in a particular patient. Also, if cost is a prime consideration, chlorpheniramine is considerably less expensive. The effect of terfenadine is maximum after 4 to 8 hours and lasts some 12 to 24 hours after stopping treatment. It is usually given in a dose of 60 mg twice per day, but it is now available as a single daily dose of 120 mg.*

Astemizole is unique in its long action and indeed it can be shown to be effective some 3 weeks after administration. It takes 1 to 2 days to reach its maximum effect and is usually given in a dose of 10 mg once per day.

The only substantiated side effect of terfenadine and astemizole is weight gain, perhaps more obvious with astemizole. This is due to an appetite stimulating effect, which was noted with some of the older antihistamines and can be controlled by diet.

Recently a number of new drugs were introduced, including cetirizine† (Zirtek†), loratadine (Claritin)†, mequitazine (Primalan)†, and acrivastine (Semprex†). These new agents are probably satisfactory drugs that usually don't have drowsy side effects, but they show little advantage over terfenadine, which has been used in vast amounts throughout the world. Because of the absence of drowsiness with terfenadine it has been possible to give very large doses. However, it has been found that doses three or even four times the usual dose of terfenadine have no more effect, presumably because mediators other than those that can be inhibited by $H_1$ antagonists play an important part in urticarial wheal production.

The efficacy of $H_1$ antagonists in urticaria largely depends on the severity of the wheal production. In severe acute attacks even large doses of $H_1$ antagonists are to a large extent swamped by the intensity of wheal production, whereas in less severe states the wheals can be completely suppressed. The $H_1$ antagonists all have other pharmacologic actions, such as an antiserotonin effect in some, but there is no clear evidence that these other pharmacologic actions are of benefit. Changing the antihistamine or giving two different antihistamines may have a use in the general management of some of these difficult cases.

---

*Only a 60-mg tablet is available in the United States.
†Not available in the United States.

## Other Antihistamines and Related Drugs

$H_2$ antagonists, cimetidine (Tagamet), and ranitidine (Zantac), when added to $H_1$ antagonists, have a slightly greater effect on the wheal of dermatographism, but there is debate as to their overall value in management of these cases or in chronic urticaria.

Beta-adrenergic agents, such as epinephrine (Adrenalin), are helpful in severe attacks and ephedrine is sometimes of value in chronic urticaria. Terbutaline (Brethine), ketotifen,* and oxatomide* have also been used, but with variable results, and are not recommended for urticaria. Tricyclic antidepressants are known to exert a potent $H_1$ antagonist effect, and amitriptyline (Elavil) and doxepin (Sinequan) are of use, particularly if there is some underlying depression.

## MANAGEMENT

### Acute Urticaria

Most cases settle down after a period of rest. $H_1$ antagonists help but in very severe attacks a course of systemic corticosteroids is indicated.

If an associated angioedema is severe or serious anaphylactic complications occur, the immediate treatment is with epinephrine (Adrenalin), 0.5 to 1.0 ml of the 1:1000 preparation intramuscularly and 0.5 ml repeated every 20 to 30 minutes as necessary.

### Chronic Urticaria

Drugs, food, and infective agents may be pinpointed as the cause, but in at least 80% of patients with chronic urticaria the essential cause is not clear. However, various agents can increase the urticarial tendency and give rise to exacerbations. For example some 30 to 40% of patients with chronic urticaria have exacerbations after taking salicylates. Azo dyes, benzoic acid preservatives, and possibly yeasts and other substances may have a similar effect. Such exacerbating factors may be determined by diet studies or the use of challenge tests. Similarly, attacks of fever from various causes frequently effect exacerbations. Often, a constitutional and nervous factor is involved and patients pass through phases when the urticaria is present. These times may well coincide with difficult or stressful periods in their lives. It is common at the menopause and often exacerbations occur in the premenstrual phase.

Many cases of chronic urticaria last for a period of 6 to 12 months and then naturally settle down.

---

*Not available in the United States.

Obviously the treatment at that point will erroneously be acclaimed as successful.

The use of $H_1$ antagonists is always indicated but in a few cases the condition drags on, sometimes with severe exacerbations. As would be expected, all sorts of drugs have been used and go in and out of fashion, but the desperate physician may well want to try some of these miscellaneous treatments, which range from autohemotherapy to calcium gluconate, heparin, tranexamic acid (Cyklokapron),* and anabolic steroids. Systemic corticosteroids will undoubtedly clear most cases of chronic urticaria but if the condition persists there are all the dangers and disadvantages of prolonged corticosteroid therapy. I believe it is much better to reserve such corticosteroid treatment for severe cases in which all other modes of treatment have failed.

### Angioedema

Although angioedema occurs commonly in association with both acute and chronic urticaria, a few patients have recurrent angioedema with no or very insignificant accompanying urticarial wheals.

In patients with recurrent angioedema it is of course important to exclude an intermittently taken drug or food.

Once angioedema has developed it is probably not affected by $H_1$ antagonists. If, however, the attacks are occurring frequently it may be worthwhile taking an $H_1$ antagonist quite regularly over long periods. This is now quite easy by virtue of the lack of sedative side effects.

### Delayed-Pressure Urticaria

In this condition deep wheals develop some 4 to 6 hours after pressure from, for example, clothing, standing on a ladder, working with tools, and carrying weights. The wheals last 1 to 2 days. Formerly this condition was considered among the physical urticarias, but it is now realized that in the majority of cases acute or chronic urticaria is also present. Once the swelling has developed $H_1$ antagonists appear to have little or no effect but are often given because of an associated chronic urticaria. Pressure urticaria may be just a minor nuisance or so severe that it requires a change of occupation or markedly limits social activities. Systemic corticosteroids are effective and may be used if the condition is very severe. They may also be given intermittently to reduce threatened attacks.

*This use of Cyklokapron is not listed in the manufacturer's official directive.

### Urticarial Vasculitis

In the past, 1 to 2% of patients with chronic urticaria have been said to have evidence of vasculitis on histologic examination, including patients with systemic lupus erythematosus. It is now known that a greater percentage show histologic changes of vasculitis, and various recent series report an incidence of 5% or even more. In severe grades of urticaria vasculitis the wheals tend to last longer, may be present for 2 to 3 days, and leave purpuric staining. Otherwise, the eruption cannot be clinically distinguished. A small group of patients with vasculitis also have a complement abnormality and in some cases have joint and renal involvement.

Urticarial vasculitis responds well to systemic corticosteroids, but large doses are often necessary and the treatment has to be continued for a long period of time. Even in the face of vasculitis, $H_1$ antagonists help to some extent. In many cases of proven vasculitis it is possible to avoid systemic corticosteroid therapy.

### Physical Urticarias

**Dermatographism.** Systematic dermatographism is associated with large wheals on scratch trauma giving rise to paroxysms of itching. Skin that has been repeatedly exposed to sunlight and weathering does not show dermatographism as readily as skin that has remained covered. Sunbathing or ultraviolet light therapy can often be helpful in management of this condition. $H_1$ antagonists reduce the whealing tendency and may need to be continued for months or years. As these patients are often young adults continuing with their jobs or study, use of the nonsedating antihistamines has been of great value.

**Cholinergic Urticaria.** Cholinergic urticaria occurs in response to exercise, general heat, or emotional stress, and occasionally after spiced foods or alcoholic drinks. Often there are mixtures of these factors and the condition is quite common in minor degrees. As with dermatographism young adults are most commonly affected. The characteristic wheals are small—2 to 3 mm in diameter—but in very severe cases they may merge together. The wheals last only 0.5 to 1 hour. They are helped a great deal by $H_1$ antagonists and if the attacks are very frequent and severe the patient may have to continue with quite regular treatment over periods of months or years.

**Cold Urticaria.** Essential acquired cold urticaria is a common disorder, especially in minor degrees. The main stimulus to the urticaria is a drop in temperature of the exposed skin and the wheals clear in 0.5 to 1 hour. If the whealing is widespread, severe syncope may occur, and loss of consciousness as a result of this has occasionally been responsible for deaths from drowning in cold water.

$H_1$ antagonists reduce the whealing and in the colder weather may need to be taken quite regularly. It has been said that cyproheptadine (Periactin) and doxepin (Sinequan) have had more effect than other $H_1$ antagonists but this is very doubtful and probably the best treatment is to use terfenadine, astemizole, and other nonsedative $H_1$ antagonists. Some cases have improved after so-called desensitization by exposure to cold water, gradually increasing the extent of the body exposed and the time of exposure. This treatment is often difficult to undertake but in a few severe cases and with a stoic patient it has helped.

### Hereditary Angioedema

This is inherited as a deficiency of the $C_1$ inhibitor. A definitive diagnosis is made in the laboratory. The swellings often arise spontaneously but may occur at the site of trauma. They also occur in the intestinal tract, giving rise to attacks of colicky pain. The danger is edema of the larynx and adjacent parts of the respiratory tract, leading to respiratory obstruction and asphyxia. Anabolic steroids taken regularly will reverse the biochemical deficiency; the use of danazol (Danocrine), 200 to 800 mg daily, or stanozolol (Winstrol), 2.5 to 5.0 mg daily, has transformed the management of these cases. For acute attacks with impending laryngeal edema, a purified preparation of $C_1$ inhibitor in serum has become available and is given intravenously.

# PIGMENTARY DISORDERS

method of
VICTOR D. NEWCOMER, M.D.
*Santa Monica, California*

Disturbances of pigmentation may result from the exogenous or endogenous deposition of chemicals or drugs in the skin. Changes in the normal pattern of melanin deposition represent the most frequently encountered disturbances of pigmentation. There may be an increase or decrease in the number of melanocytes or an increase or decrease in melanocytic activity or an impairment of pigment transfer mechanisms. The best known function of the melanocyte is the production of melanin in response to actinic radiation. However, the melanocyte is exquisitely sensitive to a variety of external and internal stimuli and its normal function may be modified by practically every disease that involves the skin. It is therefore essential to establish a definitive diagnosis before initiating therapy. Some of the more commonly encountered pigmentary changes are presented in this article.

## TANNING

Tanning is a protective physiologic hyperpigmentation that develops in response to exposure to actinic radiation or artificial sources of ultraviolet-B radiation (UVB 280 to 320 nm) and ultraviolet-A radiation (UVA 320 to 400 nm). Sun exposure has become of increasing medical concern, as it is now clearly established that it is these same UV rays that on chronic exposure play a key role in the production of photoaging changes in the skin and the development of actinic keratoses, basal cell carcinomas, squamous cell carcinomas, and melanomas. Sunbathing is currently in vogue, and individuals are living longer and spending more time out of doors and wearing less clothing. Further, the thinning of the ozone layer is permitting more ultraviolet light to reach the surface of the earth.

In addition, many individuals are exposed to a variety of drugs, cosmetics, and industrial and environmental chemicals that have phototoxic potentials. Other than the esthetic factors and the minimal amount of sunlight needed for the production of vitamin D in the elderly, tanning has few redeeming features, and excessive and chronic sun exposure more than any other single factor, is responsible for aging of the skin before its time. Redheads and blondes who do not have good melanocytic defenses against actinic radiation are most susceptible to the photoaging process, but brunettes and even blacks will develop sun-damaged skin with excessive sun exposure.

Sunbathing and the use of "sunparlors" and other sources of UV radiation should be discouraged. Tightly woven, lightweight clothing offers an excellent protection against actinic radiation. Outdoor activities may be planned before 10 a.m. or after 4 p.m., when UVB rays are less prevalent in the earth's atmosphere. A tan does not provide sufficient protection against further sun damage, and its effectiveness in preventing erythema is rated a sun protective factor (SPF) of 2 to 3.

Sunscreens offer the best currently available protection against the sun for those parts of the body that cannot be protected by clothing. They are given an SPF rating according to their ability to prevent erythema, one response of normal skin to UVB. The higher the SPF number, the greater the degree of protection against UVB.

A sunscreen with a high SPF (15 or greater), which usually contains a combination of at least two UV light absorbers, should be used. These currently usually include an ester of para-amino benzoic acid (PABA) and a benzophenone, the combination of which offers maximum protection against UVB and UVA. (Sundown, Presun 15, Total Eclipse 15, Sundare 15, and Supershade are some of the commercial preparations that are currently available.)

Until recently, available sunscreens have provided at best only limited protection against UVA. Photoplex is a newly introduced sunscreen that absorbs radiation throughout the UVA waveband and is also highly effective against UVB (SPF 15+).

Precautionary measures regarding tanning apply particularly to children because mounting evidence suggests that 50 to 80% of the total accumulative photodamage occurs during the first 20 years of life, and it has been predicted that the regular use of sunscreens with a SPF of 15 or greater during childhood and adolescence would reduce the lifetime incidence of nonmelanoma skin cancer by as much as 70 to 80%.

The ideal sunscreen is as yet not available, and the effectiveness of all sunscreens in actual use has yet to be determined, so that one must be cautious in assuring an individual that if sunscreens are used consistently, unlimited amounts of time can be spent in the sun and photoaging will be totally prevented.

There is some evidence that even chronically sun-damaged skin may improve with time if further sun damage is avoided. Recent clinical and laboratory evidence suggests that topically applied tretinoin (Retin-A) can reverse the skin damage due to excessive chronic sun exposure.

Tretinoin therapy is to be used indefinitely, starting with daily application for up to 8 months and then twice-weekly application thereafter.

However, all current information about tretinoin is still of a short-term nature, and a recently convened 14-member panel of the National Institutes of Health found that available evidence was insufficient to recommend the use of tretinoin and similar compounds for the treatment of sun-induced wrinkles.

## MELASMA

Melasma and chloasma are terms used to describe an acquired hypermelanosis involving primarily the face and, to some degree, the neck. It usually develops slowly and symmetrically and is not preceded or accompanied by inflammation.

The disease predominantly affects women who are pregnant, who are taking oral contraceptives, or who are heavy users of cosmetics, although there are many instances in which none of these factors is present.

Chloasma of pregnancy usually develops during the third trimester (50 to 70%) and will generally disappear shortly after delivery. Chloasma is the most commonly encountered skin reaction (8 to 29%) associated with the use of oral contraceptives, and the cosmetically concerned individual should be advised to discontinue their use at the earliest appearance of such pigmentary changes, as they are not as readily reversible as the chloasma of pregnancy and may be permanent; however, most disappear spontaneously after menopause.

Excessive sun exposure adversely affects melasma irrespective of the cause, and the avoidance of actinic radiation and similar radiation from artificial sources is essential for the successful management of this condition.

Most cosmetic companies offer a "cover up" line of cosmetics that not only soften the effects of the blotchy pigmentation into a more acceptable pattern but also act as a total sunscreen. Covermark is a tinted, inert, opaque makeup that is highly effective in covering pigmentary lesions and is also an effective sunscreen. If such occlusive makeup is unacceptable to the patient, sunscreens containing specific chemicals that absorb UV light are better tolerated, preferably a sunscreen with an SPF of 15, or higher, that is formulated to block out both UVB and UVA. Some of the sunscreens that fulfill these criteria are Bain de Soleil, Ultra Sun Block Creme, Super Shade, Total Eclipse Sunscreen, Presun 15 Lotion, and Photoplex.

RVPaque and Solar Cream both contain PABA in an opaque base, thus combining the benefits of opaque and chemical absorbers.

"Bleaching" preparations containing hydroquinone appear to be moderately effective in a significant number of patients. Eldopaque Forte contains 4% hydroquinone in an opaque base and Solaquin contains both 2% hydroquinone and compounds of PABA and benzophenone in an opaque base.

Depigmentation of melasma has been achieved within 6 weeks of therapy by applying a lotion containing hydroquinone 2% to 5% and 0.05% retinoic acid twice a day. Little benefit from such therapy will result if actinic radiation is continued or if the patient continues to take birth control pills.

Agents that contain monobenzyl ether of hydroquinone (Benoquin) should not be used because of the high risk of permanent depigmentation. Confetti-like permanent depigmentation and ochronosis-like pigmentary changes have rarely been associated with the use of hydroquinone, but the patient should be carefully monitored for the appearance of these disturbing side effects, and, if encountered, therapy should immediately be discontinued.

## POSTINFLAMMATORY MELANOSIS

Postinflammatory melanosis may follow inflammation produced by a variety of irritants such as thermal or chemical burns and is also associated with a variety of dermatoses. If the areas are protected from sunlight and further irritation, the hyperpigmentation will generally fade. This process can be hastened in some instances with the use of creams containing hydroquinone.

## DRUG-RELATED HYPERPIGMENTATION

Hyperpigmentation of the skin may also result from deposits of drugs in the dermis or as the result of disturbances in melanin formation or as the result of both mechanisms. The pigmentary disturbances may be either localized or generalized in nature. The early recognition of such pigmentary changes is highly desirable, as the pigmentation changes will disappear slowly upon discontinuation of drug use, but in some instances, the pigmentary changes are permanent.

The brown to bluish gray discoloration of the skin following the systemic or local administration of medicaments of silver, gold, arsenic, and bismuth is the result of the deposit of these metals in the skin, and there is currently no successful method for their removal. Hyperpigmentation has been associated with the administration of such drugs as phenytoin (Dilantin) and related compounds; the antimalarials, particularly mepacrine; oral contraceptives; chlorpromazine (Thorazine) and related compounds; busulfan (Myleran); bleomycin (Blenoxane); cyclophosphamide (Cytoxan); tetracycline; minocycline (Minocin); and amiodarone (Cordarone).

## FIXED DRUG ERUPTIONS

These eruptions frequently present with localized areas of various sizes up to 20 cm of increasing hyperpigmentation, with the preceding inflammatory changes being only slightly noticed. Numerous drugs are capable of inducing such reactions. Phenolphthalein (Ex-Lax, Modane), salicylates, tetracyclines, sulfonamides, quinidine, and phenacetin are among the more commonly encountered medications. The pigmentation will slowly fade if the offending medication is discontinued.

## CAROTENODERMA

A yellow-orange discoloration of the skin, carotenoderma results from ingestion of a diet of vegetables high in carotenoids. Discoloration is most marked on the palms and soles and the paranasal areas. Mucous membranes and sclerae are not involved. There is an increased incidence of carotenoderma in patients with diabetes mellitus and myxedema. Beta-carotene is used for the treatment of several skin diseases, and yellow discoloration of the skin is not an unusual side effect. The discoloration is only of cosmetic concern, and if the vegetables are discontinued or consumed in moderation or the medication discontinued, the discoloration will gradually disappear.

## TATTOOS

Tattoos are produced by the mechanical introduction of insoluble pigments into the skin either for decorative purposes or accidentally following explosions or accidents in which foreign material is ground into the skin. In accidental tattooing, the foreign material should be removed as soon as possible using soap and water, gentle brushing, curetting, and so on.

When feasible, surgical excision offers the most satisfactory approach to removal of decorative tattoos. Dermabrasion (rubbing salt into the area) and the use of the laser are alternative techniques also offering varying degrees of success depending on the size of the tattoo, the location of the tattoo, and the experience and skill of the operator.

## LENTIGINES

Lentigines (liver spots, solar lentigines) occur as multiple, uniform, dark brown flat lesions that may vary in size up to 1 cm in diameter. They develop predominantly in areas of sun exposure such as the face, external aspects of the forearms, and, most commonly, the back of the hands. Malignant degeneration does not occur. They rarely occur before the fifth decade and are found in more than 90% of Caucasians over 70 years of age. They are frequently of great concern to those who develop them because lentigines have been singled out as being one of the clear markers of the aging process.

There is no satisfactory method for prevention of their development. The consistent application of 2 to 5% hydroquinone cream twice daily for several months may lighten lentigines somewhat, but, in general, the use of hydroquinone creams has been disappointing. Where lesions are few in number and small, superficial ablation may be accomplished with a minimum of scarring by a single application of liquid nitrogen with a cotton-tipped applicator, just sufficient to obtain a light freeze. Similar effects may be obtained with light electrodesiccation, with a light application of 20 to 35% trichloroacetic acid, or with laser therapy.

## LEUKODERMA

Of the leukodermas, the most common is vitiligo, with an incidence of around 1 to 3%. It is inherited as a dominant trait and histologically is characterized by the absence of identifiable melanocytes. Depigmentation may be local or extensive. Patients with vitiligo are generally in good health, but vitiligo has been associated with alopecia areata, hyperthyroidism, adrenocortical insufficiency, pernicious anemia, scleroderma, and morphea. However, the treatment of associated diseases does not reverse the vitiligo but often makes it stationary. The incidence of autoimmune disease is anywhere from 8 to 15%. Sixty per cent of the patients with vitiligo exhibit various destructive lesions in the pigment cells of the retina. Vitiligo must be differentiated from vitiligo produced as a result of exogenous exposure to such chemicals as thiols, phenolic compounds, catechol and its derivatives, mercaptopurines, and several quinones.

The current treatment for vitiligo leaves a great deal to be desired. If the process is minimal and no treatment is desired, Cover-Mark (Lydia O'Leary), Vitadye, Man Tan, Q.T., or walnut stain may be used. In the early state, the use of topical steroids may limit further progression; however, prolonged treatment is usually required and side effects resulting from prolonged steroid usage have limited their use.

Small areas of vitiligo may be treated with topical application of methoxsalen (Oxsoralen) solution.* The 1% solution should be used diluted, first 1:4 and later 1:2 with equal parts of 95% ethanol and propylene glycol. The solution is painted on the vitiliginous areas with a cotton-tipped swab and exposed to a source of UVA radiation (PUVA) approximately 1 hour later. Exposure times are individualized, starting with a small exposure time (0.5 minute) and increasing by 1 minute with each subsequent exposure until the desired production of erythema in the vitiliginous skin is obtained, at which time subsequent exposure times are maintained. Three-times-weekly treatment is most desirable.

Twenty per cent of patients may attain complete repigmentation, and a total of 60% attain a cosmetically acceptable result with the use of trioxsalen (Trisoralen), 0.15 to 0.45 mg per kg taken daily 2 hours before exposure to sunlight.†

---

*Contraindicated in children under 12 years of age. This product is *not* to be dispensed to the patient, but applied by a physician knowledgeable about its use.

†Exceeds dosage recommended by the manufacturer.

A frequently used therapeutic program recommends that adults begin each summer with two Trisoralen tablets (5 mg) with exposure to the sun for 15 minutes on the first day. If the skin does not burn excessively in the vitiliginous areas, the time of sun exposure is increased 15 minutes each day up to 1 hour. At this point, three tablets of Trisoralen are given and the sun exposure is decreased to 30 minutes. If no burn is experienced, the exposures are increased by 15-minute intervals up to 1 hour. Exposure to sun and dose of drug are increased in this manner until the maximum number of tablets (4 to 5) and hours of sunlight (1 to 2) are reached. Natural sunlight appears to be superior to artificial light sources.

Care must be taken to use potent sunscreens in the vitiliginous areas at all times because they are prone to serious burns. UVA-absorbing wraparound sunglasses (noir) for the protection of the eyes must be worn for the rest of the day after treatment. (Refer to product labeling for extensive patient education to avoid eye and skin exposure to sunlight, including through windows and with cloud cover.)

Evidence of repigmentation in the perifollicular area may be seen as early as 3 months after initiation of therapy, but generally a long-term effort is required, with treatment continuing during the summer months for 5 years or more. Maintenance therapy is required to prevent recurrence, even if initial treatment results in complete repigmentation.

In small areas of vitiligo that have been resistant to therapy, 1.0- to 1.5-mm autologous grafts placed in similar holes 5 mm apart in the depigmented area have provided a source of successful repigmentation.

If the vitiligo is extensive (more than 50% of the body surface), total depigmentation with the monobenzyl ether of hydroquinone (monobenzone [Benoquin]) may be considered. This preparation is applied twice daily, and 10 to 12 months is required for complete depigmentation. Once begun, the process is irreversible.

## TINEA VERSICOLOR

Tinea versicolor is a very common condition that may produce extensive leukodermic macules and papules on the back, shoulders, and arms. The condition is easily identified by demonstrating the characteristic hyphae and spores of the etiologic agent *Malassezia furfur* in potassium hydroxide mounts of scrapings taken from the yellowish to brownish scaly macules characteristic of the disease. The fungus produces striking hypopigmentation at the sites of involvement, which may persist for weeks to months even after the disease has been eradicated.

Tinea versicolor responds to a variety of therapies. Clotrimazole (Lotrimin, Mycelex), haloprogin (Halotex), and tolnaftate (Tinactin) as well as most of the newer fungicides including naftinfine (Naftin), econazole (Spectrozole), oxiconazole (Oxistatin), ciclopirox (Loprox), and sulconazole (Exelderm) are effective against the organism of tinea versicolor. Applications are once to twice daily. As topical treatment should be applied to the entire torso from the neck to the waist, in most cases expense becomes a limiting factor in their use.

Selenium sulfide suspension (Exsel, Selsum) or zinc pyrithione (Zincon, Danex) or a solution of 25% sodium hyposulfite may be applied 15 to 20 minutes before showering for 1 to 2 weeks. Fifty per cent aqueous solution of propylene glycol is effective when applied twice daily for 2 to 3 weeks. Akrinol contains the hexylresorcinol salt of 9-aminoacridine and is applied twice daily for several (2 to 6) weeks. Tinver, containing 25% sodium thiosulfate and 1% salicylic acid, is applied twice daily for several weeks.

Recurrences are common unless therapy is thorough. One effective combination regimen includes the use of selenium sulfide suspension applied to the affected areas 20 minutes before showering, for 2 weeks; and Fostex Cake, containing 2% sulfur and 2% salicylic acid, as the bath soap in showering from the start of therapy and continuing for a period of 2 to 3 months for the prevention of relapse; together with ketoconazole (Nizoral), 200 mg twice daily for 2 days at the start of therapy. If the condition is resistant to topical therapy, ketoconazole, 200 mg a day for 30 days, may be given. The patient should be informed that the leukoderma requires several months to resolve and does not represent active disease.

## PITYRIASIS ALBA

A condition that has a striking component of leukoderma that has led to the misdiagnosis of vitiligo is pityriasis alba, a common chronic eczematous condition of unknown etiology that predominantly strikes children and adolescents of both sexes. It is characterized by the development of scaly patches involving mainly the face, the neck, and the external aspects of the arms. Early lesions may be erythematous with a fine branny scale; however, it is the subsequent leukoderma that frequently provokes concern in the patient. The condition may persist for months or years in some individuals.

Creams containing urea, such as Aquacare, Carmol 10, or U-Lactin, may reduce the scaling; mild tar preparations such as Alphosyl, Estar, or Psorigel are useful. Topical steroid preparations are effective in suppressing the erythematous stage but are not useful in reversing the leukoderma. Patients should avoid sunbathing, as tanning of the surrounding normal skin accentuates the leukodermic areas.

## HALO NEVUS

The development of an area of depigmentation around the nevus is typical of the halo nevus (leukoderma acquisitum centrifugum). It is not common and is usually seen in children or adolescents. In many lesions, the central nevus regresses. Normally no treatment is required, but if a question exists regarding the nature of the lesions, a biopsy should be performed.

# OCCUPATIONAL DERMATITIS

method of
HAROLD PLOTNICK, M.D.
*Wayne State University School of Medicine*
*Detroit, Michigan*

Occupational dermatoses include a large assortment of cutaneous abnormalities that are primarily caused or aggravated by components in the work place. Chemical agents by far are the leading cause of occupational skin disease. These agents include an array of primary irritants, allergic sensitizers, photosensitizers, and systemic intoxicants absorbed through the skin.

Despite the introduction of many protective devices, breakthroughs in controls occur. Chemicals that are used and well harnessed in one industry can become unleashed and hazardous in another. The industries with the greatest number of work-related dermatoses are machine tool production, plastic manufacturing, rubber production, food processing, leather tanning and finishing, and metal plating and cleaning.

Most work-related skin diseases affect the exposed areas of the body. The clinical picture of an acute contact eruption is characterized by the appearance of erythema, edema, vesiculation, and weeping. This reaction is the same whether the cause is a primary irritant or an allergic sensitizer.

A primary irritant source produces a direct physical change in the skin. The allergic patient must initially undergo an incubation period to develop antibodies against the specific antigen. Once antibodies are formed, subsequent exposure to the recognized antigen will elicit an eczematous response within 24 hours in the target skin area. Unlike the primary contact dermatitis that is localized to the areas of exposure, the allergic response may appear over other areas of the body besides the locus of contact.

## MANAGEMENT

### The Physician's Role in Industry

The physician's role in industry is not limited to the diagnosis and treatment of work-related skin injuries, but also includes identifying the cause and recommending protective measures to prevent future recurrences. Medical treatment must be prompt and comprehensive to lessen the degree of morbidity and hasten the recovery of the skin to its preinjury state. When possible, the worker is kept on the job while receiving treatment. If this approach is impractical, the worker should be moved to another area of the work place or given time off until the skin is clear. A worker who has developed an allergic reaction to a recognized chemical may experience a recurrence of the dermatitis even on minimal reexposure despite the employment of protective safeguards. In these selected cases, a change in job assignment is mandatory.

### Patch Testing

The patch test is not a perfect bioassay but it does possess unique and valuable features since it serves as a miniature model of the disease under investigation. The patch test is recommended for suspected allergens, not for evaluating known or suspected primary irritants. The latter would only contribute to a false-positive reaction and confuse the purpose of the test.

The majority of patch testing is performed under a closed system with the exact materials to which the worker is exposed. Dry materials can be utilized as is, but liquids should be diluted with equal parts of a compatible vehicle prior to testing. This cautionary procedure is necessary to avoid a potential primary irritation that could result in a false-positive reaction.

The test materials should be covered by a nonallergenic material and fixed in place by an allergy-free adhesive-treated paper tape (3M Micropore, Scanpor) for a period of 48 hours. The patch is then removed and a 45-minute rest period is observed prior to the reading. A positive test is recognized either as erythema and edema (2+), a weak reaction; or as erythema, edema, and vesiculation (3+), a stronger allergic reaction. A negative response indicates the absence of an allergic reaction.

### Hand Protection

Hands are the most common site of contact dermatitis. The use of protective gloves or a barrier cream is a necessary part of the working uniform in industries in which corrosive chemicals are encountered. These agents include low-pH acids, high-pH alkalis, chromates, coolants, cutting oils, some greases, free or uncombined monomers of epoxy and polyester systems, organic solvents, and biocides.

Protection is the key to the avoidance of primary irritants and allergic-sensitizing contact dermatitis in industry. Where hand protection is a must, the choice is the right type of glove for the specific job (e.g., canvas, leather, rubber, or butyl).

Canvas gloves are suitable for dry work. They do protect the hands from the rough edges on stock and from stains when handling various chemically coated materials. Leather gloves can be used in dry work as well, but their real advantage is in types of work in which there is a need for gripping objects, such as in the buffing and polishing industry.

Wet jobs require the use of rubber or butyl gloves. Rubber gloves are pliable and supple and are composed of either natural latex or synthetic materials. In some industries in which contact is with organic solvents or uncured plastic monomers, rubber gloves may allow minuscule amounts of chemicals to enter. In these situations, a butyl glove is preferred because of its alleged nonpermeable nature. The prolonged wearing of rubber or butyl gloves prevents evaporation of sweat, and retention of sweat within the interior of the glove may cause maceration of the epidermal surface. It is advisable that butyl gloves contain an inner fleece cotton lining to absorb the sweat. Unlined rubber gloves can be worn over absorbent, lightweight cotton gloves. Excessive sweat production within the interior of rubber gloves can sometimes leach out uncombined rubber accelerators and antioxidants that may cause allergic contact dermatitis in susceptible individuals. Workers who develop this problem should wear synthetic rubber (Neoprene) or butyl gloves.

Protective gloves can be hazardous to workers engaged in machine tool production; the gloves may be grabbed by the machine and cause injury to the worker. In this type of industry in which manual dexterity is essential, a suitable barrier cream (Kerodex 71) can be used as a protective agent. Kerodex 71 has been used effectively in industries in which coolants and cutting oils are the primary contactants. The barrier cream must be removed every 2 hours and the hands must be washed to free any retained residue and dried. A fresh application of the barrier cream is then applied to all contact areas.

### The Problem of Sweaty Hands

Hyperhidrosis (excessive sweat production) with its frequently accompanying pompholyx (dyshidrosis) may precede or become symptomatic from the prolonged use of protective rubber or butyl gloves. A worker with an active pompholyx may develop a hand dermatitis from materials that normally do not call for gloved protection. The reason for this is that open blisters may provide an easy access for potential irritants and sensitizers to invade the skin and initiate an inflammatory response.

Workers with pompholyx or its aggravated form (dyshidrotic eczematous dermatitis) respond favorably to appropriate local care. This includes soaking the hands in Burow's aluminum acetate 1:30 solution (Domeboro), one tablet per quart of water, for 15 minutes twice a day. Following the soaks, a midpotency glucocorticoid cream (e.g., fluocinolone acetonide 0.025% [Synalar], desonide 0.05% [Tridesilon], or betamethasone valerate 0.1% [Valisone]) can be helpful in clearing the dyshidrotic reaction. Workers with active pompholyx who cannot tolerate cotton-lined protective gloves or whose reaction is unresponsive to local medication must be assigned to a dry job.

### Physical and Climatologic Influences in Contact Dermatitis

The intact epidermis is provided with a natural lipid-wax protective mantle that can ward off the majority of irritants encountered by the skin. When lipid solvents bathe the skin's surface, the protective layer is washed away. The unprotected keratin layer is free to lose its water content to the atmosphere, a factor that results in a dry stratum corneum and a potential opening for primary irritants to enter the skin.

Climatologic conditions that influence the water content of the skin are recognized as the dew point and humidity. During the colder months of the year, when the ambient water content is low, there is an increase in the loss of water from the skin to the atmosphere. The physical change in the skin is recognized as chapping or dehydration secondary to a low dew point and humidity.

Skin dryness resulting from the coupling of the two examples just noted can evolve into an eczematous process, a problem often seen in the machine tool industry during the cold winter months. The worker's bare hands are in and out of various lipid solvents (coolants, cutting oils, degreasing agents) many times a day. This sequence of repeated exposure to lipid solvents followed by evaporation of solvent and epidermal water loss to the low water content of the ambient work atmosphere may account for the measurable increase in symptomatic hand eczema during the colder months of the year. The same exposure and work methods usually present little problem during the other seasons of the year.

### Treatment

The basic treatment for dehydration-induced eczematoid dermatitis is restoration of water to the thirsty epidermis. This phenomenon can be corrected by avoiding soaps and utilizing a water-miscible oil (Alpha-Keri) as a hand cleaner and by the after-work use of hygroscopic creams or lotions. These agents restore water to the epidermis and decrease its evaporation to the ambient water-deficient atmosphere. The following proprietary medications are suggested: a water-in-oil emollient (Eucerin), and lactic acid derivatives of azelaic acid (LactiCare Cream, Lac-Hydrin Lotion). These water-holding agents are best applied to a moist skin after work hours and at bedtime.

# SUNBURN AND PHOTOSENSITIVITY

method of
CRAIG A. ELMETS, M.D.
*Case Western Reserve University and
University Hospitals of Cleveland
Cleveland, Ohio*

Photosensitivity is the term used to describe a pathologic response of the skin to ultraviolet or visible light, or both. The distinguishing clinical characteristic of photosensitivity disorders is their predilection for sun-exposed areas of skin rather than any distinctive morphology of the cutaneous lesions. Photosensitivity diseases may arise acutely or on a chronic basis. Examples of acute photosensitivity include sunburn, drug-induced phototoxicity, and photoallergic contact dermatitis. Chronic cases are typified by photoaging of the skin, cutaneous premalignancies (actinic keratoses), and skin cancer. In addition, sunlight can act as a provocative factor for selected diseases, such as herpes simplex labialis, cutaneous lupus erythematosus, and certain types of porphyria. Although photosensitivity diseases are, in most instances, brought on by sun exposure during outdoor recreational or work-related activities, they may also be elicited by exposure to artificial ultraviolet light sources, such as those employed in tanning salons.

Ultraviolet radiation (UV), which is responsible for most photosensitivity diseases, has been divided into UVC (200 to 290 nm, short UV), UVB (290 to 320 nm, mid-UV) and UVA (320 to 400 nm, long UV) wavelengths. Solar UVC radiation is largely filtered by the ozone layer of the atmosphere and, therefore, is of little medical significance. However, UVC radiation is present in germicidal lamps and is responsible for the erythema that develops following excessive exposure to this type of light source. Wavelengths within the

UVB range are responsible for sunburn and have been strongly implicated in causing sunlight-induced skin cancer. UVA radiation is also present in the solar spectrum and is the wavelength band emitted by the sun lamps in tanning salons. Wavelengths within the UVA are primarily responsible for drug-induced photosensitivity. Large amounts of UVA may cause skin cancer, although much less efficiently than wavelengths within the UVB.

## ACUTE PHOTOSENSITIVITY

### Sunburn

Sunburn is common in lightly pigmented individuals and is caused by excessive exposure of the skin to solar UVB radiation. The disease typically begins 2 to 6 hours after sun exposure as a painful erythema in which intensity peaks 24 to 48 hours later. In more severe cases, blisters and erosions develop. Systemic toxicity, including fever, chills, nausea, and leukocytosis, accompanies very extensive reactions.

The major goal in management of the sunburned patient is to provide symptomatic relief until the inflammatory response subsides. In mild cases, this can be accomplished by applying cool compresses (Burow's solution) to the sunburned areas for 15 minutes three to four times daily. Frequent application of water-in-oil emollients (Eucerin cream) is also helpful, especially if they have been refrigerated prior to application. The widespread use of topical antihistamines and neomycin (Neosporin)–containing antibiotics is to be avoided. These agents are notorious for causing allergic contact dermatitis, especially when applied to inflamed skin. In more severe cases, topical application of corticosteroid creams (1% hydrocortisone cream to the face and intertriginous areas; 0.1% triamcinolone cream [Kenalog] to the other areas of the body) is of value in reducing inflammation. If blisters and erosions are present, polymyxin-bacitracin (Polysporin) or mupirocin (Bactroban) ointment should be applied immediately after the compresses have been removed to prevent the development of secondary bacterial infection. Aspirin and indomethacin (Indocin) are also of some benefit in decreasing pain and reducing inflammation. Systemic prednisone therapy (60 mg daily and tapered over 7–10 days) is indicated when systemic manifestations are present or extensive blistering has developed.

### Drug-Induced Photosensitivity

After sunburn, reactions to systemically administered drugs or topically applied chemicals and medications are the most common causes of acute photosensitivity. Drug-induced photosensitivity is usually elicited by UVA radiation and

TABLE 1. **Drugs Causing Phototoxicity**

Psoralen (Oxsoralen-Ultra)
Piroxicam (Feldene)
Amiodarone (Cordarone)
Nalidixic acid (NegGram)
Tetracycline
Furosemide (Lasix)
Hydrochlorothiazide (Hydrodiuril)
Chlorpropamide (Diabinase)
Tolbutamide (Orinase)
Chlorpromazine
Trifluoperazine (Stelazine)

may arise as the result of either phototoxic or photoallergic mechanisms. Phototoxic reactions classically present as exaggerated sunburn reactions to topically or systemically administered medications. Their onset is minutes to hours after ultraviolet light exposure, and they can be elicited in essentially all individuals who have received both a sufficient dose of medication and adequate exposure to ultraviolet light. Photoallergic reactions, on the other hand, represent a unique form of allergic contact dermatitis in which ultraviolet light serves to convert a topically applied chemical into an immunologically active allergen. The cutaneous eruption that develops is eczematous in nature and is confined to sun-exposed areas. Photoallergic reactions typically develop 24 to 48 hours after ultraviolet light exposure and occur in only a minority of individuals exposed to the sensitizing agent.

The major goal of therapy of both photoallergic and phototoxic reactions is removal of the offending substance. Once this has been accomplished, photosensitivity usually resolves in days to weeks. Many of the most common photosensitizing chemicals are listed in Tables 1 and 2. Patients should be informed of products likely to contain the photosensitizer and cross-reacting substances in order to avoid inadvertent readministration of the compound. This is a particular problem with topically applied chemicals because the offending agent is often only a minor component of the medication. Patients should also be instructed to avoid sun exposure as much as possible, to wear protective clothing, and to apply sunscreening agents.

Once a phototoxic reaction has occurred, man-

TABLE 2. **Topically Applied Photoallergens**

| Chemical | Use |
| --- | --- |
| Phenothiazines | Tranquilizers |
| Musk ambrette | Fragrance in men's after-shave lotion |
| 6-Methylcoumarin | Fragrance in sunscreens |
| PABA-esters | Sunscreen |
| Benzophenones | Sunscreen |
| Halogenated salicylanilides | Antibacterial agent in soaps |

agement is similar to that of sunburn, consisting of cool compresses, emollients, topical steroids, and in severe cases, oral prednisone therapy. Photoallergic reactions are best managed by the application of potent topical steroids (fluocinonide, Lidex cream) two to four times daily. In extensive cases, oral prednisone therapy (60 mg daily tapered over 2 weeks) is indicated. Hydroxyzine (Atarax), 25 mg every 4 to 6 hours, provides symptomatic relief of the pruritus.

### Polymorphous Light Eruption

Polymorphous light eruption is an idiopathic photodermatosis, generally induced by UVB radiation, which, as its name implies, may have a variety of morphologic presentations. These range from eczematous and papular eruptions to papulovesicles and plaques. Because pruritus is almost invariably present, lichenification due to scratching is often an accompanying feature. The disease is quiescent during the winter months, but characteristically recurs each spring, hours to days after initial exposure to the sun. As the summer progresses, photosensitivity often diminishes—a process known as hardening.

In all cases, avoidance of sun exposure, the use of protective clothing, and the application of sunscreening agents are valuable in minimizing the development of new lesions. When lesions do occur, they can often be managed with cool compresses (Burow's solution), emollients, and potent topical corticosteroids, such as 0.025% fluocinonide (Lidex) cream. Recent evidence indicates that oral psoralen photochemotherapy (PUVA) can be used to reduce the photosensitivity response even in severe cases. Furthermore, PUVA therapy, instituted early in the spring, is an effective preventative measure. Chloroquine (Aralen) and hydroxychloroquine (Plaquenil) also have demonstrated efficacy in polymorphous light eruption.

### Solar Urticaria

Some individuals develop urticarial reactions in sun-exposed areas of skin minutes to hours after exposure to sunlight. Wavelengths within the UVB, UVA, and occasionally in the visible spectrum have been shown to cause such reactions. Because the basic mechanism by which sunlight causes urticarial reactions is unknown, treatment is largely symptomatic. Oral antipruritic agents (hydroxyzine, Atarax 25 mg) should be administered every 4 to 6 hours to control pruritus. Topical corticosteroids, e.g., 0.1% triamcinolone cream (Kenalog), and topical antipruritic agents (Sarna lotion) are also of value in

controlling symptomatology. In resistant cases, PUVA photochemotherapy three times weekly until clearing has occurred followed by once or twice weekly maintenance therapy is an effective therapeutic option.

## CHRONIC PHOTOSENSITIVITY

### Photoaging

Repeated exposure of the skin to solar UVB and UVA radiation over a period of years leads to changes in the skin that many patients find cosmetically unappealing. These include fine and course wrinkling, a yellowish discoloration, loss of elasticity, and macular hyperpigmentation (solar lentigines). Although many of the changes are irreversible, topical application of tretinoin cream (Retin-A) may improve some of these abnormalities. Patients electing to undergo this form of therapy should be instructed to apply a thin layer of 0.1% tretinoin cream (Retin-A) daily. This concentration of tretinoin produces at least a mild irritant dermatitis in essentially all patients, which may necessitate discontinuation of the drug for a short period of time or the application of a topical corticosteroid, such as alclometasone (Aclovate) cream, 0.05% twice a day until the inflammation has resolved. Because the skin becomes less susceptible to the irritating effects of topical tretinoin with continued application, an alternative approach by which side effects can be avoided is to begin treatment with a less potent concentration of tretinoin (Retin-A cream, 0.025% or 0.05%) on an every-other-day basis. Once the skin has built up a tolerance to its irritating effects, the strength and frequency of application can be increased.

### Cutaneous Premalignancies and Skin Cancer

Chronic sun exposure is the leading cause of cutaneous squamous cell and basal cell carcinoma, and there is growing evidence that it promotes the development of malignant melanoma as well. Sunlight is also a well-recognized etiologic agent for precancerous lesions called actinic keratoses. Actinic keratoses are macules or slightly elevated papules with a tightly adherent sandpaper-like scale. They are present on sun-exposed areas of skin and are often better appreciated by palpation than by visualization.

Limited numbers of actinic keratoses can be treated with liquid nitrogen cryotherapy or with electrodesiccation and curettage. When many actinic keratoses are present, a short course of topical 5-fluorouracil (Efudex or Fluoroplex) is the preferred form of therapy. One per cent or 5% 5-fluorouracil should be applied twice daily for 2 to 3 weeks. Although this therapeutic regimen is associated with extensive inflammation, the inflammation alone should not preclude its continued application. For particularly severe reactions, a potent topical corticosteroid (fluocinonide 0.05%, Lidex cream) can be applied concomitantly.

Sunlight-induced cutaneous malignancies are usually treated with one of a variety of surgical procedures. Their treatment is discussed in more detail in other articles of this text.

## PHOTOAGGRAVATED DISEASES

A number of cutaneous diseases exist that are not caused by ultraviolet light but whose disease activity may, in certain instances, be promoted by sun exposure. Many of these diseases are listed in Table 3. Although treatment of the primary disease process is the major goal of therapy, appropriate photopreventative measures as listed below are also of value.

### Sunscreens and Other Photoprotective Measures

A number of measures may be taken to prevent the harmful effects of both acute and chronic sun exposure. The use of protective clothing, such as wide-brimmed hats and long-sleeved shirts, should be encouraged. Dark-colored, tightly woven materials are most effective in this regard. In highly photosensitive individuals, it may also be necessary to avoid sunlight between 10:00 a.m. and 3:00 p.m., the hours when sun intensity is at its peak.

Topically applied sunscreening agents (Table 4) provide photoprotection by binding to the most superficial layers of skin. In that location they are able to absorb or reflect ultraviolet light, thereby preventing its transmission to deeper layers of skin. Most sunscreening agents contain para-aminobenzoic acid (PABA) or its esters, although cinnamates and salicylates are also commonly employed. All of these compounds protect primarily against wavelengths within the UVB. Benzophenones have mild to moderate UVA photoprotective effects and are present in combination with UVB absorbing chemicals in some products to provide a broader spectrum of ultraviolet protection. Parsol 1789 is a much more efficient UVA absorbing compound that has been recently marketed in a sunscreen that also contains a

TABLE 3. **Photoaggravated Diseases**

| | |
|---|---|
| Lupus erythematosus | Herpes simplex |
| Dermatomyositis | Atopic dermatitis |
| Pemphigus erythematosus | Pellagra |
| Porphyria | |

TABLE 4. **Representative Sunscreens**

| Type of Sunscreen | Water Resistant |
|---|---|
| *UVB Protection* | |
| PreSun 8 and 15 Lotion | No |
| Total Eclipse | Yes |
| Super Shade 15 Gel | No |
| Solbar PF 15 Liquid | No |
| *UVB with Some UVA Protection* | |
| PreSun 15 and 29 Sensitive Skin | Yes |
| PreSun 8, 15, and 39 Creamy | Yes |
| SuperShade 15, 25, 30, and 44 | Yes |
| Sundown 6, 8, 15, 20, and 24 | Yes |
| Solbar PF 15 and PF 50 Cream | Yes |
| *UVB and Considerable UVA Protection* | |
| Photoplex | Yes |
| *UVB, UVA, and Visible Protection (Physical Sunblocks)* | |
| RV Paque | Yes |
| Dermablend | Yes |
| Covermark | Yes |

PABA ester (Photoplex). Physical sunblocks containing zinc oxide and titanium dioxide provide an opaque shield over the skin. Although these agents provide efficient photoprotection over a broad spectrum of wavelengths, including UVB, UVA, and visible light, they are cosmetically unacceptable to a large number of patients.

The relative efficacy of a given sunscreening agent in protecting against sunburn is expressed by its sun protective factor (SPF). The SPF represents the ratio of the time required for sunscreen-treated skin to produce a mild sunburn compared with that of untreated skin. A sunscreen with an SPF of 15 theoretically allows an individual 15 times greater sun exposure than if a sunscreen were not applied. In heavily pigmented individuals who never sunburn, a sunscreen with an SPF of 4 or 8 should be sufficient. For people with less pigmentation who are more susceptible to sunburn, sunscreens with an SPF of 15 or greater should be recommended. Although sunscreens have been marketed with an SPF of 50, sunscreens with an SPF of 15 to 29 are sufficient for most purposes.

For most individuals, sunscreens are employed to protect against sunburn and skin cancer. A UVB sunscreen works well for these purposes. However, frequent application of a combination UVA and UVB sunscreen has the added benefit of providing partial protection against photoaging. Water and sweat-resistant sunscreens should be recommended for those individuals who intend to use these agents while swimming or during vigorous physical exercise. For patients taking photosensitizing drugs, a potent UVA sunscreen should be prescribed. In patients with lupus erythematosus, a combination of UVA and UVB sunscreen should be utilized for photoprotection because the ultraviolet wavelengths capable of eliciting photosensitivity in this disease have not been clearly established. Wavelengths within the visible spectrum are responsible for porphyrin photosensitivity. Therefore, a physical sunscreen must be employed for patients with this type of photosensitivity. In extreme cases of photosensitivity of any cause, a physical sunblock should be used.

# The Nervous System

## BRAIN ABSCESS

method of
MAURY E. MULLIGAN, M.D.
*Veterans Affairs Medical Center*
*Long Beach, California*

Brain abscess is focal suppurative infection within the brain parenchyma that must be managed as an intracranial mass. Although surgery is often required, medical therapy alone may be adequate in selected cases.

### ETIOLOGY

The underlying diseases that predispose to brain abscess are the major determinants of the etiologic agents. Infection may result from direct extension from an adjacent site or direct implantation as a result of trauma (including surgical trauma), or it may be the consequence of hematogenous spread from a distant site of infection. In approximately 20% of cases, no predisposing factor can be found.

The most common predisposing conditions are infections of contiguous structures such as the sinuses and ears and, less frequently, other pericranial infections. In these settings, anaerobic bacteria, including anaerobic cocci, *Fusobacterium, Bacteroides,* and *Actinomyces,* are common pathogens as are aerobic and microaerophilic gram-positive cocci, including *Staphylococcus* and the various species of *Streptococcus.* Gram-negative bacilli may also be present, including *Haemophilus,* the Enterobacteriaceae, and *Pseudomonas.* The location of the abscess and the likely pathogens are closely related to the site of the contiguous infection. For example, *Bacteroides fragilis* and Enterobacteriaceae are commonly associated with otogenic infections. Many of these infections are polymicrobial, although certain pathogens such as *Staphylococcus aureus* are more likely to be recovered in pure culture. *Staphylococcus aureus* and gram-negative bacilli, including *Pseudomonas,* are important pathogens when brain abscess results from penetrating cranial trauma or surgical procedures. Coagulase-negative staphylococci as well as *S. aureus* are the most common organisms recovered from infections associated with intraventricular shunts.

Hematogenous spread from a distant site of infection occurs most often in association with chronic pyogenic pulmonary infections and is most often due to anaerobes and streptococci. Congenital heart disease also predisposes to brain abscess; the most common pathogens are aerobic and microaerophilic streptococci, anaerobic cocci, and, occasionally, *Haemophilus.* Brain abscess complicating infective endocarditis is relatively uncommon and most often caused by *S. aureus* or streptococci. Other distant foci of infection may also be associated with brain abscesses, but this is also uncommon. Hematogenous brain abscesses are distinct from those related to contiguous infection in that they are often multiple, commonly located in the distribution of the middle cerebral artery, and likely to have a higher mortality.

Various bacterial pathogens that are usually associated with meningitis may also cause focal infections; these include *Listeria monocytogenes* and *Neisseria meningitidis.*

In the compromised host, pathogens that are otherwise uncommon must be considered, especially yeast and dimorphic fungi; these include *Aspergillus, Candida, Cryptococcus,* and the agents of zygomycosis (mucormycosis) as well as many other fungi. *Nocardia, Mycobacterium,* and *Toxoplasma gondii* are also important pathogens for the immunocompromised patient. Toxoplasmosis is the most common cause of brain abscess in patients with acquired immune deficiency syndrome (AIDS). Other causes of mass lesions in this population are *Cryptococcus,* various mycobacteria, progressive multifocal leukoencephalopathy, *Candida, Listeria, Nocardia, Salmonella,* and *Aspergillus.* Protozoa and helminths are uncommon pathogens in this country but are of primary importance in other parts of the world, where, for example, cysticercosis is a leading cause of central nervous system (CNS) infection.

### TREATMENT

#### Medical Therapy

Specific antimicrobial therapy can be selected based on culture results from the primary site of infection, but it is important to consider that specimens must be obtained, transported, and processed properly. Without this attention, fastidious organisms, such as anaerobes, cannot be recovered. Blood cultures should be obtained but, even when positive, should not be assumed to represent all of the organisms that may be present in an abscess. Cultures of spinal fluid are positive in approximately 10% of cases, but lumbar puncture is contraindicated not only because of the poor diagnostic yield but also because the procedure is dangerous for the patient with an intracranial mass. Whenever possible, it is desirable to obtain a specimen directly from the abscess. Computed tomography (CT) with contrast or magnetic resonance imaging (MRI) is ideal for defining lesions, although early cerebritis that has not progressed to encapsulation may not be identified.

For the patient for whom surgical aspiration is not possible (for example, when an inaccessible lesion close to vital structures is identified), therapy must be empiric. Even when a surgical specimen is obtained, there should be an attempt to identify a predisposing cause because this allows prediction of the etiologic agents and guides therapy until culture results are available. Table 1 lists antimicrobial agents that may be considered. High-dose penicillin G plus metronidazole (Flagyl) represents excellent therapy for infections due to anaerobes and streptococci. A third-generation cephalosporin with good CNS penetration or trimethoprim/sulfamethoxazole (Bactrim, Septra) is often added when there is a primary otogenic focus or when the primary focus is unknown because of the possibility that Enterobacteriaceae or *Pseudomonas* may be present. When staphylococci are suspected, a semisynthetic penicillin such as nafcillin (Nafcil) or oxacillin (Bactocill, Prostaphlin) should be used. Vancomycin (Vancocin) should be substituted if methicillin-resistant staphylococci are likely, if an intracerebral shunt is in place, or if the patient is allergic to penicillin. Patients with AIDS who present with multiple lesions are most often treated with pyrimethamine (Daraprim) and sulfadiazine for presumed toxoplasmosis.

Although surgical therapy (aspiration or open drainage) has long been considered essential selected patients have been treated successfully with antimicrobial therapy alone. Medical therapy alone has been used for patients with multiple or inaccessible lesions, when the risk of surgery is excessive because of other factors, and when patients present with early infection (cerebritis without encapsulation). It is essential, however, that such patients be monitored closely for signs of neurologic deterioration and that imaging (CT or MRI) be done to document response to therapy.

Measures to control or prevent seizures and to decrease intracranial pressure may be needed. Thus, anticonvulsants (phenytoin [Dilantin] or phenobarbital [Luminal]) should be considered. The use of steroids is controversial, but in the case of rapid neurologic deterioration with increased intracranial pressure, steroids, mannitol, and forced hyperventilation have all been employed as lifesaving measures. Anticoagulants are contraindicated because of the risk of intracranial hemorrhage. The optimal duration of

TABLE 1. **Antimicrobial Agents Useful in the Treatment of Brain Abscess**

| Drug | Antimicrobial Spectrum/ Primary Indication | Dosage |
|---|---|---|
| Penicillin G | Streptococci, many anaerobes (not *Bacteroides fragilis*) | 200,000 to 300,000 U/kg/day (given IV every 4 hr) |
| Metronidazole | Anaerobes except *Actinomyces, Arachnia* | 30 mg/kg/day (given IV every 6 hr) |
| Chloramphenicol (Chloromycetin) | Anaerobes, some gram-negative bacilli | 50 to 60 mg/kg/day, then 30 mg/kg/day (given IV every 6 hr) |
| Nafcillin (Nafcil, Unipen) | *Staphylococcus aureus* | 100 to 200 mg/kg/day (given IV every 4 hr) |
| Vancomycin (Vancocin) | Staphylococci, including methicillin-resistant strains | 30 mg/kg/day (given IV every 6 hr) |
| Cefotaxime* (Claforan) | Gram-negative bacilli (not *Pseudomonas*) | 120 to 175 mg/kg/day (given IV every 4–6 hr) |
| Ceftazidime (Fortaz, Tazicef, Tazidime) | Gram-negative bacilli (including *Pseudomonas*) | 90 mg/kg/day (given IV every 8 hr) |
| Trimethoprim/Sulfamethoxazole (Bactrim, Septra) | Most *Nocardia*, gram-negative bacilli (not *Pseudomonas*) some staphylococci | 20 mg/kg/day trimethoprim plus 100 mg/kg/day sulfa (given IV or orally every 6 hr) |
| Pyrimethamine (Daraprim) | *Toxoplasma gondii* | For adults, 100 mg given orally twice a day, then 25–100 mg (given orally once a day) |
| Sulfadiazine USP | *Toxoplasma gondii* | 75 mg/kg/day then 100 mg/kg/day (given orally every 6 hr) |
| Amphotericin B† (Fungizone) | Most fungi | 1 mg test dose IV, then build up to 0.5 mg/kg/day IV |
| Flucytosine (Ancobon) | Selected fungi | 150 mg/kg/day (given every 6 hr IV or orally) |

*Other third-generation cephalosporins may be useful as well.
†New agents that may be effective against fungi are being investigated.

antimicrobial therapy is unknown, but many authorities advise parenteral therapy for 4 to 8 weeks followed by oral therapy, if there is a suitable agent, for 2 to 6 months.

### Surgical Therapy

Most patients require surgical therapy, either aspiration after burr hole placement or craniotomy with complete excision. Excision is used most often for the patient who is more stable neurologically and has an accessible lesion, whereas aspiration is often performed when there is rapid neurologic deterioration or to drain a relatively inaccessible lesion. Management must be individualized, however, for each patient.

Surgery is essential for the patient with severe and deteriorating neurologic deficits, especially when there are signs of brain stem compression. Because prognosis for the comatose patient is exceedingly poor, surgery should be attempted prior to this stage. Surgical excision is the standard therapy for posterior fossa lesions.

Surgery is also indicated for the patient receiving antimicrobial therapy who demonstrates neurologic deterioration or progression of disease based on CT or MRI.

With the availability of CT and MRI, aspiration may be attempted rather than excision. Stereotactic CT-guided aspiration has been documented to be a safe procedure and has been found to be an invaluable aid in identifying pathogens, often significantly affecting the choice of antimicrobial therapy. Indeed, the risk of this invasive procedure may be less than the risk of inappropriate empiric therapy.

If the abscess is large or multiloculated, presents in an anatomically critical location, or is progressive despite antimicrobial therapy plus aspiration, excision may be a necessity. There is some evidence that complete excision may be associated with a higher incidence of neurologic sequelae than aspiration.

There has been a dramatic decrease in mortality due to brain abscess, largely attributed to the advent of CT and the close monitoring it allows, thereby enabling individualized therapy for each patient.

# ALZHEIMER'S DISEASE

method of
LEONARD L. HESTON, M.D.
*University of Washington*
*Seattle, Washington*

Alzheimer's disease (AD) is a neurodegenerative disorder recognized clinically by failures of memory, judgment, and the ability to reason abstractly. There is no treatment for this brain failure. Several compounds are currently being investigated, most of them based on the demonstrated deficit in cholinergic neurotransmission in AD, but to date cholinomimetic agents have not demonstrated benefit. Attempts to enhance brain metabolism using ergot derivatives (e.g., Hydergine) given in doses of 3 to 6 mg daily for 6 months or more, probably do marginally benefit persons in earlier stages of dementia. However, the effect is most likely due to increased arousal or mood elevation or both, not to an effect on the underlying disease process. Chelation is a current pop remedy for AD espoused by segments of the popular press. It is aimed at removing aluminum from brain tissue. Brain tissue from AD patients does exhibit a marginal increase in aluminum, but this is regarded as an effect rather than a cause of cell death. Chelation has no proven benefit in AD; moreover, it is costly and dangerous.

## SYMPTOMATIC TREATMENTS

Drugs can effectively treat troublesome signs and symptoms of dementia of the Alzheimer type (DAT). Empirical results, not pharmacologic theory, best guide choice of agents and dosages.

Neuroleptic drugs are modestly useful for signs such as restlessness, agitation, and hostility. Suspiciousness, delusions, and hallucinations may also be targeted. Most frequently prescribed are thioridazine (Mellaril) and haloperidol (Haldol), although there is little evidence supporting those particular choices. The starting dose should be on the order of 10 mg of thioridazine and 0.5 mg of haloperidol. Because drug half-life is increased in the elderly, 2 to 3 days are needed before reasonable clinical equilibrium to given dose is attained. In stages, dosage can be increased until target signs are controlled or toxicity intervenes. "Start low and go slow" is a useful maxim in drug treatment of AD. It may be possible to pinpoint an especially troublesome time of day, for example, evening agitation ("sundowning"), and administer a single daily dose about 2 hours beforehand.

Neuroleptics have serious side effects in AD patients. Oversedation may impair a marginal brain, producing a misleading picture of confusion and disorientation. Extrapyramidal reactions are especially common among the brain-impaired elderly. Low potency neuroleptics such as thioridazine are less likely to produce extrapyramidal problems but are considerably more anticholinergic. Anticholinergic effects, coupled with age-related decreases in cholinergic functioning, can yield serious problems, including a toxic psychosis. Finally, tardive dyskinesia is a risk of extended neuroleptic use in the elderly. This is one reason among many why frequent attempts should be made to reduce or eliminate neuroleptics. It is salutary to remember that systematic studies of the administration of neuroleptics in AD have trouble demonstrating positive effects, while studies of their removal from patients who have been taking them usually have shown unequivocal benefits.

Beta blockers, such as propranalol (Inderal), in doses of 20 to 200 mg three times daily, may help control aggression. No adequate control studies have been done in AD, but an empirical trial is warranted in difficult cases. Depression, hypotension, and bradycardia are expectable side effects.

Antidepressants are of limited usefulness in AD. Although depression sometimes seems to be intimately associated with dementing illness, especially during the early stages, drug treatment has not proved helpful and severe anticholinergic side effects are frequent. Some patients benefit from nighttime sedation with doses on the order of 25 mg of nortriptyline (Aventyl).

Stimulants have likewise had limited use in AD. Occasionally, patients in the early stages of the disease exhibit lethargy and lack of initiative. A trial of methylphenidate (Ritalin), 5 to 30 mg daily in divided doses, may be helpful.

Sedative drugs, mostly benzodiazepines in modern practice, can provide useful sedation for many AD patients. The half-life of diazepam (Valium) nearly doubles in older patients; therefore, dosages should be small. All sedatives-barbiturates, "minor" tranquilizers, and alcohol interfere with memory formation. This is seldom important given a normal brain, but the loss may be critical to an impaired one. Tolerance and withdrawal are also potential problems. A starting dose of 5 mg of diazepam (Valium) or equivalent can be increased over several days until intoxication occurs. In some patients, the releasing effects of sedative drugs may increase agitation.

### Psychologic Management

Physicians can help greatly by giving caregivers a few general guidelines. Two common impediments to memory are encountered in everyday life. The first of these is fatigue. Nearly always, persons with brain impairment are at their best after a period of rest. Schedule strenuous events after a period of sleep. Encourage naps.

The second major hazard is anxiety, which powerfully interferes with memory formation. A vicious circle can be set up. Inability to respond to environmental challenges for any reason increases anxiety, which in turn further impairs memory and so on. Anxiety is a signal. Once signs develop, say at a social gathering, it is time to leave. Nothing else will effectively relieve the anxiety.

There are also positive things to do which, after practice, can become second nature to caregivers. Compensating for memory impairment is one example. For example, suppose a sudden noise comes from the next room where visiting grandchildren are playing. The healthy brain remembers instantly, "Oh, the children are in the next room; they explain the noise. It does not sound dangerous; they are just playing." But if memory fails, such noises are unexplained, a cause of alarm and anxiety. Being aware of this, caregivers should simply say softly, "That is the children playing in the next room. They are OK."

Social occasions can be difficult. Keep the number of new faces and new names to a minimum. Social conversations tend to focus on current events, the dementing person's salient weakness. Caregivers can judiciously supply answers and unabashedly steer conversations. AD patients poorly tolerate choices or decisions. Caregivers must say, "Now we must go to the store," not "Would you like to come to the store with me?" "Alan is coming to visit after lunch," not "We are going to have company today."

Extremely useful ongoing help with the myriad problems that confront caregivers is offered by the Alzheimer's Disease and Related Disorders Association. Toll free telephone numbers are 1-800-621-0379, and in Illinois 1-800-572-6037.

# PRIMARY INTRACEREBRAL HEMORRHAGE

method of
RALPH G. GREENLEE, Jr., M.D., and
HARRIS A. FRANKEL, M.D.
*University of Texas Southwestern Medical Center*
*Dallas, Texas*

Stroke remains a leading cause of disability and death. Although intracerebral hemorrhage (ICH) constitutes only 10% of all stroke episodes, early recognition, thorough etiologic evaluation, and assiduous clinical management can significantly modify mortality. It should be emphasized that the ultimate functional recovery from ICH is often better than that from a comparable initial deficit due to ischemic infarction. This is because the hematoma expands as an ovoid mass compressing adjacent neural structures. Much of the early neurologic deficit that ensues is due to increased intracranial pressure (ICP) with resultant ischemia. The hemorrhage resolves to leave a slit-like cavity lined by a glial scar. Thus, the aim of therapy is to minimize the size of the hemorrhage and to lessen the increased ICP.

TABLE 1. **Some Clinical Signs Usually Associated with Hypertensive Intracerebral Hemorrhage (ICH) Depending on Location**

| Location | Motor/Sensory | Pupils | Eye Deviation |
|---|---|---|---|
| Putamen | Contralateral hemiparesis, hemianesthesia | Normal | Contralateral conjugate gaze |
| Thalamus | Contralateral hemiparesis; hemianesthesia | Small | Conjugate downward deviation |
| Cerebellum | Ipsilateral facial weakness; ipsilateral truncal ataxia; ipsilateral limb ataxia | Small | Ipsilateral conjugate gaze paresis; sixth nerve paresis |
| Pons | Quadriparesis | Pinpoint | Ipsilateral horizontal gaze paresis, ocular bobbing |

Clinical syndromes relevant to the clinical management of ICH are predicated on the presence or absence of hypertension as well as an infratentorial or supratentorial location of the hemorrhage. Thus, the significant clinical history of coexisting hypertension and the appearance on computed tomogram (CT) can provide a framework for further diagnostic evaluation and management of ICH.

## HYPERTENSIVE ICH

Up to 80% of hemorrhagic strokes are associated with chronic hypertension. The ictus usually occurs when a person is active. The bleeding originates from the same small deep vessels that are affected in hypertensive ischemic stroke. Thus, bleeding in hypertensive ICH is almost always localized to one of four anatomic regions: (1) putamen adjacent to the internal capsule (50% of cases); (2) thalamus (22% of cases); (3) pons (10% of cases); and (4) cerebellar hemispheres (20% of cases). Each of the four locations produces a relatively distinct clinical presentation as illustrated in Table 1. Hypertensive ICH originating in the central white matter is rare.

The clinical deficit in hypertensive ICH usually develops gradually over 30 to 60 minutes and is completed by the time the patient arrives for evaluation. Unless there is a coagulopathy or underlying vascular malformation, the clot seldom enlarges. Clinical worsening after the initial hemorrhage is usually due to edema, ventricular obstruction, or both. Increased intracranial pressure is evidenced by nausea, vomiting, and a decreased level of alertness. Coma implies either a large hematoma with ventricular rupture, ventricular obstruction, or both and carries a poor prognosis for functional survival. Supratentorial hemorrhages can result in transtentorial herniation. These clinical features highlight the demand for careful and frequent re-examination of the patient. Attendant nursing personnel should be trained in assessing neurologic signs.

## NONHYPERTENSIVE ICH

ICH without an associated history of hypertension has a less predictable anatomic distribution. A wide variety of underlying pathologic conditions can produce these hemorrhages. Careful consideration should be given to the diagnosis of an aneurysm or arteriovenous malformation (AVM). Prolonged bleeding times due to systemic causes or the use of anticoagulants must be excluded. Amphetamine and cocaine substance abuse are presumed to lead to an arteritis which results in ICH. Amyloid angiopathy is a condition that involves amyloid deposition in cerebral vessels and results in

multisite recurrent hemorrhages. This condition can be familial and is a common cause of ICH in the elderly. The precise clinical presentation of nonhypertensive ICH depends on the anatomic location where the hemorrhage occurs. The bleeding produced by nonhypertensive ICH has a greater tendency to continue than that caused by hypertensive ICH. This can serve as a differential point in those patients who have mild to moderate hypertension and those with an increasingly enlarging intracerebral clot.

Clinical laboratory evaluation in all forms of ICH should be directed toward the differential diagnosis included in Table 2. CT scan should be performed as soon as the diagnosis of intracerebral hemorrhage is suspected. Hemorrhages as small as 1 cm in diameter can be localized by CT, although small pontine hemorrhages can be missed because of volume averaging or bone artifact. The CT localization is extremely useful in terms of guiding further evaluation and management. Associated vascular malformations should be sought on the CT, especially if the hematoma is immediately subcortical or if there is dissection of blood into the subarachnoid space. Frontopolar hematomas are often associated with anterior cerebral artery aneurysms. A follow-up contrasted scan at times reveals ring enhancement around the hemorrhage, providing evidence of a hemorrhage into a pre-existing tumor. If the CT scan is delayed for 10 to 14 days, the hematoma may appear isodense and can be missed. Magnetic resonance imaging (MRI) is superior to CT in identifying late stage hematomas, posterior fossa lesions, and arteriovenous malformations. When the etiology of ICH is not obvious, cerebral angiography should be performed in patients deemed appropriate to undergo the procedure. Lumbar puncture (LP) carries the risk of precipitating a herniation syndrome in ICH and should be avoided. LP can be indicated in those cases where the diagnosis of bleeding is in doubt or where associated intracranial infection is a possibility. Prognosis is best established by the level of consciousness at the onset of ICH. Patients presenting in coma

TABLE 2. **Some Common Causes of Nonhypertensive ICH**

Iatrogenic (oral anticoagulants)
Amyloid angiography
Vascular anomalies (AVM and aneurysm)
Sympathomimetic drugs
Inflammatory or autoimmune arteritis
Thrombocytopenia
Coagulopathy
Tumor

have a poor prognosis, and this can be important in selecting management strategies.

## MANAGEMENT

As with any patient who is critically ill, immediate measures of management should include establishment of adequate vascular access (including arterial line placement when indicated); ventilatory support when required; and maintenance of cardiac stability and correction of hematologic and/or electrolyte disturbances. Initially, patients should be placed on fluid restriction.

Early treatment of systemic hypertension is important in reducing the risk of rebleeding and minimizing increased intracranial pressure secondary to edema. However, lowering of blood pressure rapidly to normotensive levels or below can prove more harmful than beneficial. Brain tissue surrounding the intracerebral clot suffers impaired autoregulatory function, and rapid reduction of blood pressure can produce further ischemic infarction. We suggest lowering of blood pressure by 25% in the first 24 hours (or to a diastolic pressure of 100–110 mmHg) and further reduction to normotensive levels slowly over the ensuing days. This may be accomplished with agents given orally or intravenously. Initially, we use intravenously administered agents such as sodium nitroprusside (Nipride), nitroglycerin (Tridil), or labetalol (Trandate) as those afford easy titration of blood pressure (Table 3). These agents are potent vasodilators, which can elevate ICP.

Signs of increased ICP may be due to edema formation, hydrocephalus with cerebrospinal fluid (CSF) outflow obstruction, or both. In the setting of clinical deterioration with impending brain herniation, mannitol 20% may be given in a dose of 1.0 gram per kg intravenously as an initial bolus, followed by 20 to 25 grams every 6 hours. Serum electrolytes and urine output should be followed closely while attempting to keep serum osmolality near 310 mOsm per liter. Dexamethasone (Decadron) is of unproved value in supratentorial hemorrhage but can be given as an initial 12-mg intravenous bolus followed by

TABLE 3. **Intravenous Antihypertensive Agents**

Sodium nitroprusside (Nipride) (50 mg in 250 ml D5W): initial dose as 0.5 µg/kg/min; titration not to exceed 10 mcg/kg/min.
Nitroglycerin (Tridil): initial dose of 10 µg/min.; titration not to exceed 200 µg/min.
Labetalol (Trandate): Initial dose of 10 mg; then 20 to 80 mg every 10 min, not to exceed 300 mg total dose. Alternatively, an infusion of 2 mg/min may be used in sustained malignant hypertension.

4 to 6 mg every 4 to 6 hours for 48 to 72 hours to reduce vasogenic edema associated with the intracerebral clot. Intubation with forced hyperventilation to $PCO_2$ of 25 mmHg has an immediate effect of reducing intracranial pressure by reducing cerebral blood volume. Raised ICP secondary to CSF obstruction should receive early shunting by ventriculostomy.

Seizures can occur in ICH, and we suggest phenytoin (Dilantin) be given prophylactically, especially in lobar hemorrhages. The loading dose is 15 to 20 mg per kg. If given intravenously, it should be mixed in an isotonic solution and administered no faster than 50 mg per minute. Daily maintenance doses vary from 4 to 8 mg per kg to achieve a plasma level of 10 to 20 µg per ml.

The role of surgery in the management of supratentorial hemorrhage remains controversial, and definitive guidelines for its use do not exist. Surgical removal of lobar hematomas has been employed in the face of progressive obtundation and impending herniation. Functional outcome does not appear to be improved with surgery in patients with hypertensive ICH who present with severe neurologic impairment, stupor, or coma.

Cerebellar hemorrhages, however, are a special situation in which urgent surgical evacuation of the hematoma can be lifesaving. Patients with cerebellar hematomas less than 2 cm and no evidence of brain stem compression, hydrocephalus, or depressed sensorium can be managed medically under close observation. However, hematomas 3 cm or larger should undergo immediate surgical evacuation, especially if there is a depressed level of consciousness. Patients with cerebellar hemorrhage can have good functional recoveries after hematoma evacuation despite presenting in stupor or coma.

The general approach to management of nonhypertensive ICH does not differ from hypertensive ICH, but the subsequent search for etiology becomes paramount (see Table 2). Patients who present with a stroke syndrome and are taking oral anticoagulants should be presumed to have a hemorrhagic intracerebral event until proven otherwise. If confirmed, the anticoagulants should be stopped with the concomitant administration of vitamin K and fresh-frozen plasma. ICH associated with amyloid angiopathy can usually be managed medically. The need for meticulous hemostasis cannot be overstated when surgical intervention is deemed necessary. Hemorrhage associated with amphetamine/cocaine use is usually secondary to arteritis, and corticosteroids and/or other immunosupressant agents may be added. Aneurysms and AVMs often cause ICH. The timing of surgical clipping of an aneurysm is usually a function of patient grade and the discretion of the attending neurosurgeon. Likewise, AVMs may be amenable to surgical therapy which can usually be performed later in the clinical course since the risk for early rebleeding is less than that associated with aneurysmal hemorrhage.

# ISCHEMIC CEREBROVASCULAR DISEASE

method of
CARMELO GRAFFAGNINO, M.D., and
VLADIMIR HACHINSKI, M.D., D.Sc. (MED)
*University Hospital*
*London, Ontario, Canada*

Cerebrovascular disease ranks as the third cause of death in North America and most European countries. It inflicts considerable morbidity on survivors and is a large economic burden in health care costs and in loss of productivity.

Patient management is based on the clinical presentation. Transient ischemic attacks (TIAs) or minor strokes are focal neurologic deficits resulting from cerebral ischemia or infarction as a result of vascular factors. The deficit may clear within 24 hours (TIA), or it may persist for more than 24 hours but eventually results in either no neurologic deficit or a mild focal abnormality (minor stroke). The majority of TIAs clear within 15 minutes of presentation. About 25% of TIAs are associated with computerized tomography (CT) evidence of infarction.

A major stroke is a fixed focal neurologic deficit resulting from infarction or hemorrhage in a part of the brain.

Although patients between 16 and 45 years of age account for only 3 to 4% of strokes, these young patients have risk factors different from those of elderly patients and require more comprehensive investigation, frequently including angiography (Table 1).

## MANAGEMENT OF TIA AND MINOR STROKE

### Prevention

Primary prevention is the best form of medical care. Prevention implies awareness of the various risk factors for stroke.

TABLE 1. **Causes of Stroke in Young Patients**

1. Cardiac: valvular abnormalities, mitral valve prolapse, rheumatic valve disease, arrhythmias, cardiomyopathies, mural thrombi, post—myocardial infarction
2. Hypertension
3. Drug induced: cocaine, amphetamines, sympathomimetics
4. Oral contraceptives
5. Dissection of cerebral vessels (traumatic vs. nontraumatic)
6. Procoagulant states: antiphospholipid antibodies, protein C, protein S, or antithrombin III deficiency
7. AIDS

TABLE 2. **Differential Diagnosis of Focal Neurological Deficit**

| | |
|---|---|
| Seizure | Subdural hematoma |
| Migraine | Hypoglycemia |
| Tumor | |

Age is the most powerful risk factor. Stroke incidence doubles each decade after 60 years of age. The second most important risk factor and the most modifiable is hypertension. All levels of hypertension are significant, and isolated systolic hypertension as well as diastolic hypertension confer an increased risk for stroke.

Other significant stroke risk factors include the presence of cardiac disease (ischemic heart disease, heart failure, valvulopathy or arrhythmia, especially atrial fibrillation), smoking, and diabetes mellitus. Probable risk factors include hyperlipidemia, high-dose oral contraceptives, and genetic predisposition. Control of hypertension and cessation of smoking have the highest impact on stroke reduction.

### Differential Diagnosis

Making the correct diagnosis is one of the most important aspects of managing patients with TIAs or minor stroke. Not all focal deficits are due to strokes, and thus, a differential diagnosis must be kept in mind (Table 2).

### Investigation and Treatment

A patient presenting with TIAs or minor stroke should command urgent investigation and treatment, as this is the stage at which there is potential for preventing a catastrophic stroke or death. It is useful to localize the event to either the carotid artery territory or the vertebrobasilar artery (VBA). Features suggestive of VBA involvement include vertigo, diplopia, ataxia, or dysarthria. Lesions involving the carotid artery may present with amaurosis fugax, aphasia, neglect, hemiplegia, hemianesthesia, or homonymous hemianopia.

The separation into carotid artery or vertebrobasilar artery involvement is central to clinical management, as there is no surgical therapy available for the latter, which usually implies the omission of cerebral angiography in the investigation of these patients, unless arterial dissection is suspected.

All patients should have a computed tomography (CT) scan to rule out other lesions, which may require different management. Although magnetic resonance imaging (MRI) is superior at detecting ischemic infarcts, it is poor at detecting acute hemorrhage, and the procedure requires considerable patient cooperation, which may be difficult in the acute stroke setting. CT evidence of ischemic infarction may be delayed up to 48 hours.

All patients regardless of the vascular territory involved should be investigated for potential cardiac sources of emboli with a two-dimensional echocardiogram (mural thrombus, valvulopathy, or septal defects), a 24-hour Holter monitor to assess rhythm, and an electrocardiogram (ECG). Strokes of cardiac origin are treated by anticoagulation. Intravenous heparin, without a loading dose, is given 24 to 48 hours after the onset of stroke. The delay assures that the infarct has not become hemorrhagic, as is common in cardioembolic strokes. A CT scan will rule out significant hemorrhage. After 5 to 7 days of heparin therapy, the patient is switched over to warfarin (Coumadin). Anticoagulation is monitored by keeping the partial prothrombin time (PTT) (with heparin) or the prothrombin time (PT) (with warfarin) at 1.5 to 2.0 times control values. Patients with cardioembolic strokes following myocardial infarction are treated with anticoagulants for 3 to 6 months, allowing the injured endocardium, which leads to thrombus formation, time to heal and the thrombus time to organize, thus posing little risk for further emboli. Patients with strokes due to atrial fibrillation are treated with anticoagulants indefinitely, as are those with mitral stenosis or dilated cardiomyopathies.

Strokes in the VBA in patients with normal cardiac findings are managed by treating the known risk factors and prescribing aspirin. To date, the only proven dose effective in reducing stroke incidence is 325 mg four times daily. The dose may be titrated down if necessary to reduce adverse effects. Although the evidence for aspirin's benefit in women has been controversial, a recent large European study suggests women benefit as well as men. Dipyridamole (Persantine) is of no proven value for stroke prophylaxis.

In lesions of the carotid artery, the status of the carotid arteries is first assessed noninvasively with the use of duplex carotid ultrasonography. In the presence of a potentially significant lesion (greater than 30% stenosis), the role of surgery should be considered.

Although carotid endarterectomy has a good rationale, it remains uncertain whether carotid endarterectomy provides a better outcome in the long term than medical management alone. Two studies in progress are assessing this question (NASCET, the North American Symptomatic Carotid Endarterectomy Trial; and ACAS, the Asymptomatic Carotid Endarterectomy Trial). Surgery is considered only if the patient is medically fit for surgery and consents to the procedure. Since patients in a clinical trial have a better outcome than those not participating in the clinical trial, regardless of which modality they were randomized to, the best current management of patients with an appropriate lesion is participating in a controlled trial. Surgical candidates should be referred to a center participating in one of these trials, as surgery cannot be offered to the patient as a proven therapeutic modality. Surgical candidates require further investigations of the carotid arteries. The two forms of angiography available to assess the integrity of the carotid system include direct cerebral angiography and digital venous subtraction angiography. Although the former carries with it a small risk of stroke (less than 1%), it provides the best imaging of the cerebral vessels and is the method of choice.

Patients with greater than 30% stenosis in the appropriate location are then randomized to surgery or medical treatment. Surgery patients are also treated with aspirin and medical management of risk factors.

## MANAGEMENT OF MAJOR STROKE

### Diagnosis

As with TIAs and minor stroke, an important part in managing major stroke patients is that of making the correct diagnosis. The differential diagnosis is the same as for TIA, and for the same reasons, a CT scan of the head should be performed. This may confirm the diagnosis, and as well, it rules out intracerebral hemorrhage, which may require surgical intervention.

### Treatment of Acute Medical Complications

Acute stroke patients are subject to both neurologic and medical complications (Table 3), resulting in clinical deterioration or death. Patients with decreased level of consciousness from massive hemispheric stroke or impaired gag response from brain stem strokes require airway protection, with intubation if necessary.

Hypotension is treated aggressively, as the

TABLE 3. **Complications of Acute Stroke**

| Medical | Neurologic |
|---|---|
| Hypertension | Seizures |
| Cardiac dysrhythmias | Cerebral edema |
| Myocardial infarction | Intracerebral hemorrhage |
| Hypo/hyperglycemia | Progressing stroke |
| Aspiration | |
| Electrolyte disturbance secondary to SIADH* | |
| Deep venous thrombosis and pulmonary embolism | |

*Syndrome of inappropriate antidiuretic hormone secretion.

acutely infarcted brain tolerates hypotension very poorly. By contrast, hypertension is managed conservatively, as blood pressure tends to fall spontaneously after an initial rise. We recommend a target systolic blood pressure of 160 to 170 torr and diastolic pressure of 95 to 100 torr in patients without prior hypertension or a systolic pressure of 180 to 185 torr and a diastolic pressure of 105 to 110 torr in patients with a history of hypertension. Hypertensive emergencies should only be treated with intravenous drugs, thus permitting titration of dosage. Drugs of choice include labetalol (Trandate, Normodyne) (10 to 20 mg intravenously every 10 minutes up to 300 mg), hydralazine (Apresoline) (5 to 10 mg intravenously every 10 to 15 minutes), diazoxide (Hyperstat) (75 mg every 15 to 20 minutes), nitroprusside (Nipredin) (infusion 0.5 to 10 mg per kg per minute). Sublingual drug administration should be avoided, as titration of dosage is not possible, and a precipitous drop in blood pressure may lead to clinical deterioration.

Cardiac arrhythmias may be due to underlying heart disease or as a result of the stroke itself. All patients should have constant cardiac monitoring during the acute stage of their illness (first 5 days), and malignant arrhythmias should be treated accordingly.

Hyponatremia as a result of inappropriate antidiuretic hormone secretion can lead to seizures as well as to coma and should be followed with daily electrolyte measurements until resolution. This is a self-limiting problem and is treated by fluid restriction.

### Treatment of Acute Neurologic Complications

Seizures occur most commonly in cardioembolic or hemorrhagic strokes; however, atherothrombotic strokes may also be associated with seizures. A patient having suffered a seizure should be investigated for metabolic causes such as hypoglycemia and hyponatremia. A CT scan of the head is done to rule out hemorrhage. A single seizure does not warrant prophylactic treatment; however, if further seizures arise, phenytoin (Dilantin) at a loading dose of 18 mg per kg intravenously is given at a maximum rate of 50 mg per minute, while monitoring the heart rhythm and blood pressure regularly.

Patients with deteriorating neurologic status must be evaluated for metabolic disorders, including hypoglycemia, hyponatremia, sepsis, hypoxemia, and renal failure. Structural lesions, such as intracerebral hemorrhage, hydrocephalus, and cerebral edema, must be ruled out. If these metabolic and structural causes are all ruled out, the deterioration is considered to be the result of a progressing stroke. Although the pathophysiology of this state is not understood, traditional treatment has been to anticoagulate the patient with intravenous heparin even in the absence of evidence that this improves outcome. There is, however, evidence that hemorrhagic complications of treatment may result and the patient may worsen. Continued medical supportive care should be given in these cases, and heparin should be avoided until well-designed studies have proved its value.

Experimental studies have shown that the ischemic brain tolerates hyperthermia poorly and may benefit from hypothermia. Although hypothermia is not a clinically proven form of treatment, prevention of hyperthermia by expedient treatment of infections and control of fever may be of benefit.

Hyperglycemia in ischemic cells leads to increased production of lactate, which in animal studies has been shown to result in poorer neurologic outcome. Diabetic patients should be kept well hydrated and infections prevented, thus improving glycemic control. Intravenous insulin infusions are used when necessary, and care should be taken not to induce hypoglycemia. Optimal control would have the blood glucose between 10 and 13 mmol per liter.

Cerebellar stroke, although relatively rare, represents a particularly ominous situation in which rapid neurologic deterioration and death may occur as a result of increased intracranial pressure with downward herniation and brain stem compression. Patients are placed in a 45-degree position, and intravenous mannitol may be used if there are signs of decreasing level of consciousness. A neurosurgical consultation should be obtained early in the course of cerebellar infarction, as clinical deterioration may occur rapidly, requiring emergent surgical decompression.

### Late Medical Complications

Late medical complications include deep venous thromboses, respiratory and urinary tract infections, flexion contractures, and cutaneous ulceration. Prevention of these problems includes prophylactic use of heparin (5000 units subcutaneously every 12 hours), physiotherapy and occupational therapy, and good nursing care.

### Late Neurologic Complications

Recurrence of stroke is the most serious late neurologic complication; therefore, the patient with major stroke is investigated just as the patient with minor stroke. This includes a full cardiac and cerebrovascular assessment. Cardiac strokes are treated with anticoagulation, and atherothrombotic strokes are treated with aspirin at a dose of 325 mg four times daily. In patients with good residual function, surgical considerations are the same as those for patients with minor strokes, and investigations likewise.

## FUTURE DIRECTIONS

Prevention of stroke will always remain the most important part of management. Besides modifying lifestyle patterns and treating medical risk factors, it may be possible to screen individuals at risk for stroke genetically and perhaps institute primary prevention at an earlier stage.

For acute stroke therapy, there are currently two multicenter studies investigating the use of tissue plasminogen activator (tPA) (Activase) for clot thrombolysis.

Several groups of drugs are being investigated which may provide cerebral protection in the acute ischemic period. Nimodipine (Nimotop), a calcium-channel blocker, improved stroke outcome and reduced mortality in one study of acute stroke patients, a result that merits confirmation. More selective calcium-channel blockers are being developed. Oxygen-free radical scavengers are also being evaluated in the prevention of damage to tissues adjacent to the ischemic zone after reperfusion.

For secondary prevention, the antiplatelet agent ticlopidine has been shown to benefit both patients with TIA and patients with completed stroke, in women as well as men. Ticlopidine has not yet been approved for general use in North America.

# REHABILITATION OF THE STROKE PATIENT

method of
PAUL E. KAPLAN, M.D.
*Department of Physical Medicine, The Ohio State University*
*Columbus, Ohio*

Rehabilitation of the patient with stroke starts as the usual objectives of acute medical therapy are reached. The patient must be medically stable. This includes not only vital signs but also the function of all of the major organ systems. Dialysis patients do receive rehabilitation, but their regimen is special, as it involves close coordination of therapy and dialysis schedules. As all three types of failure reduce the patient's endurance and power, the amount of func-

tional progress made will be reduced. Eventually, it will become more difficult to justify continued inpatient rehabilitation, which should include 3 hours of therapy delivered at least 5 days a week. Many of these patients could respond better to less intense therapy delivered at skilled nursing facilities. Rehabilitation, then, would be delayed until the patient's strength reserves have been augmented. Moreover, the patient must be responsive and neurologically stable. While efforts at stimulating comatose patients have become more effective over the past 5 years, the requirement of the patient's having to respond to intensive therapy will usually prevent a trial of rehabilitation, except under strictly observed, preset conditions which have already been codified in an approved protocol. As standards regarding extra care facilities become higher and more efficiently enforced, that option will alleviate present pressures for a rehabilitative therapeutic trial in these patients. One factor that is not important in deciding when rehabilitation should begin is the duration of the stroke. Rehabilitation could, and should, start while the patient is still in the intensive care unit. Indeed, at this stage, goals are limited and endurance is low, but some form of reconditioning and orientation could be effectively started.

## REHABILITATION

The primary conditions of the rehabilitation contract do not vary either from team to team or from patient to patient. Only the expression of those principles varies. The first principle is that the patient is, in fact, a vital and central member of that team. Without his or her active participation, no information will be retained. The second includes convergence of expectations of the patient and the rest of the team. Only when the difference between them has been reasonably narrowed can good dialogue begin. The third is the feeling of confidence that the patient and the rest of the team have of both the ability and the will to perform. As long as the expectations and reality of progress are documented regularly in the patient's chart, restitution, usually served by our Utilization Review Committee, will not generate an early discharge. The patient and the team must in fact provide therapy in an effective and efficient manner. Team conferences cannot obviate this requirement. In fact, one great danger to the team process is that one professional will become convinced that he or she is carrying most of the load.

Finally, some form of standardized, clinimetric functional outcome scale must be applied to pre-screen rehabilitation patients and follow them through rehabilitation. While there are over 50 such scales, the Uniform National Data System with its Functional Independence Measure (FIM) is easily applied to stroke rehabilitation and has been the accepted screen for thousands of patients. Validity, precision, and reliability are all acceptable. Moreover, FIM measures self-care, sphincter control, mobility, locomotion, communication, and social cognition. The FIM was developed at a special national conference, but it is related to the previously existing Barthel scale. This scale has had excellent results when compared head to head with the competing Katz scale. Moreover, a recent 5-year prospective study of stroke rehabilitation in multiple rehabilitation centers has identified a Barthel window associated with a maximal response to rehabilitation. Patients too well or too ill—and, therefore, placed on either side of this window—simply did not do as well as those within the Barthel window. To implement these advances in quality control, monitoring standards have been raised. In order to meet requirements for certification by the Commission of Accreditation of Rehabilitation Facilities, rehabilitation centers need to have a system in place that will monitor functional outcome data on an organized basis.

### Self-Care Activities

This category include basic personal management skills—feeding, grooming, bathing, dressing, and toileting. With these skills intact, reintroduction of the patient into the community of his or her choice is easy. Without them, some form of involuntary care will probably be applied under the pressure of socioeconomic circumstances and limited resources. Success in activities of daily living (ADL) demands stamina and coordination. Both occupational therapy (OT) and physical therapy (PT) are necessary because ADL therapy must closely parallel progress in neuromuscular re-education. Speech therapy is also necessary to ensure two related objectives—safe communication and safe swallowing. Both involve exercise of involved muscles and then practice of the function itself.

Four complications impair progress:

1. Prolonged flaccid paralysis of the hemiplegic arm and shoulder is frequently painful and can generate traction plexopathies. The best treatment is emphasizing safety and joint protection techniques during the flaccid period, which can last over a year from ictus (Table 1).

2. Sympathetic reflex dystrophy yields hand-shoulder and at times hip-foot syndromes. The most effective and efficient treatment is working through the burning pain to restore as much function as possible to the involved limb. The knee or elbow is spared. The early stage commonly begins with swelling of the patient's hand or foot. Compression, milking-type massage, and mobilization of the shoulder or hip, if aggressive, will help reduce future edema and painful con-

tractures. Various medication or block procedures have been advocated, but all have tremendous side effects, and none have been proved effective in adequately controlled studies. One of the accepted regimens involved short, intensive courses of oral steroids, but use of these medications also can be followed by even more intensive episodes of reflex dystrophy once therapy has ceased.

3. Tendinitis progressing to bursitis of the hip or shoulder can mimic sympathetic reflex dystrophies. Vigorous deep heating and mobilization procedures are often effective here, but first, a high index of suspicion should be present for the clinician to diagnose these conditions. Arthrography and/or arthroscopy have been applied to confirm and treat tendon lacerations.

4. Spasticity is the common end response to upper motor neuron injury. It is exacerbated by infection, emotional turmoil, and decubitus ulcers. In the arm, dystonia includes both spasticity and rigidity in a plastic type of resistance. Minor tranquilizers, alone or with baclofen (Lioresal), have been used to reduce spasticity. Dantrolene (Dantrium) in large doses can generate significant liver, cognitive, and gastrointestinal side effects and is usually prescribed cautiously in these patients. Block therapy can be painful and can also weaken the involved limb. Significantly, antisympathetic medication used to treat hand-shoulder syndromes can often generate a greater reduction in spasticity than it can in sympathetic reflex dystrophy.

### Sphincter Control

Both the bowel and bladder could become hypertonic and hyperactive in patients after ictus. At first, early after ictus, the tone of both might be reduced. But this stage is transient. Retention, a medical complication, is evanescent and is followed by incontinence, a social complication. In men, an external catheter can reduce incontinence, especially at night, but can itself become a source of infection in uncircumcised patients. In women, progress must be made in transfer procedures before decatheterization and toileting programs can succeed. A wide variety of antiparasympathetic medications will reduce bladder hyperactivity. Bowel continence depends on the absence of organic brain syndrome, with its inconsistent psychosis, and the presence of regular, well-rounded dietary habits. Snack or junk foods are almost always low in roughage and will produce many small fecal movements. Impotence can be a problem, especially in combination with hand-shoulder syndrome and spasticity. Psychotherapeutic intervention and edu-

TABLE 1. **Leading Musculoskeletal Complications of Stroke**

| Complication | Importance | Preferred Treatment Plan |
|---|---|---|
| 1. Flaccid paralysis of upper extremity | 1. Delays and reduces neurologic return; increased risk of traction neuritis | 1. Careful arm placement; functional electrical stimulation |
| 2. Hand-shoulder syndrome | 2. Pain and joint contracture; delays and reduces functional return | 2. Restore function to limb—vigorous therapy despite pain |
| 3. Tendinitis, bursitis | 3. Pain and joint contracture; delays and reduces functional return | 3. Heat, strengthening exercises |
| 4. Joint contracture | 4. Pain and reduced functional return | 4. Moist heat/hydrotherapy, ranging exercises, casting technique |
| 5. Exogenous obesity | 5. Greatly reduces mobility and is often accompanied by diabetes, heart disease, renal failure | 5. Reconditioning exercises, aggressive mobility exercises, diet |
| 6. Spasticity | 6. Greatly decreases coordination and isolated volitional activity | 6. Hydrotherapy, aggressive neuromuscular re-education, casting techniques |

cation can help alleviate the discomfort of this complex condition over time.

### Mobility and Locomotion Activities

Diet also matters here as well. Obesity accompanies intake of high-calorie food. Obesity, along with spasticity, will effectively limit the capacity for functional ambulation. These patients are usually extremely deconditioned. Transfer and gait therapy involves following the developmental sequence that will help develop trunk coordination and positional ability in the patient. Mat activities are vital, and the obese, deconditioned patient has a much harder time. Working first within a therapeutic pool can reduce weight and spasticity. Later, the water can also provide resistive exercise. On the other hand, progress within the therapeutic pool must still be able at some point to be translated to work on mats or on the parallel bars. Within the past decade, plastic orthoses have become available in a wide variety of strength, flexibility, and shapes. The basic study of the physics and the physiology of these orthoses has not completely kept pace with the clinical complexity of the orthoses themselves. Consequently, prescription of these orthoses is liable to be greatly influenced by local myth and tradition.

Many stroke patients have other medical conditions, disorders, and diseases as well. Diabetes, hypertension, coronary artery disease, and chronic and acute renal failure are frequent. The majority of stroke patients will require monitoring of vital signs and heart rhythm before, during, and after therapy. Therapy orders should be specific. The diagnosis and all special medical contraindications/limitations must accompany the written therapeutic prescription. Moreover, the attending physician should often visit the patient during therapy. In this way, he or she will have a realistic appreciation for how well the patient is actually performing and also for how the patient is being treated.

### Cognitive and Communicative Therapy

For the aphasic, apraxic, and/or ataxic patient, the speech pathologist should work closely with the occupational therapist. At times, alternative communication systems will be helpful when these three problems are present. Depression, anger, and anxiety frequently accompany these conditions. Supportive psychotherapy has the fewest side effects and, when sustained, can yield lasting benefits. Applying chemical agents merely imposes chemical restraints and effects. Tricyclic antidepressants help exacerbate hypertension, cardiac work, and diabetes. They also lower the seizure threshold and can produce confusion in the stroke patient not unlike the clinical picture of the organic brain syndrome. Both major and minor tranquilizers rob the patient of spontaneous activity and can generate listlessness, fatigue, and depression. There is some clinical evidence that these drugs, especially chlorpromazine (Thorazine), could help delay the return of cognitive function. On the other hand, there is a steady incidence of late seizures. Electroencephalographic (EEG) evaluation and antiseizure medication might be required at any time.

Finally, people with stroke disorders have cerebral hemispheres that are relatively decentralized. They are usually more sensitive to medication and its side effects. In addition, organic brain syndrome is notoriously inconsistent and very arbitrary in onset. When in doubt, always try physical or psychologic interventions rather than chemical agents. Physical and psychologic therapy in the context of a multidisciplinary team approach is both effective and efficient. Therapy should be available after hours as organic brain syndrome often becomes worse after sundown. Trying to solve psychologic and emotional complications in a nonjudgmental, supportive, patient way is both professional and humanistic, effective and positive.

# EPILEPSY IN ADOLESCENTS AND ADULTS

method of
BASIM M. UTHMAN, M.D.
*Veterans Affairs Medical Center*
*Gainesville, Florida*

and

B. J. WILDER, M.D.
*Veterans Affairs Medical Center and University*
*of Florida College of Medicine*
*Gainesville, Florida*

Epilepsy is a disorder characterized by a sign and symptom complex of recurrent episodes of central nervous system (CNS) electrochemical dysfunction that results in involuntary movements and/or various sensory experiences with or without convulsions, impairment of consciousness, or inappropriate changes in ongoing behavior. With the exception of certain rare disorders such as Lafora's disease and Baltic myoclonus, epilepsy should not be considered a disease entity in itself. Every effort should be made to differentiate epilepsy from seizures associated with other underlying illnesses as decisions for management and treatment are made. Epilepsy is a common neurologic disorder, second only to stroke. According to different studies, it is estimated that the prevalence of epilepsy ranges between 0.6 to 3.4% in the general population, with more conservative rates of 0.5 to 1%. The incidence of epilepsy may be age-specific with an estimated 20 to 40 new cases per 100,000 per year through maturity and middle life. Combining the incidence rates for isolated seizures with those for epilepsy, it is estimated that 5.9% of the total population may experience at least one nonfebrile seizure in a lifetime.

## DIAGNOSIS OF EPILEPSY

Before considering a patient as epileptic, every effort to rule out nonepileptic seizures should be made. A seizure of any type could be a symptom of an underlying disease process or systemic derangement, which may or may not be directly related to CNS pathology, and thus may be treated differently. These may include cardiogenic causes, electrolyte imbalance, metabolic derangements, drug withdrawal, drug and metallic intoxication, infections, hyperthermia, and pseudoseizures (Table 1).

The diagnosis of epilepsy is established when seizures recur without an associated illness that could have directly caused convulsive or nonconvulsive seizures. However, some illness and physiologic states, such as sleep deprivation, may be factors in precipitat-

TABLE 1. **Causes of Nonepileptic Seizures**

1. Cardiogenic
   a. Simple syncope
   b. Transient ischemic attacks
   c. Arrhythmias
   d. Sick sinus syndrome
   e. Embolism
   f. Intractable congestive heart failure
2. Electrolyte imbalance
   a. Hypocalcemia
   b. Hyponatremia and water intoxication
   c. Hypomagnesemia
3. Metabolic
   a. Hypoglycemia
   b. Hyperglycemia
   c. Thyrotoxic storm
   d. Pyridoxine deficiency
   e. Porphyria
   f. Uremia, hepatic coma
4. Acute drug withdrawal
   a. Alcohol
   b. Benzodiazepines
   c. Cocaine
   d. Barbiturates
5. Drug Intoxication
   a. Cocaine
   b. Dextroamphetamine
   c. Theophylline
   d. Isoniazid
   e. Lithium
   f. Nitrous oxide anesthesia
   g. Acetylcholine esterase inhibitors
6. Metals
   a. Mercury
   b. Lead
7. Infections
   a. Gram-negative septicemia with shock
   b. Viral meningitis
   c. Bacterial meningitis (gram-negative or syphilitic)
8. Hyperthermia
9. Pseudoseizures (psychogenic)
10. Idiopathic (isolated unprovoked seizure)

ing an epileptic seizure. In about 50% of patients, the cause of epilepsy cannot be determined. Neuroimaging studies often fail to show structural abnormalities in epileptic patients. Neurophysiologic studies such as the electroencephalogram (EEG) sometimes show no interictal abnormalities. This should not exclude the diagnosis of a seizure disorder. Although the EEG is an important tool in diagnosis, abnormal findings such as paroxysmal discharges and focal sharp waves do not make the diagnosis of epilepsy, but when coupled with a seizure history, they indicate a seizure disorder. Focal and generalized EEG abnormalities associated with partial or generalized seizures represent brain electrical dysfunction and do not indicate an etiologic factor. In general, focal EEG abnormalities correlate well with seizures of partial onset, and generalized paroxysmal discharges correlate with generalized seizure disorders. The best correlation between EEG and seizures occurs in absence epilepsy (petit mal epilepsy) with the EEG showing 3 (2.5 to 4) Hz paroxysmal generalized spike and wave discharge.

With a careful history, clinical observation, and EEG, an accurate classification of seizure type can be made in most patients. The International Classification of Epileptic Seizures pivots around the onset of seizures, whether it is generalized or focal, and whether there is associated loss or impairment, or no impairment, of consciousness. "Partial" seizures denote seizures beginning locally, and these may be either simple or complex. Simple partial seizures indicate elementary signs or symptoms without impairment of consciousness. These symptoms may be somatic motor (e.g., jacksonian seizures), somatosensory, special sensory, or autonomic. Often, patients report having just auras and no seizures. These "auras" usually represent simple partial seizures with somatic and special sensory symptoms that may be isolated or may precede a complex partial seizure. The physician should carefully look for these symptoms because patients may disregard these symptoms and inadvertently not volunteer this information. Complex partial seizures (CPS) (partial seizures with complex symptoms), also known as temporal lobe or psychomotor seizures, denote seizures beginning locally with impairment of consciousness. Impairment of consciousness manifested by staring is a common symptom that is frequently described by witnesses as "glassy eyes." Other symptoms may be cognitive, affective, "psychosensory," or "psychomotor" with semipurposeful automatisms. Not infrequently, partial seizures may spread and become secondarily generalized.

Generalized seizures are associated with loss of consciousness at the onset and are bilaterally symmetric without local onset. Generalized seizures may be convulsive or nonconvulsive. Convulsive generalized seizures predominantly seen in adolescents may be tonic-clonic (grand mal), clonic, clonic-tonic-clonic, or myoclonic. Nonconvulsive generalized seizures may include absence (petit mal), atonic, and akinetic seizures. Classification of seizures is important for communication among treating physicians, treatment of specific seizure types, and prognosis. Some common seizure types may be difficult to differentiate clinically. The majority of patients that report their seizures as petit mal do not have typical absence or petit mal seizures, but they turn out to have complex partial seizures. Absence (petit mal) and complex partial seizures are commonly confused and misdiagnosed. In the majority of cases, a differential diagnosis can be made on the basis of history, duration of seizure, presence of aura and/or postictal confusion, pattern of automatic behavior, and EEG. In absence seizures there is no aura or postictal confusion; minor clonic activity (eye blinks or head nodding) is present in up to 45% of cases; mean duration is about 10 seconds; and EEG shows the typical bilateral, symmetric three-cycles-per-second spike and wave that may be easily provoked by hyperventilation. On the other hand, complex partial seizures may be preceded by an aura, followed by postictal confusion, last longer (1 to 2 minutes), are associated with more complex automatisms and less frequent clonic components, and the EEG tends to show focal slow or sharp and slow activity. The differentiation between these two types of seizures is important. Absence seizures tend to disappear in adulthood but CPS do not. Furthermore, phenytoin (Dilantin) and carbamazepine (Tegretol) are effective in CPS but may aggravate absence attacks. Another important distinction is between primarily generalized tonic-clonic sei-

zure and secondarily generalized tonic-clonic seizure. The former denotes loss of consciousness from the onset of the attack and is more common in the idiopathic epilepsies. The latter denotes focality of onset with subsequent spread of activity to involve both hemispheres and is more common in the symptomatic group. These two types respond differently to different antiepileptic drugs (AEDs). In addition, the manifestation of certain types of seizure may localize the firing focus that may not otherwise show on neuroimaging or EEG studies.

Classification of the epilepsies and the epileptic syndromes is a further effort to categorize epileptic individuals who have seizures of similar type, behavior, and natural history. Classification depends on the seizure type, specific EEG abnormality, and age at onset.

From the etiologic point of view, one has to differentiate between symptomatic (or secondary) and idiopathic (or primary) epilepsy. Symptomatic epilepsy is usually due to recent or remote focal or diffuse injury to the brain. Idiopathic epilepsy is due to a genetic predisposition. The signs of this injury are usually structural abnormalities that can often be detected by neuroimaging studies (Table 2). The most common types of seizures seen in symptomatic epilepsy are

TABLE 2. **Possible Causes of Epileptic Seizures in Adolescents and Adults**

A. Symptomatic
  1. Head trauma
    a. Perinatal
    b. Postnatal
    c. Acute head trauma
  2. Encephalopathy
    a. Hypoxic (cardiac arrest, carbon monoxide poisoning, perinatal ischemia, suffocation, or respiratory arrest).
    b. Hypertensive
    c. Infectious
      (1) Viral (herpes simplex, Jakob-Creutzfeldt disease)
      (2) Bacterial
      (3) Fungal
      (4) Parasitic (neurocysticercosis)
  3. Neoplasia
    a. Primary brain tumors (astrocytoma, glioblastoma, multiforme)
    b. Metastatic
  4. Temporal mesial sclerosis
  5. Phakomatoses
  6. Vascular
    a. Malformations
    b. Aneurysms
    c. Hemorrhage (intraparenchymal, superficial siderosis)
    d. Stroke (thrombotic or embolic infarcts)
    e. Thrombotic thrombocytopenia purpura
    f. Cortical phlebothrombosis or thrombophlebitis
  7. Degenerative
B. Idiopathic
  1. Juvenile myoclonic epilepsy (JME)
  2. Juvenile absence
  3. Myoclonic
  4. Primary generalized tonic-clonic (GTC) or clonic-tonic-clonic (GCTC)

complex partial seizures and the secondarily generalized seizures. The idiopathic type entails epilepsies of unknown etiology without underlying CNS structural abnormalities or history of brain injury. These epilepsies tend to run in families, and the mode of inheritance is variable. Seizure types in the idiopathic group of adolescent and adult epileptics are usually primary generalized convulsive or nonconvulsive seizures (Table 2). Note that classic absence epilepsy is not common in the adult age group, and absence attacks are often accompanied by generalized tonic-clonic, generalized clonic-tonic-clonic, or myoclonic attacks. The main causes of epileptic seizures with onset in the adolescent age group (10 to 18 years) are idiopathic and traumatic. In early adulthood, trauma, vascular malformation or bleeding, and idiopathic causes are common. In middle age (35 to 60 years), trauma, neoplasm, and vascular disease become more common. In late adulthood (over 60 years), vascular disease, tumor, and degenerative disease take precedence.

## TREATMENT

### Management of Acute Seizures

In situations of acute seizures the treating physician should observe the clinical manifestations from the onset, if possible, with attention to any localization-related signs. This is done with the goal of classifying the seizure type. First aid measures should be taken in order to secure patent airway, breathing, and circulation. No acute treatment with intravenous AEDs is necessary unless the seizure is prolonged or recurs repetitively within an hour. Every effort should be made to rule out nonepileptic seizures. Blood for complete blood count, serum glucose, electrolytes, calcium, albumin (to estimate free $Ca^{++}$), magnesium, blood urea nitrogen, creatinine, liver function tests, and AEDs should be obtained. Urine for urinalysis, microscopy, and drug screen should be collected. Temperature and vital signs should be monitored. Alcohol breath and signs of trauma (such as batter sign and raccoon eye) should be looked for. A careful history from witnesses, family members, inmates, or rescue squad should be taken. A lumbar puncture for CSF cell count, glucose, protein, Gram's stain, and culture may be obtained. Pleocytosis may be seen sometimes acutely after prolonged convulsive generalized seizures without underlying infection.

In some situations, the patient may be admitted to the hospital for 24-hour observation. Later on, an EEG and a CT scan or MRI of the head should be obtained even if the neurologic examination shows no abnormality. The patient should be advised to be on seizure precaution (no driving, diving, operating heavy machines, etc.) for several months, up to 1 year. Treatment with AEDs may not be initiated if the seizure was isolated

and no possible etiology was identified. Before committing a patient to long-term therapy with AEDs, the diagnosis of epilepsy should be established by documented recurrence of one or more similar or related seizures. For better compliance and success of treatment, the patient should be educated about his or her seizures and the treatment plan should be shared with him or her.

## MANAGEMENT OF PATIENTS WITH A HISTORY OF RECURRENT SEIZURES

When a patient is referred with documented history of recurrent seizures (two or more) and the diagnosis of epilepsy is established, a careful history about seizure types, age at onset, duration of seizures, frequency of seizures, time of occurrence of seizures, trends of clustering or cyclicity, and precipitating factors should be taken. Longest seizure-free period and history of best control with certain AEDs with adequate documented serum AED levels should be evaluated. Appropriate studies should be considered if prior workup was judged to be incomplete. If a patient is already treated and is taking more than one AED, every effort to treat with one drug should be made. Patients are often on unnecessary polypharmacy. Polypharmacy is more expensive, more difficult to comply with, and may produce more side effects. Above all, because of drug interactions, one may not achieve adequate effective AED levels with usual doses. This may result in toxicity and poor seizure control. The main principle in the treatment of epilepsy is to classify the seizure type and the epilepsy and treat with the most appropriate drug. Before considering another drug, monotherapy should be pushed until seizure control is achieved or toxicity occurs, whichever comes first. Often, serum AED levels above the upper "therapeutic" range may be necessary to achieve seizure control. Serum AED levels should be considered as a guide only, and dosages should be modified as dictated by the response of the patient.

### DRUG TREATMENT

The goal of treatment should be complete seizure control with minimal or no side effects. Therefore, after identifying the seizure type, therapy should be started with the least toxic single drug that is likely to produce long-term seizure control. A total daily dose may be individually "tailored" and "fine tuned" according to patient response. Serum levels serve as a guide to dosing and avoiding toxicity. They may be obtained periodically to assure compliance. A trough serum AED level is preferable in order to have a consistent method of comparison at different intervals. The physician must be aware that different AEDs interact with each other when given together and serum levels may change. AEDs may interact with other medications, too, such as antacids, antimicrobial agents (erythromycin), antifungals, oral contraceptive pills, isoniazid, disulfiram (Antabuse), propoxyphene (Darvon), calcium-channel blockers, and $H_2$-blockers. Interactions can be pharmacokinetic or pharmacodynamic. Pharmacokinetic interactions may occur at the stage of absorption, protein binding, or clearance and metabolism. Protein binding is an important property of most commonly used AEDs. For example, phenytoin is 90 to 95% protein bound. If another high protein compound is added and 10% of the protein-bound phenytoin is knocked out of its protein sites, the serum free (unbound) phenytoin level would double and the patient may experience toxic side effects. Some AEDs are inhibitors (e.g., valproic acid [Depakene]) and some are inducers (e.g., phenytoin and carbamazepine) of hepatic enzymes and thus may increase or decrease the serum levels of other drugs used concomitantly. Pharmacodynamic interactions are effects of drugs that may potentiate or antagonize the effects of the other drugs on receptor sites.

The four major AEDs used at present include phenytoin, carbamazepine, valproic acid, and ethosuximide (Zarontin). Adjunctive AEDs include clorazepate (Tranxene), clonazepam (Klonopin), phenobarbital, primidone (Mysoline), and acetazolamide (Diamox). Ethosuximide or valproic acid is the drug of choice for absence seizures. Valproic acid is the drug of choice in the treatment of absence epilepsy with tonic-clonic, absence with myoclonic (e.g., juvenile myoclonic epilepsy), generalized tonic-clonic, and generalized clonic-tonic-clonic seizures. Carbamazepine and phenytoin may be as effective as valproic acid in the convulsive generalized seizures such as grand mal (generalized tonic-clonic) seizures. Tonic and atonic seizures respond poorly to therapy; however, valproic acid remains the drug of choice, with clonazepam as an alternative. Phenytoin and carbamazepine are the drugs of choice in the symptomatic epilepsies of adolescents and adults, including seizures of partial onset. However, valproic acid may be effective in the treatment of seizures of partial onset and, in particular, those that become secondarily generalized. When the first AED is pushed to its maximum tolerated dosage without complete control of seizures, a second AED may be added. The first drug should be kept in use temporarily. After attaining good seizure control with combination therapy, the first AED may be gradually withdrawn to see if seizure control can be maintained on mono-

therapy with the second drug. Tapering the first AED should be done slowly, over several weeks, to prevent the occurrence of withdrawal seizures. If seizures recur, combination therapy with the first and second AED may be necessary. The patient should be advised not to drive during the process of AED withdrawal. When combination therapy with two AEDs fails to control seizures, a third AED may be added with the understanding that the first or second AED will be gradually withdrawn to minimize drug interactions and side effects.

A common question by patients is whether they have to be on AEDs for the rest of their lives or not. Often, patients may experiment on themselves by withdrawing their AEDs to test if they need them or not. Sometimes, the patient may remain seizure free while off medications; however, most of the time the withdrawal of AEDs is either sudden or too fast and the patient may experience recurrence of seizures. In that case it is difficult to differentiate whether the recurrent seizure was a withdrawal seizure or not. If seizures recur after appropriate slow AED withdrawal (roughly decrease dosage by one pill every 1 to 2 weeks), chances are that AED therapy should be resumed to obtain seizure control. It is important to discuss long-term plans with the patient and share the probable prognosis to the best of the physician's knowledge. It is highly recommended that AED therapy be continued for 2 to 5 years after the last seizure. At the end of that seizure-free period, an EEG is done and continuation of AED therapy is re-evaluated.

### Antiepileptic Drug Treatment and Pregnancy

Patients with childbearing potential are advised of teratogenic risks associated with the use of AEDs during pregnancy. Most AEDs have some teratogenic effects; however, these should be weighed against the risks of having seizures. The comparative teratogenicity of AEDs has not been well established. Each patient should be dealt with on an individual basis. As a general rule, if a pregnancy is planned ahead of time, discontinuation of AEDs should be considered before pregnancy occurs. Alternatively, the lowest effective dose may be administered. When a patient taking AEDs seeks advice during the second trimester of her pregnancy, discontinuation of AEDs may not be a wise decision since most of the teratogenic effects tend to occur during the first trimester. Because of some pharmacokinetic changes during pregnancy (e.g., increased metabolism, decreased absorption, increased volume of distribution), close monitoring of serum AED levels (e.g., every 4 to 6 weeks) is advised and periodic increase in dosage may be necessary. AEDs may increase the risk of third trimester and neonatal hemorrhage. Pregnant women on AEDs are advised to take folic acid and multivitamins and intramuscular vitamin K before delivery. The newborn should also be treated with vitamin K for prevention of hemorrhage. Most AEDs have been reported to cause a fetal anticonvulsant syndrome characterized by hypoplastic nails, short distal phalanges, and wideset eyes. Phenytoin has been linked with cleft palate defects.

Another concern, which is fortunately reaching the layman's awareness, is the use of generic forms of certain AEDs. The bioavailability of some generic forms of AEDs is not the same as the brand name for certain drugs, in particular phenytoin and carbamazepine. There may be several generic products of the same AED, and bioavailability among them may vary considerably.

## Methods of Treatment

**Phenytoin.** Phenytoin (Dilantin) is a drug of choice for the treatment of partial (simple or complex) seizures and primary and secondary generalized tonic-clonic seizures. Maintenance dosage is 4 to 7 mg per kg per day. A loading dose of 15 to 20 mg per kg can be given either orally in three equal doses at 2- to 4-hour intervals or intravenously at a rate not to exceed 50 mg per minute. Phenytoin is also available in 125 mg and 30 mg per 5 ml oral suspension in 8-ounce bottles and in 5-ml unit dose pouches. For parenteral use, it is available in 5 ml ampules containing sterile solution of 50 mg phenytoin sodium per ml. Rapid intravenous administration may cause severe hypotension. Phenytoin should not be given intramuscularly because injections are painful and absorption is erratic through that route. Muscle biopsy at site of phenytoin injection showed crystal formation of phenytoin and muscle fiber necrosis. The usual phenytoin dose of 4 to 5 mg per kg per day can be taken once daily by most adults. The average half-life of phenytoin is 22 to 24 hours, and it may take 1 week or more to reach a steady state level if a loading dose was not given. Some patients are naturally fast metabolizers of phenytoin and may need a higher dose than usual. Therapeutic serum levels denote the serum AED level usually associated with significant reduction in seizures or complete seizure control without evidence of toxicity. The usual therapeutic range for phenytoin is 10 to 20 $\mu$g per ml of serum. However, some patients with serum levels less than 10 $\mu$g per ml or greater than 20 $\mu$g per ml may be well controlled without

toxicity. Phenytoin toxicity may include ataxia, dysarthria, nystagmus, cognitive impairment, dystonic posturing, and in some cases of extremely high serum levels, increased seizure frequency. Allergic or idiosyncratic reactions are rare and may include Stevens-Johnson syndrome, hepatitis, nephritis, lymphoma-like syndromes, agranulocytosis, thyroiditis, and systemic lupus erythematosus. Side effects associated with chronic phenytoin use may include gingival hyperplasia, hirsutism, and coarse facial features. Peripheral neuropathy is rarely seen. Phenytoin 100 mg Kapseals are almost completely absorbed through the gastrointestinal tract over a 1-day period with peak levels at 8 to 12 hours after dose. It is 90 to 95% protein bound in the serum and is metabolized mainly in the liver. One may not be able to accurately predict serum phenytoin concentration at a certain dose from serum concentration taken at another dose. Phenytoin has dose-dependent pharmacokinetics, which may change from first order kinetics at lower doses to zero order kinetics at higher doses. This change happens to occur at serum levels that are in the therapeutic range. Therefore, if a change in dose is desired when serum levels are in the therapeutic range, fine-tuning of the dose with smaller increments or decrements should be practiced. For that reason phenytoin is also available in 50 mg tablets (Infatabs) which have the advantage of prompt absorption and the disadvantage of toxic side effects associated with serum peak level. A 30-mg capsule is also available. Periodic trough phenytoin levels are recommended, and sometimes determination of serum unbound (free) phenytoin may be necessary in cases with hepatic disease or drug interactions. Drugs that are known to increase serum phenytoin level include carbamazepine, cimetidine (Tagamet), chloramphenicol (Chloromycetin), isoniazid, chlorpromazine (Thorazine), and propoxyphene. Phenytoin may lower the serum levels of concomitant oral contraceptives and other steroids, digoxin, and thyroid hormone. Salicylates and ethanol may lower serum phenytoin level.

**Carbamazepine.** According to the VA Cooperative double-blind AED efficacy study, carbamazepine (Tegretol) and phenytoin showed no statistically significant difference in their effect on reducing generalized tonic-clonic seizures or seizures of partial onset. Both were superior to primidone and phenobarbital. The usual maintenance dose is 10 to 20 mg per kg per day given orally. Because of its relatively short half-life (8 to 20 hours) and toxic effects associated with peak levels (2 to 3 hours after ingestion), administration in 2 to 4 divided daily doses is recommended. Carbamazepine is supplied as 100-mg chewable and 200-mg scored tablets which can be divided easily for initiation of therapy. Carbamazepine is also available in 100 mg per 5 ml oral suspension. The initial dose should be small (100 to 200 mg in two daily doses for adults) to prevent gastrointestinal and other unpleasant side effects. This dosage can be increased in daily increments of 200 mg every 3 to 5 days until seizure control or therapeutic serum levels are attained. Usually patients cannot tolerate taking the full maintenance daily dose initially and titrating up is recommended; otherwise carbamazepine treatment may be dropped and prematurely considered as a failure.

Carbamazepine is approximately 75% protein bound. Valproic acid may compete for binding sites. Carbamazepine is metabolized in the liver to carbamazepine-10, 11-epoxide, and carbamazepine-10, 11-dihydroxide. The former is pharmacologically active and has an anticonvulsant activity and toxicity similar to the parent compound. The usual therapeutic range of serum carbamazepine level is from 8 to 12 $\mu$g per ml; however, higher levels may be necessary in some cases for seizure control. During long-term therapy with carbamazepine, epoxide concentrations range between 15 to 50% of the carbamazepine serum concentrations. Carbamazepine is a hepatic enzyme inducer and may reduce the effects of co-administered drugs such as oral anticoagulants and contraceptives. Other hepatic enzyme–inducing drugs such as phenobarbital and phenytoin may reduce the effects of carbamazepine, and higher doses of carbamazepine may be necessary to achieve the same serum levels. Cimetidine, propoxyphene, erythromycin, and chloramphenicol co-administration may raise serum carbamazepine concentrations and may result in toxicity. Carbamazepine causes autoinduction of its metabolism that results in a decrease in its half-life. This process may take many weeks (8 to 15) before stable steady-state serum levels of carbamazepine can be achieved; thus, close monitoring of serum carbamazepine levels in the first 2 to 4 months is advisable. A baseline CBC and serum electrolyte and liver function tests are recommended, to be followed up periodically at 2 to 3 months initially for the first 6 to 12 months then probably biannually thereafter. Carbamazepine was reported earlier to have serious hematologic toxicity; however, this is rare and the toxicity of carbamazepine is probably no greater than that of other AEDs. Side effects of carbamazepine may include gastrointestinal disturbances, drowsiness, diplopia, blurred vision, and headache. These side effects are more common with higher serum carbamazepine levels, and dose adjustment usually alleviates those symptoms. Side effects are sometimes intermittent and coincide with peak serum levels. In these situations spreading and dividing the total daily dose over a longer period of time may alleviate the symptoms. Most of the adverse reactions are usually experienced in the first few weeks of therapy and often clear in a few days to weeks without dosage adjustment. Acute overdosage of carbamazepine may result in nausea, vomiting, nystagmus, drowsiness or coma, restlessness, agitation, confusion, tremor, abnormal reflexes, mydriasis, flushing, and urinary retention. Allergic reactions to carbamazepine may include various forms of dermatitis and skin eruptions or rashes. Carbamazepine administration should be avoided in patients with history of serious blood dyscrasias or known sensitivity to tricyclic compounds. Carbamazepine should be used with caution in patients with cardiac irregularities or coronary artery disease. Carbamazepine may have an antidiuretic effect that may result in water intoxication and hyponatremia and increase in seizure activity. Neural tube defects have been reported in children of mothers receiving carbamazepine during pregnancy. The risks and benefits of carbamazepine treatment during pregnancy have to be weighed, and serum carbamazepine levels should be closely monitored to avoid excessive concentrations and exposure to the fetus.

**Ethosuximide.** Ethosuximide (Zarontin) is very effective in the treatment of absence (petit mal) seizures and well tolerated by patients. Common side effects include drowsiness and gastrointestinal upset. Leukopenia may occur in a minority of patients and is reversible if detected early and ethosuximide is withdrawn. Maintenance dose is usually 15 to 30 mg per kg per day given in two equal doses. Therapy is started initially at 500 mg per day followed by 250 mg daily increments every few days to 1 week until seizure control is achieved or intolerable side effects result. Ethosuximide is available in 250 mg capsules. It is absorbed through the gastrointestinal tract almost completely, and its binding to serum protein is minimal. Ethosuximide does not have significant interactions with other AEDs, and if toxicity associated with peak serum levels occurs, the total daily dosage should be divided into three or four equal doses.

**Valproic Acid.** Valproic acid (Depakene) has the same efficacy as ethosuximide in the treatment of absence seizures. Either AED may be used as first choice; however, in some cases, a combination of both valproic acid and ethosuximide may be necessary to control petit mal seizures. Valproic acid is as effective as phenytoin and carbamazepine in the treatment of primary generalized tonic-clonic seizures. Valproic acid is the drug of choice in the treatment of absence associated with myoclonic or generalized tonic-clonic seizures, in particular, juvenile myoclonic epilepsy. In some instances, valproic acid may be effective in the treatment of seizures of partial onset, especially secondarily generalized seizure. A controlled double-blind study comparing the efficacy of carbamazepine and valproic acid in the treatment of partial seizures is under way. The usual maintenance dose is 15 to 60 mg per kg per day in three or four divided doses. The initial dose is 15 mg per kg per day with increments of 4 to 10 mg per kg per day every week until seizure control is achieved or side effects occur.

The therapeutic serum level range is 50 to 140 μg per ml. Common side effects include gastrointestinal upset, drowsiness, tremor, and weight gain. Other side effects may include platelet dysfunction, hyperammonemia, and elevated serum transaminase. Idiosyncratic side effects may include pancreatitis, thrombocytopenia, hepatitis, coma, and hair loss. Fatal hepatic failure may occur, and the greatest risk is in younger children on polypharmacy. At particular risk are those under 2 years of age who are on other AEDs. Gastrointestinal side effects are more frequent with valproic acid (Depakene) and are much less frequent with the enteric coated divalproex sodium formulation (Depakote). Divalproex sodium is available in 125 mg, 250 mg, and 500 mg tablets. Valproic acid is not available for parenteral use in the United States at present. A slow-release 125-mg "sprinkle" formulation is available for children. The absorption of divalproex sodium is delayed, with the peak concentration occurring 3 to 4 hours after oral administration. Depakote can be given in two to three divided daily doses. Valproic acid is almost completely absorbed, and it is 75 to 90% protein bound (less protein-binding percentage at higher serum levels). Valproic acid is primarily metabolized in the liver, and minimal amounts are lost in the urine or feces. Active metabolites are formed. A 2-en metabolite is an anticonvulsant and may account for the increasing efficacy noted in some patients over a 4- to 6-week period after initiation of therapy. Neural tube defects are reported in 1 to 2% of the offspring of epileptic mothers who receive valproic acid during the first trimester of pregnancy.

Other AEDs that may be used as adjunctive therapy include phenobarbital, primidone (Mysoline), clorazepate (Tranxene), mephenytoin (Mesantoin), methsuximide (Celontin), ethotoin (Peganone), and clonazepam (Klonopin). Phenobarbital and primidone used to be widely employed in treating seizures; however, they are now avoided except in special situations. Phenobarbital is a sedative, reduces attention span, and impairs learning. The above-mentioned adjunctive AEDs may be tried when the four major AEDs are ineffective or cause intolerable and serious side effects. Diazepam (Valium) or lorazepam (Ativan) may be used orally or rectally for intermittent home treatment to stop clusters of seizures and avoid unnecessary and expensive hospitalization. In addition to phenytoin, phenobarbital, diazepam, and lorazepam may also be administered intravenously in the treatment of acute seizures, including status epilepticus.

# EPILEPSY IN INFANTS AND CHILDREN

method of
PETER CAMFIELD, M.D., and
CAROL CAMFIELD, M.D.
*Izaak Walton Killam Hospital for Children*
*Halifax, Nova Scotia, Canada*

A seizure may result from an acute brain disturbance such as hypoglycemia, or a chronic disturbance, such as a cortical scar from a head injury. Epilepsy implies a tendency for recurrent spontaneous seizures and is diagnosed only after two or more unprovoked seizures. Seventy percent of epilepsy begins in childhood. For many, the epileptic tendency is outgrown; for others, the disorder is lifelong. For some, epilepsy results from brain abnormalities which may be more disabling than the epilepsy. For others, the cause is less pervasive and normal life is possible provided that seizures are controlled.

## EPIDEMIOLOGY

There are many types of epilepsy in childhood with multiple causes. Seizure and epilepsy classification is outlined in the chapter on epilepsy in adolescents and adults. The onset of epilepsy in infants and children is most frequent between ages 6 and 8 years. The most common seizure types are partial (with or without secondary generalization) and generalized tonic-clonic. Prognosis depends on the type of epilepsy, its cause, and associated neurologic deficits.

Many children have a single unprovoked seizure but never a recurrence. After a first seizure, the overall risk of recurrence is 50%. Seizure type, neurologic well-being, and EEG "epileptic" discharge influence the risk of recurrence (Table 1). Recurrences are usually within 6 to 12 months of the first seizure. If a second seizure occurs, 80 to 90% of children will have further seizures, unless they are treated with medication.

Treatment with antiepileptic medication does not appear to significantly alter the natural history of childhood epilepsy. Medication provides seizure control, and brain maturation may result in eventual remission. In general, the chance that a child with newly diagnosed epilepsy will achieve 2 years seizure free on medication is approximately 70%. At this point, 70 to 80% will remain seizure free if medication is

TABLE 1. **Approximate Percent Risk of Recurrence Within 24 Months of a Single Unprovoked Seizure**

| | EEG Norm, Neuro Norm | EEG Abn, Neuro Norm | EEG Norm, Neuro Abn | EEG Abn, Neuro Abn |
|---|---|---|---|---|
| Generalized tonic-clonic | | | | |
| Focal with secondary generalization | 30 | 45 | 50 | 75 |
| Partial elementary | 50 | 70 | 75 | 90 |
| Partial complex | 60 | 75 | 85 | 95 |

*Abbreviations:* EEG Norm = no epileptic (spike) discharge; EEG Abn = epileptic (spike) discharge; Neuro Norm = normal neurologic examination; Neuro Abn = abnormal neurologic examination.

stopped. Thus, for a newly diagnosed patient, the chance of outgrowing epilepsy is about 50%. Prognosis can be more refined by knowledge of the specific epileptic disorder.

## WORK-UP OF A CHILD WITH NEWLY DIAGNOSED EPILEPSY

The cause of epilepsy is unknown in approximately one-half of patients. Assessment must include a history from a first-hand witness who can describe the seizure well enough to exclude diagnoses such as syncope or syncope with a secondary seizure. The physical examination should include a complete skin examination to rule out neurocutaneous syndromes such as neurofibromatosis with multiple café-au-lait spots or tuberous sclerosis with depigmented macules.

If an acute cause is suspected, initial blood work should include a complete blood count (CBC) and serum electrolytes, calcium, blood urea nitrogen, and glucose. Unless an infectious cause is likely, a lumbar puncture is of no value. An electroencephalogram (EEG), preferably with sleep, is essential for proper classification. Unless an actual seizure is recorded, the EEG can only support the diagnosis of epilepsy. Epilepsy is a clinical diagnosis, and some children with epilepsy will have a normal EEG while others without seizures may have "epileptic discharge" on EEG. Unless there are focal neurologic abnormalities, deteriorating school work or personality, or difficult to control seizures, computed tomography (CT) or magnetic resonance imaging (MRI) scans are not routinely indicated since surgically treatable lesions such as cortical brain tumors or arteriovascular malformations cause less than 1% of childhood epilepsy.

### GENERAL PHILOSOPHY OF TREATMENT

#### Starting Medication

Not all children with epilepsy require treatment, especially if the seizures are very infrequent or minor. Once the seizure and epilepsy type are clearly defined, treatment should begin with the drug anticipated to be most effective with fewest side effects (Table 2). Parents need to understand the goals of treatment and have background information about epilepsy. Side effects of drugs should be carefully explained, and written handouts are often valuable. It is appropriate to start with a single drug and gradually increase the dose until the seizures stop or side effects are noted. Treatment with more than one drug is rarely indicated, since polytherapy increases the risk of unwanted side effects and complex drug interactions.

#### Dosing Interval

In general, the clearance of antiepileptic drugs is greater in children than in adults, and the dose often must be higher on a mg per kg per day basis, sometimes with shorter dosing intervals. Nonetheless, we try to enhance compliance by avoiding more than twice daily dosing. Most patients take medication at breakfast and bedtime.

#### Baseline Laboratory Studies and Serum Drug Levels

Before the drug is started, baseline hematologic and liver function tests should be obtained. A few weeks later, the child should be examined to ensure there are no significant side effects, which occasionally are more troublesome than the epilepsy. If the child has no side effects, there is little value in routine blood work.

Serum drug levels document compliance. The "therapeutic range" for each drug is based on trough (before morning dose) levels, which are often difficult to obtain. Drug dosages should be primarily determined by clinical response rather than an arbitrary serum level. Patients may not have clinical toxicity with serum levels above "the therapeutic range" or seizure control may be satisfactory with low levels. Phenytoin (Dilantin) has notoriously variable pharmacokinetics in children, and serum phenytoin levels may be more valuable than levels for other drugs.

#### Severe Toxic Reactions

Severe toxic reactions, such as hepatitis, aplastic anemia, or Stevens-Johnson syndrome, are known for each anticonvulsant. Parents should be informed of these possible reactions and instructed to contact their physician should the early symptoms begin. There is no evidence that routine screening for toxic effects is of value, and we do not recommend it. If a child develops a symptom of a toxic reaction, testing should be tailored for that particular symptom.

TABLE 2. **Antiepileptic Medications for Infants and Children**

| Drug | Usual Dose | Half-Life (hr) | Therapeutic Range µg/ml (mmol/ml) | Side Effects |
|------|-----------|----------------|-----------------------------------|--------------|
| Carbamazepine (Tegretol) | Build up over 2 weeks to 10–20 mg/kg/day in 2–3 daily doses | 6–12 | 5–14 (13–40) | Drowsiness, diplopia, allergic skin rash, aplastic anemia, hepatitis |
| Clonazepam (Klonopin) | 0.05–0.3 mg/kg/day in 2–3 daily doses | 24–36 | | Drowsiness, behavior disturbance, drooling, ataxia |
| Ethosuximide (Zarontin) | 10–20 mg/kg/day in 1–2 daily doses | 24–36 | 40–100 (280–570) | Nausea, moodiness, aplastic anemia |
| Phenobarbital | 4–5 mg/kg/day in 1 daily dose | 48–100 | 10–30 (65–150) | Irritability, hyperactivity, allergic skin rash, cognitive deficits |
| Phenytoin (Dilantin) | 4–7 mg/kg/day in 2–4 daily doses; many patients are rapid metabolizers | 6–30 | 10–20 (40–80) | Mental dullness, gingival hyperplasia, allergic rash, hirsutism |
| Primidone (Mysoline) | Build up over several weeks to 12–25 mg/kg in 2 daily doses | Mostly metabolized to phenobarbital* | | Same as phenobarbital |
| Valproate (Depakene) | Build up over several weeks to 20–60 mg/kg/day in 2–3 daily doses | 6–12 | 50–100 (400–700)* | Nausea, vomiting, hair loss, weight gain tremor, thrombocytopenia, pancreatitis, hepatitis† |

*Therapeutic range not well known.
†Greatest risk <2 years of age with polypharmacy.

### Activity Restriction

Children with epilepsy continue to be socially stigmatized. Restrictions on the child's activity should be based on the seizure type and degree of seizure control. If seizure control is excellent, all activities should be permitted. A child with epilepsy is more likely to drown in the bathtub than in the swimming pool. Contact sports are not contraindicated for children with good seizure control. Epilepsy is often hidden from others, and parents and children need to be encouraged to share this problem with friends so that it does not become a "deep dark secret."

### Stopping Medication

If a child has had 2 or more years seizure free on medication, the epilepsy may be outgrown. It is usually reasonable to stop treatment at this point by tapering medication over 4 to 8 weeks. Medication can be restarted if seizures recur. Recurrences are generally within a few months of stopping medication.

### SELECTED TYPES OF CHILDHOOD EPILEPSY

The following are the most important types of seizure disorders in infants and small children; however, there are other specific types of epilepsy. In general, expert consultation should be sought early in the course of disease for all children with epilepsy.

### Neonatal Seizures

Seizures in the newborn are most often the result of an acute brain insult. Although hypoglycemia must be excluded, asphyxia is the most common cause. Other important causes include intracranial hemorrhage, meningitis, and congenital anomalies of the brain. Many movements in the newborn resemble, but are not true, epileptic seizures. Tonic episodes, recurrent subtle "seizures" with odd lip and mouth movements, and myoclonic jerks are usually not epileptic but rather "brain stem release phenomena" resulting from diffuse cortical insults. Rhythmic one-sided clonic movements are usually true seizures. The diagnosis of neonatal seizures is often incorrect on clinical grounds alone, and simultaneous video EEG may be necessary.

Anticonvulsants are not needed when the cause is a correctable metabolic disturbance. Postasphyxial seizures usually resolve within 24 to 48 hours and are often associated with multiorgan failure and long-term neurologic deficits. Anticonvulsant treatment is indicated when seizures are frequent because animal models of asphyxia suggest that seizures may cause further brain damage. Initially, a loading dose of phenobarbital is recommended at 20 mg per kg intravenously as a slow push, with maintenance starting 12 hours later at 4 to 5 mg per kg per day in one or two daily doses. Should phenobarbital be unsuccessful, phenytoin (Dilantin) may be given with a loading dose of 20 mg per kg intravenously and maintenance of 4 to 6 mg per kg per day in three divided doses. Lorazepam (Ativan) at 0.1 mg per kg may be given as an intravenous bolus. The pharmacology of these drugs is highly variable in the newborn, and serum level determinations are recommended.

Most causes of neonatal seizures are self-limited, and long-term anticonvulsants are rarely needed. If asphyxia was the cause, anticonvulsants usually may be stopped prior to neonatal discharge.

### Infantile Spasms

This unique form of epilepsy develops at age 4 to 8 months. An infantile spasm is a brief myoclonic seizure. Most often, the head drops, the baby flexes at the waist, and arms are extended. This position is maintained for a few seconds. The child relaxes, only to have the spasm repeat 5 to 10 seconds later in a string of attacks including 10 to 60 spasms. When a child begins to have infantile spasms, development usually halts and irritability may be prominent. The EEG typically shows a pattern of hypsarrhythmia. The cause is usually static diffuse brain damage from hypoxic ischemic encephalopathy or developmental anomalies of the brain such as lissencephaly or tuberous sclerosis. For 10 to 30% the cause is unknown; the spasms begin in a previously normal infant. With successful treatment, development may continue and personality be restored. Unfortunately, the long-range prognosis is poor, with 90% showing mental retardation. Even though treatment does not clearly alter the long-term outlook, resumption of the child's development after cessation of the spasms suggests that treatment be started promptly.

Adrenocorticotropic hormone (ACTH) gel by injection is the treatment of choice. How this drug works is unknown; however, at least 70% of patients will have a long-lasting remission induced by a short course of ACTH. Many protocols for ACTH use have been developed with similar results. We give ACTH gel 4 to 5 units per kg intramuscularly once per day for a week followed by 4 to 5 units every other day for four doses and then taper off the dose on an every-other-day schedule over 3 weeks. Parents learn the injection technique for home use. Hypertension, irritability, and overwhelming infection are rare, but important, complications. Valproate (Depakene) and benzodiazepines (especially nitrazepam*) are alternate or supplementary treatments. However, if ACTH is unsuccessful, seizure control is not likely to be easily achieved.

_____

*Investigational drug in the United States.

### Lennox-Gastaut Syndrome and Myoclonus and Akinetic Seizures

Lennox-Gastaut syndrome has its onset between ages 1 and 3 years and has much in common with infantile spasms. The classical definition includes a mixture of generalized seizure types, including akinetic "drop" attacks, myoclonus, atypical absence, and brief nocturnal tonic seizures. The EEG shows slow spike and wave (less than 3 Hz), and the child usually is or becomes mentally retarded, often with difficult behavior. Causes are similar to infantile spasms, and for 10 to 20%, the cause is unknown. Seizure control is extremely difficult. Akinetic attacks are particularly distressing because of facial injuries (a protective helmet is often needed). The most effective drugs are valproate or a benzodiazepine. ACTH may be of some benefit. The nocturnal tonic seizures are rarely improved with currently available medication.

Other children may have myoclonus, akinetic seizures, and unusual absence attacks in various combinations and severity. The prognosis is usually not as dismal for those without the complete Lennox-Gastaut syndrome.

### Generalized Absence Seizures

Absence, or typical petit mal, epilepsy is uncommon and often confused with complex partial seizures. Onset is usually between 4 to 10 years. Onset at a later age should suggest juvenile absence or juvenile myoclonic epilepsy. Multiple seizures per day begin in an otherwise normal child. Seizures last 5 to 15 seconds with sudden onset without warning. There is a blank stare with slackening of facial muscles and slight twitching of the eyelids, often with minor automatisms such as lip smacking or fumbling with clothing. It is very unusual to fall, and the seizure ends abruptly without postictal confusion. Most children are completely unconscious during the seizure and unaware that it is occurring. The EEG shows typical 3/Hz spike and wave discharge during a seizure and interictally. Because of the high frequency of attacks, an actual seizure is almost always recorded, especially during hyperventilation. No further investigation is needed as the typical attack is not caused by definable brain pathology. Generalized tonic-clonic attacks occur in 30 to 50%.

Treatment is necessary to avoid accidents (for example, crashing a bicycle) and to prevent learning problems at school. Ethosuximide (Zarontin) is a powerful medication for absence with few side effects but is ineffective against generalized tonic-clonic attacks. Valproate is effective for both generalized tonic-clonic and absence, but because of the greater incidence of serious side effects, we usually begin with ethosuximide and warn parents of the possibility of major seizures. Should these occur, the patient is switched to valproate. Seizure control can be documented by follow-up EEG. Most patients require several years of treatment, but the majority outgrow absence epilepsy, especially if there are no generalized tonic-clonic attacks and the child is intellectually normal.

### Rolandic Epilepsy

This clinical EEG syndrome, also known as jacksonian *or* Bravais-jacksonian epilepsy, is clearly defined, common, and benign. Onset is usually between age 6 and 10 years in an otherwise normal child. Seizures are typically nocturnal and infrequent. During the seizure, the child is conscious but unable to talk. There are clonic twitches of one side of the face and tongue. On occasion, the clonic movements may spread into the arm, but only rarely is there secondary generalization. The EEG shows a characteristic pattern of spikes over the rolandic fissure, especially during sleep. The disorder appears to be inherited as an autosomal dominant with variable penetrance. Rolandic epilepsy is unique because it is always outgrown in adolescence.

Anticonvulsant treatment is often not necessary once the family and child understand the benign nature of rolandic epilepsy. If treatment is chosen, carbamazepine (Tegretol) is usually effective.

### Generalized Tonic-Clonic Seizures

Generalized tonic-clonic seizures in children are of two types: primary and secondary generalized. Primary generalized seizures occur in otherwise normal children with the interictal EEG showing generalized spike and wave discharge. Some have photically induced seizures, especially from the flickering of television. A genetic cause is often postulated. Treatment with carbamazepine, phenobarbital, phenytoin or valproate is usually successful. For those with concomitant myoclonus, absence, or photosensitivity, valproate is suggested.

Children with secondary generalized tonic-clonic seizures have global neurologic deficits from a diffuse brain disorder, for example, the sequelae of a hypoxic event. The interictal EEG discharge is usually an irregular generalized spike and wave. Treatment is with the same medication as primary generalized seizures, but control is not as readily achieved.

### Partial Epilepsy in Childhood

Approximately one-third of epilepsy in childhood is partial or focal. Partial epilepsy implies a localized area of cortical abnormality from which seizures arise. Brain-imaging studies may be worthwhile, especially if there are abnormalities on neurologic examination or difficult seizure control. Nonetheless, the cause is usually not discovered. As in adults, the most common type of partial seizure in childhood is complex partial. These seizures differ from absence because of an aura, more complex automatisms, longer duration, perturbation of consciousness (1 to 2 minutes), and a postical phase of confusion or tiredness. Concomitant learning or behavior disturbances are common. Prior to treatment, the patient has often had many attacks which have not been appreciated as clearly abnormal by the family. The long-range prognosis does not appear to be as favorable as with generalized seizures.

In general, the drug of choice for partial epilepsy is carbamazepine, with phenytoin, phenobarbital, or primidone (Mysoline) as second choices. Valproate does not appear to be as effective in partial seizures.

### Febrile Seizures

Febrile seizures result from a peculiar sensitivity of the developing nervous system to fever. One or more febrile seizures will occur in 3 to 4% of all children, typically between 6 months and 4 years of age (peak age 18 months). The temperature is usually high (greater than 39° C). Seizures from central nervous system (CNS) infection are not considered to be febrile seizures. Most febrile seizures are brief and generalized.

If the seizure is ongoing at presentation, it should be promptly stopped (see section on status epilepticus). Initial assessment must exclude meningitis, either clinically or with a lumbar puncture (especially recommended for children less than 1 year of age). Other than a CBC and possibly a serum glucose, no other investigations are routinely indicated. EEG is not predictive of further problems and, like skull films, is not helpful. A brief period of observation is recommended.

There is convincing evidence that febrile seizures do not cause brain damage. Epilepsy (recurrent afebrile seizures) develops in only 2 to 3% of children with febrile seizures. The risk of epilepsy is highest in those with complex febrile seizures (more than one seizure in an illness, focal features, prolonged febrile seizures) plus developmental or neurologic abnormalities. Even if all these features are present, the risk of epilepsy is only 10 to 15%.

Following a first febrile seizure, the risk of a second febrile seizure is about 40%. Recurrence risk is highest in those whose first febrile seizure occurred at less than 1 year. Complex features of an initial febrile seizure plus a family history of febrile seizures or epilepsy and attendance at daycare also increase the risk of recurrence. With none of these features, the risk of recurrent febrile seizures is low (1 to 20%), and with all these factors the risk is high (70 to 80%).

Regardless of complex features, after a first febrile seizure no treatment is suggested. Reassurance for parents is very important because most think that their child is dying during the seizure. Vigorous attempts to monitor the child's temperature and extensive use of antipyretics do not reduce the recurrence risk but do engender "fever phobia" and should be discouraged.

If a child has had multiple febrile seizures and is still well under the age of 3 years, phenobarbital 4 to 5 mg per kg as a single daily dose is highly effective. Unfortunately, behavioral side effects and sleep disturbance limit its usefulness. Intermittent phenobarbital given at the time of fever is ineffective. Diazepam (Valium) liquid given rectally 0.5 mg per kg (up to 20 mg) every 12 hours when the child is sick has been shown to be effective in preventing febrile seizures. It can also be used at home during a seizure to stop the seizure almost as effectively as intravenous diazepam. If rectal diazepam is to be used, the child must have few caretakers. The family should be carefully taught and warned not to teach others. The child should receive a test dose in hospital.

### Status Epilepticus

Convulsive status epilepticus is defined as 30 minutes of continuous tonic-clonic seizure or multiple shorter seizures without recovery of consciousness. Prognosis is primarily related to the cause of status; however, there is compelling evidence that prolonged seizures themselves have the potential to injure the brain.

Status should be immediately stopped. The cause should be considered with a brief history and physical examination. Metabolic derangements, such as hyponatremia or hypoglycemia, must be excluded. When the cause is uncertain, initial blood work should include electrolytes, glucose, calcium, and CBC. Oxygen should be administered and the airway suctioned if necessary.

Diazepam should be the first drug given. It is best administered as an intravenous bolus of 0.2 mg per kg over 2 to 3 minutes. When venous access is difficult, the same liquid injectable diazepam can be given rectally at 0.5 mg per kg with good serum levels usually within 4 minutes. Lorazepam (Ativan) 0.05 to 0.1 mg per kg intravenously may be equally effective. Diazepam has a short period of action and should usually be followed by maintenance anticonvulsant medication, either phenytoin 20 mg per kg intravenously or phenobarbital 10 mg per kg intravenously or intramuscularly as a loading dose.

If the seizure does not stop with diazepam, intravenous phenytoin 20 mg per kg should be given in normal saline. A cardiac monitor should be used while phenytoin is infused over 10 to 20 minutes. It must not be given intramuscularly. An intravenous load of 10 mg per kg of phenobarbital may be given as an alternative to phenytoin; however, phenobarbital appears to cause greater respiratory depression than does phenytoin, especially following a benzodiazepine. If the seizure is not stopped within 30 minutes of administration of phenytoin or phenobarbital, expert consultation is needed. Several additional drugs may be of further help, including short-acting anesthetic barbiturates, phenobarbital in coma doses, lidocaine (Xylocaine), or intravenous paraldehyde.

# HEADACHE

method of
JAMES R. COUCH, M.D., Ph.D.
*Southern Illinois University School of Medicine*
*Springfield, Illinois*

Headache can be divided into functional and organic. The functional headaches include migraine and its variants, tension headache, and cluster headache and its variants. The organic headache includes any headache associated with an organic process that primarily or secondarily involves the nervous system or its associated vascular tree or meningeal coverings. Other processes involving craniofacial or cervical structures may also produce organic headaches through a pain referral mechanism or through involvement of structures in the head. Examples of this type of process would be the sinus headache or headache associated with the temporomandibular joint dysfunction or occipital neuralgia.

The term functional headache is a misnomer. The term implies that the headache has no pathophysiologic basis and is a psychosomatic disorder. Extensive research has established clues indicating that the migraine and cluster headaches indeed have an organic basis involving cerebral and cerebrovascular processes. The situation is less clear for the so-called tension (muscle contraction) headache, but it is likely that at least a significant proportion of these headaches has a pathophysiologic basis. In my opinion, the nomenclature should be changed to idiopathic headache to avoid the implication of purely psychosomatic origin. This implication has destroyed the relationship between physician and patient in many cases.

The organic headache, on the other hand, is a very important, although much less common, entity. The entities that produce organic headache include infectious, inflammatory, vascular (infarct or hemorrhage), and toxic processes as well as intracranial mass lesions (tumor, hematoma), and headache associated with fever. The extracranial processes associated with headache would include extracranial and facial infections or inflammatory processes, joint disease, neuralgias, and dental and ophthalmologic problems. Differentiating organic from functional headache requires a careful history with attention to the pattern of occurrence of a headache, including data on frequency, duration, intensity, timing, and association with trigger factors or events. This should be combined with a careful physical and neurologic examination. Any headache of recent onset or headache associated with new neurologic findings or new findings of local craniofacial or cervical abnormality should be suspect for an organic headache. On the other hand, a recurrent headache over a period of time without indication of progressive neurologic deficit would be a potential candidate for the category of functional, or idiopathic, headache.

## MIGRAINE

Migraine is the most common headache that causes people to seek help from a physician. Migraine is reported to occur in 15 to 30% of women and 3 to 13% of men. The higher estimates may be more realistic.

Migraine may be divided into categories of classic, common, migraine variants, and the migraine tension headache as outlined in Table 1. Table 2 summarizes the symptoms associated with migraine. Note that photophobia, phonophobia, nausea, and vomiting are the most common symptoms associated with migraine.

Classic migraine, in the past, has been defined as a migraine headache preceded by a prodrome,

TABLE 1. **Brief Classification of Functional (Idiopathic) Headache**

A. Migraine
   1) Classic migraine
   2) Common migraine
   3) Migraine variants
      a) Basilar artery migraine
      b) Acephalalgic migraine (migraine-sans-migraine, migraine accompagnée)
      c) Ophthalmoplegic migraine
      d) Stabs and jabs syndrome
      e) Benign exertional headache
      f) Benign orgasmic headache
B. Cluster headache
   1) Acute cyclical cluster headache
   2) Chronic cluster headache
   3) Chronic paroxysmal hemicrania
C. Tension headache (muscle contraction headache)
D. Chronic daily headache (migraine-tension headache)

TABLE 2. **Symptoms Associated with Migraine**

A. Frequently associated (seen in most headaches)

| Symptoms | % of Patients Reporting Symptom with Most Headaches |
|---|---|
| Photophobia | 90 |
| Phonophobia | 90 |
| Nausea | 80–85 |
| Vomiting | 50–60 |
| Diarrhea | 25 |
| Visual—(spots, lines, visual loss or aberration) | 50–75 |
| Blurred vision | 50–75 |

B. Occasional symptoms (symptoms occurring with some but not all headaches)

| Symptoms | % of Patients Reporting Symptom (Lifetime Experience) |
|---|---|
| Hemisensory loss | 30–35 |
| Hemisensory loss | 30–35 |
| Aphasia | approx. 25 |
| Vertigo | 20 |
| Loss of consciousness | |
| Syncope | 10 |
| Confusional state | 10 |

or aura, which usually consists of visual or other neurologic symptoms. A common migraine was defined as a migraine headache unassociated with an aura. As some migraineurs will have occurrence of neurologic or visual symptoms after the onset of the headache, classification of this headache is difficult. In the new classification of the International Headache Society, the term migraine with aura has replaced classic migraine, and it is stipulated that the aura may occur before or after onset of the headache. Common migraine, then, is defined as a migraine unassociated with visual or neurologic symptomatology. In common migraine, the patient typically has onset of a nonspecific type of headache that may develop into a migraine headache with nausea or other gastrointestinal symptomatology, but visual and neurologic symptoms are absent or very minor.

In Table 1, several diverse conditions are listed under migraine variants. Migraine-sans-migraine (acephalgic migraine) deals with the occurrence of migraine-associated neurologic or visual symptoms in the absence of headache. This problem is more common than usually realized. Fisher reviewed the problem of migraine-associated neurologic symptoms in patients over age 50 in which transient ischemic attack was a consideration and coined the term "transient migrainous accompaniment" (TMA) for this problem. In his review of 125 patients over age 50 with TMA, Fisher noted that half had migraine-sans-migraine. A significant percentage of patients with apparent transient ischemic attacks but no evidence of carotid or cardiac disease may indeed be manifesting TMA often appearing with no or minimal headache.

Exertional migraine and orgasmic migraine refer to intense migraine-like headache associated with effort or orgasm. Again, these patients tend to have a background of migraine headache in addition to the specific event-related headache.

The stabs and jabs syndrome, or "ice pick" headache, consists of brief intense jabbing pains usually around the eyes and usually occurring during a migraine headache. Etiology of these sharp exacerbations is not known, but they do tend to occur on a background of migraine headache.

Multiple humoral agents have been postulated as being the major factor in migraine. These include serotonin, histamines, prostaglandins, platelet factors, endorphins, and other monoamines. To date, no one agent has been found to be the sole factor in the occurrence of migraine. Serotonin has been under intense investigation, and many of the agents used to treat migraine affect serotoninergic and other monoaminergic systems.

The etiology of migraine has been studied by a number of investigators. On the one hand, the classic work of Wolff, postulating migraine to be a vascular disorder with cerebral vasoconstriction followed by painful vasodilatation, has held sway for many years. Recently, there has been work suggesting that the migraine headache may originate in the neural centers of the brain stem which interact with cerebral and extracranial vasculature and may affect cerebral blood flow through direct neural connections. Olesen, in studies of cerebral blood flow in migraine, found a spreading oligemia moving from the occipital cortex anteriorly in patients with classic migraine. Olesen postulated that the spreading oligemia, which did not follow usual vascular distribution boundaries, might be an epiphenomenon of the neural process of spreading depression. These conclusions have been questioned recently, and the pathophysiology of migraine still remains an enigma.

## Therapy of Migraine

Therapy of migraine can be divided into two general categories: (1) Symptomatic therapy—employed for the intermittent occasional headache occurring at two per month or less; and (2) Preventive (prophylactic) therapy—employed for the frequent migraine headache occurring once a week or more often and the chronic daily headache with a migrainous component.

## Symptomatic Therapy

**NSAIDs and Nonhabituating Combinations.** With regard to the occasional or pure intermittent headache, Table 3 summarizes the preparations that I have found useful in treating migraine symptomatically. The major principle in this approach is to use the least amount of medication with the least habit-forming potential that will give the patient adequate relief. There are a large number of patients who have only occasional migraines and who may respond quite well to aspirin or acetaminophen or may respond to stronger nonsteroidal anti-inflammatory drugs (NSAIDs) such as naproxen, fenoprofen, or ibuprofen. While larger doses of NSAIDs are usually inadvisable for long-term use, short-term use of naproxen, 375 mg every 6 to 8 hours, or fenoprofen 600 mg every 6 hours, taken for 2 to 6 doses is an acceptable method of treating migraine. This regimen may well provide patients with an effective but non–habit-forming means of controlling their headache.

Isometheptene/dichloralphenazone combination (Midrin) may be effective for a significant percentage of patients. This is taken by the same regimen outlined for oral ergot below. A combination of promethazine/aspirin/caffeine (Synalgos) may provide relief with a non–habit-forming formulation.

**Ergot Preparations.** Ergot preparations have been, for many years, the "gold standard" of symptomatic therapy of migraine. Ergot therapy is so intertwined with migraine that a number of physicians have suggested that if the headache does not respond to ergot, it is not a migraine headache. Experience has shown, however, that the concept of defining pathophysiology from knowledge of pharmacologic agents that treat a disease is one often fraught with the potential for error.

The dosage for ergotamine, the most commonly used ergot preparation, is 1 to 2 mg at onset of headache. This may be repeated in 30 minutes and then hourly, with a maximum of 6 mg per day or 10 mg per week. The ergotamine may be taken by tablet, sublingual preparation, inhaler, or suppository depending on the patient's preference. The fastest absorption of the drug is through inhalation or rectal routes. Gastroparesis associated with migraine can slow absorption by the oral route. Compounding with a barbiturate, such as pentobarbital, can enhance the effect of ergotamine and decrease the gastrointestinal side effects (see below). Caffeine is added to enhance absorption of ergot in the Cafergot preparation. This works well for some patients, but in others the caffeine will delay sleep, which is in itself therapeutic for migraine. In my expe-

TABLE 3. **Symptomatic Therapy for Migraine**

| Drug | Usual Dose | Usual Daily Maximum Dose | Potentially Habituating |
|------|-----------|-------------------------|------------------------|
| NSAIDs and analgesics | | | |
|   Aspirin | 650 mg q 4 hr | 3900 mg | ? |
|   Ibuprofen | 400–800 mg q 4 hr | 2400 mg | No |
|   Fenoprofen (Nalfon) | 200–600 mg q 6 hr | 3200 mg | No |
|   Naproxen (Naprosyn) | 250–500 mg q 6–12 hr | 1250 mg | No |
|   Acetaminophen | 650–1000 mg q 4 hr | 4000 mg | ? |
| Ergot and other vasoconstrictors | | | |
|   Ergotamine preparations | 1–2 mg at onset | 6 mg | Yes |
|   Dihydroergotamine (injection only) | 0.5–1 mg | 3 mg | ? |
|   Isometheptene preparations | 1 capsule at onset and repeat q 30–60 min, not to exceed 5 in 12 hours | 6 capsules | No |
| Barbiturate preparations | | | |
|   Butalbital and acetaminophen or aspirin | 1 tablet q 4 hr | 4–6 tablets | Yes |
|   Phenobarbital | 15–30 mg q 4 hr | 90–120 mg | Yes |
| Minor narcotics | | | |
|   Codeine | 30 mg q 4 hr | 120–240 mg | Yes |
|   Codeine and acetaminophen or aspirin | | | |
|   Propoxyphene (Darvon) | 60–100 mg q 4 hr | 400 mg | Yes |
| Major narcotics* and injectable preparations | | | |
|   Meperidine | 25–50 mg | 200–300 mg | Yes |
|   Morphine | 2–8 mg | 24–32 mg | Yes |
|   Pentazocine (Talwin) | 25 mg | 360 mg | Yes |
|   Butorphanol (Stadol) | 2–4 mg | 20 mg | Yes |
|   Nalbuphine (Nubain) | 10 mg | 160 mg | Yes |
|   Codeine | 30–60 mg | 240 mg | Yes |
| Antinausea/antianxiety agents | | | |
|   Prochlorperazine (Compazine) | 10–25 mg | 100 mg | No |
|   Hydroxyzine (Atarax) | 25–75 mg | 400 mg | No |
|   Promethazine (Phenergan) | 25–75 mg | 150 mg | No |

*Antinauseants can be combined with major or minor narcotics to enhance their effect and reduce the dosage of narcotics.

rience, 50 to 60% of patients respond very well to ergot preparations.

A significant minority of patients will have intense gastrointestinal side effects that will limit the usefulness of these agents. These side effects may relate to direct irritation of the gastric mucosa or stimulation of the emesis center in the brain stem. Occasional patients may complain of minor psychiatric side effects consisting of nervousness, racing thoughts, or dysphoria. Paresthesia and coldness in fingers or toes may occur occasionally. A large number of patients may, however, be able to take modest doses of ergot for occasional headaches and find that they can abort migraine attacks in the early phase with a minimum of side effects and discomfort.

The physician must be aware that the ergot preparations may be habit forming. This is an insidious process but one that carries a significant morbidity. Patients who become habituated to ergot may gradually develop a pattern of chronic daily headache that recurs whenever the patient goes longer than 6 to 48 hours without taking ergot. The headache usually is less specific in its features—gastrointestinal and neurologic symptoms are less prominent, and head pain is the major feature. The pain is usually bilateral, steady, and dull. These patients usually present a picture of increasing ergot usage with decreasing therapeutic effect, and when they attempt to discontinue the medication, the headaches are temporarily worse. The only definite treatment consists of withdrawing the patient from the ergot and breaking the cycle. This is usually a very difficult process. In studies that have been reported from Europe, recidivism with return to ergot usage has occurred in 40 to 50% of patients.

Patients may be treated for severe migraine headaches with dihydroergotamine (DHE 45) 1 mg intramuscularly by itself or with hydroxyzine (Atarax) (25 to 75 mg) or promethazine (Phenergan) (25 to 75 mg). Raskin has reported good success with intravenous dihydroergotamine preceded by metoclopramide (Reglan) or prochlorperazine (Compazine). For this regimen, patients are given 10 mg of either metaclopramide or prochlorperazine intravenously followed in 3 to 5 minutes by 0.5 mg of dihydroergotamine also given intravenously, both given over 60 seconds. The 0.5 mg of dihydroergotamine could be repeated in another 2 to 5 minutes. In a significant number of patients, this results in very rapid relief of the headache. This regimen can be repeated every 8 hours and has been used to treat status migrainosus by Raskin. In my experience, side effects are surprisingly few. However, a significant minority of patients develop nervousness, racing thoughts, and dysphoria and refuse to take the intravenous regimen again.

**Barbiturates and Propoxyphene.** The next group of useful drugs is the combination in which 50 mg of butalbital is compounded with either 325 mg of aspirin or 325 mg of acetaminophen. Patients may take 1 or 2 of these tablets every 4 to 6 hours but should be limited to no more than 8 tablets per day for a total dose of butalbital, not exceeding 400 mg per day. This type of regimen may work very well for patients who have only occasional migraine headaches. Butalbital is a drug that potentially can be abused, and patients may develop an abuse pattern with rebound-withdrawal headaches as described above occurring from not taking the butalbital.

Combinations of aspirin, acetaminophen, or butalbital with codeine, dihydrocodeine, or other codeine analogs have been used to provide a somewhat stronger analgesic effect. Propoxyphene (Darvon), with or without aspirin, or acetaminophen may provide relief for some patients. Use of 25 mg of an antinauseant such as hydroxyzine or promethazine may significantly increase the effectiveness for headache.

There is significant habit-forming potential with the use of barbiturates and propoxyphene. The patient should be watched carefully for possible habituation and development of rebound-withdrawal headaches.

If patients reach a point of taking ergot, butalbital, or minor narcotic preparations on a daily basis, the physician should be highly suspicious of substance abuse. The rebound-withdrawal headache is insidious in its appearance and can be treated only by withdrawing the habituating substance.

NARCOTICS. For patients with severe headaches narcotic preparations can be employed for relief (see Table 3). The concomitant use of an antinauseant/antianxiety agent, such as promethazine or hydroxyzine, in a dose of 25 to 75 mg can significantly diminish the amount of narcotic needed. Frequently, 25 mg of meperidine with 75 mg of hydroxyzine will afford adequate relief to the patient with occasional, very severe headaches. The potential for habituation, of course, is great if frequent doses are administered.

**Other Drugs.** Occasional patients may respond to an as-needed use of 25 mg of amitriptyline, 20 to 40 mg of propranolol, or 4 mg of cyproheptadine. This is more of an idiosyncratic sort of response but may be useful in some patients who have been on these agents as preventative medications and who no longer need continuous therapy.

## Preventive Antimigraine Agents

Preventive antimigraine agents should be considered in those patients who have migraine headaches occurring at least once a week or more often or who have prolonged sieges of headaches lasting a number of days such that the patient has, more than 8 days per month, a headache that significantly limits activity (by more than 50%). The advantages and disadvantages of a preventive regimen should be weighed carefully and should be discussed in detail with the patient. The advantage of a successful regimen is that the patient may become headache free or at least experience a significant reduction in days with headache, thus decreasing headache-associated morbidity and increasing the patient's ability to lead a normal and productive life. The ideal prophylactic agent would produce complete cessation of headache and have some carryover effect so that the headaches would not reoccur as soon as the medication was discontinued.

The mechanism of action of preventive antimigraine agents is unknown. It has been suggested that this activity may relate to serotonin or other monoamine systems or to prostaglandins. Migraine tends to occur in cycles, and the preventive agents appear to suppress the migraine headache during the upside of the cycles. When the cycle remits, the preventive agent can be discontinued. It is unclear as to whether the preventive agents may induce termination of the upside of the cycle. In some, but not all patients, this appears to be the case.

It is important to discuss with the patient the definition of successful preventive antimigraine therapy at the time such therapy is begun. I feel that successful preventive therapy constitutes a 50% or greater reduction in headache-associated morbidity. This can be achieved by reducing the number of days with headache, the intensity of headaches, or a combination of both. Patients may experience a successful result by the above standards but claim failure because occasional headaches have occurred. Many patients expect total relief and feel that any occurrence of headache is a sign of failure of the regimen. It is important to note that complete control of headache can be achieved in some, but certainly not all, patients.

All of the agents listed below have significant side effects. The most common side effects are sedation, loss of energy and drive, dry mouth, constipation, weight gain, and gastrointestinal cramping and distress. As noted, the preventive agents do not "cure" the migraine but appear to suppress its occurrence, and for that reason, they will not be effective unless taken on a daily basis, often requiring multiple doses per day.

The need to take medication on an ongoing basis is not infrequently a major problem for patients and may be a deterrent to the use of preventive antimigraine agents. A significant number of patients will have side effects that will result in termination of the therapy at an early date. A somewhat larger number of patients will have side effects that are tolerable in the short term but become much less tolerable for long-term usage. If the headaches have responded well to the medication, the patient may become more aware of and concerned about side effects and want to discontinue medication.

It is important to stress that preventive anti-migraine agents should be used for as short a time as feasible. I usually attempt to discontinue the medication after the patient has been head-ache free for 3 to 6 months or at a point where the incidence of headache is rather low for a 3-month period. In virtually all patients, an attempt should be made to discontinue preventive medication by the twelfth month. In most cases, the medication should be tapered over 5 to 15 days to reduce occurrence of rebound headaches. If the headache reoccurs, the preventive medication can be restarted.

For many patients there will be significant questions arising as to whether the agents retain their effectiveness over prolonged use. Development of tachyphylaxis with gradual recurrence of the headache is not an uncommon phenomenon. If this question arises, patients should be given a trial period of tapering and discontinuing medication to determine if the headache changes while off medication.

Medications that are usually employed for preventive antimigraine therapy are listed in Table 4. A comparison of the effectiveness of these agents was obtained by compiling the studies of effectiveness and assessing the number of patients who were more than 50% improved with preventive antimigraine therapy on some type of numerical scale. Using this standard, the following estimates were derived. For the most part, these percentages indicate the number of patients who were more than 50% improved on the active drug track of double-blind placebo controlled studies: methysergide 58%, amitriptyline 55%, propranolol 51%, cyproheptadine 48%, and clonidine 42%. All of the agents noted above have shown significant improvement of the drug-treated as compared with the placebo-treated patients in double-blind studies except for clonidine. Studies of clonidine have not shown significant improvement over placebo.

For newer agents, including nonsteroidal anti-inflammatory drugs and calcium-channel blocking agents, less data are available. These agents will also be reviewed.

The placebo effect is a very important one in the studies mentioned above. For most placebo controlled studies of headache therapy, 30 to 35% of placebo-treated patients show improvement of more than 50%. Indeed, in a recent study from our group, we compared headache occurrence at 0 and 4 weeks of therapy with placebo. Over the 4-week period, 63% of subjects showed more than 50% improvement in their headaches. While this may sound distressing at first, it is a factor that the physician can use in treating the headache patient.

Table 4 lists the available preventive antimigraine agents which, in my experience, have been found effective. The table lists the usual effective dose and the range of doses that have been used. For most of these agents it is necessary to begin therapy with a small dose and increase the dose on a weekly or twice weekly basis. Initial use of high doses will often result in significant side effects and rejection by the patient of a possibly effective medication.

The beta-adrenergic–blocking agents that are effective in migraine are those without intrinsic sympathetic activity, including propranolol, nadolol, timolol, atenolol, and metoprolol. These all seem to be about equally effective in treating migraine, and to date, there has been no substantial study suggesting that patients who fail therapy with one beta-blocking agent may succeed with another.

The usual doses are reviewed in Table 4. The initial dose should be small and then increased by increments every 3 to 7 days to minimize side effects. For instance, for propranolol, start with 20 mg twice a day, and increase the dose by 20 mg every third day to a dose of 120 to 160 mg per day and then re-evaluate the patient.

The beta-blocking agents are usually most effective in the pure intermittent migraine and less effective for the combination tension-migraine type of headache. Long-term therapy may be tolerated very well. Beta-adrenergic agents are not effective for pure tension headache or cluster headache.

The major side effects of the beta-adrenergic–blocking agents are those of a feeling of a loss of drive and energy and a feeling of "being slowed down." While patients usually distinguish this from simple sedation, it is a problem that produces significant distress for some patients and may result in discontinuance of the medication. Occasionally, patients complain of sedation and weight gain.

Tricyclic antidepressants are relatively more effective in patients with combination tension-migraine headaches but may be effective in the pure intermittent migraine, especially if either syndrome is associated with depression. Previous

TABLE 4. **Preventive Antimigraine Agents**

| Drug | Usual Dosage Range (per day) | Usual Maximum Dose (per day) | Most Common Side Effects of Class of Drugs | Serious Toxicity of Class of Drugs |
|---|---|---|---|---|
| Beta-adrenergic blocking agents | | | | |
| Propranolol (Inderal) | 80–160 mg | 320 mg | Loss of energy, lethargy, depression, diminished exercise tolerance, bradycardia, hypotension, exacerbate asthma, dizziness, nausea, diarrhea, withdrawal headache | Bronchospasm, exacerbate congestive heart failure, severe bradycardia, AV blockade, severe hypotension, severe depression, confusion, hallucinations, masks hypoglycemia in diabetics, bone marrow depression |
| Nadolol (Corgard) | 40–120 mg | 200 mg | | |
| Timolol (Blocadren) | 20–30 mg | 60 mg | | |
| Atenolol (Tenormin) | 50–100 mg | 100 mg | | |
| Metoprolol (Lopressor) | 50–100 mg | 400 mg | | |
| Tricyclic antidepressants and other tricyclic compounds | | | | |
| Amitriptyline (Elavil) | 75–200 mg | 300 | Sedation, lethargy, dry mouth, constipation, urinary hesitancy, weight gain, hypotension, insomnia (2–3%), decreased libido, withdrawal headache | Cardiac arrhythmia, hypotension, paralytic ileus, urinary retention, hepatic dysfunction, psychosis, manic state, confusional state, bone marrow depression |
| Doxepin (Sinequan) | 75–200 mg | 300 mg | | |
| Protriptyline (Vivactil) | 20–40 mg | 60 mg | | |
| Cyproheptadine (Periactin) | 12–24 mg | 36 | | |
| Methysergide (Sansert) | 4–8 mg | 12 | Nausea, vomiting, abdominal cramping, diarrhea, confusion, insomnia, sedation, dissociative reaction, dysphoria, paresthesia and/or coldness of extremities, edema, weight gain, postural hypotension | Inflammatory fibrosis in peritoneal area, heart, and lungs; coronary vasospasm that can lead to infarction; peripheral vasospasm |
| Calcium-channel blocking agents | | | | |
| Verapamil (Calan) | 160–240 mg | 480 mg | Hypotension, fatigue, sedation | Hepatic dysfunction, aberrant cardiac conduction, congestive heart failure, AV conduction blocks, severe hypotension |
| Diltiazem (Cardizem) | 120–240 mg | 360 mg | | |
| NSAIDs | | | | |
| Naproxen (Naprosyn) | 500–1000 mg | 1000 mg | Abdominal pain and cramping, nausea, diarrhea, constipation, dizziness, decreased appetite, peripheral edema, dry eyes | Nephritis, hematuria, hepatotoxicity, pancreatitis, bone marrow depression |
| Fenoprofen (Nalfon) | 1800–2400 mg | 3200 mg | | |

studies by Couch and Hassanein, however, showed that the antimigraine antidepressant effects were clearly dissociable, indicating separate pharmacologic action on migraine and depression.

Sedation, dry mouth, and blurred vision are probably among the most common side effects associated with these drugs. These can be minimized if therapy is initiated in small doses and the dose increased gradually. Weight gain is a not uncommon complaint and may be a distressing enough side effect that the patient will discontinue the medication.

Small doses should be employed initially and then increased slowly to avoid side effects. Large initial doses may cause significant sedation or other side effects and result in rejection of the therapy.

In my experience, amitriptyline (Elavil) is the most effective of this group. Doxepin (Sinequan) is the next most effective, and protriptyline (Vivactil) is of questionable usefulness. Imipramine (Tofranil) and nortriptyline (Pamelor) have been only marginally effective in comparison with amitriptyline.

The nonsteroidal anti-inflammatory agents are a relatively recent addition to the therapeutic armamentarium. Naproxen (Naprosyn) at a dose of 500 mg twice a day and fenoprofen (Nalfon) at a dose of 600 mg three times a day have been reported to be effective in some trials. In my experience, these medications are effective as primary prophylactic antimigraine agents in a significant number of patients, but this group would appear smaller than the group responding to beta-blocking agents or tricyclics. Some patients receive excellent relief with minimal or no side effects. Tachyphylaxis frequently develops after periods of 1 to 6 months, and patients must discontinue the medication for several months to restore responsiveness. The major side effect is that of gastrointestinal discomfort, which can be quite severe. The possibility of nephritis must be kept in mind, and the patient should be periodically tested while on these medications for changes in renal function and occurrence of hematuria.

Other NSAIDs have been tried in migraine prophylaxis, but the two mentioned above are the ones that have been tested most extensively.

Cyproheptadine (Periactin) is a tricyclic compound with a high antiserotonin potency, which is marketed as an antihistamine. Available studies suggest cyproheptadine is effective in migraine prophylaxis with better than 50% improvement in headache in 48% of patients. Cyproheptadine may be very effective for some patients, and Rothner has stated that cyproheptadine is the drug of choice for children with migraine. My experience confirms a relatively high degree of effectiveness for this medication in children and often a higher degree of effectiveness than that seen in adults.

The usual dose of cyproheptadine for adults ranges from 16 to 24 mg per day, although doses as high as 36 mg are usually tolerated well.

Weight gain is a major problem with cyproheptadine. Patients should be warned about enhancement of appetite and a possible tendency to gain weight. Sedation is less commonly a problem and usually less of a problem than with the tricyclic antidepressants.

Methysergide (Sansert) is the first preventive antimigraine agent that was introduced and still remains the agent with the best record for preventive antimigraine efficacy. The usual dose is 2 mg two or four times a day. Doses as high as 10 to 12 mg per day can be employed. In studies comprising some 1500 patients, 58% received better than 50% relief from the medication.

Methysergide has a significant side effect profile. Early onset side effects include gastrointestinal cramping, paresthesias of the hands and feet, and peripheral vasoconstriction with coldness and possibly discomfort of the hands and feet. Nausea, vomiting, and, less commonly, mental effects of nervousness, loosening of thought processes, or even hallucinations may occur. These latter mental symptoms result from the close structural similarity of methysergide and LSD.

The major and most feared side effect of methysergide is that of inflammatory fibrosis. Several reports between 1965 and 1970 documented a small number of patients who developed inflammatory fibrosis in the retroperitoneal area around the kidneys, myocardial fibrosis, and/or pulmonary fibrosis. These patients all had taken methysergide for more than 2 years without interruption. The first case reports were formulated from fatalities related to this process. Subsequently, several patients who were suspected to have the process showed normalization of renal and pulmonary function following discontinuation of methysergide. Present guidelines for use of methysergide stipulate that the patient should not be allowed to take the medication more than 6 months without interrupting the therapy for at least 1 month. Subsequent to 1970 when this regimen became widely employed, there have been virtually no cases of the inflammatory fibrosis reported that related to methysergide use.

Other, less common side effects, including edema of the legs or hands, at times accompanied by a rash, are occasionally seen with methysergide use, and these require discontinuation of methysergide. Lastly, methysergide has been associated with precipitation of angina. Methysergide should not be used in patients with a history of cardiac disease and should be used only with caution in patients over 50 years of age. If there is any doubt as to the cardiac status, the patient should have an electrocardiogram performed before therapy is initiated.

Ergonovine has been employed by Raskin in doses of 0.2 mg two or three times daily as a preventive antimigraine agent. The potential side effects are similar to those of the acute side effects listed for methysergide. In my limited experience, this regimen has not been particularly beneficial, but others have reported good results.

The monoaminoxidase-inhibiting agents were investigated by Lance in the early 1970s and found to be effective in some patients. A number of authors have employed these agents as drugs of last resort. Physicians employing these agents should take time to familiarize themselves thoroughly with the agent and with complications—primarily hypertensive crisis that may result from ingestion of a tyramine in foodstuffs while taking these medications. Examples of banned foods include red wine, aged cheeses, broad beans, and certain types of snack foods, including, most recently, "chicken nuggets" at some fast food outlets. An extensive list of incompatible foods can be obtained from the package insert.

In my experience, MAO inhibitors have been variably effective for this very difficult group of patients; however, occasional patients have responded well. The usual medication employed is phenelzine at a dose of 15 mg three times a day. Doses of up to 30 mg three times daily may be employed. Sedation and suppression of appetite may occur, especially at the higher doses.

Clonidine (Catapres) has been the subject of a number of investigations and has been employed at doses of 0.1 mg two or three times daily as a preventive migraine agent. The studies have generally shown this medication to be ineffective. The author's experience has been in concordance with these reports.

The calcium-channel–blocking agents, from a theoretical standpoint, appear to be very promising antimigraine drugs. In practice, however, they have not proved to be very effective except as therapy for migraine variants (see below) or as adjunct therapy. The medications that have shown some activity are verapamil and diltiazem. Occasional patients may resond to verapamil (Calan) at a dose of 160 to 480 mg per day or diltiazem (Cardizem) at a dose of 120 to 240 mg per day. In my experience, these medications are more often effective as adjunctive medications used in combination with tricyclic compounds, methysergide, or even beta-adrenergic–blocking agents.

The side effect profile of these agents is relatively benign, with hypotension and fatigue being the major problems, but these occur very infrequently. Sedation and weight gain have been rarely noted.

As a final comment on the problems of migraine prophylaxis, two additional points should be made. First, the physician should try to employ monotherapy as much as possible. When a new prophylactic agent is initiated, the previous agent should be discontinued. Lack of attention to this simple dictum may result in the patient's taking four or five medications, with escalation of side effects and possibly conflicting effects in terms of therapeusis.

Second, when the previous agent is discontinued, withdrawal headaches may occur unless the agent is tapered over a period of 5 to 10 days. Such rebound headaches are fairly common with tricyclic agents, beta-adrenergic–blocking agents, methysergide, and cyproheptadine but are less so with NSAIDs and calcium-channel–blocking agents.

### Therapy of Migraine Variants

Possibly the most distressing migraine variant for the patient is that situation in which migraine-associated neurologic symptomatology occurs frequently either in conjunction with a headache or in the absence of a headache (migraine-sans-migraine). Examples of this syndrome are transient visual symptomatology of teichopsia or hemianopsia or transient hemiparesis or hemisensory loss associated with migraine. The calcium-channel–blocking agents are uniquely effective in therapy of this syndrome with a very high degree of blockade of the migraine-associated neurologic symptomatology. Again, verapamil and diltiazem in the doses noted above appear to be the drugs of choice. Nifedipine not infrequently causes cerebral vasodilatation which, in turn, may result in worsening of the headache. Other preventive antimigraine agents may be effective if they prevent migraine occurrence.

The exertional headache and coital headache are two very distressing syndromes for the unfortunate individuals afflicted. In some patients, use of nonsteroidal anti-inflammatory agents, particularly indomethacin, may be effective in preventing these headaches. In other patients, the standard preventive antimigraine therapy mentioned above may have some benefit for the patient.

### MIGRAINE STATUS

Migraine status refers to that situation in which the patient has a severe and ongoing migraine headache which necessitates multiple visits to the emergency room or admission to the hospital. When faced with this problem, the physician must first be absolutely certain the problem is status migrainosus and not a headache of organic origin.

One of the more common causes of status migrainosus is the habituation-withdrawal headache related to daily use and abuse of barbiturates, ergotamine, or minor narcotics (codeine, propoxyphene). At times, abuse of aspirin or acetaminophen may contribute to status migrainosus. In these cases, withdrawal of the abused drug is an essential part of the therapeutic approach.

The cornerstones of treatment of this syndrome are rest, sleep, antinauseant medication, and judicious use of pain medication. In most cases, the use of a preventive antimigraine medication will be required to help break the cycle. Initial therapy with the dihydroergotamine/prochlorperazine (Compazine) or dihydroergotamine/metoclopramide regimen is often very useful. I find that combining this with high doses of amitriptyline or doxepin is frequently very effective. The amitriptyline provides sedation as well as antinauseant and antimigraine effect. Cyproheptadine, methysergide, or a beta-blocking agent may be useful at other times. NSAIDs are also useful adjuncts here. The dihydroergotamine will produce temporary relief of the headache, but the headache will frequently recur after 2 to 8 hours. Judicious use of doses of meperidine (25 mg) along with hydroxyzine (75 mg) given every 4 to 6 hours may be employed if the dihydroergotamine is not effective. Some authorities use steroids beginning with the equivalent of 100 mg of prednisone and then tapering rapidly over 4 to 10 days.

In treating status migrainosus, it is very important to investigate associated factors. The major associated factors are usually emotional or psychiatric stress, hormonal factors associated with a missed menstrual period or other estrogen/progesterone interactions, minor head injury, or occasionally, occurrence of infection such as influenza or aseptic meningitis. If psychologic stress and depression or anxiety are major factors, often the hospitalization and temporary removal of the patient from a stressful environment are major therapeutic factors.

## CLUSTER HEADACHE

The cluster headache is the most intense of all the functional headaches and is one that produces tremendous distress for the patient. This headache has had numerous names. The term cluster headache was suggested by Kunkle, based on the pattern of occurrence of the headaches. Subsequently, the term has been generally adopted. In England, however, this syndrome is termed the migrainous neuralgia.

The headache is characterized by unilateral location which virtually always involves the orbit. The pain may spread to the temple, forehead, or face, or even down to the neck or shoulder from the orbit, but in virtually all cases a component of pain involves the orbit. The pain comes on rapidly over a period of a few minutes reaching a plateau of high intensity. This plateau lasts for 15 to 60 minutes for the most part and then the pain remits rapidly. During the headache, patients almost always feel better in an upright position, whether sitting or standing and will indicate that lying down makes the headache worse. Patients frequently pace or rock back and forth during the headache. The headache is usually so intense that the patient is unable to carry on any other activity.

Symptoms associated with the cluster headache include rhinorrhea and lacrimation on the side of the headache and, often, unilateral photophobia on the side of the headache. Miosis may occur on the affected side during the headache. Nausea and/or vomiting occur in about 30%.

Headaches tend to occur in cycles that last from 4 to 24 weeks (average 12 weeks). The headaches may occur from one to three times per day, and often the onset is around the same time each day during a cluster. The headaches typically last for less than an hour, although occasionally durations of 2 to 4 hours may be seen. There is a strong male predominance, with ratios quoted from 4:1 to 9:1 in the literature.

The only consistent precipitating factor for cluster headache is alcohol. The cluster patient not infrequently is a heavy alcohol user in between his cycles of cluster headache, but during the cycle, any alcohol at all will precipitate a headache. Smoking has been postulated as a factor, but the evidence is less convincing here.

Therapy of cluster headache presents fewer possibilities than that for migraine. Symptomatic therapy of cluster headache is generally less than satisfactory. The cluster attack is usually so brief that it is difficult to know whether an analgesic or narcotic medication actually was effective or whether the natural history of the headache was such that the headache would have remitted anyway. The cluster headache is associated with gastroparesis which further slows absorption of any medication taken by mouth. Ergot preparations may be effective in symptomatic therapy but need to be given by routes other than through the gastrointestinal tract. The ergot inhaler (Medihaler) may be very effective. Sublingual ergot may also be effective but is probably less effective than the ergot inhaler. Kudrow has shown that the headache may be relieved in approximately 10 minutes with use of ergot.

Inhalation of pure oxygen has been shown to be effective in aborting the acute migraine attack. For some patients this is very effective. Other patients find that the cluster headache will be suppressed while the oxygen is being inhaled but as soon as inhalation is stopped, the headache reoccurs. Other types of analgesic medication are relatively ineffective as noted above.

For preventive therapy, methysergide and calcium-channel–blocking agents have both been found effective; however, systematic studies have been relatively few. Methysergide in doses of 6 to 8 mg per day is effective in about 70% of patients. The only study on therapy of subsequent cycles done by Kunkle suggested that the effectiveness of methysergide declined over time. Of the calcium-channel–blocking agents, verapamil is the only agent that has been studied to any extent. Verapamil is often effective in doses of 240 to 320 mg per day, but good statistical studies are so far lacking.

Therapy with a short course of steroids is

highly effective in aborting or suppressing the cluster headache. The effective dose may vary from 20 to 100 mg. The headaches usually recur when the dose of prednisone is dropped below 10 to 20 mg per day. I have found it useful to combine steroids with either verapamil or methysergide, using an initial dose of prednisone at 80 mg per day, with tapering over 10 days. Either methysergide or verapamil may be started at the same time and then continued for 2 to 3 months after steroid therapy is stopped. The usual preventive antimigraine agents, including beta-adrenergic–blocking agents, tricyclic antidepressants, antihistamines, and nonsteroidal anti-inflammatory agents are generally ineffective in treating cluster headache.

The syndrome of chronic cluster headache is one in which cluster type headaches occur over a period longer than 6 months and usually at a lower frequency than the acute cyclical type of cluster headache. Frequencies of 1 a day to 1 a week over a long period of time may be seen. Chronic cluster headaches may be treated with the same types of medication. However, effectiveness is variable. Lithium carbonate at doses necessary to obtain a blood level of 0.6 to 1.2 mEq per liter may be effective in this syndrome. Lithium has also been reported effective in acute cyclical cluster headache, but most authorities agree that its major usefulness is in chronic cluster headache. Patients not infrequently may develop tachyphylaxis to lithium over a period of 6 to 12 months. Effectiveness may be restored in some patients by using drug holidays of 1 to 3 months.

Another variant of cluster headache is chronic paroxysmal hemicrania, which is a problem seen primarily in women and consists of occurrence of cluster-like headaches many times per day, usually lasting approximately 15 minutes. This is a very rare syndrome and is said to be absolutely responsive to indomethacin at doses up to 150 mg per day.

## TENSION HEADACHE

The tension headache is the most common type of headache. The tension headache is generally defined as a steady, aching, bilateral headache that occurs in a band-like distribution around the head. The tension headache may also have a prominent occipital component with radiation of pain down the back of the neck. In some patients, this is the major aspect of the headache. The headache is generally bilateral, although it may occasionally be unilateral. Probably the most important factor making this diagnosis is that the headache is a recurrent head pain not associated with progressive neurologic disease and not associated with the gastrointestinal, visual, or neurologic symptoms of the migraine syndrome.

The genesis of the term tension headache came from the theory that the headache was due to excessive muscle tension in the occipital frontalis muscle and suboccipital muscles. Proving this has been difficult, and there has been relatively little evidence to suggest that this may be the mechanism for a sustained or ongoing head pain. In certain definable syndromes, such as myofascial pain associated with temporomandibular joint disease or muscle spasm due to cervical radiculopathy or greater occipital neuralgia, muscle tension may in fact be the etiology of part of the pain. For the usual patient, however, it is difficult to demonstrate that the pain is actually due to tense muscles. The pain is equally often due to psychiatric tension.

Therapy of the tension headache is usually oriented more toward associated conditions rather than the headache itself. It is important to rule out physical processes such as greater occipital neuralgia, high cervical radiculopathies at the C-3, C-4, or C-5 level, cervical vertebral abnormalities, intrinsic processes within the cervical musculature, or myofascial pain associated with this temporomandibular joint syndrome.

The physician should search for psychiatric processes that may contribute to pain, including depression and anxiety. A large percentage of those patients who report a tension headache to a physician are actually depressed or have an agitated depression.

Many of patients who have tension headaches will need only very simple therapy with a nonhabituating analgesic or nonsteroidal anti-inflammatory agent in modest doses. The physican should be very careful about prescribing medication that is potentially habit forming. Barbiturates and minor narcotics should be used only with great caution and often are no more effective than NSAIDs. Long-term usage of benzodiazepines should be strictly avoided in these patients because of the habituating potential of these agents. The patients will often claim to have effective relief from use of benzodiazepines, but at the same time, these patients are usually very susceptible to habituation to benzodiazepines, and this represents a very real danger for the patient. Any patient who is using benzodiazepines on a daily basis or who is using more than 30 minor narcotic-analgesic (codeine, acetaminophen, etc.) or barbiturate analgesic preparations per month should be considered possibly habituated to the medication.

The patients with more chronic "tension" headaches usually will be found to have chronic daily headaches (summarized below) which may also be considered a combination of migraine or tension headache.

The patient with chronic tension headache often represents a very good candidate for biofeedback therapy. Biofeedback therapy and relaxation techniques should be pursued whenever possible. Last, these patients are often excellent candidates for physical therapy and exercise programs. It is often quite useful to get the patient involved in some type of regular exercise program which, in turn, may be very beneficial to the patient from the therapeutic standpoint.

## CHRONIC DAILY HEADACHE (TENSION-MIGRAINE HEADACHE)

The chronic daily headache is a headache that usually has features of both tension and migraine headache. The usual pattern is one of a headache occurring daily or almost daily which is of mild or moderate intensity with periodic intensification of the headache into a migraine type of pattern with gastrointestinal and/or neurologic symptomatology. The migraine-like phase may last for 2 to 24 hours and then will remit, leaving the baseline, less well-defined type of headache. Various reports of this type of headache consider it to be a migraine headache with interposed tension headache or a tension headache with a secondary vascular component. Work on this type of headache has shown that most sufferers have a background of migraine headache. In the usual situation, the patient evolves from a pattern of intermittent migraine into a pattern of chronic daily headache in association with some intercurrent event. This intercurrent event may include things such as a head injury, alteration in hormonal status with pregnancy, abortion, missed periods, or hysterectomy or an infectious event with some degree of involvement of the nervous system, such as an aseptic meningitis. On the other hand, chronic daily headaches may also evolve during periods of psychologic stress associated with marriage, family, or occupation.

Various viral and autoimmune etiologies have been proposed. Diaz-Miatoma and Vanast have presented evidence suggesting that the chronic daily headache may represent a form of chronic Epstein-Barr virus infection. Confirmatory proof is so far not available.

Therapy of the chronic daily headache again involves a two-pronged approach. The physician must first look for associated conditions such as the type mentioned above and provide appropriately directed therapy. The drug therapy of the chronic daily headache usually involves the preventive antimigraine agents. Amitriptyline and other tricyclic agents have been the most effective in this syndrome, although all of the major preventive antimigraine agents have also been effective. Combinations of agents may sometimes give a better result than a single agent alone. The combination of amitriptyline and beta-blocking agents has been the most frequently employed. Amitriptyline in doses of 150 to 200 mg per day along with propranolol in doses of 80 to 160 mg per day may be effective for some patients. Other modalities, such as biofeedback and relaxation therapy, may be very useful adjuncts in this syndrome. The amount of analgesic and narcotic medication the patient takes should be strictly limited. These patients are at high risk for habituation. Long-term use of benzodiazepines should be strictly avoided.

# EPISODIC VERTIGO

method of
THOMAS BRANDT, M.D.
*University of Munich*
*Munich, Germany*

Vertigo, the unpleasant distortion of static gravitational orientation or the erroneous perception of self- or object-motion, is not a clinical entity, but a multisensory syndrome which is induced by either physiologic motion stimulation or pathologic dysfunction. It is characterized by a combination of phenomena involving perceptual, oculomotor, postural, and vegetative manifestations: vertigo, nystagmus, ataxia, and nausea. Vertigo usually implies a mismatch between the inputs from the three sensory systems, visual, vestibular, and somatosensory. These systems are mutually interactive and redundant in that orientation and balance are guided by simultaneous reafferent cues. The functional ranges of the individual systems overlap, enabling them to compensate partially for each other's deficiencies. The intensity of the vertigo is a function of the mismatch and is increased if one intact sensory system is eliminated, as with eye closure during pathologic vestibular vertigo, for example. Management includes pharmacologic and physical therapy as well as surgery and psychotherapy.

### GENERAL MEDICAL THERAPY

Physicians tend to overestimate the benefits provided by antivertiginous drugs as a result of their strong promotion by the pharmaceutical industry. There are only three clear indications for the use of these drugs to provide symptomatic relief of nausea and vertigo: (1) acute peripheral vestibulopathy (vestibular neuritis); (2) acute brain stem or archicerebellar lesions near the vestibular nuclei; and (3) prevention of motion sickness. There is no indication for these drugs in patients suffering from chronic dizziness or most forms of positional vertigo.

When nausea is a prominent symptom of a vestibular vertigo syndrome, vestibular sedatives, such as the antihistamine dimenhydrinate (Dramamine), 50 mg every 6 hours, or the anticholinergic scopolamine (Transderm-Scop), 0.6 mg, can be administered parenterally for symptomatic relief, with the major side effect of general sedation. Alternative choices include the antihistamines promethazine hydrochloride (Phenergan), 50 mg; cyclizine (Marezine), 50 mg; meclizine (Bonine), 25 mg; flunarizine (Sibelium),* 10 mg; or cinnarizine (Stutgeron),* 15 mg; as well as the phenothiazines prochlorperazine (Compazine), 5 mg; thiethylperazine (Torecan), 10 mg; buclizine (Bucladin-S),* 50 mg; or diphenhydramine (Benadryl), 50 mg.

The capacity to act as acetylcholine antagonists by competitive inhibition is the only known similarity among the drugs used to counter labyrinthine vertigo and motion sickness. The most probable sites of primary action are the synapses of the vestibular nuclei, which exhibit a reduced discharge and diminished neuronal response to body rotation.

## PERIPHERAL LABYRINTHINE VERTIGO SYNDROMES

### Vestibular Neuritis

Acute unilateral (idiopathic) vestibular paralysis, also known as vestibular neuritis, is the second most common cause of vertigo. The chief symptom is the acute onset of prolonged severe rotational vertigo, associated with spontaneous horizontal/rotatory nystagmus, postural imbalance, and nausea without concomitant auditory dysfunction. Caloric testing invariably shows ipsilateral hypo- or nonresponsiveness (horizontal semicircular canal paresis). The cause may be a viral infection of the vestibular nerve with a partial rather than a complete vestibular paresis. The condition mainly affects those aged between 30 and 60 and has a natural history of gradual recovery over 1 to 6 weeks. Recovery is produced by the combination of central compensation of the vestibular tone imbalance (aided by physical exercise) and peripheral restoration of labyrinthine function.

During the first 1 to 3 days, when nausea is prominent, vestibular sedatives (Dramamine or Transderm-Scop) can be administered parenterally for symptomatic relief. These drugs should not be given longer than nausea lasts because they prolong the time course of central compen-

---

*Not available in the United States.

sation of the peripheral vestibular tone imbalance. Further management is physical therapy using exercises according to current knowledge of vestibular physiology (Table 1). Vestibular exercises consist mainly of eye, head, and body movements designed to provoke a sensory mismatch; they enhance compensation by facilitating central recalibration, although the symptoms initially are uncomfortable. Active sensory stimulation is necessary during the critical recovery period, and this implies that patients with acute peripheral vestibular lesions should not be immobilized but should perform exercises.

Pharmacologic and metabolic studies in animals suggest (as stated by Zee) that the state of central compensation for peripheral vestibular lesions is both dynamic and fragile: alcohol, phenobarbital, chlorpromazine (Thorazine), diazepam (Valium), and adrenocorticotropic hormone (ACTH)-antagonists retard compensation; caffeine, amphetamines, and ACTH accelerate compensation; cholinomimetics, cholinesterase inhibitors, adrenergic agents, γ-aminobutyric acid (GABA)-agonists, and alcohol may (re)produce decompensation. The use of drugs for acceleration of compensation in patients has still to be proved.

### Benign Paroxysmal Positioning Vertigo (BPPV)

In benign paroxysmal positioning vertigo—the most common form of vertigo—attacks of rotational vertigo and concomitant rotatory nystagmus are precipitated by head extension as well as with lateral head tilt toward the affected ear. Cupulolithiasis in the posterior semicircular canal is mainly causative, in that the "heavy cupula" creates an oversensitivity of the posterior canal to angular acceleration. Thus, in a strict sense, BPPV constitutes an enhanced postrotatory positioning response, but not a positional response. The natural history for BPPV is spontaneous recovery in weeks or months, but in some patients, the condition persists for years. The histologically proven explanation of cupulolithiasis led us (Brandt and Daroff) to construct a most effective form of mechanical therapy for these patients in order to promote the loosening and ultimate dispersion of the degenerated otolithic material from the cupula (Fig. 1).

**Therapeutic Protocol.** Patients are seated, with their eyes closed, and first tilt laterally with the lateral aspect of their occiputs resting on the bed to ensure proper plane-specific stimulation of the posterior semicircular canal. They remain in this position until the evoked vertigo subsides or for at least 30 seconds, and then sit up for another 30 seconds before assuming the opposite head-down position for another 30 seconds. The se-

TABLE 1. **Physical Therapy for Acute, Unilateral Labyrinthine Lesions**

| Clinical Stage | Physical Exercise | Strategy |
|---|---|---|
| I. Approximately days 1–3<br>Nausea | No exercise; bedrest | Prevent falls |
|    Spontaneous nystagmus with fixation | Head immobilization | Avoid active head accelerations leading to "cross-coupled" effects |
| | Eyes closed | Avoid visual-vestibular mismatch |
| II. Approximately days 3–5<br>   No spontaneous nausea<br>Incomplete suppression of spontaneous nystagmus by fixation straight ahead | Exercise in bed (supine and sitting)<br>1. Fixation straight ahead; voluntary saccade and eccentric gaze-holding (10, 20, and 40° horizontal/vertical); reading exercise<br>Smooth pursuit (finger movements or pendulum ±20–40°; 20–60°/sec)<br>Active head oscillations with fixation of a stationary target at 1 meter distance (0.5–2 Hz; ±20–30°; yaw > pitch > roll) | Visual control of stabilization of gaze in space by suppressing spontaneous nystagmus through voluntary fixation impulse (retinal slip)<br>Visually guided control of target fixation<br>Provoke vestibular stimuli for recalibration of VOR under visual control of retinal slip of the viewed target |
| | 2. First balance exercise—free sit and stance and guided gait (eyes open, eyes closed) | Circulatory training, prophylaxis of thrombosis |
| III. Approximately days 5–7<br>Suppression of spontaneous nystagmus with fixation straight ahead, but continued gaze nystagmus in the direction of fast phase, and spontaneous nystagmus with Frenzel's glasses | 1. Static stabilization:<br>Four-point stance;<br>Stance on one knee and one foot<br>Upright stance (eyes open/eyes closed; head upright/head extension) | Recalibrate visuovestibulospinal reflexes for postural control and eye-head coordination at free body movements |
| | 2. Dynamic stabilization:<br>Smooth pursuit and head oscillation exercises at free stance as described in preceding section<br>Exercises with rope, ball, and club under fixation (eye and head) of the instrument (sitting/standing/walking) | |
| IV. Approximately weeks 2–3<br>No spontaneous vertigo<br>Weak spontaneous nystagmus with Frenzel's glasses | Complex balance exercise, successive increase in difficulty, above the demands for postural control under daily life conditions | Expose the subjectively "recovered patient" increasingly to unstable body positions in order to facilitate rearrangement and recruitment of control capacities |

quence of positioning is repeated about five times at each session. The maneuvers are carried out by the patients themselves every 3 hours while awake and are terminated after 2 consecutive vertigo-free days. In extreme cases, when patients are subject to nausea or in particularly anxious patients, vestibular sedative drugs, such as dimenhydrinate, are given during the first 1 to 3 days of the physical therapy. This simple physical approach leads to relief in the majority of cases within 1 to 4 weeks, even if the vertigo had lasted for months before the initiation of the therapy. In some patients, particularly in the elderly and in severe post-traumatic forms, a slight but minimally distressing BPPV may persist, which is unresponsive to physical training. The time course of individual recovery, undulating and with abrupt remissions, supports a purely physical mechanism rather than central compensation by habituation.

In the rare patients not responding even to prolonged physical therapy, surgical transection of the posterior ampullary nerve via a middle ear approach can be considered. This operation provides relief of vertigo. It is, however, not easy to locate the particular semicircular canal nerve surgically, and sensorineural hearing loss is a possible complication.

### Meniere's Disease

Meniere's disease is discussed separately (p. 847). Only three aspects of therapy are mentioned here.

1. Nowadays, less than 3% of patients ultimately require surgical treatment, such as middle fossa vestibular nerve section or labyrinthectomy, since the success of regular "endolymphatic sac shunt operation" has been shown to be placebo effect. Spontaneous permanent fistulization is a possible explanation for permanent recovery in Meniere's disease.

2. The histamine derivative betahistine hydrochloride (Vasomotal, Aequamen),* 8 mg three

---

*Not available in the United States.

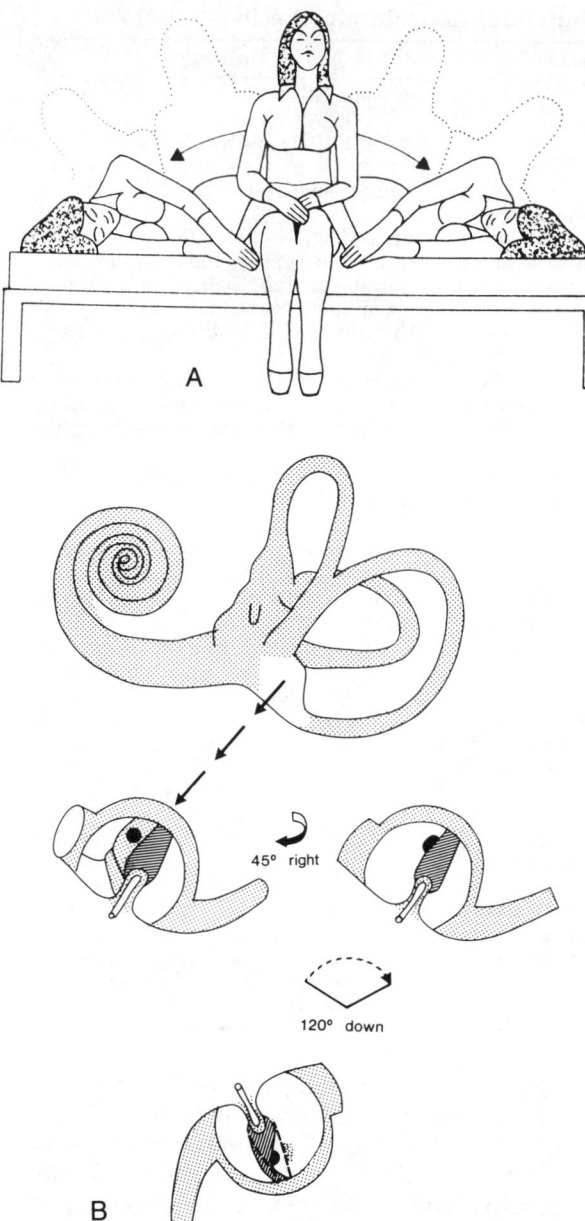

**Figure 1.** *A,* Sequence of repetitive positionings in patients with benign paroxysmal positioning vertigo in seated position, with eyes closed. *B,* Mechanism of cupulolithiasis. Inorganic "heavy particles" detached from the otoconial layer (by degeneration or head trauma) gravitate to and become settled on the cupula of the posterior semicircular canal. The heavy material causes a specific gravity differential between the cupula and the endolymph with postrotatory overexcitability following head extension or rapid head tilts toward the affected ear.

times daily, has been advocated as the drug of first choice.

3. Intratympanic treatment with ototoxic antibiotics, such as gentamicin sulfate (Garamycin), 8 to 24 mg instilled daily via a plastic tube inserted behind the anulus by a transmeatal approach, is obviously able to selectively damage

the secretory epithelium (and thereby to improve endolymphatic hydrops) before significantly affecting vestibular and cochlear function. Instillations (up to 10 days), therefore, should be stopped when daily audiograms or a check of spontaneous nystagmus by use of Frenzel's glasses indicate end-organ dysfunction.

### Vestibular Drop Attacks (Tumarkin's Otolithic Crisis)

Rarely, in early or late stages of endolymphatic hydrops, vestibular drop attacks may occur when sudden changes in endolymphatic fluid pressure cause inadequate end-organ stimulation with a reflex-like vestibulospinal loss of postural tone. The prognosis of vestibular drop attacks is relatively benign. Pharmacologically, administration of fentanyl and droperidol (Innovar) has been tried with questionable success. Drop attacks disappear after gentamicin (intratympanally) treatment. Selective section of the vestibular nerve (in order to preserve serviceable hearing of the affected ear) may be the latest thinking.

### Perilymph Fistula

Perilymph fistulas may lead to episodic vertigo and sensorineural hearing loss owing to a pathologic elasticity of the otic capsule, usually at the oval and round windows, which permits abnormal transfer of ambient pressure changes to maculae and cupulae receptors. Despite some typical clinical fistula tests, a definite diagnosis can be made only by exploratory tympanotomy.

In the acute case, medical treatment is universally recommended since most fistulas heal spontaneously. Medical care consists of absolute bedrest with the head elevated for 5 to 10 days. Avoidance of straining, sneezing, or coughing, or head hanging positions and the use of stool softeners are important for reduction of further explosive and implosive forces, which may activate perilymph leakage. If symptoms clear, the patient is sent home and advised to limit physical activity and to do no lifting or straining for another 2 weeks.

When symptoms persist for over 4 weeks or a hearing loss worsens, exploratory tympanotomy is indicated under local anesthesia, with the Valsalva maneuver or gentle palpation of the footplate to make the leak apparent. The results of surgical interventions are not encouraging, especially with respect to improvement of the hearing defect.

### Miscellaneous Peripheral Vestibular Vertigo Syndromes

**Vestibular Paroxysmia.** There is some evidence that neurovascular compression of the eighth cranial nerve can cause a paroxysmal and persistent vertigo/ataxia syndrome (with or without tinnitus and hearing loss) by local demyelination and axonal hyperactivity. The proposed name of the disease "disabling positional vertigo" is misleading and can be applied to a variety of forms of vertigo. Carbamazepine (Tegretol), the drug of first choice for trigeminal neuralgia, was indeed effective in a few vertigo patients in whom we suspected a neurovascular compression syndrome. Further information is required if the clinical picture presented by "vestibular paroxysmia" is to be accurately defined. Hesitation is highly justifiable since retromastoid craniotomy with microvascular decompression is the recommended procedure once the diagnosis has been established. This surgical procedure is still associated with a mortality of about 1% and a considerable morbidity of about 10%, even though others report lower rates.

**Hyperviscosity Syndrome.** Otologic symptoms—hearing loss and especially vertigo—are among the most frequent manifestations of the hyperviscosity syndrome associated with polycythemia, hypergammaglobulinemia, or Waldenström's macroglobulinemia. Vertigo is probably predominantly produced by vascular obstructions in the venules of the peripheral labyrinthine organ, comparable to retinal vein congestions. Symptomatic improvement occurs with a reduction in blood hyperviscosity, regardless of the underlying cause.

## CENTRAL VESTIBULAR VERTIGO SYNDROMES

### Vestibular Epilepsy

Vestibular seizures are secondary to focal discharges from either the temporal lobe or the parietal association cortex receiving vestibular projection from the thalamus. For effective medical treatment with anticonvulsants, such as carbamazepine and phenytoin, see the epilepsy chapter.

### Basilar Insufficiency and Basilar Artery Migraine

Transient attacks of vertigo of central origin are the most common early symptom of basilar insufficiency because of the steep pressure gradient from the aorta to the terminal pontine arteries. These are long, tenuous, circumferential arteries and, therefore, provide a most vulnerable blood supply for the vestibular nuclei. Whereas basilar insufficiency is a disease of the elderly (see cerebral vascular disease), sudden attacks of basilar artery migraine occur predominantly in adolescent girls (see headache). The benign paroxysmal vertigo of childhood (BPV) with onset within the first 4 years of life is probably related to migraine. The sudden attacks of BPV last seconds to minutes and do not require drug therapy. The natural history is spontaneous relief within months or years.

### Downbeat and Upbeat Nystagmus/Vertigo Syndromes

Downbeat or upbeat nystagmus in the primary position of gaze with oscillopsia and postural instability are well-defined clinical syndromes, almost specific for structural lesions of the paramedian cranial cervical junction (e.g., Arnold-Chiari malformation). It is our recent experience that the GABA-ergic baclofen (Lioresal) can effectively suppress downbeat as well as upbeat nystagmus and distressing oscillopsia in some patients. In Arnold-Chiari malformation a surgical suboccipital decompression because of the compression of the herniating cerebellum against the caudal brain stem may gradually improve nystagmus.

### Familial Periodic Ataxia

This is a rare, disabling condition, which commonly manifests either as recurrent attacks of unsteadiness of gate and stance or as attacks of vertigo and nystagmus, among several members of a family. Acetozolamide (Diamox) is effective in preventing periodic ataxia/vertigo; the calcium-entry blocker flunarizine (Sibelium)* can also be tried.

### Physiologic Stimulation Vertigo

**Motion Sickness.** This is induced during passive locomotion in vehicles and is generated either by unfamiliar accelerations to which a person has not adapted or by an intersensory mismatch involving conflicting vestibular and visual stimuli.

Physical prevention of motion sickness involves vestibular training to promote central habituation, as well as head fixation and head position during stimulation to avoid cross-coupling effects. Motion sickness is significantly reduced when ample peripheral vision of the stationary surroundings is provided during vehicle accelerations. Conversely, the symptoms are heightened in closed ship cabins or while reading and, to a lesser extent, while simply sitting in the back seat of a moving vehicle. This creates a visual-vestibular conflict, with the vestibular signals of acceleration being contradicted by visual information of a seemingly stationary environment.

---

*Not available in the United States.

Anti-motion sickness drugs, such as scopolamine (Transderm-Scop) or dimenhydrinate (Dramamine), are effective in preventing both vestibular and optokinetic motion sickness.

**Physiologic Height Vertigo.** Height vertigo, a visually induced syndrome commonly experienced atop high structures, is manifested by a subjective instability of posture and locomotion, coupled with a fear of falling and vegetative symptoms, which spontaneously remit after termination of the inducing stimulus. Physiologic postural instability under height vertigo conditions is secondary to a geometrically explainable, visually induced postural imbalance, when the distance between the observer and the nearest stationary contrasts in the environment becomes critically large.

Susceptible subjects should avoid the free upright stance in critical situations at high altitudes. This is done intuitively by grasping for stationary framework or leaning against a wall for support. When looking down, one should obtain stationary cues from nearby contrasts in the peripheral visual field. Staring at moving objects such as clouds increases the danger of falling because additional postural destabilization through linearvection may be induced. One should avoid long exposure times because height vertigo usually takes several seconds to develop. Looking through binoculars is very dangerous because it restricts the visual field and introduces the unusual and therefore unadapted-to magnification factor. Body and head position should be adjusted to the gravitational vector because vision will receive a relatively greater sensorial weight (which is undesirable) if the otoliths are displaced beyond their optimal working range by extreme head tilt. It may also be true on the basis of our observations that the feet should be firmly planted on an "earth horizontal" surface.

## Psychogenic Vertigo

**Acrophobia.** Panic attacks in acrophobia require a neurotic personality as well as the eliciting stimulus situation, which is often uncomfortable even for healthy subjects. Although the dissociation between the objective and subjective risk of falling is typically realized by acrophobic patients, they cannot overcome their avoidance behavior.

Psychotherapy is dominated by behavioral approaches that can be classified as either systematic or in vivo desensitization procedures. Systematic desensitization is based on the construction of a graduated hierarchy of anxiety-provoking visual scenes, which, after a training phase in muscle relaxation, are subsequently visualized by the patient while in a relaxed state. Although therapist- or self-directed (tape-recorded) desensitization has been widely used, in vivo desensitization is more effective in the treatment of phobia. In vivo desensitization techniques aim to reduce avoidance behavior or anxiety by increasing contact with real life rather than the patient's imaging provoking stimuli. Successive approximation to the feared situation is supported by instructions and reinforcement. Contact desensitization stresses the advantage of joint participation and physical contact with the therapist model (participant modeling). Flooding, an alternative technique, also uses exposure to real phobic stimuli but without a graduated approach. It is based on getting the patient into the feared situation and maintaining the exposure for prolonged periods of times.

Drugs used for symptomatic relief from panic attacks in phobic patients are either tranquilizers or antidepressants like imipramine (Tofranil). The long-term course of untreated anxiety neurosis, however, indicates that during a 5-year interval, most children and 50% of adults have either recovered from their phobias or substantially improved.

**Phobic Postural Vertigo.** A syndrome of phobic postural vertigo attacks has been described by us which is distinguishable from agoraphobia and acrophobia. It is the third most common form of vertigo and is characterized by the combination of initial vertigo with subjective postural and gait instability and the fear of impending death. Because patients express fears of an organic disease, we usually carry out detailed neurologic diagnostic procedures. Our therapeutic regimen consists mainly of relieving the patients of their fear of an occult organic disease and of giving a detailed explanation of the mechanism that causes the factors that provoke phobic reactions. We recommend a controlled "self-desensitization"—within the context of behavioral therapy—by repeated exposure to situations that evoke the condition.

## Drugs and Vertigo

The list of drugs that may have adverse effects on hearing or balance is impressive. It includes analgesics, anesthetic agents, anticonvulsants, antidepressants, antidiabetic agents, antihypertensive agents, anti-inflammatory drugs, contraceptives, cytotoxic agents, cardiovascular drugs, sedatives, and tranquilizers. There is no common syndrome or mechanism of drug vertigo. Aminoglycoside antibiotics can permanently damage the cochlea or the vestibular labyrinth. The reversible ototoxicity of high-dose salicylate (aspirin) is characterized by bilateral hearing loss, tinnitus, and vertigo. The loop diuretics ethacrynic acid (Edecrin) and furosemide (Lasix) are ototoxic as well as alkylating chemotherapeutic (anticancer) agents. The antiepileptic phenytoin is the prototype of a cerebellotoxic drug. Other toxic compounds, such as alcohol or mercury, can affect both the peripheral vestibular labyrinth and the central cerebellar pathways.

# MENIERE'S DISEASE

method of
GALE GARDNER, M.D.
*University of Tennessee—Memphis*
*Memphis, Tennessee*

Meniere's disease is *not* simply an instance of dizziness or vertigo. It is a specific disorder of the labyrinth (inner ear) that produces a combination of complaints including vertigo (sensation of spinning), hearing loss (of a particular type), tinnitus (ear noise, usually roaring), and frequently a sensation of fullness in the ear. To qualify as true Meniere's disease, all these symptoms must occur, followed by varying periods with no attacks. During the attacks, the patient is frequently nauseated, may vomit, and is clearly ill and probably apprehensive.

Meniere's disease is *not* any of these symptoms occurring singly. It is not dizziness alone, although many patients have this symptom, nor is it hearing loss or tinnitus alone. These isolated symptoms must be evaluated separately.

## ETIOLOGY

A number of disease processes may produce the combination of vertigo, hearing loss, and tinnitus. The most important is an acoustic neuroma, usually arising in the internal auditory canal and apparently producing symptoms by causing pressure on the neurovascular contents of the canal. It is crucial for the physician to think of this possibility whenever treating a patient with the symptoms of Meniere's disease. Primary care physicians should think of the possibility of a tumor when dealing with a patient who has unilateral hearing loss or tinnitus, with or without dizziness or vertigo. In the presence of these symptoms, and if the hearing loss is of the sensorineural type (nerve dysfunction rather than conductive or mechanical dysfunction), an imaging study is indicated.

Other disorders that may produce this combination of symptoms are syphilis (usually localized in the inner ear and central nervous system), hyperlipidemia, food allergy, hypothyroidism, and others.

The condition that we refer to as "true" Meniere's disease is believed to be caused by an increase in the amount of inner ear fluid (endolymph), producing hydrops of the labyrinth. We do not yet know the cause of this condition or the mechanism whereby it occurs, which, of course, makes treatment difficult.

## DIAGNOSIS

True Meniere's disease is diagnosed by the history of attacks of vertigo, with associated hearing loss (that usually fluctuates in severity) and tinnitus, with initial involvement of usually only one ear. The severity of the attack is helpful in differentiating true Meniere's disease from other labyrinthine disorders. A hearing test (audiogram) is needed to show that the hearing loss involves nerve dysfunction (sensorineural hearing loss). If the hearing loss is caused by mechanical factors such as dysfunction of the eardrum, ear bones (ossicles), or ear canal, it is referred to as conductive, and Meniere's disease may be ruled out. Tuning fork tests, if performed properly, can also help in making this determination, but the diagnosis should be confirmed with audiometry. A caloric test, or more desirably an electronystagmographic examination, may also help to make the diagnosis. These tests are likely to show spontaneous or positional nystagmus during attacks, and perhaps a reduction in caloric response on the involved side. At some point, I obtain a computed tomography scan or a magnetic resonance imaging scan with gadolinium of every patient who I believe has Meniere's disease because some of them will be found to have an acoustic tumor instead.

## TREATMENT OF THE ACUTE ATTACK

Those who have never had Meniere's disease frequently underestimate the impact of the attack on a patient. Lacking medical knowledge, the patient is at the mercy of imagination and suspects everything from a stroke to a heart attack. Reassurance and support are therefore essential in managing the acute attack. Fortunately, the patient can be told that attacks rarely last longer than 2 or 3 hours. Supportive treatment during this time is all that is required.

For a mild attack without nausea or vomiting, meclizine (Antivert or Bonine), 25-mg tablets, or cyclizine lactate (Marezine), 50-mg tablets, may be given every 4 to 6 hours for dizziness.

For a more severe attack with nausea and vomiting, one may use cyclizine lactate, 50 mg (1 ml) intramuscularly, immediately and every 4 to 6 hours thereafter. Prochlorperazine (Compazine) may be given as a 25-mg suppository immediately and then used twice daily. For emergency room settings with severe attacks, I use atropine sulfate, 0.0125 mg per kg intravenously or intramuscularly; it can be repeated in 2 hours. Atropine should be used with caution in patients with a history of cardiac disease, particularly in the presence of supraventricular tachycardia. Diazepam (Valium) may also be given intravenously or intramuscularly, at a dosage of 5 to 10 mg, and may be repeated in 3 to 4 hours.

In an unusually severe attack or in the presence of complicating factors, it may be necessary to admit a patient to the hospital and to provide fluid replacement.

## PREVENTION OF ATTACKS

To list the medications and treatment programs that have been used and advocated in the past for Meniere's disease would exceed the space limitations of this section. Suffice it to say that the following general types of treatment may be considered: tranquilizers, vagal blockers (such as atropine), antihistamines, vasodilators, diuretics, vitamins, histamine, steroids, low-salt diet, special head exercises, and avoidance of alcohol, caffeine, and tobacco, to name only a few.

My own medical maintenance regimen is fairly simple. Primarily, the patient is repeatedly reassured that if worst comes to worst the disease can be controlled surgically, but that 80 to 90% of individuals can be controlled successfully with nonsurgical measures. For individuals less than 60 years of age, I use a combination of (1) belladonna-ergotamine-phenobarbital (Bellergal), one tablet given twice daily, (2) meclizine, one 25-mg tablet given at bedtime, and (3) diazepam, one 2-mg tablet (or even less if necessary) three times a day, unless contraindications to any of these regimens exist.

For patients over the age of 60 years, I generally use a combination of (1) meclizine and (2) diazepam, as indicated previously, as well as (3) nicotinic acid, 50-mg tablets, in a flushing dose before breakfast and at bedtime.

Certain qualifications are necessary. In my office, we spend a great deal of time counseling patients on reducing the amount of these medications to below the point at which sedation or other side effects occur. We also spend time determining any contraindications to their use, either because of other conditions that may be present (e.g., glaucoma in the case of belladonna-ergotamine-phenobarbital) or because of incompatibility of these medications with other medications the patient may be taking.

## SURGERY

Surgery should be considered when medical treatment has failed; when there are no medical, age-related, or other contraindications; and when the condition is significantly affecting the patient's life.

### Types of Surgery

Generally, surgery takes two forms. In situations in which hearing remains relatively good,

conservative surgery that does not sacrifice hearing function is preferred. If the hearing has gradually deteriorated with the passage of time, which is not uncommon, a destructive procedure is indicated. The rationale is that this type of surgery is generally more effective than the conservative type, and there is no valid reason to preserve hearing that is no longer useful.

Without discussing surgical details that are of little interest to the primary care physician, here are the procedures I prefer to offer these patients. These procedures are performed by approaching the labyrinth either from behind the auricle (postauricular), from above, or directly through the ear canal. The conservative procedure I prefer to use initially is to place a shunt tube between the endolymphatic sac of the labyrinth and the adjacent subarachnoid space (endolymphatic sac—subarachnoid shunt) through a postauricular incision. A variation is to place the shunt tube between the endolymphatic sac and the mastoid space. Should these operations fail, I prefer to cut the balance (vestibular) nerve while preserving the hearing nerve, using either a posterior fossa approach (retrolabyrinthine vestibular nerve section) or a middle fossa approach (middle fossa vestibular nerve section).

When hearing in the involved ear is not considered useful to the patient, but the balance problem is incapacitating and medication has not controlled the problem, I prefer to destroy the balance end organ with nerve endings, with sacrifice of hearing (labyrinthectomy). In a younger patient I do this through a postauricular incision, drill away the three balance canals, open the vestibule of the labyrinth, and remove the membranous end organs for balance (transmastoid labyrinthectomy). In an elderly patient I do the operation through the ear canal, open the vestibule, connect the oval and round windows in the middle-ear space, and remove the membranous end organs (transcanal labyrinthectomy).

### Effectiveness of These Procedures in Relieving the Effects of Meniere's Disease

Nothing in life is perfect, but as surgical procedures go, labyrinthectomy is highly effective, eliminating balance problems or significantly alleviating them 95% of the time, but with sacrifice of hearing. The conservative sac procedures allow preservation of hearing and improve the patient's balance function (in my experience, in approximately 80% of cases) but do little, if anything, to improve the hearing, which usually continues to deteriorate slowly.

The retrolabyrinthine and middle fossa nerve section procedures appear to offer the best of both worlds, controlling vertigo as effectively (95% or better) as labyrinthectomy but preserving hearing as well. Yet these are both intracranial procedures and carry greater risks than the other procedures, which are all relatively low-risk operations.

None of these procedures has a high or even a predictable rate of success in stabilizing or improving hearing or in controlling tinnitus; however, in some cases, dramatic improvement in these areas occurs. Because of the tendency for this disease to fluctuate in severity, it is difficult, if not impossible, to know with certainty whether to attribute postoperative improvement to the effects of surgery or to the fluctuating nature of the disease.

### Bilateral Involvement

Unfortunately, 20 to 40% of patients may ultimately develop bilateral Meniere's disease. In this situation, conservative surgery may be indicated, but the use of streptomycin may also be considered to reduce balance dysfunction nonsurgically. This must be done with care to avoid undue injury to the labyrinth by following the hearing and balance function with testing during the course of treatment.

# VIRAL MENINGOENCEPHALITIS

method of
RONALD S. MURRAY, M.D., and
JACK S. BURKS, M.D.
*Rocky Mountain Multiple Sclerosis Center*
*Englewood, Colorado*

Encephalitis and meningitis are inflammatory syndromes of the brain and meninges, respectively. Although meningitis may occur in isolation, inflammation of the brain and spinal cord is often accompanied by meningeal inflammation. Terms such as meningoencephalitis and meningomyelitis are often used to describe this association. Meningitis is characterized by headache, stiff neck, photophobia, and nonspecific constitutional signs such as fever, vomiting, and lethargy. Encephalitis is indicated when focal neurologic deficits, seizures, and change in level of consciousness and/or cognition accompany the aforementioned signs and symptoms.

Many infectious and noninfectious etiologies produce meningitis and/or encephalitis, and a prudent search for treatable causes is mandatory. These causes may be bacterial, fungal, viral, parasitic, postinfectious, postvaccinal, allergic, vasculitic, or neoplastic. In addition, an ever-increasing proportion of patients are immunosuppressed (AIDS, chemotherapy, steroid therapy, hypogammaglobulinemia) and may be prone to

unusual and persistent central nervous system (CNS) infections from single or multiple organisms.

Clues to the etiologic agent may be apparent on general physical examination. Tests of value in the acute setting are brain imaging with CT or magnetic resonance (MRI) scan, cerebral spinal fluid (CSF) analysis, chest x-ray, white blood count with differential, electrolytes, glucose, and renal and liver function tests. Once the spinal fluid and other tests are obtained, empiric therapy with antibiotic, antiviral, or antifungal medications should not be withheld while the diagnostic evaluation is in progress.

## VIRAL MENINGITIS

Viral (aseptic) meningitis is usually a benign and self-limited illness complicating respiratory or intestinal tract infections. The patient usually has a clear sensorium and a nonfocal neurologic examination. CSF analysis should include cell count, protein and glucose levels, Gram's stain, India ink prep, AFB stain, and cultures for nonviral infectious agents. Aseptic meningitis is indicated by finding a CSF lymphocytic pleocytosis of up to 2000 cells per ml, normal to slightly reduced CSF glucose, normal to slightly elevated CSF protein, normal to slightly elevated increased intracranial pressure (ICP), and negative bacterial and fungal cultures. Acute and convalescent serologies may be helpful in identifying the inciting virus. Bedrest, minor analgesics, fever prophylaxis, and reassurance generally suffice as treatment. Recovery is often complete within 1 to 2 weeks, although some patients may complain of headache and fatigue for several months.

## VIRAL ENCEPHALITIS

Worsening neurologic status in a patient with meningeal signs and symptoms heralds the onset of viral encephalitis. Encephalitis is indicated when focal neurologic deficits, seizures, and change in level of consciousness and/or cognition accompany constitutional symptoms. Unlike viral meningitis, encephalitis is associated with high morbidity and mortality. A high index of suspicion for herpes simplex encephalitis (HSE) is warranted, as early antiviral therapy can minimize mortality and morbidity. Definitive early diagnosis of HSE is accomplished by virus isolation or viral antigen demonstration by immunofluorescent techniques in brain biopsy material. The involved temporal lobe is the preferred biopsy site. However, empiric early therapy with acyclovir (Zovirax), foregoing brain biopsy, has gained favor owing to the benign and infrequent side effects of this antiviral agent. We recommend brain biopsy prior to treatment as follows: acyclovir (Zovirax) 10 mg per kg infused intravenously over 1 hour, every 8 hours for 10 days.

Supportive therapy can minimize the morbidity associated with encephalitis and is applicable regardless of the specific pathogen. Even with very severe infections, remarkable recoveries occur and physical therapy should be instituted early to prevent joint contractures. Meticulous nursing care will prevent the complications associated with bedrest. Bladder atony/hypotony frequently occurs and requires catheterization. Patients with protracted courses may develop malnutrition and require hyperalimentation.

Respiratory failure from concomitant tracheo-bronchopulmonary infection, airway obstruction, or poor ventilatory drive may complicate management. An artificial airway, assisted ventilation, and tracheal toilet all may be necessary.

Fluid/electrolyte imbalance due to dehydration, dilutional hyponatremia, or inappropriate secretion of antidiuretic hormone (ADH) is common. Electrolytes and urine/serum osmolality should be monitored and fluid input adjusted regularly.

Brain edema with concomitant elevated ICP may result in a deteriorating neurologic picture. A computed tomography (CT) or magnetic resonance imaging (MRI) scan may be helpful, and an intracranial pressure monitor will confirm and quantitate the elevated pressure and facilitate management. Fluid input should be adjusted to avoid overhydration. Mannitol (1.0 gram per kg of 20% solution given over 20 minutes intravenously) osmotically removes excess CNS fluid and should be given in repeat doses every 4 to 12 hours as needed. Glycerol given orally in a dose of 3 grams per kg divided into six doses per 24 hours is an alternative osmolar agent. Hyperventilation is helpful early to constrict CNS blood vessel caliber and is generally used until osmotic agents have decreased the ICP. The response is usually brisk if $Pco_2$ is maintained at 25 mmHg but may diminish after 24 hours. The use of glucocorticoids is controversial but useful in patients with ominous cerebral edema. We recommend dexamethasone (Decadron) 10 mg intravenously initially, followed by 4 mg intravenously every 4 hours until the infection is under control. Steroids are then tapered over 5 to 7 days.

Seizures may result from direct viral or inflammatory damage of neurons, increased intracranial pressure, or fluid and electrolyte (hyponatremia) imbalance. Phenytoin (Dilantin), 20 mg per kg given intravenously as a loading dose at a rate not to exceed 50 mg per minute,* while monitoring blood pressure and electrocardiogram (ECG), is the drug of choice. Maintenance dose is

3 to 5 mg per kg daily for adults and 4 to 8 mg per kg for children. Phenobarbital, 5 mg per kg intravenously every 30 minutes, at a rate not to exceed 100 mg per minute, until seizures cease or blood pressure falls (total loading dose not more than 20 mg per kg) is an alternative. Maintenance dose of phenobarbital is 2 to 3 mg per kg daily for adults and 3 to 5 mg per kg for children. Status epilepticus requires intravenous treatment with 5 or 10 mg of diazepam (Valium) and phenytoin. Additional antiepileptics or paralysis (to prevent hyperthermia and increased metabolic requirements) may be needed in a few patients. We do not recommend prophylaxis against seizures with viral CNS infection.

To summarize, it is extremely important to search for treatable causes of meningitis and encephalitis. Specific therapy can lessen morbidity and mortality in afflicted patients. For patients with severe infections, i.e., encephalitis, supportive therapy in the anticipation of an excellent outcome is of utmost importance to the patient's long-term rehabilitation.

# REYE'S SYNDROME

method of
JOHN C. PARTIN, M.D.
*State University of New York at Stony Brook*
*Stony Brook, New York*

Reye's syndrome (RS) is a metabolic encephalopathy and hepatopathy that usually occurs in community outbreaks in association with influenza or influenza-like respiratory illness and chickenpox. The onset of RS is signaled by unexpected and unusually severe vomiting, the onset of which begins 3 to 5 days after the beginning of the antecedent viral infection. About one-third of cases progress through a stage of agitated delirium to coma, and of these, one-third die or sustain severe brain damage.

The epidemiology of RS has changed over the past 5 years. The total number of cases has diminished since aspirin use was identified as a possible risk factor, and the average age has increased, perhaps owing to self-medication with aspirin-containing products by older children. Most important, it has been proven that many children under the age of 36 months who were formerly diagnosed as having RS in fact had RS "mimickers," prominent among which are disorders of fatty acid oxidation, such as medium-chain acyl CoA dehydrogenase deficiency; disorders of urea production such as ornithine transcarbamylase deficiency; disorders involving carnitine metabolism; and other genetic defects. The Centers for Disease Control diagnostic criteria for RS now require the exclusion of at least 20 genetic disorders of metabolism in addition to exclusion of bacterial meningitis and viral encephalitis. RS should be considered in the differential diagnosis of

---

*Exceeds dosage recommended by the manufacturer.

older children or adolescents presenting with agitated delirium who are suspected of taking drugs.

The pathogenesis of RS involves injury to liver and brain mitochondria, which results in severe depletion of tissue glycogen, impaired ammonia metabolism, and defective metabolism of unesterified fatty acids. Cerebral edema, a complication of the metabolic encephalopathy in severe cases, may be uncontrollable in spite of intensive therapy.

## TREATMENT

### Treatment of Noncomatose (CDC Stage 0, I) Cases

Prompt vigorous treatment of early RS with intravenous 10% glucose and maintenance fluids can restore tissue glycogen, reduce lipolysis, and may prevent the progression of Stage I cases to coma. Noncomatose cases are identified by a history of the unexpected onset of vomiting within 1 week of an appropriate antecedent illness, alanine amino transferase (ALT) greater than 200 IU (mean 900 IU); normal or prolonged plasma prothrombin time, and normal or elevated blood ammonia. Noncomatose, Stage I patients are treated with 2000 ml per $M^2$ per 24 hours of intravenous fluids containing 10% glucose, 50 mEq per $M^2$ per 24 hours sodium chloride (NaCl), 40 mEq per $M^2$ per 24 hours potassium chloride (KCl), started immediately in the emergency room. Initial urine should be examined for ketones and saved for analysis by gas chromatography mass spectrography for fatty acid metabolites. The blood sugar should be measured 4 to 6 hours after glucose infusion is begun to assure that high-normal values are obtained. ALT, ammonia ($NH_3$), and prothrombin time (PT) should be measured every 12 hours for the first 36 hours or more frequently if neurologic signs advance. All Stage I cases should be observed closely, since some will progress to coma. Noncomatose children admitted with prolonged prothrombin times or elevated blood ammonia are at risk of progression and should be kept under particularly close observation. Return of full appetite is a reliable sign of recovery.

Patients who present with agitated delirium or frank coma should be managed in a qualified intensive care unit. We do not use prolonged deep sedation with barbiturates or morphine or protracted muscle paralysis because these methods make meaningful neurologic examination impossible. We use moderate doses of pentobarbital (Nembutal) or morphine and intermittent pancuronium (Pavulon) to control patients during endotracheal intubation, lumbar puncture, and performance of painful procedures and when struggling against the ventilator adversely affects intracranial pressure (ICP). The goals of management are (1) to assure adequate brain oxygen by early elective endotracheal intubation; (2) to restore tissue glycogen and reduce lipolysis; (3) to prevent severe hypophosphatemia; (4) to maintain appropriate intravascular volume to support cerebral perfusion pressure (PP) and the integrity of renal function; and (5) to control cerebral edema if present.

Lumbar puncture (LP) should be performed soon after the airway is secured to exclude bacterial meningitis, viral encephalitis, and cerebral hemorrhage. We have experienced no adverse complications of LP in 250 cases. Patients are nursed in a 30-degree head-up position on a cooling blanket to control hyperpyrexia and with a nasogastric tube in place. Urine output is monitored by indwelling catheter. In severe cases, central vein catheters and arterial cannulas are placed to monitor blood pressure and estimate cerebral PP. An ICP monitor may be of some help in managing increased intracranial pressure. Most comatose cases of RS demonstrate centrally mediated respiratory alkalosis often with blood pH of 7.5 and $P_{CO_2}$ of 24 torr; those requiring mechanical ventilation should have $P_{CO_2}$ maintained at about 24 torr. Blood sugar should be measured frequently enough to assure levels in the range of 110 to 140 mg per dl. Extreme dehydration through fluid restriction or the excessive use of osmotic diuresis should be avoided. Dehydration should be corrected if present initially, and intravenous fluids should be administered at the rate of 1600 to 1800 ml per $M^2$ per 24 hours (maintenance fluids in most cases). Hypophosphatemia may occur, and phosphate 15 to 20 mEq per liter may be required after glucose infusion is begun.

Cerebral edema is managed by hyperventilation to reduce $P_{CO_2}$ to 24 torr and intravenous mannitol beginning with a dose of 250 mg per kg administered over 5 to 15 minutes. Higher doses of mannitol may be employed, but a hyperosmolar state must be avoided; the serum osmolality should be maintained between 312 and 320 mOsm. In situations refractory to mannitol, furosemide can be tried, and some have advocated the use of intragastric 20% glycerol.

One large series of comatose RS patients was treated with exchange transfusion using fresh whole blood with a mortality of about 20%. It is unclear whether exchange transfusion has anything to add to the above treatment regimen. Cranial decompression has been thought to be lifesaving, but at the cost of significant morbidity.

Deep barbiturate coma with or without hypothermia appears to be associated with an unacceptable morbidity and mortality. Corticosteroids have not proved helpful. The use of citrulline* to

---

*Not available in the United States.

enhance ureagenesis or carnitine (Carnitor) to facilitate unesterified fatty acid metabolism has been suggested, but these modalities are unproved.

# MULTIPLE SCLEROSIS

method of
MARIA V. LOPEZ-BRESNAHAN, M.D.,
and STEPHEN L. HAUSER, M.D.
*Massachusetts General Hospital and Harvard
Medical School
Boston, Massachusetts*

Multiple sclerosis (MS) is a disease of the central nervous system characterized by inflammation, demyelination, and gliosis. Excluding trauma, MS is the most common cause of neurologic disability arising in young and middle adulthood. While the etiology of MS is not known, indirect evidence suggests that MS is an autoimmune disease and that a genetic predisposition and an environmental exposure contribute to susceptibility.

## THE COURSE OF THE DISEASE

The clinical course of MS may be stratified into three general categories. The first, relapsing-remitting MS (RRMS), is characterized by recurrent attacks of neurologic dysfunction. MS attacks generally evolve over days to weeks and may be followed by complete, partial, or no recovery. The second, chronic progressive MS (CPMS), is characterized by gradually progressive worsening without periods of stabilization or remission. Most cases of CPMS evolve in individuals with known RRMS, although in 20% of CPMS patients no prior history of RRMS is present. The third, inactive MS (IMS), is characterized by fixed neurologic deficits of variable magnitude. Most patients with IMS have an earlier history of RRMS.

## THE PROGNOSIS OF MS

The choice of therapy in MS is influenced by the expected prognosis, in addition to considerations of efficacy and toxicity. It is generally stated that, at the time of diagnosis, one-third of patients have a favorable, one-third a poor, and one-third an intermediate long-term prognosis. Prognosis in these terms is defined by the presence or absence of functional impairment and interference with independence. Survival tables indicate only a small effect of MS on life expectancy, and thus the major consideration relates to neurologic incapacity.

Although the course of MS may be uncertain in individual patients, some general rules help to select patients for different treatments. For patients with RRMS, the clinical status 5 and 10 years from onset of initial symptoms provides a useful index of the long-term course. RRMS tends to be most active during the first decade of symptoms, and disability is likely to develop in patients who have frequent relapses and accumulating disability or in patients whose course evolves to CPMS. CPMS represents the most predictable form of MS; 90% of CPMS patients are disabled within 10 years of the onset of the progressive phase.

MS treatment may be divided into two categories consisting of (1) treatment designed to arrest the disease process, and (2) symptomatic treatment.

## TREATMENT DESIGNED TO ARREST THE DISEASE PROCESS (Figure 1)

### Adrenocorticotropic Hormone (ACTH) and Corticosteroids

Long the mainstay of MS therapy, ACTH and corticosteroids are used for their anti-inflammatory and other immunosuppressant properties. While these agents have not been shown to alter the long-term course of MS, they appear to expedite recovery from acute attacks. Thus, they are most useful as short-term therapy for patients with RRMS.

When neurologic symptoms arise in RRMS, it is important to decide whether they result from new inflammatory lesions or extension of preexisting lesions or if a recurrence of old symptoms has occurred as a result of infection or other intercurrent illness. The latter must be excluded and treated specifically. Treatment of acute attacks with new or extended neurologic symptoms depends on severity. Mild deficits, which do not impede functioning, can go untreated, while moderate attacks, causing some disability to the patient, can be treated on an outpatient basis with a tapering course of prednisone (Table 1). Severe attacks, which are functionally disabling, warrant hospitalization for intravenous treatment with ACTH (Table 2). This is the only medication proved in controlled studies to hasten recovery. Many clinicians believe that ACTH is more effective than prednisone, although no clinical trials have compared the two.

Intravenous methylprednisolone (Solu-Medrol) has recently gained favor as a relatively safe method of high dose, short-term corticosteroid therapy (Table 3). When compared with ACTH, studies have shown that methylprednisolone more rapidly improves the cerebrospinal fluid (CSF) profile. However, it is not known whether methylprednisolone is clinically more effective than ACTH. Thus, we reserve methylprednisolone for cases in which ACTH has failed previously or for severe attacks with rapid neurologic deterioration.

Because of the high incidence of hypomanic reactions to ACTH or corticosteroid therapy in the MS population, lithium carbonate (Eskalith),

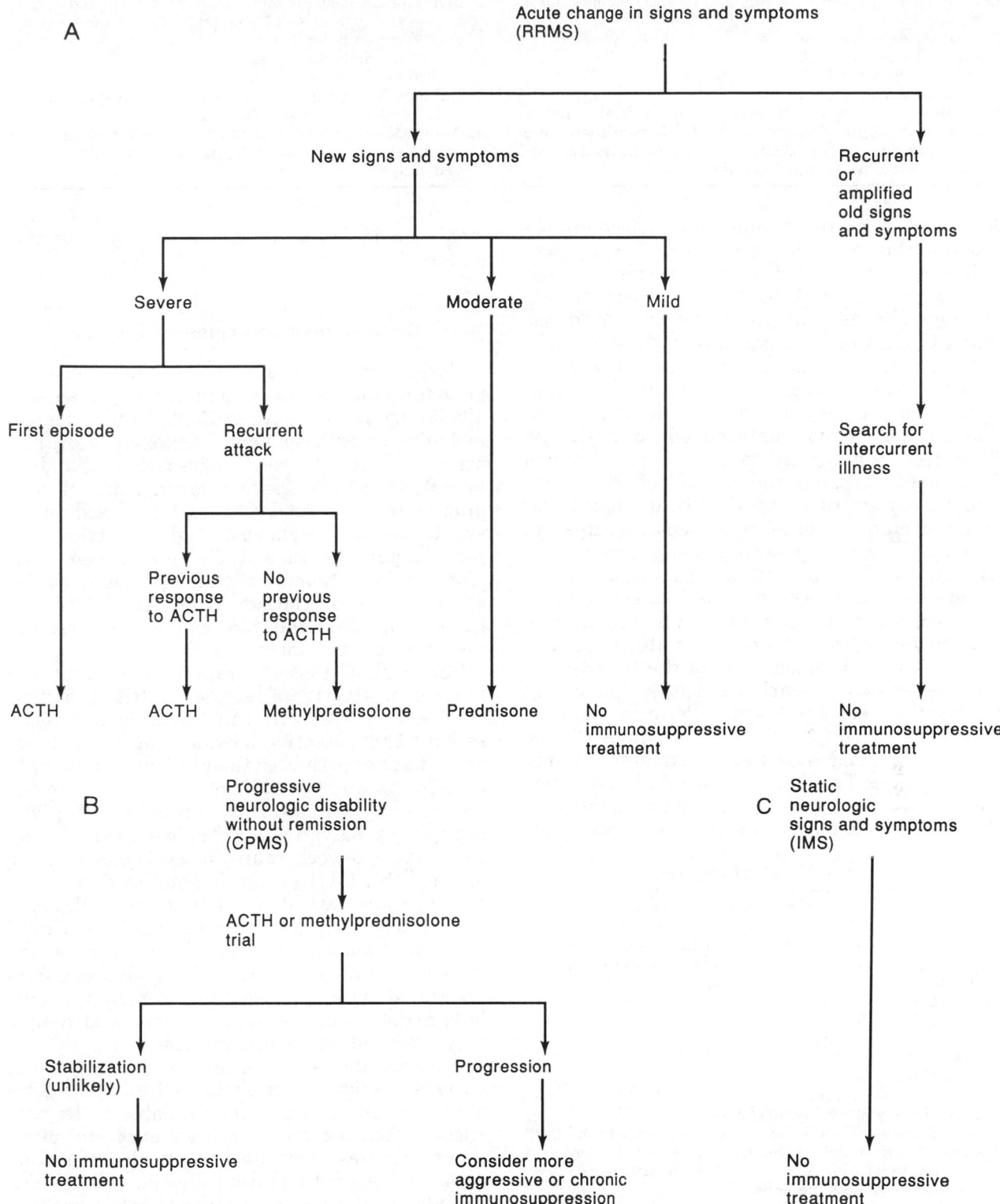

**Figure 1.** Treatment options for patients at different stages of the disease course (*A, B,* or *C*) are presented. *Abbreviations:* RRMS = relapsing-remitting multiple sclerosis; CPMS = chronic progressive multiple sclerosis; IMS = inactive multiple sclerosis.

## TABLE 1. **Prednisone Protocol**

1. Prednisone is given as a single daily morning dose for 4 weeks:
   - 80 mg daily for 1 wk
   - 60 mg daily for 1 wk
   - 40 mg daily for 1 wk
   - 20 mg daily for 1 wk
2. Lithium, 300 mg tid, is given prophylactically during treatment, as are antacids or $H_2$ blockers. Patients are encouraged to increase their intake of bananas and orange juice to avoid potassium depletion.

---

300 mg two or three times daily, is routinely added to the treatment regimen.

The chronic use of corticosteroids has not proved to be useful in the treatment of MS, although clinical trials have used only low doses. Patients frequently experience a sense of well-being on steroids, having increased energy and motivation and decreased spasticity. Thus, patients often request chronic steroid administration, but these symptomatic benefits do not justify their use. Some patients may become steroid dependent, with recrudescence of neurologic symptoms each time tapering is attempted. Patients on chronic steroid treatment are subject to suppression of the hypothalamic-pituitary-adrenal axis, weight gain, and cushingoid appearance. Other adverse effects include susceptibility to infection, cataract formation, and aseptic necrosis of bone. Bone loss should be monitored; quantitative computed tomography of the lumbosacral spine is sensitive to early changes and need only be checked every 2 to 3 years. Parathyroid levels may be required to exclude other causes of bone loss. Calcium and vitamin D treatments have not been shown to be advantageous. Although alternate day dosing may help to minimize the adverse effects of steroid treatment, chronic steroid treat-

## TABLE 2. **ACTH Protocol**

1. Aqueous ACTH (20 U/ml), 80 U, is given IV in 500 ml of 5% dextrose and water over 6–8 hr for 3 days.
2. ACTH gel (40 U/ml) is then given IM in a dose of 40 U q 12 hr for 7 days. The dose is then reduced every 3 days as follows:
   - 35 U bid for 3 days
   - 30 U bid for 3 days
   - 50 U q d for 3 days
   - 40 U q d for 3 days
   - 30 U q d for 3 days
   - 20 U q d for 3 days
   - 20 U every other day for 3 doses

   Improvement, when it occurs, can be expected from 2–12 days after initiation of therapy. Some patients may need a slower taper over several months. In such cases, every-other-day dosing is preferred.
3. Potassium chloride, 20–40 mEq tid, is given during ACTH therapy, and potassium level should be checked periodically.
4. Lithium 300 mg tid, should be used prophylactically during ACTH treatment.

## TABLE 3. **Methylprednisolone**

1. Methylprednisolone is mixed in 500 ml D5W and administered slowly, over 4–6 hours, preferably in the morning:
   - 1000 mg daily for 3 days
   - 500 mg daily for 3 days
   - 250 mg daily for 3 days
2. Lithium, 300 mg tid, is given during treatment. Antacids or $H_2$ blockers are recommended.
3. A low-sodium diet is given to avoid fluid retention. At 48 hours laboratory values are checked: CBC, electrolytes, and glucose.

---

ment should not be routinely employed in this disease.

### Cytotoxic Immunosuppressive Therapy

Various cytotoxic agents have been used to provide more aggressive immunosuppression in MS. Many studies have evaluated these agents, including cyclophosphamide (Cytoxan),* azathioprine (Imuran),* and cyclosporine (Sandimmune)* in both relapsing-remitting and chronic progressive disease. Protocols have used intravenous and oral regimens, single induction, and periodic pulse treatment. They have been given alone or in combination with corticosteroids or other therapies. The actual clinical benefits of these drugs and the risk-benefit ratio remain uncertain at this time.

The goal of these therapies is to limit the number or severity of relapses in RRMS or halt CPMS in patients with rapid neurologic deterioration. The potential adverse effects of these drugs has not permitted their lenient use in early or mild disease. Cyclophosphamide has been the most extensively used, and, at present, it is given in rapidly progressive MS (Table 4). Studies suggest that a 3-week course of cyclophosphamide given with ACTH results in stabilization of disease in some patients for 1 to 2 years. Patients most likely to respond are young, have CPMS with rapid worsening, and are ambulatory at the time of treatment. There are many adverse effects associated with this treatment, including hair loss, a risk of hemorrhagic cystitis, and temporary profound immunosuppression.

Azathioprine given orally on an outpatient basis is a relatively safe and well-tolerated form of chronic immunosuppression (Table 5). Its beneficial effect, a decrease in frequency and duration of relapses, is modest in controlled trials and must be weighed against potential risks which include hepatitis, susceptibility to infection, and, potentially, an increase in cancer risk.

---

*This use of these drugs for MS is not listed in the manufacturers' official directives.

## Investigational Treatments

More than 100 other experimental therapies have been proposed for MS. These modalities are in various stages of investigation and are not yet practically applicable.

## SYMPTOMATIC TREATMENT

A larger part of treatment in patients with MS targets complications of the disease.

### Spasticity

Spasticity with stiffness, flexor spasms, and clonus can be functionally disabling and painful. Spasticity may be worsened by underlying infections such as urinary tract infections, obstipation,

TABLE 4. **Cyclophosphamide with ACTH Protocol**

1. Patients are admitted to the hospital after infections, such as urinary tract infections, are excluded.
2. On admission, a CBC, blood chemistries, including liver function tests, and urinalysis are checked.
3. An indwelling catheter is recommended only if there is significant urinary retention or if urinary frequency or urgency are difficult to handle with the large fluid intake required during treatment.
4. The dose of cyclophosphamide (CTX) is determined by the patient's weight: over 115 lbs., 500 mg/day; under 115 lbs., 400 mg/day. Most patients receive a total dose between 5 grams and 7.5 grams (some patients have required as much as 10 grams and as little as 4 grams). These doses are aimed at producing leukopenia within 10–14 days of treatment. Cyclophosphamide is mixed in 1 L of ½ normal saline and is given in four divided doses daily. Each dose is given over 1–2 hr.
5. Fluid intake should be 3–4 L daily (while the patient is receiving CTX) to ensure proper dilution of CTX in the bladder.
6. CBC should be checked every other day for 1 wk, then daily.
7. The WBC should begin falling on day 8–14. If it does not fall by day 15, increase the daily CTX dose by 100 mg. CTX is stopped and the patient is generally discharged from the hospital when the WBC drops below 4500/mm³. Close follow-up care is essential. Most patients reach a nadir at between 600–1800 WBC/mm³. In approximately 25% of patients there will be a neutropenia below 1000/mm³. At the first sign of infection (e.g., a shaking chill, fever), patients are evaluated and treated immediately.
8. Daily urinalyses are obtained during therapy. Treatment should be stopped for microscopic hematuria (greater than 5 RBC/HPF) on 3 consecutive days. If hematuria develops and the patient has not been drinking enough fluid, IV fluids should be given.
9. The patient should expect to lose all hair, but it will all grow back 4–6 mo after treatment.
10. Synthetic IV ACTH is given concomitant with CTX: 25 U for the first 3 days, then reduced by 5 U every 3 days for a total of 15 days of treatment; then ACTH gel, 40 U IM for 3 days, 20 U IM for 3 days, then discontinue. The IV ACTH is usually given while the patient sleeps. Antacid therapy, lithium prophylaxis, and potassium repletion should be given as recommended in the ACTH protocol.

TABLE 5. **Azathioprine and Prednisone Protocol**

1. Azathioprine is started at 150 mg daily. Baseline laboratory tests are obtained prior to treatment, including CBC, platelets, and liver function tests. These are rechecked at 2 wk, 4 wk, 8 wk, and then every 8 wk for 6 mo, then every 6 mo while treatment continues.
2. If liver function tests become abnormal, the dose should be decreased to 100 mg daily, and if liver function does not improve at this lower dose after several weeks, the medication should be discontinued.
3. Chronic azathioprine is initiated with a tapering dose of prednisone as follows:
   - 80 mg daily for 1 wk
   - 60 mg daily for 1 wk
   - 60 mg alternating with 40 mg daily for 1 wk
   - 60 mg alternating with 20 mg daily for 1 wk
   - 60 mg every other day for 1 wk
   - 40 mg every other day for 1 wk
   - 20 mg every other day for 1 wk
4. Lithium, 300 mg tid, and antacids or $H_2$ blockers are given during prednisone treatment.

and other painful lesions imperceptible to the patient. These precipitants must be sought out and treated specifically. All medications for spasticity result in an increase in weakness. This may be incapacitating to some weak patients who depend on stiffness for ambulation.

Baclofen (Lioresal) is the most useful medication for spasticity in MS. It can be started at 5 mg three times a day and increased by 5 mg per dose every 3 days to a maximal dose of 20 mg four times daily. In some patients, doses as high as 240 mg* daily in divided doses are used, although the incidence of side effects increases at such high doses. Baclofen should not be discontinued abruptly but tapered over 4 weeks as there is a small chance that hallucinations, anxiety, and tachycardia may accompany rapid drug withdrawal. Recently, intrathecal baclofen delivered via an indwelling catheter has been used experimentally and found to be effective at low doses with few side effects and few complications.

Diazepam (Valium) may also be useful for spasticity in some patients. Initial dose is 2 mg given 1 to 3 times daily. However, its use is limited by its sedative effect. It is especially effective for nocturnal spasms which may respond to a dose of 2 mg at bedtime.

Dantrolene (Dantrium), which decreases spasticity by inhibition of muscle contractility, also frequently causes weakness. It is best reserved for nonambulatory patients. Dantrolene may be started at 25 mg daily and increased to 25 mg four times daily, then by increments of 25 mg to a total dose of 100 mg four times a day. Hepatotoxicity is a serious complication of dantrolene therapy, and liver function tests must be monitored.

---

*Exceeds dosage recommended by the manufacturer.

Steroids, when given for treatment of an acute attack, will improve pre-existing spasticity. Therefore, in exceptional cases where other causes for worsening have been excluded and other agents have failed, a course of steroids may be given; their effect may last for several months.

Surgical procedures such as myelotomies, dorsal rhizotomies, and nerve blocks interrupt the reflex arc, thus modulating spasticity. These extreme procedures may be considered in medically recalcitrant, severe, nonambulatory cases.

## Pain

Neuritic pain, including trigeminal neuralgia and radicular pain, may respond to carbamazepine (Tegretol) or phenytoin (Dilantin). Carbamazepine is started at 100 mg twice a day and increased daily by 100 mg twice a day up to 1200 mg daily; the minimum effective dose should be used. Phenytoin may be given as 100 mg three times a day and increased up to 200 mg three times a day. Other patients may respond to amitriptyline (Elavil), 50 to 150 mg in divided doses or at bedtime.

## Paroxysmal Symptoms

Paroxysmal phenomena are transient, repetitive, and usually stereotyped neurologic symptoms. They may occur many times in a day and last generally from 15 seconds to 1 minute each. They include unpleasant tonic movements, dysesthesias, focal weakness, pain, itching, dysarthria, or ataxia. Generally spontaneous, they may in some instances be triggered by sensory or motor stimuli or by hyperventilation. Acetazolamide (Diamox), 125 to 250 mg three times a day, or carbamazepine (Tegretol), up to 1200 mg in divided doses, may abolish or markedly diminish these symptoms.

## Tremor

Tremor in MS may be incapacitating, and in our experience no effective treatments are available. Isoniazid (isonicotinic acid hydrazide [INH]) starting at 200 mg twice daily and increasing to 1200 mg in divided doses is reported to benefit postural tremor. Pyridoxine 50 mg daily must be administered concomitantly to prevent peripheral neuropathy. Clonazepam (Klonopin) may be of limited help in some patients; 0.5 mg twice daily may be given initially and increased gradually to 2 to 5 mg daily in divided doses. Propranolol (Inderal), up to 40 mg four times daily, is frefquently tried though rarely effective.

## Bladder Dysfunction

Bladder dysfunction is common in MS. The type of dysfunction may change over time, and specific urinary symptoms correlate poorly with the results of urodynamic studies.

Bladder hyperreflexia responds to anticholinergic treatment such as oxybutynin (Ditropan), 5 mg two to three times daily. Alternatively, propantheline (Probanthine), another anticholinergic, may be used at doses of 7.5 mg to 15 mg four times daily.

Urinary retention due to bladder hyporeflexia may respond to bethanecol (Urecholine), a cholinergic agent, 10 to 50 mg three to four times a day. Dyssynergia between detrussor and external sphincter muscles is a common problem that is difficult to treat and may require a combination of anticholinergic medication to decrease bladder contractions as well as intermittent catheterization. In more extreme cases, supravesical urinary diversion or a chronic indwelling catheter may be required. Because of the increased risk of urinary tract infection with an indwelling catheter, ascorbic acid should be given chronically to acidify the urine.

## Bowel Dysfunction

Bowel dysfunction includes constipation and urge incontinence. Regimentation of bowel function with laxatives and enemas may be helpful in both conditions, and a low fiber diet to decrease bulk may be useful for patients with incontinence.

## Sexual Dysfunction

Sexual dysfunction may occur in both men and women. Penile implants are available, and erections may be pharmacologically achieved using papaverine (Pavaloid) and phentolamine (Regitine) injections in the corpora cavernosa. Women may experience vaginismus, which may respond to antispasticity medications; decreased vaginal lubrication leading to dyspareunia, which may be simply treated with lubricants; or vaginal anesthesia.

## Psychiatric Disturbances

Psychiatric disturbances are frequent in patients with MS. Depression is common. Imipramine (Tofranil) can be helpful in doses of 75 to 200 mg daily. This should be initiated at a lower dose and increased as tolerated and may be given as a single dose at night. Plasma levels may be used to monitor dose requirements. Other antidepressants may be more useful in particular patients. Some studies suggest that psychotherapy may be beneficial to depressed patients with MS.

The incidence of bipolar affective disorder may be increased in patients with MS. Lithium carbonate is useful when treatment is required.

Pathologic laughing and weeping can occur independent of affective illness. This disturbing symptom may respond to amitriptyline (Elavil) 25 to 75 mg daily.

Psychosis is less common but has been reported in MS independent of steroid treatment. Antipsychotic agents such as perphenazine (Trilafon) at doses between 4 and 8 mg three times a day may be effective. Steroid treatment must be curtailed if it precipitates psychosis.

Cognitive impairment with memory loss and slowed thinking may develop in MS. Although currently untreatable, recognition of this disability is important for both patient and family.

### Fatigue

Fatigue that can be profound occurs in 80% of MS patients. As it is most prominent in the late afternoon, a shift to an earlier work schedule or a regular afternoon nap may be helpful. Amantadine (Symmetrel), 100 mg twice a day, may transiently benefit a small proportion of patients.*

### Health Maintenance

Health maintenance should be emphasized to all patients with MS. This includes maintaining a nutritious diet and avoiding rapid weight loss. Regular sleep and moderate exercise as practical is strongly recommended. Swimming is an ideal form of exercise as it provides support for patients with weakness and it is a cool exercise for those with heat sensitivity. Avoidance of stress or use of relaxation techniques such as meditation and biofeedback may be useful for patients struggling with psychosocial issues.

---

*This use of amantadine for fatigue is not listed in the manufacturer's official directive.

# MYASTHENIA GRAVIS

method of
CHRISTIAN HERRMANN, JR., M.D.
*University of California*
*Los Angeles, California*

Present findings indicate that autoimmune myasthenia gravis is an acquired immune complex disorder of neuromuscular transmission in voluntary striated muscle. Elevated titer of antibody to acetylcholine receptor is detectable in the serum of most patients. There is a break in immunologic tolerance with blocking and degradation of acetylcholine receptors; widening of the synaptic cleft; and partial destruction, simplification, and shortening of the postjunctional membrane. Thymic hyperplasia and/or thymoma may be associated.

Clinically, myasthenia gravis is characterized by variable weakness and easy fatigability. After a short rest of the muscles, there is partial to total recovery of strength. Extraocular, facial, and oropharyngeal muscles are usually affected early, but any of the voluntary striated muscles of the body may be involved. Commonly, its onset in women occurs before the age of 40 years and in men after the age of 40. Either sex may be affected at any time. About 12% of infants born to myasthenic mothers have a transient transmitted form of neonatal myasthenia gravis that remits permanently in days or weeks. Pregnancy is not generally contraindicated in myasthenia gravis.

## TREATMENT

### Anticholinesterase Therapy

Anticholinesterase drugs are the usual first line of treatment for myasthenia gravis. Their action is attributed to inhibition of cholinesterase at the neuromuscular junction, allowing acetylcholine to accumulate and facilitate remaining neuromuscular transmission. The three most frequently used are (1) neostigmine bromide (Prostigmin), (2) pyridostigmine bromide (Mestinon), and (3) ambenonium chloride (Mytelase). These partially reduce the defect in neuromuscular transmission and improve strength but are not a cure.

A fourth, very short-acting anticholinesterase agent, edrophonium chloride (Tensilon), is used to aid in the diagnosis of myasthenia gravis and to assess the effectiveness of the dosage of anticholinesterase drugs noted before. It is not useful for ongoing treatment. The diagnostic edrophonium test is best done when the patient has stopped taking all anticholinesterase drugs for 8 to 12 hours. A detailed test of muscle strength is done throughout the body, with areas of weakness noted, including cranial, oropharyngeal, and respiratory muscles. This is followed by a control injection or protective placebo injection of atropine sulfate, 0.4 mg intravenously. This acts to protect the patient from muscarinic side effects of the edrophonium to be given subsequently, as well as to assess psychologic effects of an intravenous injection. A detailed test of muscle strength of the areas previously noted to be weak is done again. This is followed by edrophonium, 2 mg intravenously, with repeated muscle testing in 30 seconds to 2 minutes, as after the atropine

TABLE 1. **Anticholinesterase Drugs Used in Diagnosis and Management of Myasthenia Gravis**

| Drug | Form | Adult Single Dose and Route | Usual Effective Duration and Range |
|---|---|---|---|
| Tensilon (edrophonium chloride) | 10 mg/ml | 2–10 mg IV | 10 min (2 min to 2 hr) |
| Prostigmin (neostigmine methylsulfate) | 0.25, 0.5, and 1 mg/ml | 1 mg IM | 2 hr (2–4 hr) |
| Prostigmin (neostigmine bromide) | 15-mg tablet | 15 mg PO | 3 hr (2–5 hr) |
| Mestinon (pyridostigmine bromide) | 10 mg/2 ml | 2 mg IM | 2 hr (2–4 hr) |
| Mestinon (pyridostigmine bromide) | 60-mg tablet | 60 mg PO | 4 hr (3–7 hr) |
| Mestinon Timespan (pyridostigmine bromide) | 180-mg tablet (slow release) | 90–180 mg PO | 8 hr (6–12 hr) |
| Mestinon Syrup (pyridostigmine bromide) | 60 mg/5 ml syrup | 60 mg/5 ml (1 tsp PO) | 4 hr (3–7 hr) |
| Mytelase (ambenonium chloride) | 10-mg tablet | 5–10 mg PO | 6 hr (4–8 hr) |

injection. Not all areas of weakness may respond equally to the edrophonium. A second injection of edrophonium, 4 to 8 mg intravenously, may be given in 3 to 5 minutes after the first if the first was not definitive and detailed muscle testing of weak areas is done again. In most myasthenics there is a clear-cut, although transient, improvement in strength that may not be uniform in all areas of weakness. This lasts usually 2 to 5 minutes and occasionally longer.

A list of commonly used anticholinesterase drugs and comparable dosage forms and routes of administration is given in Table 1. Anticholinesterases do not occur naturally in humans. Excessive anticholinesterase therapy may have adverse effects, increasing weakness and provoking other unpleasant and potentially dangerous side effects. These are listed under the column "Cholinergic Crisis" in Table 2.

Oral anticholinesterase therapy may be started gradually with one-half of a 15-mg tablet of neostigmine (7.5 mg) or one-half of a 60-mg tablet of pyridostigmine (30 mg) at 4-hour intervals or two or three times daily. Patients with weakness

in chewing and swallowing will find it helpful to take the drug 30 to 60 minutes before meals and refrain from talking while eating. Gastrointestinal effects will be fewer if a small amount of milk, bread, crackers, or other bland food is eaten before the anticholinesterase. Foods such as coffee, fruit, tomato juice, or carbonated or alcoholic beverages tend to increase the parasympathetic side effects on the gut, bladder, bronchi, and mucous glands. They are best avoided or taken at the end of a meal.

The dosage of anticholinesterase drug may be increased gradually at about 2-day intervals and the dose intervals shortened to 3 hours only if these changes are followed by objective improvement in symptoms and signs. Increases of one-fourth to one-half tablet per dose are recommended. Both the physician and patient must realize that anticholinesterase drugs seldom restore muscle strength to more than 80% of normal strength with optimal dosage. Weakness of extraocular, oropharyngeal, respiratory, and other muscles at times selectively or together may show little improvement with anticholinesterase drugs.

TABLE 2. **Symptoms and Signs of Myasthenic and Cholinergic Crises**

| Myasthenic Crisis | Cholinergic Crisis | |
|---|---|---|
| Ocular ptosis | *Muscarinic Symptoms and Signs:* | *Nicotinic Symptoms and Signs:* |
| Dysarthria or anarthria | | |
| Dysphagia or aphagia | Sweating | Muscle fasciculations |
| Dyspnea or apnea | Salivation | Dysarthric speech |
| Facial weakness | Lacrimation | Dysphagia |
| Masticatory weakness | Abdominal cramping | Trismus |
| Difficulty handling secretions | Nausea | Muscle cramps and spasms |
| General weakness | Vomiting | General weakness |
| | Diarrhea | |
| | Urinary frequency | *CNS Symptoms and Signs:* |
| | Incontinence of bowel and bladder | |
| | Miosis | Restlessness |
| | Blurred vision | Anxiety |
| | Bradycardia | Vertigo |
| | Bronchorrhea | Headache |
| | Substernal pressure | Confusion and stupor |
| | Dyspnea and wheezing | Coma |
| | Bronchospasm | Convulsions |
| | Pulmonary edema | |

Neostigmine and pyridostigmine are quite similar in their action and effectiveness. Some patients note more muscarinic side effects such as abdominal cramps, diarrhea, nausea, salivation, tearing, and sweating with neostigmine than with pyridostigmine. The action of neostigmine is about 30 to 45 minutes shorter than that of pyridostigmine. A few patients find that neostigmine gives more prompt and slightly greater improvement in muscle strength than pyridostigmine.

There are additional helpful forms of pyridostigmine. The syrup contains 60 mg in 5 ml (approximately 1 teaspoonful). This is palatable and easily administered and adjusted for young myasthenic children. Patients with swallowing difficulty may handle this form more easily and with greater safety than the tablets. It is also easily given by nasogastric tube. The other useful form of pyridostigmine is Mestinon Timespan tablets. Each contains 180 mg of pyridostigmine. About one-third of the dosage is released promptly, and the remainder is released over the next 6 to 12 hours. When a tablet is given at bedtime, it allows the moderate to severe myasthenic to sleep through the night without awakening to take regular anticholinesterase medication. Usually, only patients with moderate to severe myasthenia require medication during sleeping hours, and the dosage may be reduced to one-half or two-thirds of that taken during waking hours. Since the regular forms of pyridostigmine give more prompt and dependable release and absorption, Mestinon Timespan is not recommended for daytime use.

When patients are temporarily unable to take anticholinesterase drugs by mouth or are unable to swallow, parenteral forms of neostigmine methylsulfate or pyridostigmine bromide may be substituted. The equivalent of a 15-mg tablet of neostigmine is 1 to 1.5 mg of neostigmine methylsulfate intramuscularly. The equivalent of a 60-mg tablet of pyridostigmine bromide is 2 mg of pyridostigmine bromide intramuscularly. Parenteral anticholinesterase therapy is seldom more effective than oral therapy. It is not practical for long-term care.

Ambenonium chloride is the third available oral anticholinesterase drug. It is used much less frequently than neostigmine and pyridostigmine. It may be more effective against weakness of the extremities than of the cranial muscles. Duration of action is a bit longer than that of pyridostigmine. Patients not responding well to neostigmine or pyridostigmine may be tried carefully on ambenonium. Muscarinic toxic effects are less prominent, but nicotinic and central nervous system symptoms and signs of toxicity may appear. The nicotinic manifestations include muscle twitching and weakness. The central nervous system manifestations include headache, restlessness, and anxiety. Between 5 and 7.5 mg of ambenonium chloride is equivalent to 15 mg of neostigmine or 60 mg of pyridostigmine (tablets) given orally. One may start with 5 mg of ambenonium every 4 to 6 hours and increase by 2.5 mg per dose if there is objective improvement and no undesirable side effects.

To assess effects of anticholinesterase drugs, it is useful to examine patients just before the next dose of drug and 45 to 75 minutes after it. Helpful areas to test include the following:

1. The patient's inability to sustain upward gaze can reveal fatigue of the lid levators or extraocular muscles.
2. Continuous counting on a single breath gives a rough estimate of respiratory muscle strength and vital capacity.
3. The time the patient is able to keep the arms or legs elevated is an indication of the fatigability of these muscles.
4. The number of times the patient is able to cross and uncross one thigh over the other, squat, and arise or repeatedly compress a partially inflated blood pressure cuff or hand dynamometer is a simple test of strength and fatigability of neuromuscular transmission in these areas.
5. The patient's abilities to close the jaw tightly against resistance, to protrude the tongue into each cheek against resistance, to elevate the soft palate, to cough, to swallow, and to speak are useful signs that aid in assessing oropharyngeal strength.

Measurement of the vital capacity is a simple test of respiratory muscle function and reserve. It is weakness in oropharyngeal and/or respiratory muscle strength that constitutes the greatest threat to the myasthenic's life. Treatment should be directed to achieve optimal improvement in these areas.

The edrophonium chloride test may also be used in an attempt to determine how adequate ongoing anticholinesterase therapy is. One hour after the oral dose of the drug, the patient's strength is tested. The patient is then given 2 mg (0.2 ml) of edrophonium chloride intravenously, and strength is retested in 30 seconds to 2 minutes. If strength is significantly improved, the dosage of oral anticholinesterase may be increased. If strength is unchanged or declines, the oral anticholinesterase dosage is not changed. If muscarinic and nicotinic effects appear after 2 mg of edrophonium chloride, along with increased weakness, the oral anticholinesterase dosage should be lowered.

Although some differences are noted among

the effects of neostigmine, pyridostigmine, and ambenonium, overall results are quite similar. Of the three, currently pyridostigmine is the most frequently used oral anticholinesterase drug.

### Crisis

Muscle weakness leading to inability to maintain a patent airway free of secretions and/or adequate respiratory exchange constitutes crisis in the myasthenic. It may be caused by increase in the myasthenia gravis itself, too much anticholinesterase drug, or both. Rapid distinction among myasthenic, cholinergic, or mixed or insensitive crises may be difficult in the acute situation, if not impossible. Promptly providing an adequate airway with tracheal intubation, if necessary, suctioning of excessive tracheobronchial secretions to clear the airway, and positive-pressure assisted or controlled respiration may be lifesaving. Bilateral weakness of the abductors of the vocal cords may obstruct the airway, thus limiting exchange. Factors often associated with myasthenic crisis are infections, especially upper respiratory tract infections, menses, omitting anticholinesterase medication, vigorous physical activity, certain drugs, and emotional upsets.

Drugs having an adverse effect on neuromuscular transmission include most hypnotics, tranquilizers, and antihistaminics, as well as thiazides, quinine, quinidine, procainamide, calcium channel blockers, beta-blockers, ether, d-tubocurarine, pancuronium, succinylcholine, magnesium sulfate, D-penicillamine, adrenocorticotropic hormone (ACTH), adrenocorticosteroids, and aminoglycoside antibiotics. The latter include colistimethate, colistin, dihydrostreptomycin, kanamycin, neomycin, novobiocin, polymyxin B, gentamicin, streptomycin, and tobramycin.

Cholinergic crisis may be caused by too much anticholinesterase medication. It may develop in the course of a spontaneous remission, or following thymectomy or an overenthusiastic use of anticholinesterase drugs by the physician or patient. Some patients become unresponsive, insensitive, or resistant to anticholinesterase drugs. This happens particularly when the dosage is gradually increased to high levels over a long period of time. It must be remembered that both the antibodies to acetylcholine receptor and anticholinesterase drugs are attacking and acting on the postjunctional membrane of the neuromuscular junction. Each may adversely affect neuromuscular transmission. The symptoms and signs of myasthenic and cholinergic crises are listed in Table 2.

In the presence of cholinergic crisis or an un-responsive, resistant, or insensitive state, the anticholinesterase drug is stopped for 3 days or more. This is best done in a hospital, since the patient frequently initially becomes still weaker and may require an airway and mechanical ventilation for a time before strength spontaneously improves. This allows junctions that may be damaged and depolarized by excessive prolonged administration of an anticholinesterase drug to recover. Fluid balance and nutrition are maintained parenterally or by nasogastric tube.

If endotracheal intubation is required for more than 3 to 4 days, tracheostomy will be more comfortable for the patient, provide better tracheobronchial toilet, and reduce risk of damage to the larynx. A short, low-pressure cuffed tube is used. At times, patients withdrawn from anticholinesterase drugs and supported improve to the point that they may function for days or weeks without anticholinesterase medication.

Atropine is best used only sporadically or in an emergency to counteract muscarinic side effects of anticholinesterase drugs. Regular use may obscure the signs of cholinergic intoxication. Oral and tracheobronchial secretions are reduced and become thick, tenacious, inspissated, and difficult to aspirate. Bronchial plugging with atelectasis may result. Sedative and tranquilizing drugs are best avoided in the anxious apprehensive myasthenic. These symptoms and signs may be those of failing respiratory function rather than a psychologic reaction to illness. Such drugs may aggravate hypoxia and hypercapnia, setting up a vicious circle of more respiratory depression with vagal activity already increased by the anticholinesterase drug, leading to arrhythmia and asystole.

The patient in crisis should be turned frequently and given postural drainage, percussion to the chest, and meticulous tracheobronchial toilet. Auscultation of the chest, chest x-rays, and fiberoptic bronchoscopy may help to remove mucous plugs. Smears, cultures, and sensitivities of tracheobronchial secretions, along with appropriate antibiotics, aid in recovery and reduce mortality. Periodic determination of arterial blood gases aids evaluation of adequacy of mechanical ventilation, need for supplemental oxygen, and adjustment of depth and rate of respiration. Automatic periodic sighing, available on some respirators, may help prevent atelectasis and contractures of the chest wall from lack of full range of movement because of weakness. The lung in most myasthenics is normal and compliant once infection and atelectasis are overcome. For this reason, compressed air is best used for long-term operation of the positive pressure respirator.

## Thymectomy

Improvement or remission of autoimmune myasthenia gravis following thymectomy has been reported in up to 80% from several centers dealing with large numbers of myasthenic patients. It is most apt to occur in patients without thymoma. However, thymoma, which may occur in 15% of patients with myasthenia gravis, is also an indication for thymectomy, since about 35% of thymomas may become invasive or malignant. Exactly why improvement or remission occurs is not known. Results cannot be predicted in advance in the individual patient. Thymectomy is not helpful in congenital myasthenia. It may be less effective in patients older than 60 years of age, in whom the thymus is usually atrophic. It is not recommended for debilitated patients or those showing malignant spread of thymoma. It is not done as an emergency procedure or in the presence of active pulmonary infection, pregnancy, or rapidly worsening myasthenia. Improvement following thymectomy may not occur for weeks or months. Operative risk is small in the hands of a competent thoracic surgeon in a facility where neurologic and medical staff are familiar with the disorder and have intensive care facilities including respiratory support available. The transcervical or suprasternal approach to the thymus has been used at a few centers, but this is not usually satisfactory for removal of thymomas and may not allow removal of all thymic tissue, since the surgeon's operative field is restricted. Most centers continue to use a median sternotomy, which avoids these problems.

Treatment with alternate-day corticosteroid therapy for a few weeks or months before thymectomy is helpful in myasthenic patients with moderate to severe oropharyngeal and/or respiratory muscle weakness. It is not recommended for all patients having thymectomy.

Preoperatively, the patient is allowed to take usual doses of anticholinesterase medication with small sips of water up to the time of surgery. Postoperatively, anticholinesterase medication is resumed in 12 to 24 hours as weakness occurs, and dosage requirements are usually less. About one-half to three-quarters of the preoperative dose is given to start with. Close cooperation with postoperative follow-up by the neurologist is essential. Meperidine (Demerol) rather than morphine is used to relieve pain.

## Corticosteroid Therapy

Although some physicians have used alternate-day prednisone as the first choice of treatment even in essentially limited ocular myasthenia gravis, we have generally reserved its use for patients with more generalized weakness not responding favorably to anticholinesterases or thymectomy or both. This regimen may be considered in older patients who are not suitable candidates for thymectomy. However, both the patient and physician should be aware of the long-term commitment, side effects, risks, and complications of chronic use of corticosteroids, since fewer than 10% of patients are able to discontinue them completely in most cases. Strength may greatly improve, but the majority of patients remain dependent upon the corticosteroids for their improvement. Withdrawal is usually followed by recurrent weakness in weeks or months and by the need for even higher doses to reverse the weakness. In some, the improvement may be maintained on a relatively low dose, compared with amounts required to initiate the improvement. Improvement takes place over weeks or months.

Since there may be some paradoxical worsening of the myasthenia gravis when corticosteroids are first begun, they are best started in a hospital setting with staff familiar with this form of treatment in myasthenia gravis and with facilities for mechanical respiratory support and intensive care, should these be needed.

Patients with obesity, hypertension, and/or diabetes mellitus are best not treated with steroids. Patients who are anergic or who have positive skin tests for tuberculosis are best given simultaneously prophylactic isoniazid and pyridoxine with the corticosteroids.

We recommend that patients taking corticosteroids maintain a diet high in protein, potassium, and calcium; moderate in complex carbohydrates; and low in fat with no added free sugars. Supplemental 10% potassium chloride may be needed to keep the serum potassium in the upper normal levels. We recommend that patients receiving corticosteroids take antacid or nonfat milk 1 to 2 hours after each meal and at bedtime. We prefer to avoid chronic cimetidine or ranitidine therapy.

The blood count, serum potassium, and blood glucose are determined at office visits. Liver function tests are recommended for those on isoniazid; progress chest films are recommended at 6- to 12-month intervals.

We prefer to start alternate-day prednisone at 20 to 25 mg and increase this by 5 mg every second or third dose cycle. When strength begins to improve (which is usually not immediately), the dosage may be maintained at that level. We have seldom needed to exceed 100 mg on alternate days. If the patient already requires mechanical respiratory support, a higher initial starting dose, up to 100 mg, may be used in an attempt to reverse severe weakness sooner. This seldom happens before the second or third week. Methylprednisolone, 60 mg intramuscularly, or dexamethasone, 12 mg orally, in divided doses daily, has also been used in such states.

### Nonsteroidal Immunosuppressive Therapy

Azathioprine (Imuran),* cyclophosphamide (Cytoxan),* and methotrexate* have been used for long-term treatment in some patients. Those not responding to thymectomy or corticosteroids or those in whom corticosteroids are unacceptable because of side effects or contraindications may find these drugs helpful. These agents may also be used to reduce the dosage of corticosteroids required when side effects of these are troublesome. They are useful to provide ongoing immunosuppression in conjunction with plasmapheresis. The major long-term experience with them has been abroad rather than in the United States. Azathioprine, 2 to 3 mg per kg daily, is given in single or divided oral doses. Significant response may not be noted for 2 months to 1 year. Maximal improvement may not occur for up to 24 months, but once it is achieved it is quite even, with little fluctuation from day to day. When the patient is stable, dosage may be tapered slowly. Side effects and complications include nausea, vomiting, leukopenia, thrombocytopenia, anemia (often megaloblastic), and hepatotoxicity. Patients receiving this are best followed initially with weekly blood counts and a monthly blood chemistry panel, with particular attention to liver function tests. Lowering or discontinuing the drug usually reverses these effects. A comparable dose of cyclophosphamide is used. Results and side effects are the same except for the added risks of hemorrhagic cystitis and alopecia. Azathioprine and cyclophosphamide are not recommended for women in childbearing years because of possible developmental defects in the fetus. A risk of malignancy, as well as increased susceptibility to infection, is another consideration. The use of cyclosporine is currently under investigation.

### Plasmapheresis Therapy

Exchange of 2 liters of plasma for equal amounts of human albumin and saline every other day three times a week may relieve weakness temporarily. Long-term benefit from this regimen usually requires combining it with corticosteroids, other immunosuppressants, and/or thymectomy. It may be helpful in preparing moderately to severely weak patients for thymectomy or to shorten the time of crisis. Since plasma-

pheresis requires special facilities and skills and entails other risks, it is best done at centers familiar with both myasthenia gravis and pheresis.

### Adjuvant Therapy

Ephedrine sulfate, 25 mg orally two or three times daily, is helpful to some patients. It may make patients wakeful if given late in the day or evening. It should be avoided in men with prostatism, since it inhibits micturition. Potassium chloride, 1 to 2 grams given orally in 10% solution two or three times daily with meals, is helpful to other patients who function better with serum potassium levels at high normal. A few patients appear to benefit from calcium gluconate or lactate, 1 to 2 grams taken orally two to four times daily.

### Care for Surgery

Myasthenics may require surgery apart from thymectomy. Preoperative cathartics and enemas are avoided. The patient may take usual anticholinesterase drugs with small sips of water up to the time of surgery. If necessary, this may be converted to a parenteral dose of neostigmine or pyridostigmine. Muscle relaxants and sedatives are best avoided. Spinal, local, or regional anesthesia is preferable. When general anesthesia is necessary, ether is avoided—although it is seldom used for patients at present. Sodium pentothal and inhalation agents, such as nitrous oxide or enflurane, may be used. In those with significant oropharyngeal and/or respiratory weakness preoperatively, the endotracheal tube may be left in place postoperatively until the patient is well awake and demonstrates stable respiratory function by adequate measured vital capacity. Meperidine is given to relieve pain. Meticulous care should be given to the respiratory tract to promote full expansion of the lungs using intermittent positive-pressure breathing (IPPB), assisted coughing, and careful tracheobronchial toilet to prevent atelectasis and pulmonary infection. Since patients with myasthenia gravis tend to fatigue with repeated voluntary effort, incentive spirometry is usually counterproductive as compared with IPPB to expand the lungs in someone with pre-existing respiratory muscle weakness. If antibiotics are needed, those listed earlier that are known to interfere with neuromuscular transmission are avoided. Dosage requirements for anticholinesterase are often lower postoperatively. Therapy may be started parenterally as weakness develops. When the patient is able to swallow and is no longer nauseated and bowel

---

*This use of these agents is not listed by the manufacturers.

sounds are normal, medication may be given by nasogastric tube or orally.

### Associated Disorders

The presence of one autoimmune disease increases the likelihood of another in the same patient. As a consequence, one may see such conditions as Graves' disease, Hashimoto's thyroiditis, rheumatoid arthritis, polymyositis, dermatomyositis, scleroderma, vitiligo, pernicious anemia, lupus erythematosus, pemphigus, idiopathic thrombocytopenic purpura, red cell aplasia, autoimmune hemolytic anemia, autoimmune secondary amenorrhea, and multiple sclerosis. The most common are disorders of the thyroid, especially hyperthyroidism. Periodically, tests of thyroid function as well as determinations of creatine phosphokinase levels are desirable.

### OUTLOOK

Better and newer forms of treatment, including improved mechanical respiratory support, antibiotics to combat infection, corticosteroids, other immunosuppressants and current discoveries, and understanding of the immunopathophysiology of neuromuscular transmission have all helped to reduce mortality and morbidity as well as increase longevity. It is important for patients to learn to pace their physical activities. Patients and their families benefit from learning the nature of myasthenia gravis and general principles of management to reduce unnecessary anxiety, to allow them more control of their care, and to promote a smoother course. Most patients with myasthenia gravis are able to lead gainful, productive, satisfying lives.

# TRIGEMINAL NEURALGIA

method of
GARY G. FERGUSON, M.D.
*University Hospital and the University of*
*Western Ontario*
*London, Ontario, Canada*

"Idiopathic" trigeminal neuralgia, or tic douloureux, is a distinctive clinical entity characterized by the occurrence of brief, provokable paroxysms of pain in the distribution of the trigeminal nerve. This pain is uniquely intense and is often described by patients as having the quality of an electrical shock. If the pain occurs at all frequently, a patient will be rapidly incapacitated and insistent on treatment. The pain usually arises at or near a trigger point on the face or in the mouth and may spread to other divisions of the trigeminal nerve, but it remains strictly ipsilateral during any given paroxysm.

The annual incidence of new cases of tic douloureux is estimated to be 4 to 5 per 100,000 population. Women are afflicted twice as often as men. Two-thirds of patients have their first symptoms after age 50. Pain is more common on the right than the left side. A small percentage of patients develop bilateral tic. Pain occurs most commonly in the mandibular division and least commonly in the ophthalmic division. Tic pain tends to occur in episodic bouts with totally pain free intervals. A single paroxysm of lancinating pain may last only a few seconds. A few paroxysms may occur in rapid succession to be followed by minutes, hours, or even days of relief from pain. Bouts of intermittent pain may last for weeks or months, resolving either spontaneously or following treatment. Remission may occur for months or years, but the usual tendency is for recurrence. Permanent spontaneous remission is not to be anticipated.

Tic pain is characteristically triggered by a nonnoxious stimulus to the face or the mouth, such as that produced by talking, eating, brushing the teeth, shaving, combing the hair, or even a gentle breeze. During a paroxysm of pain, a patient may wince, as if receiving an electrical shock. Patients often try to protect their face and the trigger area from the slightest disturbance. Patients generally avoid touching their faces, although an occasional patient finds relief by applying pressure to the painful area.

### DIAGNOSIS

The diagnosis of tic douloureux depends entirely on the description of the pain given by the patient (see Table 1). The neurologic examination is normal, although occasionally minor changes in trigeminal sensory function are observed. Abnormalities on neurologic examination suggest "symptomatic" trigeminal neuralgia due to an underlying structural lesion of the trigeminal nerve or its pathways, such as may occur with cerebellopontine angle tumors, posterior fossa aneurysms, arteriovenous malformations, or multiple sclerosis (MS). About 1% of patients with MS develop typical symptoms of tic douloureux. The younger the patient, the greater is the likelihood of an underlying structural lesion.

Tic douloureux is differentiated from other facial pains by the unique characteristics of the pain. Other causes of facial pain with which it may be confused include dental pain, temporomandibular joint dysfunction, sinusitis, cluster migraine, postherpetic neuralgia, atypical facial pain, and the rare syndromes of glossopharyngeal or geniculate neuralgia.

Extensive and costly investigations are not warranted in an older patient with typical tic douloureux and a normal neurologic examination. It is reasonable, however, to obtain a high-resolution CT scan in most patients, with particular attention to the structures of the posterior fossa and skull base. MR scanning provides exquisite resolution of posterior fossa anatomy and is a reasonable alternative if competitively priced.

## TREATMENT

### Medical Treatment

A patient with other than short-lived pain will insist on treatment. Any symptomatic cause of trigeminal neuralgia should be dealt with in its own right, which generally results in resolution of the pain. Patients with MS and tic douloureux are treated in a similar fashion to other patients with "idiopathic" trigeminal neuralgia. In all such patients, the initial therapy is medical (Table 1).

The drug of choice is carbamazepine (Tegretol). The effectiveness of this tricyclic anticonvulsant is so pronounced that many regard the clinical response as a diagnostic test. Although some patients will be relieved of their pain with a first dose, carbamazepine is not effective in all patients, and as a general rule, its effectiveness decreases with time. Carbamazepine is generally well tolerated by patients and may be used for prolonged periods of time if necessary. Nonetheless, a number of precautions are necessary. This drug may suppress bone marrow function dramatically and cause hepatic dysfunction and adverse skin reactions. Prior to treatment, baseline hematologic and hepatic function tests should be obtained. These should be repeated monthly during treatment, which should be discontinued at the first sign of abnormality. Bone marrow

TABLE 1. **A Plan for the Management of Patients with Idiopathic Trigeminal Neuralgia (Tic Douloureux)**

**Diagnosis**
1. History—provokable paroxysms of unilateral pain in the distribution of the trigeminal nerve
2. Neurologic examination—normal
3. Investigation—CT or MR scan—normal

**Medical Treatment** (always the first line of therapy)
1. Carbamazepine (Tegretol)—begin with 100–200 mg twice daily and increase as necessary to a maximum daily dose of 800–1200 mg, in divided doses
2. Phenytoin (Dilantin)—300 to 400 mg daily
3. Baclofen (Lioresal)—begin with 5–10 mg three times a day; may increase to 15–20 mg four times a day
4. Combinations of the above drugs

**Surgical Treatment** (to be considered only if medical treatment fails; the choice depends on the age, general health, and wishes of the patient)
1. Peripheral procedures
   a. V1—supraorbital and supratrochlear neurectomies
   b. V2—infraorbital neurectomy or alcohol block
   c. V3—inferior alveolar neurectomy
2. Percutaneous retrogasserian rhizotomy (contraindicated in V1 tic)
   a. Radiofrequency thermocoagulation
   b. Glycerol rhizolysis
3. Open intracranial procedures
   a. Microvascular decompression of the trigeminal nerve in the posterior fossa
   b. Partial trigeminal sensory root section

suppression is a relatively rare occurrence and is generally rapidly reversible. Fatal aplastic anemia is very rare.

Initially, many patients will feel unwell on carbamazepine. Common complaints are nausea, loss of appetite, drowsiness, mental dulling, and unsteadiness. These symptoms are most prominent if the initial dose is too high, in more elderly patients, and in patients with MS. Treatment should begin with a relatively low dose and be increased gradually to the minimum dosage that effectively controls the pain. An appropriate starting dose in younger patients is 100 to 200 mg twice daily with meals. The maximum tolerable dose is in the range of 800 to 1200 mg per day, although an occasional patient may tolerate higher dosages for short periods in a crisis. As major bouts of pain tend to be episodic, the dosage should be gradually reduced and the drug ultimately discontinued when the pain is no longer present. Carbamazepine should not be used prophylactically during periods of long remission. In elderly patients or patients with MS, starting dosages may be as little as 50 mg once or twice daily, and maximum tolerable dosages are unlikely to exceed 600 mg per day.

Other medications are not as effective in controlling tic douloureux but should be considered in patients who have become refractory to carbamazepine, have developed toxicity, or are intolerant of the side effects. Phenytoin (Dilantin) in a divided daily dosage of 300 to 400 mg is generally well tolerated and, if ineffective alone, may be tried in combination with carbamazepine. More recently, baclofen (Lioresal) has been observed to be useful in some patients, either alone or in combination with carbamazepine or phenytoin. A dosage of 5 to 10 mg three times a day should be given initially and can be increased gradually to a maximum of 15 to 20 mg four times a day.

### Surgical Treatment

Neurosurgery plays an important role in the management of patients with tic douloureux in whom medical therapy has proved ineffective (see Table 1). It is generally possible, by one surgical means or another, to relieve pain with an acceptable risk. The choice of the procedure to be used must be individualized to the particular circumstances and wishes of the patient. The risks and benefits of the various procedures to be considered should be carefully reviewed with the patient, with whom the choice ultimately resides.

In general, three categories of procedures are available: (1) procedures involving the peripheral branches of the trigeminal nerve, either alcohol block or nerve avulsion; (2) percutaneous procedures to produce a lesion of the retrogasserian rootlets of the trigeminal nerve, either by radiofrequency rhizotomy or glycerol rhizolysis; and (3) open intracranial procedures to either decompress or section the trigeminal sensory root or its components.

Procedures on the peripheral branches of the trigeminal nerve (first division—supraorbital and supratrochlear nerves; second division—infraorbital nerve; third division—inferior alveolar nerve) are attractive because of a high degree of initial success and low morbidity. They are most useful in elderly or frail patients, in patients with MS, or in patients unwilling to accept a procedure with higher risk. For the rare patient with isolated first division tic, a peripheral procedure is preferable to a percutaneous retrogasserian procedure, as there is no risk of corneal anesthesia or neuroparalytic keratitis. The disadvantages of the peripheral procedures are that facial numbness is an inevitable consequence, and pain relief is relatively short-lived, averaging 6 to 12 months for alcohol blocks and 2 to 4 years for nerve avulsion. An alcohol block can be performed quickly as an outpatient procedure. The certainty of success with an alcohol block is not as great as with nerve avulsion, but the procedure may easily be repeated. This technique is most commonly used for pain in the infraorbital nerve distribution. Peripheral neurectomies are certain to relieve pain but usually require a general anesthetic and a short hospital stay.

Percutaneous procedures on the retrogasserian rootlets of the trigeminal nerve are the most widely practiced surgical procedures to treat tic douloureux. These procedures are well tolerated, carry virtually no risk of mortality or morbidity beyond trigeminal nerve dysfunction, have a high initial success rate, and relieve pain on average for longer than the peripheral procedures. This may be 5 years or more with radiofrequency thermocoagulation. The duration of pain relief is generally proportional to the extent of the sensory loss, which tends to lessen with the passage of time. Like the peripheral procedures, these procedures are well suited to elderly patients, patients who are poor risks for major surgery, patients with MS, patients who will not accept higher risks, or who have pain in more than one division. Percutaneous rhizotomy is best suited to patients with third division pain and is contraindicated in first division pain. The disadvantage of these procedures relates to facial numbness. If the numbness is extensive and severe, it may be poorly tolerated in contrast to the more limited numbness of peripheral procedures, which is generally well tolerated. Patients complain bitterly of an unpleasant dysesthetic sen-

sation in the face. If there is a dense sensory loss, there is a significant risk of anesthesia dolorosa, an agonizing, unremitting, and untreatable facial pain, which may totally obsess the patient. Inadvertent first division sensory loss with corneal anesthesia runs the risk of neuroparalytic keratitis with potential loss of vision.

Percutaneous rhizotomy is performed under neuroleptic anesthesia by placing the tip of a fine bore needle through the foramen ovale and into the retrogasserian rootlets of the trigeminal nerve under fluoroscopic control. Two methods are currently used to produce a lesion. The greatest experience exists with radiofrequency thermocoagulation, the aim of which is to produce analgesia without anesthesia in the division of pain. Limiting the sensory loss to a single division may be a problem. The more recently described alternative procedure of glycerol rhizolysis involves the stepwise injection of absolute anhydrous glycerol, a mildly neurotoxic agent that produces relatively little or no sensory loss but is associated with a higher early recurrence rate. Both procedures can be repeated after early or late recurrence of pain.

A wide variety of intracranial procedures have been described for the treatment of tic douloureux. Currently, the most widely used procedure is microvascular decompression of the trigeminal nerve by a posterior fossa approach (Jannetta procedure). The rationale is Jannetta's hypothesis that tic douloureux is caused by vascular compression of the trigeminal sensory root at its entry zone on the side of the pons, usually by an exaggerated loop of the superior cerebellar artery. Definitive treatment is to identify the offending vascular compression and to separate the vessel permanently from the nerve by a prosthetic implant, such as a patch of Dacron. This is thought to produce permanent relief of pain without facial numbness, an ideal management result. In my experience, this procedure does result in the greatest overall patient satisfaction of any surgical procedure for tic douloureux.

Microvascular decompression should be performed only by an experienced microsurgeon and should be reserved for patients under 65 to 70 years of age, who are otherwise excellent surgical risks. In expert hands, the risk of perioperative death or lasting and major morbidity is under 1%, while the risk of injury to adjacent cranial nerves is likewise extremely low. Convincing vascular compression will be found in 90% of patients, and lasting relief of pain will occur in 70 to 80%. In patients in whom no vascular compression is found, a partial sensory root section provides an excellent chance of prolonged pain relief with an acceptable degree of sensory loss.

# OPTIC NEURITIS

method of
ALFREDO A. SADUN, M.D., PH.D.
*Doheny Eye Institute/USC School of Medicine*
*Los Angeles, California*

Optic neuritis is a clinically defined entity of unknown etiology. It is characterized by an acute impairment of optic nerve function sometimes accompanied by pain that usually shows at least partial resolution over a matter of weeks. The term is not used when the optic nerve deficit is due to a congenital, traumatic, or toxic etiology. Although some investigators include vascular and infectious causes, most consider optic neuritis to be a result of inflammation associated with local and sometimes multiple demyelination. Usually, the optic disk appears normal on fundoscopy (retrobulbar optic neuritis); when disk hyperemia is noted, the term papillitis is used. It is important to remember that, although recent articles have demonstrated a high level of association with positive findings in certain laboratory tests, the diagnosis of optic neuritis remains a clinical one.

The onset of optic neuritis almost always occurs between the ages of 20 and 50. Before 20 or after 50, the clinician should take the attitude that he or she is dealing with a different disease. There is a predilection for women (3:2) and a known association with multiple sclerosis (MS). The vast majority of patients with MS will have an attack of optic neuritis (sometimes subclinical and demonstrable only by laboratory tests). The likelihood that symptoms of MS will develop later is greater for those in whom optic neuritis occurs when young, and greater among women than men.

Classically in optic neuritis there is an abrupt loss of vision unilaterally occurring over several hours. The visual deficit is often characterized as fogginess or cloudiness of central vision and may vary from a minimal loss of acuity (20/25) to no light perception. This visual loss is often preceded or accompanied by retrobulbar pain aggravated by ocular movement, especially horizontal ductions. Occasionally, the patient will also describe bright flashes of light and dim illumination with eye movement or eyelid closure. Rarely, there may be photopsia or photophobia. In addition to a loss of visual acuity, there is a characteristic desaturation of color perception and a loss of brightness sense. Uncommonly, there may be other ocular findings including venous sheathing and, rarely, uveitis. The most characteristic aspect of the disease is its tempo. Visual loss generally reaches its climax within 5 days of onset; after several weeks, visual acuity begins to improve. The return of visual function is usually incomplete and may take several months.

## TREATMENT

Before treatment is initiated, the physician needs to feel confident with the diagnosis. Unlike many other opthalmologic disorders, the diagnosis cannot be based on an objective observation. Indeed, the classic description of optic neuritis is: "The patient sees nothing; the doctor sees nothing." Therefore, it is incumbent upon the physician to rule out other entities. Fortunately, the characteristic tempo of optic neuritis is of great aid. A triad of optic nerve function tests—afferent pupillary defect, color vision, and measurement of brightness sense—is particularly useful. Additionally, the central visual field should be measured either by Amsler's grid or tangent screen. Contrast sensitivity of high spatial frequencies is almost always impaired in optic neuritis. These office tests usually suffice. However, with atypical presentations of history or examination, other testing may be appropriate. Blood tests that include a collagen vascular battery (complete blood count, erythrocyte sedimentation rate, rheumatoid factor, antinuclear-antibody, and total complement) are appropriate if vision is 20/200 or worse. If the visual loss is down to no light perception or if there is a history of sinus disease, a computed tomographic (CT) scan is prudent. In cases of skin rash and papillitis, syphilis serologic testing should be performed. In most circumstances, magnetic resonance imaging (MRI) is *not* necessary or desirable. Although a course of oral corticosteroids probably shortens the acute illness, this treatment has not been demonstrated to improve the ultimate visual outcome. The risks of treating with corticosteroids include (1) obfuscating the natural course of the disease and thus the diagnosis, and (2) the side effects of systemic steroid treatment. In cases when steroids are given, improvement in vision may be consistent not only with the diagnosis of optic neuritis but also with the effects of steroids on other inflammations, infections, and space occupying lesions. Therefore, in most cases steroids should not be used; however, if they are used, a more extensive work-up, including CT scan of head and orbit, is necessary. In general, there are three circumstances that justify the use of systemic steroids: (1) when visual acuity is worse than hand motion; (2) when the patient has both eyes affected and therefore would profit most from prompt resolution of symptoms; and (3) when the patient has had several previous attacks of optic neuritis and a diagnosis of MS is already established. However, the decision to treat with steroids needs to be made with the patient after presenting the relative risks and benefits and taking into consideration such issues as whether the patient is pregnant, has a history of gastric ulcer, etc. I usually do not treat with steroids, but when I do my regimen is prednisone beginning with 80 mg per day and then tapering by 20 mg approximately every 5 to 10 days. This tapering schedule also needs to take into account the patient's age, general health, etc.

## COURSE

Optic neuritis is a self-limiting disease in which improvement generally occurs within days to weeks. Almost 90% of patients will have ultimate visual acuities of 20/40 or better. Even patients who are down to no light perception often regain vision to better than 20/200. If there is no improvement in visual acuity after 1 month, reconsider the diagnosis. Two months after the onset of optic neuritis, most patients have visual acuities of 20/25 or better. However, even those with 20/20 vision often complain that they still have definite vision sequelae, including some color desaturation; a sense of dimness in illumination; a sense of visual fatigue when looking at objects of high contrast in bright light; complaints of mottled areas of darkness in the central field; and problems with depth perception, especially when looking at moving targets.

An important issue for the patient is the relationship of optic neuritis to MS. MS is a remitting disease characterized by lesions separated in space and time. The patient with MS may, in addition to having optic neuritis, demonstrate nystagmus, gaze palsies, cranial nerve palsies, and internuclear ophthalmoplegia. About 20% of patients with MS will have optic neuritis as the presenting sign. However, most patients who present with acute optic neuritis will later develop other neurologic symptoms consistent with the diagnosis of MS. Nonetheless, I think it is important not to make the premature diagnosis of MS in patients with optic neuritis. The diagnosis should not be made until the patient has had neurologic symptoms separated in space and time. Recent studies indicate that MRI will reveal unidentified bright objects in almost every optic neuritis patient, thus suggesting an even stronger correlation with MS. However, many asymptomatic patients will show unidentified bright objects on MRI studies. In addition, autopsy series have shown that from 4 to 7% of normals will have demyelination plaques. Therefore, it is important to emphasize to the patient that the diagnosis of MS is a clinical diagnosis. An MRI study on most patients with optic neuritis is not only unjustified but also does a disservice to the patient in that it suggests a laboratory diagnosis that has little prognostic meaning. Other laboratory tests such as oligoclonal banding of the CSF fluid can be useful, but not definitive in predicting MS. There are several studies that suggest that the course of MS is more likely to be benign when the presentation is with optic neuritis. Because of the complexities of the many issues in relating optic neuritis to MS, it is important that the physician establish a good line of communication with the patient and only then approach the subject in a cautious and circumspect fashion.

# GLAUCOMA

method of
RONALD L. GROSS, M.D.
*Cullen Eye Institute, Baylor College of Medicine*
*Houston, Texas*

Glaucoma is the leading cause of irreversible blindness in the world. In the United States alone, 600,000 people have been blinded by glaucoma. It is the leading cause of irreversible blindness among blacks and among the three most common causes overall. In the U.S., 1.5 million people are affected by glaucoma, and another 1.0 million may have the disease but are not yet diagnosed.

Increasing age is a major risk factor for glaucoma, affecting 4% of the population over age 65, and nearly 15% of the population over age 80. Blacks are affected 10 times more frequently than caucasians; in blacks, glaucoma has an earlier onset and more aggressive course. Immediate family members have a 10- to 15-fold increased risk of developing glaucoma compared with the general population. Patients with myopia, diabetes, and systemic hypertension are also more likely to be affected by glaucoma.

The term *glaucoma* refers to several conditions characterized by typical visual field loss due to optic nerve damage as a result of elevated intraocular pressure. The progressive damage to the optic nerve can be halted by an adequate reduction in intraocular pressure. In most cases, the elevated pressure is due to obstruction of the outflow of aqueous humor. This fluid is produced in the posterior chamber and normally passes between the iris and the lens through the pupil into the anterior chamber of the eye. It exits through the trabecular meshwork into the episcleral venous circulation. An obstruction to outflow increases aqueous humor volume, raising the intraocular pressure and damaging individual axons of the optic nerve in a typical manner. Visual field testing evaluates the function of the optic nerve and exhibits characteristic abnormalities in glaucoma. Although intraocular pressure plays an important role in glaucoma, the site of damage is the optic nerve. Its appearance and function are key factors in diagnosis and treatment.

Patients with elevated intraocular pressure without change in optic nerve appearance or visual field abnormality are *glaucoma suspects*. Only 10 to 20% of these patients will develop glaucoma, but they are at increased risk compared with the general population.

### PRIMARY OPEN-ANGLE GLAUCOMA

The most common form of glaucoma, affecting nearly two-thirds of patients, is *primary open-angle glaucoma* (POAG). The disease is bilateral but may be asymmetrical. It is caused by increased resistance to aqueous humor outflow through the trabecular meshwork resulting in a mild to moderate elevation of intraocular pressure.

It is a chronic disease, and because intraocular pressures are not elevated markedly, it is asymptomatic. There is no pain or redness of the eye. The visual field loss tends to be peripheral and slowly progressive such that the patient may have no visual complaint. When central vision is affected, it is far progressed and difficult to control.

Because POAG is insidious, early diagnosis is the most important factor in preventing visual loss. Patients over 35 years old should be evaluated every 3 years. Older adults, blacks, individuals with a family history of glaucoma, and those with other ocular or systemic problems (ocular trauma, myopia, diabetes, systemic hypertension) are at an increased risk and should be evaluated more frequently.

Glaucoma screening consists of four components: (1) medical and family history, (2) visual acuity testing, (3) examination of the optic nerve, and (4) measurement of intraocular pressure.

Examination of the optic nerve is greatly enhanced by pupillary dilation. The optic nerve is composed of the retinal ganglion cell axons. The majority of axons enter the optic nerve from the superior and inferior poles. The surface of a normal optic nerve is generally flat or slightly elevated with a small, central, pale, depressed physiologic cup. This cup is surrounded by a neural rim that normally has an orange-red color. Appearance of the normal optic nerve and its cup varies. It is important to document the appearance of the optic nerve such that any change can be recognized. In glaucoma, early damage to nerve fibers at the inferior and superior pole of the disk result in a vertical elongation of the optic cup with narrowing of the neural rim and pallor of the optic nerve. The vessels of the optic disk tend to be displaced nasally.

Glaucoma should be suspected if cupping represents greater than one-third of the surface of the disk, extends to the rim of the disk, results in an optic cup that is larger vertically than horizontally; or there is asymmetry between the optic disks of the two eyes, a flame-shaped hemorrhage in the nerve fiber layer near the border of the optic disk, or a definite change in the appearance of the optic disk from a previous evaluation.

Intraocular pressure measurement is also important in screening for glaucoma. There are many ways to measure intraocular pressure; the simplest is Schiøtz's tonometry. This requires topical anesthetic but is painless and accurate. A level above 22 mmHg is suspicious for glaucoma, and further evaluation is warranted. Intraocular pressure fluctuates in all patients, more so in those with glaucoma. Therefore, patients with damage may not have elevated pressures at any one time of measurement. Conversely, glaucomatous damage is not always present in those with elevated intraocular pressures.

## Treatment

Treatment consists of reducing intraocular pressure. Medical therapy is instituted initially using the minimum concentration, frequency, and number of medications to control the disease and minimize side effects.

Topical glaucoma medications affect the autonomic nervous system. These include the following:

1. *Beta blockers:* Beta blockers decrease intraocular pressure by reducing the secretion of aqueous humor. The potential side effects from ocular drops are the same as for systemic usage and include exacerbation of reactive airway disease, bradycardia, systemic hypotension, decreased libido, and altered mentation. These agents should not be used in patients with heart block or failure, asthma, or obstructive lung disease.

2. *Sympathomimetic agents:* Epinephrine or dipivefrin (Propine) 0.1% increases aqueous outflow. Potential side effects include systemic hypertension, headache, cardiac palpitations and arrhythmias. Most common is development of a topical allergic response.

3. *Miotics:* Parasympathomimetic agents such as pilocarpine improve aqueous outflow through the trabecular meshwork. Often these result in ocular side effects due to the ciliary body spasm and pupillary miosis. Systemic cholinergic effects are rare. Cholinesterase inhibitors, such as echothiophate iodide (Phospholene Iodide), are topical agents that can inhibit systemic cholinesterase. Patients taking these drugs should not receive agents such as succinylcholine during general anesthesia.

To decrease the systemic absorption of all topical ophthalmic drops, nasal lacrimal duct compression or simple eyelid closure should be performed for 3 to 5 minutes following instillation of each drop.

The chronic use of systemic carbonic anhydrase inhibitors is controversial. These reduce intraocular pressure by inhibiting aqueous production. However, they can cause urinary frequency, anorexia, nausea, depression, malaise, peripheral neuropathy, kidney stones, and rarely aplastic anemia. These drugs are sulfonamides and are contraindicated in patients allergic or sensitive to these medications. They may lower serum potassium concentrations and should be used with caution in patients on non–potassium sparing diuretics or digoxin.

For POAG, treatment is advanced until intraocular pressure has been reduced by a significant amount compared with the level at which damage occurred. If this level is reached, the patient is followed closely with evaluation of the optic nerve and visual field to be sure that no further progression has occurred. If medical therapy is unsuccessful in adequately lowering intraocular pressure, surgical methods are considered. Argon laser is used to treat the trabecular meshwork to increase aqueous outflow. It is successful in approximately 80% of POAG patients, with 50% lasting 5 years. In addition, there are several other surgical procedures designed to provide alternative aqueous outflow or reduce aqueous production.

### PRIMARY ANGLE-CLOSURE GLAUCOMA

Primary angle-closure glaucoma is an ocular emergency. The onset is acute with severe symptoms. Patients at risk are those with "narrow angles," usually in an eye that is hyperopic, resulting in close apposition of the lens and iris. When an attack occurs, flow between the lens and iris is stopped. Aqueous humor continues to be secreted, forcing the iris anteriorly, covering the trabecular meshwork and preventing any outflow of aqueous humor. Within a very short period of time, intraocular pressure can rise to a dangerous level.

The acute attack may be precipitated by physical or emotional stress, dilation of the pupil due to dim lighting, or eyedrops. The predisposition to angle closure is uncommon (1% of the population), and the majority of patients at risk never have an attack. Physicians should not hesitate to dilate pupils to facilitate examination of the posterior segment of the eye. Antihistamines and other medications with autonomic effects may dilate the pupil slightly, which could precipitate an attack in a predisposed patient. Used in their recommended dosage, this is rare.

Unlike patients with open-angle glaucoma, a patient with acute angle-closure exhibits severe symptoms, including ocular pain and redness, blurred vision, rainbow-colored halos around lights, headaches, and frequently nausea and vomiting. Usually only one eye is affected. On examination, that eye is red, the pupil mid-dilated and oval, and the cornea cloudy, and on tactile tension the eye is very firm.

If acute angle-closure glaucoma is suspected, the patient should be immediately referred to an ophthalmologist; prior to this or if this is not possible, treatment should be begun. Treatment should include a topical beta blocker, 1 drop every 30 minutes, and pilocarpine 2%, 1 drop every 15 minutes for 1 hour; also acetazolamide (Diamox) 500 mg if not contraindicated. Osmotic diuretics, such as glycerin (Osmoglyn) or isosorbide (Ismotic) orally or mannitol intravenously, 1 to 1.5 grams per kg of body weight, can be given if necessary. Medical therapy is usually effective in lowering intraocular pressure and breaking the attack. Following this, a laser peripheral iridotomy is performed to make an opening in the iris, allowing aqueous humor flow to the trabecular meshwork and preventing future attacks. In some patients, all the effects of the angle-closure attack cannot be reversed and chronic therapy is required.

### PRIMARY DEVELOPMENTAL GLAUCOMA

This is a rare condition in which glaucoma is caused by abnormal development of the anterior segment, including the outflow channels. In 75% of patients, the condition is bilateral. Patients with developmental glaucoma usually present within 1 year of life initially with excessive tearing. In addition, the infant with developmental glaucoma may have enlarged eyes as a result of the increased intraocular pressure in eyes that are immature and relatively elastic. Photophobia or light sensitivity is a common symptom, as is frequent blinking or blepharospasm. The treatment of developmental glaucoma is primarily surgical. Developmental glaucoma must also be considered as one of the causes of a cloudy cornea at birth.

### SECONDARY GLAUCOMAS

One of the most common forms of secondary glaucoma is steroid-induced glaucoma. This occurs when corticosteroid eyedrops or rarely systemic corticosteroids are used for several weeks. Up to 15% of normal patients and 95% of POAG patients may have a 15-mmHg increase in intraocular pressure after being treated with long-term topical corticosteroids. Once this is identified, discontinuation of the steroid with treatment of the glaucoma will reverse the effect. However, it may take 2 to 3 months. There is no concentration or type of corticosteroid that will avoid the pressure rise. Other ocular complications can also result from steroid use, including cataract formation and exacerbation of viral infections. Therefore, great care should be exercised when prescribing these drops for patients.

Secondary glaucoma may also be caused by

ocular trauma, retinal vein occlusion, intraocular inflammation, intraocular tumors, diabetes, and cardiovascular disease. Any patient suspected of having secondary glaucoma should be referred to an ophthalmologist for evaluation as soon as possible.

# ACUTE FACIAL PARALYSIS

method of
KEDAR KARIM ADOUR, M.D.
*Kaiser Permanente Medical Care Program*
*Oakland, California*

Facial paralysis is an alarming symptom to the treating physician as well as the patient. This, in association with outdated erroneous data found in the literature, often leads to unnecessary, costly diagnostic tests and extensive, potentially life-threatening surgical procedures. The fault can be traced to overuse of the generic term "Bell's palsy" for all cases of facial paralysis. Bell's palsy has also been synonymous with and defined as idiopathic facial paralysis affecting only the facial nerve within the confines of the temporal bone. In the past 15 years, Bell's palsy, the most common cause of facial paralysis, has been redefined as a viral cranial polyneuritis, probably caused by herpes simplex reactivation, and its diagnosis is no longer reached by exclusion. We suggest that the term idiopathic facial paralysis be replaced with that of "Antoni's palsy" in honor of the man who, in 1919, correctly labeled the disease as "acute infectious polyneuritis cerebralis acusticofacialis."

Obtaining an accurate medical history and performing a complete physical examination can often yield sufficient information to provide the diagnosis or suggest which diagnostic tests are needed. However, complacency and reassurance alone are to be condemned.

## CLASSIFICATION

Successful diagnosis necessitates a valid classification system. We suggest a pathologic classification (Table 1) because recent use of gadolinium-DPTA–enhanced magnetic resonance scanning demonstrates brain stem involvement in viral facial paralysis and because the distinction between central and peripheral lesions is not well defined. For clarification, when there is sparing of forehead function, inequality of the voluntary and emotional facial muscle motion, ipsilateral motor weakness of the arm or leg, dysarthria, or confusion, a "central" lesion is indicated. Viral facial paralysis, which accounts for 90 to 95% of all cases, is considered "peripheral," although there often is inflammation from the brain stem to the stylomastoid foramen.

Consideration of the onset of paralysis as acute and progressive is mandatory. Acute cases include patients with paralysis reaching maximum severity within 2 weeks of onset. These cases include patients with

TABLE 1. **Proposed Pathologic Classification of Facial Paralysis in Order of Frequency***

| Acute Paralysis† | Progressive or Chronic Paralysis‡ |
|---|---|
| Polyneuritis | Malignancies |
|   Bell's palsy |   Primary parotid and |
|     (probably herpes simplex) |     adnexa |
|   Herpes zoster |     Adenocystic |
|   Guillain-Barré syndrome |     Acinic cell |
|   Idiopathic autoimmune |     Squamous cell |
|     disease |     High-grade |
|   Lyme disease |       mucoepidermoid |
| Trauma |     Undifferentiated |
|   Skull fracture or concussion |     Malignant mixed tumor |
|   Surgery |   Metastatic |
|   Facial and penetrating |     Breast |
|     injury |     Lungs |
|   Birth trauma |     Kidney |
| Otitis media |     Colon |
|   Acute bacterial |     Skin |
|   Chronic |   Congenital |
|     Bacterial |   Benign tumors |
|     Cholesteatoma |     Schwannoma |
| Sarcoidosis |     Neurofibroma |
| Cerebrovascular accident |     Hemangioma |
| Neurologic disorders |     Glomus tumor |
| |     Cholesteatoma |

*From Adour KK, Hilsinger RL Jr, and Callan EJ: Am J Otol, 7[suppl], 68–73, 1985.
†Cases usually sudden in onset, reaching maximum severity within 2 weeks.
‡Cases increasing in severity after 2 weeks or persisting as flaccid paralysis beyond 4 months.

Guillain-Barré syndrome or newly recognized Lyme disease and exclude neurologic disorders, such as multiple sclerosis and amyotrophic lateral sclerosis. Progressive facial paralysis can occur over weeks, months, or years in patients who, if they do show recovery, never recover completely. These progressive cases challenge our diagnostic acumen and justify extensive evaluation.

## CRANIAL POLYNEURITIS

Cases of cranial polyneuritis of herpes simplex (Antoni's palsy) are similar in history, natural course, and outcome. The onset of paralysis is often preceded by a viral syndrome. The symptoms and signs during the early phase of facial paralysis include facial numbness, epiphora, pain, dysgeusia (aberrant taste), hyperacusis (dysacusis), and decreased tearing (Table 2). The facial

TABLE 2. **Frequency of Early Symptoms and Signs of Bell's Palsy***

| Symptom or Sign | Percent (n = 446) |
|---|---|
| Epiphora | 68 |
| Pain | 62 |
| Facial numbness | 60 |
| Dysgeusia | 57 |
| Hyperacusis | 29 |
| Decreased tearing, Schirmer's test | 17 |
| Decreased tearing, subjective | 15 |

*From Adour KK, Hilsinger RL Jr, and Callan EJ: Am J Otol 7[suppl], 68–73, 1985.

numbness is diagnostic for trigeminal nerve involvement because no somatic sensory fibers have been found in the facial nerve. The pain is usually retroauricular, indicating inflammation of the second or third cervical nerve, but can and does radiate into the face (cranial V) or into the neck and arm (cervical 4, 5, and 6). Dysgeusia suggests dysfunction of the geniculate ganglion, which contains the cell bodies of the chorda tympani nerve and is probably the site of reactivation of the herpes simplex virus. These symptoms are usually unilateral but can be contralateral. The hyperacusis is better labeled as dysacusis because it reflects intolerance to noise and not more acute hearing. Dysacusis is not related to stapedial muscle paralysis but probably represents loss of inhibition to the cochlea. After evaluating more than 4000 patients with all forms of facial paralysis, we have concluded statistically that the presence of dysgeusia or dysacusis in a patient with acute facial paralysis is sufficient for a definitive diagnosis of cranial polyneuritis.

Physical findings can include inflammation of the fungiform and circumvallate papilla of the tongue and hypesthesia of cranial V and IX and of cervical 2. Motor paralysis of branches of the vagus nerve are seen as unilateral shift of the palate or shortening of one vocal cord with rotation of the posterior larynx to the affected side.

Thus, Antoni's palsy (Bell's palsy) can be diagnosed when facial paralysis is peripheral in origin, systemic disease is not evident, the history is of acute onset, and concomitant sensory cranial polyneuritis is evident. No further diagnostic tests are needed. The diagnosis must not be made when symptoms have been slowly progressive or when there is evidence of "central" cerebral vascular accident.

Because Antoni's palsy occurs 4.5 times more frequently in diabetics than in nondiabetics, tests for fasting glucose level should be considered in all patients more than 40 years of age and in patients with recurrent Antoni's palsy. The disease is expressed as viral sensory polyganglionitis with secondary autoimmune demyelination, and the motor nerves are affected as they traverse the affected sensory ganglions.

Cranial polyneuritis of herpes zoster with facial paralysis (herpes zoster oticus, Ramsay Hunt syndrome) is differentiated from the herpes zoster simplex form (Antoni's palsy) by increased severity of symptoms, presence of auricular vesicles, and a rising titer of antibody to varicella-zoster virus. There is a "zoster-like form" of Antoni's palsy without auricular vesicles or rising titers of antibody to varicella-zoster virus. Patients with either form of this syndrome have a higher risk of nerve degeneration.

## TREATMENT OF CRANIAL POLYNEURITIS

Discussing diagnosis and prognosis is essential to treatment. The more the physician knows about the pathophysiology, natural course, and eventual prognosis, the better the treatment will be.

Protection of the eye is paramount. Dark glasses should be worn during the day, artificial tears instilled at the slightest evidence of drying, and a bland eye ointment (i.e., Lacri-Lube S.O.P.) used during sleep. Taping the eye is not recommended.

Corticosteroids remain the best treatment for viral inflammatory autoimmune disease. Prednisone (Deltasone) relieves the pain of Antoni's palsy so dramatically that analgesics are not necessary. Because the disease can progress from a mild, incomplete paresis to a severe, complete paralysis we recommend that *all* patients be started on treatment. There is no way to predict which patients will progress to the severe form. If treatment is delayed until the severity is determined, irreversible nerve damage may occur. We treat our patients with both prednisone and acyclovir (Zovirax) and tailor the treatment to the degree of severity. For adults, a daily total of 1 mg per kg body weight of prednisone, taken in divided doses in the morning and evening, is suggested for both Antoni's palsy and Ramsay Hunt syndrome. Acyclovir, 200 to 400 mg orally five times per day, is given for Antoni's palsy. Because absorption of acyclovir from the gut is poor, the dose should be increased to 800 mg five times per day for Ramsay Hunt syndrome; one should even consider intravenous treatment.

The patient should be seen on the fifth or sixth day after onset of paralysis. If paralysis is incomplete, the prednisone can be tapered to zero during the next 5 days and the acyclovir discontinued. If any question arises about the severity or the progression of severity, the full dose of prednisone and acyclovir should be continued for a total of 10 days and the prednisone tapered to zero during the next 5 days.

Electrotherapy is of no benefit and may be harmful. Experimental research has shown that electrical stimulation of denervated muscle retards ingrowth of neurofibrils to the motor endplates.

Predicting prognosis is an integral part of therapy. Any practitioner who elects to evaluate patients with facial paralysis should have electrical tests available. Percutaneous nerve excitability tests are simple, reproducible, and reliable prognostic indicators. Elaborate electrical tests, such as electroneurography, evoked electromyography, and strength-duration curves, are used by those who perform facial nerve decompression for viral facial paralysis.

### Surgery

Surgical facial nerve decompression is unnecessary and harmful in treating viral autoimmune neuritis and facial paralysis attributable to acute otitis media. Facial nerve exploration may be necessary in traumatic facial paralysis and mandatory in chronic otitis media with cholesteotoma.

# PARKINSON'S DISEASE

method of
ROGER KURLAN, M.D., and
IRA SHOULSON, M.D.
*University of Rochester School of Medicine and
    Dentistry
Rochester, New York*

## DIAGNOSIS

"Shaking palsy," later called *idiopathic Parkinson's disease* (PD), was described by James Parkinson in 1817 and is characterized neuropathologically by loss of pigmented neurons in the substantia nigra and accumulation of cytoskeletal deposits or Lewy bodies. The characteristic clinical features of PD include tremor, rigidity, bradykinesia, and postural instability. This constellation of clinical signs is referred to as "parkinsonism" or the "parkinsonian syndrome." Idiopathic PD is one of a variety of disorders (Table 1) associated with parkinsonism; they may have differing treatments and prognoses. Thus, diagnostic considerations are important prior to undertaking drug therapy.

There is a large group of disorders, often referred to collectively as *atypical parkinsonism*, that may have clinical features virtually indistinguishable from the idiopathic disorder. Metabolic disorders, drugs, encephalitis, and a variety of degenerative conditions may induce parkinsonism (Table 1). Atypical parkinsonian syndromes may require interventions other than antiparkinsonian drugs. For example, drug-induced parkinsonism predictably improves or resolves following withdrawal of the offending agent.

Certain clinical clues may be helpful in distinguishing patients who have atypical parkinsonism from those with the idiopathic disorder. Atypical parkinsonism is often associated with symmetrical motor involvement; tremor may be minimal or absent; and there may be additional neurologic signs not usually associated with idiopathic PD, including prominent autonomic dysfunction (e.g., orthostatic hypotension, urinary incontinence or retention, impotence), oculomotor abnormalities, early speech and swallowing difficulties, cerebellar signs, and dementia. The idiopathic type of PD tends to have asymmetrical involvement of motor signs, affecting one side of the body more than the other particularly early in its course; resting tremor; "lead-pipe" rigidity; and a more predictably favorable response to antiparkinsonian medications. Because hereditary factors do not appear to be central to the pathogenesis of idiopathic PD, the presence of a family history of parkinsonism would suggest one of the atypical parkinsonian syndromes. Most importantly, a failure to respond to antiparkinsonian medications should raise the possibility of an atypical parkinsonian variant.

*Akinetic-rigid syndromes* are generally associated with paratonic (or unpredictable) rigidity, apraxia of gait that may appear short-stepped and shuffling (rather than truly bradykinetic), and postural (rather than resting) or absent tremor. Because this constellation of neurologic signs may be mistaken for the truly rigid, slow, and tremulous features of parkinsonism, akinetic-rigid syndromes are also referred to as "pseudoparkinsonism." These disorders are often due to bihemispheric cortical dysfunction rather than nigral degeneration. Akinetic-rigid syndromes rarely respond favorably to antiparkinsonian medications.

Thus, distinguishing between conditions most appropriately treated with antiparkinsonian medications (idiopathic PD and certain forms of atypical parkinsonism) and those requiring other therapeutic interventions (reversible causes of parkinsonism or pseudoparkinsonism) is a necessary diagnostic prelude to treatment. In practice, however, therapeutic trials of antiparkinsonian medications are often required to clarify diagnosis.

## INFORMING THE PATIENT WITH PARKINSON'S DISEASE

It is helpful to review the clinical features, course, and pathogenesis of PD in accordance with individual's education and preconceptions. It is usually desirable that one or more family members receive information regarding the status of the patient and be instructed in the administration of medications. Currently available medications for PD should be discussed, including efficacy and adverse effects in the context of anticipated advances in pharmacotherapy. The variability of illness and response to treatment makes it difficult to be precise in providing prognostic information. Some pa-

TABLE 1. **Differential Diagnosis of Parkinsonism**

I. Idiopathic Parkinson's disease
II. Atypical parkinsonian syndromes
   A. Drug-induced
   B. Postencephalitic
   C. Metabolic
      1. Wilson's disease
      2. Hypoparathyroidism, pseudohypoparathyroidism
      3. Basal ganglia calcification (Fahr's syndrome)
   D. Degenerative
      1. Early onset Huntington's disease
      2. Progressive supranuclear palsy
         (Steele-Richardson-Olszewski)
      3. Multiple system atrophies
         a. With autonomic failure (Shy-Drager syndrome)
         b. Olivopontocerebellar degeneration
         c. Striatonigral degeneration
         d. Corticobasalganglionic degeneration
      4. Hallervorden-Spatz disease
III. Akinetic-rigid (pseudoparkinsonian) syndromes
   A. Alzheimer's disease
   B. Multiple cerebral infarctions
   C. Normal pressure hydrocephalus
   D. Brain tumor
   E. Post-traumatic
   F. Posthypoxic

tients are able to maintain an active independent life for decades, while others experience a more malignant course of illness. Patients are encouraged to remain active and maintain a regular but realistic exercise schedule for as long as possible.

Parkinson's disease associations sponsor a variety of educational programs and newsletters regarding medications, exercise, diet, and research. Support groups may be helpful in ameliorating the isolation of the patient and caregiver.

## PHARMACOTHERAPY

### Levodopa

Degeneration of dopaminergic neurons in the nigrostriatal pathway, arising in the substantia nigra of the midbrain and terminating rostrally in the putamen and caudate, results in the dopamine deficiency state that is the neurochemical hallmark of Parkinson's disease. Administration of levodopa (Larodopa), the immediate precursor of dopamine, represents rational "replacement" therapy for this neurodegenerative disorder. Levodopa is absorbed in the small intestine and crosses the blood-brain barrier by a facilitated active transport mechanism for amino acids. In the brain, levodopa is presumably taken up by nigrostriatal neurons and decarboxylated to form dopamine, which is the active transmitter at the nigrostriatal synapse.

Although nausea and vomiting may accompany plain levodopa therapy, these side effects can be virtually eliminated by the co-administration of levodopa with a peripheral decarboxylase inhibitor such as carbidopa (Sinemet). Because carbidopa does not cross the blood-brain barrier, the conversion of levodopa to dopamine is prevented in the periphery. When combined with carbidopa, levodopa can be used in lower doses; less dopamine is formed systemically, thereby diminishing many side effects; and more dopamine enters the brain to produce the desired antiparkinsonian effects.

Prior to the availability of levodopa, the expected duration from diagnosis of PD to death was less than 10 years. With the advent of levodopa and other dopaminergic therapies, survival of patients with PD approaches normal age-adjusted life expectancy. Levodopa has had a remarkably favorable impact on the illness of PD, including reduced mortality, lessened morbidity, and an improved quality of life.

Unfortunately, several limitations of levodopa therapy have become evident since its introduction in the late 1960s. Neurologic disability gradually worsens despite levodopa therapy, and the beneficial response to the drug is lost steadily over several years. Although levodopa represents effective symptomatic therapy, this intervention has not been demonstrated to favorably influence the progressive degeneration of nigral neurons. In addition, levodopa therapy is accompanied by a variety of acute and chronic adverse effects, including cardiovascular (orthostatic hypotension, cardiac arrhythmias), gastrointestinal (nausea, vomiting, anorexia), mental (hallucinations, illusions, paranoia, delirium), involuntary movements (dyskinesias), and fluctuations in motor performance (see later discussion).

There are general guidelines for levodopa treatment that appear useful in prolonging efficacy and minimizing adverse effects. Most clinicians withhold levodopa until significant functional impairment appears, often initiating treatment with adjunctive parkinsonian medications (see later). Carbidopa/levodopa (Sinemet) is available in three dosage formulations: 10/100, 25/100, and 25/250. The numerator indicates the amount of carbidopa in each tablet, and the denominator indicates the amount of levodopa. Levodopa is prescribed initially in the 25/100 carbidopa/levodopa (Sinemet) formulation because it usually causes fewer adverse gastrointestinal side effects than levodopa alone or formulations containing a smaller proportion of carbidopa. Sinemet 25/100 is started at very low dosage (e.g., one-half tablet) and increased gradually but steadily according to a written schedule (Table 2). Doses may be taken with meals to minimize nausea. Dosage titration schedules need to be individualized for each patient. For example, a patient with associated dementia may require more gradual dosage increments and a lower maximal dosage to minimize the risk of adverse mental effects. Virtually all patients are able to tolerate initiation of carbidopa/levodopa therapy using this "start low, go slow" approach.

Close clinical monitoring is an important aspect of carbidopa/levodopa initiation. The patient is instructed to call to provide a progress report in 7 to 10 days or earlier if problems arise. Further adjustments in the levodopa dosing schedule may be required. For example, individual doses may need to be reduced if bothersome dyskinesias or hallucinations appear.

The goal of therapy is to achieve the lowest carbidopa/levodopa dosage that is sufficient for

TABLE 2. **Example of Initiation Schedule with Carbidopa/Levodopa 25/100 (Sinemet) Tablets**

| Days | Breakfast | Lunch | Dinner | Bedtime |
|------|-----------|-------|--------|---------|
| 1–4 | None | None | ½ | None |
| 5–8 | ½ | None | ½ | None |
| 9–12 | ½ | ½ | ½ | None |
| 13–16 | 1 | ½ | ½ | ½ |
| 17–20 | 1 | ½ | 1 | ½ |
| 21 on | 1 | 1 | 1 | 1 |

alleviating functional impairment. The patient's ability to perform daily activities, such as working, arising from bed or chair, walking, dressing, and eating, serves as the primary end point for dosage adjustments. In practice, these functional capacities generally reflect the intensity of bradykinesia, rigidity, and imbalance. More conspicuous parkinsonian signs, such as a tremor, are generally less helpful in gauging the adequacy of treatment. Tremor may be very resistant to dopaminergic therapy.

### Anticholinergics

Anticholinergic drugs, such as trihexyphenidyl (Artane) and benztropine mesylate (Cogentin), have been used in an attempt to rectify the imbalance between reduced dopaminergic and relatively heightened cholinergic neurotransmission of PD. However, treatment with anticholinergics is attended by a variety of adverse effects (e.g., constipation, visual blurring, urinary retention, dry mouth, and altered mentation) that may be particularly disturbing to elderly patients. Anticholinergic-induced memory impairment, confusion, hallucinations, and personality change may produce features of dementia. Subtle adverse effects on mentation may be appreciated only after withdrawal of the drug. Anticholinergics appear most helpful early in the course of illness, particularly for younger patients with prominent resting tremor. Anticholinergic medications are initiated at low dosages with gradual increments (usually two to three doses per day) in order to achieve the lowest effective dosage. Although several anticholinergic medications are available, ethopropazine (Parsidol) has a particularly wide dosage range and therefore can be titrated with relative ease.

### Amantadine

Amantadine (Symmetrel) enhances release of presynaptic dopamine, produces anticholinergic effects, and stimulates dopamine receptors. Amantadine may be useful as initial treatment (prior to levodopa), especially in mildly affected and younger patients; and in combination with levodopa in patients with early motor fluctuations, particularly end-of-dose deterioration. Some patients with prominent imbalance (retropulsion and propulsion) and an occasional patient with atypical parkinsonism may respond to amantadine. The drug should be initiated in low dosages, with gradual increments to achieve the lowest effective dosage. Initiation of treatment with the syrup formulation (50 mg per 5 ml) may help avoid adverse effects and optimize dosage

titration. Once an individual dosage of 100 mg is achieved, the capsule formulation can be substituted. A total daily dosage of 200 mg per day (divided into two doses) is generally not to be exceeded. Common adverse effects include confusion, hallucinations, dry mouth, livedo reticularis, and peripheral edema. Because amantadine is largely metabolized by renal excretion, caution should be taken in administering this drug to patients with impaired renal function, including those taking diuretics and prone to prerenal azotemia.

### Dopamine Receptor Agonists

Bromocriptine (Parlodel) and pergolide (Permax) are the directly acting dopamine receptor agonists that are currently marketed in the United States. Dopamine agonists possess several theoretical advantages over levodopa. Because they directly stimulate postsynaptic dopamine receptors, their action should not be dependent on the integrity of degenerating presynaptic dopaminergic neurons. In addition, they have the potential for exerting more potent and long-lasting effects than levodopa, and agonists directed toward specific dopamine receptor subtypes (e.g., $D_1$ and $D_2$) might theoretically produce more specific therapeutic effects and minimize untoward effects related to generalized dopaminergic activation. Despite these theoretical advantages, dopamine agonists are relatively ineffective when administered alone and most useful when given as adjunctive therapy to levodopa. Only a minority of patients have been able to tolerate high daily dosages on a long-term basis. Adverse effects include orthostatic hypotension, nausea, vomiting, hallucinations, and involuntary movements. Beneficial effects may be short lived, possibly related to dopamine receptor down-regulation. Some of these problems have been obviated by the use of low dosages of dopamine agonists (see later). The agonist drugs are most helpful for patients experiencing a declining response to levodopa, those with motor fluctuations, and the occasional patient with atypical parkinsonism. Some studies suggest that adding low doses of bromocriptine or pergolide to levodopa in the early phases of PD (early combination treatment) may forestall the appearance of dyskinesias and motor fluctuations.

Dopamine receptor agonists are initiated at low dosages with gradual increments, and adverse effects may be avoided by low maintenance dosages (5 to 20 mg per day for bromocriptine and 0.75 to 3.0 mg per day for pergolide). Bromocriptine is administered three or four times daily,

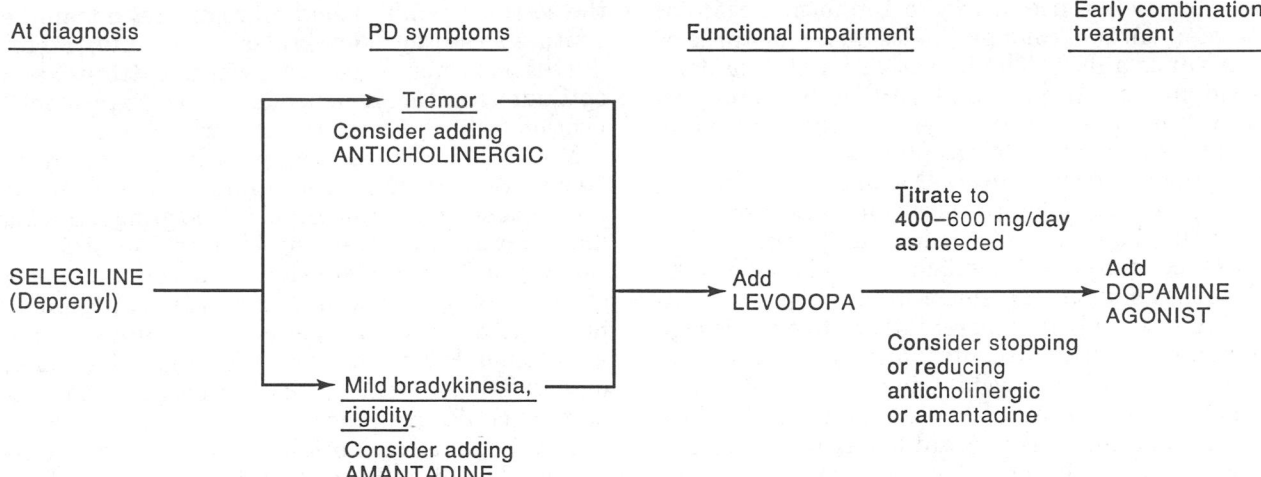

**Figure 1.** Therapeutic considerations in early Parkinson's disease (PD).

whereas pergolide is usually given in two or three daily doses.

### Selegiline (Deprenyl; Eldepryl)

Selegiline (Deprenyl) is a relatively selective type-B monoamine oxidase (MAO) inhibitor that retards the breakdown of dopamine without risking the adverse pressor reactions that might occur when administering levodopa in combination with nonselective or type A MAO inhibitors. Selegiline prolongs the duration of action of levodopa and allows a reduction in levodopa dosage by 10 to 25%. This effect may be particularly helpful in patients with motor fluctuations, particularly end-of-dose deterioration. Recent controlled clinical trials indicate that when used in the earliest stages of illness, selegiline therapy slows functional decline and extends the time until levodopa is required. This beneficial effect of selegiline may in part be related to inhibition of oxidative processes that predispose patients to neuronal dysfunction and death.

The usual dosage of selegiline is 5 mg twice a day but a lower dosage (2.5 to 5.0 mg per day) may be as effective; dosages greater than 10 mg per day afford no additional benefit and may be attended by risks of adverse pressor effects. Elderly patients and those suffering levodopa-induced dyskinesias may better tolerate initiation of selegiline therapy with a single morning dose of 2.5 mg (one-half tablet) or 5 mg. Levodopa dosage reduction may be required prior to achieving a full dosage of selegiline. Accentuation of dyskinesias, nausea, dizziness, orthostatic hypotension, and insomnia due to heightened dopaminergic activity are the most frequently encountered side effects of selegiline therapy.

### CARE PROBLEMS

#### Choice of Pharmacologic Treatment (Figure 1)

Most clinicians withhold levodopa therapy until significant functional impairment appears. Based on the observed benefit of selegiline in early PD, consideration should be given to initiating this drug at the time of diagnosis. Some patients may experience a mild improvement of symptoms with selegiline alone, and monotherapy with this drug may be adequate for months or years. For younger patients with prominent tremor, addition of an anticholinergic should be considered. Mild bradykinesia, rigidity, and postural imbalance may respond well to amantadine therapy. When indicated, levodopa/carbidopa (Sinemet) is initiated at very low dosages and increased gradually but steadily in order to achieve the lowest dosage that is effective in alleviating functional impairment. Generally a maintenance dosage of the 25/100 formulation, one tablet three or four times daily, will prove satisfactory for patients with early disease. The dosage may be increased as functional disability dictates. Once a daily dosage of about 600 mg of levodopa (1½ tablets four times a day) has been achieved, dopamine receptor agonists may be added and adjusted in response to disability.

#### Adverse Effects of Drug Treatment

**Nausea.** Anorexia, nausea, and vomiting are infrequent when a decarboxylase inhibitor is used in combination with levodopa (i.e., as Sinemet). However, gastrointestinal side effects may still be a problem for some patients.

Nausea can be minimized by slow initiation of carbidopa/levodopa therapy, administration with or after meals, use of the 25/100 formulation, or supplemental carbidopa (Lodosyn, 25 mg three or four times a day). The investigational drug domperidone, a peripheral dopamine receptor ($D_2$ type) antagonist, may lessen nausea induced by levodopa or dopamine receptor agonists.

**Psychiatric Disturbances.** Dopaminergic therapy may be associated with confusion, hallucinations, illusions, delirium, agitation, and paranoia. The presence of dementia, which occurs in about 30% of patients with PD, seems to predispose an individual to adverse psychiatric effects. Dosage reduction or drug discontinuation (see later) may be required when psychiatric symptoms develop. Neuroleptic therapy should be avoided, since these dopamine receptor antagonists may worsen parkinsonism. In patients on a combination of antiparkinsonian drugs, consideration should be given to sequential systematic discontinuation of medications. However, the benefit of such changes must be balanced against the problem of increasing immobility.

Depression occurs in about 40% of patients with PD and may have a profound influence on functional abilities. Most depressed PD patients respond favorably to tricyclic antidepressant medications. The anticholinergic properties of some antidepressants may benefit parkinsonian features; however, cumulative anticholinergic central toxicity may develop when tricyclic antidepressants are added to existing anticholinergic agents, especially in the elderly patient with cognitive impairment. Antidepressants can also exacerbate hypotension or hypertension. Nonspecific monoamine oxidase inhibitors are contraindicated in patients receiving levodopa because profound adverse pressor effects may develop from increased catecholamines.

**Dyskinesias.** Drug-induced involuntary movements (dyskinesias) typically take the form of chorea, choreoathetosis, or dystonia; usually reflect high plasma levels of levodopa; and may be lessened following levodopa dosage reduction. When dosage reduction of levodopa is accompanied by unacceptable immobility, some patients will respond to the addition of or an increase of a dopamine agonist.

**Motor Fluctuations.** Initially, levodopa produces a smooth antiparkinsonian effect in most patients. Fluctuations in motor performance, between periods of satisfactory mobility usually accompanied by dyskinesias ("on" time) and periods of parkinsonian immobility ("off" time), are one of the most troublesome long-term problems associated with levodopa therapy. The majority of patients will develop some form of motor fluctuations within 5 years of beginning levodopa therapy. Such on-off phenomena are in part related to fluctuating plasma levels of levodopa in the setting of diminished nigrostriatal dopamine synthesis, storage, and release capacity. Motor fluctuations may occur in several patterns, and optimum treatment depends on accurate identification of the particular pattern (Table 3).

Motor fluctuations that parallel plasma dopa levels are most amenable to adjustments in the levodopa dosing regimen. Early morning akinesia may improve by advancing levodopa administration 30 to 60 minutes prior to the planned time of awakening, or the use of longer acting dopaminergic agents (e.g., pergolide or amantadine) at bedtime. Peak-dose dyskinesia and end-of-dose deterioration ("wearing off") often occur in tandem. Such fluctuations can be lessened by reducing individual doses or shortening dosage intervals while maintaining about the same total daily dosage of levodopa (e.g., Sinemet 25/250 at 9 a.m., 1 p.m., 5 p.m., 11 p.m. can be modified to 25/100, 1½ tablets every 3 hours, 7 a.m. to 10 p.m.). It is important to note the times that the patient takes medication in relation to the times when motor fluctuations develop. An hourly diary of the patient's motor function recorded for several days may be helpful. Random or unpredictable fluctuations in motor performance ("yo-yoing"), transient freezing episodes, and start-hesitation do not closely parallel plasma dopa levels and are less responsive to adjustments in levodopa dosing schedules. Transient freezing, a common cause of falls in Parkinson's disease, sometimes improves following levodopa dosage reduction.

Modest improvement in motor fluctuations may be achieved for some patients with the use of a "low-protein" diet, whereby the patient ingests no more than 7 grams of protein *before* the evening meal and can have free protein intake at supper and through the rest of the day. Compliance with this diet is very difficult, and some patients develop severe and prolonged off periods after supper.

TABLE 3. **Common Patterns of Motor Fluctuations**

I. Closely related to plasma dopa levels
  A. Early morning akinesia—parkinsonian immobility on arising due to long duration since bedtime levodopa dose and resultant low plasma dopa level
  B. End-of-dose deterioration ("wearing off")—declining mobility at end of levodopa dosing interval reflecting declining plasma dopa level
  C. Peak-dose dyskinesia—involuntary movements occurring usually 30–60 min after levodopa and reflecting high plasma dopa level
II. Poorly related to plasma dopa levels
  A. Transient freezing—sudden appearance of short-stepped gait or inability to walk
  B. Start-hesitation—inability to initiate walking
  C. Random oscillations—on-off fluctuations unrelated to timing of levodopa doses

**Loss of Efficacy.** Although most patients with PD benefit initially from levodopa therapy, declining efficacy is typically observed after a few years of treatment. Loss of response has been ascribed to progressive degeneration of dopaminergic nigral neurons, but alterations in levodopa pharmacokinetics and dopamine receptors (pharmacodynamics) may be contributing factors. Transient discontinuation of levodopa in a supervised setting ("drug holiday") is based on a pharmacologic strategy designed to restore dopamine receptor sensitivity. A drug holiday carries definite risks of medical complications, and evaluations of its efficacy have yielded mixed results. In our hands, levodopa drug holiday appears to be most beneficial for patients who experience both otherwise unremediable loss of response to levodopa and unacceptable levodopa-induced side effects, such as excessive dyskinesias or hallucinations. A complete discontinuation of levodopa should be carried out in hospitalized patients by a physician experienced with this procedure. Some patients will develop autonomic instability (tachycardia, fever, excessive perspiration) during the first few days of drug holiday. We observe the patient closely off of antiparkinsonian drugs until the nadir of parkinsonian immobility is reached, usually within 4 to 7 days. Intensive support is provided, including physical therapy for range of motion exercises, respiratory therapy (incentive spirometry, chest percussion, and postural drainage), and measures to prevent venous thrombosis (subcutaneous low-dose heparin, elastic stockings, foot board) and aspiration pneumonia (soft or puréed diet or nasogastric feedings). Respiratory and swallowing functions are monitored closely, and drug holiday is aborted if significant respiratory dysfunction supervenes. Once the nadir of parkinsonian immobility is reached, levodopa therapy is reinstituted using the "start low, go slow" method. Following drug holiday, patients usually require a lower daily dosage of levodopa (50 to 75%) in comparison with their dosage prior to withdrawal of antiparkinsonian medications. With the wider variety of antiparkinsonian agents, including selegiline and dopamine receptor agonists, the need for levodopa drug holidays may be declining.

### Associated and Intercurrent Problems

Several problems that may arise during the course of PD are amenable to specific treatments (Table 4). Seborrheic dermatitis can be treated with selenium sulfide (Selsun) shampoo one to three times per week or fluocinolone (Synalar) solution. Orthostatic hypotension (disease-related or drug-induced) may improve with me-

**TABLE 4.** **Associated or Intercurrent Problems with Parkinson's Disease**

I. Cutaneous—seborrhea, edema
II. Autonomic—orthostatic hypotension
III. Genitourinary—impotence, incontinence
IV. Gastrointestinal—constipation, ileus, dysphagia, sialorrhea
V. Visual—diplopia, accommodation disturbance
VI. Pulmonary—aspiration
VII. Trauma—fractures, nerve compression
VIII. Neuropsychiatric—depression, panic/anxiety, personality change, dementia

chanical measures including elevation of the bed to about 30 degrees and the use of thigh-length elastic stockings. The addition of sodium chloride supplementation (1 to 3 grams per day) and fludrocortisone (Florinef), 0.1 to 1.0 mg per day in two to four divided doses, will usually restore blood pressure and alleviate symptoms if mechanical maneuvers alone fail. Constipation will usually improve following an increase in daily fluid intake (to 2 to 3 liters per day), the addition of bulk-forming agents (e.g., psyllium hydrophilic mucilloid [Metamucil]), and/or stool softeners (e.g., docusate sodium [Colace]). Methscopolamine (Pamine), 2.5 mg two to four times daily, may be helpful for troublesome sialorrhea. Urinary frequency, hesitation, or retention may require urologic examination (such as cystometrics) and specific uropharmacologic therapy (e.g., oxybutynin hydrochloride [Ditropan]).

### FUTURE DIRECTIONS IN THERAPY

Because parkinsonian motor fluctuations are closely related to fluctuating levels of plasma levodopa, research efforts are being directed toward measures to produce more steady and sustained central dopaminergic stimulation. Studies of sustained-release oral and parenteral preparations of levodopa are in progress. Furthermore, continuous and prolonged delivery of levodopa via mechanical infusion pumps utilizing both peripheral (intravenous, intraduodenal) and central (intrathecal, intraventricular) routes is under investigation. Some patients have responded to continuous subcutaneous delivery of the experimental dopamine receptor agonist lisuride. A variety of other dopamine agonists are under study as drugs that may provide better therapeutic indices. Surgical implantation or transplantation of catecholamine generating tissue (such as adrenal medulla and fetal cells) into the striatum of advanced PD patients is an approach that has proved disappointing in pilot studies. However, implantation techniques may eventually prove effective. As new insights are gained into the mechanisms of neuronal degeneration, preventive strategies aimed at forestalling nerve cell loss will likely take on increasing importance.

# PERIPHERAL NEUROPATHIES

method of
E. PETER BOSCH, M.D.
*University of Iowa College of Medicine*
*Iowa City, Iowa*

A stepwise systematic approach consisting of careful history taking, physical examination, and nerve conduction studies not only confirms the presence of a neuropathy but also limits the large number of possible etiologies. A wide range of potential causes are to be considered in polyneuropathies, including inherited disorders, diabetes, and other systemic diseases; inflammatory demyelinating conditions; plasma cell dyscrasias; malignancy; alcohol and nutritional deficiencies; drugs; heavy metals and industrial agents; infections; connective tissue diseases; and vasculitis. Electrodiagnostic studies play a key role in the evaluation by confirming the diagnosis of neuropathy, providing precise localization of focal nerve entrapments, and giving clues as to the nature of the underlying nerve pathology. Response to therapy and potential for recovery depend in part on the primary pathologic process involving the peripheral nerves.

In axonal neuropathies, which comprise the majority of peripheral nerve disorders, axonal degeneration occurs, starting at the most distal part of the nerve fiber and gradually progressing toward the nerve cell body. In general, an axonal neuropathy presents with symmetrical, distal, graded sensory loss; distal muscle weakness with prominent atrophy; and early loss of ankle jerks. Nerve conduction velocities are only slightly affected, but the axonal loss results in reduced nerve action potential amplitudes. If the cause leading to axonal degeneration is removed, recovery may be delayed and often incomplete because axonal regeneration proceeds at a slow rate of 2 to 3 mm per day. Gangliosides and adrenocorticotropic hormone (ACTH) and several of its peptide fragments are reported to enhance axonal regeneration in experimental studies, but to date clinical trials have been largely disappointing. Administration of purified brain gangliosides (Cronassial*) failed to show any therapeutic effect in chronic neuropathies. In demyelinating neuropathies an insult to the myelin sheath and the Schwann cells or changes in axonal caliber lead to the breakdown of myelin with relative sparing of axons. Early generalized loss of reflexes, disproportionately mild muscle atrophy in the context of weakness affecting both proximal and distal limb muscles, and the presence of tremor or palpably enlarged nerve trunks are clinical clues pointing to a demyelinating process. Marked slowing of nerve conduction confirms demyelination, which is most commonly seen in immune-mediated inflammatory polyradiculoneuropathies, hereditary

---

*Not available in the United States.

neuropathies, and dysproteinemias. Recovery depends on remyelination and thus dramatic improvement may occur within weeks. The distinction between demyelinating and axonal disorders often becomes blurred on close inspection because many neuropathies produce mixed pathologic features. In neuronopathies, loss of the neuronal cell bodies occurs, with consequent degeneration of their entire axons. Collateral sprouting from adjacent surviving axons is limited, which accounts for the poor recovery in this situation.

Despite intensive investigation, the cause of about 20 to 25% of chronic neuropathies remains undetermined. When the diagnosis remains elusive or specific therapy is not available, certain general measures will help to reduce the disability of patients with peripheral nerve disorders.

## GENERAL SUPPORTIVE MEASURES

Physical therapy plays an important part in the treatment of *motor weakness* and should be started early in the course of the illness. It is helpful in preserving the range of motion of joints, preventing contractures, maintaining optimal motor function, and assisting in gait training. Foot drop is a common problem that may result in falls with subsequent injuries. Light plastic foot-ankle orthoses, which aid in dorsiflexion of the feet, often improve the patient's gait and provide mechanical support for ankle stability. When weakness of wrist extension is present, wrist extension splints may be necessary for optimal hand function. Patients should be referred for occupational therapy if their disabilities interfere with the tasks of daily living.

*Severe sensory loss* predisposes an individual to unnoticed trauma, leading to callus formation, nonhealing ulcerations complicated by secondary infections, and osteomyelitis. These complications are, to a large extent, preventable by avoiding trauma to the insensitive distal parts of the limbs. Careful attention should be paid to having well fitting shoes and meticulous care of the feet and toes. Patients should not walk barefoot and are encouraged to inspect their shoes daily for foreign bodies as well as their feet for the presence of irritated skin lesions. Dry, atrophic skin may be protected from breakdown with a moisturizing cream. If foot ulcers develop, weight bearing should cease until healing occurs.

The *management of pain* that occurs in peripheral neuropathies is discussed in the section on diabetic neuropathy but can be applied to any neuropathic pain irrespective of etiology. *Treatment of autonomic dysfunction* is also described under diabetic neuropathy because postural hypotension and other symptoms are most often associated with chronic polyneuropathies resulting from diabetes and amyloidosis.

## ACUTE INFLAMMATORY DEMYELINATING POLYRADICULONEUROPATHY OR GUILLAIN-BARRÉ SYNDROME

Guillain-Barré syndrome (GBS) is the most frequent cause of acute generalized paralysis. Although its annual incidence is only 1.8 cases per 100,000 in the United States, about one-sixth of all patients develop respiratory failure and thus GBS is among the most common neurologic causes of admission to an intensive care unit. Despite advances in intensive care, mortality remains at 3%. GBS is characterized by progressive, mostly symmetrical weakness and areflexia that may be associated with cranial nerve paralysis, autonomic instability, and respiratory failure. The maximal deficits develop within days to at most 4 weeks and after a variable plateau period begin to improve over months. About two-thirds of patients have a preceding event, such as a viral upper respiratory infection or gastrointestinal illness, immunization, or surgical procedure. GBS may follow infection with human immunodeficiency virus (HIV), either during seroconversion or as the only indication of a chronic, silent HIV infection. Therefore, GBS patients who have conceivable risk factors, suspicious laboratory results such as cerebrospinal fluid (CSF) pleocytosis or positive hepatitis B serology, or require treatment with plasmapheresis should be screened for the presence of HIV-1 antibody. Elevated CSF protein with normal cell count and abnormal nerve conduction studies consisting of focal slowing, or motor conduction block and prolongation of F wave or distal latencies confirm the diagnosis but may be nondiagnostic within the first week of the onset of symptoms. A large body of evidence supports an immunologically mediated peripheral nerve injury leading to intense inflammation and demyelination of the peripheral and cranial nerves. Peripheral nerve myelin glycolipids appear to be the targets of the immune attack, recruiting both the cellular and humoral arms of the immune system.

Most patients in whom the diagnosis of GBS is considered require hospital admission for monitoring on a well-staffed general care unit until the tempo of their individual disease progression is established. Baseline studies must include an accurate forced vital capacity (FVC) determination, chest radiograph, electrocardiogram, serum electrolytes, and chemistries. During the progressive phase it is important to closely monitor respirations, the patient's ability to cough and swallow, and cardiovascular functions. If the initial FVC is at or below 25 ml per kg in a patient whose weakness is progressing, transfer to an intensive care unit is mandatory to avoid the risk of precipitous respiratory failure. In a deteriorating patient FVC should be measured at least every 4 hours while awake and every 6 hours at night until the patient is stable. Maximal inspiratory and expiratory pressures are another useful, although less readily available, method to follow respiratory muscle weakness. Signs of impending respiratory failure include a downward trend in FVC measurements; deterioration in blood gases (i.e., hypoxemia as the result of atelectasis); and clinical signs of respiratory muscle fatigue, such as brow sweating, tachycardia, tachypnea, and paradoxical inward movements of a lax abdominal wall during inspiration. I favor early, elective endotracheal intubation and assisted ventilation when the FVC falls below 20 to 15 ml per kg. In a patient with severe oropharyngeal weakness, even earlier intubation is considered to protect the airway. Tracheostomy can usually be delayed until the end of the second week of mechanical ventilation. By waiting until the second week about one-third of patients can be extubated and spared the tracheostomy. Careful respiratory toilet, chest physical therapy, and incentive spirometry aid in preventing atelectasis in patients with impaired cough and sigh.

Autonomic dysfunction among severely afflicted patients ranges from fixed tachycardia and episodic or sustained hypertension to orthostatic hypotension, sinus bradycardia, sudden arrhythmias, and even cardiovascular collapse. Continuous electrocardiogram (ECG) and blood pressure monitoring will allow early detection of life-threatening situations that may require specific treatment. Postural hypotension is best managed by use of elastic stockings, avoidance of giving nursing care in the upright or sitting position, and judicious use of volume expansion.

*Meticulous supportive care* and the prevention of complications provide the best chance for a favorable outcome. Regular repositioning; attention to pressure areas, eyes (particularly in the presence of facial diplegia), mouth, bowel, and bladder; and nutrition are essential. Once a patient becomes bed-bound, elastic stockings and subcutaneous heparin 5000 U twice daily are used to lower the risk of venous thrombosis and pulmonary embolism. During the paralytic phase, emphasis should be placed on positioning patients to avoid nerve pressure palsies. Passive movements of all major joints twice daily and padded plastic boots aid in maintaining limb flexibility and preventing ankle contractures. Pulmonary and urinary tract infections are important potential complications, occurring in one of four patients in intensive care units. Careful respiratory toilet, care in maintaining a closed urinary drainage system, and surveillance for nosocomial infections with sputum and urine cultures may aid in their prevention. Relief of back and limb pain occurring frequently in bedridden patients is initially attempted with nonsteroidal anti-inflammatory agents, but often codeine containing analgesics, synthetic analogues of morphine, or a single dose of corticosteroids (methylprednisolone [Solu-Medrol], 20 to 40 mg intramuscularly) is necessary. Psychologic support and constant reassurance about the potential for excellent recovery are very important in patients who are paralyzed over prolonged periods. About 80% of patients make a good recovery with no or only minimal residual deficits. In the recovery phase, active physical therapy will hasten the return of useful limb function.

Until recently, *specific immune interventions* have failed to modify the natural course of GBS. Although various preparations of corticosteroids have been used with occasional, anecdotal benefit, a controlled trial of prednisolone (Delta-Cortef) in acute GBS suggested a trend toward longer hospitalization, greater residual deficits, and higher relapse rate among treated patients. Corticosteroid use is currently not recommended. Three multicenter randomized studies have shown that plasmapheresis improves the outcome in severely affected patients with GBS. In the North American trial, patients randomized to the plasma exchange arm had significantly greater improvement at 4 weeks and 6 months, spent less time on the respirator, and recovered to independent walking in less time. Beneficial results were most evident when plasmapheresis was begun early in the course (preferably within 2 weeks of onset of symptoms) and performed on continuous flow machines. Factors that predict poorer outcome, such as prolonged recovery beyond 6 months, include abnormally low amplitudes of distal compound muscle action potentials (i.e., less than 20% of normal values), older age, rapid progression of maximal deficits in less than 7 days, and the need for ventilatory support. Plasma exchange therapy should be instituted for patients with moderate to severe weakness (defined as the ability to walk only with support or worse) or rapidly deteriorating patients with poor-risk factors within the first 3 weeks of onset of symptoms. Initially, about 5 plasma exchanges are performed on an alternate-day schedule to achieve a cumulative plasma exchange of 200 to 250 ml per kg. The treatments may be extended to 10 exchanges over a 3-week period in the event of clinical worsening. Plasmapheresis should be performed only in centers with experienced blood bank and intensive care unit staff. Under these circumstances the risks of the procedure are small, but they include hypotension, cardiac arrhythmias, citrate-induced hypocalcemia, and

complications arising from the sites of venous access.

## CHRONIC INFLAMMATORY DEMYELINATING POLYRADICULONEUROPATHY

Chronic inflammatory demyelinating polyradiculoneuropathy (CIDP) is thought to be an immune-mediated peripheral nerve disorder distinguished from acute GBS by its clinical course. Typically, its onset is insidious, developing over weeks to months, and its course is one of slow or stepwise progression for longer than 2 months, or relapsing. CIDP presents as a predominant motor neuropathy leading to proximal and distal muscle weakness; generalized hypo- or areflexia; and sensory impairment of large fiber modalities with CSF protein elevation, electrodiagnostic abnormalities indicative of demyelination (i.e., slowing of motor conduction velocity below 70% of normal, or motor conduction block), and sural nerve biopsy features of demyelination and large fiber loss. The diagnosis should be considered only after systemic disorders associated with polyradiculoneuropathies have been excluded by thorough investigations. There are patients who may acquire a CIDP-like syndrome together with certain concurrent illnesses, such as monoclonal gammopathies, chronic active hepatitis, inflammatory bowel disease, hereditary motor and sensory neuropathy, and HIV infection. From a practical, therapeutic standpoint, this group of patients may respond to immunosuppressive therapy like those with the idiopathic form. Timely recognition is extremely important because CIDP represents one in five cases of initially undiagnosed, chronic polyneuropathy, and a significant proportion of these respond to immunosuppressive therapy.

Corticosteroids have become the standard of care in either relapsing or chronic CIDP of sufficient clinical severity. This is supported by the randomized controlled study of Dyck and colleagues in which prednisone (Deltasone) (starting dose 120 mg every other day with 5 mg on alternate days) used for 3 months produced moderate improvement when compared with the placebo group. In my practice, I begin corticosteroid therapy in patients with moderate to severe clinical involvement (Figure 1). Daily, single-dose prednisone (80 to 100 mg) is taken for 4 to 6 weeks. If an initial response is achieved after 4 weeks, a gradual switch to alternate-day dosing is begun by reducing the even-day dose by 10 mg every week over the next 10 weeks to 100 mg on alternate days. When major improvement has occurred, the dose is gradually tapered by 10 mg per month followed by 5-mg decrements at doses

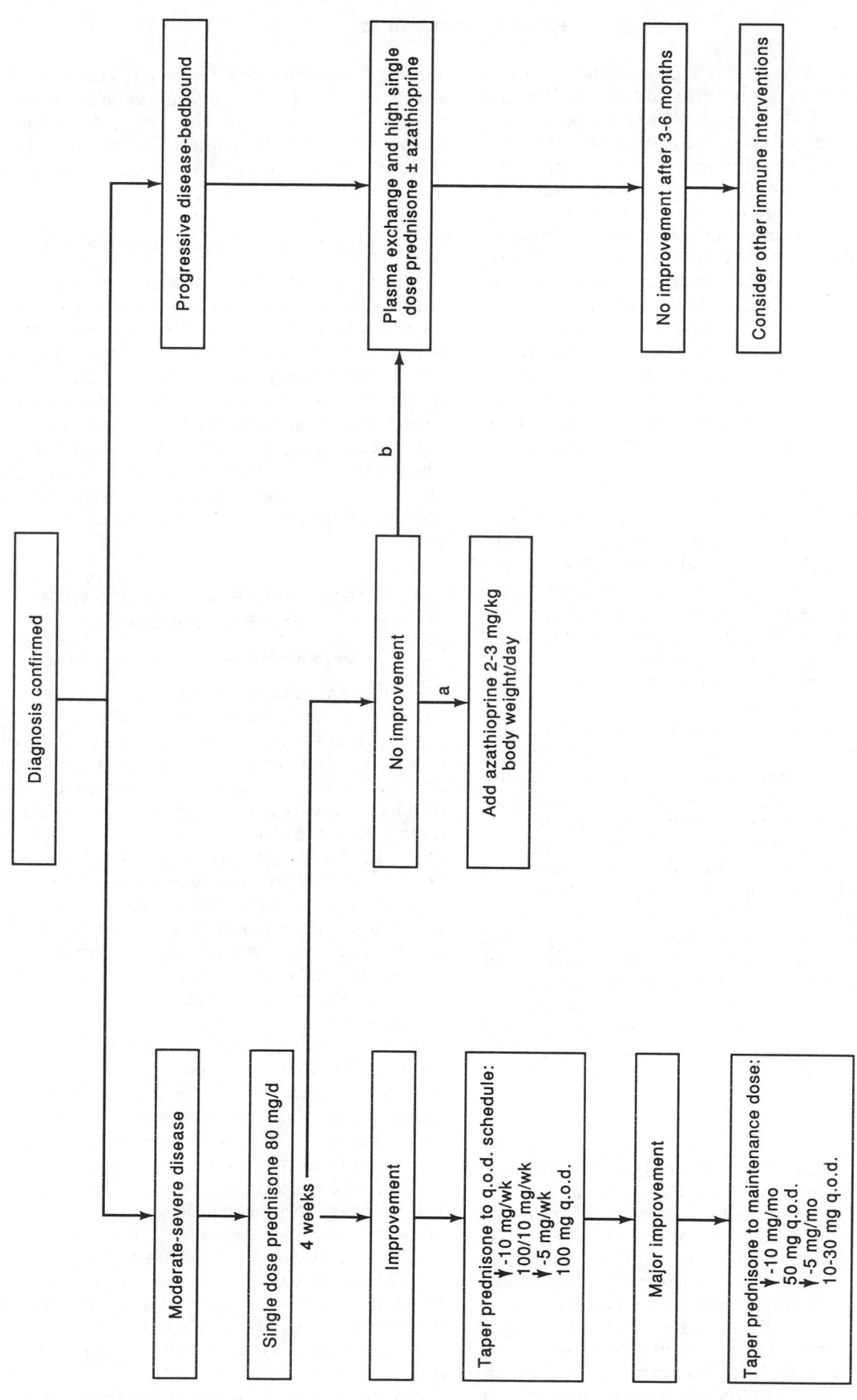

**Figure 1.** Steps in the management of chronic inflammatory demyelinating polyradiculoneuropathy (CIDP). (From Bosch EP, and Mitsumoto H: Disorders of peripheral nerves. *In* Bradley WG, Daroff RB, Fenichel GM, and Marsden CD (eds): Neurology in Clinical Practice. Stoneham, MA, Butterworth Publishers, 1990. Reprinted by permission.)

below 50 mg. The individual patient's clinical response serves as a guideline to the rapidity and completeness of the taper. Many patients continue prednisone, 10 to 30 mg, on alternate days for years to avoid recurrences. Side effects from prolonged use of prednisone are many but may be reduced by a single alternate-day dosing schedule. Precautions taken to diminish complications include a low-sodium (2 grams) and low-carbohydrate diet, $H_2$-receptor antagonists for patients with peptic ulcer diathesis, calcium supplementation, and vitamin D for elderly patients at risk for osteoporosis. Patients are followed for and informed about the potential development of cataracts, glaucoma, truncal obesity, hypertension, hyperglycemia, osteoporosis, aseptic hip necrosis, peptic ulcer disease, and susceptibility to infections.

Clinical response is assessed monthly. For patients with inadequate response to corticosteroids or those who require high prednisone maintenance doses with unacceptable side effects, azathioprine (Imuran), at 2 to 3 mg per kg per day, is added to potentiate the immunosuppressive effects. Because one in five patients may develop toxicity requiring discontinuation of therapy, the patients need careful monitoring of blood counts and liver function tests.

Plasmapheresis has been used with transient improvement and subsequently its benefit was confirmed by a randomized controlled study. Plasma exchange is usually combined with azathioprine together with prednisone at full or reduced doses for patients who fail to respond after 4 weeks of initial therapy, who continue to worsen, or who develop unacceptable side effects. In severely affected patients who are nonambulatory at the initial evaluation I initiate plasma exchange along with prednisone to achieve rapid improvement before immunosuppressive agents can take effect. The optimal schedule for exchanges has not been established; an initial series of five exchanges on alternate days is followed by two exchanges during the third week, and the subsequent intervals are dictated by the individual clinical response.

The majority of patients will show some initial improvement within 3 to 6 months of therapy. If neither prednisone in combination with azathioprine nor plasmapheresis is effective, other immune intervention may be considered; cyclophosphamide (Cytoxan, Neosar) (2 mg per kg per day) for limited periods, cyclosporine (Sandimmune), and total lymphoid irradiation have been used with benefit in such refractory patients. High-dose intravenous human gamma globulin (Gammagard, Sandoglobulin) (0.4 gram per kg for 3 to 5 consecutive days) holds promise; we and others have observed occasionally remarkable but short-lasting improvements. Some patients remain unresponsive or have residual deficits despite all efforts. To identify all the responders, immunosuppressive therapy should be continued at least 6 months before treatment is judged as ineffective and abandoned.

## MULTIFOCAL MOTOR NEUROPATHY

These patients present with progressive multifocal lower motor neuron signs masquerading as motor neuron disease. Electrophysiologic studies demonstrating multifocal motor conduction block distinguish this acquired demyelinating motor neuropathy from motor neuron disease. The majority of patients have high serum antibody titers to gangliosides. Treatment with cyclophosphamide is reported to result in substantial clinical improvement and has been correlated with a reduction of antiganglioside antibody titers.

## NEUROPATHIES ASSOCIATED WITH SYSTEMIC DISORDERS

### Diabetic Peripheral Neuropathies

Peripheral neuropathies are among the most common complications of diabetes mellitus, which, in turn, is the most frequent identifiable cause of polyneuropathies in the United States, and as such they have a considerable clinical impact. It is estimated that about 8% of diabetics have neuropathy at the time of diagnosis, increasing with the duration of diabetes to 50% after 25 years. The highly heterogeneous clinical manifestations of diabetic neuropathies are grouped into three major syndromes: symmetrical distal polyneuropathies; symmetrical proximal neuropathies; and focal, asymmetrical neuropathies. In many of these syndromes sensory, motor, and autonomic fibers are concomitantly involved. Recent experimental, clinical, epidemiologic, and electrophysiologic studies support the premise that persistent hyperglycemia with its consequent metabolic alterations contributes to the pathogenesis of diabetic neuropathy. Hyperglycemia leads to increased nerve glucose, fructose, and sorbitol concentrations by activating the polyol pathway, enhanced glycosylation of structural proteins, and reduced nerve myoinositol, all of which may have adverse effects on nerve function. Hyperglycemia also leads to reduced nerve blood flow, endoneurial hypoxia, and basement membrane thickening of vasa nervorum, which eventually results in ischemia and nerve fiber loss.

Several lines of evidence support the concept that metabolic control of hyperglycemia influences onset and ameliorates symptomatic neuropathies in diabetic patients. The frequency of overt neuropathy is related to both the duration and the degree of hyperglycemia; nerve conduction velocity is inversely correlated with glycosylated hemoglobin, and strict metabolic control improves nerve conduction and lowers sensory thresholds. Therefore, I strive for optimal glucose control and normal plasma lipids in conjunction with ideal body weight. The chosen method for glucoregulation must be tailored for each individual patient. There is still no definite evidence that strict control achieved by multiple daily insulin injections or continuous administration of insulin with a pump is superior to good conventional control. However, recurrent hypoglycemia must be avoided during intensive insulin treatment because it too may cause a motor neuropathy. The question of whether intensive insulin treatment may prevent the development or progression of overt neuropathy cannot be answered until the results of the ongoing Diabetes Control and Complications Trial are known. It is important to consider aggravating factors or agents that might contribute to the peripheral nerve damage. Patients who drink excessively are encouraged to reduce or abstain from alcohol, and those who smoke are advised to stop. There is no basis to justify the routine use of B vitamins unless there is reason to suspect a coexisting vitamin deficiency.

Recent attempts to correct abnormalities of nerve metabolism hold considerable promise for future management. Clinical trials with aldose reductase inhibitors, such as sorbinil,* which prevent the accumulation of alcohol sugars in nerve tissue, have resulted in modestly improved nerve conduction, some clinical benefit, and a burst of regenerating fibers in follow-up nerve biopsies. None of the aldose reductase inhibitors is currently approved for clinical use. Dietary supplementation of myoinositol has yielded disappointing results.

Diabetes predisposes a patient to entrapment neuropathies. Nerve conduction studies are necessary to localize coexisting single or multiple entrapment neuropathies. Diabetic mononeuropathies occur at the common sites of nerve compression, including the wrist (median nerve), the elbow (ulnar nerve), and the fibular head (common peroneal nerve). When of short duration, symptomatic entrapment neuropathy is treated in a manner similar to that for patients without polyneuropathy.

Cranial mononeuropathies, including the pupil sparing third nerve palsy, have an excellent prog-

nosis, spontaneous recovery occurring within 6 to 12 weeks. Despite severe weakness, the asymmetrical proximal motor neuropathy generally resolves to some degree within 6 to 12 months. Once pain control is achieved in these patients and their frequently associated depressive symptoms abate, we encourage them to participate in aggressive physical therapy.

The *control of pain and dysesthesias* constitutes a challenge in the management of patients with diabetic neuropathy. In some patients, striking improvement in pain occurs after control of hyperglycemia, which, by itself, is reported to modify pain perception. Analgesics, such as aspirin, acetaminophen, or nonsteroidal anti-inflammatory agents, are preferred to narcotic agents, which should be avoided because of the risk of addiction. In more than half of the patients, shooting or stabbing pains will respond to carbamazepine (Tegretol). The initial dose of 100 mg twice daily is gradually increased until pain relief or therapeutic anticonvulsant levels (4 to 8 μg per ml) are achieved. Tricyclic antidepressants (e.g., amitriptyline [Elavil, Endep], 25 to 150 mg at bedtime), alone or in combination with fluphenazine (Prolixin) (1 mg three times daily), may bring relief from constant, deep aching pain. Amitriptyline is started at a 25-mg dose at bedtime and increased slowly to avoid lethargy, and anticholinergic side effects, such as urinary retention, which are more likely to develop in patients with coexisting autonomic neuropathy. Desipramine (Norpramin), which causes urinary retention and sedation less frequently than does amitriptyline, can be substituted in patients with unacceptable side effects. Combination therapy of a tricyclic agent with fluphenazine is restricted to patients with persistent pain who fail to respond, and its use is limited to 1 to 3 months to avoid tardive dyskinesias produced by phenothiazines. Mexiletine (Mexitil), an orally active lidocaine antiarrhythmic agent (initial dose 600 mg per day, advancing to 1200 mg per day), is said to benefit some patients. Topical capsaicin cream (Axsain), which depletes substance P from nociceptive nerve endings, is reported to be effective and best suited for patients with painful focal neuropathies, such as truncal mononeuropathy. Counterstimulation by bathing the feet and hands in cold or warm water, or transcutaneous nerve stimulation, may produce temporary relief.

*Autonomic neuropathy,* which may affect several organ systems, can be detected in most diabetic patients with neuropathy by using specialized tests. Symptomatic postural hypotension is initially managed by such simple measures as (1) the avoidance of psychotropic, diuretic, or other drugs that might aggravate the condition; (2)

---

*Investigational drug in the United States.

sleeping with the head elevated by 5 to 20 degrees; (3) liberal dietary salt intake (at least 150 mEq per day); and (4) waist-high elastic stockings. If these measures fail, fludrocortisone (Florinef) (starting dose 0.1 mg daily to be increased gradually up to 0.5 mg twice daily) is begun. With high doses one should watch closely for side effects, such as fluid overload, supine hypertension, or hypokalemia. Indomethacin (Indocin) (25 to 50 mg three times daily), which acts by inhibiting prostaglandin synthesis, in combination with fludrocortisone may be helpful in patients with refractory disease. The combination of dihydroergotamine (DHE-45) and caffeine (6.5 to 10 μg* subcutaneously plus 200 mg caffeine orally 30 minutes before breakfast) is reserved for patients with severe symptomatic hypotension in whom other forms of treatment have failed.

Delayed gastric emptying is often relieved with metoclopramide (Reglan), a dopamine antagonist (usual dosage is 10 mg before each meal and at bedtime). Increasing gait problems as a result of drug-induced parkinsonism may develop in such patients and should not be mistaken for deterioration due to the neuropathy. Tetracycline (Sumycin) is frequently effective in diabetic autonomic diarrhea and it is given at the onset of an attack (one to two doses of 250 mg). If tetracycline fails, routine antidiarrheal agents or clonidine is used until episodes remit. Disturbing facial sweating after food intake may be suppressed by propantheline bromide (Pro-Banthine) at a single dose of 15 mg half an hour before meals at social occasions.

In patients with bladder dysfunction, the principal goals of management should be to improve bladder emptying and to reduce the risk of urinary tract infection. This requires close cooperation with a urologist. Sexual dysfunction in men may include erectile impotence or ejaculatory failure. There is no conservative treatment for neuropathic erectile failure but surgical insertion of semirigid or inflatable penile prostheses is available.

*Meticulous foot care* is extremely important in preventing unnoticed mechanical or thermal injuries, which set the stage for ulcerations, secondary infections, and distal joint destruction. Neuropathic edema develops as the result of sympathetic denervation leading to vasodilatation and arteriovenous shunting. Ephedrine (30 mg three to four times daily) may reduce this form of edema by stimulating vasoconstriction.

### Uremic Neuropathy

A mixed sensorimotor polyneuropathy commonly occurs in patients undergoing chronic hemodialysis. The diagnosis of uremic polyneuropathy should be made only in the context of end-stage renal failure (e.g., creatinine clearance less than 10 mL per min) of several months' duration. If the neuropathy worsens during hemodialysis, increasing the frequency and duration of dialysis is required. Rapid improvement follows successful renal transplantation. Uremic and diabetic patients with occlusive vascular disease are at risk to develop a serious, often unrecognized, ischemic complication of arteriovenous shunt placement. Causalgia-like pain develops abruptly together with a distal, graded sensory loss in the territory of all major nerves of the involved upper limb, hence the term *ischemic monomelic neuropathy*. Prompt ligation of the arteriovenous fistula is required to prevent permanent sequelae. Drug toxicity should be considered as an offender in rapidly progressive neuromuscular syndromes in patients with renal insufficiency. For instance, a severe neuropathy may follow the use of nitrofurantoin (Macrodantin). Colchicine, given at conventional doses, may cause a neuromyopathy with proximal weakness and elevated creatine kinase levels that mimics polymyositis.

### Hypothyroidism

Carpal tunnel syndrome, or less frequently, a mainly sensory polyneuropathy, occurs in hypothyroidism. Thyroid function should be checked in all patients presenting with carpal tunnel syndrome. Thyroid replacement may make surgical decompression of the median nerve unnecessary.

### Malignancy

Peripheral neuropathies in patients with cancer or lymphomas may occur as a result of direct invasion or neurotoxic chemotherapeutic agents, or as a remote effect. Persistent numbness of the chin secondary to involvement of the mental nerve should alert the clinician to disseminated cancer with metastatic lesions to the jaw or bone marrow infiltration. Acute polyradiculoneuropathies of the GBS type occur more commonly in association with lymphomas, particularly Hodgkin's disease, than with other malignancies. GBS and lymphoma should be treated independently according to their respective indications.

Clinical recognition of the rare but distinct paraneoplastic syndrome of *subacute sensory neuronopathy* assumes therapeutic significance, as its symptoms often precede those of the underlying cancer by several months. Characteristically, the clinical picture consists of the subacute onset of severe pansensory loss, total areflexia, and

---

*Exceeds dosage recommended by the manufacturer.

marked sensory ataxia with relative preservation of motor strength. Autoantibodies directed against nuclei of the central nervous system (CNS) and dorsal root ganglia neurons (called anti-Hu antibodies) have been detected in serum and CSF. The great majority of cases have occurred in association with small-cell lung carcinoma, which potentially responds to chemotherapy. With few exceptions, the clinical course of the neuropathy is not altered by either successful treatment of the tumor or treatment with plasmapheresis and immunosuppressive drugs.

### Plasma Cell Dyscrasias

All patients with chronic undiagnosed polyneuropathies, particularly those having CIDP-like features or autonomic failure, should be evaluated for underlying plasma cell dyscrasias as outlined in the decision tree (Figure 2). Up to 10% of patients with chronic idiopathic polyneuropathy harbor a monoclonal gammopathy, which in some way may be directly involved in the pathogenesis of the neuropathy. I order both serum and urine immunofixation electrophoresis (IF) because a small monoclonal (M) protein may be obscured in the serum protein electrophoresis (SPEP) pattern. If an M protein is detected, hematologic studies, including bone marrow biopsy, radiographic metastatic skeletal surveys, and tissue biopsies (e.g., rectum or nerve and muscle) are indicated to arrive at a diagnosis.

About one-half of these patients will have a polyneuropathy in association with an IgG, IgM, or IgA monoclonal gammopathy of undetermined significance (MGUS; formerly called benign monoclonal gammopathy). The IgM group is of particular interest because in one-half of these patients the IgM protein binds to carbohydrate epitopes of glycolipids (e.g., myelin-associated glycoprotein, or MAG) on the myelin sheath. Considerable evidence indicates that the IgM monoclonal protein with anti-MAG activity causes the neuropathy. A causal relationship, if any, between IgG and IgA MGUS and the associated polyneuropathy is less clear. If the coexisting neuropathy has CIDP-like features and its severity warrants intervention, the patients with MGUS are treated in the same manner as that for CIDP patients—with prednisone, azathio-

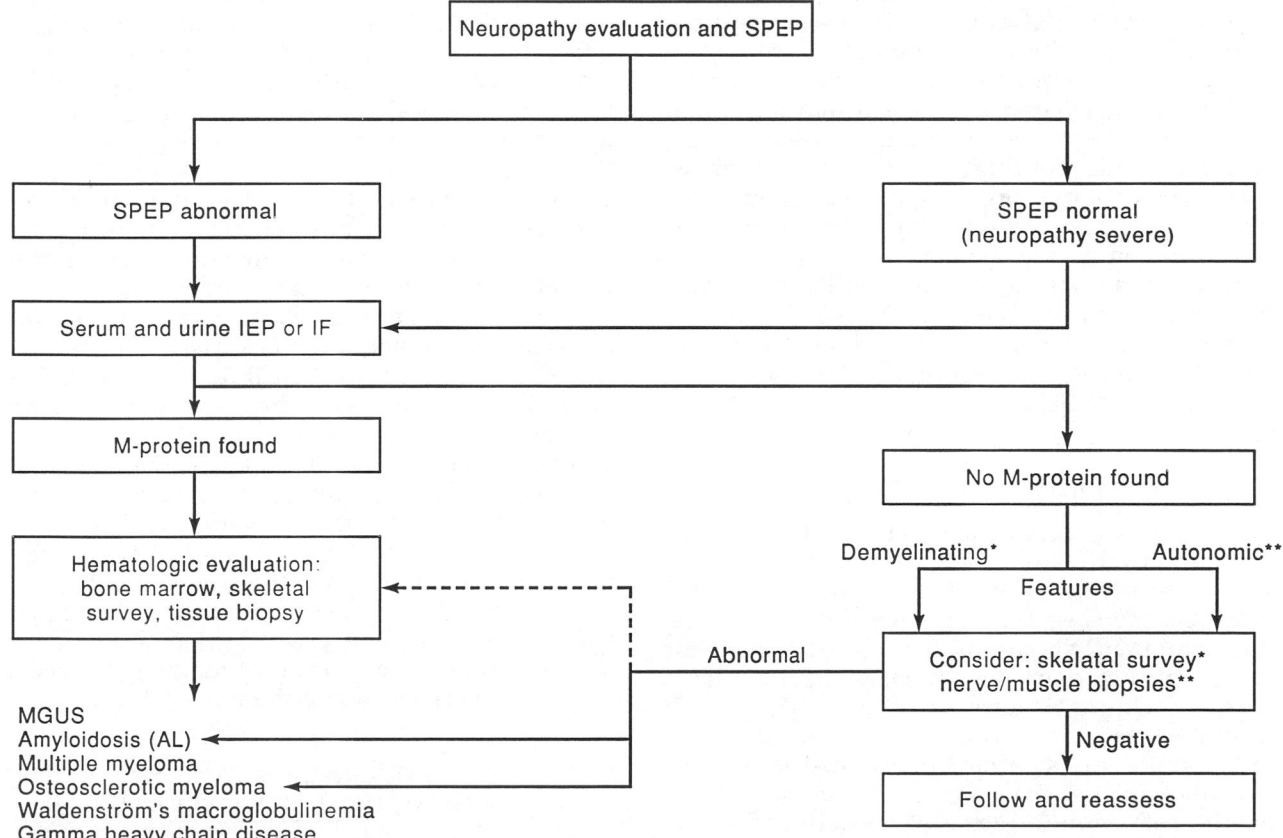

**Figure 2.** Decision tree in the evaluation of polyneuropathies associated with plasma cell dyscrasias. *Abbreviations:* SPEP = serum protein electrophoresis; IEP = immunoelectrophoresis; IF = immunofixation electrophoresis; M = monoclonal; MGUS = monoclonal gammopathy of undetermined significance.

prine, or plasmapheresis, or all of these, as outlined earlier in this article. Those patients with IgM anti-MAG activity and progressive neuropathy may respond to aggressive immune interventions that aim to lower the M protein concentration by 50%. This is best achieved by a combination of intermittent plasmapheresis and prednisone plus cyclophosphamide or chlorambucil.

*Amyloid neuropathy* occurring in association with primary systemic amyloidosis is related to the deposition of monoclonal light chain fragments in peripheral nerve tissue and presents as a sensorimotor polyneuropathy of axonal type with prominent autonomic features. Attempts at treatment with chemotherapy, usually melphalan (Alkeran) and prednisone or treatment with colchicine, or all three, have been disappointing. Symptomatic management of autonomic failure has been discussed earlier.

An axonal polyneuropathy is rarely associated with *multiple myeloma*. Treatment of the underlying myeloma does not affect the course of the neuropathy.

In contrast to typical osteolytic multiple myeloma, about 50% of patients with *osteosclerotic myeloma* develop a demyelinating, mainly motor polyneuropathy. Its clinical features closely resemble CIDP and consideration of this diagnosis mandates serum protein studies and a metastatic skeletal survey. Treatment depends on the extent of the plasmacytoma. If solitary, surgical extirpation or radiation therapy may result in remission of the neuropathy. In multiple lesions, chemotherapy using melphalan and prednisone occasionally provides benefit.

The demyelinating polyneuropathy in patients with *Waldenström's macroglobulinemia* may respond to chemotherapy or plasmapheresis, or both, but the response appears to be less predictable than in MGUS.

### Peripheral Nerve Vasculitis

Vasculitis is a clinicopathologic process characterized by inflammation and necrosis of blood vessels resulting in ischemia in the distribution of the damaged vessels. Peripheral nerve involvement frequently occurs in the context of systemic vasculitic disorders, as in classic polyarteritis nodosa, Churg-Strauss syndrome, Wegener's granulomatosis, and collagen vascular diseases, or in apparent isolation. In isolated peripheral nerve vasculitis, the peripheral neuropathy may be the sole manifestation of vasculitis. The peripheral nervous system lesions of necrotizing vasculitis typically result in multiple mononeuropathy or mononeuritis multiplex by affecting

several noncontiguous major nerve trunks in sequential order. However, overlapping mononeuropathies and asymmetrical or distal symmetrical sensorimotor polyneuropathies of the axonal type are not uncommon presentations. Diagnosis of such cases can be difficult without a high index of suspicion. Diagnosis depends ultimately on identifying vasculitis in nerve and muscle biopsy samples, or both. The combination of affected nerve and adjacent muscle sampling often increases the chance of visualizing characteristic arterial lesions.

In systemic vasculitis with multiple organ involvement the combination of prednisone and cyclophosphamide provides the best approach for rapidly suppressing disease activity and achieving clinical remission. Cyclophosphamide is started orally at 1 to 2 mg per kg of body weight per day in a single dose together with prednisone (1.5 mg per kg per day in three to four divided doses). The initial divided dose steroid schedule is consolidated to a single morning dose within 10 days, and after 4 to 8 weeks prednisone is switched to single alternate-day therapy. Complete blood counts are closely monitored during treatment and the dose is adjusted to maintain the total leukocyte count above 3000 per mm$^3$. Patients should be kept on both drugs until significant improvement occurs, at which time prednisone may be gradually tapered. Cyclophosphamide is maintained for 1 year after the disappearance of all traces of active disease. This combination therapy is reported to result in an 80 to 90% remission rate in patients with Wegener's granulomatosis or systemic necrotizing vasculitis. The most serious toxic effects from cyclophosphamide include bone marrow suppression resulting in major infections, herpes zoster, gonadal failure, hemorrhagic cystitis, and increased risk of malignancy. Liberal fluid intake and frequent voiding may lessen the risk of hemorrhagic cystitis, which develops in about 15% of patients on oral cyclophosphamide. Intravenous bolus cyclophosphamide therapy (0.5 to 1.0 gram per M$^2$ of body surface area given every 1 to 3 months) is said to avoid the bladder complications associated with continuous oral therapy. Patients with isolated peripheral nerve vasculitis are treated with high single-dose prednisone alone because their favorable prognosis may not justify the risks associated with cyclophosphamide therapy.

## ALCOHOLIC NEUROPATHY AND NUTRITIONAL DEFICIENCIES

Alcoholic neuropathy is one of the most common causes of peripheral neuropathy. Alcoholism may not be suspected at the initial evaluation unless a high index of suspicion is maintained in any painful sensorimotor polyneuropathy of undetermined cause. Deficiency of thiamine and other B vitamins due to inadequate dietary intake, impaired absorption, and greater metabolic demand, and possibly a direct toxic effect of alcohol, may all contribute to the distal axonopathy. Abstinence from alcohol, expert counseling, and a nutritionally balanced diet supplemented by B vitamins constitute the principal therapy. Supplemental B vitamins are given in the following daily dosages: thiamine 50 mg, niacin 100 mg, riboflavin 10 mg, pantothenic acid 10 mg, and pyridoxine 50 mg. In patients with vomiting or gastrointestinal complications, the vitamins are added to intravenous fluids.

Deficiencies of folate, vitamin $B_{12}$, thiamine, pyridoxine, pantothenic acid, and vitamin E have been associated with peripheral neuropathies. Most nutritional deficiencies in the United States result from the lack of multiple B vitamins caused by alcoholism, self-imposed fad diets, gastric bypass procedures for morbid obesity, and malabsorption. Adequate vitamin replacement is essential in these patients.

Isolated pyridoxine deficiency neuropathy may occur in patients treated with isoniazid and hydralazine and can be prevented by supplementary pyridoxine (100 mg daily). Excessive doses of pyridoxine (500 to 3000 mg daily) must be avoided, as such megadoses cause a toxic sensory neuronopathy.

Peripheral neuropathy is part of the general nervous system involvement in *vitamin $B_{12}$ deficiency*. Treatment is initiated with 100 μg of vitamin $B_{12}$ given intramuscularly on alternate days for 2 weeks, followed by twice-weekly injections, until neurologic symptoms have improved or stabilized and the hematologic abnormalities have been corrected. Replacement requires monthly vitamin $B_{12}$ injections (100 μg intramuscularly) for the remainder of the patient's life. The practice of prescribing vitamin $B_{12}$ supplementation for undiagnosed neuropathies lacks a rationale and is discouraged.

## TOXIC NEUROPATHIES

Industrial and environmental agents, heavy metals, and drugs are known to produce peripheral neuropathies. Today, drugs, particularly chemotherapeutic agents, are by far the most common offenders. Table 1 lists those drugs that have been repeatedly incriminated in inducing peripheral neuropathy. Most neurotoxic agents produce distal axonal degenerations in a dying-back pattern. This leads to early sensory loss in the feet, loss of ankle jerks, and later distal leg weakness

**TABLE 1. Some Drugs That Induce Neuropathies**

| **Antineoplastic** | **Central Nervous System** |
|---|---|
| Cisplatin (Platinol) | Lithium (Lithobid) |
| Vincristine (Oncovin) | Nitrous oxide |
| **Antimicrobial** | Thalidomide* |
| Chloroquine (Aralen) | **Other** |
| Dapsone | Cimetidine (Tagamet) |
| Isoniazid | Colchicine |
| Metronidazole | Disulfiram (Antabuse) |
| (Flagyl) | Gold (Solganal, Myochrysine) |
| Nitrofurantoin | Phenytoin |
| (Macrodantin) | Pyridoxine (megadoses) |
| **Cardiovascular** | |
| Amiodarone (Cordarone) | |
| Hydralazine (Apresoline) | |
| Perhexiline* | |

*Not available in the United States.

and atrophy with a gradual spread of the deficits more proximally with time. Myelin damage resulting in segmental demyelination occurs in only a few toxic conditions, such as amiodarone, perhexiline, and hexacarbon intoxications. Considerable slowing of nerve conduction velocity is found in these situations. A detailed history probing for a background of occupational exposure and the use of drugs, inclusive of vitamins and folk remedies, is important in the evaluation of suspected toxic neuropathies. In few instances, telltale signs, such as hair loss in thallium poisoning, white transverse nail lines (Mees' lines) in arsenic poisoning, or blue gum lines in lead intoxications, will provide specific diagnostic clues. In exceptional cases a nerve biopsy may be helpful in establishing the diagnosis of hexacarbon neuropathy by revealing typical neurofilamentous axonal swellings.

The treatment strategy common to all toxic neuropathies involves recognition of the toxic agent, elimination of sources of its exposure, and expectant supportive care. Despite removal of the toxin, worsening of clinical symptoms may continue for several weeks before recovery begins. Specific therapy is not available for most cases. There is insufficient evidence that chelating agents increase the rate of clinical recovery in established arsenic, gold, lead, and thallium neuropathy. The neurotoxicity of cisplatin (Platinol) is considered a dose limiting side effect of this cytotoxic agent. A mainly sensory neuropathy usually develops in patients who have received a total cumulative dose of 300 to 600 mg per M². Severely affected patients become markedly disabled by sensory ataxia. A new ACTH analogue that enhances nerve regeneration holds promise in delaying or preventing cisplatin-induced neuropathy. A distal sensorimotor polyneuropathy occurs almost universally as a dose limiting side effect of treatment with vincristine.

## HEREDITARY NEUROPATHIES

The hereditary neuropathies, a complex and heterogeneous group of disorders, have in common an insidious onset and indolent course over years to decades. Most of these disorders are rare, with the exception of *hereditary motor sensory neuropathy (HMSN, or Charcot-Marie-Tooth disease),* which is a leading cause (up to 40%) of chronic, undiagnosed neuropathies. Skeletal abnormalities such as hammer toes or high arches, a thorough family history, and the examination of relatives aid in recognition.

Management of the inherited neuropathies is mainly supportive. Genetic counseling is undertaken after proper clinical evaluation, inclusive of nerve conduction studies of available family members. Fortunately, the rate of progression in Charcot-Marie-Tooth disease of both types (i.e., the hypertrophic form, or HMSN, type I, with very slow conduction velocity; and the neuronal form, or HMSN, type II, with fairly normal conduction velocities) is slow and disability occurs relatively late in life. Patients are instructed in proper foot care and advised to wear broad, well-fitting shoes. Heat-molded insoles may be used to distribute the body weight more evenly in patients with foot deformity. Braces or orthopedic procedures are sometimes indicated for severe footdrop or progressive deformities. The prevention of acromutilations, which appear to be related to trauma and abuse of insensitive limbs and to neglect of injuries, is of utmost importance in the *hereditary sensory and autonomic neuropathies.* This can be achieved by meticulous foot care, avoiding walking barefoot, and daily inspection of shoes and feet for foreign bodies or any sores on the feet. Those hereditary neuropathies for which specific therapy is available are briefly mentioned.

A concurrent CIDP-like syndrome may develop in some patients with hereditary motor and sensory neuropathy. These patients typically have a positive family history of affected kin and have had pes cavus or hammer toes since an early age but develop subacute worsening with proximal muscle weakness and raised CSF protein level. The newly acquired symptoms often respond to corticosteroid therapy, hence the term *prednisone-responsive hereditary motor and sensory neuropathy* (see Chronic Inflammatory Demyelinating Polyradiculoneuropathy).

Large doses of vitamin E (100 to 300 U per kg per day) have been reported to prevent the onset, or arrest the progression, of the sensory ataxic neuropathy associated with *abetalipoproteinemia. Fabry's disease,* an X-linked lysosomal disorder, leads to angiokeratomas, vascular disease, and a small fiber neuropathy. The associated paresthesias and lancinating pains that are typically intensified by physical exertion or in a hot environment respond to carbamazepine. *Refsum's disease,* a rare disorder of phytanic acid metabolism, leads to night blindness, a chronic hypertrophic neuropathy, and ataxia. Chronic dietary restriction of phytanic acid is said to improve the condition, and plasmapheresis may be helpful in acute deteriorations.

### Porphyric Neuropathy

The acute hepatic porphyrias (acute intermittent porphyria, variegate porphyria, and hereditary coproporphyria) are the result of genetic defects in hepatic heme synthesis. These gene defects remain latent until precipitating factors, such as certain drugs, most notably barbiturates, or alcoholic beverages, or fasting, trigger acute attacks of central and peripheral nervous system manifestations. Symptoms include severe abdominal pain, constipation, and sinus tachycardia; more severe attacks are followed by a rapidly progressive, predominantly motor neuropathy of axonal type or encephalopathy with seizures, or both. The diagnosis is confirmed by the marked elevation of the porphyrin precursors, porphobilinogen and aminolevulinic acid, in urine.

The attack must be treated promptly to correct the metabolic insult before neuronal damage becomes permanent. All offending drugs are removed. The administration of a high-carbohydrate diet (at least 400 grams daily, or the equivalent in glucose or levulose infusions) results in reduced porphyrin precursor production and may be associated with clinical improvement. Persistent symptoms or progressive neurologic deficits for 24 hours after carbohydrate loading are indications for treatment with hematin (hemin; Panhematin). In clinical studies, hematin therapy, at the recommended dose of six infusions of 4 mg per kg body weight at 12-hour intervals, has resulted in consistent reduction of porphyrin precursors by the repression of aminolevulinic acid (ALA) synthase, and clinical improvement in most attacks. Abdominal pain is controlled by chlorpromazine (Thorazine), antiemetics, and analgesics (codeine, meperidine) when necessary. All family members should be screened for the gene defect. Ideally, all attacks should be prevented in susceptible carriers by avoiding inducing drugs and circumstances.

# ACUTE HEAD INJURIES IN ADULTS

method of
THOMAS G. SAUL, M.D.
*Mayfield Neurological Institute*
*Cincinnati, Ohio*

The diagnostic and therapeutic approach to acute head injury in adults should consist of logical procedures that can be rapidly executed. The procedures should be flexible enough to allow sound clinical decision making, especially if the patient has multiple trauma.

The primary goals of treatment of the head-injured patient are: (1) immediate resuscitation and medical stabilization; (2) early recognition and surgical treatment of intracranial mass lesions; and (3) aggressive medical therapy to prevent the detrimental effects of shock, hypoxia, and hypercarbia.

## ASSESSMENT

A severe head injury is one that renders the patient unable to open his eyes and talk or move appropriately in response to a painful stimulus. This is equivalent to a score of 7 or less on the Glasgow Coma Scale (Table 1). The emergency room personnel should evaluate the neurologic status before any necessary sedation is administered or intubation is performed. One can do this by answering the following questions: (1) does the patient open his eyes and to what stimulus? (2) does the patient utter recognizable words? (3) does the patient follow commands? (4) does the patient move each extremity equally and to what stimulus? and (5) what are the size and reactivity of the pupils? In addition, someone on the admitting team should be obtaining information in regard to time of injury, mechanism of injury, and clinical changes that occurred during the patient's transfer. This information will enable the neurosurgeon to determine the severity of the injury, the presence of any lateralizing neurologic findings compatible with an intracranial mass lesion, and the progression of the patient's condition from the time of injury.

## STABILIZATION

The stabilization of the patient begins and is simultaneous with the assessment. This is done according to the well-accepted principles of assuring an adequate airway, ventilation, and circulation. A basic principle in resuscitating the injured brain is to get oxygen to the brain and keep intracranial pressure (ICP) normal. Therefore, patients with severe head injury should be

TABLE 1. **The Glasgow Coma Scale**

| | |
|---|---|
| Verbal response: | |
| None | 1 |
| Incomprehensible sounds | 2 |
| Inappropriate words | 3 |
| Confused | 4 |
| Oriented | 5 |
| Eye opening: | |
| None | 1 |
| To pain | 2 |
| To speech | 3 |
| Spontaneously | 4 |
| Motor response: | |
| None | 1 |
| Abnormal extensor | 2 |
| Abnormal flexion | 3 |
| Withdraws | 4 |
| Localizes | 5 |
| Obeys | 6 |

intubated and hyperventilated as soon as possible. Baseline arterial blood gases should be drawn, and frequent serial determinations should be made routinely thereafter. A neurologic deficit can increase as a result of hypoxia.

All patients should have their systemic blood pressure watched closely. This has a twofold purpose. First, a decrease in cerebral perfusion pressure (CPP) leads to further cerebral dysfunction. CPP is a balance between mean arterial pressure and ICP. Therefore, we must know the arterial pressure to have an accurate assessment of brain perfusion. Second, 50 to 60% of the patients with severe head injury will have multiple injuries. In these patients, maintenance of adequate perfusion of all organ systems is mandatory. One should attempt to maintain the patient in a normotensive state with systolic pressure between 100 and 170 mm Hg. Pressures higher than 170 mm Hg can cause increased cerebral blood volume, leading to increased ICP, as well as aggravate the formation of vasogenic edema. Initially hyperventilation is instituted to achieve a $PaCO_2$ of approximately 25 mm Hg. This causes constriction of the cerebral vasculature with resultant decreases in cerebral blood volume (not cerebral blood flow), which will decrease intracranial pressure. This initial stabilization process is directly aimed at disrupting pathophysiologic processes and thus preventing secondary brain injury.

## DIAGNOSIS

After the patient has been stabilized and assessed, the neurodiagnostic work-up should commence and proceed rapidly. Two important facts should be remembered: (1) any unconscious head-injured patient may be harboring a spine injury, as 5 to 20% of patients with head injury will have a fracture of their spinal column; and (2) if a patient with a head injury has a neurologic status characterized by not following commands or even greater impairment, there is an approximately 25% chance that he has an intracranial surgical lesion.

A lateral cervical spine film should be obtained immediately after stabilization of the patient to rule out a cervical spine injury, which if unrecognized could result in additional neurologic deficit due to spinal cord injury.

Anteroposterior and lateral skull films should be obtained immediately in those patients who have penetrating wounds of the skull and those suspected of having a depressed skull fracture. Plain skull films are of value in localizing the position of foreign bodies inside the calvaria and the amount of depression of the skull. In severe closed-head injuries, the skull film may be deferred until after computed tomography (CT) of the head is performed and in many cases may not be required.

A patient with an intracranial mass lesion (epidural or subdural hematoma) has the potential for sudden clinical deterioration at any time. Therefore, the burden is on the physician to diagnose or rule out these lesions as rapidly as possible. There is no question that the CT scan is the diagnostic test of choice to identify these lesions. The basic advantages of CT scanning are: (1) it is rapid, noninvasive, and safe to perform; (2) CT gives an actual picture of the pathology, thus avoiding some of the "guess work" necessary with other diagnostic tests; and (3) CT differentiates between intraparenchymal blood and brain swelling or edema. There are several other equally significant benefits of CT scanning these patients. CT can diagnose coexisting or dual pathology (e.g., the combination of subdural hematoma and intracerebral hemorrhage or a depressed skull fracture associated with an intracerebral hemorrhage). CT fully delineates the extent of intracranial pathology. Thus, the CT scan can aid in planning a more precise surgical treatment and increases the likelihood that the correct surgical procedure will be selected.

The indications for obtaining a CT scan are simple considering the high incidence of surgical lesions (at least 25 to 30%). Any patient who has sustained head trauma and presents with any sign of neurologic abnormalities in the emergency room should probably undergo CT scanning. Neurologic abnormalities include any alteration in mental status (i.e., disorientation, drowsiness), as well as localizing or lateralizing signs (e.g., hemiparesis, pupillary dilatation). A patient who will not speak, follow commands, open his eyes when told to do so, or move purposefully to avoid pain should unequivocally undergo CT scanning.

Included in the diagnostic work-up of these patients are various laboratory tests that are relevant to a patient's neurologic status. These specimens are obtained during the initial resuscitation and sent immediately to the laboratory while the above regimen is being instituted. Laboratory tests should include toxic screen (both urine and blood), serum alcohol level, electrolytes, blood urea nitrogen (BUN), hemoglobin and hematocrit, glucose, and serum osmolarity.

## TREATMENT

### Surgical Treatment

After diagnostic work-up, surgery should be performed immediately if indicated. If another body system injury also requires immediate surgery, the procedures can be performed simultaneously.

The vast majority of emergency intracranial surgery for head trauma is done to decompress the brain. This is true for depressed skull fracture, an expanding hematoma, or a swollen hemorrhagic lobe. Therefore, the goals of this surgery are to relieve the pressure adequately and to prevent its recurrence. Additional goals are to clean, debride, and prevent infection in wounds that are contaminated.

### Medical Treatment

After surgery is completed, the care of both surgical and nonsurgical patients is essentially the same and consists of aggressive medical therapy. Maintaining intracranial pressure within normal ranges is the mainstay of medical therapy. Although the basic therapy is the same, the institution of more aggressive medical therapy can be guided by the ICP levels.

Three techniques are available for the clinical application of ICP monitoring: intraventricular, subarachnoid, and epidural. Each has its advantages and disadvantages. The intraventricular catheter technique is popular and probably the most reliable in regard to ICP recordings. The major advantages of the intraventricular technique are that it is a direct ventricular fluid pressure reading, and with an intraventricular catheter in place one can drain cerebrospinal fluid (CSF) in order to treat ICP elevations. The disadvantages are the risk of CNS infection and intracerebral hemorrhage, since the brain tissue has to be penetrated to gain entry into the ventricle.

A subarachnoid screw is a hollow bolt that is implanted via a burr hole into the subdural space. The advantages of the subarachnoid screw apparatus are a lower infection rate and ease of insertion. The disadvantage is the inability to drain CSF in order to treat intracranial hypertension.

Epidural monitors are also available. These include a fiberoptic epidural probe and an epidural bolt functioning on the same principle as the subarachnoid screw. The advantages of these devices are the extremely low risks of CNS infection and ease of insertion. The disadvantages are that some physicians question the reliability of epidural recordings and the CSF cannot be drained.

Selection of patients for ICP monitoring is not always clearcut. Most neurosurgeons would agree that any patient who is arousable and purposeful probably would not require ICP monitoring. Conversely, a patient who is comatose and does not have purposeful movement to a painful stimulus should have ICP monitoring.

Comatose patients who have abnormal CT scans on admission are at high risk for developing intracranial hypertension. Therefore, routine ICP monitoring in these patients may be justified. Patients with normal CT scans at admission have a low incidence of intracranial hypertension unless they demonstrate two or more of the following features: (1) systolic blood pressure under 90 mmHg, (2) motor posturing, and (3) age over 40 years. These patients have a high risk of elevated ICP and may benefit from ICP monitoring. It is strongly recommended that patients who are not monitored routinely have a follow-up CT scan within 12 to 14 hours to rule out any delayed intracranial abnormality that could alter the intracranial pressure.

By monitoring ICP, one knows when to begin

and stop treatment and whether the treatment is effective in reducing ICP. The empirical use of some of the regimens described later in this chapter without knowing the patient's ICP is questionable. These are not benign treatments and are not without complications. Moreover, the treatment modalities available should be used in a logical fashion based on varying levels of ICP.

Normal ICP is generally accepted to be equal to or less than 15 torr. Numerous reports in the literature document that pressures consistently between 20 and 30 torr are associated with a high mortality rate. However, when ICP monitoring was first employed, pressures of 20 to 40 torr were tolerated by the neurotraumatologists because it was thought that cerebral perfusion was still adequate at those levels. However, we are now appreciating the correlation between the level of ICP and its responsiveness to treatment. There seems to be a "point of no return" in regard to ICP levels, i.e., pressures greater than 25 torr are much more difficult to reduce than ICP less than 20 torr. Therefore, over the years, the level of ICP at which specific treatment is instituted has been lowered. I begin specific treatment when ICP is consistently greater than 16 torr. The majority of neurosurgeons would definitely treat pressure greater than 20 torr.

The medical treatment of intracranial hypertension can be categorized into general and specific measures. The general measures are techniques and drugs instituted at all levels of intracranial pressure to maintain intracranial homeostasis. Specific measures are those aimed at returning elevated ICP to normal levels.

### General Measures

The general measures include the following: (1) head and neck positioning, (2) hyperventilation, (3) sedation, (4) fluid balance, (5) normotension, (6) steroids, and (7) nursing care.

**Head and Neck Positioning.** Elevating a patient's head 30 to 45 degrees facilitates venous drainage out of the intracranial vault and thus prevents unnecessary elevations of ICP. It is important to maintain the head and neck in a neutral position. This keeps the head from falling forward or to one side and thus impeding flow through the internal jugular veins, which would decrease venous drainage and would ultimately lead to increased intracranial venous pressure and increased ICP. Sometimes a cervical collar can be used, and if needed, the head may be taped in a neutral position when in an elevated state.

**Hyperventilation.** All patients who are comatose are intubated and should be continued on hyperventilation so that the $PaCO_2$ is between 25 to 30 mm Hg. It is well accepted that hypocarbia in the acute phase will decrease ICP by a reduction in the cerebral blood volume. Because this ultimately improves cerebral perfusion pressure, the mild decrease in cerebral blood flow is not deleterious, and the net effect is beneficial in regard to ICP dynamics. The chronic use of hyperventilation (greater than 3 days) is somewhat more controversial. Therefore, if after 24 to 36 hours ICP has remained normal, hyperventilation may be withdrawn and the $PaCO_2$ allowed to increase. It is important to leave the ICP monitor in during the time of weaning from hyperventilation because if ICP increases as $PaCO_2$ increases, hyperventilation therapy should be reinstituted. After 24 hours with normal intracranial pressure at higher $PaCO_2$, the monitor may be removed if there are no other indications for continued monitoring.

**Sedation.** A patient may require sedation in order to facilitate ventilatory treatment. Also, sedation may diminish the patient's adverse response to noxious external stimuli. A patient may be hypertensive owing to painful stimuli from nursing maneuvers, diagnostic tests, associated injuries, and other factors. As has been discussed, hypertension has detrimental effects on ICP. Abnormal posturing (decerebration and/or decortication) may result from or be aggravated by stimulation. This can increase systemic blood pressure and subsequently increase intracranial pressure. Proper sedation may abort these responses. Paralytic drugs may also be used as needed to achieve the desired results. The drugs used should be chosen on the basis of how much they would interfere with neuro-assessment, whether their effects can be reversed with an antagonist, or whether they have a short half-life. If a well-functioning ICP monitor and access to CT scanning are available, one should not hesitate to employ drugs such as fentanyl citrate (Sublimaze), morphine, chlorpromazine (Thorazine), and pancuronium bromide (Pavulon).

**Fluid Balance.** Patients with severe head injuries should not be fluid overloaded. Intravenous fluids should be administered cautiously. Increasing the vascular volume with large volumes of fluids will engorge the brain, increase its bulk, and increase ICP. Therefore, normovolemia is conducive to maintaining normal ICP. Furthermore, the *proper* intravenous fluid is just as important as the rate of infusion. Large amounts of hypotonic fluids can have a detrimental effect of brain function, not only by decreasing osmolarity but also by exacerbating edema formation.

**Normotension.** Two facts must be remembered regarding the management of systemic arterial blood pressure. First, cerebral perfusion pressure is determined by both intracranial pressure and mean arterial pressure. Therefore, maintenance of an adequate level of systolic pressure is imperative. All efforts must be made to avoid hypotensive states (systolic pressure less than 100 torr). Second, post-traumatic edema is a vasogenic type and may be exacerbated by increases of hydrostatic pressure in the capillary beds, as is seen with the hyperemia caused by profound hypertension (systolic pressure greater than 170 torr). Systolic pressures should be kept between 100 and 170 mm Hg. Pharmacologic means can be employed to maintain acceptable blood pressure and cardiac function. If hypotension continues to be a problem, hemodynamic monitoring with a Swan-Ganz catheter may be indicated for proper management. Systolic pressures greater than 170 should be avoided. First, external factors causing increased blood pressure must be ruled out. Pain, abnormal posturing, and increased ICP can cause elevated blood pressure. After dealing with these aspects, one should treat the blood pressure with an appropriate antihypertensive agent, e.g., nitroprusside (Nipride), methyldopa (Aldomet), hydralazine hydrochloride (Apresoline), and labetalol (Trandate, Normodyne).

**Steroids.** The use of steroids in the management of severe head injuries is controversial and probably always will be. There has never been well-accepted scientific proof that steroid therapy decreases morbidity and mortality of severe head injuries. The results of both experimental and clinical investigations have been contradictory. Studies can be found that support the beneficial effect, no effect, and, in some instances, the adverse effect of steroid therapy.

The beneficial effect that is documented in some studies is probably due to the anti-edema properties of steroids. Edema formation may occur at any time within weeks of the injury. Therefore, there is a logical rationale behind instituting steroid therapy early (on admission) and continuing treatment for 3 to 10 days. Any beneficial effect of steroids is not due to an ability to rapidly decrease high levels of ICP. Because of this, steroid therapy is not included in the armamentarium of specific treatments for intracranial hypertension. It is included in the general measures because it seems to be more of a prophylactic treatment design to maintain intracranial homeostasis.

**Nursing Care.** The best friend that a patient with severe head injury has is the nurse at the bedside. The primary goal of all of the general measures to control ICP is maintenance of cerebral homeostasis. This demands a holistic approach to the patient's care. This approach is best provided by a competent nurse, knowledgeable in the principles of ICP and attuned to the above-mentioned measures.

Since much of brain function and intracranial pressure dynamics depend on good oxygenation and pulmonary care, the nursing duties of suctioning, chest percussion, and postural drainage are important aspects of the patient's care. These maneuvers should be done regularly and frequently, as indicated by arterial blood gases and chest films. Frequent careful turning of the patient to prevent atelectasis and the development of infiltrates and infection is imperative.

Hyperthermia and systemic infection can also alter brain function and lead to difficulty in assessing the patient and managing the treatment. Therefore, the nurse should consistently monitor temperature and white blood cell count and notify the appropriate persons for treatment intervention.

Close nursing observation of a patient's patterns of agitation and responses to nursing maneuvers will facilitate judicious use of sedation and paralytic agents, as outlined above. The nurse should be well trained in neuro-assessment skills. The detection of early neurologic changes in the coma scale parameters and the levels of ICP may indeed allow for treatment intervention in time to avoid the permanent detrimental effects of these events.

### Specific Treatment for ICP Control

As stated before, specific therapeutic regimens are instituted when the ICP reaches levels that cannot be tolerated. There is a well-accepted armamentarium of drugs and techniques available able to reduce elevated ICP. The efficacy of this armamentarium is maximized if it is used in an organized step-wise fashion. No one drug is the answer to ICP problems. The treatment must be viewed as "balanced therapy" in which drugs can be alternated and in which timing of an individual drug is important to derive the maximum benefit from all of them. The most commonly used modalities at the present time include (1) hyperventilation, (2) hyperosmolar agents (mannitol), (3) loop diuretics (furosemide), (4) CSF drainage, and (5) barbiturates.

**Hyperventilation.** The use of controlled hyperventilation to produce hypocarbia has been discussed earlier, and it is included in this section to emphasize its importance. It is generally accepted that hyperventilation decreases intracranial pressure during the acute phase of a head injury (within the first 24 hours). The value of more prolonged periods is a bit more controversial. However, recent studies have recommended continuation of hyperventilation therapy for as long as ICP remains abnormal. Also, hyperventilation should be reinstituted if ICP increases again several days into the patient's course. Hyperventilation to a $Paco_2$ of 25 to 30 torr is continued in all patients whose ICP is above acceptable levels.

**Hyperosmolar Agents.** Intravenous solutions containing high-molecular-weight substances do not cross the blood-brain barrier. This creates an osmotic gradient between brain tissue and blood through which water leaves brain tissue and enters the vascular tree. This decreases brain bulk and therefore decreases ICP. Mannitol is the agent of choice in this group of drugs at the present time; however, mannitol therapy is not free of problems. Patients requiring frequent administration often develop significant hyperosmolar electrolyte imbalances. These derangements threaten the patient from a cardiovascular and renal standpoint and ultimately limit the drug's use. Doses of 0.25 to 1.0 gram per kg have been shown to be effective in reducing the patient's ICP. Therefore, recommended doses of mannitol for control of ICP are 0.25 to 0.5 gram per kg bolus administration every 4 to 6 hours as needed for ICP control. Mannitol may also be given as a continuous infusion, which is generally indicated when bolus doses are being required at shorter intervals. Neither a maximum dose of mannitol nor an optimum dose has ever been described. It has been shown that serum osmolarity must be raised by 10 mOsm to have a decrease in ICP. Serum osmolarity of 310 to 320 is associated with a good decrease in ICP; however, osmolarities greater than 320 are dangerous and mark the limit of mannitol therapy. Frequent electrolyte and osmolarity determinations are mandatory.

**Diuretics.** Recently furosemide (Lasix) has been shown by some to be effective in reducing intracranial hypertension. However, the use of this loop diuretic in decreasing ICP is not as well established as that of mannitol. The mechanisms by which furosemide and others like it (ethacrynic acid) reduce ICP may be multiple. By decreasing total body water, brain water will move out into the vascular tree and be excreted. This decreases brain bulk. These agents are also known to decrease the production of CSF and therefore to decrease ICP. Finally, some reports maintain that furosemide may have a direct effect on brain edema. The theoretical advantage of employing furosemide is that it will thwart or help to avoid hyperosmolar states. At the present time, furosemide is not a first-choice agent to be used alone to decrease ICP in a patient with a severe head injury. However, we include it and use it in an alternative fashion with mannitol. This seems to decrease mannitol requirements and stave off electrolyte imbalances. Furosemide can be started with mannitol on an alternating basis.

**CSF Drainage.** If an intraventricular catheter is used to measure ICP, one has the opportunity to decrease ICP by removing CSF from the ventricle. This CSF drainage is effective in decreasing ICP because of the pressure volume relationship within the cranium. There are commercially available ventricular drainage systems that provide continuous drainage if the ICP goes above a certain level. This is done under manometric control. Intermittent drainage can also be accomplished with such systems. Whatever system is employed, CSF drainage is an effective adjunct to controlling ICP. Strict sterile technique should be employed when handling the intraventricular catheter and external ventricular drainage. The more manipulations of this apparatus, the greater the chances for infection.

**Barbiturates.** In recent years, high-dose intravenous barbiturate therapy has proved to be effective in controlling high levels of ICP that are refractory to the aforementioned modalities. The mechanism by which barbiturates decrease ICP remains controversial and unknown. Many patients with intracranial hypertension will respond to high-dose intravenous barbiturates with a drop in ICP. The question of the efficacy of barbiturates in reducing morbidity and mortality of severe head injuries is not completely answered yet. Controlled randomized trials are being conducted throughout the United States at the present time. Preliminary studies indicate that this is certainly an acceptable treatment to lower ICP.

Barbiturate therapy is a major endeavor that should be administered only in an intensive care environment. Most reports have recommended the use of pentobarbital or pentothal. Pentobarbital is used more often, probably because it has a more sustained effect on decreasing ICP. Pentothal is a faster acting barbiturate and has been employed to abort ICP elevations associated with nursing maneuvers. Loading doses of 5 to 10 mg per kg have been recommended to achieve a decrease in ICP to levels of 15 to 20 torr and to maintain serum levels of approximately 4 mg per dl. Maintenance doses of 1 to 2 mg per kg every 1 to 2 hours will maintain these effects in the majority of patients. All patients undergoing barbiturate treatment should have arterial lines inserted for constant mean arterial pressure recordings, and ICP monitors should also be inserted. In addition, these patients should have Swan-Ganz catheters placed for constant monitoring of the true volume status, cardiac output, and pulmonary status. Barbiturates can have a marked depressive effect on cardiopulmonary function. Such monitoring can detect early changes and help avert the deleterious effects on the heart and lungs and subsequently on brain function.

Any increase in ICP while barbiturate therapy is being given warrants an immediate CT scan after a search for other causes of increased ICP (e.g., fluid overload, hypercarbia). Finally, as a point of emphasis, barbiturate therapy is an aggressive treatment modality that should not be embarked upon in a cavalier fashion. It involves large expenditures of funds, time and energy. Certainly, direct ICP recordings should be an indication of the need for this treatment.

# ACUTE HEAD INJURIES IN CHILDREN

method of
YOON S. HAHN, M.D.
*Stritch School of Medicine, Loyola University*
*Maywood, Illinois*

In the vast majority of cases, the injury to the nervous system is insignificant; however, impact to the skull and brain with severe injury is an inevitable part of childhood play.

Occasionally, the brain is the primary site of injury or processes are set in motion that will secondarily injure the central nervous system. Little can be done about primary injury to the brain, but a great deal can now be done about the secondary damage. The secondary brain damage can result from cerebral ischemia, raised intracranial pressure, intracranial mass lesions, such as epidural hematoma, and associated systemic hypotension. These will compound the primary damage to the brain and can initiate a process leading to irreversible brain damage or death if medical-surgical intervention is not prompt.

Trauma accounts for about one-third of all pediatric surgical admissions, and one-half of these children have incurred a head injury. One child in 10 will suffer a significant head injury during school years, and one-third of these children will be hospitalized. Mortality figures for head injury in children vary widely. There are about 100,000 accidental deaths per year in North America and approximately 25,000 are in children. Studies at one time showed that of those children admitted in a comatose state, one-half to three-quarters died. However, recent studies paint a somewhat more optimistic picture, with a mortality rate of 20 to 40%.

## GENERAL MANAGEMENT

In our study on 738 children with minor head injuries (Glasgow coma scale 13 to 15), 13% of them had a surgical lesion such as epidural hematoma, acute subdural hematoma, or depressed skull fractures and various types of scalp laceration, etc. Two children from this study, both assigned Glasgow coma scale value 13, had a so-called talk and die event. Therefore, the fact that some children who eventually die of a head injury are awake at the time of injury or when admitted to the hospital supports the use of more liberal criteria for computed axial tomography scan or admission for observation. In most of these cases, a delayed mass lesion or cerebral edema occurs in the first 48 hours. No perfect set of criteria exists for deciding who should be hospitalized for observation, which results in admission of a large number of children who recover completely without any surgical treatment. This is done in the hope that the children who will deteriorate later are included in this larger group so that the impending intracranial disaster can be promptly and appropriately taken care of.

Effective criteria for admission of a child with acute head injury should include the following:

1. A history of loss of consciousness or lethargy
2. Skull fracture
3. Labile physiologic response such as vomiting, irritability, or behavioral change
4. Convulsion
5. Cerebrospinal fluid leak
6. Caretakers who do not appear able to observe the child at home adequately
7. The lack of an adequate history, which should influence the decision in favor of admitting

Admission to the hospital of a child with a head injury requires that the hospital have an area for constant observation, personnel knowledgable in care of trauma, emergency equipment available for pediatric patients, a computed tomography scanner, and a readily available neurosurgeon. Pediatric endotracheal tubes and volume respirators are essential for the care of some of these children. The absence of any of these capabilities precludes admission and demands transfer of the patient to another hospital.

Children not admitted should be watched closely at home and their caretakers (parents) should be instructed to return to the hospital if the child's level of consciousness deteriorates or he or she develops signs or symptoms such as seizures, persistent vomiting, irritability, or headaches; however, one should remember that not all caretakers will follow up with the instructions given. Studies have questioned the reliability of the caretakers.

Our study discloses that only one of three caretakers carries out the instructions given. Again, this observation stresses the policy of admission—if there is any question raised about the caretakers (parents), admit the patient and observe the child yourself.

Children can be divided into two groups after admission:

*Group I:* Includes children who are alert to

lethargic and have stable vital signs and no focal neurologic deficits.

*Group II:* Includes children who show any of the following—stupor or coma, unstable vital signs, focal neurologic findings such as weakness on one side of the arm or leg, open or penetrating wound at head, and depressed skull fracture with or without leaking cerebrospinal fluid.

Although the policy is controversial, I believe that all children admitted with the diagnosis of head injury, whether minor or severe, should be examined with CT scans of the head. Skull films are useful for assessment of problems such as fracture(s) and its extent, involvement of the portion of calvarium, whether the fracture is depressed or crossing the area of middle meningeal artery, or pneumatized sinuses. However, obviously the radiographic findings contribute little to the patient's management because neither the extent nor the shape of skull fractures depicts the severity of brain injury. Therefore, it is prudent, when possible, to obtain computed scans in all head injuries that require hospital admission.

The immediate care for children in Group I should include close observation at a care facility where vital signs and neurologic status can be checked frequently and a proper nurse/patient ratio is available. Observations should include:

1. Level of consciouness
2. Size, equality, reactions of pupils
3. Movement of the extremities
4. Of course, vital signs such as blood pressure and pulse rate.

Until the child is determined to be stable, frequent observations should be recorded. A pulse monitor with an alarm is very useful. A shock-like state with hypotension and tachycardia is very unusual in head-injured children except if systemic injury (major organ injury) has occurred. However, very young children can lose enough blood into the subgaleal space (cephalhematoma, subperiosteal hematoma) or intracranial space to produce a shock-like state. Obviously, other sources of blood loss should be sought when this occurs in older children. Conversely, hypertension and bradycardia (Cushing's phenomenon) are early indicators of an expanding intracranial mass lesion or diffuse cerebral edema with increased intracranial pressure.

The changes in blood pressure and pulse usually are progressive. Therefore, when Cushing's phenomenon is noted one should not only increase the frequency of vital signs check but also repeat the CT scan to rule in or out intracranial hematoma (epidural or acute subdural) or diffuse cerebral edema or post-traumatic hydrocephalus.

Some children may require intravenous fluids because of persistent vomiting. The intake, output, and electrolytes of these children should be watched closely. Inappropriate antidiuretic hormone (SIADH) syndrome is seen occasionally after a head injury in children. Confusion, alterations in level of consciousness, and seizures can be precipitated by the ensuing hyponatremia. Profound hyponatremia with seizures can cause irreversible damage to the central nervous system. If profound hyponatremia exists and the child is symptomatic, 3% saline may be used to restore normal serum osmolality. Occasionally, diabetes insipidus occurs following a head injury. It is usually transient and seldom requires the use of antidiuretic hormones.

Group II patients include those children who have obvious or suspected surgical lesions and need immediate further diagnostic studies to determine whether a surgical lesion exists. A delayed hematoma (usually subdural, rarely epidural) can occur, usually within the first 24 to 48 hours following head injury.

Little can be done to correct diffuse axonal injuries of brain. Damage is already done, but expanding hematomas, advancing cerebral edema, cerebral ischemia, hypoxia, hypercarbia, open wounds, and depressed skull fractures can be controlled and corrected.

The initial management of comatose or unconscious children is designed to resuscitate the child and prevent further damage of the brain due to hypoxia, ischemia, or intracranial mass lesions. Obviously, the first step is to establish an *airway*! Essentially all comatose children should have an endotracheal tube placed immediately. All children who are in a coma or with a history of multiple or associated neck injury should be managed as if they have spine instability or spinal cord injury until proved otherwise. One should choose an appropriate size of endotracheal tube. A quick reference is the size of the patient's nostril. The child's head should be held and a slight traction should be applied in line with the long axis of the body while intubation is performed. Slight or minimum extension with a small roll under the shoulder is permissible in the young child, but flexion must be avoided. Immobilization of the neck should be carried out at the scene of the accident. A firm collar should be applied, or the child should be placed on a hard board with sandbags on either side of the head and tape across the forehead to immobilize the head and neck. When endotracheal intubation is deemed not to be the best route for an airway in a situation such as associated maxillofacial injury, one should not hesitate to perform tracheostomy. Tissue hypoxia and hypercarbia compound any intracranial insult. One should make sure that the patient is breathing well or is ventilated properly.

The next step is to make sure the heart is beating properly. Obtain venous access and begin fluid resuscitation and send blood for typing and cross-matching. Isotonic crystalloid should be given in amounts necessary to make the child euvolemic. Children with head injury should not be kept dry.

Cerebral vasculature dilates in response to the fall in pH. As the $PCO_2$ increases, so does intracranial pressure, and a previously delicate balance may shift toward rapid deterioration. Hyperventilation leads to a decline in the $PCO_2$, an increase in the pH, and cerebro vascular constriction.

Hyperventilation is an effective way to rapidly reduce intracranial pressure. Unlike in the adult, the cerebral vasculature of children remains sensitive to hyperventilation for several days, and controlled ventilation may be used to reduce intracranial pressure for long periods of time.

If the airway is well established and the vital signs are stable, the next step is to get a CT scan of the head to determine if there is an intracranial mass.

Magnetic resonance imaging (MRI) is another valuable tool in the evaluation of traumatic lesions of the brain. In view of its precise anatomic and pathologic sensitivity, MRI is useful in patients with head injury in whom CT scans fail to demonstrate anatomic substrate for the degrees of coma or neurologic deficits. MRI can define a small subdural hematoma not detectable on CT scans or show axonal injuries in the white matter of the brain. However, many of these lesions may not be of any clinical significance. MRI with its current prolonged scan time is unlikely to supplant the CT scan for the diagnosis of acute head injury or to improve the outcome of injured patients. Rather, it is of great prognostic value, and permits an appreciation of the spectrum of diffuse axonal injuries.

The Glasgow coma scale (GCS) has been widely accepted and used as an objective neurologic assessment of head injury patients (Table 1). However, this scale has a limited usefulness for children under 3 years of age. The assessment of the "eye opening response" is applicable for patients of any age. However, in assessing a "best motor response," caution is required with infants to differentiate "withdrawn" or "flexion" of all extremities from true "localization to pain."

A more obvious problem is the "verbal response" in neonates and infants. The subscoring system of the GCS "best verbal response" needs modification for use in children under 36 months of age.

### TABLE 1. Glasgow Coma Scale (Recommended for Age 4–Adult)

|  | Score |
|---|---|
| **Eyes** | |
| *Open* | |
| Spontaneously | 4 |
| To verbal command | 3 |
| To pain | 2 |
| No response | 1 |
| **Best Motor Response** | |
| *To Verbal Command* | |
| Obeys | 6 |
| *To Painful Stimulus* | |
| Localizes pain | 5 |
| Flexion-withdrawal | 4 |
| Flexion—abnormal | 3 |
| Extension | 2 |
| No response | 1 |
| **Best Verbal Response** | |
| Oriented and converses | 5 |
| Disoriented and converses | 4 |
| Inappropriate words | 3 |
| Incomprehensible sounds | 2 |
| No response | 1 |
| **GCS Total** | 3–15 |

The Children's Coma Scale (modified GCS) is given in Table 2.

The GCS should be used at a reasonably early time after the injury or at the initial neurologic assessment as soon as the care for the airway, establishment of circulation, and venous access are achieved.

### TABLE 2. Children's Coma Scale (Modified Glasgow Coma Scale; Recommended for Age 3 and Younger)

|  |  | Score |
|---|---|---|
| **Eye Opening** | | |
| Spontaneous | | 4 |
| Reaction to speech | | 3 |
| Reaction to pain | | 2 |
| No response | | 1 |
| **Best Motor Response** | | |
| Spontaneous (obeys verbal command) | | 6 |
| Localizes pain | | 5 |
| Withdraws in response to pain | | 4 |
| Abnormal flexion in response to pain (decorticate posture) | | 3 |
| Abnormal extension in response to pain (decerebrate posture) | | 2 |
| No response | | 1 |
| **Best Verbal Response** | | |
| Smiles, oriented to sound, follows objects, interacts | | 5 |
| **Crying** | **Interacts** | |
| Consolable | Inappropriate | 4 |
| Inconsistently consolable | Moaning | 3 |
| Inconsolable | Irritable, restless | 2 |
| No response | No response | 1 |
| **CCS Total** | | 3–15 |

The lack of cooperation by a child makes the neurologic examination difficult. The initial examination is most crucial. Be sure to watch for spontaneous reactions of the child. You can obtain a great deal of findings by careful observations. Make brief but repeated examinations rather than one long perfect examination.

After the child has been resuscitated and it is determined that the child does not have a surgical lesion yet the GCS scoring is 3 to 8 (severe head injury), intracranial pressure (ICP) monitoring is indicated. This monitoring has potential benefit and very little risk to the child. The effectiveness of the various treatments for children with severe head injury, such as hyperventilation and osmotherapy, may be impossible to evaluate without an ICP monitor, and the deterioration due to a slowly expanding epidural or subdural hematoma or cerebral edema cannot be detected without ICP monitoring in comatose patients or medically paralyzed patients. Monitoring ICP has demonstrated that the clinical state of a patient does not always reflect the ICP. Although almost all patients who are developing midbrain dysfunction show a simultaneous elevation of ICP, many patients with elevated ICP and even with plateau waves do not show signs of neurologic deterioration. As cerebrovascular tone begins to fail, systemic arterial pressure, which is usually elevated at this point, gains impeached entry into the intracranial compartment. If the resistance vessels are capable of response to a decrease in blood $PCO_2$, hyperventilation or osmotherapy may reduce ICP and rescue the child. However, if the resistance vessels are permanently damaged as a result of ischemia, vasoconstrictor tone is lost, vasoparalysis ensues, and vessels dilate passively to the systemic blood flow. Ultimately, mean systemic arterial pressure and ICP become equal, whereupon cerebral blood flow ceases and the child dies.

The dose of mannitol (usually 0.25 to 1.5 grams per kg of body weight) or the effect of hyperventilation (usually keeping $PCO_2$ at approximately 25 mEq) can be determined only by monitoring ICP. An arterial line allows the monitoring of systemic arterial pressure so that the cerebral perfusion pressure (the difference between ICP and systemic arterial pressure) can be maintained at a level sufficient to ensure brain perfusion. The most important early factors of the traumatic pathophysiology are brain compression and distortion rather than changes in ICP per se. The speed or rate at which such changes in brain shape occur is a major factor in determining brain dysfunction. Brain shift causes distortion of the vasculature, with edema and subsequently a decrease in cerebral blood flow. Later, as ICP approaches systemic arterial pressure, cerebral perfusion pressure falls and cerebral blood flow diminishes further.

Children with evidence of dangerously increased intracranial pressure without a surgical lesion benefit from controlled ventilation and prolonged use of hyperosmotic agents. Mannitol is usually effective only for about 72 hours because it leaks slowly across the blood-brain barrier and decreases the effective osmotic gradient.

The efficacy of barbiturates in doses to induce coma (barbiturate coma) to protect the brain is yet to be established. However, barbiturates can lower ICP in cases when hyperventilation and/or hyperosmotic agents have failed.

Before one determines if a patient has a surgical lesion, osmotic agents to reduce ICP are indicated only if the patient is deteriorating and is not responding to hyperventilation. A neurosurgeon must be available before giving mannitol. The administration of mannitol to all patients with severe head injuries is definitely contraindicated and rather dangerous. Hyperosmolar agents dehydrate the damaged brain and may allow hematomas to expand. Unless prompt surgical decompression is carried out, the rebound associated with these agents makes the state of the child with a mass lesion even worse.

If the child is in status epilepticus, this is a medical emergency. Anticonvulsant(s) such as lorazepam (Ativan), diazepam (Valium), or phenobarbital (Luminal) is indicated in doses appropriate to stopping seizures. The physician should be prepared to deal with the depressed respirations that frequently follow as a result of the postictal state and/or direct action of the medications given. Phenytoin (Dilantin) is a better drug in the awake child but has a delayed effect if given orally and is absorbed poorly from intramuscular depots. Therefore, it is most useful given as a slow intravenous infusion. Seizure medication obviously is needed; however, it would be a mistake to sedate a child to make him or her more comfortable, thereby altering the level of the child's mental state and losing this useful vital and important aspect of the observation to assess neurologic deterioration. Therefore, analgesics or narcotics that alter the child's state of consciousness should be used only when absolutely necessary.

Not everyone who develops seizure needs an anticonvulsant. The seizure that occurs right at the time of impact (impact seizure) is usually not consequential. Therefore, an anticonvulsant is indicated for children with the following:

1. Severe head injury (GCS or CCS score of 3 to 7)
2. Acute subdural hematoma
3. Diffuse cerebral edema

4. Compound depressed skull fracture (not all depressed skull fractures)

5. Seizing or past history of seizure disorder

It is essential that the acutely injured child receive adequate calories. All too often, we focus on the injury and neglect the child's nutritional needs. The caloric requirements of the injured child are increased over the normal state. If these nutritional demands are met, the rate of recovery improves and complications can be fewer.

# BRAIN TUMORS

method of
DAVID R. MACDONALD, M.D.
*University of Western Ontario and London
Regional Cancer Centre
London, Ontario, Canada*

Brain tumors may be primary (arising from the skull, meninges, intracranial blood vessels, cranial nerves, or brain) or metastatic (arising from an extracranial systemic cancer). Primary brain tumors are classified histologically according to the presumed cell of origin (Table 1). Almost two-thirds of primary brain tumors are gliomas, and most of these (almost one-half of all primary brain tumors) are histologically malignant (glioblastoma multiforme, gliosarcoma, anaplastic astrocytoma, anaplastic oligodendroglioma, anaplastic ependymoma, mixed malignant glioma). Gliomas are classified as well differentiated, anaplastic

TABLE 1. **Histologic Classification
of Primary Brain Tumors**

Gliomas
    Glioblastoma multiforme
    Gliosarcoma
    Astrocytoma
    Oligodendroglioma
    Ependymoma
    Mixed gliomas
    Optic nerve glioma
    Brain stem glioma
    Cystic cerebellar astrocytoma
Meningioma
Pituitary adenoma
Pineal tumors
    Pinealomas (pineocytoma, pineoblastoma)
    Germ cell (e.g., germinoma)
Primitive neuroectodermal tumors
    Medulloblastoma
    Cerebral neuroblastoma
Primary cerebral lymphoma (microglioma)
Choroid plexus papilloma
Craniopharyngioma
Dermoid and epidermoid tumors
Colloid cyst
Sarcoma
Nerve sheath tumors
    Neurofibroma
    Schwannoma (acoustic neuroma)

(malignant), or glioblastoma multiforme, by using the criteria of Burger and Vogel, on the basis of the degree of cellularity, pleomorphism, anaplasia, and the presence or absence of mitotic figures, vascular endothelial proliferation, and necrosis.

In North America the incidence of primary brain tumors is approximately 8 to 10 per 100,000 persons per year. There is a bimodal distribution, with an early peak in childhood (ages 5 to 10 years) and a subsequent peak in adulthood (ages 55 to 65 years). In children, two-thirds of primary brain tumors arise in the posterior fossa (cystic cerebellar astrocytomas, medulloblastomas, brain stem gliomas, ependymomas) and one-third arise supratentorially (e.g., astrocytomas, ependymomas, pineal tumors, and craniopharyngiomas). In adults the overwhelming majority of primary brain tumors arise supratentorially.

The cause of most primary brain tumors is unknown. Primary brain tumors may occur as part of a well-recognized hereditary disorder such as neurofibromatosis, tuberous sclerosis, or von Hippel–Lindau disease. Rarely, several members in one family may have primary brain tumors in the absence of one of these disorders, which raises the suspicion of a hereditary factor. In most cases, however, primary brain tumors occur sporadically, and the relatives of patients with brain tumors do not seem to be at increased risk of developing a tumor. Environmental factors, especially exposure to chemicals such as vinyl chloride, have been postulated to increase the risk for primary brain tumor, but the evidence is weak and most patients do not have a history of chemical exposure. Long-term survivors of childhood cancer who have been treated with radiotherapy or chemotherapy and children who have been treated with cranial radiation for benign disorders such as tinea capitis may also have a slightly increased risk for primary brain tumor in later life.

The incidence of most primary brain tumors is slightly higher in male than in female individuals and may be slightly higher in white than in black persons (although unequal access to health care may make apparent racial differences inaccurate). Meningiomas and pituitary adenomas occur more frequently in women than in men.

Most gliomas present subacutely, over several weeks, with signs and symptoms of increased intracranial pressure (ICP) (headaches, nausea and vomiting, confusion, altered consciousness, and papilledema) and focal neurologic deficits (e.g., seizures, aphasia, and hemiparesis) depending on the location of the tumor. Tumors may occasionally present acutely, with seizures, hemorrhage, or stroke-like events. Rarely, subfrontal, temporal lobe, or midline tumors may present insidiously, with personality change, confusion, and memory loss, and may mimic a dementing process. In children, posterior fossa tumors may present with increased ICP, obstructive hydrocephalus, cerebellar ataxia, or multiple cranial nerve palsies from brain stem dysfunction. Occasionally, a child with morning headaches, vomiting, and impaired school performance is labeled as having "school phobia" and is referred for psychologic therapy until more specific signs or symptoms develop.

Pituitary adenomas and other parasellar tumors (e.g., craniopharyngioma) may present insidiously with endocrine dysfunction (e.g., amenorrhea, galactorrhea, hypothyroidism, growth delay, acromegaly, and altered thirst) and only later produce visual impairment, cranial nerve palsies, or obstructive hydrocephalus from suprasellar extension of tumor. Pineal region tumors may present either with obstructive hydrocephalus or a dorsal midbrain syndrome (large, poorly reactive pupils and abnormal vertical gaze). Cerebellar-pontine angle tumors (acoustic neuromas, meningiomas) may present with hearing loss long before ipsilateral cerebellar ataxia, other cranial nerve palsies, or increased ICP develops.

## TREATMENT

The optimal conventional treatment for malignant gliomas is summarized in Table 2. An accurate diagnosis is vital. Patients with appropriate signs and symptoms should have a computed tomography (CT) scan of the head with and without intravenous contrast. Almost all patients who have symptomatic primary brain tumors have readily visible lesions on contrast-enhanced CT scans. Small tumors that present early with seizures and tumors in the temporal lobe tip or low in the posterior fossa may be difficult to visualize on CT scan. The diagnostic yield can sometimes be increased by using fine cuts through the appropriate area or direct coronal cuts. A magnetic resonance imaging (MRI) scan is likely more sensitive than the CT scan but may be less specific. Sagittal $T_1$-weighted, axial $T_1$-weighted, and axial $T_2$-weighted images may be required to adequately visualize tumors on the MRI scan. It may be difficult to differentiate the tumor from peritumoral edema without the use of a paramagnetic contrast agent (gadolinium-DTPA). Plain skull x-ray films, pneumoencephalography, and radionuclide brain scanning seldom provide useful additional information; in addition, lumbar puncture may be hazardous in the presence of intracranial mass lesions. Cerebral angiography is seldom required, although it may be needed to exclude vascular malformations or to determine the vascular supply of tumors before experimental therapies such as intra-arterial chemotherapy.

Corticosteroids are used to control cerebral edema and increased ICP that are associated with brain tumors. Dexamethasone (Decadron), 4 mg four times daily, is the standard initial dose. Oral

TABLE 2. **Optimal Conventional Treatment for Malignant Glioma**

Accurate localization (CT scan, MRI scan)
Corticosteroids
Anticonvulsants, anticoagulants (as needed)
Maximum feasible surgical resection
Radiotherapy (6000 cGy to tumor)
Chemotherapy (BCNU)

and intravenous doses are equivalent. The dose should be adjusted as required to control symptoms, and the lowest possible dose should be used to minimize side effects. The side effects are related to total dose, duration of therapy, and individual susceptibility. Common side effects include cushingoid face and body habitus, weight gain, fluid retention, hypertension, hyperglycemia, hypokalemia, proximal muscle weakness, oral candidiasis, osteoporosis, and aseptic bone necrosis. Acute neurologic deterioration from cerebral edema or from increased ICP may require higher doses of corticosteroids (up to 100 mg* dexamethasone intravenously) as well as intravenous mannitol (0.5 to 2 grams per kg, repeated every 6 hours) or intubation with hyperventilation. Mannitol is used only in acute situations because long-term use is precluded by loss of effectiveness and fluid and electrolyte disturbances. A ventriculoperitoneal shunt may be needed to control obstructive hydrocephalus.

Anticonvulsants are used to control seizures. Approximately 25% of patients with gliomas have seizures as part of the initial presentation, and up to 50% have seizures at some time. The use of prophylactic anticonvulsants is controversial. Phenytoin (Dilantin) is the most commonly used anticonvulsant because it is inexpensive, effective, available in oral and intravenous preparations, and can be given in a large initial loading dose. The initial loading dose is 18 mg per kg (orally or intravenously), usually about 1000 mg for an average adult, given no faster than 50 mg per minute intravenously. Most patients can be maintained on 300 to 400 mg daily, given either as a single daily dose at bedtime or as divided doses in the morning and evening. The blood level of phenytoin should be monitored and maintained in the suggested therapeutic range (10 to 20 $\mu$g per ml; 40 to 80 $\mu$mol per liter). Side effects include rash, gum hypertrophy, liver dysfunction, and intoxication (dysarthria, ataxia, and diplopia). Carbamazepine (Tegretol) is as effective as phenytoin and may have somewhat fewer side effects, but it is not available in a parenteral form, cannot be loaded, must be given in three or four divided doses, and is more expensive. The usual maintenance dose is 600 to 1200 mg daily. The therapeutic level is 4 to 12 $\mu$g per ml (17 to 40 micromoles per liter). Myelosuppression and hepatotoxicity are rare but potentially serious complications. Phenobarbital is effective and inexpensive but is not usually used as a first line anticonvulsant because of its sedative properties. The usual dose is 60 to 200 mg daily, as a single bedtime dose. The therapeutic blood level is 15

---

*This dose may exceed manufacturer's recommended dose.

to 40 μg per ml (65 to 170 μmol per liter). Primidone (Mysoline), clonazepam (Rivotril), and valproic acid (Depakene) may be useful if the above-mentioned drugs are ineffective or cannot be tolerated.

Patients with primary brain tumor are at high risk for deep vein thrombosis and pulmonary embolism, especially in the perioperative period. Prolonged bed rest should be avoided. Antiembolic stockings, intermittent pneumatic compression leggings, or subcutaneous heparin (5000 units twice daily) may help prevent deep vein thrombosis postoperatively. Most neurosurgeons are reluctant to use anticoagulants during the immediate perioperative period. Patients with deep vein thrombosis or pulmonary embolism require anticoagulation, initially continuous intravenous heparin and then warfarin (Coumadin). Excessive anticoagulation should be avoided. Optimal anticoagulation (partial thromboplastin time twice control; prothrombin time 1.5 times control) is safe in primary brain tumor patients and does not seem to increase the risk of hemorrhage in tumors.

### Surgery

The goals of surgery for primary brain tumor include determination of a histologic diagnosis to guide further therapy; maximal tumor removal; improvement of symptoms by tumor debulking and reduction of increased ICP; and provision of additional time for other treatments such as radiotherapy or chemotherapy. Some benign tumors such as meningioma, acoustic neuroma, or pituitary adenoma may be completely resectable and cured surgically. Surgery may be curative for cystic cerebellar astrocytomas, but most intraaxial tumors cannot be completely removed. In these cases the goal is to remove as much of the tumor as possible without increasing the patient's neurologic deficit. Gross total tumor resection may be possible in polar tumors that arise in the tips of the frontal, temporal, or occipital lobes; lobectomy may be appropriate in some patients. Major resections are often possible in tumors occurring centrally in the frontal, temporal, and parietal lobes. Major resections may not be possible in deep-seated tumors; however, almost any tumor can be biopsied by using stereotactic techniques. Accessible tumors should be resected rather than biopsied because survival is increased by increasing completeness of resection.

### Radiation Therapy

After surgery, radiation therapy is the primary mode of treatment for most intraparenchymal brain tumors. Although most primary brain tumors are not curable by radiotherapy alone, this treatment increases the total and tumor-free survival for most patients with incompletely resected brain tumors. Standard treatment for malignant glioma is external beam radiotherapy, 6000 cGy (rad) in 6 weeks to the tumor plus an adequate margin. Whole-brain radiotherapy for malignant glioma has generally fallen out of favor because of concerns about long-term side effects. Stereotactic radiation implants (brachytherapy) and radiosurgery (using either a linear accelerator or the Gamma-Knife) are new experimental radiotherapy techniques that are designed to deliver highly focused radiation to small brain tumors or vascular malformations. The aim is to deliver a high dose to a small area while sparing the surrounding normal brain.

The role of radiotherapy in the treatment of well-differentiated astrocytomas (low-grade gliomas) is controversial. Some retrospective studies suggest that survival is increased with focal radiotherapy (usually 5000 to 5500 cGy in 5 to 6 weeks). Radiotherapy may also prolong tumor control and increase survival in incompletely resected, recurrent, or malignant meningiomas. Focal radiotherapy is also recommended for incompletely resected pituitary adenomas or craniopharyngiomas. Radiotherapy may be curative treatment for pineal germinomas, although it is controversial whether focal or craniospinal treatment is required.

Radiotherapy prolongs survival and may be curative in patients with medulloblastoma, after surgical removal of the tumor. Standard treatment is craniospinal radiation with 5500 cGy to the posterior fossa, 3500 to 4500 cGy to the whole brain, and 3500 to 4500 cGy to the spinal neuraxis. These doses are reduced for young children. In good-risk patients (complete resection of the primary tumor and no evidence of systemic or leptomeningeal metastases), the 5-year survival is 50 to 70%.

### Chemotherapy

Chemotherapy may be given as part of the treatment for some malignant primary brain tumors, especially malignant glioma or medulloblastoma. Chemotherapy can be given as an adjuvant at the time of initial treatment or later at the time of tumor recurrence. Many chemotherapeutic agents have been tried, either singly or in combination. The standard chemotherapeutic agents for malignant glioma are the nitrosoureas, either BCNU (carmustine) or CCNU (lomustine). BCNU is given intravenously, 200 mg per $M^2$, every 6 to 8 weeks, often starting at the beginning of radiotherapy. A cumulative dose of 1500 mg per $M^2$ should not be exceeded. Common side effects include local vein irritation during infusion, transient nausea and vomiting on the days of treatment, myelosuppression (which may be delayed 4 to 6 weeks after treatment and which tends to be cumulative with increasing total dose), and pulmonary fibrosis (risk increases with increasing total cumulative dose, especially more than 1500 mg per $M^2$). CCNU is given orally at a dose of 130 mg per $M^2$ every 6 weeks. The toxicity is similar to that of BCNU. Several other agents have shown some effectiveness including AZQ (diaziquone), PCNU, procarbazine (Matulane), cisplatin (Platinol), and carboplatin (Paraplatin). We have found the combination of procarbazine, CCNU, and vincristine (Oncovin), termed PCV-3, effective. In PCV-3, CCNU is given at 110 mg per $M^2$ orally on day 1, procarbazine is given at 60 mg per $M^2$ orally daily for 14 days beginning on day 8 (days 8 to 21), and vincristine is given at 1.4 mg per $M^2$ (maximum 2.5 mg) intravenously on days 8 and 29. Cycles are repeated every 6 to 8 weeks according to blood cell counts. Gliomas vary in their chemosensitivity; anaplastic oligodendroglioma is a particularly chemosensitive tumor, especially to PCV-3.

Chemotherapy is being increasingly used in combination with radiotherapy in the treatment of children with brain tumors, especially high-risk medulloblastoma or malignant glioma, and in very young children (younger than 3 years of age) instead of cranial radiotherapy. Effective combinations include: PCV-3; cisplatin plus etoposide (VP-16); CCNU, vincristine, and cisplatin; and the "8 in 1" (eight drugs in 1 day) regimen.

Experimental chemotherapy includes intra-arterial chemotherapy (usually BCNU or cisplatin), high-dose chemotherapy (sometimes with autologous bone marrow transplantation), osmotic opening of the blood-brain barrier with mannitol followed by chemotherapy, intralesional infusion chemotherapy, and the use of new agents. Biologic response modifiers, such as interferon (especially interferon-alpha), interleukin-2, lymphokine-activated killer cells, and monoclonal antibodies, are under study. None of these new approaches has yet proved to be more effective than standard systemic chemotherapy.

## PROGNOSIS

Malignant glioma is almost always fatal. Data from published multicenter clinical trials (which may be more optimistic than "real life" because of selection bias that favors good-risk patients in many clinical trials) indicate that the median survival after surgery alone is 3 to 4 months and that few patients survive more than 6 months. The median survival for surgery followed by radiotherapy is 8 to 10 months, but only 5 to 10% of patients survive 18 months. The addition of BCNU chemotherapy to surgery and radiotherapy increases the median survival modestly, to approximately 12 months, but increases the 18-month survival to 25 to 30%. The survival is better for anaplastic astrocytoma than for glioblastoma. Favorable prognostic features include young age (under 45 years) at diagnosis, anaplastic astrocytoma (versus glioblastoma), major or complete surgical resection (versus biopsy alone), good functional status after surgery (Karnofsky's performance status 80 or better), presentation with seizures, and a history of prior low-grade glioma.

In most patients, the tumor eventually recurs. Possible treatments at the time of recurrence include repeat resection (especially if the functional status is good), brachytherapy, and alternate chemotherapy. Radiation necrosis of brain may mimic recurrence of malignant glioma both clinically and radiologically. Neither the CT nor the MRI scan can reliably differentiate radiation necrosis from recurrent tumor; positron-emission tomography may be able to make this distinction. Surgical resection or corticosteroids may be effective therapy for radiation necrosis.

## BRAIN METASTASES

Brain metastases may occur in up to 15 to 20% of all patients with systemic cancer. As the treatment for systemic cancer has improved and survival has increased, the incidence of metastatic brain tumor has also increased. The most common sites of primary cancer that are metastatic to brain are lung, breast, skin (melanoma), kidney, and colon. Up to 40% of patients with small cell carcinoma of lung (oat cell carcinoma) develop brain metastases, and up to 70% of patients dying of metastatic melanoma have at least autopsy evidence of brain metastases. Brain metastasis is usually a late manifestation of systemic cancer but may occasionally produce the initial presenting symptoms of cancer.

Metastatic tumors present as any other intracranial mass, with signs and symptoms of increased ICP or focal neurologic disturbances, or both. Seizures are common. Metastatic brain tumors are single in one-half of patients affected; approximately 80% occur supratentorially, 15% in the cerebellum and 5% in the brain stem. The initial treatment is dexamethasone to control cerebral edema and increased ICP. Patients with a single accessible brain metastasis who are stable or have no systemic disease often benefit from surgical resection followed by postoperative whole-brain radiation. Patients with multiple brain metastases or patients in whom surgical resection is inappropriate are treated with whole-brain radiotherapy. Standard treatment regimens include 2000 cGy in 5 fractions or 3000 cGy in 10 fractions. Most patients respond to corticosteroids and cranial radiation; however, the survival is poor because most patients die of progressive systemic cancer. The median survival is 3 months after radiation therapy for patients with nonresected tumors (1-year survival is 15%). Rarely, brain metastases can be cured after radiotherapy. The median survival for patients with a resected single metastasis followed by radiotherapy is approximately 12 months.

Systemic chemotherapy has been attempted in some patients with brain metastases, especially those from carcinoma of the breast or small cell carcinoma of the lung. The response and survival rates are similar to those for cranial radiation therapy. No prospective randomized trials comparing radiotherapy with chemotherapy or radiotherapy plus chemotherapy have been reported. Chemotherapy would be feasible only for tumors for which effective systemic chemotherapy is available.

## CENTRAL NERVOUS SYSTEM LYMPHOMA

Systemic lymphomas seldom spread to the parenchyma of the brain. Non-Hodgkin's lymphoma may involve the leptomeninges or the spinal or intracranial epidural space. Hodgkin's disease rarely involves the central nervous system.

Primary central nervous system lymphomas (microglioma, reticulum cell sarcoma) were once considered to be extremely rare. These tumors present with clinical and radiologic features similar to those of malignant gliomas. They often involve the deep periventricular regions, may be multifocal, and may occur with ocular lymphomas. The incidence is increased in patients with chronic immunosuppression (such as after renal transplantation), and most are B cell in origin. Primary central nervous system lymphomas develop in 2 to 3% of all patients with acquired immunodeficiency syndrome (AIDS). The incidence of these primary lymphomas seems to be increasing in both the AIDS and non-AIDS populations. These tumors are often responsive to corticosteroids, and prolonged remissions may occur after use of steroids only, although the tumors eventually recur despite steroid therapy. Surgery is diagnostic but not curative. Cranial radiation therapy, usually 5000 to 6000 cGy in 6 weeks, is standard. Patients with clinical or cerebrospinal fluid evidence of leptomeningeal seeding are treated with craniospinal radiation or with intrathecal or intraventricular (via an Ommaya reservoir) chemotherapy with methotrexate or cytarabine (ara C). These tumors may be chemosensitive. A variety of chemotherapeutic regimens, usually similar to those used for systemic lymphoma (e.g., MOPP, CHOP), have been reported to have at least some effectiveness. Combinations of chemotherapy and radiotherapy may be more effective than radiotherapy alone. The average survival after radiotherapy for non-AIDS patients with central nervous system lymphoma is 1 to 2 years but is less than 6 months in AIDS patients, usually because of concurrent systemic illnesses.

# The Locomotor System

## RHEUMATOID ARTHRITIS

method of
NANCY JOSEPH LANCE, M.D., and
MICHAEL H. ELLMAN, M.D.
*Michael Reese Hospital and Medical Center*
*Chicago, Illinois*

Rheumatoid arthritis is a chronic disease with a prevalence of 0.3 to 1.5% in the United States. It affects women two to three times more often than men and can occur at any age, with the peak incidence between 30 and 60 years of age. The etiology remains unknown. The disease is characterized by symmetric inflammation of the peripheral joints, especially the small joints of the hands and the wrists. The inflammation almost always leads to joint destruction. Treatment is directed toward suppressing the inflammation early in the course of the disease with disease-modifying medications, thereby delaying joint destruction and deformities.

### DIAGNOSIS

The physical examination reveals symmetrical polyarticular arthritis with palpable synovial thickening, especially of the wrists and the small joints of the hands and the feet. The distal interphalangeal joints of the hands are spared early in the course of the disease. Large joint involvement usually occurs late. Axial skeleton involvement other than atlantoaxial subluxation is unusual. Subcutaneous nodules, especially on the extensor surface of the forearm, are often present. Other findings include a positive rheumatoid factor test in approximately 75% of patients and characteristic radiographic changes consisting of periarticular osteopenia, joint space narrowing, and bony erosions. Systemic symptoms such as fatigue and morning stiffness are usually present.

Extra-articular manifestations may include pericarditis, pleural effusions, the sicca complex, and episcleritis. A Baker's or popliteal cyst is common and may leak synovial fluid into the calf, producing leg swelling and inflammation mimicking thrombophlebitis. Diagnosis of this "pseudothrombophlebitis" can be made with ultrasound examination or arthrography. Treatment includes intra-articular steroids and rest. Vasculitis may occur, often presenting with mononeuritis multiplex and digital and leg ulcers. Felty's syndrome is uncommon. It is characterized by leukopenia, thrombocytopenia, splenomegaly, and leg ulcers. These patients are at high risk for developing gram-positive cocci infections.

Atlantoaxial subluxation may occur in rheumatoid arthritis. The most common early symptom is pain radiating upward into the occiput. Later symptoms include paresthesias of the arms and hands, slowly progressive spastic quadriparesis, and transient episodes of medullary dysfunction that may result in changes in the level of consciousness and syncope. Diagnosis is established with lateral x-ray films of the cervical spine in flexion. Magnetic resonance imaging can confirm the high spinal cord compression and detect superior migration of the odontoid process into the foramen magnum. Asymptomatic patients and those with mild symptoms may be treated with a soft cervical collar; firm collars should be used for better stabilization when symptoms and signs progress. Surgical stabilization should be considered for severe or progressive neurologic involvement.

### TREATMENT

After rheumatoid arthritis is diagnosed, it is essential to discuss the disease process and management approach with the patient. There are no cures; response to medications may be maddeningly slow. Patient literature, self-help and support group information, exercise tapes, etc., are available from the local and national chapters of the Arthritis Foundation. Also essential is a multidisciplinary approach to patients, consisting of physical and occupational therapy, social work, orthopedic surgery, and nursing. It is our observation that primary care physicians often neglect the essential role of the team approach in the management of rheumatoid arthritis.

Rest is essential for relief of fatigue and reduction of joint inflammation. We ask our patients to try to spend 30 to 60 minutes lying down during the late morning or early afternoon. We also recommend a well-balanced diet, although there is no causal relationship between diet and the development or outcome of rheumatoid arthritis.

Pain management without medications may be employed by physical and occupational therapists. This may include application of hot packs, hydrotherapy, and infrared treatments. Ultrasound may also be used to provide heat therapy. Cold therapy is often used to relieve muscle spasm and reduce joint swelling. Application of electrical stimuli with a transcutaneous electrical nerve stimulation (TENS) unit has also been used to decrease pain; it is noninvasive and safe.

Physical and occupational therapists help guide the patient through exercise programs that aid in muscle strengthening and increase joint range of motion. Splints are important in reducing pain and preserving function. There are few rheumatoid patients in our practice who do not require wrist splinting. The splints are placed to help relieve pain and maintain wrist extension and to treat carpal tunnel syndrome, if present. Devices such as walkers and canes that aid in ambulation when lower extremity joints are painful are helpful in maintaining independence.

Patients with rheumatoid arthritis are no longer admitted to the acute care hospital for bed rest and physical therapy during disease flares, although bed rest is beneficial. Most hospitalizations occur when a patient has complications of the disease, such as new onset of pleural effusion, vasculitis, and pericarditis. Many patients are receiving immunosuppressive medications, so that infections must be promptly diagnosed and treated.

### Medical Therapy

Current medical therapy encompasses a pyramidal system that institutes first-line agents such as aspirin or other nonsteroidal anti-inflammatory medications (NSAIDs) at the base (Table 1) and ends with experimental therapies. Aspirin and NSAIDs are generally not considered remittive agents. If the patient has joint erosions on x-ray films, progressing disability, and pain, disease-modifying agents should be started (Table 2). These medications include gold sodium thio-

TABLE 1. **Nonsalicylate Nonsteroidal Anti-inflammatory Drugs Frequently Used in Rheumatoid Arthritis**

| | |
|---|---|
| Propionic acid | |
|   Fenoprofen (Nalfon) | 400–600 mg qid |
|   Ibuprofen (Motrin) | 400–800 mg qid |
|   Naproxen (Naprosyn) | 250–750 mg bid |
|   Ketoprofen (Orudis) | 50–75 mg tid |
| Indolacetic acid | |
|   Indomethacin (Indocin) | 25–50 mg tid |
|   Indomethacin SR (Indocin SR) | 75 mg once or twice per day |
|   Sulindac (Clinoril) | 150–200 mg bid |
|   Tolmetin (Tolectin) | 400–600 mg tid |
| Oxicam | |
|   Piroxicam (Feldene) | 10–20 mg/day |
| Phenylacetic acid | |
|   Diclofenac sodium (Voltaren) | 50–75 mg bid |

*Note:* We recommend that nonsteroidals be taken with food or antacids.

TABLE 2. **Disease-Modifying Antirheumatic Drugs***

| Medications | Dosage | Comments |
|---|---|---|
| Gold sodium thiomalate (Myochrysine) Aurothioglucose (Solganal) | 50 mg/week IM | Usually our first-line agent |
| Auranofin (Ridaura) | 3 mg bid PO | Used in early disease; not as effective as IM gold |
| Hydroxychloroquine (Plaquenil) | 200 mg/day PO | Used in early disease; well tolerated |
| Penicillamine (Cuprimine, Depen) | 250–750 mg/day PO | Used in more advanced disease or in gold failure |
| Sulfasalazine (Azulfidine) | 1–2 grams/day PO | Effective anti-inflammatory agent |
| Methotrexate (Rheumatrex) | 5–20 mg/week PO or IM | Used first in severe disease and when other drugs fail |
| Azathioprine (Imuran) | 1.5–2.5 mg/kg/day PO | Effective in refractory rheumatoid arthritis; used often as a steroid-sparing agent |
| Cyclophosphamide (Cytoxan) | 1–2 mg/kg/day PO 500–750 mg/M²/month IV | Effective in refractory arthritis; usually used in arthritis complicated with vasculitis; toxic |

*Complete drug information must be read before use of these medicines.

malatin (Myochrysine), hydroxychloroquine (Plaquenil), penicillamine (Cuprimine, Depen), and sulfasalazine (Azulfidine). Low-dose corticosteroids (prednisone [Deltasone], 5 mg) may be initiated during this period to decrease inflammation, reduce morning stiffness, and "bridge" the time until the disease-modifying drugs become effective. If a patient fails to respond to a trial of these agents, immunosuppressive agents may be used. These include azathioprine (Imuran), methotrexate, and cyclophosphamide (Cytoxan). Patients who do not respond to this therapy may undergo more experimental forms of treatment. These include use of total lymph node radiation or combination medical therapy with agents such as methotrexate and azathioprine or hydroxychloroquine.

Newer and unconventional therapies are being used more frequently. Rather than initiate therapy with gold or hydroxychloroquine, immunosuppressive drugs, especially methotrexate, may be used early in the disease process to prevent further joint damage. If there is no response or disease progression occurs, another immunosuppressive agent or remittive agent may be added to methotrexate. Multiple drugs in lower dosages may decrease potential toxicities of each specific medication. Combination chemotherapy also allows for the use of multiple drugs with different mechanisms of action to be used simultaneously. Cyclophosphamide or even cyclosporine (Sandimmune) may be used if other medications fail. As opposed to conventional therapy, this protocol, described earlier, may decrease inflammation quicker and more completely.

It is our policy to use conventional drug regimens in rheumatoid arthritis patients, starting with gold or hydroxychloroquine and later using penicillamine as the second-line treatment after nonsteroidal agents; only if these fail do we use immunosuppressive medications. Patients seen initially with advanced or rapidly progressive disease may be treated earlier with immunosuppressive medications, especially methotrexate.

### Medications

**Salicylates.** Aspirin may be used as the initial anti-inflammatory agent. There are many properties of aspirin that make it attractive. It is relatively inexpensive, it is easily available, serum levels are easily measurable, and it is well tolerated in most patients.

The usual initial adult dosage is 3.6 grams in four divided daily doses. This should be taken with meals and snacks. The dosage may be increased after 5 to 7 days by one or two tablets until relief is obtained or tinnitus occurs.

The most common side effect is gastrointestinal discomfort. Enteric-coated aspirin (Ecotrin) or aspirin combined with antacids may reduce these symptoms. Another common side effect is tinnitus, which is especially frequent in elderly patients. This may be reversed by decreasing the dosage. Contraindications to salicyclates include a history of a peptic ulcer, upper gastrointestinal bleeding, and allergy. We use the prostaglandin $E_1$ analogue misoprostol (Cytotec) for gastric protection in patients with a history of gastrointestinal bleeding who require aspirin or other anti-inflammatory agents. Aspirin hypersensitivity remains an infrequent but serious problem. The clinical presentation of hypersensitivity includes asthma, nasal polyps, and even anaphylaxis. Compliance is a potential problem with aspirin because of the large doses and frequent dosing necessary for its anti-inflammatory effect.

Nonacetylated salicylates have less prolonged effects on platelets and may have fewer gastrointestinal complications. These drugs include sodium salicylate, salsalate (Disalcid), and choline magnesium trisalicylate (Trilisate). We generally do not find these drugs to be as effective as aspirin. In patients with aspirin hypersensitivity, these drugs must be used with caution.

Laboratory testing should be performed periodically and includes complete blood and platelet counts, serum creatinine determinations, and liver enzyme tests.

**Nonsteroidal Anti-inflammatory Drugs.** The NSAIDs are effective anti-inflammatory agents. They inhibit prostaglandin synthesis as effectively as aspirin. They are usually better tolerated than aspirin, but are more expensive.

Side effects of all of the NSAIDs are generally the same because of their inhibition of prostaglandin synthesis. The most common side effect is gastrointestinal toxicity. These drugs, however, may produce significantly less gastrointestinal bleeding than aspirin. However, gastric ulceration and perforation may occur. The incidence of gastrointestinal bleeding increases with the duration of treatment.

The NSAIDs decrease renal blood flow and may cause renal insufficiency in patients with pre-existing renal diseases, those receiving diuretic medicines, and patients with hypertension, cirrhosis, or congestive heart failure. Direct drug toxicity may cause nephrotic syndrome, interstitial nephritis, or renal papillary necrosis. Central nervous system toxicity with NSAIDs includes confusion, headache, drowsiness, depression, anxiety, and dizziness.

Mild hepatic dysfunction with asymptomatic elevation of aminotransferase levels is common. Rarely does severe hepatitis occur. The hepatic dysfunction usually reverses on discontinuation of the drug. Rarely reported side effects are pancreatitis; blood dyscrasias, including aplastic anemia; and dermatologic toxicities, including toxic epidermal necrolysis.

**Gold.** Gold salts have been used for more than 50 years to retard the progression of disease in rheumatoid arthritis. Parenteral forms of gold, gold sodium thiomalate (Myochrysine) and aurothioglucose (Solganal), are given intramuscularly. The regimen we use includes a 5-mg, and then a 25-mg, test dose, which is followed by a weekly 50-mg dose. This is administered until a total dose of 1000 mg is achieved. If there is no improvement at this time, we stop the medication. The dosing interval is decreased to every 2 weeks, then every 3 weeks, and finally once every 4 weeks in those patients with good responses. If there are no side effects and good response continues, we continue gold therapy indefinitely.

Drug toxicity occurring with gold is relatively common. Gold sodium thiomalate may cause a "nitritoid" reaction characterized by flushing, fainting, headache, and nausea. This usually occurs immediately after injection. The most common side effect with gold is a dermatitis that is mild and usually preceded by pruritus. We make it a habit to ask about itching prior to each gold injection. Exfoliative dermatitis is rare. Stomatitis, which is also relatively common, usually occurs after the rash. These adverse reactions are usually reversible with cessation of the drug. At times, lower dosages of gold may be reinstituted while closely monitoring for recurrence of side effects.

Proteinuria is a manifestation of renal toxicity. Mild proteinuria may occur, but nephrotic syndrome, although rare, can happen. These manifestations are usually reversible with discontinuation of the drug.

Other toxicities due to gold administration include leukopenia, thrombocytopenia, aplastic anemia, interstitial pneumonitis, anaphylaxis, and angioneurotic edema. These require prompt discontinuation of therapy. Hepatitis, cholestatic jaundice, colitis, and pancreatitis have also been reported.

Oral gold, auranofin (Ridaura), is also available for use. We usually start with one tablet daily for the first 1 to 2 weeks. The maintenance dose is 3 mg twice daily. The most common side effect is diarrhea. Other toxicities such as nephrotic syndrome and hematologic abnormalities occur less often than with injectable gold. We think oral gold is less effective than injectable gold, and to be effective, it must be started early in the course of rheumatoid arthritis.

For both injectable and oral gold, complete blood and platelet counts and urinalysis should be monitored frequently, usually every 2 weeks initially for injectable gold and then once a month. Monthly testing is suggested for patients taking oral gold.

It is our opinion that gold therapy remains the mainstay of the treatment of rheumatoid arthritis. We think it should be used early and often in patients. Family members can be trained in the administration of the parenteral forms.

**Hydroxychloroquine.** The antimalarial hydroxychloroquine (Plaquenil) is easy to administer, is well tolerated, and has relatively few side effects. The maintenance dosage is usually 200 mg per day. It takes about 1 to 3 months before a response is noticed.

The major potential side effect of hydroxychloroquine is retinal toxicity. This manifests with loss of vision to red light and decreasing visual fields, potentially progressing to blindness. Patients being evaluated for the use of hydroxychloroquine require a baseline ophthalmologic examination. This evaluation must include visual field examination and color vision acuity. This should be repeated every 6 months. If any visual changes occur, the drug must be discontinued. Patients may even be given an Amsler's grid for home eye examination to measure visual fields, field distortions, and the size of the blind spot. Other eye involvement includes corneal deposits and ciliary body dysfunction. These usually resolve with discontinuation of hydroxychloroquine.

Side effects with hydroxychloroquine, such as hematologic abnormalities, central nervous system dysfunction, and dermatologic reactions, are serious but usually occur with higher dosages than those used in rheumatoid arthritis and are uncommon in our experience.

**D-Penicillamine.** D-Penicillamine is an effective medication that we consider more toxic than gold or hydroxychloroquine. The recommended initial dosage is 125 or 250 mg orally once a day. The dosage is slowly increased by 250 mg every 6 weeks to 750 mg daily in divided doses. Because of decreased absorption with food, D-penicillamine is usually taken between meals.

There are multiple drug toxicities that have been noted with D-penicillamine. The most common side effect is dermatitis. Other common side effects include a decrease in taste (hypogeusia), gastric irritation, fever, rash, and oral ulcers. These effects are usually reversible with discontinuation or reduction of medicine.

Hematologic abnormalities, including leukopenia and thrombocytopenia, may occur. Proteinuria occurs relatively frequently, usually with losses of less than 500 mg of protein in 24 hours. The drug may be continued, but frequent monitoring is required. At higher levels of proteinuria, the drug should be discontinued. The proteinuria is usually reversible, but may take months to resolve.

Other less common side effects include myasthenia gravis, Goodpasture's syndrome, pemphigus, bronchiolitis obliterans, cholestatic jaundice, and a lupus-like illness.

Laboratory data that should be monitored include complete blood and platelet counts and urinalysis every 2 weeks initially. When results are stable, laboratory testing should be monitored every 4 weeks.

**Sulfasalazine.** Sulfasalazine (Azulfidine) has been used primarily in the treatment of inflammatory bowel disease. It has been found to be an effective anti-inflammatory agent in rheumatoid arthritis. The sulfa moiety confers its activity. The usual dosage is 2 grams per day. We start at 500 mg daily and increase by 500 mg on a weekly basis until response or 2 grams per day is reached. Side effects include dermatitis and gastrointestinal disturbances. Sulfa allergy is a contraindication to its use. Renal stones may occur. Hematologic abnormalities and hepatitis may occur, but are uncommon. We advise monthly complete blood and platelet counts, urinalysis, and liver enzyme tests for monitoring.

**Methotrexate.** Methotrexate is an immunosuppressive drug that is effective in treating rheumatoid arthritis. This drug often is effective quickly (about 2 to 6 weeks). It is given orally (or intramuscularly) once a week. We start with 5 to 7.5 mg orally initially. If no response is obtained, we increase the dosage by 2.5 mg every 2 to 3 weeks until a maximal dosage of 20 mg per week is attained.

When immunosuppressive medication is required, we use methotrexate first. This drug is usually well tolerated. Compliance is good. It is our drug of choice for moderate to severe rheumatoid arthritis that has not responded adequately to other medications.

Methotrexate binds dihydrofolate reductase, causing depletion of active intracellular folate. Low folate levels may account for such side effects as pancytopenia, gastrointestinal intolerance, and stomatitis. We provide folic acid supplementation (1 mg per day) to patients with low or low-normal folate levels.

Methotrexate has many potential serious side effects. Because of its predominantly renal excretion, it is contraindicated in patients with renal impairment. The most feared side effect is hepatic toxicity. The most common finding has been transient increases in aminotransferase levels. On liver biopsy specimens, fatty infiltration and inflammation may be found. Rarely has severe fibrosis occurred, and cirrhosis due solely to once-weekly methotrexate dosing is rare.

Other side effects that occur include mucositis and gastrointestinal bleeding due to ulceration. Nausea is common on the day of drug administration. Bone marrow suppression, interstitial pneumonitis, headache, and alopecia may occur, but are uncommon. Methotrexate is a known teratogen and should be avoided in pregnancy.

Laboratory values that should be obtained monthly are complete blood and platelet counts and liver enzyme tests.

**Azathioprine.** Azathioprine (Imuran) is also an immunosuppressive drug that is effective in treating refractory rheumatoid arthritis. The dose is usually 1.5 to 2.5 mg per kg per day. We usually start with 50 mg daily and do not increase it until 4 to 6 weeks later and then at 25- or 50-mg increments. Onset of action is slow, usually 3 months. We usually prescribe azathioprine in patients failing to respond to, or who are intolerant of, methotrexate.

Azathioprine is converted to 6-mercaptopurine, and this purine analogue inhibits nucleic acid synthesis. Metabolism of 6-mercaptopurine involves oxidation by xanthine oxidase, which is inhibited by allopurinol (Zyloprim), a reversible xanthine oxidase inhibitor. Caution and reduction of azathioprine dosages are needed if allopurinol use is required.

Azathioprine has potentially serious side ef-

fects in the dosage range used for rheumatoid arthritis. Gastrointestinal toxicities include nausea, vomiting, pancreatitis, and hepatitis. Bone marrow depression leading to pancytopenia may occur. Although rare, there is the possibility of malignancy developing with the use of azathioprine.

We monitor drug toxicity with complete blood and platelet counts every 2 weeks initially and then every month when the patient and the drug dosage are stable.

**Cyclophosphamide.** Cyclophosphamide (Cytoxan) is an immunosuppressive agent that is also used in patients with refractory arthritis. Although we use it infrequently, it often ameliorates rheumatoid arthritis when other drugs have failed. This drug is most commonly used by us in the treatment of rheumatoid vasculitis. Cyclophosphamide may be given orally at a dosage of 1 to 2 mg per kg per day or as an intravenous monthly pulse dose of 500 to 750 mg per $M^2$ of body surface area.

There are many serious toxic side effects. These include bone marrow depression, hemorrhagic cystitis, bladder cancer, and other malignancies. Other potential side effects include sterility and renal and hepatic toxicity. Alopecia is common.

Careful monitoring of laboratory data is essential. We recommend complete blood and platelet counts every 2 weeks initially and then once a month. It is our opinion that a rheumatologist should be consulted prior to using cyclophosphamide.

**Corticosteroids.** Corticosteroids are effective for the short-term treatment of rheumatoid arthritis, but, because of serious side effects, they should be used with caution. As systemic anti-inflammatory agents, they may be used as a "bridge" until the disease-modifying medications work. We use 5 mg of prednisone in most of our patients. After the disease-modifying agent has attained effect, the corticosteroids should be tapered and discontinued if possible. This is often difficult. Patients with vasculitis and other extra-articular manifestations require higher dosages of corticosteroids, often in combination with a cytotoxic agent.

Multiple adverse effects are associated with the long-term use of corticosteroids. These include gastrointestinal bleeding, cataracts, weight gain, and poor wound healing. Higher dosages are associated with hypertension, glucose intolerance, psychosis, avascular bone necrosis, and increased infections. The long-term use of corticosteroids in rheumatoid arthritis patients is particularly associated with osteoporosis. Calcium and vitamin D supplementation should be considered.

Intra-articular steroids are exceptionally beneficial in active persistent synovitis. The dosage varies from 10 to 30 mg of a long-acting preparation, such as prednisone tebutate (Hydeltra-T.B.A.) or triamcinolone hexacetonide (Aristospan) diluted in 1% lidocaine. The latter steroid especially provides long-term anti-inflammatory effect. The injection must be performed using sterile technique. Joint infection must always be excluded before its use. We advise no more than two or three injections per year in a single joint. Intra-articular corticosteroids work best in the patient whose disease is under good control except for one or two joints. We rarely instill corticosteroids into the hip joint.

### Surgical Management

An experienced orthopedic surgeon is an essential part of the team that treats rheumatoid arthritis. Patients who have joint subluxations, tendon ruptures, and painful joint destruction benefit from surgical intervention. Hips and knees are now regularly replaced with artificial prostheses, allowing patients to continue to ambulate and maintain their independence.

There is a higher rate of infection in prosthetic joints in patients with rheumatoid arthritis as compared with patients with osteoarthritis. Rheumatoid arthritis patients should be monitored carefully for infections and treated aggressively if they arise. Prophylactic antibiotics should be given with surgical procedures that may cause significant bacteremia in patients with total joint prostheses.

Wrist and hand surgery are often required. These usually involve tendon repositioning or reconstruction, wrist synovectomy, joint fusion, metacarpophalangeal joint prostheses, and surgical release for nerve entrapment in the carpal tunnel syndrome. Neurosurgical intervention may be required in patients with neurologic deficits secondary to atlantoaxial subluxation.

### Goals of Therapy

Rheumatoid arthritis is a chronic disease that may cause severe joint destruction and systemic complications. Early diagnosis and the early use of disease-modifying treatment are essential. Patient education facilitates treatment decisions and patient compliance. We review medication dosing schedules and side effects with patients on a regular basis. We start occupational and physical therapy early. Gold and hydroxychloroquine are our standard drugs for early and mild disease. If immunosuppressive agents are to be used, a rheumatology consultation is suggested. Methotrexate has become the drug of choice for patients failing to respond to gold or hydroxychloroquine or those with severe disease. A multidisciplinary approach, including physical and occupational therapy, nursing, orthopedic surgery, and social work, is essential for the optimal management of patients. Maintenance of independence and good quality of life are the goals of therapy.

# JUVENILE RHEUMATOID ARTHRITIS

method of
CAROL B. LINDSLEY, M.D.
*University of Kansas Medical Center*
*Kansas City, Kansas*

Although there are more than 100 different types of arthritis in children, by far the most common form of chronic arthritis is juvenile rheumatoid arthritis (JRA). Juvenile rheumatoid arthritis is a disease characterized by arthritis of variable patterns and may be associated with nonarticular manifestations. It is estimated to affect up to 250,000 children in the United States. The disease onset can be from infancy to adulthood, but peak incidence occurs between 1 and 4 years of age and 9 and 14 years of age. The cause of JRA remains unknown. Onset frequently follows an upper respiratory tract infection or sometimes trauma, but no causative relationship between these events and the subsequent disease has been identified. Current areas of research with regard to etiology focus on an as yet unidentified viral agent, an exaggerated or abnormal immune response, genetic predisposition, or a combination of these factors. In JRA in general, there is a 2 to 3:1 female/male ratio, although the sex ratio varies with different subtypes. There are three onset subtypes of JRA defined by the clinical manifestations present during the first six months of illness; systemic onset, polyarticular onset (many joints), and pauciarticular onset (few joints). The onset may be insidious or fulminant, and any joint can be involved initially.

*Systemic-onset JRA* affects 10 to 20% of the children with JRA, has a male predominance, and is characterized by persistent, intermittent fever with elevations to 103 to 106° F and an evanescent rash. Between the fever spikes, there is typically a drop to normal or subnormal levels. Usually, the spikes are in the late afternoon or early evening and are associated with periods of joint discomfort. In the majority of patients with systemic-onset JRA, a rash is associated with the high fever. Occasionally, a child has rash alone. The evanescent rash is characterized by small salmon-pink lesions, generally 3 to 4 mm in diameter and often with central clearing. The rash is usually present over the anterior chest, axillae, and buttocks, and, to a lessor extent, on the extremities. It is generally nonpruritic. Fever and rash are often accompanied by hepatosplenomegaly, lymphadenopathy, and pericarditis. As the fever and rash subside over a period of weeks or months, the joint symptoms become more prominent. Over half of these children develop polyarticular involvement, with about 25% progressing to severe deforming arthritis.

*Polyarticular-onset JRA* is characterized by involvement of five or more joints during the first 6 months of disease. It is more common in females and is characterized by symmetrical small joint involvement of the hands and feet. This subtype represents from 30 to 40% of all patients with JRA. Children may show mild systemic symptoms, such as low-grade fever and malaise, and morning stiffness is often present. The younger children may also have involvement of the tendon sheath (tenosynovitis), which causes diffuse swelling of the involved area, usually the hand or the foot. Frequently, there is early involvement of the cervical spine, wrists, and hips. A subgroup of polyarticular JRA involves children that are seropositive for rheumatoid factor. They tend to have an older age of onset, a higher incidence of rheumatoid subcutaneous nodules, and progressive arthritis manifested by articular erosions and joint deformity. Except for age of onset, this small subgroup (5 to 10% of all those with JRA) have a disease course similar to that of adult rheumatoid arthritis.

*Pauciarticular-onset JRA* involves four or fewer joints during the first 6 months of disease. As in the polyarticular type, there is a female predominance. The most commonly affected joints are weight-bearing joints, most frequently knees and ankles. Pauciarticular JRA represents 40 to 50% of children with this disease and is divided into two subgroups. One subgroup includes boys with peripheral arthritis and the presence of the HLA-B27 histocompatability antigen. Children with JRA in this subgroup are at increased risk for ultimate development of spondylitis. The other subgroup of pauciarticular JRA involves young girls (less than 6 years of age) with increased risk for chronic iridocyclitis. Chronic iridocyclitis is a prime cause of morbidity in this group and involves inflammation of the anterior uveal tract of the eye. If untreated, it may result in blindness. At least 80% of the chronic iridocyclitis that occurs in JRA occurs in this relatively small group and is often also associated with the presence of antinuclear antibodies (ANA). Thus, the ANA test is a marker for increased risk of eye disease. As eye disease in young children may be entirely asymptomatic, regular examinations for the early detection of inflammation are critical (see Table 2).

## DIAGNOSIS

The diagnosis of JRA is dependent on the objective demonstration of chronic inflammation in one or more joints for a minimum of 6 weeks in a person younger than 16 years of age. Inflammation is characterized by swelling or limitation of motion associated with pain, tenderness, or increased warmth. Pain alone (arthralgia) is not adequate for the diagnosis. Other diseases must be excluded. The specific exclusions considered in an individual patient depend on the type of onset and general clinical presentation, but should include viral and bacterial infections, malignancy, osteone-crosis, and other inflammatory joint diseases. There is no specific diagnostic laboratory test for JRA. The majority of patients with active disease have an elevated erythrocyte sedimentation rate. However, it may be normal or mildly elevated in pauciarticular disease. The white blood cell count may be normal or elevated. Marked leukocytosis is often present in children with systemic disease (40,000 to 80,000 cells per $\mu$l) and may be accompanied by thrombocytosis. A positive ANA test occurs in 30 to 40% of patients. The rheumatoid factor is found in only 5 to 15% and denotes a high-risk subgroup described earlier. By far, the majority of patients with JRA are seronegative for rheumatoid factor and, thus, the absence of rheumatoid factor is not helpful in excluding the diagnosis of JRA. Synovial fluid analysis is particularly helpful in monoarticular arthritis to rule out bacterial infection and to document the presence of an inflammatory fluid.

Characteristic radiographic changes in patients with JRA often occur late. Initially, only periarticular swelling and juxta-articular osteoporosis are present. These are followed at variable intervals by joint space narrowing, erosive changes, and finally joint fusion. The earliest radiographic changes often occur in the wrist.

## TREATMENT

There is no cure for JRA. The goal of treatment is to relieve pain, to preserve joint function, and to minimize the extra-articular manifestations. The four main components of long-term treatment are drug therapy, physical and occupational therapy, education of the patient and the family about the disease, and the use of appropriate community services.

### Drug Therapy

**First-Line Agents.** This group of agents provides anti-inflammatory, antipyretic, and analgesic effects and includes aspirin and more than 20 nonsteroidal anti-inflammatory drugs (NSAIDs). Traditionally, aspirin has been the drug of choice in the treatment of JRA and still continues as such in many centers. It is readily available and the least expensive of all NSAIDs. It should be used in the dosage of 75 to 90 mg per kg per 24 hours (maximum 4 grams per day). The initial dosage and aggressiveness of treatment obviously depend on the severity of the child's symptoms. For an acutely ill child, 90 mg per kg per 24 hours (weight <25 kg) is the starting dosage and occasionally needs to be increased to control severe symptoms. However, high-dose salicylate therapy must be closely monitored with serum salicylate levels (therapeutic range 15 to 30 mg per dl) 7 to 10 days after initiation of therapy and then periodically. In an individual patient, a small increment in blood level may make a significant difference in the control of symptoms.

Moreover, a small increment in oral dosage can result in a relatively large increase in serum level. Children should be carefully monitored for signs of salicylism (lethargy, lability, tinnitus, or hyperpnea). As the serum level increases, the risk of hepatotoxicity increases, and liver function tests, aspartate aminotransferase (AST) and alanine aminotransferase (ALT) levels should be monitored closely. The salicylate therapy should be discontinued or the dosage reduced if AST and ALT values consistently exceed 100 IU. A variety of salicylates are available, including enteric-coated aspirin (Ecotrin), choline magnesium trisalicylate (Trilisate), and salsalate (Disalcid), which are generally well tolerated. Salicylates adequately control the clinical symptoms in the majority of the patients with JRA. Because of the high incidence of gastrointestinal (GI) side effects, salicylates should be taken with food to minimize irritation. Antacids or sucralfate (Carafate) may also be helpful. Because of the possible risk of Reye's syndrome, salicylates should be discontinued during serious viral illness, especially influenza, and on exposure to chickenpox.

The U.S. Food and Drug Administration (FDA) has approved other NSAIDs for use in children younger than 14 years of age, including tolmetin sodium (Tolectin), naproxen (Naprosyn), and ibuprofen (Advil, Motrin, Nuprin, Rufen). Naproxen, choline magnesium trisalicylate, and ibuprofen are available in liquid preparation (Table 1).

Other NSAIDs that are used in the treatment of children with JRA include sulindac (Clinoril), 5 to 7 mg per kg per day, and indomethacin (Indocin), 1.5 to 3 mg per kg per day (maximum 150 mg daily*). These other drugs should be used in special circumstances. There is some evidence that sulindac may have fewer renal side effects, and indomethacin is often particularly effective in treating HLA-B27–positive pauciarticular JRA. Six to 12 weeks may be required for optimal response to NSAID therapy. Thereafter, a different NSAID may be tried.

The most common side effect of the NSAIDs is GI toxicity, including abdominal pain, dyspepsia, peptic ulcer disease, and GI bleeding. Hepatic and renal toxicity can also occur. Urinalysis should be obtained every 3 to 4 months, and, if abnormalities are noted, further evaluation should be done. Central nervous system effects are rare, but necessitate discontinuation of NSAIDs. Photosensitivity reactions have been reported. Long-term multiple NSAID therapy should be avoided.

**Second-Line Agents** (Slow-Acting Antirheumatic Drugs). Those patients who have persistent poly-

TABLE 1. **Nonsteroidal Anti-inflammatory Drugs**

| | Dosage (mg per kg per day) | Doses Per Day |
|---|---|---|
| Tolmetin sodium (Tolectin) | 20–50 | 3–4 |
| Naproxen (Naprosyn) | 10–20 | 2 |
| Ibuprofen (Advil, Motrin, Nuprin, Rufen) | 30–40 | 3–4 |

articular disease, unresponsive or only partially responsive to NSAID therapy for 6 months or longer, are candidates for therapy with second-line agents. Unresponsiveness is judged by persistence of patient's symptoms, particularly stiffness, swelling, or fever, and usually radiographic evidence of progressive joint disease. Approximately 50% of patients respond to treatment with gold, hydroxychloroquine, or penicillamine. Response often requires a minimum of 8 to 12 weeks, and treatment is associated with significant risk for toxicity. Thus, treatment should not be initiated without clear indications. Gold treatment can be in the form of either oral medication, auranofin (Ridaura), or parenteral gold salts, aurothioglucose (Solganal) or gold sodium thiomalate (Myochrysine). Auranofin is usually well tolerated in the dosage of 0.1 to 0.2 mg per kg per day, but may be less effective than a parenteral preparation and is not currently approved by the FDA for use in young children. Parenteral gold salts should be given by weekly intramuscular injections. Following test injections of 0.25 mg per kg, then 0.5 mg per kg, 0.75 mg per kg per week initially is given to a weekly maximum of 50 mg and continued for 20 weeks. If good response occurs, the injections are maintained at less frequent intervals of every 2 to 3 weeks for at least one year or longer if clinical response continues and toxicity is avoided. Both oral and parenteral gold require baseline hematologic, hepatic, and renal studies followed by weekly (parenteral gold salts) or biweekly (auranofin) complete blood count (CBC), urinalysis, and clinical examination for toxicity (rash, mouth ulcers). Patients with systemic JRA may be at increased risk for toxicity. Hydroxychloroquine* (Plaquenil), 5 to 7 mg per kg per day, is well tolerated and is effective in about 50% of the patients. Regular ophthalmologic monitoring for retinal toxicity must be done initially and then every 3 to 6 months. Penicillamine* (Cuprimine, Depen) has had limited testing in children, but appears to be effective about 50% of the time. It is initiated in a dosage of 5 mg per kg per day and is

*Exceeds dosage recommended by the manufacturer.

*Manufacturer's warning: Efficacy in the treatment of JRA has not been established.

increased gradually to a maximum of 10 mg per kg per day. Close monitoring for renal toxicity, dermatitis, or a lupus-like syndrome must be done.

Sulfasalazine* (Azulfidine) has received limited experience in children, although it has been shown to be effective in adults with rheumatoid arthritis (RA). The initial course is 40 to 60 mg per kg per day in divided doses with meals for 6 to 12 weeks, followed by a gradual reduction of dosage to approximately 25 mg per kg per day. Sulfasalazine appears to be most useful in those with persistent polyarthritis or spondyloarthritis unresponsive to other regimens, but is associated with bone marrow toxicity, dermatitis, and GI irritation and is contraindicated in patients with prior salicylate or sulfa toxicity or glucose-6-phosphate dehydrogenase deficiency.

**Methotrexate.*** Preliminary studies of methotrexate in children with JRA show efficacy in the treatment of polyarthritis unresponsive to conservative regimens and slow-acting antirheumatic agents. Efficacy has been shown at dosages below those known to be associated with toxicity, and safety for long-term oncogenesis and sterility has been demonstrated. However, methotrexate can be associated with increased susceptibility to infection, bone marrow suppression, GI ulceration, hepatitis and cirrhosis, pulmonary insufficiency, and pneumonitis. Therefore, baseline hematologic, hepatic, renal, and pulmonary studies should be done prior to the institution of therapy. The usual dosage is 10 mg per $M^2$ orally once a week in the morning with water or clear liquids. Periodic CBC, urinalysis, and AST and ALT determinations should be performed and periodic serum levels of methotrexate monitored. One-hour levels should be approximately $6 \times 10^{-7}$ M, followed by a 24-hour level of less than $2 \times 10^{-8}$ M.

The NSAID should be continued during the use of any of the second-line drugs. Caution and careful monitoring should be used when an NSAID is used in combination with methotrexate, as toxicity of the latter may be increased.

**Other Agents.** Immunosuppressive agents, including cyclophosphamide (Cytoxan), azathioprine (Imuran), and chlorambucil (Leukeran), are not approved for the treatment of JRA. However, azathioprine has been used in adult RA. There is ongoing research into the use of plasmapheresis and intravenous gamma globulin therapy, but use of these remains experimental.

**Corticosteroids.** Oral corticosteroids may be required for severe systemic disease or progressive

---

*Manufacturer's warning: Efficacy in the treatment of JRA has not been established.

chronic uveitis. As low a daily dosage as possible (usually 1 mg per kg per day) should be used initially, with slow tapering to alternate-day treatment as symptoms permit. Significant toxicity, including growth retardation, increased susceptibility to infection, and iatrogenic Cushing's syndrome, is associated with prolonged daily therapy. Intravenous steroid pulse therapy may be used to control life-threatening systemic disease or a serious flare of polyarticular disease. There is limited experience with this in the pediatric population. Methylprednisolone acetate, 10 to 30 mg per kg per dose in a single pulse given over 60 minutes every day for 3 days, or every other day for 3 doses, has been used. Close monitoring of fluid balance, electrolyte levels, and cardiovascular functions should be done during infusion in a hospital setting. Potential toxicities of such therapy include acute fluid and electrolyte imbalances, sudden death from arrhythmia, hypertensive crisis, GI hemorrhage, seizure disorder, osteonecrosis, hyperglycemia, ketosis, and increased risk of infection.

Selective use of intra-articular corticosteroids (triamcinolone hexacetonide [Aristospan], 20 mg per ml, 25 mg for large joints, and 10 mg for small joints) can be beneficial. Particular caution is needed with regard to serial injections (more than three) and hip joint injections. Close follow-up regarding overuse of the injected joint and increased risk for infection is needed.

### Physical and Occupational Therapy

Each child needs a balanced rest/activity program tailored to current disease activity. Physical and occupational therapy are an important component of JRA treatment. Almost all children with JRA require an exercise program at one time or another. Painful joints are held in flexion and used with decreased frequency, often leading to flexion contractures within a short time. The longer the duration of symptoms without adequate therapy, the more difficult it is to reverse the changes. Inflamed joints should receive range of motion at least once daily. With active inflammation, the exercise program consists initially of passive range of motion and thereafter a progressive program should be instituted under the direction of a physical or occupational therapist. As disease activity diminishes, passive exercises can be replaced by active ones and ultimately by progressive strengthening exercises. Emphasis is almost always on joint extension rather than flexion, as flexion contractures are common problems. In addition to prescribed exercises, swimming and bicycle or tricycle riding are excellent all-around activities. Many children have shoulder and hip girdle involvement that particularly benefits from swimming. Normal play or sport activities, however, do not take the place of prescribed exercises. Many small aids are helpful in selected patients, such as doorframe pulleys, tilt tables, writing spacers, and self-help devices. Heat is good in relieving morning stiffness and muscle spasm and can be accomplished with an early morning shower, the use of an electric blanket or sleeping bag, or the use of a heated water bed. Adequate rest is important, but prolonged bed rest is contraindicated.

Splinting is helpful in maintaining functional position, particularly of wrists and knees. Splints can be made from either plaster or plastic material; appropriate fit is important. Splints are most beneficial when worn at night to rest the joints. Dynamic splints and serial casting are helpful in selected patients. Elastic joint supports help protect knees or ankles during vigorous activity. Fitted soft cervical collars may relieve cervical spine discomfort and help maintain good posture. Firm collars may be required in the child with C1-2 subluxation. Crutches or a cane temporarily reduce the load on a painful hip or knee to permit continued mobility. Orthotic devices such as metatarsal bars, heel cushions, and medial arch supports are often useful.

### Surgery

A small number of children ultimately require artificial joint replacement. Hip and knee replacements are the most common and successful. Other surgical procedures, such as soft tissue release of contractures, correction of micrognathia, synovectomy, and cervical spine stabilization, may be helpful in selected patients.

### Eye Disease

Periodic eye examination by an ophthalmologist, including slit lamp examination, is required to prevent injury from chronic iridocyclitis, which is often asymptomatic in the young child and is associated with JRA in 10 to 15% of patients. Known risk factors for iridocyclitis include young age (less than 6 years), arthritis pattern (pauciarticular onset), and a positive ANA. Table 2 presents recommended frequency of examination based on these factors. Activity of eye disease does not correlate with arthritis activity. If detected early, iridocyclitis usually responds to topical corticosteroids and mydriatic agents. Progressive eye disease may require oral corticosteroids. Adjunctive NSAID therapy may reduce the eye disease activity. Complications of chronic iridocyclitis include cataracts, glaucoma, and blindness.

TABLE 2. **Recommended Frequency of Ophthalmologic Examination**

Patients with three risk factors—every 3 to 4 months
Patients with two risk factors—every 6 months
Patients with one risk factor—yearly
Patients older than 12 years of age who have not experienced iridocyclitis anytime in the course of their disease—yearly
Patients with documented eye inflammation, whether active or not, should follow an individual regimen as indicated by the ophthalmologist

### GENERAL ISSUES OF CHRONIC DISEASE

JRA is a chronic disease, and there are several generic issues important to optimal management. Compliance with the medical regimen, including medication, exercise program, and splinting, is a problem. Most children respond to simple behavior management strategies, particularly if instituted early. Parents should be encouraged to treat their children with JRA as normally as possible. Extremes should be avoided, such as being insensitive to the child's needs or being overindulgent. Depression and low self-esteem may require specific psychosocial intervention, especially in the teen-ager. Family counseling may be indicated.

The nutritional aspects of chronic disease are best addressed with careful monitoring of the child's growth variables and periodic dietary surveillance. Children with severe disease may require iron, calcium, or caloric supplementation. No special diet is needed, but a well-balanced one with adequate calories to account for any increased metabolic need is appropriate.

Education is an ongoing need for both the parent and the child. The child needs to have information regarding the disease and its treatment, and the goals of the treatment should be reiterated and modified as age appropriate. The child should attend school regularly and participate in a regular or alternative physical education program if at all possible. Federal law requires that schools provide adequate programs for children with special needs (Public Law 94-142). Communication between the family and the school is of major importance to optimize the child's educational experience. Individual education programs (IEPs) or privileges such as an elevator pass, two sets of books (home and school), use of a tape recorder, or assistance at lunch may be needed. Educational materials are available from the Arthritis Foundation and American Juvenile Arthritis Organization.

The multiple aspects of care of the child with JRA are best dealt with by close cooperation between the primary physician and a health care team with expertise in the care of the child with arthritis.

## PROGNOSIS

The overall prognosis for a child with JRA is good. Ten to 15 years after disease onset, approximately 75% of the children are in remission. Most of these children have a polycyclic course with periods of disease remissions and exacerbations. The highest risk for long-term deformity is in patients with seropositive polyarticular disease or persistent polyarticular disease following systemic onset. Deformity involving wrists and hips is of particular concern and may progress in spite of relatively good disease control.

Other complications include growth disturbances, particularly leg length discrepancy, micrognathia, and scoliosis. The mortality from JRA in the United States is less than 1%, usually secondary to systemic infection associated with immunosuppressive therapy or rarely amyloidosis.

# ANKYLOSING SPONDYLITIS

method of
T. DOUGLAS KINSELLA, M.D.
*University of Calgary*
*Calgary, Alberta, Canada*

Ankylosing spondylitis (AS) is an inflammatory arthropathy that causes variable degrees of vertebral ankylosis. It is reputed to occur in 1.0% of the population, but, more credibly, probably affects no more than 0.2% with clinical disease. Ankylosing spondylitis is expressed clinically more frequently in adults than in children and three to four times more often in males than in females. The disease typically occurs as an isolated primary syndrome (primary AS), but also in association with various genitourinary, gastrointestinal, and cutaneous disorders (secondary AS) (Table 1).

TABLE 1. **Classification of Ankylosing Spondylitis**

1. Primary (idiopathic) ankylosing spondylitis
2. Secondary (reactive) ankylosing spondylitis
   a. Gastrointestinal disease
      Ulcerative colitis
      Regional enteritis
      Whipple's disease
      Gram-negative dysentery
      Yersiniosis
   b. Genitourinary disease
      Chlamydial infection
      Mycoplasma infection
   c. Cutaneous disease
      Psoriasis
      Acne conglobata
      Hidradenitis suppurativa

TABLE 2. **Diagnostic Criteria for Primary Ankylosing Spondylitis***

1. Axial skeleton stiffness: relieved by exercise; at least 3 months' duration
2. Lumbar pain: persists at rest; at least 3 months' duration
3. Thoracic cage pain: persists at rest; at least 3 months' duration
4. Past or current iritis
5. Decreased lumbar range of motion
6. Decreased chest expansion (age related)
7. Bilateral, symmetrical radiographic sacroiliitis

*Diagnosis requires No. 7 and any one of No. 1 through 5, or any five of the six clinical criteria

## PATHOLOGIC CHARACTERISTICS

There are three lesions that characterize the pathologic changes in AS: sacroiliitis, axial spine involvement, and enthesitis. Less frequently, there may occur inflammation of small central and large peripheral joints and involvement of extra-articular tissues, including the eye, the heart, the lung, the spinal cord, and the kidneys.

For the certain pathologic and clinical diagnosis of AS, sacroiliitis must be present (Table 2). In primary disease, sacroiliitis is usually bilateral and symmetrical; in secondary disease, it is often unilateral and asymmetrical. Both the lower synovial (diarthrosis) and upper nonsynovial (synchondrosis) portions of the sacroiliac (SI) joints are inflamed in AS. Involvement of the synovial segment causes para-articular osteopenia at onset and may progress to cartilaginous erosion and, eventually, fibrotic ankylosis. Histologically, the synovitis of AS is similar to that of rheumatoid arthritis (RA) but shows a sparser infiltrate containing more mononuclear cells (macrophages and lymphocytes).

Axial spine involvement in AS can cause a variety of lesions, including vertebral erosions and osteopenia and synovitis of apophyseal and costovertebral joints. In addition, periosteal inflammation, at sites of contact of ligaments and tendons with bone, causes enthesitis, which frequently results in ligamentous calcification and ossification. Thus, the net result of sacroiliitis, spondylitis, and enthesitis in AS is both acute and chronic mechanical restriction of spinal movement.

There is frequent inflammation of small central joints (e.g., manubriosternal and sternoclavicular joints) in primary AS, and synovitis of large peripheral joints (hips and shoulders) in about 25% of patients. Although the anterior eye is the site of recurrent acute iritis in about one-third of patients, chronic inflammation characterizes other extra-articular lesions of AS. The latter include proximal (root) aortitis and heart block in about 5%, apical pulmonary fibrosis in about 1%, and the rare lesions of caudal adhesive leptomeningitis and IgA nephropathy.

In the secondary (reactive) forms of AS, any of the foregoing lesions may occur. However, secondary AS usually displays milder disease and more restricted articular involvement than primary AS. In addition, of course, the pathologic features of the accompanying disorder are present.

## ETIOLOGY AND PATHOGENESIS

The etiology of AS is unknown. Although its pathogenesis is also unknown, there is an incontrovertible link between AS and the presence of the human leukocyte antigen HLA-B27 in both primary and secondary forms of the disease (Table 3). The effect exerted by B27 in AS is not known, except that B27 does not cause the disease. Thus, the majority of B27-positive subjects (6 to 7% of the normal population) do not have AS; a small percentage of typical primary AS occurs in B27-negative caucasians, as does a larger percentage in B27-negative blacks; and fewer patients with secondary AS express B27 (see Table 3). Because of such considerations, the pathogenetic relationship between HLA-B27 and AS remains unknown and, to date, provides no therapeutic assistance.

## CLINICAL FEATURES

Ankylosing spondylitis characteristically begins during early adult life, with a male/female ratio of about 4:1. The reason for this male preponderance is not known and is also perplexing because males and females inherit HLA-B27 in equal proportions and, therefore, should equally express spondylitis. One explanation for the latter might be an equal prevalence of AS in both sexes, but different degrees of clinical severity, as a result of which more severe disease in males falsely appears as an increased male prevalence.

The classic symptoms at onset of AS are low back pain and stiffness worsened by inactivity and improved by activity (see Table 2). As time passes, similar symptoms may involve other spinal segments sequentially, as well as small anterior central joints of the thorax. In adults, hips and shoulders are the most frequently involved peripheral joints, whereas in children and adolescents knees and feet are most commonly involved.

Physical examination of the spine at onset of AS is invariably within normal limits. However, usually within 3 years of symptomatic onset, postural defects, local tenderness, and restricted range of motion appear in the lumbar spine and, subsequently, may appear in other spinal segments and peripheral joints. Restricted chest expansion may indicate chest wall or costovertebral joint disease. Thus, physical examination is of minor assistance in the diagnosis of new and early disease, but is of diagnostic and prognostic aid in established disease.

For the certain clinical diagnosis of AS, radiologic evidence of sacroiliitis is a sine qua non (see Table 2). In primary disease, sacroiliitis is bilateral and usually symmetrical, but is often unilateral and/or asymmetrical in secondary AS. Radiologic sacroiliitis also may take 3 to 5 years to become apparent, thereby causing further diagnostic delay and confusion at onset. In established disease, typical changes are easily seen radiologically in SI joints and the axial skeleton; peripheral joint disease shows no radiologic specificity.

Laboratory studies never establish the diagnosis of AS. Nevertheless, typing for HLA-B27 in a patient with compatible symptoms, but normal or inconclusive x-ray findings in SI joints, can be of diagnostic assistance. An elevated erythrocyte sedimentation rate (ESR) usually accompanies active disease, as does an elevated serum IgA level.

The course of primary AS is usually one of mild to moderate progression over decades, causing some limitation of movement, but no severe morbidity and no significant mortality. In secondary AS, the worst prognosis occurs with psoriatic spondylitis, in which there often occurs severe erosive and ankylotic disease of axial and peripheral joints. In general, symptoms of active primary AS are uncommon after the age of 50 years, but, of course, pre-existing functional abnormalities persist. Extra-articular disease most frequently appears as acute anterior iritis, and about one-third of such patients experience two or three unilateral or bilateral recurrences.

The number of conditions that may be confused with primary AS is not large, and the prevalence of mechanical problems of the lumbar spine far exceeds that of AS. Differentiation between primary and secondary forms may be difficult at onset, but reactive disorders eventually declare themselves, causing no therapeutic disadvantage to patients in the interval. Finally, because AS invariably displays a striking complex of pain and stiffness relieved by exercise and worsened by inactivity, persistence of such a complex in a young male demands appropriate radiologic examination.

## TREATMENT

Four therapeutic modalities underlie the management of AS: patient education, physiotherapy, pharmacologic therapy, and surgical therapy.

*Education* concerning all facets of AS must be given to all patients at diagnosis. The importance of this cannot be overstated, given the anxiety engendered in young persons by a diagnosis of arthritis. Excellent educational materials are available from the Arthritis Foundation in the United States and the Arthritis Society in Canada. As well, lay support groups, such as the recently formed Ankylosing Spondylitis Association, provide both didactic and applied continuing education. The content of educational programs in AS must be such as to emphasize, at diagnosis,

TABLE 3. **Correlations Between Clinical Spondylitis and Prevalence of HLA-B27**

| Clinical Group | HLA-B27 Prevalence (%) |
|---|---|
| Normal subjects (caucasian) | 6–7 |
| Normal subjects (black) | 2–3 |
| Primary ankylosing spondylitis | >95 |
| Secondary ankylosing spondylitis | |
|    Inflammatory bowel disease | 50 |
|    Gram-negative dysentery | >80 |
|    Yersiniosis | >80 |
|    Urethritis/dysentery (Reiter's syndrome) | >70 |
|    Psoriasis | >50 |

the usual good prognosis and, after diagnosis, the need for a continuing exercise regimen at home.

*Physiotherapy* should be initiated in all AS patients at diagnosis, practiced twice daily, and reviewed at intervals to provide both educational and therapeutic regimens. The latter include breathing, postural, and range-of-motion exercises for appropriate spinal segments. Particular emphasis should be given to proper posture of the cervical spine because its typical anterior flexion contracture, when pronounced, significantly restricts activities of daily living. Similarly, exercises to prevent postural deficits caused by work habits and sleeping postures should also be given at diagnosis and reviewed at intervals throughout a patient's lifetime.

Physical modalities, such as heat, ice, and nerve stimulation, seem to help some AS patients during exacerbations. As in other rheumatic diseases, however, there is controversy concerning the benefit of such modalities in AS. Regardless, most patients do experience at least transient benefit from these modalities during exacerbations, when daily therapeutic exercises are best curtailed or eliminated. Overall, proper programs of physiotherapy, particularly therapeutic exercises, bring major benefit to the long-term prognosis of AS.

*Pharmacologic therapy* in AS requires both acute and chronic regimens. The rationale for this approach derives from numerous pathologic studies that show that inflammation in AS is both acute and chronic. Thus, anti-inflammatory therapy is required during the active clinical course of AS, which usually ceases before age 50 years, to impede the natural progress of the disease.

Nonsteroidal anti-inflammatory drugs (NSAIDs) are the only agents essential to the treatment of AS. Of the many NSAIDs, indomethacin (Indocin) has had the longest and safest clinical experience. Prior to the use of indomethacin, phenylbutazone (Butazolidin) provided comparable benefit but such severe hematologic toxicity (marrow aplasia) that it is now contraindicated. Similarly, there are no indications for the use of potent anti-inflammatory or immunosuppressive measures, such as radiotherapy, corticosteroids, and methotrexate, which bring significant morbidity and mortality to this relatively benign disease.

The availability of long-acting NSAIDs has further simplified the management of AS. The combination of therapeutic exercises twice daily and sustained-release indomethacin (Indocin SR) nocturnally allows most AS patients to pursue essentially normal lives. During exacerbations, which typically occur two or three times per year, lessening of exercise and increased dosages of indomethacin usually produce remissions within 2 weeks, subsequent to which patients should return to their maintenance regimen. Occasionally, because of toxicity or inefficacy of indomethacin, the use of another long-acting NSAID may be needed to produce the desired benefit. Overall, the therapeutic outcome of AS is usually excellent when the principles of patient education, physiotherapy, and pharmacologic therapy are pursued with diligence and constancy.

*Surgical therapy* is often required for 10 to 15% of AS patients with hip involvement. When conservative therapy fails, such patients usually benefit from joint replacement. There was early controversy concerning a high frequency of postoperative hip ankylosis in AS patients, although this seems to have been negated by longer experience with new surgical techniques. In the past, there was some interest in correcting spinal (postural) deformities by various spinal osteotomy procedures, but these have been abandoned because of high morbidity and mortality rates. Although atlantoaxial subluxation is a rare complication of primary AS, it is not uncommon in psoriatic spondylitis and may require surgical reduction and stabilization.

**Miscellaneous Therapeutic Considerations.** Acute anterior uveitis is an emergency, requiring immediate mydriatics, analgesics, and local corticosteroids, preferably under ophthalmologic supervision. Peripheral arthritis, other than in the hip, usually responds to physiotherapy, oral NSAIDs, and/or intra-articular steroids. Other, uncommon manifestations of AS (in heart, lung, and central nervous system) should be managed by interventions specific for the particular problem encountered. With occasional exceptions, the arthritis of secondary AS proceeds independently of the underlying disorder and, therefore, requires no unusual therapeutic interventions.

Ethical principles must shape all medical acts. With respect to therapeutic interventions, the determinative ethical principle is primum non nocere—"above all, do no harm." This principle, also described as nonmaleficence, must guide the therapy of AS. Thus, because primary AS causes only rare mortality and minimal morbidity, potent corticosteroids and immunosuppressants are not ethically warranted for this disorder.

# TEMPOROMANDIBULAR DISORDERS

method of
JEFFREY P. OKESON, D.M.D.
*University of Kentucky*
*Lexington, Kentucky*

In 1983 the American Dental Association adopted the term "temporomandibular (TM) disorders" to include all functional problems associated with the masticatory structures. Structures considered to be masticatory are the teeth, the periodontal ligaments, the bones that support the teeth (the maxillae and mandible), the TM joints, and the muscles that mobilize the mandible (muscles of mastication). Other terms that are commonly used to describe masticatory problems are "temporomandibular joint dysfunction," "craniomandibular disorders," and "myofascial pain dysfunction syndrome."

It is estimated that between 5 and 20% of the population suffer from TM disorders. Epidemiologic studies reveal even a greater percentage of signs related to masticatory dysfunction. For example, the prevalence of TM joint sounds is reported to be between 25 and 50% of the general population. At this time, there is controversy regarding the clinical significance of some of these signs.

Approximately 5% of the population actively seek treatment for TM disorders. The majority of this group are female (80 to 85%), although epidemiologic studies reveal a more equal male/female ratio for signs and symptoms.

## ANATOMY

The area where craniomandibular articulation occurs, called the TM joint, is one of the most complex joints in the body. It provides for hinging movement in one plane and therefore can be considered a ginglymoid joint. However, at the same time, it provides for gliding movements, which classifies it as an arthrodial joint. Thus, it is technically considered a ginglymoarthrodial joint.

The TM joint is formed by the mandibular condyle fitting into the mandibular fossa of the temporal bone. Separating these two bones from direct articulation is the articular disk (sometimes called the "meniscus"). The disk is attached to the condyle both medially and laterally by collateral ligaments. These ligaments permit rotational movement of the disk on the condyle during opening and closing of the mouth. This so-called condyle-disk complex translates out of the mandibular fossa during mouth opening.

Unlike other synovial joints, the articulator surfaces of the TM joints are lined with dense fibrous connective tissue (not hyaline cartilage). This is an important feature in the management of many TM disorders. Dense fibrous connective tissue has a greater ability to repair itself than does hyaline cartilage. This implies that management of arthritic conditions of the TM joint may be different from that of other synovial joints. The TM joint has a fair ability to adapt or remodel when proper joint conditions are introduced (see the treatment sections).

Although there are many types of TM disorders, the two most common categories are masticatory muscle disorders and disk-interference (internal derangement) disorders. Because the majority of TM disorders fall into one of these two categories, they will be discussed in more detail.

## MASTICATORY MUSCLE DISORDERS

Masticatory muscle disorders are a group of disorders associated with functional problems of the muscles that move the mandible. They present as a group of symptoms that arise from an extracapsular source (outside the TM joint). Muscle spasms and pain are the most common complaints.

**Etiology.** It is thought that both malocclusion and emotional stress can play a significant role in masticatory muscle disorders. Muscle hyperactivity such as bruxism and clenching of the teeth greatly contributes to muscle spasms and pain. It is presently believed that nocturnal bruxism is more closely associated with increased emotional stress than with occlusal factors. Dental malocclusion or a poor dental prosthesis may contribute to these muscle pain disorders, especially when there is a history of pain beginning with dental therapy.

**Clinical Findings.** The most common complaint reported by patients with masticatory muscle disorders is myalgia. The muscles of mastication (temporalis, masseter, and medial pterygoid) are often tender to palpation. The patient's ability to open the mouth widely is frequently restricted. The normal range of jaw opening is approximately 4 cm, or about the width of three fingers.) Many of the symptoms are similar to those reported by patients suffering from fibrositis or fibromyalgia. Functions of the jaw such as chewing and talking usually increase the symptoms. Symptoms are most commonly bilateral and are relatively diffuse over several muscles, although this may not always be true.

Because muscle pain is deep, it can produce referred pain. A common secondary complaint of patients who experience constant muscle pain is muscle tension headache. This type of headache is frequently produced by cervical and masticatory muscle involvement. Palpation of these muscle groups is indicated to determine whether the source of the headache pain is masticatory or cervical.

**Treatment.** The initial therapy for masticatory muscle disorders should be conservative and reversible. Mild analgesics (ibuprofen [Motrin], 600 mg three or four times a day) are helpful in decreasing pain and lessening the likelihood of cyclic muscle pain. The patient should be instructed to begin a soft diet and to limit jaw movement to painless motions. The patient should be encouraged to keep the jaw muscles relaxed and not to allow the teeth to contact unless chewing (avoid clenching the teeth). If nocturnal bruxism is suspected, an occlusal appliance can be fabricated and worn during sleep to decrease this muscle activity. If a change in the dental condition created the symptoms, dental correction may be indicated. When increased emotional stress is suspected, various behavior modification therapies such as relaxation techniques assisted with biofeedback may be helpful. When muscle pain is present, physical therapy can also be useful (e.g., moist heat, ultrasound, electrogalvanic stimulation). Muscle relaxants are not generally effective, although they can be used on a short-term basis for acute conditions (e.g., cyclobenzaprine [Flexeril], 10 mg two or three times a day).

### DISK-INTERFERENCE (INTERNAL DERANGEMENT) DISORDERS

Disk-interference disorders are a group of TM disorders that result from functional problems between the mandibular condyle and the articular disk. These problems are considered to be intercapsular disorders (within the TM joint). Mechanical alteration of joint movement and joint pain are common disk-interference complaints.

**Etiology.** Disk-interference disorders result from a mechanical disruption of normal condyle-disk function during opening and closing of the mouth. The most common cause of this disorder is trauma. Trauma, especially gross macro-trauma, can quickly elongate ligaments that support the condyle-disk complex, causing disruption in normal biomechanical relationships. Micro-trauma received over time as a result of muscle hyperactivity (bruxism) or an unstable dental condition can also contribute to this disorder.

**Clinical Findings.** The most common reported clinical symptom of disk-interference disorders is clicking or popping of the TM joint during jaw movement. These joint sounds are created by abnormal movement between the condyle and the disk during opening and closing. On occasion, multiple grating sounds or crepitation can be heard. Crepitation is often closely associated with degenerative joint disease. On occasion, the articular disk can be dislocated anteromedially to the condyle, inhibiting normal translation of the involved joint. This condition is clinically referred to as a "closed lock" because the patient cannot open the jaw wider than 25 to 30 mm interincisally (width of one to two fingers). Joint pain may or may not be present. When pain is present, it is arthralgic and associated with joint movement. Symptoms are usually unilateral (although not always), and the patient locates the discomfort specifically to the involved TM joint. Ear pain on the same side as the involved TM joint is a common complaint.

**Treatment.** Treatment of disk-interference disorders is directed toward re-establishing normal condyle-disk function. In some instances, a dental appliance can be used to re-establish a normal condyle-disk relationship and therefore eliminate the joint symptoms. This appliance is generally worn 24 hours a day for at least 8 weeks to allow adaptation or healing of the intracapsular structures. The appliance is then slowly eliminated in an attempt to return the joint to its normal position and function.

If painful symptoms return, alteration of the dental condition may be indicated. When pain is present, the patient is instructed to minimize joint sounds by decreasing jaw function. Analgesics such as ibuprofen, 600 mg as needed for pain, may be helpful. If inflammation of the joint structures is suspected, an anti-inflammatory medication such as ibuprofen, 600 to 800 mg three times a day for 3 weeks, is indicated. Sometimes physical therapy is helpful in decreasing pain and increasing joint mobility.

On occasion, occlusal appliance therapy, physical therapy, and medications may not be successful in reducing symptoms. When pain persists, surgical therapy may be considered. Surgery is directed toward re-establishing normal condyle-disk function. In most cases, conservative therapy is relatively successful; therefore, surgery is indicated only in about 5% of patients with intercapsular disorders.

Asymptomatic clicking of the TM joint is a relatively common finding (25 to 50% of the general population). Presently, therapy to eliminate it is relatively unsuccessful and therefore is not indicated. Only joints with painful clicking or with signs of progressing intercapsular problems should be considered for treatment.

# FIBROSITIS, BURSITIS, AND TENDINITIS

method of
JAMES J. CURRAN, M.D.
*University of Chicago Medical Center*
*Chicago, Illinois*

### FIBROSITIS (FIBROMYALGIA)

Fibromyalgia is a common entity characterized by fatigue, pain, and stiffness. Clinically, the syndrome is more common in women (mean age of 40 years) than in men by a 10:1 ratio. Fibrositis is considered "primary" if there are no associated disease states accompanying it. Major criteria employed in diagnosing fibrositis include pain, achiness, and morning stiffness in three or more locations for 3 months or longer; the absence of underlying systemic disease; and multiple trigger points (usually 12 of 14 anatomically defined sites). Common locations of these focally painful areas include the medial aspect of the knees, the medial aspect of the ankles, multiple points along the superior border of the trapezius muscles bilaterally, the lumbosacral spine, and bilateral wrist involvement. Minor criteria for the diagnosis of fibrositis include nonrestorative sleep dysfunction, chronic fatigue, chronic headache, diffuse pain in the neck or shoulders, and the irritable bowel syndrome.

Pain is the dominant symptom in fibrositis. Additionally, mental stress, anxiety, depression, subjective joint swelling, generalized achiness, and paresthesias are all common complaints of patients with this disorder. Physical factors such as weather changes (usually cold and dampness), strenuous physical exertion, and lack of sleep tend to exacerbate these symptoms. Most patients report that rest, modest exercise, heat applications, and massage ameliorate their symptoms.

The physical examination findings are generally normal, with no evidence of arthritis or synovitis unless there is an associated connective tissue disease. Skin hypersensitivity and diffuse muscle discomfort may be present. Occasionally, patients may have Raynaud's phenomenon. Local points of tenderness may exhibit hyperemia. A reticulate appearance of the skin over the extremities may be noted. The laboratory data usually are normal. However, a weakly positive antinuclear antibody may be found in as many as 20% of fibrositis patients.

Diagnostically, the history and physical examination are characteristic. The differential diagnosis of systemic myalgias and arthralgias with chronic pain include such entities as thyroid disease, parathyroid disease, collagen vascular disease, paraneoplastic syndromes, polymyalgia rheumatica, brucellosis, osteoporosis, osteomalacia, and myositis. Costly diagnostic evaluations are not indicated. A rational baseline screening, when considering the diagnosis of fibrositis, would include thyroid functions, muscle enzyme levels, complete blood count with platelet count, C-reactive protein determination, erythrocyte sedimentation rate, serum chemistry profile, and urinalysis.

### Treatment

Therapeutically, fibrositis is a chronic condition, whose symptoms are variable. Patients should be reassured that fibrositis is nonerosive, nondeforming, and nonprogressive. Patient education to attain insight into their disease process and its chronicity are vital. Several placebo-controlled studies have found that medications such as amitriptyline (Elavil), in dosages of 10 to 50 mg at bedtime (starting with a low dosage and titrating for systemic improvement), have been helpful in restoring normal sleep patterns and decreasing pain and stiffness. Likewise, cyclobenzaprine (Flexeril), in a dosage of 10 mg in the evening, has been found to be effective. Anti-inflammatory medications alone or in combination with tricyclic compounds have not been found to be efficacious. Biofeedback, physical therapy in the form of ultrasound, muscle-stretching exercises, massages, and occasionally ice applications have been helpful in alleviating symptoms.

## BURSITIS AND TENDINITIS

### Bursitis

Bursa are fluid-filled sacs that overlie bony prominences to minimize friction. Clinically important bursa that may become inflamed and painful include subacromial (shoulder), anserine (medial knee), olecranon (elbow), trochanteric (hip), calcaneal (heel), and prepatellar and infrapatellar (knee) bursae.

Common causes of bursitis include trauma; overuse; crystal-induced diseases, such as gout, apatite deposition disease, and chondrocalcinosis; connective tissue diseases, such as rheumatoid arthritis; and infections. Diabetics also have an increased incidence of bursitis and tendinitis, especially involving the shoulders.

Shoulder bursitis or tendinitis is a common cause of acute and chronic shoulder pain. Clinically, patients complain of nocturnal, diffuse shoulder pain as well as specific pain on abduction from 70 to 110 degrees ("painful arc") of the shoulder. The pain is poorly localized about the deltoid muscle mass and may radiate down the arm. Prolonged tendinitis may eventuate into a frozen shoulder (adhesive capsulitis). Trochanteric bursitis may be interpreted by the patient as being either hip discomfort or sciatica. On examination, however, the hip range of motion is intact and there is point tenderness over the greater trochanter. The straight leg–raising test is negative. The olecranon bursa is frequently traumatized. If there is acute pain, erythema, and warmth, the bursa must always be aspirated to assess for the possibility of crystal-induced disease and/or bacterial infection of the bursa. Septic bursitis is commonly caused by *Staphylococcus aureus*. Occasionally, patients may not have constitutional symptoms early in the course of septic bursitis. The prepatella bursa is a frequent site for tophaceous gout. It, along with the infrapatella bursa and the anserine bursa, is also subject to overuse and trauma.

## Tendinitis

Tendinitis or tenosynovitis is inflammation of the cellular lining membrane of the fibrous sheath in which tendons move. The commonest causes of tenosynovitis are overuse and trauma. The most frequent sites of involvement are the extensor tendons of the wrist and thumb and the dorsiflexors of the ankle. Tendinitis clinically manifests with pain, crepitation, and swelling over the tendon sheath. Stenosing tenosynovitis is a result of local sheath fibrosis, tendon enlargement, and subsequent entrapment of the enlarged tendon distal to the site of fibrosis. This results in a trigger finger.

Common clinical tendinitis syndromes include rotator cuff tendinitis of the shoulder, which is usually degenerative in nature. The supraspinatus tendon is involved most frequently. Clinically, cuff tendinitis presents as a dull ache, which is exacerbated by abduction or pressure on the shoulder. Rotator cuff tendinitis is more common in the dominant shoulder and in male patients. Bicipital tendinitis presents with pain in the anterior shoulder, which may radiate down to the forearm. Yergason's sign (pain on resisted supination of the hand) is indicative of bicipital tendon inflammation. Frequently, there is tenderness over the bicipital groove on palpation of the anterior shoulder. Epicondylitis is more common in males than in females, usually in the dominant arm. The lateral epicondyle is more frequently involved. There is pain on forced extension of the wrist. Pain may radiate from the forearm down to the hand. The cause of tenosynovitis of the elbow is usually overuse or trauma. Achilles' tendinitis presents with pain in the ankle and pain on dorsiflexion of the foot.

Diabetes mellitus is associated with increased frequency of flexor tenosynovitis of the hands and wrists with carpal tunnel syndrome, Dupuytren's contractures, and trigger fingers being the commonest entities. Diabetics are also prone to calcific tendinitis and periarthritis of the shoulder with adhesive capsulitis. Rheumatoid arthritis patients may frequently develop tenosynovitis of the extensor tendons of the wrists bilaterally. Trigger fingers and carpal tunnel syndrome are also common in rheumatoid patients. They may develop tarsal tunnel syndrome with extensor tenosynovitis of the tendons on the medial aspect of the ankle. Seronegative spondyloarthropathies, specifically Reiter's syndrome, may involve the Achilles' tendon. Crystal-induced arthropathies, such as hydroxyapatite disease, gout, and pseudogout, may present as tendinitis involving the shoulders.

The commonest infectious agent that presents as a tenosynovitis (usually involving the hands and the wrists) is caused by *Neisseria gonorrhoeae*. Tenosynovitis is the commonest manifestation of the gonococcal arthritis-dermatitis syndrome. Idiopathic tenosynovitis of the abductor pollicis longus and the extensor pollicis brevis as they pass over the radial styloid process is called de Quervain's disease. Patients complain of wrist and thumb pain on motion. Finkelstein's test is positive (place the thumb in the palm, clasp the fingers around the thumb, then forcibly move the wrist in an ulnar direction).

### Treatment

Therapy for tendinitis and bursitis consists of ice applications and administration of nonsteroidal anti-inflammatory medications. For patients with de Quervain's tenosynovitis, a thumb spica splint is helpful. Patients with a painful shoulder related to tendinitis or bursitis usually respond to ice and anti-inflammatory medications; other modalities such as range-of-motion exercises, physical therapy, and ultrasound are helpful in relieving pain. Occasionally, patients require local corticosteroid injections; 20 to 30 mg of a steroid preparation, prednisolone tebutate (Hydelra-T.B.A.) or methylprednisolone acetate (Depo-Medrol), combined with 1 or 2 ml of 1% lidocaine (Xylocaine) is usually sufficient to relieve the symptoms. Patients should be advised of the risks of corticosteroid injections, which include infection and possible tendon rupture. Joints should be rested for 7 days after an injection. Patients with recurrent tendinitis should embark on a program of muscle strengthening and stretching to ameliorate their symptoms. Tendinitis pain usually subsides within 4 to 6 weeks. Prolonged pain may indicate a tendon tear. Surgical intervention may be helpful in calcific tendinitis or if there has been complete tendon rupture.

# OSTEOARTHRITIS

method of
DAVID H. NEUSTADT, M.D.
*University of Louisville School of Medicine*
*Louisville, Kentucky*

and

JEFFREY B. NEUSTADT, M.D.
*Georgetown University*
*Washington, D.C.*

Osteoarthritis (osteoarthrosis, degenerative joint disease) is the most commonly encountered rheumatic disorder and the major cause of disability and reduced activity in the elderly. Radiographic evidence of osteoarthritis is found in up to 85% of people older than age 85. Autopsy examination discloses bony alterations in most weight-bearing joints of almost all persons after the age of 45 years. The pathologic process of the disease is characterized by loss of cartilage with subchondral bone alterations, including osteophyte formation. Associated para-articular ligament and musculotendinous weakening may lead to development of angular deformities and joint instability. There is increasing recognition of a definite inflammatory component in many patients with symptomatic osteoarthritis. The traditional belief that osteoarthritis is simply a "wear and tear" disease is no longer tenable.

The onset and course of nontraumatic osteoarthritis are insidious and gradually progressive and are manifested by variable pain and soreness, loss of function, bony enlargement, occasional synovitis, and ultimately end-stage disabling features, especially when advanced involvement of the knee or the hip develops.

Osteoarthritis may be classified into primary (idiopathic) and secondary (local) forms, though management is similar. Secondary osteoarthritis occurs as an aftermath of an etiologic or specific underlying provocative factor, such as a congenital hip dysplasia, or an inflammatory form of arthritis, such as rheumatoid arthritis. Joints commonly affected in osteoarthritis include the weight-bearing and frequently used joints such as the hips, the knees, the spine, the distal interphalangeal joints, and the first carpometacarpal and the first metatarsophalangeal joints. Joints rarely involved in osteoarthritis include the metacarpophalangeals, the wrists, the shoulders, and the ankles.

Special forms of osteoarthritis and significant associated conditions include inflammatory or cystic erosive osteoarthritis, crystal deposition disease, and diffuse idiopathic skeletal hyperostosis (DISH).

## MANAGEMENT

The management program for osteoarthritis should be individualized in accordance with the specific symptomatic problems presented by each patient (Table 1).

**General Considerations.** Education of the patient and the family is the basic foundation of the treatment program. Realistic reassurance that the patient does not have a serious, potentially crippling disease, such as rheumatoid arthritis, and providing an understanding of what to expect are of great importance in successful manage-

TABLE 1. **Comprehensive Management of Osteoarthritis**

Patient education
Realistic reassurance and coping measures
Measures for reduction of joint loading
Physical therapy and assistive equipment
Drug therapy and chondroprotective therapy
Intra-articular therapy
Surgery

ment. Patient education material, such as the "Osteoarthritis" booklet, available from the Arthritis Foundation is a useful supplement to patient education.

Reducing the impact of the load force and stress on the malaligned joint may not only help decrease symptoms, but also retard progression of the disease. Explaining the biomechanical factors involved help the patient to understand the importance of rest and protection of the affected joints. Bioengineering research studies have demonstrated that the weight load on the knee when rising from a low seated to a standing position is an astounding nine times the total body weight. Weight reduction by dietetic means is strongly encouraged in the obese patient. Protective and preventive measures for knee involvement include limited standing, walking, and stair climbing and avoidance of jogging. Knee bending and weight bearing during rising can be avoided by using a high chair or stool and an elevated toilet seat.

**Physical Therapy.** Physical therapy deserves emphasis as part of a comprehensive management program. Heat modalities, chiefly in the form of moist hot packs, soaks, and underwater pool therapy, are palliative, as well as effective in facilitating the therapeutic exercise program.

Specific instructions should be given for exercise. Exercises should be chiefly isometric (quadriceps-strengthening exercises) rather than isotonic, to avoid stressing the joint. Active range-of-motion exercises and mild stretching improve joint function and flexibility.

Instructions and advice should be given on the use of assistive aids and devices, such as canes, crutches, proper shoes with needed corrections, back supports, braces, and cervical supporting collars.

Diathermy, shortwave, and ultrasound are rarely of value in the management of patients with osteoarthritis. Transcutaneous electrical nerve stimulation (TENS) may be used to help patients cope with chronic pain associated with osteoarthritis, especially in pain problems involving the cervical and lumbar spine.

### Pharmacotherapy

The basic program of education, reassurance, joint rest and protection, and physical therapy may adequately control symptoms in some patients with early or mild osteoarthritis. The majority of patients, however, require drug therapy. Currently, no available drugs predictably halt the progression of the disease, but the drugs used do reduce pain and inflammation. The two major groups of drugs available for patients with osteoarthritis include the analgesics and anti-inflammatory agents.

**Analgesics.** In some patients with osteoarthritis, the joint problem is mainly or entirely mechanical and an anti-inflammatory effect is not needed. Analgesic compounds currently available include acetaminophen (Tylenol), propoxyphene (Darvon), pentazocine (Talwin), and codeine or codeine congeners. Effective dosages of acetaminophen are 0.5 to 1 gram, given at 4- to 6-hour intervals. Side effects are rare and minimal. Propoxyphene (Darvon) is effective, especially in preparations in combination with acetaminophen (e.g., Darvocet-N 100), given in a dosage of up to one tablet every 4 to 6 hours as needed for pain. Pentazocine (Talwin), available in 50-mg tablets, is highly effective for pain relief, but is poorly tolerated, causing frequent nausea, vomiting, dizziness, ataxia, and sedation. Codeine and other narcotic congeners are usually avoided owing to the potential for developing tolerance and dependence from long-term administration.

**Anti-inflammatory Agents.** The anti-inflammatory drugs used for osteoarthritis also possess analgesic properties. These drugs, categorized as nonsteroidal anti-inflammatory drugs (NSAIDs) include aspirin, other salicylates, and a host of newer agents (Table 2). These NSAIDs provide effective relief from pain and inflammation.

Aspirin is inexpensive, effective, and frequently the first anti-inflammatory agent prescribed. It is given as needed in 650-mg doses at 4- to 6-hour intervals, and with this dosage schedule it seldom causes serious undesirable effects. If the plain soluble aspirin causes gastrointestinal (GI) upset, the drug can be given as enteric-coated preparations (Ecotrin, 325 or 500 mg), or in a new sophisticated delivery system form, zero-order–release aspirin 800-mg tablets (ZORprin), which permits twice daily dosing and avoids disintegration in the stomach. Salicylism with significant tinnitus and hearing impairment is a relatively frequent adverse reaction, particularly in the elderly, necessitating discontinuance of the drug. Rarely, confusion may result from aspirin in older patients.

Nonacetylated salicylates are widely used as a substitute for aspirin in osteoarthritis. Nonacetylated salicylate compounds currently available include magnesium salicylate (Magan), choline magnesium trisalicylate (Trilisate), and salsalate (Disalcid). These preparations may be conveniently administered in a dosage of 1 to 1.5 grams twice daily. Nausea and GI upset occur occasionally and salicylism rarely. These agents are weak prostaglandin inhibitors. Toxicity is relatively minor, and adverse events are infrequent. Diflunisal (Dolobid) is also a nonacetylated salicylate, but it has prostaglandin-inhibiting properties similar to those of a typical NSAID.

A number of NSAIDs are currently available in the United States, with several additional agents waiting in the wings at the U.S. Food and Drug Administration (FDA). The drugs now approved for use in the treatment of osteoarthritis can be divided into five chemical families: propionic acid derivatives (ibuprofen [Motrin], fenoprofen [Nalfon], naproxen [Naprosyn], ketoprofen [Orudis], and flurbiprofen [Ansaid]); indolacetic acids (indomethacin [Indocin], sulindac [Clinoril], and tolmetin [Tolectin]; anthranilic acid (meclofenamate [Meclomen]; oxicams (piroxicam [Feldene]); and phenylacetic acids (diclofenac [Voltaren]). All NSAIDs can provide varying degrees of pain relief and suppression of inflammation. The drugs are similar in their major proposed mechanism of action (i.e., inhibition of the cyclo-oxygenase enzyme in the prostaglandin synthesis pathway), but vary in their pharmacokinetics, dosage, response, and side effects (see Table 2). Patients' beneficial responses to a trial of a particular NSAID varies considerably and is not predictable. Clinical and pharmacokinetic differences, as well as possible multifarious differences in their mechanism of action, may help explain the variability of efficacy from patient to patient.

Cost and compliance also must be considered in selecting an NSAID. If a patient finds it difficult to be compliant on a four-times-daily regimen, an NSAID with a longer half-life may be prescribed, permitting once- or twice-daily administration.

The chief limiting factor in the use of NSAIDs is the occurrence of adverse effects. Prostaglandin (cyclo-oxygenase) synthesis inhibition is the major cause of NSAID-induced gastric pathologic changes, potential coagulopathy, and disturbed renal function. Some side effects, such as skin eruptions, hepatitis, and interstitial nephritis, are probably due to hypersensitivity or idiosyncrasy.

TABLE 2. **Summary of Nonsteroidal Anti-inflammatory Drugs**

| Drug | Half-Life (hours) | Usual Daily Dosage (mg) |
|---|---|---|
| Aspirin | 3–5 | 650 qid |
| Diclofenac (Voltaren) | 2 | 75 bid |
| Diflunisal (Dolobid) | 8–12 | 500 bid |
| Fenoprofen (Nalfon) | 3 | 600 qid |
| Flurbiprofen (Ansaid) | 5 | 100 bid |
| Indomethacin (Indocin) | 4.5 | 25 qid |
| Ketoprofen (Orudis) | 2.5 | 75 bid |
| Meclofenamate (Meclomen) | 3 | 100 qid |
| Naproxen (Naprosyn) | 13 | 250 bid |
| Piroxicam (Feldene) | 30–80 | 20 qd |
| Sulindac (Clinoril) | 16 | 200 bid |
| Tolmetin (Tolectin) | 1.5 | 400 qid |

Estimates indicate that more than 30 million people take NSAIDs on a daily basis. Side effects arising from these drugs are reputed to occur more frequently than with any other form of drug treatment. The incidence of GI symptoms related to NSAIDs remains extremely variable. Not infrequently, endoscopy demonstrates gastric ulcers in patients who are without GI complaints. The most serious potential side effects of NSAIDs are peptic ulcer disease (with GI bleeding) and renal failure. Both of these adverse events are caused by the same mechanism that produces the anti-inflammatory effect—inhibition of prostaglandin synthesis. A history of peptic ulcer disease is a relative contraindication to NSAIDs, although they can be taken with antacids and after meals in an attempt to avoid recurrent ulceration and upper GI bleeding. If peptic ulceration does occur, NSAIDs should be discontinued and appropriate antiulcer treatment initiated. Concomitant prophylactic use of misoprostol (Cytotec), an analogue of prostaglandin E1 has been recommended to protect gastric mucosa. Other GI side effects of NSAIDs, including dyspepsia, nausea, and diarrhea, may be controlled by symptomatic measures. Inhibition of renal tissue prostaglandin synthesis is thought to cause the rare renal complications of NSAIDs. These include peripheral edema, transient acute renal insufficiency, hyperkalemia, and renal papillary necrosis. Patients at special risk for renal complications include those with decreased intravascular fluid volume (from diuretic drugs, congestive heart failure, and cirrhosis). Acute renal failure is characterized by a rise in serum blood urea nitrogen, creatinine, and potassium levels. Withdrawal of the NSAID and adequate hydration reverse the renal failure. A nephrotic syndrome (tubulointerstitial nephropathy) has also been seen with NSAID use, most frequently with fenoprofen. This problem is probably an idiosyncrasy of the drug, unrelated to prostaglandin inhibition. Although usually reversible on withdrawal of the NSAID, it sometimes requires treatment with corticosteroids when a frank nephrotic syndrome has occurred.

The hypothesis has been proposed that certain NSAIDs may accelerate the progression of osteoarthritis by inhibiting the synthesis of vasodilator prostaglandins, thereby reducing joint perfusion. In so-called indomethacin hip, the affected hip disclosed greater loss of joint space than did the contralateral hip, which served as a treated control for the affected hip. However, at this time, the evidence suggests that the clinical benefits of NSAIDs outweigh the possible chondrotoxic effects. Additional studies are in progress to assess the question of potential deterioration of cartilage and osteoarthritis with different NSAIDs.

## Intra-articular Therapy

Intra-articular corticosteroid therapy in osteoarthritis is of considerable value when administered judiciously and when indicated. This form of treatment must always be considered as an adjunct to a conventional management program.

A fairly large or painful knee effusion is the strongest indication for arthrocentesis, followed by a corticosteroid injection. The potential deleterious effect of developing instability of the knee can be avoided by giving infrequent injections and prescribing a strict rest regimen after each injection. Infection is avoided by adhering to a meticulous aseptic technique.

Intra-articular superoxide dismutase (Orgotein)* has been shown to have anti-inflammatory properties in animal models of osteoarthritis. In a recent multicenter trial of osteoarthritis of the knee, intra-articular Orgotein was effective in reducing symptoms for up to 3 months after injection. Additional trials with intra-articular Orgotein in osteoarthritis of the knee are underway in an effort to confirm the initial favorable clinical results.

## Specific and Investigational Forms of Therapy

Although no available therapeutic agent predictably alters the underlying pathogenesis of osteoarthritis, research has been carried out with certain noteworthy approaches. Arteparon, an investigational drug, a mixture of proteoglycans (a glycosaminoglycan polysulfate), has been reported to "refresh" the cartilage. It may inhibit neutral proteases, hyaluronidase, and other enzymes that play a role in the degradation of cartilage. Rumalon (marketed in Europe) is another treatment aimed at restoring the disturbed cartilage metabolism to normal. This calf costal cartilage and bone marrow extract is thought to benefit osteoarthritis by causing a regeneration of cartilage. Further controlled trials are required to confirm the beneficial claims for these substances.

## Special Forms and Problems Related to Osteoarthritis

**Cystic Erosive Osteoarthritis.** Although the lumpy-bumpy nodes of the distal interphalangeal joints (Heberden's nodes) and proximal interpha-

---

*Available as an orphan drug from Pharmacia or Bristol-Myers Company.

langeal joints (Bouchard's nodes) are unsightly, discomfort is minimal, except during the early developing stage. It is important to strongly reassure the patient that this is not a generalized serious crippling disease, stressing the distinction from rheumatoid arthritis. Occasionally, when nodes are acutely inflamed, it is necessary to administer a local steroid injection. Generally, symptomatic measures such as warm soaks followed by massage of a topical analgesic balm are adequate to control symptoms. If the thumb base (trapeziometacarpal) joint is troublesome, local injection and sometimes splinting are necessary to provide relief.

**Crystal Deposition Disease.** Calcium pyrophosphate or hydroxyapatite crystals may be found in association with osteoarthritis and may be responsible for acute inflammatory flares (pseudogout). Diagnosis is made by x-ray findings of chondrocalcinosis and polarized light microscopic identification of crystals. Treatment includes arthrocentesis with aspiration and intra-articular corticosteroids for acute synovitis and a therapeutic trial with one of the NSAIDs.

**Diffuse Idiopathic Skeletal Hyperostosis.** DISH is a not uncommon skeletal disorder involving chiefly the spine and enthesis sites with exuberant bone formation and a characteristic flowing calcification, particularly affecting the dorsal spine. There is giant osteophyte formation and frequently large calcaneal spurs. The striking clinical symptom is overall stiffness, especially in the thoracic spine. Treatment is symptomatic, with strong reassurance that the disease is not a serious form of spondyloarthropathy, such as ankylosing spondylitis, which it frequently resembles.

### Surgery

Surgical treatment of osteoarthritis is indicated when drug therapy and other conventional measures fail to adequately control symptoms, which prevent the patient from coping with the activities of daily living. Intractable hip or knee pain at rest, particularly at night, deserves serious consideration for surgical intervention. The four methods of orthopedic management for osteoarthritis currently include osteotomy for joint realignment, arthroplasty (joint replacement), arthrodesis (fusion), and arthroscopic procedures.

When arthritic involvement is limited chiefly to one compartment of the knee, a high-tibial or distal femoral osteotomy, which shifts the weight-bearing load to the uninvolved compartment, may provide relief of pain and postpone the need for total knee replacement.

Total joint replacement is reserved for the patient with refractory pain and disability involving the hip or the knee and occasionally the shoulder. Complications of total joint arthroplasty include infection, prosthetic failure or loosening, instability, and fractures. Failed total joint replacement can be revised, but revision is not uniformly successful, especially after infection. Newer techniques using porous-ingrowth prostheses and press-fit noncemented prostheses may decrease the failure rate, particularly in younger patients who want to return to more aggressive physical activity.

Arthrodesis provides relief of pain, with the obvious sacrifice of joint motion. It is reserved for the patient with incapacitating pain or the relatively young patient with an infected joint or severe post-traumatic osteoarthritis such as may result from a fracture or a dislocation of the hip. Fusion of the cervical or lumbar spine is considered for severe neck or back pain associated with significant mechanical instability of the spine.

Arthroscopic joint débridement with removal of calcified loose bodies, cartilage fragments, and bony spurs may be a useful procedure for the patient without end-stage disease but with pain and/or locking of the joint.

# POLYMYALGIA RHEUMATICA AND GIANT CELL ARTERITIS
method of
ALAN HOWARD COHEN, M.D.
*Kaiser Permanente*
*San Diego, California*

### POLYMYALGIA RHEUMATICA

Polymyalgia rheumatica (PMR) is a relatively common disease of unknown etiology characterized by aching and stiffness in the neck, the shoulder girdle, and/or the pelvic girdle. PMR usually occurs in people older than the age of 50 years, with women predominating in a ratio of 2:1. There is a striking predilection for caucasians.

The onset of myalgias and arthralgias may be sudden or insidious. Proximal musculoskeletal discomfort is usually persistent and is often accompanied by constitutional symptoms, including fever, weight loss, malaise, and fatigue. Symptoms of depression may be prominent. Pain, swelling, and morning stiffness of peripheral joints may be present.

Although the physical examination results are often unremarkable, pain can be elicited frequently by passive or active motion of the shoulders, the hips, and the neck. A careful examination may reveal active synovitis of peripheral joints, primarily in the knees and the wrists. Findings suggestive of carpal tunnel syndrome are seen occasionally.

A markedly elevated Westergren's erythrocyte sedimentation rate (ESR) (typically >50 mm per hour) is characteristic of PMR, although modestly elevated or normal values may be seen. Other laboratory findings include a normochromic, normocytic anemia, elevated C-reactive protein (CRP) level, abnormal liver function test results, increased alpha globulin concentration, and hypoalbuminemia. Levels of muscle enzymes are normal, and tests for rheumatoid factor and antinuclear antibodies are generally negative. Synovial fluid is mildly inflammatory.

The differential diagnosis of PMR includes connective tissue diseases, such as rheumatoid arthritis, systemic lupus erythematosus, and polymyositis; hypothyroidism or hyperthyroidism; malignancies; chronic infections; and systemic vasculitides. Giant cell arteritis (GCA) coexists in approximately 15% of patients with PMR.

### Treatment

Although some patients with PMR respond to nonsteroidal anti-inflammatory drugs, the mainstay of treatment is corticosteroids. Prednisone, given as a single morning dose of 10 to 15 mg, is the recommended initial treatment. A rapid clinical response and normalization of the ESR or CRP are characteristic. Musculoskeletal and constitutional symptoms are typically diminished significantly within the first 24 to 48 hours of therapy, and patients are often 90 to 100% improved after the first week. Although the ESR is usually reduced markedly after 1 week and is often normalized within 4 weeks, it may remain modestly elevated indefinitely. When the patient is clinically stable for 2 to 4 weeks, the daily dose of prednisone may be reduced by 1 mg every 2 to 4 weeks. The subsequent clinical response and ESR should be monitored on a regular basis. Control of symptoms can usually be maintained with 5 to 7.5 mg of prednisone daily. Relapses are common during periods of steroid reduction. Because most patients require a minimum of 18 months of therapy, therapeutic measures to prevent corticosteroid-related osteoporosis should be considered.

### GIANT CELL ARTERITIS

Giant cell arteritis is a systemic vasculitis involving both large and medium-sized arteries that affects the same population as PMR. The vessels that originate from the arch of the aorta are involved most prominently, although other arteries, including those in the extremities, may be affected. Inflammation of the vessels tends to occur in a discontinuous fashion, with involved segments showing infiltration of lymphocytes, macrophages, histiocytes, and multinucleated giant cells.

The onset of GCA may be abrupt or insidious. Clinical manifestations include constitutional symptoms, symptoms of PMR (approximately 50% of patients), and symptoms related to the specific arteries affected. Headaches, often temporal or occipital in location, occur in most patients and are frequently accompanied by jaw claudication and/or scalp tenderness. Sudden, irreversible loss of vision due to narrowing of the ophthalmic or posterior ciliary arteries occurs in approximately 10% of patients. Other symptoms include limb claudication, tongue pain, upper respiratory tract complaints (hoarseness, sore throat, and cough), diplopia, and unilateral weakness.

Physical findings include tender and thickened temporal arteries, scalp and tongue ulcers, arterial bruits, diminished pulses, visual field deficits, transient ophthalmoplegias, and signs of PMR. Myocardial infarctions, brain stem strokes, and peripheral neuropathies have been reported.

Except for the characteristic histologic findings seen on arterial biopsy in patients with GCA, laboratory results in GCA are identical to those in PMR.

The diagnosis of GCA should be considered in any patient older than the age of 50 years who has either a new form of headache or sudden loss of vision, accompanied by symptoms of PMR, constitutional symptoms, and/or a markedly elevated ESR. Histologic confirmation should be obtained by a timely biopsy of an involved temporal artery. Because the arteritis is segmental, a 4- to 6-cm specimen should be excised and sectioned meticulously for histologic examination. If the initial biopsy specimen is normal, biopsy of the contralateral temporal artery may be performed. When the diagnosis of GCA is strongly suspected on the basis of clinical features, but the arterial biopsy specimens are normal, corticosteroid therapy should not be withheld.

### Treatment

When the diagnosis of GCA is entertained or established, prednisone, 40 to 60 mg per day, should be started immediately. Higher dosages of corticosteroids have been used successfully to treat arteritic ischemic neuropathy. Reversible symptoms and findings usually remit, and laboratory abnormalities usually normalize within 2 to 4 weeks. The initial dosage of prednisone should be maintained for at least 4 weeks. Afterwards, the daily dose may be decreased by 10% per week until a dosage of 10 to 15 mg is reached. Prednisone should then be tapered by 1 mg per month. As in PMR, most disease flares occur during steroid tapers. Clinical symptoms as well as the ESR or CRP are good measures to follow to assess disease activity in both GCA and PMR. Most patients with GCA require between 18 months and 4 years of treatment. Complications of high-dose corticosteroid therapy include adrenal suppression, infections, compression fractures, osteopenia, and proximal myopathy. Methotrexate (Mexate) and azathioprine (Imuran) have been used recently to treat patients with refractory GCA as well as those who could not tolerate high-dose prednisone therapy.

# OSTEOMYELITIS

method of
LAYNE O. GENTRY, M.D.
*Baylor College of Medicine*
*Houston, Texas*

## PATHOPHYSIOLOGY

Bacterial invasion of bone can occur through three different routes: hematogenous spread of blood-borne infection, direct spread from a contiguous source of infection, or direct inoculation.

Hematogenous spread of bacteria to bone, usually invasive gram-positive cocci such as *Staphylococcus aureus* or *Streptococcus viridans,* is more often noticed in the long bones of children, which are highly vascularized and growing. In adults, the vertebrae remain vascularized throughout life and are susceptible to bacterial invasion from seeding associated with intravenous catheters or intravenous drug abuse. Bacteremic patients are often severely ill, and it is difficult to suspect the concurrent involvement of bone from the clinical presentation alone.

Bone may also become infected from the spread of infection from a contiguous focus, such as a postoperative wound infection or an infected plantar ulcer in a diabetic patient. Both gram-positive and gram-negative organisms, as well as anaerobes and even fungi and other atypical pathogens, may be associated with osteomyelitis resulting from contiguous spread of infection. This route of transmission actually favors the less vascularized long bones in adults, as these patients may be undergoing antibiotic therapy for the contiguous infection and bone would provide a "safe" medium for bacterial growth owing to either inadequate antibiotic penetration or the presence of devitalized tissue. As with hematogenous osteomyelitis, the patient may be acutely ill from the initial infection, yet with few

or no symptoms of bone involvement. Unlike cases resulting from hematogenous spread, there is little accuracy associated with an empiric diagnosis; there may be a lack of correlation between the microbiologic etiology of the primary infection and that of the osteomyelitis. Frequently, the contiguous infection is polymicrobial, whereas the secondary osteomyelitis is monomicrobial.

Osteomyelitis due to direct inoculation, such as from an open fracture or perioperative contamination, may not become clinically apparent until weeks or months after the bone is contaminated. *Pseudomonas aeruginosa* and coagulase-negative *Staphylococcus,* respectively, are often implicated. Only infrequently are blood cultures positive in these patients, as the lack of vascularization in adult bone precludes bacterial seeding of the blood stream. Patients with direct osteomyelitis are rarely ill and often complain only of erythema or mild pain. A detailed medical history usually reveals risk factors for osteomyelitis, such as previous osteomyelitis, recent contiguous infection, or underlying diabetes mellitus.

Osteomyelitis is characterized as acute when signs and symptoms have been present for less than 3 months, and chronic when signs and symptoms have been present for more than 3 months. Acute osteomyelitis is most often diagnosed in children with bacteremia and may respond favorably to a short-term regimen of parenteral antibiotics followed by oral therapy. Chronic osteomyelitis in adults often follows trauma or major orthopedic surgery, and the current standard therapy includes 4 to 6 weeks of parenteral antibiotics.

Despite published assumptions that anaerobic osteomyelitis is more common than reported, in most series in which anaerobic cultures are performed, anaerobes are rarely found in bone. Anaerobes may be suspected in infected plantar ulcers in diabetic patients, in victims of human bite, or when gas or a foul-smelling exudate is noted. As the number of immunocompromised patients continues to grow, owing to increased survival from cancer, organ transplantation, and acquired immune deficiency syndrome (AIDS), we should see more fungal osteomyelitis and osteomyelitis due to opportunistic pathogens such as Mycobacteriaceae.

## DIAGNOSIS

For patients in whom osteomyelitis is suspected, laboratory data may be suggestive or inconclusive for infection. Elevations of the leukocyte count and sedimentation rate should support an infectious explanation for mild, nonspecific symptoms. For many patients with osteomyelitis, however, laboratory values remain normal despite active infection.

Radiographic or radionuclide findings are crucial to the diagnosis of osteomyelitis. Radiologic evidence of destruction (lytic lesions) and new bone formation (periosteal elevation with increased density) are usually the earliest evidence of infection, even though diagnostic radiologic findings may not be detectable for 10 to 14 days after injury and infection. Computed tomography (CT) has been shown to offer an improved image of the surrounding soft tissue and any sequestrum, albeit at much greater expense. Magnetic resonance imaging, the most sensitive yet most expensive technique available, may offer superior data for vertebral osteomyelitis and is capable of defining the extent of bony involvement. However, in long-bone infection, this technique may not add to less expensive data from radiography or tomography.

Radionuclide scans offer the earliest reliable evidence of an acute inflammatory process in bone. Technetium polyphosphate scanning has been extensively used as a sensitive early indicator of osteomyelitis and, when combined with a detailed history and physical examination and careful radiography, constitutes a comprehensive diagnostic strategy for most types of chronic osteomyelitis. Newer radionuclide studies such as gallium and indium scans have been proposed as significant developments; however, results have not been consistent in the hands of various investigators, and these newer scans are significantly more expensive than technetium scans.

Radiographic and radionuclide data are sensitive, yet not specific for osteomyelitis. The differential diagnosis for a patient with erythema, pain, and radiographic or radionuclide findings of an acute inflammatory process in bone includes tumor, infarction, injury, and infection.

In bacteremic patients, a positive blood culture combined with positive radiographic or radionuclide evidence is diagnostic of osteomyelitis. For patients with a contiguous infection to an area of acute inflammation of bone, osteomyelitis is the diagnosis until proved otherwise. For these cases, however, the precise microbiologic etiology of the infection is yet to be established.

Biopsy of bone, either open or percutaneous, is the only reliable means of confirming the diagnosis. This procedure can be completed in less than 20 minutes and is relatively risk free (apart from biopsy of the small bones of the hands and feet). Because biopsy is a surgical procedure with a nontrivial expense to the patient, site-specific radiographic evidence prior to biopsy should clearly imply an infectious etiology for what are often benign symptoms. Fluoroscopic or CT control greatly improves the sensitivity and accuracy of bone biopsy.

## MANAGEMENT

Chronic osteomyelitis is often accompanied by the presence of a sequestrum, which must be surgically débrided for antimicrobial therapy to be successful. Evidence of inadequate surgical débridement is the most frequent underlying factor in failures of therapy for chronic osteomyelitis.

Under the present diagnosis-related financial system, hospitals are reimbursed the equivalent of 10 to 12 days of care for chronic osteomyelitis. As there is no evidence to suggest that less than 4 weeks of antimicrobial therapy will be successful for these patients, it is obviously not economical for osteomyelitis patients to receive their care as inpatients. In fact, hospitalization is rarely appropriate, as most patients with chronic

osteomyelitis have no problems that would preclude them receiving care as outpatients.

Long-term intravenous access catheters have been demonstrated to be safe for outpatients. Patients receiving home care should be visited weekly by a nurse, who inspects the catheter site. Laboratory monitoring, including white blood cell count, serum creatinine determination, erythrocyte sedimentation rate, and tests for tolerance of antimicrobial therapy (e.g., serum creatinine level with aminoglycosides) should be performed every 2 to 4 weeks. Improvement in any abnormal laboratory findings should parallel clinical progress. Routine radiographs and radionuclide scans are not necessary and are optional at 4- to 6-month intervals for follow-up, with suggestive clinical findings.

Although parenteral therapy can usually be stopped prior to 6 weeks, oral fluoroquinolone therapy may continue longer. An early return to a full range of motion is essential to rehabilitation. Unless there is the danger of pathologic fracture, patients should maintain a normal schedule of activities during therapy.

### Antimicrobial Therapy

In acute osteomyelitis, the patient may be severely ill, and therapy for the primary infection (bacteremia or contiguous focus) should be the primary concern. _S. aureus_ is the dominant pathogen, usually susceptible to the β-lactamase–resistant penicillins (Table 1). Osteomyelitis itself rarely causes fever or troublesome sequelae such as septic shock. Most primary infections can be resolved with 1 week or less of aggressive parenteral antimicrobial therapy. Following resolution of the major signs and symptoms of infection, antimicrobial selection, dosing, and duration of therapy can be adjusted to account for the osteomyelitis. The initial interval of therapy can count toward the 4-week minimum required to minimize the risk of recurrence.

As noted, most cases of gram-positive osteomyelitis are caused by strains of _Staphylococcus_ and _Streptococcus_ susceptible to the β-lactamase–resistant penicillins, although _Enterococcus faecalis_ is an increasingly troublesome pathogen which requires ampicillin (Omnipen, Polycillin). These antimicrobial agents penetrate exceedingly well into bone and are thus highly effective in regimens of 4 to 6 weeks in facilitating a complete cure of the osteomyelitis. Rifampin (Rifadin, Rimactane) may be added in combination, to increase antistaphylococcal activity against less susceptible strains. In troublesome cases of recurrent gram-positive osteomyelitis, long-term suppressive therapy with an oral agent such as

TABLE 1. **Antimicrobial Therapy**

| Pathogen | Preferred Therapy | Dosage | Comments |
|---|---|---|---|
| **Gram-Positive** | | | |
| *Staphylococcus aureus* (methicillin suscep-tible) | β-Lactamase–resistant penicillin | | |
| | Nafcillin (Nafcil) | 2 grams IV q 6 hr | |
| | Oxacillin (Prostaphlin) | 2 grams IV q 6 hr | |
| | *or* | | |
| | First-generation cephalo-sporin | | Penicillin hypersensitive |
| | Cefazolin (Kefzol) | 2 grams IV q 8 hr | |
| | *or* | | |
| | Oral fluoroquinolone | | Less proven for *S. aureus* |
| | Ciprofloxacin (Cipro) | 750 mg PO q 12 hr | |
| | Ofloxacin (Floxin) | 400 mg PO q 12 h | FDA approval pending |
| *S. aureus* (methicillin-resistant) or coagu-lase-negative *Staphyloccus* | Vancomycin (Vancocin) | 1 gram IV q 12 hr | Possible combination with rifampin (Rifacin) |
| *Streptococcus* spp. | Ampicillin (Principen) | 2 grams IV q 6 hr | Vancomycin (Vancocin) for resistant *Enterococcus* or penicillin hypersensitivity |
| **Gram-Negative** | | | |
| *Pseudomonas aerugi-nosa* | Third-generation cepha-losporin | | |
| | Ceftazidime (Fortaz) | 2 grams IV q 12 hr | |
| | Ceftriaxone (Rocephin) | 2 grams IV q 24 hr | |
| | *or* | | |
| | Oral fluoroquinolone | | Many advantages |
| | *or* | | |
| | Semisynthetic penicillin | | If resistant |
| | Piperacillin (Pipracil) | 3 grams IV q 6 hr | |
| | Mezlocillin (Mezlin) | 3 grams IV q 6 hr | |
| | *or* | | |
| | Aminoglycoside | | For highly resistant strains only, owing to possible nephrotoxicity |
| | Amikacin (Amikin) | 15 mg/kg/day | |
| | Tobramycin (Nebcin) | 5 mg/kg/day | |
| *Enterobacteriaceae* and other gram-negative organisms | Oral fluoroquinolone | | Clear first choice |
| | *or* | | |
| | Third-generation cepha-losporin | | |
| | *or* | | |
| | β-Lactamase inhibitor | | |
| | Ticarcillin–clavulanic acid (Timentin) | 3.1 grams IV q 6 hr | Proven in mixed infection |
| | Imipenem-cilastatin (Primaxin) | 1.0 gram IV q 6 hr | |
| Anaerobes | Clindamycin (Cleocin) | 0.9 gram IV q 8 hr | Anti-*Staphylococcus* activity as well |
| | Metronidazole (Flagyl) | 0.5 gram IV q 8 hr | |

amoxicillin–clavulanic acid (Augmentin) or di-cloxacillin (Dynapen) following completion of par-enteral therapy may be necessary.

Many other antimicrobial agents, such as the first- and second-generation cephalosporins and the oral fluoroquinolones, demonstrate in vitro activity against susceptible gram-positive cocci at concentrations achieved by these agents in bone. However, the clinical results have been inconclusive for these agents in *S. aureus* osteo-myelitis, and there have been reports of untoward microbiologic events, including superinfection and emergence of resistance. Apart from penicil-lin hypersensitivity, there are no obvious reasons to select the more expensive and possibly less effective cephalosporins or oral fluoroquinolones for susceptible gram-positive osteomyelitis.

Increasingly, however, osteomyelitis may be caused by more resistant staphylococci (including coagulase-negative strains) and *E. faecalis*. For acute cases, the potentially serious nature of the bacteremia dictates aggressive therapy, such as vancomycin (Vancocin) in combination with gen-tamicin (Garamycin) or rifampin, until there is resolution of the major symptoms and blood cul-tures become negative. Unfortunately, continua-tion of vancomycin therapy for a prolonged regi-men, to cure the osteomyelitis, may predispose the patient to ototoxic reactions. For those strains of cross-resistant gram-positive cocci that are susceptible in vitro to the oral fluoroquinolones, it may be worthwhile to attempt suppressive therapy with an oral fluoroquinolone after the initial septic episode has resolved.

Recently, newer broad-spectrum antimicrobial agents have gained widespread acceptance for serious gram-negative infections. These agents include the third-generation cephalosporins, such as ceftazidime (Fortaz, Tazidime) and ceftriaxone (Rocephin); monobactams, such as aztreonam (Azactam); β-lactamase inhibitors, such as sulbactam-ampicillin (Unasyn), ticarcillin–clavulanic acid (Timentin), and imipenem-cilastatin (Primaxin); and the oral fluoroquinolones, such as ciprofloxacin (Cipro). These agents have all been shown to be effective not only for osteomyelitis, but also for many of the types of infection that may predispose to osteomyelitis through hematogenous or contiguous spread as well. In particular, ticarcillin–clavulanic acid is well suited as monotherapy for mixed gram-positive and gram-negative osteomyelitis.

The selection of antimicrobial agents for gram-positive osteomyelitis should be based on susceptibilities of the infecting pathogens, any history of patient hypersensitivity, and cost. Aminoglycosides may be added in combination for resistant gram-negative pathogens such as *Pseudomonas,* although these agents are frequently nephrotoxic if administered for a prolonged period. For patients with underlying diabetes mellitus, aggressive therapy for frequently mixed aerobic and anaerobic, gram-positive and gram-negative infection is required, as amputation is a frequent result of failure of an initial course of antibiotics. The serum bactericidal test may be useful in predicting the efficacy of the antibiotic therapy selected. In osteomyelitis patients, it has been shown that peak titers of 1:8 or greater and trough titers of 1:4 or greater are associated with clinical success, whereas lower values are associated with clinical failure and recurrence.

The oral fluoroquinolones provide the hope for effective oral therapy for many cases of osteomyelitis and a reduction in both the economic impact and the inconvenience to the patient that are associated with prolonged intravenous infusion of antibiotics.

Improved radiologic and radionuclide techniques have enhanced our ability to detect the early stages of osteomyelitis. Biopsy of bone is usually required to provide an exact microbiologic diagnosis and the susceptibilities that dictate selection of therapy. Newer antimicrobial agents have been developed that are effective against a broad spectrum of the pathogens responsible for osteomyelitis and that are safe when administered for an extended course. Oral agents such as the fluoroquinolones may eventually replace parenteral therapy for a majority of cases. The prognosis for acute osteomyelitis remains excellent, and, for chronic or recurrent osteomyelitis, the infection can usually be managed through a combined surgical (débridement) and medical (antimicrobial therapy) approach, although 20% of the cases may be expected to relapse each year.

# COMMON SPORTS INJURIES

method of
BRIAN C. HALPERN, M.D.
*Marlboro, New Jersey*

Sports injuries occur basically in two settings, organized and recreational. Organized sports at the high school level alone account for more than 1 million injuries per year. All of these result from either

1. Chronic trauma (overuse), which develops from repetitive forces on anatomic structures, causing inflammation, pain, and disability, or

2. Acute trauma (contact and noncontact), which signifies immediate failure of a bone, ligament, musculotendinous unit, or other body system, with resulting impairment of function.

Overuse syndromes comprise the greatest number of sports injuries seen clinically. Accurate diagnosis, followed by activity modification with appropriate rehabilitation, is essential to their treatment. A functional classification helps to stage the overuse injury (Table 1), and sports specificity better defines the biomechanical cause.

## SHOULDER

Sports requiring overhead use of the upper extremity, such as throwing sports, racket sports,

TABLE 1. **Classification of Overuse Syndromes**

Grade I
  Postactivity pain
  Symptoms of less than 2 wk duration
  Generalized soreness

Grade II
  Pain during late activity and immediately afterward
  Symptoms of 2–3 wk duration
  Localized pain

Grade III
  Pain during early activity
  Symptoms of 3–4 wk duration
  Point tenderness with evidence of inflammation
    (erythema, swelling, crepitus)

Grade IV
  Pain with activities other than training that prevent
    or affect performance
  Symptoms of more than 4 wk duration
  Grade III signs plus disturbance in function, decreased range of motion, muscle atrophy

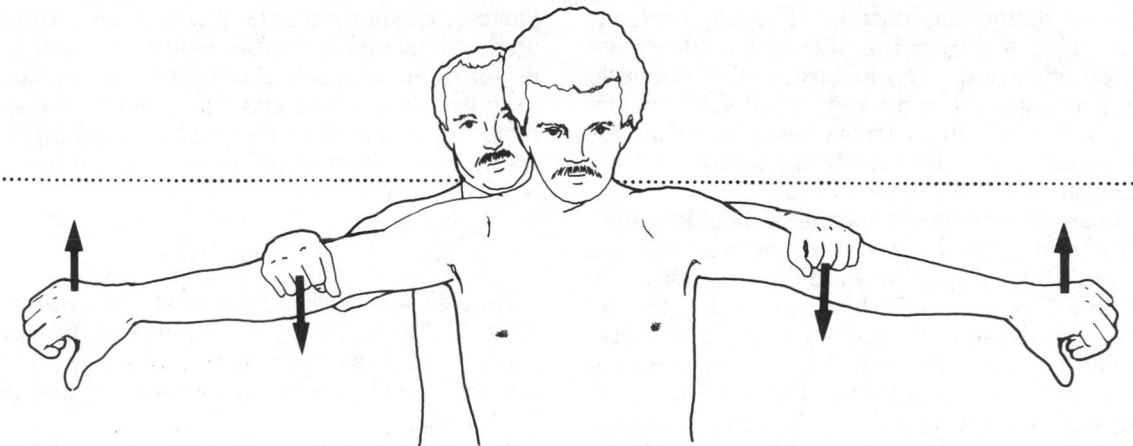

**Figure 1.** Supraspinatus test.

and swimming, commonly cause overuse injuries of the shoulder, followed in frequency by overuse injuries of the elbow. In the shoulder, the posterior rotator cuff muscles suffer chronic inflammation when impinged against the coracoacromial ligament and the anterior part of the acromion in overhead motion. Physical examination often reveals a positive supraspinatus test (pain, and/or weakness, elicited by applying downward force to the shoulder at 90 degrees of abduction, 30 degrees of forward flexion, and full internal rotation; see Figure 1) and/or a positive impingement test (pain elicited by internal rotation of the humerus in the forward flexed position; see Figure 2). As this syndrome progresses, refractory tendinitis, wearing of the supraspinatus muscle and the biceps tendon, and partial or complete thickness rotator cuff tears can occur.

**Treatment.** Early treatment consists of rest, strengthening and flexibility exercises, and anti-inflammatory medications. This can be followed

by physical therapeutic modalities such as ultrasound and electrical stimulation. An injection of a corticosteroid can be used after failure of the initial therapeutic regimen, but it should be reserved for the seasoned athlete and not used in the very young participant.

## ELBOW

Elbow pain commonly evolves from tension overload on the medial aspect, compression overload on the lateral aspect, or irritation and weakness of the wrist extensors or flexors.

**Treatment.** Treatment is the same as that for the shoulder, plus correction of any biomechanical fault in the throwing mechanism or arm stroke.

## KNEE

Sports requiring increased lower extremity loading, as in running, jumping, and biking, commonly result in overuse injuries of the knee, followed in frequency by overuse injuries of the lower leg. In the knee, patellofemoral pain predominates, with such problems as patellar tendinitis and synovial plica irritation. Other possible diagnoses include pes anserine bursitis, iliotibial band syndrome, popliteal or biceps femoris tendinitis, meniscal tear, subluxated patella, and osteochondral damage. Physical examination usually reveals tenderness over the affected structures, and radiographs are usually normal. When evaluating the knee, a history of effusion within 2 hours of injury indicates a hemarthrosis, whereas effusion occurring 12 hours or more after injury indicates fluid of synovial origin. A hemarthrosis suggests an anterior cruciate tear, osteochondral fracture, peripheral meniscal tear, incomplete ligament tear, or sub-

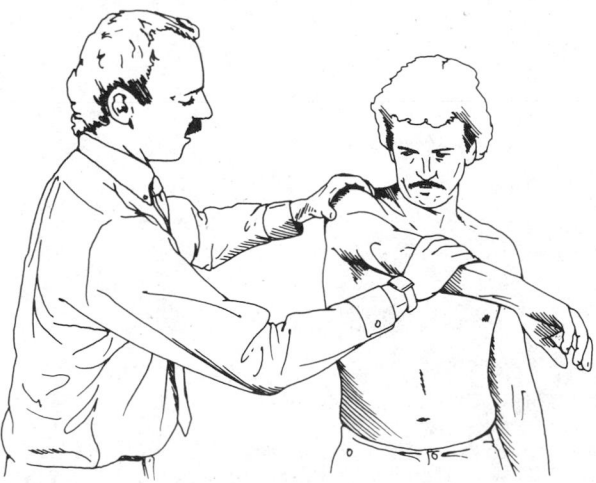

**Figure 2.** Impingement test.

luxated or dislocated patella. The physical examination, at a minimum, should include range of motion with palpation for areas of tenderness, anterior and posterior drawer, pivot shift or jerk test, valgus and varus stress tests, external rotation recurvatum test, Lachman's test, and attempted patellar subluxation test.

**Treatment.** Immediate treatment should include rest, ice and immobilization, compression, and elevation. Rehabilitation should begin as early as possible. Treatment is the same as that for the upper extremity but does not include corticosteroid injection into the patellar tendon, because this can result in local atrophy and increased risk of subsequent rupture. The same risks of corticosteroid injection are seen with tendinous injections at other sites in the body as well.

## LOWER LEG

In the lower leg (exclusive of the ankle and foot), the majority of syndromes are tibial periostitis (shin splints), stress fractures, and com-

TABLE 2. **Classification of Sprains and Strains**

| Grade I |
| Microtear with some fiber tear |
| Grade II |
| Greater fiber tear |
| Grade III |
| Complete tear |

partment syndromes. It is sometimes difficult to distinguish among these conditions without the use of radiographs, bone scans, and compartment pressure measurements. Treatment consists of rest, immobilization as needed, flexibility exercises, and correction of any biomechanical fault with orthotics.

## ANKLE

Lateral ankle sprains remain ubiquitous and occur biomechanically during inversion and plantar flexion. They often result in immediate swelling and disability to the extent of inability to bear weight.

**Treatment.** Ankle sprains are treated with ice, immobilization, rest, elevation, compression, and rapid rehabilitation to restore normal ankle motion and strength. Return to participation hinges on the athlete's ability to run and cut without pain or instability. Some type of external support, such as taping or bracing, should be used for early return to sport participation. As in every injury, rehabilitation is the key.

Acute traumatic injuries are classified, in decreasing order of frequency, as sprains or strains, contusions, and fractures or dislocations. A grading system for sprains (injury to ligaments) and strains (injury to muscles or tendons) is presented in Table 2. Most injuries resulting from acute trauma are to the knee, followed by the ankle or foot; wrist, hand, or fingers; and shoulder.

# Obstetrics and Gynecology

## ANTEPARTUM CARE

method of
VAL CATANZARITE, M.D., PH.D.
*Sharp Memorial Hospital*
*San Diego, California*

The role of prenatal care has shifted dramatically during the past several decades as the technology for predicting, detecting, and treating abnormalities of pregnancy and of the embryo or the fetus has evolved. The improved education of the patient and increasing capabilities of the obstetrics care system have combined to make prenatal care an ever more dynamic and active process.

Optimally, prenatal care begins with a preconception visit—a get acquainted visit between obstetrics care provider and the couple planning pregnancy—during which potential risks to the pregnancy may be reviewed and discussed, baseline laboratory tests may be obtained, and prenatal care planned.

It is during this visit that the expectations of the couple for the pregnancy can be explored and a realistic view reinforced and potential exposures to drugs or chemicals minimized or prevented. The groundwork for the relationship between the couple and the obstetrics care provider is often established within the first few minutes of contact, therefore the first visit should be relaxed and pleasant.

### PRECONCEPTION OR FIRST PRENATAL VISIT

#### History

**Obstetric and Gynecologic History.** A history of the couple's reproductive health should include maternal age, gravidity, parity, and outcomes of all prior pregnancies. Obstetric history tends to repeat itself! Obtaining full records for prior pregnancies may have a tremendous yield of information relevant to current pregnancy. Particular attention must be paid to abnormal fetal outcomes, such as miscarriage, intrauterine death, large-for-gestational-age or small-for-gestational-age infants, episodes of preterm labor in the prior pregnancy, or preterm rupture of the membranes. Pre-eclampsia or pregnancy-induced hypertension, particularly remote from term, severe, or with atypical features, carries a recurrence risk of 30 to 50%.

Currently, in the United States, the rate of cesarean section is between 20 and 30%. Most women who have had a prior, low-transverse cesarean section are candidates for a trial of labor during subsequent pregnancies.

The gynecologic history is also important. Past and current birth control methods and plans for contraception following pregnancy can be explored. The regularity of menstrual cycles is used in dating the pregnancy. For the patient who is seen while planning a pregnancy, use of a menstrual calendar can be initiated.

The couple should be specifically questioned regarding any history of sexually transmitted diseases. Syphilis, gonorrhea, and chlamydiosis can have adverse fetal effects and are easy to test for and treat—particularly before pregnancy. The patient who has a history of herpes often has unrealistic fears about potential adverse fetal or neonatal effects of herpes. The patient with a history of pelvic inflammatory disease should be made aware of the risk of ectopic pregnancy, and sonography should be planned early to confirm an intrauterine gestational sac.

**Acquired Immune Deficiency Syndrome.** The specter of acquired immune deficiency syndrome (AIDS) looms large in the thinking of many reproductive-aged women. The American College of Obstetricians and Gynecologists has recently recommended that all high-risk women be offered screening for human immunodeficiency virus (HIV). In certain areas of the country, HIV seropositivity is found in up to 3% of newborn babies, 30% to 50% of whom develop neonatal or pediatric AIDS and die of this disease. Given the grave implications of HIV seropositivity for pregnancy, and the spread of the virus from the traditional high-risk groups (Haitians, intravenous drug abusers, prostitutes, and female partners of males who are bisexual or members of high-risk groups), many obstetricians now offer HIV screening to all women planning pregnancy or seen during the early part of pregnancy.

**Medical Conditions.** A complete past medical history is an essential component of the preconception or first prenatal visit. This should include allergic reactions to drugs or medications, operations, hospitalizations, and any conditions requiring a physician's care. A "check list" patient information form, specifically listing such conditions as hypertension, cardiac problems, tuberculosis, pneumonia, asthma, kidney disease or kidney infections, bladder infections, gastrointestinal diseases, hepatitis, endocrine diseases, anemia, and neurologic or neuromuscular complaints, can be completed by the patient prior to the office visit to streamline the history-taking process.

**Medications.** Relatively few drugs or medications are known teratogens (Table 1), but it is not unusual for patients to use over-the-counter drugs on a routine basis. The patient who is taking a potential teratogen can often be switched to a different drug. I encourage my patients to discontinue all nonprescription drugs except for acetaminophen during the preconception period and also during the pregnancy.

**Alcohol.** Exposures to "illicit" drugs and environmental toxins are an integral part of the medical history. Heavy alcohol consumption is not uncommon in women of childbearing age. Full-blown fetal alcohol syndrome, with symmetrical growth retardation, craniofacial and central nervous system abnormalities, and, in some cases, cardiac and musculoskeletal abnormalities, occurs in 30 to 50% of offspring of women who drink 2 oz of absolute alcohol (four to five mixed drinks) per day. Alcohol effects are present in more than 10% of women drinking even 1 oz of absolute alcohol daily. The recommendation is for pregnant women to abstain as much as possible from alcohol; however, no fetal risk has been associated with the consumption of an occasional glass of wine—and this information may be extremely comforting to the woman who consumed small amounts of alcohol before she knew that she was pregnant.

**Nicotine.** Cigarette smoking has been clearly linked to increased rates of preterm delivery and growth disturbances in the fetus. In addition, children who grow up in homes where tobacco is smoked have an increased rate of respiratory disease. All pregnant women, and their husbands, should be advised to minimize or quit smoking.

**Drug Abuse.** The use of "street drugs" is a source of increasing concern to the obstetrician. Although the rate of intravenous drug use in most areas of the country is relatively low, potent amphetamines ("crank") and highly refined cocaine ("crack") are readily available and commonly abused by women of all social classes. These can cause growth retardation and preterm delivery, as well as placental abruption. In addition, cocaine is increasingly seen as a cause of serious neonatal complications and neurodevelopmental problems in childhood.

**Family History and Pedigree.** Significant health problems among parents, siblings, and nephews or nieces should be identified. In particular, details of any stillbirths, babies with birth defects, or babies who died or required an operation during the first year of life should be obtained. The ethnic background of the parents is important. Blacks in the United States have a 10% rate of carriage of sickle cell trait, and screening for sickle cell trait is a routine part of prenatal care. Hemoglobinopathies are also relatively common in patients of Southeast Asian origin. Alpha- and beta-thalassemias are seen in individuals of Asian, African, and Southern European (Greek and Italian) ancestry. Tay-Sachs disease, uniformly lethal to the neonate, is an autosomal recessive condition with a carrier rate of about 1 in 30 among people in Jewish ancestry and 1 in 150 in the general population; carrier testing is recommended for all couples of Jewish ancestry and can be considered for all couples in which one partner is Jewish.

Consanguinity, or history of birth defects in the immediate family, may be an indication for detailed genetic counseling.

**Social History.** The living circumstances, employment, and exercise and "lifestyle" habits of a couple may need to be modified as pregnancy progresses.

## Physical Examination

Vital signs, including blood pressure, pulse, and respirations, as well as the general appearance of the patient are noted.

**Head, Eyes, Ears, Nose, and Throat Examination.** Dental pathologic changes are commonly noted. The patient should be encouraged to continue regular dental care, and her dentist reassured that procedures under local anesthesia, including fillings and extractions, can be safely undertaken during pregnancy.

TABLE 1. **Human Teratogens Commonly Used by Women in Reproductive Years**

| | |
|---|---|
| Carbamazepine (Tegretol) | Tetracycline |
| Ethanol | Trimethadione |
| Isotretinoin (Accutane) | Valproic acid (Depakene) |
| Lithium | Warfarin (Coumadin) |
| Phenytoin (Dilantin) | |

The thyroid is slightly enlarged in size during normal pregnancy and may have a somewhat "mushy" feel.

**Breasts.** Breasts enlarge in size during pregnancy, and become tender. With the glandular proliferation, the texture of the breasts may become difficult to evaluate. However, any firm masses should be evaluated for the possibility of malignancy; breast cancer is among the most common cancers seen during pregnancy.

**Respiratory System.** The respiratory rate and depth of breathing increase during pregnancy. The lungs should remain clear.

**Cardiovascular System.** A soft (I-II/VI) systolic ejection murmur in the pulmonic area reflects the increased cardiac output of pregnancy. An $S^3$ may also be heard in the normal patient. An $S^4$, or any diastolic or loud systolic murmur, should be further investigated.

**Abdominal Examination.** Abnormal physical findings in the upper abdomen, such as hepatosplenomegaly, are uncommonly encountered during pregnancy. These may be obscured in late pregnancy by the growing uterus.

The uterus rises out of the pelvis at approximately 14 weeks' gestation, but may be palpable abdominally in the very slim patient as early as 12 weeks or so. From about 18 to 38 weeks, the size of the uterus, measured in centimeters from the pubic symphysis to the top of the fundus, should be within about 2 cm of the gestation age in weeks.

**Pelvic Examination.** During even very early pregnancy, the vaginal walls and cervix soften and take on a bluish or "cyanotic" appearance (Chadwick's sign).

The uterine size is not appreciably increased until 6 to 8 weeks' gestation; Hegar's sign (softening of the isthmic portion of the uterus [the part between the cervix and the fundus]) is usually appreciated at 6 to 8 weeks.

Clinical sizing by an experienced examiner during the first trimester is a fairly accurate means of confirming menstrual dates in gestational age assessment. The uterine diameter, in centimeters, matches the gestational age fairly well from 8 to 12 weeks. Beyond the 12- to 14-week range, however, clinical uterine sizing becomes less accurate.

Evaluation of the adnexa is obscured by the growing uterus after 10 to 12 weeks. The corpus luteum may be palpable at 6 to 10 weeks as a slightly tender, 4- or 5-cm adnexal mass. Any adnexal mass larger than about 5 cm should be evaluated by sonography.

In addition to uterine sizing, evaluation of pelvic architecture is part of the initial examination. The "obstetric conjugate"—the distance from the underside of the pubic symphysis to the sacral promontory—is normally 11 cm or more. The bi-ischial diameter in most patients exceeds 8.5 cm. The angle of the pubic arch, the convergence of the pelvic side walls and of the sacrum, and the prominence of the ischial spines allow a determination of pelvic type (gynecoid, anthropoid, android, or platypelloid), and, in rare cases, reveal an abnormality or deformity that precludes a trial of vaginal delivery.

### Laboratory Evaluation

Routine laboratory tests performed at the preconception or first prenatal visit are summarized in Table 2. A complete blood count (CBC) includes a hematocrit and red blood cell indices; in cases of anemia, the red blood cell indices may suggest a cause. A severely microcytic anemia is seen in thalassemias as well as iron deficiency states. Platelet counts are routinely included in CBCs performed by some laboratories. The lower limit of normal for platelet count during pregnancy is 150,000 per $mm^3$. Any count below 100,000 per $mm^3$ deserves further investigation.

Determination of the blood type, Rh antigen, and antibody screen (indirect Coombs' test) is important for two reasons. First, the Rh-negative patient whose spouse is Rh positive is at risk to become sensitized during the pregnancy or at the time of delivery. $Rh_0(D)$ immune globulin (RhoGAM) prophylaxis is indicated after any significant bleeding episode, at 26 weeks, and after delivery if the baby is Rh positive. The presence of irregular antibodies may place the fetus at risk for erythroblastosis fetalis, or hemolytic disease of the newborn, and require further evaluation and/or treatment of the fetus during the latter half of gestation.

Finally, obstetrics is a "bloody business." The patient whose antibody screen is negative can be safely transfused, in the event of heavy bleeding, with type specific, non–cross-matched blood. If

TABLE 2. **Laboratory Tests During Pregnancy**

**First Visit**
Blood type, Rh, and antibody screen
CBC
Urinalysis
Rubella titer
VDRL or RPR
Hepatitis B surface antigen
Pap smear
Gonococcus and chlamydial cultures
HIV (?)
Glucola 50-gram screen (high-risk patients)
**Subsequent Testing**
15–19 wk: MSAFP
26–28 wk: Glucola 50-gram screen (low-risk patients)
         Glucose tolerance test (high-risk patients)
36–38 wk: Hemoglobin and hematocrit

the antibody screen is positive, blood must be cross-matched before administration, and this may be considered even prior to vaginal delivery.

A urinalysis is performed routinely at the first prenatal visit. Asymptomatic bacteriuria occurs in 5 to 10% of pregnant (and nonpregnant) women; however, during pregnancy, the rate of progression from asymptomatic bacteriuria to pyelonephritis is much higher than in the nonpregnant state, and eradication of asymptomatic bacteriuria is recommended. The presence of other abnormalities on the urinalysis, such as proteinuria or red blood cell casts, suggests the possibility of chronic renal disease.

The rubella titer is determined at the first visit. For the patient who is being seen prior to pregnancy and who does not plan pregnancy for the next 6 months, rubella vaccination is in order. Otherwise, the nonimmune patient can be vaccinated after delivery.

Syphilis is again increasing in prevalence during pregnancy; congenital syphilis can be prevented by prompt treatment. A positive screening test (rapid plasma reagin [RPR] or Venereal Disease Research Laboratory [VDRL]) should trigger a fluorescent treponemal antibody absorption (FTA-ABS) test and further evaluation.

Papanicolaou's (Pap) smear, gonococcus culture, and *Chlamydia* culture are routinely performed during pregnancy by most obstetricians. Gonorrhea can be treated with oral or intramuscular penicillins or cephalosporins. Chlamydial carriage is treated with tetracycline in the nonpregnant patient and with erythromycin during pregnancy. The abnormal Pap smear is evaluated as in the nonpregnant state.

Some obstetricians routinely perform hepatitis B surface antigen screening during pregnancy, and some also offer routine screening for HIV.

## PREGNANCY DATING

Accurate dating of the pregnancy is critical in planning prenatal care.

**Menstrual Dates.** In women who have regular cycles, and who have not been using birth control pills, ovulation occurs 2 weeks before the beginning of each menstrual period. The majority of women with regular cycles have a menstrual period every 26 to 30 days; for these women, it is accurate enough to calculate the estimated date of confinement and the gestational age by counting the number of weeks since the last menstrual period. "Dating wheels" can be used for this purpose.

In women who have longer or shorter cycles, it is more accurate to calculate from the probable date of ovulation by subtracting 2 weeks from the date of the *missed* menstrual period and adding 38 weeks.

Few patients have regular cycles with lengths of more than 35 days or less than 21 days. In these patients, menstrual dating is generally unreliable.

The timing of ovulation after quitting oral contraceptives is unpredictable. Thus, menstrual dating is not accurate until regular cycles have been re-established.

Many patients who have had fertility problems know their conception date, either because they have tested their urine on a daily basis for ovulation, or because they have been doing "basal body temperature" charting. For these patients, the estimated date of confinement is 38 weeks from the date of conception.

**Pregnancy Testing.** Pregnancy tests not only confirm pregnancy, but may also be valuable in dating. The blood pregnancy test (serum human chorionic gonadotropin-beta [hCG-beta]) turns positive at $1\frac{1}{2}$ to 2 weeks following conception. Monoclonal urine pregnancy tests turn positive within about 3 weeks of conception (i.e., 5 weeks from the last menstrual period).

**Physical Examination.** The combination of regular cycles and known last menstrual period, or conception dating, together with the pelvic examination by an experienced examiner between 6 and 13 weeks, is a good way of establishing the gestational age. However, first-trimester examination alone, even by an experienced examiner, has an error range of 2 to 3 weeks.

**Auscultation of the Fetal Heart.** Fetal heart beat is a confirmatory test in determining gestational age. Except for very obese patients, fetal heart tones should be audible with a Doppler device between 9 and 12 weeks' gestation; if not, it is possible that the pregnancy is not so far along as was thought, a molar pregnancy is present, or the embryo has died. Sonography is indicated if heart tones are not heard by 12 to 13 weeks.

In most patients, the fetal heart tones can be first heard using a fetoscope between 18 and 21 weeks' gestation. If the heart tones are heard before 18 weeks or cannot be heard by 22 weeks, ultrasonography is indicated.

**Ultrasound Examination.** Ultrasonography is the most accurate means of establishing gestational age in pregnancies in which the menstrual history is irregular, the last menstrual period is unknown, or the menstrual history does not match other clinical information. The accuracy of ultrasound examination in dating pregnancies is much better early in gestation than late. Ultrasound examination performed at 8 to 13 weeks is accurate within 7 days. A scan before 22 weeks establishes a gestational age with an error range of about 10 days. If the scan is done between 22 and 26 to 28 weeks, the gestational age estimate is accurate within 2 weeks. A single scan performed after 28 weeks' gestation has an error range of ±3 weeks, and, therefore, is not particularly useful in judging gestational age. The reason for this is that ultrasound simply assesses the size of the fetus. There is much more variation in fetal growth during the third trimester than in the first or second trimester.

Some patients present late in pregnancy, and without any solid criteria for dating. In these cases, either clinical or ultrasound dating can be used, but the unreliability of either method must be recognized in obstetric decision making.

## SUBSEQUENT PRENATAL VISITS

The first prenatal visit is usually scheduled shortly after a positive pregnancy test. If the patient has already had a preconception visit, the baseline laboratory and clinical evaluation has already been performed; if not, it can be done at this time. If the patient is at risk for ectopic pregnancy, this can be excluded by means of an ultrasound examination performed at about 6 weeks' gestation.

Subsequent visits in the normal pregnancy are scheduled at monthly intervals until 32 weeks, then every other week until 36 weeks, and then weekly until delivery. At each prenatal visit, the patient's weight, blood pressure, and urinary protein and glucose determinations are recorded. The fetal heart is auscultated, either with a Doppler device or with a fetoscope. After 14 weeks, the fundal height is measured from the symphysis to the top of the uterus. The patient is questioned regarding contractions, fetal movement, and bleeding. Late in the pregnancy, the extremities are examined for evidence of edema.

**Weight Gain.** There is a wide range of normal for weight gain during pregnancy. For women who are underweight before the pregnancy, many gain 15 to 20 lb or more by the twentieth week of pregnancy; large women may gain substantially less. Most patients gain between ½ and 1 lb per week during the last 20 weeks of gestation. The frequency of poor pregnancy outcomes is increased in underweight women of low or normal weight with poor weight gain (Table 3).

Accelerated weight gain may be due to edema, particularly in the third trimester, or simply from overeating. Poor weight gain is most often due to either morning sickness or self-imposed dietary restriction; particularly when the patient was slim before the pregnancy and has gained little weight by the twentieth week, a dietary consultation may be in order.

Concordance of the gestational dating and

TABLE 3. **Weight Gain During Normal Pregnancy**

| | |
|---|---|
| **Fetal Compartment** | |
| Fetus | 3500 grams |
| Amniotic fluid | 500 grams |
| Placenta | 500 grams |
| | 4500 grams |
| **Maternal Compartment** | |
| Blood volume | 2000 grams |
| Extravascular fluid | 2000 grams |
| Uterine hypertrophy | 1000 grams |
| Breast enlargement | 500 grams |
| | 5500 grams |

measurement of the uterus is used to screen for growth abnormalities. If the fundal size lags significantly behind gestational dating (3 cm discrepancy or greater, between 20 and 38 weeks' gestation), the possibility of either a small-for-gestational age fetus or decreased amniotic fluid is evaluated by sonography. If the fundal height is significantly ahead of dates, multiple gestation, macrosomia, and polyhydramnios may be the cause, and, again, ultrasound examination differentiates among these.

**Fetal Activity.** Fetal movement is first perceived by most multiparous patients between 15 and 18 weeks and by primiparous patients between 18 and 20 weeks. Beyond 24 weeks' gestation, maternal perception of fetal movement is the best screening tool for potential fetal jeopardy.

The normal fetus has a 20- to 40-minute sleep/wake cycle. Thus, the normal fetus should be moving for part of every hour; a simple way to screen for normal fetal activity is to ask the mother to count fetal movements for an hour each day. If she feels less than four kicks in the first hour, she is asked to count for a second hour. If she has felt less than eight kicks by the end of 2 hours, she is asked to call and further testing can then be arranged. If good fetal health cannot be demonstrated by means of either a nonstress test, a biophysical profile, or a contraction stress test, and the fetus is at a viable gestational age, intervention may be indicated.

The fetal heart is auscultated at each visit beyond 12 weeks' gestation. The baseline fetal heart rate is normally between 120 and 160 beats per minute; this declines from early gestation toward term. Occasional irregularities in the fetal heart rate are normal, just as occasional premature beats in the adult heart are normal. However, frequent "missed beats" suggest an abnormality of the cardiac conduction system. This can be evaluated by real-time, M-mode, and Doppler sonography.

**Edema.** Edema of the legs is common during late pregnancy. This is due to compression of the venous return from the legs by the gravid uterus. It improves with rest in the recumbent position and tends to recur late during the day. Edema of the hands or the face is always pathologic and may be indicative of pre-eclampsia.

**Blood Pressure.** The blood pressure is measured at each prenatal visit. Normal blood pressure during pregnancy ranges from 90/50 to 130/80. Pressures in the first trimester of 130/80 or more suggest mild chronic hypertension.

Normally, the blood pressure falls from pre-pregnant and first-trimester values to reach a nadir during the late second trimester, and then rises back to the prepregnant values near term. About 10% of patients during their first pregnancy develop pregnancy-induced hypertension, defined as a rise in the blood pressure of 30 mmHg systolic and 15 mmHg diastolic above first-trimester or prepregnant values, after the twentieth week of pregnancy. If this blood pressure rise is accompanied by proteinuria or generalized edema, the patient is said to have pre-eclampsia. Pre-eclampsia, when it develops, resolves only after delivery and may present significant threats to both maternal and fetal health.

**Urinary Glucose and Protein.** At each prenatal visit, a dipstick determination of urinary protein and glucose is also performed.

During normal pregnancy, renal blood flow increases to such an extent that the capacity of the kidney to reabsorb filtered glucose may be exceeded, even in the presence of normal blood glucose levels. Thus, 1+ or 2+ glycosuria is not uncommon during pregnancy. Glycosuria in the 3+ or 4+ range is uncommon and may be indicative of hyperglycemia. For the patient with persistent 2+ dipstick determinations, or any value of 3+ or 4+, I perform a serum glucose determination.

Urinary protein is also checked at each visit. Trace proteinuria is common and generally innocuous. Values of 1+ occasionally occur during normal pregnancy, but may be indicative of early pre-eclampsia. Urinary protein dipstick determinations of 2+ or greater are always abnormal. As mentioned above, elevation in blood pressure, generalized edema, and proteinuria are the cardinal signs of pre-eclampsia.

### Common Complaints

A variety of discomforts are reported by the normal pregnant patient. Many of these relate to physiologic changes and can be managed with reassurance and symptomatic treatment. In an occasional patient, the complaints are persistent or severe enough to require further intervention.

"Morning sickness" is nearly universal during the first trimester. Patients usually report a "queasy" or "unsettled" feeling to the stomach on arising. This may be accompanied by occasional or even daily vomiting, most often occurring early in the day. Small, dry carbohydrate feedings immediately on arising, and holding off on intake of liquids until later in the day, are usually effective in controlling these complaints. Occasionally, an antiemetic medication may be required, although, given the medicolegal furor over alleged teratogenic effects of doxylamine (Bendectin), most obstetricians are reluctant to prescribe such medications for morning sickness.

Danger signs in morning sickness are steady weight loss of more than 5 lb, the development of orthostatic symptoms suggestive of hypovolemia, or persistent ketonuria. Patients who are significantly dehydrated, or who are not responding to the measures described earlier, generally do well with hospital admission, intravenous hydration, and placing the gut at rest for 24 to 48 hours. An occasional patient has severe and protracted nausea and vomiting, hyperemesis gravidarum. These patients require hospital admission, with vigorous replacement of vitamin, fluid, and electrolyte losses. If the nausea and vomiting persist, a careful evaluation of potential underlying causes should be undertaken; if no cause is found, parenteral nutrition may be used to tide the patient over through the period of hyperemesis. Fortunately, the nausea and vomiting associated with pregnancy tend to resolve by 10 to 12 weeks of gestation.

Gastrointestinal reflux also occurs commonly during pregnancy, usually in the third trimester. With rising progesterone levels, the tone of the lower esophageal sphincter decreases. This, together with pressure on the stomach by the growing uterus, increases the tendency toward gastric reflux. Some patients complain of a sour taste in the mouth; others actually notice regurgitation of food from the stomach back into the mouth. These symptoms may be controlled between meals through the use of antacids. Most patients respond well to dietary changes, including eating multiple small meals rather than two or three larger ones and remaining upright for several hours after meals.

Gastrointestinal reflux is most marked and most disturbing when the patient lies down. Elevating the head of the bed by 4 to 6 inches by placing wooden blocks or bricks underneath the bedposts is helpful; some patients need to sleep in a reclining chair, in a semiupright posture.

A general feeling of fatigue or loss of energy occurs in many pregnant women, particularly those who are active. This is usually due to the demands of the pregnancy asking mother to "slow down." However, patients who report severe limitation of activity need to be evaluated for cardiac or pulmonary disease.

Numbness and tingling of the medial aspect of the hand (thumb, index finger, and the middle half of the middle finger) occurs in about 5% of pregnant women. This is related to compression of the median nerve in the carpal tunnel on the volar aspect of the wrist. The complaint is most pronounced in the dominant hand and may be quite severe at night and during the early morning hours, improving during the day. The diagnosis is usually apparent by history, but may be confirmed on physical examination by the finding of a positive Tinel's sign (a tingling or shock-like sensation in the affected areas on percussion of the median nerve), or the findings of sensory loss or wasting of the thenar muscles of the affected hand. Splinting, injection of the carpal tunnel with corticosteroids, or even surgical carpal tunnel release may be necessary during pregnancy. Symptoms abate over 2 to 6 months after delivery.

Varicose veins are a common complaint during pregnancy, are more common in multigravid women, and tend to increase in severity with advancing gestation. Elastic support hose are used to control the associated discomfort. Because the varicosities are at least in part due to the compression of the venous return from the legs by the gravid uterus, surgical treatment of varicose veins is not recommended during pregnancy.

Leg cramps, particularly occurring at night, may be troublesome. The physiologic basis of these cramps is unclear. Most patients respond to calcium supplements. However, in a rare patient, the cramps may be so persistent or severe as to require medication.

### Laboratory Testing Later in Pregnancy

**Maternal Serum Alpha-Fetoprotein (MSAFP) Screening.** Alpha-fetoprotein (AFP) determination is recommended, between 15 and 19 weeks' gestation, for the detection of narrow tube defects and other congenital anomalies. Alpha-fetoprotein is one of the dominant plasma proteins in the fetus. The level of AFP rises with gestational age from the end of the second trimester until 20 weeks' gestation. Elevation in maternal serum AFP level may be caused by either underestimation of gestational age, multiple pregnancy, or intrauterine demise or threatened abortion with release of AFP from the fetal to the maternal compartment. In addition, elevation of MSAFP occurs in open neural tube and ventral wall defects and a variety of other fetal abnormalities. MSAFP screening is performed by drawing a blood sample from the mother at 15 to 19 weeks' gestation. The AFP value is then corrected for gestational age and for maternal weight. Values

in excess of 2.5 multiples of the median (MOM) (or slightly lower in some laboratories) are considered to be elevated. When a first value returns as "high," dating criteria for the pregnancy are reviewed, and, if they are felt to be uncertain, an ultrasound examination to confirm gestational dates is performed. If the dates are accurate, a subsequent determination is performed. After two elevated MSAFP values (or a single value ≥ 3 MOM), sonography is performed to confirm a singleton pregnancy, check the accuracy of gestational dating, and exclude the possibility of an intrauterine demise. Then, careful examination of the fetus for a neural tube or ventral wall defects is performed. If the fetus appears to be normal, or if an abnormality is suspected on scan but not confirmed, amniocentesis for AFP and acetylcholinesterase (AChE) testing is performed. Significant elevation of the AFP value from the amniotic fluid strongly suggests a fetal anomaly. Elevation of the AChE level occurs only when an open neural tube defect is present; increased AFP with a normal AChE occurs with ventral wall and other fetal abnormalities.

Even if the amniotic fluid AFP and AChE levels are normal, the pregnancy is at increased risk for the subsequent development of preterm labor, preterm rupture of the membranes, growth retardation, and other adverse outcomes and must be followed carefully.

Maternal serum AFP screening programs, in which all pregnant women are screened between 15 and 19 weeks, have been shown to detect 80 to 90% of open neural tube defects, 70 to 90% of ventral wall defects, and a substantial proportion of misdated and twin pregnancies.

Experience has also shown that low MSAFP values represent a risk factor for chromosomal trisomies. Most laboratories provide an estimate of the risk for trisomies based on maternal age and weight-adjusted MSAFP value. If the risk figure exceeds the risk for trisomy associated with maternal age of 35, ultrasound examination to confirm gestational dating is performed. If the dates are confirmed, genetic counseling and amniocentesis for chromosome testing are recommended.

**Glucose Screening.** The hormonal changes of pregnancy, particularly the production by the placenta of human placental lactogen (hPL), make pregnancy a "diabetogenic" state. In turn, elevated glucose levels during pregnancy have adverse effects on the fetus.

For patients at low risk for carbohydrate intolerance—patients below age 30, who have no family history of diabetes, who are not obese, and who have not previously had a macrosomic infant, glucose screening by means of a 50-gram "glucola" test at 26 to 28 weeks is performed. For these patients, a glucose determination is performed 1 hour following ingestion of a 50-gram glucose load. Depending on the laboratory, a threshold value between 130 and 145 mg per dl triggers further evaluation for gestational diabetes, by means of a 3-hour glucose tolerance test (see below).

For patients at high risk (older than 30, family history of diabetes, obese, or previous macrosomic infant), a glucola screen is performed shortly after the first prenatal visit, and then either a subsequent glucola screen or a full glucose tolerance test is done at 26 to 28 weeks.

The glucose tolerance test includes a fasting blood glucose determination, followed by a 100-gram oral glucose load. Then, blood glucose levels are determined at 1, 2, and 3 hours. The upper limits of normal for plasma glucose are fasting, $\leq105$ mg per dl; 1 hour, $\leq190$ mg/dl; 2 hour, $\leq165$ mg/dl; 3 hour, $\leq145$ mg/dl. If two or more values are abnormal on the 3-hour glucose tolerance test, the patient is diagnosed as having gestational diabetes and is treated accordingly.

**Rh-Negative Patients.** In patients who are Rh negative (that is, who lack the $Rh_0$ (D) antigen), the blood type of the husband is determined. If the husband is Rh positive, and the antibody screen is negative, a dose of $Rh_0$ (D) immune globulin (RhoGAM) is given after any significant bleeding episode, or after amniocentesis to prevent sensitization. In addition, at 26 to 28 weeks, a subsequent antibody screen is performed. As long as the patient has remained Rh negative, a prophylactic dose of RhoGAM is administered to prevent sensitization, which occasionally occurs in the absence of maternal bleeding during the third trimester. In addition, RhoGAM is given after delivery to the Rh-negative, nonsensitized patient who has delivered an Rh-positive baby.

## Obstetric Sonography

The development of high-resolution ultrasound devices has virtually revolutionized the practice of obstetrics. Ultrasound examination has no known adverse fetal effects; screening sonography, performed at 16 to 20 weeks, has proved to be cost effective in numerous studies. It results in early diagnosis of intrauterine deaths and multiple gestations, accurate dating of pregnancy, and the detection of a number of fetal anomalies.

At the present time, universal screening is not performed in the United States. Indications for scanning are summarized in Table 4.

**Ectopic Pregnancy.** In normal pregnancy, a gestational sac is seen with vaginal ultrasound at $5\frac{1}{2}$ weeks, and is seen in more than 90% of

TABLE 4. **Indications for Sonography**

Ectopic pregnancy
Adnexal masses
Uncertain dates
Suspected multiple gestation or fetal demise
At risk for sonographically detectable anomalies
Size/dates discrepancy
Third-trimester bleeding
Suspected malpresentation
Guidance for invasive procedures (CVS, amniocentesis, percutaneous umbilical blood sampling)
Assessment of fetal health (biophysical profile scoring, Doppler velocimetry)

patients in whom the quantitative hCG level exceeds 2000 mIU per liter. The gestational sac is seen with abdominal scanning at about 6 weeks' gestation, or when the quantitative hCG-beta level exceeds 6000. Occasionally, an extrauterine gestational sac or even an extrauterine embryo is seen with ultrasound. However, the primary importance is to demonstrate an intrauterine pregnancy. Then, the risk of ectopic pregnancy is reduced to about 1 in 10,000 (the rate of coexistent ectopic and intrauterine pregnancies).

**Adnexal Masses.** Ultrasound examination is recommended whenever an adnexal mass of larger than 5 cm is palpated during pregnancy. Depending on the size and on the appearance of the mass on ultrasound, laparotomy and surgical removal of the mass may be indicated.

**Pregnancy Dating.** When sonography is performed between 7 and 12 weeks, the gestational age, as inferred from the crown rump length of the embryo, is accurate within 7 days. Between 13 and 22 weeks, the gestational age inferred from measurements of biparietal diameter, femur length, and abdominal circumference is accurate within 10 days. Between 22 and 26 weeks, the gestational age is accurate within approximately 2 weeks.

**Structural Defects.** A wide range of congenital anomalies can be diagnosed by the experienced sonographer. Examples include anencephaly, open neural tube defects, ventral wall defects, cardiac abnormalities, renal anomalies, and skeletal dysplasias. In our hands, anatomic sex determination between 15 and 20 weeks is possible in more than 50% of patients with an accuracy rate in excess of 95%. An experienced sonographer can exclude even minor defects, such as cleft lip or polydactyly, as the pregnancy advances.

**Growth Abnormalities.** Ultrasound examination can also be used to evaluate patients with size/date discrepancy. A variety of formulas and tables for estimation of fetal weight using ultrasound have been developed and, in general, are accurate within 15% of the actual weight. In the patient with size less than dates, oligohydramnios can be readily diagnosed from ultrasound. If the fetal weight estimate is less than the tenth percentile for confirmed gestational age, the diagnosis of intrauterine growth retardation is strongly suspected.

In the patient with size greater than dates, ultrasound can be used to diagnose polyhydramnios; after the diagnosis is made, the fetus can be evaluated for the possibility of a causative anatomic abnormality (e.g., duodenal atresia). An estimated fetal weight in excess of the ninetieth percentile for dates raises a high level of suspicion for a macrosomic infant.

**Third-Trimester Bleeding.** Ultrasound examination is highly accurate in determination of placental location and can be used to make the diagnosis of placenta previa. In the patient in whom placenta previa is excluded, the finding of a retroplacental lucency may support the clinical diagnosis of placental abruption.

Ultrasound examination can also be used to assess the health of the fetus in utero. The biophysical profile as a means of antenatal fetal assessment and Doppler velocimetry are discussed elsewhere in this text.

## GENETIC STUDIES

For the patient who is at increased risk for chromosomal abnormalities or for any of the steadily increasing numbers of congenital diseases that can be diagnosed by a biochemical or "gene probe" technology, genetic counseling and either chorionic villus sampling (CVS) or amniocentesis may be offered.

Amniocentesis has been the mainstay of chromosomal diagnosis for decades. With amniocentesis, after ultrasound examination to evaluate fetal and placental location, a sterile preparation of the abdomen is performed, and a 20- or 22-gauge needle is introduced into the amniotic cavity. Fluid is withdrawn. Fetal fibroblasts from the amniotic fluid can be induced to proliferate in the laboratory, and, after 7 to 10 days, chromosome preparations can be made, or biochemical or gene probe tests performed.

In the past, amniocentesis was usually performed at 16 to 20 weeks. However, with the use of ultrasound in guiding the needle into the amniotic cavity, and with improvements in the technology for culturing fibroblasts from amniotic fluid, amniocentesis can be performed in many patients as early as 12 to 13 weeks' gestation. The rate of fetal loss in relation to amniocentesis appears to be in the range of 1 pregnancy loss per 200 to 300 amniocentesis tests.

Chorionic villus sampling is a recently developed technique that offers an earlier alternative to amniocentesis testing for chromosomal and other genetic defects. Here, a small amount of placental tissue is aspirated under direct ultrasound guidance, via either transabdominal or transcervical approach. The sample of chorionic villi can be used for direct chromosome preparations or cells can be grown in culture (as for amniotic fluid fibroblasts) for gene probe or biochemical testing. Chorionic villus sampling is offered in an increasing number of prenatal diagnostic centers. The pregnancy loss rate in relation to CVS appears to be only slightly higher than that for amniocentesis.

## RECORD KEEPING

It is both sound medical practice and an essential medicolegal protection to clearly document care provided during the course of pregnancy. Standardized prenatal record forms provide a compact, convenient, and legible format for record keeping. I document any serious complications of pregnancy, and even initial visits for potentially complex pregnancies, by means of dictated narrative reports. A xerographic copy of the full prenatal flow sheet is provided to the patient prior to any out-of-area travel, on transfer of care to another physician, and during the mid–third trimester.

It is presently recommended that records be stored for at least 7 years after delivery; in fact, if space permits, it is probably prudent to keep records for a full 21 years after delivery.

## FAMILY-ORIENTED CARE

In the face of the growing complexity of the technical aspects of obstetric care, it is easy to lose the primary focus of good antenatal care—the relationship between the family and the obstetric care provider. I have found it helpful to schedule an uninterrupted 30- to 60-minute visit for the initial examination and to plan a second, relaxed visit in the consultation room during the mid–third trimester, at which time the process of intake to the hospital maternity unit can be explained, and any questions or worries about the labor and delivery process can be answered.

# ABORTION

method of
HOOSHANG M. NIKOO, M.D.
*Episcopal Hospital*
*Philadelphia, Pennsylvania*

*Incidence*

The true incidence of *spontaneous abortion* is difficult to assess, but the generally accepted rate is 10%.

However, if fertilization and elevation of human chorionic gonadotropin (hCG) hormone is considered to be true pregnancy, more than 60% of fertilized ova do not reach viability and end as abortuses.

The incidence of *induced abortion* in the United States has almost tripled since the Supreme Court's 1973 decision that legalized abortion. Before 1973, almost 500,000 induced abortions were performed yearly in the United States. More than 1.3 million legal abortions were reported in 1987.

## Etiology

Although there is no conclusive etiologic factor for spontaneous abortion, certain factors are known to contribute to the incidence of spontaneous abortion.

*Genetic Factors.* Between 40 and 60% of the abortuses in the first 12 weeks of gestation have abnormal chromosomal arrangement, the most common being numeric aberration, monosomies, trisomies, or polyploidies. Parents usually have normal karyotypes, but, in 4 to 6% of the parents with more than two spontaneous abortions, some balanced translocation has been reported. Maternal and paternal age have been reported to be an important factor in chromosomal abnormalities, but this has not yet been proved.

*Infectious Disease.* Any viral or bacterial infection that causes high fever could interfere with normal fetal development and become a factor in spontaneous abortion. Moreover, certain infectious diseases such as mycoplasmal infection of the genital tract, rubella, toxoplasmosis, and *Listeria monocytogenes* have been specifically related to an increased spontaneous abortion rate, with mycoplasma gaining more attention as a specific etiologic factor.

*Endocrine Disorders.* Thyroid dysfunction and Cushing's disease have been reported to cause spontaneous abortion, but not diabetes mellitus. Progesterone deficiency in early pregnancy is always considered an etiologic factor; indeed, in luteal phase defect, in which the corpus luteum has a shorter-than-normal life span, repeated early spontaneous abortion is seen. This condition is diagnosed by endometrial biopsy in the luteal phase. If a discrepancy of 48 hours or more exists between histologic and calendar dating of the cycle, a short luteal phase is suspected. In some instances, this condition is due to high levels of serum prolactin, and, in these cases, the possibility of pituitary microadenomas should be investigated.

*Abnormalities of the Genital Tract.* Abnormal müllerian development is a cause for mid-trimester pregnancy loss. Diethylstilbestrol (DES)-exposed patients have a specific uterine abormality, which is either a T-shaped uterine cavity or an incompetent cervix; the rate of pregnancy loss is high. Submucosal fibroids and, rarely, intramural or subserosal fibroids also cause spontaneous abortion. Incompetent cervix due to cervical trauma or congenital maldevelopment is a known factor in second-trimester losses. Hysterosalpingography, a simple test, is usually sufficient for diagnosis, and corrective surgery is indicated if no other cause for repeated spontaneous abortion is found.

*Environmental Factors.* Exposure of pregnant women to chemical and industrial wastes, especially to those with high levels of arsenic and lead compounds, has been shown to cause a high rate of spontaneous abortion. Chronic exposure to radiographic and anesthetic agents (occupational hazards) also correlates with an increased incidence of spontaneous abortion.

*Maternal Habits.* Drug, alcohol, and tobacco usage during pregnancy has been correlated with an increased incidence of spontaneous abortion. The effect of lysergic acid (LSD) usage on chromosomal breakage is well known. Cigarette smoking also has some known effect on placental development and increases the abortion rate. The effect of surgery and emotional and physical trauma in the etiology of spontaneous abortion is unclear, but laparotomies and removal of organs close to a pregnant uterus have increased the rate of abortion.

## Clinical Classification

Spontaneous abortion has different clinical stages: threatened abortion, inevitable abortion, incomplete abortion, complete abortion, missed abortion, habitual abortion, and septic abortion.

**Threatened abortion** is the appearance of bleeding during the first half of pregnancy. Bleeding during pregnancy is abnormal, but some nonpregnancy-related bleedings are from the cervix (polyps, cervicitis, tumors), vagina, or urethra and should be differentiated by careful examination. Some small amount of bleeding in early pregnancy is due to the implantation of the zygote and is considered normal. Dark brown bleeding, usually due to necrosis of the decidua after fetal death, is abnormal. Mild abdominal cramping usually accompanies the bleeding.

**Therapeutic Considerations.** A thorough pelvic examination is done to rule out other causes for the bleeding.

A pelvic ultrasound examination is done not only to rule out bleeding due to ectopic pregnancy but also to confirm fetal viability. If, with the ultrasound, the fetus is seen to be alive, the prognosis for the continuation of the pregnancy is excellent, with 90% of the patients able to carry the pregnancy, regardless of treatment. If no viable fetus and only an empty gestational sac are seen in the ultrasound examination, the outcome of the pregnancy is poor, regardless of treatment. Bed rest and repeat ultrasound examination in 1 week will differentiate a blighted ovum or missed abortion from a very early normal gestation.

If repeat ultrasound examination fails to reveal a viable fetus, a dilatation and evacuation (D & E) is probably necessary to terminate the pregnancy, thus preventing complications of missed abortion and septic abortion. The appearance of a living fetus will indicate a normal pregnancy with a good prognosis.

Hormones should not be used to treat threatened abortion. They are not effective and could cause prolongation and retention of a dead fetus or adverse effect on organogenesis of a living one.

Bed rest, avoiding sexual activity, and taking vaginal precautions are psychologically beneficial to the patient, but they do not have medical therapeutic value.

**Inevitable abortion** is the appearance of ruptured membrane, uterine contractions, vaginal bleeding, and cervical dilation. Treatment is the same as for incomplete abortion.

**Incomplete abortion** involves a partially expelled fetus and placenta. Because the retained portion of the product of conception usually prevents the involution of the uterus, abdominal cramps, vaginal bleeding, cervical dilation, and the appearance of portions of the product of conception from the cervical canal characterize this condition.

**Therapeutic Considerations.** After proper diagnosis, the aim should be the prompt evacuation of the uterus. This could be accomplished best by transferring the patient to the operating room (OR) or short procedure unit with OR facilities. An intravenous fluid with 1000 ml of 5% glucose and 10 to 20 U of oxytocin (Pitocin) is started. An analgesic such as 50 mg of meperidine (Demerol) is given intravenously. A paracervical block is done by injecting 7 ml of 1 or 2% lidocaine to the paracervical areas at the 4 and 8 o'clock positions.

No surgical dilation is needed, because the cervix is already dilated. A suction catheter is inserted into the canal, and, with mild negative pressure of 30 to 40 mmHg, the suction is completed and the bleeding and pain stop. Rarely, a sharp curette is used to ascertain the completeness of the evacuation.

A whole dose of $Rh_o$ (D) immune globulin (RhoGAM) is given to Rh-negative patients.

A blood count is performed after the procedure to rule out anemia and excessive blood loss.

Methylergonovine (Methergine), 0.2 mg by mouth every 6 to 8 hours for 2 days, may be given.

The patient should be observed for a few hours, followed by discharge with a follow-up visit scheduled in 2 weeks. A method of contraception should be discussed at the time of discharge.

**Complete abortion** occurs when the entire product of conception is expelled spontaneously, the uterus contracts, and bleeding stops without interference. This usually happens at 6 to 10 weeks of gestation, after an episode of bleeding and abdominal cramps. The patient passes the sac of pregnancy and the fetus. The bleeding and abdominal cramps diminish thereafter and finally stop.

**Therapeutic Considerations.** The product of conception should be examined grossly and microscopically to rule out incomplete abortion or ectopic pregnancy.

An ultrasound examination should be done to rule out the possibility of retained placenta. The endometrial cavity seen as a regular line indicates the completeness of the abortion with no dilatation and curettage necessary, but a shadow that is irregular or not identifiable indicates an incomplete abortion with treatment as such.

Methylergonovine is prescribed. A whole dose of RhoGAM is given for RH-negative patients.

A repeat serum hCG level determined 48 to 72 hours after the abortion shows a very low level or becomes negative. This is a reassuring sign of complete abortion and rules out the possibility of ectopic pregnancy.

**Missed abortion** is the condition wherein the product of conception is retained in the uterus for 8 weeks or longer after the death of the fetus. Usually there is no vaginal bleeding. The early pregnancy symptoms, including morning sickness and breast enlargement and tenderness, disappear and a previously positive pregnancy test may become negative. Pelvic examination fails to reveal uterine growth, and the uterus even becomes smaller when compared with previous examinations. Ultrasound examination reveals no evidence of fetal viability, and the sac of pregnancy is usually irregularly shaped.

Carrying a dead fetus may be psychologically intolerable to some patients, even though this could facilitate the spontaneous expulsion of the fetus; but when the pregnancy is more advanced and spontaneous expulsion has not occurred within 1 month, a coagulation defect may occur. The rate of this serious complication of missed abortion could be as high as 25% if missed abortion continues longer than 2 months. To prevent this complication, the uterus should be evacuated either by a suction curettage if the pregnancy is less than 14 weeks or by medical induction if the pregnancy is more advanced. The medical induction could safely be accomplished by instillation of prostaglandin $F_{2\alpha}$ or vaginal insertion of prostaglandin $E_2$, and intravenous infusion of oxytocin.

**Treatment.** Treatment of the coagulation defect is usually accomplished by evacuation of the uterus after stabilization of the patient. If the phenomenon is severe, serious bleeding may occur. The bleeding should be treated with an infusion of fresh-frozen plasma; a transfusion of fresh blood, if available; the administration of cryoprecipitate; a platelet transfusion; and, rarely, when the previously mentioned measures fail, a lifesaving heparin infusion.

**Habitual abortion** refers to three or more spontaneous, consecutive losses of pregnancy.

The most common cause for early (first trimester) abortions is genetic disorders. Other etiologic factors are short luteal phase and mycoplasmal infection of the genital tract. Mid- and third-trimester pregnancy losses are usually due to genital tract anomalies and incompetent cervix.

**Therapeutic Considerations.** For early habitual abortions, therapeutic measures include a complete work-up, including endometrial biopsy, *Mycoplasma* culture, and chromosomal testing of parents. In the case of luteal phase defect, treatment includes 25 to 50 mg of progesterone given intramuscularly every other day, with 2500 to 5000 U of hCG given intramuscularly biweekly. The treatment should start at mid-cycle and continue until 6 to 12 weeks of gestation if pregnancy occurs. Mycoplasmal infection is treated with erythromycin or doxycycline. Some physicians recommend a medical treatment of early habitual abortion with a 14-day course of 100 mg of doxycycline (Vibramycin) given by mouth twice daily, but the value of this method is still unclear.

TREATMENT OF INCOMPETENT CERVIX. This is defined as the spontaneous, painless opening of the cervical os and the loss of pregnancy. This typically occurs in the second trimester. The cause is either traumatic with previous mechanical dilation of the cervix or is congenital due to abnormal cervical development.

The best-accepted treatment for incompetent cervix is a cerclage procedure. The easiest technique is the McDonald operation, which involves placing a suture at the level of the internal os. The suture is left in place until the last few weeks of pregnancy; then it is removed and a vaginal delivery is allowed. The Shirodkar procedure involves placing a permanent suture at the cervix; delivery is performed by cesarean section. This procedure is more complicated and should be performed only by experienced personnel.

The success rate in correction of true incompetent cervix is more than 85% with either cerclage procedure. Concomitant use of 250 to 500 mg of 17-medroxyprogesterone caproate in weekly injections is also recommended and may enhance the success rate.

**Induced abortion** is the deliberate termination of the pregnancy prior to survivability of the fetus. It is called *therapeutic abortion* when the termination is performed to safeguard the mother's health (for example, termination of a pregnancy in a cancerous uterus); it is called *elective abortion* when the termination is requested by the mother for social, economic, or other reasons.

**Septic abortion** is the development of infection with incomplete abortion. Typical signs of infection are present and include fever, chills, and abdominal tenderness. In more severe cases,

signs of septic shock and acute renal failure may develop. Septic complication is the most common cause of death in second-trimester abortion, and it is considered to be a more severe complication if the pregnancy was accompanied by an intrauterine device (IUD) in situ.

**Therapeutic Considerations.** Prompt evacuation of the uterus and use of proper antibiotics and adequate hydration of the patient usually prevent more serious complications.

### Elective Abortions

The primary factor in choosing the particular method is gestational age. Ninety per cent of elective abortions are performed in the first trimester, and the primary means of abortion at this stage is the suction curettage. Suction curettage is, at best, to be performed under local anesthesia, and, if preceded by the insertion of a *Laminaria* tent to the cervix, is relatively simple and very safe. The adverse effect concerning the patient's future pregnancies is minimal.

A *Laminaria* tent is a device made from the stems of a special seaweed called *Laminaria digitata*. Through its hydrophilic action, the device, if inserted properly into the cervix, will gradually dilate the cervical canal and will reduce the cervical trauma and laceration due to mechanical dilation. The *Laminaria* is usually inserted 6 to 8 hours prior to the scheduled procedure and is removed just before starting the suction curettage.

Suction curettage is performed under aseptic conditions. If the *Laminaria* is not used, the cervix is dilated using Pratt dilators and under paracervical anesthesia. A plastic curette is inserted into the cavity. The diameter, in millimeters, of the suction curette is usually chosen to correspond to the gestation age by week; for example, a 6-mm curette is used for a pregnancy of 6 weeks, an 8-mm-curette for a pregnancy of 8 weeks. The curette is then connected to the pump, and, using negative pressure created by the pump, the evacuation is started and completed. The negative pressure, at between 30 and 50 mmHg, should not exceed 50 mmHg. Some physicians perform a sharp curettage after the completion of suctioning, but this practice should be limited, because too vigorous a curettage could cause intrauterine synechiae and future infertility.

The intravenous use of 10 to 20 U of oxytocin (Pitocin) in 1000 ml of 5% dextrose in Ringer's lactate solution is recommended to lower the blood loss. No prophylactic antibiotic is usually necessary, but if a patient has a history of pelvic inflammatory disease or with teen-age patients who are at risk of developing infection, a single dose of 500 mg of doxycycline is given a few hours prior to the procedure. This significantly lowers the rate of postoperative infection.

A proper contraception should be prescribed, since ovulation occurs usually 17 to 22 days after the D & E.

### Mid-trimester Abortion

The morbidity and mortality rates for second-trimester abortion are at least four times higher than for the first trimester. The methods for mid-trimester abortion are medical, surgical, or mechanical.

The medical method for mid-trimester abortion includes the instillation technique with hypertonic saline. Amniocentesis is performed under aseptic conditions. Two hundred milliliters of commercially available 20% saline solution is then instilled into the amniotic cavity. After the completion of the procedure, the patient is kept under observation, and, in 85 to 90% of patients, spontaneous labor starts and the fetus is expelled. In more than 50% of patients, the placenta is also expelled spontaneously; it should be removed surgically if not expelled spontaneously.

Injecting 40 mg of prostaglandin $F_{2\alpha}$ into the amniotic cavity is also a very effective way of inducing mid-trimester abortion. The technique is more effective if it is combined with the intravenous infusion of oxytocin (Pitocin) after the labor is started.

Prostaglandin $E_2$ also has been used to induce midtrimester abortion. This product is in the form of vaginal suppositories, and the insertion of one suppository every 6 to 8 hours will start the labor in 8 to 24 hours.

Complications of the saline instillation include the development of clotting defect, water intoxication, hypernatremia, and myometrial necrosis due to extravasation of the hypertonic saline during the injection. Infection and bleeding are seen in more than 4% of patients owing to placental retention. Rarely, the fetus is born alive. A very stressful condition for both patient and hospital personnel, this creates a hard medicolegal problem.

Complications related to the prostaglandin administration most commonly include diarrhea, nausea, vomiting, and hyperthermia. The most serious complication, however, is uterine rupture or expulsion of the fetus from the lower uterine segment, which may cause uterovaginal fistula formation. The complication occurs more commonly if the prostaglandins are used with an intravenous oxytocin infusion, especially if the infusion is started before the rupture of the membranes. Care should be taken to avoid this very serious complication.

Surgical methods for mid-trimester abortions include the use of suction curettage to terminate pregnancies of more than 12 weeks. Currently, there is enough evidence to show this to be a safe technique when done by experienced personnel. The basic technique is similar to that of the suction curettage performed for first-trimester abortion. The complication rate is less than that of the instillation techniques.

Hysterotomy is used in about 1% of abortions performed in the United States. Hysterotomy, in fact, is a miniclassic cesarean section and has very high rates of mortality and morbidity compared with suction curettage. The mortality rate is almost 40 times higher, and future pregnancies should be delivered by cesarean section. Hysterotomy should be used only if other methods have failed; routine use is discouraged!

Pregnant hysterectomy could be used as a means of abortion if serious uterine pathology coexists with pregnancy and warrants a hysterectomy. It must be emphasized that such an occasion occurs rarely and should be evaluated on an individual basis.

Mechanical methods used to induce abortion include the use of bougies, bags, catheters, and other mechanical means. There is a high rate of infection with these techniques and in general they are disadvantageous.

### Effect of Induced Abortion on Future Pregnancies

The effect of induced abortion on subsequent pregnancies is unclear. Studies are divided equally in reporting no adverse effect and adverse effects, which include increased chance of pregnancy loss, premature ruptured membrane, growth retardation, increased rate of placenta previa by threefold, infertility, increased rate of ectopic pregnancy by fivefold, increased rate of first-trimester vaginal bleeding, and incompetent cervix.

It is reasonable to assume that if induced abortion is performed early, if cervical trauma is minimized by using *Laminaria,* and if there is no postoperative infection, the effect of induced abortion in future pregnancies should not be significant. However, the rates of infertility and ectopic pregnancy will increase if other than the just-stated ideal conditions, especially no postoperative infection, occurs.

# ECTOPIC PREGNANCY

method of
MARY ANN McRAE, M.D.
*Southern Illinois University School of Medicine*
*Springfield, Illinois*

The incidence of ectopic pregnancy in the United States has increased fourfold during the past 15 years, reaching almost 88,000 cases in 1987. Fortunately, the mortality associated with ectopic pregnancy has not increased at the same rate, reflecting improvements in both diagnosis and therapy. In 1987, the mortality rate from ectopic pregnancy in the United States was 0.034%.

This increase in the incidence of ectopic pregnancy is due to many factors, including current intrauterine device use, history of infertility, history of pelvic inflammatory disease, and prior tubal surgery. Between 15 and 50% of all pregnancies occurring in women after tubal ligation are ectopic. Increased sexual activity and number of sexual partners may also make tubal disease more common. Advances in tubal surgical techniques permit the salvage of previously irreparable tubes. More widespread use of drugs for ovulation induction with the stimulation of multiple follicles allows for potential combined uterine and ectopic pregnancies. Finally, many ectopic pregnancies that would have previously gone undetected as they spontaneously resorbed or aborted into the pelvis are now being detected with sensitive human chorionic gonadotropin-beta (hCG-beta) assays.

Signs and symptoms of ectopic pregnancy include abnormal vaginal bleeding, pelvic pain, and a palpable pelvic mass, usually in the presence of a positive pregnancy test result. With current sensitive hCG-beta measurements and ultrasonography, the diagnosis is often made before clinical symptoms occur.

The quantitative hCG-beta radioimmunoassay is the most useful diagnostic test, detecting the presence of a pregnancy in 99% of patients. In addition to detecting intrauterine and extrauterine pregnancies, hCG-beta levels, measured serially, allow assessment of the viability of the pregnancy. Both ectopic pregnancies and spontaneous abortions produce hCG at a decreased rate. Eighty-five per cent of normal uterine pregnancies are associated with a mean increase of hCG of at least 66% every 48 hours. On the other hand, ectopic pregnancies, and 87% of pregnancies that spontaneously abort, are associated with a less rapid rate of hCG increase.

Progesterone production is also impaired in ultimately nonviable pregnancies. A single value of less than 15 ng per ml suggests either an impending abortion or an ectopic pregnancy, but does not discriminate between the two.

The diagnosis of ectopic pregnancy is strengthened by an ultrasound scan of the uterus, demonstrating the absence of an intrauterine gestational sac. Using transabdominal ultrasonography, it is possible to identify a gestational sac in 94% of intrauterine pregnancies in which the hCG-beta titer is greater than 6000 to 6500 mIU per ml (discriminatory zone). This level of hCG is usually reached by 6 weeks' gestation. A lower discriminatory zone can be utilized with vaginal ultrasonography. Visualization of the actual ectopic pregnancy within the fallopian tube is not yet routinely possible with current sonography equipment. Sonography can provide additional valuable information, such as the presence of free fluid in the pelvis, suggesting intraperitoneal hemorrhage. Although the demonstration of a gestational sac within the uterus does not exclude the possibility of ectopic pregnancy, it makes it extremely unlikely. Traditionally, the in-

cidence of combined ectopic and intrauterine pregnancy has been thought to be 1 in 30,000 pregnancies. More recently, combined pregnancies have been reported as frequently as 1 in 3000 to 4000 pregnancies.

## TREATMENT

Management of ectopic pregnancy has changed dramatically over the past 25 years. Previously, ectopic pregnancy was treated by salpingectomy or hysterectomy. While lifesaving in cases of ruptured ectopic pregnancy, the procedure resulted in infertility in a substantial number of patients. Historically, salpingectomy has been followed by a subsequent term birth rate of only 30%. More conservative surgical procedures, such as linear salpingostomy, fimbrial expression, and segmental excision, have been utilized recently in the treatment of ectopic pregnancy, increasing the subsequent term pregnancy rate to 60%. However, these are associated with a 30 to 50% repeated ectopic pregnancy rate, depending on the health of the contralateral tube. These conservative procedures can be performed safely via laparoscopy in certain cases. Such conservative procedures are indicated if the patient wishes to conceive, is hemodynamically stable, and has a tube that can be repaired. Conservative tubal surgery, whether performed laparoscopically or via laparotomy, is technically demanding and yields best results when performed by surgeons experienced in these surgical techniques. Investigators in some centers are experimenting with pharmacologic treatment of early unruptured ectopic pregnancies with high-dose methotrexate* administration followed by leucovorin rescue. Potential risks and subsequent fertility rates are still being assessed.

Regardless of the treatment regimen, but especially with more conservative procedures, it is necessary to demonstrate that no viable chorionic tissue remains. Persistent ectopic pregnancy is being described more frequently, up to 5% of cases in some reports, with the advent of conservative surgical treatment. This condition usually resolves without sequelae, as the residual trophoblastic tissue regresses. Occasionally, recurrent bleeding and pain require additional treatment. Persistent ectopic pregnancy is treated with surgery or chemotherapy and requires close follow-up until hCG titers are negative.

A role for close observation of early ectopic pregnancies with low and falling hCG titers has been suggested. A number of untreated ectopic pregnancies may spontaneously regress or undergo abortion into the peritoneal cavity. Oth-

---

*This use of methotrexate is not listed in the manufacturer's official directive.

ers may form chronic ectopic pregnancies, resulting in significant tubal distortion. What role observation has in the treatment of early ectopic pregnancy with falling hCG levels still needs to be established with controlled studies and adequate follow-up fertility data.

# VAGINAL BLEEDING IN LATE PREGNANCY

method of
PHILLIP J. GOLDSTEIN, M.D.
*Sinai Hospital of Baltimore*
*Baltimore, Maryland*

Vaginal bleeding in late pregnancy is a common complaint. By far, the most common reasons for such bleeding are local causes such as cervicitis and postcoital trauma. What makes the complaint so important, however, is the differential diagnosis between vaginal bleeding of benign nature and vaginal bleeding associated with other pathologic entities with high morbidity and mortality, such as placenta previa and abruptio placentae (premature separation of the placenta). The identification, differential diagnosis, and management of third-trimester bleeding is the subject of this article.

## LOCAL CAUSES

Vaginal bleeding in late pregnancy is commonly reported by pregnant women. The most important initial information obtained by the physician should be an estimation of the amount of bleeding, if possible. Because vaginal bleeding is difficult to self-assess, one approach is to ask the patient whether the amount of bleeding is more or less than that of a menstrual period. Bleeding associated with major pathologic alteration tends to be associated with more aggressive bleeding than that associated with menstruation. If the bleeding is less than this, the patient still must be evaluated with a careful appraisal, including a history of recent intercourse, and a physical examination.

Changes in the cervix during pregnancy result, not uncommonly, in eversion of the endocervical glands. The endocervical tissue (columnar epithelium) is easily infected by the normal vaginal bacterial flora. As a consequence, it is easily traumatized during intercourse. Whether or not there has been recent coital trauma, the patient still may have some sloughing of the epithelium of the endocervical glands as a result of minor infections. Cultures should be obtained in such symptomatic women to identify specific organisms, especially if abnormal discharge is present. Should an active infection be identified, therapy should be instituted with an appropriate antibiotic known to be safe in pregnancy.

Rarely the pelvic examination reveals a cervical lesion suggestive of neoplastic disease. All such women should have a Papanicolaou's (Pap) smear performed if they have not already had a Pap smear in pregnancy. Any lesion that looks suspicious should undergo biopsy. Colposcopy-directed biopsy may be performed of abnormal white epithelial areas or otherwise suspicious lesions after application of 3% acetic acid to the entire cervix and squamocolumnar junction. Management of the abnormal Pap smear in pregnancy requires a more extensive evaluation and is not discussed in this section. The pregnant cervix may bleed vigorously after biopsy, but direct pressure, and application of Monsel's solution (ferric subsulfate) or silver nitrate will usually control the bleeding.

Vaginal bleeding of a mild degree may be associated with cervical dilation. Such dilation may occur in the absence of perceived labor ("bloody show"). Occasionally, minor vaginal bleeding occurs in women who are in preterm labor and who are not aware of the uterine contractions. They often believe symptoms are due to either gastrointestinal or genitourinary upset. In any case, one needs to examine these patients and not assume that minor vaginal bleeding is of no consequence. Should the patient be preterm, manifesting signs of incompetent cervix, or in preterm subclinical labor, management plans for each should be devised. Preterm labor, in and of itself, may be associated with abruptio placentae (see later).

## DIFFERENTIAL DIAGNOSIS: ABRUPTIO PLACENTAE AND PLACENTA PREVIA

Placenta previa and abruptio placentae constitute the two most common, potentially lethal causes of antepartum bleeding. In both, coagulopathy may result from excessive utilization of endogenous coagulation products due to exuberant bleeding, including platelets, fibrinogen, and Factor VIII. Placental disruption at the maternal-fetal surface produces a space-occupying lesion. In abruptio placentae, blood may dissect along the planes of least resistance, leading to a progressive disruption of the maternal-fetal interface. The increased pressure associated with this disruption results in rupture of the decidua cells, with consequent elaboration of prostaglandins, leading to pain and uterine contractions. Because the placenta may have implanted high in the uterus, an abruption may be "occult," or associated with no visible vaginal bleeding. Indeed, in about 20 to 25% of cases, clinical abruption is not associated with profuse vaginal bleeding.

Contrasting placental abruption and placenta previa, one can readily see that because of the ease with which blood can egress from the maternal-fetal surface through the cervix in a placenta previa, a space-occupying lesion need not develop. Second, because the decidua is less well developed in the lower uterine segment than in the fundus and because no high pressure mass lesion develops, there is less stimulation of prostaglandin elaboration that leads to labor. Hence, the term "painless vaginal bleeding" is often applied to placenta previa. In fact, uterine irritability to some degree is common even though labor-like contractions are not. Occult abruptio placentae may cause the patient to present with shock or hemodynamic instability, out of proportion to blood loss. The same is usually not true of placenta previa. In fact, the patient's hemodynamic status is likely to correspond to the amount of blood loss described. Suffice it to say that in management of placenta previa versus abruptio placentae, awareness of their clinical similarity leads to a flexible but structured plan of action.

## GENERAL MANAGEMENT CONSIDERATIONS

Both entities require consideration of rapid replacement of blood. Both require maternal and intensive fetal monitoring. Both require evaluation for coagulopathy. In abruptio placentae, the uterus tends to be irritable so that, even in the absence of contractions, by palpating the uterus one can stimulate a contraction. In classic severe abruption, the uterus has a board-like feeling. This is seldom true with placenta previa.

### Placenta Previa

Placenta previa occurs in 0.5 to 1% of all pregnancies after 20 weeks. The incidence seems to be higher early in pregnancy. Placenta previa may be classified according to whether it completely overlies the cervix (complete) or has merely an edge of the placenta near the cervix (low lying or marginal). The diagnosis is made by ultrasound. Clues that might help in the diagnosis of placenta previa include a fetal malpresentation, such as a transverse or a breech position. Placenta previa is associated with a twofold increase in congenital fetal malformations. In addition, the majority of investigators believe that intrauterine growth retardation is common in this condition.

The major presenting symptom of placenta previa, as previously stated, is painless vaginal bleeding. The earlier in pregnancy this bleeding occurs, especially if more than 100 ml, the worse the prognosis is, especially for preterm birth. Active bleeding in a patient with placenta previa requires admission to the hospital. At the time of admission, she should have a large-bore intravenous line inserted and fluids started. Intake and output must be monitored precisely. (It may not be necessary to insert a Foley's catheter at the time of admission.) Blood should be drawn at the time of the venipuncture to assess hemoglobin concentration, hematocrit, and coagulation variables. The initial evaluation may be factitious because the patient may have hemoconcentration and vasoconstriction due to severe hemorrhage. Therefore, initial blood work should be repeated at frequent intervals until the patient's stability is ensured. Blood pressure and pulse should be taken at frequent intervals—e.g., every 15 minutes until stable, every ½ hour for 2 hours, and then hourly. Orthostatic blood pressure and pulse

measurements are useful. If at the time of admission, the patient is hemodynamically fragile, central venous pressure and/or Swan-Ganz catheter monitoring is useful. The complete blood count and coagulation profile, including serum fibrinogen level, platelet count, and partial thromboplastin time, should be re-evaluated at appropriate intervals, depending on the patient's clinical status.

Obviously, in association with maternal monitoring, fetal monitoring should be employed. Electronic fetal monitoring can indicate patterns of concern, such as fetal tachycardia, the absence of reactivity, and late decelerations. If the patient is actively bleeding, tocolysis is contraindicated. If the patient is not actively bleeding after a few hours of observation, one can consider inhibiting any uterine irritability that might have been identified. Should the patient stabilize with no evidence of fetal or maternal distress, one can consider using steroids to accelerate maturation of fetal pulmonary function. It has been demonstrated that respiratory distress is increased in the face of fetal asphyxia as well as secondary to prematurity, thus warranting use of steroids. If placenta previa is documented between 28 and 32 weeks, such a management plan would be indicated. There are few data to support the use of steroids after 34 weeks, but we use the drug weekly to 34 weeks.

### Vasa Praevia

Vasa praevia is a variant of placenta previa. This entity occurs usually with marginal insertion of the cord and is more common in multiple gestations. Essentially, the cord inserts at the lateral aspect of the placenta, and the blood vessels that course through the cord, rather than being invested in Wharton's jelly, are exposed in the fetal membranes. This represents a potentially catastrophic situation for the fetus, but only rarely is one able to make the diagnosis of vasa praevia at the time of actual bleeding.

However, vasa praevia may be found on ultrasound with careful evaluation. Should the diagnosis of marginal or partial placenta previa be made, one should carefully examine the ultrasound or ask the consultant ultrasonographer to evaluate the patient for vasa praevia. Should the diagnosis be made, increased surveillance is necessary even beyond that associated with placenta previa. These patients should have a cesarean section essentially as soon as diagnosis is made after 32 weeks because the dependent blood vessels are easily traumatized and ruptured. Steroid therapy for pulmonary maturation can also be used here. It may be useful to look for fetal red blood cells in the vaginal blood using either an Apt test or a Kleihauer-Betke test.

### Double Set-up Examination

If the pregnancy is 36 weeks or greater at the time of third-trimester bleeding, bleeding is not terribly significant, and there is uterine contractility, one may consider a double set-up examination. The double set-up examination is a *predelivery* examination, not an examination for curiosity only. In the double set-up, the patient is prepared as though for cesarean section and is placed in the lithotomy position; only then, with the scrub nurse present, anesthesia immediately available, and adequate blood in the blood bank, can one proceed with a gentle pelvic examination. The first examination is done by speculum for evaluation of the cervix. Occasionally, one can see the presenting part with the cervix reasonably well dilated. Under these circumstances, one may then proceed with expectant management to allow the baby to act as a tamponade for the low-lying or marginal placenta previa. If in fact bleeding of a moderate degree is coming from the cervix, and the cervix seems to be undilated visually, gentle palpation can be accomplished. One can occasionally feel a boggy mass in the anterior vaginal or lateral fornices of the portio vaginalis. These maneuvers usually confirm the diagnosis of placenta previa. Under emergency conditions, ultrasound is not as precise as we would like in making this diagnosis. The double set-up examination can be eliminated in circumstances in which bleeding is extremely brisk, if the ultrasound clearly demonstrates placenta anteriorly and posteriorly over the cervical os, and, of course, if there is any evidence of fetal instability or maternal hemodynamic instability.

The primary cause of perinatal morbidity and mortality in the case of placenta previa is prematurity. After a patient is stabilized, the management plan should be aimed at achieving 36 weeks of gestation. To this end, bed rest with bathroom privileges and diminished activity should be prescribed. Obviously, there should be no coitus. Iron stores should be replaced with 300 mg of ferrous sulfate orally three times daily. The blood bank needs to be alerted to keep a blood sample available until delivery. Hematocrits should be obtained at frequent intervals. Most of these patients need to be maintained in the hospital unless they become absolutely "dry." Placenta previa is seductive because the magnitude of bleeding can be unrecognized. If one bleeds 100 ml a day for 5 days, 500 ml of blood may be lost in less than a week! Biweekly nonstress testing is indicated. A biophysical profile is also useful in assessing fetal growth and fetal behavior.

Conceivably, one can manage such patients as outpatients. However, strict criteria need to be employed, in writing. For instance, the patient must live less than 15 minutes away. Transportation must be readily available for an emergency drive to the hospital.

At cesarean section, the operator should try to avoid the placenta if possible. It is occasionally useful to have an ultrasound examination prior to surgery as a marker. I have not found ultrasound to be terribly useful because the upper limit of the placenta sometimes is not well defined by this technique. Without accurate measurement from cervix to top of placenta, one is left, at best, with an estimate. A classic cesarean section may be done, but I generally employ a low-transverse cervical cesarean section with good results. One of the difficulties with a low-transverse cesarean section may be the malpresentation of the fetus; therefore, the position of the fetus should be well established prior to section so that no delay is encountered in removing the fetus either by the breech or by the vertex. Because so many of these fetuses are transverse, technical difficulty may be encountered at the time of the hysterotomy, and the incision may need to be extended.

### Abruptio Placentae

Abruptio placentae occurs in approximately 1 in 80 pregnancies. Associated findings include the presence of maternal essential hypertension or pre-eclampsia. It is more common in primigravid patients and is increased in multiple gestation. Another high-risk factor is cocaine abuse.

Should a patient present to a labor room with vaginal bleeding of a severe nature with a board-like abdomen and a dead fetus, the diagnosis of abruptio placentae is essentially made. The management of patients with different grades of abruptio cannot be expectant as with the case of placenta previa. The patient should be set up similarly to the placenta previa patient with a large-bore needle intravenous line; appropriate blood studies drawn, including complete blood count and coagulation profile; and precise evaluation of intake and output. Once again, the use of a central venous pressure or Swan-Ganz catheter should be considered. In addition, a separate tube of blood is drawn at the time of the routine laboratory tests and taped to the patient's head board to evaluate for coagulability of the patient's blood. Continuous fetal heart monitoring as well as maternal monitoring is critical. In this condition, as compared with placenta previa, fetal compromise may be extremely rapid.

The management of these patients is aimed at vaginal delivery; however, cesarean section occurs in approximately 40 to 50% of all cases. If ultrasound examination confirms a fundal placenta and/or the presenting part is deep in the pelvis, the diagnosis of abruptio placentae rather than placenta previa is likely. This is especially true in the presence of extraordinary abdominal discomfort. If there are uterine contractions occurring at frequent intervals, and the patient seems to have a board-like abdomen, the diagnosis is essentially made. Once again, a double set-up examination may be conducted in the operating room, where it is likely that the cervix will be seen to be dilated and the bleeding coming from inside the uterus. At that point, membranes should be ruptured, and an internal scalp electrode and an internal uterine pressure catheter should be applied. The absence of fetal heart rate variability, or the presence of bradycardia or tachycardia mandates immediate delivery. If fetal heart rate variability seems reasonable, fetal heart rate is normal, and decelerations are minimal, observation is indicated. If the patient is not in efficient labor after 30 minutes of observation, a dilute solution of oxytocin (Pitocin) should be employed. High doses of oxytocin may be needed under these circumstances. Any delay in progress of labor, manifested by lack of either cervical dilation or descent should lead to cesarean section.

At the time of cesarean section, one occasionally notices the uterus to be mottled and purple in color. This condition is called a "Couvelaire's uterus," and the uterus contracts well after the cesarean section is performed. There is no fear in making an incision through these areas even though they do contain extravasated blood. It is critical not to close the incision after the cesarean section until hemostasis is ensured. Occasionally, the coagulopathy manifested by these patients does not appear until shortly after surgery starts. Although in most cases the surgery relieves the coagulopathy, the operative field should be constantly observed to make certain that any blood vessels that need to be tied are in fact tied. Because the patient may be in shock, bleeding may not occur until the blood pressure attains normal levels. These patients should be monitored closely post partum because some become pre-eclamptic or even eclamptic after delivery, despite essentially "normal" blood pressures during the acute event.

# HYPERTENSIVE DISORDERS OF PREGNANCY

method of
FREDERICK P. ZUSPAN, M.D.
*The Ohio State University*
*Columbus, Ohio*

High blood pressure in pregnancy remains one of the leading causes of maternal and fetal morbidity and mortality. There are substantial controversies regarding therapy and classification of disease. The majority of this article focuses on management of pre-eclampsia and eclampsia with regimens that I have advocated for the past 35 years, some of which are accepted as the standard of care in this country.

## PRE-ECLAMPSIA

### Incidence, Description, Etiology, and Classification

Pre-eclampsia is a syndrome of unknown etiology that is characterized by the sequential development of hypertension (blood pressure of 140/90) and proteinuria (> 300 mg per liter) after the twentieth week of gestation. After the disease progresses in a patient with pre-eclampsia who develops a seizure, the patient is then known to have eclampsia. Eclampsia portends the possibility of death for the mother (0.5 to 17%) and for the fetus (10 to 37%). The higher figures are observed in developing countries, and survival and condition of the newborn depend on the length of gestation. Eclampsia can occur ante partum, intra partum, or during the first 5 days post partum.

The demographic variables and potential profile of a patient who may experience pre-eclampsia are as follows: pre-eclampsia occurs in 6 to 8% of pregnancies; is principally a disease of the first term pregnancy (85%); occurs in 14 to 20% of multiple gestations; occurs in 30% of patients with major uterine anomalies; and occurs in 25% of patients with chronic hypertension and 25% with chronic renal disease; some women have repetitive, severe disease, which most likely has a recessive genetic origin.

Pathogenesis is well understood, even though the etiology is obscure, and the major goal of prenatal care is to detect early onset of pre-eclampsia and then activate aggressive therapy to prevent severe complications. All severe complications of pre-eclampsia and eclampsia should be prevented or ameliorated.

Pre-eclampsia occurs only in humans, and there is no acceptable animal model. It is not preventable because its origin is at the time of implantation.

The classification and nomenclature used on both the international and the American scene vary, and authorities cannot agree on how to make a diagnosis of gestational hypertension, pregnancy-induced hypertension, and pre-eclampsia. These words should not be used interchangeably. Definitions have been proposed by the American College of Obstetricians and Gynecologists in 1972, the World Health Organization in 1987, the International Society for the Study of Hypertension in Pregnancy in 1987 and 1988, and, most recently, the National Blood Pressure Council in 1990.

"Gestational hypertension" is defined as a pregnant woman at more than 20 weeks' gestation with a blood pressure of 140/90 (sustained), and no proteinuria or less than 300 mg per liter. This patient may be treated as an outpatient and should be seen at least weekly or biweekly. "Pre-eclampsia" is defined as more than 20 weeks' gestation with a blood pressure of at least 140/90 (sustained) and proteinuria that is persistent and greater than 300 mg per liter. This classification may be mild or severe. In any event, the patient should be hospitalized and treated. The statistics in gestational hypertension and mild pre-eclampsia for the outcome of mother and baby are identical to those of a normal pregnancy. *(There is no single test that identifies the hypertensive diseases of pregnancy and/or pre-eclampsia. Objective measures are blood pressure and proteinuria.)*

### Objective Measures

**Blood Pressure.** It is best to use the first, fourth, and fifth Korotkoff sounds with the patient consistently either in the sitting position or the lateral recumbent position, which I prefer. An increase of 30 mmHg systolic and an increase of 15 mmHg diastolic does *not* make the diagnosis of pre-eclampsia. It only alerts the health care team to a change.

**Proteinuria.** A voided or catheterized specimen is observed for the presence or absence of red blood cells or white blood cells, which may cause an erroneously high protein value. On dipstick testing, this would be more than a 2+ for significance (i.e., >300 mg per liter).

**Edema.** Edema is not an objective measure, as it is subjective and observed in normal pregnancy. If edema is present, it should involve the hands and face, to be of any significance. It is associated with a weight gain of more than 5 lb in 7 days or less when present.

### Pathophysiology

Pathophysiology includes specific target organ involvements. The major target organs are the cardiovascular system (elevated blood pressure), the renal system (proteinuria), and the placenta (intrauterine growth retardation). The minor target organs for disturbed pathophysiology include the reticuloendothelial system (decreased platelets), the liver (jaundice), and the brain (edema and hemorrhage).

Study of the major target organ, the placenta, has taught us that this defect begins at the time of conception (i.e., birth-implantation defect); hence, it is probably not preventable. The defect is a failure of the trophoblastic tissue to invade the maternal spiral arteries, which results in less dilation of the spiral arteries. In conjunction with this, I have shown that there is a lack of adrenergic denervation at the base of the spiral artery. It has been known for some time that the endothelial injury is the deposition of fibrin products on the renal glomeruli, causing endotheliosis. More recently, studies have shown a disruption of the arachidonic acid system with production of less prostacyclin and more thromboxane.

### Management

A patient with mild pre-eclampsia should be hospitalized and given bed rest and observed. If the cervix is favorable and she is at more than 36 weeks' gestation, induction of labor is by far the simplest solution to the problem. If her gestational age is less than 36 weeks, evaluation of fetal status is most likely necessary and selective induction or delivery would take place if the condition worsens, depending on maternal and fetal status.

The management of the patient with severe pre-eclampsia demands decisive thought and attention. This patient may have one or more of the following findings:

Blood pressure of 160 mmHg systolic or 110 mmHg diastolic
Oliguria, less than 500 ml per day
Decreased platelet count, less than 100,000 per $mm^3$
Increased liver enzyme levels and/or jaundice
Proteinuria of greater than 3 grams per liter or 4+ on random sample
Pulmonary edema
Coma

One should assume that this patient constitutes a medical emergency and needs to be stabilized with the following regimen: Intravenous magnesium sulfate, 4- to 6-gram load, is given over 5 minutes, then 1 to 2 grams per hour. The blood pressure is controlled if the diastolic is persistently greater than 100 to 110 mmHg using intravenous hydralazine (Apresoline), 5-mg bolus. In 20 minutes, if blood pressure is not stabilized, one should add 100 mg of hydralazine to 200 ml of normal saline and infuse by automated device. A dynamap or similar blood pressure recording apparatus should be used to monitor the blood pressure, which should be maintained between 80 and 100 diastolic.

After appropriate laboratory data are obtained (complete blood count, platelet and electrolyte concentrations, liver battery, and serum creatinine, blood urea nitrogen, and uric acid levels) and results are evaluated, one should consider termination of pregnancy, as the patient most likely will not improve. Pregnancy can most likely be terminated by induction of labor using oxytocin (Pitocin), starting at levels of 0.5 mU per minute. If cesarean section is utilized, general anesthesia is probably the anesthesia of choice, but epidural anesthesia may be used in selected patients. I do not recommend spinal anesthesia becase of the physiologic disruption in the mother. If magnesium sulfate is utilized, it should be continued for at least 24 hours following delivery.

After magnesium sulfate is started, if an overdose occurs, calcium chloride or gluconate (1 gram) may be given intravenously. When magnesium sulfate is administered, the patient should be monitored by bioassay, utilizing the following:

1. Deep tendon reflexes: These should be hypoactive, but present, and should be checked on an hourly basis. Reflexes become absent if the serum magnesium concentration is greater than 5 mmol per liter.

2. Respirations: These should be observed on an hourly basis and should exceed 12 per hour. When the magnesium concentration exceeds 6.5 mmol per liter, respirations may become obtunded and cardiac arrest occurs at concentrations greater than 12 mmol per liter.

3. Urinary output: This should be monitored on an hourly basis utilizing a Foley's catheter. At least 100 ml should be observed in a 4-hour period or approximately 25 ml per hour. If oliguria is present, the dosage of magnesium sulfate may need to be decreased, as it is excreted principally by the kidney.

4. Serum magnesium levels: These may be obtained as a guidepost to therapy, but are usually not needed. Cord blood magnesium level may help the pediatrician, as it takes approximately 48 hours for the newborn to excrete the magnesium. Magnesium cord levels and maternal levels are almost identical.

I do not advocate the use of other agents in treating severe pre-eclampsia or eclampsia, as this simple method has stood the test of time and

has resulted in the best survival rate for the fetus and the least maternal mortality in the world literature for severe disease.

*The standard of care in the United States is utilizing magnesium sulfate to control convulsions and hydralazine to control blood pressure.* Other drugs may be used to control the blood pressure, but parenteral hydralazine has stood the test of time. Neither of these drugs cures the patient, but they control the condition until intervention takes place.

### Decision for Delivery

After the patient's seizure tendency and blood pressure are controlled, a decision can be made as to whether or not delivery should take place. The more serious the condition of the patient, the greater is the need to proceed to delivery. If the patient is less than 34 weeks' gestation, she should be referred to a tertiary care center for the availability of a neonatal intensive care unit.

Delivery is the definitive care for this disease, and all medications and therapy that have been identified are only temporizing measures. The following may seem appropriate.

1. One should establish gestation by history, lung maturity, or ultrasound.

2. Delivery should be achieved as soon as possible in severe disease—there is no magic waiting period for stabilization, but laboratory test results should be evaluated prior to this decision.

3. Laboratory tests should include electrolyte determinations, uric acid, liver function battery, and complete hemogram and clotting profile, including platelets and fibrin split products and urinary protein.

4. The condition of the cervix can be evaluated, and, if a favorable Bishop's score is present, oxytocin induction should be attempted.

5. Appropriate monitoring of the fetus is necessary, utilizing external monitoring until membranes are ruptured, and then a scalp clip is applied. If the patient is to be induced, an intrauterine pressure catheter should be inserted. If the fetus is less than 1500 grams, I usually consider a cesarean section, unless the cervix is most favorable.

One should remember to continue the magnesium sulfate for at least 24 hours post partum and then gradually diminish the dosage. The blood pressure should continue to be controlled during this period, and the patient may actually need to go home while receiving blood pressure medications. Diuresis most likely occurs within 72 hours post partum.

### Prevention

The potentially high-risk patient—e.g., first term pregnancy, diabetes, chronic renal or cardiovascular disease, and multiple gestations—should be identified and seen at more frequent intervals after the twentieth week of gestation. Bed rest is encouraged: at least ½ hour at noon and 1 hour before the evening meal, as rest is the only thing that increases uterine blood flow; if hypertension intercedes, the restriction of activities is increased.

It is also advantageous for the patient to have a well-balanced, nutritious diet in which at least 1 gram of protein per kg of body weight per day is consumed to prevent a negative nitrogen balance, and there is some recent evidence that 2 grams of calcium per day may also be beneficial in prevention.

In the United States, there are seven centers doing a multicenter study on the use of children's aspirin as a preventive measure for severe complications of pre-eclampsia. The value of this has yet to be decided, and until these studies are completed I would not encourage people to utilize daily children's aspirin in high-risk patients.

Additionally, there are multicenter studies taking place on the use of at least 2 grams of calcium per day, and these have not yet been completed. These are to be looked at in the future, and the use of calcium may well help prevent the serious complications of pre-eclampsia.

## CHRONIC HYPERTENSION IN PREGNANCY

Chronic hypertension in pregnancy is usually not seen during the first pregnancy or in younger women; however, it may be, because approximately 8 to 10% of high school adolescents have hypertension. There is usually an antecedent history of hypertension in the patient, and most often there is a positive family history of the disease.

Early diagnosis of chronic hypertension is important to make certain that pre-eclampsia is not the offending agent. The main goal in taking care of the patient who has chronic hypertension in pregnancy is to prevent or diagnose early superimposed pre-eclampsia.

Chronic hypertension in pregnancy may well cause intrauterine growth retardation, and serial ultrasounds are needed. I would recommend an ultrasound prior to the twentieth week of gestation, another at 30 weeks, and a third at approximately 34 weeks of gestation to rule in or rule out intrauterine growth retardation.

The randomized prospective studies that have been done are few, and none of them show any benefit of antihypertensive drugs on fetal salvage. The use of antihypertensive drugs in these patients is to prevent maternal complications and to stabilize blood pressure fluctuations.

### Diagnosis

I have utilized home blood pressure monitoring techniques for the past 12 years to understand the true value of the blood pressure. Utilizing home blood pressure evaluations decreases the need for antihypertensive drugs by 40% and decreases the need for hospitalization sixfold. Patients are taught to take the first, fourth, and fifth Korotkoff sounds and record all three at least two times per week.

I currently prefer a digital electronic blood pressure monitor, even though the aneroid manometer is more accurate. The reason for this is that it is simpler for the patient to lie on her side in the left lateral recumbent position. She should then take the blood pressure in the upper arm as it lies across the chest and record the values. It is advisable for her to take her blood pressure, if possible, in the sitting and then in the lateral recumbent position on each occasion.

The use of home blood pressure monitoring provides the patient with a mechanism for diagnosing early pre-eclampsia (i.e., an increase over her baseline blood pressures at specific times of the day). Additionally, if she is permitted to have urine dipsticks for protein, she should also use these each time she takes her blood pressure. An increase in protein in the urine and elevated blood pressure should be viewed as early signs of impending pre-eclampsia, and the patient needs to be hospitalized. Prevention and early diagnosis of pre-eclampsia in the chronic hypertensive patient is the main theme of management.

### Drug Therapy

There is no specific standard of care for the type of drug to be utilized to control the blood pressure. Alpha-methyldopa (Aldomet) has been used in the past in the two randomized prospective studies that have been done, but beta blockers and alpha and beta blockers have also been used (Table 1). Studies in Europe have shown that intrauterine growth retardation is associated with beta-blocker therapy. The choice of drug and the dosage depend on patient response.

TABLE 1. **Commonly Used Drugs**

| Drug Name | Type | Usual Dosage |
|---|---|---|
| Propranolol (Inderal) | Beta blocker (off patent) | 20–40 mg bid to qid |
| Atenolol (Tenormin) | Beta blocker | 25–50 mg bid to tid |
| Labetalol (Trandate, Normodyne) | Beta blocker with alpha component | 100 mg bid to tid |
| Hydralazine (Apresoline) | Direct action, not alpha or beta blocker | 20–30 mg bid to qid |

There is controversy surrounding when antihypertensive therapy should be started, utilizing the diastolic pressure of between 84 and 90 mmHg.

The work-up is dictated by the severity of the hypertension. If the patient is taking diuretics, these should be gradually eliminated over a period of 4 to 6 weeks and then discontinued. It is necessary for the chronically hypertensive patient to be seen at least every 2 weeks in the physician's office. It has been previously stated that at least three ultrasounds should be done during the pregnancy to rule out intrauterine growth retardation, as this does not usually begin until after the thirtieth week of gestation. It is necessary to do antepartum testing beginning at 30 to 32 weeks, and this should be done on a weekly or biweekly basis. The nonstress test and the vibra-acoustic stimulation test are preferred. If either is not satisfactory, an oxytocin challenge test is used. Additionally, fetal activity counts are started at 34 to 36 weeks' gestation, and, if these are begun earlier, spurious results may often be obtained. The patient is asked to lie on her side twice a day and count movements of the baby. As long as there are more than six movements per 1-hour observation period, this is considered normal.

The patient is not permitted to go beyond term because of the potential for placental pathologic change, and oftentimes delivery takes place before term and usually by cesarean section because the cervix is often not favorable. Ninety per cent of cases of patients who have chronic hypertension in pregnancy should end up with a good fetus and a normal mother, but the remaining 10% pose major problems for health care.

Contraception post partum should not include oral contraceptives, but any other form is acceptable. Many of these patients seek surgical sterilization.

# OBSTETRIC ANESTHESIA

method of
MARSHA L. WAKEFIELD, M.D.
*Medical College of Georgia*
*Augusta, Georgia*

In obstetric circles the comment is often made that the ideal anesthetic would be the one that best benefits the patient, the passenger, and the power (to effect delivery). All of these factors must be considered in choosing the most appropriate anesthetic technique for an obstetric procedure.

"Natural" childbirth encompasses many methods (e.g., those of Read, Jacobson, and Lamaze). It is most effective when "prepared" childbirth allows an informed parturient and her partner to participate in a satisfying birth experience. However, it is important to remember that this concept does not mean a denial of regular medical care or an endurance test, and that pain medications or regional anesthesia may be used without the feeling of failure.

## SYSTEMIC MEDICATIONS

Systemic medications have long been used for pain relief in childbirth. However, the emphasis has shifted from the era of total oblivion (i.e., twilight sleep) to the current recommendations to use the minimal drug dose that is effective. The primary concerns of excessive systemic medication include (1) maternal respiratory depression, (2) diminished maternal consciousness and cooperativeness, and (3) neonatal depression. The selection, timing, mode of administration, and dose of drug administered to the parturient should be based on knowledge of the effect of the drug on the mother and the fetus.

The dose and site of administration, the maternal distribution and metabolism of the drug, and the physiochemical properties of the drug itself (e.g., pH, lipid solubility, molecular weight) influence the amount of drug transferred to the fetus. Narcotics are the most widely used systemic medications for labor analgesia. Because they are lipid soluble and have molecular weights less than 500, they all cross the placenta easily by diffusion. Incremental intravenous injection is preferred to intramuscular injection because of its more prompt, predictable, and smoother action.

Meperidine (Demerol) is still the most popular narcotic for labor analgesia. Meperidine is usually administered in doses of 50 to 100 mg intramuscularly or 10 to 50 mg intravenously. When the drug is given intramuscularly, the peak analgesic effect occurs 40 to 45 minutes after injection. When the drug is administered intravenously, analgesia begins within 30 seconds and peaks at 5 to 10 minutes. The duration of action is 2 to 4 hours. Because meperidine rapidly crosses the placenta, the maternal and fetal equilibrium occurs within 6 minutes after intravenous administration. The incidence of neonatal respiratory depression is greatest in the second, third, and fourth hours after administration. This corresponds to the time of maximal fetal uptake of meperidine. The half-life of meperidine is 3 hours in the mother but 23 hours in the neonate. Other analgesics that have been used are morphine, pentazocine (Talwin), and fentanyl (Sublimaze). More recently, the narcotic agonist-antagonists butorphanol (Stadol) and nalbuphine

(Nubain) have gained some popularity because of potentially less respiratory depression.

Morphine administered in doses of 5 to 10 mg intramuscularly or 2 to 3 mg intravenously has not been as popular as meperidine because it has been shown to cause more neonatal respiratory depression at equipotent doses. Pentazocine, usually administered in doses of 20 to 30 mg intramuscularly or 10 to 20 mg intravenously, never gained widespread use because of its psychomimetic properties. Fentanyl, although widely used in general anesthetic procedures, has not been as useful as an analgesic in obstetrics because of the rapid onset of respiratory depression and its shorter duration of action. The usual dose administered is 50 to 100 µg intramuscularly and 25 to 50 µg intravenously.

Butorphanol is usually administered in doses of 1 to 2 mg intramuscularly or intravenously during labor. A potential advantage with butorphanol is the mild sedative effect in addition to the narcosis. This effect would otherwise be achieved only by giving a tranquilizer with the other narcotics. Nalbuphine can be administered in doses of 10 to 15 mg intramuscularly. Smaller incremental doses may be given intravenously.

If a narcotic antagonist is needed, the preferred one is naloxone (Narcan). This drug is a pure antagonist and reverses the analgesic effect of narcotics as well as the respiratory depression. If respiratory depression in the neonate is a concern, it is best to administer naloxone directly to the neonate at birth. There is unreliable placental transfer of naloxone when administered to the mother shortly before delivery. Also, administering naloxone just before delivery leads to loss of analgesia in the mother. The maternal dose of naloxone is 0.1 to 0.4 mg intravenously. The neonatal dose is 0.01 mg per kg intravenously or intramuscularly (only with adequate tissue perfusion).

Phenothiazines are also widely used in combination with the narcotics because of their anxiolytic and antiemetic activities. Promethazine (Phenergan) is frequently used in combination with meperidine for labor analgesia and has been noted to reduce the dose requirement of meperidine. If it is given alone, promethazine may have a mild antianalgesic effect. Promethazine crosses the placenta rapidly and reaches equilibrium within 15 minutes. Promethazine and propiomazine (Largon) are the most commonly used phenothiazines in obstetrics. Others such as promazine (Sparine), chlorpromazine (Thorazine), and prochlorperazine (Compazine) are seldom used because of their greater alpha-adrenergic blocking properties and thus the potential for hypotension to occur. Neonates whose mothers had received meperidine (50 mg) plus promethazine (50 mg) intramuscularly or meperidine (50 mg) plus propiomazine (20 mg) intravenously had Apgar scores similar to those whose mothers received only meperidine.

## ANESTHESIA FOR VAGINAL DELIVERY

### Continuous Lumbar Epidural Analgesia for Labor and Vaginal Delivery

Continuous lumbar epidural analgesia is the most effective means of pain relief for labor. Once continuous epidural anesthesia has been established, it can be used for either spontaneous or operative delivery as the need arises. Epidural analgesia has been shown to decrease the level of circulating maternal catecholamines and, in the absence of hypotension, may actually improve uteroplacental blood flow.

Once the patient has been committed to delivery and the fetus has been evaluated, the epidural block may be administered. To prepare the parturient for the anesthetic, the physician must be able to monitor both the mother and the fetus. It is important to remember that aspiration pneumonitis is still a major cause of maternal morbidity and mortality. Although regional anesthesia has the advantage of maintaining the maternal protective airway reflexes, loss of consciousness is a remote possibility with an unintentional subarachnoid or intravenous placement of an epidural dose of local anesthetics. Therefore, it is important that measures be taken to minimize the hazard of aspiration by administering a nonparticulate antacid such as 0.3 M sodium citrate (Bicitra). Because epidural anesthesia causes sympathetic blockade with vasodilation, it is important that the patient be acutely hydrated with 500 to 1000 ml of a non–dextrose-containing intravenous solution. Rapid increases in maternal blood glucose level, as with rapid volume expansion with dextrose-containing intravenous fluids, may put the neonate at increased risk for hypoglycemia. Adequate preloading helps to maintain venous return and, therefore, to prevent maternal hypotension and decreased uteroplacental perfusion. Aortocaval compression or supine hypotensive syndrome occurs in 15 to 20% of parturients at term. This syndrome is a result of compression of the aorta and vena cava by the gravid uterus when the parturient is supine, which impedes venous return to the heart and may cause hypotension, nausea, vomiting, and changes in cerebration. Most women can compensate by vasoconstriction in the lower extremities. The sympathetic blockade of regional anesthesia may exacerbate supine hypotensive syndrome if the mother is not kept in the lateral or semilateral position (left uterine displacement) after the epidural anesthesia is established. In addition to preparing the mother, it is important that proper resuscitation equipment be in good working order and readily available in the area where the block is being placed. This equipment should include an oxygen flowmeter, Ambu bag and masks, suction apparatus, and intubation supplies.

After appropriate preparation of the mother and the equipment, the epidural space may be identified from either the caudal or the lumbar approach. The lumbar epidural approach has advantages over the caudal approach for labor, including (1) ability to achieve a segmental block of specific pathways for each stage of labor; (2) finer control of autonomic blockade; (3) higher success rate; (4) smaller drug doses; (5) quicker uterine pain relief because injection is nearer to T11-12; (6) less maternal discomfort; (7) no risk of puncturing the rectum or fetal head; and (8) less risk of infection. Potential disadvantages of the lumbar or caudal epidural approach compared with spinal anesthesia (for delivery) include (1) delayed onset of anesthesia, usually 10 to 20 minutes; (2) "patchy" or incomplete pain relief; (3) a more difficult technique to master; and (4) larger doses of drug needed.

In the adult the spinal cord usually ends at the L1 level, occasionally extending as far as the vertebral body of L2. The dural sac extends as far as the level of S1-2. The epidural space extends from the foramen magnum rostrally to the sacral hiatus caudally. The L2-5 interspaces are usually chosen for obstetric epidural block. The landmarks for epidural anesthesia are the same as those for spinal anesthesia. A line between the left and right iliac crests crosses either the spinous process of the L4 vertebra or the L4-5 vertebral interspace. The patient may be in either the lateral decubitus position or the sitting position.

After positioning the patient, the lumbar area is prepared and draped in sterile fashion. The interspace is identified and a small-gauge needle is used to make a skin wheal. The epidural needle is then inserted into the intervertebral space 1.2 to 3.7 cm until the needle is anchored in the interspinous ligament. The stylet is then removed and the needle is slowly advanced by using the loss-of-resistance technique (saline or air-filled syringe) or "hanging drop" method to identify the epidural space. After identification of the epidural space has been confirmed by negative aspiration for blood or cerebrospinal fluid, a test dose of local anesthetic may be administered.

The most appropriate test dose in the obstetric setting is controversial. The addition of epinephrine 1:200,000 (15 μg in a 3-ml test dose) has been recommended to rule out possible intravascular placement. However, in the patient in active labor, the maternal heart rate and blood pressure may change as much or more with a contraction than may be noted in response to the epinephrine test done. The physician should also usually wait 3 to 5 minutes for evidence of spinal blockade before administering additional drug. The most effective means of preventing the sequelae of unintentional intravenous or subarachnoid placement is to use incremental dosing. Only 3 to 5 ml of drug should be given at a time and verbal contact should be maintained with the patient. Early detection is the key to preventing serious reactions.

For continuous lumbar epidural block, a catheter is usually inserted and the needle carefully removed leaving 3 to 4 cm of catheter in the epidural space. The catheter should then be aspirated to detect the presence of cerebrospinal fluid or blood. If the aspiration is negative, incremental dosing can continue via the catheter until an adequate level of analgesia is obtained. My initial dose of local anesthetic is usually 8 to 15 ml of 0.25% bupivacaine with an onset of action of 5 to 10 minutes and an expected duration of action of 1½ to 2 hours. Each repeat dose or "top up" is usually about two-thirds of the initial dose. Other local anesthetics may be used. Lidocaine, 1 to 1.5%, usually is effective for about 60 minutes, but it has been associated with tachyphylaxis when used for prolonged periods. 2-Chloroprocaine (Nesacaine), 2%, may also be used with an expected duration of action of only 45 minutes.

Use of the continuous infusion technique for epidural analgesia has become popular especially in busy obstetric suites. It has been suggested that a continuous infusion would cause fewer episodes of hypotension and more constant analgesia. Continuous infusion has not been found to result in lower total drug requirements or greater maternal satisfaction when compared with regularly administered intermittent top-up doses. The larger volumes and more dilute solutions of local anesthetics may be used to provide suitable analgesia with the least amount of motor blockade. It is important to regularly evaluate the patient being infused because the catheter could potentially migrate into a blood vessel (noted by decreasing analgesia with or without systemic signs from the low doses of local anesthetic) or it could migrate into the subarachnoid space (noted by increasing sensory level and motor block). After epidural anesthesia has been established with the initial loading dose, the infusion is usually begun at a rate of 10 ml per hour. The rate is then adjusted to maintain a T10 sensory level. The most commonly used solutions are 0.25% bupivacaine, 0.125% bupivacaine, and 1% lidocaine.

Epidural narcotics are beginning to be widely used, not only for postcesarean pain relief, but also as an adjunct to local anesthetics for labor. The potential advantages include additional analgesia and a decrease in total dose of local anesthetic used. Because of their site of action at opiate receptors in the spinal cord, motor function and sympathetic blockade are not affected by the use of epidural narcotics. Epidural narcotics alone have not been as effective in providing adequate analgesia for labor and delivery as has the combination of local anesthetics and epidural narcotics. Morphine (Duramorph) is the only narcotic for epidural use currently approved. Morphine has the greatest potential for late respiratory depression (8 to 12 hours) and a delayed onset of action (60 minutes). Therefore, it has limited usefulness as an adjunct to labor analgesia. However, fentanyl has been widely studied and used as either an addition to the initial dose (50 μg in 10 ml of 0.25% bupivacaine) or an addition to a continuous infusion (2 to 5 μg per ml of 0.125% bupivacaine infused). Butorphanol, in doses of 1 to 2 mg (initial bolus), and sufentanil (Sufenta), in doses of 20 to 30 μg (initial bolus) or 2 μg per ml infusion, have also been used. There has been no noted increase in neonatal effects as reflected in the Apgar scores by the addition of these low-dose epidural narcotics. As for all narcotics, there may occasionally be side effects such as pruritus, nausea, and urinary retention.

During the second stage of labor, pain from the pelvis and perineum is carried by the pudendal nerve (S2, S3, and S4). The most difficult root to block is S2 because of its large diameter. Therefore, it may be necessary in the second stage to reinforce a block with a "delivery" dose. Usually, 10 to 15 ml is needed with the mother in the semisitting position to ensure good perineal analgesia. Lidocaine, 2%, or 2-chloroprocaine, 3%, may be useful just before delivery because of their more rapid onset of action.

Because epidural analgesia for labor is almost exclusively an elective procedure, it is imperative that the safety of the mother and the fetus be given primary consideration. Proper equipment, monitors, and personnel must be available to ensure the safest and most satisfying birth experience.

### Spinal Block for Vaginal Delivery

Spinal anesthesia for vaginal delivery is usually administered just before delivery. It is not a useful technique for prolonged labor analgesia. Spinal anesthesia is less popular now than it was previously. The occurrence of post–dural puncture headache, the increased risk of hypotension, and the greater use of continuous epidural anesthesia in obstetrics account for this decline in popularity. However, the ease with which spinal anesthesia may be induced and its rapid onset make this method an attractive option in certain situations.

Spinal anesthesia produces excellent analgesia for spontaneous and instrumental vaginal delivery, for a cerclage operation, for manual removal of the placenta, and for cesarean section. A T10 level suffices for vaginal deliveries and cerclage procedures; a T4 level is required for a cesarean section.

A saddle block or a low spinal block produces adequate anesthesia for vaginal delivery. The saddle block anesthetizes only the sacral roots, but the low spinal block extends also to the T10 level. With the patient sitting, a 25-gauge or 26-gauge spinal needle is placed in the subarachnoid space. After return of cerebrospinal fluid, a hyperbaric solution of local anesthetic is injected and the patient is kept in a sitting position for 1 to 2 minutes and is then returned to the lithotomy position. The most commonly used drug is hyperbaric solution with 5% lidocaine. Typically, a dose of 40 mg (range 30 to 60 mg) for an average-size patient is used. Other solutions such as hyperbaric tetracaine (average dose 4 to 5 mg) or hyperbaric bupivacaine (average dose 8 mg) may be used for low spinal anesthesia with longer duration of action. Because of the more rapid onset of sympathetic block, an appropriate fluid preload is necessary to avoid hypotension.

### Peripheral Nerve Blocks

For the first stage of labor, the pain is transmitted by afferent fibers, which travel along with sympathetic fibers to T10-L1. These may be blocked peripherally by either a lumbar sympathetic or a paracervical block. To give effective analgesia for first stage of labor, the lumbar sympathetic block must be bilateral and even with bupivacaine provides only 2 to 3 hours of analgesia. With this block it is important to aspirate the needle before giving local anesthetic to avoid unintentional subarachnoid or intravenous injection. Lumbar sympathetic block may also produce systemic hypotension.

The visceral afferent fibers that transmit labor pain lie in the paracervical area where they are known as Frankenhäuser's plexus. Paracervical block gives good analgesia for first stage of labor, does not impair motor power, and does not cause systemic hypotension. It was very popular in the 1950s and 1960s until the occurrence of fetal bradycardia and fetal hypoxia was reported.

There are several mechanisms proposed for the bradycardia. It may result from excessive absorption of local anesthetic into the fetal circulation, which causes fetal myocardial depression. It might also result either from uterine artery vasoconstriction or from an increase in uterine tone, both of which are caused by a high concentration of the local anesthetic. The degree and duration of fetal bradycardia correlate with fetal hypoxia and acidosis.

The pudendal nerve (S2-4) is a branch of the sacral plexus. The pudendal block is performed to relieve pain from the second stage of labor and to provide anesthesia for episiotomy and low forceps delivery. A pudendal block does not provide adequate analgesia for midforceps rotations or extractions. The transvaginal approach is the more widely used and practical route in the obstetric patient. It is performed just before delivery, and although it is a relatively easy and uncomplicated block for the obstetrician, it results in adequate anesthesia only about 50% of the time.

### General Anesthesia for Vaginal Delivery

Rarely, general anesthesia may be required for delivery, for example, when the baby is in distress or when uterine relaxation may be needed for a difficult breech delivery or delivery of a second twin. Endotracheal anesthesia is necessary under those circumstances. A nonparticulate antacid should be administered, if possible, and a rapid-sequence induction must be performed using cricoid pressure until the trachea has been secured with a cuffed endotracheal tube. General anesthesia may also occasionally be needed for manual removal of the placenta and may be the technique of choice in the rare event of uterine inversion.

### ANESTHESIA FOR CESAREAN SECTION

#### Regional Anesthesia: Epidural

As previously mentioned in the discussion of epidural anesthesia for labor and delivery, proper preparation is important to prevent potential side effects. The potential for supine hypotension to be exacerbated by sympathetic blockade is even more significant when surgical levels of anesthesia are necessary. Sympathetic blockade has been reported to be from two to six dermatomal levels higher than the level of sensory block. Because of the higher level of sensory block needed for cesarean section (i.e., T4-2), there is limited ability to compensate for the near-complete sympathetic blockade by vasoconstriction in unblocked segments or increased heart rate.

Two simple precautions can minimize the cardiovascular effects of high epidural block: the intravenous administration of 1.5 liters of a non–dextrose-containing intravenous fluid just before the block and maintaining left uterine displacement. Likewise, it is important to remember to administer 30 ml of a nonparticulate antacid such as 0.3 M sodium citrate as a prophylaxis against acid aspiration.

The effects of epidural anesthesia on respiratory muscle activity are not clinically significant in the healthy parturient. A sensory level of T3 is not usually accompanied by a change in vital capacity, and even at a T1 sensory level there is no blockade of the phrenic nerve. Apnea from a high epidural block is not caused by direct blockade of the phrenic nerve but by the decreased perfusion of the medullary centers related to systemic hypotension. However, a total spinal block affects the respiratory center as well as the respiratory muscles. During an epidural block with a high thoracic sensory level, the patient may complain of dyspnea because of the lack of sensory input from the intercostal muscles. Slow diaphragmatic breathing should be encouraged, and patients should be reassured that such a feeling is to be expected.

Especially when the epidural block is used for an elective cesarean delivery, it is important to use an epinephrine-containing test dose. In this instance the epinephrine is a more reliable marker of intravascular injection, and the toxicity risk is greater because of the higher doses (volume and concentration) needed for surgical anesthesia. After proper placement of the catheter has been confirmed, incremental doses of 2% lidocaine with epinephrine, 0.5% bupivacaine, or 3% 2-chloroprocaine may be administered to achieve an adequate sensory level for surgery. Blood pressure and pulse should be checked frequently, and any hypotension (systolic less than 100 mmHg) should be treated with 5- to 10-mg increments of ephedrine. Proper intravenous fluid preloading helps to offset the potential for a decrease in maternal arterial pressure. Also, the mother should be maintained in the left tilt position to avoid aortocaval compression. It is important to maintain maternal blood pressure (systolic of 100 mmHg or mean of 70 mmHg) because of its direct influence on uterine perfusion. During the surgery the mother should receive supplemental oxygen to optimize fetal oxygenation before delivery.

After delivery of the infant, epidural narcotics may be used to provide both intraoperative and postoperative analgesia. It has also been noted that epidural fentanyl (onset of action 5 to 6 minutes) provides additional analgesia during the exteriorization of the uterus. The delayed

TABLE 1. **Epidural Opioids**

| Narcotic | Dose | Onset of Action (min) | Duration of Action (hr) |
|----------|------|----------------------|------------------------|
| Morphine | 3–5 mg | 30–60 | 16–24 |
| Fentanyl | 50–100 µg | 6–9 | 3–5 |
| Sufentanil | 15–50 µg | 2–8 | 3–6 |
| Butorphanol | 2–4 mg | 10–15 | 6–12 |
| Hydromorphone | 1–2 mg | 10–13 | 6–8 |

onset of action of epidural morphine (30 to 60 minutes) makes it less useful for this purpose. The more fat-soluble opiates such as fentanyl have a shorter duration of action and therefore require repeated dosing or a continuous infusion with the catheter left in place for at least 24 hours. A single dose of epidural morphine lasts 12 to 24 hours. The most common side effects of the epidural opioids are respiratory depression, pruritus, nausea, and urinary retention. Intraspinal morphine has the highest incidence of respiratory depression. The risk of respiratory depression is greater in patients with underlying lung disease and those receiving additional parenteral narcotics. Because morphine is the least lipid-soluble narcotic, a higher concentration of free drug remains in the cerebrospinal fluid and slowly moves rostrally in the cerebrospinal fluid. This concentration of free drug accounts for the late respiratory depression (6 to 12 hours) as the drug reaches the brain stem. These effects can be treated with small doses (0.1 to 0.4 mg) of naloxone (Narcan). The usual doses of the most commonly used epidural opioids are given in Table 1.

### Regional Anesthesia: Spinal

Spinal anesthesia may be used for cesarean section with the advantages of rapid onset of anesthesia, more profound sensory and motor blocks, and the least maternal and fetal drug exposure. Potential disadvantages include a more unpredictable sensory level, greater incidence of significant hypotension, and the risk of post–dural puncture headache. It has been noted that even with adequate fluid preload (1.5 to 2 liters) and left uterine displacement, there may be sig-

nificant hypotensive episodes in up to 40% of parturients with spinal anesthesia. These hypotensive episodes are usually effectively treated by aggressive use of ephedrine. Some physicians have even advocated the use of prophylactic intramuscular ephedrine (25 to 50 mg). There is no untoward effect on the neonate as long as hypotension is avoided. Hyperbaric formulations of the spinal agents are used because they give the most reliable and predictable thoracic levels when compared with isobaric or hypobaric solutions. Lidocaine (5% in 7.5% dextrose), tetracaine (0.5% in 5% dextrose), tetracaine (1%) and procaine (10%) in a 1:1 mixture, and bupivacaine (7.5% in 8.25% dextrose) are the most commonly used spinal preparations. Recent comparisons of hyperbaric bupivacaine, hyperbaric tetracaine, and the mixture of tetracaine and procaine for cesarean section suggest that there may be less hypotension with the hyperbaric bupivacaine. A suggested dosing regimen is shown in Table 2.

More recently, spinal opiates such as morphine or fentanyl in small doses (0.2 mg and 6.25 µg, respectively) have been added to the group of spinal local anesthetic agents to provide postoperative analgesia. Respiratory depression is a potential side effect, but the most frequently noted side effect is itching.

### General Anesthesia for Cesarean Section

General anesthesia is necessary in cases of fetal distress, in patients who refuse regional anesthesia, or in patients with contraindications for regional anesthesia (i.e., coagulation abnormalities, anatomic spinal anomalies, or hemodynamic instability). All the monitors that are available

TABLE 2. **Spinal Anesthetic Doses in Parturients**

| Anesthetic | Dose (mg) for Heights of | | | | |
|------------|-----------|-----------|-----------|-----------|-----------|
| | *152 cm* | *160 cm* | *168 cm* | *176 cm* | *182 cm* |
| Hyperbaric lidocaine, 5%* | 60 | 65 | 70 | 75 | 80 |
| Hyperbaric tetracaine, 0.5%† | 7 | 8 | 9 | 10 | 11 |
| Hyperbaric bupivacaine, 0.75%* | 7.5 | 10 | 12 | 14 | 15 |
| Mixture‡ of tetracaine and procaine, 1% in 10% | 6 in 60 mg | 7 in 70 mg | 8 in 80 mg | 9 in 90 mg | 10 in 100 mg |

*Both lidocaine and bupivacaine are marketed in a premixed formulation with dextrose.

†Tetracaine is available in a 1% solution and in a lyophilized form made hyperbaric by mixing with 10% dextrose.

‡Tetracaine 1% mixed with procaine 10% results in a hyperbaric solution.

in the surgical suite should also be available in the area where a cesarean section is performed. Preparation for general anesthesia includes adequate assessment of the airway, prophylactic antacid administration, left uterine displacement, adequate intravenous access for hydration, and preoxygenation. Preoxygenation is important for increasing both the maternal and fetal oxygen stores. Because of a decreased functional residual capacity and increased oxygen consumption, the pregnant patient develops arterial desaturation faster than the nonpregnant patient. Likewise, because of the enlarged breasts and venous engorgement of the airway in the pregnant patient, laryngoscopy may be more difficult. With a potentially longer period of apnea before intubation, it is imperative that all pregnant patients be adequately preoxygenated.

Because of the high risk of aspiration pneumonitis, all pregnant patients receiving general anesthesia must be considered to have a full stomach. Therefore, use of a rapid-sequence induction, with cricoid pressure until the airway has been secured with a cuffed endotracheal tube, is preferred. Thiopental (Pentothal) is the most commonly used induction agent in a dose of 3 to 4 mg per kg. Alternatively, ketamine (0.75 to 1 mg per kg) can be used in patients in whom hypovolemia or bronchospasm may be a concern. Succinylcholine is still unsurpassed at offering the best intubating conditions in the shortest time. The usual dose of succinylcholine is 1 to 1.5 mg per kg. Cricoid pressure must be applied correctly to avoid distorting the airway. When pressure is applied correctly, the esophagus is compressed between the back of the cricoid cartilage and the anterior surface of the body of the sixth cervical vertebra. Thus, passive regurgitation is prevented. It is important to maintain the cricoid pressure until the airway has been secured. The surgical incision should not be made until the endotracheal tube has been verified to be in the trachea. This verification allows the option of awakening the mother and securing the airway in the event of a failed intubation. After the trachea has been successfully intubated, the anesthesia is maintained with nitrous oxide and oxygen (a minimum of 50% oxygen until delivery). Lower doses of a volatile agent (0.5% halothane, 0.75% isoflurane, 1% enflurane) can be added without a significant increase in uterine relaxation or in blood loss. The addition of the volatile agent does decrease the chance of maternal recall, which may be present when nitrous oxide and oxygen are used alone. Muscle relaxation may be maintained with either a succinylcholine drip or the nondepolarizing relaxants. Although all of these agents cross the placenta and can be detected in fetal blood, at the usual

clinical doses the amount is not sufficient to cause any neonatal problems. Unnecessary haste to deliver the infant is not warranted just because of the use of general anesthesia. However, an interval from induction to delivery of more than 8 to 10 minutes may have some neonatal effect from the equilibration of the nitrous oxide. This effect is dealt with by oxygen administration and ventilation of the neonate. An interval from uterine incision to delivery of more than 3 minutes has also been shown to be associated with fetal acidosis and lower 1-minute Apgar scores. This interval delay must be limited regardless of whether a regional or general anesthetic is used.

Once the infant has been delivered, oxytocin (Pitocin) is added to the intravenous fluids (20 U per liter), and the volatile agent is decreased or discontinued while narcotics are added. If the oxygen saturation is acceptable, the nitrous oxide may be increased to 70%. Either very-low-dose volatile agents or a small dose of a benzodiazepine (1 to 2 mg of midazolam* [Versed] or 2 to 5 mg of diazepam [Valium]) may be used to supplement anesthesia. The addition of narcotics after the delivery allows for decreased use of volatile agents, thus reducing the concern about their potential for uterine relaxation and increased blood loss. Narcotics such as fentanyl (1 to 3 μg per kg), morphine (0.1 to 0.2 mg per kg), and meperidine (1 to 2 mg per kg) can be used. The narcotics also provide some analgesia in the postanesthesia care unit and allow for a smoother and potentially more rapid emergence from anesthesia. On emergence from anesthesia, the mother should demonstrate complete reversal of neuromuscular blockade, ability to maintain her airway, and the ability to follow verbal commands. It is important that she be awake and able to cooperate before extubation because of the risk of vomiting and aspiration if protective reflexes are still depressed.

---

*Product labeling states that this drug is not recommended for obstetric use.

# POSTPARTUM CARE

method of
DAVID E. MILLER, M.D., PH.D.
*Wake Medical Center*
*Raleigh, North Carolina*

Ideally, postpartum management affords the opportunity for caregivers to monitor a maternal-infant pair for early obstetric and neonatal complications, to provide educational experiences for new parents, and to help launch the family unit in a relatively stress-free environment. Prior to the hospitalization of obstetrics, the latter needs were met by extended family. Now that extended families are rarely available and pressure from third-party payers for early discharge constrains traditional surveillance for obstetric complications, it is important to incorporate more of our educational and social interventions into the prenatal care of our patients.

The major maternal killers continue to be hemorrhage, hypertension, and sepsis. Although a significant percentage of eclamptic seizures occur post partum and delivery room procedures are certainly relevant to introduction of organisms to the patient, by far the greatest immediate risk following delivery of an infant is hemorrhage. The potential blood flow from the placental implantation site is on the order of 500 ml per minute. It is crucial to have a well-rehearsed plan for preventing or correcting such rapid blood loss.

Fortunately, common things are common! Patients bleed from lacerations of the birth canal or failure of the uterus to contract. The uterus fails to contract because something is still in it or because of atony. Other possible causes of hemorrhage such as uterine rupture, lower segment lacerations, and disseminated intravascular coagulation are rare in the absence of obstetric complications, which should already be evident by the time of delivery, or of obstetric manipulations by the physician, also obvious.

The birth canal is best inspected immediately after handing the infant to the parents and before placental separation begins. The patient is distracted and already numbed to some degree by passage of the infant. Bleeding is usually modest before placental separation, allowing easy visualization. Depression of the perineal body with three fingers of the pronated hand while pushing the cervix side to side with a sponge stick permits rapid and adequate evaluation of the vaginal walls and fornices. The cervix is then grasped at the 12 o'clock position with the ring clamp and gently pulled caudally and anteriorly for inspection. Rarely, it may be necessary to grasp it with a second ring clamp at the 6 o'clock position as well.

The placenta is delivered spontaneously or by maternal Valsalva's maneuver, an abdominal hand serving only to detect shape and firmness of the uterine fundus. Prior to separation, the uterus has a discoid shape, which becomes distinctly globular as the placenta passes into the vagina. The placenta should be inspected while held in the hands, maternal side up and flattened out rather than draped over one hand. In this position, it is easy to detect missing cotyledons. Finally, the perimeter of the fetal membranes is carefully inspected for truncated vessels that would suggest a succenturiate placental lobe yet to be delivered. Routine manual exploration of the uterine cavity is cruel, dangerous, and futile compared with careful inspection of the placenta as described.

With these observations accomplished in the first few moments after delivery of the infant, it becomes a reasonable assumption that subsequent excessive bleeding is due to uterine atony and attention can be immediately directed toward uterine massage and administration of oxytocin (Pitocin), 20 U per liter of 5% dextrose in Ringer's lactate solution, 10 U intramuscularly, or slow intravenous push. If control is not prompt and unequivocal, it is crucial to re-evaluate prior assumptions and move promptly toward fluid replacement (through large-bore access lines) and surgical intervention (dilatation and curettage, hypogastric or uterine artery ligation, hysterectomy). One must watch out for significant blood loss accumulating as a series of individual, easily controlled episodes of atony. In this situation, the sustained tetanic contraction induced by an ergot preparation is useful (methylergonovine maleate [Methergine], 0.2 mg intramuscularly or orally). When significant lacerations of the cervix or of vaginal walls or vulva are noted, one should not "putter about." Adequate anesthesia and exposure are essential to provide humane patient management and to avoid simply converting a bleeder to a hematoma. I recommend a gloved assistant and a pudendal block as a minimum. Lacerations of the anterior vulva often require general anesthesia for repair.

The 1 or 2 hours after delivery are devoted to keeping a running tally of accumulated blood loss (usually significantly more than the 500 ml commonly described), frequent monitoring of maternal vital signs, and careful observation of the newborn infant's color, airway patency, and temperature. The perineum is inspected frequently for any signs of hematoma or onset of bleeding from small lacerations previously thought not to require repair. Sterile vaginal examination is performed for bladder distention with inability to void, complaints of pain not explained by known lacerations, or deterioration of vital signs out of proportion to observed blood loss. Pelvic hematomas can sequester large amounts of blood and/or distort the urethra without being visible at the perineum. It is important not to interfere unnecessarily in the family interaction, but crucial to remain obstetrically alert.

Postpartum stays for a normal vaginal delivery currently vary between 12 hours and 3 to 4 days. The longer stays allow time for initiation of lactation and for instruction and assistance with breast-feeding or for supportive care for those who do not. A tight breast binder, ice pack, and analgesic as necessary until the discomfort has passed are usually sufficient to suppress lactation. It is important not to stimulate the nipples for several days. In general, 20% or fewer have significant difficulty suppressing lactation, even in the absence of expensive and potentially dangerous potions administered to "dry up" their breasts.

Most urinary tract infections and cases of endometritis have become evident by day three. The patient will have passed her nadir of anemia as her fluid compartments re-equilibrate, and the infant will be safely past the peak of hyperbilirubinemia. The patient will have developed rapport and skills with her infant to ease integration into the home environment and will be rested from the labor of labor.

The minimal stay is barely enough to give reasonable assurance of continued hemostasis and to demonstrate normal urinary function. For such an early discharge to be safe, it is necessary that blood type, Rh factor, and rubella status have been previously documented. Initial hematocrit and observed blood loss must project to an ultimate hematocrit that is reasonable and the patient must have a support system adequate to ensure that late complications will be recognized and properly responded to. She should be extensively counseled regarding what to expect in the next few days and be sophisticated enough to comprehend and to recognize significant deviations from that norm.

I tell a patient to expect bleeding from 10 days to 3 weeks, which is initially red and smells like the meat department of the grocery store but which will gradually become brown or pink then clear. She is to report any persistent bleeding more than a normal period or any foul odor of the lochia. She demonstrates her ability to take her temperature and is to report any reading over 100.4° F. Afterbirth cramps and other aches and pains may persist for several days, but she should feel distinctly better from one day to the next. If she is feeling persistently bad (or blue) for any reason, she is to call me about it.

Intercourse and douching are proscribed until all bleeding has ceased, usually after 2 to 3 weeks. Bathing and showers are allowed. Activity should be gradually increased over 2 or 3 weeks—in general, "If it doesn't hurt, it won't injure." Contraceptive method is decided on. I recommend that iron supplements be continued for at least 3 months or for the duration of breast-feeding. She will be contacted from the office or by a visiting nurse in 2 weeks and is to return for an examination and Papanicolaou's (Pap) smear in 6 to 8 weeks from delivery. Pelvic support is evaluated, and the value of Kegel's exercises re-emphasized if indicated.

# RESUSCITATION OF THE NEWBORN

method of
SUSAN E. DENSON, M.D.
*The University of Texas Medical School at Houston*
*Houston, Texas*

### PATHOPHYSIOLOGY OF ASPHYXIA

In utero, the fetus is totally dependent upon the placenta, which is of dual origin with two separate circulations. Optimal status in the fetus is dependent upon normal function of both the fetal and maternal circulations to allow transfer of nutrients and exchange of critical gases including oxygen and carbon dioxide. Oxygen is transferred to the fetus via the process of diffusion from the maternal venous blood, and as a result, the oxygen level of umbilical venous blood is only approximately 30 mmHg. This relatively low oxygen level is compensated for in three ways: a relative increase in fetal hematocrit; a shift to the left in the oxygen-hemoglobin dissociation curve, giving a higher oxygen saturation and therefore a higher oxygen content at this low oxygen; and the fetal circulation, which selectively perfuses the myocardium and the brain with the most highly saturated blood available in utero. Although when maternal and fetal circulations are unimpaired, this system works effectively, alterations in either system result in problems with the fetus.

Because the human fetus and placenta are relatively inaccessible for direct study, the animal model has answered questions about the sequence of events that can occur in asphyxia. The animal model has been subjected to complete asphyxia by cord clamping without access to an oxygen-enriched atmosphere and has been studied for respiratory response, cardiovascular response (heart rate and blood pressure), and biochemical changes. After approximately 1 minute of gasping, the animal enters primary apnea, a period characterized by apnea, a fall in heart rate, a rise in blood pressure, and the onset of respiratory effort with stimulation or spontaneously after about 1 minute. This is followed by the onset of spontaneous gasping efforts, which become progressively weaker and which end as the animal enters secondary apnea. During secondary apnea, in addition to apnea, the heart rate continues to fall, the blood pressure falls, the animal will not begin respirations when stimulated, and death will ensue if ventilation is not initiated. These physiologic changes, which occur in less than 10 minutes, are accompanied by marked biochemical changes. The $PaO_2$ falls rapidly from 30 to 0, the $PaCO_2$ rises from 45 to greater than 150, and the pH falls from 7.3 to 6.8. These studies demonstrate that asphyxia with its alteration in the respiratory function of the placenta results in severe acidosis in addition to the hypoxic-ischemic event.

This same pattern of events is felt to occur in the human fetus, and although asphyxia may not be complete as in the animal model, the end result is a compromised fetus that may require a resuscitative response.

## ADAPTATION AT BIRTH

Successful adaptation at birth is dependent upon exchanging the lung for the placenta as the organ for gas exchange. The lung, which was atelectatic and fluid filled in utero, must expand. The fetal circulation, which bypassed the lung in utero, must be replaced with new blood flow patterns incorporating the lung in order to support effective gas exchange. Situations that interfere with the ability to expand the lung postnatally or interfere with the transition from the fetal circulation will result in problems at birth and may require a resuscitative response.

## RISK FACTORS AND INDICATORS OF COMPROMISE

The problems that may result in the need for resuscitation at birth can be of maternal, placental, or fetal origin. Approximately two-thirds of the compromised fetuses can be recognized prenatally or intrapartum by being aware of certain risk factors or indicators of fetal compromise.

Maternal risk factors include maternal diabetes, pregnancy-induced hypertension, maternal drug abuse, infection, and bleeding. Placental risk factors include abruptio placentae, placenta previa, and prolapsed cord. Fetal risk factors include polyhydramnios, oligohydramnios, foul smelling amniotic fluid, intrauterine growth retardation, prolonged rupture of membranes, prematurity, and postmaturity. Indicators of fetal compromise include meconium-stained amniotic fluid and abnormal fetal heart rate patterns.

## PREPARATION FOR RESUSCITATION

Preparation for resuscitation can be divided into two stages—advance and immediate preparation. For the two-thirds of patients who can be recognized in advance and more so for the one-third who cannot be anticipated, advance preparations must be made. These include acquisition of appropriate equipment and education of personnel.

Education of hospital personnel to make available a person trained in neonatal resuscitation at every delivery is now an attainable goal and needs to be addressed at the hospital level. One successful approach is to use the American Heart Association–American Academy of Pediatrics Neonatal Resuscitation Course, which can be used in any hospital, large or small, for training of all staff. The immediate preparation of personnel involves identifying the team and assigning roles. At least two people need to be made responsible for the infant—one to manage the airway, and the other to assist in evaluation and management. A third person is necessary if medications are required.

Advance preparation of equipment consists of making certain the essential elements are always available and located conveniently (Table 1). This requires a regular "check" system whereby the equipment is checked routinely for function and availability, and to make certain no items are out of date. Immediate preparation of equipment involves making certain of the availability of the equipment and preparing the equipment for use, including preheating the warmer, preparing the appropriate size endotracheal tube, and checking all equipment for function.

## APPROACH TO RESUSCITATION

Decisions about the approach to neonatal resuscitation in the past have been made based on the Apgar score. This score, which came to be used as an indicator of asphyxia, was not initially

TABLE 1. **Neonatal Resuscitation: Essential Equipment**

**Environment**
Radiant warmer
Blankets
Gloves

**Suction**
Bulb syringe
DeLee's suction apparatus (#10)
Suction catheters (#6, #8, #10)
Wall suction
Meconium aspirator
Feeding tube (#8)
Syringe (20 ml)

**Airway Management**
General
  Oxygen
  Flowmeter and tubing
  Oral airway
Bag and mask ventilation
  Infant resuscitation bag capable of delivering 90–100% oxygen with pressure release valve or pressure gauge
  Masks—premature and newborn size
Intubation
  Laryngoscope with interchangeable blades (size 0 for premature, size 1 for term)
  Replacement bulbs and batteries
  Endotracheal tubes (sizes 2.5, 3.0, 3.5, 4.0)
  Stylet
  Scissors
  Tape

**Medications**
Epinephrine (1:10,000)
Naloxone hydrochloride (Narcan) (1 mg/ml)
Normal saline (250 ml)
Albumin—5% solution
Sodium bicarbonate (4.2%, 0.5 mEq/ml)
Dextrose (10%)
Sterile water (20 ml)
Normal saline (10 ml)

**Miscellaneous**
Stethoscope
Umbilical catheterization tray
Umbilical catheters (3.5 Fr, 5 Fr)
Stopcock
Syringes
Needles

developed for this purpose and has probably been erroneously used. There is not always a correlation between the degree of asphyxia and the Apgar score, as the Apgar score may be more related to gestational age and other factors. The Apgar score is more useful as an indicator of the effectiveness of resuscitation and the infant's response to resuscitation. As a result, it should still be assigned at 1 and 5 minutes in all infants and every 5 minutes until 20 minutes if the 5-minute score remains less than 7. The infant can be evaluated and a course of action more effectively developed based on the assessment of respiratory effort, heart rate, and color. If evaluated in this order followed by an appropriate response, most infants will be effectively resuscitated.

## INITIAL STEPS

The initial management of all infants at birth is similar and consists of preventing heat loss and establishing an airway. The importance of preventing heat loss cannot be overemphasized. If this step is not addressed and the infant becomes hypothermic, resuscitation is made more difficult as oxygen consumption increases, acidosis develops, and metabolic consequences ensue. Heat loss is prevented or minimized by employing three simple steps: place the infant on a preheated radiant warmer; dry the amniotic fluid thoroughly with special attention to the head with its increased surface area; and remove the wet blankets and replace them with dry materials.

The airway is initially established by positioning of the equipment and the infant. The warmer is placed in slight Trendelenburg's position, and the infant is positioned with the neck slightly extended. Appropriate positioning of the neck is essential because the infant's airway is pliable due to incomplete development of the cartilaginous structures of the trachea. Any flexion of the neck can result in tracheal compression and obstruction of air movement. At the same time, care should be taken to avoid overextending the neck, as spinal cord injuries have occurred and it is proposed that tracheal compression can occur in this position. The airway is further established by removal of secretions by suctioning. The removal of normal secretions can be accomplished by the use of a bulb syringe, suctioning first the mouth, followed by the nose. Suctioning of the meconium-stained baby to prevent meconium aspiration, a disorder that can have a mortality rate as high as 30%, is more involved. Meconium aspiration is felt, in most cases, to involve the postnatal aspiration into the airway of meconium from the mouth, nose, and pharynx. As a result,

removal of this meconium is the goal. This is best done by the individual delivering the infant by suctioning the infant's mouth, nose, and pharynx while the head is on the perineum and before the chest is delivered. Removal of meconium from the airway before passive expansion of the chest or the first breath should prevent this disorder in most cases. When the infant is placed on the warmer, the mouth is suctioned and if meconium is present, the trachea must be directly suctioned. This can be done with a No. 10 DeLee suction trap or an endotracheal tube. Either of these methods should be adapted for use with one of the commercially available meconium aspirators to allow wall suction to be used. Oral contact with either the DeLee or the endotracheal tube is discouraged because the risk of infection is significant for both the infant and the caregiver. Infections in both groups have been reported after the use of such techniques. Some investigators would recommend the suctioning of the meconium-stained fluid to take precedence over the previously mentioned initial steps. If this is done, one should then return to those steps (i.e., suction for meconium, prevent heat loss, position, in that order).

## EVALUATION OF RESPIRATIONS

The previous step has cleared the airway; the next step is to evaluate respirations. The stimulation of drying and suctioning will have been adequate to establish respirations in most infants, but for those who have not responded, tactile stimulation may be tried. If tactile stimulation is chosen, it should be done appropriately by slapping the sole of the foot, flicking the heel, or rubbing the infant's neck. Tactile stimulation should be tried only briefly with a maximum of two attempts. If this does not result in effective respirations, ventilation with a bag and mask is to be initiated.

## VENTILATION

Successful ventilation with a bag and mask occurs when the appropriate equipment is used properly. The bag should be attached to a mask of appropriate size for the infant (either premature or newborn). There are two types of bags available for infant resuscitation: a self-inflating bag, and a flow inflating or anesthesia bag. The self-inflating bag is easier for most to use and is perhaps better in settings where the need for resuscitation occurs less frequently. Whichever bag is selected, it should be capable of delivering an oxygen concentration of 90 to 100%. It should also have either a pressure release valve or a pressure gauge as a safety measure. This will protect the infant's lung from excess pressure by either automatically "popping off" at a set pressure (pressure release valve) or by making the individual aware of the pressure being used (pressure gauge). Ventilation is initiated by placing the mask over the infant's nose and mouth after the neck has been slightly extended. The infant should then be ventilated at a rate of 40 to 60 breaths per minute. The amount of pressure required depends both on the size of the infant and on the compliance of the lungs. The initial breath should be delivered with at least 30 to 40 cm of $H_2O$ pressure. Subsequent breaths should be with a pressure as low as 15 to 20 cm $H_2O$ if the lungs are normal, or as high as 40 cm $H_2O$ if lung disease is present. One can evaluate the effectiveness of ventilation by observing chest wall movement. If the chest wall is moving, most likely adequate ventilation is being provided. If the chest wall is not moving, one should re-evaluate the airway for blockage (secretions, position), check the seal of the mask, and increase the pressure if the first steps are not effective.

## EVALUATION OF HEART RATE

After ventilation is initiated, either spontaneously by the infant or by bag and mask ventilation, the next evaluation is of the heart rate. If the baby is breathing spontaneously but the heart rate is less than 100, ventilation by bag and mask is initiated. If the infant is ventilated either for apnea or for bradycardia, he or she should be ventilated as described earlier for 15 to 30 seconds, at which time the heart rate should be evaluated.

## CARDIAC COMPRESSIONS

If the heart rate is below 60 or between 60 and 80 and not rising despite adequate ventilation, external cardiac compressions should be instituted. There are two acceptable techniques for cardiac compression in the neonate. The "thumb technique" is one in which the two thumbs are placed parallel or overlapping over the sternum for compression with the hands encircling the torso to support the back. The "two-finger technique" is one in which the tip of the middle finger and either the index finger or the ring finger of one hand are used to compress the sternum with the other hand used to support the back. Both techniques provide the infant with firm support for the back and allow the neck to be slightly extended. Compressions are done at the same location, depth, and rate. Compressions should be over the lower third of the sternum to a depth of one-half to three-quarters of an inch and at a rate of 120 per minute. The compressions at 120 per minute are to be accompanied by positive-pressure ventilation at a rate of 40 to 60 per minute. This can be done either simultaneously, i.e., compressions and ventilations done at the same time with no attempt at coordination; or interposed, with ventilations occurring during the "pause" after each third compression. There are no data to support either method as being superior in neonatal resuscitation at this time. The person involved in resuscitation should use the technique that works best in his or her own setting. There is one exception, as one should consider interposing ventilations if cardiac compressions are being done in the infant supported with bag and mask ventilation. In this setting, simultaneous ventilations may be less successful in inflating the lung because air will tend to enter the stomach.

After 30 seconds of chest compressions with ventilation, the heart rate should be checked. If the heart rate is greater than 80, compressions can be discontinued and ventilation continued until the heart rate is greater than 100 and the infant is breathing spontaneously. If the heart rate is less than 80, medications are indicated in addition to continuing ventilation and cardiac compressions.

## MEDICATIONS

The need for medications occurs infrequently in delivery room resuscitations, as the cause of the arrest is diminished respiratory function and instituting ventilation is usually successful. When medications are used, it is important that the correct dose be given by the correct route. This requires that the correct concentration be available at the bedside and the dose known. It is helpful to have medication sheets readily available at each delivery site with the correct concentration, amount to prepare, and the dose for neonates of different sizes. This will minimize errors during the emergency situation, especially when these medications are infrequently used (Table 2).

Drugs can be administered in the delivery room by three potential routes: the umbilical vein, peripheral veins, and intratracheal instillation. The optimal route for most drugs is the umbilical vein, because all drugs can be given by this route. The umbilical catheter, when placed, needs to be passed through the vein to a level just below the skin to avoid infusing the solutions directly into the liver. Peripheral veins can be utilized, but these are difficult to access and are not practical during most emergency situations. The intratra-

TABLE 2. **Medications for Neonatal Resuscitation**

| Drug | Indication | Preparation | Dose | Route* | Sample Total Dose | | | |
|------|-----------|-------------|------|--------|-------------------|---|---|---|
| | | | | | 1 kg | 2 kg | 3 kg | 4 kg |
| Epinephrine | HR 0 or <80 after ventilation | 1:10,000 | 0.1–0.3 ml/kg | IT IV (rapidly) | 0.1–0.3 ml | 0.2–0.6 ml | 0.3–0.9 ml | 0.4–1.2 ml |
| Volume expander | Blood loss proved or suspected Evidence of hypotension | Normal saline Ringer's lactate 5% albumin | 10 ml/kg | IV (slowly) | 10 ml | 20 ml | 30 ml | 40 ml |
| Sodium bicarbonate | Proved or suspected metabolic acidosis | 4.2% (0.5 mEq/ml) | 2 mEq/kg (4 ml/kg) | IV (slowly) | 4 ml | 8 ml | 12 ml | 16 ml |
| Naloxone (Narcan) | Respiratory depression and maternal narcotic administration <4 hr prior to delivery | 1 mg/ml | 0.1 mg/kg (0.1 ml/kg) | IV IT IM SQ | 0.1 ml | 0.2 ml | 0.3 ml | 0.4 ml |

*Route: IV = intravenous; IT = intratracheal; IM = intramuscular; SQ = subcutaneous.

cheal route is a good choice in situations in which the infant is intubated and the drug needed can be given by this route. Drugs can be given directly into the endotracheal tube but may be more effective when injected through a No. 5 French catheter passed beyond the tip of the endotracheal tube followed by a normal saline flush. Studies have shown good absorption of appropriate drugs with this technique.

The choice of drugs for neonatal resuscitation is simpler than for adults. The goals for chemical resuscitation are to stimulate the heart rate, improve blood pressure, and correct metabolic acidosis. This requires the use of few drugs.

The first drug used is epinephrine. It has several points of action, including an increase in coronary artery perfusion, an increase in myocardial contractility, an increase in heart rate, and an increase in systemic blood pressure. It is used when bradycardia persists despite adequate ventilation and cardiac compressions. A reasonable guideline is to use epinephrine when the heart rate is 0 or less than 80 after 30 seconds of adequate ventilation and compression. The concentration to be used is 1:10,000 with a dose of 0.1 to 0.3 ml per kg. It can be used intravenously or intratracheally. If the infant is intubated, it can be given intratracheally while awaiting umbilical venous catheter placement. In many cases, the infant will respond to the intratracheal route and avoid the need for a venous catheter. If given intratracheally, the larger dose (0.3 ml per kg) should be given and is best either diluted 1:1 with normal saline or undiluted followed by a normal saline flush. The infant should respond to the epinephrine within 3 seconds with an increase in heart rate. If the infant remains bradycardic, consider repeating the epinephrine dose, as it may be repeated every 5 minutes.

The next group of drugs to be considered are volume expanders, as hypovolemia due to blood loss will frequently result in the need for resuscitation. Volume expanders should be considered when blood loss is known to be present (abruptio placentae, placenta previa, prolapsed cord, etc.) or when it is presumed to be present based on clinical findings, including hypotension, poor perfusion, or poor response to resuscitation. Volume expanders available in the delivery room may include crystalloid preparations (normal saline, Ringer's lactate) and colloid preparations (5% albumin). The dose is 10 ml per kg given intravenously over 5 to 10 minutes. If there is no response in blood pressure or perfusion, the dose can be repeated.

The next drug to be considered is sodium bicarbonate, which is intended to correct acidosis. As demonstrated in the animal model, asphyxia results in a severe acidosis that is both metabolic and respiratory in origin. The respiratory component must be treated with ventilation, and in a prolonged episode the metabolic component may require treatment to counteract the adverse effects of this acidosis on myocardial and peripheral circulatory function. Sodium bicarbonate should be given for a documented or presumed metabolic acidosis only after ventilation has been established. The preparation recommended is the 4.2% solution (0.5 mEq per ml), which is commercially available. If the 8.4% solution is the only one available, it must be diluted 1:1 with sterile water to make a 4.2% solution before use in the neonate. The dose is 2 mEq per kg (4 ml per kg of 4.2% solution) given slowly by the intravenous route.

The last drug to be discussed is naloxone (Narcan), a narcotic antagonist, which will reverse respiratory depression caused by narcotics administered to the mother before delivery. Its use is to be considered when the infant presents with respiratory depression in a clinical setting in which the mother received narcotics usually within 4 hours of delivery. The recommended concentration is 1 mg per ml (neonatal Narcan is no longer used). The dose to be given is 0.01 to 0.1 mg per kg naloxone. It can be given intravenously, intratracheally, intramuscularly, or subcutaneously. It will result in spontaneous respirations in the infant if drug depression was the cause. There are two precautions when considering this drug. First, the duration of action of most narcotics is longer than naloxone's duration of action. As a result, the infant may become apneic again and must be observed for this possibility. Second, naloxone can initiate withdrawal in the infant of a drug abusing mother. This must be a consideration in certain clinical settings.

Two drugs previously used in neonatal resuscitation have been removed from consideration. There is no current evidence that atropine or calcium is useful in the acute phase of neonatal resuscitation. The removal of atropine is unique to the neonate, as it continues to be used in pediatric and adult resuscitations. This is understandable because its major impact is in heart block, which is virtually never the cause of an arrest or depression in the newborn. The removal of calcium is not unique, as it was removed from adult and pediatric guidelines as well. Calcium had been advocated in the past in cardiac arrest with asystole or electromechanical dissociation. However, poor salvage rates; high serum calcium levels; and the concern about cellular accumulation of calcium within the myocardium, which is implicated in cell death, have removed it from consideration. It really has no role except in an arrest due to hypocalcemia or an overdose of calcium channel blockers, neither of which is likely to be the case in the delivery room.

## ENDOTRACHEAL INTUBATION

Most infants can be successfully resuscitated with bag and mask ventilation, but some will require endotracheal intubation. Intubation should be initiated when bag and mask ventilation is not effective and the infant is not responding to resuscitation. Other indications include the need for tracheal suction for meconium and the presence or suspicion of a diaphragmatic hernia, both of which can be aggravated by bag and mask ventilation. Successful intubation requires good technique. The equipment preparation for intubation includes choosing the appropriate blade for the laryngoscope (size 0 for most infants, premature or term; size 1 for large term infants) and choosing the appropriate size endotracheal tube (2.5 for infants less than 1000 grams or under 28 weeks of gestation, 3.0 for infants 1000 to 2000 grams or 28 to 34 weeks' gestation, 3.5 for infants 2000 to 3000 grams or 34 to 38 weeks' gestation, 4.0 for infants more than 3000 grams or older than 38 weeks' gestation). A stylet should be placed if desired. Intubation is best done by two people—the assistant and the person performing the intubation.

The assistant has two goals: to assist in visualization and to assist in evaluation. Good visualization is accomplished by several steps. The infant should be placed on a flat surface with the head stabilized in the midline and slightly extended. The child should be suctioned to clear the airway of secretions. Evaluation includes assessing tube position by listening to breath sounds and assessing the heart rate after the tube is placed.

The person intubating must be aware of the anatomy of the airway and must have adequate visualization to be successful. The laryngoscope is held with the thumb and index finger of the left hand, and the last three fingers are placed on the chin for support. The laryngoscope blade is inserted into the mouth and passed over the tongue, and the tip of the blade is placed in the vallecula, the area just anterior to the epiglottis. When the blade is pulled forward, the vocal cords will be in sight and the trachea can be intubated with the appropriate size endotracheal tube. If a guidewire is used, it should be removed at this point and ventilation begun. The infant should be assessed for symmetry of breath sounds, chest wall movement, and response in heart rate. If there is a poor response to intubation, consider mechanical problems, including tube malposition (esophageal intubation, right mainstem bronchus intubation), inadequate pressure when ventilating, or pulmonary problems preventing response (pneumothorax, diaphragmatic hernia).

## EVALUATION OF COLOR

Because of the low oxygen levels in the fetal blood stream, all infants will have cyanosis at birth. As the lungs expand and the infant establishes respirations, this rapidly resolves in most infants, usually by 1 to 2 minutes after birth. Occasionally the infant will remain cyanotic despite adequate respirations and a normal heart rate. In this situation, it is appropriate to administer free-flow oxygen to the infant. Oxygen can be delivered by face mask or by the use of an oxygen tube held closely (about one-half inch) to the nose. This will deliver about 80% oxygen, and most infants will respond to this measure.

## IMMEDIATE STABILIZATION

The period immediately following resuscitation should focus on dealing with the consequences of the experience as well as considering the cause of the event.

Pulmonary effects of asphyxia are indirect as well as direct. The indirect effect is depression of the central nervous system resulting in apnea that will require ventilation. The direct effects are related to gestational age. The premature infant who is asphyxiated is at greater risk for respiratory distress syndrome, whereas the full-term infant is at risk for persistent pulmonary hypertension (persistent fetal circulation) or meconium aspiration syndrome. These can be evaluated by obtaining a chest x-ray and an arterial blood sample. The chest x-ray will show characteristic changes in respiratory distress syndrome, meconium aspiration syndrome, pneumonia, or surgical problems such as diaphragmatic hernia or pneumothorax. The ventilatory and oxygen requirements can be determined only by obtaining the arterial blood gas sample to assess the pH, $PaO_2$ and $PaCO_2$. Noninvasive transcutaneous oxygen and carbon dioxide monitors can be helpful in following the infant; however, these cannot replace the arterial blood gas sample. Prompt response to abnormalities can minimize ongoing problems. The cardiac effects of asphyxia may be manifested by transient myocardial ischemia, which can be diagnosed by electrocardiogram or echocardiogram. Clinically these infants may have hypotension unresponsive to volume expansion. The use of an inotropic agent such as dopamine may be required to correct hypotension. It can be used as a continuous infusion in a dosage of 5 to 20 μg per kg per minute.

The renal complications of asphyxia are primarily ischemic and may result in acute tubular necrosis. Although less of a concern in the immediate postresuscitation period, it can become a problem over the next few hours because the infant is at risk for fluid overload, hyponatremia, and hyperkalemia. The infant must be monitored for weight, and urine output and electrolyte levels must be followed.

The most common metabolic complication of asphyxia is hypoglycemia because the stress of asphyxia depletes the infant's glycogen stores. Glucose levels must be monitored in the immediate stabilization period and intravenous fluids given to minimize this problem. A glucose infusion of at least 5 to 7 mg per kg per minute will usually be adequate. This can be achieved by infusing 10% dextrose at 100 ml per kg per day. Glucose screening should continue to ensure normoglycemia. If hypoglycemia occurs, it should be treated aggressively. A bolus of 2 ml per kg of 10% dextrose will correct most hypoglycemia, but this must be followed with a continuous infusion of glucose as described earlier to maintain the glucose level.

Infection must be considered as a possible cause of stress resulting in the need for resuscitation. The history must be looked at for risk factors and the infant "screened" for infection. However, these may be negative even in the presence of infection. Strong consideration should be given to treating the infant with broad-spectrum antibiotics after obtaining appropriate cultures (usually blood and cerebrospinal fluid).

# CARE OF AT-RISK NEONATES

method of
WILLIAM H. TOPPER, M.D., and
ALLEN ERENBERG, M.D.
*University of Kansas Medical Center*
*Kansas City, Kansas*

Specialized care of newborns with unusual needs or problems began in the United States at the turn of the century when Couney introduced his "child hatcheries" in the fashion used by Tarnier and Budin in Europe. The first permanent preterm nursery began at Michael Reese Hospital in Chicago under the direction of Julius Hess in 1922, and the first neonatal intensive care units appeared in the 1960s. The 1970s and 1980s brought the most extensive change and development in neonatal intensive care. The basis of neonatal care continues to be environmental warmth and nutrition, although much of the most visible "success" has been in respiratory care.

The use of terms such as "high-risk" or "at-risk" emphasizes the immense value of identification, anticipation, and prevention, or at least early intervention, in perinatal and neonatal care. The rationale is to assess jeopardy and thereafter intervene to attempt to reduce the hazards of death (mortality) or disability (morbidity). A number of well known factors place the neonate in jeopardy, with the consequences of this jeopardy often being worse for the infant than for the mother. Identifiable risk factors are listed in Table 1. These risk factors place approximately 3 to 4% of newborns at high risk, and another 15 to 20% are at moderate or "some risk." Annually, perinatal deaths in the United States exceed all other causes of death combined until age 55 years.

In the 1940s, as specific texts devoted to newborn care appeared, prematurity was defined only by birthweight (under 2500 grams). A decade later, the distinction of low birthweight versus prematurity had been made. The prognosis for extreme immaturity has changed over time, and viability is now considered possible at 23 to 24 weeks of gestation. Gestational age is a more important predictor of survival than birthweight, although data are often presented by birthweight because it can be more accurately deter-

TABLE 1. **Identifiable Neonatal Risk Factors**

| Family-Socioeconomic | Maternal | Prenatal | Fetal-Neonatal |
|---|---|---|---|
| Occupational status | Prolonged infertility | Multiple fetuses | Fetal distress |
| Poverty | Age <18 or >35 yr | Abnormal presentation | Intrauterine infection |
| No transportation | Substance abuse | Abnormal gestational age | Pre- or post-term |
| Mental health problems | Previous abortion | Inadequate prenatal care | Asphyxia |
| History of child abuse | Previous preterm infant | Conception soon after previous | Low Apgar scores |
| Single parent, divorce, separa- | Previous infant death | delivery | Birthweight <2500 grams |
| tion | Unplanned pregnancy | Exposure to radiation | Birthweight >4500 grams |
| No phone | Use of therapeutic drugs | Exposure to viral illness | Intrauterine growth retardation |
| No housing | Emotional stress | Stress—physical or mental | Macrosomia |
| No social supports | Sexually transmitted | Abnormal weight gain | Congenital anomalies |
| Lives >50 miles away | disease | Prolonged rupture of | Infant morbidity |
| Poor education | Previous cesarean section | membranes | Hyperbilirubinemia |
| Parental anxiety | Race | Abnormal fetal growth | Apnea |
| Poor bonding pattern | Rh sensitization | Placental anomalies | Hypoglycemia |
| Advanced parental age | Diabetes mellitus | Polyhydramnios | CNS infection |
| Foreign language | Short stature | Oligohydramnios | Sepsis |
| Medical indigence | 5 + pregnancies | Vaginal bleeding | CNS hemorrhage |
| Many siblings | Abnormal weight | Poor diet | Seizures |
| Siblings with developmental | Major maternal disease | Abnormal fetal heart rate | Enterocolitis |
| disabilities | Malnutrition | Decreased activity | Hyperviscosity |
| Very young children at home | Congenital anomalies | Maternal fever | Pneumothorax |
| Family history of serious he- | Abnormal obstetric history | Abnormal labor duration | Respiratory distress |
| reditary problems-anomalies | Inborn metabolic error | Meconium-stained fluid | Mechanical ventilation |
| | Hypertension | | Surgery |
| | Anemia | | Anemia |
| | Thrombocytopenia | | Abnormal head size |
| | History of previous infant | | Abnormal neurologic |
| | with jaundice or | | examination |
| | respiratory distress | | |

mined. Survival improves significantly with advancing gestational age, rising from less than 50% at 24 to 26 weeks to more than 90% by 30 weeks' gestation.

In the 1970s, the concept of regionalization was advanced, becoming the model for organization of perinatal care and promoting a cooperative effort to reduce perinatal morbidity and mortality. Levels of neonatal care were defined along the low-, moderate-, and high-risk categories as levels I, II, and III, respectively. Economy of services and consolidation of expertise were used as justifications for this model. This concept of regionalization, with current concerns about possible "deregionalization," is being re-examined in an effort to ensure optimal perinatal care in the 1990s.

This article outlines important general care issues applied to all levels of risk and provides definitions and descriptions of specific care routines and problems for those infants at more than low-risk.

## GENERAL CARE

Whether at high, medium, or low risk, all neonates share some universal problems and care needs. As the problems that an infant has or is at risk for increase, these general care measures must intensify (e.g., low-birthweight infants) and management of specific problems such as respiratory distress may need to be instituted.

### Long-Range Planning and Preparation

Each perinatal health care system must assess its needs. Planning and preparation must be done

to ensure that the intended level or type of care is provided and that emergencies and situations beyond the intended care level can be expeditiously addressed. Each facility must know what it can do and where to get help if needed. This maintains the original regional concept introduced in the 1970s. The American Academy of Pediatrics and American College and Obstetricians and Gynecologists provide a readily available basis for many of these considerations in the current edition of *Guidelines for Perinatal Care*.

The perinatal health care institution must address and regularly re-evaluate the readiness, as well as the effectiveness, of the facility and personnel. This can be done through a perinatal committee that ensures that the appropriate policies and procedures are developed and maintained. Preparation and continuing education of the staff are the most important issue. It is in this area that the proper organization and cooperation within the region are so fundamentally effective. The physical plant or facility for neonatal care should be convenient to the labor and delivery area and particularly close to the postpartum rooms. These should be easily accessible to families, and the area must provide a means of continuous observation of all infants; maintenance of proper infection control standards; and attention to environmental standards of space, noise, and light.

There is currently some conflict in the popular

and generally laudable trend toward single-room care of the prenatal population, along with the trend toward shorter hospital stays. It may now be more difficult to ensure provision of the appropriate mechanism for screening, problem identification, continuing assessment, and discharge planning for mothers and infants. Whether hidden or disguised, equipment and supplies for thermal support and resuscitation must still be immediately available in these single-room situations.

### Laboratory and Services Support

Laboratory facilities and nursery monitoring tools must be available to provide the necessary measurements involved in well baby care and assessment. The studies needed for problem assessment in the at-risk population must also be accessible. As intensity of care provided increases, so must the laboratory support. All newborn care facilities must provide the means to weigh infants, screen hematocrit, measure blood glucose and bilirubin levels, assess blood gases, perform x-ray examinations, and initiate intravenous fluid support. In addition, state-mandated screening and cord blood testing are necessary. If any at-risk infants are to be maintained in the nursery setting, the laboratory and support requirements increase to include complete blood counts, serum electrolyte and calcium concentrations, urine testing, continued intravenous and medication therapy, gavage feeding, respiratory care, serial blood gas determinations, transcutaneous blood gas monitoring, and enhanced thermal support with either incubators or overhead warmers.

### Immediate Preparation

Even after the facility is equipped, staffed, and prepared for its planned level of care and handling of emergencies, the patients who receive care must benefit from continued risk assessment, triage, and communication within the system. Risk assessment and management are a continuum, ideally involving prepregnancy evaluation and counseling, prenatal screening, pregnancy-related care and serial assessments, intrapartum screening and monitoring, and delivery and continued postpartum evaluation of mother and infant. Not all high-risk factors are discernible prior to delivery, but 75 to 80% of poor outcomes result from the 25 to 30% of pregnancy and labor patients identified as at risk prior to delivery.

### Delivery Room Care and Resuscitation

The basic equipment needed for all delivery rooms is listed in numerous publications available through the American Academy of Pediatrics. Currently, the American Heart Association and the American Academy of Pediatrics have at least two programs available that are designed to improve quality of infant care and resuscitation in the delivery room (Neonatal Resuscitation Program) and other settings (Pediatric Advanced Life Support). All institutions delivering care to perinatal patients should incorporate these or similar programs into the continuing education of all staff involved with the delivery and care of newborns.

The steps involved for the newborn care staff in the initial care of all neonates include the following:

1. Readiness and anticipation through continued risk assessment. In the acute delivery crisis, the three critical questions to be answered are whether there is meconium-stained amniotic fluid, what the anticipated gestational age is of the newborn, and whether there are multiple fetuses.

2. Physiologic assessment—commonly by the Apgar scoring method.

3. Resuscitation procedures, as necessary.

4. Maintenance of normal body temperature via appropriate thermal environment.

5. Physical observation and brief examination (Table 2).

6. Parent-infant bonding.

7. Reflection on relationship of maternal or placental conditions with the infant problems that have been identified and request for appropriate testing (further screening of the mother, placenta examination).

### Newborn Care

The minimal care standards for all newborn infants include a thorough examination by a physician upon admission and discharge so that a perspective can be obtained, prophylaxis of eyes with appropriate material, prophylaxis with vitamin K, state-mandated screening tests (now universally thyroid and hyperphenylalaninemias), and screening of cord blood for Rh and Coombs' testing if the mother is Rh negative (or for syphilis and Rh, type, and Coombs' if mother is untested). Many infants at risk by perinatal assessment or history must be screened by hematocrit and glucose levels, and many state screening systems now include conditions such as galactosemia, hemaglobinopathies, and other inborn errors of metabolism.

TABLE 2. **Physical Examination of the Newborn**

**General**

1. Observe infant's posture and usual position; handle the infant to get a feel for tone and responsiveness; check for major congenital anomalies or obvious syndromes; measure vital signs (heart rate, respiratory rate, temperature, blood pressure); measure weight, length, and head circumference; assess gestational age.
2. Consider whether infant is relaxed, lethargic, or distressed; compare size with gestational age and determine whether small, appropriate, or large for gestational age.
3. *Note:* The overall feel one gets about an infant is often as important as the detailed examination; infants requiring intensive care will not tolerate an extensive examination.

**Skin**

1. Observe color, perfusion, and pigmentation; look for rashes, lesions, meconium staining, and evidence of trauma.
2. Consider whether rashes are benign newborn types (e.g., toxic erythema) or pathologic.
3. *Note:* The skin, like the general and neurologic examinations, can give a quick impression of the general health of an infant.

**Head**

1. Examine fontanelles, sutures, overall shape, and scalp.
2. Consider presence of trauma (scalp lesion, cephalohematoma, caput succedaneum, forceps mark), increased intracranial pressure, and anomalies.
3. *Note:* Extensive molding may make the initial head circumference inaccurate.
4. *Eyes*
   a. Observe gaze and fixation, pupils, and red reflex; look for discharge and puffiness.
   b. *Note:* The infant may open eyes if held in an upright position; the ophthalmoscopic examination can be used for gestational age assessment (pupillary membrane remnants).
5. *Ears*
   a. Evaluate size, shape, and position; look for evidence of trauma.
   b. *Note:* External ear malformations raise the question of associated renal anomalies.
6. *Nose*
   a. Pass a catheter into each nostril to assess patency.
   b. *Note:* Nasal obstruction can cause or aggravate respiratory distress.
7. *Mouth*
   a. Examine the palate and tongue.
   b. Consider anomalies that may complicate feeding or breathing.
   c. *Note:* The mucous membranes give a more accurate assessment of oxygenation than do the peripheral extremities.
8. *Neck*
   a. Examine for mobility and masses.
   b. Consider the possibility of birth trauma and spinal cord injury in the inactive infant.

**Thorax**

1. Examine the shape, ventilatory pattern, and breathing rate and regularity; look for features of respiratory distress (nasal flaring, grunting, air hunger, retractions).
2. Consider symmetry of chest and adequacy of ventilation; differentiate between pathologic apnea and periodic breathing.
3. *Lungs*
   a. Listen to breath sounds
   b. Consider equality of breath sounds and presence of rales and rhonchi.
   c. *Note:* Auscultation of lungs in a otherwise healthy infant will yield little useful information.
4. *Heart*
   a. Feel the point of maximal impulse (PMI) (location and intensity); feel the pulses in all extremities; auscultate the heart for rate, rhythm, murmurs, and heart sounds; assess perfusion by capillary refill.
   b. Consider whether a murmur is pathologic or benign; evaluate cardiac output, cyanosis; assess for congestive heart failure, or arrhythmia.
   c. *Note:* Perform this part of the examination early or when infant is quiet.

**Abdomen**

1. Observe shape and size, along with color of abdominal wall; listen to bowel sounds; palpate gently to assess for tenderness and guarding; attempt to palpate liver, spleen, and kidneys; check stool and urine output.
2. Consider size, shape, and location of major organs; investigate the presence of masses, lesions, or obstruction.
3. *Note:* Responsive infants are sensitive and "guarding" may be overdiagnosed.
4. *Cord*—count vessels and look for infection.
5. *Anus*—determine patency.
6. *Genitals*—determine gender and appropriateness of features for gestationial age; evaluate for anomalies or ambiguity; look for hernias, hydroceles, imperforate hymen, phimosis, or hypospadias.

**Musculoskeletal**

1. Examine back, extremities, and major joints; perform Ortolani's examination of hips.
2. Consider trauma.

**Neurologic**

1. Examine state, responsiveness, reactivity, consolability, tone, spontaneous movements; perform Moro's examination; catalogue primitive reflexes if status is chronically impaired.
2. Consider general status, maturity level, degree of distress, and focal neurologic signs (e.g., brachial plexus or facial nerve injury).
3. *Note:* Attention to the timing of the last feeding will improve judgment of infant's state; the general neurologic status of an infant tells the observer a great deal about the health and maturity of the child.

The examination of the infant must include an overall evaluation, screening for various acute problems, and a gestational age assessment. Even if the infant is physically normal in appearance and without acute problems, the continuum of risk assessment and care needs must be maintained by establishing the relationship of size (weight, head circumference, and length) to gestational age. Gestational age is established from the history and obstetric techniques (last menstrual period, serial obstetric assessment, ultrasound) and neonatal examination. The Ballard modification of the Dubowitz scoring system is almost universally applied, and forms for the procedure are readily available as a service by infant formula companies. Anticipated problems and care needs can then be identified once the infant is assessed as being small, appropriate, or large for gestational age at preterm, term, or post-term delivery. The brief neonatal examination (see Table 2) can be used by infant care personnel to assess the infant's status, serially screen for problems, and facilitate communication with other staff members who are not physically present.

The concept of the transition period needs emphasis. Newborns, of course, do not immediately adapt to their external environment, and the time required for the most dramatic change is the "transition" period, which often lasts for up to 12 hours. With time, the infant usually becomes progressively more adapted, and most transition-related problems appear fairly early, especially in the first 4 hours with problems such as respiratory distress and hypoglycemia. The environment must provide for optimal heat support and observation during the transition period. Single-room care and efforts to promote parent-infant bonding can potentially reduce the ability to meet these environmental needs, and at-risk infants need to be observed in the traditional nursery setting. Screening and identification of risk factors, of course, will prepare the staff for problems that may arise in the transition period.

Over the years, neonatal care has included a variety of feeding routines and methods. Currently, we are enjoying re-emphasis of two basic principles: introduction of enteral feedings after delivery as soon as they are safe and use of maternal breast milk. Even at-risk infants should have "nutrition" listed as a major problem from the onset of their care. In the absence of any other problems, these nutritional needs often influence where care can be provided, initially or on back transport from higher levels of care. Although major illnesses and catheters may prevent or delay enteral feedings, several rules apply: nipple feedings are reasonable with infants of 34 or more weeks' gestation; gavage feeding must be available (at least initially) for infants less than 34 weeks' gestation; and intravenous therapy is usually necessary in infants born at less than 1800 to 2000 grams because of their notoriously slow transition period and high frequency of other problems such as ileus, hypoglycemia, and specific fluid and electrolyte needs.

The skin care and hygiene practices for neonates can no longer reflect only the needs and interests of the individual infant, but now must incorporate the necessities of universal blood and body secretion policies related to a number of infectious diseases. Infants technically do not need bathing, although removal of amniotic fluid, blood, meconium, and vernix is esthetically desirable, but these materials must now be removed to reduce their infectious risk. Gloves should be used until after the infant's first bath, which should be done only after thermal stability is documented. The cord should be kept dry and serially assessed for infection. Various substances such as alcohol and triple dye have their proponents, although there is concern that these may desiccate the cord, perhaps prolonging its retention. The use of antibiotic substances such as bacitracin (Baciguent) on the cord has no place in the routine care of newborns.

Families demand and deserve active participation in the care of their newborns. Although the use of single-room care complicates observation and serial assessment of at-risk infants, the numerous problems associated with parenting and bonding with at-risk infants can often be prevented, reduced, or better assessed when parents are actively involved, even when the infant is in an intensive care nursery.

Ideally, at the point of delivery of any infant, the subsequent caretakers should have enough risk assessment information to benefit from planning, anticipation, and triage. This is a reasonable goal, since most perinatal problems can be assessed prior to delivery. Thereafter, unanticipated problems must be quickly addressed, solved or stabilized, treated on site, or transferred expeditiously. When the immediate future cannot be predicted, appropriate assessment and monitoring must be continued until the course is better defined. Neonatal transport is of great utility but is no substitute for maternal transport to the appropriate center for care before delivery. Delivery in the hospital where the infant most likely will get optimal care is very valuable, since up to 30% of all neonatal deaths (50% of those in infants with birthweights of less than 1000 grams) occur in the first 4 hours of life.

The essential aspects of stabilization of all at-risk or ill neonates include the following:

1. Thermal environment

2. Glucose management

3. Fluid management

4. Respiratory support

5. Assessment and initial management of specific problems as defined in the next section.

No matter where the newborn is in the at-risk continuum, the principles of discharge preparation and management are often the same and include:

1. Physiologic stability—thermal and in primary diseases

2. Feeding program in place—usually nipple feedings but alternative methods on occasion

3. Weight gain—unless this goal cannot be achieved (i.e., terminal care)

4. Freedom from apnea and other acute life-threatening events, or treatment for the same

5. Confirmed parental competence, comfort, and acceptance

6. Adequate home situation—aimed at maximizing infant safety and parental success

7. Elaboration and scheduling of follow-up care needs

Beyond the usual well baby care routines, at-risk infants requiring specialized follow-up are those who have had problems such as birthweight less than 1500 grams, small size for gestational age, perinatal asphyxia, need for mechanical ventilation, central nervous system abnormalities (abnormal neurologic examination, seizures, intracranial hemorrhage, abnormal head size), unresolved hyperbilirubinemia, exchange transfusion, bronchopulmonary dysplasia, apnea, special medical care needs (feedings, oxygen, medications), anomalies or other genetic problems, and significant risk for sensorineural and developmental handicaps.

## SPECIAL PROBLEMS AND CARE

This section expands upon the general care measures raised in the previous section. Its purpose is to allow the reader to provide care as necessary in emergencies, predict what help will be necessary, understand what may be done elsewhere, and participate as a knowledgeable asso-

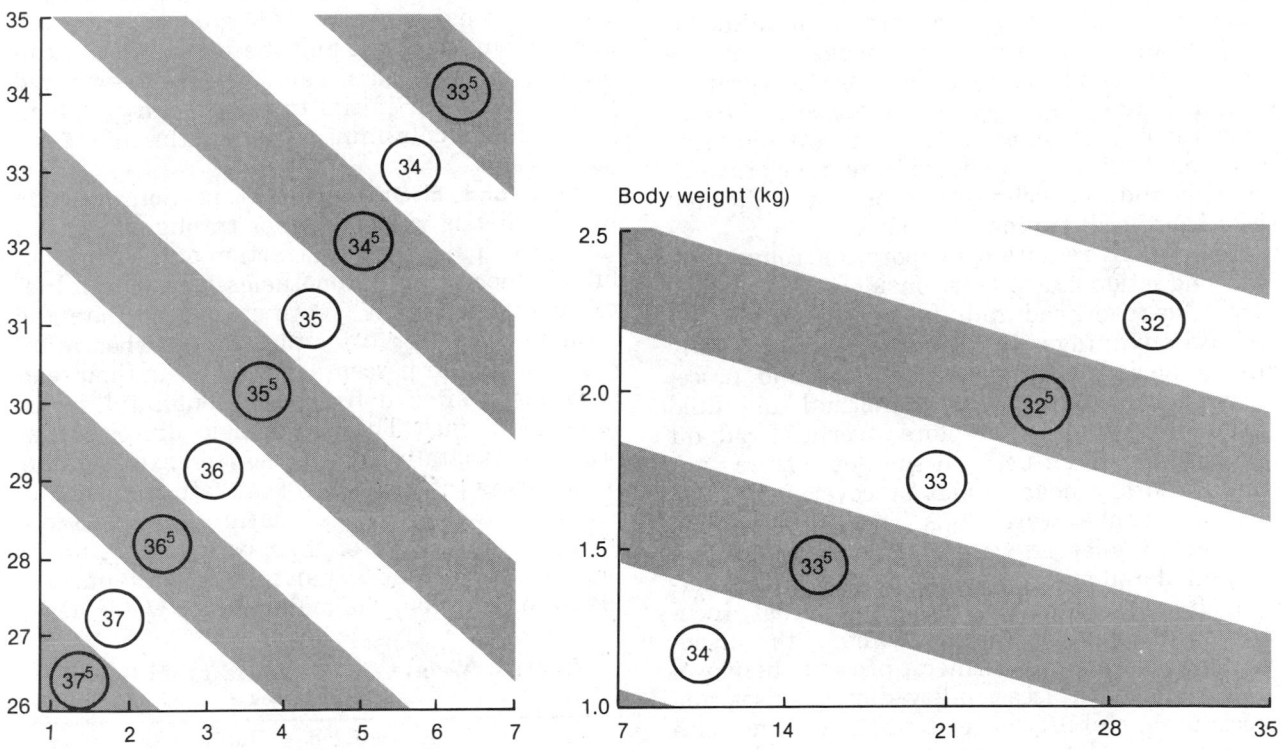

**Figure 1.** Impact of gestational age, body weight, and postnatal age on neutral thermal environmental temperatures. (From Sauer PJJ, Dane HJ, and Visser HKA: New standards for the thermoneutral environment of the very low birth weight (VLBW) infant. Pediatr. Res. *17*(4):334A, 1983.)

ciate in the counseling of families whose infants are being cared for by others.

## Impact of Birthweight and Gestational Age on General Care

With decreasing gestational age or birthweight, there are mandatory adjustments necessary in the environment, screening measures (routine and state-mandated), fluid and electrolyte management, and nutritional needs and techniques. The incidence of specific disease and abnormal behavior is higher as well.

**Environment.** The needs, limitations, and risks of the environment increase inversely with birthweight and gestational age. The neutral thermal environment is the temperature range in which a homeotherm has the lowest oxygen consumption (or metabolic rate) to maintain a normal body temperature. Figure 1 is a useful representation of the impact of gestational age or birthweight on neutral thermal environmental temperatures. Although core temperature is the "bottom line" for the homeotherm, surface temperatures are useful in assessing adequacy of environment versus stress on the infant attempting to maintain a normal core temperature. Axillary temperatures are the preferred value for temperature measurement in neonates because they are safe and usually reflect core temperature well, although they may be influenced by surface temperature. In small infants, rectal temperatures are not equivalent to core temperatures anyway, and this technique poses some additional risks from local trauma.

Heat flux by radiation, evaporation, convection, and conduction must all be considered in neonatal care. The overhead radiant warmer has some definite advantages in intensive care, especially during periods of close assessment and procedures, but it has potential thermal and fluid disadvantages also. Therefore, overhead radiant warmers are often used on smaller infants with supplementary heat shields or coverings, warm mist, and heated water pads. The temperature of the heated mist or water pad must be closely controlled and monitored to avoid unwanted thermal effects (cooling, overheating, burns). Incubators, although not having some of the disadvantages of radiant warmers, present their own limitations with accessibility during crises and procedures, stability of heat while working with the infant, and ability to maintain an adequate temperature in the most diminutive infants.

Infants with lower birthweights and gestational ages also suffer an increased susceptibility to additional hazards in the environment, giving rise to the current concerns about the ill effects of noise, light, and the quantity and quality of handling and stimulation.

**Screening Routines.** Alteration of timing of obtaining the samples may be necessary for the commonly state-mandated screens in at-risk infants. Thyroid function or thyroxine ($T_4$) levels may be low at first in ill infants, and therefore the initial screening should be performed later. Screens in preterm infants often need to be repeated because of the frequently low $T_4$ concentrations (with normal thyroid stimulating hormone levels), resulting apparently from low thyroid binding globulin levels. The impact of large numbers of preterm infant samples on the laboratory results when normative neonatal value ranges are established must also be considered.

Hyperphenylalaninemia screening is dependent somewhat on protein intake; therefore, ideally a nutritive protein source should be provided before screening, which may delay the optimal timing of this screen as well. Occasionally we encounter interference from antibiotics administered to infants and must repeat the study. Many of the other screens (galactosemia, hemoglobinopathies) are based upon red blood cell assays, so transfusion may be a problem. For these reasons, we screen for galactosemia and hemoglobinopathies using the initial blood sample drawn upon admission to the nursery and then perform our initial thyroid and hyperphenylalaninemia determination when the infant is 7 days of age.

**Fluids and Electrolytes.** The portion of body weight that is water declines throughout gestation, principally from contraction of the extracellular compartment. Nonetheless, the normal fetus has a higher body water content than the neonate will after transition. All newborns approach a similar percentage of water in their lean body mass after delivery (although full-terms have more fat). The physiologic diuresis that occurs postnatally is this loss of extracellular fluid during the transition from fetus to neonate. Therefore, we expect less mature infants to lose a higher percentage of their body weight under normal circumstances than full-term infants (Table 3). In addition, the maintenance water needs

TABLE 3. **Weight Changes and Fluid Needs in Neonates**

| Birthweight (grams) | Predicted Weight Loss (%) | Initial Intravenous Fluid Rate (ml/kg/day) |
|---|---|---|
| <1000 | 10–15 | 120–140 |
| 1000–1750 | 5–10 | 100–120 |
| 1750–2500 | 5 | 100 |
| >2500 | 3–5 | 80 |

vary inversely with gestational age and birthweight because of differences in surface area, integrity of the integument, and renal function. Birthweight is used for all calculations until about 1 week of age. This avoids calculation difficulties induced by large weight changes.

The electrolyte needs vary with clinical condition and time. We do not stock electrolyte solutions (only $D_5$ or $D_{10}W$), and we custom-order or mix each intravenous solution in the unit. Because the extra (fetal) fluid that the neonate will have before physiologic diuresis is predominately extracellular, the sodium content is high. Potassium may have "other" sources early in life, such as tissue damage, transfusions, and medications, but is not in similar excess as sodium after delivery. Serum calcium regulation is complex, and the preterm child is notoriously impaired with homeostasis. Therefore, the temporal hierarchy of electrolyte additions in the at-risk newborn on intravenous fluid therapy is usually calcium, potassium, and finally sodium.

Serial monitoring of the fluid and electrolytes status must include the following:

1. Serial weights
2. Input (by type and total)
3. Output (by compartment and total)
4. Serial electrolytes—Na, K, Cl, total carbon dioxide, Ca, glucose
5. Urine assessment—particularly volume and concentration
6. Blood urea nitrogen (BUN), creatinine—if an abnormality of hydration or renal function is suspected

**Nutrition.** Illness, low birthweight, and prematurity abridge the rule "introduce feeds, preferably breast milk, as soon as safe," but only from the safety and not the need aspect. Ileus, catheters, concurrent illness, and risk of necrotizing enterocolitis oppose the apparent benefits of early gut stimulation and the ever present need to maximize nutrition. High-risk infants are now usually managed with a combined approach or parenteral nutrition and enteral feeding. The limitation of parenteral nutrition is usually glucose tolerance, since we are rigid about protein-calorie relationships (not introducing protein until protein sparing calories are provided, maintaining proper protein to carbohydrate ratios). In the very-low-birthweight infant, we often must use insulin to control glucose levels, which then allows provision of more generous calories and earlier introduction of protein. Lipid is, of course, an excellent caloric and essential nutrient source but has some limitations and risks of its own. Careful attention to these details while "pushing hard" to maximize overall nutrition can yield excellent results, especially for such monitors as the integrity of the skin in the second week of life in extremely-low-birthweight infants. Optimal nutrition can be given in this manner without many problems from cholestasis or necrotizing enterocolitis. Enteral feedings are not started until umbilical artery catheters are removed (5 to 7 days) and only then if the umbilical artery catheter course was uneventful (which may necessitate an aortic ultrasonographic examination to confirm no thrombus). Endotracheal intubation is not a contraindication to gavage feedings. The decision to use naso- versus orogastric tubes is based on management of the airway and the significance of the gag reflex in each particular infant. Small bowel cannulation is no longer used. Gavage feedings are intermittent (every 2, 3, or 4 hours), and the tube is allowed to remain in place. Initial feedings are with full-strength formula or breast milk at approximately 40 ml per kg per day. Progress is made slowly thereafter. Many authors recommend smaller volumes and diluted formula, but our almost negligible incidence of necrotizing enterocolitis supports the multifactorial etiology of this disease and the conclusion that it is not simply "overaggressive feeding."

Breast milk, or formulas similar to it, is an excellent material for feeding preterm infants, especially early in the course or when supplementary materials are being used intravenously. The nutrient limitations of breast milk and breast milk–like formulas, such as electrolyte content (especially calcium and phosphate) and high lactose loads, often need to be addressed by using one of the common "preemie formulas." An alternative is the supplementation of mothers' breast milk with breast milk fortifiers. At-risk infants who are being enterally fed only are often given vitamin supplements (after considering the intake of vitamins in their formula) using a "neonatal vitamin preparation" of commercial liquid multivitamins with extra vitamin D, vitamin E, and folate.

### Evaluation of Abnormal Behavior

Neonates, especially less mature ones, have a limited number of ways in which they can react or express signs and symptoms of illness. The presentation of disease is often very nonspecific and may include temperature instability, changes in activity (agitation or lethargy), feeding problems, unusual skin color, abnormality of cardiac rate or output (shock, poor perfusion, pallor), abnormalities of respiratory effort (distress) and rate, delays of stooling and/or voiding, and episodic events or "spells." Focal or very specific problems may produce generalized symptoms, and generalized or global problems may have fairly focal presentations.

The most common problems that present in previously healthy neonates include hypoglycemia, sepsis, respiratory distress from a variety of causes, impaired transition (respiratory and/or cardiac), hyperbilirubinemia, and inability to take adequate feedings. Sepsis and hypoglycemia are the great masqueraders in the newborn and should be seriously considered with any abnormal sign or symptom. The assessment of the above signs and symptoms should include the following:

### In General

1. History: Re-examine the risk factors toward predicting problems.

2. Examination: Always generalize and examine the whole infant (see Table 2).

3. Evaluation: One should select from the following group of nonspecific "screens": complete blood count, hematocrit, glucose, blood gas evaluation, weight, urine output, and assessment of urine concentration (specific gravity or osmolality).

### For Specific Findings

1. Respiratory distress: Consider the wide range of etiologies, as to be discussed, especially that nonpulmonary diseases can produce respiratory distress. The response to oxygen can be helpful in determining a pulmonary origin for documented hypoxemia. Pertinent laboratory tests include arterial blood gas analysis, complete blood count, chest x-ray, blood glucose, and cultures.

2. Possible sepsis: Although a complete culture evaluation is very desirable, the work-up is never curative and therapy may be warranted before culturing is completed, typically before urine is obtained or lumbar puncture is successful. It is important to remember that both of these sites can yield supportive data even after antibiotics are initiated because of the presence of white blood cells (pyuria or pleocytosis) or bacterial antigens. Appropriate septic work-up studies may include complete blood count, coagulation studies, arterial blood gas analysis, cultures (blood, CSF, urine, respiratory tract), urinalysis, lumbar puncture, and antigen screens. Screening infants with acute phase reactant studies may be useful, but negative results should not discourage treatment in the ill infant.

3. Hyperbilirubinemia: Because this a frequent "physiologic" problem, the purpose of the work-up is to find any pathologic cause. Most neonates with pathologic icterus have an increased production of unconjugated bilirubin, and findings

on the initial examination (bruising, pallor) and testing (hematocrit, reticulocyte count, nucleated RBC count, Rh type–Coombs' total-direct bilirubin) reflect that likelihood.

4. Poor feeding: The major concerns pursued are whether some life-threatening illness (sepsis, adrenal insufficiency, hypoxia) is making the infant too ill to feed and whether the poor feeding has resulted in the common consequences of dehydration and hypoglycemia.

5. Evidence of poor cardiac output: Since this may be the emergent consequence of any severe neonatal problem, rapid and complete assessment is mandatory for a wide variety of problems including sepsis, hypovolemia, hypoglycemia, congenital heart disease, metabolic disease, and metabolic acidosis.

### Special Care Modalities

The at-risk infant's care often requires attention to vascular access, medications, and transfusions.

**Vascular Access.** This is not a minor issue in neonatal intensive care. Abuse, misuse, or inadequacy of lines and vascular access is a frequent problem in the treatment of illness or as a cause of iatrogenic disease. The optimal time to plan and place appropriate lines is well before their need arises.

1. Peripheral venous lines: These are now placed with 22- or 24-gauge "plastic" catheters, rather than butterflies, in the extremities or scalp. Shaving of the hair is rarely needed, since it can be parted and matted flat with a tape adhesive such as benzoin. Risk of infiltration or damage from sclerosing solutions (calcium, hyperalimentation, medications) is real, and any infiltration that is tightly swollen and/or discolored should be considered for treatment with hyaluronidase (Wydase) injected through multiple punctures.

2. Arterial catheters: The umbilical artery catheter (UAC) is still the major line used in neonatal intensive care. There are proponents of both high ($T_6$–$T_{10}$) and low ($L_3$–$L_4$) placement, but we generally always use high lines initially, using a Silastic or polyurethane catheter. The infusate is heparinized (1 U per ml, or less in very small infants receiving high fluid rates), but the flushes are not heparinized, to avoid accidental heparinization. We do not infuse anything but simple crystalloid or parenteral nutrition solutions with 10% or less glucose through these catheters, using heparin locks in peripheral veins for transfusions, medications, and other intermittent infusions.

3. Central venous catheters: There are two

types and circumstances of use. First, the umbilical venous catheter (UVC) is used in acute delivery-related resuscitations as well as in the early management of the extremely-low-birthweight infant (usually less than 750 grams) as an accessory to the UAC to replace the peripheral vein line or heparin lock. In both cases, the UVC is ideally placed with its tip just outside the right atrium or "barely in" if the ductus venosus cannot be entered. Second, central venous catheters placed through a peripheral vein using a commercially available percutaneous device have essentially eliminated the use of Broviac-type central line cutdowns in the neonatal intensive care unit (NICU). These are usually inserted near the end of the useful life of the UAC. Both of these venous lines are managed with heparin, as are the UACs.

**Medications.** The most commonly used medications, the doses, and the role of monitoring are very important topics. The most commonly used drugs are listed in Table 4. The provision of care to at-risk neonates mandates familiarity with these topics, and the appropriately equipped nursery must have one of the numerous texts available as a reference.

For the unknown bacterial agent, the initial choice of antibiotics remains a penicillin and an aminoglycoside. We prefer to use caffeine rather then theophylline for treatment of apnea of prematurity in the hospital but use theophylline after discharge because of the availability of supplies and level monitoring. The pharmacokinetics of all medications varies widely with gestational age and associated illnesses. In general, the interval between doses is increased as the gestational age decreases.

**Transfusions.** The use of blood products is commonplace in the NICU, and efforts must be made to minimize the potential consequences of infections and exposure to many donors. The basic red blood cell supply for the unit comes from the city blood bank's best known, O-negative donors, drawn into multipack containers so that several infants can use the pack at the same time and several transfusions can be given to the same infant from each donor. The donors are thoroughly screened for hepatitis B virus, human immunodeficiency virus, and cytomegalovirus. In the ill neonatal population, the early transfusions are given as specific volumes are removed, but later transfusions are given to correct the hematocrit when blood is removed less frequently. Transfusions are usually administered in the first month of life to reduce the later impact on the infant's marrow response.

### TABLE 4. **Common Medications for Newborns**

*Antibiotics*
  Ampicillin (or alternative penicillin) (Omnipen)
  Cefotaxime (Claforan)
  Gentamicin (or alternative aminoglycoside) (Garamycin)
  Methicillin (Staphcillin) or nafcillin (Nafcil)
  Vancomycin (Vancocin)
*Diuretics*
  Chlorothiazide (Diuril)
  Furosemide (Lasix)
*Cardiovascular Agents*
  Atropine
  Digoxin (Lanoxin)
  Dopamine (Intropin) and dobutamine (Dobutrex)
  Epinephrine (Adrenalin)
  Indomethacin (Indocin)
*Anticonvulsants*
  Phenobarbital (Luminal)
  Phenytoin (Dilantin)
*Sedatives-Analgesics*
  Chloral hydrate (Noctec)
  Morphine
*CNS Agents*
  Aminophylline and theophylline
  Caffeine
  Naloxone (Narcan)
*Other*
  Calcium
  Dexamethasone (Decadron, Hexadrol)
  Ferrous sulfate (Feosol)
  Glucagon
  Insulin
  Sodium bicarbonate
  Vitamins

### Specific Problems and Disease Entities

**Asphyxia.** Because of the frequent consequences and concerns that accompany this diagnosis, it should follow strict definitions. The complex of perinatal asphyxia is a collection of findings, including evidence of fetal distress (fetal heart rate tracing abnormalities, meconium staining of the amniotic fluid), need for resuscitation, low Apgar scores, metabolic acidosis detected by cord blood or the first postnatal blood gas analysis, and/or neonatal disease consistent with asphyxial injury. The diagnosis should not rest solely on low Apgar scores or any other single finding. Asphyxial injury can affect a number of systems in the neonate and usually affects more than one. These include central nervous system (hypoxic-ischemic encephalopathy [HIE], intracranial hemorrhage, seizures, abnormal activity, cerebral edema), pulmonary (aspiration syndromes, shock lungs), cardiac (persistent fetal circulation, myocardial ischemia), gastrointestinal (necrotizing enterocolitis, hepatic injury), renal (delayed urine output, acute tubular necrosis), and hematologic (disseminated intravascular coagulation, depressed marrow function). The management must be directed at evaluation of all these possibilities, although long-term prognosis is mostly dependent upon central nervous system injury.

**Respiratory Distress.** The initial work-up, differential diagnosis, and evaluation, although often influenced by clinical history, follow the "rule of fives," which states that there are five most common pulmonary diseases and five major systems involved in the etiology of respiratory distress: (1) pulmonary (hyaline membrane disease, transient tachypnea of the newborn, pneumonia, aspiration syndromes, and extrapulmonary collections of air or "pneumos"), (2) cardiac (congenital heart disease, persistent fetal circulation), (3) metabolic (hypoglycemia, metabolic acidosis, hypothermia, inborn errors of metabolism), (4) central nervous system (hemorrhage, infection, depression), and (5) hematologic (anemia, polycythemia).

**Metabolic Problems.** In addition to the conditions mentioned earlier, common metabolic disorders in at-risk neonates are metabolic acidosis and glucose and calcium abnormalities.

Metabolic acidosis is a common "sign," especially in less mature infants. Its morbid significance often increases with gestational age of the infant. The differential diagnosis includes renal tubular acidosis, late metabolic acidosis, sepsis, intracranial hemorrhage, hypovolemia, hypoperfusion, hypoxia, congestive heart failure, increased muscle work, necrotizing enterocolitis, hypothermia, asphyxia, inborn metabolic errors, protein overload, malnutrition, and many other conditions. It is of great value to determine whether an anion gap exists by drawing electrolytes carefully and anaerobically (to avoid ventilating the $CO_2$ off and creating a false gap), and essential to assume the worst and rule out serious causes before relying only on symptomatic therapy with base salts. The commonplace renal tubular acidosis in the diminutive preterm infant can be palliated with routine use of cations in the form of base salts (bicarbonates, citrates, or acetates) and avoidance of chloride salts until the base deficit normalizes.

Glucose abnormalities, both hyper- and hypo-, are very common. Hypoglycemia is the more important because of a higher incidence and more severe consequences. Preterm and growth-retarded infants frequently suffer hypoglycemia because of inadequate stores and intake relative to their glucose utilization. Large-for-gestational-age infants often have hyperinsulinemia and thereby increased glucose utilization and clearance. Bolus therapy and hyperglycemia need to be avoided in these latter infants if possible so that they do not produce excessive insulin. Low glucose monitoring stick results must be checked with serum or blood glucose levels, but if the infant is symptomatic, the level seems very low, or there is any question, therapy should be instituted immediately. Miniboluses of glucose (2 ml per kg of $D_{10}W$) are effective, although the constant delivery of glucose may need to be instituted. Glucagon is effective in emergencies when no intravenous line is in place, provided that the patient has some hepatic glycogen stores. Early feedings can often prevent or treat very mild cases of hypoglycemia. Diazoxide has replaced steroids as the drug of choice for long-term management of refractory cases.

Hyperglycemia is a common management problem in the extremely-low-birthweight infant because of apparent pancreatic immaturity. Insulin, at insulin to glucose ratios (0.3 U per gram of glucose) published for the treatment of hyperkalemia, is initiated to cover some of the infused glucose, aimed at returning the blood sugars to a level at which osmotic diuresis is not a problem. We do not use intravenous solutions of less than 5% dextrose because of the problems of hypotonic fluids and the eventual futility of inadequate nutrition. Hypo- and hyperglycemia must be considered important signs of infection and other forms of stress in newborns.

The acute and long-term management of calcium, along with phosphorus and magnesium, requires a great deal of thought. The in utero acquisition of calcium is related to gestational age and the content in the fetus quadruples after 28 weeks' gestation; therefore, the premature infant is very dependent upon postnatal therapy to recover from this congenital deficiency. Acutely, hypocalcemia is a frequent problem needing treatment. Phosphate levels may rise in certain conditions, such as asphyxia, renal failure, or use of older formulas with inappropriate Ca to P ratios, but are seldom an acute management problem. Hypomagnesemia rarely occurs in the absence of severe or resistant hypocalcemia. Therefore, phosphorus and magnesium are considered almost exclusively in the context of calcium.

The inherent deficiencies of bone mineralization in preterms are aggravated by chronic disease (chronic lung disease, necrotizing enterocolitis, cholestasis, acidosis, renal disease); calciuric drugs (furosemide); poor intake of calcium, phosphorus, or vitamin D; use of soy formulas; and aluminum excess. It can be assumed that not enough calcium and phosphorus can be given intravenously because of solubility problems, so chronic parenteral alimentation alone is a problem. Modern premature infant formulas maximize the amount of these minerals in the proper ratios, but careful attention must be given to monitoring Ca, P, and alkaline phosphatase levels, as well as estimating bone mineralization by serial bone x-rays or other methods. Infants who have renal or hepatic disease should receive 1,25-dihydroxy vitamin D.

**Cardiac Problems.** The peripartum transition of the cardiovascular system is a frequent concern in neonatal care, involving a spectrum from the "transitional murmurs" that raise the question of congenital heart disease to the "worst disease" in neonates (persistent fetal circulation [PFC] or, more properly, persistent pulmonary hypertension [PPH]). The cardiac transition is dependent upon an effective pulmonary transition in which the lungs are inflated properly with the appropriate gas rather than fetal lung liquid; the pulmonary vascular resistance falls because of the establishment of negative intrathoracic pressure and the relaxed pulmonary vasoconstriction as a result of rising $PO_2$; and the systemic vascular resistance rises, in part, from the loss of the low-resistance placental circuit. These events are followed by functional closure of the ductus arteriosus and foramen ovale. The essential preventive measures during the delivery room and early postpartum care of newborns are the institution of effective ventilation and lung inflation and the provision of adequate oxygenation.

The treatment of PFC-PPH is complicated and often very frustrating. The condition itself is often associated with other major problems such as asphyxial injury, severe pulmonary disease, or sepsis. The mainstays of therapy in our unit are aggressive normalization of ventilation, generous oxygenation, sedation, careful attention to cardiovascular status, and alkalinization with base infusions. Paralysis, hyperventilation, pulmonary vasodilators, and extracorporeal membrane oxygenation are occasionally needed.

The patent ductus arteriosus can be regarded as a transitional problem in the preterm infant. Its incidence is inversely related to gestational age. This problem is most commonly seen as a complication of respiratory distress and should be considered when the course includes deterioration of pulmonary function, heart murmur, widening of pulse pressure and finding of full or bounding pulses, or cardiomegaly and engorged pulmonary vasculature on chest x-ray. Signs of classic "congestive heart failure" are unusual unless presentation is fulminant or diagnosis delayed, although findings may include pulmonary edema, metabolic acidosis, or decreased cardiac output. Digoxin (Lanoxin) is now rarely used, and management includes time, careful control of fluid administration (especially avoiding excesses or overload), ventilatory support, indomethacin, and ligation. Indomethacin is the preferred method of closure, but we are very willing to have the ductus surgically ligated if there are any contraindications to medical therapy. Presence of intracranial hemorrhage is one of the most common reasons to defer to ligation.

Congenital heart disease is the most common major anomaly dealt with in the neonatal population. Of the five major syndromes, two usually manifest as decreased perfusion (hypoplastic left heart syndrome and aortic arch anomaly–coarctation group) and three are seen predominately as cyanosis (transposition of the great vessels, hypoplasia of right heart structures, and tetralogy of Fallot). The initial work-up includes history, physical examination, four-extremity blood pressures, evaluation of response to oxygen and continuous distending pressure to differentiate from lung disease, x-ray examination, echocardiography with Doppler ultrasound, and cardiac catheterization.

**Infectious Diseases.** Newborns, especially preterms and those receiving intensive care, are notoriously susceptible to infections. The host-related reasons for this are both abnormal nonspecific defenses (defective white blood cell function, abnormal serum opsonin activity, and deficiencies in complement pathways) and impaired specific host defenses (defective antibody response, abnormalities in circulating immunoglobulins). The major risk factor is prematurity, but others include intensive care, foreign bodies, anomalies, and multiple maternal and environmental factors.

Of the numerous conditions involved, the major ones can be grouped into bacterial infections, congenital infections known by the acronym TORCH,* and the issues raised by sexually transmitted diseases (STDs). The patterns of etiologic agents in bacterial infections continue to change, but group B streptococci and *Escherichia coli* remain the chief causative agents of primary infections, with nursery-acquired problems from staphylococci and gram-negative organisms (as well as yeasts).

TORCH infections often have ubiquitous presentations and should be considered in the evaluation of pneumonitis, thrombocytopenia, hepatosplenomegaly, chorioretinitis, growth retardation, hepatic dysfunction, anomalous development, cerebral calcifications, bone changes, delayed development, and cutaneous lesions. Many infants with TORCH infections have asymptomatic shedding of viruses. The highly publicized STDs are frequent issues in neonatal units, not so much from a major occurrence of serious disease as from the infection control point of view with associated risks to other infants and staff.

**Gastrointestinal Problems.** Feeding-related issues have been reviewed earlier. Nutrition is an issue in all patients and has many associated problems. Feeding intolerance, to variable de-

---

*Toxoplasmosis, rubella, cytomegalovirus, and herpes simplex.

grees, is a very frequent occurrence and one of the dilemmas in the differential diagnosis of necrotizing enterocolitis (NEC). NEC is still a major cause of morbidity and mortality in NICUs and is reported to occur in as many as 15% of admissions, usually in the very-low-birthweight population. It should be considered a "final common pathway" disease with a very wide variety of associated clinical settings, possibly initiated through the routes of infection, mucosal injury, and/or compromised gut perfusion.

**Renal Disorders.** The renal manifestations of immaturity are major issues involved in the management of preterm infants and include altered drug metabolism and excretion, renal tubular acidosis, problems with conservation and excretion of sodium and water, numerous other fluid and electrolyte disorders, and propensity for renal failure. The vast majority of cases of renal failure in the neonatal population are prerenal in origin, and the primary cause of renal hypoperfusion must be resolved if there is to be hope of recovery of renal function.

**Neurologic Disease.** When neurologic injury occurs in the perinatal period, the manifestations and location of the lesions are often gestational age dependent. In very immature infants, the developmental orientation of the brain is central and the periventricular area often suffers, whereas the cerebral cortex is frequently the damaged area of full-term gestation. Acute manifestations of central nervous system insult include abnormal behavior and tone, cerebral edema, seizures, and intracranial hemorrhage. Fluid retention in an asphyxiated infant is often a difficult diagnostic problem but should not be assumed to be the syndrome of inappropriate antidiuretic hormone secretion because renal insults are very common, as is inadequate hydration from pre-existing placental insufficiency. Intracranial hemorrhage is more often a "marker" of central nervous system stress or injury in the preterm than the full-term, and its absence in the asphyxiated full-term child should not be taken as definitive reassurance. The long-term sequelae of cerebral insult can be the result of neuronal injury (seizures, microcephaly, mental retardation), glial and support tissue injury, and/or hemorrhage (hydrocephalus, proencephaly). Cerebral palsy seems to be related closely to periventricular leukomalacia, a lesion of apparent perfusion failure in the periventricular white matter usually accompanied by hemorrhage.

By far, the major type of intracranial hemorrhage seen in newborns is of the periventricular-intraventricular type. Although problems may result from the least severe grades, most concern with long-term outcome is for those patients who have dilated ventricles or intracerebral extension of their hemorrhage. Primary subarachnoid hemorrhage occasionally occurs and can be associated with the signs and symptoms of apnea, irritability, fever, or seizures.

Seizure types seen in newborns include subtle, tonic, multifocal clonic, focal, and myoclonic. Two difficulties for diagnosis are the high incidence of irritability and tremors in stressed neonates and the high frequency of subtle seizures, especially in less mature infants. The more common causes include the following:

1. Acquired brain injury—asphyxia, HIE, hemorrhage; may include direct trauma
2. Metabolic problems—chiefly hypoglycemia and hypocalcemia; may also be caused by pyridoxine deficiency or dependency, hypomagnesemia, hyponatremia, hypernatremia, and aminoacidurias
3. CNS infection—either chronic (TORCH) or acute (meningitis)
2. Developmental anomalies
3. Other—drug intoxications (local anesthetics) or withdrawal (narcotics)

The most commonly used anticonvulsant is still phenobarbital, but specific therapy of any specific cause is important.

**Special Syndromes.** Maternal diabetes remains a fairly important influence on perinatal management and outcome. The many problems associated with this syndrome include high fetal wastage and intrauterine death, polyhydramnios, prematurity, macrosomia (or growth retardation in advanced maternal vascular disease), birth trauma, congenital anomalies, hypoglycemia, hypocalcemia, hypomagnesemia, respiratory distress, hyperbilirubinemia, hyperviscosity, small left colon syndrome, renal vein thrombosis, and inheritance of diabetes.

A new problem potentially induced by the effective obstetric management of premature-prolonged rupture of the amniotic membranes is acquired oligohydramnios syndrome. After weeks in utero without adequate amniotic fluid, these infants may be born with findings similar to those originally described with Potter's syndrome. The major acute medical problem usually is pulmonary hypoplasia.

## Long-Term Needs of At-Risk Infants

At-risk neonates need and benefit from careful attention to their long-term care needs. Many of these are addressed while they are still in intensive care, during their convalescent hospitalizations (which may be after back transfer), and as outpatients. The caretakers must address the following issues:

**Growth and Nutrition.** Growth of NICU patients and graduates should be carefully monitored by serial assessment of weight, length, and head circumference. These should be plotted regularly on growth charts, preferably ones that combine in utero and postnatal curves, with correction for the infant's prematurity. Impaired growth may be related to concomitant problems causing increased energy utilization (bronchopulmonary dysplasia) [BPD], cardiac disease) or impaired intake (CNS disorders, parenting, cardiac disease, BPD). As intake is increased, the caretaker must ensure adequacy of all nutrients, particularly protein. Therefore, simple caloric supplements with materials such as carbohydrate or medium-chain triglyceride oil should not be given until intake of appropriate, nutritionally complete infant formula is adequate (usually calculated in terms of 110 to 120 calories per kg per day).

**Developmental Assessment.** This is an essential issue in follow-up care, if for no other reason than to reassure a worried family of the usual healthy and normal outcomes in survivors of neonatal intensive care. The neurologic and developmental assessment should be corrected for prematurity for the first 2 or 3 years. General neurologic examination and physical-occupational therapy assessments may reveal abnormalities of tone that are usually transient and often insignificant. Formal developmental measurements, such as the Bayley scale, are usually begun at about 9 months corrected age. Cerebral palsy, hydrocephalus, delayed developmental milestones, and sensorineural impairment are the major long-term sequelae.

**Sensorineural Testing.** Various factors in the care and environment of the newborn put vision and hearing at risk. The criteria for eye examinations by an experienced ophthalmologist now include prematurity and any significant exposure to oxygenation. Hearing may soon be screened in all patients staying in the intensive care nursery for more than a few days, but assessment at least should meet the minimum standards of the American Otologic Society's criteria for infant screening, including family history of hearing deficits, craniofacial anomalies, evidence of CNS infection, TORCH infections, severe hyperbilirubinemia, asphyxia, and exposure to excessive levels of ototoxic drugs.

**Special Medical Problems.** Bronchopulmonary dysplasia (BPD), anemia, apnea, risk for hypertension, and sequelae of iatrogenic disease are often the problems that need attention in the early follow-up visits after discharge. The major predisposing disease for BPD is the respiratory distress syndrome, although it may occur after severe meconium aspiration and viral pneumonias. Controversy over specific etiology may exist, but functionally BPD is the summation of the effects of oxygen, positive-pressure ventilation, endotracheal intubation, infection, and immaturity. Most infants with BPD eventually recover and do fairly well, particularly if they can escape the ill effects of the two compromising problems of malnutrition and repeated respiratory infection. Most will likely require periodic attention to or even rehospitalization for lower respiratory tract infections. Oxygen therapy is important, and overzealous weaning can aggravate the problems of cor pulmonale and poor weight gain. Other common, although not universal, therapies for BPD include fluid restriction, diuretics, and bronchodilators (oral and inhalation). Steroids may have a role in some patients.

Graduates of neonatal intensive care are frequently mildly anemic. This problem relates to large iatrogenic blood losses for laboratory samples, potential deficiencies of essential nutrients, and rapid growth while marrow is still fairly quiescent. The low point of the hemoglobin level usually occurs by 8 to 12 weeks of age. Supplementation should be given early with vitamin E and folate, and dietary iron is added by at least 1 month of age when transfusions are no longer given unless anemia is severe. The hemoglobin or hematocrit should be monitored frequently, with occasional reticulocyte counts.

Blood pressure should be measured during follow-up because of the occasional problem of hypertension, presumably the result of UAC-related problems and/or other insults to the kidneys. Infants with BPD seem more prone to hypertension.

The immature infant often manifests apnea, either isolated or secondary to another specific problem. It may be precipitated by infection; thermal instability; metabolic derangements such as hypoglycemia or hypocalcemia; drugs given to the mother or infant; acute or chronic CNS problems; and impaired oxygenation through hypoxemia, hypovolemia, or anemia. The precipitating factor should be sought out and corrected, if present. Thereafter, caffeine and theophylline are often used. Relatively healthy preterm infants may not resolve their propensity for apnea prior to discharge. Although there may be controversy on the management of asymptomatic preterm babies, those who have active clinical symptoms (reflux, hypoxia, and seizures) warrant evaluation as well as consideration of methylxanthine therapy and home monitoring.

SEQUELAE OF IATROGENIC DISEASE. These are frequently cosmetic in nature and, if appropriately addressed, can reduce the negative impact for the patient and family. Care and planning of therapy during the acute phases of illness can reduce the incidence of iatrogenic sequelae of neonatal intensive care.

**Immunizations.** The recommended schedule of childhood immunizations should be followed as closely (by calendar and not corrected age) as possible. Some of the issues that arise are avoiding giving live virus immunizations while infant is still in the NICU, concerns about aggravation of other problems such as seizures or apnea, and size of the patient relative to the possibly intense local reactions to injections. Although concerns about the safety of some vaccines may be real, the threat of the diseases being prevented is usually even greater in the NICU graduate than in the low-risk population.

**Parenting—Acceptance-Bonding, Skills, Stress, and Fatigue.** It is hoped that the family and socioeconomic circumstances can be clarified early in the neonate's course and an outpatient management plan formulated to promote acceptance, stability, and optimal outcomes at home. Active involvement of the family in the acute care unit is a great foundation for success after discharge, but the better the accommodation of a family to the inpatient caretakers, the more dependent they usually are to continued contact and support after discharge.

# NORMAL INFANT FEEDING

method of
ROBERT P. DILLARD, M.D., and
WILLIAM F. BALISTRERI, M.D.
*Children's Hospital Medical Center*
*Cincinnati, Ohio*

Infant feeding regimens reflect a combination of science, tradition, and folklore. Nevertheless, there are pitfalls to be avoided and general principles to be followed that clearly support optimal health in infants. Simply stated, the goals of infant feeding are to maintain life, promote growth, allow the development of physical and mental potential, prevent or correct nutritional deficiencies, and repair injury. In addition, adverse effects must be avoided, either those of toxic substances or those due to an excess of normal nutrients. Nutritional practices established in early life are also thought to play a role in degenerative disease, such as coronary atherosclerosis. Although the influence of infant feeding on those processes is unknown, it remains a major concern.

## BREAST-FEEDING

These nutritional goals are best met through the feeding of human milk from a healthy mother. That being the case, infant nutrition, in a greater sense, begins at conception and is influenced by the general health of the mother and her nutrition during pregnancy. Maternal nutrition is often influenced by the overall health status of the community and by the availability of adequate food. All women should receive prenatal care and be instructed in a diet appropriate for pregnancy. Less advantaged women should be referred to public assistance programs. Regardless of their diets, it is clear that women must avoid alcohol and other so-called recreational drugs during pregnancy.

An environment supportive of breast-feeding and educational efforts should be provided throughout pregnancy, labor, delivery, and the postpartum period. Childbirth preparation may decrease medication use, resulting in a mother and infant more alert and ready to initiate breast-feeding. The physician should not be coercive in promoting breast-feeding, but it is reasonable to provide information about this optimal method of infant nutrition. Breast milk provides a high-quality, whey-predominant protein that forms a fine, flocculent curd and is easily digested. Breast milk lipase, as well as the structure of triglycerides in breast milk, provides for optimal fat absorption. All essential fatty acids are provided, and the high percentage of monounsaturated fatty acids may be beneficial. Lactose, the predominant carbohydrate, aids calcium absorption, and all minerals exist in an ideal balance for absorption and utilization. The renal solute load is low, and ample free water is provided to the nursing baby.

Fears and myths should be addressed. Breast-feeding may be thought impossible because of breast size, or because a relative did not successfully breast-feed, or because it may be thought to ruin breast shape. To identify any problems, the breast should be examined during routine prenatal care. Fortunately, the breast usually adapts for nursing without difficulty and anatomic problems are rare. A more important issue is that even though an increased number of women are breast-feeding, role models are not readily available. Consequently, prenatal classes may be useful in teaching details of breast-feeding.

The infant should be offered the opportunity to nurse as soon as possible. This may occur in the delivery room, which should be suitably warm. Little nutrition is provided by this initial nursing, but stimulation of milk production is thought to be enhanced.

Once in the postpartum unit, mother and infant should be separated as seldom as possible. Optimal nursing frequency and length will vary from one mother-infant pair to another. Factors such as maternal fatigue and infant alertness must be taken into account. Nursery protocol should be flexible enough to accommodate individual variation. It is known that early frequent nursing is associated with greater milk production and sustained successful breast-feeding. "Rooming in" affords the best opportunity for mother and infant to achieve synchrony in wakefulness, nursing times, and sleeping. Some infants may wish to nurse as often as every 2 hours. However, one must be careful to avoid maternal fatigue. A more dangerous situation is the lethargic or passive baby, who may sleep for long periods of time, miss feedings and become dehydrated, but not cry or otherwise complain. These babies must not be overlooked. Therefore, a maximum duration between feeding or observation, such as 3 to 4 hours, must be observed in the postpartum unit. A rigid 4-hour schedule is not physiologic and does not attend to the needs of either group of babies.

Nursing length must be sufficient to stimulate milk production and flow. Let-down may take several minutes to occur; therefore, approximately 10 to 15 minutes on each breast is a reasonable duration in the first days after delivery. Both breasts should be used with each feeding. Often, as nursing progresses, the baby will empty the breast nursed first and partially empty the breast nursed second. To even out, the next feeding should begin at the "second" breast.

Enough of the areola should be in the infant's mouth to allow the baby to empty the collecting ductules with sucking. When first placed to the breast, the infant's tongue should be positioned over the lower gingival ridge. At the end of nursing, suction can be released by slipping the little finger into the baby's mouth.

Soap should not be used on the nipples and the breast should be dried well following a bath or shower. Most mothers, for comfort, will want to wear a nursing brassiere 24 hours a day, but breast pads should be changed frequently. Air exposure after nursing or the use of a hair dryer or 40-watt bulb (at least 18 inches from the breast) will protect the nipple and help relieve soreness. Leaving a small amount of milk on the nipple to dry seems protective. If nipple soreness occurs, beside the aforementioned measures, it is useful to have nursing occur more frequently, but following let-down, for only 5 to 10 minutes per breast. Nursing should begin on the more comfortable breast, but once let-down occurs, the baby should be switched. Nursing can subsequently be finished by changing back to the comfortable side. A small amount of hydrous lanolin may be applied to the nipple and need not be washed off prior to the next feeding. Other creams and lotions may not be safe, and any that require washing are not helpful.

Uterine cramping may occur with nursing. Usually, education and reassurance to the mother of the normalcy of this phenomenon and that breast-feeding aids uterine involution are all that is required. If necessary, simple pain medication, such as acetaminophen (Tylenol), may be used.

The majority of nursing problems during the neonatal period revolve around inadequate mother-infant contact time, "nipple confusion," and interference with the let-down reflex. Milk production usually occurs readily, but let-down is easily interfered with by such factors as pain, embarrassment, and anxiety. Often, with minor nursing difficulties, a nursing is skipped and a bottle feeding is given to the infant. Some infants quickly become confused, since mouth position for the artificial nipple is different from that for the breast. The resulting scenario is that of a mother with a swollen, engorged breast, who has an infant who bites once or twice, turns away, and cries. This is devastating to the mother, quickly leading to the vicious cycle of impaired let-down, engorgement, pain, anxiety, further impaired let-down, engorgement, possible mastitis, and a crying, unhappy infant throughout. Once this occurs, treatment is difficult. Prompt recognition of this situation and explanation to the mother is necessary. Measures such as warm packs and breast pumping sufficient to allow proper positioning of the infant on the breast are necessary. Nasal oxytocin spray (Syntocinon) prior to nursing may also be helpful. To promote let-down, the mother may use a single spray into one or both nostrils 2 to 3 minutes before putting the infant to the breast. Some infants may need gavage or dropper feedings till nursing is re-established.

The problem of nipple confusion, along with decreased milk production, alteration of gut flora, and introduction of unnecessary foreign antigen, is among the cited reasons to avoid early supplemental or complemental bottle feedings.

Once mother and baby are home, nursing length can vary considerably. Infant personality plays a large role, with some babies nursing quickly and efficiently. Others are more casual, and nursing may last as long as 40 minutes. Some infants nurse briefly, rest, and nurse again. Others require coaxing; these babies cannot be hurried. Other babies are excitable and may even have difficulty holding onto the breast. They may need gentle restraint with swaddling to facilitate nursing. Maternal fatigue must be avoided during this adjustment period, as it is a major cause of decreased milk production.

Monitoring the adequacy of nutrition in a breast-fed infant may be accomplished by checking weight gain, the number of wet diapers per day, and the number and quantity of stools. Usually, the breast-fed infant will recieve at least six feedings a day and sleep well between feedings. There should be at least six wet diapers a day. Birthweight should be regained, at the latest, by 3 weeks, and there should be no weight lost beyond 10 days of age. Subsequently, weight gain should be approximately 20 to 30 grams daily. Infrequent stooling in a breast-fed infant should alert the physician to the possibility of inadequate intake. Only a minority of breast-fed infants have an interval of greater than 24 hours between stooling. The more observed pattern is several stools daily, usually associated with nursing.

### Maternal Diet During Lactation

The quantity and some components of human milk are altered by the nutritional status and diet of the mother. Poorly nourished mothers may have lactation failure. This may be prevented or reversed by adequate nutrition. Human milk variation and mineral content can be improved with diet and supplementation. However, certain components of breast milk are unaltered and remain constant as long as lactation is sustained. Those include human milk protein, carbohydrate, and iron. Maternal energy needs are great during lactation and are met by diet and utilization of fat stored during pregnancy. Mothers may gradually attain pre-pregnancy weight while consuming an additional 400 to 600 kcal daily. Caloric restriction in order to lose weight during early lactation may lead to decreased milk production and should be avoided.

A diet similar to that eaten during pregnancy should be continued. It is appropriate to use the traditional four food groups—(1) meat, fish, poultry, egg, and high-protein meat substitute; (2) dairy products, such as milk, cheese, and milk products; (3) fruit and vegetables; (4) cereal, grains, potatoes, and rice—as a basis for dietary advice. Large amounts of milk need not be consumed by a lactating mother; they are unnecessary and may cause considerable discomfort to lactase-deficient women. Many women prefer to continue their prenatal vitamin and mineral supplements. These, in general, are not necessary in the well-nourished mother and will not alter breast milk in any beneficial fashion. Although breast milk iron will be unchanged, it is difficult for women to replete iron stores by diet alone; therefore, iron supplementation is advisable. If concern over the nutritional status of the mother exists, continuation of her supplement is advisable.

Maternal fluid intake should be at least 2 liters of water a day. In general, other fluids tend to have either excessive caffeine or nutrient-sparse

calories. The effect of sugar substitutes during lactation is unknown.

Considerable speculation but little information exists on the influence of maternal diet on breast milk flavor, on colic, or on other infant problems. Many pediatricians believe that removing cow milk from the mother's diet will, in some infants, relieve colic. Excessive chocolate (greater than 16 grams a day) consumption by a mother has been reported to cause irritability and increased bowel activity in her infant. Maternal fava bean consumption may cause hemolysis in the glucose-6-phosphate (G6PD)–deficient infant, and excessive caffeine intake has been associated with irritability and poor sleeping patterns. Generally, it is safe for the mother to avoid food that she feels is an annoyance to her nursing infant, as long as adequate overall nutrition is not compromised.

### Contraindications to Breast-Feeding

Relatively few contraindications to breast-feeding exist. Absolute contraindications include active tuberculosis, syphilis, and AIDS. Uncertainty remains in the United States whether the hepatitis B–positive mother should breast-feed her infant. We feel, with proper vaccination, that breast-feeding should be permitted.

Certain drugs are contraindicated during breast-feeding. These include all the chemotherapeutic agents, such as cyclophosphamide (Cytoxan); the immunosuppressant agent cyclosporine (Sandimmune); lithium (Lithobid); a drug used for psychosis; the anticoagulant phenindione;* migraine medications containing ergotamine; and drugs that suppress lactation, such as bromocriptine (Parlodel) and chlorothiazide (Diuril). The use of amphetamines, heroin, marijuana, and phencyclidine is a contraindication to breast-feeding. Smoking should also be discouraged, because, besides its other harmful actions, it is known to decrease milk production.

Drugs requiring temporary cessation of breast-feeding include radioactive isotopes, varying in excretion time from 15 hours to 3 days (technetium-99m) to as long as 2 weeks (iodine-131). It is best to consult with a nuclear medicine physician about the use of a particular agent in a breast-feeding mother. The majority of other drugs are excreted to some extent in breast milk but generally may be used. This decision must be made on an individual basis. Particular caution is required with the use of sulfonamides, which probably should not be used in the neonatal period in the presence of jaundice or with any

---

*Not available in the United States.

suspicion of G6PD deficiency. Metronidazole (Flagyl) use requires cessation of breast feeding for 12 to 24 hours to allow excretion. Details of drug precautions for nursing mothers are available (Pediatrics, *84*:924, 1989).

Upon returning to work, mothers may still nurse in some modified manner. They may pump their breasts and store milk by freezing in plastic bottle liner bags. Milk to be used within 24 hours may simply be refrigerated. Formula may replace some feedings. The mother should introduce bottle feeding 1 to 2 weeks before returning to work. Substituting a bottle feeding every few days for a nursing should ease the transition and help avoid engorgement. She may need to empty her breast once or twice during the day. The success of continued nursing depends mainly on the work environment of the mother and her endurance.

## FORMULA FEEDING

Commercial infant formulas provide an alternative acceptable method of feeding. The formulas currently available in the United States meet the American Academy of Pediatrics Committee on Nutrition's recommended range of nutrient composition. They include all necessary vitamins and major and trace minerals. Iron-fortified formula contains sufficient iron. In the United States, the standard infant formula preparations most used are produced by Mead Johnson (Enfamil), Ross Laboratories (Similac), and Wyeth (SMA): Recently, Carnation and Gerber have entered the formula market. There appear to be no substantial practical differences among these formulas. All standard formulas are available as cans of concentrated liquid (50% of product sold), ready-to-feed (40% of product sold), and powder. At normal concentration they provide 20 kcal per fluid ounce.

The formulas are based on cow milk or soy protein. Cow milk–based formulas comprise the majority of formula used in the United States for infants during the first 6 months. These formulas are modified to resemble human milk. The protein base is either casein from skimmed milk or a mixture of skimmed milk and demineralized cow milk whey protein. There appears to be no advantage of one protein composition over another for healthy term infants. Recently, Wyeth Laboratory has added nucleotides to its formula. It is unknown if this provides any advantage over other formulations. Lactose is most commonly used as the carbohydrate source. Vegetable oil, including soy, coconut, corn, oleo, and safflower, is used as a fat source. This results in a cholesterol content that is lower in these commercial formulas than that found in breast milk.

Protein hydrolysate formulas such as Nutramigen, Pregestimil, and Alimentum are also cow milk based. They are lactose-free and may use sucrose, tapioca, and corn syrup solids as carbohydrate sources. Fat is commonly provided by vegetable oils and may supply a higher percentage of medium-chain triglycerides. These formulas may be useful in special situations, such as documented cow and soy protein allergy, postenteritis diarrhea, and cystic fibrosis. Although these formulas have been promoted for use in infants with colic, this indication remains in question. They are more expensive and have no advantage over standard formula for feeding healthy term infants.

Soy formulas are based on soy protein isolates. Methionine is added to improve protein quality. They are all lactose-free and use sucrose, corn syrup solids, or a mixture of sucrose and corn syrup solids as the carbohydrate source. They use soy, oleo, coconut, and safflower oil in various combinations to resemble human milk fat. They are all cholesterol-free. All of these formulas are fortified with iron. Soy formulas have been improved over the last 60 years and are considered to be safe for normal infant feeding. There remains some concern regarding the effect of soy phytic acid and its effect on mineral and trace element absorption. For term infants who are advanced to solids at the usual time, there appear to be no adverse effects. However, soy formula is inappropriate for premature infants and children with digestive disorders, such as cystic fibrosis. Soy formulas are usually promoted as a substitute for cow milk formulas in potentially allergic infants, in primary and secondary lactase deficiency, and in galactosemia. Indications are clear-cut as far as carbohydrate intolerance and galactosemia are concerned; however, the proper management of the possibly allergic infant remains controversial. Of infants allergic to cow milk, 10 to 20% may also develop soy allergy. However, soy formula availability and cost continue to make it a reasonable initial alternative to cow milk formula in most situations. If not tolerated, a protein hydrolysate may be used.

### Formula Volume

Initially, infants should be offered 60 ml at each feeding. An appropriate frequency is every 2 to 3 hours. There is no particular advantage to a strict 4-hour schedule. Variability in infant temperament, as in the breast-fed baby, must be taken into account when considering feeding schedules. Most infants will gradually begin to skip night-time feedings and take larger amounts of formula during daytime hours. The exact volume of formula cannot be predicted because of variability in energy requirements. In general, infants will consume between 150 and 180 ml per kg per day. The adequacy of nutrition is monitored as for the breast-fed infant.

### Feeding Technique

The infant should be held for all feedings. Bottle propping and supine feeding should not be done. Burping may be attempted following 2 to 3 ounces of formula or if the infant seems uncomfortable. Some infants resent being interrupted and manifest their displeasure through crying. For these infants burping is best left to the end of the feeding. All babies reflux or "spit" to some degree. This is generally harmless and can be monitored for spontaneous resolution as long as growth remains normal and the baby is otherwise well.

### Formula Preparation

If desired, formula can be warmed; however, most infants show no preference. There have been reports of uneven warming with microwave ovens, and we prefer that they not be utilized. Formula temperature should always be tested prior to feeding. The traditional drop on the back of the wrist remains a satisfactory method.

Most municipal water supplies are safe, and water from these sources need not be boiled. All other water should be boiled. Nipples and bottles should be washed thoroughly in hot, soapy water with a bottle and nipple brush. Colored bottles, those representing cartoon characters, and those with uneven internal contours should be avoided. An automatic dishwasher may also be used to clean bottles. Details of formula preparation are readily available from formula manufacturers.

### EVAPORATED MILK

Evaporated milk formula has many disadvantages, including an excessive mineral and protein load and a high content of butter fat, which is more difficult to digest. The levels of linoleic and arachidonic acid may be inadequate, and vitamin C, vitamin E, and occasionally vitamin D must be provided from another source. Seamed cans, with improper handling, may be an inadvertent source of lead.

Nevertheless, an occasional parent may request an evaporated milk formula, and it must be recognized that many infants have been satisfactorily fed with these formulas. The traditional method of formulation is 13 ounces (standard size can) of evaporated milk with the addition of 1 to 1.5 cans (19 ounces) of water and two tablespoons of table sugar. Corn syrup was the traditional carbohydrate used, but recently it has been recommended that it be avoided because of the possible presence of *Clostridium botulinum* in corn syrup preparations.

### WHOLE MILK, SKIM MILK, AND 2% MILK

The feeding of unmodified whole milk during the first 6 months of infancy is inappropriate. Even when modified with boiling, dilution, and the addition of carbohydrate, it presents the same disadvantages of evaporated milk formula. Whole milk may be safe to use during the second 6 months, but some children will experience an unacceptable gastrointestinal occult blood loss. Whole milk is appropriate during the second year of life, but should be considered as a small part of a mixed diet and should not exceed 20% of the total caloric intake.

Skim milk does not allow adequate energy intake during infancy. Although growth may continue, it has been well demonstrated that energy stores are sacrificed. Two per cent milk has not been as well studied, but it appears best to avoid low-fat milk during the first 2 years of life.

Various companies have marketed follow-up formulas. No advantage to these formulas over standard infant formula and the usual introduction of solid foods has been demonstrated.

### INTRODUCTION OF SOLIDS

There are several indications that an infant is ready for the introduction of solids. The child should in some way be able to indicate when hungry, demonstrate satiety, or refuse further food. The infant should be able to sit readily with minimal support and participate actively in feeding. Food should be received with a spoon and be efficiently moved from the front of the mouth to the hypopharynx. In most infants, these requirements are not met until 4 to 6 months of age. Although solids can be introduced earlier, with difficulty, there is no advantage in doing so. As long as adequate growth is maintained, the breast-feeding infant may nurse exclusively well into the second half of the first year of life. Cow milk- and soy-based formulas also appear adequate for 6 months. Some prefer a somewhat earlier introduction of solids, at around 4 months, in conjunction with soy formula, because of concern about its nutritional adequacy. Cereal is often added to formula in an attempt to induce night-time sleeping. Sleeping at longer intervals during the night is a complex behavioral event and is poorly understood. However, the use of solids to achieve that goal has not been shown to alter sleeping behavior. Moreover, as has been observed by Foman, use of food to induce sleepiness and the early use of widely spaced feedings may not be in the best interest of the infant. Decreased glucose tolerance and increased serum cholesterol have been observed with infrequent feeding of large amounts of food.

After 6 months of age, the order of introduction of solid foods is not of critical importance. Rice cereal is usually introduced first because of its low cost, convenience, low antigenicity, fortification with iron, and easy digestibility. We prefer the avoidance of gluten containing cereal (wheat, rye, oats, barley) until 9 months of age. The risk of gluten-sensitive enteropathy may be lessened or the effects delayed. Otherwise, the traditional method of adding a single-ingredient food at intervals of 5 to 7 days seems to work well. It makes little difference if fruits or vegetables are introduced first. They may be added in an alternate fashion. There is no urgency in the introduction of meats, since formula and breast milk provide high-quality protein.

Traditional concerns about allergic potential or food intolerance have led many pediatricians to recommend caution in the introduction of milk products, egg white, wheat, semolina, buckwheat, rhubarb, corn, peanuts and other nuts, cocoa, fish and shellfish, oranges and other citrus fruits, pork, berries, and tomatoes. Since true immunoglobulin E (IgE)–mediated allergy has been documented with consumption of many of these foods, these concerns seem reasonable and we recommend that introduction be delayed until the infant is 9 months of age.

Cucumbers, onions, cabbage, and broccoli are also usually avoided during the first year of life because they are considered difficult to digest.

Home-prepared spinach, beets, and collard greens should be avoided in the young infant, because they may contain sufficient nitrite to cause methemoglobinemia.

Foods such as uncut hot dogs, nuts (especially peanuts), grapes, raw carrots, and round candies must be avoided throughout early childhood because of the potential danger of aspiration. Otherwise, home preparation of infant food is perfectly acceptable if done properly. However, commercially available pureed food has greatly improved over the past several years and, with a few exceptions, can be recommended. The elaborate phase systems marketed by some manufacturers are overdone and needlessly complicated, but are otherwise harmless. Glass containers are safe and nutrient information is available on labels. Dehydrated baby food has recently been marketed and is a safe and acceptable form of pureed food. Desserts are totally unnecessary, and mixed dinners provide less nutritional value per dollar than does simply mixing meats and vegetables.

During the second 6 months, foods of increasing texture may be tolerated as the child becomes more adept at feeding himself with fingers and spoon. By the second year, the child should be able to drink from a cup and eat a modified table food diet. Various toddlers' foods may be continued for the parents' convenience.

Originally, fruit juices were fed to infants as a source of vitamin C. This is no longer necessary, but juice may be added in the second 6 months to provide variety in the diet. It is best to offer juice in a cup, as juice containing bottles may promote caries. There has been considerable concern about daminazide in apple juice, but all commercially available infant apple juice is daminazide-free. Fruit drinks should be avoided, and those in seamed cans may be contaminated with lead.

## VITAMINS AND MINERALS

The formula-fed infant obtains all necessary vitamins and need not have additional supplementation. We strongly recommend iron-fortified formula. Several studies have demonstrated no adverse effects from iron fortification. Conversely, the benefits from iron fortification have been well documented.

The use of iron supplementation in the breast-fed infant is more controversial. In general, an exclusively breast-fed term infant will not need iron supplementation. However, other foods interfere with breast milk iron absorption, so when possible, they should be iron fortified. Newborn iron stores exist mainly in circulating hemoglobin. Therefore, low-birthweight infants or any infant who has had blood loss will require additional iron. The addition of 7 mg per day of elemental iron will usually suffice.

Breast milk is low in vitamin K and puts the nursing infant at risk for hemorrhagic disease of the newborn. It is efficient and safe for all newborn infants to receive 1 mg of natural vitamin K at birth.

The vitamin D content of human milk is low—about 22 IU per liter—and rickets has been reported in nursing infants. However, this is extremely rare and has usually been associated with nontraditional or unusual lifestyles, including deficient diets and inadequate sun exposure for both mother and infant. During winter in northern climates, particularly for dark-skinned infants, vitamin D supplementation is recommended. Otherwise, the healthy term infant needs no supplemental vitamin D. Ready-to-feed and liquid concentrations of formula are uniformly low in fluoride—approximately 0.1 mg fluoride per kg in the final product. If the community water supply is fluoridated and used in formula preparation, other fluoride supplementation should not be used. Even with ready-to-feed formula, in a community with fluoridated water, there is evidence that adequate fluoride is obtained from other sources. With nonfluoridated water supplies, infants should receive 0.25 mg of fluoride daily. There are different opinions about the need for supplemental fluoride in the nursing infant. Supplement is probably not necessary in communities with fluoridated water supplies, but should be given otherwise. Fluoride supplementation is also advisable, at a dose of 0.25 mg daily, if exclusive breast-feeding is continued beyond 6 months of age.

# DISEASES OF THE BREAST

method of
D. L. WICKERHAM, M.D., and
NORMAN WOLMARK, M.D.
*University of Pittsburgh*
*Pittsburgh, Pennsylvania*

The visible breast extends from the second or third rib to the sixth or seventh costal cartilage and from the sternal border to the anterior axillary line. The extension of the breast tissue into the axilla (the tail of the breast) is common and may be visible. Accessory breast tissue and nipples may occur anywhere along the embryologic milk line. Normal breast development begins at the time of puberty. The initial sign of this development is often a tender nubbin of breast tissue in the subareolar area. This is frequently unilateral and should not be biopsied, as this may remove the entire developing breast. Significant breast development in a child prior to puberty with or without other signs of sexual development should be referred for endocrinologic evaluation.

True amastia is rare. Hypoplasia of the breast may be associated with congenital absence of the pectoral muscle or bony deformities of the thorax. More common is an asymmetrical development of the breast. In adolescents, this is best treated by observation alone, and over time the magnitude of any difference frequently diminishes.

## NEOPLASTIC DISEASES

### Screening

Breast cancer is the most common life-threatening malignancy in adult women in the United States. It is estimated that over 140,000 new cases will be diagnosed this year. It has been contended that the most effective method of decreasing the mortality from breast cancer is the detection of the disease at an early stage. Although not definitive, several large-scale, randomized clinical trials using mammograms and physical examination have demonstrated as much as a one-third reduction in the mortality rate from breast cancer in the screened populations. The National Cancer Institute recommends yearly screening for women 50 years of age and older. For women 40 to 49 years of age, annual or biennial examinations are suggested, depending on the specific risk factors of that particular patient. The American Cancer Society has advocated a baseline examination sometime between the age of 35 and 40. Breast self-examination on a monthly basis beginning at age 20 is also encouraged, although its benefit in mortality reduction is not established.

### Benign Lesions

Tender nodular breast tissue that increases in prominence during the luteal phase of the menstrual cycle is often inappropriately referred to as fibrocystic disease of the breast. This is a nonspecific term, is not a risk factor for the development of breast cancer, and the use of the term to describe *clinical* findings would probably be best avoided altogether. Breast pain (mastodynia) is very common in premenopausal women and is most often cyclical. Although in a rare patient the pain may be incapacitating, most women can tolerate the discomfort if they are reassured that it is not a symptom of cancer or other serious disease. Therapy with low-salt, low-caffeine diets supplemented by prostaglandin inhibitors has provided inconsistent results. In severe cases, suppressing ovarian function with medications, such as Danazol (Danocrine), is thought to be effective. However, the medication is expensive, causes virilization, and is occasionally hepatotoxic. In the majority of patients, breast pain resolves completely after menopause, but may continue if estrogen replacement therapy is prescribed.

Mammary epithelial hyperplasia is a *histologic* diagnosis of benign disease that is associated with a one- to twofold increased risk of subsequent invasive breast cancer. If this hyperplasia has atypical features present, the risk elevation is four to five times that of the general population.

Gross cysts of the breasts become common in women in their late thirties and forties. They are uncommon in women after menopause except for patients on estrogen replacement therapy. Without other histologic abnormalities, cysts do not carry an increased risk of subsequent breast cancer. Cysts are easily diagnosed by needle aspiration or sonography. Biopsy of the cyst should be considered even if the cytology is benign, if the mass does not fully resolve or recurs, or if the aspirated fluid is bloody.

The most common breast tumor in teenagers and women in their twenties is a fibroadenoma. These masses are firm, smooth-bordered, well-demarcated, nontender, mobile lesions. Because breast cancer is rare under the age of 25, these lesions may be followed over time. A fine-needle aspiration cytology at the initial evaluation is also appropriate. Mammograms in young women do not aid in the evaluation of fibroadenomas because the breast tissue is so dense. Most of these lesions are slow growing and may well involute over time. Should an enlargement be noted, the putative fibroadenoma should be excised.

Bilateral nonbloody nipple discharge from multiple ducts is associated with benign duct ectasia or medications, such as tricyclic antidepressants and some antihypertensive medications. Benign intraductal papillomas may cause a unilateral nipple discharge that may be from a single duct and that is often spontaneous. The discharge may be clear, serous, or bloody. Cytologic examination of the fluid is indicated, but excision of the subareolar major duct system may be required to exclude a breast cancer even if the cytology is benign or acellular. A serum prolactin level should be obtained in women with galactorrhea if they have not breast-fed within the last 5 years. If the prolactin level is elevated, further evaluation for a tumor of the pituitary is indicated.

### Noninvasive Carcinoma

The incidence of noninvasive intraductal carcinoma—ductal carcinoma in situ—appears to be on the rise, perhaps due to the increasing use of screening mammograms. In the past, the standard treatment for this disease was simple mastectomy with or without an axillary dissection. The concern was that biopsy without mastectomy resulted in a 10-year risk of subsequent ipsilateral invasive cancer, which ranged from 20 to 50%. These data were obtained from small retrospective series of patients in whom the tumors were palpable at the time of presentation. The natural history of intraductal cancers detected by mammogram alone is not known and may be quite different from data published in the older literature. An increasing trend is to treat such minimal intraductal cancers with lumpectomy with or without axillary dissection and with or without radiation therapy. A current National Surgical Adjuvant Breast Project (NSABP) trial is evaluating lumpectomy in this disease and will determine if radiation is of benefit in reducing risk of ipsilateral breast tumor recurrence.

Lobular carcinoma in situ is also called lobular neoplasia. It is not considered a malignancy or even a precursor of cancer by some authors. It does appear to be a marker of an increased risk of subsequent carcinoma (25% at 20 years). The risk is bilateral and the subsequent invasive cancer may be of lobular or ductal origin. The treatment is surgical but the extent of the procedure varies from bilateral mastectomies to local excision. The latter is becoming more frequently performed, but requires follow-up examinations two to four times per year and annual mammograms.

### Invasive Carcinoma

Invasive carcinomas arise from both the lobular and ductal components of breast tissue. Approximately 85% of these cancers are infiltrating ductal; 10% are infiltrating lobular; and the remaining 5% include medullary, mucinous, tubular, and adenoid cystic carcinomas. The standard diagnostic technique remains excisional biopsy. Fine-needle aspiration cytology of palpable masses is a simple, accurate technique that is being used more frequently. Nonpalpable lesions detected mammographically require needle localization prior to operative excision. Stereotactic aspiration cytology for nonpalpable lesions is performed routinely in Europe, and several centers in North America have begun to use this technique.

Once a diagnosis is obtained, the surgical options may be discussed with the patient and her family to allow informed decisions to be made.

The treatment options and the local management of invasive breast cancer range from radical mastectomy to lumpectomy and axillary node dissection followed by radiation therapy. True radical mastectomy is performed in less than 2% of cases each year in the United States and is generally limited to patients with locally advanced tumors in which the pectoral muscle(s) have been invaded. Modified radical mastectomy—total mastectomy plus axillary dissection—remains the most common procedure and allows for the option of breast reconstruction either immediately or at a delayed time. Based largely on the results of NSABP protocol B–06, which demonstrated that the survival of patients with lumpectomy—including axillary dissection—and radiotherapy was the same as patients with modified radical mastectomy, an increasing number of breast conserving procedures are being performed. In June 1990, the NIH Consensus

Development Conference on the Treatment of Early Stage Breast Cancer concluded that breast conservation treatment is an appropriate method of primary therapy for the majority of women with Stage I and II breast cancer, and is preferable because it provides survival equivalent to that of total mastectomy and axillary dissection while preserving the breast. Current NSABP guidelines for lumpectomy include (1) tumor less than or equal to 5 cm clinically, (2) clinical Stage I or Stage II, (3) free margins histologically, and (4) breasts of sufficient size to allow a satisfactory cosmetic outcome. At present, outside of clinical trials, breast radiation following lumpectomy is recommended regardless of tumor size. A radiation boost to the tumor bed is frequently performed, but its benefit has not been established.

### Prognosis

The traditional clinical tumor, nodes, and metastases (TNM) staging of breast cancer allows a standardized characterization of the extent of a patient's tumor and a generalization of prognosis. Five-year survival rates are as follows: In situ, greater than 95%; Stage I (clinically negative axillary nodes), 85%; stage II (clinically involved axillary nodes), 66%; stage III (locally advanced disease), 41%; stage IV (metastases), 10%. With additional staging procedures, a more precise assessment of prognosis is possible. The presence or absence of histologic nodal involvement and the number of nodes involved remain the most accurate predictors of outcome. Within nodal categories, tumor size, histologic grade, and hormonal receptor status are also of prognostic importance. Additional new markers, including flow cytometry evaluation of DNA content and S-phase percentage, amplification of oncogenes, epidermal growth factor receptor, and cathepsin D, have been reported by some investigators to be of value in predicting prognosis.

### Adjuvant Therapy

Only 50% of patients with operable breast cancer will be cured by the resection of the tumor. The goal of systemic adjuvant therapy is to reduce the risk of tumor recurrence and improve overall survival. Because the risk of recurrence is greatest in patients with node-positive tumors, the initial trials were conducted in this group. Numerous studies comparing various therapies with untreated controls have shown improved disease-free survival and survival for the patients receiving treatment. The magnitude of benefit is greatest in premenopausal women. In 1985, the NIH Consensus Conference on Adjuvant Chemother-

apy for Breast Cancer recommended the routine use of combination chemotherapy for node-positive premenopausal women. Standard combinations include cyclophosphamide (cytoxan), methotrexate, and 5-FU (CMF); cyclophosphamide, methotrexate, 5-fluorouracil, vincristine (Oncovin) and prednisone (CMFVP); and 5-fluorouracil, doxorubicin (Adriamycin), and cyclophosphamide (FAC), which are given for up to 12 months. The same Consensus Conference recommended that postmenopausal, node-positive, estrogen receptor (ER)–positive women can be treated with the oral antiestrogen tamoxifen (Nolvadex). It was thought that ER-negative, node-positive postmenopausal women should be considered for adjuvant chemotherapy but that it was not a routine recommendation. Since that conference, increasing evidence has demonstrated that combination chemotherapy with or without tamoxifen is superior to tamoxifen alone in this population of postmenopausal women.

Because patients with node-negative breast cancer were considered to have a "good prognosis," systemic adjuvant therapy was not initially tested in this group. The results of four randomized, large-scale clinical trials have recently demonstrated an improvement in disease-free survival at 3 to 5 years of follow-up. ER-negative patients received combination chemotherapy, and ER-positive, node-negative women received tamoxifen. Controversy remains over routinely recommending such therapies, due to the lack of a survival benefit, the small magnitude of benefit demonstrated, the toxicity incurred, and the cost of such therapy.

The optimal adjuvant therapy for node-negative and node-positive patients has yet to be determined. It is appropriate for all patients to be considered for entry into ongoing clinical trials to improve the therapy of this disease.

### Posttherapy Follow-up

Regardless of the initial local and systemic care, structured follow-up examinations and testing are a vital part of the care of all breast cancer patients. Patients should be seen by a physician every 3 months for the first 2 to 3 years and every 6 months until year 10, at which time yearly examinations should be conducted. Mammograms should be obtained yearly and chest x-rays obtained once per year until the fifth year. Blood counts, liver function studies, serum calcium, and alkaline phosphatase should be obtained at least twice a year. Bone scans and other scans are not routinely required unless symptoms or biochemical abnormalities are apparent. A careful history eliciting symptoms of recurrence is of paramount importance.

## Locally Advanced Cancer

Patients with large, bulky tumors are increasingly being treated, first with combination chemotherapy even if their tumors are technically resectable at the time of presentation. Most combinations include doxorubicin (Adriamycin). Depending on the magnitude of response, the sequence of subsequent care may be surgery followed by radiation therapy with or without additional chemotherapy. Radiation alone (without surgery) may be considered for those patients who have had a complete response to chemotherapy. Inflammatory carcinoma occurs in 1 to 4% of patients and is the result of tumor involving dermal lymphatics causing erythema, swelling, and peau d'orange (skin edema) of the breast. Combination chemotherapy is the standard treatment, again followed by operation or radiation therapy, depending on the tumor response to chemotherapy.

## Recurrent Breast Cancer

Localized chest wall recurrence following mastectomy is felt by many to be a marker of subsequent systemic disease. A complete metastatic evaluation is appropriate to rule out detectable disease elsewhere in the body. After the treatment of the recurrence by excision or radiotherapy, or both, consideration of systemic therapy may be appropriate.

Ipsilateral breast recurrence following lumpectomy and radiation therapy is not thought to have the same ominous significance as does a chest wall recurrence. Mastectomy is an effective treatment for the vast majority of such patients; however, increasingly, re-excision (relumpectomy) is performed when a satisfactory cosmetic result can be achieved. The benefit of systemic therapies following ipsilateral breast tumor recurrence is not known.

## Systemic Recurrence

Whenever possible, histologic or cytologic confirmation of the recurrence should be obtained. Hormone receptors should be determined on excised tumor tissue. Therapy remains largely palliative, and survival benefits have not been clearly demonstrated. However, long survival times with good quality of life are possible. Hormone-responsive tumors are treated initially with endocrine therapies, including tamoxifen, megestrol acetate (Megace), medroxyprogesterone (Provera), aminoglutethimide (Cytadren), and oophorectomy. Combination chemotherapy is given to patients with tumors that are hormone independent or at the time of tumor progression in patients initially treated with endocrine therapies. Chemotherapy may also be given to ER-positive tumors when the recurrence becomes life-threatening, for instance, in the event of lymphangitic spread to the lung or liver metastases.

# ENDOMETRIOSIS

method of
W. PAUL DMOWSKI, M.D., PH.D., and
CARLOS ROTMAN, M.D.
*Institute for the Study and Treatment of
Endometriosis and Rush Medical College
Chicago, Illinois*

Endometriosis traditionally has been considered a gynecologic disorder limited to the female reproductive system and only occasionally spreading to the other organs. This concept has been challenged recently by reports that suggest systemic changes and involvement of the immune system. Furthermore, the presenting symptoms of endometriosis may originate from outside of the reproductive system and the lesions may not be limited to the female pelvis (e.g., catamenial hemoptysis and pneumo- or hemothorax in pulmonary endometriosis). In such circumstances, pelvic endometriosis may or may not be present and if present, may be asymptomatic. Endometriosis, therefore, may be a diagnostic and therapeutic challenge to physicians treating women between menarche and menopause.

**Definition.** The disease is characterized by ectopic (i.e., outside of the uterus) growth and function of the endometrial cells.

**Pathogenesis.** It is generally accepted that endometriosis begins with the retrograde transport through fallopian tubes of endometrial cells or fragments desquamated during the menstrual period (transplantation theory of Sampson). These cells (or tissue fragments) then implant, proliferate, and develop into characteristic endometriotic lesions under cyclic stimulation by the ovarian hormones. From the peritoneal cavity, endometriosis may spread through lymphatic and vascular channels into distant locations. It is also possible that endometrial cells may disseminate from the uterus through lymphatic or vascular channels, giving origin to endometriosis in the pelvic cavity, as well as in distant locations. The retrograde menstrual flow and dissemination of the endometrial fragments into the peritoneal cavity occur in women with, as well as without, endometriosis. It is unknown why endometriotic fragments implant in ectopic locations and develop into endometriosis in only some women. Recent studies indicate that this process may be under the control of the immune system and that endometriosis may be a result of an altered immune function.

**Incidence.** In the absence of noninvasive diagnostic techniques, true incidence of endometriosis is unknown. The prevalence of endometriosis among women of reproductive age is estimated as at least 2%.

**Risk Factors.** Women with shorter menstrual cycles (less than 27 days) and longer flow (greater than 7 days) are more than twice as likely to develop endometriosis than those with longer cycles and shorter flow. If a first-degree relative suffers from endometriosis, the prevalence of endometriosis is seven times higher and the disease more likely to be severe.

**Symptoms and Findings** (Table 1). Although pelvic pain syndrome is characteristic of endometriosis, any symptom that occurs during, or that is exacerbated by, menses should raise a suspicion. Similarly, any lesion, regardless how distant from the female pelvis, that increases in size or bleeds cyclically should be suspect of endometriosis.

**Laboratory Tests.** There are no laboratory tests diagnostic of endometriosis. Antiendometrial and antiphospholipid autoantibodies are present in about two-thirds of the patients, and CA–125 antigen is mildly elevated (10 to 60 U per ml). Ultrasound may demonstrate pelvic endometriomas.

**Diagnosis.** The diagnosis can only be confirmed by laparoscopy, laparotomy, or biopsy of a suspected lesion.

**Staging.** Endometriosis is staged according to the revised American Fertility Society Classification into Stages I to IV, depending on the extent and location of the lesions.

## TREATMENT

Several approaches to the treatment of endometriosis are currently available, and their advantages and disadvantages are outlined in Table 2. The specific selection should be based on individual indications and contraindications. Consideration should be given to the patient's age, type and intensity of symptoms, location and extent

TABLE 1. **Endometriosis: Symptoms and Findings**

**Symptoms***
1. Pelvic pain complex: dysmenorrhea, dyspareunia, pelvic pain, dysuria, painful defecation
2. Prostaglandin-related symptoms, such as diarrhea, nausea, vomiting, or general malaise occurring during menses
3. Bleeding abnormalities: premenstrual staining, menorrhagia or metrorrhagia, rectal bleeding, hematuria
4. Any pain symptom or abnormal bleeding of catamenial pattern
5. Infertility: primary or secondary; recurrent spontaneous abortions

**Findings**
1. Cul-de-sac: Exquisitely tender nodularities
2. Uterus: Fixed in retroversion
3. Adnexa: Enlargement, tenderness, fixation
4. Local swelling or hemorrhagic lesions of catamenial pattern
5. Ultrasound: characteristic, echogenic cysts

*Symptoms variable, not related to the extent of the disease.

of lesions, response to previous therapy if any, her family status, desire for fertility, and in infertile patients, the presence of other infertility factors. In discussing with the patient different therapeutic approaches, we like to present preferred and alternative methods as they apply in her individual situation. The patient then participates actively in the selection of treatment.

*Symptomatic management* is recommended in Stage I or II symptomatic endometriosis in a young woman not interested in pregnancy who would like to preserve her reproductive potential. It consists of (1) prostaglandin synthetase inhibitors administered on a time-contingent rather than pain-contingent basis, beginning 1 to 2 days before the onset of symptoms; (2) analgesics administered also on a time-contingent basis; (3) strongly progestational oral contraceptives administered cyclically; and (4) pain management, counseling, support, and patient education. The purpose of management is to alleviate symptoms and arrest progression of the disease.

*Medical management* is recommended in women with Stage I and II endometriosis who do not respond to symptomatic management, in Stage I and II endometriosis and infertility, and in stage III and IV endometriosis with or without post-treatment surgical intervention. A variety of hormonal preparations currently available for the management of endometriosis present a challenge to the physician but offer to the patient a chance for a more individualized approach. It should be kept in mind that there is no drug available to "eradicate" endometriotic lesions. Suppression of ovarian estradiol secretion is the mechanism of action for all therapeutic regimens. The degree and length of ovarian suppression determine, therefore, the effectiveness of the therapy. This can be easily monitored by the clinical response (development of amenorrhea and hypoestrogenic changes) as well as by the laboratory tests. Peripheral estradiol levels during treatment should be between 20 and 40 pg per ml and not above 60 pg per ml. In the absence of estrogenic stimulation, uterine and ectopic endometrium undergo atrophy and endometriosis resolves.

*Danazol-induced pseudomenopause* effectively suppresses the ovarian function and endometriosis. The drug binds to steroid receptors in a variety of tissues, inducing direct (at the ovarian level) and indirect (through pituitary gonadotropins) ovarian suppression. It is also possible that danazol binding to androgen and progesterone receptors in the endometrium as well as the effect on the immune system plays a role in the suppression of endometriosis. Danazol-induced ovarian suppression and resolution of endometriosis are optimal at the daily dose of 10 to 15 mg per kg

TABLE 2. **Endometriosis: Advantages and Disadvantages of Major Therapeutic Approaches**

| Treatment | Main Advantages | Main Disadvantages |
|---|---|---|
| Symptomatic | Control of symptoms and progression of the disease without alteration of the menstrual cycle | Variable effectiveness; progression of the disease may continue |
| Hormonal | Has effect on microfoci; simple; cost effective | Little or no effect on endometriomas and adhesions; long treatment; side effects and risks of hormones |
| Laparoscopic cautery or laser | Treatment at the time of diagnosis | No effect on microfoci; resection of endometriomas, and adhesions may be incomplete; complex equipment; potential risks; high surgical skills needed |
| Conservative surgery | Effect in severe disease with adhesions; short treatment | Requires microsurgical skills; no effect on microfoci; postoperative adhesions |
| Hormonal followed by conservative surgery | Effect on microfoci, endometriomas, and adhesions; facilitates and limits surgery; improves results | Long treatment; side effects of hormones; requires microsurgical skills; postoperative adhesions |
| Definitive surgery | The only treatment that is effective and prevents recurrence | Terminates reproductive function |

(about 800 mg per day), but less than adequate at lower doses (below 600 mg per day). Side effects of danazol can be categorized as hypoestrogenic, androgenic-anabolic, and general. The androgenic-anabolic side effects paradoxically appear to be more frequent and more intense at the lower dose of the drug, which is also less effective clinically. At the lower dose of danazol, ovarian steroidogenesis of estrogens and androgens continues. Androgens are then converted to testosterone. Free testosterone levels are increased because of decreased sex hormone binding globulin (SHBG) and displacement of testosterone from SHBG by danazol. Recent studies indicate that danazol can suppress autoantibodies against cell-derived antigens (i.e., phospholipids, histones, and polynucleotides), which are present in approximately 50% of women with endometriosis. Suppression of these autoantibodies may play a role in improved reproductive performance (improved fertility, decreased frequency of spontaneous miscarriages) after treatment.

*Gonadotropin releasing hormone agonist (GnRH-a)-induced medical hypophysectomy* is a new and promising alternative to danazol treatment. GnRH-a administered continuously downregulates GnRH receptors in the pituitary, resulting in follicle stimulating hormone (FSH) and luteinizing hormone (LH) suppression. In the absence of FSH and LH, ovarian steroidogenesis is suppressed and peripheral estradiol levels are in the menopausal range. There is probably no direct effect of GnRH-a on the ovary. The degree of ovarian suppression depends on the type, the route of administration, and the dose of the agonist, but in general is more profound than that induced with danazol. With suppression of the ovarian function prompt endometrial atrophy and resolution of endometriosis occur. Several GnRH-a agents have been clinically evaluated. Available for clinical use are intranasal nafarelin and leuprolide (Lupron) for daily subcutaneous or monthly depot injections. Buserelin and Zoladex (goserelin) may soon become available. Side effects of GnRH-a are primarily related to the hypoestrogenic state. Oversuppression with GnRH-a (estradiol levels below 20 pg per ml) may predispose to the increased calcium mobilization from the bones.

*Estrogen-progestogen–induced pseudopregnancy* is considered less effective in the management of endometriosis than the other regimens. Estrogen/progestogens bind to estradiol and progesterone receptors in the endometrium, inducing decidual rather than atrophic changes. They should be administered continuously, and the dose individually adjusted to maintain amenorrhea. Most effective are combination-type birth control pills with strongly progestational properties. In some patients, especially at the beginning of treatment, the symptoms of endometriosis may increase and endometriotic lesions may enlarge. Side effects of pseudopregnancy are the same as of birth control pills and potentially serious.

*Oral or parenteral progestogens* have inconsistent suppressive effect on the ovarian function. Acting synergistically with endogenous estrogens, they induce decidual changes in the endometrium similar to those observed with estrogen-progestogens. Clinically, they seem to be less effective than regimens inducing endometrial atrophy. Side effects of progestogens alone are fewer and better tolerated than estrogen-progestogen preparations. It should be kept in mind that absorption and metabolic clearance of long-acting, depot-type progestogens may be delayed for several years, interfering with the reproductive function.

*Laparoscopic laser vaporization or electrocoagulation* offers several advantages over medical therapy and conservative surgery. In most hands, this technique should be limited to Stage I and II endometriosis without large endometriomas or extensive adhesions. Laparoscopic surgery seems to be followed by fewer adhesions than laparotomy.

*Conservative surgery* is recommended in patients with Stage III and IV endometriosis when adhesive disease and endometriomas are present. It should be performed using microsurgical techniques, and all efforts should be concentrated on (1) complete resection of endometriotic lesions and (2) restoration of pelvic anatomy. Prevention of postoperative adhesions is of major concern. Adjuvants, such as dextran (Hyskon), dexamethasone (Decadron), and promethazine (Phenergan), administered intraperitoneally and intramuscularly after surgery, are of questionable value. Recently introduced, Interceed, an adhesion-preventing membrane, as well as similar products currently under investigation, may prove to be of value.

*Combined medical and surgical treatment* offers several advantages over conservative surgery alone in the management of advanced endometriosis. Hormonal suppression before treatment leads to the resolution of microfoci and small endometriotic lesions and may decrease the size of large endometriomas. The surgery is less extensive, and more ovarian tissue can be preserved. Furthermore, surgical procedures are facilitated by the decreased vascularity of the endometriotic lesions and a relative ischemia of the reproductive system secondary to ovarian suppression.

*Definitive surgery*—i.e., total abdominal hysterectomy and bilateral oophorectomy—is the only procedure that prevents recurrence. It should be reserved, however, only for older patients who have completed their families and have severe symptomatic disease. Estrogen replacement therapy in the dose equivalent to 0.625 mg of conjugated estrogens daily will not reactivate residual disease and will prevent metabolic changes associated with castration.

# DYSFUNCTIONAL UTERINE BLEEDING

method of
JEFFREY M. GOLDBERG, M.D., and
MOON H. KIM, M.D.
*Ohio State University Hospitals*
*Columbus, Ohio*

Dysfunctional uterine bleeding (DUB) accounts for approximately 85% of abnormal uterine bleeding. It results from anovulation with chronic unopposed estrogenic stimulation of the endometrium. Normally, sequential exposure to progesterone after ovulation serves to stabilize and limit proliferation of the endometrium as well as to effect a uniform endometrial slough with prostaglandin-induced vasoconstriction for hemostasis at menses. In chronic anovulation, the endometrium becomes thickened and friable with areas of breakdown causing bleeding. Continued estrogen-induced endometrial proliferation brings about repair of the raw surface but also leads to further breakdown and bleeding from other areas. Thus, DUB is characterized by periods of oligomenorrhea or amenorrhea punctuated by irregular episodes of bleeding that are very variable in interval, duration, and amount of flow. Also, the menstrual molimina commonly associated with ovulatory cycles—i.e., dysmenorrhea, breast tenderness and swelling, fluid retention, and emotional lability—are usually absent. As anovulation is more common at the extremes of reproductive life, DUB occurs most frequently at these times. Approximately 50% of patients with DUB are perimenopausal and another 20% are postmenarcheal.

## DIAGNOSIS

DUB is a diagnosis of exclusion. Other causes of abnormal bleeding that must be ruled out are listed in Table 1. It is helpful to categorize patients as adolescent, of reproductive age, and perimenopausal because the etiology and treatment of abnormal bleeding differ among these groups. Evaluation begins with a detailed menstrual and obstetric history and inquiry about

TABLE 1. **Causes of Abnormal Genital Bleeding**

**Dysfunctional uterine bleeding (DUB):** anovulation
**Pregnancy complications:** ectopic, threatened or incomplete abortion, retained secundines, placental polyp, hydatidiform mole
**Uterus:** submucosal myoma, polyp, endometritis, malignancy
**Cervix:** polyp, eversion, cervicitis, malignancy
**Vagina:** vaginitis (infectious and atrophic), foreign body, trauma, malignancy
**Vulva:** infection, trauma, benign and malignant neoplasias
**Extragenital lesions:** urethral caruncle, hemorrhoids
**Blood dyscrasia:** idiopathic thrombocytopenic purpura (ITP), von Willebrand's disease, leukemia
**Systemic disease:** hypothyroidism, cirrhosis, renal failure
**Iatrogenic:** sex steroids, anticoagulants, IUD
**Other:** luteal phase deficiency, persistent corpus luteum

systemic diseases, general bleeding tendencies, family history of bleeding disorders, and medication usage, especially sex steroids and anticoagulants. The general physical examination requires a thorough inspection of the entire perineum to diagnose vulvar, GI, and GU sources of bleeding. A vaginal speculum is inserted to confirm that the bleeding is of uterine origin and to exclude lesions of the vagina and cervix. A bimanual examination is performed to document uterine size, shape, and consistency; and the presence of adnexal masses.

In most cases the history and physical examination will greatly limit the differential diagnosis and lead to a logical and cost-efficient selection of laboratory tests to confirm the suspected etiologic factor(s). Useful tests and procedures that should be considered are listed in Table 2. A minimal laboratory evaluation includes a sensitive assay for β-hCG, a Pap smear, and a complete blood count (CBC). A clotting profile should be considered, particularly in adolescents with heavy bleeding, because up to 25% of these patients may have an underlying bleeding diathesis. A biphasic basal body temperature chart (BBT) and serum progesterone level greater than 3 ng/ml will establish that the patient is ovulatory. On the other hand, the finding of cervical mucus with preovulatory characteristics—i.e., copious, watery, good spinnbarkeit, and ferning during what should be the luteal phase—is a good office bioassay to support a diagnosis of anovulation. We advocate obtaining serum prolactin and thyroid stimulating hormone (TSH) levels, as hyperprolactinemia and hypothyroidism are easily correctable causes of anovulation. Pelvic ultrasonography is useful in confirming the clinical impression of uterine myomas and adnexal masses. An endometrial biopsy performed early in the bleeding episode may yield useful diagnostic information. It is indicated in all patients over 35 years of age or with chronic anovulation to exclude endometrial hyperplasia and adenocarcinoma resulting from prolonged unopposed estrogenic stimulation. Various in-office techniques are available. We prefer the Pipelle device (Unimar, Inc., Wilton, CT) because it is inexpensive and disposable, technically easy to use (no tenaculum is required in most cases), is better tolerated by the patients, and provides a good specimen for histologic examination. Approximately 25% of patients with a presumed diagnosis of DUB will have intrauterine pathology, such as a polyp or submucous myoma, which may be missed with endometrial sampling. Hysterographic or hysteroscopic examination of

the endometrial cavity is indicated when bleeding persists despite hormonal therapy or dilation and curettage (D&C), or both.

## TREATMENT

Treatment is individualized based on the patient's age, desire for contraception or fertility, and the severity and chronicity of the bleeding. The goals of treatment are to arrest the acute episode, prevent recurrences, provide cyclic withdrawal bleeding for prophylaxis against endometrial hyperplasia and adenocarcinoma, and induce ovulation in the infertile patient. In the face of uncontrollable profuse hemorrhage, rapidly insert an intravenous line and a Foley catheter; obtain blood for β-hCG, CBC with platelets and clotting studies, and a type and cross-match; and transfuse as needed. An operative D&C should be performed, as this is the quickest way to stop bleeding. It is effective in almost all cases except those due to blood dyscrasia, submucous myomas, and genital malignancy. If bleeding continues, one should consider hysteroscopy for diagnosis. Possible hysteroscopic resection of a myoma or endometrial ablation with various techniques (neodymium–yttrium aluminum garnet [YAG] laser or urologic resectoscope with or without "roller-ball" coagulation) may be done as indicated. Another technique that may be attempted is embolization of the hypogastric or uterine arteries by placing a catheter into the femoral artery in retrograde fashion under fluoroscopic guidance and injecting Gelfoam, Silastic beads, or autologous clot. Alternatively, surgical ligation of these vessels may reduce the arterial pressure enough to achieve hemostasis via normal clotting mechanisms. If these modalities are unsuccessful or unavailable, or if the patient does not desire future fertility, a hysterectomy can always be performed as a last resort.

For the acute bleeding episode that is heavy but not life-threatening, medical treatment should be offered. High-dose estrogen therapy, conjugated estrogens (Premarin), 2.5 mg orally every 6 hours, will bring about cessation of bleeding due to all causes of estrogen-progestin imbalances within 12 to 24 hours by stimulating rapid endometrial proliferation for healing. It has been shown to be as effective as Premarin, 25 mg intravenously every 4 hours. The same dose is continued for a total of 21 days with the addition of medroxyprogesterone acetate (Provera), 10 mg orally daily during the last 10 days to allow for a withdrawal bleed. Alternatively, an oral contraceptive pill (containing 50 μg of ethinyl estradiol) orally four times daily for 1 week may also be used, but it may not be as effective due to the antiestrogenic properties of the progestin. After

TABLE 2. **Evaluation of Dysfunctional Uterine Bleeding (DUB)**

Beta-human chorionic gonadotropin (Beta-hCG)
Complete blood count (CBC) ± platelet count, coagulation profile, iron studies
Papanicolaou's (Pap) smear
Basal body temperature (BBT) chart, serum progesterone
Serum prolactin
Thyroid function studies
Liver function studies
Endometrial biopsy
Hysterosalpingogram or hysteroscopy
Pelvic ultrasonography

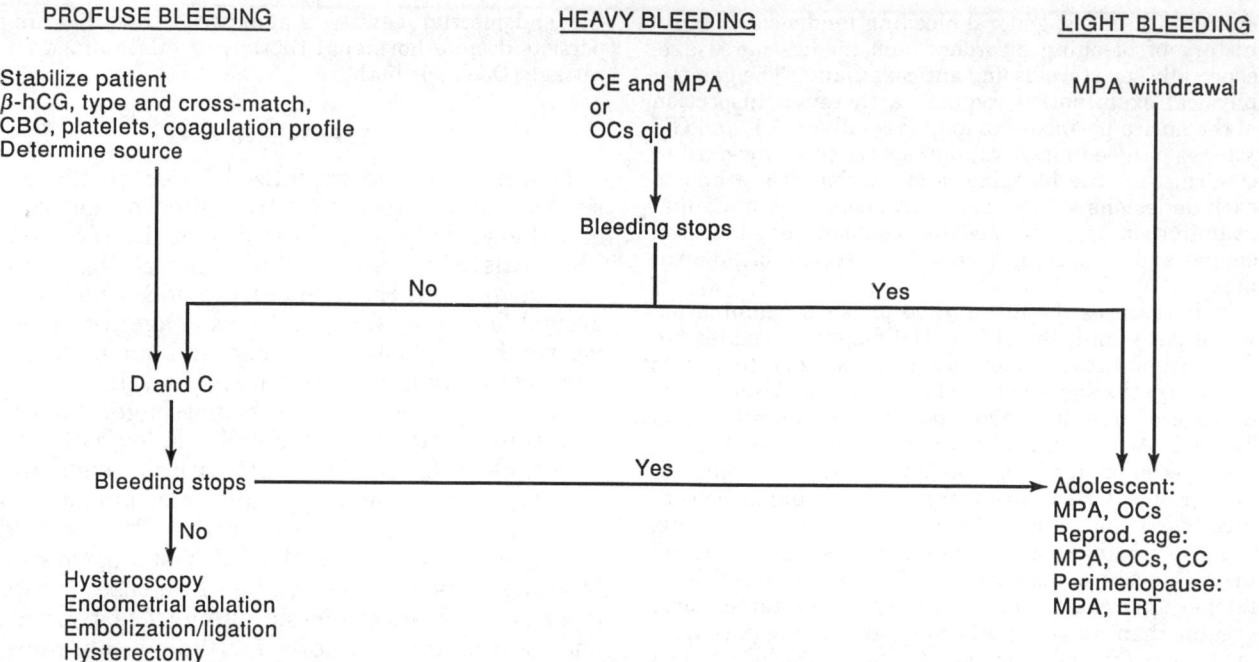

**Figure 1.** Treatment of dysfunctional uterine bleeding (DUB). *Abbreviations:* CE = conjugated estrogen; MPA = medroxy-progesterone acetate; OCs = oral contraceptives; CC = clomiphene citrate; ERT = estrogen replacement therapy.

this week the patient can be switched to a low-dose oral contraceptive pill in cyclic fashion for a minimum of three cycles. Unlike the long-term use of pharmacologic doses of estrogens, the acute administration does not elicit any alterations in the hemostatic mechanism. If hormonal therapy is unsuccessful a D&C with or without hysteroscopy is indicated. One should be aware that high-dose estrogen therapy and D&C, although usually effective in controlling the acute episode, do not correct the underlying problem and if untreated recurrent episodes should be anticipated.

Several options are available after the acute episode has been resolved and for patients with mild to moderate bleeding. Observation only is a reasonable approach for adolescents without anemia, as regular ovulatory cycles should ensue in most cases within 2 years. When treatment is necessary in the adolescent who is not sexually active, Provera, 10 mg orally daily for 10 days every 1 to 2 months, is preferred because it will not delay hypothalamic maturation as oral contraceptives may. However, if the patient is sexually active oral contraceptives should be offered. Oral contraceptives are also a good choice for the reproductive-age woman who requires contraception. In addition, they will also help to reduce the elevated circulating androgen levels in patients with anovulation as part of the polycystic ovarian syndrome. If the patient does not want or has a contraindication to oral contraceptives, she can also be managed with cyclic medroxypro-gesterone (Provera) to provide regular withdrawal bleeding. When fertility is desired, ovulation induction is indicated, with clomiphene citrate (Clomid) being the first line of therapy. Finally, the perimenopausal patient can be maintained on cyclic medroxyprogesterone (Provera) until withdrawal bleeding ceases to occur, at which time she can be switched to a standard regimen for estrogen replacement therapy (ERT). Alternatively, she can be managed with ERT initially. Endometrial biopsy is indicated for any unscheduled bleeding in these patients. A flow diagram of this management algorithm is presented in Figure 1.

# AMENORRHEA

method of
RANDALL BARNES, M.D.
*The University of Chicago*
*Chicago, Illinois*

Amenorrhea is usually defined as the absence of menses for 6 months in a previously normal menstruating woman. However, evaluation of amenorrhea is straightforward and relatively inexpensive and may be initiated before 6 months. One must realize that amenorrhea is one manifestation of anovulation, and pathologic processes causing anovulation may result in oligomenorrhea as well as amenorrhea. Patients whose menstrual cycles are 35 days or longer are often anovulatory and should be evaluated, unless they are perimenarcheal or perimenopausal.

Amenorrhea may be categorized as primary or secondary. Primary amenorrhea is defined as the failure to menstruate spontaneously by age 16, or the absence of breast development by age 14. Primary amenorrhea can be a great diagnostic challenge. I limit this discussion for the most part to the evaluation and treatment of secondary amenorrhea, as it is much more commonly encountered and the principles of therapy are similar for both primary and secondary amenorrhea.

## EVALUATION

Rational therapy of amenorrhea requires adequate diagnostic evaluation. The most common cause of amenorrhea in reproductive-aged women is pregnancy. The newer generation urinary pregnancy tests can detect human chorionic gonadotropin (hCG) at levels of 25 mIU per ml and are a rapid, reliable test to exclude pregnancy.

Amenorrhea may be associated with chronic illness. Because it is most unusual for debilitating illness to present as amenorrhea, and because the appropriate therapy is that directed at the specific disease, no further consideration will be given here to the amenorrhea of chronic disease.

Amenorrhea is not uncommon while taking oral contraceptive pills because the progestin component of the pill induces endometrial atrophy. It is not necessary to prescribe a higher dose estrogen pill simply to re-establish withdrawal bleeding. One should only reassure the patient that she need not worry about pregnancy in the absence of withdrawal bleeding, if the pill is taken faithfully.

Once pregnancy is excluded as a cause of the condition, one should measure prolactin and follicle stimulating hormone (FSH) in all patients with oligomenorrhea or amenorrhea. One should also measure total testosterone, free testosterone, and dehydroepiandrosterone sulfate (DHAS) if hirsutism or acne is present. If amenorrhea is present, one should give a progesterone challenge to determine estrogen status: progesterone in oil, 200 mg intramuscularly, or medroxyprogesterone acetate (Provera), 10 mg orally per day for 5 days, may be used. Any vaginal bleeding within 2 weeks is a positive test and indicates that estrogen levels are adequate.

If FSH is elevated in a woman age 40 or younger, the diagnosis is premature ovarian failure. Premature ovarian failure may be preceded by a "premature perimenopause," and a positive progesterone challenge test may occur during the transition to the menopausal state.

A negative progesterone challenge test and a normal or low FSH suggest hypothalamic-pituitary failure (hypogonadotropic hypogonadism). One may measure serum estradiol to confirm the hypoestrogenic state. If the estradiol is normal or the history is suggestive of Asherman's syndrome, a hysterosalpingogram or hysteroscopy is necessary to determine if intrauterine adhesions are present; otherwise, the diagnosis is hypothalamic-pituitary failure. These patients require computed tomography or magnetic resonance imaging of the pituitary and hypothalamus to rule out a mass lesion.

If the radiologic studies are negative, the hypothalamic-pituitary failure is almost certainly due to suppression of the hypothalamic gonadotropin-releasing hormone (GnRH) pulse generator. GnRH is secreted by the hypothalamus in pulses about every 60 to 90 minutes in follicular phase women. This in turn results in luteinizing hormone (LH) pulses in the peripheral blood occurring with the same frequency. Women with hypothalamic-pituitary failure have few if any measurable LH pulses, suggesting suppression of GnRH release. This may occur with weight loss, stress, or strenuous exercise, or it may be idiopathic.

In women without androgen excess if the progesterone challenge test is positive and the prolactin level is normal, the diagnosis is hypothalamic-pituitary dysfunction. These patients may be regarded as being intermediate between normal ovulatory function and hypothalamic-pituitary failure. GnRH pulses are frequent enough that some gonadotropin secretion occurs, resulting in follicular development and estrogen secretion, but not in ovulation. The cause may be weight loss, stress, exercise, or idiopathic.

In a patient with hyperprolactinemia, a careful drug history is important. Pituitary prolactin secretion appears to be under tonic hypothalamic dopamine inhibition. Drugs that are dopamine antagonists, such as phenothiazines; dopamine synthesis inhibitors, such as α-methyldopa (Aldomet); or drugs that affect dopamine release or re-uptake, such as reserpine or tricyclic antidepressants, may cause hyperprolactinemia. One should measure thyroid stimulating hormone (TSH) in all women with hyperprolactinemia to rule out hypothyroidism. If the drug history is negative and if TSH is normal, patients should have computed tomography or magnetic resonance imaging of the pituitary and hypothalamus to rule out a pituitary adenoma or hypothalamic lesion.

In women with androgen excess, a serum testosterone level greater than 200 ng per dl is suspicious for a tumor. A DHAS level greater than 6 μg per ml suggests an adrenal tumor. If the testosterone alone is elevated, an ovarian tumor is more likely. One should carefully evaluate the patient's history and physical examination together with serum androgen levels when considering the diagnosis of tumor. An abrupt onset of rapidly worsening symptoms at a time distinct from menarche is more typical of an androgen secreting tumor. A long history of stable or gradually worsening symptoms with a perimenarcheal onset is typical of polycystic ovary syndrome (PCOS) or "late-onset" 21-hydroxylase deficiency. Acne and hirsutism may be present in patients with or without an androgen secreting tumor. However, breast atrophy, voice changes, increase in upper body muscle mass, and clitoromegaly suggest severe androgen excess and a tumor.

Androgen secreting ovarian tumors are usually palpable in reproductive-aged women. Transvaginal ultrasound can demonstrate small ovarian tumors and is a valuable diagnostic test in women suspected of having a nonpalpable tumor. If one suspects an adrenal tumor, a computed tomography or magnetic resonance imaging of the adrenal should be done.

The great majority of women with androgen excess

will have only mild elevations of testosterone and no evidence of tumor. In these patients one must distinguish between adrenal and ovarian causes of androgen excess. This is best accomplished by measuring testosterone and free testosterone before and after dexamethasone suppression of adrenal androgen secretion. If testosterone levels do not suppress to normal, the diagnosis is PCOS. If testosterone levels fall into the normal range after 4 days of dexamethasone 0.5 mg four times a day, the source of androgen excess is the adrenal. An ACTH test can then be performed after giving 1 mg of dexamethasone the night before. Cortisol and 17-hydroxyprogesterone are measured basally and 1 hour after 250 μg of ACTH. A basally suppressed cortisol level (less than 5 μg per dl) rules out Cushing's syndrome. A rise of 17-hydroxyprogesterone to greater than 10 ng per ml is diagnostic of 21-hydroxylase deficiency.

## THERAPY

Ideally one should treat amenorrhea by treating the underlying disease process. In cases of hypothalamic-pituitary failure or dysfunction caused by stress, exercise, or weight loss, it is sometimes possible for the patient to alter her lifestyle or habits and become eumenorrheic. In obese women with PCOS, weight loss may result in the return of ovulation and resolution of androgen excess. Hysteroscopic lysis of intrauterine adhesions is the treatment for Asherman's syndrome.

In the majority of cases of amenorrhea, the underlying cause is unknown, not amenable to therapy, or the patient is unwilling or unable to modify her behavior. One must then treat the specific problem or potential problem associated with the amenorrhea. Almost all patients with amenorrhea require at least one of the following therapies at one time or another: (1) progestin therapy to prevent endometrial hyperplasia; (2) estrogen replacement therapy to prevent short- and long-term sequelae of hypoestrogenism; (3) ovulation induction for infertility; (4) treatment of hirsutism.

### Progestin Therapy

Women with amenorrhea who have withdrawal bleeding after progesterone challenge have endogenous estrogen production adequate to stimulate endometrial growth. These patients require periodic progestin withdrawal to prevent endometrial hyperplasia and carcinoma. This is particularly important in women with PCOS, who have normal estradiol levels and elevated estrone levels that result in relatively high total estrogen levels. In general, 5 mg of medroxyprogesterone or its equivalent should be used for at least 13 days of every other month.

Spontaneous menses during the progestin-free month suggests return of ovulatory function. If menses occur, one should measure serum progesterone on about cycle day 21. A progesterone level greater than 3 ng per ml confirms ovulation and suggests that progestin therapy is no longer needed. In women with hypothalamic-pituitary dysfunction or hyperprolactinemia, no withdrawal bleeding after progestin therapy suggests that the patient has become hypoestrogenic. Such patients may require further evaluation (FSH, prolactin, radiologic studies) and possible estrogen replacement therapy.

The low-dose oral contraceptive pill (OCP) may be a better alternative than progestin therapy in women with hypothalamic dysfunction or PCOS who desire contraception but are unwilling to use barrier methods. In PCOS the OCP may also improve acne and hirsutism. It should not be used in women with hyperprolactinemia because the high estrogen content may stimulate growth of prolactinomas.

### Estrogen Replacement Therapy

Women with hypothalamic-pituitary failure or premature ovarian failure should receive estrogen replacement therapy. Estrogen replacement effectively treats immediate symptoms of hypoestrogenism, such as hot flashes and vaginal dryness. It decreases the long-term risk of osteoporosis, and good evidence exists, particularly in younger women, that physiologic replacement doses of estrogen decrease the risk of cardiovascular disease. Estrogen replacement therapy is also appropriate for hyperprolactinemic women who are hypoestrogenic and do not require or tolerate a dopamine agonist, such as bromocriptine. Estrogens should be restricted to women without a macroadenoma.

A commonly used estrogen replacement regimen is 0.625 mg of conjugated estrogens (Premarin) daily for the first 25 days of each month and 5 mg of medroxyprogesterone from the thirteenth to the twenty-fifth. Withdrawal bleeding usually occurs during the pill-free interval. In women who wish to avoid withdrawal bleeding, 0.625 mg of conjugated estrogens and 2.5 mg of medroxyprogesterone can be given daily. After 3 months of therapy, about 80% of women become amenorrheic on this regimen. A progestin should always be given with estrogen replacement therapy to prevent endometrial hyperplasia.

### Ovulation Induction

In anovulatory women with positive progestin withdrawal and without hyperprolactinemia, clomiphene citrate (Clomid, Serophene) is the drug of choice for ovulation induction. Clomiphene is an antiestrogen that blocks estrogen-negative feedback at the pituitary and the hypothalamus. This results in increased GnRH pulse frequency and increased pituitary secretion of FSH. Ovulation occurs in about 90% of women appropriately treated with clomiphene, and about one-half of those become pregnant within six ovulatory cycles.

The initial dose of clomiphene is 50 mg per day for 5 days, starting at day 3 of progestin-induced withdrawal bleeding. Patients ovulate about 7 days after taking the last pill. Couples without male factor infertility should have intercourse every other day from 5 days after the last clomiphene pill until a rise in the basal body temperature occurs. This avoids the use of expensive urinary LH surge detection kits to time ovulation. Serum progesterone should be measured 14 days after taking the last pill to confirm ovulation. If the serum progesterone is less than 10 ng per ml, the clomiphene dose in the next cycle should be increased by 50 mg per day to a maximum of 250 mg per day for 5 days. Once ovulation occurs, a postcoital test should be performed in a subsequent cycle to check the quality of cervical mucus, as it may be adversely affected by an antiestrogen, such as clomiphene. If cervical mucus is poor, intrauterine insemination should be performed, using washed sperm timed by a qualitative urinary LH kit.

One should monitor women requiring 200 or 250 mg of clomiphene daily with serial ultrasound measurement of follicular diameter and serial serum estradiol levels. When the maximum mean follicular diameter is 20 to 25 mm, give 10,000 U of human chorionic gonadotropin (hCG). Ovulation will occur about 36 hours later. To reduce the risk of ovarian hyperstimulation, do not give hCG if estradiol is greater than 2000 pg per ml.

In women with PCOS who do not respond to to the maximum dose of clomiphene citrate, serum DHAS should be measured. If DHAS is elevated, give 0.5 mg of dexamethasone daily for 2 weeks, induce withdrawal bleeding with a progestin, and then add 250 mg of clomiphene daily for 5 days. If DHAS is not elevated, adding dexamethasone to clomiphene is probably not helpful.

Human menopausal gonadotropin (hMG; Pergonal) is the appropriate agent for ovulation induction in women with hypothalamic-pituitary failure or in women who do not respond to clomiphene. hMG therapy is expensive, requires intensive monitoring, and carries the risk of ovarian hyperstimulation and multiple gestation. Only physicians specifically trained in its use should administer hMG.

One may begin hMG therapy at any time in women with hypothalamic-pituitary failure or begin day 3 after progestin withdrawal in women unresponsive to clomiphene. The usual starting dose is two 75-U ampules per day given intramuscularly. In women with PCOS, who are particularly at risk of ovarian hyperstimulation, begin with one ampule per day. hMG is given in the evening to allow for dosage adjustment based on that day's monitoring results.

After 4 days of hMG therapy, one should begin ultrasound and estradiol monitoring. hMG dose may be altered according to monitoring results. Monitoring is continued until the maximum mean follicular diameter is about 18 mm and the estradiol level is 1000 to 2000 pg per ml. Then 10,000 U of hCG is then given to induce ovulation, which occurs about 36 hours later. If numerous follicles are present or if estradiol is greater than 2000 pg per ml, do not give hCG, as the risks of hyperstimulation and multiple gestation are unacceptably high. Virtually all women with hypothalamic-pituitary failure ovulate with hMG and about 80% become pregnant in three or so cycles. About 80% of pregnancies are a single gestation, and of the 20% multiple gestation, about three-fourths are twins.

Two recent modifications of hMG therapy in PCOS have attracted wide interest. The first is the use of pure human FSH (hFSH; Metrodin) for ovulation induction in PCOS unresponsive to clomiphene. In PCOS, elevated endogenous serum LH levels stimulate theca cell androgen production; thus, pure hFSH has the theoretical advantage that no LH is administered to further stimulate ovarian androgen secretion. However, in clinical studies hFSH has no practical advantage over hMG. Ovarian response, incidence of hyperstimulation, and pregnancy rates are the same for hMG and hFSH in women with PCOS.

The second modification is to treat PCOS with GnRH agonists (GnRHa, Lupron) prior to ovarian stimulation with hMG. Two to 4 weeks of daily subcutaneous GnRHa injections result in a paradoxical down-regulation of the pituitary-ovarian axis. LH and FSH secretion are inhibited, and estradiol falls to menopausal levels. Ovarian androgen production is also effectively inhibited. Thus the hormonal milieu comes to resemble that of hypothalamic-pituitary failure. hMG therapy is then initiated while continuing GnRHa administration. It was hoped that a PCOS patient so treated would respond to hMG in a manner similar to hypothalamic-pituitary failure patients—i.e., a smooth response without hyperstimulation and a high pregnancy rate. Unfortunately, the PCOS ovary is still hyperresponsive to hMG after GnRHa treatment. However, pregnancy rates are probably improved because GnRHa treatment prevents premature pituitary secretion of LH in response to rising estradiol levels. Premature rises of LH, occurring before hCG injection, result in premature luteinization of the follicle and a dysmature ovum that is not fertilizable.

Pulsatile administration of GnRH by portable pump is an alternative to hMG therapy. GnRH may be administered by intravenous catheter or subcutaneous needle. Pulses of 5 to 25 µg are administered every 90 to 120 minutes, the subcutaneous route requiring higher pulse doses. GnRH cycles should be monitored by ultrasound and estradiol measurements. Spontaneous ovulation usually occurs after 10 to 20 days of GnRH. The pump can then be discontinued and 2500 U of hCG given every 5 days to support the corpus luteum. Almost all patients with hypothalamic-pituitary failure ovulate with GnRH therapy, and pregnancy rates are 60 to 75%. Although ovarian hyperstimulation and multiple gestation have been reported with GnRH use, the incidence is probably less than with hMG. However, the pump is inconvenient and there is much less experience with GnRH than with hMG for ovulation induction.

The drug of choice for ovulation induction in hyperprolactinemia is a dopamine agonist, such as bromocriptine (Parlodel). The starting dose is 2.5 mg given at bedtime to minimize side effects of nausea and orthostatic hypotension. The dose is continued for 2 weeks and the prolactin level checked. One should increase the dose in 2.5-mg increments as necessary until prolactin normalizes and ovulation occurs. Rarely doses of bromocriptine as high as 20 mg per day will not be sufficient to normalize prolactin levels. About 80% of women treated with bromocriptine achieve pregnancy. A sensitive urinary pregnancy test should be performed if menses are more than 2 days delayed or if the BBT is elevated more than 14 days. Although bromocriptine does not appear to increase the incidence of congenital malformation, women without radiologic abnormality or with a microadenoma should stop bromocriptine as soon as pregnancy is diagnosed. If a macroadenoma is present, one should continue bromocriptine throughout pregnancy to prevent tumor enlargement.

## Treatment of Hirsutism

Hirsutism, which is the excessive growth of androgen-sensitive hair in women, can be a socially disabling condition. The severity of hirsutism depends on both production of and sensitivity of the skin to androgens. Thus, it may be severe in women with only mild androgen excess.

In women with an androgen secreting tumor, removal of the tumor results in amelioration of hirsutism over a period of months. In women with mild degrees of hirsutism, mechanical or cosmetic measures such as plucking, bleaching, waxing, or electrolysis often provide effective control.

Many women will require medical therapy to adequately control hirsutism. If the site of excessive androgen production is clearly the adrenal, such as in "late-onset" 21-hydroxylase deficiency, low-dose corticosteroids effectively treat hirsutism and induce ovulation. In 21-hydroxylase deficiency, 5 to 10 mg of prednisone a day or its equivalent is usually sufficient to inhibit excess adrenal androgen and 17-hydroxyprogesterone production and still maintain adequate adrenal reserve.

In PCOS the ovary is the source of androgen excess and the preferred therapy is the OCP together with an androgen receptor antagonist. OCPs inhibit LH-dependent theca cell androgen production by suppressing pituitary LH secretion. The estrogen component of the pill increases serum sex hormone binding globulin, so that more testosterone is tightly protein bound and unable to diffuse into cells and exert a biologic effect. OCPs that contain norgestrel should not be used to treat hirsutism, because they do not increase sex hormone binding globulin levels. To treat hirsutism, give OCPs cyclically, as for contraception. The pill also provides contraception and prevents the possible feminization of a male embryo by concomitantly administered androgen antagonists.

The drug most used in the United States to treat hirsutism is probably spironolactone (Aldactone), which is an aldosterone antagonist approved for use as a potassium sparing diuretic. Spironolactone is an androgen antagonist, and it inhibits 5a-reductase, the enzyme that converts testosterone to the more potent dihydrotestosterone. Spironolactone should be given together with the OCP, starting at a dose of 200 mg per day. Continue therapy for at least 6 months before determining efficacy, as that period of time is needed for the thick, pigmented, long hair produced by an androgen-stimulated follicle to grow out and be replaced by a thinner, less pigmented, shorter, and less noticeable hair. Studies report that hirsutism significantly improves with spironolactone and oral contraceptive pills in about 75% of women. After a response has occurred, the dose of spironolactone can be gradually reduced to the lowest dose that maintains the improvement. Some patients can be maintained on oral contraceptive pills alone.

Flutamide (Eulexin), a pure androgen antagonist, has recently been approved for the treatment of prostatic cancer in the United States. Preliminary studies using flutamide, 250 mg twice a day, and the oral contraceptive pill to treat hirsutism have yielded impressive results. Because of the preliminary nature of these studies and the high cost of flutamide, it should only be considered in hirsute women unresponsive to other therapies.

A final treatment option for hirsutism is GnRHa. Daily subcutaneous leuprolide (Lupron, 0.5 to 1 mg) or monthly depot-leuprolide (depo-Lupron 3.75 mg) administration inhibits ovarian androgen as well as estrogen production. Preliminary studies suggest that GnRHa used alone is effective in about 75% of hirsute women. One may give estrogen replacement therapy to hirsute women receiving GnRHa to prevent complications of hypoestrogenism. Again, the studies are preliminary and the drug is expensive; however, GnRHa may prove to be an effective alternative treatment in women unresponsive to other therapies or in women in whom the OCP is contraindicated.

# DYSMENORRHEA

method of
RONALD NELSON, M.D.
*White Memorial Medical Center*
*Los Angeles, California*

Dysmenorrhea is a common menstrual symptom. A majority of women (70%) experience pain during menstruation at some time during their reproductive years. For many, this pain is a tolerated burden of menstruation and medical attention is infrequently sought; they rely on simple analgesics for relief. However, in about 25%, the pain is significant enough to require professional assistance. Severe dysmenorrhea with incapacitation and a loss of normal daily activity is experienced by 10 to 15% of women.

In recent years, there has been a significant increase in our understanding of the underlying etiology and pathophysiology for the development of dysmenorrhea. As a result, more rational and effective medical approaches have been developed that have improved dramatically the lives of these women.

## PRIMARY DYSMENORRHEA

Primary dysmenorrhea occurs in the absence of pelvic pathology and almost invariably occurs with ovulatory cycles. Adolescent females make up the large proportion of women with primary dysmenorrhea. The menstrual pain usually begins some 6 to 12 months after menarche, coinciding with the onset of ovulation cycles. The prevalence of primary dysmenorrhea declines with advancing age.

The pain usually begins with the onset of menstrual flow but may precede it by several hours. It typically lasts from several hours to 1 to 2 days but seldom persists for more than 2 to 3 days. Systemic complaints (nausea, vomiting, diarrhea, and headaches) frequently accompany the menstrual pain.

A number of studies of dysmenorrhea in women have revealed an increased production and concentration of prostaglandin in the endometrium during the luteal and menstrual phases of the cycle. Analyses of secretory endometrium, endometrial washings, and menstrual fluid have demonstrated significantly higher levels of prostaglandin in women with dysmenorrhea. These findings correlate well with the observation of hypercontractility of uterine muscle during menses in dysmenorrhea. The inhibition of prostaglandin production by several different prostaglandin synthetase inhibitors has been shown to be very effective in relieving the symptom of dysmenorrhea.

## SECONDARY DYSMENORRHEA

Menstrual pain associated with detectable pelvic pathology is secondary dysmenorrhea. It is more frequently seen in the older woman and often associated with endometriosis, leiomyomata, adenomyosis, pelvic infection, and use of the intrauterine device (IUD). Secondary dysmenorrhea in the adolescent may be caused by congenital obstructive defects of the genital tract.

For therapeutic reasons, it is important to distinguish between primary and secondary dysmenorrhea. Primary dysmenorrhea is approached more commonly with conservative medical management, whereas secondary dysmenorrhea is more frequently treated surgically. The pain of secondary dysmenorrhea usually worsens with time and may not be restricted to the menses. Dyspareunia is a common complaint.

A detailed history and pelvic examination are usually sufficient to differentiate secondary causes. Laboratory tests are generally of little value. A pelvic ultrasound and diagnostic laparoscopy should be considered when pelvic pathology is suspected or there is no response to conservative medical management.

## MEDICAL MANAGEMENT OF PRIMARY DYSMENORRHEA

The two medical approaches that have been most successful in the treatment of primary dysmenorrhea are the inhibition of ovulation with oral contraceptives and of prostaglandin production by prostaglandin synthetase inhibitors. The choice between these approaches depends on whether the woman desires oral contraception for birth control and whether there may be a con-

TABLE 1. **Treatment of Dysmenorrhea with Prostaglandin Synthetase Inhibitors**

| Prostaglandin Inhibitor | Dosage |
| --- | --- |
| Mefenamic acid (Ponstel) | 250–500 mg qid |
| Ibuprofen (Motrin) | 400 mg qid |
| Naproxen sodium (Anaprox) | 275 mg qid |

traindication to the use of oral contraceptives or prostaglandin synthetase inhibitors.

**Ovulation Inhibition.** Combined oral contraceptives would be the treatment of first choice if the patient desires birth control. Oral contraceptives produce a marked reduction in the concentration of prostaglandin in the menstrual fluid and result in a considerable decrease in uterine muscle contractility. With combined oral contraceptives, most women find relief from primary dysmenorrhea. If there is an incomplete response to oral contraceptives, a prostaglandin synthetase inhibitor can be added.

Ovulation may be inhibited with danazol (Danocrine) and gonadotropin releasing hormone agonist (GnRHa). Although extremely effective, these drugs have limited application for primary dysmenorrhea. Either approach is expensive, associated with significant side effects, and not recommended for long-term therapy.

**Prostaglandin Synthetase Inhibitors.** If oral contraception is not acceptable, the drug of choice for treatment of primary dysmenorrhea is a prostaglandin synthetase inhibitor. Commonly used inhibitors are outlined in Table 1. Nonsteroidal anti-inflammatory agents (NSAIDs) have proved to be extremely effective in eliminating significant menstrual pain. They are rapidly absorbed and act quickly in reducing prostaglandin concentration in the endometrium. The effect of NSAIDs on menstrual pain is so rapid that treatment prior to the onset of menstruation is usually unnecessary.

Side effects associated with these nonsteroidal anti-inflammatory agents are generally relatively mild. The most common symptoms are heartburn, nausea, dizziness, visual disturbances, bronchospasm, and allergic reactions. The medication is usually well tolerated because of the short duration of therapy usually required. Contraindications to these drugs would include a history of previous ulcer disease or bronchospastic reactions to ingestion of aspirin or aspirin-like drugs.

## SURGICAL MANAGEMENT

Surgical approaches in the management of primary dysmenorrhea are rarely indicated. Presacral neurectomy is not indicated in the absence of pelvic pathology. Recently there has been an enthusiasm for transection of the uterosacral ligaments by laser at the time of diagnostic laparoscopy for refractory dysmenorrhea. This approach remains controversial and should not be recommended until further studies have documented its usefulness and long-term effectiveness.

Treatment of secondary dysmenorrhea is directed toward the underlying cause. In most instances medical management is less successful, except when the dysmenorrhea is associated with IUD use.

# PREMENSTRUAL SYNDROME (PMS)

method of
WILLIAM R. KEYE, JR., M.D.
*William Beaumont Hospital*
*Royal Oak, Michigan*

Premenstrual syndrome (PMS) is the presence of recurring emotional and physical symptoms and behavioral changes that are limited to the premenstrual (luteal) phase of the menstrual cycle and that disappear within several days of the onset of menstruation. The symptoms are severe enough to affect the quality of the woman's life, diminish her functional level, and perhaps cause her to seek medical care. There also must be the absence of underlying emotional or physical disease or recurring environmental stress to account for the symptoms.

It is possible to separate women with a true premenstrual syndrome from those with the following:

1. A premenstrual exacerbation of an underlying physical or emotional disorder.
2. Chronic emotional or physical disorders that are not cyclic.
3. Recurring social, environmental, or personal stresses.

The prevalence of PMS has been reported to range from 5% to 95%. However, using the definition above, it appears that fewer than 10% of women of reproductive age meet the diagnostic criteria for PMS. Apparently, reports suggesting a much higher prevalence of PMS have included women with extremely mild symptoms or women who suffer from chronic symptoms that are more severe during the premenstrual phase of the menstrual cycle. Although 20% to 25% of women may experience troublesome and disturbing premenstrual symptoms at some time during their reproductive years, we estimate that fewer than 10% suffer such severe symptoms that their lives are significantly affected.

## CLINICAL FEATURES

Although women who seek care for PMS average about 35 years of age, they have usually experienced symptoms for 10 or more years. They frequently report that their premenstrual symptoms began during adolescence, following the birth of a child, or after a major life stress. They experience 1 to 14 days of symptoms that typically begin after ovulation but before the onset of their menstrual period and that disappear within 24 to 48 hours of the onset of their menstrual flow.

The premenstrual symptoms experienced by women with PMS are physical, emotional, and behavioral. The most common physical symptoms are fatigue, headache, abdominal bloating, breast tenderness and swelling, acne, joint pain, decreased urination, constipation, and incoordination. The most common emotional symptoms are depression, anxiety, hostility, and anger. In addition, many women complain of an intolerance of others; a sensitivity to rejection; the desire to be alone, as well as paranoia; panic attacks; fear; decreased sexual desire; sensitivity to noise, light, and touch; confusion; a decreased ability to concentrate; or impaired judgement and memory. Many of these women also complain of a tendency to be verbally critical of others, to be violent toward their husbands or children, and to experience increased appetite and a craving for sugar, chocolate, salt, or alcohol.

In addition to these monthly physical, emotional, and behavioral symptoms, many women with long-standing or severe premenstrual syndrome also experience marked psychologic reactions to these monthly premenstrual symptoms, including feelings of guilt, shame, decreased self-esteem, unassertiveness, decreased self-confidence, worthlessness, a distorted and negative body image, and hopelessness.

Finally, some of the women with long-standing, moderate-to-severe premenstrual syndrome also have disturbed interpersonal relationships because of their PMS. In addition, they may experience frequent job changes or a poor work record because of recurring outbursts of anger and poor impulse control during the luteal phase of the menstrual cycle. For many women, PMS may disrupt their marital and family relationships.

## ETIOLOGY

The etiology of PMS is unknown. Since its medical description by Frank in 1931, there have been many hypotheses promoted to explain PMS. Unfortunately, none has withstood careful scientific investigation. However, recent studies suggest that the normal fluctuation in estrogen and progesterone during the luteal phase triggers symptoms by some unknown mechanism. It also appears that genetic, biologic, or psychologic factors may predispose some women to PMS. Finally, anecdotal experience has demonstrated that psychosocial stress can intensify the severity of the syndrome.

## CLINICAL EVALUATION

Women with mild or moderate symptoms can be evaluated and treated in one or two visits. However, women with long-standing or severe premenstrual syndrome often require a more extensive evaluation, including a multidisciplinary survey of their monthly symptoms, psychologic reactions, and interpersonal problems. Regardless of the severity of the problem, the evaluation of all patients with PMS includes a history, a prospective recording of daily symptoms, an evaluation of the impact of these symptoms on the patient and her family, an evaluation of the psychologic consequences of her PMS, and a search for underlying medical and psychiatric conditions that may mimic PMS. This evaluation can usually be accomplished in two or three sessions.

*Initial Assessment*

The initial evaluation should explore the patient's menstrual and obstetric history, age, circumstances surrounding the onset and/or exacerbation of PMS, timing of the PMS symptoms, most severe symptoms, and previous therapies and their outcomes. Other factors that should be explored include the impact of PMS on self-esteem, self-image, assertiveness, ambition, and general psychologic state; the impact of PMS on family, friends, coworkers, colleagues, and patients; and the expectations regarding therapy.

The PMS history should then be followed by a standard medical history, a review of systems, a family history, and a physical examination designed to rule out underlying disease. The patient is then instructed to record daily the presence and severity of her symptoms. A simple grid with the days of the cycle listed across the top and the symptoms down the left side of the grid is a useful tool for recording the presence and severity of symptoms.

*Additional Studies*

In addition to charting her symptoms, the patient may also be instructed to seek evaluation of predisposing or complicating medical or psychosocial problems. This may involve an interview with a social worker, psychologist, or psychiatrist, perhaps supplemented by formal psychologic testing.

Each physical symptom should be thought of as a "chief complaint" for which a differential diagnosis should be established and a detailed examination performed. PMS should be a diagnosis by exclusion and should be considered as the explanation for individual symptoms only after underlying diseases have been ruled out. Therefore, an extensive physical examination of all body systems in patients with possible PMS should be performed. The importance of such a complete examination becomes obvious when one considers the most common physical symptoms described by women with PMS; fatigue, headache, breast pain, heart palpitations, joint pain, incoordination, bowel problems, and abdominal bloating are nonspecific and often secondary to other conditions.

Although laboratory and radiologic studies may be necessary to rule out underlying diseases, there is no one study that is indicated. Numerous previously undetected diseases, including systemic lupus erythematosus, meningiomas, gliomas, hypertension, endometriosis, attention deficit disorder, and hyperprolactinemia, have been diagnosed with this approach.

This lengthy discussion of the evaluation of PMS emphasizes the fact that effective therapy requires a correct diagnosis.

## TREATMENT

Fortunately, treatment of PMS can begin during the evaluation of premenstrual syndrome. For most patients therapy should include medical therapy and counseling designed to

1. reduce the number and severity of premenstrual symptoms.

2. restore the patient's psychologic health.

3. deal with social and interpersonal problems resulting from PMS.

Thus, the patient may be offered a combination of the following therapies: education; medication; peer support groups; individual psychotherapy; group psychotherapy in such areas as stress management, impulse control, or assertiveness training; and sex, marital, or family therapy. By offering help in these areas, the PMS health care provider has the greatest opportunity to interrupt the seemingly self-perpetuating nature of PMS in which premorbid personality characteristics and the psychosocial consequences of the premenstrual symptoms act as stressors that may exacerbate the severity of the premenstrual symptoms.

### Medical Therapy

Medical therapies for PMS can be classified into three major groups:

1. those that are designed to relieve one or more specific symptoms without attempting to modify the underlying disease process.

2. those that presumably correct a proposed underlying pathophysiologic disorder.

3. those that alter the normal ovulatory menstrual cycle.

#### Symptomatic Therapy

**Over-the-Counter Drugs.** Over-the-counter medications for PMS commonly contain acetaminophen or acetylsalicylic acid in combination with caffeine or other mild diuretics and an antihistamine, such as pyrilamine maleate. These agents have been chosen to relieve the common premenstrual symptoms of headache, joint pain, cramps, tension, irritability, bloating, and anxiety. Although women with mild or moderate PMS may experience some relief, women with severe symptoms may not report significant therapeutic effect from over-the-counter drugs.

**Psychoactive Drugs.** Because anxiety, depression, irritability, and hostility are prominent symptoms of PMS, psychoactive drugs are frequently prescribed for PMS. Unfortunately, clinical trials have generally failed to demonstrate a consistent therapeutic effect. In selected cases anxiolytics, such as alprazolam (Xanax), or antidepressants, such as fluoxetine (Prozac), are useful in reducing anxiety, irritability, or depression.

#### Therapy Based on Presumed Etiology

**Progesterone.** Thirty years ago, Green and Dalton reported the efficacy of pharmacologic doses of progesterone in the treatment of premenstrual syndrome. Recently a double-blind, placebo-con-trolled study reported by Dennerstein and colleagues demonstrated benefit from the oral administration of micronized progesterone, 100 mg each morning and 200 mg each evening in the luteal phase.

Although the mechanism by which progesterone decreases premenstrual symptoms is unclear, no evidence exists that it replaces a hormone deficiency. More likely, progesterone or its metabolites exert a direct pharmacologic effect on the central nervous system, inducing anxiolytic, sedative, and hypnotic effects.

Hand-made capsules of micronized progesterone are now available in many pharmacies in the United States, as are candied lozenges or troches for buccal or sublingual administration.

**Prostaglandin Inhibitors.** In an attempt to explain the wide variety of symptoms and organ systems involved in premenstrual syndrome, investigators have looked at a possible role for prostaglandins in the etiology of PMS.

Recently, Mira and colleagues reported significant improvement in many physical (fatigue, headache, and general aches and pains) and emotional (mood swings, pessimism, irritability) symptoms using 250 to 500 mg of prostaglandin inhibitors three times a day for 10 days in the luteal phase. No improvement in breast symptoms, food cravings, tension, sleeping difficulty, inefficiency, or inability to concentrate occurred.

No consistent relief appears to be provided by thyroid replacement therapy, antifungal agents, herbs, nutritional supplements, or diuretics.

#### Anovulation Therapy

The third category of medical therapies are those that are neither symptomatic in nature nor designed to treat an underlying biochemical abnormality. These therapies are designed instead to abolish ovulation, menstruation, and the cyclic changes in gonadotropins and ovarian steroids.

**Oral Contraception.** The obvious choice of an agent to cause anovulation is the birth control pill because of its widespread use and relative safety. However, a large subgroup of women have symptoms that are worse, not better, on oral contraceptives. In spite of these observations, some women with premenstrual symptoms report a benefit from either combination estrogen-progestin or progestin-only oral contraceptives.

**Depomedroxyprogesterone Acetate.** Depomedroxyprogesterone acetate (Depo-Provera) is used by 15 million women in 80 countries as a means of contraception.* In addition, many physicians use depomedroxyprogesterone acetate to treat pre-

---

*This use of Depo-Provera is not listed in the manufacturer's official directive.

menstrual or menstrual symptoms. The suppression of ovulation and menstruation by 30 mg of medroxyprogesterone acetate or 150 mg every 2 to 3 months of depomedroxyprogesterone acetate can be extremely helpful in severe and otherwise unresponsive cases.

**Hysterectomy and Oophorectomy.** If premenstrual syndrome is truly dependent upon the fluctuations in ovarian hormones in the luteal phase of the menstrual cycle, one would predict that a bilateral oophorectomy would eliminate the symptoms of PMS. In fact, a recent study by Casson and colleagues has demonstrated that anovulation induced by danazol, 800 mg per day, and subsequent oophorectomy in the positive responders to danazol had a lasting beneficial effect on premenstrual symptomatology.

### Nonmedical Therapies

**Validation.** Many women with PMS experience personal rejection by friends, family, and health care professionals. This situation can create increased feelings of inadequacy and self-doubt and trigger suspicion of mental illness. When a physician verifies the symptoms as PMS, women generally experience a reduction in the severity of their premenstrual symptoms. The physician may validate the PMS by simply listening to the patient's story in an empathic and nonjudgmental way to make the confirmation or by determining PMS through the use of a prospective calendar or diary.

**Education.** A woman with PMS must learn that not all uncomfortable feelings are the result of PMS and that PMS cannot explain all mood changes, depression, anxiety, anger, malaise, or fatigue. It is imperative that the PMS sufferer and her family and friends be educated regarding the personal and social complications of PMS. By reassuring the patient and her family that anger, resentment, and feelings of inadequacy are common reactions to PMS, it is hoped that friends and family can gain an acceptance of their involvement and become supporters and defenders, not critics, of the woman with PMS.

**Self-Help: Lifestyle Changes.** Aerobic exercise for 20 to 30 minutes a day for 3 to 7 days each week during the premenstruum often reduces the severity of symptoms. Another self-help measure is the institution of a modified "hypoglycemic" diet. This diet avoids simple carbohydrates; prescribes frequent small meals; eliminates white flour, salt, caffeine, and alcohol; focuses on fiber, protein, and complex carbohydrates; and recommends moderation of the intake of calcium and dairy products.

In light of the harmless, inexpensive, and health-promoting aspects of these self-help measures, it seems reasonable to recommend these measures early in the course of treatment to most women with PMS, even in the absence of well-designed scientific studies demonstrating their benefit.

**Achieving Cooperation of Family and Friends.** Many women with PMS can recount that family and "friends" have undermined their therapy by refusing to pay for medication or follow-up visits, to acknowledge the reality of PMS, or to assume responsibility for tasks or job responsibilities that could ease the burden of PMS. In addition, family members may complicate the life of the PMS sufferer through their alcohol abuse or by physical or psychologic trauma.

The PMS sufferer should be taught to stand up for her rights and expect and obtain cooperation from others.

**Eliminating Predisposing Factors.** In many cases, recovery from PMS is dependent upon such factors as attitudes, expectations, coping styles, attributional style, motivation, ambitions, social support, and family dynamics. For example, it may be more important to deal with the alcoholic and abusive husband than to prescribe medication to the wife with PMS. It may be more important to deal with the psychologic scars of childhood sexual abuse than to recommend exercise and a hypoglycemic diet.

# MENOPAUSE

method of
LILA E. NACHTIGALL, M.D.
*New York University School of Medicine*
*New York, New York*

We entered the 1990s with 43 million women over the age of 50 in the United States. The last menstrual period occurs at an average age of 51.4, meaning that many of those 43 million women are past menopause, and over 30 million of these women will live half their lives postmenopausally. In addition, 1.9% of women will have premature menopause (defined as menopause before 40 years of age) and will live more than half of their lives after menopause. All these statistics imply that menopause has become a major health issue to be dealt with in the 1990s.

The question of whether menopause is a physiologic occurrence or whether it is an endocrine deficiency state has been discussed for at least the 40 years that hormone replacement therapy has been available. A lack of true scientific data had kept us from a consensus. However, during the last decade many controlled scientific studies have been completed that help to answer that question. The answer is that each woman has to be individually evaluated, as with any endocrinopathy, to determine if therapy is indicated.

The most common and universal symptom of menopause is the "hot flush," or "hot flash." These are part of a complex of vasomotor symptoms that also include paresthesias, formication, irritability, sweats, sleep disturbances, and occasionally even cold chills. The pathogenesis of this vasomotor instability has been poorly understood, and only since 1983 have researchers been searching for answers. The relationship of the high follicle stimulating hormone (FSH) level (pathognomonic for menopause) and peaks of luteinizing hormone (LH) level to the flush has been studied but discounted. The best theory appears to be that estrogen receptors, normally present in varying numbers in the hypothalamus of women, play a major role in the temperature control and catecholamine release. This explains both the variation in symptoms from woman to woman and why no other medication is as effective as estrogen in relieving these vasomotor symptoms. Therefore, unless there is an absolute contraindication to its use, estrogen replacement should be given to any woman with flushes, insomnia, irritability, or difficulty with temperature control. Treatment for this type of instability is usually short term (2 to 5 years) and can be withdrawn gradually with no return of symptoms. In cases in which a patient cannot or will not take hormone replacement therapy, alternate treatment includes clonidine in doses of 1 to 2 mg daily, which is effective in less than 50% of women; or megestrol* 40 mg daily, which is an antimitotic progesterone and is the only progesterone approved for women who have had breast cancer.

Over the last 2 decades data have been accumulated that indicate that natural or surgical menopause is directly related to bone loss. The 1984 NIH Health Consensus Conference on Osteoporosis noted the high risk of fractures in postmenopausal caucasian women and suggested that these women are candidates for hormone replacement therapy for the prevention of osteoporotic fractures. Trabecular bone osteoporosis, which leads to reduced height, spinal compression fractures, and "dowager's hump," is familiar to most women. However, the more serious osteoporosis involves cortical bone, which leads to fracture of the hip, affects one out of three women over the age of 85, has a 20% mortality rate, and a 50% permanent incapacitation rate. Therefore,

because no treatment for osteoporosis exists once it occurs, a serious attempt must be made at prevention.

Effective prevention requires the assessment of risk factors, which are listed in order of importance in Table 1. Any woman having two or more risk factors should be considered for treatment with hormone replacement therapy. To prevent bone loss, therapy should begin within 3 years from the last menstrual period and should continue somewhere between 10 and 15 years, depending on the patient's age at menopause and the degree of risk. Adequate calcium intake, preferably in the diet, should be encouraged as well. Women who are either producing or receiving estrogen require about 1000 mg of calcium daily. A study by Ettinger and colleagues demonstrated that women continued to lose bone when calcium was given without estrogen but increased bone density when these were given in combination. Estrogen replacement therapy started any time after menopause stabilizes bone density but does not increase it once 3 years have elapsed from the last menstrual period.

Alternate therapy includes calcitonin, to which patients become refractory and which has to be given parenterally, and fluorides, which stimulate bone formation but can lead to fluorosis and gastrointestinal disturbances and have not yet been approved for this purpose. Recently, diphosphonates such as etidronate (Didronel) have been found to halt osteoporosis in several studies and were approved for this purpose by the FDA in 1990.

TABLE 1. **Risk Factors for Osteoporosis***

Menopause before age 40
Family history of osteoporosis
Family origin in British Isles, northern Europe, China, or Japan
Heavy cigarette smoking (½ pack or more per day)
Loss of height, especially in upper body
Fracture with no known cause
Hyperparathyroid disease
Uremia
Increased cortisone production or previous long-term cortisone ingestion
Vitamin D deficiency state
Very fair skin
Small bones
Consumption of more than 5 ounces of alcohol per day or known liver disease
Diet low in calcium
Lactase deficiency
Malabsorption problem
Hyperthyroidism
Underweight
Sedentary life style
Previous high-protein, low-carbohydrate diet for more than 1 year in adulthood

---

*This use of megestrol is not listed in the manufacturer's official directive.

*From Nachtigall LE, and Heilman J: Estrogen: The Facts Can Change Your Life. Los Angeles, Price Stern Sloan, 1986.

Urogenital atrophy, almost entirely related to estrogen deficiency, will eventually occur in all untreated postmenopausal women. The time of occurrence is extremely variable, with a range of between 1 and 15 years. As a result of estrogen deprivation, the vagina loses its rugae and its cornified epithelium becomes thin and nonelastic. This leads to diminution in vaginal lubrication, resulting in dyspareunia and eventually total inability to have intercourse. The lack of cornification leads to increased incidence of bacterial, fungal, or trichonomonal vaginitis. The lack of cornification around the urethra leads to increased incidence of urethritis and cystitis. Fortunately, all urogenital atrophy can be reversed by estrogen replacement therapy given orally, transdermally, parenterally, or intravaginally. This reversal can be accomplished even many years postmenopausally.

Cardiovascular disease, a major cause of death in the United States, accounts for 355,000 deaths per year in women. The possible role of estrogen in decreasing the cardiovascular disease mortality has been assumed, but is still controversial. Certainly the epidemiology of cardiovascular disease points to a protective effect of endogenous estrogen. The male to female ratio is 4:1 at age 35 and still is 3:1 at the time of menopause. In addition, premenopausal oophorectomy is associated with the increased risk of cardiovascular disease. Of dozens of case-control and cohort studies of estrogen replacement on the cardiovascular system, all but one show a decreased mortality rate in women on estrogen replacement as opposed to women on no replacement. The one study in which there was an increased incidence of cardiovascular disease in women on estrogen replacement therapy was confounded by an exceptionally high evidence of cigarette smoking.

The most likely explanation of the beneficial effects of estrogen on cardiovascular risk derives from its ability to favorably alter lipid and lipoprotein levels. The median high-density lipoproteins (HDLs) are 10% higher in estrogen users and the median low-density lipoproteins (LDLs) are 11% lower. This magnitude of change has been associated with a 50% reduction of cardiovascular disease. However, in the Lipid Research Clinic Study, when HDL and LDL alterations were analyzed, there was an additional 30% decrease in cardiovascular disease mortality. This suggests that other factors may be involved—i.e., increased cardiac output, better elasticity of blood vessels, or altered regional blood flow.

An epidemiologic study from the Netherlands actually showed a 12% incidence in atherosclerosis in untreated postmenopausal women as compared with a 3% incidence in women of the same age on hormone replacement.

It is now generally accepted that postmenopausal hormone replacement with estrogens alone raises HDL and lowers LDL, resulting in a favorable lipid profile. Whether the addition of progestogens changes this profile or if there are differences with doses, preparations, and duration of use is still being actively debated. For the most part, studies using low-dose medroxyprogesterone acetate, micronized progesterone, and medrogestone show little change in the beneficial effect derived from estrogen alone. Table 2 shows the multifactorial risk factor improvements on estrogen alone versus estrogen plus progesterone.

TABLE 2. **Calculated $t$ Values\***

| Variable | Effects of CEE Alone (Matched Pairs $t$ Test) | CEE Interaction (Effect of Whether Administered First or Second) (Two-Sample $t$ Test) | Differential Effect of Medrogestone (Matched Pairs $t$ Test) | Medrogestone Time Interaction (Carryover) (Two-Sample Analysis) |
|---|---|---|---|---|
| Total cholesterol | 2.855† | −0.223 | 1.605 | −0.242 |
| HDL-C | −6.620† | −1.800 | 1.154 | 1.080 |
| % HDL-C | −7.649‡ | −1.634 | 0.735 | 0.799 |
| HDL$_3$-C | −1.749 | −0.820 | −0.224 | 1.143 |
| HDL$_2$-C | −5.199‡ | −2.040 | 1.625 | 0.721 |
| Triglycerides | −1.937 | −0.167 | 1.144 | −1.378 |
| LDL-C | 6.352‡ | 0.227 | 0.707 | 0.031 |
| VLDL-C | −1.036 | 0.165 | 1.358 | −1.129 |
| LDL-C/HDL-C | 7.051‡ | 0.265 | 0.715 | −1.168 |
| Apolipoprotein A-I | −1.290 | 0.215 | 0.987 | 0.415 |
| Apolipoprotein A-II | 0.372 | −1.029 | 0.133 | 0.299 |
| Apolipoprotein B | 0.525 | 2.412† | 0.226 | −1.092 |

\*From Sonnendecker EWW, Polakow ES, Benade AJS, and Simchowitz E: Serum lipoprotein effects of conjugated estrogen and a sequential conjugated estrogen-medrogestone regimen in hysterectomized postmenopausal women. Am J Obstet Gynecol *160:* 1132, 1989.

$CEE$ = conjugated equine estrogens.

†$p < 0.01.$

‡$p < 0.001.$

For now, women who develop an unfavorable lipid pattern after menopause or have a strong family history of ischemic heart disease or atherosclerosis should be given hormone replacement.

After considering the multiple benefits of treatment for specific indications in the menopausal and postmenopausal woman, it is necessary to examine the risks. The strong association of unopposed estrogen and development of endometrial cancer is well accepted. Progestogens protect the endometrium against excessive estrogen-induced stimulation, and an inverse relation exists between the proliferative features under microscopy and progesterone dose. Because of lipid pattern alteration in high doses and adverse symptomatic effects, the minimum dosage that leads to consistent endometrial transformation should be used. Daily low doses of micronized estradiol (0.7 to 1.05 mg) combined with daily micronized progesterone (200 to 300 mg) have been shown to give minimal side effects, total symptomatic improvement, an improved lipid profile, and amenorrhea without endometrial hyperplasia in all menopausal patients in one clinical trial and may be the drugs of choice in the future.

The epidemiologic literature on breast cancer and estrogen replacement therapy is confusing. Although most studies have found little or no increase in breast cancer risk, a study done in Sweden seems to show a slightly increased risk in certain subgroups, even though they represented small enough total numbers to be related to chance only. The current intelligence is that estrogen is not a carcinogen for breast cancer, but can be a growth accelerator factor, and for this reason it is important for women to have a careful breast examination as well as a mammography to rule out early malignancy before going on hormone replacement prescription. Breast examination and mammography should be performed annually thereafter.

This leads to the conclusion that menopausal women need to be carefully evaluated. If they have vasomotor instability, a high risk for development of osteoporosis, vaginal or urogenital atrophy, high risk of ischemic or atherosclerotic heart disease, or premature ovarian failure, they should begin hormone replacement therapy. This is usually accomplished with a dose of conjugated estrogen 0.625 mg daily or its equivalent but can be up to 1.25 mg daily in surgical menopause or early menopause with severe symptoms. Women who have not had hysterectomies should receive medroxyprogesterone 10 mg daily for 10 days a month or its equivalent, but an individual dose can be determined with an endometrial biopsy after therapy is instituted. Recent studies have shown low-dose progesterone—i.e., medroxypro-gesterone (Provera) 2.5 mg or megestrol (Megace) 10 mg on a daily basis—to be successful.

Although the oral route is the most common form of estrogen replacement therapy, the transdermal route has the advantage of avoiding the first hepatic pass, which is beneficial in women with previous liver disease and also prevents the concentration of gallbladder bile, avoiding gallstones and gallbladder disease associated with the oral medication. If urogenital atrophy is the only symptom being treated, vaginal conjugated estrogen creams of 1 gram, 1 to 2 times per week, are most effective. However, vaginal routes are notorious for their absorption variability.

Women with previous breast cancer should usually not be given hormone replacement therapy. At one time the same was said for women with previous endometrial cancer. However, now the feeling is that if the cancer was Stage 0 or Stage I and 2 years have passed without sequelae, these patients can be treated.

# VULVOVAGINITIS

method of
MARK C. MABERRY, M.D.
*University of Texas Southwestern Medical Center*
*Dallas, Texas*

The symptoms of vulvovaginitis are some of the most common reasons for outpatient gynecologic visits. They include discharge, vulvar pruritis, and vaginal odor. The patient often presents with a prior history of vulvovaginitis, with the infection frequently representing a recurrence or treatment failure of a previous infection. Therefore, it is important for the physician to take a thorough history, including past history of infection, sexual history, menstrual history, as well as the consistency, color, and odor of the discharge. Physical examination should include a detailed examination of the vagina, cervix, vulva, and perineal area. The next step involves determining the vaginal pH with nitrazine paper and then obtaining an appropriate sample of the discharge for microscopic examination using both saline and potassium hydroxide (KOH) solutions. The symptoms, signs, and criteria for diagnosis of the most common forms of vaginitis are summarized in Table 1.

## CANDIDA

*Candida* species are among the most common etiologic agents of vulvovaginitis. Although *Candida* may be present in small amounts, the growth is usually checked by the various lactobacilli and corynebacteria normally present in the vagina of reproductive age women. However, under certain circumstances, notably pregnancy

TABLE 1. **Symptoms, Signs, and Laboratory Findings in Women with Vaginitis***

| | Discharge | pH | Microscopic Findings | Symptoms |
|---|---|---|---|---|
| Monilial | White, thick | 4.0 to 5.0 | Pseudohyphae | Pruritis |
| Trichomonas | Thin, copious, yellow | 5.0 to 7.0 | Motile trichomonads | Copious discharge, pruritis |
| Nonspecific | Scant, gray | 5.0 to 6.0 | Clue cells | Fishy odor, discharge |
| Atrophic | Scant, purulent, bloody | 6.0 to 7.0 | White blood cells | Bleeding |

*Adapted from Friedrich EG, Jr: Vaginitis. In Friedrich EG, Jr: Vulvar Disease. Philadelphia, WB Saunders Co, 1976.

and diabetes mellitus, both states of decreased cellular immunity, overgrowth results in candidal vulvovaginitis.

The majority of cases of monilial vulvovaginitis are caused by *Candida albicans,* a yeast-like fungus that may be found throughout the gastrointestinal tract as well as the vulva and the vagina. *Candida glabrata* (formerly *Torulopsis glabrata*) may also be responsible for monilial vaginitis as well as other species of *Candida.* Although *Candida albicans* is seen in over 95% of women with monilial vulvovaginitis, the other species of *Candida* may be responsible for recurrent infections or treatment failures.

The main clinical manifestations of monilial infection are a thick, white, "cottage cheese" discharge and pruritis, especially if the vulvar area is involved. Physical examination may reveal marked erythema and edema of the perineum, buttocks, and intertrigal regions, with chafing and cracking of the involved skin areas.

The diagnosis is usually suspected on the basis of history and physical examination and can be confirmed by placing the discharge on a microscopic slide and adding 10% KOH. In over 80% of cases, the KOH preparation, which lyses the vaginal epithelial cells, will reveal the branched and budding pseudohyphae of the candidal organisms when viewed under low power. Occasionally it may be necessary to culture the discharge for *Candida* using Nickerson's media. The vaginal pH is usually between 4.0 and 5.0.

There are numerous regimens available for the treatment of monilial vulvovaginitis. A commonly used antifungal agent, nystatin (Mycostatin), is available in vaginal suppositories, cream, or ointment, and the usual dose is either one suppository or 1 gram of the cream applied intravaginally two times a day for 7 days. However, the newer imidazoles, including miconazole (Monistat) and clotrimazole (Lotrimin), may be more effective in eradicating infection (Table 2). The usual dose for both agents is one suppository or application every night for 7 days. The cream may also be applied to the vulva to relieve the pruritis associated with monilial infection. Terconazole is a relatively new triazole antifungal reported to be effective for the treatment of *Can-*

*dida albicans.* The usual dose is one applicator full of cream intravaginally once daily for 7 days or one vaginal suppository once daily for 3 days. Gentian violet, a topical 1% aqueous dye, has also been reported to be effective when "painted" on the cervical and vaginal mucosa of patients with monilial vulvovaginitis. Potential drawbacks include local irritation as well as staining of clothing. Boric acid, given as gelatin capsules containing 600 mg of boric acid powder intravaginally once at night for 2 weeks, may be useful in recurrent fungal infections.

## TRICHOMONAL INFECTION

Trichomonal vaginitis results from infection with the flagellar parasite *Trichomonas vaginalis.* This parasite is most often sexually transmitted and commonly exists in vaginal and cervical secretions in females and seminal fluid in males. It has been estimated that approximately one in five women will experience trichomonal infection during her lifetime.

The primary symptom is a profuse discharge, which may require a pad and may vary from white and watery to green, thick, and frothy. Patients may experience intense pruritis. In contrast to monilial infections, the discharge is generally malodorous. The vaginal pH is usually between 5.0 and 7.0.

Examination of the vagina and cervix may reveal characteristic red punctate lesions known as "strawberry patches," although this finding is actually seen in less than 5% of women with

TABLE 2. **Suggested Regimens for the Treatment of *Candida* Vulvovaginitis***

| Agent | Dose |
|---|---|
| Nystatin (Mycostatin) | One vaginal suppository or 1 gram of cream bid for 7 days |
| Miconazole (Monistat) | One vaginal suppository or one application of cream every night for 7 days |
| Clotrimazole (Lotrimin) | (Same as for miconazole) |
| Terconazole (Terazol) | One vaginal suppository every night for 3 days or one application of cream every night for 7 days |

*Refer to manufacturer's guidelines and recommendations.

active trichomonal infection. In cases of severe infection, there may be vulvar and vaginal erythema and edema.

In 80 to 90% of cases, *Trichomonas* can be easily demonstrated on microscopic examination of a small aliquot of the vaginal discharge mixed with saline. Motile trichomonads with characteristic single flagella are easily identified under low microscopic power. Trichomonads may also be identified on Papanicolaou's smears but not as reliably as with the wet saline preparation. The presence of white blood cells (greater than 10 per high-power field) on the wet mount is statistically associated with *Trichomonas* infection, even in the absence of obvious motile trichomonads.

The cornerstone of treatment for *Trichomonas* vulvovaginitis is metronidazole (Flagyl). The currently recommended dosage is a single 2-gram oral administration (Table 3). Patients may experience less gastrointestinal disturbance if the dosage is divided into two 1-gram administrations, usually one in the morning and one at bedtime. For women with frequent recurrences, it may be necessary to treat the patient for a longer period of time, such as 250 mg three times a day for 5 days. One important side effect of metronidazole therapy, especially with longer courses, is the development of monilial infections, probably secondary to the eradication of specific vaginal bacteria.

Significant controversy exists regarding whether to treat the male partner of a patient with trichomonal vulvovaginitis. Because the organism only survives in the male genital tract for short periods of time and because of the potential Antabuse (antialcohol) effect of metronidazole, treatment of the male sexual partner is probably not warranted. Instead, the female should be advised to refrain from intercourse during the treatment period or else use a condom to prevent reinfection.

TABLE 3. **Suggested Treatment Regimens for** *Trichomonas* **and Nonspecific Vaginitis**

| |
|---|
| **Trichomonas** |
| Metronidazole (Flagyl) |
|  Single, 2-gram oral dose |
|  250 mg tid for 5 to 7 days |
| Clotrimazole* (Lotrimin) |
|  One vaginal suppository daily for 7 days |
| **Nonspecific Vaginitis** |
| Metronidazole |
|  250 mg tid for 5 to 7 days |
| Ampicillin |
|  250 mg qid for 5 to 7 days |
| Cephalosporin |
|  250 mg qid for 5 to 7 days |

*For symptomatic treatment only (see text).

## BACTERIAL INFECTIONS

Another common cause of vaginitis is bacterial infection of the vagina, usually associated with the organism *Gardnerella vaginalis* (formerly *Haemophilus vaginalis* or *Corynebacterium vaginalis*). This facultative anaerobe along with a motile rod-shaped bacterium called *mobiluncus* in association with other anaerobic bacteria produces the signs and symptoms of "nonspecific vaginitis."

The discharge commonly seen with nonspecific vaginitis or "bacterial vaginosis" is usually of grayish watery consistency associated with a "fishy" or malodorous smell, most pronounced after sexual intercourse. In contrast to monilial and trichomonal infections, there are few if any symptoms of vulvar or vaginal inflammation or edema.

The vaginal pH is usually between 5.0 and 6.0. If a small drop of 10% KOH is added to the discharge of patients with bacterial vaginosis, a "fishy" odor is often released ("positive whiff test"). This odor is the result of amines released by degradation of amino acids by the potassium hydroxide. Microscopic examination usually reveals a small number of white blood cells and desquamated epithelial cells with clusters of bacteria attached to them, the so-called clue cells. However, the cells may not be present in all patients with bacterial vaginosis.

Numerous agents have been used to treat nonspecific vaginitis, including local agents, such as sulfa creams and tetracycline vaginal tablets, as well as systemic agents like tetracycline, ampicillin, and most recently, metronidazole. Vaginal sulfa creams have been shown not to be effective against *G. vaginalis,* and tetracycline is contraindicated in pregnancy. The treatment of choice is probably metronidazole (Flagyl), 250 mg three times a day for 5 to 7 days in mild cases and 500 mg twice a day in severe infections or recurrences, although this regimen has not yet been approved by the Food and Drug Administration (FDA). Other less effective regimens are ampicillin or a cephalosporin 250 mg four times a day for 5 to 7 days. As with metronidazole, protracted therapy with either ampicillin or cephalosporins may be associated with *Candida* overgrowth.

## VAGINITIS DURING PREGNANCY

Although vaginitis is a relatively common disorder during pregnancy, it sometimes is difficult to diagnose because vaginal "discharge" (or leukorrhea) is also a common symptom of pregnancy per se. The salient features of vaginitis during pregnancy include an odorous discharge and pruritis.

The diagnosis of vulvovaginitis in pregnant women is the same as for nonpregnant women as outlined previously. Treatment, however, presents a therapeutic dilemma to the clinician, especially when treating patients in the first trimester. This is especially true with regard to the use of metronidazole for the treatment of either *Trichomonas* or nonspecific vaginitis during pregnancy. Although metronidazole is an FDA Category B drug—i.e., "relatively safe"—it is not recommended for use in the first trimester of pregnancy because of concern of possible oncogenic and mutagenic effects. Although there are no studies to date that would implicate metronidazole as a teratogenic agent, because of the fear of litigation many clinicians use clotrimazole for symptomatic relief in patients with *Trichomonas* infection in the first trimester of pregnancy. Both clotrimazole and miconazole are relatively safe for use during pregnancy and are FDA Category B drugs, as are ampicillin and cephalosporins (Table 4). Terconazole is relatively new and is thus an FDA Category C drug (i.e., little or no information is available regarding use in pregnancy). According to its manufacturer, terconazole is not teratogenic in laboratory animals. It, however, should probably be avoided in the first trimester.

### ATROPHIC VAGINITIS

Both preadolescent and postmenopausal females share the relative lack of estrogen on the genital tract. In the preadolescent state, the labia are underdeveloped, and the vaginal mucosa is fine and similar to the postmenopausal state with friable, "atrophic" vaginal tissue as well as loss of rugae. In both situations, the vaginal pH is usually above 5.0, owing to a relatively small number of lactobacilli.

Atrophic vaginitis is a common cause of physician consultation in postmenopausal women. They present with a purulent vaginal discharge, often bloody, as well as vulvar and vaginal irritation. In addition, these patients may report dyspareunia and urinary urge incontinence. On examination, the vagina is pale and adhesions may be noted, which bleed when probed. The discharge is usually scant, yellowish in color, with a pH above 5.0. Wet mount reveals red blood cells, large numbers of white blood cells, and frequent exfoliated parabasal cells. Papanicolaou smear and a bimanual examination must be performed to rule out a genital tract carcinoma.

In the absence of malignancy, the mainstay of

**TABLE 4. FDA Categories of Antimicrobial Agents for Treatment of Vulvovaginitis During Pregnancy**

| Agent | Category |
| --- | --- |
| Metronidazole* | B |
| Clotrimazole | B |
| Miconazole | B |
| Terconazole | C |
| Ampicillin | B |
| First-generation cephalosporin | B |
| Pyrantel pamoate | C |

*Not recommended for use during first trimester.

treatment for atrophic vaginitis in a postmenopausal women is hormonal therapy. Intravaginal estrogen cream, which is inserted two to three times per week, is usually sufficient to relieve the symptoms. In addition, if the patient is not already on oral hormone replacement therapy, one may want to add this to her regimen.

### OTHER CAUSES

The most common cause of vaginal discharge in the preadolescent female is the presence of a foreign body in the vagina. The discharge is usually malodorous and often bloody. Diagnosis can usually be made via a gentle pelvic examination (which may have to be performed under general anesthesia) with demonstration of the foreign object in the vagina. Bacterial cultures can be taken and appropriate antimicrobial therapy begun. Cleaning of the vagina with iodophor may be done following the removal of the foreign object.

Less commonly, vaginitis in the prepubescent female may be secondary to the pinworm *Enterobius vermicularis*. *Enterobius* vaginitis results from migration of the adult worm from the anus to the vaginal area. Symptoms include vaginal discharge, perineal erythema, and pruritis, which is usually most severe at night. The diagnosis can be made by applying cellophane tape to the perianal-perineal region and then placing the tape, adhesive side down, on a microscopic slide. Demonstration of the characteristic double-walled *Enterobius* ova are pathognomonic for the disease. One dose of pyrantel pamoate (Antiminth) suspension is sufficient to cure the infestation, although other family members should be treated as well.

Finally, in the presence of possible sexual abuse, one should be alert to the presence of gonorrhea, herpes simplex, or *Chlamydia trachomatis* as the etiology of vaginitis in the pediatric age group.

# TOXIC SHOCK SYNDROME

method of
ARTHUR L. REINGOLD, M.D.
*University of California*
*Berkeley, California*

Toxic shock syndrome (TSS) is a distinctive, acute, multisystem illness caused by infection with *Staphylococcus aureus*. The most prominent clinical manifestations of TSS include high fever; hypotension; a diffuse scarlatiniform rash; vomiting and diarrhea; myalgias; and mucous membrane hyperemia, including a "strawberry" tongue. Dysfunction of multiple other organ systems, including the renal, hepatic, cardiovascular, hematologic, and central nervous systems, also can be seen and, at times, dominate the clinical picture. Patients who survive the acute illness experience desquamation, which can be generalized or limited to the extremities. Because no diagnostic test for TSS exists, the diagnosis is made on clinical grounds, based on meeting the criteria of a complex case definition (Table 1). Although this case definition has been useful for epidemiologic studies, it only captures the most severe cases of TSS and it is evident that many patients have milder cases that do not meet all of these criteria. In the absence of a diagnostic test for TSS, however, the spectrum of illness remains unknown. Among cases meeting the strict criteria, the fatality rate is in the range of 2 to 4%.

## ETIOLOGY AND PATHOGENESIS

As noted previously, TSS is caused by infection with *S. aureus*. Cases of TSS have been associated with *S. aureus* infections at a wide array of body sites, including the vagina; cutaneous and subcutaneous lesions (e.g., abscesses, surgical wounds, burns, insect bites, and other wounds); joint spaces; bone and soft tissue; and the respiratory tract, among others. *S. aureus* infection of the vagina resulting in TSS is most commonly seen during menstruation, particularly in the presence of tampon use, but can also occur in the absence of menstruation, when it may be associated with the use of barrier contraceptives (e.g., a diaphragm or contraceptive sponge). Bacteremia is extremely rare in TSS, and the disease is almost certainly toxin mediated; in most cases, a newly described staphylococcal exoprotein toxin, toxic shock syndrome toxin–1 (TSST–1), appears to be responsible for most, if not all, of the clinical manifestations. In rabbits, purified TSST–1 can produce most of the signs and symptoms of TSS. However, in a number of TSS cases, particularly nonmenstrual cases associated with focal cutaneous and subcutaneous wounds, other staphylococcal toxins, such as enterotoxin B, may play a primary role. The mechanisms and pathways whereby TSST–1 and other staphylococcal toxins produce their effects on various organ systems remain ill defined, although endogenous mediators, such as interleukin–1 and tumor necrosis factor, appear to play a role. Whatever the sites and mechanisms of cellular injury, capillary leakage of intravascular fluid contributes in a substantial way to the observed derangements in volume status and the functioning of multiple organ systems. Most of the adult population (more than 90%) has measurable antibodies to TSST–1, which are believed to be protective against TSST–1–induced TSS.

## EPIDEMIOLOGY

At present, approximately 50 to 60% of diagnosed TSS cases in the United States occur in menstruating women, virtually all of whom are using tampons. Cases of TSS with onset during menstruation occur more commonly in younger women (15 to 24 years of age) than in older women of reproductive age, and appear to occur at a higher rate among white women, probably due to the fact that a higher proportion of them use tampons. Cases of TSS also occur in postpartum women. Early postpartum TSS (onset in the first week) is generally due to use of tampons to control the flow of lochia or to infection of a C-section surgical incision. Later postpartum onset is generally due to breast infections (abscesses or mastitis) or to tampon use once menstruation resumes. Cases of nonmenstrual TSS can occur at any age, and have been documented in newborns and in those over 80 years of age. The incidence of TSS associated with wounds and with other *S. aureus* infections outside the female reproductive system appears not to differ substantially by sex or by race. TSS cases have been reported from all 50 states in the U.S. and from most other developed countries.

## DIAGNOSTIC APPROACH

TSS should be considered in the differential diagnosis of any patient with the acute onset of otherwise unexplained high fever, hypotension, or a diffuse macular erythematous rash. Patients in whom it is particularly important to consider the diagnosis of TSS include menstruating and postpartum women and postoperative patients (Table 2). Among postoperative

TABLE 1. **Simplified Case Definition
of Toxic Shock Syndrome**

1. Fever: temperature ≥38.9° C (102° F)
2. Rash: diffuse macular erythroderma
3. Hypotension: systolic blood pressure ≤90 mmHg or orthostatic changes in blood pressure
4. Desquamation 1 to 2 weeks after onset of illness
5. Evidence of involvement of ≥3 body systems (gastrointestinal, muscular, mucous membrane, renal, hepatic, hematologic, and central nervous systems)
6. No evidence of another cause for the illness

TABLE 2. **Patients in Whom to Suspect
Toxic Shock Syndrome**

Young women who are menstruating, particularly those using tampons or barrier contraceptives—i.e., a contraceptive sponge or diaphragm
Postpartum women
Patients with recent surgery, particularly nasal surgery or procedures that require nasal packing
Patients with or at high risk of cutaneous/subcutaneous staphylococcal infections—e.g., burn patients, patients with furuncles, etc.)

patients, those who have undergone nasal surgery and/or have nasal packing appear to be at the highest risk of developing TSS. A careful physical examination, including a pelvic examination in women and a thorough search for possible sites of focal staphylococcal infection, is mandatory in any patient in whom the diagnosis of TSS is being considered. Surgical wounds and other focal cutaneous/subcutaneous lesions infected with a TSS inducing strain of *S. aureus* may appear uninflamed and innocuous. Re-exploration of a surgical wound is advisable whenever TSS is suspected in the postoperative interval, even if the wound appears uninfected. Even if TSS appears to be the most likely cause of the illness, other diagnoses should be considered (Table 3) and cultures of blood, urine, wounds, and the vagina, cervix, or used tampon should be obtained before presumptive antimicrobial therapy is initiated. In addition, specimens should be obtained for baseline determinations of hepatic, renal, and hematologic function. Similarly, a chest radiograph should be obtained to serve as a baseline for monitoring changes in cardiopulmonary function.

## TREATMENT

Treatment of TSS should focus on immediate resuscitation/stabilization of the patient, minimizing further release and uptake of staphylococcal toxins, and prevention/treatment of complications.

### Resuscitation/Stabilization

By definition, patients meeting the strict case definition for TSS are severely ill and require hospitalization; those with disturbances in their hemodynamic function should be in an intensive care unit setting where they can be monitored closely until stable. All patients admitted to the hospital with TSS should have a widebore intravenous catheter inserted, and restoration of fluids should begin immediately. Intravascular volume depletion in TSS patients typically is due to a combination of reduced intake of fluids; losses due to vomiting and diarrhea; increased insensible losses due to high fever; and leakage of fluids into extravascular compartments. Colloid containing intravenous fluids should be infused rapidly and blood pressure monitored frequently; fluid requirements in the first 12 to 24 hours can be prodigious. A urinary catheter should be inserted and urine output monitored closely. Ad-

TABLE 3. **Differential Diagnosis of Toxic Shock Syndrome**

| | |
|---|---|
| Scarlet fever | Rocky Mountain spotted fever |
| Kawasaki disease | Meningococcemia |
| Stevens-Johnson syndrome | Septic shock |
| Measles | Leptospirosis |

ministration of oxygen is also reasonable at this stage.

Many patients will respond promptly to volume repletion, as evidenced by improvements in blood pressure and/or urine output. In those patients who do not respond to volume replacement, who develop evidence of pulmonary edema, or who are in shock at the time of admission, treatment with a vasopressor agent like dopamine hydrochloride should be considered. In such instances, there should be closer monitoring of hemodynamic parameters and titration of the dose of the pressor agent via a Swan-Ganz catheter and an intra-arterial catheter. If hemodynamic parameters indicate low cardiac output, rather than the high cardiac output usually observed in such cases, cardiomyopathy and depressed myocardial contractility, which have been seen in some TSS cases, should be considered the likely cause. Treatment of this complication requires restricting fluid volume, reducing cardiac afterload, and substituting dobutamine for dopamine.

Some experts also suggest giving high-dose corticosteroids (e.g., methylprednisolone [Solu-Medrol], 10 to 20 mg per kg every 6 to 8 hours for 2 or 3 days) to patients with severe TSS. Prospective studies of high-dose corticosteroids for TSS have not been done, although one retrospective analysis of cases has suggested that they are beneficial in this setting when administered early in the course of the illness. In treating the majority of patients with TSS, however, high-dose corticosteroids are probably unnecessary.

### Minimizing Further Uptake of Toxin

Minimizing the uptake and systemic distribution of additional staphylococcal toxins is accomplished by a combination of draining and removing any focus of infection and treating with antimicrobial agents active against *S. aureus*. Thus, at the time of the initial pelvic examination, any intravaginal device (e.g., tampon, diaphragm, contraceptive sponge, etc.) should be removed (and cultured). Irrigation of the vagina with saline or povidone-iodine, which has been employed in some cases, is of unknown benefit, although it is unlikely to be harmful. A thorough search should be made in all patients for other possible sites of a staphylococcal infection. If found, focal lesions should be drained. In postoperative patients, particular attention should be paid to the surgical wound, which should be re-explored even if it appears grossly uninfected. Adequate drainage of the surgical wound must be ensured.

Antimicrobial therapy should be included in the treatment of all patients with suspected TSS,

TABLE 4. **Complications in Toxic Shock Syndrome**

Acute renal failure
Adult respiratory distress syndrome
Metabolic acidosis
Electrolyte disturbances (hypocalcemia, hypophosphatemia, hypomagnesemia)
Disseminated intravascular coagulation
Encephalopathy
Cardiomyopathy
Hair and nail loss

even though the effect of such therapy on the outcome of the acute illness is unproved. The majority of TSS-associated strains of *S. aureus* are resistant to penicillin and ampicillin (Omnipen), but sensitive to most other antimicrobial agents, including β-lactamase–resistant penicillins (e.g., nafcillin [Nafcil] or cloxacillin [Tegopen]) and cephalosporins (e.g., cefazolin [Ancef, Kefzol]). Antistaphylococcal therapy should be given intravenously in doses similar to those employed for other life-threatening systemic staphylococcal infections (e.g., 100 mg per kg per day of the previously named drugs, divided into four doses and given every 6 hours). Other agents active against *S. aureus,* such as vancomycin (Vancocin) (30 mg per kg per day every 6 hours) or clindamycin (Cleocin) (25 mg per kg per day every 8 hours) also can be used. Many physicians choose to add an aminoglycoside as empiric antimicrobial coverage against gram-negative organisms until the results of blood cultures are available. As for most infectious diseases, the minimum duration of antimicrobial therapy required to treat TSS adequately is unknown. In general, most patients receive a 10- to 14-day course of treatment with an antistaphylococcal agent, with the route of administration being changed from intravenous to oral when the patient is stable and an intravenous line is no longer required.

### Treatment of Complications

A number of complications can arise during the course of TSS (Table 4). Those requiring the most urgent attention are adult respiratory distress syndrome, electrolyte disturbances, metabolic acidosis, and acute renal failure. Thus, patients with severe TSS may require intubation and ventilatory support; close monitoring and correction of abnormalities in the level of serum calcium, other electrolytes, and pH; and short-term hemodialysis or peritoneal dialysis. Seizures and arrhythmias, which can be seen in TSS, generally are secondary to the preceding metabolic disturbances and will respond to treating the underlying cause(s). Late sequelae of TSS, including hair and nail loss and persistent neuropsychiatric problems—e.g., lingering depression, neuromyasthenia, inability to concentrate, difficulty with memory, and so forth—are not amenable to medical intervention; patients with these complications require support and counseling while the complications resolve spontaneously.

### PREVENTION

Women can substantially reduce the risk of TSS associated with menstruation by using sanitary napkins rather than tampons. However, because the risk of TSS is low (approximately 1 to 2 per 100,000 menstruating women per year), even among tampon users, and because many women want the advantages and convenience offered by tampons, it is unlikely that many women will choose to stop using tampons altogether. Women who wish to minimize their risk of TSS while continuing to use tampons should be advised to use the lowest absorbency product compatible with their needs (uniform absorbency labeling of all tampons is now required) and to consider using napkins at night. Frequent changing of tampons, although reasonable on other grounds and intuitively appealing as a means of reducing risk of menstrual TSS, has not been shown to be associated with a reduced risk. Neither routine vaginal cultures nor use of antimicrobial agents to treat or prevent vaginal colonization with *S. aureus* can be recommended or justified as reasonable prevention strategies for TSS.

Women who have had menstrual TSS are at increased risk of recurrent TSS during subsequent menstrual periods. Recurrences can be more or less severe than the initial episode, and multiple recurrences are possible. Appropriate antistaphylococcal treatment of the acute episode of TSS is associated with a markedly reduced risk of subsequent recurrences. In addition, however, women who have had menstrual TSS can reduce their risk of recurrences further by avoiding tampon use. Although many physicians have employed follow-up vaginal cultures to monitor women with a history of menstrual TSS, the appropriate use of and response to such culture results remain uncertain and their value unclear.

# CHLAMYDIA TRACHOMATIS INFECTION

method of
SEBASTIAN FARO, M.D., PH.D.
*Baylor College of Medicine*
*Houston, Texas*

*Chlamydia trachomatis* is one of the most common sexually transmitted microorganisms and is associated with a number of infections in both males and females, including nongonococcal urethritis or urethral syndrome, epididymitis, sterility, cervicitis, endometritis, salpingitis, possible postpartum endometritis, and transmission to the neonate resulting in conjunctivitis and pneumonia. *C. trachomatis* is also responsible for endemic trachomata. This bacterium has also been implicated as a possible etiologic agent that causes abortion, preterm labor, and premature rupture of membranes.

## EPIDEMIOLOGY

The Centers for Disease Control estimates that there are 3 to 4 million cases of chlamydial infection in the United States annually. Chlamydia is more common than the combined estimated number of new cases of gonorrhea, syphilis, and herpes infection. The incidence of cervical colonization is dependent upon the patient population involved. The range is from 2 to 20%. The higher carriage rates are found in the more sexually promiscuous population.

*C. trachomatis* is the leading cause of pneumonia in infants less than 6 months of age and has also superseded *N. gonorrhoeae* as a leading cause of neonatal conjunctivitis. Chlamydial pneumonia is thought to affect 3 to 10 per 1000 live births. In populations with a high prevalence of cervical infection, the incidence may be as high as 50 to 60 per 1000 live births.

## MICROBIOLOGY

*C. trachomatis* is a gram-negative, obligate parasite that has a specific requirement for adenosine triphosphate and amino acids. The organism has the ability to synthesize DNA and RNA as well as a cell wall. However, the obligate requirement for adenosine triphosphate and certain amino acids makes this organism a parasite. There are two stages in the life cycle of this organism. The infective stage, known as the elementary body, attaches to the host cell and is ingested by phagocytosis. Once inside the cell, the elementary body undergoes a metamorphosis to become a reticulate body or initial body, which is the metabolic phase of the life cycle. The initial body duplicates by binary fission and then changes into the elementary body. The host cell, containing elementary bodies, undergoes lysis, liberating infectious organisms. The organism is now capable of reinfecting new cells to repeat its life cycle.

Serotypes L1, L2, and L3 are responsible for lymphogranuloma venereum (LGV), a disease not common in the U.S. However, an increase in the incidence of this disease has been noted, due to the migratory patterns of peoples from South America and far east Asia.

Serotypes D through K are responsible for the more commonly sexually transmitted chlamydial infections. It is estimated that between 20 and 40% of sexually active females have been exposed to this bacterium and have antibody titers to *C. trachomatis*. The colonization rate may be as high as 20% in sexually promiscuous women, whereas the rate drops below 5% in low-risk populations. Patients with a high-risk pro-

file, for instance, those who are young, promiscuous, indigent, unmarried, or live in the inner city, and those who are infected with or who have a prior history of other sexually transmitted diseases, are likely to acquire *C. trachomatis*. Patients with documented chlamydial cervicitis should also be screened for *Neisseria gonorrhoeae*, because it is not uncommon for patients to be co-infected with these two bacteria. Although cervicitis due to *C. trachomatis* frequently accompanies gonorrhea, the incubation period for infection with *C. trachomatis* is 2 to 5 days longer than that for gonorrhea. Thus, the physician may miss identifying a chlamydial infection if the patient is treated with an antibiotic that is not active against *C. trachomatis*—e.g., penicillin and cephalosporins. The fact that the patient has a purulent discharge may make it even more difficult to develop a clinical impression that *Chlamydia* exists. The patient should be cultured specifically for *Chlamydia*. Clinical indications of chlamydial infection are presented in Table 1. However, when coinfections exist, such as *N. gonorrhoeae*, *T. vaginalis*, or herpes simplex, it may be more difficult to utilize the clinical clues indicating chlamydial infection, making it more necessary to obtain an appropriate specimen for detection of *C. trachomatis*.

Chlamydial infection may be asymptomatic in up to 80% of women and 25% of men. It is estimated that approximately 20 to 30% of cases of pelvic inflammatory disease are due to *C. trachomatis*. The incidence of infertility as a sequela of chlamydial infection is not known. However, many infertility patients who come to laparoscopic examination are found to have pelvic adhesions and tubal occlusion secondary to that seen with chlamydial infection, even though these patient have never had symptomatic infections. Therefore, it is important to consider chlamydial infection in patients with vague lower abdominal pain or irregular uterine bleeding.

## DIAGNOSIS

*C. trachomatis* infection can be diagnosed by traditional tissue culture methods or by one of the new rapid tests—i.e., enzyme immunoassay (EIA) (Chlamydiazyme or Testpack [Abbott]), or by direct immunofluorescence—several of which are commercially available. Approximately 60% of cases can be detected by Papanicolaou's smear; however, this is not a good, reliable method. If none of the methods are available, a tentative diagnosis may be achieved by microscopic examination of an endocervical specimen, as outlined in Table 1.

The clinical clues to chlamydial infection are puru-

TABLE 1. **Clinical Clues to Chlamydial Infection**

1. Presence of mucopus in the endocervical canal
2. Microscopic examination
   a. Presence of white cells
   b. Absence of bacteria on Gram's stain
   c. <10 squamous epithelial cells per high-powered field
3. Hypertrophy of columnar epithelium of endocervix
4. Pyuria but no bacteria on Gram's stain or culture of urine

lent urethral discharge, endocervical mucopus, spotting after intercourse, intermenstrual spotting, vague lower abdominal pain, cervical atypia, or infertility. Chlamydial infection should also be searched for in patients with premature rupture of amniotic membranes.

## TREATMENT

Once a diagnosis is established or strongly suspected, antibiotic therapy should be instituted for the patient and her sexual partner (Table 2). Erythromycin administered to pregnant women has been associated with a cure rate of approximately 90%. Erythromycin in the ethyl succinate form (EES) seems to be well tolerated, with better compliance and less nausea than those with erythromycin base.

Because neonatal infection rates among offspring of untreated infected women approach 50%, all women who have chlamydial infections diagnosed during pregnancy should receive treatment. Their sexual partners must be treated simultaneously. In cases of a positive initial culture, the follow-up culture should be performed within 7 to 14 days after completing therapy.

In cases of suspected salpingitis, the patient should be re-examined within 72 hours after receiving antibiotic therapy. If the patient's condition is not improving, she should be hospitalized and parenteral therapy instituted. Consideration should also be given to performing laparoscopy to establish a correct diagnosis. It is important to remember that patients with pelvic inflammatory disease receiving a cephalosporin, such as cefotetan (Cefotan) or cefoxitin (Mefoxin), do not have activity against *Chlamydia,* and therefore doxycycline (Vibramycin) or erythromycin should be given.

New agents that have not yet been released for the treatment of *Chlamydia,* mainly the quinolones, have demonstrated good activity against *Chlamydia.* These, when they become available, will offer alternatives to using tetracyclines, doxycycline, or erythromycin, especially in those patients who cannot tolerate these agents. Quinolones are contraindicated in pregnant and breast-feeding mothers. Recent data suggest that

### TABLE 2. Treatment of *Chlamydia trachomatis* Infection

Tetracycline, 500 mg PO qid for 7 days
*or*
Doxycycline, 100 mg PO bid for 7 days

**During Pregnancy**
Erythromycin, 500 mg PO qid for 7 days
*or*
Erythromycin ethyl succinate, 400 to 800 mg PO qid for 7 days

penicillins, such as ampicillin (Amcil, Omnipen), amoxicillin (Amoxil, Larotid), ticarcillin (Ticar), and piperacillin (Pipracil) may have activity against *Chlamydia.* Data are not yet available from good control studies demonstrating the efficacy of these agents. Clindamycin (Cleocin) has also been shown to be effective against *Chlamydia.* Therefore, treating patients with pelvic inflammatory disease with a combination of clindamycin and an aminoglycoside should provide adequate coverage for *Chlamydia.*

# PELVIC INFLAMMATORY DISEASE

method of
R. PHILLIP HEINE, M.D., and
WILLIAM DROEGEMUELLER, M.D.
*University of North Carolina School of Medicine*
*Chapel Hill, North Carolina*

Pelvic inflammatory disease (PID) is a term used to refer to infection of the upper genital tract, including the endometrium, the oviducts, the ovary, the uterine wall and serosa, the broad ligaments, and the pelvic peritoneum. Salpingitis, infection of the oviducts, is a term used interchangeably with PID. Oviduct involvement is characteristic of PID and results in the most long-term sequelae. Chronic PID is no longer used because pelvic infections are not chronic in duration. The exceptions to this are actinomycosis and tuberculosis; either may produce both acute and chronic infection.

The growing epidemic of sexually transmitted diseases (STDs), the antecedents of PID, is a major concern in today's society. The annual cost of PID and its sequelae is estimated at $3.5 billion a year in 1990. Pelvic inflammatory disease accounts for 2.5 million office visits, 267,000 inpatient hospital admissions, and 119,000 operative procedures annually in the United States. To counteract this problem, an emphasis must be placed on prophylaxis and aggressive therapy of lower and upper genital tract infections.

One to two per cent of young sexually active women develop PID annually. In women 16 to 25 years of age, PID is the most prevalent serious infection. One of four women experiences serious long-term sequelae, including a 10-fold increase in ectopic pregnancy and a fourfold increase in chronic pelvic pain. Reproductive difficulties are increased, with an 11.4%, 23.1%, and 54.3% incidence of infertility following one, two, and three episodes of PID, respectively. After one infection women are more susceptible to reinfection. It is not known whether subsequent infections result from increased susceptibility of damaged mucosa or from reinfection by a high-risk cohort.

## ETIOLOGY

Acute PID is created by organisms that ascend from the vagina and the cervix to infect the mucosa of the endometrium and/or the oviduct. Eighty-five per cent of cases are spontaneous infection; 15% represent breaks in the cervical mucus following procedures such as endometrial biopsy, curettage, intrauterine device (IUD) insertion, and hysterosalpingography. Organisms commonly isolated from culture of tubal fluid include *Neisseria gonorrhoeae, Chlamydia trachomatis,* and endogenous aerobic and anaerobic bacteria. The role of *N. gonorrhoeae* in PID is well known; 15% of women with untreated cervical infection develop acute PID. *N. gonorrhoeae* produces a rapid onset, intense inflammatory reaction in the tubes, with cellular destruction much more extensive than that of chlamydial infection. Chlamydia, which has supplanted *N. gonorrhoeae* as the most common cause of STD, produces a disease of insidious onset, with tubal damage mediated by an immunopathologic mechanism rather than by direct cytotoxicity. The role of genital mycoplasma in the genesis of PID is unclear, but most evidence points to a commensal rather than a pathologic relationship. Infection of the upper genital tract is frequently caused by endogenous aerobic and anaerobic organisms. Aerobic organisms commonly implicated are nonhemolytic *Streptococcus, Escherichia coli,* group B *Streptococcus,* and coagulase-negative *Staphylococcus.* Anaerobes include *Bacteroides* species, *Peptococcus,* and *Peptostreptococcus.*

A rare cause of upper genital tract infection is actinomyces, and, in most cases, it is associated with IUD use. It is not known whether actinomyces plays a primary or secondary role in the infectious process.

Tuberculosis of the upper genital tract primarily produces a chronic salpingitis. Tuberculosis should be suspected in patients who have chronic abdominal and pelvic pain, irregular bleeding, and infertility and who are from areas in the world where tuberculosis is endemic.

## RISK FACTORS

Gross indicators of exposure to STD include marital status, age at first intercourse, coital frequency, and number of sexual partners. The chance of having PID is increased fivefold in women having multiple sexual partners. Sexually active adolescent women have a 1 in 8 chance of acquiring disease; those older than 25 years have a 1 in 80 chance. Sexual habits play a role in this difference, but lack of antibody protection may also be important. Oral contraceptives and barrier methods are protective against PID. An IUD increases the risk approximately twofold, but only for the first 2 months after insertion. Pelvic inflammatory disease is exceedingly rare in a patient with a previous tubal ligation. Transcervical penetration from a break in the cervical mucous barrier via instrumentation is a risk factor, and in high-risk patients antibiotic prophylaxis is encouraged.

## SYMPTOMS AND SIGNS

Patients with PID have many clinical symptoms: The most common is a dull aching lower abdominal and pelvic pain, usually of less than 1 week's duration. Other symptoms include vaginal discharge, fever, irregular bleeding, urinary tract symptoms, nausea and

vomiting, and proctitis. Of interest, only one in three patients has a temperature greater than 38° C. A late symptom is infertility, as 50% of women with tubal obstruction do not remember having symptoms of acute disease. *N. gonorrhoeae*–related PID is usually rapid in onset, with pain beginning a few days after the start of menses. Chlamydial infection, on the other hand, has a slow onset, less pain, and less fever.

The hallmark of PID is lower abdominal and pelvic tenderness. Most patients have direct tenderness to palpation of the abdomen and some have rebound tenderness. Pelvic examination reveals a purulent cervical discharge with tenderness of the parametrium and adnexa, especially with movement of the uterus or the cervix. Fullness in the adnexa is a common finding, most likely because of inflammatory adhesions or edema. The true incidence of adnexal abscess is approximately 10%. Fitz-Hugh–Curtis syndrome with right upper quadrant tenderness occurs in 5 to 10% of cases of acute PID and is caused by *N. gonorrhoeae* or chlamydial perihepatic inflammation.

## DIAGNOSIS

PID is diagnosed clinically, but even with strict criteria the disease is confirmed in only 65% at laparoscopy. Table 1 outlines the Obstetrical and Gynecologic Infectious Disease Society's clinical criteria for diagnosis of PID. The differential diagnosis includes lower genital tract infection, ectopic pregnancy, torsion or rupture of an adnexal mass, appendicitis, and endometriosis. It is important to culture the endocervix for *N. gonorrhoeae* and obtain either an antigen detection test or a direct culture for *Chlamydia*. The mucus should be examined for inflammatory cells, and a gram's stain should be performed. Also recommended are a sensitive pregnancy test to evaluate for a potential ectopic pregnancy and a complete blood count for leukocytosis. Only 50% of women with acute PID have a white blood cell count of greater than 10,000 cells per mm³. Ultrasound is of limited value, except when the examiner cannot determine the presence or absence of an abscess. Although laparoscopy is considered the

TABLE 1. **Salpingitis: Clinical Criteria for Diagnosis***

| Criteria | |
|---|---|
| Abdominal direct tenderness, with or without rebound tenderness | All 3 necessary for diagnosis |
| Tenderness with motion of cervix and uterus | |
| Adnexal tenderness | |
| *plus* | |
| Gram's stain of endocervix positive for gram-negative, intracellular diplococci | 1 or more necessary for diagnosis |
| Fever (temperature >38° C) | |
| Leukocytosis (>10,000 white blood cells/mm³) | |
| Purulent material (white blood cells present) from peritoneal cavity by culdocentesis or laparoscopy | |
| Pelvic abscess or inflammatory complex on bimanual examination or on sonography | |

*From Hager WD, Eschenbach DA, Spence MR, et al: Obstet Gynecol *61:*114, 1983. Reprinted with permission from The American College of Obstetricians and Gynecologists.

"gold standard" for diagnosis of PID, its routine use is not feasible. Laparoscopy should be used only when diagnosis is uncertain or if the patient is not responding to therapy.

## TREATMENT

The resolution of symptoms and preservation of tubal function are the primary goals in the management of PID. Ideally, all patients would be hospitalized to ensure patient compliance and adequate levels of antibiotics. As hospitalization is economically impractical, many patients are treated on an outpatient basis. Table 2 lists the most recent Centers for Disease Control (CDC) recommendations for outpatient treatment. This treatment includes a one-time intramuscular injection of either cefoxitin or ceftriaxone followed by an oral course of doxycycline or tetracycline for 10 to 14 days. Ceftriaxone may be the preferred drug because cefoxitin-resistant strains of *N. gonorrhoeae* are now being isolated. The 14-day course of either doxycycline or tetracycline is important because *Chlamydia* coexist in 25 to 40% of cases with *N. gonorrhoeae*. The patient should be re-examined within 48 to 72 hours and hospitalized if response is suboptimal. Additional admission criteria include nulliparity, presence of a tubo-ovarian complex or abscess, pregnancy, peritoneal signs, and uncertain diagnosis. CDC recommendations for treatment of inpatients with PID are outlined in Table 3. Regimen A includes cefoxitin or an equivalent cephalosporin in combination with doxycycline. This regimen is an excellent choice against community-acquired disease because it is active against both *N. gonorrhoeae* and *Chlamydia*. Regimen B is a combination of clindamycin and gentamicin, and it is highly active against anaerobes and facultative gram-negative rods. Regimen B is preferred in

TABLE 2. **Recommended Regimen for Ambulatory Management***

---

Cefoxitin (Mefoxin), 2 grams IM, plus probenecid, 1 gram PO, concurrently, or ceftriaxone (Rocephin), 250 mg IM, or equivalent cephalosporin

*plus*

Doxycycline (Vibramycin), 100 mg PO bid for 10–14 days

*or*

Tetracycline 500 mg PO qid for 10–14 days

Alternative for patients who do not tolerate doxycycline: Erythromycin, 500 mg PO qid for 10–14 days, may be substituted for doxycycline or tetracycline. This regimen, however, is based on limited clinical data.

---

*From Centers for Disease Control. MMWR *38* (S-8):31–33, 1989.

TABLE 3. **Recommended Regimen for Inpatient Treatment***

---

One of the following:

**Regimen A**
Cefoxitin (Mefoxin), 2 grams IV q 6 hr, or cefotetan† (Cefotan), 2 grams IV q 12 hr,

*plus*

Doxycycline, 100 mg q 12 hr PO or IV
This regimen is given for at least 48 hr after the patient clinically improves.
After discharge from hospital, continuation of doxycycline, 100 mg PO bid for a total of 10–14 days

**Regimen B**
Clindamycin (Cleocin), 900 mg IV q 8 hr,

*plus*

Gentamicin (Garamycin), loading dose IV or IM (2 mg/kg) followed by a maintenance dose (1.5 mg/kg) q 8 hr
This regimen is given for at least 48 hr after the patient improves.
After discharge from hospital, continuation of doxycycline, 100 mg PO bid for 10–14 days total

---

*From Centers for Disease Control. MMWR *38* (S-8):31–33, 1989.

†Other cephalosporins, such as ceftizoxime (Cefizox), cefotaxime (Claforan), and ceftriaxone (Rocephin), which provide adequate gonococcal, other facultative gram-negative aerobic, and anaerobic coverage, may be utilized in appropriate doses.

patients with IUD-related infection, suspected abscess, or procedure-related infection. New antibiotics were developed because of increases in penicillinase-producing and tetracycline-resistant *N. gonorrhoeae* as well as chromosomally mediated resistance to multiple antibiotics. This new generation of antibiotics has excellent activity against pelvic pathogens. These new antibiotics include second- and third-generation cephalosporins (in the CDC Regimen A) and β-lactamase resistant antibiotics, such as ampicillin-sulbactam and ticarcillin–clavulanic acid. Imipenem-cilastatin also has outstanding activity in PID. As outlined in CDC inpatient Regimen A, doxycycline should be administered concurrently with these antibiotics and continued to complete a 14-day course. Intravenous therapy with any regimen should be continued for at least 4 days and at least 48 hours after the patient's condition has improved.

Surgical intervention in PID is restricted to life-threatening infection, ruptured tubo-ovarian abscess, drainage of a pelvic mass that is pointing into the cul-de-sac, persistent mass in older women for whom fertility is not a question, and removal of a persistent symptomatic mass. In women for whom ovarian function and future fertility are desirable, conservative surgery with unilateral removal of a tubo-ovarian complex or abscess is recommended.

# LEIOMYOMAS OF THE UTERUS

method of
SUSAN M. LOBEL, M.D.,
ANDREW J. FRIEDMAN, M.D., and
ISAAC SCHIFF, M.D.
*Harvard Medical School*
*Boston, Massachusetts*

Uterine leiomyomas (also known as fibroids) develop from single myometrial cells that proliferate after undergoing neoplastic change. Estrogen appears to be important for the development and growth of these benign tumors, as revealed by the fact that leiomyomas arise only during reproductive years and often show increased growth rates during high-estrogen states (e.g., pregnancy) and regression following estrogen withdrawal (e.g., menopause). Leiomyomas are the most common female solid pelvic tumor, occurring in approximately 25% of reproductive-age women. Moreover, black women have a prevalence rate that is three to nine times that of caucasians. Multiple leiomyomas are encountered in the majority of women with these tumors. They are firm, spheric, and white or tan with a whorled trabecular pattern visible on cross-section.

Uterine leiomyomas may be submucosal, intramural, or subserosal. Occasionally, they are found in extrauterine locations, including the broad ligament, the fallopian tubes, the vagina, the vulva, and the bowel. Rarely (i.e., less than 0.1%), leiomyomas may undergo sarcomatous degeneration.

## DIAGNOSIS

Approximately 20 to 50% of women with leiomyomas have symptoms attributable to these tumors. Common symptoms include menorrhagia (with subsequent social debilitation and iron deficiency anemia), pelvic pressure (causing discomfort, urinary frequency, and/or constipation), and increased abdominal girth. Less commonly, dyspareunia and reproductive complications may result (e.g., recurrent abortions, abnormal fetal presentation, abruptio placentae, premature labor, outlet obstruction, and tubal obstruction). Fibroids that grow rapidly may outgrow their blood supply or undergo torsion and degeneration, which is associated with severe, acute abdominal pain.

On physical examination, uterine leiomyomas can usually be appreciated as an enlarged, often irregular, firm pelvic mass contiguous with the uterus. The diagnosis may be confirmed (and the possibility of an adnexal mass ruled out) by ultrasonography or magnetic resonance imaging. Hysteroscopy or hysterosalpingography are often helpful in the detection of submucosal fibroids. Of note, this type of fibroid may present with menorrhagia or hypermenorrhea in the absence of uterine enlargement. Fibroids may compress the ureters, leading to hydronephrosis detectable by intravenous pyelogram or ultrasound.

## TREATMENT

The treatment of uterine fibroids is influenced by their size, the symptoms, and the patient's age and reproductive interests. Small asymptomatic fibroids may be managed expectantly with biannual pelvic examinations to ensure size stability. A baseline ultrasound to document uterine size and check for hydronephorosis is advisable in these cases.

The one definitive treatment for uterine leiomyomas is hysterectomy. More than 175,000 hysterectomies for leiomyomas are performed annually in the United States. When uterine fundal size exceeds 12 cm, palpation of adnexa is usually difficult, symptoms may worsen, and the risk of compression of adjacent visceral structures increases. Hysterectomy is therefore often recommended.

In women wishing to preserve fertility or to avoid hysterectomy for other reasons, myomectomy (selective removal of the fibroids) may be performed. In a small number of cases, owing to leiomyoma location and bleeding complications, this is not feasible. The need for further major surgery for recurrent fibroids is approximately 20 to 30%. Some small submucous fibroids can be resected with the hysteroscope, thereby avoiding laparotomy and its attendant risks.

Medical management of fibroids is limited. Progesterone may be used to regulate menorrhagia after appropriate endometrial sampling has ruled out neoplasia. Many physicians avoid the use of oral contraceptives in women with fibroids out of concern that the estrogen will stimulate fibroid growth. Current research is focusing on the use of gonadotropin-releasing hormone agonists (GnRH-a), which have the ability to decrease uterine volume by approximately 50% within 3 months through the creation of a hypoestrogenic state. However, fibroids return to pretreatment size often within 3 to 6 months following cessation of therapy. Because long-term GnRH-a use may be associated with hypoestrogenic complications (e.g., osteoporosis), these agents should not be used for longer than 6 months. Some preliminary data suggest that preoperative GnRH-a treatment may decrease intraoperative blood loss at hysterectomy and myomectomy.

# CANCER OF THE ENDOMETRIUM

method of
JOHN H. MALFETANO, M.D.
*The Albany Medical College*
*Albany, New York*

Carcinoma of the body of the uterus is the most common gynecologic malignancy and has remained so for the past decade. Throughout the 1970s, there was a 1.5-fold increase in the number of endometrial cancer patients. In 1975, 27,000 new cases were reported, reaching a high of 40,000 cases in 1986; the estimated number of new cases annually now appears to be stable at 34,000. Endometrial carcinoma is the sixth leading cause of death in females after breast, colorectal, lung, ovarian and cervical carcinomas.

## EPIDEMIOLOGY

Uterine cancer is a disease of the postmenopausal female (75% of cases), with a peak incidence at 58 years of age. Some 25% of the patients are premenopausal, 5% of whom are under the age of 40 at the time of diagnosis. Endometrial carcinoma is more common is caucasian women than in black or Asian persons. The apparent rise in the incidence of carcinoma of the corpus is attributed primarily to two factors: obesity and the use of unopposed exogenous estrogens for menopausal symptoms. Other associated risk factors include living in a highly industrialized Western country, familial history, upper socioeconomic class, history of anovulation, nulliparity, estrogen-producing ovarian neoplasms, and the coincident disorders of adult-onset diabetes mellitus and hypertension. The high-risk woman characterized by obesity, failure of ovulation, or prolonged estrogen administration produces continuous, unopposed estrogen stimulation to the endometrium and appears to be causally subject to subsequent development of endometrial carcinoma. This continuous endometrial stimulation in susceptible individuals leads to hyperplastic states within the endometrium and thereafter to frank carcinoma.

## DIAGNOSIS AND DETECTION

The first symptom in virtually all women with carcinoma of the endometrium is abnormal bleeding, spotting, or discharge. The frequency, amount, and duration of bleeding are of no consequence, and all forms of bleeding demand investigation, especially in the postmenopausal female. Nearly 30 to 50% of postmenopausal bleeding is caused by carcinoma. Papanicolaou's smear, which has been so successful in detecting early cervical carcinoma, is not reliable for detection of endometrial carcinoma. The false-negative rate of cervical and vaginal smears in endometrial carcinoma ranges from 50 to 80%.

A variety of sampling techniques, both cytologic and histologic, are available for the detection of endometrial carcinoma. It is axiomatic that any woman with postmenopausal bleeding must have the endometrial cavity sampled, either by an office endometrial biopsy or by formal curettage of the endometrium. Only with an office biopsy that is positive for carcinoma can the physician be certain about the etiology of the abnormal bleeding. Any other pathologic result from the office sampling necessitates a formal dilatation and curettage of the uterus. A small carcinoma within atypical adenomatous hyperplasia may be missed by office biopsy alone. Repeat sampling is also necessary if symptoms persist without any etiology, and in rare circumstances, hysterectomy is indicated for diagnosis.

Carcinoma of the uterine corpus was previously clinically staged. In 1988, the International Federation of Gynecology and Obstetrics revised the staging completely to comply with surgical staging (Table 1). This process depends on the physical examination, chest and x-ray roentgenograms, and blood chemistry. The stage is influenced by the subsequent surgical pathologic findings. This change in staging was based on the extensive data available on the surgical-pathologic spread pattern of endometrial cancer and established prognostic factors. These prognostic factors include the depth of myometrial invasion, status of the cervix, presence or absence of pelvic and/or para-aortic nodal disease, peritoneal cytology, and extrauterine metastases.

TABLE 1. **FIGO Classification of Carcinoma of the Corpus Uteri***

| Stage | Characteristics |
|---|---|
| IA G123 | Tumor limited to endometrium |
| IB G123 | Invasion to less than one-half the myometrium |
| IC G123 | Invasion to more than one-half the myometrium |
| IIA G123 | Endocervical glandular involvement only |
| IIB G123 | Cervical stromal invasion |
| IIIA G123 | Tumor invades serosa and/or adnexa, and/or positive peritoneal cytology |
| IIIB G123 | Vaginal metastases |
| IIIC G123 | Metastases to pelvic and/or para-aortic lymph nodes |
| IVA G123 | Tumor invasion of bladder and/or bowel mucosa |
| IVB | Distant metastases, including intra-abdominal and/or inguinal lymph nodes |

**Histopathology: Degree of Differentiation**

Cases of carcinoma of the corpus should be classified (or graded) according to the degree of histologic differentiation, as follows:

G1 = 5% or less of a nonsquamous or nonmorular solid growth pattern

G2 = 6–50% of a nonsquamous or nonmorular solid growth pattern

G3 = >50% of a nonsquamous or nonmorular solid growth pattern

**Rules Related to Staging**

1. Because corpus cancer is now staged surgically, procedures previously used for determination of stages are no longer applicable, such as the findings from fractional D&C to differentiate between stage I and stage II.

2. It is appreciated that there may be a small number of patients with corpus cancer who will be treated primarily with radiation therapy. If that is the case, the clinical staging adopted by FIGO in 1971 would still apply but designation of that staging system would be noted.

3. Ideally, width of the myometrium should be measured along with the width of tumor invasion.

*Reprinted with permission from The American College of Obstetrics and Gynecologists. (OBSTETRICS AND GYNECOLOGY, Vol 75, No. 2, February 1990.

TABLE 2. **Five-Year Survival in Carcinoma of the Uterine Corpus**

| Stage | 5-Year Survival (%) |
|-------|---------------------|
| I | 63–94 |
| II | 50–65 |
| III | 25–35 |
| IV | 5–10 |

## TREATMENT

Adenocarcinoma of the endometrium remains one of the most treatable gynecologic malignancies despite a previous lack of unanimity concerning the best treatment. Nearly 70% of patients with endometrial cancer present with Stage I disease, which portends a favorable prognosis. Survival ranges from 63 to 94% for patients with Stage I cancer; however, extrauterine disease is more difficult to control (Table 2).

The treatment of endometrial carcinoma is based on the surgical pathologic findings at operation. Treatment planning and prognosis are related to the risk factors of tumor grade, myometrial invasion, extension to the cervix or adnexa, and possibly positive peritoneal cytology. These virulence factors are helpful in selecting women who are at risk for pelvic and para-aortic nodal metastasis and, therefore, who are to be candidates for postoperative radiation therapy. As the tumor becomes more undifferentiated, with deeper invasion into the myometrium, the incidence of nodal disease increases (Tables 3 and 4).

The approach to Stage I carcinoma of the uterine corpus is surgical. In opening the abdominal cavity, pelvic and paracolic washings are obtained by instilling 100 to 150 ml of saline and sending the specimens for cytologic evaluation and cell block. The entire abdomen is then explored. An extrafascial hysterectomy and bilateral salpingo-oophorectomy are performed. Bilateral pelvic lymph nodes, as well as aortic lymph nodes, are sampled and sent for histologic evaluation, followed by resection or biopsy of any other sites that may harbor metastatic disease.

## POSTOPERATIVE MANAGEMENT

The radiation fields are tailored to the surgical and pathologic findings at surgery. Standard pel-

TABLE 3. **Endometrial Cancer Grade Versus Positive Pelvic and Para-Aortic Nodal Disease**

| Grade | Pelvic Nodes (%) | Para-Aortic Nodes (%) |
|-------|------------------|------------------------|
| 1 | 3 | 0–2 |
| 2 | 10 | 4.0–13.6 |
| 3 | 36 | 28–37.5 |

TABLE 4. **Depth of Myometrial Invasion and Pelvic and Para-Aortic Nodal Disease**

| Myometrial Invasion | Pelvic Nodes (%) | Para-Aortic Nodes (%) |
|---------------------|------------------|------------------------|
| Endometrium only | 1–3.6 | 1–1.8 |
| Inner one-third | 5–11.5 | 3–9.8 |
| Middle one-third | 6–10 | 0–1 |
| Outer one-third | 25–43 | 17–21 |

vic fields should deliver midplane doses of 4500 to 5000 cGy and cover the upper one-third of the vagina. The upper extent of the radiation field should cover the L4-5 vertebral interspace. Extended para-aortic fields to cover T10 and deliver 4500 to 5000 cGy are necessary if there is paraaortic nodal disease. Patients with Grade 3 lesions, positive pelvic nodes, extension to the cervix, or tumor of any grade with myometrial invasion of 50% or more are candidates for postoperative therapy.

Endometrial cancer patients with no risk factors can be considered for postoperative vaginal treatment. Vaginal cylinders produce a surface dose to the vaginal apex of 6000 cGy and reduce vaginal cuff recurrences to approximately 1%.

Patients with para-aortic nodal disease represent a difficult problem because they probably have systemic disease. To date, there is no known effective therapy for this group; however, extended-field radiation therapy to the para-aortic chain, with or without chemotherapy, has been quite promising.

Patients with occult clinical Stage II endometrial carcinoma should be treated in the same manner as other Stage I patients. Postoperative pelvic radiation is indicated if there is stromal involvement of the cervix. Patients with gross Stage II carcinoma of the uterus are treated like patients with Stage IB carcinoma of the cervix. This includes radical hysterectomy and bilateral salpingo-oophorectomy, pelvic and para-aortic lymphadenectomy, or pelvic radiation therapy plus an interstitial implant combined with extrafascial hysterectomy and bilateral salpingo-oophorectomy. The experienced pathologist may have difficulty distinguishing Stage II carcinoma of the endometrium from adenocarcinoma of the endocervix, and the final diagnosis may be discovered only postoperatively.

## GROUP II PATIENTS (MEDICALLY INOPERABLE)

Some patients, because of advanced stage or a poor medical condition that prevents surgery, fall into the Group II category. This relatively rare group of patients can be treated with external pelvic radiation and intracavitary therapy. The overall survival rate with radiation therapy alone in Stage I disease ranges from 28 to 78% at 5 years.

## STAGE III AND STAGE IV ENDOMETRIAL CANCER

Adequate treatment of advanced endometrial cancer is not available and must be individualized. Depending on the sites of metastatic disease, surgery, radiation therapy, and chemotherapy may be used.

## RECURRENT DISEASE

Cytotoxic chemotherapy for endometrial cancer has been slow to evolve because of high cure rates with surgery and radiation therapy. Hormonal therapy had been the mainstay of treatment of recurrent disease. Estrogen and progesterone receptors are contained in endometrial cancers, and tumors should be sent for determination of these receptors at the time of initial operation. Tumors can be hormonally manipulated if the receptor status is known. Progestational agents alone or with tamoxifen, which may increase progesterone receptors, can be used.

Recent studies have shown that progestational agents are not nearly as effective as earlier studies had suggested and that pulmonary lesions may be the only ones to respond. Ongoing present clinical trials using systemic agents, cisplatin (Platinol), doxorubicin (Adriamycin), and cyclophosphamide (Cytoxan) are encouraging.

# CANCER OF THE UTERINE CERVIX

method of
JOANNA M. CAIN, M.D.
*University of Washington Medical Center*
*Seattle, Washington*

The average age of women with invasive cervical cancer is 53 years. However, there is concern that the age of women with invasive cervical cancer is decreasing, with more patients in the 20- to 40-year old age group. The risk factors associated with this disease are those associated with exposure to an infectious agent—e.g., early age at first intercourse, multiple sexual partners, and infection with herpes virus Type 2 or papillomavirus—and with exposure to potential carcinogens, such as smoking.

## DIAGNOSIS

Cervical cytologic sampling (Papanicolaou's [Pap] smear) remains the best form of early detection of cervical invasive cancers and those lesions that may be precursors of invasive cervical cancer, cervical intraepithelial neoplasia (CIN) I through III. The appro-

priate frequency interval for Pap smears is controversial, but studies in the United States suggest that the number of invasive cervical cancers increases when the sampling interval has lengthened to 3 years or longer. For those patients with one or more high-risk factors listed earlier, including any previously abnormal Pap smear findings, yearly Pap smear follow-up is recommended. A single normal Pap smear finding has a false-negative rate of 15 to 30%. It is important to remember that a grossly evident invasive cancer may have a normal Pap smear appearance. A Pap smear is not a histologic diagnostic tool, only a screening device to indicate who needs further evaluation. Patients with an abnormal cervical area should undergo biopsy regardless of the Pap test results. With no high-risk factors and three consecutive normal Pap smears, women should have a repeat Pap smear every 2 years.

## STAGING

The International Federation of Gynecology and Obstetrics (FIGO) has defined the stages of cervical cancer as outlined in Table 1. This staging system (1985) represents a departure from the previous system in the definition of subgroups of Stage I. Although the overall system remains clinical, with stages assigned prior to operative intervention, the accurate measurements demanded in Stage IA1 and IA2 may require a cone biopsy specimen with careful pathologic preparation to clarify.

The work-up prior to treatment of this disease always includes a careful history and physical examination, chest x-ray, and serum evaluation of renal, hepatic, and hematologic status. The use of intravenous pyelography is generally recommended. This may be replaced in advanced disease by a computer tomography study or magnetic resonance imaging, which

TABLE 1. **FIGO Classification of Cervical Cancer**

| Stage | Characteristics |
| --- | --- |
| 0 | Carcinoma in situ, intraepithelial carcinoma |
| I | Carcinoma confined to the cervix |
| IA1 | Minimal microscopically evident stromal invasion |
| IA2 | Stromal invasion less than 5-mm deep and less than 7-mm wide |
| IB | Limited to the cervix but not meeting requirements for IA |
| II | The carcinoma extends beyond the cervix, but has not extended onto the pelvic wall, or the cancer involves the vagina, but not the lower third |
| IIA | No obvious parametrial involvement |
| IIB | Obvious parametrial involvement |
| III | The carcinoma has extended onto the pelvic wall; on rectal examination, there is no cancer-free space between the tumor and the pelvic wall, or the tumor involved the lower third of the vagina |
| IIIA | No extension to the pelvic wall |
| IIIB | Extension onto the pelvic wall and/or hydronephrosis or nonfunctioning kidney |
| IV | The carcinoma has extended beyond the true pelvis or has clinically involved the mucosa of the bladder or rectum |
| IVA | Spread of growth to adjacent organs |
| IVB | Spread to distant organs |

assesses potential nodal involvement as well as renal and ureteral status. Cystoscopy and sigmoidoscopy may be of value in some patients with large lesions or unusual histologic types.

## TREATMENT

Stage 0 lesions are those described as carcinoma in situ without any evidence of invasion. Therapy for these lesions focuses on removal of the involved epithelium either surgically or by ablation with cryotherapy, laser vaporization, or hot cautery. All of these are effective (90%), with the surgical removal of the area by cervical conization slightly more effective (97%). When there is any question of the extent of disease, the involvement of the endocervix, or a major discrepancy with the Pap smear finding, cervical conization is warranted, despite the slightly higher morbidity, including cervical imcompetence, stenosis, and bleeding.

### Stage I

Stage IA cervical cancer has the potential of being treated less aggressively than the other stages of cervical carcinoma. The ability to limit the surgical resection to a cone biopsy with wide margins or a hysterectomy (preferred) is predicated on identifying factors that suggest that the risk for metastatic disease is low. The FIGO staging system implies a decision point by the definition of stage IA2, however, this is neither universally accepted nor utilized in this country. The more generally accepted rule for definition of microinvasive disease is that set by the Society of Gynecologic Oncologists—i.e., less than 3 mm invasion and no lymphatic or vascular invasion. The decision about risk of metastasis and selection of therapy should be made only after review of the pathologic findings.

Patients with Stage IA lesions who are thought to be at higher risk for metastatic disease, and those with IB and early IIA lesions, have two alternatives for therapy that are equally effective, radiation therapy and radical hysterectomy with node dissection. Five-year survival is 50 to 90% and is based on risk factors such as the presence of positive nodes, cell types such as "glassy cell" or adenocarcinoma, and occult parametrial involvement. The decision between these options is based on the ability of the patient to safely undergo radical surgery and the potential benefits to the patient of avoiding radiation or identifying metastatic disease. Generally, patients with significant medical illness or the physically infirm are better served by radiation. There

are subgroups of patients with disease greater than 4 cm in diameter (or barrel shaped) or with pathologic features suggesting a high risk for recurrence who are appropriately treated by combinations of surgery and/or radiotherapy and/or chemotherapy. Those decisions should be made by a physician knowledgeable in the field.

### Stage II, III, and IVA

Patients with Stage IIA and more extensive cancer are primarily treated with radiation therapy. For patients with large bulky disease, adjuvant chemotherapy or radiosensitizer protocols are often utilized to attempt to improve an otherwise poor prognosis (20 to 50% 5-year survival). The design of the external beam radiation fields is done on an individual basis to include all areas suspected of having involved nodes plus an echelon of nodes above. The adequate treatment of pelvic central disease requires an additional local implant, afterloaded with cesium, generally done after the completion of external beam therapy. The incidence of complications of radiation therapy increases with dosage and with certain anatomic attributes, such as pelvic adhesions that do not allow small bowel to move out of the field. These complications include injury to the bowel wall, the ureter, the bladder wall, and the vaginal wall, resulting in stenosis, obstruction, or fistula formation. Long-term radiation cystitis and proctitis can be difficult to treat and can cause hemorrhage and dysfunction.

### Metastatic and Recurrent Disease

The treatment of distant metastases, whether Stage IVB or recurrent disease, is generally chemotherapy. The agents utilized have been Cisplatin (Platinol), mitomycin (mitomycin-C, Mutamycin), bleomycin (Blenoxane), and methotrexate. Each has been used alone and in combination, but the long-term results are poor.

The treatment of recurrent disease is based on the prior therapy and the location of the disease. If no previous radiation has been given, radiation therapy is the first choice. If previous radiation therapy has been given and the disease is central, pelvic exenteration is the first consideration. The other options for treatment include intraoperative radiation if disease is localized but not appropriate for exenteration, or reirradiation if the initial dose allows this or sufficient time has elapsed from the initial treatment. The use of chemotherapy in this setting has had a poor response.

# NEOPLASMS OF THE VULVA

method of
IRA R. HOROWITZ, M.D.
*Johns Hopkins University School of Medicine*
*Baltimore, Maryland*

Vulvar neoplasia is the fourth most common genital tumor in women, accounting for 3 to 5% of genital tumors and 0.3% of all female malignancies. The majority of patients present in the sixth decade of life. Unfortunately, vulvar disease and its treatment have altered the psychosocial well-being of women. The surgery is frequently disfiguring and is fraught with complications, such as leg edema, vaginal stenosis, dyspareunia, wound separation, and lack of a cosmetic vulva. Recent changes in treatment protocols have helped to decrease the procedural morbidity and improved the patient's self-image.

## PREINVASIVE LESIONS

The Ninth Congress of the International Society for the Study of Vulvar Disease (1987) in conjunction with the International Society of Gynecological Pathologists changed the nomenclature for preinvasive vulvar disease. Non-neoplastic epithelial disorder of the skin and mucosa is the new term for vulvar dystrophy (Table 1). Hyperplastic dystrophy is classified as squamous cell hyperplasia, and atypical hyperplastic dystrophy is categorized as vulvar intraepithelial neoplasia (VIN.) Mixed dystrophies are reported as lesions containing both lichen sclerosus and squamous cell hyperplasia.

### Non-Neoplastic Epithelial Disorders

On gross examination, lichen sclerosus and squamous cell hyperplasia present as white plaques (leukoplakia), the former being an atrophic lesion with the microscopic appearance of a thin squamous epithelium and flattened rete ridges. On microscopic examination of squamous cell hyperplasia, the squamous epithelium has a thick superficial layer of parakeratosis or hyperkeratosis and elongated rete ridges. Mixed lesions demonstrate the histologic features of both lesions. Occurring in 20% of non-neoplastic epithelial disorders, mixed lesions are more difficult to treat. Early studies have suggested that mixed lesions have a predisposition to transform into vulvar malignancies. However, this issue continues to be debated and should not alter treatment protocols.

**Diagnosis.** Patients with non-neoplastic epithelial disorders frequently present with pruritus and vulvodynia. Often, patients are treated by practitioners for atrophic vulvitis and/or monilial vulvitis only to have their symptoms persist. The key to making a correct diagnosis is a thorough medical history followed by a comprehensive inspection of the female genitalia, including the cervix, the anus, and the vagina. Non-neoplastic epithelial disorders and intraepithelial neoplasia are multifocal and may be present on all anogenital mucosal surfaces. After completing visual and digital examination, 3% acetic acid is placed on the vulva, the anus, the vagina, and the cervix and a colposcopic evaluation performed. Areas of raised white plaques as well as increased vascularity, punctation, and mosaicism should undergo biopsy to identify histologic changes. If colposcopy is not available or additional diagnostic tests are warranted, the vulva and the anus are painted with a 1% aqueous solution of toluidine blue, which is allowed to stain for 3 minutes. The epithelium is then decolorized with 1% acetic acid for 1 minute. Surface nuclei of dysplastic or anaplastic lesions retain the blue stain and should undergo biopsy. Biopsies are easily performed using 1% lidocaine (Xylocaine) injected circumferentially around the lesion with a 25-gauge needle. A Keyes punch enables the physician to circumscribe the lesion and incise the epidermis. Forceps and scissors are then required to free the remainder of the specimen from the underlying tissue. The vagina and the cervix can also be evaluated with Shiller's or Lugol's solution, which does not stain intraepithelial neoplasia.

**Treatment.** Lichen sclerosus is treated with 2% testosterone propionate in stearin lanolin cream.* The cream is applied to the vulva three times daily for 6 to 8 weeks followed by a daily application for 1 week and then weekly application. Testosterone's androgenic side affects such as clitoromegaly, hirsutism, voice changes, acne, and dermal hypertrophy may not be accepted by all patients. Alternatively, 1 or 2% progesterone† cream has been substituted in patients who could not tolerate testosterone. Results have been com-

TABLE 1. **Non-Neoplastic Epithelial Disorders of the Skin and Mucosa***

| Old Terminology | New Terminology |
|---|---|
| Lichen sclerosus et atrophicus | Lichen sclerosus (LS) |
| Hyperplastic dystrophy (without atypia) | Squamous cell hyperplasia (SCH) |
| Mixed dystrophy | LS and SCH |

*From Ridley CM, Frankman O, Jones SC, et al: New nomenclature for vulvar disease, International Society for the Study of Vulvar Disease. Human Pathol 20(5):495, 1989.

*This use of testosterone is not listed in the manufacturer's official directive.

†This use of progesterone is not listed in the manufacturer's official directive.

parable, but without the androgenic side affects; 75 to 90% of patients treated with either regimen have reported symptomatic relief.

Squamous cell hyperplasia is best treated with a fluorinated corticosteroid cream. I use a 1% hydrocortisone ointment applied three times daily for 6 to 8 weeks, after which the patient is weaned to daily applications. Corticosteroid administration results in dermal atrophy, unlike testosterone, which causes hypertrophy. Mixed lesions are initially treated with a course of fluorinated corticosteroid and then the remaining lichen sclerosus treated with 2% testosterone propionate. Non-neoplastic epithelial disorders frequently recur and require long-term administration of topical agents as described earlier. Surgical procedures such as laser vaporization, simple lesion excision, and cryotherapy have also been utilized in treating non-neoplastic epithelial disorders, but should be reserved as second-line therapy after treatment with topical compounds has failed. Vulvectomy and skinning vulvectomy should be avoided in these patients because of the recurrence rate and disfiguration secondary to the procedure unless all conservative measures have failed. The pruritus and vulvodynia that plague patients with non-neoplastic epithelial disorders can be controlled by administering benzocaine (Americaine) or lidocaine (Xylocaine) ointment topically during the initial steroid therapy. Palliation of more severe and recalcitrant disease can be accomplished with intradermal alcohol or triamcinolone diacetate (Aristocort) injections in a grid distribution on the vulva.

### Vulvar Intraepithelial Neoplasia

Mild and moderate dysplasias of the vulva epithelium are designated VIN I and II, respectively. Bowen's disease, erythroplasia of Queyrat, and carcinoma simplex have been classified as VIN III, which also includes in situ disease and severe dysplasia (Table 2). Vulvar intraepithelial neoplasia is multifocal, with 50% of the patients presenting in the third and fourth decades of life. An association has been found between VIN and human papillomavirus subtypes 6, 11, 16, 18, and 31. Human papillomavirus subtypes 16 and 18,

however, are responsible for the majority of VIN III and invasive neoplasia. Patients with atypical or flat condyloma acuminatum should have biopsy of their lesions prior to conservative chemical desiccation to rule out intraepithelial neoplasia. In addition, 20 to 30% of patients with VIN III have associated genital tract neoplasia, with the preponderance being intraepithelial neoplasia of the anus, the vagina, and the cervix followed by cervical, vaginal, and endometrial carcinoma. The diagnostic evaluation of VIN is identical to that described for non-neoplastic epithelial disorders of the skin and the mucosa.

**Treatment.** Small focal lesions of VIN may be treated with local excision, cryotherapy, or laser vaporization. Extensive and multifocal lesions, however, are best treated with laser vaporization, skinning vulvectomy, or simple vulvectomy. Laser vaporization is performed under regional or general anesthesia with a carbon dioxide laser attached to a colposcope and microslad. The laser is set with a 2.0-mm spot size and power of 20 to 25 watts, and vaporization is performed to a depth of 3 mm. On completing vaporization of the lesion, the operative field is dressed with 1% silver sulfadiazine (Silvadene) cream. Ample quantities of analgesic medications must be prescribed postoperatively because the patient may experience excruciating discomfort. Unfortunately, many physicians frequently forget that laser vaporization results in a third-degree burn and requires special care.

Skinning vulvectomy may be partial or complete, with its advantage over laser vaporization being a specimen sent for histologic evaluation. Unfortunately, this procedure carries increased morbidity when compared with laser therapy. Split-thickness skin grafts are also required on completion of the skinning vulvectomy. Carbon dioxide laser vaporization and skinning vulvectomy both offer cosmetic and functional results without mutilation of the female genitalia. Hair dryers and heat lamps provide valuable assistance in keeping the surgical field dry after either procedure.

Local chemotherapeutic agents such as 5% fluorouracil (Efudex) cream, bleomycin sulfate (Blenoxane), and interferon (Roferon-A) have met with limited success. Clinical trials are currently under way using porphyrin compounds systemically or topically followed by photoirradiation with an argon–rhodamine dye laser; this provides another method for treating these patients in the future.

TABLE 2. **Vulvar Intraepithelial Neoplasia***

| Old Terminology | New Terminology |
| --- | --- |
| Mild atypia (dysplasia) | VIN I |
| Moderate atypia (dysplasia) | VIN II |
| Severe atypia (dysplasia) | VIN III |
| Carcinoma in situ | VIN III |

*From Ridley CM, Frankman O, Jones SC, et al: New nomenclature for vulvar disease, International Society for the Study of Vulvar Disease. Human Pathol 20(5):495, 1989.

### Paget's Disease

Paget's disease of the breast was first described by James Paget in 1874. Its manifestation on the vulva was reported in 1901 by W. Dubrewilh. Twenty per cent of patients with Paget's disease of the vulva have an underlying adenocarcinoma versus more than 90% of patients with a Paget's breast lesion, who have occult carcinomas. Grossly, Paget's disease has an eczematoid scaly appearance, is well demarcated, and frequently presents as a raised velvety lesion. The most common symptoms, as with most vulvar lesions, are pruritus and vulvodynia. It is imperative to obtain a vulvar biopsy to make the diagnosis definitively. Microscopically, cells are large and round, with abundant cytoplasm, few mitotic figures, and hyperchromatic or vesicular nuclei.

**Treatment.** After diagnosis is confirmed, a thorough evaluation should be made to rule out breast, vaginal, cervical, bladder, or gastrointestinal adenocarcinoma. Wide local excision with 3-cm margins is suggested in treating Paget's disease. This affords the surgeon the opportunity to evaluate the surgical specimen for an underlying adenocarcinoma. In addition, Paget's disease spreads laterally beyond the lesion and requires extensive margins. As a result of this lesion's behavior, its mode of spread, and frequency of occult carcinomas, Paget's disease should not be treated primarily with laser vaporization. Recent studies using monoclonal cytokeratin antibodies have enabled pathologists to distinguish Paget's disease of the vulva from Bowen's disease (VIN III) and superficial spreading melanoma (Table 3).

### Follow-Up

All patients treated for preinvasive disease of the vulva require a minimum of follow-up at 1 month postoperatively, quarterly examinations for 1 year, and then semiannual evaluations. Patients with procedure-related morbidity or recurrence require more comprehensive and frequent evaluations.

### INVASIVE CARCINOMA

Vulvar carcinoma accounts for 3 to 5% of all female genital cancers, with approximately 90% being squamous cell carcinoma. The most com-

TABLE 3. **Cytokeratin Expression***

| Histology | Cytokeratin | | |
| --- | --- | --- | --- |
| | *54 kDa* | *57 kDa* | *66 kDa* |
| Paget's disease | Positive | Variable | Negative |
| Bowen's disease (VIN III) | Negative | Positive | Positive |
| Melanoma | Negative | Negative | Negative |

*Modified from Shah KD, Tabibzadeh SS, and Gerber MA: Am J Clin Pathol *88*(6):689, 1987.
kDa = kilodaltons.

TABLE 4. **TNM Classification of Vulvar Carcinoma***

| T | Primary Tumor |
| --- | --- |
| TIS | Vulvar intraepithelial neoplasia III |
| T1 | Confined to vulva and/or perineum, diameter ≤2 cm |
| T2 | Confined to vulva and/or perineum, diameter >2 cm |
| T3 | Adjacent spread to urethra and/or vagina and/or anus |
| T4 | Infiltration of upper urethral mucosa and/or bladder mucosa and/or rectal mucosa and/or fixed to the bone |
| N | Regional lymph nodes |
| N0 | No nodes palpable |
| N1 | Unilateral lymph node metastasis |
| N2 | Bilateral lymph node metastasis |
| M | Distant metastasis |
| M0 | No clinical metastasis |
| M1 | Distant metastasis (including pelvic node metastasis) |

*Modified from FIGO News: Int J Gynecol Obstet *28*:189, 1989.

mon presenting signs and symptoms are pruritus and pain followed by vulvar lesions, bleeding, and dysuria. The International Federation of Gynecology and Obstetrics (FIGO) clinical staging of vulvar carcinoma is based on the TNM classification (Tables 4 and 5). This system evaluates lesion size, location, and inguinal node spread and metastasis. Clinical staging includes physical examination, chest x-ray examination, vulvar biopsy, node biopsy, serum chemistry determination, hematologic profile, intravenous pyelography, cystoscopy, and sigmoidoscopy (the latter three if required by location of the lesion). Additional studies obtained but not used for staging are magnetic resonance imaging (MRI), computed tomography (CT), ultrasonography, and lymphangiography. Lymphangiography has not proved efficacious in vulvar disease, having a sensitivity of less than 20% and a specificity of

TABLE 5. **FIGO Clinical Staging of Vulvar Carcinoma***

| Stage | TNM | | |
| --- | --- | --- | --- |
| 0 | TIS | | |
| I | T1 | N0 | M0 |
| II | T2 | N0 | M0 |
| III | T3 | N0 | M0 |
| | T1 | N1 | M0 |
| | T2 | N1 | M0 |
| | T3 | N1 | M0 |
| IVA | T1 | N2 | M0 |
| | T2 | N2 | M0 |
| | T3 | N2 | M0 |
| | T4 | N2 | M0 |
| | T4 | N0 | M0 |
| | T4 | N1 | M0 |
| IVB | Tx | Nx | M1 |

*Modified from FIGO News: Int J Gynecol Obstet *28*:189, 1989.
*Abbreviations:* x = any T and/or N.

less than 70%. DNA hybridization has revealed the presence of human papillomavirus 6, 11, 16, 18, and 31 in VIN and invasive carcinoma; the majority of the anaplastic lesions are subtype 16, 18, and 31.

**Treatment.** The standard treatment of vulvar carcinoma has been en bloc resection of the vulva, including the clitoris, and a bilateral superficial and deep inguinal femoral lymphadenectomy. In the past, more extensive lymph node dissections, including pelvic lymphadenectomy, were performed in patients with positive inguinal lymph nodes. Presently, radiation therapy rather than lymphadenectomy is preferred to treat the pelvic nodes, as demonstrated by a recent Gynecologic Oncology Group study. Several clinical trials are presently under way to compare inguinal node dissection and radiation therapy. The preliminary results thus far are encouraging and suggest that treatment modalities may be equally efficacious in treating inguinal lymph nodes. Some surgeons report up to a 90% wound separation in patients undergoing an en bloc resection of the vulva and inguinal nodes. Recent modifications advocate a radical vulvectomy or radical hemivulvectomy with inguinal femoral lymphadenectomy through separate incisions. This has resulted in decreased incidence of wound separations and infections and shortened hospital stays. The number of positive inguinal nodes is a prognostic factor in determining survival (Table 6). Radiation therapy, however, has been successful in obtaining local control in advanced disease. Surgery is more efficacious than primary radiation in the treatment of vulvar carcinoma. Radical vulvectomy and bilateral inguinal femoral lymphadenectomy have accrued 5-year survivals of 60 to 65% versus 25 to 30% in patients treated with definitive radiation therapy. Teletherapy and iridium needle placement in large tumors have been utilized to decrease tumor burden and permit a less radical procedure. This has helped to decrease the number of exenterations for lesions extending into the urethra and/or the anus. Unfortunately, the vulva has a poor tolerance to high doses of radiation, and therefore marked skin toxicity results, especially in the menopausal patient.

TABLE 6. **Correlation of Positive Inguinal Lymph Nodes and Survival***

| Positive Lymph Node (N) | Estimated 2-Year Survival |
|:---:|:---:|
| >4 | 27% |
| 2–3 | 66% |
| 1 | 80% |

*Reprinted with permission from The American College of Obstetricians and Gynecologists. (OBSTETRICS AND GYNECOLOGY, *68*(6), 1986, p. 733.)

### Stage I and II Lesions

Stage I lesions are defined as being 2 cm or less in largest diameter with no inguinal nodes palpable. Several studies to date have not found positive inguinal nodes in patients with less than 1 mm of invasion, and therefore many gynecologic oncologists have advocated not doing lymphadenectomies in patients with less than 1 mm of invasion. Superficial lymphadenectomy in patients with less than 5 mm of invasion carries a nodal positivity of 10 to 30%. This has enabled alteration of therapy by performing radical local excisions of the primary lesion to the inferior fascia of the urogenital diaphragm and ipsilateral superficial inguinal lymphadenopathies. The lymph nodes are then sent for frozen section examination, and, if nodes are positive, a more thorough dissection of the deep femoral lymph nodes below the cribriform fascia and adjacent to the femoral vessels is performed. Superficial lymphadenectomy consists of the removal of the nodal tissue above the cribriform fascia and adjacent to the greater saphenous and superficial epigastric veins. In patients with lesions invading greater than 5 mm, an ipsilateral superficial and deep femoral lymphadenectomy is recommended.

Recently, treatment protocols have been modified in patients with lateralizing lesions 2 cm or less in greatest diameter. Radical hemivulvectomy and ipsilateral inguinal femoral lymphadenectomy are performed versus a complete vulvectomy and bilateral inguinal femoral lymphadenectomy. This modification has markedly decreased the incidence of wound separation and bilateral lymphedema. In addition, a hemivulvectomy frequently preserves the clitoris, thereby improving sexual function postoperatively. Midline and Stage II lesions (>2 cm) are treated with a radical vulvectomy and bilateral inguinal femoral lymphadenectomy through separate incisions to decrease morbidity. The perineal defects can be closed in a multitude of fashions, including primary closure, secondary granulation, Z-plasty (rhomboid flap), gracilis myocutaneous graft, and tensor fascia lata myocutaneous graft. If two or more nodes are positive, the patient should receive radiation therapy to the ipsilateral groin, the ipsilateral pelvis, and the contralateral groin. Alternatively, the patient can choose to have a radical vulvectomy and bilateral inguinal femoral radiation consisting of 45 to 50 Gy over a 5-week interval rather than lymphadenectomy. In addition to the above, radiation therapy is utilized to provide a perineal boost in patients with positive surgical margins. Complications of a radical inguinal femoral lymphadenectomy can be divided into immediate postoperative and delayed complications (Table 7).

TABLE 7. **Complications of Radical Vulvectomy and Inguinal Lymphadenectomy***

| Immediate | % | Delayed | % |
|---|---|---|---|
| Wound separation infection | 85 | Leg edema | 69 |
| Urinary tract infection | 18 | Lymphangitis, phlebitis, cellulitis | 13 |
| Thromboembolic disease | 9 | Vaginal stenosis | 13 |
| | | Pelvic relaxation | 11 |
| | | Stress urinary incontinence | 11 |
| | | Hernia | 5 |

*Reprinted with permission from The American College of Obstetricians and Gynecologists. (OBSTETRICS AND GYNECOLOGY, *61*, 1983, p. 63.)

### Stage III and IV Disease

Stage III tumors can be lesions of any size with adjacent spread to the urethra, the anus, or the vagina (T3 lesions) and/or unilateral lymph node metastasis (N1). Patients with T1 or T2 lesions with N1 nodes are treated as described earlier with a radical vulvectomy and bilateral inguinal femoral lymphadenectomy. As for patients with Stage I and II lesions, the patient undergoes pelvic radiation if inguinal nodes are positive. Stage III lesions with minimal spread to organs adjacent to the vulva can be treated by extending the surgical margins of the vulvectomy to include the distal one-third of the urethra, the distal vagina, or the anus as long as the lesion does not involve the anal sphincter. For extensive T3 lesions and T4 (Stage IV lesions) invading the bladder or the bowel mucosa, treatment consists of an exenterative procedure, radiation, or a combination of radiation and surgery. Recent studies have advocated the combination of chemotherapy and teletherapy to treat cervical and vulvar carcinomas.

### Recurrence

Recurrence and survival are directly correlated with lesion size and the number of positive lymph nodes. Table 8 summarizes the survival statistics from the gynecologic oncology literature for the past 2 decades as well as the 1985 FIGO Annual Report. Small local recurrences can be treated with wide local excision or radiation therapy.

TABLE 8. **Five-Year Survival in Patients Treated for Vulvar Carcinoma***

| FIGO Stage | 5-Year Survival |
|---|---|
| I | 70–90% |
| II | 45–80% |
| III | 30–50% |
| IV | 10–20% |

*From Copeland LJ: Neoplasms of the vulva. *In* Rakel RE (ed): Conn's Current Therapy 1989. Philadelphia, WB Saunders Co, 1989.

Extensive recurrences, however, require exenterative procedures and/or a combination of radiation therapy and extensive resection of the perineum. Chemotherapy thus far has limited use in the treatment of vulvar carcinoma. Chemotherapeutic agents such as doxorubicin (Adriamycin), cisplatin (Platinol), bleomycin sulfate (Blenoxane), methotrexate, mitomycin (mitomycin-C, Mutamycin), 5-fluorouracil, and etoposide (VePesid) have had minimal success in controlling recurrent or systemic disease.

## OTHER VULVAR NEOPLASMS

### Verrucous Carcinoma

Unlike invasive squamous cell carcinoma of the vulva, verrucous carcinoma is an indolent, locally invading, cauliflower-like tumor that rarely metastasizes. The verrucous lesion is frequently mistaken for a giant condyloma of Buschke-Löwenstein, and therefore it is imperative that the surgeon obtain multiple biopsy specimens to ensure the diagnosis. Treatment consists of radical local excision for small lesions and radical vulvectomy for larger lesions. In light of the tumor's indolent nature, lymphadenectomy is rarely required unless palpable and suspicious lymph nodes are present. If lymph nodes are positive on frozen section examination, the patient should undergo a radical vulvectomy and bilateral inguinal femoral lymphadenectomy. Radiation therapy may transform this lesion into a more anaplastic lesion and is contraindicated in its treatment.

### Melanomas

Melanomas are the second most common vulvar malignancy. Two-thirds of the patients with melanomas are postmenopausal and fair skinned. There are three histologic types of melanomas: superficial spreading, lentigo maligna, and nodular. The most aggressive is the nodular melanoma. Unlike squamous lesions, melanomas are not staged by the FIGO classification but by the depth of invasion (Table 9). Preoperative evalu-

TABLE 9. **Staging Systems for Vulvar Melanoma**

| Level | Clark | Breslow | Chung |
|---|---|---|---|
| I | Intraepithelial | <0.76 mm | Intraepithelial |
| II | Into papillary dermis | 0.76–1.50 mm | <1 mm superficial penetration |
| III | Filling dermal papillae | 1.51–2.25 mm | 1–2 mm into subepithelial tissue |
| IV | Into reticular dermis | 2.26–3.0 mm | Penetration >2 mm |
| V | Into subcutaneous fat | >3 mm | Into subcutaneous fat |

ation should include a chest x-ray film and a CT scan or MRI of the abdomen and pelvis to rule out retroperitoneal, hepatic, or pelvic disease.

**Treatment.** Treatment is tailored to the depth of invasion. Melanotic Level I or II lesions (<1 mm) can be treated with wide local excision without lymphadenectomy. To date, no studies have reported Level I or II lesions with positive inguinal lymph nodes. Patients with Level III, small lateralizing lesions can be treated with a radical hemivulvectomy and ipsilateral inguinal femoral lymphadenectomy. Larger lesions and Level IV and V lesions require radical vulvectomy and bilateral inguinal femoral lymphadenectomy. Occasionally, large lesions necessitate perineal resection, vaginectomies, or exenterations to adequately resect the tumor. Poor results have been obtained using radiation and chemotherapy to control this disease. Responses to tamoxifen citrate (Nolvadex) have been reported, but necessitate prolonged administration as long as the patient's condition is stable. The prognosis of melanoma patients is dependent on the depth of invasion, tumor volume, and lymph node metastasis, with an overall 5-year survival of 30%.

### Bartholin's Gland Carcinoma

Patients with Bartholin's gland carcinomas account for 3 to 5% of all those with vulvar carcinomas, with a mean age of 57 years and a range of 14 to 85 years of age. Ninety per cent of the histologic cell types are equally divided between adenocarcinoma and squamous cell carcinoma, with the remaining 10% adenoid cystic, transitional, and mixed cell types.

**Treatment.** Treatment consists of radical hemivulvectomy or radical local excision and an ipsilateral inguinal femoral lymphadenectomy. Postoperative pelvic and contralateral groin irradiation should be performed if ipsilateral groin nodes are positive. If the tumor is adherent to the pubic ramus, preoperative radiation may permit future surgical resection. Occasionally, large Bartholin's gland carcinomas invading the rectum require exenterative procedures to obtain adequate surgical margins.

### Basal Cell Carcinoma

Basal cell carcinoma accounts for approximately 2% of all vulvar lesions and usually presents with vulva pruritus and/or ulceration. This tumor is locally invasive and is treated with a wide local excision of the lesion. Basal cell carcinomas rarely metastasize to lymph nodes and therefore do not require lymphadenectomy unless suspicious lymph nodes are palpated.

### Sarcomas

Vulvar sarcomas account for 1 to 3% of all vulvar malignancies. The most common histologic type is leiomyosarcomas, which occur in the third and fourth decades of life. The patient frequently has a rapidly growing tumor. Prognostic features include lesion size, contour, and mitotic figure index.

**Treatment.** Treatment consists of a radical local excision, with lymphadenectomy required only if a suspicious lesion is present. Recurrences are treated with a wide local excision. More aggressive rhabdomyosarcoma can also manifest itself on the vulva. Treatment consists of radical local excision followed by VAC chemotherapy with vincristine sulfate, dactinomycin (Actinomycin D), and cyclophosphamide (Cytoxan). In patients with positive surgical margins, nodal metastasis, and recurrence, radiation therapy can be helpful in controlling central disease.

### Nongynecologic Metastasis to the Vulva

Although rare, several nongynecologic primary tumors have been reported to metastasize to the vulva. They include non-Hodgkin's lymphoma and melanoma as well as breast, pulmonary, gastric, and renal carcinomas. Therapy consists of treating the primary tumor and excision of the metastatic lesions.

# THROMBOPHLEBITIS IN OBSTETRICS AND GYNECOLOGY

method of
RIAD CACHECHO, M.D.
*Boston University School of Medicine*
*Boston, Massachusetts*

Deep venous thrombosis (DVT) is a serious disorder, which can be life-threatening, especially if untreated. Its occurrence in the general population is greater than 200,000 patients per year. The incidence in pregnant women is estimated at 1 per 250 deliveries; compared with other women of the same age, pregnant women have a fivefold increased incidence of DVT. This risk increases further with cesarian sections. The risk of DVT in the gynecologic population is comparable with that in general surgical patients. Table 1 presents the incidence of DVT in surgery. Table 2 gives risk factors for DVT.

## ETIOLOGY AND PATHOPHYSIOLOGY

More than a century ago, Virchow described the classic pathologic changes that predispose to DVT:

TABLE 1. **Incidence of Deep Venous Thrombosis in Surgical Patients**

| Group | Age | Surgical Procedure | Incidence of Deep Venous Thrombosis (%) |
|---|---|---|---|
| Low risk | <40 yr | Minor surgery (<30 min) | <3 |
| Moderate risk | 40–60 yr | Major surgery (>30 min) | 10–40 |
| High risk | Patients with risk factors listed in Table 2 | | 50 |

venous stasis, endothelial injury, and hypercoagulability. Today, these remain the inciting factors. All may be implicated in DVT formation in the obstetric and gynecologic population.

Venous stasis occurs during pregnancy as the enlarged uterus compresses the iliac veins. A large pelvic tumor may also compress the iliac veins, producing a low-flow state. Prolonged bed rest in both groups exacerbates this problem.

Endothelial injury occurs during labor and surgical procedures. This injury triggers a cascade of events, including initiation of platelet aggregation, activation of coagulation pathways, and release of vasoactive mediators, resulting in clot formation.

Estrogens inhibit antithrombin III and Factor X inhibitor, both of which are naturally occurring anticoagulants. This inhibition produces a hypercoagulable state, which is especially pronounced during the third trimester of pregnancy. Congenital deficiencies of antithrombin III, protein-C, or protein-S exacerbate this predisposition to venous thrombosis. Protein-C is normally increased in pregnancy and reduced post partum.

## DIAGNOSIS

Calf pain and tenderness, ankle edema, a palpable venous cord, and pain on ankle dorsiflexion (Homan's sign) are the classic signs of thrombophlebitis. However, these signs are present in only approximately 50% of patients who have deep venous thrombosis. Thus, the clinical examination is insensitive, and a careful medical history becomes vital in determining which patients are at risk for development of DVT.

TABLE 2. **Risk Factors for Deep Venous Thrombosis**

Previous DVT
Oral contraceptives and estrogens
Pregnancy
Immobilization
Obesity
Cancer
Trauma
Long-bone or pelvic fracture
Age >60 yr
Hypercoagulability
Pelvic or abdominal surgery
Congestive heart failure
Dehydration

*Noninvasive Methods of Detection*

**Doppler Ultrasound.** This method uses sound waves to evaluate venous blood flow and its alteration with the respiratory cycle. When DVT develops, there is loss of blood flow, with absence of respiratory fluctuations in the involved vein. Although Doppler ultrasound is an accurate method of detection, results vary markedly with different examiners, making interpretation inconsistent.

**Impedance Plethysmography.** Impedance plethysmography (IPG) uses a high-frequency electrical current and records variations in electrical resistance, or impedance, of the extremity. Because blood is an excellent conductor, test results depend on the blood volume in the extremity and its fluctuation in response to temporary occlusion with a pressure cuff. Impedance plethysmography is especially sensitive in popliteal, femoral, and iliac veins. It is of little value, however, in calf vein thrombosis and cannot distinguish between old and fresh blood clots. External compression of the venous outflow by a gravid uterus or a pelvic tumor and congestive heart failure produce false-positive test results. Hence, IPG has limited value in such circumstances.

**Phleborrheography.** Phleborrheography (PRG) evaluates changes in the venous blood flow related to the respiratory pattern. It has many of the same advantages and limitations as IPG. In addition, PRG does not localize the site of venous thrombosis.

In patients who are at high risk for DVT, IPG and PRG are useful as serial monitoring studies. These tests are also helpful in the follow-up assessment of patients who are recovering from DVT and those who are undergoing treatment with anticoagulants.

**Duplex Venous Imaging.** This recently popularized technique uses simultaneous ultrasound imaging and Doppler signals to evaluate anatomic and functional changes in the venous system. Its sensitivity in detecting clots in the major veins of the calf, the thigh, and the groin approaches 100%. Differentiation between old and new thrombi is also possible.

**Triplex Venous Imaging.** This modern technique adds the advantage of a color flow signal to the duplex technique to improve accuracy in detecting DVT.

*Invasive Methods of Detection*

**Radioactive Fibrinogen Imaging.** This method uses radiolabeled fibrinogen (with $^{125}$I) and follows its incorporation into an actively forming thrombus. This study is extremely sensitive and can detect clots that may be clinically insignificant. The radioactive isotope crosses the placenta and is excreted in breast milk. Thus, this method is contraindicated in pregnant women and nursing mothers.

**Contrast Venography.** This method is the "gold standard" of DVT diagnosis, and all other methods of detection are compared with venography when assessing efficacy. Venography requires injection of intravenous contrast medium to look for filling defects in the involved vein. It is highly sensitive and can differentiate both between old and new clots and between thrombosis and external compression. If this test is performed during pregnancy, appropriate protection (lead apron on the lower abdomen) for the fetus is required. The discomfort, the difficulty in repeating the study, and the risk of phlebitis make this method less acceptable for physicians and patients than non-invasive methods.

An algorithm for DVT diagnosis is illustrated in Figure 1.

## TREATMENT

### General Treatment

Patients with DVT are initially treated with rest and leg elevation. This treatment continues for several days, usually until a therapeutic level of anticoagulation is achieved. Warm soaks and wraps with elastic (Ace) bandages are used to alleviate local inflammatory symptoms.

### Anticoagulation Therapy

The purposes of anticoagulation therapy are to stop formation and propagation of the thrombus and to prevent embolization to the lungs. Pulmonary embolism (PE) may be fatal and can be prevented with proper anticoagulation.

The acute phase of anticoagulation extends 3 to 7 days from the time of DVT diagnosis. The recommended therapy during this initial period is intravenous heparin, beginning with a loading dose of 5000 to 10,000 IU. This bolus is followed by a maintenance dosage of 1000 IU per hour as a continuous intravenous infusion. Subsequent dosage is adjusted to maintain the activated partial thromboplastin time (APTT) at one and one-half to two times the control level. The half-life of heparin is 90 minutes, and its effect can be reversed with protamine sulfate, 1 mg per 100 IU of heparin.

After the patient is adequately heparinized, I recommend initiation of oral therapy with warfarin (Coumadin). A daily dose of 10 mg is administered for the first 2 to 3 days, followed by 2.5 to 7.5 mg daily to maintain the prothrombin time at one and one-half times the control level.

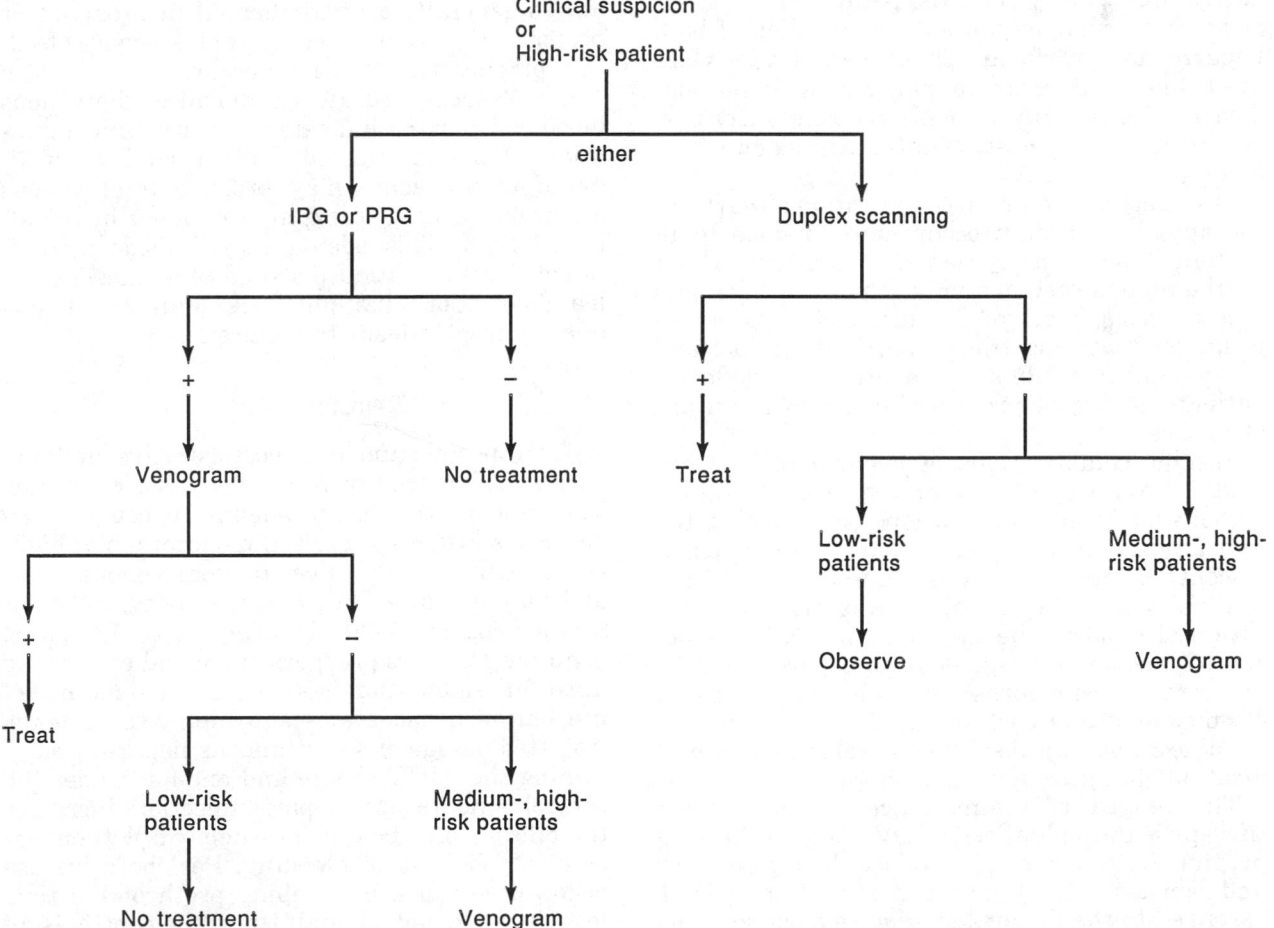

**Figure 1.** Algorithm for diagnosis of deep venous thrombosis (DVT). *Abbreviations:* IPG = impedance plethysmography; PRG = phleborrheography.

When the prothrombin time is adequate, heparin is discontinued and the patient is discharged while receiving warfarin. Warfarin's half-life is approximately 48 hours, and its action on the coagulation system is detected 36 to 72 hours after the initial dose. The effect of warfarin is reversed in 6 to 8 hours with vitamin K (AquaMEPHYTON) administration or promptly with fresh-frozen plasma. Fresh-frozen plasma is used to treat bleeding complications or to prepare patients for urgent surgery.

Warfarin crosses the placenta and may cause fetal or neonatal hemorrhage, as well as central nervous system deformities. It is contraindicated in pregnancy. Therefore, I recommend using heparin for the chronic phase of anticoagulation in pregnant women. One may administer 5000 IU of heparin every 8 to 12 hours subcutaneously, or continuously infuse heparin intravenously to maintain the APTT at one and one-half times the control level. Continuous infusion requires a pump and a tunneled central line. Either treatment option is suitable for outpatients.

Bleeding into the central nervous system, the gastrointestinal system, the genitourinary tract, or the retroperitoneum is a complication of both heparin and warfarin. These complications are most likely to occur in patients with platelet disorders, especially patients concomitantly taking aspirin or nonsteroidal anti-inflammatory agents.

Skin necrosis is a rare complication of warfarin therapy, but it may occur more frequently in protein-C–deficient patients. It presents as an erythematous rash evolving into a full-thickness skin necrosis. Treatment consists of stopping the drug, resuscitating the patient with fluids, and using topical antibiotics. In protein-C–deficient patients, it may be prevented by concomitant use of heparin.

Specific complications of heparin therapy include thrombocytopenia and arterial thromboembolism. These complications occur during the first 2 weeks of therapy and may require heparin discontinuation. Osteopenia caused by inhibition of renal vitamin D metabolism is also a complication of heparin therapy. This inhibition is observed especially if high doses of heparin are used for more than 4 months. Patients with osteopenia often complain of back pain.

Table 3 lists the absolute and relative contraindications to anticoagulation therapy.

The length of maintenance anticoagulation therapy is individualized. If DVT occurred during pregnancy, treatment is stopped during delivery and reinstated for 3 months post partum. If DVT extended to the femoral or iliac veins or resulted in PE, therapy is continued for at least 6 months. Warfarin is used after delivery in non-breastfeed-

**TABLE 3. Contraindications to Anticoagulation Therapy**

*Absolute*
 Central nervous system surgery or trauma
 Eye surgery or trauma to the eye
 Bleeding gastrointestinal ulcer
 Drug allergy
 Active bleeding after trauma

*Relative*
 Recent major surgery
 Recent major trauma
 Gastrointestinal ulcer
 Necrotic tumor

ing mothers and in gynecologic patients. Follow-up is accomplished by IPG testing, which is an easy, cost-effective method of detecting resolutions or propagation of the clot and, therefore, of determining the duration of anticoagulation therapy.

**Fibrinolytic Therapy.** Streptokinase (Streptase, Kabikinase) and urokinase (Abbokinase) activate the plasminogen system, resulting in clot dissolution. This activation prevents both acute and chronic complications of DVT. Fibrinolytic therapy is generally contraindicated in pregnant or postoperative women because of the severe bleeding complications that may occur.

**Thrombectomy.** Surgical removal of the venous blood clot may be indicated in rare clinical situations. For example, an ileofemoral DVT if allowed to propagate may produce total venous occlusion, leading to extensive edema in the affected limb. This edema may impede arterial inflow. This condition is called phlegmasia cerulea dolens, or blue phlebitis. Failure to adequately treat it leads to gangrene.

## PROPHYLAXIS

Early postpartum and postoperative ambulation is the key to prevent DVT in at risk patients. The perioperative use of pneumatic compression devices is also warranted in moderate- and high-risk groups. These devices prevent venous stasis and may enhance fibrinolytic activity. Subcutaneous heparin, 5000 IU every 8 to 12 hours, beginning 2 hours preoperatively and continuing until full ambulation is an alternative method of prevention in moderate- and high-risk patients. Adjusted dosage of subcutaneous heparin (maintaining the APTT at one and one-half times the control, 6 hours after heparin injection) increases the efficacy of subcutaneous heparin without increasing the risk of bleeding. Perioperative use of low-dose warfarin, keeping prothrombin time less than one and one-half times the control is an alternative, effective method of prevention in the high-risk group. However, bleeding complications are greater with warfarin than with other methods.

Discontinuation of contraceptive pills and estrogen before elective surgery is recommended.

Improvement of blood rheologic measures, increased plasminogen release, and inhibition of von Willebrand's factor, as well as the antithrombotic activity of lidocaine, if used, may be responsible for the prophylactic effect of epidural anesthesia against DVT.

Pregnant women with history of DVT and PE are given subcutaneous heparin antenatally and post partum until full ambulation.

In protein-C–deficient patients, I recommend continuing prophylaxis with heparin or warfarin for 3 to 6 months post partum or postoperatively.

## COMPLICATIONS

**Pulmonary Embolism.** Pulmonary embolism is a serious, life-threatening complication of DVT. It may present with shortness of breath, tachycardia, tachypnea, chest pain, and hypoxia, all of which are nonspecific signs or symptoms. Pulmonary embolism may also be asymptomatic. Chest x-ray films and electrocardiograms are usually nonspecific and nonsensitive.

The pulmonary arteriogram is the "gold standard" diagnostic test. Because of its invasiveness, it is usually preceded by an isotope lung scan. If the isotope scan is completely normal, no further work-up is needed. If the scan indicates a low or moderate probability of PE, an abnormal arteriogram is needed to confirm the diagnosis. A highly suggestive lung scan does not require a confirmatory pulmonary arteriogram before proceeding to anticoagulation therapy.

The treatment of PE is similar to that of DVT, except that the treatment is continued for at least 6 months. Patients who have a contraindication to or a complication of anticoagulation, or who develop PE while receiving full anticoagulation, require inferior vena cava disruption. This disruption is achieved by either surgical application of a venocaval clip or percutaneous insertion of a venocaval filter.

**Postphlebetic syndrome.** Occlusion of the deep veins of the lower extremities or destruction of the venous valves by local inflammatory reactions to venous thrombosis results in venous pooling in the affected limb. This pooling leads to chronic swelling, hyperpigmentation, and ulceration, which may be a debilitating, crippling process. If simple leg elevation and properly fitted stockings fail to alleviate the edema, surgical removal of dilated varicose veins, repair of the incompetent valves, or ligation of the perforating veins is indicated.

# CONTRACEPTION

method of
JANET P. REALINI, M.D.
*University of Texas Health Science Center*
*San Antonio, Texas*

Many contraceptive options are available; each has advantages and disadvantages. Choice of a contraceptive method should be tailored to the woman's (or the couple's) situation and preferences. Patients should be helped to understand the risks and benefits of each method so that they may make an informed choice. When reversibility is no longer desired, vasectomy and tubal sterilization become options.

The effectiveness of a contraceptive method depends not only on the inherent fallibility of the method itself, but also on how well the couple is able to use the method (Table 1).

## HORMONAL CONTRACEPTION

*Oral contraceptives* are highly effective when used properly. Many "combination" estrogen-progestogen products are available. One should be-

TABLE 1. **Effectiveness of Contraceptive Methods***

| Method | Failure Rate† | |
| --- | --- | --- |
| | *Lowest Expected* | *Typical* |
| Chance | 85 | 85 |
| Spermicides | 3 | 21 |
| Periodic abstinence | | 20 |
| Calendar | 9 | |
| Ovulation (cervical mucous) method | 3 | |
| Symptothermal‡ | 2 | |
| Postovulation (basal body temperature) | 1 | |
| Withdrawal | 4 | 18 |
| Cap (with spermicide) | 6 | 18 |
| Sponge | | |
| Parous women | 9 | 28 |
| Nulliparous women | 6 | 18 |
| Diaphragm (with spermicide) | 6 | 18 |
| Condom (without spermicide) | 2 | 12 |
| Intrauterine device | | 3 |
| Progesterone T | 2.0 | |
| Copper T380A | 0.8 | |
| Oral contraceptives | | 3 |
| Combination | 0.1 | |
| Progestin only | 0.5 | |
| Depot medroxyprogesterone acetate | 0.3 | 0.3 |
| Implants (Norplant) | 0.04 | 0.04 |
| Female sterilization | 0.2 | 0.4 |
| Male sterilization | 0.1 | 0.15 |

*Adapted from Trussell J, Hatcher R, Cates W, Stewart F, and Kost K: Stud Fam Plann *21*(1), 1990, Table 1.
†Percentage of women experiencing an accidental pregnancy during the first year of use.
‡Cervical mucous method supplemented by calendar in the preovulatory phase and basal body temperature in the postovulatory phase.

TABLE 2. **Oral Contraceptives: Contraindications**

**Absolute**
Thromboembolism
Cerebrovascular disease
Coronary artery disease
Undiagnosed abnormal genital bleeding
Known or suspected pregnancy
Estrogen-dependent malignancy (including breast, endometrium, melanoma)
Benign or malignant liver tumor that developed during estrogen use

**Relative**
Hypertension
Diabetes mellitus, or history of gestational diabetes
Hyperlipidemia
Liver disease
Cholestatic jaundice of pregnancy
Smokers older than 35 years
Severe migraine
Age older than 40 years (unless at low cardiovascular risk)

gin with a preparation containing 35 μg or less of estrogen. It is theoretically desirable to minimize the progestogen dose as well; triphasic pills do this most effectively.

A woman takes the first pill of the packet on day 1 (the day her menses starts) or day 5 of her menstrual cycle, or on the first Sunday after her menstrual period starts. If pills are begun after day 5, a back-up method of contraception should be used for at least 10 days. Missed pills are "made up" by taking two pills a day. If two or more pills are missed in a cycle, a back-up contraceptive method should be used. If three or more pills are missed, the pills should be discontinued, another method used, and the pills restarted at the next menses.

Oral contraception is associated with increased risks of cardiovascular events, but mortality risks appear to be concentrated in those older than 35 years who smoke. Current recommendations allow for prescribing oral contraceptives to nonsmoking women older than 40 when they are carefully screened for cardiovascular risk factors (Table 2).

Long-term use of oral contraceptives reduces the risks of endometrial and ovarian cancers. Research continues about breast and cervical cancer risks. Papanicolaou's (Pap) smears should be performed annually for oral contraceptive users. Abnormalities of glucose and lipid metabolism may be minimized by using preparations containing low doses of progestin.

Break-through bleeding in the first few months of use is usually self-limited. When persistent bleeding occurs after several months, one may change to another 30- or 35-μg estrogen pill or give brief small doses of supplemental estrogen. Occasionally, it is necessary to switch to a 50-μg estrogen preparation. Lack of withdrawal bleed-

ing should prompt exclusion of pregnancy and may necessitate changing preparations to one with stronger progestin—or even to 50 μg of estrogen for several cycles.

*Progestin-only minipills* are chiefly used for lactating women; they are taken every day and require excellent compliance for effectiveness. Irregular bleeding and amenorrhea are common problems.

*Long-acting hormonal methods* require little patient compliance and effectively inhibit ovulation. Depot medroxyprogesterone acetate, 150 mg intramuscularly every 3 months, is not approved by the U.S. Food and Drug Administration (FDA), but it is widely used in other countries. A system of 6-norgestrel–containing capsules inserted surgically under the skin (Norplant) is highly effective for 5 years or until surgically removed. Long-acting progestins cause menstrual irregularities, amenorrhea, and weight gain in some users.

## INTRAUTERINE DEVICES

The intrauterine device (IUD) is an option for parous women who are at little risk of sexually transmitted diseases (Table 3). IUDs apparently prevent fertilization of the ovum. The T380A intrauterine copper contraceptive (ParaGard; [GynoPharma]) is effective for 4 years, whereas the intrauterine progesterone contraceptive (Progestasert [Alza]) must be replaced yearly.

Proper insertion of the IUD high in the uterine fundus with sterile technique ensures optimal effectiveness. Insertion may be performed at any time of the menstrual cycle as long as pregnancy is excluded. Insertion is ordinarily delayed until

TABLE 3. **Intrauterine Devices: Contraindications**

**Absolute**
Pregnancy, known or suspected
Undiagnosed abnormal genital bleeding
Gynecologic malignancy, known or suspected (including unresolved abnormal Pap smear)
Acute cervicitis
Previous major pelvic surgery
Abnormalities of the uterus with distorted uterine cavity
History of ectopic pregnancy
Presence or history of pelvic infection
Presence or history of sexually transmitted disease
Presence or history of postpartum endometritis or infected abortion

**Relative**
Dysmenorrhea
Hypermenorrhea
Multiple sexual partners
Nulliparity
Anemia
Coagulopathy
Congenital or rheumatic heart disease
Corticosteroid therapy

6 to 8 weeks post partum to avoid expulsion of the device.

Complications of IUD use include uterine perforation, bleeding, pain, and pelvic inflammatory disease. Ectopic pregnancy is prevented less well than intrauterine pregnancy. If a pregnancy occurs with an IUD in place, the device should be removed to reduce the risk of miscarriage (including septic mid-trimester abortion) and later complications.

## BARRIER METHODS

Barrier methods offer safety and protection from many sexually transmitted diseases, but require proper use for effectiveness. Condoms and vaginal spermicides, used together, are the most effective of the barrier methods. Of the vaginal spermicides, foam products disperse the best in the vagina. Proper technique is essential for effective use of condoms. Petrolatum-based lubricants must be avoided because they rapidly destroy latex condoms.

Diaphragms and cervical caps prevent pregnancy by holding spermicide against the cervical os at the time of intercourse; they must be fitted by a professional, and special training is required to fit caps. The largest diaphragm size that fits comfortably behind the pubis and in the posterior vaginal fornix is prescribed. A normal Pap smear must be obtained before prescribing a cap; the smear should be repeated after 3 months of cap use. The sponge, which is less effective in parous than in nulliparous women, is effective for up to 24 hours. The cap may be left in place for up to 48 hours, and the diaphragm for up to 24 hours. Reapplication of spermicide before repeating intercourse is necessary with vaginal spermicides and with the diaphragm, but not with the cap or sponge. The diaphragm should not be removed in this situation; rather, additional spermicide should be inserted into the vagina.

A history of toxic shock syndrome contraindicates use of a diaphragm, a cap, or a sponge. A few people cannot use barrier methods because of sensitivity to either latex or spermicide. Anatomic abnormalities or inability to learn the method may limit diaphragm use.

## PERIODIC ABSTINENCE

The calendar "rhythm" method proscribes intercourse on fertile days of a woman's cycle. The earliest fertile day is the length of her shortest cycle minus 18; the latest fertile day is the length of her longest cycle minus 11. Limiting intercourse to at least 3 days after the ovulatory basal body temperature rise is more effective. The character of cervical mucus may also be followed to help determine the fertile period.

## POSTCOITAL METHODS

After inadvertent mid-cycle exposure to pregnancy, several methods effectively reduce the risk of pregnancy, although none is FDA approved. In carefully selected patients, two ethinyl estradiol–norgestrel (Ovral) tablets are taken within 72 hours of the unprotected coitus, and two more tablets taken 12 hours later. High-dose estrogens cause more side effects. Copper IUDs, inserted within 5 days of the unprotected intercourse, are also effective.

Menstrual extraction and therapeutic abortion are procedures a woman may consider in the event of an established, unplanned pregnancy. Progesterone antagonists (e.g., RU 486) may be available in the future.

# Section 16
# Psychiatric Disorders

## ALCOHOLISM

method of
**A. WODAK, M.D.**
*St. Vincent's Hospital*
*Darlinghurst, New South Wales, Australia*

Although patients labeled "alcoholics" are familiar to all medical practitioners, few physicians are confident about the diagnosis and management of this important condition. In the United States alone, 18 million persons 18 years of age and older are estimated to have problems associated with the use of alcohol. The difficulties that both society and the medical profession have in responding to alcoholism may be partly explained by the protean nature of alcohol-related disabilities, uncertainty regarding the etiology and definition, and the acceptance of alcohol as a social beverage. In recent decades, much progress has been made in defining concepts and expanding knowledge of the biologic and psychosocial consequences of alcohol consumption.

### THE NATURE OF ALCOHOLISM

In the traditional view, alcoholism has been regarded as a unitary phenomenon with overtones of moral turpitude and irreversibility. Alcoholism has been considered to be a disease of unknown etiology with an assumed physical cause, in addition to psychologic and spiritual elements. The concept of "loss of control" has been regarded as a central and absolute component of alcoholism, with total and permanent abstinence therefore regarded as indispensable for salvation. However, in recent years, the term "alcoholism" has fallen somewhat into disfavor, both because of the association with this somewhat subjective conceptualization and because of its perjorative overtones. The term "problem drinker," referring to any person with any problem consequent on alcohol consumption, is being increasingly adopted. A fundamental component of the contemporary approach is the delineation of an alcohol dependence syndrome, which can be crudely summarized as a scientific description of alcohol addiction and alcohol-related problems, which include any harmful consequences regarded as resulting from alcohol use.

Alcohol-related disabilities are now increasingly regarded as biopsychosocial phenomena with both etiology and consequences involving biologic, physiologic, and social domains. Problem drinkers are characterized by:

1. A heavy pattern of drinking that may be either persistent or sporadic.

2. A pattern of abnormal drinking behavior, such as secrecy or a preoccupation with drinking.

3. Harmful consequences of drinking, which may be psychologic (such as tolerance or dependence), physical (such as liver cirrhosis), or social (such as marital or employment problems).

### THE ALCOHOL DEPENDENCE SYNDROME

The term "syndrome" emphasizes the clustering of phenomena with no assumption that all elements are invariably present. The alcohol dependence syndrome is regarded as a graded continuum from mild to severe. As with many other sequelae of alcohol abuse, there is a poor correlation between the quantity and duration of hazardous alcohol consumption and the risk of development of alcohol dependence. The assessment of the alcohol dependence syndrome is based on the recognition and summation of its composite parts. The components of this syndrome are now discussed and are summarized in Table 1.

#### Narrowing of the Drinking Repertoire

As alcohol dependence becomes more firmly established, the ability to choose from among a range of alcoholic beverages and to vary the quantity consumed according to the social occasion lessens. Instead of a few dry sherries in genteel surroundings or a couple of cans of beer after sport, the alcohol-dependent drinker insists on an excessively generous consumption of a preferred beverage on all occasions.

#### Salience of Drink-Seeking Behavior

With increasing alcohol dependence, alcohol consumption gains priority over all other competing claims for attention. Even when faced with potentially

TABLE 1. **Components of the Alcohol Dependence Syndrome**

| |
|---|
| Narrowing of the drinking repertoire |
| Salience of drink-seeking behavior |
| Increased tolerance to alcohol |
| Repeated withdrawal symptoms |
|   Tremor |
|   Nausea |
|   Sweating |
|   Mood disorders |
| Relief or avoidance of withdrawal symptoms by further drinking |
| Subjective awareness of a compulsion to drink |
| Reinstatement after abstinence |

catastrophic consequences if discovered drinking, such as divorce or dismissal from employment, the alcohol-dependent drinker increasingly ignores all warnings and continues to imbibe.

### Increased Tolerance of Alcohol

This is demonstrated by the need for ever-increasing quantities of alcohol to achieve the same desired effect. The development of tolerance has a predominantly neurologic basis, with only a trivial contribution from increased metabolism. Tolerance is often described by alcohol-dependent patients in terms of the curious observation that no quantity of alcohol produces intoxication, with the convenient assumption that this represents greater resistance to the baleful consequences of alcohol abuse. Cross-tolerance extends to some other sedative drugs.

### Repeated Withdrawal Symptoms

At first, withdrawal symptoms are mild and intermittent. With increasing dependence, the frequency and severity of symptoms increase, as does the likelihood of their occurrence after a decrease or cessation of alcohol consumption. The symptoms are often first apparent in the early morning soon after waking (when the blood alcohol level is at its nadir), but with increasing dependence, withdrawal symptoms may develop at any time of day and may even wake the patient at night.

The common symptoms of alcohol withdrawal consist of:

1. Tremor of the hands. This symptom may be a minor inconvenience but in severe cases can be incapacitating.

2. Nausea. In mild cases, morning anorexia may be the only manifestation. Later, nausea may develop, followed by the onset of retching or vomiting. Many patients pay little attention to the fact that breakfast has been lost from the daily routine. Later, they may notice that an attempt to brush their teeth in the morning results in dry retching.

3. Sweating. This may consist merely of clamminess on waking in patients with mild dependence. More severely dependent patients may complain of drenching sweats.

4. Mood disturbance. Initially, patients may complain of being "frightened" or "edgy." When dependence is severe, agitation or depression, or a combination of the two, may be vividly described.

### Relief or Avoidance of Withdrawal Symptoms by Further Drinking

As alcohol dependence increases in severity, the first drink of the day is taken earlier and earlier. In severe alcohol dependence, alcoholic beverages may be kept in the bedroom to relieve withdrawal symptoms that interrupt sleep. Often the daily routine is planned in advance to allow access to alcohol to prevent the onset of distressing withdrawal symptoms.

### Subjective Awareness of a Compulsion to Drink

This is a subjective preoccupation with the consumption of alcohol and is often referred to by patients as a "craving" for a drink. Although it is often thought that control is lost entirely, it is probably more accurate to consider that control is intermittently impaired and to a variable degree.

### Reinstatement After Abstinence

Individuals who have developed dependence may notice that if alcohol consumption begins after a prolonged period of abstinence, the development of alcohol dependence for the second time is telescoped into a brief period.

## ALCOHOL-RELATED PROBLEMS

The consequences of alcohol abuse are as diverse as the range of professionals and organizations from which help is subsequently requested. Alcohol-related problems in an individual may exist singly or in combination. An individual who has consumed alcohol steadily for many years may have developed only mild alcohol dependence, whereas a neighbor with an identical pattern of alcohol consumption may have suffered irreversible organ damage, unemployment, and social disgrace. Much of the harm related to alcohol abuse in a community is associated with alcoholic intoxication. Impaired psychomotor function and judgment resulting from acute ingestion of alcohol are associated with high morbidity and mortality from automobile crashes and often violent deaths, including suicide. Acute intoxication is also associated with behavioral manifestations that may result in marital and family disharmony or loss of employment. Recent consumption of alcohol is also linked to a wide variety of crimes, expecially crimes of violence such as assault, rape, and homicide. The records of patients presenting with alcohol-related problems in middle age often show a history of several "driving while intoxicated" offenses one or two decades earlier.

The range of organic conditions associated with excessive chronic alcohol consumption covers all of the major systems of the body, with the gastrointestinal system bearing the brunt of the damage. Chronic excessive alcohol ingestion often results in financial hardship and sometimes homelessness.

## EPIDEMIOLOGY

Approximately two-thirds of adults in Western countries consume alcohol; one-half of the alcohol is consumed by the heaviest-drinking 10% of the society. For the entire U.S. population 14 years of age or older, the estimated per capita consumption in 1987 was the equivalent of 2.54 gallons of pure alcohol per person, which is the eighteenth highest per capita consumption in the world. Per capita consumption has been declining in recent years in the United States and a number of other Western countries. It is generally recognized that the extent of alcohol-related harm in a community varies with the per capita alcohol consumption. Seven per cent of adult U.S. drinkers surveyed in 1984 experienced moderate dependence symptoms; 10% (14% male, 6% female) experienced moderate social or personal consequences associated with alcohol abuse. Women generally have fewer drinking-related problems and fewer dependence symptoms than men, but when allowance is made for the fact that they consume far less alcohol and weigh considerably less, women may be more susceptible to the harmful consequences of alcohol than men.

High alcohol consumption tends to be found in a number of occupations, including all sections of the alcohol beverage industry, business and administration, the armed forces and police, occupations associated with lengthy separations from home, and the medical profession. Alcohol consumption generally declines with age. It is far higher in men than in women and in persons who live alone.

## DIAGNOSIS

The diagnosis of problem drinking is now discussed and is summarized in Table 2.

### The Drinking History

A small minority of patients with a drinking problem spontaneously volunteer this information to their physician. Usually a constellation of nonspecific symptoms forms the presenting complaint, and the diagnosis is missed without a high index of suspicion on the part of the clinician. The experienced diagnostician may be alerted by the combination of seemingly unrelated, vague findings, such as diarrhea, Monday absenteeism, and hypertension in a divorced person known to be experiencing difficulties at work.

A drinking history should be obtained from all adult patients and can usually be ascertained with surprising ease in a few minutes. The supposed unreliability of the information gained generally reflects a poor interview technique with leading questions and judgmental overtones. Questions should be framed in a neutral fashion, beginning with "On how many days a week do you usually drink alcohol?" rather than "Do you drink?" It is helpful to prompt answers, beginning with the top of the range (e.g.,"Seven days a week?") and then prompting with the bottom of the range

### TABLE 2. Diagnosis of Problem Drinking

History of persistent consumption of six or more standard drinks a day (males) or four or more standard drinks a day (females)
History of injury caused by driving a car or operating equipment while intoxicated
History of abnormal drinking behavior (e.g., secrecy)
Harmful consequences of alcohol abuse
  Alcohol dependence syndrome
  Alcohol-related problems
    Medical
    Social
    Family
    Employment
    Criminal
    Legal
    Financial

(e.g.,"Less than once a week?"). The beverage of preference is ascertained and then the number of drinks consumed per day is established, again providing high and then low prompts to give the patient "permission" to reveal high levels of consumption. This information can be extended by ascertaining the drinking history over several years or even decades. Depending on the information obtained, further questioning regarding symptoms of alcohol dependence or specific alcohol-related problems may be required. The primary care physician is often well informed about the patient's family and background and thus is often well placed to draw on various sources of information for the diagnosis. This is significant because in many countries almost 80% of the population see their primary care physician at least once a year.

A number of questionnaires have been devised in recent years to assist in the diagnosis of alcohol-related disabilities in different medical settings. One of the best-known of these questionnaires is the Michigan Alcoholism Screening Test, which was devised for an inpatient psychiatric population. General health questionnaires have also been devised with disguised alcohol-related content and adapted for personal computers with simplified controls operated by patients. The use of pen-and-paper and computer-assisted questionnaires is still largely confined to research.

The history obtained should also include an attempt to establish precipitating or related factors such as the presence of psychiatric conditions or factors causing undue stress.

### The Physical Examination

Once again, the remarkable feature is the diversity of physical abnormalities and the paucity of pathognomonic anomalies associated with hazardous alcohol consumption. The combination of physical findings is usually of more assistance than any individual findings. The detection of alcohol on the breath during the day, especially if alcohol consumption has been categorically denied, clearly supports a suspicion based on the history alone. Normal cognitive function in the presence of strong alcoholic fetor is evidence of tolerance to alcohol reflecting dependence.

### Laboratory Investigations

Estimation of blood (or urinary) alcohol levels is a simple test that can often assist the clinician. A high blood alcohol level in the presence of either denial of drinking or normal cognitive function must be regarded as strong evidence supporting the physician's suspicions. The results of a number of standard hematologic and biochemical tests are elevated in the presence of sustained, excessive alcohol consumption, but lack of sensitivity and specificity when used individually remains a problem. These tests include alanine transaminase, aspartate transaminase, alkaline phosphatase, gamma-glutamyltransferase, erythrocyte mean corpuscular volume, uric acid, and high-density-lipoprotein cholesterol. A low platelet count that returns to normal over several days is often found in heavy drinkers admitted to the hospital. The likelihood of abnormality in any of these tests increases with the quantity of alcohol consumed and the duration of heavy drinking. Combinations of tests improve the sensitivity and specificity of single tests, and composite indices based on discriminant function analysis show promise but are still mainly confined to research.

## MANAGEMENT

The first step in management is to assemble the evidence compiled covering the drinking history, alcohol dependence, and alcohol-related problems. Judgments can then be made about whether the patient is at risk because of a persistent or sporadic pattern of heavy drinking or has already developed alcohol-related disabilities. The severity of the problems and the existence of any primary disorders should be considered. Questionnaires are available to facilitate assessment of some of these aspects, but they are not yet in widespread use.

The next step in management is to give the patient a succinct summary of the assessment so that an informed and responsible choice for the future can be made by the patient. Some patients may be ambivalent about their objectives or may even strive for contradictory aims. However, many patients are clear about their intentions. Some wish to abstain permanently, whereas others desire a period of abstinence followed by a review of the situation. Still others do not wish to abstain for any period but seek to control their alcohol consumption by reducing it to a safe level. The task for the physician in this instance is to attempt to reconcile the patient's aims with the medical reality. There is little to be gained by encouraging a severely jaundiced patient with cirrhosis in the belief that a mere reduction in alcohol consumption is sufficient. However, a patient who has had many unsuccessful attempts to achieve total abstinence may be best advised to seek a middle alternative and attempt a meaningful reduction in alcohol consumption. The consumption of six or more standard drinks a day for men or four or more standard drinks a day for women should be regarded as harmful.

Patients who wish to achieve total abstinence generally experience great difficulty in attempting to stop while carrying out their normal routine and should be encouraged to seek admission to a detoxification center. Detoxification is the process of providing a safe, caring environment for the duration of the body's metabolism of a drug of dependence and the associated withdrawal symptoms in order to facilitate subsequent rehabilitation. The patient should be nursed in a quiet, nonthreatening environment with subdued, even lighting. The staff should have a sympathetic and sensitive manner. In many cases, detoxification is conducted in a psychiatric clinic or general hospital. Outpatient detoxification should be reserved for carefully selected patients.

Sedative medication to which the patient is cross-tolerant prevents the development of withdrawal symptoms. A variety of oral agents with long half-lives have proved to be satisfactory, including the benzodiazepines diazepam (Valium) and chlordiazepoxide (Librium). Diazepam has the advantage of having additional anticonvulsant properties and can be conveniently administered in 20-mg doses hourly while the patient is agitated until a state of sedation has been achieved. Uusually the end point occurs with three or fewer doses. No futher doses are then required. Alternatively, diazepam can be administered in 10- to 20-mg doses every 4 to 6 hours, tapering down to zero over several days. Another agent used is chlormethiazole (Hemineurin), which itself is associated with the development of dependence. The intravenous administration of chlormethiazole is effective but also dangerous, as it can result in respiratory depression. The major tranquilizer haloperidol (Haldol) lowers the seizure threshold and may cause hypotension. Therefore, it should be reserved for patients with delirium tremens who have not responded to benzodiazepines.

However, detoxification can also be achieved satisfactorily without any medication and without undue discomfort, using a tranquil environment and a carefully selected and trained staff (who need not be health professionals). The experience of overcoming a major life problem without recourse to a psychoactive substance may even be an important learning experience.

Detoxification should be accompanied by a plan for future management that includes follow-up by a family physician, referral to a psychiatrist or other specialist, or referral to Alcoholics Anonymous.

The family must not be neglected at this time of crisis, and medical support is an important ingredient in management. The spouse may be advised to attend Alanon, a community-based organization established for the close relatives of alcoholics and based on a philosophy similiar to that of Alcoholics Anonymous. Another organization resembling Alcoholics Anonymous, Alateen, has been established for the benefit of teenage children of alcoholics.

Alcoholics Anonymous is a remarkable organization that exists in many countries and was established more than 50 years ago. It is a self-help organization, but many patients are unable to accept its quasi-religious nature. Every encouragement should be provided for attendance at the meetings of Alcoholics Anonymous, although it must be acknowledged that the organization does not suit everybody. Alcoholics Anonymous is free, has no waiting list or bookings, and keeps no records. Many large towns and cities have several meetings a week that follow a standard format. Identification with the central tenets of the organization is an important ingredient in its success. There are, without question, many people today who owe their lives and sobriety to Alcoholics Anonymous. However, it has not been possible to devise satisfactory research methods to assess the efficacy of Alcoholics Anonymous scientifically.

The role of pharmacologic agents in the management of patients with problems resulting from alcohol abuse is surprisingly limited. Multivitamins, especially vitamin B, should be used generously and may reduce the incidence of the Wernicke-Korsakoff syndrome. Intravenous rehydration with aqueous solutions containing dextrose can precipitate Wernicke's encephalopathy in thiamine-deficient patients and should therefore be initiated only after administration of adequate doses of parenteral thiamine. Hypokalemia is common in severe alcohol withdrawal and should be managed by administration of oral potassium. Anticonvulsants are frequently prescribed for alcohol withdrawal, but because of hepatic enzyme induction, therapeutic levels of phenytoin (Dilantin) are difficult to maintain after cessation of drinking. In the long-term management of patients with epilepsy who also have fluctuating alcohol consumption, the administration of anticonvulsants often causes more problems than it solves because of erratic compliance. Antidepressant medication is also frequently prescribed, but the evidence of its efficacy in the depressed alcohol-dependent patient is doubtful. Although depression is common in persons who consume excessive quantities of alcohol, it is often limited to the period of alcohol withdrawal or may be secondary to the social sequelae of drinking. It is difficult to achieve therapeutic plasma levels with tricyclic antidepressants because of hepatic enzyme induction. The monoamine oxidase inhibitors are not recommended because of the risk of precipitating a hypertensive crisis, as many alcoholic beverages contain tyramine.

Alcohol-sensitizing drugs have been available for almost 40 years. More experience has been gained with disulfiram (Antabuse) than any other similar agent, although the mode of action of all of them is identical. The inhibition of aldehyde dehydrogenase results in the build-up of the primary alcohol metabolite acetaldehyde, which is a toxic substance that causes a flushing reaction consisting of extreme dizziness, hypotension, nausea, vomiting, and sweating. The sensitizing reaction after administration of disulfiram can even

occur several days after the last dose and can result from minimal quantities of alcohol. This agent should be used only after the patient has been fully informed about its interaction with alcohol. It is probably best reserved for situations where administration of the drug can be supervised. It may be considered for patients who need to get through a difficult period of festivities or anniversaries of personal loss or bereavement. In general, disulfiram should be prescribed for at least several months only in carefully selected patients who are medically fit. Only in recent years has the efficacy of this drug been scientifically evaluated. Some studies indicate a small to modest effect when disulfiram is included in a comprehensive treatment program. A new form of pharmacotherapy involving serotonin uptake blockers appears encouraging in animal research and limited clinical studies, but these agents are still restricted to research.

### Inpatient Alcoholism Treatment Programs

Until recently, programs involving 3 to 4 weeks of hospital admission were the major form of treatment. However, they have not been demonstrated to be more effective than far cheaper and simpler outpatient treatment. The high relapse rates after both intensive inpatient and outpatient treatment appear similar. The inpatient programs typically include education regarding the effects of alcohol, individual and group therapy, stress management and assertiveness training, an introduction to Alcoholics Anonymous, and special sessions with health professionals. The goal of treatment is generally abstinence, with admission contingent on a satisfactory assessment of motivation. Despite high relapse rates after completion of treatment, a number of studies have found a positive outcome in terms of cost/benefit analysis.

### Early Intervention and Controlled Drinking

Discouraging evaluations of the effectiveness of prolonged inpatient programs for severely alcohol-dependent patients have been followed by an interest in early intervention for less severely dependent patients for whom goals other than abstinence may be more appropriate. The choice between controlled drinking (i.e., a reduction from previous high levels) and abstinence should be made jointly by the patient and the physician. It is generally considered that younger patients who are only mildly dependent on alcohol do better with controlled drinking, whereas older more dependent patients achieve more satisfactory results when they aim for abstinence. However, these guidelines are not universally accepted and lack precision. Moreover, many patients agree to reduce their alcohol consumption, but not to the degree suggested by their physician. The culmination of the negotiation between patient and physician may be written into the patient's notes, suggesting a form of a contract.

The results of several early intervention studies with a controlled drinking approach are promising, but the area remains extremely controversial. The techniques used in controlled drinking begin with setting goals agreed to by the patient and clinician. The next step is to monitor alcohol consumption, often using a daily diary to record drinking and its context. A set of rewards and punishments is often established for success or failure in complying with the targets. Simple principles to be followed include never drinking alcohol to quench thirst; alternating alcoholic and nonalcoholic beverages; not gulping alcoholic drinks; and setting a minimum time for consuming each alcoholic drink. Textbooks and self-help manuals with various degrees of sophistication, length, and expense are available.

A variety of psychologically based techniques for outpatient management have been developed in the last decade. In recognition of the fact that abstinence is usually relatively easy to achieve, even in severely dependent patients, with failure attributed almost always to relapse, new techniques have been devised. These techniques anticipate situations likely to lead to relapse by developing successful coping strategies to prevent a return to drinking. These cognitive techniques emphasize the distinctions among cognition, feeling, and action to provide patients with power to change their behavior. These forms of therapy can include the spouse and the entire family. At present, cognitive-behavioral techniques with controlled drinking objectives are still developing and expanding. Impressive evidence is accumulating regarding the effectiveness of these approaches. The remaining unresolved question is, For whom are these techniques most suitable?

### Prevention

The first element of any intervention should be an attempt to prevent, if possible, the occurrence of the condition. In the case of alcohol abuse, the relationship between per capita alcohol consumption and alcohol-related disabilities has already been noted. Although a number of factors influence per capita alcohol consumption, the increasing price and decreasing availability of alcohol are generally regarded as the most important measures. The development of national health policies on alcohol has been encouraged by the World Health Organization as part of the movement for Health for All in the Year 2000. Medical practitioners who would like to see the incidence of alcohol-related disabilities decline should support the implementation of national alcohol strategies designed to reduce either per capita alcohol consumption or alcohol-related harm without reducing consumption (e.g., safety belt legislation). Improving the quantity and quality of treatment services provides additional benefits. Noting that members of the medical profession have a high risk of developing alcohol-related disabilities, physicians should consider supporting efforts to assist their impaired colleagues.

The renewed interest in preventing alcohol-related problems follows partly from the failure of treatments to deliver expected results. However, it also follows from the evolving view of alcohol dependence and alcohol-related problems that emphasizes a public health application more than previously. Support for prevention has also followed from the recognition that a treatment system adequate to manage all persons with alcohol-related problems would bankrupt the health system.

It is generally assumed that most alcohol-related problems in the community are caused by the few individuals who have the highest consumption of alcohol. However, from a community perspective, it is the drinker who consumes far more than average but less than the maximum who is responsible for more problems simply because there are so many "heavy social drinkers" and so few "alcoholics." Lowering the per capita alcohol consumption can reduce the number of heavy social drinkers at risk, to the benefit of the whole community. The provision of earlier intervention with goals more specifically developed for less dependent populations can also be of benefit.

In 1990, alcohol cost the United States almost $136 billion, of which 61% was attributed to lost employment and reduced productivity. In an era of increasing concern about economic growth, the development of improved treatment and more effective prevention strategies has a new and urgent meaning.

# NARCOTIC POISONING

method of
LOUIS J. LING, M.D.
*Hennepin Regional Poison Center*
*Hennepin County Medical Center*
*Minneapolis, Minnesota*

Narcotic poisoning has been a constant problem for many years in both illegal and therapeutic misadventures. There are many natural and synthetic narcotics available (Table 1), and many poisonings will be combined with other drugs such as ethanol, cocaine, other hypnotics, and adulterants or contaminants in street drugs. A recent popular combination, known as speedball, has been the addition of heroin to cocaine to decrease the side effects of each. Unintentional poisoning may occur in novice or occasional users, in those whose tolerance has waned, or because of variability in the strength of street drugs. Inadvertent poisoning may occur, especially in older patients or those with decreased liver function given normally therapeutic doses of narcotics.

## CLINICAL PRESENTATION (Table 2)

The classic presentation is the triad of miosis, respiratory depression, and central nervous system (CNS) depression; however, this may not always be present depending on concomitant poisonings and other medical conditions. Several opiates have unique problems. Meperidine (Demerol) and diphenoxylate (Lomotil) can cause miotic pupils. Seizures may occur with propoxyphene (Darvon), meperidine, and codeine poisoning. Pulmonary edema can occur after intravenous use. Nausea and vomiting and hypotension may occur.

Cardiac arrhythmias are not direct results but may occur from hypoxia or pulmonary edema. Narcotic abusers are at risk for other complications such as endocarditis, head trauma, anoxia, and hypoglycemia, which may also confuse the clinical presentation.

## AGENTS

Heroin and morphine are the classic drugs of abuse. Diverse narcotics such as hydrocodone cough suppressant or "Ts and blues," a combination of Talwin (Pentazocine) and tripelennamine (PBZ) have been popular narcotics of abuse.

In recent years, designer drugs have become popular. Most of these are derivatives of fentanyl (Sublimaze), an anesthetic 200 times more potent than morphine. They are best known by illicit users for their color and are called China White, named for its off-white appearance; Persian White, for its pure white appearance; or Mexican Brown, for its light brown color. Corresponding drugs are alpha-methylfentanyl, p-fluorofentanyl, and the most potent 3-methylfentanyl, which is reportedly 7000 times stronger than morphine. Inadvertent deaths occur when the user is not familiar with the potency and because the potency can vary widely. Because the lethal dose is measured in

TABLE 1. **Representative Narcotic Preparations***

| Generic Name | Trade Names | Street Names | Toxic Dose (mg)† | Plasma Half-Life (hr) | Comments |
|---|---|---|---|---|---|
| Morphine | | Dreamer, Miss Emma | 10 | 2.5–3.0 | Oral, subcutaneous, intramuscular, intravenous routes. |
| Heroin (diacetylmorphine) | | Smack, H, Scag, Dope, Junk, DooJee, Horse (caballo, manteca, tecaté), Speedball (with cocaine) | 3 | 2.5–3.0 | Snorted, smoked; subcutaneous, intravenous, intramuscular routes. Appears in urine as morphine. |
| Hydromorphone | Dilaudid | Little D | 1.5 | 3 | Oral, rectal, subcutaneous, intramuscular, intravenous routes. |
| Meperidine | Demerol | Pethidine, Big D | 75 | 3 | May cause seizures and mydriasis. |
| Opium | Pantopon | Big O, Black stuff | PO or RR only | | May be smoked as powder. Overdose usually oral. |
| Codeine | Codeine | Cough medicine | 120 | 2.5–3.0 | Oral, subcutaneous, intramuscular routes. |
| Oxycodone | Percodan, Percocet | Perks | 15 | 3 | Oral route only; abuse common. |
| Hydrocodone | Hycodan | Hyke | 5–10 (oral only) | 2–4 | Common cough syrup. |
| Propoxyphene | Darvon | Dummies | | 10–12 | Oral only. Seizures in overdose. |
| Methadone | Dolophine | Meth, Fizzies | 10 | 24–48 | Common mixed overdose. Extended treatment necessary. |
| L-α-Acetylmethadol | LAAM | LAAM | 10 | 48–72 | Ultra–long-acting methadone congener. Extended treatment necessary. |
| Diphenoxylate | Lomotil | | 300 (oral only) | | Overdose seen in children. Concomitant atropine poisoning. |
| Fentanyl | Sublimaze | Sub, China white | 0.1 | 0.5 | Common anesthetic. |

*From Manual of Toxicologic Emergencies, edited by Noji and Kelen. Chicago, Year Book Medical Publishers, 1989.
†Dose based on equivalent to 10 mg of morphine subcutaneously.

TABLE 2. **Opiate Overdose: Symptom Summary***

| Clinical Presentation | Effect | Treatment |
|---|---|---|
| Pinpoint pupils | Stimulation of nerve III nucleus | None |
| Coma | Agonist at opioid receptors | Naloxone |
| Respiratory depression | Depression of medullary respiratory center and of central nervous system | Naloxone; assisted ventilation |
| Bradycardia | Decrease in sympathetic tone; increase in parasympathetic tone | Naloxone |
| Hypotension | Dilation of peripheral arteriolar and venous blood vessels | Fluids Naloxone |
| Hypothermia | External cooling; peripheral vasodilation; central nervous system depression | Rewarming if temperature is less than 90° F |
| Pulmonary edema | Increase in pulmonary vascular permeability | Positive end expiratory pressure; assisted ventilation as required |
| Seizures Morphine Meperidine Propoxyphene | Epileptogenic effects of parent compound and metabolites | Naloxone; oxygen; anticonvulsants, if necessary |

*Reprinted by permission of the publisher from Ellenhorn MJ, and Barceloux DJ: Medical Toxicology. Copyright 1988 by Elsevier Science Publishing Co., Inc.

micrograms, most of these compounds are missed in routine toxicology analysis.

The synthesis of meperidine and meperidine analogues in illicit labs has resulted in contamination by an impurity known as MPTP (1-methyl–4-phenyl–1,2,3,5-tetrahydropyridine). Intravenous use of MPTP has been associated with a Parkinson-like syndrome in users, initially intermittent but chronic and irreversible after chronic exposure.

Methadone (Dolophine) is used as a substitute for heroin and other opiates in maintenance programs for people addicted to opiates. Because they have a high tolerance, they often take doses of 50 to 180 mg per day, doses that may be lethal in nontolerant patients. Because methadone has a half-life that may be as long as 25 hours, treatment of this poisoning requires prolonged observation and use of antagonistic agents.

## TREATMENT

Respiratory support, maintaining an open airway, and adequate ventilation are the most important components of treatment. Narcotic poisoning has a specific and safe antidote, naloxone (Narcan) which rapidly reverses the narcotic effect. It reverses morphine poisoning most readily, but synthetic narcotics such as codeine, methadone, pentazocine, and propoxyphene require larger doses for a response. It should be given as soon as possible after intravenous access is established or, if necessary, through an endotracheal tube. The initial dose should be at least a 2-mg bolus, and if a synthetic narcotic is suspected, naloxone should be repeated until 10 mg is given or until it is clear there is no response. Caregivers need to be ready to restrain patients who respond to naloxone and suddenly become agitated. Because of the safety of naloxone, even in high doses, it should be used along with intravenous D50 in all comatose patients since a response is diagnostic of narcotic poisoning and can eliminate further diagnostic procedures. It is important to remember that patients who respond to naloxone require continued treatment, since the naloxone effect is shorter than that of all of the narcotics. An intravenous naloxone drip, which gives the total naloxone dose necessary to awaken the patient every hour, will prevent relapse of the narcotic effect. The naloxone should be stopped if the patient develops withdrawal symptoms.

Poisoning with some combination analgesics with acetaminophen or aspirin may need simultaneous treatment for the nonnarcotic component.

## Withdrawal (Table 3)

Those who are physically dependent on opiates undergo a withdrawal syndrome when the drug is withheld. Onset depends on the half-life of the particular drug. Initial symptoms are purposeful attempts to get more drug through manipulation,

TABLE 3. **Withdrawal from Narcotics**

| | Nonpurposive Withdrawal Symptoms (hr) | Peak (hr) | Time in Which Majority of Symptoms Terminate (d) |
|---|---|---|---|
| Morphine | 14–20 | 36–48 | 5–10 |
| Heroin | 8–12 | 48–72 | 5–10 |
| Methadone | 36–72 (2nd day) | 72–96 (6th day) | 14–21 |
| Codeine | 24 | | |
| Hydromorphone (Dilaudid) | 4–5 | | |
| Meperidine | 4–6 | 8–12 | 4–5 |

*Reprinted by permission of the publisher from Ellenhorn MJ, and Barceloux DJ: Medical Toxicology. Copyright 1988 by Elsevier Science Publishing Co., Inc.

pleas, and mimicking of physical symptoms. Shortly after, physical symptoms independent of the patient's control appear and include lacrimation, rhinorrhea, perspiration, and yawning. Anorexia, restlessness, irritability, abdominal pain, and nausea can be seen. Piloerection, mydriasis, diarrhea, tachycardia, hypertension, twitches or tremors, and flushing are physical signs. With morphine and heroin, withdrawal begins 8 to 10 hours after the last dose, is most intense from 36 to 72 hours, and gradually resolves over 7 to 10 days. Mild withdrawal can be treated with diazepam for restlessness or with methadone, which is rapidly tapered. Severe withdrawal with objective signs should be treated in a controlled setting where there is a supportive aftercare program to prevent relapse. Clonidine (Catapres*) at a dose of 6 μg per kg every 6 hours† has been used successfully to blunt withdrawal and is used by addicts who know its effects. Side effects such as hypotension need to be anticipated.

---

*This use of Clonidine is not listed in the manufacturer's official directive.

†Exceeds dosage recommended by the manufacturer.

# ANXIETY DISORDERS

method of
DAVID V. SHEEHAN, M.D., and
B. ASHOK RAJ, M.D.
*University of South Florida*
*Tampa, Florida*

There are seven diagnoses clustered under the category of anxiety disorders in the 1987 edition of the *Diagnostic and Statistical Manual* (DSM-III-R), published by the American Psychiatric Association. These are:

1. Panic disorder
   a. Without agoraphobia
   b. With agoraphobia
2. Agoraphobia without panic disorder
3. Social phobia
4. Simple phobia
5. Obsessive-compulsive disorder
6. Post-traumatic stress disorder
7. Generalized anxiety disorder

## PANIC DISORDER WITH OR WITHOUT AGORAPHOBIA AND AGORAPHOBIA WITHOUT PANIC DISORDER

These two diagnostic categories will be considered together since they are so similar.

### Clinical Description

The disorder starts in 50% of all cases with unexpected attacks of symptoms conventionally regarded as autonomic manifestations of anxiety, e.g., palpitations, shortness of breath, lightheadedness, choking spells, chest pain/pressure, sweating, trembling, hot flashes, paresthesias, derealization, or fear of dying or going crazy. In many cases panic attacks begin with four or more of the above symptoms occurring suddenly and unexpectedly. The disorder can begin with one intense panic attack, usually followed by limited-symptom attacks. This is often followed by a stage of health fears with frequent visits to emergency rooms and medical specialists. Reassurance that nothing is seriously wrong medically does not allay patients' fears for long, and for this reason, physicians are likely to view them as hypochondriacs. When patients have severe unexpected panic attacks in a particular situation, e.g., driving a car, they begin to fear and avoid the situations they associate with their bad attacks. At this stage they begin to have some limited phobic avoidance. If the attacks persist over time, the patient progresses to a stage of extensive phobic avoidance, at which stage many are labeled agoraphobic. Agoraphobia (from the Greek word *agora,* meaning marketplace) means a fear of crowded places. This is one of the most characteristic phobias patients develop as a complication of either limited-symptom attacks or panic attacks. As a terminal stage of the disorder as many as 60% of all such patients develop a secondary depression.

### Treatment

This disorder is multidimensional. Effective treatment therefore attempts to control as many of the component dimensions as fully as possible. It is necessary to control the limited-symptom attacks, the panic attacks, the phobias, and the depression and to manage any aggravating life stresses. These can be dealt with in four stages.

**Stage 1.** Control the unexpected limited-symptom attacks. The unexpected limited symptom attacks are the lowest common denominator clinically in this disorder. Even after the panic attacks are reduced to zero, limited-symptom attacks frequently remain. As long as they persist, recovery is incomplete. If the physician focuses on eliminating these unexpected limited-symptom attacks, the panic attacks will be blocked in the process. Effective treatment of these attacks requires medication. Five classes of medications are useful. The benzodiazepines are the most widely prescribed, most rapidly acting, the safest, and most thoroughly studied class of drugs for this condition. The high potency benzodiazepines are effective if used correctly. In the case of alprazolam (Xanax), or clonazepam (Klonopin), start with 0.5 mg three times daily (after each meal) and increase the total daily dose by 0.5 mg every 2 to 3 days until the patient reaches a safe balance between side effects and benefit. Over the first 3 months of treatment, usually two further dose adjustments are required to keep pace with short-term tolerance. The final effective doses by the end of the third month are usually between 4 and 6 mg per day. When the benzodiazepines are tapered after a treatment period of 6 to 12 months, it should be done very, very slowly, at a rate not faster than 0.5 mg every 2 to 3 weeks of alprazolam or clonazepam or matched equivalent doses for the other benzodiazepines. This minimizes withdrawal problems.

The monoamine oxidase inhibitors (MAOIs), particularly the hydrazine MAOIs, are the most effective class of drugs for severe cases of panic disorder, particularly when complicated by extensive phobic avoidance and depression. Their successful use requires experience and skill. MAOIs should always be considered in refractory cases.

The tricyclic antidepressants are effective in panic disorder even in the absence of depression, although they are not as effective as MAOIs or as safe as benzodiazepines. Recent data suggest that trazodone, a novel antidepressant and the class of 5-HT reuptake inhibitors (of which fluoxetine is the first and only one currently available in the U.S.) may also be effective and more safe than the tricyclic antidepressants.)

The benzodiazepines are not effective antidepressants. The antidepressant classes take 4 to 6 weeks to provide good, stable clinical benefit, while the benzodiazepines are effective in the first week. Most patients will respond to at least one of these drug classes.

**Stage 2.** Overcome the phobias. Although some of the medications help reduce phobic anxiety, they usually do not do so completely. Doing in vivo exposure behavior therapy is usually necessary to extinguish all phobias. This requires bringing patients in direct contact with their phobia, maintaining this contact for 2 to 3 hours at each exposure session, and practicing this exposure frequently. Patients quickly learn that their anxiety attacks are blocked by medication and become less anxious and even comfortable remaining in situations that previously made them anxious.

**Stage 3.** Deal with the psychosocial problems. Psychosocial problems are important aggravating factors in any illness, including panic disorder. When present they need to be addressed with psychosocial treatments. However, sometimes they are not present to a significant degree. It is

therefore not necessary to routinely impose psychotherapy on all patients with this condition since some don't need it.

**Stage 4.** Consider long-term management and education. Provide the patient with practical information about their illness and its management, particularly recent data about its biologic underpinnings and newer pharmacologic treatments. More than 70% of all patients get some relapse of their original symptoms within 3 months of coming off medication. Many will require long-term treatment over many years if they are to remain free of disability.

## SOCIAL PHOBIAS

Social phobic patients fear being the focus of attention. Examples include fears of being watched eating, writing in front of others, or speaking publicly, to such an extent that it produces social, personal, or occupational disability. Not all social phobias respond to the same kind of treatment. Some social phobias occur as a complication of panic disorder or of limited-symptom attacks. Such patients require the same treatment as panic disorder described above. They respond particularly well to MAO inhibitors. Other patients have never had a panic attack or a limited-symptom attack in the course of their illness and have an "uncomplicated" social phobia. Such uncomplicated social phobias respond to in vivo exposure behavior therapy. In difficult cases, this may be assisted by the use of a benzodiazepine or beta blocker, 1 to 1 ½ hours before the exposure to facilitate the extinction of the phobic anxiety. With increasing confidence and success, patients can then be encouraged to manage without any medication.

## SIMPLE PHOBIA

A simple phobia is a special kind of fear that leads to crescendo anxiety on exposure to the feared stimulus (e.g., cats, spiders, airplanes), is out of proportion to the reality of the situation, and leads to subsequent fear and avoidance of the situation. These phobias occur in the absence of any history of panic disorder or limited-symptom attacks and lead to some disability in the patient's life. Such uncomplicated single phobias do not normally require medication treatment unless they are a complication of another psychiatric disorder such as panic disorder. They respond best to in vivo exposure behavior therapy. Patients are gradually brought in direct contact with the phobic stimulus, they are kept in contact with it for 2 to 3 hours at each exposure session, they are not allowed to make their usual avoidance response, and they are encouraged to practice this exposure frequently. This usually leads to extinction of the phobias. Occasionally in severe cases a benzodiazepine or beta blocker is used to facilitate this exposure treatment.

## OBSESSIVE-COMPULSIVE DISORDER

The essentials of diagnosis are the presence of recurrent obsessions and compulsions. Obsessions are thoughts, ideas, images, or impulses that intrude into consciousness and are experienced as being senseless or repugnant. Compulsions are repetitive, purposeful behaviors which when resisted produce anxiety and when indulged in provide a release of tension. Obsessive fears of contamination with dirt or germs may lead to compulsive-like cleaning or hand washing. The obsessive doubter fears he has forgotten to turn off the gas or latch the door, and this may lead to compulsive checking behaviors. Obsessive-compulsive persons may exhibit compulsive rituals designed to prevent an obsessive fear from happening. As a consequence of these intrusive thoughts or beliefs, they may develop avoidance of places or people, or they may be extremely slow in completing tasks. Obsessions and compulsions are often seen in the clinical picture of panic disorder and depression, and these entities should be ruled out before a diagnosis of primary obsessive-compulsive disorder is made.

### Treatment

This consists of using behavior therapy techniques and medication.

**Behavior Therapy.** The techniques usually used are as follows: (1) *Exposure therapy coupled with response prevention.* This technique is particularly effective against obsessions of contamination. Patients are exposed to the feared object (e.g., dirt) for increasing lengths of time and are then prevented from making their usual response (e.g., washing their hands). (2) *Imaginal flooding with response prevention.* In this technique the patient is asked to keep thinking about an obsessive fear (e.g., gas leaking) and is not allowed to go and check. (3) *Thought-stopping or substitution.* Obsessive worriers without rituals attempt to substitute a more acceptable thought for the intrusive one when it occurs or distract themselves by another activity, e.g., snapping a rubber band on their wrists. Rituals generally respond better to behavior therapy than do the obsessional features, and the effects of behavior therapy appear to be longer-lasting. To achieve maximum benefit, the patient should practice the exposure techniques even in situations outside

the therapist's office, and a friend or spouse can be trained to help with response prevention.

### Medication Management

This is an area of growing research interest. The tricyclic antidepressant clomipramine (Anafranil), which was approved by the FDA in February 1990 and is now available in the United States, is effective in 66% of patients. Its antiobsessional effect occurs even in the absence of depression in the clinical picture. Pure obsessionals as well as ritualizers get benefit. The dosage is from 75 mg to 300 mg per day, and it takes from 4 weeks to as long as 12 weeks to exert its effect. Patients typically will relapse even after 1 year of treatment and experience the side effects common to the tricyclics. MAO inhibitors, such as phenelzine (Nardil), and tricyclic antidepressants are sometimes effective. The benzodiazepine alprazolam (Xanax) is effective if panic attacks complicate the clinical picture, the doses required being the same as those for panic disorder. Fluoxetine (Prozac), which is a serotonin reuptake blocker, produces benefit in doses ranging from 20 to 80 mg per day. Common side effects are nausea, headache, nervousness, and insomnia. Other serotonin reuptake blockers such as sertraline and fluvoxamine, not yet approved for marketing in the U.S., show promise with doses ranging from 100 mg to 300 mg daily. Their side effects are similar to those of fluoxetine.

## POST-TRAUMATIC STRESS DISORDER

This occurs in response to an event outside the range of usual human experience that would be markedly distressing to almost anyone. War, natural disasters, and rape are examples of such experiences. Symptoms may occur immediately after the event (acute) or express themselves after a latent period (delayed). Clinically, the subject re-experiences the event in the form of intrusive thoughts, dreams, flashbacks, or distress in situations that remind him of the trauma; avoids thoughts, feelings, or activities that arouse recollections of the trauma; exhibits constriction of activities and relationships; and has poor sleep, irritability and anger, hypervigilance, startle, and poor concentration—all suggestive of abnormal arousal.

The treatment of this condition consists of individual stress-oriented psychotherapy, group psychotherapy, and pharmacotherapy.

The goal of individual psychotherapy is to explore in detail the content of the specific traumatic experience, its meaning, and the feelings it arouses. Repeated, direct exploration of events and feelings sometimes leads to resolution so that the trauma no longer dominates the patient's behavior. Group therapy is helpful in promoting change resulting from mutual trust, understanding, and support provided by the group. Medications are useful in controlling extreme symptoms or, if there is concurrent diagnosable panic disorder, generalized anxiety disorder, or major depression. Flashbacks experienced by these patients may meet criteria for panic attacks. Benzodiazepines are helpful in reducing anxiety and insomnia but should be used with caution as drug and alcohol abuse and dependence are common complications of post-traumatic stress disorder. Phenelzine (Nardil) and imipramine are both effective in reducing flashbacks and decreasing nightmares. This is a complex disorder requiring major psychotherapeutic effort and judicious use of medications.

## GENERALIZED ANXIETY DISORDER

Generalized anxiety disorder is an excessive anxiety and worry about two or more life circumstances for 6 months or longer, during which the person has been bothered by these concerns more days than not. It is often accompanied by symptoms from the following areas: (1) *motor tension*—shakiness, jitteriness, tension, inability to relax, and easily startled; (2) *autonomic hyperactivity*—sweating, heart-pounding, dry mouth, dizzy spells, tingling in hands and feet, upset stomach, flushing, and tachycardia; (3) *apprehensive expectation*—anxious worrying that something bad will happen to himself or to others; and (4) *vigilance and scanning*—manifested by being on edge, impatient, or irritable, or having problems falling asleep or staying asleep. Generalized anxiety may occur spontaneously or in relation to psychosocial stressors and persist even after the stressors have abated. It may occur in association with other psychiatric disorders such as panic disorder, depression, and obsessive-compulsive disorder. Abuse of alcohol, barbiturates, and antianxiety medication is common, and it is important to rule out intoxication, withdrawal syndromes, or underlying endocrine or pulmonary conditions as the cause of the chronic anxiety.

### Treatment

In milder cases, psychotherapy alone may be effective. It consists of educating patients about their illness and exploring the role of past experiences in present emotional, cognitive, and behavioral reactions. Patients should be encouraged to develop strategies to deal with anxiety-provoking situations. If the anxiety largely stems from interpersonal social difficulties, group therapy may help. The more severe states require the use of medications. The most frequently used drugs are the benzodiazepines. These drugs sedate, relax muscle tension, and reduce reactivity to anxious situations. They have varying durations of action and so require careful attention to the dosing schedule. The major drawback is the development of tolerance and dependence. The long-acting benzodiazepines are diazepam (Valium), clorazepate (Tranxene), and chlordiazepoxide (Librium). They are a good choice if a regular schedule is needed as they are less frequently associated with the peaks and valleys experienced with the shorter-acting benzodiazepines such as alprazolam (Xanax), and oxazepam (Serax). In the elderly or those with liver disease, the long-acting drugs may accumulate and cause excessive sedation or ataxia. In this group the short-acting medications, especially those metabolized by conjugation such as oxazepam (Serax) and lorazepam (Ativan), may be better. Ideally, treatment should be of short duration (3 to 4 weeks). In practice, many patients require a regular dosing schedule for several months or even longer. If these drugs are used on a regular basis for more than 2 weeks, they should not be stopped abruptly but tapered slowly at the rate of half a tablet every 2 weeks. This will minimize the risk of withdrawal phenomena such as rebound anxiety or seizures. Tricyclic antidepressants and monoamine oxidase inhibitors are often effective when the benzodiazepines fail. To minimize the subjective disruption they induce, start with small doses of 25 mg of imipramine (Tofranil) at bedtime and increase the dosage by 25 mg every 3 days. It takes about 4 to 6 weeks to work effectively. Beta-adrenergic blockers, antihistamines, and neuroleptics are not indicated in this condition. Buspirone (BuSpar) is a nonbenzodiazepine anxiolytic that might be useful in doses of 10 to 60 mg a day. It takes about 2 weeks to work and does not interact with alcohol or have a withdrawal syndrome. It is worth trying in patients at risk for addiction and has a good safety profile.

# BULIMIA NERVOSA

method of
B. TIMOTHY WALSH, M.D.
*College of Physicians and Surgeons*
*Columbia University*
*New York, New York*

Bulimia nervosa refers to an eating disorder whose salient characteristic is frequent episodes of binge-eating, usually followed by self-induced vomiting. While various patterns of excessive food intake have been noted for centuries, this syndrome was only formally recognized and defined about a decade ago. Bulimia nervosa occurs primarily among young — women, and epidemiologic studies suggest that between 1 and 5% of the young adult female population of the United States may suffer from this disorder. Although patients with bulimia nervosa recognize that their eating behavior is grossly abnormal and typically are very concerned about their lack of control over eating, they are usually also very ashamed of the disturbance and may come to medical attention only inadvertently or with great reluctance.

## DIAGNOSIS

Diagnostic criteria for bulimia nervosa are presented in Table 1. The essential behavioral characteristic of this syndrome is the presence of recurrent episodes of binge-eating. Most patients with bulimia nervosa consume impressive amounts of food during binges, ranging from one to several thousand calories per episode. The current criteria require a minimum frequency of two episodes of binge-eating per week for at least 3 months in order for patients to receive a diagnosis. Although patients may plan their eating binges, once the eating has begun, they feel a limited amount of control over their eating behavior, and it is this sense of loss of control that is particularly distressing. Patients with bulimia nervosa regularly engage in activities intended to prevent the weight gain that would otherwise result from the binge-eating. Self-induced vomiting is the compensatory technique most frequently employed, occurring in 90% of patients with bulimia nervosa seen in eating disorder clinics. Other commonly employed techniques are the abuse of laxa-

### TABLE 1. **Diagnostic Criteria for Bulimia Nervosa***

A. Recurrent episodes of binge-eating (rapid consumption of a large amount of food in a discrete period of time).
B. A feeling of lack of control over eating behavior during the eating binges.
C. The person regularly engages in either self-induced vomiting, use of laxatives or diuretics, strict dieting or fasting, or vigorous exercise in order to prevent weight gain.
D. A minimum average of two binge-eating episodes per week for at least 3 months.
E. Persistent overconcern with body shape and weight.

*From the Diagnostic and Statistical Manual of Mental Disorders, Third Edition, Revised (DSM-III-R), American Psychiatric Association, Washington, D.C., 1987.

tives, diuretics, and diet pills; vigorous exercise; and severe food restriction when not binge eating. Patients with bulimia nervosa are intensely concerned with their shape and weight and often base their self-esteem primarily on how much they weigh.

If the patient provides a full history, the diagnosis of bulimia nervosa is usually not difficult. However, because of the shame and embarrassment associated with this illness, patients, particularly when they visit their general physician, may not be forthcoming. Therefore, the physician should consider the diagnosis of bulimia nervosa in young women who express an intense desire to lose weight, who request prescriptions for diet pills or diuretics, or who exhibit some of the physical signs or symptoms or the laboratory abnormalities noted below. In such cases, the physician should gently but directly inquire about the occurrence of binge-eating and whether the patient has ever had the need to resort to the use of self-induced vomiting or the use of laxatives or diuretics out of fear of gaining weight.

For patients with bulimia nervosa of several years' duration, treatment via one of the established methods described below is indicated and should be initiated as soon as the diagnosis is established. However, the physician should also be aware that there are probably many individuals with mild variants of bulimia nervosa, for example, young people who, for a few months, binge-eat and occasionally induce vomiting. Although definitive information is not available, it is possible that brief interventions and counseling based on the approaches described below may be sufficient to prevent such behavioral problems from progressing into full-blown bulimia nervosa.

## CLINICAL CHARACTERISTICS

Most patients with bulimia nervosa are women in their late teens to mid-twenties. Most have had the disorder for several years before presenting for treatment and report that episodes of binge-eating occur five or more times weekly. The patients who present to clinics for treatment are usually of normal body weight. However, there is a significant overlap with the syndrome of anorexia nervosa. Approximately one-quarter of patients of normal body weight who present for treatment of bulimia nervosa have past histories of anorexia nervosa. Conversely, about half of the patients hospitalized for anorexia nervosa also meet criteria for bulimia nervosa. There is a significant frequency of bulimia among the obese, but the exact frequency and its clinical significance are as yet undetermined.

## PHYSICAL SIGNS AND COMPLICATIONS

There are no physical signs that are invariably present among patients with bulimia nervosa. However, in some individuals, the behavior may result in physical abnormalities which may be noted during physical examination and may alert the physician to the presence of this syndrome.

Significant dental problems have been reported in patients with bulimia nervosa, particularly among those who repeatedly induce vomiting. The lingual surfaces of the upper anterior teeth may become eroded and more sensitive to changes in temperature. As the biting edges deteriorate, the teeth may also take on a "moth-eaten" appearance. These dental problems appear to be caused by the repeated exposure of the teeth to stomach acid, gradually leading to decalcification and erosion of the lingual surfaces.

Some patients with bulimia nervosa, again primarily those who induce vomiting, may develop painless bilateral salivary gland enlargement which is occasionally quite striking. The glandular enlargement appears to be due to hypertrophy, not to inflammatory cell infiltration, and usually will diminish if eating behavior normalizes.

Occasionally, patients who induce vomiting by stimulating the gag reflex develop calluses on the dorsal surface of their hands, known as Russell's sign. Severe gastrointestinal complications in bulimia nervosa appear to be rare. Nonetheless, life-threatening complications have been reported, including esophageal tears and gastric rupture following binge-eating. There is a higher frequency of menstrual disturbance among women of normal weight with bulimia nervosa compared with their peers, although it is not clear which features of the illness, such as the abnormal eating patterns or weight fluctuations, are responsible for these reproductive disturbances.

Some patients with bulimia nervosa have resorted to the use of syrup of ipecac to induce vomiting, and some such patients may be vulnerable to the development of myopathy because of toxic effects of absorbed emetine.

## LABORATORY ABNORMALITIES

Patients who induce vomiting or abuse laxatives or diuretics are prone to develop the expected fluid and electrolyte disturbances. A significant fraction of patients who repeatedly induce vomiting develop hypokalemic alkalosis, which can occasionally be profound. Extensive laxative abuse has been associated with the development of metabolic acidosis.

About one-quarter of patients with bulimia nervosa have elevations of serum amylase, which is largely of salivary origin and, presumably, is a reflection of the binge-eating and vomiting. A moderate elevation of total amylase in an otherwise healthy young person may therefore suggest the presence of bulimia nervosa.

## ASSOCIATED PSYCHOLOGIC DISTURBANCES

It is now amply documented that patients with bulimia nervosa frequently exhibit disturbances of mood, typically a fluctuating level of depression accompanied by significant anxiety. It remains unclear to what degree such mood disturbances should be viewed as etiologic factors in the development of bulimia and to what degree as the result of a significant behavioral problem. However, it is important for the physician to inquire about the presence of depression.

Many patients with bulimia nervosa have current or past histories of drug abuse, particularly alcohol and stimulants which may initially have been used for weight reduction. In addition, patients may abuse, in large quantities, over-the-counter appetite suppressants and laxatives.

As noted earlier, there is a significant overlap between bulimia nervosa and anorexia nervosa. The physician should inquire about a past history of anorexia nervosa and should seriously consider a current diagnosis of anorexia nervosa in underweight patients with bulimia nervosa. If the patient meets current criteria for anorexia nervosa, management of this illness, because of the potentially life-threatening nature of the weight loss, takes precedence.

## TREATMENT

In the past decade, two major forms of treatment have been developed for bulimia nervosa. One is a form of psychologic treatment, usually referred to as cognitive behavioral therapy, and the second is the use of antidepressant medication. Both forms of treatment appear effective for many patients with bulimia nervosa, but definitive guidelines are not currently available to predict which patients respond preferentially to which form of treatment. The cognitive behavioral therapy has the advantage of being time-limited, usually requiring between 2 and 5 months and, of course, does not entail the risk of medication side effects. On the other hand, this form of treatment is best conducted by therapists with specific training and experience and requires a significant commitment of time and energy from the patient. The use of antidepressant medication is more straightforward for most physicians; its major disadvantages are the risk of side effects and lack of certainty about how long antidepressant medication needs to be continued in patients who respond to it.

The cognitive behavioral psychotherapy that has been developed for bulimia nervosa focuses specifically on the disturbed eating behavior. This form of treatment is pragmatic and relatively atheoretical—it does not assume any deep-seated psychologic cause for the eating disturbance. Rather it focuses on the abnormal behavior and on maladaptive patterns of thinking which appear to perpetuate the eating disorder. Typically, patients in this form of therapy meet with the therapist once or twice a week for the first month of treatment. The patient is required to record the details of episodes of binge-eating, both the foods consumed and the environmental and emotional circumstances. The therapist first helps the patient to identify the factors that appear to trigger episodes of binge-eating and then to devise alternative coping methods. For example, most patients with bulimia nervosa are intensely and overly concerned with their weight and believe that the consumption of a "normal" diet will produce uncontrolled and unacceptable weight gain. They therefore frequently attempt to rigidly restrict their caloric intake and expect to remain in perfect control of their diet at all times. The constant caloric deprivation and psychologic pressure appear to set the stage for binge-eating, particularly at times of emotional stress. Cognitive behavioral treatment attempts to educate the patient about the importance of maintaining caloric intake, to clarify the distortions of thinking, and to develop a more flexible and realistic approach to eating. It should be emphasized that the therapist in cognitive behavioral treatment is active and directive, and in these ways, such therapy differs substantially from traditional psychoanalytic forms of psychotherapy.

There are now compelling data to suggest that many patients with bulimia nervosa have impressive and lasting responses to cognitive behavioral treatment. This form of treatment is best delivered by a mental health practitioner who has experience with cognitive behavioral techniques and specifically with their application to patients with eating disorders.

The second major treatment modality for patients with bulimia nervosa is the use of antidepressant medication. The association between mood disturbance and bulimia nervosa described above has prompted over a dozen double-blind, placebo-controlled trials which have demonstrated conclusively that, at least in the short term, antidepressant medication is more effective than placebo in the treatment of bulimia nervosa. Most classes of antidepressant medication have been demonstrated to be effective. The use of antidepressant medication in the treatment of bulimia nervosa is, at present, virtually identical to the use of such medication in the treatment of depressive illness. Treatment may be initiated with one of the tricyclic antidepressants, particularly one with few anticholinergic side effects such as nortriptyline (Pamelor) or desipramine (Norpramin). Nortriptyline, at a dose of 75 mg per day, is sufficient for many patients. Treatment may be started at a dose of 25 mg daily, and the dose can be raised over a period of 1 week to 75 mg daily. After 1 week at this dose, a plasma level of nortriptyline should be obtained and the dose adjusted to achieve a nortriptyline level between 50 and 150 ng per ml, 8 to 12 hours after an oral dose. Alternatively, desipramine can be prescribed at a starting dose of 50 mg daily, gradually building to a full dose of 200 mg daily over a 1-week period. If there is insufficient symptom relief after 2 weeks at 200 mg, the dose can be gradually raised to 300 mg daily. Blood level determination is also useful in the use of desipramine; the desipramine dose should be ad-

justed so that the steady state desipramine level is above 150 ng per ml but less than 500 ng per ml. In at least one-half of patients with bulimia nervosa, significant symptom reduction will occur by the end of 3 to 4 weeks of antidepressant medication at the appropriate dose. Tricyclic antidepressants are generally well tolerated. Common side effects include dry mouth, constipation, and orthostatic hypotension. Since tricyclic antidepressants prolong cardiac conduction and can be dangerous in individuals with conduction disease, an electrocardiogram (ECG) should be obtained before initiating treatment.

Fluoxetine (Prozac) is a recently introduced antidepressant medication that appears to be effective for many patients with bulimia nervosa. Some clinicians prefer to initiate drug treatment with fluoxetine while others reserve its use for patients who fail to respond to a trial of a tricyclic antidepressant; such patients can be switched to fluoxetine several days after the tricyclic antidepressant has been discontinued. While a dose of 20 mg per day of fluoxetine is sufficient for the treatment of many patients with depression, 60 mg daily appears to be required for effective treatment of bulimia nervosa. Treatment with fluoxetine can be begun at 20 mg daily and rapidly increased to 60 mg daily. The outcome of treatment with fluoxetine should not be assessed until at least 3 weeks at 60 mg daily. Fluoxetine is usually well tolerated by patients with bulimia nervosa; common side effects include nausea, insomnia, and mild nervousness. Rarely, patients may develop a serious allergic reaction with features of serum sickness; the appearance of a skin rash should therefore prompt immediate consideration of discontinuing the fluoxetine.

Patients who fail trials of both a tricyclic antidepressant and fluoxetine should be referred for treatment with cognitive behavioral psychotherapy as described above if this has not already been attempted. Patients who have failed adequate trials of a tricyclic antidepressant, fluoxetine, and cognitive behavioral therapy may be considered for treatment with MAO inhibitors. Such drugs can be safely used in some patients with bulimia nervosa, but patients must be carefully screened for their ability to adhere to a tyramine-free diet and to avoid the use of stimulants, including over-the-counter cold preparations. In addition, MAO inhibitors cannot be initiated for at least 5 weeks after the discontinuation of fluoxetine, since there is a potentially dangerous interaction between MAO inhibitors and fluoxetine. Tranylcypromine (Parnate) at a dose of 30 to 60 mg daily and phenelzine (Nardil) at a dose of 45 to 60 mg daily have been successfully employed in the treatment of otherwise refractory patients with bulimia nervosa. Because of the frequent side effects and risks of MAO inhibitors, these compounds are usually the last resort for outpatient treatment. Although only rarely necessary, hospitalization should be considered for patients who have failed to respond to both structured forms of psychotherapy and antidepressant medication on an outpatient basis, as well as for patients with severe or unstable medical complications.

# DELIRIUM

method of
BENJAMIN LIPTZIN, M.D
*Harvard Medical School*
*Boston, Massachusetts*

Delirium is a generalized disorder of brain functioning that can have serious consequences. Key features include a disturbance of attention, orientation, memory, perception, sleep/wake cycle, and/or activity level. The disorder is most common in general hospital settings, particularly in elderly patients. Some studies have found the prevalence to be as high as 80% in elderly medical/surgical patients. Symptoms may develop over several hours or over several days. Once the symptoms appear, they may persist for days or weeks, even when the presumed underlying causes have been treated. The presence of delirium is often associated with a longer hospital stay or a higher probability of dying during the hospitalization or in the following year. A new onset of delirium is often the first sign of acute illness (e.g., infection, dehydration, or myocardial infarction) in an elderly patient. Despite its importance, delirium often goes undetected by physicians and nurses, especially when the patient is quietly confused rather than agitated, combative, paranoid, or hallucinating.

The key differential diagnosis is that of dementia. Delirious patients can present with severe cognitive impairments, including disorientation to time and place, poor memory, and inability to give a coherent history. If the onset is acute or the patient is cognitively intact at some point during the day, delirium should be assumed rather than dementia. Even in demented patients, a rapid change in cognitive status is probably due to delirium and not worsening dementia. Elderly patients who present acutely with psychotic features such as delusions or hallucinations should also be assumed to have a delirium unless they have a past history of schizophrenia, mania, psychotic depression, or delusional disorder.

## EVALUATION

Careful observation and history taking is the key to making a diagnosis of delirium. Patients should be asked their name and what brought them to the hospital. Patients may seem pleasant and cooperative but give a rambling, incoherent story and have no idea they are in a hospital or sick. Other useful questions include "Where do you live?" "Who do you live with?" and "Who is in your family?" As part of a standardized mental status exam, the patient should also be asked to perform serial 7 substractions and to remember three objects after a 5-minute delay. The patient should also be observed for restlessness, suspiciousness, somnolence, hyperalertness, labile mood, belligerence, or distractibility. Even if a patient seems completely intact, one should talk to the nursing staff and read any written notes about the patient's behavior over the previous 48 hours. Any abnormalities should be checked with family members to determine if they were present before the acute illness which led to hospitalization.

Delirium is a final common pathway for many different disorders (Table 1), and these need to be systematically inquired about through history taking, physical examination, and laboratory evaluation. Prescribed and nonprescribed medications (including alcohol) frequently lead to delirium in an older person who has reduced metabolism of the drug or increased sensitivity to its effects because of age or drug-disease or drug-drug interactions. If there is no obvious medication causing the delirium, it is necessary to carefully evaluate each organ system. Often, multiple pathologies will be uncovered, and it will not be obvious that any one was the specific cause of the delirium. In addition to a standard laboratory assessment that includes a complete blood count, chemistry profile, and urinalysis, if the clinical history warrants it, other sources of infection should be sought and a chest x-ray and electrocardiogram performed. If a central nervous system disorder is suspected, an electroencephalogram, CAT or MRI scan, and lumbar puncture should be considered.

TABLE 1. **Causes of Delirium**

Drug intoxication
  Psychotropic drugs
    Antidepressants, sedative/hypnotics, neuroleptics, lithium
  Other prescribed medications:
    Cardiac: digitalis, antiarrhythmics, antihypertensives
    GI: cimetidine, ranitidine
    Anti-inflammatory
    Narcotic analgesics
  Over-the-counter drugs: alcohol, antihistamines
Drug-withdrawal
  Alcohol, sedative/hypnotics
Metabolic disorders
  hypoxia, hypoglycemia, fluid/electrolyte imbalance, acid-base imbalance, kidney failure, hepatic failure, anemia, vitamin deficiencies, endocrinopathies
Cardiovascular disorders
  congestive heart failure, myocardial infarction, cardiac arrhythmia, shock
CNS disorders
  head trauma, seizures, cerebrovascular diseases, infections, space-occupying lesions (tumor, subdural hematoma, abscess)
Infections
Sleep deprivation
Postoperative states

## TABLE 2. Management of Delirium

Hospitalization unless mild
Careful monitoring
Consultations: psychiatric, geriatric, neurologic
Physiologic support: adequate hydration, adequate nutrition, treatment of underlying illness
Environmental support
Supportive nursing care
Psychotropic drugs: short-acting benzodiazepine, neuroleptic

### TREATMENT (Table 2)

Discovering the underlying medical cause for the delirium and reversing it, if possible, is the key to treating the delirious patient. Until that can be accomplished, the patient needs to be closely observed in a safe environment, usually a hospital. Whatever the underlying etiology, general supportive measures can be helpful. The patient should be kept in a quiet room with lights on in the daytime and a night light after bedtime. Stimulation should not be excessive, but some gentle music or television program may be soothing. Orientation cues, such as a calendar or clock, should be visible. Sensory impairments should be corrected with eyeglasses or a hearing aid. Family members should be encouraged to spend time with the patient for reassurance and orientation. Staff interventions should be carefully explained in a firm but caring manner. Patients should be encouraged to do as much for themselves and be as active as possible. Physical restraints should be used only if the patient is unsupervised and at risk of falling or pulling out intravenous lines or other tubes.

In the quietly confused patient, the above interventions along with careful monitoring may be sufficient to get the patient safely through the period of delirium. The highly agitated or psychotic patient may need pharmacologic intervention. In a delirium due to withdrawal from alcohol or other central nervous depressants, standard detoxification should be done. In other cases of delirium, short-acting benzodiazepines, such as lorazepam (Ativan) 0.25 to 2 mg depending on the patient's size or frailty, can be given at bedtime or every 4 hours if needed up to a maximum of 8 mg per day. If this does not provide enough sedation or if the patient is clearly psychotic, an alternative is to use a neuroleptic. The butyrophenones are preferable to most phenothiazines since the latter have anticholinergic effects that can cause delirium. Haloperidol (Haldol) 0.5 to 5 mg can be given orally or intramuscularly every 4 hours up to a maximum of 20 mg per day and titrated to the patient's response. The drug should be tapered over several days as the delirium resolves.

# AFFECTIVE DISORDERS

method of
GARY D. TOLLEFSON, M.D., PH.D.
*St. Paul–Ramsey Medical Center and University of Minnesota Medical School
Minneapolis, Minnesota*

The spectrum of affective disorders represents one of the more common challenges facing the practicing physician. Major affective disorders occur with a point prevalence in excess of 8 million Americans. Affective disorders represent extremes on a normal continuum ranging from elation to melancholia. Like extremes of blood pressure, cholesterol, or glucose, affective illnesses are characterized by symptom severity and chronicity. Thus, these diagnoses are disease states, not routine variations. The affective disorders often vex the clinician. Such patients may manifest a syndrome consisting of mood, somatic, cognitive, and psychomotor symptoms in the context of a high concurrence of physical disease and environmental distress. This patient group manifests a high utilization rate of health care services and may account for up to 20% of the primary care physician's workload. Despite their prevalence, these clinical problems go unrecognized and untreated in 75% of victims. As a multifaceted diagnosis, the affective disorders are truly biopsychosocial problems.

## TYPES OF DEPRESSION

Primary affective disorders, like other medical syndromes, come in different forms. The following will briefly describe the four major diagnostic types.

### Major Depressive Disorder

Within the accepted nosology of the *Diagnostic and Statistical Manual of Mental Disorders,* Third Version: Revised (DSM-III-R), major depression consists of a series of core symptoms in the context of a minimum of 2 weeks of sadness. The core symptoms include:
1. Depressed mood.
2. Diminished interests or pleasure in activities.
3. Significant change in appetite and/or weight.
4. Insomnia or hypersomnia.
5. Psychomotor agitation or retardation.
6. Fatigue and /or loss of energy.
7. Lack of concentration or indecision.
8. Diminished self-esteem /feelings of guilt.
9. Thoughts of death or suicide.

Despite a number of advances in understanding the neurobiology of depression, there are no sensitive/specific diagnostic markers available for the clinician. The differential diagnosis rests on a comprehensive data base. The physician's index of suspicion should be aroused in cases where the patient reports fatigue, pain, chronic sleep disturbances, and anxious features, or in the context of irritable bowel or fibromyalgia.

Precipitating factors in major depression may include prior episodes, a positive family history, concurrent illness, postpartum state, and/or severe or unanticipated stress. The course of major depression is variable. Some individuals may experience a single episode with a full or near full recovery to their premorbid level of function. However, the majority will experience recurrent episodes. The greater the frequency of these recurrences in their history, the more extended maintenance pharmacotherapy may have to be. (See discussion in the pharmacotherapy section.) The frequency of recurrent episodes is positively related to age. While most individuals recover fully from recurrent major depression, one in three may experience a more chronic course with considerable residual symptoms. This has been referred to as a major depression of a chronic type or a so-called double depression, major depression superimposed upon a dysthymic disorder. While major depression is not restricted to any one segment of the population, certain individuals may represent a high-risk profile: alcoholism, somatization, anxiety, Alzheimer's and related organic mental syndromes, and so forth.

Types of major depression include bipolar (associated with at least one previous episode of hypomania), unipolar:single, and unipolar:recurrent. Bipolar depression may often manifest itself with psychomotor retardation, hypersomnia, seasonal mood differences, a more robust familial history, and as a whole, an earlier age of onset. Within a bipolar cohort, some 10% will experience at least four discrete affective episodes within 1 year. This subgroup has been referred to as "rapid cyclers" and, as will be discussed, may require a specialized treatment package.

The differential diagnosis of the depressive syndrome is broad; however, it should commence with a careful medical history, physical examination, drug history, and appropriate cost-effective use of the laboratory. Physical diseases such as hypothyroidism that occur without intellectual compromise are classified as organic affective syndromes (physical diseases mimicking depression; Table 1).

The cardinal associated feature of a major depressive episode is anxiety. It has been estimated that up to 50% of patients with major depression may present with concomitant anxious symptoms. In our current nomenclature, when a patient demonstrates anxious features that have occurred within 3 months of the onset of a major depression and with no prior history of anxiety, the diagnosis is major depression alone. In other cases, co-morbid diagnoses of major depression and anxiety (e.g., panic disorder) may be justified if the latter clearly occurred independent of the change in mood. Other anxious features observed in depressive states include obsessive rumination, hypochondriasis, phobia, or somatization. Depressed patients may also develop psychotic features. Their delusions or hallucinations often are "mood congruent"—that is, associated with a low or diminished self-esteem. Thus, delusional themes may include persecution owing to perceived individual weaknesses, past moral transgressions, or other self-denigration. Their treatment package may also differ from conventional major depression without psychotic features.

Major depression may emerge in any age group. We are increasingly cognizant that depression may even affect prepubertal children. Such children often mani-

TABLE 1. **Examples of Medical Conditions Presenting with Depression**

| **Infections** | **Malignancies producing paraendocrine products** |
|---|---|
| Intracranial | |
| Viral pneumonia (postacute phase) | Bronchogenic (ACTH) |
| Hepatitis | Lymphoma (PTH) |
| Viral mononucleosis | Hepatoma (insulin) |
| | Lung (IADH) |
| **CNS Impairment** | **Others** |
| Tumor | Wilson's disease |
| Demyelination | Collagen vascular disease |
| Uremia | (e.g., lupus cerebritis) |
| Hypoxia | |
| Hepatic encephalopathy | **Drugs that can induce depression** |
| **Deficiencies** | Steroids |
| Niacin | Centrally active antihypertensives |
| Pyridoxine | |
| $B_{12}$ and/or folic acid | Narcotics |
| Electrolyte | Anticonvulsants |
| | Antineoplastics |
| **Endocrine** | Dopamine agonists |
| Pituitary insufficiency | Prostaglandin inhibitors |
| Hypothyroidism | Hormonal agents |
| Adrenal excess or insufficiency | Histamine blockers |
| | Sedative hypnotics |
| Diabetes mellitus | |
| Hyperparathyroidism | |
| Hypoglycemia | |

fest somatic complaints or psychomotor agitation (hyperkinesis). Among adolescents, major depression may be demonstrated via behavioral changes, e.g., antisocial behavior. Concomitant use or abuse of alcohol and illicit drugs may also be a heralding factor. Of course, suicide is a significant risk in preadult depression.

On the other end of the age continuum, major depression may influence the geriatric patient. Depressive equivalent symptoms here may include a change in cognitive function (pseudodementia). It is important to recognize that major depression may exist alone or in concert with a primary organic dementia. Major depression alone will often be associated with a personal or familial past history, denial, significant loss of interest or pleasure in normal activities, concentration difficulties exceeding memory deficits, retained insight into cognitive liabilities, and loss of future orientation.

When a major depressive syndrome accompanies a primary dementia, e.g., Alzheimer's disease, there remains a significant value in an empiric antidepressant trial. Often, the degree of cognitive dysfunction (superimposed impairment secondary to the depression) is reversible upon effective pharmacotherapy and may enhance the patient's degree of independent living skills and intellectual function.

The duration of a major depressive episode is quite variable. Without an effective therapeutic intervention, it can run a course of many months or years. While the predisposing factors for an episode of major depression are multifactorial, particularly of note for the primary care physician are concomitant chronic medical disorders and drug abuse/dependency. Major depression may also occur in the context of profound psychosocial stressors or in the postpartum or postmenopausal period. Certain patients may take on a seasonal attribute to their depression, e.g., at least 3 months of mood disturbance in 3 consecutive years that have a temporal seasonal relationship (e.g., beginning in October/November). It is yet unclear whether these represent a distinct entity or a variant of a major depressive disorder. This pattern has been referred to as a seasonal affective disorder (SAD). The SAD syndrome most often occurs in bipolars (so-called bipolar II or hypomania or "mild" mania by history) in women, during the second to third decade of life, and includes atypical symptoms of hyperphagia (carbohydrate craving), hypersomnia, fatigue, and social withdrawal. While responsive to conventional pharmacotherapy, it may also respond to bright light (2000 lux full-spectrum lighting at least 2 hours per day during the at-risk season, e.g., October through April). The pathophysiology of this disorder is unknown; however, it is likely that it is interdigitated with light/temperature sensitive bodily rhythms.

## Bipolar Illness (Mania)

The essential feature of mania is a distinct period characterized by either an elevated or expansive mood or, alternatively, irritability. This change in mood and the associated symptoms must be of sufficient severity to lead to an impairment in normal psychosocial function. As with other psychiatric diagnoses, a primary manic depressive or bipolar diagnosis is not made if a mediating organic factor can be established.

The diagnosis of a "manic syndrome" includes the following points: 1. A distinct period of abnormally and persistently elevated, expansive, or irritable mood. 2. At least three of the following symptoms have been present to a significant degree: (1) inflated self-esteem or grandiosity; (2) decreased need for sleep; (3) more talkative than usual or pressured speech; (4) flight of ideas/racing thoughts; (5) distractibility; (6) psychomotor agitation or increased time in goal-directed activities; (7) excessive involvement in pleasurable activities with potential for negative consequence/poor impulse control.

Changes in self-esteem are in the opposite direction of depression. They are associated with a continuum from being uncritical and highly self-confident to frank grandiosity (which may become delusional). The sleep pattern of the individual experiencing mania is often decreased. It is not unusual for the patient to awaken several hours early and be full of energy. In more severe manifestations, the individual may go for several days without any sleep, yet minimally complain of fatigue. During the course of the mental status examination, someone experiencing mania will typically manifest loud, rapid, and difficult to interpret speech patterns. Speech includes humorous content, e.g., jokes or puns. The thought process in someone experiencing mania is associated with what has been referred to as "flight of ideas." This implies a continuous flow of an accelerated thought process/speech, often covering numerous topics. Distractibility often characterizes the manic patient. As part of the profile of increased energy, the individual frequently will pursue numerous activities. In the milder phases, increased sociability emerges; however, the individual's appreciation of these intrusive contacts is minimal. Last but not least, this syndrome is typified by poor impulse control. Poor judgment through the spending of large amounts of cash, poor business decisions, hypersexuality, aggression, and so forth emerge and may take on a flamboyant or bizarre quality. It is important to re-emphasize that mania may also be complicated by delusions or hallucinations. Typically their content will be congruent with the patient's predominant mood. In the manic patient, mood-congruent delusions are often associated with inflated self-esteem, e.g., themes of persecution are linked to the individual's having a special relationship or attribute.

Bipolar disorder may begin in the early twenties or manifest itself anytime thereafter. Typically, the course of this disorder is a relatively rapid onset with symptomatic crescendo over several days. The episode may last anywhere from days to months. It is usually cyclic or recurrent. Most often complications of this disorder include concomitant substance abuse and/or associated social, legal, and financial difficulties. The estimated prevalence of bipolar disorder is from 0.4 to 1.2% of the adult population. In general, the disorder is equally common in males and females. A familial pattern is quite robust among first-degree biologic relatives of patients with this diagnosis.

In the assessment of the suspected manic patient, strong consideration should be given to organic mood syndromes induced by psychoactive substances, e.g., psychostimulants. Also, several organic disease states may mimic mania (Table 2). Historically, many patients with probable manic-depressive disorder had been diagnosed as schizophrenic. Schizophrenia still represents a challenging differential diagnosis in that the acute psychotic features are difficult to distinguish. It is best to rely on the associated features of bipolar disorder, e.g., a family history of mood disorder, good premorbid adjustment, previous track record of good interepisode recovery, and the nonpsychotic symptom constellation previously described.

## Cyclothymia

Cyclothymia is a chronic mood disorder. Under the current DSM-III-R, the diagnosis is based on a course of at least 2 years' duration (1 year for children and adolescents). Cyclothymia resembles a bipolar disorder. It includes hypomania (e.g., no psychotic features/hospitalization not required) alternating with periods of depressed mood or loss of interest. Patients evaluated during either of these mood cycles would not manifest sufficient criteria or duration to be classified as having either major depressive disorder or bipolar in their first 2 years. The cyclothymic patient should not have more than a 2-month interval where he or she has been asymptomatic. The precise threshold between cyclothymia and true bipolar illness is not always clear.

Cyclothymia may occur in individuals with a family history of bipolar disorder and, at least in some quarters, represent either a mild or prodromal form of bipolar disorder. Like most of the affective disorders, cyclothymia usually begins in adolescence or early

TABLE 2. **Organic Causes of Manic and Hypomanic Symptoms***

**Drug related**
Steroids and ACTH†
Isoniazid†
Bromides†
L-Dopa†
Antidepressants
Hallucinogens (marijuana, LSD, mescaline, psilocybin, STP, cocaine)
Sympathomimetic amines (dexedrine, methedrine, Preludin, Ritalin)
Disulfiram (Antabuse)
Alcohol
Barbiturates
Anticholinergics (Symmetrel, Pagitane, Akineton, Cogentin, Artane)
Anticonvulsants (Phenurone, Zarontin, Milontin)
Benzodiazepines

**Neurologic conditions**
Tumors (parasagittal meningioma, diencephalic glioma, suprasellar craniopharyngioma)†
Epilepsy
Infection (postviral encephalitis, influenza)†
General paresis
Multiple sclerosis
Huntington's disease
Postcerebrovascular accident
Right temporal lobectomy
Post-traumatic confusion
Postelectroconvulsive therapy
Deliriform organic brain disease

**Metabolic conditions**
Postoperative states†
Hemodialysis†
Hyperthyroidism
Postinfectious hypomania
Cushing's disease
Addison's disease

**Other conditions**
Postisolation syndrome

*From Lazare A: Manic behavior. In Lazare A (ed): Outpatient Psychiatry: Diagnosis and Treatment. © 1979, the Williams & Wilkins Co., Baltimore.
†Meets criteria of Krauthammer and Klerman (1978) for secondary mania.

adulthood. It typically has an insidious onset and pursues a chronic course. The degree of psychosocial impairment is variable. Prevalence estimates of cyclothymia range from 0.4 to 3.5%. As with bipolar affective disorder, males and females are at equal risk. Since mood cycles are the predominant feature of the cyclothymic patient, differential diagnoses include bipolar disorder or a number of the Axis II personality disorders typified by marked shifts in mood, e.g., borderline, histrionic, and antisocial. The mood lability of these personality disturbances are often reactive to environmental stressors and typically would not include other features consonant with a primary major mood disorder.

## Dysthymia (Depressive Neurosis)

Like cyclothymia, dysthymia is a chronic disorder of mood. However, the dysthymic experience is a prolonged period of depressed mood only. The essential criteria for dysthymia include:

1. Predominant depression for at least 2 years (1 year for children and adolescents).

2. At least two of the following symptoms while depressed: (a) poor appetite or overeating; (2) insomnia or hypersomnia; (3) low energy or fatigue; (4) low self-esteem; (5) poor concentration and difficulty with decision-making; (6) feelings of hopelessness.

3. During a 2-year period the patient has not been without symptoms for more than a 2-month interval.

4. No evidence of a previous unequivocal major depressive episode in the first 2 years while the diagnosis of dysthymia is being established.

Longitudinal studies reveal that dysthymia is a frequent complication of a number of pre-existing primary medical and/or psychiatric disorders. These are often referred to as secondary manifestations of dysthymia. Dysthymia may often be co-morbid with personality disorders as well. Dysthymic disorder usually begins in childhood or adolescence. While psychosocial impairment is present, it is usually not as severe as that seen in major depression. Hospitalization is rare. While the predisposing factors to the development of a dysthymic disorder are not well delineated, chronic psychosocial stressors in childhood or early adolescence may predispose to either primary or secondary types. Epidemiologic studies of dysthymia would suggest it to be frequent, although exact figures are not available. It may occur more commonly among first-degree biologic relatives of patients with major depressive disorder and equally in males and females. The major factors to differentiate from a diagnosis of dysthymia would be a discrete episode of major depression that has only partially remitted with treatment or, conversely, nonpathologic normal fluctuations in mood that have minimal or no interference with psychosocial functioning.

## Atypical Depression

The term atypical depression has been used to describe a mood syndrome that differs from more conventional major depression along at least one of several critical variables. These variables include age of onset, course, family history, clinical phenomenology, response to treatment, and ultimate prognosis. While clearly the clinical criteria of "atypical depression" merit greater precision, patients with an atypical disorder may manifest (a) reverse of vegetative signs, e.g., hypersomnia/hyperphagia; (b) an admixture of both depressive and anxious features; or (c) mild severity/chronicity. A number of investigators argue that atypical depression may preferentially respond to monoamine oxidase inhibitors (MAOIs). Other literature suggests that newer second-generation agents, including those with selective serotinergic reuptake blockade, may also be effective. When using a tricyclic antidepressant, the literature would support achievement of a routine therapeutic blood level in atypical patients as well.

## PHARMACOLOGIC TREATMENT OF DEPRESSION

### Heterocyclic Antidepressants

As has been mentioned in the preceding sections, the clinician should approach major depression as a medical syndrome. Table 3 portrays a comparison of depression, as a neurochemical entity, with a more conventional model—Parkinson's disease. Consonant with this concept is the perspective that initiation of pharmacologic therapy should be based on some degree of symptom severity, i.e., along a continuum. A rational approach to the pharmacologic management of major depression is similar to that of hypertension:

1. Accurate differential diagnosis.
2. Identification of target symptoms in order to assess response patterns.
3. Selection of optimal treatment agents.
4. Titration of dose to maximize efficacy and minimize side effects.
5. Avoidance of abrupt discontinuation of treatment (a gradual, several weeks to months tapering recommended).
6. Follow-up for complications.
7. Ongoing assessment of prognosis/need for maintenance treatment.
8. Encouragement of concurrent environmental modifications.

Selection from the pharmacologic menu of current antidepressant agents should be based on a risk-benefit analysis, that is, selection of an agent most likely to be effective (based on clinical presentation) and best tolerated regarding side effect potential (based on medical history of the patient). Side effects of pharmacotherapy compromise patient compliance and thus reduce the likelihood of a successful outcome. Further, emergent side effects may prevent appropriate dose titration in order to achieve an effective therapeutic response. The menu of pharmacologic agents available to the clinician includes both

TABLE 3. **Major Depression as Neurochemical Disorder**

|  | MDD | Parkinson's |
|---|---|---|
| Suspected brain focus (foci) | Yes | Yes |
| Corresponding clinical signs and symptoms | Yes | Yes |
| Neurotransmitter irregularity | Yes | Yes |
| Pharmacotherapy is oriented to restore a biochemical equilibrium | Yes | Yes |
| Maintenance pharmacotherapy may be necessary | Yes | Yes |
| Pharmacologic agents may potentiate or antagonize the clinical picture | Yes | Yes |

MDD = major depressive disorder.

TABLE 4. **The Antidepressants Comprise a Pharmacologic Menu**

| First Generation | Second Generation |
|---|---|
| 1. 3°Amine<br>  Ex. AMI | 5. 5-HT Reuptake<br>  Ex. fluoxetine |
| 2. 2°Amine<br>  Ex. DMI | 6. Novel<br>  Ex. bupropion |
| 3. MAOI<br>  Ex. phenelzine | 7. 5-HT Related<br>  Ex. trazodone |
| 4. Lithium | 8. GABA-Related<br>  Ex. adinazolam |

AMI = amitriptyline; DMI = desipramine; MAOI = monoamine oxidase inhibitor; 5-HT = serotonin; GABA = gamma-amino butyric acid.

first- and second-generation agents (Table 4). The newer second-generation agents are structurally different molecules, i.e., nontricyclic. While they apparently do not work any faster and are of comparable efficacy with the conventional tricyclic antidepressants, their safety profile is usually more favorable. These newer agents demonstrate a higher specificity on select neurotransmitter systems relevant to depression and minimize concomitant risks associated with the tricyclic's multireceptor profile, i.e., anticholinergic, antihistaminic, hypotensive, and cardiovascular effects. In addition, the second-generation agents demonstrate a higher therapeutic index and thus may be associated with a reduced probability of morbidity and mortality in a toxic scenario.

**Fluoxetine Hydrochloride (Prozac).** Fluoxetine is one of the second-generation antidepressants not chemically related to the tricyclic or other available agents. It is a propylamine derivative. It is the first available of a group of highly selective reuptake blockers of serotonin. Fluoxetine is extensively metabolized in the liver. Fluoxetine's elimination half-life is 2 to 3 days and that of its active metabolite norfluoxetine, 7 to 9 days. Ease of administration is one of the advantages of this agent. It is usually initiated at 20 mg once daily with meals in the morning. The majority of patients respond to this starting dose. Occasionally titration in the range of 40 to 60 mg per day may be necessary.

In contrast to the conventional tricyclic agents, fluoxetine has minimal binding activity at cholinergic, histaminic, or alpha-adrenergic receptors. Thus, the associated side effects of tricyclics already discussed are infrequently seen with fluoxetine. Where it is not well tolerated, patients on fluoxetine may experience anxiety, restlessness, or insomnia. Approximately 4% of fluoxetine recipients experience a skin rash or urticaria. Fatigue, nausea, or other gastrointestinal complaints, headache, and lightheadedness have also been reported. Concomitant administration of MAOIs or the serotonin precursor tryptophan is discouraged. A further advantage of fluoxetine has been the usual lack of associated weight gain with extended therapy. Approximately one in eight patients will experience weight loss. Most others maintain a stable weight. The relationship of therapeutic effect and plasma levels of fluoxetine or its metabolites is unknown at this time.

**Bupropion Hydrochloride (Wellbutrin).** Bupropion is structurally similar to phenylethylamine. In contrast to classic tricyclic antidepressants, it is a very weak blocker of acetylcholine, serotonin, norepinephrine, or dopamine. The actual mechanism of action of bupropion is unknown. The relationship of therapeutic effect in plasma levels of bupropion or its metabolites is unknown.

Bupropion is rapidly absorbed and hepatically metabolized. Half-life on the initial phase is 1 to 2 hours; half-life of the second phase is 14 hours. Bupropion manifests four basic metabolites: morpholinol, threoamino alcohol, erythroamino alcohol, and erythroamino diol. These metabolites have been found to be some one-half as potent as the parent drug in screening for antidepressant agents. The elimination of bupropion may be affected by reduced renal or hepatic function as it is a moderately polar compound that is conjugated in the liver prior to urinary excretion. Like all antidepressants, it has a 2- to 3-week latency before its onset of action is manifested. Bupropion is routinely started at the dose of 75 mg, three times a day. It may need to be titrated to a single maximum dose of 150 mg three times a day or a total of 450 mg per 24 hours. Bupropion appears to have efficacy comparable with that of antidepressants such as amitriptyline.

Bupropion was voluntarily withdrawn by the manufacturer in 1986 for further study on its association with seizure. The drug is associated with generalized tonic-clonic seizure at an approximate incidence of 0.4% (4/1000). Controlled prospective studies of the incidence of seizures with conventional tricyclic antidepressants are lacking. However, this may represent an increase over their relative risk. There are no direct comparative studies in the literature.

The most frequently encountered adverse events with bupropion have included agitation, dry mouth, insomnia, headache, nausea and vomiting, constipation, or tremor. As with fluoxetine, the advantage of bupropion is the much lower anticholinergic, antihistaminic, or hypotensive risks associated with conventional tricyclic antidepressants. Escalation of dosage of bupropion should be done in gradual increments. One of the major advantages of bupropion is the limited risk of postural hypotension and its minimal cardiovascular profile. It has been reported that tricyclic recipients who have experienced orthostatic hypotension do not experience recurrence of or-

thostasis when receiving bupropion. Bupropion also reportedly has no clinically significant effect in cardiac conduction. As with the above discussion of fluoxetine, another important difference between bupropion and the conventional tricyclics is the effect on body weight. Of bupropion recipients, 28% are reported to have lost weight, and in total some 90% experience either weight loss or no gain. To my knowledge, there are no fatal overdoses reported with bupropion.

Iatrogenic orthostatic hypotension is among the most problematic of the side effects, especially in the elderly or medically ill patient. The conventional tricyclic antidepressants are relatively more common offenders. Orthostatic hypotension often develops at therapeutic blood levels (nontoxic). Thus, this side effect may limit their therapeutic utility. In such cases, newer second-generation agents should be considered. The best candidates are fluoxetine (Prozac), bupropion (Wellbutrin), and perhaps the tricyclic antidepressant nortriptyline (Pamelor/Aventyl). In the screening assessment, minimal cardioacceleration (less than ten beats per minute) in the face of a 10 to 15 mm drop suggests a heightened predisposition to a further drug-induced alteration of the baroreceptor reflex.

A number of investigators have attempted to come up with both descriptive and laboratory parameters for predicting pharmacologic response. Unfortunately at this time, the utility of these models is quite limited. Choice of an individual agent should be dictated by the patient's complete clinical picture. This includes select psychiatric symptomatology (Table 5) and predisposing medical history (Table 6).

Figure 1, in the absence of a more refined system, offers one model for a rational approach to drug selection. First-line therapies should include either the secondary amine tricyclics desipramine or nortriptyline (which are relatively

TABLE 5. **Prediction of Response**

**Treatment Selection Based upon a Subclassification of Mood Disorders**

| Target Symptoms | Agent(s) |
| --- | --- |
| Agitated | BDZ + AD buspirone + AD |
| Psychotic | NL + AD amoxapine/ECT |
| Obsessive | Fluoxetine/clomipramine |
| Retarded | Bupropion |
| BP: rapid cycler | Carbamazepine/verapamil |
| "Atypical" | Phenelzine |
| Partial response | Lithium/thyroid + AD |
| Insomnia | BDZ + AD |
| BP: depressed | Lithium |
| Obesity | Bupropion/fluoxetine |
| PUD | Doxepin/trimipramine |

BDZ = benzodiazepine; AD = antidepressant; NL = neuroleptic; PUD = peptic ulcer disease; BP = bipolar.

TABLE 6. **TCA Risks**
**(Lack Specificity/"Dirty Drug")**

| Class | Example | Reference | At-Risk Patient |
|---|---|---|---|
| Anticholinergic | AMI | ATR | BPH/AD |
| Antihistaminic | DOX | Dph. | Obese/alert |
| Anti-adrenergic | DOX | Phentol. | DM/elderly |
| Cardiovascular | IMI | Quin. | Heart block, MI |

Overdose: ↑ Morbidity: Mortality
*Risks*—Only a 10–14 day supply

BPH = benign prostatic hypertrophy; AD = Alzheimer's dementia; DM = diabetes mellitus; MI = recent myocardial infarction. Quin. = quinidine; Dph. = diphenhydramine; ATR = atropine; DOX = doxepin; IMI = imipramine; AMI = amitriptyline; Phentol. = phentolamine.

safer than the tertiary tricyclics) or the novel serotonin reuptake blocker fluoxetine (Prozac). The atypical antidepressant bupropion can also be used as a first-line intervention or certainly should be considered if any of the above agents have not been clinically effective and before pursuing the other alternatives outlined. If the client has failed in trials with several distinct heterocyclic antidepressants, augmentation therapy with lithium for at least 2 to 3 weeks is recommended. Effective lithium levels should be in the

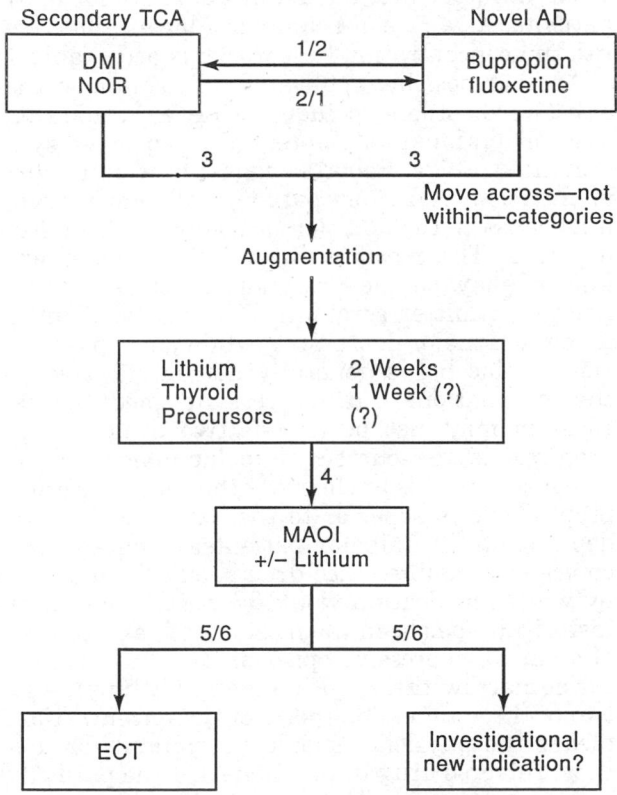

**Figure 1.** An approach to depression pharmacology. *Abbreviations:* TCA = tricyclic antidepressant; DMI = desipramine; NOR = nortriptyline; AD = Alzheimer's dementia; MAOI = monoamine oxidase inhibitor; ECT = electroconvulsive therapy.

0.5 to 0.9 mEq per liter range. Thereafter, if clinical response is not seen, further consideration of MAOIs, electroconvulsive therapy, or newer investigational compounds may be necessary. Clearly, depressed patients in a primary care setting who do not demonstrate a robust response to initial antidepressant pharmacotherapies should be considered for psychiatric referral. Tricyclic antidepressants have also been used in nondepressive conditions.

The original theories of antidepressant activity were based on the assumption that these drugs were actually blocking the reuptake of one or more monoamines. However, while this effect occurs within several days in vitro, the depressed patient typically requires 2 to 4 weeks to respond. This observation, coupled with advances in our ability to assess drug-receptor interactions, led to an alternative interpretation. Clinical efficacy appears to be related to changes in receptor sensitivity subsequent to subacute administration of a number of the antidepressant drugs. Three separate theories have emerged: (1) beta-adrenergic receptor down-regulation; (2) alpha$_2$-receptor down-regulation; and (3) the enhancement of central serotonin neurotransmission. A wide variety of tricyclic, second-generation, and monoamine oxidase inhibitors have been associated with beta-adrenergic receptor down-regulation. Electroconvulsive treatment is similarly classified. However, several novel or atypical antidepressants such as bupropion are discordant with this model. The second theory asserts that antidepressants alter the presynaptic inhibitory alpha$_2$-adrenergic receptor, yielding a net increase in synaptic norepinephrine (yohimbine-like). It is important to remember that the alpha$_2$-adrenergic receptor is an inhibitory site. While many antidepressants demonstrate this property, several investigators have revealed that trazodone (Desyrel), bupropion (Wellbutrin), and several other novel agents have no presynaptic alpha-adrenergic profile.

Perhaps the most intriguing of these three hypotheses centers on the enhancement of synaptic serotonin. A wide spectrum of antidepressants is associated with an alteration of serotonin receptor sensitivity. Conventional tricyclic antidepressants work at postsynaptic serotonin receptors. Conversely, the newer selective serotonin reuptake blockers such as fluoxetine (Prozac), the MAOIs, and the partial I-A agonist/antagonist buspirone (Buspar) work presynaptically and produce subsensitivity at the *inhibitory* serotonin autoreceptor. The common denominator, albeit through different pathways, is enhanced synaptic serotonin.

Unfortunately, none of these theories totally explains the activity of the full spectrum of antidepressants currently available. Other systems implicated in the development of new antidepressants include selective enhancement at the gamma-aminobutyrate or dopamine receptors and beyond the postsynaptic receptor at the second messenger adenosine 3,5-monophosphate.

Initiation of antidepressants should include patient education regarding the biologic aspects of the disease, awareness of the 2- to 4-week response latency, knowledge that antidepressants are not addictive nor need to be taken life-long (most patients), and an informed discussion of alternatives and the risk of no treatment.

### Lithium

The therapeutic toxic potential of lithium was not recognized until the late 1940s when Cade announced discovery of lithium's antimanic effect. Lithium (atomic number 3) demonstrates a number of unique chemical properties. It bears similarities to the cations sodium, potassium, calcium, and magnesium in its central nervous system profile. The precise mechanism of action in the major affective disorders remains unknown. However, at least 15 to 20 biochemical profiles have been described. At present, the only approved indications for the use of lithium are in the treatment of acute mania or in the maintenance therapy of bipolar affective disorders. Studies of lithium in the treatment of acute mania demonstrate that it is significantly superior to placebo. It does, however, manifest a latent period of 5 to 14 days from the initiation of drug treatment to the onset of its antimanic effect. Thus, lithium alone may be inadequate for the severely manic patient, particularly where hospitalization and mood-congruent psychosis occur. In such cases the short-term addition of a neuroleptic and/or benzodiazepine (antiagitation strategies) may be utilitarian. A thorough medical and psychiatric history should be obtained before the initiation of lithium therapy. Patients must have baseline renal function testing. In most cases, measurement of serum creatinine will be adequate. Because lithium may suppress thyroid function, pretreatment screening, e.g., thyroid stimulating hormone, is recommended. Additional laboratory testing such as electrolytes, chemistry panel, and an electrocardiogram (ECG) should be pursued where clinically indicated. The preparation of choice is the sustained release forms of lithium (Lithobid; Eskalith CR) that come in 300 mg or 450 mg sizes, respectively. In the absence of any renal compromise, initial dosages of lithium for acute mania are approximately 1200 mg per day. Lithium is rapidly and completely absorbed from the gastrointestinal

tract. Depending on the formulation, it reaches a peak serum level within 1 to 5 hours. Unlike other agents used in the treatment of affective disorders, lithium has no metabolites, is not protein bound, and is excreted by the kidney. Traditional guidelines suggest levels between 0.8 to 1.2 mEq per liter in the acute manic. Because lithium has a half-life of approximately 24 hours, 5 days may be necessary to reach a steady-state blood concentration. Thus, serum lithium levels need not be determined in less than 5 to 7 days after a dose change unless toxicity is suspected. In the medically ill or older patient, the half-life of lithium may be increased in relationship to diminished ability to excrete the drug (renal). A serum lithium level should be obtained as close to 12 hours after the last dose as possible.

Lithium is also a well-established strategy for maintenance of patients with bipolar or manic-depressive disorder. In general, a history of relapse or recurrence should be present in order to establish appropriate indications for maintenance therapy beyond 6 to 12 months after the initial episode. Maintenance therapy is often accomplished at lower dosages and accompanying drug concentrations. Maintenance levels from 0.4 to 0.9 mEq per liter should be adequate for most patients. As a rule of thumb, the lowest effective lithium concentration that works is acceptable.

Another possible application of lithium in the affective disorders includes using it in addition to a conventional antidepressant, a so-called synergistic strategy. Reports suggest that up to 50% of previously refractory patients will demonstrate a response to the addition of lithium within 2 to 3 weeks. The mechanism of action, while unknown, may be the presynaptic release of the neurotransmitter serotonin. The use of lithium alone in a major depressive, while perhaps superior to placebo, is generally not as effective as the conventional antidepressant medications. Lithium may also be an effective drug for the prophylaxis of recurrent unipolar major depressive disorder. It is unclear whether or not lithium prophylaxis is superior to the heterocyclic antidepressants in unipolar patients. Generally the choice of a maintenance drug should be dictated by which medication would be best tolerated or historically has been the most effective in control of an acute depressive episode.

The narrow therapeutic index of lithium, e.g., two to three times the therapeutic concentration, means the physician should be vigilant for toxicity. Adverse drug interactions are one pathway to lithium toxicity. The thiazide diuretics reduce the net clearance of lithium (relative to other monovalent cations) and may cause a substantial increase in serum lithium concentrations. Other diuretics not active in the proximal convoluted tubule may be safer. Recent evidence also suggests that the nonsteroidal anti-inflammatory drugs decrease lithium clearance as well. Any agent that alters glomerular filtration rate or renal clearance may lead to toxicity. In contrast, those agents that enhance filtration/clearance, such as aminophylline or caffeine, have the reverse effect of lowering serum lithium concentrations. Accordingly, the amount of dietary sodium and fluid intake should be held relatively constant during lithium pharmacotherapy.

Like all psychotropic medications, lithium has a profile of side effects and toxicity. The common side effects include sedation, thirst, weight gain, tremor, diarrhea, and fluid retention. Less common, but noteworthy, reactions include hair loss, euthyroid goiter or hypothyroidism, sinus node dysfunction/ectopy, anorexia, polyuria/polydipsia of diabetes insipidus, and aggravation of preexisting dermatologic conditions such as acne or psoriasis.

Bipolar patients with a history of a rapid cycle (more than four episodes per 12 months) appear to respond less well to lithium. In patients with a rapid cyclic course, consideration should be given to substituting one of the newer second-generation agents, such as bupropion, for any conventional tricyclic; confirming that the patient is euthyroid; and discontinuing lithium with initiation of an alternative anticycling agent (see next section).

## NONLITHIUM ALTERNATIVES IN BIPOLAR DISORDER

For the patient with a history of rapid cycling or episodes characterized by mixed manic and depressive features, alternatives to lithium may be necessary. Options include anticonvulsants such as carbamazepine or valproate or a calcium-channel blocker such as verapamil. Carbamazepine has a molecular structure that actually resembles that of imipramine. It was introduced into neurologic practice in 1959 and soon was observed to have beneficial effects on behavior and psychologic functioning. As many as two-thirds of bipolar patients may show some improvement on this drug. Its greatest utility appears in the rapid cycler or the lithium-resistant patient. Where liver function is normal, carbamazepine can be started in doses of 200 mg twice a day. Once at steady state (approximately 5 days), therapeutic drug monitoring is encouraged. Often patients are maintained in the range of 6 to 12 µg/ml. There may be an even tighter correlation between clinical response and one of the carbamazepine metabolites, 10,11-epoxide. Side effects include drowsiness, visual disturbance, motor disturbance, diarrhea, nausea, rash,

weight gain, and mild hyponatremia. Of special importance is the periodic screening for hematologic or hepatic reactions. The former include aplastic anemia, neutropenia, thrombocytopenia, or anemia. The prevalence of these events range from 10% (transient neutropenia) to 0.5 per 100,000 per year (aplastic anemia). Idiosyncratic non-dose–related hypersensitivity reactions have been reported and include fever, rash, hepatic tenderness, and eosinophilia. Overdose should be treated similarly to that for imipramine.

Electroconvulsive therapy (ECT) is clearly effective in both bipolar and unipolar patients. ECT is particularly effective when these diagnoses are complicated by psychotic features. However, controlled studies of ECT as a prophylactic treatment are lacking. ECT techniques have become considerably refined in electrode placement, stimulus waveform, and so forth. Increased intracranial pressure and mass effect continue to be the principal contraindications. In addition, any patient considered a poor risk for general anesthesia may not be appropriate for ECT. While mechanisms are yet unknown, the receptor-neurotransmitter profiles of ECT closely resemble those of the tricyclic antidepressants, especially in noradrenergic profiles.

Other treatment alternatives include valproate, clonazepam, verapamil, and possibly acetazolamide. Lithium added to one of these may provide even greater efficacy.

## THERAPEUTIC DRUG MONITORING

Therapeutic drug monitoring should be a strategy designed to improve both the safety and efficacy of pharmacotherapy. Many of the therapeutic and adverse reactions associated with psychotropic drugs are concentration-dependent, i.e., different actions predominate at different concentrations. One of the major reasons for nonresponse to pharmacotherapy is inadequate dosing, i.e., not achieving a therapeutic concentration of the drug. This may occur in at least 50% of antidepressant drug nonresponders referred to tertiary centers. This can be partly explained by the wide interindividual differences in concentration-dose relations. Pharmacokinetic variance is related to the so-called first pass metabolism of these drugs, i.e., differing hepatic degradation rates prior to the drug's systemic availability.

Through the use of therapeutic drug monitoring, the physician has available (at least for some of the psychotropic drugs) a technique to assist in dosage adjustment, to maximize therapeutic efficacy, and to minimize potential toxic effects. The percent of responders to conventional tricyclic therapy by dose is only in the range of 40 to

60%. With the use of concurrent plasma level monitoring, tricyclic response rates can be maximized to 70 to 80% of recipients. Obviously, psychotropic medications are not without risk. Lithium, carbamazepine, and the tricyclic antidepressants possess a relatively narrow therapeutic index. Clinical studies in tricyclic recipients suggest that one in 50 physically healthy individuals receiving 100 mg of a reference tricyclic antidepressant may generate a toxic concentration. These drugs also represent one of the leading causes of death from drug overdose. Among the more common serious toxic effects associated with these agents are cardiovascular arrhythmia, conduction delay, sudden death, seizure, and delirium. With the possible exception of orthostatic hypotension, many psychotropic side effects are dose dependent. When tricyclic levels exceed 450 ng per ml, the majority of patients are at risk for such complications.

Thus, therapeutic drug monitoring has merit as a standard of care issue. Therapeutic drug level monitoring can provide valuable information in the following areas: (a) patient compliance; (b) maximizing clinical response; (c) avoiding toxicity. It is a quantitative index for the practitioner. However, it is important to recognize limitations. Therapeutic monitoring may not reflect pharmacodynamics (receptor site activity), nor does it always account for multiple active metabolites. Psychotropic drugs with useful concentration-response relationships include the tricyclic antidepressants, lithium, anticonvulsants, possibly haloperidol/fluphenazine/thiothixene, and indirectly the MAOIs via platelet monoamine oxidase activity. The utility in maximizing treatment outcome amongst several of the so-called "second generation" agents is limited.

## PREGNANCY

The risk of fetal malformation (e.g., the cardiovascular system) is greater with lithium than with the tricyclic antidepressants. Evidence suggests that the incidence of teratogenicity with mothers receiving tricyclics is no greater than that of chance. Data regarding the second-generation agents appear to show similar results, albeit available data are scant. Reproductional studies with fluoxetine have generally been limited to animal models. Doses from nine to 11 times the maximum human daily dose have revealed no evidence of fetal harm. However, adequate or well-controlled studies in pregnant women are lacking. Thus the drug should be used during pregnancy only if clearly indicated. Fluoxetine is detectable in breast milk. Bupropion also crosses the placental barrier. The concentration

in fetal tissue is reportedly less than that of the placenta or other maternal tissues. In animal studies there is no evidence of impaired fertility or fetal harm in bupropion recipients. Data on human teratogenicity are lacking. It may be detected in breast milk. The use of any medication should be avoided whenever possible during the first trimester of pregnancy. However, lithium does represent a relatively higher risk. A further complicating factor is that the hemodynamics/volume changes that occur during pregnancy may complicate the maintenance of a normal therapeutic lithium level. Breast-feeding by mothers who are taking lithium is also discouraged. Lithium appears to enter breast milk and can obtain a meaningful concentration in the infant. Data on whether lithium exposure adversely affects growth and development or could manifest any behavioral liabilities are as yet unavailable. Carbamazepine also crosses the placenta, achieving a drug concentration of 60% of the mother's serum; transfer is also seen in breast milk. Among the array of anticonvulsants, carbamazepine may actually be the safest.

## PSYCHOTHERAPEUTIC STRATEGIES

A significant advance in the nonpharmacologic treatment of depression has been the emergence of structured, time-limited, cognitive, interpersonal, and behavioral psychotherapeutic techniques. These strategies are effective in reducing the symptoms of depression in ambulatory patients. These newer psychotherapeutic strategies have several common denominators. They allow the therapist to individualize treatment for the patient, are time limited, focus on the present, embellish patient education and information, and provide concrete objectives. These strategies have been demonstrated by some investigators to be as effective as pharmacotherapy in certain outpatient populations. The overall rate of response to treatment in nonpsychotic, mild to moderately symptomatic patients enrolled in such trials has approached 60 to 70%.

The keys to effective psychotherapy include discussion of a diagnosis, prognosis, and treatment plan, including a definite statement of the objectives of treatment. This allows the psychotherapist and, for that matter, the referring physician, the ability to assess therapeutic efficacy or lack thereof over a defined period. The success of these short-term psychotherapies is based on establishment of a close therapeutic alliance or relationship. Succinctly, application of these newer behavioral strategies assists the patient in defining particular problems in terms of either interpersonal or cognitive styles. The patient is actively encouraged to become involved in a process of change that diminishes risk factors for more serious and/or chronic disturbance in mood. This model is time limited and entirely consistent with a cost-effective health care model.

Factors that may predict a good response to these forms of psychotherapy alone may include:

1. Shorter duration of the current episode (less than 1 year.

2. History of good interepisode recovery (if past history present).

3. Absence of major concurrent personality disorder.

4. Illness of mild to moderate severity.

5. Nonpsychotic, nonbipolar forms of depression.

Psychotherapy and concomitant management with medication are not mutually exclusive. In certain individuals with moderate to severe symptoms in whom medication is indicated, psychotherapy may also assist in dealing with current psychosocial stressors, predisposing psychologic factors, psychologic adjustments consequent to a course of a major affective disorder, and a forum for provision of patient and family education.

## WHEN TO REFER TO A PSYCHIATRIST

The physician's initial ability, willingness, and comfort in the detection and discussion of a psychiatric disorder are critical in a successful referral. Referral has been associated with cost efficiency through the earlier identification and effective management of patients with complicated mental disorders. Consultation within the affective disorders can be useful when the differential diagnosis includes questions around possible organic etiology (disease or drug), psychosomatic versus psychologic factors affecting a concurrent physical condition, failure to respond after a 4-week trial of a conventional antidepressant, initiation of nonpharmacologic treatments of depression, the potentially suicidal patient, the bipolar patient, affective disorders complicated by psychosis, and other complicated co-morbid disorders, such as panic, obsessional eating, and alcoholism. Consultation for mood disorder should also be considered for children and adolescents. Acute behavioral changes, academic difficulties, a change in peer or family relationships, or a continued pattern of psychosomatic complaints may be indicative of major depression within this age group.

In order to carry out an effective referral, the physician should be aware of possible reasons for patient resistance. These can include the social stigma of a psychiatric label, self-esteem, failure to understand the role of emotion in physical complaints, lack of education about the biologic aspects of mental disorders, or belief that mental disorders are chronic and untreatable. Thus, it is essential that the referring physician assist the patient in understanding the motive behind the referral, desire to continue to be a part of the case management, and minimize the patient's perception of a loss of credibility in the referral process. The simple explanation that the use of a psychiatrist as a specialist, analogous to consultation with other medical specialists, and patient education regarding the biologic basis of mental disorders will enhance patient follow-through.

# SCHIZOPHRENIA

method of
SAMUEL J. KEITH, M.D.
*National Institute of Mental Health*
*Rockville, Maryland*

Schizophrenia remains one of the world's most significant public health problems. It affects over 1% of the population of the United States during the course of a lifetime and evidence would suggest that this same percentage is affected worldwide. Its etiology is presumed to be a biologic abnormality of the function or structure of the brain. Its symptoms are devastating disruptions of the cognitive, emotional, and behavioral aspects of life. Millions of people will have their lives interrupted in late adolescence or early adulthood at a time when they are trying to complete an education or enter a career. Many will never return to this life course. Up to 10% will commit suicide rather than to continue with a life so distorted from what they had planned. To consider the treatment of schizophrenia, however, one must face this massive human suffering on an individual patient basis. Each person brings a unique set of assets and liabilities to his or her illness and life experience in general. The response to the illness of schizophrenia may have included psychotic elements of hallucinations or delusions and/or a thought disorder making the expressing and consequently the understanding of their experience difficult. They may also be suffering from varying degrees of "negative symptoms"—a loss of will and drive, a withdrawal from social activities, or a reduction in emotional range. But it will be the integration of the response to the illness with the assets and liabilities of the individual person that leads us to the guiding principles of treatment.

Viewpoints expressed herein do not necessarily reflect the opinions, official policy, or position of the National Institute of Mental Health. This article was prepared by a U.S. Public Health Service officer and is therefore in the public domain.

## ACUTE PSYCHOTIC PHASE

For many clinicians, the first contact with someone with schizophrenia will be in a hospital emergency room when the person is in the acute psychotic state. From a history taken from the patient and especially informative others, from a toxicology screen, x-ray, and electroencephalogram (EEG) when indicated, many other conditions that can present as acute psychosis should, of course, be ruled out. With a presumptive diagnosis of schizophrenia, in most situations hospitalization should be instituted. There are some environments, family or other, in which a person experiencing acute psychosis can be managed, but if there are any concerns of safety for either the patient or others, hospitalization is usually indicated.

### Pharmacotherapy

The initiation of neuroleptic medication should take place after as thorough a discussion of the benefits and risks of the medication as the patient's condition will allow. Further, this "informed consent" should not be seen as a one-time opportunity, but rather a process in which education about the medication is provided over time. It is important to establish this openness in communication from the onset as the patient's full participation in his or her treatment will be essential for a successful outcome.

The selection of a neuroleptic should be based on any history of effective neuroleptic medication with a given patient and, failing that, should be one with which the physician has experience. There is no evidence to suggest that any particular type of neuroleptic is superior to any other. The differences between the neuroleptics is mainly in their side effects, and without any history of neuroleptic use, it is difficult to predict which side effects a given patient will tolerate well. Flexibility in the early days of treatment to change neuroleptics for a more tolerable side effect profile or the use of medication to combat side effects is to be encouraged.

Anticholinergic medication such as benztropine mesylate (Cogentin) in the range of 2 to 6 mg per day may be initiated for side effects such as "pseudoparkinsonism," dystonia, akinesia, or akathisia. These latter two side effects are particularly persistent. Anticholinergic medication should be given only if side effects develop, not prophylactically as many patients will not require them and therefore do not need the additional exposure to medication.

Dosage of the neuroleptic agent should be initiated in the range of 400 to 800 mg per day of chlorpromazine (Thorazine) equivalents. There is no indication that higher dosages or "rapid neuroleptization" provides any benefit beyond perhaps sedation, and if sedation is needed, a benzodiazepine such as lorazepam (Ativan) in the range of 2 to 6 mg a day is suggested. In addition to providing better sedation, it may reduce the amount of neuroleptic required. The benzodiazepine should be phased out after the initial agitation period is past, generally several days to 2 weeks.

There is an undeniable, and frequently irresistible, urge to increase the neuroleptic dosage in the early phase of treatment, particularly in the patient who does not appear to be responding rapidly. There is an equally pressing need to *change* the type of neuroleptic under the same circumstances. If only to give pause, two points should be considered:

1. There is some evidence both clinical and biologic that the full antipsychotic response to neuroleptics may take up to 6 weeks.
2. Changing a neuroleptic in the 4- to 6-week range may indeed be followed by clinical improvement, but post hoc does not mean propter hoc—it may mean that a full recovery requires 6 weeks regardless of the neuroleptic.

While early flexibility in changing the medication for side effect issues is encouraged, clinical rationales for changing the neuroleptic early in the first month of treatment are otherwise hard to come by.

### Psychosocial Approaches

There are three psychosocial concerns during this period—the patient, his or her family or significant others, and the general environment. Each of these must be given full attention by the clinician when designing the treatment plan.

**The Patient.** The experience of psychosis is without doubt the most confusing ordeal a person can have. Certain internal and external stimuli are poorly differentiated, distorted, or disorganized leading to the hallmark symptoms of schizophrenia—hallucinations, delusions, or thought disorder. There is relatively little evidence to suggest that any form of intensive interpersonal therapy or, for that matter, intensive interaction of any kind is helpful at this time. Interactions with the patient, therefore, should be structured, straightforward, time limited, and delivered by one person at a time. This should not be interpreted as encouraging avoidance of the patient; the provision of good clinical management will require interactions of many kinds. The principles noted above will make these interactions more productive and helpful for the patient.

**Environment.** The principles involved in the one-to-one interaction with the patient are also important in establishing the milieu strategy for the inpatient unit itself. Intense, multifaceted, multidirectional stimuli that one would attempt to control in the individual interaction should be controlled on the inpatient unit. Prior to initiating such modalities as "community meeting" or group psychotherapy, their role should be considered in this context. For the acutely psychotic patient, we do not recommend them. The patient may frequently remain at a distance from the ward community and does so for distinct and adaptive reasons. He or she should not be forced to enter the social milieu but should be approached individually and in a low intensity manner. Family visits should also follow this pattern, and a straightforward explanation of these principles to the family—that they are being asked to apply the same principles as the professional staff—is much more acceptable and morale enhancing than the unexplained or, worse yet, accusatory implication of a no visiting by family rule.

## THE RECOVERY PHASE

We use this term to represent the period following the acute psychosis. The absolute end point of this phase is difficult to describe and for some patients the end of this phase may never be reached. It is perhaps better described in terms of its treatment goals: stabilization; prevention of relapse; reduction of pharmacologic intensity; and incremental progress toward social, vocational, and financial independence. Each of these represents a desirable, if sometimes extremely difficult goal to reach.

Stabilization is a critical first step in the process toward recovery. As discussed below it is a slow, complex process that should be allowed to progress at its own pace. Further, the process is not like the healing of a broken arm in which once the cast comes off, the major problems are over and the arm will be "as good as new." Strategies for directly intervening in this stage are discussed below.

Prevention of relapse represents a complex interaction between the virulence of the illness, the capacity to ensure treatment, and the assistance from the psychosocial environment. Maintaining patient stability is desirable as each relapse represents a destructive interval with potential for demoralization for everyone involved—the patient, the family or significant others, and the clinician.

Reduction of pharmacologic intensity has become an important treatment goal over the past decade as it has become increasingly apparent that standard dosages (chlorpromazine [CPZ] equivalents in the range of 400 to 800 mg) do not provide absolute protection from relapse even in guaranteed delivery regimens (injectable depot); and further, these medications are not without problems of side effects like tardive dyskinesia and treatment-influencing, pharmacologically induced "negative symptoms." Balanced against the goal of reducing pharmacologic intensity, however, are several significant issues discussed below.

Incremental progress toward social, vocational, and financial independence is an obvious, if difficult to obtain goal. The emphasis is on *incremental steps* as progress needs to be slow, and focused on specific attainable goals, since an accelerated, overstimulating treatment regimen runs a high risk of failure and potentially increased stress for the patient, family, and others. Independence is perhaps the most frequently discussed concern of families as they consider one of their major fears: what will happen after they can no longer provide support.

Once again, the treatment should be considered from the model of pharmacologic and psychosocial principles, with the focus on the patient, the family, and the environment. It should be emphasized, however, that these issues are separated for the purpose of clarity of the discussion, not because in the real world they exist separately any more for the clinician than for the family or patient.

### Pharmacotherapy

The major pharmacologic goal of this period is to achieve a solid clinical stabilization with the least pharmacologic intensity. For approximately 70% of patients experiencing a psychotic episode, stabilization can be obtained with standard neuroleptic treatment. We will discuss general strategies for the remaining 30% in a later section.

**Stabilization.** Stabilization is a process that will take up to 6 months. During this period we discourage reduction of the daily dosage below 400 to 800 mg of CPZ equivalents. Once stabilization is achieved, however, a dosage reduction should be considered. A growing body of research suggests that up to an 80% reduction can be accomplished without adverse clinical consequences when compared with standard maintenance levels. It should be borne in mind, however, that these reductions and subsequent clinical management have taken place in the context of an excellent follow-up program in major centers of research. Lacking the capacity to provide a high level of follow-up (and that will include not only the clinic capacity but the cooperation of the patient and significant others as discussed below), dosage reduction should be approached conservatively. Even with an excellent follow-up program we strongly recommend that reduction in dosage be attempted no more frequently than every 6 months—to do so more rapidly invites a process that will not give the opportunity to observe the results of one reduction before the next one is attempted. The pharmacokinetics of neuroleptics are not completely understood; furthermore, the clinical response of completely stopping medication is usually not immediate and may take from 3 to 6 months before appearing. Therefore, lowering the dose again after 3 months of no unfavorable response may only serve to hasten adverse consequences. Further, the clinician must be prepared to intervene at the earliest possible point should the reduction in medication be followed by an increase in symptomatology.

**Nonstabilized Patients.** As noted above, approximately 30% of patients will not achieve stabilization on standard neuroleptic treatment. Three explanations should be considered for these patients: poor compliance; unusual metabolism; and true nonresponder or incomplete standard neuroleptic responder. The amount of time before one should consider a patient nonresponsive is variable, but 6 to 8 weeks of neuroleptic treatment (if compliance is not an issue) should be sufficient to see some improvement.

Difficulties with compliance are to be expected. These are not easy medications to take. The side effect profile is not pleasant; the implications of taking medication for psychiatric conditions are frequently seen as stigmatizing. To make the medication easier to remember to take, it is recommended to not divide the daily dose if it is in the standard range but to ask the patient to take the dose at bedtime. Under the best of circumstances, it is difficult to remember to take a medication three or four times a day; when a person is suffering from an illness like schizophrenia with its potential for disorganized thinking, remembering to take medication is made all the more difficult. The consideration of guaranteed medication regimens using injectable depot neuroleptics should also be considered. For many patients this is much easier to accept and to accomplish with an every-2-weeks fluphenazine (FPZ decanoate [Prolixin]) or monthly haloperidol (HPD decanoate [Haldol]) injection than with daily pill taking. Further areas of compliance will be addressed in the psychosocial arm of the treatment.

Studies of serum levels of neuroleptics to provide the clinician with guidance on potential "rapid metabolizers" who are not responding to standard doses of neuroleptics have not proven to be anywhere near as useful as they have with such medicines as lithium or tricyclic antidepressants. For the time being, serum levels of neuroleptics remain in the domain of the research scientist and do not appear to be ready for clinical use.

True standard neuroleptic nonresponders (or incomplete responders) require careful additional treatment considerations. Until recently, we have had only neuroleptic augmentation to consider. Now with the release of the "novel" or atypical neuroleptic, clozapine (Clozaril), we have two separate courses to consider.

Neuroleptic augmentation is a positive term that seems to have replaced the pejorative term "polypharmacy." It seems that all things go in cycles, and while there does not appear to be a full return to a symptomatic "Chinese menu" type of pharmacologic response system, there are a number of additive treatments that should be considered. Currently, the three most popular augmentations for neuroleptic treatment in the nonresponsive patient are lithium, (Lithobid), carbamazepine, (Tegretol), and benzodiazepines. The body of scientific literature supporting the use of these medications as neuroleptic augmenters is small, and before using any of them the clinician should become familiar not only with the clinical outcome literature, but also with the use of these medications in general, as they are not without their own sets of requirements for good clinical practice.

The role of the augmenting medication in clinical practice will no doubt decrease proportional to the increased use of clozapine, recently released for general use in the United States. Clozapine is a medication that is not new. It has been used in Europe for over 15 years and has been the focus of intensive research in the United States over the past several years. It is a dopamine-receptor blocker like other standard neuroleptics, but it differs from the standard neuroleptic in a differential blockade of $D_1$ over $D_2$ receptors and in having serotonergic $S_2$ blocking properties. Whether this is the difference responsible for its mechanism of action and side effect profile (less tardive dyskinesia has been reported) is not known.

On the positive side for clozapine are the clinical outcome results; even in relatively short-term (6 weeks) studies of neuroleptic nonresponders, clozapine produced significant improvement (30%). On the negative side are the side effects, the most significant of which is bone marrow suppression leading to agranulocytosis in approximately 1% of patients taking the medication. The peak risk period for agranulocytosis is from 6 weeks to 6 months after the initiation of treatment, but cases of agranulocytosis have been reported after 5 years. In introducing the medication, the pharmaceutical firm, Sandoz, has developed an extensive monitoring process unparalleled in medicine. Clozapine will not be available except through this monitoring process, which involves weekly blood drawing before the next week's supply of medication will be dispensed. All data will be centrally stored and reported back to the prescribing physician. It should be clearly noted, however, that even with weekly blood counts, the monitoring will not prevent agranulocytosis. The circulating half-life of a granulocyte is too short in relation to the time spent developing in the bone marrow. What the monitoring procedure will do, however, is to provide early detection of bone marrow suppression and thereby permit discontinuation of the medication and important "reverse isolation" in the hospital to be initiated.

The clinical use of clozapine, particularly in the outpatient setting in the United States, has not been extensive, and the interested clinician should carefully follow developments in the clinical research literature. For now it is recommended only for patients who are nonresponsive to standard neuroleptics.

Initiation of treatment should be at a low dose (25 mg), and the patient should be under good clinical observation. The dosage may be increased by 50 mg every 3 to 4 days depending on side effects, which include sedation, postural hypotension, sialorrhea, and seizures, the latter seen particularly with rapidly increasing or high dosages. The target dose range is between 300 to 500 mg per day, although higher dosages have been used. There is currently considerable debate over whether to discontinue other medications before starting clozapine or whether decreasing other medications while increasing clozapine is satisfactory. The conservative approach is the former, but it would, in many instances, require hospitalization for clinical and safety reasons. A potential compromise may well involve the use of the day hospital. Additional research and clinical use will provide answers to these questions.

## Psychosocial Treatment

The psychosocial treatment in the recovery period needs to involve the patient and members of his or her social environment. Schizophrenia is a complex illness, poorly understood and clinically difficult to manage. The interaction of the psychotic process, its inherently thought-disordered presentation, and the concomitant social withdrawal and loss of will create a condition that is difficult to comprehend. It is for these reasons that the treatment team needs to be composed of the patient and family as well as the designated clinician(s). The treatment of an illness like schizophrenia is prolonged and may span many years. It is critical to have everyone working together from a common set of blueprints. This is not to say that everything is done in a rigidly prescribed pattern nor that it is all done through a group process or in a family context. Each member of this "treatment team" will have his or her own clinical needs which must be considered. A shared set of principles is, however, helpful.

Our approach would be classified under psychoeducational. We use our capacity to teach about schizophrenia and its incumbent problems as a means of treatment. It has been our experience that intensive interpersonal treatments do not work for the broad spectrum of schizophrenic patients. In fact, for many, the intensive, interpersonal, unstructured quality of many dynamic therapies is deleterious for someone suffering from schizophrenia. Treatment should begin with an educational focus and use common problem-solving techniques and basic communication skills.

**The Patient.** Much of the early phase of treatment involves education about the effect of medication and what it is intended to do. Consistent, regular contact in a nonthreatening environment is particularly important for the disorganized and frightened patient. It is helpful to identify reasonable goals that are obtainable in the near future and to explain how the medication will aid in achieving these goals. Education about what schizophrenia is and the important role of the family in the treatment process are also presented. Other areas to be addressed include the basic techniques of problem solving within the context of the therapy session itself. Problem solving will take on more significance when working with the patient and family together, but most patients require some additional work in order to be able to hold their own in a family setting. This is particularly true in highly functioning families.

**The Social Environment.** For most patients discharged from a hospital setting, the social environment is their family. There have been many who argue that this is not the best of all possible worlds for either the family or the patient, but that aside, this is the most common situation. Even in those situations where the patient does not return to his or her family, there is quite frequently family involvement. We feel that family involvement is a positive addition to the treatment, and where it is not possible, we try to identify friends or significant others to serve in that role.

It is important in working with families that

the patient be clearly aware of the open lines of communication among the patient, family, and clinician. This should be explained to the patient so that he or she will understand that the clinician will also be talking to the family, including the patient, from time to time—not about the specifics of what he or she discusses with the clinician but about goals that either the family, the patient, or clinician find important for everyone to work on together.

The education program should be initiated early and should convey what is known about schizophrenia. In the clinic situation it may be possible to use a workshop format. With the individual family, it should be done during office visits. It is recommended that the patient and family sessions on education be held separately, as this leads to increased candor in questions from the family and the patient's condition may make it impossible to tolerate long or complex educational presentations at this point. While it is important to review what we know from the biologic, genetic, and neurophysiologic perspectives, in their daily lives patients and families struggle with much more mundane issues such as stress, interactions, and treatment problems. Much more time needs to be spent working on these areas. For many families, this educational experience may be their first exposure to someone willing to talk about schizophrenia with them. They will have many questions, and the process that is established will repay itself manyfold. Don't take anything for granted. In talking about stress, for example, it is important to note that stress takes many forms. There are a number of specific stresses or vulnerabilities that affect someone prone to psychosis. Stresses are those external factors that affect someone from the outside world. Vulnerabilities are those internal factors to which we as individuals are uniquely susceptible. We all, of course, experience stress, and we all have our vulnerabilities. For the person who is vulnerable to psychosis, however, stresses that might make someone else anxious or depressed or which they might shrug off may have considerably more impact and may even lead to psychosis. Further, certain types of stresses have been identified which many people who are vulnerable to psychosis find particularly difficult. These are important to identify and understand, as reducing them becomes central in the success of a treatment program.

First, setting therapeutic expectations at too high a level is stressful to patients who are vulnerable to psychosis. Therapists, family members, friends, and even the patient can often set expectations that are too high or currently unattainable. These then hold the potential of producing either high levels of anxiety or will lead to failure and resultant depression, too often progressing on to psychosis. Indeed, frequently one of the early signs of relapse is an overextension into too many or too difficult areas or the development of overvalued ideas. A "small steps" approach that provides both a measure of success and a direction is preferred. Encouragement to recognize these small steps and a positive response should be given, even if the progress is still well below where everyone would like to be. Taking a single course in school and working part time or on a volunteer basis are the kinds of steps that help a person regain some confidence. For others even these steps may be too large, and a focus on getting out of bed or coming to the dinner table may be important to work on. Once this foundation of success is established, small additional increments can be attempted. It is important to recognize failure early so that the patient can be assisted in defining new strategies to accomplish the goal or even withdrawing from it for the present and making the withdrawal a positive learning experience.

Second, an overinvolved or overintrusive attitude on the part of others close to them is difficult for people vulnerable to psychosis. Becoming involved in the details of a person's decision-making seems to undermine his or her confidence, and in addition, the interpersonal closeness involved is threatening to the person. Unless there is a high risk anticipated, it is usually better to save interventions for critical times. Remaining on the sidelines is, of course, difficult for all of us as there certainly have been periods when it was absolutely necessary to become intricately involved because of the psychotic process taking place. In general, an approach that supports good decisions with encouragement and enthusiasm and leaves the others alone insofar as possible is favored. Everyone has differing levels of tolerance, but the principle is clear; its application will vary. An exception to this principle comes when the family is asked for input on solving some problem. In this situation, neither solving the problem nor telling the person that it's up to them is as effective as the stepwise problem-solving exercise in which any number can participate as outlined below:

1. Identify specifically what the problem is.
2. Generate a list of potential solutions with no value judgment placed on them at this point.
3. Discuss the pros and cons of each of the proposed solutions.
4. Choose the solution based on the discussion.
5. Plan and sometimes rehearse the implementation of the solution.
6. After it has been tried, review its success or failure and plan accordingly.

As noted above, the patient will have already experienced this problem-solving exercise in the course of his or her treatment and during family sessions so neither the patient nor the family will find this unusual.

Third, life events, both those that happen (e.g., an automobile accident or incident) and those that were expected to happen (e.g., acceptance of a date, a high grade that was not achieved) can be stressful. It is difficult, if not impossible, to identify which events are going to be particularly stressful. One particular kind, however, deserves noting and that is the type of life event that may involve a comparison between the person and a friend, colleague, or family member. The success of the other person—employment, academics, social life, getting married—or how another person would have handled something differently or better seems to highlight how far behind the person who has experienced psychosis may be with his or her life plan. There is no way either to predict or prevent these life events from happening. The point here is to maintain sensitivity—not all of us experience life events in the same way.

It is important to explain that medication is a critical element in the treatment approach. The clinician should explain that he or she will monitor the medication and if, for example, the patient is taking lithium, will from time to time get serum levels to ensure the therapeutic level. It should also be explained that the clinician needs to have the family's support on the medication, not in violation of the second point above—being overintrusive—but if asked, the family should be supportive by pointing out how much has been accomplished when the patient has been taking the medication. A focus on the positive aspect—he or she has accomplished a lot—is more useful than becoming overinvolved, intrusive, or critical of the patient's not taking medication or in taking it. If the clinician senses that the patient is having some difficulty in taking it, he or she may suggest that the patient work with the family in helping to remember. It is sometimes easier for a clinician to suggest the family's becoming involved than it may be for them to do it on their own. The problem-solving exercise above may be a helpful way to become involved without undermining the patient's independence.

Finally, it should be explained that research and clinical experience has identified early signs of impending relapse which can often be avoided with a vigorous pharmacologic intervention. Examples of such areas would be losing interest or becoming increasingly depressed, difficulty concentrating, social withdrawal, difficulties with decisions, sleep or sleep pattern difficulties, or, as noted above, becoming overcommitted or feeling overexpansive. Families and patients should be asked to try to become aware of when these early signs begin to change, both to assist in the clinical management but also to attempt to expand the patient's insight. Of particular importance are the possible additional feelings or actions that may be unique to the particular patient.

The concept of the clinical team (the patient's family, significant others, the patient, and the clinician or clinical staff) in this psychoeducational approach requires much reinforcement. Any techniques that give an increasing sense of involvement and control over the illness of schizophrenia will be significant. There will, of course, be times when the symptoms of schizophrenia will dominate and a sense of control difficult to achieve, and it is important that this be well understood also.

## LONG-TERM OUTCOME

There are probably many factors that remain unknown and at best uncertain about the long-term outcome of schizophrenia. The range of long-term outcome studies in the literature goes from encouraging to discouraging with virtually every intermediate outcome as well.

It is a frequently observed pattern of schizophrenia that the florid psychotic symptoms seem to "burn out" in many patients after the age of 35. Whether this represents some alteration or decline in the dopamine receptors is debated in the research field. What remains clear and what may eventually determine the long-range outcome, however, is the pattern of negative symptoms that persist as the positive symptoms decline. Currently, there are no known pharmacologic treatments for negative symptoms, although early studies of clozapine have shown some improvement in this area. (It should be remembered that the seminal study of clozapine was only a 6-week study and that the comparison group was receiving such substantial doses of CPZ that negative symptoms would not be likely to improve.) We are unable at this point to recommend a specific psychosocial strategy that will work in all patients. The capacity to withstand interpersonal involvement will need to be individualized with each patient to avoid too rapid an immersion which then leads to relapse. On the other hand, we are convinced that retaining this interpersonal involvement in life may well play a major role in eventual outcome once psychotic symptoms fade. Involvement in community programs of rehabilitation, halfway houses, transitional employment, or independent living will need to be carefully adjusted through what unfortunately will be a trial-and-error process. We know of no way to predict the outcome of these forays and have frequently been surprised in both directions. We encourage the smallest increments possible at each step of the process. The speed of the process is not important; the direction is.

# PANIC DISORDER AND AGORAPHOBIA

method of
ROBERT POHL, M.D.
*Wayne State University School of Medicine
Detroit, Michigan*

A panic, or anxiety, attack is characterized by a surge of fear or discomfort along with physical and psychologic symptoms of anxiety. Most people have had similar symptoms subsequent to a near-miss accident or to a sudden startle: there is a wave of anxiety, the heart pounds, and respiration accelerates. These episodes, however, are very brief and occur for an obvious reason. Panic attacks usually last minutes to hours. Panic disorder refers to recurrent panic attacks that occur unexpectedly or in response to a trivial stress. Many panic disorder patients also develop a fear of being trapped, alone, or away from home during an attack. Fears of travel, restaurants, and standing in line are common, and once these phobias develop, panic attacks may be more likely to occur in these situations. This pattern of phobias is called agoraphobia.

## HISTORY

Anxiety symptoms and phobias were generally thought to be byproducts of intrapsychic conflict (neurosis) until the early 1970s. At that time, antidepressants were discovered to block panic attacks, and it was noted that agoraphobia almost always followed the development of panic attacks. There is often a family history of similar illness. These discoveries led to the present model of panic attacks as a hereditary, primarily biologic phenomenon, with agoraphobia a psychologic response to recurrent attacks.

## DIAGNOSIS

In addition to the surge of fear or discomfort, patients have four or more typical symptoms listed in the DSM-III-R. These symptoms include shortness of breath, dizziness, palpitations or tachycardia, trembling or shaking, sweating, choking, nausea, feeling unreal, paresthesias or numbness, hot or cold flashes, chest pain or discomfort, a fear of dying, and a fear of going crazy or doing something uncontrolled. Most patients seek nonpsychiatric medical attention first, usually from a general physician or an emergency room. Individual patients may focus on certain symptoms and visit a corresponding specialist (e.g., a cardiologist for heart pounding). Although the syndrome can start late in life, the typical patient is a young to middle-aged adult. Diagnosis is generally straightforward in the absence of drug toxicity, substance abuse, hyperthyroidism, or obvious cardiac disease. The presence of mitral valve prolapse does not affect treatment response. The lifetime prevalence of panic disorder is 2%.

## COURSE AND COMPLICATIONS

Panic disorder has a fluctuating course, and spontaneous remissions and exacerbations can occur. The frequency of panic attacks varies from multiple attacks daily to one or fewer attacks per week. However, even infrequent and mild attacks can have disabling psychologic effects. The most common complications are interpanic anxiety and agoraphobia. Many patients also develop significant depression. Substance abuse may occur as a form of self-treatment. Untreated panic disorder patients have a high rate of suicide, even higher than that of patients with a primary diagnosis of depression.

## TREATMENT

The primary goal of treatment is to treat the panic attacks. This can be done with either high potency benzodiazepines or with antidepressants. Benzodiazepines have the advantage of an immediate effect but are potentially addicting, have anxiety as a withdrawal effect, and tolerance may develop to the therapeutic effects over extended periods of time. Antidepressants generally have more side effects and a delayed onset of action, but they lack abuse potential and can be safely and effectively used over long periods of time. Because panic disorder is often a chronic illness, antidepressants are usually the treatment of choice, with low doses of benzodiazepines sometimes given as an adjunctive treatment until the antidepressant works.

The treatment standard is imipramine (Tofranil), although other tricyclic antidepressants appear to be equally effective (desipramine, Norpramin). Some panic disorder patients are unusually sensitive to these drugs and become more anxious and jittery during initial treatment. For this reason, start with a very low dose of 10 mg at bedtime and increase in daily 10-mg increments up to 100 mg at bedtime. If there is no response in 2 weeks, the dose can be increased in 10-mg increments to 300 mg. The average dose required is 150 to 200 mg at bedtime. Almost all patients develop moderate anticholinergic side effects and an increase in resting heart rate. Symptoms of postural hypotension may occur.

Fluoxetine (Prozac) is a relatively new antidepressant that appears to be effective for panic disorder. Although it can also cause initial anxiety and jitteriness, it lacks the anticholinergic and sedative effects of tricyclic antidepressants and has a simpler dosing schedule. The patient takes one 20-mg tablet in the morning. This dosage is often effective and should not be increased for 3 to 4 weeks because there is a delayed onset of action and a long half-life that results in accumulating drug levels over a period of weeks. Because of the long half-life, it is possible to start sensitive patients on a lower dose by giving it every other day.

Monoamine oxidase inhibitors (MAOIs) are a very effective treatment, but they are inconvenient to take and are therefore used as a second- or third-line treatment. The usual therapeutic dosage is between three and six 15-mg phenelzine (Nardil) or 10-mg tranylcypromine (Parnate) tablets daily. One tablet can be given as a starting dose for 3 to 4 days, and then the dosage can be increased by one tablet every few days to three daily. If the patient does not respond in 3 weeks, the dosage can be increased by one tablet each week, up to a maximum of six daily. The dosage should be divided during the day, and evening or bedtime doses should be avoided.

MAOIs such as phenelzine and tranylcypromine interact with a variety of other drugs and foods to increase blood pressure and are safe to use only if the patient is given a written list of foods to avoid and instructed to check on the safety of all medication, including over-the-counter medication, before use. Substances to be avoided include common foods such as cheese and any sympathomimetic amines such as deconges-

tants. A list of foods to avoid can be found in the product labelling. MAOIs cannot be started for 1 to 2 weeks after a tricyclic antidepressant is discontinued or for 5 weeks after fluoxetine has been discontinued. In addition, the dietary restrictions must be followed for 10 days after stopping a MAOI. MAOIs also have anticholinergic and postural blood pressure effects similar to those of tricyclic antidepressants.

High potency benzodiazepines, such as alprazolam (Xanax), clonazepam (Klonopin), and lorazepam (Ativan), are also effective. The doses required to block panic attacks are moderate to high, for example 3 to 6* mg daily of alprazolam (given in a divided dosage). Long-term use is problematic, and when the dosage is decreased, it is difficult to distinguish benzodiazepine withdrawal anxiety from a return of the patient's anxiety disorder. Abrupt discontinuation can cause grand mal seizures. If benzodiazepines are used, it is often better to use lower doses as an adjunctive treatment with antidepressants and to gradually discontinue their use once the patient has responded.

Panic disorder patients also benefit from information about their illness. Because a fear of dying, going crazy, or doing something uncontrolled is part of the syndrome, reassurance that none of these things will happen is helpful. Phobic symptoms generally subside once panic attacks have ceased. Patients who remain agoraphobic should be instructed to expose themselves gradually to feared situations.

---

*Exceeds the maximum dose recommended by the manufacturer.

# Physical and Chemical Injuries

## BURNS

method of
C. GILLON WARD, M.D.
*University of Miami School of Medicine*
*Miami, Florida*

Burn trauma crosses all socioeconomic barriers. It can occur as a result of a true accident over which the victim has no control, such as a hotel fire. Burns also occur as a result of ignorance, such as using a brush and gasoline to clean tile, not realizing the brush can generate heat sufficient to ignite the gasoline. Burns occur as a result of stupidity, such as looking into a gas tank with a match. And burns occur as a wanton act of aggression, such as when a child is abused by being dipped in hot water. But no matter how a burn occurs, when a patient is seen in an emergency room, a standard therapy regimen should be set into motion that can lead to a predictable outcome for the victim. For the inexperienced, the most difficult aspect at first seeing a burn patient is getting beyond the visual impact of the injury and realizing that burning is a specific trauma and should be dealt with as any general trauma situation. There are guidelines unique to burn patients, but the overall guide is the same as in any trauma unit.

### INITIAL EVALUATION

When a burn patient is first evaluated, the primary consideration is the ABCs of resuscitation. An airway must be intact and, if not so, must be established. The patient should be able to breathe and, if not, must be assisted. Cardiac status must be evaluated and an adequate blood pressure maintained. In establishing an airway for a burn patient, a primary question is, "Does the patient require intubation?" If so, for what length of time? Soft cuffed endotracheal tubes are best, for they can remain in place for several weeks. The manner by which the endotracheal tube is secured is important. There are negative aspects to the technique, but the best way is to have the endotracheal tube passed through the nose. This allows for better securing of the tube. The disadvantage is that if the tube is too large, it can obstruct sinuses and eustachian tubes, leading to sinusitis or inner ear infections, which subsequently are the sources of occult infections and sepsis. These taken into account, however, the preferred method is still the nasal route for prolonged intubation of these patients. Additional support, whether the patient is intubated or not, is the addition of oxygen by mask or the respirator. If there is a question of carbon monoxide poisoning in association with the burn, the oxygen will help wash out the unwanted gas, disassociating it from hemoglobin and lowering the carboxyhemoglobin levels. Once the airway is established, the patient is breathing, and the cardiovascular system is known to be functioning, a further evaluation as to the presence of other additional trauma can be made, particularly if the patient has been involved in an explosion, a fall, or a vehicular accident.

### ADMISSION

The criteria for admitting a critical patient are moot. There are, however, indications for admission when a patient does not have an obviously critical injury. Admission should be considered when there is:

1. Child abuse.
2. Electrical injury.
3. Inhalation injury.
4. Involvement of the major joints, such as the elbow and the knee, and the hands, the face, and the genitalia.
5. Circumferential extremity injury.
6. A 10 to 15% total body surface area burn.
7. A 2% or greater total body surface area third-degree burn.
8. A history of diabetes or vascular insufficiency.
9. Associated traumatic injury.

### MANAGEMENT

#### Fluid Resuscitation

Once respiratory function is secured, the major early intervention for a burn victim is replacement of fluids being lost through the burn wound. This is best done by peripheral lines rather than central lines. If intravenous lines can be placed in areas not burned, it is preferable. Do not hesitate, however, to cannulate veins through the burn wound if no others are available. The volume of fluid required by a patient during the first 24 to 36 hours postinjury is determined by the patient's weight and the size of the injury. For this reason, the admission weight is documented, the burn is mapped, and the size is estimated. A standard formula is Ringer's lactate of which the first 24-hour total volume requirement is based upon 4 ml per percentage of burn per kg of weight. The 24-hour volume is divided by 24, giving an hourly estimated volume requirement. The fluid is started at the calculated hourly rate and subsequently adjusted depending on the amount of urine the patient produces. The required urine output is based on a formula of 600 to 800 ml per square meter per day, which translates into 24 to 35 ml per square meter per hour. An alternative formula is one half ml per kg per hour. If fluids are infused at a rate to produce such urine volume, there is little concern for early renal failure or renal shutdown.

The body surface area of the burned adult can be calculated by the estimated rule of nines: arm = 9%; leg = 18%; chest & abdomen = 18%; back and buttocks = 18%; head = 9%; and genitalia (male) = 1%. The surface area of children has different proportions, and standard charts give better estimates of wound size.

The resuscitation volume for patients as described using Ringer's lactate is adequate for people 60 pounds or over. However, in children under 60 pounds, the resuscitation volume must include that required by the burn and the 24-hour maintenance. For example, a 22-pound child with a 20% total body surface area burn would require 800 ml for the first 24 hours. Normal maintenance for such an individual, based on 1500 ml per square meter, is 750 ml per day. Therefore, such a child would receive only 50 ml over maintenance volume for the burn. The correct first 24-hour requirement would be 750 ml maintenance plus 800 ml, totaling 1550 ml (Figure 1). Evaluation of urine production is most accurate with the Foley catheter draining the bladder.

In the very young child, less than 1 year of age, resuscitation fluid with glucose should be considered. The very young have a limited store of glycogen, and they do not easily convert protein and fat to glucose. The addition of glucose to resuscitation fluid, however, must be carefully watched because it can cause more problems than it's worth. There may be an associated glucosuria that is not tolerated because it causes an osmotic diuresis, giving a false sense of adequate resuscitation in the face of dehydrating the patient. In such cases, glucose is removed from the resuscitation fluid. Ketones may be present in the urine, but this has no clinical consequences during the early stages of resuscitation of a burn victim, provided the individual is not a known diabetic in the premorbid state.

If there is concern about an excess volume of resuscitation fluid, hypertonic solutions can be used. It is the sodium that resuscitates the patient. One hundred mEq of sodium acetate added to a liter of Ringer's lactate gives a solution with 230 mEq of sodium per liter. Therefore, if the volume being infused can cause clinical problems, such as edema of the lungs or edema of the extremities leading to escharotomies, hypertonic solution can reduce the swelling associated with the resuscitation. Another variation of fluid resuscitation is done with patients who have sustained high-voltage–associated electrical injury. Myoglobin and hemoglobin released as a result of the accident can precipitate in the kidneys if the urine is acid. These patients are given large volumes of fluid to produce 100 ml of urine per hour and medications that will make the urine alkaline, such as sodium bicarbonate. Diuretics such as mannitol are used if necessary. Once a diuretic is used, however, the ability to judge adequate total body resuscitation by urine output is compromised.

### Emergency Room Care

While in the emergency room, there are standard procedures for admission diagnostic studies for immediate use and in preparation for long-term problems. Standard blood work such as complete blood counts, electrolytes, blood urea nitrogen, platelets, clotting studies, and liver function studies are ordered. It is normal for the hematocrit to rise during the first 18 to 24 hours; it is an indication of intravascular loss of fluids as a consequence of the burn injury. Typically, patients with burns do not require blood transfusions unless there is a loss from other traumatic lesions. There is no clinical indication for typing and cross-matching these patients unless there is blood loss from other trauma. An electrocardiogram should be done on any patient 35 years or older; cardiac monitoring must be considered for patients who have sustained electrical injuries. Cardiac enzyme studies are not helpful for patients with electrical injuries because these enzymes are released from muscle and are abnormally high without cardiac damage being present.

The patient with a known or suspected inhalation injury typically has normal arterial blood gases on admission. Though carbon monoxide levels do not necessarily correlate with clinical problems, they can be informative and help substantiate inhalation injuries. The chest radiograph of a person who has sustained an inhala-

## Conversion: POUNDS to Sq METERS

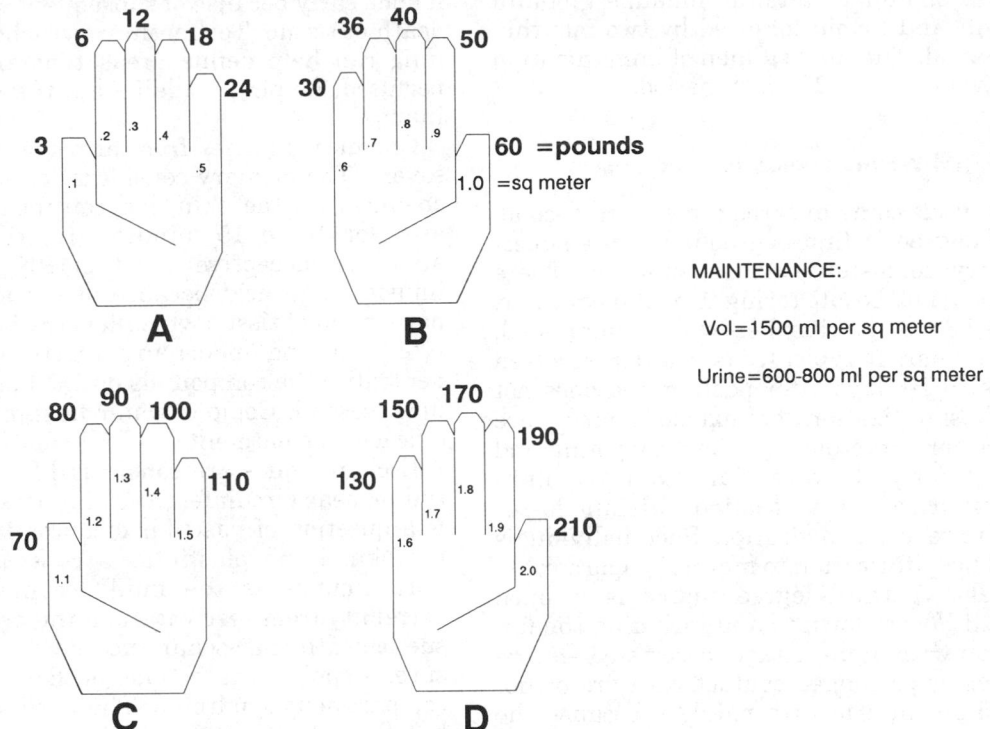

MAINTENANCE:

Vol=1500 ml per sq meter

Urine=600-800 ml per sq meter

**Figure 1.** Rule of thumb for calculating 24-hour volume, maintenance, and urine output.

tion injury is typically normal and shows only preburn pathology. A standard set of films should be a posteroanterior, lateral, and anteroposterior (AP) views. The AP view is important in a patient who will be in an intensive care unit, flat on his back. All subsequent films will be portable, and a baseline study at the time of admission is valuable. The classic signs and symptoms of an inhalation injury are singed nasal hairs, sputum that contains carbon, hoarseness, and facial burns. A patient can have all of these, yet not have an inhalation injury. In a reverse corollary, a patient can have none of the classic signs and yet have a severe inhalation injury. The most important component of the diagnosis of an inhalation injury is that the burn occurred within an enclosed space. Respiratory insufficiency usually does not occur until after the patient has received resuscitation fluid, usually 18 hours into the process. At this time the blood gases begin to deteriorate, the first parameter to decrease being the $PO_2$.

Giving pain medication should be resisted when a patient is first seen in the emergency room. If given, it should not be given intramuscularly. When a patient is in severe hypovolemic shock, medication given in a muscle is not mo-

bilized until after fluid resuscitation. In the burn patient, this is after 18 to 36 hours of receiving fluids. If the drug is morphine, there may be respiratory depression and hypotension when least anticipated. A restless and uncooperative patient has hypovolemic shock and hypoxia as the primary diagnosis, not pain. The treatment is fluid volume and oxygen, not pain medication.

The wound is assessed while the patient is in the emergency room, but not to the point of delaying activities of higher priority. A patient who can be discharged has the wounds cleaned and a topical agent of choice applied. Silver sulfadiazine (Silvadene) is the most common topical agent in use in the United States today. It is applied twice a day with a light occlusive dressing to hold it on the wound. Discharged patients are followed with clinic or office visits within 24 to 48 hours. Prophylactic antibiotics are not prescribed.

Tetanus is a persistent problem, and therefore, all major burn patients receive a booster of tetanus toxoid, even if they are known to have been immunized in the past. If a patient has a small injury and has not been immunized, the guidelines from the American College of Surgeons are followed. Patients never immunized or in whom immunization history is unclear should receive a full immunization against tetanus with an appropriate dose of human tetanus immune globulin (Hyper-Tet) and toxoid followed by two monthly doses of toxoid. The full regimen of immunization must be given over a 3-month period.

### Initial Wound Evaluation and Care

Burn wounds come in three types: first, second, and third degree. A first-degree injury is a superficial injury consistent with a sunburn. There may or may not be blistering 1 or 2 days later. The skin is red, it blanches when compressed, and it is tender. It typically is a lesion resolved in a week to 10 days after peeling and does not require hospitalization or extraordinary care other than for symptoms. In the very young and the very elderly, however, an extensive first-degree sunburn can be associated with fluid losses that lead to severe dehydration. Such individuals may need hospitalization to maintain appropriate fluid levels. A third-degree injury is a burn through all layers down to and including the fat. This is seen with high-voltage–associated electrical injuries or prolonged contact with fire or hot objects. These injuries are painless because the nerve endings have been destroyed. The blood vessels are coagulated, and there is no blanching when the wound is compressed.

A second-degree injury is between a first and third degree injury. It is subdivided into superficial and deep. By the nature of the injury, a second-degree burn has intact hair follicles and sweat glands which allows it to close by a secondary intention from the epithelial cells growing out from these organs. Second-degree wounds are painful, red, and blister immediately.

A special type of burn is one caused by hot tar. This produces a deep second- or third-degree injury. While there is no immediate need to remove the tar, a full evaluation of the wound cannot occur until it is. Commercial tar remover such as Goop, Tween–80, and Medi-Sol, a citric acid derivative, can be used. Silver sulfadiazine (Silvadene) or polymyxin B sulfate–bacitracin zinc–neomycin sulfate (Neosporin) ointment will remove tar over a 24-hour period because of the propylene glycol content.

There are three components in the mechanism of burn wounds associated with high-voltage electricity of 500 volts or greater. There is direct damage from the current, causing coagulation and direct cellular destruction; there is an arc of electrical current which has a temperature in excess of 2500° C; there is an ignition of clothing by the arc, resulting in a typical thermal burn. It takes 5 days to a week to recognize the full extent of a high-voltage–associated electrical injury. Débridement is necessary but is frustrating if done early because of subsequent and continued death of tissue. Technetium pyrophosphate scanning can help define areas that are vascularly perfused, helping to delineate the extent of the injury.

Chemical injuries from acid and alkali can be severe. The primary consideration is to wash the chemical off the skin and continue to flush the area for 10 to 15 minutes. Injuries caused by alkali are deceptive and typically cause deeper injuries than acid because of the associated denaturation of tissue which lets the base penetrate into tissue and underlying structure. Attempts to neutralize the compounds on the burn wound are unsuccessful. Copious water flushing is the most efficacious treatment.

Escharotomies are considered for circumferential or near circumferential injuries where there is a question of vascular compromise. Typically, the skin is nonelastic as a consequence of the burn injury. As the fluid accumulates in the extremity from resuscitation, the pressure in tissue beneath the eschar exceeds the venous pressure, stopping the venous outflow, similar to a compartment syndrome. The outflow is shut off, but the arterial system continues to supply the extremity with blood, causing a rapid increase in the subeschar pressure. This eventually leads to pressures equal to or in excess of the arterial pressure and subsequent nonflow states of the extremity. The eschar must be cut to reduce the pressure and allow limb perfusion. Such conditions are seen with high-voltage–associated electrical injury but also occur with deep second-degree injuries and some superficial second-degree injuries. Similar situations happen with an infiltrated intravenous line maintained on a perfusion pump, particularly in small children, but occasionally in adults. The diagnostic test is to palpate the pulse and feel the extremity to see if it is tense and hard. Pressures beneath the eschar can be measured. If it is 30 mmHg or greater, an escharotomy should be done. Though a cold knife is adequate, bleeding is controlled best with cautery. An escharotomy is a bedside procedure. Short-acting general anesthetics, such as ketamine, are effective and easily used in environments outside the operating room.

### Vascular Access

A patient on ventilatory support usually has an arterial line placed. The radial artery is the most common and easily maintained. It is used for frequent arterial blood gas sampling as well as other standard clinical tests. An occasional arterial blood gas can be done with arterial sticks always using a No. 25 needle.

Venous sites tend to have more frequent infections than arterial sites. Theoretically, these lines should be changed every 72 hours. With long-term patients, however, this becomes impractical. Intravenous lines should be avoided through the burn eschar unless there is no other site available. Suppurative thrombophlebitis is the result of an infected vein, the mortality from which is 100% if untreated and unrecognized. It can be a difficult diagnosis to make since the suppurative vein may be at an intravenous site of several weeks past. Treatment is excision of the infected vein. The vessel bed is packed with a topical antibiotic.

### Additional Care

Burn patients are injured not only in the physical but also in the psychologic sphere. Though wounds may be closed by secondary intention or skin grafting, the process of rehabilitation therapy continues. The beginning of the therapy starts at the day of admission. Emphasis is placed on maintaining range of motion, regaining strength, and acquiring activities of daily living required at the time of discharge. Patients with very extensive burns require 1 to 2 years of therapy interspersed with reconstruction surgery. Psychologic rehabilitation, however, may take a number of years, and one should not anticipate an early discharge from this aspect of care. A burn injury does not temper an individual's personality, but rather tests it to the core. Premorbid defects remain and are accentuated. Children continue their normal psychologic development, but it is difficult when there is a psychologic detour as a consequence of a burn. The ultimate goal, both physically and mentally, is to return a functioning individual back into the community who is productive and living a happy, useful life. With these in mind, the burn team of occupational therapists, physical therapists, psychologists, social workers, physicians, and nurses comes together to act as a united force.

# DISTURBANCES DUE TO COLD

method of
JAMES B. REULER, M.D.
*Veterans Administration Medical Center*
*Portland, Oregon*

The primary clinical syndromes associated with exposure to the cold are frostbite, immersion foot, and systemic hypothermia. Frostbite is due to the effects of freezing of tissues whereas immersion foot results from exposure to nonfreezing temperatures and water. Hypothermia is generally the result of several insults to the thermoregulatory system, leading to a depression of the core body temperature. Previously encountered in military or outdoor recreational activities, these problems are seen increasingly in urban areas owing to the expanding size of the homeless population.

## FROSTBITE

All local cold injury is a continuum of frostbite. The varying degrees of cold injury are caused by exposure to freezing temperatures, usually less than $-7°$ C, for at least 12 hours.

Tissue injury is due to ice crystal formation in the extracellular space, causing cellular dehydration and denaturation of proteins. Release of thromboxane mediates progressive dermal ischemia, a result of sludging and microvascular occlusion. At any ambient air temperature level, the rapidity of onset and the extent of tissue injury are magnified by the addition of wind velocity and exposure to water or metal, both of which cause rapid heat loss through conduction. Duration of cold exposure, increasing age, other medical problems, and previous cold injury all increase the risk of development of local cold injury.

## FROSTNIP

Frostnip, the mildest of local cold injuries, does not imply tissue loss. Most commonly involved are those areas with greatest exposure and where blood flow is most variable due to arteriovenous anastomoses. These include the nose, ears, hands, and feet. Clinical features include decreased sensation of the involved area and blanching of the skin. Treatment is simple and includes removal from exposure and warming the involved area with gloves, scarf, or other insulating material.

## SUPERFICIAL AND DEEP FROSTBITE

Frostbite may be viewed as a form of thermal injury and staged as a burn, for example, Stage 1—erythema and swelling; Stage 2—blister formation with sloughing of some epidermal tissue; Stage 3—full-thickness injury with gangrenous skin and subcutaneous tissue; and Stage 4—complete necrosis and loss of the affected part. A simpler classification divides frostbite into superficial and deep. Superficial frostbite affects the skin and subcutaneous tissues. The involved area appears white and does not blanch, but the tissue below the surface is soft and resilient. Within 24 hours after warming, blisters may form and, if hemorrhagic, suggest structural damage to the subdermal tissue vascular plexus. This stage generally begins to resolve by 10 days from the injury. An eschar, present for several weeks, subsequently sloughs leaving viable skin.

Deep frostbite is characterized by the involved area's feeling hard and solid, and underlying tissues cannot be depressed. These features denote involvement of the skin, subcutaneous tissues, muscles, tendons, nerves and bones. After rewarming, the involved area remains cool, mottled, and cyanotic, and blisters may take weeks to form and may be associated with significant edema. As superficial frostbite injury is replaced by deeper injury, the skin becomes hard and painless. Gradually, dexterity diminishes, ultimately replaced by paralysis, and pain gives way to numbness and anesthesia.

Ultimately, a line of demarcation becomes evident, and viable tissue separates from the mummified part composed of nonviable tissue. Regardless of the classification system used, experience has demonstrated that early clinical evaluation of frostbite injury is often inaccurate and overestimates the extent of irreversible injury. This difficulty in accurately predicting the extent of ultimate tissue loss during the early recovery phase of frostbite injury underlies the surgical dictum "frostbite in January, amputate in July" and highlights the importance of conservative management and expectant observation.

## MANAGEMENT

The primary goals for treatment of severe frostbite injury are to minimize tissue loss and salvage potentially viable tissue, realizing that it may take weeks to assess the success of management. Because partial thawing and then refreezing causes the most severe injury, greater than having the involved area remain frozen for a longer period of time, attempts to rewarm the involved extremity in the field should be avoided and treatment delayed until the patient can be transported to a facility where definitive management can be initiated. It is preferable for a frostbite victim to walk out on a frozen extremity rather than to attempt partial thawing in the field prior to evacuation to a medical facility.

The critical aspect of treatment for severe frostbite injury is rapid rewarming. Clothing should be removed, the entire extremity exposed, other concomitant medical problems identified, and the core body temperature raised if hypothermia is present prior to institution of definitive management for frostbite. The involved extremity should be handled with great care to avoid further trauma. Rapid rewarming is accomplished by submerging the entirety of the involved area in a water bath with a temperature maintained between 39 to 42° C, a whirlpool bath unit being ideal for this therapy. The extremity should remain in the water bath at this temperature range until the frostbitten tissue develops a flushed appearance, usually evident within 15 to 30 minutes of bath rewarming. Complete thawing occurs within 30 to 60 minutes, often accompanied by a return of sensation to the frozen area.

Subsequent to thawing, blood flow resumes but small vessels are occluded with platelet aggregates. There are four degrees of changes noted in the post-thaw period. First-degree changes are characterized by hyperemia and edema; second-degree changes are evident in the form of vesicles. These changes are indicative of superficial frostbite injury. Third-degree changes include necrosis of the entire skin thickness and part of the subcutaneous supporting structure, and fourth-degree changes include full-thickness necrosis of the skin as well as the underlying muscle and bone with inevitable gangrene. These latter changes are indicative of deep frostbite injury. A gradual demarcation develops between viable and dead tissue in the form of dry gangrene and mummification. It is important to re-emphasize the importance of conservative nonsurgical management as the prediction of the extent of viable tissue remaining is very difficult and premature amputation is to be avoided.

Once bath rewarming is completed, the involved extremities should be suspended in a protective cradle to minimize further trauma, adequate tetanus prophylaxis should be assured, and whirlpool treatments should be continued at least twice daily. Resulting pain may require narcotic analgesia.

Recent studies suggest that white blisters, containing prostaglandins and thromboxane $A_2$, should be unroofed and débrided, as these chemical mediators are felt to play a primary role in the pathogenesis of frostbite injury. However, hemorrhagic blisters reflect greater structural damage to the subdermal plexus and should be left intact to avoid further damage to this vascular network and to maximize the viability of surrounding tissue. Because of the above-mentioned pathophysiology, the use of antiprostaglandin agents has been advocated as a means of decreasing the dermal ischemia in frostbite. Oral administration of aspirin or ibuprofen along with aloe vera cream, a topical inhibitor of thromboxane, applied every 6 hours to blistered areas, has been used in several protocol studies.

Other therapies have been advocated during the initial management of severe frostbite, although uniformity of opinion does not exist regarding their efficacy. These include heparin, warfarin (Coumadin), intravenous dextran, and surgical or medical sympathectomy, the latter including the use of intra-arterial reserpine or oral phenoxybenzamine (Dibenzyline).

Long-term sequelae of frostbitten areas that have been salvaged include cold sensitivity, manifested as a Raynaud's-type phenomenon, and dysesthesias. Sympathetic blockade and vasodilitation may be useful as treatments for these late complications.

## PREVENTION

Prevention of cold injury is a paramount consideration for any person venturing into subfreezing environmental conditions. These precautions include adequate clothing to assure maintenance of core body temperature and protection of the hands, feet, and head from wind and moisture. In these conditions, particular attention must be given to avoidance of direct contact of the skin with metal objects and liquid fuels, as both conduct heat at rapid rates and can cause precipitous freezing of tissues.

## IMMERSION FOOT

Trench foot and immersion foot are both conditions of nonfreezing cold injury. The former is due to exposure of the feet to wet, cold footgear, whereas the latter condition is a result of direct immersion. Both occur with exposure to water less than 10° C for periods exceeding 10 hours, are hastened by the limb being in an immobilized, dependent position, and represent disordered sympathetic tone and vasospastic changes in the blood vessels.

There are three stages to trench or immersion foot. The ischemic, or vasospastic, phase, also known as the prehyperemic phase, is characterized by a cold, swollen extremity that feels numb, is white or bluish in coloration, and has decreased palpable pulses. This phase is due to vasoconstriction and tissue anoxia leading to damaged small vessels and nerve endings. The second, or hyperemic, phase is characterized by a warm, dry, swollen, and erythematous extremity. This phase may last 2 to 6 weeks after rewarming, during which time peripheral pulses are bounding. The recovery, or posthyperemic, phase may last weeks to months after recovery and is characterized by increased sensitivity to cold and skin depigmentation and may give way to chronic pain and hyperhidrosis.

## TREATMENT

As with freezing injuries, rewarming is critical but at a slower rate and at lower temperatures. Rewarming at room temperature, which can be initiated in the field, is adequate. Overheating of the tissue may actually enhance small vessel occlusion and extend the area of injury. Elevation of the feet decreases edema and will minimize further vascular insult in areas that are in jeopardy. Bullae should be left intact, and antibiotics should be considered when there is extensive tissue sloughing to minimize risk of infection. Surgical intervention, when required, usually is limited to superficial débridement.

## HYPOTHERMIA

Hypothermia, defined as a core temperature of less than 35° C, develops when heat loss, through conduction, convection, radiation, and evaporation, outstrips the body's ability to generate heat. An attempt to lower the core temperature is met by the mobilization of a number of forces, shivering being the most obvious, which prevent heat loss and increase heat production. The body's core is protected by outer layers that modulate this heat loss and gain. The superficial zone is composed of the skin, subcutaneous tissue, and thermoreceptors and is the most important aspect of the heat exchange mechanism. Temperature at the skin may drop to near environmental temperatures in an attempt to conserve heat. The skeletal muscle mass, comprising the intermediate zone, generates large amounts of heat by shivering when the core temperature is in danger of dropping. The preoptic anterior hypothalamus choreographs the various components of this mechanism, with the autonomic nervous system providing rapid control of heat dissipation and the neuroendocrine aspect of thermogenesis involving a more delayed increase in heat production.

Physiologic effects of hypothermia include a gradual decline in heart rate and cardiac output, with hypotension becoming clinically significant below 25° C. Sinus bradycardia, T wave inversions, and advanced conduction changes as well as the pathognomonic Osborne or J wave, may be evident on the electrocardiogram as body temperature drops. Atrial fibrillation is commonly seen at temperatures of less than 30° C, and below 25° C, ventricular fibrillation is an immediate hazard. In severe hypothermia, pneumonia is frequently a complication owing to depression of the respiratory center, decreased cough reflex, and cold-induced bronchorrhea. The oxyhemoglobin disassociation curve is shifted to the left, increasing affinity for oxygen, although usually this is not clinically significant because of the concomitant decrease in oxygen requirements in hypothermia. Acid-base disturbances are common and complex, but no uniform pattern is seen. Fluid shifts and a cold-induced diuresis may cause severe volume depletion and hemoconcentration. Disseminated intravascular coagulation is a feature in severe cases. Cerebral blood flow decreases 6 to 7% per degree drop in core temperature and, combined with decreases in microcirculation due to viscosity, may cause decreased mentation. The electroencephalogram (EEG) is flat below 20° C, and clinical features are frequently indistinguishable from death. Therefore, the dictum, "no one is dead until warm and dead," is applicable.

Most patients with hypothermia have experienced multiple insults to the thermoregulatory mechanism. Cold water immersion and exposure to environmental extremes, particularly in military or recreational activities, are common clinical settings for hypothermia. However, extremes of environmental temperatures are not required to cause significant heat loss, but rather the combination of ambient air temperature, wind velocity, and moisture may lead to heat loss through several mechanisms. The elderly are particularly vulnerable to the development of hypothermia owing to decreased physiologic response to the cold, autonomic dysregulation, and medication that may impair thermoregulation and increase the risk of falls and exposure. In the elderly, hypothermia may have a very subtle presentation, often manifested only as a confusional state.

In the hospital setting, hypothermia may develop in the perioperative period owing to heat loss from low operating room temperatures, use of cold infusion and irrigation fluids, ventilation with cold gases, anesthetic-induced alterations of thermoregulation, preparation of the skin with cold liquids, and exposure of the body cavities. Other causes of hypothermia include hypothyroidism, severe burns or erythrodermas, and sepsis.

Mortality is related more to underlying medical problems than to the level of core temperature depression. Most physicians will encounter hypothermia in patients who are hemodynamically stable, such as the elderly, alcoholic, or trauma victim in the emergency room. Initial management should focus on prevention of further heat loss, determination of true core temperature using a low-reading thermometer or rectal probe, assessment of cardiac rhythm by monitor, and fluid resuscitation. Correction of arterial blood gas measurements for body temperature is not necessary as uncorrected values (measured in the laboratory at a standard temperature of 37° C) are as reliable in a setting of rapidly changing body temperature and acid-base status during rewarming.

Hemodynamic stability rather than core temperature per se should be the determinant of which rewarming methods to use. For stable patients admitted to the hospital with core temperatures less than 32.2° C, cardiac monitoring should be maintained. Most important, serial core temperatures must be recorded to assure that the temperature is rising.

Most patients who are hemodynamically stable can be managed safely with a combination of rewarming techniques, including standard blankets, warming blankets, warmed intravenous fluids, heated inspired oxygen, and possibly, whole-body bath rewarming. Core rewarming should be reserved for patients who are in asystole or refractory ventricular fibrillation whose body temperatures must be raised in order to convert to a stable rhythm.

Controversy surrounds the role of infield cardiopulmonary resuscitation (CPR) in the comatose, apparently pulseless, and apneic hypothermic patient, the "hypothermic code." Arguments against in-the-field CPR of unmonitored hypothermic patients include difficulty in accurate assessment of vital signs, chest compressions may precipitate ventricular fibrillation, hypothermic patients can tolerate anoxia and hypoxia for extended periods, CPR may impede rescue efforts, and once begun, CPR must be continued. Recently adopted recommendations by the American Heart Association state that CPR is indicated and should be done in a pulseless, unmonitored hypothermic patient in the field, but that a longer time to check for a pulse (up to 1 minute) may be required. This recommendation highlights the fact that coma, areflexia, extreme bradycardia, and slow respiratory rate induced by profound hypothermia may make the distinction from death difficult.

Because the only definite criterion for the diagnosis of death in hypothermia is failure to respond to rewarming and resuscitation, CPR, once instituted, should be continued until it can be demonstrated that the cardiac rhythm is stabilized or that there is no response after raising the core temperature to over 30° C. Even prolonged asystole does not represent irreversible cardiac compromise and reports have documented successful resuscitation after prolonged (several hours) CPR in this setting.

For the patient with an arrested cardiac rhythm in whom CPR has been initiated, a method for core rewarming must be instituted while resuscitation continues. The most effective method to achieve this goal in this setting is partial femoral-femoral cardiopulmonary bypass (CPB) using a heat exchanger. Where CPB is not available, peritoneal dialysis, using warm dialysate and rapid exchanges, may be substituted.

It is likely that hypothermia-related mortality in the United States is underreported because physical signs are not recognized and may mimic other conditions, hospitals often do not use low-reading thermometers, medical personnel are not aware of the significance of hypothermia, and the autopsy cannot definitively prove hypothermia as a cause of death. Attention to preventive measures is critical, including well-conditioned and equipped parties with knowledgeable leaders when venturing into back country wilderness areas, use of thermal suits and flotation devices for individuals involved in cold water work or recreational activities, and increased availability of low-income housing, shelter space, and low-income energy assistance programs in urban areas, particularly for the elderly.

# DISTURBANCES DUE TO HEAT

method of
DOUGLAS S. DIEKEMA, M.D., and
GREGORY L. LANDRY, M.D.
*University of Wisconsin School of Medicine*
*Madison, Wisconsin*

Heat-related illnesses have plagued humankind since the beginning of time. They currently take 1000 to 2000 lives each year and have played a role in several wars. Indeed, much of what we know about heat illness comes from the military where it remains a significant problem today. In addition, heat illnesses pose a particular problem for athletes, laborers, and the elderly.

Under normal conditions, human temperature is maintained between 36.4 and 37.6° C through a variety of mechanisms that balance heat load and heat loss. Heat production rises dramatically with muscle activity, increasing as much as twelvefold during intense physical activity. Body core temperature may rise to 40° C during strenuous exercise. Heat may also be gained through radiation from the sun, ambient temperatures above 33° C, and contact with objects that are sources of large radiant heat loads (such as asphalt surfaces, metals, or hot tubs).

Heat loss is accomplished through four mechanisms. As long as body temperature exceeds ambient temperature, heat loss can occur via radiation, convection, and conduction. Radiation (50 to 65%) and convection (15%) account for most of the body's heat loss while conduction accounts for very little under normal circumstances.

The fourth mechanism for heat loss, evaporation, becomes essential when ambient temperatures exceed body temperature. At rest, insensible water loss through the lungs and skin account for about 25 to 30% of cooling. As ambient temperature or activity increases, however, sweating becomes the major mechanism of heat loss. With training and acclimatization a person can produce up to 4 liters of sweat per hour and is capable of dissipating up to 1700 kcal per hour for brief periods of time.

Relative humidity may limit evaporative heat losses. When humidity exceeds 75%, evaporation decreases, and less heat is dissipated per unit of sweat produced. When humidity exceeds 90%, very little evaporation occurs, and sweat simply remains on the skin or drips off.

Under normal circumstances both sweating and respiratory rate increase in response to heat load. Dilation of cutaneous blood vessels, constriction of splanchnic blood vessels, and increased cardiac output serve to increase blood flow through the skin where heat can be lost to the environment. While these mechanisms

effectively optimize heat loss, a delicate balance exists between the body's attempt to maintain temperature balance and its attempt to maintain central blood volume. As body temperature rises, cellular metabolic needs and oxygen demand increase. In the face of decreased perfusion, especially to splanchnic organs, tissue ischemia may occur. In addition, core temperatures of 106° C or greater may lead to direct cellular damage.

The spectrum of heat-related illness occurs as a consequence of these efforts to maintain a normal body temperature in the face of excessive internal or environmental heat load.

## TREATMENT OF MINOR HEAT-RELATED PROBLEMS

Several minor heat-related problems occur within the context of normal temperature regulation.

*Heat edema* is a self-limited, mild swelling of the hands and feet occurring during the first few days of exposure to a warm environment. It requires no treatment.

*Heat tetany* manifests itself as carpopedal spasm (rather than cramping of heavily used muscles) during exposure to heat and may accompany heat stroke or heat exhaustion. It is thought to be caused by hyperventilation and the alkalosis that results. It resolves as heat stress is alleviated and hyperventilation ceases.

*Heat syncope* occurs shortly after heat exposure, especially in unacclimatized individuals. It may occur after long periods of standing or with hard physical work and is probably caused by hypotension resulting from decreased plasma volume combined with cutaneous vasodilation. Treatment includes rest and removal from the heat. Consciousness returns once the patient is placed supine. An individual with heat syncope should not be permitted to resume activity until the following day.

*Prickly heat* or *heat rash* is an acute inflammatory response caused by the blockage of sweat pores and secondary infection, usually with Staphylococci. It is most common in hot, tropical climates. Treatment includes chlorhexidine (Hibiclens) in a light cream or lotion (antibacterial) and 1% salicylic acid (desquamation) applied to affected areas three times a day. Large areas of involvement should not be treated with salicylic acid because of the risk of toxic absorption. If the rash becomes pustular, oral erythromycin stearate (Erythrocin, Wyamycin) (250 mg by mouth four times daily) or dicloxacillin (Dynapen) (250 mg by mouth four times daily) may be added.

*Anhidrotic heat exhaustion* may occur after several weeks of prickly heat. Symptoms of mild heat exhaustion develop with physical exertion. This disorder is marked by the relative lack of sweating of the trunk and limbs in combination with excessive sweating of the forehead and face. Treatment includes avoidance of physical exertion and removal from the heat until the plugs are shed from the sweat pores, a process which may take weeks. Normal activity should not resume until the patient is able to sweat normally.

*Heat cramps* occur in heavily exercised muscles, most commonly the calves and abdominal muscles, under conditions of heat stress. Persons performing heavy work who sweat profusely and replace their fluid losses with hypotonic solutions appear particularly susceptible. Lack of sleep, poor diet, lack of acclimatization, and recent alcohol ingestion may predispose to heat cramps. Onset of cramping may occur during exertion or several hours later. Contact with cold water or air, rapid voluntary contraction of a muscle, or passive extension of a flexed limb may initiate cramping. Most cramps are intermittent and painful, lasting less than a minute. Though a laboratory work-up is not indicated in straightforward cases, serum sodium and chloride are occasionally found to be low.

Treatment consists of fluid and salt replacement along with rest and removal from the heat. An oral solution consisting of ¼ to ½ tsp sodium chloride per liter of water is usually adequate to replace salt and water deficiencies. Persistent or frequent cramping may require intravenous normal saline, 10 ml per kg of which can be administered over 1 to 2 hours. Increased use of table salt on foods and the use of electrolyte replacement drinks will prevent future episodes. Salt tablets often pass through the gastrointestinal tract undigested and should be avoided because of their propensity to cause vomiting, pooling of oral fluids, and potassium depletion.

## HEAT EXHAUSTION

Heat exhaustion, the most common of the heat illnesses, comprises a continuum which lies between minor heat-illnesses and heat stroke. Heat exhaustion occurs in the setting of successfully maintained thermoregulation and usually involves a combination of volume and salt depletion.

Body core temperatures are usually below 40° C and may be normal. Sweating often continues. Patients present with lethargy and intense thirst, followed by headache, giddiness, anorexia, nausea, vomiting, and muscle cramps or tetany. Orthostatic hypotension, tachycardia, hyperventilation, and syncope may be present. In contrast to those with heat stroke, patients with heat exhaustion will have unimpaired mental func-

tion. Coma, seizures, and bizarre behavior are not seen in heat exhaustion.

### Treatment

Treatment of heat exhaustion includes rest in a cool environment. When body temperature is elevated, active cooling with wet towels, fans, or skin wetting may be helpful. Dehydration should be treated with an oral electrolyte solution in mild cases or, in more severe cases, intravenous 5% dextrose in half normal sodium chloride solution. Healthy adults can be rehydrated over 1 to 2 hours, whereas elderly patients, those with cardiovascular disorders, and those with hypernatremia should be rehydrated more slowly and assessed frequently. Patients with hypotension may require a 20 ml per kg intravenous bolus of Ringer's lactate or normal saline. This should be followed by intravenous rehydration. Serum electrolytes should guide selection of the proper intravenous solution.

### HEAT STROKE

Heat stroke is a medical emergency, with mortality rates from 17 to 70%. In contrast to other forms of heat illness, loss of temperature regulation characterizes heat stroke.

The diagnosis of heat stroke requires exposure to a heat load, elevated body temperature, and significant central nervous system (CNS) dysfunction (confusion, delirium, seizures, or coma). A high index of suspicion is necessary since any delay in treatment may result in permanent tissue damage or death.

The classic form of heat stroke occurs most frequently in infants and the elderly, and it tends to develop over days in those unable to obtain fluids and a sufficiently cool environment. Initial symptoms include malaise, headache, and dizziness followed by decreased mental performance. At body temperatures greater than 42° C, confusion, gait disturbance, combativeness, coma, and seizures commonly occur. Muscle rigidity, transient hemiplegia, tremor, and dystonia may also be seen. These patients are usually dehydrated and may have lost the ability to sweat. The skin is hot, flushed, red, and often dry. Body temperatures are nearly always elevated above 40° C. Tachycardia is usually present, and hypotension may occur. Hyperventilation is also common and may lead to hypokalemia or tetany.

Exertional heat stroke occurs more commonly in fit, young athletes. It develops over hours and onset tends to be abrupt. These patients are not severely dehydrated and often continue to sweat profusely. Initially, the person experiences a sense of physical deterioration. Inability to concentrate, chills, throbbing pressure in the head, nausea, unsteadiness, and piloerection on the chest and arms may occur next. If the process continues, irritability and irrationality result. Muscle cramps and paresthesias of the hands and feet may occur. Shortly thereafter, the face becomes ashen gray, and confusion and collapse follow. It should be noted that CNS dysfunction can be very sudden, with loss of consciousness being the first indication of a problem.

### Treatment

Treatment of heat stroke must begin immediately. Any patient with altered mental function under conditions of heat stress should have a rectal temperature recorded. If greater than 41° C, aggressive cooling should begin immediately. Ice packs should be placed on the skin in areas of large blood vessels such as the neck, abdomen, axilla, and groin. Clothing should be removed and water splashed on the skin. Fans, if available, will provide increased evaporation. The patient must be taken to a cool environment as soon as possible, but active cooling should not be delayed in order to accomplish this. Transport should occur in a vehicle with air conditioning or open windows to maximize convection.

Cooling should continue in the emergency room. Evaporation should be maximized by keeping the patient's skin wet with tepid water (less than 28° C) while moving air over the skin using fans. This method maximizes heat loss by enhancing cutaneous blood flow while at the same time avoiding a shivering response. Consciousness usually returns rapidly with cooling, and hypoglycemia should be considered if prolonged mental impairment results. An alternative technique, submersion in a cold water bath combined with vigorous muscle massage, has not proved more effective than evaporative cooling. Furthermore, the cold water is noxious to patients, results in shivering, and may cause cutaneous vasoconstriction which minimizes heat loss from body to ice water. We prefer the former method while recognizing that further studies are necessary.

Cooling should continue until body temperature falls to 39° C at which point it should be discontinued to avoid hypothermia. Cold intravenous solutions, cold gastric lavage, and cold inhaled air probably contribute little when added to effective evaporative cooling.

Endotracheal intubation should be performed in patients who need airway protection, such as those with coma or seizures. Supplemental oxygen (4 to 6 liters per minute) helps meet high oxygen needs of tissue. Cardiovascular support is essential. In the patient with flushed skin, frequent checks of blood pressure and pulse and an electrocardiogram during cooling may be sufficient.

Those with pale skin, tachycardia, and low blood pressure require aggressive support. Hypotension often responds to cooling, and large fluid volumes should be avoided since they can cause pulmonary edema once cutaneous vessels constrict with cooling. If severe hypotension persists after cooling has begun, fluid challenge with 10 ml per kg of normal saline should be given intravenously. A central venous pressure line and a urinary catheter may be necessary to moniter fluid status. Pressor agents, such as isoproterenol or dopamine, may be required if fluid therapy and cooling fail to resolve profound hypotension.

Severe shivering should be suppressed using 25 to 50 mg of intravenous chlorpromazine (Thorazine). Seizures can be managed acutely with 5 to 10 mg intravenous diazepam (Valium). Phenytoin (Dilantin) is not effective in the presence of heat stroke.

Laboratory studies should include arterial blood gas, complete blood cell and platelet counts, electrolytes, blood urea nitrogen, creatinine, glucose, serum glutamic-oxaloacetic transaminase, serum glutamic-pyruvic transaminase, lactate dehydrogenase, creatine phosphokinase, uric acid, lactic acid, calcium, prothrombin time, partial thromboplastin time, and fibrin degradation products.

Acute tubular necrosis occurs in as many as 35% of patients, and rhabdomyolysis may occur and lead to acute renal failure. Early fluid replacement in hypotensive patients may help prevent renal sequelae. Intravenous furosemide (Lasix) (20 to 40 mg) or mannitol (0.2 grams per kg) may be used for inadequate urine output in the face of normal volume status.

Acidosis is common in heat stroke, and those patients with a pH less than 7.2 should be treated with bicarbonate. In interpreting blood gas results, pH must be corrected for body temperature. Each 1° C rise in body temperature decreases the pH by 0.0147.

Transient hypokalemia may result from respiratory alkalosis and resolves spontaneously. In the presence of acidosis, however, a low potassium level represents a true deficit and requires replacement. High potassium levels reflect cellular damage or renal failure and should be treated in the usual manner.

A hypocoagulable state exists in heat stroke which may lead to diffuse intravascular coagulopathy in severe cases. This usually occurs in the first 48 to 72 hours and should be treated in the usual manner.

Late complications include persistent CNS

symptoms, the most common of which are cerebellar defects. Many survivors have permanently increased susceptibility to heat stroke. Massive liver damage with eventual liver failure may also occur.

### PREVENTION

The prevention of heat illness includes a recognition of risk factors. Those at increased risk of heat illness include those who are obese, elderly, physically disabled, or alcoholic. Infants have less ability to sweat than adults and have increased heat transfer between their bodies and the environment owing to an increased surface to mass ratio. Persons with cystic fibrosis are also at risk for heat illness and can lose large amounts of salt in their sweat. Fever, nausea, vomiting, and diarrhea create conditions under which heat illness may be more likely. Congenital absence of the sweat glands is a rare disorder which also increases the risk of heat illness.

Preventive measures seek to reduce heat load and enhance heat loss. Light-colored clothing reflects radiant heat and thus decreases heat load. Clothing permeable to moisture will allow increased heat loss via evaporation. Phenothiazines, antihistamines, and other drugs with anticholinergic effects impair sweating ability and should be avoided if heat stress is a possibility. Patients with cystic fibrosis may require increased salt intake during warm weather.

Young athletes should take special care to replenish fluid losses regularly, drinking more frequently than thirst dictates. Weight may be used to moniter fluid losses. A 5% decrease in weight should disqualify the athlete from any further participation until rehydration has occurred. It is important for coaches, parents, and athletes to recognize the early signs of heat stress and promptly remove those athletes from the heat. Activities should be scheduled to avoid the hottest part of the day.

Though the ideal oral rehydration fluid for athletes remains under investigation, we recommend that cool liquids containing less than 2.5 grams of glucose per 100 ml be used for hydration. Those exercising regularly in warm weather should salt their food to replenish sweat losses.

Acclimatization via gradual conditioning in the heat is also an important element in the prevention of heat illness. This usually requires 5 to 14 days of training in hot (greater than 30° C) weather. Acclimatization leads to increased sweat production, decreased salt concentration in sweat, increased cardiac output, decreased peripheral resistance, and increased blood volume.

Saunas, steam rooms, and hot tubs present special problems. While evaporative heat losses can occur in a sauna, the high temperature may result in heat illness when volume depletion leads to decreased sweating. Steam rooms use lower temperatures than saunas (which means slower heat accumulation), but the higher humidity reduces heat dissipation via sweating. Hot tubs create two problems. Heat is gained from the hot water, and evaporative cooling cannot occur. In all three cases, prolonged exposure should be avoided, and use should be terminated when one feels "too" hot, lightheaded, nauseated, or otherwise uncomfortable.

# SPIDER BITES AND SCORPION STINGS

method of
JOSEPH G. PHANEUF, M.D.
*The University of Texas Southwestern Medical Center*
*Dallas, Texas*

### BROWN RECLUSE SPIDER BITES (LOXOSCELISM)

At present, there is a tendency for many physicians to make a diagnosis of a possible brown recluse bite when a necrotic skin lesion is noted. However, a necrotic skin lesion is not equivalent to a brown recluse spider bite. Trauma, infection, and bites from other spiders may produce a necrotic skin reaction easily mistaken for a brown recluse bite (cutaneous loxoscelism). Spiders commonly found in the United States whose bite may result in some cutaneous necrosis include most notably *Chiracanthium* (three species of common house and garden spiders), as well as *Argiope aurantia* (black-and-yellow garden spider), *Lycosa* (wolf spider), *Phidippus* (black jumping spider), and *Tegenaria agrestis* (a spider recently identified in the northwest United States). It is rare for a brown recluse spider bite to cause a large infarct of the skin. When cutaneous necrosis is greater than 10 cm in diameter, or if the patient is very toxic early on, as in septicemia, consider alternative diagnoses such as a necrotizing bacterial infection, trauma (including factitious ulceration), or pyoderma gangrenosum.

*Loxosceles reclusa*, known as the brown recluse or "fiddle back" spider, has a leg span of 1 to 5 cm and may be recognized by the dark violin shaped marking on the dorsal thorax. In the United States five other species of *Loxosceles* have been reported to cause necrotic arachnidism, and on some species, the violin marking is very faint or absent. *L. reclusa* bites are the most common and severe of all "brown spider bites." *L. reclusa* is a common spider in the central and southern United States, but bites are possible outside its natural habitat as a result of spider transport during household moves. The brown recluse spider is commonly found indoors in closets, storage boxes, basements, and attics. In warmer climates this spider may also be found outdoors under trees, rocks, wood piles, and debris. It is not an aggressive spider, and its habits are nocturnal. Patients are usually bitten while sleeping or when putting on shoes or clothing that have been left in the spider's territory. Bites usually occur during the spring, summer, and early fall.

Most bites are insignificant, usually painless, and rapid uncomplicated healing is the rule. Patients having a significant reaction will develop considerable pain and erythema at the bite site which rapidly progresses to a dusky cyanosis within several hours. A "halo" or ring of pallor due to vasoconstriction is frequently noted around the bite with reactive erythema peripheral to the "halo." Lymphangitis is common and a generalized morbilliform eruption may occur a few days after the bite. One to 2 days after the bite, a hemorrhagic blister may develop and within 1 week a small (2 to 5 cm) area of necrosis may be evident. The hemorrhagic blister and subsequent area of necrosis may be eccentrically shaped as determined by the gravitational spread of the venom.

A patient rarely will develop systemic loxoscelism. A mild systemic reaction may manifest as fever, fatigue, chills, nausea, and arthralgias. Intravascular hemolysis may occur, and this rarely progresses to disseminated intravascular coagulation, renal failure, and coma. The first sign of severe hemolysis is a gradual drop in hemoglobin or hematocrit associated with the development of free hemoglobin in the plasma or urine. If a systemic reaction is suspected, serial urinalyses and hematologic evaluations (including complete cell count with platelet count, prothrombin time, and partial thromboplastin time) should be done.

At present, confirmation of cutaneous or systemic loxoscelism can be made only by the recovery and expert identification of the actual biting spider. Lacking this evidence, recovery of additional brown recluse spiders at the location where the bite occurred will add precision to what is usually only a presumptive diagnosis. In the future, an ELISA test may be available to help confirm the clinical diagnosis of a brown recluse bite.

### Treatment

Early wide excision of the bite is *not indicated*. Clinical experience (University of Missouri, Co-

lumbia, Missouri) and clinical studies (Veterans Administration and Vanderbilt University, Nashville, Tennessee) have shown that early excision within the first 2 weeks is not necessary, may have complications, and may be potentially disabling or disfiguring. Conservative treatment is the mainstay of therapy. Conservative therapy consists of rest, good hydration, frequent cleansing of the bite site, and tetanus prophylaxis as indicated. An involved extremity will benefit from immobilization, splinting or padding, and elevation. Prophylactic antibiotics are not necessary because secondary bacterial infection is uncommon for bona fide *L. reclusa* bites, but infection may occur days after the bite in areas of necrosis. If an infection develops, treatment is best directed by culture and sensitivity results. Heat should not be applied to the bite site. Cooling the bite site may increase patient comfort and decrease the enzymatic reaction of the venom, but caution is advised since ice packs applied to an area of already damaged skin may add cold-induced injury. Systemic and intralesional steroids are not helpful in preventing or treating cutaneous necrosis.

Since almost all bites heal uneventfully with conservative management, it is not surprising that most treatment programs have favorable outcomes. A currently popular treatment is dapsone (50 mg every 12 hours for 2 to 3 weeks).* Caution is encouraged because dapsone commonly causes mild hemolysis and methemoglobinemia. However, in rare instances, it may cause severe hemolysis, agranulocytosis, or dapsone hypersensitivity syndrome. A glucose–6-phosphate dehydrogenase level should be obtained before therapy, and dapsone is contraindicated if this level is abnormally low. Serial blood counts should also be obtained to monitor for significant hemolysis during therapy. No random prospective clinical trials comparing dapsone with conservative management have been published to date. In the past, systemic corticosteroids (prednisone 1 to 2 mg per kg per day for 3 to 5 days) have traditionally been administered to prevent and treat hemolysis. In vitro corticosteroids prevent hemolysis of red blood cells exposed to *L. reclusa* venom. However, neither dapsone nor systemic corticosteroids have been compared with conservative treatment alone. Scientific validation of their efficacy awaits further studies. Antivenin is not currently available, and previous clinical studies have suggested that antivenin does not prevent cutaneous necrosis. Presumed brown recluse bites should not be excised nor débrided for the first 3 to 6 weeks because natural

---

*This use is not listed by the manufacturer.

healing is excellent. For those very rare bites that have not healed uneventfully after 6 to 8 weeks, repair by plastic surgery may be undertaken if necessary or desired.

Hospitalization is necessary for proper monitoring and treatment for the extremely rare patient who develops severe hemolysis, disseminated intravascular coagulation, and renal failure. Caution regarding transfusion is important since the venom may make cross-matching of blood difficult. If transfusions are needed, packed red blood cells are preferable to whole blood since complement or other factors in the serum may react with venom components and contribute to hemolysis. Hemodialysis or peritoneal dialysis may be needed to treat renal failure. The venom is rapidly inactivated in tissue. Therefore, the overall strategy is to help the patient survive the consumptive coagulopathy and renal failure, which are usually short-term and reversible phenomena.

### Prevention

The best preventive measure is the shaking out of boots, shoes, clothing, and blankets before using them. Making noise or vibrations prior to entering attics, basements, seldom-used closets, or wood piles may also provide some benefit since *L. reclusa* prefers to avoid human contact. Pesticides cannot be used safely to rid a building of brown recluse spiders, and spiders will easily re-enter buildings after chemical treatment.

### BLACK WIDOW SPIDER BITES (LATRODECTISM)

Envenomation by the black widow spider causes very little local reaction but may cause severe pain in several muscle groups 30 minutes to 3 hours after the bite. Several species of *Latrodectus* are found throughout the United States and are particularly prevalent in the southeast, southwest, and California. *Latrodectus mactans* has the greatest notoriety, but all members of this species have a similar venom and neuromuscular toxicity. Mature females are glossy black with an abdomen about 6 mm in width, 15 mm in length, and a leg-spread of 40 mm. The ventral abdomen usually has a red marking which may consist of red blotches or the typical hourglass-shaped red marking. This marking is highly variable and depends on the age and the number of moltings. The black widow is commonly found outdoors in barns, garages, and storerooms and may spin its web just outside of homes where outdoor lighting attracts insects. Most bites occur in late summer and early fall.

Serious black widow bites are uncommon in most areas of the United States, and well-documented bites may not cause systemic reactions. However, there is significant regional variability, and physicians in areas such as Arizona and California report that black widow bites (*L. hesperus,* western species) with associated systemic symptoms are not uncommon.

The black widow venom is a very potent neurotoxin stimulating the release of acetylcholine and epinephrine, as well as other neurotransmitters. Systemic reactions have classically been described as generalized spasm of several voluntary muscle groups. However, deep musculoskeletal pain may occur in the absence of muscle spasm. The bite itself is commonly felt as a pin prick sensation, and normally the bite site does not develop any edema, ecchymosis, or necrosis. Within 30 minutes the victim may note pain in local muscle groups that spreads to other voluntary muscle groups, especially the abdominal musculature. Pain in the back, groin, and thighs is also common. The symptoms may mimic the findings seen with an acute abdomen or renal colic. However, the absence of abnormal peritoneal signs and the presence of pain in several muscle groups should help in the differential diagnosis. Anxiety, restlessness, and hypertension are commonly seen with severe envenomations. Tachycardia is usually present, but a normal pulse rate or bradycardia is occasionally noted. Death is rare, but cardiovascular collapse may occur in children, the elderly, physically debilitated patients, and those with cardiovascular disease. Black widow envenomations may mimic metabolic, neurologic, or psychiatric disorders. Thus, expert advice from appropriate consultants, including a regional poison control center, may be helpful.

### Treatment

A warm bath and muscle relaxants may be effective in mild cases. Calcium gluconate (10 ml of a 10% solution) given intravenously over 10 to 20 minutes with cardiac monitoring may be an effective treatment for severe muscular cramping or pain, but the duration of relief is usually very short. Muscle relaxants such as diazepam (Valium) or methocarbamol (Robaxin) may also be helpful. Tetanus toxoid should be administered if indicated. Intravenous narcotics may be necessary to treat severe pain. Patients with severe envenomations and those at highest risk should be closely monitored in the hospital. Black widow spider antivenin (antivenin *Latrodectus mactans,* equine origin) is probably the most effective treatment for black widow bites but may cause anaphylaxis, serum sickness, or a hypersensitivity reaction. Treatment with antivenin is rarely indicated; however, it should be considered for high-risk patients, all patients with severe pain not responsive to other treatments, and in life-threatening circumstances. The recommended dose is one vial (2.5 ml) of antivenin in 10 to 50 ml of saline solution given intravenously over a 15-minute period. Skin testing should be done before using antivenin to determine if the patient is allergic to horse serum.

## SCORPION STINGS

Most scorpion stings in the United States are not medically significant and, at most, cause local burning pain, occasional swelling, and no systemic symptoms. *Centruroides sculpturatus*, found mainly in Arizona, has a neurotoxic venom that can cause a life-threatening crisis. Parts of Texas, New Mexico, Nevada, and small areas of California also have colonies of this scorpion. Envenomation outside this area is possible due to unknowing transport of scorpions by travelers and during household moves. *C. sculpturatus*, also known as the "bark scorpion," is unique in that it is a climbing species preferring to be on or near trees and, unlike other scorpions, never burrows in the ground. Scorpions are nocturnal and only sting man when handled or threatened.

Most stings by *C. sculpturatus* result in pain and paresthesias only. Adults are stung more often than children; however, children (10 years of age and younger) are more likely to have a serious reaction and require intensive supportive care. Serious envenomations can cause cranial nerve dysfunction such as blurred vision, rotary eye movements, fasciculations of the tongue, and loss of control of pharyngeal muscles resulting in respiratory distress and even respiratory arrest. Excessive neuromuscular activity may manifest as uncontrollable jerking of the extremities and thrashing about that may be mistaken for centrally mediated seizure activity. Besides excessive neuromuscular activity, the venom may also cause parasympathetic and sympathetic discharge resulting in increased salivation, restlessness, hypertension, tachycardia, and hyperthermia.

### Treatment

Analgesics, local applications of a cool compress, and tetanus toxoid as indicated are all that is necessary for most stings that cause local pain and paresthesias. Severe envenomations, especially in the young, need prompt supportive care with special attention to the airway. Administration of *C. sculpturatus* antivenin is the treatment of choice for severe envenomations, but only after the initiation of appropriate supportive care. This antivenin is made from goat serum, and as with horse serum, hypersensitivity reactions and serum sickness may occur. It is only available to licensed physicians in Arizona from the Antivenin Production Laboratory, Department of Microbiology at Arizona State University.

Corticosteroids, antihistamines, atropine, and calcium have all been used to treat serious envenomations, but have not been found to be effective. Barbituates and narcotics have been used to control excessive skeletal neuromuscular activity (jerking of extremities and thrashing about). Caution is advised since sedating a person with poor airway control and marginal respiratory muscle control can result in respiratory arrest.

# SNAKEBITE

method of
LODEWYK H. S. VAN MIEROP, M.D.
*University of Florida College of Medicine*
*Gainesville, Florida*

The annual mortality worldwide among about 1 million cases of venomous snakebite is conservatively estimated to be about 40,000. However, fewer than 12 individuals die from snakebite in the United States every year among approximately 8000 cases of snakebite. The low mortality and similarly low morbidity are primarily due to excellent roads and availability of modes of transportation, which allow the great majority of victims to be seen in a medical facility within a few hours after the bite has occurred. Moreover, high-quality antivenin is available for intravenous use.

Only about 10% of the species of snakes in the United States are venomous, and of these the great majority are pit vipers (Crotalidae), so named because of a heat-sensing facial pit on either side of the head between the eye and the nostril. There are three genera: *Crotalus*, or large rattlesnakes with about 30 species, including the large and dangerous Eastern and Western diamondback rattlesnakes; *Sistrurus*, or ground rattlers, with two species, the massasauga and the pygmy rattlesnake; and *Agkistrodon*, or moccasins, with two species, the cottonmouth and the copperhead. All have long hollow fangs, which are movable.

The family Elapidae to which the Old World cobras, mambas, and kraits belong, as well as all of the venomous snakes in Australia, is represented in the United States by two genera of coral snake (*Micrurus* and *Micruroides*), each with one species. Of these, only the Eastern subspecies of coral snake (*Micrurus fulvius*) is dangerous to humans. It is small, only about 2 to 3 feet long, and its fangs are short and fixed. The venom, however, is highly toxic.

Of increasing importance and concern are bites by exotic venomous snakes that are kept as "pets." Antivenin against the bites by such exotic snakes is not always readily available. Zoologic parks usually have a supply of (imported) antivenin for the species that they keep, and the Oklahoma Poison Control Center, 405–271–5454, has information concerning antivenins to exotic venomous snakes.

The great majority of victims in the United States are male, young, and caucasian, and many of the bites are inflicted while the victims are handling the snakes or are trying to catch them. Most are bitten in the upper extremity, particularly the fingers or the hand.

## VENOMS

The venoms of vipers and pit vipers are often classified as being hematotoxic and vasculotoxic, whereas those of elapids, including the coral snake, are said to be neurotoxic and cardiotoxic, causing paralysis and cardiac dysfunction. It must be recognized, however, that this is an oversimplification. Some viper-type snakes—e.g., the South American rattlesnake and some populations of Mojave Desert rattlesnake—may produce a strongly neurotoxic venom, whereas some elapid bites can cause a great deal of necrosis. Snake venoms are mixtures of mostly hydrolytic enzymes and a few inherently toxic substances. The venom of some U.S. pit vipers—e.g., the Eastern diamondback rattlesnake (*Crotalus adamanteus*)—contains a procoagulant, which, through a thrombin-like action, produces a rather pure and by itself usually benign defibrination, without affecting other clotting factors. This venom-induced defibrination only superficially resembles disseminated intravascular coagulation and should not be treated as such. Antivenin is effective in reversing defibrination.

## SYMPTOMS AND SIGNS

The symptoms and signs of pit viper bites include immediate pain, which rapidly intensifies, and swelling, which in all but the mildest cases is progressive and often involves an entire limb. Significant neurovascular embarrassment necessitating fasciotomy is uncommon. Bluish discoloration, ecchymoses, blebs, and blisters may develop. Local necrosis may occur even in optimally treated patients. Nausea, vomiting, abdominal cramps, and diarrhea are common in moderate or severe envenomation, and there may be weakness, dizziness, and cold and clammy skin associated with hypotension and shock. Hematemesis, hematuria, bloody diarrhea, and bleeding in internal organs are rare in the United States, as in acute renal failure. Fasciculations (fine muscular contractions) commonly occur after bites by some of the large rattlesnakes, including the Eastern diamondback rattlesnake. They usually begin near the site of the bite and around the mouth and may become generalized.

The initial symptoms and signs of coral snake bite are unimpressive. There is little or no pain, and swelling, if present at all, is mild and localized. Local necrosis does not occur. Systemic symptoms are almost always delayed for 8 to 12 hours, sometimes even longer, and are initially manifested by a picture of bulbar paralysis. The paralysis may progress to involve the musculature of the trunk and the extremities and may become near total. Unfortunately, after symptoms appear they tend to progress rapidly, and treatment with antivenin becomes less effective.

## TREATMENT

### First Aid

The first aid and definitive treatment of venomous snakebite continues to be controversial. Incision and suction as first aid measures are no longer recommended. If a medical facility cannot be reached within a few hours a tourniquet of nonstretchable material may be used. It should be applied loosely enough to allow several fingers to be passed underneath it because only the lymphatics and superficial veins need to be occluded. It should be remembered that an initially loose tourniquet of this type may become tight as swelling increases and progresses proximally to the tourniquet. Frequent inspections are therefore mandatory. It is doubtful that tourniquets are useful in coral snake bites unless applied tightly. Under these circumstances, the aim is to preserve life, realizing that the bitten part may be lost because of total and prolonged interruption of the blood supply.

### Forms of Treatment Not Recommended

Cryotherapy (the use of ice to cool the bitten part) was at one time popular, but is only mentioned here to point out that it often causes more damage owing to superimposed frostbite than the venom itself and should *never* be used in cases of snakebite.

Recently, high-voltage, low-current electrical shock therapy administered at the site of the bite and derived from stun guns, outboard motors, or lawn mowers has received a great deal of publicity in the lay press. Several experimental studies, however, have failed to demonstrate any beneficial effect, and electrical shock therapy cannot be recommended at this time.

### Emergency Room Management

Venomous snakebite should and usually does remain a medical problem. The bitten part should be cleaned and elevated as much as possible. An arm or a hand can be suspended from an intravenous catheter pole by means of a stockinette in which a window has been cut out at the site of the bite to allow for inspection. A leg can be kept elevated on pillows or by means of some type of orthopedic suspension device.

Although surgical intervention is usually not necessary, even in cases with marked swelling, it is useful to have a member of the surgical staff see patients who have been bitten by pit vipers so that they may have a basis for comparison by which to judge conditions at a later time. The swelling usually begins to recede in 2 to 4 days. Fasciotomy may occasionally be necessary, but it should not be used as a primary, preventive procedure. Because of the highly compartmentalized nature of fingers, some surgeons advocate longitudinal, lateral incisions in some cases of pit viper bite.

### Laboratory Studies

In moderately severe or severe cases of pit viper bite, blood should be drawn as soon as possible for routine tests, clotting studies, platelet count, and determination of fibrinogen levels and fibrin split products, as well as typing and cross-matching. Cross-matching may become difficult or impossible if not done early, presumably because of the effects of the venom. If results of clotting studies are normal on admission, they should be repeated 3 or 4 hours later. If defibrination occurs, clotting studies may be repeated every 4 to 10 hours, depending on severity of the case.

### Antivenin

Most experts at present agree that the mainstay of therapy is antivenin. In the United States, two kinds are available: one against bites by pit vipers (Antivenin [Crotalidae] Polyvalent), the other a monovalent antivenin for the treatment of coral snake bites (Antivenin [*Micrurus fulvius*]). Both are of high quality and should be used intravenously only.

By no means all cases of venomous snakebite need to be treated with antivenin. Venomous snakebite does not always produce envenomation, and in many more cases envenomation is only local. Antivenin is rarely indicated in cases of copperhead or pygmy rattlesnake bite, particularly if 2 hours or more have elapsed after the bite has occurred. It should be considered only in the case of small children or in cases seen early after the bite, particularly if it involves fingers or hand. Even bites by the larger pit vipers may be so mild, producing only local symptoms, that antivenin may not be indicated. Although antivenin is effective in the treatment of generalized envenomation, its benefits in the treatment of the local damage at the bite site are uncertain, particularly if the bite has occurred 2 hours or more earlier. In such cases the doubtful advantages of its use do not outweigh it disadvantages. As in the case of copperhead or pygmy rattle-snake bite, the use of antivenin in relatively mild cases without systemic symptoms may be justified if the bite has occurred in the hand, particularly if it is the dominant one, and the patient is seen within a short time.

Intravenous access should be established. In severe or potentially severe cases, it is advisable to establish two intravenous routes, one in each of two different limbs. One of these is available at all times for antivenin infusion and the other for blood, plasma, medications, etc.

If a decision is made that antivenin treatment is necessary, it should be given early, in adequate amounts, and always intravenously (exception: some foreign-manufactured antivenins should not be given intravenously). Skin testing for hypersensitivity to horse serum should be carried out as described in the package insert. The conjunctival test is not recommended. Epinephrine 1:10,000 should be kept ready, drawn up in a syringe for immediate intravenous use if there is a hypersensitivity reaction to either the skin test or the subsequent administration of antivenin. A negative skin test result does not guarantee that the patient will not have a hypersensitivity reaction and antivenin infusion should be started slowly and cautiously. Except for the most severe and peracutely progressing cases, intravenous administration of reconstituted, but undiluted antivenin directly into the intravenous tubing by push is not recommended because such rapid administration may produce a nonspecific kind of anaphylactoid-like reaction. If antivenin treatment is decided on, it should *not* be given in one-vial increments over many hours. At least 5 vials (50 ml) and more usually 8 to 10 vials (in bites by pit vipers) may be diluted with 250 to 500 ml of suitable diluent, such as Ringer's lactate solution, and, if possible, infused over a period of 2 to 4 hours. Rarely is it necessary to give more than 30 vials of antivenin. Fluid overloading may be a problem in small children. All patients bitten by coral snakes, even if asymptomatic, should receive at least five vials of antivenin if definite fang marks are present, if there is a history that the snake "hung on" or "chewed," or if there are swelling and tenderness at the site of the bite. If itching, hives, or other evidence of hypersensitivity to horse serum occurs, infusion should be stopped and the patient should be given diphenhydramine or hydroxyzine at a dosage appropriate for age and size. Antivenin treatment may then be restarted at a slower rate with careful observation. Pronounced hypersensitivity (anaphylactic) reactions are uncommon, but if they occur further administration of antivenin is contraindicated, unless the severity of the bite is judged to likely lead to death of the patient if antivenin is withheld. In this event, the options should be discussed in detail with the patient and the family and, if possible, a written consultation should be obtained from another physician. Difficulties may be avoided by the use of intravenous epinephrine diluted 1:10 to a final concentration of 1:10,000 in saline, given slowly intravenously as necessary. Mixing the antivenin with ephedrine prior to administration has also been recommended.

### Supportive Measures

Pain in pit viper bite is usually severe enough to require analgesics. Salicylates should not be used. Fluid loss into the extravascular compartment may be considerable, and intravenous fluid therapy, including blood in some cases, may be necessary. Tetanus prophylaxis is necessary, and antibiotics should be given in all but the mildest cases.

# ACUTE POISONINGS

method of
HOWARD C. MOFENSON, M.D.,
THOMAS R. CARACCIO, PHARM.D., and
JOSEPH GREENSHER, M.D.
*Long Island Regional Poison Control Center
East Meadow, New York*

### BASIC MANAGEMENT OF POISONINGS

The severity of the manifestations of acute poisoning exposures varies greatly with the age and intent of the victims. Accidental poisoning exposures make up 80 to 85% of all poisoning episodes and are most frequent in children under 5 years of age. Many of these episodes are actually ingestions of relatively nontoxic substances that require minimal medical care. Intentional poisonings constitute 10 to 15% of poisonings, and often these patients require the highest standards of medical and nursing care and the occasional use of sophisticated equipment for recovery. Suicide attempts

The assistance of Lauren Leader and Helene Jacobs in the preparation of this manuscript is gratefully acknowledged.

are of a significant number, and the use of toxic substances is often involved. The majority of the drug-related suicide attempts involve a central nervous system depressant, and "coma management" is vital to the treatment.

Sixty per cent of patients who take a drug overdose do so with their own prescribed medication and 15 per cent with drugs prescribed for relatives. The top poisoning categories for all ages are over-the-counter analgesics, sedative-hypnotics, benzodiazepines, cleaning agents and petroleum products, alcohol and substance abuse, pesticides, tricyclic antidepressants, plants, carbon monoxide, and opioids.

### ASSESSMENT AND MAINTENANCE OF VITAL FUNCTIONS

*Upper airway obstruction* is the most common cause of death in intoxicated patients outside the hospital. Any patient who is comatose and has absent protective airway reflexes is able to tolerate an endotracheal tube (cuffed for those over ages 7 to 9 years) and should have it inserted as soon as possible.

*Ventilation* is required if the respiratory rate and depth are inadequate.

*The circulatory status* is best assessed by the blood pressure and heart rate and rhythm. The circulatory clinical status and tissue perfusion may be inferred from the skin temperature, the return of color after pressure blanching (capillary filling), and the urine output. Intra-arterial blood pressure measurements are essential for adequate monitoring.

If the circulation fails to improve after adequate ventilation and oxygenation, then a 15- to 20-cm elevation of the foot of the bed may aid by increasing the venous return to the heart. A fluid challenge also may improve the circulatory status if hypovolemia is the cause. If these measures fail, plasma expanders and similar products may be required. As a last resort vasopressors may be needed. If these measures fail to produce a response, a central venous pressure or a pulmonary artery wedge pressure (PAWP) line should be inserted to monitor for heart failure and fluid overload.

TABLE 1. **Level of Consciousness (Reed Coma Scale)**

| Stage | Conscious Level | Pain Response | Reflexes | Respiration | Circulation |
|---|---|---|---|---|---|
| 0 | Asleep | Normal | Normal | Normal | Normal |
| 1 | Coma | Decreased | Normal | Normal | Normal |
| 2 | Coma | None | Normal | Normal | Normal |
| 3* | Coma | None | None | Normal | Normal |
| 4† | Coma | None | None | Abnormal | Abnormal |

*Patients in Stages 3 and 4 require intubation and placement in an intensive care unit.
†Patients in Stage 4 need intervention to sustain life.

*The level of consciousness* of all intoxicated patients should be assessed and the time of assessment recorded. The Glasgow Coma Score used in head trauma is not useful in intoxications, as alcohol, depressant drugs, and hypotension may give falsely lowered scores. The Reed Coma Scale is preferred (Table 1).

## PREVENTION OF ABSORPTION AND REDUCTION OF LOCAL DAMAGE

*Ocular exposure* should be immediately treated with water or saline irrigation for 20 minutes with eyelids fully retracted. Do not use neutralizing chemicals. All caustic and corrosive injuries should be evaluated by an ophthalmologist.

*Dermal exposure* is treated immediately with rinsing, not a forceful flushing in a shower, which might result in deeper penetration of the toxic substance. The skin should be rinsed with copious amounts of water for at least 30 minutes. Hair shampoo, cleansing of fingernails and navel, and irrigation of the eyes are necessary in an extensive exposure. The clothes may have to be discarded. Leather goods are irreversibly contaminated and must be abandoned. Caustics (alkali) often require hours of irrigation until the "soapy" feeling of the burn is gone. Dermal absorption may occur with pesticides, hydrocarbons, and cyanide.

*Injected exposures* to drugs and toxins or those introduced by envenomation may require a proximal tourniquet and early suction. (See Antidotes 4 through 6 in Table 4.)

*Inhalation exposures* to toxic substances are treated by immediately removing the victim from the contaminated environment.

*Gastrointestinal exposure* is the most common route of poisoning, and an estimate of what, when, and how much of the toxic substance was ingested must be made. If there is a possibility of potential intoxication, gastrointestinal decontamination is performed rather than waiting for symptoms to develop.

### Gastrointestinal Decontamination

To decrease gastrointestinal absorption, emesis should be induced or gastric aspiration and lavage performed. Neither of these methods is completely effective; each removes only 30 to 50% of the ingested substance. They are recommended up to 3 to 4 hours postingestion; however, there are few indications for induced emesis in the emergency department in an adult, since it delays the administration of more effective activated charcoal.

### Emesis

*Relative contraindications* to the induction of emesis are (1) petroleum distillate ingestion of high-viscosity agents; (2) agents that are likely to rapidly produce coma (short-acting barbiturates) or convulsions (propoxyphene, camphor, isoniazid, strychnine) in less than 30 minutes and therefore may predispose to aspiration during emesis; and (3) prior significant vomiting.

*Absolute contraindications* to the induction of emesis are (1) caustic (alkali) or corrosive (acid) ingestions; (2) convulsions because of the danger of aspiration and possible induction of laryngospasm; (3) coma because of the possibility of aspiration with the loss of protective airway reflexes; (4) absence of a cough reflex—absence of the gag reflex is not a reliable indication of lack of airway protection, since a number of healthy people lack gag reflexes; (5) hematemesis, in which vomiting may produce additional damage; (6) an infant under 6 months of age, because of immature protective airway reflexes; and (7) foreign bodies—emesis is ineffective and risks obstruction or aspiration.

**Inducing Emesis.** *Syrup of ipecac* is the preferred agent, but never fluid extract of ipecac, which is too potent, or salt water, which has produced fatal hypernatremia. Emesis is not recommended to be induced at home in children under 1 year of age but can be performed in a medical facility under supervision when indicated. The dose of syrup of ipecac in the 6- to 9-month-old infant is 5 ml; in the 9- to 12-month-old, 10 ml; and in the 1- to 12-year-old, 15 ml. In children over 12 years and in adults, the dose is 30 ml. The dose may be repeated *once* if the child does not vomit in 15 to 20 minutes. The vomitus should be inspected for remnants of pills or toxic substances and the appearance and odor noted.

*Apomorphine* is a parenteral emetic that must be freshly prepared. Its use is fraught with complications, although it produces more rapid onset of emesis than syrup of ipecac. We do not recommend its use in the cooperative patient. Naloxone should be available to reverse central nervous system (CNS) depression.

*Gastric aspiration and lavage* may be preferable to the induction of emesis in cooperative adolescents or adults because a large tube can be introduced through the oral cavity. *Contraindications* to gastric aspiration and lavage in intoxicated patients are (1) caustic (alkali) and corrosive (acid) ingestions, because of the risk of esophageal perforation; (2) uncontrolled convulsions, because of the danger of aspiration and injury during the procedure; (3) petroleum distillate products; (4) coma or absent protective air-

TABLE 2. **Substances with Enterohepatic Recirculation**

Chloral hydrate
Colchicine
Digitalis preparations (digoxin, digitoxin)
Glutethimide
Halogenated hydrocarbons (DDT derivatives)
Isoniazid
Methaqualone
Phenothiazines
Phenytoin
Salicylates
Tricyclic antidepressants

way reflexes, which require the insertion of an endotracheal tube to protect against aspiration; (5) significant cardiac dysrhythmias, which should be controlled first; and (6) hematemesis, which may be a relative contraindication.

The best results with gastric aspiration and lavage are obtained with the largest possible orogastric tube that can be reasonably passed (nasogastric tubes are not large enough for this purpose). In adults, use a large-bore orogastric Lavacuator hose or a No. 36 French Ewald tube; in children, use a No. 22–28 French orogastric-type tube.

The amount of fluid used will vary with the patient's age and size, but in general 300 ml per lavage is used in an adult and 100 ml in a child.

Continuous gastric suction has been used for substances that have an enterohepatic recirculation or are actively secreted into the gastrointestinal tract, such as tricyclic antidepressants (imipramine [Tofranil]) and local anesthetics such as mepivacaine (Carbocaine) (Table 2).

*Activated charcoal* is produced by combustion of organic material in the absence of air until the carbon particle is formed. There are few *relative contraindications* to the use of activated charcoal: (1) it should not be administered prior to, concomitantly with, or shortly after syrup of ipecac because it may adsorb the ipecac and interfere with its emetic properties; (2) it should not be given prior to, concomitantly with, or shortly after oral antidotes unless proved not to interfere significantly with their absorption; (3) it does not effectively adsorb caustics and corrosives and may produce vomiting or cling to the esophageal or gastric mucosa and falsely appear as a burn on endoscopy; and it should not be given if there are no bowel sounds. Activated charcoal has no *absolute contraindications,* but it does not effectively adsorb alcohols, boric acid, caustics, corrosives, cyanide, metals, and drugs insoluble in aqueous acid solution (Table 3). Activated charcoal is a stool marker, indicating that the toxin has passed through the gastrointestinal tract and that no further significant absorption from the original ingestion will occur.

The dose of activated charcoal is 1 gram per kg per dose orally with a minimum of 15 grams. The usual adolescent and adult dose is 60 to 100 grams. It is administered as a slurry mixed with water or by orogastric tube. It is too thick to get down by nasogastric tube. It should not be mixed with milk, marmalade, or starch because these interfere with charcoal's adsorptive action. Charcoal is administered with a cathartic initially. Subsequently, cathartics should be given every 12 to 24 hours.

Activated charcoal may be administered orally every 4 hours as long as bowel sounds are present, and it may be especially beneficial in intoxications that have an enterohepatic recirculation (see Table 2). Repeated dosing with oral activated charcoal has been shown to increase the clearance of many drugs without enterohepatic recirculation (see individual poisonings).

*Catharsis* is used to hasten the elimination of any remaining toxin in the gastrointestinal tract. Cathartics are *relatively contraindicated* (1) when ileus is indicated by absence of bowel sounds, (2) in intestinal obstruction or evidence of intestinal perforation, and (3) in cases with a pre-existing electrolyte disturbance. Magnesium sulfate (Epsom salts) is contraindicated in renal failure; sodium sulfate (Glauber's salts), in heart failure or diseases requiring sodium restriction. Magnesium sulfate or sodium sulfate is administered in doses of 250 mg per kg per dose as 20% solutions. The adolescent and adult dose is 30 grams. Sorbitol is given at 2.8 ml per kg to a maximum of 214 ml of a 70% solution, for adults. The cathartic should be given with the initial dose of activated charcoal. Sorbitol in children under age 3 years should be used with caution and is not recommended under 1 year of age.

*Dilutional treatment* is indicated for the immediate management of caustic and corrosive poisonings but is otherwise not useful. *Contraindications* to dilution are (1) inability of the patient to swallow, resulting in aspiration of the diluting fluid, and (2) signs of upper airway obstruction, esophageal perforation, and shock. The administration of large quantities of diluting fluid—above 30 ml in children and 250 ml in

TABLE 3. **Toxic Substances Not Effectively Adsorbed by Activated Charcoal**

Alcohols
Aliphatic hydrocarbons
Boric acid
Caustic alkali
Corrosive acids
Cyanide
Glycols
Metals—iron, lead, lithium, mercury
Mineral acids
Saline cathartics—sodium, magnesium

adults—may produce vomiting, re-exposing the vital tissues to the effects of local damage and possible aspiration.

*Neutralization* has not been proved to be scientifically effective.

## THE USE OF ANTIDOTES

Antidotes are available for only a relatively small number of poisons. An available antidote should be administered only after the vital functions are established. Table 4 summarizes the commonly used antidotes and their indications and methods of administration. Most informational, so-called first aid measures and antidotes on commercial product labels are notorious for their inaccuracy; it is preferable to contact the regional poison control center rather than follow recommendations on these labels.

## ENHANCEMENT OF ELIMINATION

The medical methods for elimination of the absorbed toxic substances are diuresis, dialysis, hemoperfusion, exchange transfusion, plasmapheresis, enzyme induction, and inhibition. The methods to increase urinary excretion of toxic chemicals and drugs are being studied extensively, but the other modalities have not been well evaluated.

In general, these methods are needed in only a minority of instances and should be reserved for life-threatening circumstances or when a definite benefit is anticipated.

**Diuresis.** Diuresis increases the renal clearance of compounds that are partially reabsorbed in the renal tubules. *Forced-fluid diuresis* is based on the principle that it will shorten exposure for reabsorption at the *distal* renal tubules. The risks of diuresis are fluid overload, with cerebral and pulmonary edema, and disturbances in acid-base and electrolyte balance. Failure to produce a diuresis may imply prerenal or renal failure. If renal failure is present, dialysis should be considered.

*Osmotic diuresis* is meant to increase the osmotic gradient and prevent reabsorption from the *proximal* loop and *distal* tubules. Mannitol is used to initiate this type of diuresis, and then fluids are added in sufficient amounts to produce a diuresis similar to forced-fluid diuresis.

*Acid and alkaline diuresis* is based on the principle that to inhibit reabsorption of certain toxic agents the urinary pH can be adjusted so that the substance is maintained in its ionized form, which interferes with its passage back into the blood. Electrolyte and acid-base monitoring is necessary. Hypokalemia and hypocalcemia are frequent complications. *Acid diuresis* is accomplished by using ammonium chloride (Antidote 2, Table 4). Although it may enhance the elimination of weak bases, such as amphetamines and fenfluramine (Pondimin), it is not recommended. Ammonium chloride is contraindicated if rhabdomyolysis is present. *Alkaline diuresis* with sodium bicarbonate can be utilized in the therapy of weak acids, such as salicylates, and long-acting barbiturates, such as phenobarbital (Antidote 35, Table 4).

**Dialysis.** Dialysis is the extrarenal means of removing certain toxins from the body and can substitute for the kidney when renal failure occurs. Dialysis is never the first measure instituted; however, it may be lifesaving later in the course of the severe intoxication. It is needed only in a small minority of intoxications (Table 5). *Peritoneal dialysis* is only one-twentieth as effective as hemodialysis. It is easier to use and less hazardous to the patient but also less reliable in removing the toxin. *Hemodialysis* is the most effective means of dialysis but requires experience with sophisticated equipment. *The patient-related criteria for dialysis* are anticipated prolonged coma and the likelihood of complications, renal impairment, and deterioration despite careful medical management.

**Hemoperfusion.** Hemoperfusion is the extracorporeal exposure of the patient's blood to an adsorbing surface (charcoal or resin). This procedure has extended extracorporeal removal to a large range of substances that were either poorly dialyzable or nondialyzable. Hemoperfusion may be used for agents that have high protein binding, low aqueous solubility, and poor distribution in the plasma water. In these cases hemodialysis is relatively ineffective. Hemoperfusion has proved useful in glutethimide (Doriden) intoxication, barbiturate overdose even with short-acting barbiturates, theophylline, cyclic antidepressants, and chlorophenothane (DDT). The commonly used types are activated charcoal and resin cartridges. In general, supportive care is all that is required. Analysis of studies with hemodialysis and hemoperfusion does not indicate that they reduce morbidity or mortality substantially except in certain cases (Table 6).

## SUPPORTIVE CARE, OBSERVATION, AND THERAPY OF COMPLICATIONS

*The comatose patient* is on the threshold of death and must be stabilized initially by establishing an airway. Intubation should be accomplished in any comatose patient.

An intravenous line should be inserted in all comatose patients and blood collected for appro-
*Text continued on page 1101*

TABLE 4. **Antidotes***

| Medications | Indications | Comments |
|---|---|---|
| 1. **N-Acetylcysteine** (NAC, Muco-myst), Mead Johnson. Glutathi-one precursor that prevents accu-mulation and helps detoxify acetaminophen metabolites.<br>**Dose:** *Adult*, 140 mg/kg PO of 5% solution as loading dose, then 70 mg/kg PO q 4 hr for 17 doses as maintenance dose. *Child*, same as adult.<br>**Packaged:** 10 and 20% solution in 5-, 10-, and 30-ml vials. | Acetaminophen toxicity. Most effective within first 8 hr (to make more palatable, administer through a straw inserted into closed container of citrus juice).<br>**AR:** Stomatitis, nausea, vomiting. See Acetaminophen in text.<br>The full course of therapy is required in any patient whose level falls in the toxic range. | IV preparation experimental. The dose of NAC should be repeated if the patient vomits within 1 hr after administration. Methods to stop vomiting of the NAC are (1) placement of a tube in the duodenum, (2) slow administration over 1 hr, (3) ½ hour before NAC dose use metoclopramide (Reglan), 1 mg/kg IV over 1–2 min (max dose 10 mg) every 6 hr or droperidol (Inapsine), 1.25 mg IV; for extrapyramidal reactions use diphenhydramine (see 18. Diphenhydramine). |
| 2. **Ammonium chloride**, USP, usually given via nasogastric tube.<br>**Dose:** *Adult*, 2 grams q 6 hr in 60-ml dose to maximum of 12 grams/day or 1.5 grams as 1–2% IV q 6 hr up to 6 grams/day. *Child*, 75 mg/kg (2.75 mEq/kg) 4 times/day to maximum of 2–6 grams IV or PO.<br>**Packaged:** 325-, 500-, and 1000-mg tablets: 2.14% in 500 ml, 21.4% in 30 ml, 26.75% in 20 ml. | Acidification of urine may enhance the elimination of phencyclidine and other weak bases (amphetamines and strychnine), but the danger of rhabdomyolysis and precipitation of myoglobin in the renal tubules in an acid milieu indicates that this therapy is too dangerous to recommend routinely. | Goal in acid diuresis is to keep urine pH 4.5–5.5 and output 3–6 ml/kg/hr. Monitor blood pH, keep at 7.2–7.3.<br>A diuretic may be used to enhance acid diuresis.<br>Contraindications: weak acid drugs, rhabdomyolysis and myoglobinuria, liver dysfunction, renal dysfunction, closed-head injury. |
| 3. **Amyl nitrite.** | See 14. Cyanide antidote kit | |
| 4. **Antivenin Black Widow Spider** (*Latrodectus mactans*)<br>**Dose:** 1–2 vials infused over 1 hr.<br>**Packaged:** 6000 U/vial with 2.5 ml sterile water and 1 ml horse serum 1:10 dilution. | Black widow spider; all *Latrodectus* species with severe symptoms. Most healthy adults will survive with supportive care. Used in elderly or infants or if there is underlying medical condition causing hemodynamic instability.<br>**AR:** Same as antivenin polyvalent because derived from horse serum. | Preliminary sensitivity test.<br>Supportive care alone is standard management. |
| 5. **Antivenin Polyvalent** for Crotalidae (pit vipers), Wyeth. IV only.<br>**Dose:** depends on degree of envenomation: minimal: 5–8 vials; moderate: 8–12 vials; severe: 13–30 vials. Dilute in 500–2000 ml of crystalloid solution and start IV at a slow rate, increasing after the first 10 min, if no reaction occurs.<br>**Packaged:** 1 vial (10 ml) lyophilized serum, 1 vial (10 ml) bacteriostatic water for injection, 1 vial (1 ml) normal horse serum. | Venoms of crotalids (pit vipers) of North and South America.<br>**AR:** (Shock anaphylaxis) reaction occurs within 30 min. Serum sickness usually occurs 5–44 days after administration. It may occur in less than 5 days, especially in those who have received horse serum products in the past.<br>Symptoms include fever, edema, arthralgia, nausea, and vomiting, as well as pain and muscle weakness. | Consider consulting with Regional Poison Control Center and herpetologist.<br>Administer IV.<br>Preliminary sensitivity test.<br>Never inject in fingers, toes, or bite site. |
| 6. **Antivenin**, North American coral snake. Wyeth. IV only.<br>**Dose:** 3–5 vials (30–50 ml) by slow IV injection. First 1–2 ml should be injected over 3–5 min.<br>**Packaged:** 1 vial antivenin, 10 ml. 1 vial bacteriostatic water 10 ml for injection. | *Micrurus fulvius* (Eastern coral snake); *Micrurus tenere* (Texas coral snake)<br>**AR:** Anaphylaxis (sensitivity reaction). Usually 30 min after administration. Signs/symptoms: Flushing, itching, edema of face, cough, dyspnea, cyanosis. Neurologic manifestations: Usually involve the shoulders and arms. Pain and muscle weakness are frequently present, and permanent atrophy may develop. | Same as for Antivenin polyvalent for Crotalidae. Will not neutralize the venom of *Micrurus euryxanthus* (Arizona or Sonoran coral snake). |

*This is for informational purposes and is not intended to substitute for independent judgment. It is always advisable to review the package insert for the most up-to-date information. Contact Regional Poison Control Center for additional details on use.

*Abbreviations:* AR = adverse reactions to antidotes; MP = monitor parameters; FDA = U.S. Food and Drug Administration; ECG = electrocardiogram; CNS = central nervous system; GI = gastrointestinal.

TABLE 4. **Antidotes*** *Continued*

| Medications | Indications | Comments |
|---|---|---|
| 7. **Atropine** (various manufacturers). Antagonizes cholinergic stimuli at muscarinic receptors.<br>**Dose:** *Adult*, Initial dose 2–4 mg IV. Dose every 10–15 min as necessary until cessation of secretions. Severe poisoning may require doses up to 2000 mg. *Child*, Initial dose of 0.02 mg/kg to a maximum of 2 mg every 10–15 min as necessary until cessation of secretions.<br>Use preservative-free atropine for infusion.<br>**Packaged:** 0.3 mg/ml in 30 ml; 0.4 mg/ml in 0.5-, 1-, 20-, and 30-ml vials; 1 mg/ml in 1- and 10-ml vials. | Therapy in carbamate and organophosphate insecticide poisonings. Rarely needed in cholinergic mushroom intoxication (*Amanita muscaria, Clitocybe, Inocybe* spp.). Lack of signs of atropinization confirms diagnosis of cholinesterase inhibition.<br>**Diagnostic Test:** *Child*, 0.01 mg/kg IV. *Adult*, 1 mg total.<br>**AR:** Flushing and dryness of skin, blurred vision, rapid and irregular pulse, fever, and loss of neuromuscular coordination. | If cyanosis, establish respiration first because atropine in cyanotic patients may cause ventricular fibrillation.<br>If severe signs of atropinization, may correct with physostigmine in doses equal to one-half dose of atropine.<br>If symptomatic, administer until the end point of drying secretions and clearing of lungs. Hallucinations, flushing of the skin, dilated pupils, tachycardia, and elevation of body temperature are not end points and do not preclude atropine administration. Atropinization should be maintained for 12 to 24 hours; then taper dose and observe for relapse.<br>Atropine has been administered successfully by IV infusion, although this method has not received FDA approval.<br>**Dose:** Place 8 mg of atropine in 100 ml D5W or saline.<br>Conc. = 0.08 mg/ml.<br>Dose range = 0.02–0.08 mg/kg/hr or 0.25–1 ml/kg/hr.<br>Severe poisoning may require supplemental doses of IV atropine intermittently in doses of 2–4 mg until drying of secretion occurs. |
| 8. **BAL** | See 17. Dimercaprol | |
| 9. **Bicarbonate** | See 35. Sodium bicarbonate | |
| 10. **Botulism antitoxin**, Connaught Medical Research Laboratories.<br>**Dose:** *Adult*, 1 vial IV stat, then 1 vial IM; repeat in 2–4 hr if symptoms appear in 12–24 hr. *Child*, Check with state health department. | Prevention or treatment of botulism. | Contact local or state health department for full management guidelines. |
| 11. **Calcium disodium edetate** (EDTA, Disodium Versenate), Riker.<br>**Dose:** *Adult*, Maximum 4 grams. *Child*, 1 gram maximum. Moderate toxicity, IM or IV, 50 mg/kg/day for 3–5 days. Severe toxicity, IV or IM, 75 mg/kg/day for 4–5 days, divided into 3–6 doses daily. Dilute 1 gram in 250–500 ml saline or D5W, infuse over 4 hr twice daily for 5–7 days. *Child*, Maximum 1 gram.<br>For lead levels over 69 µg/dl or if symptoms of lead poisoning or encephalopathy: Add BAL alone initially, 4 mg/kg, then combination BAL and EDTA at different sites. EDTA dose: 12.5 mg/kg IM. | For chelation of cadmium, chromium, cobalt, copper, lead, magnesium, nickel, selenium, tellurium, tungsten, uranium, vanadium, and zinc.<br>**AR:**<br>1. Thrombophlebitis.<br>2. Nausea, vomiting.<br>3. Hypotension.<br>4. Transient bone marrow suppression.<br>5. Nephrotoxicity, reversible tubular necrosis (particularly in acid urine).<br>6. Fever 4–8 hr after infusion.<br>7. Increased prothrombin time. | Hydrate first and establish renal flow.<br>Avoid plain sodium EDTA, since hypocalcemia may result.<br>Procaine 0.25–1 ml of 0.5% for each ml of IM EDTA to reduce pain.<br>Do not use EDTA orally.<br>Limit use to 7 days (otherwise loss of other ions and cardiac dysrhythmias may occur).<br>**MP:** Calcium levels, urinalysis, renal profile, erythrocyte protoporphyrin, blood lead, and liver profile.<br>Contraindicated in iron intoxication, hepatic impairment, and renal failure. |

*This is for informational purposes and is not intended to substitute for independent judgment. It is always advisable to review the package insert for the most up-to-date information. Contact Regional Poison Control Center for additional details on use.

*Abbreviations:* AR = adverse reactions to antidotes; MP = monitor parameters; FDA = U.S. Food and Drug Administration; ECG = electrocardiogram; CNS = central nervous system; GI = gastrointestinal.

*Table continued on following page*

TABLE 4. **Antidotes*** *Continued*

| Medications | Indications | Comments |
|---|---|---|
| (See Lead in text for latest recommendations.) Modify dose in renal failure. **Packaged:** 200 mg/ml, 5-ml ampules. | | |
| 12. (A) **Calcium gluconate**, various manufacturers. **Dose:** *Adult,* 10 grams in 250 ml of water PO or by nasogastric tube; 30 grams maximum daily dose. **Packaged:** 500-, 650-mg, 1-gram tablets. | To precipitate fluorides, magnesium, salts, and oxalates after oral ingestion. | |
| (B) **Calcium gluconate** 10%. **Dose:** IV 0.2–0.5 ml/kg of elemental calcium up to maximum 10 ml (1 gram) over 5–10 min with continuous ECG monitoring. Titrate to adequate response. **Packaged:** 10% in 10-ml vial. | Calcium channel blocker poisoning, e.g., nifedipine (Procardia), verapamil (Calan), diltiazem (Cardizem). It improves the blood pressure but does not affect the dysrhythmias. Hypocalcemia as result of poisonings. Black widow spider envenomation. | Repeat dose as needed. Monitor calcium levels. Contraindicated with digitalis poisoning. |
| (C) **Calcium chloride.** **Dose:** IV 0.2 ml/kg up to maximum 10 ml (1 gram) with continuous IV monitoring. Titrate to adequate response. | Hydrofluoric acid (if irrigation with cool water fails to control the pain). AR: IV bradycardia, asystole, necrosis with extravasation. | Infiltration with calcium gluconate should be considered if hydrofluoric acid exposure results in immediate tissue damage, and erythema and pain persist following adequate irrigation. |
| (D) **Infiltration of calcium gluconate.** **Dose:** Infiltrate each square cm of the affected dermis and subcutaneous tissue with about 0.5 ml of 10% calcium gluconate using a 30-gauge needle. Repeat as needed to control pain. **Packaged:** 10% in 10-ml vial. | | |
| (E) **Calcium gel** 3.5 grams USP, calcium gluconate powder added to 5 oz of water-soluble lubricating jelly. | Dermal exposures of hydrofluoric acid less than 20%. | Gel must have direct access to burn area. If pain persists, a calcium gluconate injection may be needed. |
| 13. **Chlorpromazine,** various manufacturers. Phenothiazine derivative. **Dose:** *Adult,* 1 mg/kg dose† IV/IM or 0.5 mg/kg dose if taken with barbiturate. **Packaged:** 25 mg/ml in 1-, 2-, and 10-ml vials. | Only in *pure* amphetamine overdose, with life-threatening manifestations. (Diazepam [Valium] is preferred.) Toxicity: CNS depression, coma, hypotension, extrapyramidal syndrome, agitation, fever, convulsions, dry mouth, cardiac arrhythmias, ECG changes. | Do not use if any signs of atropinization or "street drug" amphetamines are present. Watch for hypotension. In general, it is safer to use diazepam (Valium) or haloperidol (Haldol). |
| 14. **Cyanide antidote kit**, Lilly. Nitrite-induced methemoglobinemia attracts cyanide off cytochrome oxidase, and thiosulfate forms nontoxic thiocyanate. **Doses:** Amyl nitrite.‡ Inhale for 30 sec of every min. Use a new ampule every 3 min. Reapply until sodium nitrite can be | Cyanide poisoning. AR: Hypotension, methemoglobinemia. | *Note:* If a child is given the adult dose of sodium nitrite, a fatal methemoglobinemia may result. *Do not use methylene blue* for methemoglobinemia in cyanide therapy. Observe for hypotension and have epinephrine available. Cyanide kits should have amyl nitrite changed annually. |

*This is for informational purposes and is not intended to substitute for independent judgment. It is always advisable to review the package insert for the most up-to-date information. Contact Regional Poison Control Center for additional details on use.

†This dose may exceed the manufacturer's recommended dose.

‡This use is not listed by the manufacturer.

*Abbreviations:* AR = adverse reactions to antidotes; MP = monitor parameters; FDA = U.S. Food and Drug Administration; ECG = electrocardiogram; CNS = central nervous system; GI = gastrointestinal.

TABLE 4. **Antidotes*** Continued

| Medications | Indications | Comments |
|---|---|---|
| given. Then inject IV 300 mg (10 ml of 3% solution) of sodium nitrite at a rate of 2.5 to 5 ml/min. Then inject 12.5 grams (50 ml of 25% solution) of sodium thiosulfate. *Child*, Use the following chart for children's dosage.<br>**Packaged:** 2- to 10-ml ampules sodium nitrite injection: 2- to 50-ml ampules sodium thiosulfate injection; 0.3-ml amyl nitrite inhalant. | | Administer 100% oxygen between inhalations of amyl nitrite.<br>Monitor hemoglobin, arterial blood gases, methemoglobin concentration (nitrite given to obtain a methemoglobin of 25%). Some add nitrite ampule to resuscitation bag. |

| Hemoglobin | Initial Child Dose of Sodium Nitrite 3% (do not exceed 10 ml) | Initial Child Dose of Sodium Thiosulfate (do not exceed 12.5 grams) |
|---|---|---|
| 8 grams | 0.22 ml/kg (6.6 mg/kg) | 1.10 ml/kg |
| 10 grams | 0.27 ml/kg (8.7 mg/kg) | 1.35 ml/kg |
| 12 grams | 0.33 ml/kg (10 mg/kg) | 1.65 ml/kg |
| 14 grams | 0.39 ml/kg (11.6 mg/kg) | 1.95 ml/kg |

If signs of poisoning reappear, repeat above procedure at one-half the above doses.

| Medications | Indications | Comments |
|---|---|---|
| 15. **Deferoxamine mesylate** (DFOM, Desferal), Ciba. Has a remarkable affinity for ferric iron and chelates it.<br>**Therapeutic Dose:** *Adult*, 90 mg/kg† IM or IV q 8 hr to a maximum of 1 gram per injection; may repeat to maximum of 6 grams in 24 hr. *Child*, Same as adult. IV administration can be given by slow infusion at rate not exceeding 15 mg/kg/hr.<br>**Packaged:** 500 mg/ampule (powder). | DFOM is useful in the treatment of symptomatic iron poisoning or cases where the serum iron level > 350 µg/dl.<br>A positive result of a DFOM challenge test is not a definite indication that therapy is necessary in the asymptomatic patient. Oral DFOM is not recommended.<br>Iron intoxication.<br>Therapeutic: See dose in left column.<br>*Diagnostic trial*: Give deferoxamine, 50 mg/kg IM (up to 1 gram). If serum iron exceeds total iron-binding capacity, unbound iron is excreted in urine, producing a "vin rosé" color of chelated iron complex in the urine (pink-orange). However, may be negative with high serum iron exceeding total iron-binding capacity.<br>**AR:** Flushing of the skin, generalized erythema, urticaria, hypotension, and shock may occur. Blindness has occurred rarely in patients receiving long-term, high-dose DFOM therapy. Contraindicated in patients with renal disease or anuria. | Therapy is usually continued until urine color and/or iron levels are normal. Therapy is rarely required over 24 hr.<br>Establish a good renal flow.<br>To be effective, DFOM should be administered in first 12–16 hr.<br>In mild to moderate iron intoxication, IM or IV route. In severe intoxication or shock, IV route only.<br>Monitor serum iron levels, urine output, and urine color. |
| 16. **Diazepam** (Valium), Roche.<br>**Dose:** *Adult*, 5–10 mg IV (maximum 20 mg) at a rate of 5 mg/min until seizure is controlled. May be repeated 2 or 3 times. *Child*, 0.1–0.3 mg/kg up to 10 mg IV slowly over 2 min.<br>**Packaged:** 5 mg/ml, 2- to 10-ml vials. | Any intoxication that provokes seizures when specific therapy is *not* available, e.g., amphetamines, PCP, barbiturate and alcohol withdrawal.<br>Chloroquine poisoning.<br>**AR:** Confusion, somnolence, coma, hypotension. | IM absorption is erratic. Establish airway and administer 100% oxygen and glucose. |

*This is for informational purposes and is not intended to substitute for independent judgment. It is always advisable to review the package insert for the most up-to-date information. Contact Regional Poison Control Center for additional details on use.

†This dose may exceed the manufacturer's recommended dose.

*Abbreviations:* AR = adverse reactions to antidotes; MP = monitor parameters; FDA = U.S. Food and Drug Administration; ECG = electrocardiogram; CNS = central nervous system; GI = gastrointestinal.

*Table continued on following page*

TABLE 4. **Antidotes*** *Continued*

| Medications | Indications | Comments |
|---|---|---|
| 17. **Dimercaprol (BAL),** Hynson, Westcott, and Dunning.<br>**Dose:** Recommendations vary; contact Regional Poison Control Center. Prevents inhibition of sulfhydryl enzymes. Given deep IM only. For *severe lead poisoning:* see 11. EDTA. For *mild arsenic or gold:* 2.5 mg/kg q 6 hr for 2 days, then q 12 hr on the third day, and once daily thereafter for 10 days. For *severe arsenic or gold:* 3–5 mg/kg q 6 hr for 3 days, then q 12 hr thereafter for 10 days.† For *mercury:* 5 mg/kg initially, followed by 2.5 mg/kg 1 or 2 times daily for 10 days.<br>**Packaged:** 100 mg/ml 10% in oil in 3-ml ampules. | For chelation of antimony, arsenic, bismuth, chromates, copper, gold, lead, mercury, and nickel.<br>**AR:** 30% of patients have reactions: fever (30% of children), hypertension, tachycardia; may cause hemolysis in glucose-6-phosphate dehydrogenase deficiency patients. Doses greater than recommended may cause various adverse effects: nausea, vomiting, headache, chest pain, tachycardia, and hypertension. | Contraindicated in instances of hepatic insufficiency, with the exception of postarsenic jaundice.<br>Should be discontinued or used only with extreme caution if acute renal insufficiency is present.<br>Monitor blood pressure and heart rate (both may increase), urinalysis, qualitative urine excretion of heavy metal.<br>Contraindicated in iron, silver, uranium, selenium, and cadmium poisoning. |
| 18. **Diphenhydramine (Benadryl),** Parke-Davis. Antiparkinsonian action.<br>**Dose:** *Adult,* 10–50 mg IV over 2 min. *Child,* 1–2 mg/kg IV up to 50 mg over 2 min. Maximum in 24 hr, 400 mg.<br>**Packaged:** 10 mg/ml in 10- and 30-ml vials. 50 mg/ml in 1-, 5-, 10-, and 30-ml vials. Capsules, tablets 25 mg. Elixir, syrup 12.5 mg/5 ml. | Used to treat extrapyramidal symptoms and dystonia induced by phenothiazines and related drugs.<br>**AR:** Fatal dose, 20–40 mg/kg. Dry mouth, drowsiness. | Continue with oral diphenhydramine 5 mg/kg/day to 25 mg 3 times a day for 72 hr to avoid recurrence. |
| 19. **EDTA** | See 11. Calcium disodium edetate | |
| 20. **Ethanol (ETOH).** Competitively inhibits alcohol dehydrogenase.<br>**Loading Dose:** Administer 7.6–10.0 ml/kg of 10% ETOH in D5W over 30 min IV or 0.8–1.0 ml/kg 95% ETOH PO in 6 oz of orange juice over 30 min. While administering loading dose, start maintenance.<br>**Maintenance Dose:** Volume of 10% ETOH needed IV or 95% oral solution (not in dialysis). (See table of maintenance dose below.) If patient is on dialysis, add 91 ml/hr in addition to regular maintenance dose. See comments to prepare 10% solution if not commercially available.<br>**Packaged:** 10% ethanol in D5W 1000 ml; 95% ethanol. May be given as 50% solution orally. | Methanol, ethylene glycol.<br>Ethanol infusion therapy may be started in cases of suspected methanol and ethylene glycol poisoning presenting with increased anion gap and osmolal gap, or if the urine shows the crystalluria of ethylene glycol poisoning or the hyperemia of the optic disk of methanol intoxication.<br>**AR:** CNS depression, hypoglycemia. | Monitor blood ethanol 1 hr after starting infusion and every 4–6 hr. Maintain a blood ethanol concentration of 100–200 mg/dl. Monitor blood glucose, electrolytes, blood gases, urinalysis, and renal profile at least daily. Continue infusion until safe concentration of ethylene glycol or methanol is reached. Ethanol-induced hypoglycemia may occur. Dialysis, preferably hemodialysis, should be considered in severe intoxication not controlled by ethanol alone.<br>To prepare 10% ethanol for infusion for infusion therapy: Remove 100 ml from 1 liter of D5W and replace with 100 ml of tax-free bulk absolute alcohol after passing through 0.22 μm filter. 50-ml vials of pyrogen-free absolute ethanol for injection are available from Pharm-Serve, 218–20 96th Avenue, Queen's Village, NY 11429. Telephone 718-475-1601. |

*This is for informational purposes and is not intended to substitute for independent judgment. It is always advisable to review the package insert for the most up-to-date information. Contact Regional Poison Control Center for additional details on use.

†This dose may exceed the manufacturer's recommended dose.

*Abbreviations:* AR = adverse reactions to antidotes; MP = monitor parameters; FDA = U.S. Food and Drug Administration; ECG = electrocardiogram; CNS = central nervous system; GI = gastrointestinal.

TABLE 4. **Antidotes** *Continued*

| Medications | Indications | Comments |
|---|---|---|

*Maintenance Dose:*

| Patient Category | ml/kg/hr using 10% IV | ml/kg/hr using 50% oral |
|---|---|---|
| Nondrinker | 0.83 | 0.17 |
| Occasional drinker | 1.40 | 0.28 |
| Alcoholic | 1.96 | 0.39 |

21. **Fab** (antibody fragment) (Digibind).
    **Dose:** The average dose used during clinical testing was 10 vials. Dosage details are specified by the manufacturer. It should be administered IV over 30 min. Calculate on basis of body burden either by known amount ingested or by serum digoxin concentration.
    *Calculation of dose of Fab:*
    1. Known amount ingested multiplied by bioavailability (0.8) = body burden. Body burden divided by 0.6 = number of vials.
    2. Known serum digoxin (obtained 6 hr postingestion) multiplied by volume distribution (5.6 liters/kg) and weight in kg divided by 1000 = body burden. Body burden divided by 0.6 = number of vials.

Digoxin, digitoxin, oleander tea with life-threatening intoxications, refractory dysrhythmias, hyperkalemia. 40 mg binds 0.6 mg digoxin.

Contact Regional Poison Control Center.
Preliminary sensitivity test.
Administer through a 0.22-μm filter. It causes a rise in measured bound digoxin but a fall in free digoxin.

22. **Glucagon.** Works by stimulating production of cyclic adenyl monophosphate.
    **Dose:** 50–150 μg/kg over 1 min IV followed by a continuous infusion of 1–5 mg/hr in dextrose and then taper over 5–12 hr. 2 mg of phenol is in 1 mg of glucagon; 50 mg is the maximum amount of phenol recommended and therefore toxicity may result when high doses of glucagon are used.
    **Packaged:** 1-mg (1-unit) vial with 1-ml diluent with glycerin and phenol; also in 10-ml size.

Propranolol and other beta-blocker intoxication.
**AR:** Generally well tolerated—most frequent are nausea, vomiting.

Do not dissolve the lyophilized glucagon in the solvent packaged with it when administering IV infusion, because of possible phenol toxicity. Use 0.9% saline or D5W.
Effects of single dose observed in 5–10 min and last for 15–30 min.
A constant infusion may be necessary to sustain desired effects.

23. **Labetalol hydrochloride** (Normodyne), Schering; (Trandate), Glaxo. Nonselective beta and mild alpha blocker.
    **Dose:** IV 20 mg over 2 min. Additional injections of 40 or 80 mg can be given at 10-min intervals until desired supine blood pressure achieved. Maximum dose 300 mg. Alternative: Slow IV infusion: 200 mg (40 ml) is added to 160 or 250 ml of D5W and given at 2 mg/min. Titrate infusion according to response.
    **Packaged:** Solution 5 mg/ml in 20 ml.

Hypertensive crises secondary to cocaine.
**AD:** GI disturbances, orthostatic hypotension, bronchospasm, congestive heart failure, atrioventricular conduction disturbances, and peripheral vascular reactions.

Concomitant diuretic enhances therapeutic response. Patient should be kept in a supine position during infusion.
**MP:** Monitor blood pressure during and after administration.

---

*This is for informational purposes and is not intended to substitute for independent judgment. It is always advisable to review the package insert for the most up-to-date information. Contact Regional Poison Control Center for additional details on use.

*Abbreviations:* AR = adverse reactions to antidotes; MP = monitor parameters; FDA = U.S. Food and Drug Administration; ECG = electrocardiogram; CNS = central nervous system; GI = gastrointestinal.

*Table continued on following page*

TABLE 4. **Antidotes*** *Continued*

| Medications | Indications | Comments |
|---|---|---|
| 24. **Methylene blue**, Harvey and others. Physiologically transformed to reduced form, leukomethylene blue, which is then oxidized to methylene blue in the presence of methemoglobin. The methemoglobin is converted to hemoglobin.<br>**Dose:** *Adult*, 0.1–0.2 ml/kg of 1% solution (1–2 mg/kg over 5 min IV). *Child*, Same as adult.<br>**Packaged:** 1% 10-ml ampules. May repeat in 1 hr if necessary, only once. | Methemoglobinemia.<br>**AR:** GI (nausea, vomiting), headache, hypertension, dizziness, mental confusion, restlessness, dyspnea when IV dose exceeds 7 mg/kg. Also, hemolysis, dysuria, blue skin or urine, burning sensation in vein.<br>Treatment is unnecessary unless methemoglobin is over 30% or respiratory distress. | Saliva, urine, and other body fluids may turn blue.<br>*Contraindications:* Renal insufficiency; cyanide poisonings when sodium nitrite is used to induce methemoglobinemia; in glucose-6-phosphate dehydrogenase deficiency patients.<br>Monitor hemolysis, methemoglobin level, and arterial blood gases.<br>Avoid extravasation because of local necrosis. |
| 25. **Naloxone** (Narcan). Pure opioid antagonist.<br>**Dose:** *Adult*, 0.4–2.0 mg IV and repeat at 3-min intervals until respiratory function is stable. Before excluding opioid intoxication on the basis of a lack of naloxone response, a minimum of 2 mg in a child or 10 mg in an adult should be administered. *Child*, Initial dose is 0.1 mg/kg.<br><br>**Packaged:** 0.02 and 0.4 mg/ml ampules, and 10-ml multidose vial. | Narcotic, opiate, CNS depression.<br>This drug is relatively free of adverse reactions. Rare report of pulmonary edema.<br>Should be administered with caution in pregnancy. It is used only to reverse depression and hypoxia. | Naloxone infusion therapy should be used if a large initial dose was required, repeated boluses are necessary, or a long-acting opiate is involved. In infusion therapy the initial response dose is administered every hour and may need to be boostered in ½ after starting. The infusion may be tapered after 12 hr of therapy. Naloxone infusion: Calculate daily fluid requirements, add initial response dose of naloxone multiplied by 24 to the solution. Divide fluid by 24 to determine ml/hr of naloxone infusion.<br>Does not cause CNS depression.<br>Routes: IV or endotracheal are preferred routes.<br>Pentazocine (Talwin), dextromethorphan, propoxyphene (Darvon), and codeine may require larger doses. |
| 26. **Nicotinamide** (various manufacturers).<br>**Dose:** *Adult*, 500 mg IM or IV slowly, then 200–400 mg q 4 hr. If symptoms develop, the frequency of injections should be increased to every 2 hr (maximum 3 grams/day). *Child*, One-half suggested adult dose.<br>**Packaged:** 100 mg/ml: 2-, 5-, 10-, 30-ml vials; 25- and 50-mg tablets. | Vacor poisoning: phenylurea pesticide intoxication. *Note:* Vacor 2% is now available only to professional exterminators. 0.5% Vacor is available to the general public and can be toxic to children if swallowed.<br>**AR:** Large doses: flushing, pruritus, sensation of burning, nausea, vomiting, anaphylactic shock. | Nicotinamide is most effective when given within 1 hr of ingestion.<br>Do not use niacin or nicotinic acid in place of nicotinamide.<br>Monitor liver profile. |
| 27. **Oxygen** 100%.<br>**Dose:** *Adult*, 100% oxygen by inhalation or 100% oxygen in hyperbaric chamber at 2–3 atm. *Child*, Same as adult. | Carbon monoxide, cyanide, methemoglobinemia. Any inhalation intoxication. | Half-life of carboxyhemoglobin is 240 min in room air 21% oxygen; if a patient is hyperventilated with 100% oxygen, half-life of carboxyhemoglobin is 90 min; in chamber at 2 atm, half-life is 25–30 min. |
| 28. **Pancuronium bromide** (Pavulon). Nondepolarizing (competitive) blocking agent.<br>**Dose:** *Adults and children*, Initially, 0.1 mg/kg IV; for intubation, 0.1 mg/kg IV, repeated as required (generally every 40 to 60 min).† | Neuromuscular blocking agent.<br>Used for intubation and seizure control, acts in 2 min, lasts 40–60 min.<br>**AR:** Main hazard is inadequate postoperative ventilation. Tachycardia and slight increase in arterial pressure may occur owing to vagolytic action. | The required dose varies greatly and a peripheral nerve stimulator aids in determining appropriate amount. Should monitor electroencephalogram, since motor effect may be abolished without decreasing electrical discharge from brain. |

*This is for informational purposes and is not intended to substitute for independent judgment. It is always advisable to review the package insert for the most up-to-date information. Contact Regional Poison Control Center for additional details on use.

†This dose may exceed the manufacturer's recommended dose.

*Abbreviations:* AR = adverse reactions to antidotes; MP = monitor parameters; FDA = U.S. Food and Drug Administration; ECG = electrocardiogram; CNS = central nervous system; GI = gastrointestinal.

TABLE 4. **Antidotes**\* *Continued*

| Medications | Indications | Comments |
|---|---|---|

**Packaged:** Solution 1 mg/ml in 10 ml; 2 mg/ml in 2- and 5-ml containers.

29. D-**Penicillamine** (Cuprimine), Merck; (Depen), Wallace. Effective chelator and promotes excretion in urine.

    **Dose:** 250 mg 4 times daily PO for up to 5 days for long-term (20–40 days) therapy; 30–40 mg/kg/day in children. Maximum 1 gram/day. For chronic therapy, 25 mg/kg/day in 4 doses.

    **Packaged**: 125- and 250-mg capsules.

Heavy metals, arsenic, cadmium, chromates, cobalt, copper, lead, mercury, nickel, and zinc.

**AR:** Leukopenia (2%); thrombocytopenia (4%); GI: nausea, vomiting, diarrhea (17%); fever, rash, lupus syndrome, renal and hepatic injury; anaphylactic shock.

This is not considered standard therapy for lead poisoning after chelation therapy.

May produce ampicillin-like rash, allergic reactions, neutropenia, and nephropathy. Contraindication: hypersensitivity to penicillin.

**MP:** Routine urinalysis, white differential blood count, hemoglobin determination, direct platelet count, renal and hepatic profiles. Collect 24-hr urine; quantify for heavy metal.

30. **Physostigmine salicylate** (Antilirium), Forest. Cholinesterase inhibitor. A diagnostic trial is not recommended.

    **Dose:** *Adult*, 1–2 mg IV over 2 min: may repeat every 5 min to maximum dose of 6 mg. *Child*, IV, 0.02 mg/kg over 2 min to a maximum dose of 2 mg.† Once effect accomplished, give lowest effective dose every 30–60 min if symptoms recur.

    **Packaged:** 1 mg/ml in 2 ml/ampule.

Used if conventional therapy fails for coma, convulsions, severe cardiac dysrhythmias, severe hypertension, hallucinations secondary to anticholinergics, antihistamines, and anticholinergic plants.

**AR:** Death may result from respiratory paralysis, hypertension/hypotension, bradycardia/tachycardia/asystole, hypersalivation, respiratory difficulties/convulsions (cholinergic crisis).

Do not consider for the following: antidepressants, amoxapine, maprotiline, nomifensine, bupropion, trazodone, imipramine.

IV administration should be at a slow controlled rate, not more than 1 mg/min.

Rapid administration can cause adverse reactions.

Can be reversed by atropine.

Lasts only 30 min.

Contraindicated in asthma, cardiovascular disease, intestinal obstruction.

31. **Pralidoxime chloride** (2-PAM, Protopam) Ayerst. Cholinesterase reactivator by removing phosphate.

    **Dose:** *Adult,* 1–2 grams in 100–250 ml saline IV over 15–30 min. Repeat in 1 hr if needed. May repeat every 8–12 hr. If severe, can give 0.5 gm/hr infusion. *Child,* 25–50 mg/kg IV over 15–30 min, no faster than 10 mg/kg/min. Maximal dose 12 grams/day.

    **Packaged:** 1 gram/20 ml vials.

Organophosphate insecticide (OPI) poisoning. Not usually needed in carbamate insecticide poisoning.

Most effective if started in first 24 hr before bonding of phosphate.

**AR:** Rapid IV injection has produced tachycardia, muscle rigidity, transient neuromuscular blockade. IM: conjunctival hyperemia, subconjunctival hemorrhage, especially if concentrations exceed 5%. Oral: nausea, vomiting, diarrhea, malaise.

Should be used only after initial treatment with atropine. Draw blood for erythrocyte cholinesterase level prior to giving 2-PAM. The use of 2-PAM may require a reduction in the dose of atropine.

**MP:** Monitor renal profile and reduce dose accordingly t½ = 1–2 hr. Reversal of OPI effects at 4 µg/ml of 2-PAM. Start early because "aging" of $PO_4$ on acetylcholinesterase makes it more difficult to reverse.

32. **Propranolol** (Inderal). Nonselective beta blocker.

    **Dose:** *Adult*, 0.1–0.15 mg/kg IV, administered in increments of 0.5 to 0.75 mg every 1–2 min with continuous ECG and blood pressure monitoring up to 10 mg. *Child*, 0.01–0.15 mg/kg per dose slow IV with repeat dose q 6–8 hr as needed.

    **Packaged:** 1 mg/ml; tablets: 10, 20, 40, 60, 80, 90 mg; capsules: 20, 80, 160 mg.

Cocaine intoxication.

Has not been scientifically proved to be safe and effective. Anecdotal reports only. Labetalol is theoretically preferred agent for cocaine intoxication.

**AR:** Bradycardia, hypotension, pallor; neurologic effects include hallucinations, coma, and seizures.

Not a specific antidote; used for catecholamine storm and dysrhythmias.

Increased mortality has been reported in animals that received propranolol for cocaine poisoning, and hypertension has occurred in humans following its use in cocaine intoxication.

---

\*This is for informational purposes and is not intended to substitute for independent judgment. It is always advisable to review the package insert for the most up-to-date information. Contact Regional Poison Control Center for additional details on use.

†This dose may exceed the manufacturer's recommended dose.

*Abbreviations:* AR = adverse reactions to antidotes; MP = monitor parameters; FDA = U.S. Food and Drug Administration; ECG = electrocardiogram; CNS = central nervous system; GI = gastrointestinal.

*Table continued on following page*

TABLE 4. **Antidotes*** *Continued*

| Medications | Indications | Comments |
|---|---|---|
| **33. Protamine sulfate.**<br>**Dose:** 1 mg neutralizes 90–115 U of heparin. Maximum dose 50 mg IV over 5 min at 10 mg/ml.<br>**Packaged:** 5 ml = 50 mg; 25 ml = 250 mg. | Heparin overdose.<br>**AR:** Rapid administration causes anaphylactoid reactions. | **MP:** Monitor thromboplastin times. Doses of up to 200 mg have been tolerated over 2 hr in an adult. |
| **34. Pyridoxine (Vitamin B₆).**<br>Gamma-aminobutyric acid agonist.<br>**Dose:** *Unknown amount ingested:* 5 grams over 5 min IV. *Known amount:* Add 1 gram of pyridoxine for each gram of INH ingested IV over 5 min.<br>**Packaged:** 50 and 100 mg/ml; 10 and 30 ml. | Isoniazid (INH), monomethylhydrazine mushrooms.<br>**AR:** Unlikely owing to the fact that vitamin B₂ is water soluble. However, nausea, vomiting, somnolence, and paresthesia have been reported from chronic high doses. | Pyridoxine is given as 5–10% solution IV mixed with water. It may be repeated every 5–20 min until seizures cease. Some administer pyridoxine over 30–60 min.<br>**MP:** Correct acidosis, monitor liver profile, acid-base parameters.<br>Lethal dose of pyridoxine is 1 gram/kg. |
| **35. Sodium bicarbonate.**<br>**Dose:** IV 1–3 mEq/kg as needed to keep pH 7.5 (generally 2 mEq/kg q 6 hr). When alkalinization is desired to correct acidosis to a pH of 7.3, use 2 mEq/kg to raise pH 0.1 unit.<br>**Packaged:** 50 ml, 44.6 mEq, 50 mEq ampule. | To promote urinary alkalinization for salicylates, phenobarbital (weak acids with low volume of distribution excreted in urine unchanged).<br>To correct severe acidosis.<br>To promote protein-binding and supply sodium ions into Purkinje cells in cyclic antidepressant intoxication.<br>**AR:** Large doses in patients with renal insufficiency may cause metabolic alkalosis. In patients with ketoacidosis, rapid alkalinization with sodium bicarbonate may result in clouding of consciousness, cerebral dysfunction, seizures, hypoxia, and lactic acidosis. | Alkaline diuresis. The assessment of the need for bicarbonate should be based on both the blood and urine pH. Maintain the blood pH at 7.5. Keep the urinary output at 3–6 ml/kg/hr.<br>May use a diuretic to enhance diuresis. Potassium is necessary to produce alkaline diuresis.<br>Monitor electrolytes, calcium, pH of both urine and blood, arterial blood gases. |
| **36. Sodium nitrite.** | See 14. Cyanide antidote kit. | |
| **37. Sodium thiosulfate.** | See 14. Cyanide antidote kit. | |
| **38. Vitamin K (AquaMEPHYTON)** Merck. Promotes hepatic biosynthesis of prothrombin and other coagulation factors. Competitive antagonist of warfarin. It may be administered orally in the absence of vomiting.<br>**Dose:** *Adult,* 2.5–10 mg IV, depending on potential for hemorrhage. Oral dose is 15–25 mg/day. Severe bleeding, 5–25 mg slow IV push. Rate 1 mg/min. Repeat q 4–8 hr depending on prothrombin time. *Child,* 1–5 mg IV may be given orally when vomiting ceases at a dose of 5–10 mg/day.<br>**Packaged:** 2 mg/ml in 0.5-ml ampules. 2.5- or 5-ml vials. | Warfarin (coumarin), superwarfarins, salicylate intoxication. | Fatalities from anaphylactic reaction have been reported following IV route. It takes 24 hr for vitamin K to be effective. The need for further vitamin K is determined by the prothrombin time test. If severe bleeding, fresh blood or plasma transfusion may be needed. |

*This is for informational purposes and is not intended to substitute for independent judgment. It is always advisable to review the package insert for the most up-to-date information. Contact Regional Poison Control Center for additional details on use.

*Abbreviations:* AR = adverse reactions to antidotes; MP = monitored parameters; FDA = U.S. Food and Drug Administration; ECG = electrocardiogram; CNS = central nervous system; GI = gastrointestinal.

TABLE 5. **Indications and Contraindications for Dialysis**

**Immediate Consideration of Dialysis**
Ethylene glycol with refractory acidosis
Methanol with refractory acidosis and levels consistently over 50 mg/dl
Lithium levels consistently elevated over 4 mEq/liter
*Amanita phalloides*

**Indications on Basis of Patient's Condition** (coma greater than Stage 3 of Reed Coma Scale)

| | |
|---|---|
| Alcohol* | Iodides |
| Ammonia | Isoniazid* |
| Amphetamines | Meprobamate |
| Anilines | Paraldehyde |
| Antibiotics | Potassium* |
| Barbiturates* (long-acting) | Quinidine |
| Boric acid | Quinine |
| Bromides* | Salicylates* |
| Calcium | Strychnine |
| Chloral hydrate* | Thiocyanates |
| Fluorides | (Certain other drugs also dialyzable) |

**Indicated for General Supportive Therapy**
Uncontrollable metabolic acidosis or alkalosis
Uncontrollable electrolyte disturbance, particularly sodium or potassium
Overhydration
Renal failure
Hyperosmolality not responding to conservative therapy
Marked hypothermia
Nonresponsive Stage 3 or greater coma (Reed Coma Scale)

**Contraindicated on Pharmacologic Basis Except for Supportive Care**
Antidepressants (tricyclic and monoamine oxidase inhibitors)
Antihistamines
Barbiturates (short-acting)
Belladonna alkaloids
Benzodiazepines (Valium, Librium)
Digitalis and derivatives
Hallucinogens
Meprobamate (Equanil, Miltown)
Methyprylon (Noludar)
Opioids (heroin, Lomotil)
Phenothiazines (Thorazine, Compazine)
Phenytoin (Dilantin)

*Most useful.

priate tests, including toxicologic analysis (10 ml of clotted blood, initial gastric aspirate, 100 ml of urine). The initial management of the comatose patient should include the administration of 100% oxygen, 100 mg of thiamine intravenously, 50% glucose as an intravenous bolus, and 2 to 10 mg of naloxone (Narcan) intravenously. Other causes associated with coma and mimicking intoxications should be eliminated by examination and laboratory tests (trauma, infection, cerebrovascular accident, hypoxia, and endocrine-metabolic causes).

*Pulmonary edema* complicating poisoning may be cardiac or noncardiac in origin. Fluid overload during forced diuresis may cause the cardiac variety, particularly if the drugs have an antidiuretic effect (opioids, barbiturates, and salicylates). Some toxic agents produce increased pulmonary capillary permeability, and other agents may cause a massive sympathetic discharge resulting in neurogenic pulmonary edema (opioids and salicylates). Management consists of minimizing the fluid administration; diuretics; and oxygen. If renal failure is present, dialysis may be necessary. The noncardiac type of pulmonary edema occurs with inhaled toxins such as ammonia, chlorine, and oxides of nitrogen, or with drugs such as salicylates, opioids, paraquat, and intravenous ethchlorvynol (Placidyl). This type does not respond to cardiac measures, and oxygen with intensive respiratory management using mechanical ventilation with positive end-expiratory pressure (PEEP) is necessary.

*Hypotension and circulatory shock* may be caused by heart failure due to myocardial depression, hypovolemia (fluid loss or venous pooling), decrease in peripheral vasculature resistance (adrenergic blockage), or loss of vasomotor tone caused by central nervous system depression.

*Renal failure* may be due to tubular necrosis as a result of hypotension, hypoxia, or a direct effect of the poison on the tubular cells (salicylate, paraquat, acetaminophen, carbon tetrachloride). Hemoglobinuria or myoglobinuria may precipitate in the renal tubules and produce renal failure.

*Cerebral edema* in intoxications is produced by hypoxia, hypercapnia, hypotension, hypoglycemia, and drug-impaired capillary integrity. Computed tomography may aid in diagnosis. Therapy consists of correction of the arterial blood gas and metabolic abnormalities and the hypotension. Re-

TABLE 6. **Plasma Concentrations Above Which Removal by Extracorporeal Means May Be Indicated***

| Drug | Plasma Concentration (mg/dl) | Method of Choice |
|---|---|---|
| Phenobarbital | 10 | HP>HD |
| Other barbiturates | 5 | HP |
| Glutethimide | 4 | HP |
| Methaqualone | 4 | HP |
| Salicylates | 80 | HD>HP |
| Ethchlorvynol | 15 | HP |
| Meprobamate | 10 | HP |
| Trichloroethanol | 5 | HP |
| Paraquat | 0.1 | HP>HD |
| Theophylline | 6 (chronic), 10 (acute) | HP |
| Methanol | 50 | HD |
| Ethylene glycol | Unknown | HD |
| Lithium | 4 mEq/liter | HD |
| Ethanol | 500 | HD |

*Modified from Haddad L and Winchester JF (eds): Clinical Management of Poisoning and Drug Overdose. Philadelphia, W. B. Saunders Co., 1983, p 162.

*Abbreviations:* HP = hemoperfusion; HD = hemodialysis.

duction of the increased intracranial pressure may be accomplished by 20% mannitol, 0.5 gram per kg, run in over a 30-minute period, and hyperventilation to reduce the $Pa_{CO_2}$ to 25 mmHg. The head should be elevated, and intracranial pressure monitoring should be considered. Fluid administration should be minimized.

*Seizures* are caused by many substances, such as amphetamines, camphor, chlorinated hydrocarbon insecticides, cocaine, isoniazid, lithium, phencyclidine, phenothiazines, propoxyphene, strychnine, tricyclic antidepressants, and drug withdrawal from ethanol and sedative-hypnotics. Recurring or protracted seizures require intravenous diazepam (Valium) and phenytoin.

*Cardiac dysrhythmias* occur with poisoning. A wide QT interval occurs with phenothiazines and a wide QRS interval occurs with tricyclic antidepressants, quinine, or quinidine overdose. Digitalis, cocaine, cyanide, propranolol, theophylline, and amphetamines are among the more frequent toxic causes of dysrhythmias. Correction of metabolic disturbances and adequate oxygenation will correct some of the dysrhythmias; others may require antidysrhythmic drugs or a cardiac pacemaker or cardioversion.

*Metabolic acidosis* with an increased anion gap is seen with many agents in overdose. Assessment of the arterial blood gases, electrolytes, and osmolality may be a clue to the etiologic agent. Intravenous sodium bicarbonate may be needed when the pH is below 7.1 if there is adequate ventilation.

*Hematemesis* can be produced by caustics and corrosives, iron, lithium, mercury, phosphorus, arsenic, mushrooms, plant poisons, fluoride, and organophosphates. Therapy consists of fluid and blood replacement and iced saline lavage if there is no esophageal damage.

## TOXICOKINETICS FOR THE PRACTICING PHYSICIAN

Toxicokinetics is clinical pharmacokinetics from the viewpoint of the toxicologist. Pharmacokinetics is a mathematical description of what the body does to a drug. Knowledge of the toxicokinetics of a specific toxic agent will allow the physician to plan a rational approach to the definitive management of the intoxicated patient after the vital functions have been stabilized.

The *LD*$_{50}$ (the lethal dose for 50% of experimental animals) and the *MLD* (the minimum lethal dose) are seldom relevant in human intoxications but indicate potential toxicity of the substance. *Protein binding* of toxic agents influences the volume distribution, elimination, and action of the drug. Diuresis and dialysis are usually reserved for drugs with less than 50% protein binding. The *therapeutic blood range* is the concentration of any drug at which the majority of the treated population can be expected to receive therapeutic benefit. The *toxic blood range* is the concentration at which this majority would be expected to have toxic manifestations. The range is not an absolute value. *Blood concentrations* are a quantitative aid in determining whether more specific measures need to be instituted in correlation with the clinical manifestations. The *apparent volume distribution (Vd)* is the percentage of body mass in which the drug is distributed. It is determined by dividing the amount absorbed by the blood concentration. When a substance has a large volume distribution, as in most lipid-soluble chemicals (above 1 liter per kg), and is concentrated in the body fat, it will not be available for diuresis, dialysis, or exchange transfusion. *Elimination routes* of detoxification will allow the physician to make therapeutic decisions, such as using ethanol to interfere with the metabolism of methanol and ethylene glycol into more toxic metabolites. *Urine identification* is usually qualitative and allows only the identification of an agent.

*Never manage a poisoned patient solely by laboratory tests, and always treat according to the manifestations of poisoning, not the laboratory test results.* The laboratory toxicology analyst should be given whatever historical information is available so that the agent can be sought and identified as rapidly as possible. Toxicologic analysis is like a miniresearch project, unlike most other laboratory tests. *Specimens* for toxicologic analysis require the patient's name, date, time of exposure, time specimen was drawn, therapeutic drugs administered, patient's manifestations, and other relevant data. The toxicologic specimens that should be obtained for analysis are (1) vomitus or initial gastric aspiration, (2) blood, 10 ml (ask the analyst about the type of container and anticoagulant), and (3) urine, 100 ml.

## COMMON POISONS AND THERAPY

*Abbreviations Used in Following List of Common Poisons*

| | |
|---|---|
| t½ | = half-life (time required for blood level to drop by 50% of the original value) |
| Vd | = volume of distribution (liter per kg) |
| TLV | = threshold limit value in air |
| TWA | = time-weighted average |
| PPM | = parts per million in air and water |

*Conversion Factors*

| | |
|---|---|
| 1 gram | = 1000 milligrams (mg) |
| 1 milligram (mg) | = 1000 micrograms (μg) |
| 1 microgram (μg) | = 1000 nanograms (ng) |

Standard International Units:

| 1 mole | = mol wt in grams per liter |
| 1 millimole | = mol wt in milligrams per liter |
| 1 micromole | = mol wt in micrograms per liter |

Blood levels:

| 1 microgram per ml | = 100 micrograms per dl |
| | = 1 milligram per liter |
| | = 1000 nanograms per ml |
| 100 mg per dl | = 0.1 gram per dl |
| | = 1000 mg (1 gram) per liter |
| | = 1 mg per ml |

**Acetaminophen, APAP** (Tylenol). *Toxic dose:* Child, 3 grams or more; adult, 7.5 grams or more. Liver toxicity, 140 mg per kg. *Toxicokinetics:* Absorption time, 0.5 to 1 hour. Vd, 0.9 liter per kg. Route of elimination by liver. Draw peak blood level after 4 hours in overdose. *Manifestations:* First 24 hours: malaise, nausea, vomiting, and drowsiness, followed by a latent period of 24 hours to 5 days; then hepatic symptoms, disturbances in clotting mechanism, and renal damage. *Management:* (1) Activated charcoal may be given when *N*-acetylcysteine is contemplated. In these circumstances, the loading dose of *N*-acetylcysteine is given twice. (2) *N*-Acetylcysteine for toxic overdose (Antidote 1, Table 4). Start and give a full course if a toxic dose has been ingested or if blood concentrations are above the toxic line on the nomogram shown in Figure 1. (3) In this instance, a saline sulfate cathartic is preferred to sorbitol. *Laboratory aids:* APAP level, optimally at 4 to 6 hours. Plot levels on nomogram in Figure 1 as a guide for treatment. Monitor liver and renal profiles daily.

**Acids.** See Caustics and Corrosives.

**Alcohols**

1. **Ethanol** (grain alcohol). *Manifestations:* Blood ethanol levels over 30 mg per dl produce euphoria; over 50, incoordination and intoxication; over 100, ataxia; over 300, stupor; and over 500, coma. Levels of 500 to 700 mg per dl may be fatal. Chronic alcoholic patients tolerate higher levels, and the correlation may not be valid. *Management:* (1) Gastrointestinal decontamination up to 1 hour postingestion. Activated charcoal and cathartics are not indicated. (2) Give 0.25 gram per kg of dextrose, 25 to 50%, intravenously if the blood glucose level is less than 60 mg per dl. (3) Thiamine, 100 mg intravenously, if chronic alcoholism is suspected, to prevent Wernicke-Korsakoff syndrome. (4) Hemodialysis is indicated in severe cases when conventional therapy is ineffective (rarely needed). (5) Treat seizures with diazepam (Valium) followed by phenytoin (Dilantin) if unresponsive. (6) Treat withdrawal with hydration and chlordiazepoxide (Librium) or diazepam. Large doses of sedatives may be required for delirium tremens. *Laboratory aids:* Arterial blood gases, electrolytes, blood ethanol levels, glucose; determine anion and osmolar gap and check for ketosis. Chest radiograph to determine whether aspiration pneumonia is present. Liver function tests and bilirubin levels.

2. **Isopropanol** (rubbing alcohol). Normal propyl alcohol is related to isopropanol but is more toxic. *Manifestations:* Ethanol-like intoxication with acetone odor to breath, acetonuria, acetonemia without systemic acidosis, gastritis. *Management:* (1) Gastrointestinal decontamination. Activated charcoal and cathartics not indicated. (2) Hemodialysis in life-threatening overdose (rarely needed). *Laboratory aids:* Isopropyl alcohol levels, acetone, glucose, and arterial blood gases.

3. **Methanol** (wood alcohol). *Toxic dose:* One teaspoonful is potentially lethal for a 2-year-old child and can cause blindness in an adult. The toxic blood level of methanol is above 20 mg per dl, the potentially fatal level over 50 mg per dl. *Manifestations:* Hyperemia of optic disk, violent abdominal colic, blindness, and shock. *Management:* (1) Gastrointestinal decontamination. Activated charcoal and cathartics are not indicated. (2) Treat acidosis vigorously with sodium bicarbonate intravenously. (3) If clinically suspect methanol because of metabolic acidosis, with an anion gap if methanol concentration above 20 mg per dl, immediately initiate ethanol IV or PO to produce a blood ethanol concentration of 100 to 150 mg per dl (Antidote 20, Table 4). (4) Folinic acid and folic acid have been used successfully in animal investigations. Administer leucovorin, 1 mg per kg up to 50 mg IV every 4 hours for six doses. (5) Consider hemodialysis if the blood methanol level is greater than 50 mg per dl or if significant metabolic acidosis or visual or mental symptoms are present. *Note:* The ethanol dose has to be increased during dialysis therapy. (6) Continue therapy (ethanol and hemodialysis) until blood methanol level is preferably undetectable and there are no acidosis and no mental or visual disturbances. This will often require 2 to 5 days. (7) Ophthalmology consultation. *Laboratory aids:* Methanol and ethanol levels, electrolytes, glucose, and arterial blood gases.

**Alkali.** See Caustics and Corrosives.

**Amitriptyline** (Elavil). See Tricyclic Antidepressants.

**Amphetamines** (diet pills, various trade names). *Toxicity:* Child, 5 mg per kg; adult, 12 mg per kg has been reported as lethal. *Toxicokinetics:* Peak time of action is 2 to 4 hours. t½, 8 to 10 hours in acid urine (pH less than 6.0) and 16 to 31 hours in alkaline urine (pH, 7.5). *Route of elimination:* Liver, 60%; kidney, 30 to 40% at alkaline urine pH; at acid urine pH, 50 to 70%. *Manifestations:* Dysrhythmias, hyperpyrexia, convulsions, hypertension, paranoia, violence. *Management:* (1) Gastrointestinal de-contamination. Avoid induced emesis because of rapid onset of action. (2) Control extreme agitation or convulsions with diazepam. Chlorpromazine (Thorazine) may be dangerous if ingestion is not pure amphetamine. (3) Treat hypertensive crisis with nitroprusside. (4) Acidification diuresis is not recommended. (5) Treat hyperpyrexia symptomatically. (6) If focal neurologic symptoms, consider cerebrovascular accident. Obtain computed axial tomography scan. (7) Observe for suicidal depression that may follow intoxication. (8) In life-threatening agitation use haloperidol (Haldol). (9) Significant life-threatening tachydysrhythmia may respond to the alpha and beta blocker labetalol (Normodyne; Antidote 23, Table 4) or other appropriate antidysrhythmic agents. In a severely hemodynamically compromised patient, use immediate synchronized cardioversion. *Laboratory aids:* Monitor for rhabdomyolysis (creatine phosphokinase [CPK]), myoglobinuria, hyperkalemia,

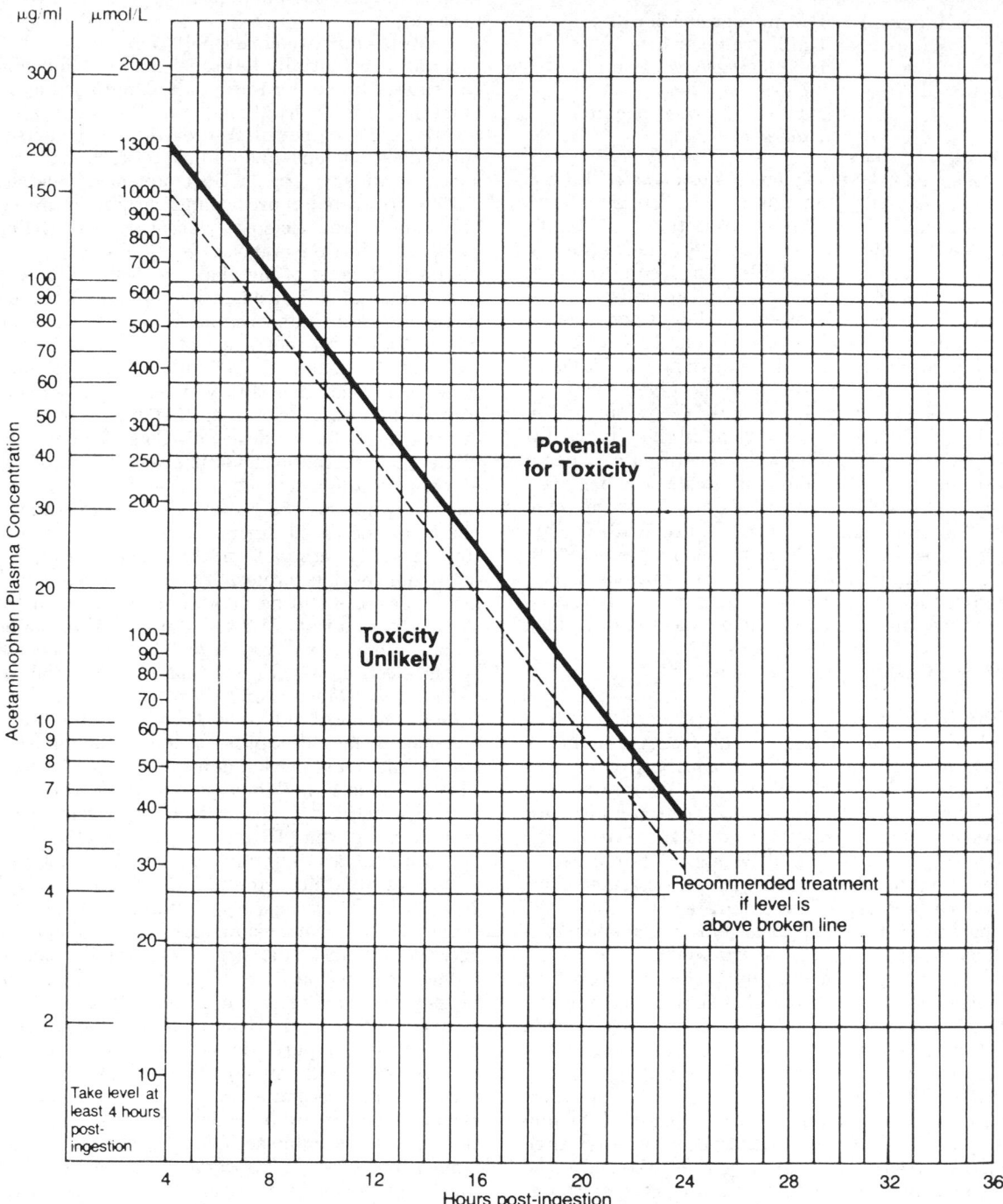

**Figure 1.** Nomogram for acetaminophen intoxication. Start *N*-acetylcysteine therapy if levels and time coordinates are above the lower line on the nomogram. Continue and complete therapy even if subsequent values fall below the toxic zone. The nomogram is useful only in acute, single ingestions. Serum levels drawn before 4 hours may not represent peak levels. (From Rumack BH and Matthew H: Acetaminophen poisoning and toxicity. Reproduced by permission of Pediatrics *55*:871, 1975.)

TABLE 7. **Toxicokinetics of Anticholinergic Agents**

| Drug | Potential Fatal Dose | Peak Effect | Vd (Liters/kg) | t½ (hr) | Excretion Route (%) |
|------|----------------------|-------------|----------------|---------|---------------------|
| Atropine | Child: 10–20 mg; adult: 100 mg | 1–2 hr, may be prolonged in overdose | 2.3 | 2–3 | Renal (30–50) hepatic (50–70) |
| Diphenhydramine | 20–40 mg/kg; 2 oz has been fatal in 2-year-old child | 3–4 hr, may be prolonged in overdose | 3–4 | 5–8 | Renal (some hepatic) |

and disseminated intravascular coagulation. Toxic blood level, 10 µg per dl.

**Aniline.** See Nitrites and Nitrates.

**Anticholinergic Agents.** Examples are antihistamines—hydroxyline (Atarax), diphenhydramine (Benadryl); antipsychotics (neuroleptics)—phenothiazines (Thorazine); antidepressant drugs (tricyclic antidepressants)—imipramine (Tofranil); antiparkinsonian drugs—trihexyphenidyl (Artane), benztropine (Cogentin); over-the-counter sleep, cold, and hayfever medicine (methapyrilene); ophthalmic products (atropine); plants—jimsonweed *(Datura stramonium),* deadly nightshade *(Atropa belladonna),* henbane *(Hyoscyamus niger);* and antispasmodic agents for the bowel (atropine). *Toxicokinetics:* See Table 7. *Manifestations:* Anticholinergic signs—hyperpyrexia, dilated pupils, flushing of skin, dry mucosa, tachycardia, delirium, hallucinations, coma, and convulsions. *Management:* (1) Gastrointestinal decontamination up to 12 hours postingestion. (2) Control seizures with diazepam. (3) Control ventricular dysrhythmias with lidocaine. (4) Physostigmine (Antidote 30, Table 4) for life-threatening anticholinergic effects refractory to conventional treatments. (5) Treat urinary retention. (6) Treat cardiac dysrhythmias only if tissue perfusion is not adequate or if the patient is hypotensive.

**Anticonvulsants.** See Table 8. *Toxic dose:* Specific anticonvulsant blood levels and the clinical manifestations will indicate toxicity. In general, the ingestion of five times the therapeutic dose is expected to have the potential for toxicity. *Management:* (1) Gastrointestinal decontamination up to 12 hours postingestion. Repeated doses of activated charcoal will shorten t½ of carbamazepine, phenobarbital, primidone, phenytoin, and possibly others. (2) Monitor specific anticonvulsant blood levels. (3) The effectiveness of hemoperfusion and dialysis has not been established.

**Antidepressants.** See Tricyclic Antidepressants.

**Antifreeze.** See Alcohols (Methanol) and Ethylene Glycol.

**Antihistamines (H₁ Receptor Antagonists).** See Anticholinergic Agents.

**Arsenic and Arsine Gas.** *Toxic dose:* In humans, the inorganic arsenic trioxide toxic dose is 5 to 50 mg; the potential fatal dose is 120 mg or 1 to 2 mg per kg. Sodium arsenite is nine times more toxic than arsenic trioxide. Organic arsenic is less toxic. The maximum allowable concentration for prolonged exposure is 0.05 PPM. See Table 9. Humans are more sensitive than rodents to arsenic. Acute poisoning results from accidental ingestion of arsenic-containing pesticides. (Ant traps sold in some states contain arsenic.) *Toxicokinet-*

TABLE 8. **Anticonvulsants**

| Drug | Peak Time of Action/Hr (Steady State) | Vd (Liters/kg) | t½ (hr) | Route of Elimination (%) | Protein Binding (%) | Blood Level (µg/ml) | Comment* |
|------|----------------------------------------|----------------|---------|--------------------------|---------------------|---------------------|----------|
| Carbamazepine (Tegretol) | 8–24 (2–4 days) | 1.0 | 18–54 | Liver (98) | 70 | Therapeutic, 5–12 | Related to tricyclic antidepressants, can cause dysrhythmias |
| Ethosuximide (Zarontin) | 24–48 (5–8 days) | 0.8 | 36–56 | Liver (80–90) Renal (10–20) | 0 | Therapeutic, 40–100 | |
| Phenytoin (Dilantin) | PO, 6–12 IV, 1 (5–10 days) | 0.6–1.0 | 20–30; varies in toxic doses: zero-order kinetics | Liver (95) | 87–93 | Therapeutic, 10–20; toxic, 20–30; nystagmus only, 30–40; ataxia, 40+; coma, convulsions | Dysrhythmias with parenteral use only |
| Primidone (Mysoline) | 3–4? (4–7 days) | 0.6 | Parent, 3–12; metabolites, 30–36 | Liver | 60 | Therapeutic, 6–12 primidone and 15–40 phenobarbital (PB); toxic, over 50 primidone and over 40 PB (see Barbiturates) | Metabolized to active metabolites phenylethylmalonamide and PB; overdose gives white crystals in urine† |
| Valproic acid (Depakene) | ? (1–2 days) | 0.4 | 5–15 | Liver (80–100) | 20 | Therapeutic, 60–100 | Produces nausea and vomiting, changes in liver function |
| Clonazepam (Clonopin) | ? (4–12 days) | | 20–60 | Liver (98) | 90 | Therapeutic, 20–70 ng/ml | |

*Manifestations: The major manifestations of these agents are depression of consciousness and respiratory depression. Other significant manifestations are mentioned in this column.

†Primidone produces whorls of shimmering white crystals in the urine from precipitation of intact primidone in massive overdose.

TABLE 9. **Comparative Acute Toxicities of Some Common Arsenicals***

| Arsenical | Oral LD$_{50}$ in Rats (mg/kg) | Estimated Mortality in Human Poisoning (%) |
|---|---|---|
| Arsenic trioxide | 385 | 12 |
| Sodium arsenite | 42 | 65 |
| Calcium arsenite | ca. 275 | ? |
| Lead arsenite | 1500+ | 5 |
| Ortho Crabgrass Killer† | 3719 | None known |

*From Done AK: . . . And old lace. Emerg Med 5:246, 1973. Used by permission.

†Product containing 8% each of only mildly toxic octyl NH$_4$ and dodecyl NH$_4$ methanearsonate.

ics: Rapidly absorbed by inhalation and ingestion. Crosses placenta and can cause fetal damage. Distributes into spleen, liver, kidneys. *Excretion:* In urine, 90%. Following acute ingestion, it takes 10 days to clear a single dose; chronic ingestion takes up to 70 days. *Arsine gas:* Forms when active hydrogen comes in contact with arsenic. This may occur when zinc, antimony, lead, or iron is contaminated with arsenic and comes in contact with acid. This causes arsine inhalation intoxication characterized by a latent period of 2 to 48 hours and a triad of abdominal pain, jaundice (due to hemolysis), and hematuria. *Manifestations:* Gastroenteritis, neurologic and cardiac abnormalities, subsequent renal involvement. A garlic odor to the breath may be a clue. Smaller doses and prolonged low-level exposure produce subacute (stomatitis) and chronic (peripheral neuropathy) symptoms.

*Management:* (1) Gastrointestinal decontamination. Follow with abdominal radiographs, as arsenic is radiopaque. Consider whole-bowel washout if usual methods fail to remove arsenic. (2) Intravenous fluids to correct dehydration and electrolyte deficiencies. (3) Treat shock with oxygen, blood, and fluids as needed. (4) In severe cases, administer BAL (dimercaprol) (Antidote 17, Table 4). (5) In chronic poisoning, D-penicillamine (Antidote 29, Table 4) may be used to chelate arsenic. Therapy should be continued in 5-day cycles until the urine arsenic is less than 50 μg per liter. (6) Hemodialysis is effective in acute poisoning and can be used concurrently with chelation therapy in severe cases, especially if renal failure develops. (7) Arsine intoxication is treated by exchange transfusion and hemodialysis if renal failure occurs. BAL is ineffective. *Laboratory aids:* Blood arsenic and 24-hour urine arsenic levels. Excessive exposure is indicated by a level of 50 μg per liter of arsenic in urine, but persons whose diets are rich in seafood may excrete 200 μg per day. View values over 100 micrograms per day with suspicion. Monitor electrocardiogram (ECG) and renal function. A blood arsenic level above 1.0 mg per liter is toxic and one of 9 to 15 mg per liter is potentially fatal (false values occur in inexperienced laboratories).

**Aspirin.** See Salicylates.

**Atropine.** See Anticholinergic Agents.

**Barbiturates.** See Table 10. *Management:* (1) Gastrointestinal decontamination up to 8 to 12 hours. Avoid emesis in short-acting barbiturates. Activated charcoal and a cathartic in repeated doses have been

TABLE 10. **Barbiturates: Examples and Elimination***

| | Long Acting | | Intermediate | Short Acting | |
|---|---|---|---|---|---|
| Generic name | Barbital | Phenobarbital | Amobarbital | Pentobarbital | Secobarbital |
| Trade name | Veronal | Luminal | Amytal | Nembutal | Seconal |
| Slang name | — | Purple hearts | Blue heaven | Yellow jackets | Red devils |
| pKa | 7.74 | 7.24 | 7.25 | 7.96 | 7.9 |
| Detoxification | Renal | Renal 30%, hepatic 70% | Hepatic 98% | Hepatic 90–100% | Hepatic 90–100% |
| Onset: IV | 22 min | 12 min | — | 15–30 min | 10–30 min |
|     PO | Over 1 hr | 20–60 min (peak 6–18 hr) | 15–30 min (peak 3–4 hr) | 10–15 min (peak 2–4 hr) | 10–15 min (peak 2–4 hr) |
| Protein binding (%) | 5 | 20–40 | — | 35 | 44 |
| Hypnotic dose (mg) | 300–500 | 100–200 | 50–200 | 50–100 | 50–100 |
| Fatal dose (grams) | 10 | 8 | 5 | 3 | 3 |
| Toxic dose (mg/kg) | 8 | 15–35 | Over 6 | 3–5 | 3–5 |
| Therapeutic level (μg/ml) | 5–8 | 15–40 | 5–6 | 1–4 | 3–5 |
| Toxic level (μg/ml) | Over 30 | Over 40 | 10–30 | Over 10 | Over 10 |
| Lethal level† (μg/ml) | Over 100 | Over 100 | Over 50 | Over 35 | Over 35 |
| Duration of action (hr) | Over 16 | Over 6 | 6 hr | 6 hr | 6 hr |
| Half-life (hr) | 58–96 | 50–120 | 8–42 | 15–48 | 19–34 |
| Rate of metabolism (hr) | — | 0.7 | 2.5 | — | — |
| Volume distribution (liters/kg) | — | 0.75 | 0.5–1.1 | 0.65–1.5 | 0.65–1.5 |

Manifestations

  Low dose: Euphoria, ataxia, incoordination, nystagmus on lateral gaze

  High dose: Flaccid coma, hypotension, respiratory depression, pulmonary edema (particularly with the short-acting barbiturates), subcutaneous bullae (6%), dermatographia

*Classification into long acting, intermediate, and short acting has no relationship to the duration of coma.

†These levels are not absolute, and tolerance occurs.

shown to reduce the serum half-life and increase the nonrenal clearance over 50%. Give every 4 hours while the patient is comatose. (2) Supportive and symptomatic care is all that is necessary in the majority of cases. (3) Alkalinization with sodium bicarbonate, 2 mEq per kg IV during the first hour, followed by sufficient sodium bicarbonate (Antidote 35, Table 4) to keep the urinary pH at 7.5 to 8.0, enhances excretion of long-acting barbiturates. Forced diuresis should be used with caution because of fluid overload. At present, alkalinization without diuresis is advocated. (4) In severe cases that do not respond to conservative measures, consider hemodialysis and hemoperfusion. (5) Treat any bullae as a local second-degree skin burn. (6) Give intensive care monitoring to the comatose patient. *Treatment of withdrawal: In an emergency,* use thiopental pentothal (2/2) or diazepam intravenously. If the patient is stable, a pentobarbital tolerance test may be given; 200 mg of pentobarbital is given orally and the patient examined after 1 hour for signs of intoxication (nystagmus, slurred speech, and ataxia). If none are present, the dose is repeated every 3 hours until these signs develop. This is the stabilizing dose; the patient is maintained on this dose for 72 hours and then changed to phenobarbital, 30 mg substituted for each 100 mg of pentobarbital. The pheno-

barbital is tapered, decreasing by 10% or 30 mg every 3 to 5 days. *Laboratory aids:* Emergency plasma barbiturate concentrations rarely alter management.

**Benzene.** See Hydrocarbons.

**Benzodiazepines** (BZP). See Table 11. *Toxicity:* Low toxic potential. More than 500 mg has been ingested without respiratory depression. Benzodiazepines have an additive effect with sedatives such as alcohol and barbiturates. Most patients intoxicated with benzodiazepines alone recover within 24 hours. Many of these agents have active metabolites with a long plasma t½, so performance in skilled tasks such as driving may be impaired. Withdrawal may be delayed. *Manifestations:* CNS depression. Deep coma leading to respiratory depression suggests presence of other drugs. *Management:* (1) Gastrointestinal decontamination. (2) Supportive and symptomatic care. (3) Withdrawal, if it occurs, is treated with a long-acting benzodiazepine on a tapering schedule. *Laboratory aids:* Document benzodiazepines in urine. Quantitative blood levels are not useful.

**Bleach.** Household bleaches are 4 to 6% sodium hypochlorite. Commercial types are 10 to 20%. *Manifestations:* Difficulty in swallowing; pain in mouth, throat, chest, or abdomen. General household strength bleach does not produce burns; commercial strength bleach

TABLE 11. **Benzodiazepines (BZP)**

| Drug | Oral Dosage Range | Peak Oral Plasma Levels (hr) | Half-Life (hr) | Major Active Metabolites (Half-life in hr) | Elimination Rate |
|---|---|---|---|---|---|
| **ANXIOLYTICS** | | | | | |
| Diazepam (Valium) | 6–40 mg/day | 1–2 | 20–50 | Desmethyldiazepam (30–60) | Slow |
| Chlordiazepoxide (Librium, Libritabs, various others) | 15–100 mg/day | 2–4 | 5–30 | Desmethylchlordiazepoxide, demoxepam, desmethyldiazepam | Slow |
| Clorazepate (Tranxene) | 15–60 mg/day | 1–2.5 | 30–60 | Desmethyldiazepam | Slow |
| Prazepam (Centrax) | 20–60 mg/day | 6 | 78 | 3-Hydroxyprazepam, desmethyldiazepam | Slow |
| Halazepam (Paxipam) | 60–160 mg/day | 1–3 | 7 | N-3-Hydroxyhalazepam, desmethyldiazepam | Slow |
| Oxazepam (Serax) | 30–120 mg/day | 1–2 | 3–10 | None | Rapid to intermediate |
| Lorazepam (Ativan) | 2–6 mg/day | 2 | 10–20 | None | Intermediate |
| Alprazolam (Xanax) | 0.75–4 mg/day | 0.7–1.6 | 12–19 | α-Hydroxyalprazolam | Intermediate |
| **HYPNOTICS** | | | | | |
| Flurazepam (Dalmane) | 15–60 mg | 3–6 | 50–100 | Desalkylflurazepam (50–100) | Slow |
| Midazolam (Versed) | 5–30 mg/day IV | 0.3–0.8 | 3–5 | None | — |
| Flunitrazepam (Rohypnol— investigational, Roche) | 1–2 mg | <1 | — | 7-Aminoflunitrazepam (23), N-desmethylflunitrazepam (31) | — |
| Temazepam (Restoril) | 15–30 mg | 2–3 | 9–12 | None | Intermediate |
| Triazolam (Halcion) | 0.125–0.5 mg | 0.5–1.5 | 2–3 | α-Hydroxytriazolam | Rapid |
| **ANTICONVULSANT** | | | | | |
| Clonazepam (Klonopin) | 1.5–20 mg/day | 1–4 | 24–48 | None | — |

TABLE 12. **Kinetics and Other Actions of Calcium Channel Blockers**

| Parameter | Nifedipine (Procardia) | Verapamil (Calan, Isoptin) | Diltiazem (Cardiazem) |
|---|---|---|---|
| Bioavailability (%) | 65 | 20 | <40 |
| Dose | | | |
|   Adult, PO (mg/day) | 30 | 240 | 90 |
|   Maximum mg/day | 120–180 | 480–720 | 240–360 |
|   IV (mg/kg) | 0.1 | — | |
| Preparations | 10- and 20-mg tablets | 80- and 120-mg tablets | 30-, 60-, 90-, and 120-mg tablets |
| Slow release | 480-mg capsules | | |
| Onset of action (min) | | | |
|   PO | <20 | <30 | <15 |
|   IV | <1 | <1 | — |
|   Sublingual | 3 | — | — |
| Peak effect | | | |
|   PO | 1–2 hr | 5 hr | 1–2 hr |
|   IV | | 5–15 min | |
|   Sublingual | 20 min | | |
| Peak blood concentration (min) | 30–60 | 90–120 | 120–180 |
| $t\frac{1}{2}$ (hr) | 3–5 | 3–7 | 4–9 |
| Protein binding (%) | 90 | 90 | 90 |
| Vd (liters/kg) | 3 | 4.5–7 | 4–5 |
| Elimination | Hepatic | Hepatic | Hepatic |
| Toxic blood concentration (ng/ml) | >100 | >300 | >200 |
| Coronary vasodilation | + + + | + + | + + |
| Peripheral vasodilation | + + + | + + | + |
| Negative inotropy | − | + | + |
| Slow atrioventricular conduction | − | + + | + |
| Preload | Decrease | — | Decrease |
| Heart rate | Increase | Decrease | Decrease |

may. Inhalation of gases produced by mixing chlorine bleach with acids (toilet bowl cleaner and rust removers—chlorine gas) or with household ammonia (chloramine gas) is irritating to mucous membranes, eyes, and upper respiratory tract. *Management:* (1) Ingestion—Avoid GI decontamination procedures. Dilute with small amounts of water or milk. Avoid acids. (2) Esophagoscopy only if unusually large amounts have been ingested, the patient is symptomatic, or the product was stronger than the average household bleach. (3) Inhalation—Remove from contaminated area. Observe for pulmonary edema. (4) Ocular exposure requires immediate gentle irrigation with water for at least 15 minutes, followed by fluorescein dye stain for damage.

**Botulism.** See article Food-Borne Illness in Section 2.

**Brake Fluid.** See Ethylene Glycol.

**Calcium Channel Blockers.** Used in treatment of effort angina and supraventricular tachycardia. See Table 12. *Manifestations:* Hypotension, bradycardia within 1 to 5 hours, CNS depression, and gastric distress. *Management:* (1) Gastrointestinal decontamination. (2) Treat hypotension and bradycardia with positioning, fluids, and calcium gluconate or chloride (see Antidote 12B, Table 4). Dopamine or norepinephrine may be used if necessary. (3) Heart block—may respond to intravenous calcium (Antidote 12B, Table 4) or atropine sulfate, 0.5 to 1 mg, if no response. (4) Ventricular pacing may be required in the severely intoxicated patient. (5) Patients receiving digitalis run the risk of toxicity and should be carefully monitored. *Laboratory*

*aids:* Specific drug levels, blood sugar and calcium, electrocardiogram (ECG).

**Camphor** (External analgesic rubs, Vicks Vaporub 4.8%, Campho-Phenique 11%). Many camphorated oil products were removed from the marketplace in September, 1982. Five milliliters of camphorated oil (20% camphor) equals 1 gram of camphor. *Toxicity:* Adult, 5 grams; child, 1 gram has been fatal. *Toxicokinetics:* Onset of manifestations, 5 to 90 minutes. Readily and rapidly absorbed through the skin, mucous membranes, and gastrointestinal tract, and crosses the placenta. Route of elimination: Rapidly metabolized in liver to the glucuronide form, which is excreted in urine. Pulmonary excretion causes a distinctive odor on the breath. *Manifestations:* Nausea, vomiting, and burning epigastric pain. Seizures may occur suddenly and without warning within 5 minutes of ingestion. Apnea and vision disturbances may occur. *Management:* (1) Induction of emesis is contraindicated because of early seizures. (2) Remove residual drug by gastric lavage. (3) Administer activated charcoal and a saline cathartic. Avoid giving oils or alcohol. (4) Treat seizures with intravenous diazepam. (5) Treat apnea with respiratory support.

**Carbon Monoxide (CO).** This is an odorless gas produced from incomplete combustion; it is found also as an in vivo metabolic breakdown product of methylene chloride (paint removers). Observe for the symptoms described in Table 13. Contrary to popular belief, the skin rarely shows a cherry-red color in the live patient. *Toxicokinetics:* CO is rapidly absorbed through the

TABLE 13. Carbon Monoxide (CO)

| CO in Atmosphere (PPM) | Duration of Exposure | Saturation of Blood (%) | Symptoms |
|---|---|---|---|
| Up to 0.01 | Indefinite | 1–10 | None |
| 0.01–0.02 | Indefinite | 10–20 | Tightness across forehead, slight headache, dilation of cutaneous vessels |
| 0.02–0.03 | 5–6 hr | 20–30 | Headache, throbbing temples |
| 0.04–0.06 | 4–5 hr | 30–40 | Severe headache, weakness and dizziness, nausea and vomiting, collapse, leukocytosis |
| 0.07–0.10 | 3–4 hr | 40–50 | Above, plus increased tendency to collapse and syncope, increased pulse and respiratory rate |
| 0.11–0.15 | 1.5–3 hr | 50–60 | Increased pulse and respiratory rate, syncope, Cheyne-Stokes respiration, coma with intermittent convulsions |
| 0.16–0.30 | 1–1.5 hr | 60–70 | Coma with intermittent convulsions, depressed heart action and respirations, death possible |
| 0.50–1.00 | 1–2 hr | 70–80 | Weak pulse, depressed respirations, respiratory failure, and death |

lungs. The rate of absorption is directly related to alveolar ventilation. Elimination occurs through the lungs. The $t\frac{1}{2}$ in room air equals 5 to 6 hours; in 100 per cent oxygen, 90 minutes; in hyperbaric oxygen, 20 minutes. The nomogram pictured in Figure 2 can be used to decide quickly whether serious CO intoxication is likely to have occurred and to select patients at high risk or who need early management in the intensive care unit or hyperbaric oxygen.

*Management:* (1) Remove the patient from contaminated area and expose to fresh air. Establish vital functions. (2) Give 100% oxygen to all patients until the carboxyhemoglobin level falls to 5% or less. Assisted ventilation may be necessary. The exposed pregnant woman should be kept in 100% oxygen for several hours after the carboxyhemoglobin level is zero because carboxyhemoglobin concentrates in the fetus and oxygen are needed five times longer to ensure elimination of CO from fetal circulation. CO or hypoxia may be teratogenic. (3) Monitor arterial blood gases and carboxyhemoglobin levels. Determine carboxyhemoglobin level at time of exposure by using nomogram. *Note:* A near-normal carboxyhemoglobin level does not rule out significant CO poisoning. (4) Only if pH is below 7.1 after correction of hypoxia and adequate ventilation, give sodium bicarbonate to correct acidosis. (5) Indications for 100% oxygen and if possible therapy with hyperbaric oxygen: (a) carboxyhemoglobin level higher than 25%; (b) carboxyhemoglobin level higher than 15% in a child or in a patient with cardiovascular disease; (c) carboxyhemoglobin level higher than 10% in a pregnant woman (and monitor fetus); (d) abnormal or ischemic chest pain or ECG abnormality; (e) abnormal chest x-ray; (f) presence of hypoxia, myoglobinuria, or abnormal renal function; (g) history of unconsciousness, syncope, or neuropsychiatric symptoms. A list of hyperbaric oxygen chambers can be obtained by contacting a regional poison control center. (6) Treat seizures with intravenous diazepam. (7) Monitor ECG, chest radiograph, and serum CPK and lactate dehydrogenase levels. (8) Treat cerebral edema with elevation of the patient's head,

minimizing intravenous fluid, hyperventilation, and, if needed, mannitol and intracranial pressure monitor. (9) Re-evaluate after recovery for neuropsychiatric sequelae. *Laboratory aids:* Arterial blood gases show metabolic acidosis and normal oxygen tension but reduced oxygen saturation.

**Carbon Tetrachloride.** See Hydrocarbons.

**Caustics and Corrosives.** Common acid substances are hydrochloric acid, sulfuric acid (battery acid), carbolic acid (phenol), nitric acid, oxalic acid, hydrofluoric acid, and aqua regia (mixture of hydrochloric and nitric acids). These are used as cleaning agents. Common alkali substances are sodium or potassium hydroxide (lye), sodium hypochlorite (Clorox) (bleach), sodium carbonate (nonphosphate detergents), potassium permanganate, ammonia, electric dishwashing agents, cement, and flat disk batteries. *Toxicity:* Acids produce mucosal coagulation necrosis. They usually do not penetrate deeply (exception: hydrofluoric acid). The gastric mucosa is the primary site of injury. Alkalis produce liquefaction necrosis and saponification and penetrate deeply. Oropharyngeal and esophageal damage by solids is more frequent than by liquids. Liquids are more likely to produce gastric damage. *Toxic dose:* Adult potential fatal dose of concentrated acid/alkali is 5 ml. The absence of oral burns does not exclude the possibility of esophageal burns (10 to 15%).

*Management:* (1) Dilute with milk or water immediately up to 30 ml in children or 250 ml in adults. Neutralization with acidic or alkalinic agents is contraindicated. Dilute only if patient can swallow. (2) Gastrointestinal decontamination is contraindicated. However, in acid ingestions some authorities advocate nasogastric intubation and aspiration in the early postingestion phase. Patient should receive only intravenous fluids following dilution until surgical consultation is obtained. Dermal and ocular decontamination should be carried out. (3) Endoscopy at 12 to 48 hours may be indicated postingestion to assess severity of burn. (4) Steroids are controversial. Some recommend administration of steroids if burns are found or esophagoscopy is not performed. (5) Antibiotics are not useful

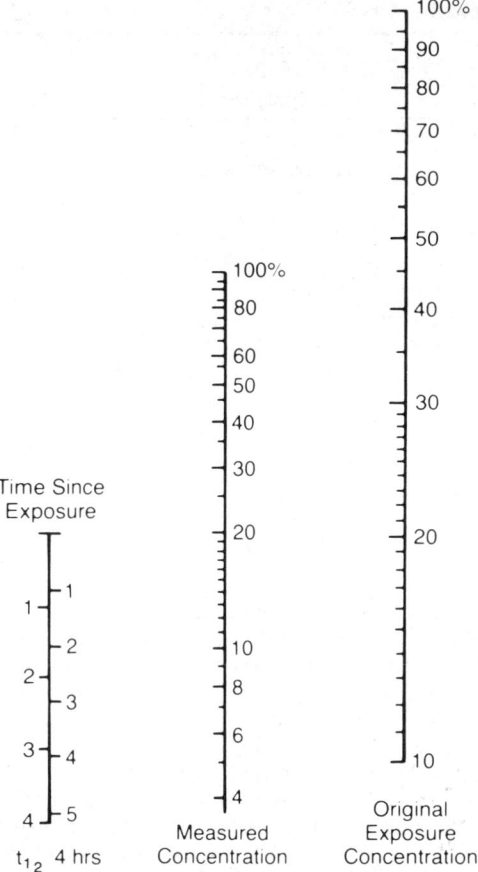

**Figure 2.** Nomogram for calculating carboxyhemoglobin concentration at time of exposure. The time since exposure is given on two scales to allow for the effects of previous oxygen administration on the half-life of carboxyhemoglobin (left-hand scale assumes a half-life of 3 hours). *Note:* The nomogram assumes a half-life of carboxyhemoglobin of 4 hours in a subject breathing room air. Most patients will not have received supplementary oxygen before admission, and at best this will have been administered via a face mask, giving a maximum fractional inspired oxygen concentration of 50 to 60% with little effect on carboxyhemoglobin elimination. The scale on the left side of the time column makes allowances for prior oxygen supplements by assuming a short half-life of 3 hours. The nomogram may help decide quickly whether serious carbon monoxide intoxication is likely to have occurred and may help select patients at high risk for early management in the intensive care unit. The nomogram may be an oversimplification because patients usually are not resuscitated with constant concentrations of oxygen, and many patients may hyperventilate, thus changing elimination characteristics. (Redrawn from Clark CJ, et al: Blood carboxyhaemoglobin and cyanide levels in fire survivors. Lancet *1*:1332, 1981.)

prophylactically. (6) Barium swallow may be necessary at 10 days to 3 weeks to assess severity of damage. (7) Esophageal dilation may need to be performed at 2- to 4-week intervals if evidence of stricture is found. (8) Intraposition of the colon may be necessary if dilation fails to provide an adequate-sized esophagus. (9) Inhalation management requires immediate removal from the environment, and clinical, x-ray, and arterial

blood gas evaluation when appropriate. Oxygen and respiratory support may be required.

**Chloral Hydrate.** See Sedative Hypnotics.

**Chlordane.** See Organochlorine Insecticides.

**Chlordiazepoxide** (Librium). See Benzodiazepines.

**Chlorine Gas.** Chlorine gas is a yellow-greenish gas with an irritating odor used in bleach, in manufacture of plastics, and for water purification. Exposure usually results from transportation mishaps, industrial accidents, chemistry experiments, the mixing of household cleaners with bleach containing hypochlorite, and accidental release around swimming pools. Its density is greater than that of air, and an odor is detected at concentrations of less than 0.5 PPM. Chlorine acts as an oxidizing agent and also acts with tissue water to form hypochlorite and hydrochloric acid and generate free oxygen radicals. *Toxic dose:* The threshold limit value is less than 1 PPM; 4 PPM is tolerated for 0.5 hour; 15 PPM immediately irritates mucous membranes of eyes, ears, nose, and throat; 30 PPM produces choking and chest pain; 60 PPM produces pulmonary edema; 400 PPM for 30 minutes is lethal; and 1000 PPM is fatal in a few minutes.

*Management:* (1) Remove the patient from contaminated environment and stabilize vital functions. Decontamination procedures for dermal and ocular contamination as indicated. Protect rescue personnel with breathing apparatus. Classification—If symptomless or with a cough that clears up in less than 1 hour, rest for 12 hours and report if symptoms occur; no vigorous exercise for 24 hours. If symptoms persist beyond period of exposure, admit to hospital and treat with bronchodilators (use theophylline, not epinephrine) and humidified oxygen. Noncardiac pulmonary edema is treated with PEEP; corticosteroids are controversial; furosemide (Lasix) may be used. For conjunctival irritation, copious water irrigation and fluorescein stain for corneal damage. For dermal burns, copious water irrigation and conventional treatment of burns. *Laboratory aids:* Chest radiograph (may not reflect damage for 24 hours), arterial blood gases, cardiac monitor for dysrhythmias.

**Chlorpromazine** (Thorazine). See Phenothiazines and Other Major Neuroleptics.

**Clinitest Tablets.** See Caustics and Corrosives.

**Cocaine** (Benzoylmethylecgonine). Toxic dose: The potential fatal dose is 1200 mg, but death has occurred with 20 mg parenterally. *Toxicokinetics*: See Table 14. *Manifestations*: Hypertension, convulsions, hyperthermia, and cardiac dysrhythmias. *Management:* (1) Supportive care. Avoid induction of emesis or gastric lavage because of rapid onset of action of cocaine. Blood pressure and thermal monitoring. Phenytoin may be effective for ventricular dysrhythmias, whereas lidocaine may be ineffective and enhance toxicity. Nitroprusside infusion, 0.5 to 10 μg per kg per minute, may be used for severe hypertension. Avoid propranolol. Control anxiety and convulsions with diazepam. Labetalol intravenously (Antidote 23, Table 4) has been used to control life-threatening hypertension and tachycardia. A nonthreatening environment to reduce all sensory stimuli and protect patient from injury is required. Apply precautions against suicide attempts and monitor the fetus if patient is a pregnant woman.

TABLE 14. **Pharmacotoxicokinetics of Cocaine**

| Type | Route | Onset | Peak | Duration t½ (min) | Possible Fatal Dose (Adult) |
|------|-------|-------|------|-------------------|------------------------------|
| Hydrochloride | Insufflation | 1–5 min | 15–60 min | 60–75 | 750–800 mg |
| | Ingested | Delayed | 50–90 min | Sustained | 1.4 grams |
| | IV | 30–120 sec | 5–11 min | 60–90 | 20–800 mg |
| Coca paste | Smoked | | | Not known | |
| Crack and free base | Smoked | (Fastest) 5–10 sec | 5–11 sec | Up to 20 min | Not known |

The management of the "body packer" and "body stuffer" is to administer repeated doses of activated charcoal (except plastic vials), secure venous access, and have drugs readily available for treating life-threatening manifestations until contraband is passed in the stool. Surgical removal may be indicated if material does not pass the pylorus. Endoscopy may be used to remove hard plastic vials, but not the bags, containing crack.

**Codeine.** See Opioids.

**Corrosives.** See Caustics and Corrosives.

**Cyanide.** See Table 15. Hydrocyanic acid and sodium and potassium salts act rapidly and are extremely poisonous. The acid is extremely volatile, producing cyanide, which has a distinctive odor of bitter almonds and can produce death within minutes after inhalation. Cyanide interferes with the cytochrome oxidase system. *Classes of cyanides and derivatives:* (1) Hydrogen cyanide and simple salts in large doses act to produce death in 15 minutes. (2) Halogenated cyanides such as cyanogen chloride produce irritant and vesicant gases that may cause pulmonary edema. (3) Nitriles such as acrylonitrile and acetonitrile. Cyanides are used as fumigants (hydrogen cyanide), in synthetic rubber (acrylonitrile), in fertilizers (cyanamide), in metal refining (salts), and in the home in some silver and furniture polishes. Cyanide in the seeds of fruit stones is harmful only if the capsule is broken. *Manifestations:* Seizures, stupor, cardiac dysrhythmias, pulmonary edema, lactic acidemia, decreased arterial venous oxygen difference. Bright red venous blood.

*Management:* Attendants should not administer mouth to mouth resuscitation. (1) Immediately, 100% oxygen. If inhaled, remove patient from contaminated atmosphere. (2) Cyanide antidote kit (Antidote 14, Table 4). Use antidote only if certain of diagnosis and (a) significant toxicity (impairment of consciousness); (b) manifestations not corrected by oxygen and out of proportion to carboxyhemoglobin level; and (c) lactic acidosis and bright red venous blood with high or normal $Pa_{O_2}$. (3) Gastrointestinal decontamination by gastric lavage. *No* syrup of ipecac. Activated charcoal not very effective (1 gram binds only 35 mg of cyanide). (4) Treat seizures with intravenous diazepam. (5) Correct acidosis. (6) Other antidotes: In Europe, dicobalt edetate, 600 mg, is used intravenously, followed by 300 mg if the response is not satisfactory. Hydroxycobalamin (vitamin $B_{12}$) is a useful antidote but must be given immediately after exposure in very large doses.

Dose: 1800 mg of vitamin $B_{12}$ per dl of KCN is usually required (forms cyanocobalamin).

**DDT and Derivatives.** See Organochlorine Insecticides.

**Desipramine** (Norpramin, Pertofrane). See Tricyclic Antidepressants.

**Diazepam** (Valium). See Benzodiazepines.

**Digitalis Preparations.** See Table 16. *Manifestations:* Abdominal pain, nausea, vomiting, diarrhea, dysrhythmias, heart block, CNS depression, colored-halo vision. *Management:* (1) Gastrointestinal decontamination. Avoid ipecac syrup; it may increase the vagal effect if patient is symptomatic. Repeated doses of activated charcoal may interrupt enterohepatic recirculation. (2) Treat ventricular premature contractions, including bigeminy, trigeminy, quadrigeminy, ventricular tachycardia, and atrial tachycardia, with phenytoin. Lidocaine also may be administered for ventricular dysrhythmias. (3) Treat bradycardia and second- and third-degree atrioventricular block with atropine or isoproterenol. External pacing may be needed. (4) Treat hyperkalemia (above 6 mEq per liter) with intravenous glucose 5 to 10%, intravenous sodium bicarbonate, intravenous insulin (insulin is not used in children), and Kayexalate retention enema (25% in sorbitol 25%) in severe cases. If hyperkalemia is present (ominous sign), insertion of a pacemaker should be seriously considered. Hemodialysis is treatment of choice for severe or refractory hyperkalemia. (5) Direct current countershock may cause life-threatening dysrhythmias. (6) Specific Fab antibody fragments (Digibind) (Antidote 21, Table 4) have been used for life-threatening cardiac dysrhythmias, hyperkalemia, and cases refractory to conventional measures. Contact Poison Control Center for calculation of Fab or use package insert. *Laboratory aids:* Monitor ECG and potassium and digitalis levels. Draw digoxin levels 6 to 8 hours postingestion. An endogenous digoxin-like substance that cross-reacts with most common immunoassay antibodies, with values as high as 4.1 ng per ml, has been reported in newborns, patients with chronic renal failure, and patients with abnormal immunoglobulin levels. The bound digoxin blood concentrations rise after use of Fab, but the free (usually unmeasured) digoxin level falls.

**Diphenhydramine** (Benadryl). See Anticholinergic Agents.

**Doxepin** (Sinequan, Adapin). See Tricyclic Antidepressants.

**Ethchlorvynol** (Placidyl). See Sedative Hypnotics.

TABLE 15. **Sources of Cyanide and Their Toxicity**

### PLANTS CONTAINING CYANIDE GLYCOSIDES

| Common Name | Part of Plant | Botanical Name |
|---|---|---|
| Apple | Seeds | *Malus* spp. |
| Apricot | | *Prunus armeniaca* |
| Arrow grass | | *Triglochin* spp. |
| Bamboo | Sprouts, stems | Tribe Bambuseae |
| Bermuda grass | | *Cynodon dactylon* |
| Bird's-foot trefoil | | *Lotus corniculatus* |
| Bitter almond | | *Prunus amygdalus amara* |
| Blackthorn, sloe | | *Prunus spinosa* |
| Calabash tree | | *Crescentia cujete* |
| Cassava | Beans and roots | *Manihot esculenta* |
| Catclaw | | *Acacia greggi* |
| Cherry laurel | | *Prunus laurocerasus* |
| Chokecherry | | *Prunus virginiana* |
| Cotonester | | *Cotoneaster* spp. |
| Cycad nut | | *Zamia pumila* |
| Elderberry | Leaves and shoots | *Sambucus* spp. |
| Eucalyptus | | *Eucalyptus cladocalyx* |
| False sago palm | | *Cycas circinalis* |
| Flax | | *Linum usitatissimum* |
| Hyacinth bean | Bean | *Dolichos lablab* |
| Hydrangea | Leaves and bulb | *Hydrangea* spp. |
| Jetbead | | *Rhodotypos tetrapetala* |
| Johnson grass | | *Sorghum halepense* |
| Lima bean | | *Phaseolus lunatus* (not in United States) |
| Mountain mahogany | | *Cercocarpus montanus* |
| Passionflower (African) | | *Adenia volkensii* |
| Peach | | *Prunus persica* |
| Pear | Seeds | *Pyrus communis* |
| Plains bahia | | *Bahia oppositifolia* |
| Plum | | *Prunus domestica* |
| Poison suckleya | | *Suckleya suckleyana* |
| Queen's delight | | *Stillingia sylvatica* |
| Sudan grass | | *Sorghum* spp. |
| Velvet grass | | *Holcus lanatus* |
| Vetch | Seed | *Vicia sativa* |

### HYDROGEN CYANIDE LIBERATED FROM SAMPLES OF CARCINOGENIC GLYCOSIDES

| Sample | HCN (mg/gram or ml) |
|---|---|
| Laetrile (amygdalin) | |
|   Sigma | 55.9 |
|   Tablet yellow | 400 |
| Kemdalin | 14.1 |
| Apricot seeds | 2.92 |
| Peach seeds | 2.60 |
| Apple seeds | 0.61 |

Laetrile is 500-mg tablet for oral use, which is 6% cyanide by weight.

### FORMS OF CYANIDE AND THEIR TOXICITY

| Product | Toxicity (Potential Lethal Dose) |
|---|---|
| Hydrocyanic acid | 50 mg (1.0 mg/kg) |
| Potassium/sodium cyanide | 150–300 mg (2 mg/kg) |
| Ferriferrocyanide (Prussian blue) | 50 grams |
| Sodium nitroprusside | 5 mg/kg causes toxicity |
| Bitter almonds | |
|   Oil | 2 oz |
|   Almonds | 50–60 (each contains 0.001 grams of cyanide) |
|   Pulp | 240 grams |
| Apricot | |
|   Wild | 100 grams of moist seed = 217 mg of cyanide |
|   Cultivated | 100 grams = 8.7 mg of cyanide |

TABLE 16. **Digitalis Preparations**

| | Digoxin | Digitoxin |
|---|---|---|
| Trade name | Lanoxin | Crystodigin |
| Onset time PO, min | 15–30 | 25–120 |
| Peak, hr | 1.5–6 | 4–12 |
| Half-life | 31–40 hr | 4–6 days |
| Protein bound (%) | 25 | 90 |
| Vd, liters/kg | 7–8 | 0.6 |
| Route of elimination | Renal, 75% | Liver, 80% |
| Toxic blood levels, ng/ml | 2.4 | >30 |
| Enterohepatic route | 30% | 14% |

**Ethyl Alcohol.** See Alcohols.

**Ethylene Glycol** (solvent, antifreeze). *Toxic dose*: Death has occurred after a 60-ml ingestion; fatal dose = 1.4 ml per kg of 100% solution. The TLV is 50 PPM. *Toxicokinetics*: Time of onset, 30 minutes to 12 hours for CNS and metabolic abnormalities to occur (Phase I). Twelve to 36 hours postingestion, cardiopulmonary depression (Phase II). In Phase III (2 to 3 days postingestion), renal failure occurs. The $t\frac{1}{2}$ is 3 hours (during ethanol therapy this is prolonged to 17 hours). *Management*: (1) Gastrointestinal decontamination up to 2 to 4 hours postingestion. Activated charcoal and cathartics are not indicated. (2) Treat seizures with intravenous diazepam. Exclude hypocalcemia. (3) Correct acidosis with intravenous sodium bicarbonate. (4) Initiate ethanol therapy to block metabolism (Antidote 20, Table 4) if the blood ethylene glycol level is higher than 20 mg per dl, or if the patient is symptomatic or acidotic with increased anion gap or osmolar gap. Ethanol should be administered intravenously or orally to produce a blood ethanol concentration of 100 to 150 mg per dl. (5) Early hemodialysis is indicated if the ingestion was large; if the blood ethylene glycol level is greater than 50 mg per dl; if severe acid-base or electrolyte abnormalities occur despite conventional therapy; or if renal failure occurs. (6) Thiamine and pyridoxine have been recommended for 48 hours but have not been extensively studied. *Laboratory aids*: Complete blood count, electrolytes, urinalysis (look for oxalate crystals), and arterial blood gases. Obtain ethylene glycol and ethanol levels, plasma osmolarity (use freezing point depression method). Calcium, creatinine, and blood urea nitrogen studies. An ethylene glycol level of 20 mg per dl is usually toxic (levels are very difficult to obtain).

**Flurazepam** (Dalmane). See Benzodiazepines.

**Glutethimide** (Doriden). See Sedative Hypnotics.

**Hallucinogens**

1. **LSD** (lysergic acid diethylamide). *Toxic dose*: ≥ 35 μg. Street doses are typically 50 to 300 micrograms. *Toxicokinetics*: Peak effect, 1 to 2 hours. Duration, 12 to 24 hours. $t\frac{1}{2}$, 3 hours. Route of elimination, hepatic.

2. **Morning-Glory Seeds** (*Rivea corymbosa* or *Ipomoea*). These have one-tenth the potency of LSD.

3. **Mescaline/Peyote** (trimethoxyphenylethylamine or *Lophophora williamsii*). *Toxic dose*: ≥ 5 mg per kg. Each button of mescaline contains 45 mg (4 to 12 produce symptoms). *Toxicokinetics*: Peak effect, 4 to 6 hours. Duration, 14 hours.

4. **Psilocybin**. Similar in effect to LSD but short acting. Peak effect, 90 minutes. Duration, 5 to 6 hours.

5. **Nutmeg** *(Myristica)*. *Toxic dose*: 5 to 15 grams (1 to 3 nutmegs). Peak effect, 3 to 6 hours. Duration, up to 60 hours.

6. **Marijuana** *(Cannabis sativa)* (Δ⁹-tetrahydrocannabinol, THC). One joint equals 500 mg of marijuana; when smoked, 50% is destroyed. *Toxicokinetics*: Time of onset, 2 to 3 minutes (smoked). Duration, 2 to 3 hours. t½, 28 to 47 hours (shorter for chronic user). *Note*: 1 per cent of the metabolite can be detected in urine up to 2 weeks after use. *Manifestations*: Visual illusions, sensory perceptual distortions, depersonalization, and derealization. *Management*: "Talk-down" technique.

7. **Inhalants**. Nitrites (amyl and isobutyl nitrite)—act immediately; aromatic hydrocarbon in airplane model glues, plastic cements (benzene, toluene, xylene)—see Hydrocarbons; *nitrous oxide* and *halogenated hydrocarbons*.

8. **Tryptamine Derivatives** (DMT, *N*-dimethyltryptamine; DET, diethyltryptamine; DPT, dipropyltryptamine). Rapid onset of action, but duration is only 1 to 2 hours.

9. **STP** or **DOM** (2,5-dimethoxy-4-methylamphetamine). Acts like LSD but lasts 72 hours or longer.

10. **MDA** (3-methoxy-4,5-ethylenedioxyamphetamine). Related to amphetamine, produces a mild LSD-like reaction lasting 6 to 10 hours ("love pill").

See also Alcohols, Amphetamines, Anticholinergic Agents, Barbiturates, Cocaine, Opioids, Phencyclidine, Phenothiazines and Other Major Neuroleptics, and Tricyclic Antidepressants.

**Haloperidol** (Haldol). See Phenothiazines and Other Major Neuroleptics.

**Heroin**. See Opioids.

**Hydrocarbons**

1. **Petroleum Distillates**. Gasoline (petroleum spirit), 2 to 5% benzene; kerosene (coal oil, kerosene, jet aviation fuel No. 1, charcoal lighter fluid); petroleum naphtha (cigarette lighter fluid, ligroin, racing fuel); petroleum ether (benzine); turpentine (pine oil, oil of turpentine); and mineral spirits (Stoddard solvent, white spirits, varsol, mineral turpentine, petroleum spirit). *Manifestations*: Materials aspirated during the process of ingestion may produce pneumonitis. Hypoxia associated with aspiration is the cause of CNS depression, not absorption. It is *unlikely* that a child accidentally or an adult during siphoning would ingest a sufficient quantity to warrant the induction of emesis.

2. **Aromatic Hydrocarbons**. *Benzene*, a solvent used in manufacturing dyes, phenol, and nitrobenzene, has a TLV of 10 PPM by inhalation according to the Occupational Safety and Health Administration (OSHA). The National Institute for Occupational Safety and Health (NIOSH) value is 1 PPM. The adult ingested toxic dose is 15 ml. Chronic exposure may cause leukemia. Two hundred PPM is fatal in 5 minutes. *Toluene*, used in manufacturing TNT, has an OSHA TLV of 200 PPM by inhalation; the NIOSH figure is 100. The adult ingested toxic dose is 50 ml. *Styrene* has an OSHA TLV of 100 PPM by inhalation. *Xylene*, used in the manufacture of perfumes, has an OSHA TLV of 100 PPM by inhalation. The adult ingested toxic dose is 50 ml. *Manifestations*: Asphyxiation, CNS depression, defatting dermatitis, and aspiration pneumonitis. A bite into a tube of household plastic cement by a young child does not warrant the induction of emesis. Ingestion of hydrocarbon with a benzene fraction over 5% may warrant induction of emesis.

3. **Aliphatic Halogenated Hydrocarbons**. See Table 17 for common examples. *Manifestations*: Myocardial sensitization and irritability, hepatorenal toxicity, and CNS depression. Dichloromethane may be converted into carbon monoxide in the body. Trichloroethylene concentrates in the fetus (pregnant women should not be exposed) and causes a disulfiram (Antabuse) reaction ("degreaser's flush") when associated with ingestion of ethanol. The decision to induce emesis must be based on the toxicity of the agent.

4. **Dangerous Additives**. Dangerous additives to the hydrocarbons, such as heavy metals, nitrobenzene, aniline dyes, insecticides, and demothing agents, may warrant the induction of emesis.

5. **Heavy Hydrocarbons**. These have high viscosity, low volatility, and minimal absorption, so emesis is unwarranted. Examples are asphalt (tar), machine oil, motor oil (lubricating oil, engine oil), diesel oil (engine fuel, home heating oil), petrolatum liquid (mineral oil, suntan oils), petrolatum jelly (Vaseline), paraffin wax, transmission oil, cutting oil, and greases and glues.

6. **Products Treated as Petroleum Distillates**. Essential oils (e.g., turpentine, pine oil) are treated as petroleum distillates. Mineral seal oil (signal oil), found in some furniture polishes, is a heavy, viscous oil that *never* warrants emesis; it can produce severe pneumonia if aspirated. It has minimal absorption. *Management*: Dermal decontamination. Removal from the environment in inhalation.

*First Aid Treatment*. See Table 18. *The use of activated charcoal, oils, and cathartics is not advised in petroleum distillate ingestions. General management*: (1) In the asymptomatic patient: observe several hours for development of respiratory distress. (2) In the symptomatic patient: supportive respiratory care for respiratory distress. Bronchospasm may be treated with intravenous aminophylline. Avoid epinephrine. Monitor ECG; arterial blood gases; liver, pulmonary, and renal function; serum electrolytes; serial radiographs. Observe for intravascular hemolysis and disseminated intravascular coagulation. If cyanosis is present that does not respond to oxygen or the arterial $Pa_{O_2}$ is normal, suspect methemoglobinemia that may require therapy with methylene blue. Steroids have not been shown to be beneficial. Antimicrobial agents are not useful in prophylaxis. (Fever or leukocytosis may be produced by the chemical pneumonitis itself.) It is not necessary to treat pneumatoceles. Most infiltrations resolve spontaneously in 1 week except for lipoid pneumonia, which may last up to 6 weeks.

TABLE 17. **Common Examples of Aliphatic Halogenated Hydrocarbons**

| Hydrocarbon | Estimated Fatal Dose (Ingested) | TLV-TWA (PPM) | Synonyms |
|---|---|---|---|
| 1,1,1-Trichloroethane | 15.7 grams/kg | 50 | Methyl chloroform, Triethane, chlorethane, Glamorene Spot Remover, Scotchgard |
| 1,1,2-Trichloroethane | 580 mg/kg | 10 | Vinyl trichloride |
| Trichloroethylene | Controversial, 3–5 ml/kg | 50 | — |
| Tetrachloroethanene | Not known | 5 | Acetylene tetrachloride |
| Dichloromethane | 25 ml | 100 | Methylene chloride |
| Tetrachloroethylene | 5 ml | 50 | Tetrachloroethene Perchloroethylene |
| Dichloroethane | 0.5 ml/kg | 200 | — |
| Carbon tetrachloride | 3–5 ml | 5 | — |

**Imipramine** (Tofranil). See Tricyclic Antidepressants.

**Iron.** The iron content of some preparations appears in Table 19. *Toxic dose*: Range, 20 to 60 mg per kg or greater of elemental iron. Dose to induce emesis, ≥ 20 mg per kg. The potential fatal dose is 180 mg per kg (600 mg of elemental iron). *Toxicokinetics*: Absorption occurs chiefly in the small intestine. For excretion there is no normal route except blood loss or gastrointestinal desquamation. *Manifestations*: Phase I—Mucosal injury possibly with hematemesis (1 to 6 hours postingestion). Phase II—patient appears improved (6 to 48 hours). Phase III—cardiovascular collapse and severe metabolic acidosis. Phase IV—sequelae of intestinal stricture and obstruction or anemia (weeks to months). Patients asymptomatic for 6 hours rarely develop serious intoxication manifestations.

*Management:* (1) Gastrointestinal decontamination. Emesis should be induced in ingestions of elemental iron of over 20 mg per kg. Emesis should be followed by gastric lavage. The solution to be used for lavage is 1 to 1.5% sodium bicarbonate to form ferrous carbonate salts, which are poorly absorbed. One hundred milliliters of this solution should be left in the stomach (prepared by dilution of a sodium bicarbonate ampule with saline). The use of deferoxamine (Desferal) in the gastrointestinal tract is not recommended. The use of diluted Fleet's enema solution risks severe hypertonic phosphate poisoning. (2) Postlavage abdominal radiograph—if significant amounts of residual radiopaque material are present, consider removal by endoscopy or surgery, since coalesced tablets have produced hemorrhagic infarction and perforation peritonitis. (3) Whole-bowel washout with polyethylene glycol solution. (4) Diagnostic chelation test—deferoxamine not reliable. (5) Indications for chelation therapy with deferoxamine are serum iron level greater than total iron binding capacity; serum iron level over 500 mg per dl; or systemic signs of intoxication independent of serum iron level. Chelation should be performed within 12 to 18 hours to be effective.

*Laboratory aids*: Serum iron levels correlate with the clinical course. Iron levels taken at 2 to 6 hours that are below 350 mg per dl predict an asymptomatic course; levels of 350 to 500 are associated with mild gastrointestinal symptoms (rarely serious); and levels greater than 500 suggest the possibility of serious Phase III manifestations. White blood cell counts greater than 15,000 per μl, blood glucose levels over 150 mg per dl, radiopaque material present on abdominal radiograph, vomiting, and diarrhea predict iron

TABLE 18. **Initial Management of Hydrocarbon Ingestions**

| Symptoms | Contents | Amount | Initial Management |
|---|---|---|---|
| None | Petroleum distillate only | <5 ml/kg | None |
| None | Heavy hydrocarbon Mineral seal oil Petroleum distillate | Any amount >60 ml | None* None ? Emesis |
| None | Petroleum distillate with dangerous additive (heavy metals, pesticides) | Depends on toxicity of additives | Emesis |
| | Aromatic | >1 ml/kg | Emesis |
| | Halogenated hydrocarbons Trichlor compound Tetrachlor compound | >1 ml/kg Any amount ingested | Emesis Emesis |
| Loss of protective airway reflex, seizures | Petroleum distillate with dangerous additive, aromatic or halogenated hydrocarbon | Depends on toxicity | Use endotracheal tube before gastric lavage |

*Emesis may be necessary if machine oil contains triorthocresyl phosphate (TOCP), which causes weakness, sensory impairment, and "partially reversible damage to the spinal cord."

TABLE 19. **Iron Content of Some Preparations**

| Salt | Elemental Iron Content (%) | Average Tablet Strength (mg) | Iron Content Per Tablet (mg) |
|---|---|---|---|
| Ferrous sulfate | 20 | 300 | 60 |
| Ferrous sulfate (dried) | 29.7 | 200 | 65 |
| Ferrous gluconate | 11.6 | 320 | 36 |
| Ferrous fumarate | 33 | 200 | 67 |

levels greater than 300 mg per dl. Monitor complete blood counts, blood glucose, serum iron, stools, and vomitus for occult blood; electrolytes; acid-base balance; urinalysis and urinary output; liver function tests; blood urea nitrogen; and creatinine. Obtain type and match of blood in severe cases. Abdominal radiographs. Follow-up is necessary for sequelae in significant intoxications—gastrointestinal series for intestinal strictures and anemia secondary to blood loss. Patients who develop fever or toxic symptoms following iron overdose should have blood and stool cultures checked for *Yersinia enterocolitica.*

**Isoniazid** (INH, Nydrazid). This is an antituberculosis drug frequently used in suicide attempts by American Indians and Eskimos. *Mechanism of toxicity:* It produces pyridoxine deficiency (doubles excretion of pyridoxine). *Toxic dose:* 1.5 grams, 35 to 40 mg per kg, produces convulsions; severe toxicity is seen at 6 to 10 grams; 200 mg per kg is an obligatory convulsant. *Toxicokinetics:* Absorption is rapid, with a peak in 1 to 2 hours (clinical symptoms may start in 30 minutes). Volume distribution is 0.6 liter per kg. It passes the placenta and into breast milk at 50% of the maternal serum level. Not protein bound. Elimination is by the liver, which produces a hepatotoxic metabolite, acetylisoniazid. The t½: Slow acetylators (2 to 4 hours) may develop peripheral neuropathy (50% of blacks and whites). Fast acetylators (0.7 to 2 hours) may develop hepatitis (90% of Orientals and a majority of patients with diabetes). Excreted unchanged, 10 to 40%. *Major toxic manifestations:* Visual disturbances, convulsions (90% or more with one or more seizures), coma, resistant severe acidosis (due to lactate secondary to hypoxia, convulsions, and metabolic blocks). *Management:* (1) Control seizures with large doses of pyridoxine, 1 gram for each gram of isoniazid ingested (Antidote 34, Table 4). If the dose ingested is unknown, give at least 5 grams of pyridoxine intravenously. (2) Correct acidosis with fluids and sodium bicarbonate (pyridoxine may spontaneously correct the acidosis). (3) Diazepam may be used as a supplement to control the seizures. (4) After patient is stabilized, or if asymptomatic, gastrointestinal decontamination procedures may be carried out, keeping in mind the rapid onset of convulsions. Asymptomatic patients should be observed for 4 hours. (5) Hemodialysis is rarely needed but may be used as an adjunct for uncontrollable acidosis and seizures. Hemoperfusion has not been adequately evaluated. Diuresis is ineffec-

tive. *Laboratory aids:* Isoniazid toxic levels are above 10 to 20 µg per ml. Monitor the blood glucose (often hyperglycemia), electrolytes (often hyperkalemia), bicarbonate, and arterial blood gases. Monitor the temperature closely (often hyperpyrexia).

**Isopropyl Alcohol.** See Alcohols.

**Kerosene.** See Hydrocarbons.

**Lead.** *Acute* lead poisoning is rare. *Acute toxic dose:* 0.5 gram. *Management:* (1) Gastrointestinal decontamination. (2) Supportive care, including measures to deal with the hepatic and renal failure and intravascular hemolysis. (3) Ethylenediaminetetraacetic acid (EDTA) in all severe cases if lead levels confirm absorption. *Chronic* lead poisoning occurs most often in children 1 to 6 years of age who are exposed in their environment and in adults in certain occupations or from illicit whiskey. *Chronic toxic dose:* Determined by blood lead level and clinical findings. Over 10 to 15 µg per dl indicates excess body burden. A chronic dose of 0.6 mg a day will increase the body burden, 2.5 mg a day will result in toxicity in 4 years, and 3.5 mg a day will cause toxicity in a few months.

*Toxicokinetics:* Absorption—10 to 15% of the ingested dose is absorbed in adults; in children up to 40% is absorbed with iron deficiency anemia. Inhalation absorption is rapid and complete. Vd—95% present in bone. In blood, 95% is in red blood cells. t½, 35 days; in bone, 10 years. The major elimination route for inorganic lead is renal. Organic lead is metabolized in the liver to inorganic lead; 9% is excreted in the urine per day. *Manifestations of acute symptoms of chronic lead poisoning* (ABCDE): Anorexia, apathy, anemia; behavior disturbances; clumsiness; developmental deterioration; and emesis. Manifestations of encephalopathy are "PAINT": *P,* persistent forceful vomiting; *A,* ataxia; *I,* intermittent stupor and lucidity; *N,* neurologic coma and convulsions; *T,* tired and lethargic. In adults one may see peripheral neuropathies and "lead gum lines."

*Management:* (1) Gastrointestinal decontamination with enemas if radiopaque foreign bodies are noted. Do not delay therapy until clear. (2) Remove from exposure. For children, see Table 20. *Laboratory aids:* (1) Provocation mobilization test—500 mg per M² of EDTA for one dose given deeply intramuscularly with 0.5% procaine diluted 1:1 and collect the urine for 6 to 8 hours. A ratio of micrograms excreted in the urine to milligrams of Ca-EDTA administered greater than 0.6 represents an increased lead body burden, and chelation should be administered. (2) Evaluate complete blood count, levels of serum iron, or ferritin; repeat blood lead levels and erythrocyte protoporphyrin. (3) Flat plate of the abdomen and long bone radiographs (knees usually). (4) Renal function tests. (5) Monitor electrolytes, serum calcium, phosphorus, blood glucose.

**Lindane.** See Organochlorine Insecticides.

**Lithium** (Eskalith, Lithane). Most cases of intoxication have occurred as therapeutic overdoses. The toxic dose is determined by serum levels, although intoxication has occurred with levels in the therapeutic range.

*Toxicokinetics:* Absorption is rapid, with complete peaking in 1 to 4 hours. Vd is 0.5 to 0.9 liter per kg.

TABLE 20. **Choice of Chelation Therapy Based on Symptoms and Blood Lead Concentration***

| Clinical Presentation | Treatment | Comments |
|---|---|---|
| *Symptomatic children* | | |
| Acute encephalopathy | BAL†, 450 mg/M²/day<br>CaNa₂-EDTA, 1500 mg/M²/day (EDTA not used alone if blood Pb > 72 μg/dl or symptoms present) | Start with BAL, 75 mg/M² IM q 4 hr<br>After 4 hr, start continuous infusion of CaNa₂-EDTA, 1500 mg/M²/day<br>Therapy with BAL and CaNa₂-EDTA should be continued for 5 days<br>Interrupt therapy for 2 days<br>Treat for 5 additional days, including BAL if blood Pb remains high<br>Other cycles may be needed depending on blood Pb rebound |
| Other symptoms | BAL, 300 mg/M²/day<br>CaNa₂-EDTA, 1000 mg/M²/day<br>Monitor BUN, creatinine, AST, ALT, urine | Start with BAL, 90 mg/M² IM q 4 hr<br>After 4 hr, start CaNa₂-EDTA, 1000 mg/M²/day, preferably by continuous infusion, or in divided doses IV (through a heparin lock)<br>Therapy with CaNa₂-EDTA should be continued for 5 days<br>BAL may be discontinued after 3 days if blood Pb < 50 μg/dl<br>Interrupt therapy for 2 days<br>Treat for 5 additional days, including BAL if blood Pb remains high (>50 μg/dl)<br>Other cycles may be needed depending on blood Pb rebound |
| *Asymptomatic children*<br>BEFORE TREATMENT, MEASURE VENOUS BLOOD LEAD | | |
| Blood Pb > 70 μg/dl | BAL, 300 mg/M²/day<br>CaNa₂-EDTA, 1000 mg/M²/day | Start with BAL, 50 mg/M² IM q 4 hr<br>After 4 hr, start CaNa₂-EDTA, 1000 mg/M²/day, preferably by continuous infusion, or in divided doses IV (through a heparin lock)<br>Treatment with CaNa₂-EDTA should be continued for 5 days<br>BAL may be discontinued after 3 days if blood Pb < 50 μg/dl<br>Other cycles may be needed depending on blood Pb rebound |
| Blood Pb 56–69 μg/dl | CaNa₂-EDTA, 1000 mg/M²/day | CaNa₂-EDTA for 5 days, preferably by continuous infusion, or in divided doses (through a heparin lock)<br>Alternatively, if lead exposure is controlled, CaNa₂-EDTA may be given as a single daily outpatient dose IM or IV<br>Other cycles may be needed depending on blood Pb rebound |
| Blood Pb 25–55 μg/dl<br>PERFORM CaNa₂-EDTA PROVOCATION TEST TO ASSESS LEAD EXCRETION RATIO | | |
| If ratio > 0.70 | CaNa₂-EDTA, 1000 mg/M²/day | Treat for 5 days IV or IM, as above |
| If ratio 0.60–0.69 | | |
|   Age < 3 yr | CaNa₂-EDTA, 1000 mg/M²/day | Treat for 3 days IV or IM, as above |
|   Age > 3 yr | No treatment | Repeat blood Pb and CaNa₂-EDTA provocation test periodically |
| If ratio < 0.60 | No treatment | Repeat blood Pb and CaNa₂-EDTA provocation test periodically |
| *Guidelines for chelation of excess lead in adults*<br>*Inorganic lead*<br>*Symptomatic cases* | | |
| Acute encephalopathy | BAL-EDTA | Same as for children |
| Abdominal pain, weakness, and colic | BAL-EDTA | Course for 3–5 days followed by oral penicillamine until urine lead is <500 μg/24 hr or 2 months, whichever less |
| Painless peripheral neuropathy | D-Penicillamine | For 1–2 months<br>If blood lead >100 μg/dl, BAL-EDTA first<br>Course 3–5 days, followed by oral penicillamine |
| *Asymptomatic cases*<br>*Blood lead concentrations* | | |
| 100 μg/dl | BAL-EDTA | |
| 80–100 μg/dl | Penicillamine alone | |
| 40–79 and EP <60μg/dl | Provocative test | |
| *Organic lead* | No chelation therapy | |

Note: OSHA requires that workers be removed from the work environment when lead levels exceed 50 μg/dl and until they are below 40 μg/dl.

*From Piomelli S., et al.: Management of childhood lead poisoning. J. Pediatr. *105*:523–532, 1984. Used by permission.
†Dimercaprol.

It is not protein bound. The t½ therapeutically is 18 to 24 hours. Eighty-nine to 98% is excreted by the kidney unchanged, one-third to two-thirds in 6 to 12 hours. Excretion is decreased in the presence of hyponatremia and dehydration. The cerebrospinal fluid concentration is one-half the plasma concentration. The breast milk level is 50% of the maternal serum level—toxic to the nursling.

*Manifestations:* The first sign of toxicity may be diarrhea. Fine tremor of hands, lethargy, weakness, polyuria and polydipsia, goiter and hypothyroidism, and fasciculations are side effects. Severe toxicity is manifested by ataxia, impaired mental state, coma, and seizures (limbs held in hyperextension with eyes open in "coma vigil"). Cardiovascular manifestations are dysrhythmias, hypotension, flat T waves, and increased QT interval.

*Management:* (1) Gastrointestinal decontamination may not be useful after 2 hours because of rapid absorption. In slow-release preparations, decontamination may be useful up to 24 hours postingestion. Activated charcoal is not indicated. (2) Hospitalize if intoxication is suspected, because seizures may occur unexpectedly. (3) Restore normothermia and fluid and electrolyte balance, particularly sodium. If diabetes insipidus is present, an infusion of sodium may cause hypernatremia. Current evidence supports saline infusion as enhancing excretion of lithium. (4) Forced diuresis has no role, unless the glomerular filtration rate is low. Consider only when the lithium level is not above 2.5 mEq per liter and fails to fall below 1 mEq per liter within 30 hours. (5) Hemodialysis is the treatment of choice for severe intoxication. Lithium is the most dialyzable toxin known. Long runs of 12 hours or longer should be used until the lithium level is less than 1 mEq per liter because of extensive reequilibration rebound. Follow levels every 4 hours after dialysis. Dialysis may have to be repeated. Expect a time lag in neurologic recovery. If hemodialysis is not available or delayed, peritoneal dialysis can be used but is less effective. (6) Monitor ECG. Refractory dysrhythmias may be treated with magnesium sulfate and sodium bicarbonate. (7) Aminophylline may increase lithium excretion and decrease lithium reabsorption but has not been extensively studied. (8) Avoid thiazides and spironolactone diuretics, which increase lithium levels.

*Laboratory aids:* Lithium level determinations should be performed every 4 hours. Although they do not always correlate with the manifestations at low levels, they are predictive in severe intoxications. Levels of 0.6 to 1.2 mEq per liter are usually therapeutic. Levels over 4.0 mEq per liter are severely toxic. Other tests to be monitored are complete blood count (lithium causes leukocytosis), renal function, thyroid, ECG, and electrolytes. Factors that predispose to lithium toxicity are febrile illness, sodium depletion, concomitant drugs (thiazide and spironolactone diuretics), impaired renal function, advanced age, and fluid loss in vomiting and diarrheal illness.

**Lomotil** (Diphenoxylate and Atropine). See Opioids and Anticholinergic Agents.

**LSD** (Lysergic Acid Diethylamide). See Hallucinogens.

**Marijuana.** See Hallucinogens.

**Meperidine** (Demerol). See Opioids.

**Meprobamate** (Equanil, Miltown). See Sedative Hypnotics.

**Mercury.** *Management:* (1) Inhalation of elemental mercury—remove from exposure. (2) Ingestion of mercuric salt—gastrointestinal decontamination. A protein solution such as egg white or 5% salt-poor albumin can be given to reduce salt to mercurous ion (less toxic). Give activated charcoal and cathartic. (3) Chelating agents (do not use Ca-EDTA because of nephrotoxicity): Dimercaprol (BAL) enhances mercury excretion through the bile as well as the urine and would be the choice if there were renal impairment from the mercury (Antidote 17, Table 4). Penicillamine (Antidote 29, Table 4) or *N*-acetyl-DL-penicillamine (investigational use). Use of BAL in methyl mercury intoxication increases the brain mercury and appears to be contraindicated; penicillamine and its analogue should be used (decreases mercury in brain). A new chelator, 2,3-dimercaptosuccinic acid, holds promise of less toxicity and more specific therapy and is now available under the Orphan Drug Program.* (4) Monitor fluid and electrolyte levels, renal function, hemoglobin levels. Obtain blood and urine mercury levels (consult the laboratory for proper collection technique and containers). (5) Hemodialysis early in the symptomatic patient is useful. (6) New but not established approaches are Polythiol resin to bind the methyl mercury excreted in the bile; heat and sauna treatment to increase mercury excretion through perspiration; and a regional dialyzer system using L-cysteine. (7) Surgical excision of *local injection sites.*

*Laboratory aids:* (1) Blood levels are below 2 to 4 µg per dl and urine levels below 10 to 20 µg per liter in 90% of the adult population. Levels above 4 µg per dl in blood and 20 micrograms per liter in urine probably should be considered abnormal. Blood levels are not always reliable. Exposed industrial workers' urine levels are 150 to 200 µg. (2) In asymptomatic patients with urine levels under 300 µg per liter, a chelating challenge with BAL or penicillamine may bring a significant increase that may aid in establishing the diagnosis. (3) Approximately 150 µg per liter of mercury in urine is equivalent to 3.5 µg per dl in blood. (4) Methyl mercury is excreted mainly through the feces, so urine mercury would not be a reliable measurement. (5) Mercury is also excreted in the sweat and saliva. The parotid fluid level is approximately two-thirds that of the blood. Since the hair is porous, it may absorb mercury from the atmosphere; however, hair concentrations of 400 to 500 µg are likely to be associated with neurologic symptoms.

**Methadone.** See Opioids.

**Methanol.** See Alcohols.

**Methaqualone.** See Sedative Hypnotics.

**Methyprylon** (Noludar). See Sedative Hypnotics.

**Narcotic Analgesics.** See Opioids.

**Neuroleptics.** See Phenothiazines and Other Major Neuroleptics.

**Nitrites (NO₂) and Nitrates (NO₃).** These are readily

---

*Inquiries can be made to the National Information Center for Orphan Drugs and Rare Diseases, 800–336–4797.

### TABLE 21. Organic Nitrates for Angina Pectoris

| Drug and Route | Trade Name | Onset (min) | Duration (hr) |
|---|---|---|---|
| Nitroglycerin | | | |
|   Oral | Many | Varies | 4–6 |
|   Sublingual | Many | 1–3 | ¼–½ |
|   2% ointment | Nitrobid Nitrol | Varies | 3–6 |
| Isosorbide dinitrate | Isordil | | |
|   Sublingual | | 1–3 | 1.3–3 |
|   Oral | | 2–5 | 4–6 |
|   Chewable | | 2–5 | 2–3 |
|   Timed release | | Varies | — |
| Pentaerythritol tetranitrate, oral | Peritrate | 2–5 | 3–5 |
| Erythrityl tetranitrate, oral | Cardilate | 2–5 | 4–6 |

available in both inorganic and organic forms. Organic nitrates used for angina pectoris are listed in Table 21. Inorganic nitrates have more toxicologic importance in natural foods and contaminated well water. *Potential fatal doses:* Nitrite, 1 gram; nitrate, 10 grams; nitrobenzene, 2 ml; nitroglycerin, 0.2 gram; and aniline dye (pure), 5 to 30 grams. *Toxicokinetics:* Onset of action of nitroglycerin sublingually is 1 to 3 minutes, with a peak action of 3 to 15 minutes and a duration of 20 to 30 minutes. Other routes have a slower onset (2 to 5 minutes) and longer duration of action (1.5 to 6 hours). Nitrites are potent oxidizing agents converting ferrous to ferric iron, which cannot carry oxygen. Normally, humans have 0.7% of methemoglobin, which is converted by methemoglobin reductase into oxygen-carrying hemoglobin. Liver detoxification by dinitration is the route of elimination. *Toxic manifestations* depend on the level of methemoglobinemia. At 10%, "chocolate cyanosis" occurs; at 10 to 20%, headache, dizziness, and tachypnea occur; and at 50%, mental alterations are present and coma and convulsions may occur. Headache, flushing, and sweating are due to the vasodilatory effect; hypotension, tachycardia, and syncope may also occur. Severe hypoxia may produce pulmonary edema and encephalopathy. Levels above 50% produce metabolic acidosis and ECG changes; cardiovascular collapse occurs at levels of 70%.

*Management:* (1) Dermal decontamination, if indicated. Aniline dyes may be removed with 5% acetic acid (vinegar). (2) Gastrointestinal decontamination if ingested. (3) Hypotension can be treated by the Trendelenburg position and fluid challenge. Vasoconstrictors (dopamine or norepinephrine) are rarely needed. (4) Methylene blue (Antidote 24, Table 4) is indicated for methemoglobin levels above 30%, dyspnea, metabolic acidosis (lactic acidosis), or an altered mental state. (5) Oxygen, 100%, or a hyperbaric chamber should be used in symptomatic patients if methylene blue fails or is not effective, e.g., as in chlorate intoxication or glucose-6-phosphate dehydrogenase deficiency. *Laboratory aids:* Methemoglobin levels, arterial blood gases. Blood has a chocolate-brown appearance and fails to turn red on exposure to oxygen.

**Nortriptyline** (Aventyl, Pamelor). See Tricyclic Antidepressants.

**Opioids** (Narcotic Opiates). See Table 22. The major metabolic pathway differs for each opioid but they are 90 per cent metabolized in the liver. Patients should be observed for CNS and respiratory depression and hypotension. Pulmonary edema is a potentially lethal complication of mainlining (intravenous use). *Manifes-*

### TABLE 22. Opioids (Narcotic Opiates)*

| Drugs | | Equivalent IM Dose† (mg) | Oral† (mg) | Peak Action (hr) | Half-life (hr) | Duration of Action (hr) | Potential Toxic Dose (mg) |
|---|---|---|---|---|---|---|---|
| *Generic* | *Trade* | | | | | | |
| Alphaprodine | Nisentil | 45 | — | 0.5 | — | 1–2 | — |
| Butorphanol | Stadol | 2 | 12 | 0.5–1.0 | 3 | 3–4 | — |
| Camphorated tincture of opium | Paregoric | — | 25 ml | — | — | 4–5 | — |
| Codeine | Various | 120 | 200 | — | 3 | 3–6 | 800 |
| Diacetylmorphine | Heroin | 3.0 | 60 | — | 0.5 | 3–4 | 100 |
| Dihydrocodeine | Hycodan | 5–10 | — | — | — | — | 100 |
| Diphenoxylate | Lomotil | — | 10 | Delayed by atropine | — | — | — |
| Fentanyl | Sublimaze | 0.2 | — | 0.5 | 1.5 | 1–2 | — |
| Hydromorphone | Dilaudid | 1.5 | 6.5 | 0.5–0.75 | 2–3 | 4–5 | 100 |
| Meperidine | Demerol | 75–100 | 300 | 0.5–1 | 0.5–5 | 4–6 | 1000 |
| Methadone | Dolophine | 10.0 | 20 | 4 | 22–97 | 4–6 | 120 |
| Morphine | Various | 10.0 | 60 | 0.75–1.5 | 2–3 | 4–6 | 200 |
| Nalbuphine | Nubain | 10.0 | — | — | 5 | 3–6 | — |
| Oxycodone | Percodan | — | 30 | — | — | 3–4 | — |
| Oxymorphone | Numorphan | 1.0 | — | 1 | 2–3 | 4–5 | — |
| Pentazocine | Talwin | — | 50–100 | 0.75 | 2 | 4–7 | — |
| Propoxyphene | Darvon | — | 65–100 | 2–4 | 8–24 | 2–4 | 500 |

*"Ts and blues" are a combination of pentazocine (Talwin) and tripelennamine (Pyribenzamine) used intravenously. Pentazocine now has naloxone added to it to counter this abuse. Innovar is fentanyl plus droperidol, used as an IV anesthetic.

†Dose equivalent to 10 mg of morphine.

*tations:* All opiate agonists produce miotic pupils (except meperidine and Lomotil early), respiratory and CNS depression, physical dependence, and withdrawal.

*Management:* (1) Supportive care, particularly an endotracheal tube and assisted ventilation. (2) Gastrointestinal decontamination up to 12 hours postingestion, as opiates delay gastric emptying time, but this is of no benefit if overdose is by injection. Convulsions occur rapidly with propoxyphene (Darvon) and codeine overdose, and this may be an indication not to use an emetic for gastrointestinal decontamination in this drug overdose. (3) Naloxone (Narcan) (Antidote 25, Table 4) may be given in bolus intravenous doses and by continuous drip. Naloxone must be titrated against the clinical response and precipitation of withdrawal in narcotic addicts. It should be repeated as often as necessary, since many opioids in overdose can last 24 hours to 48 hours, whereas the action of naloxone lasts only 2 to 3 hours. *Larger doses are needed for codeine, pentazocine, and propoxyphene.* (4) Pulmonary edema does not respond to naloxone and needs respiratory supportive care. Fluids should be given cautiously in opioid overdose, because these agents stimulate antidiuretic hormone effect and pulmonary edema is frequent. (5) *If the patient is comatose, give 50% glucose* (3 to 4 per cent of comatose narcotic overdose patients have hypoglycemia). (6) *If the patient is agitated,* consider hypoxia rather than withdrawal and treat as such. (7) *Observe for withdrawal* (nausea, vomiting, cramps, diarrhea, dilated pupils, rhinorrhea, piloerection). If these occur, stop naloxone.

OPIOID ADDICT WITHDRAWAL SCORE. Symptoms of withdrawal are diarrhea, dilated pupils, gooseflesh, hyperactive bowel sounds, hypertension, insomnia, lacrimation, muscle cramps, restlessness, tachycardia, and yawning. Each sign or symptom is given 0, 1, or 2 points, depending on the severity. A score of 1 to 5 is mild; 6 to 10, moderate; and 11 to 15, severe. Seizures are very unusual with withdrawal. They indicate severity regardless of the rest of the score. *Management:* Mild withdrawal is treated with diazepam orally, 10 mg every 6 hours; moderate withdrawal, with intramuscular diazepam; and severe withdrawal, with diazepam and diphenoxylate (Lomotil) for the diarrhea. Methadone orally may be used, 20 to 40 mg every 12 hours, decreased by 5 mg every 12 hours. When 10 mg is reached, add Lomotil. Clonidine (Catapres), 6 μg per kg every 6 hours, can be used with informed consent. (This is an unlisted use of clonidine; the manufacturer states that relief from withdrawal symptoms has been reported with 0.8 mg per day.)

*Laboratory aids:* For acute overdose obtain levels of blood gases, blood glucose, and electrolytes; chest x-ray; and ECG. Blood opioid levels confirm diagnosis but are not useful for making a therapeutic decision. For drug abusers, consider testing for hepatitis B, syphilis, and HIV antibody (HIV testing usually requires consent).

PROPOXYPHENE (Darvon). *Manifestations:* Onset may be as early as 30 minutes after ingestion. Convulsions occur early. Patients may develop diabetes insipidus, pulmonary edema, and hypoglycemia. *Elimination:* Metabolism is 90% by demethylation in the liver. Peak plasma level of 1 to 2 hours after oral dose. Half-life

is 1 to 5 hours. As little as 10 mg per kg has caused symptoms, and 35 mg per kg has caused cardiopulmonary arrest. Therapeutic blood level is less than 200 μg per ml. *Treatment* (in addition to the general management): (1) Emesis can be dangerous because of the rapid onset of seizures. (2) Indications for naloxone are respiratory depression, seizure activity, coma, and miotic pupils. Signs of naloxone effect are dilation of pupils, increased rate and depth of respirations, reversal of hypotension, and improvement of obtunded or comatose state. Larger doses of naloxone are often required and can be continued as an infusion of the initial response dose every hour. (3) Naloxone and intravenous glucose should be tried first to control seizures. If these fail, diazepam may be tried.

**Organochlorine Insecticides** (DDT Derivatives). See Table 23 for a listing of these agents. The *toxic dose* varies greatly. Chlorophenothane (DDT), 200 to 250 mg per kg, is fatal; 16 mg per kg causes seizures. Methoxychlor, 500 to 600 mg per kg, is fatal. Chlordane, 200 mg per kg, is fatal (chlordane house air guidelines are below 5 μg per m³; the occupational TLV is 500 μg per m³). These insecticides interfere with axon transmission of nerve impulses. Metabolism varies; they resist degradation in human tissue and the environment. They accumulate in adipose tissue; the elimination route is via the liver. *Manifestations:* CNS stimulation, convulsions, late respiratory depression, increased myocardial irritability. Endrin produces liver toxicity with guarded prognosis. Chronic exposure causes liver and kidney damage. *Management:* (1) Dermal decontamination, discard contaminated leather goods. Protect personnel. Gastrointestinal decontamination, no oils. Emesis can be dangerous, owing to rapid seizures. Many of these agents are dissolved in petroleum distillates, presenting an aspiration hazard. (2) No adrenergic stimulants (epinephrine) should be used because of myocardial irritability. (3) Cholestyramine, 4 grams every 8 hours, has been reported to increase the fecal excretion. (4) Anticonvulsants, if needed.

**Organophosphate and Carbamate Insecticides** (OPI). These may cause (1) irreversible inhibition of cholinesterase, either direct (TEPP) or delayed (parathion or malathion), or (2) reversible inhibition of cholinesterase (carbamates). Examples of OPI are listed in Table 24. Absorption is by all routes. The onset of acute toxicity is usually before 12 hours and always before 24 hours. *Toxic manifestations:* Early, cholinergic crisis—cramps, diarrhea, excess secretion, bronchospasms, bradycardia. Later, sympathetic and nicotine effects occur—twitching, fasciculations, weakness, tachycardia and hypertension, and convulsions. CNS effects are anxiety, confusion, emotional lability, and coma. Delayed respiratory paralysis and neurologic disorders have been described.

*Management:* (1) Basic life support and decontamination with careful protection of personnel. (2) Atropine (Antidote 7, Table 4), if symptomatic, every 10 to 30 minutes until drying of secretions and clearing of lungs occur. Maintain for 12 to 24 hours, then taper the dose and observe for relapse. (3) Intravenous pralidoxime (2-PAM) is required after atropinization (Antidote 31, Table 4). It should be given early. Its use

TABLE 23. **Organochlorine Pesticides (DDT Derivatives)**

| Chemical Name | Trade Name | Toxicity Rating | Elimination Time | Comment |
|---|---|---|---|---|
| Endrin | Hexadrin | Highest | hr–days | Banned |
| Lindane | 1% in Kwell; Benesan; Isotox; Gamene | Moderate to high | hr–days | Scabicide; general garden insecticide |
| Endosulfan | Thiodan | Moderate | hr–days | |
| Benzene hexachloride | BHC, HCH | Moderate | wk–mo | Banned, produces porphyria (cutanea tarda) |
| Dieldrin | Dieldrite | High | wk–mo | |
| Aldrin | Aldrite | High | wk–mo | |
| Chlordane (10% is heptachlor) | Chlordan | High | wk–mo | Restricted; termiticide |
| Toxophene | Toxakil Strobane-T | High | hrs–days | |
| Heptachlor | — | Moderate | wk–mo | Malignancy in rats |
| Chlorophenothane | DDT | Moderate | mo–yr | Banned in 1972 |
| Mirex | — | Moderate | mo–yr | Banned; red anticide |
| Chlordecone | Kepone | Moderate | mo–yr | Tidewater, Virginia, contamination |
| Methoxychlor | Marlate | Low | hr–days | |
| Perthane | — | Low | hr–days | |
| Dicofol | Kelthane | Low | hr–days | |
| Chlorobenzilate | Acaraben | Low | hr–days | Banned |

may require reduction in the dose of atropine. (4) Careful dermal and gastrointestinal decontamination when stable. (5) Suction secretions until atropinization drying is achieved. Intubation and assisted ventilation may be needed. (6) *Do not* use morphine, aminophylline, phenothiazine, or reserpine-like drugs or succinylcholine. *Laboratory aids:* Draw blood for red blood cell cholinesterase determination before giving pralidoxime. Levels are usually more than 50% depressed for severe symptoms. Monitor chest radiograph, blood glucose, arterial blood gases, ECG, blood coagulation status, liver function, and the urine for the metabolite alkyl phosphate *p*-nitrophenol. *Note:* If the diagnosis is probable, do not delay therapy until it is confirmed by laboratory tests. Atropine is both a diagnostic and a therapeutic agent. A test dose of 1 mg in adults and 0.01 mg per kg in children may be administered parenterally. In the presence of severe cholinesterase inhibition, the patient fails to develop signs of atropinization.

It is not medically advisable to administer atropine or pralidoxime prophylactically to workers exposed to organophosphate pesticides.

CARBAMATES (esters of carbonic acid). Carbamates cause reversible carbamylation of acetylcholinesterase. Pralidoxime is usually not indicated in the management but atropine may be required. The major differences from OPI are (1) toxicity is less and of shorter duration; (2) they rarely produce overt CNS effects because of poor penetration; and (3) cholinesterase returns to normal rapidly so that blood values are not useful in confirming the diagnosis. Some common examples of carbamates are Ziram, Temik (alkicarb) (taken up by plants and fruit), Matacil (aminocarb, carazol), Vydate (oxamyl), Isolan, furadan (Carbofuran), Lannate (methomyl, Nudrin), Zectran (mexacarbate), and Mesural (methiocarb). These agents are all highly toxic. Moderately toxic are Baygon (pro-

poxur) and Sevin (carbaryl). Some of these agents may be formulated in wood alcohol and have the added toxicity of methyl alcohol.

**Paradichlorobenzene.** See Hydrocarbons.

**Paraquat and Diquat.** Paraquat is a quaternary ammonia herbicide rapidly inactivated in the soil by clay particles. Nonindustrial preparations of 0.2% are unlikely to cause serious intoxications. *Toxic dose:* Commercial preparations such as Gramoxone 20% are very toxic; one mouthful has produced death. Systemic absorption in the course of occupational use is apparently minimal. Paraquat on marijuana leaves is pyrolyzed to nontoxic dipyridyl. *Toxicokinetics:* "Hit and run" toxin. Less than 20% is absorbed. The peak is 1 hour postingestion. The route of elimination is the kidney. Most of the dose is eliminated in the first 40 hours; it is detected in urine for 15 days. Volume distribution is over 500 liters per kg. *Manifestations:* Local corrosive effect on skin and mucous membranes. Acute renal failure in 48 hours (often reversible). Pulmonary effects in 72 hours are progressive, and oxygen aggravates the pulmonary fibrosis. Diquat does not produce effects on the lungs but produces convulsions and gastrointestinal distention. Long-term exposure may cause cataracts. Chlormequat's target organ is the kidney.

*Management:* (1) Gastrointestinal decontamination despite corrosive effects should be done cautiously with a nasogastric tube. Repeated doses of activated charcoal are recommended. Dermal and ocular decontamination as needed. (2) Hemodialysis and hemoperfusion may be carried out in tandem. Hemoperfusion with charcoal alone is the present choice; however, the results are still poor. Continue hemoperfusion until blood paraquat levels cannot be detected. (3) Diuresis may be of value but consider the risk of fluid overload. (4) Niacin and vitamin E have not been effective. (5) Avoid oxygen unless absolutely necessary (Pa$_{O_2}$ below 60 mmHg) because this aggravates fibrosis. Some use

TABLE 24. **Examples of Organophosphate Insecticides (OPI)**

| Common Name | Synonym | EFD* |
|---|---|---|
| *Agricultural Products* (highly toxic; $LD_{50}$ is 1–40 mg/kg) | | |
| Tetraethyl pyrophosphate | TEPP, Tetron | 0.05 |
| Phorate | Thimet | |
| Disulfoton† | Di-Syston | 0.2 |
| Demeton† | Systox | |
| Terbufos | Counter | |
| Chlortriphos | Calathion | |
| Mevinphos | Phosdrin | 0.15 |
| Parathion | Thiophos | 0.10 |
| Methamidophos | Monitor | Delayed neuropathy |
| Monocrotophos | Azodrin | |
| Octamethyl-diphosphoramide | OMPA, Schradan | |
| Azinphosmethyl | Guthion | 0.2 |
| Ethyl–nitrophenyl thiobenzene $PO_4$ | EPN | |
| *Animal Insecticides* (moderately toxic; $LD_{50}$ is 40–200 mg/kg) | | |
| DEF | DeGreen | |
| Dichlorvos | DDVP, Vapona | |
| Coumaphos | Co-ral | |
| Trichlorfon | Dylox | |
| Ronnel | Korlan | 10.0 |
| Dimethoate | Cygon, De-Fend | |
| Fenthion | Baytex | Long acting |
| Leptophos | Phosvel | |
| Chlorfenvinophos (tick dip) | Supona, Dermaton | |
| *Household and Garden Pest Control* (low toxicity; $LD_{50}$ is 200–1400 mg/kg) | | |
| Malathion | Cythion | 60.0 |
| Diazinon‡ | Spectracide, Dimpylate | 25.0 |
| Chlorpyrifos‡ | Lorsban, Dursban | |
| Temephos | Abate | |

*Estimated fatal dose (grams/70 kg).
†Most OPI degrade in the environment in a few days to nontoxic radicals. These are taken up by the plants and fruits.
‡Some classify these as moderately toxic.

hypoxic air, $FI_{O_2}$ 10 to 20%. (6) Corticosteroids may help prevent adrenocortical necrosis. *Laboratory aids:* Blood levels above 2 μg per ml at 4 hours or above 0.10 μg per ml at 24 hours are usually fatal. Blood level testing and advice may be obtained from ICI American, 800–327–8633. Monitor renal, liver, and pulmonary functions and chest radiographs. Urine test for paraquat exposure: alkalinization and sodium dithionite give an intense blue-green color in exposure.

**Parathion.** See Organophosphate Insecticides.

**Pentazocine** (Talwin). See Opioids.

**Perphenazine.** See Phenothiazines and Other Major Neuroleptics.

**Petroleum Products.** See Hydrocarbons.

**Phencyclidine** (Angel Dust, PCP, Peace Pill, Hog). This is the "drug of deceit" because it is substituted for many other drugs, such as THC and mescaline. There are now at least 38 analogues. Smoking may give cyanide poisoning. Improper mixing has caused explosions. *Toxic dose:* Two to 5 mg smoked or "snorted" produces drunken behavior, agitation, and excitement. Five to 10 mg produces stupor, coma, and myoclonus convulsions. Ten to 25 mg smoked, snorted, or taken orally results in prolonged coma and respiratory failure. It is usually fatal over 25 mg (250 ng per ml blood concentration). *Toxicokinetics:* Weak base. Rapidly absorbed when smoked, snorted, or ingested and secreted into stomach gastric juice. Absorbed in alkaline intestine, but ion trapping takes place in acid gastric media. Half-life is 30 to 60 minutes. Lipophilic drug with extensive Vd. The onset of action if smoked is 2 to 5 minutes (peak in 15 to 30 minutes); orally, 30 to 60 minutes. The duration at low doses is 4 to 6 hours and normality returns in 24 hours. At large overdoses coma may last 6 to 10 days (waxes and wanes). An adverse reaction in overdose occurs in 1 to 2 hours. *Route of elimination:* By liver metabolism (50%). Urinary excretion of conjugates and free PCP. *Manifestations:* Sympathomimetic, cholinergic, cerebellar. Observe for violent behavior, paranoid schizophrenia, self-destructive behavior. Clues to diagnosis are bursts of horizontal, vertical, and rotary nystagmus, coma with eyes open.

*Management* (avoid overtreatment of mild intoxications): (1) Gastrointestinal decontamination up to 4 hours postingestion, but this may not be effective because PCP is rapidly absorbed. Insert nasogastric tube into stomach for administration of activated charcoal every 6 hours, because PCP is secreted into the stomach even if it is smoked or snorted. (2) Protect patient and others from harm. "Talk down" is usually ineffective. Low sensory environment. Diazepam (Valium) may be used orally or intramuscularly in the uncooperative patient. (3) For behavioral disorders and toxic psychosis—haloperidol (Haldol), 2 to 5 mg, or diazepam or both. (4) Seizures and muscle spasm—control with diazepam, 2.5 mg, up to 10 mg (Antidote 16, Table 4). (5) Dystonia reaction—diphenhydramine (Benadryl) intravenously (Antidote 18, Table 4). (6) Hyperthermia—external cooling. (7) Hypertensive crisis (dopaminergic)—use nitroprusside, 0.5 to 10 μg per kg per minute. (8) Acid diuresis ion trapping (controversial). Ammonium chloride use is not routinely recommended. If rhabdomyolysis occurs, myoglobin may precipitate in the renal tubules (Antidote 2, Table 4). (9) No phenothiazines in the acute phase of intoxication because they lower the convulsive threshold. May be needed later for psychosis.

*Laboratory aids:* (1) CPK level will be clue to the amount of rhabdomyolysis occurring and the chance of myoglobinuria developing. Values up to 20,000 units have been reported. (2) Test urine for myoglobin and pigmented casts. Test urine with ortho-toluidine; a positive test without red blood cells on microscopic examination suggests myoglobinuria. (3) Monitor urine and blood pH and urinary output if acidifying patient. (4) Measure PCP level. (5) Evaluate blood urea nitrogen, ammonia, electrolytes, blood glucose levels (20% of patients have hypoglycemia). (6) Test for PCP in gastric juice; levels are 40 to 50 times higher than in blood. *Complications:* Rhabdomyolysis, myoglobinuria, and renal failure. Dopaminogenic-hypertensive crisis, cerebrovascular accident, encephalopathy, and malignant hyperthermia. Schizophrenic paranoid psychosis (induced in chronic users or precipitated in acute users). Loss of memory for months. Teratogenic cases have been reported. Children have been intoxicated from inhalation in a room where adults were smoking PCP. PCP-induced depression and suicide.

**Phenobarbital.** See Barbiturates.

**Phenothiazines and Other Major Neuroleptics.** Phenothiazines are represented by aliphatic compounds: chlorpromazine (Thorazine), promethazine (Phenergan), promazine (Sparine), triflupromazine (Vesprin), methoxypromazine (Tentone); piperazine compounds (dimethylamine series); acetophenazine (Tindal), fluphenazine (Prolixin), prochlorperazine (Compazine), perphenazine (Trilafon), trifluoperazine (Stelazine); and piperidine compounds: mepazine (Pacatal), mesoridazine (Serentil), thioridazine (Mellaril), pipamazine (Mornidine). Nonphenothiazines are the thioxanthines: chlorprothixene (Taractan), thiothixene (Navane); butyrophenones: haloperidol (Haldol), droperidol (Inapsine); dibenzoxazepines: loxapine (Loxitane, Daxolin); and dihydroindolones: molindone (Moban, Lidone). These have pharmacologic properties similar to those of the phenothiazines. *Manifestations:* Clues to phenothiazine overdose are miosis, tremor, hypotension, hypothermia, respiratory depression, radiopaque pills on radiograph of abdomen, and increased QT waves in the ECG. Anticholinergic actions are also present. Major problems are respiratory depression, myocardial toxicity (quinidine-like), neurogenic hypotension (antidopaminogenic), and idiosyncratic reaction, which may occur at therapeutic levels. Idiosyncratic reaction consists of opisthotonos, torticollis, orolingual dyskinesis, and oculogyric crisis (painful upward gaze) and can be mistaken for a psychotic episode. Extrapyramidal crisis is frequent in children and women. Death is usually due to cardiac effects. Phenothiazines are metabolized by the liver into many metabolites. Some remain in the body longer than 6 months.

*Management:* (1) Gastrointestinal decontamination. Emesis induction may be useful if symptoms have not occurred. If symptoms are already present, many of these agents have antiemetic action, so lavage may be required. Always provide gastric lavage to comatose patients after the airway is protected regardless of the time of ingestion because of inhibition of gastric motility. (2) Extrapyramidal signs (idiosyncratic reaction) can be treated with diphenhydramine (Benadryl) (Antidote 18, Table 4), or benztropine (Cogentin), 1 to 2 mg intravenously slowly. Symptoms recur, and these drugs should be continued orally for 2 to 3 days. *This is not the treatment of overdose,* only of the idiosyncratic reaction. (3) Monitor ECG for dysrhythmias and treat with antidysrhythmic agents. (4) Hypotension is treated with the Trendelenburg position or fluid challenge or both. Vasopressors are used only if these fail. Dopamine (Intropin) should not be used to treat the hypotension because these drugs are antidopaminogenic. If a pressor agent is needed, use norepinephrine (Levarterenol, Levophed). (5) Treat neuroleptic malignant syndrome by discontinuing the offending agent, reducing temperature with external cooling, and correcting any metabolic imbalance. Dantrolene, bromo-

criptine, and amantadine are agents that have been shown to be useful pharmacologic adjuncts for the management of this syndrome. (6) Treat hypo- or hyperthermia with external physical measures (not drugs).

*Laboratory aids:* A ferric chloride test of urine can confirm exposure to phenothiazines if there is a sufficient blood level. Blood levels are *not* useful in management. A radiograph of the abdomen is useful to detect undissolved tablets, which may be radiopaque. Monitor arterial blood gases, renal and hepatic function, and levels of electrolytes and blood glucose for creatinine kinase and myoglobinemia in neuroleptic malignant syndrome.

**Phenylpropanolamine** (PPA). See Amphetamines.

**Primidone.** See Anticonvulsants.

**Propoxyphene.** See Opioids.

**Propranolol and Beta Blockers.** Some of these agents available in the United States at this time are listed in Table 25. *Toxic dose:* Varies considerably. *Toxicokinetics:* Peak action is 1 to 2 hours orally and lasts 24 to 48 hours. In drugs with long half-lives, e.g., nadolol, it may take many days to recover from overdose toxicity (Table 25). *Manifestations:* Observe for bradycardia and hypotension. Fat-soluble drugs have more CNS effects. Partial agonists may produce tachycardia and hypertension (oxprenolol, pindolol).

*Management:* (1) Gastrointestinal decontamination with gastric lavage and activated charcoal/cathartic. Before gastric lavage, treatment with atropine, 0.01 mg per kg for a child and 0.5 mg for an adult, has been suggested to decrease the vagal effect in patients with bradycardia or significant intoxications. Avoid induced emesis because of early onset of seizures and vagal stimulation. Asymptomatic patients may be discharged after 12 to 24 hours of observation. (2) Treat hypoglycemia (frequent in children) and hyperkalemia. (3) Control convulsions. (4) Cardiovascular manifestations: Bradycardia—if hemodynamically stable and asymptomatic, no therapy. If unstable (hypotension or atrioventricular block), use atropine, isoproterenol, glucagon, and pacemaker. Ventricular tachycardia or premature beats—use lidocaine, phenytoin, or overdrive pacing. Myocardial depression and hypotension—correct dysrhythmias, institute Trendelenburg positioning, and fluids. Monitor with PAWP catheter. If low cardiac output with low PAWP, give more fluids. If low cardiac output with normal PAWP, use glucagon (Antidote 22, Table 4). Avoid quinidine, procainamide, and disopyramide (Norpace). Glucagon is probably the drug of choice, since it works through an adenyl cyclase mechanism not affected by the beta blockers. It is given as a bolus and may be continued as an infusion (Antidote 22, Table 4). If bronchospasm, give aminophylline. Hemodialysis or hemoperfusion for low volume distribution drugs that are low protein binding and water soluble (nadolol and atenolol), particularly with evidence of renal failure. If hypoglycemia, give intravenous glucose. *Laboratory aids:* Monitor blood glucose, potassium, ECG, PAWP. Fatal blood level of propranolol is 0.8 to 1.2 mg per dl (8 to 12 µg per ml).

**Quinidine and Quinine** (Antidysrhythmic and Antimalarial Agents). *Toxic dose* in child is 60 mg per kg; in adult, 2 to 8 grams. There is 95 to 100% absorption,

TABLE 25. **Pharmacokinetic Properties of Beta Blockers**

| Drug Name | Solubility and Absorption (%) | Plasma t½ (hr) | Elimination Route | Peak Concentration (hr) | Protein Bound (%) | Vd (Liters/kg) | Beta₁ Cardiac Selective |
|---|---|---|---|---|---|---|---|
| Acebutolol* (Sectral) Dose: 400–800 mg MDD: 800 mg TPC: 200–2000 ng/ml | Moderate, lipid (90) | 3–4, metabolite diacetolol | Hepatic, active metabolite | — | 26 | 1.2 | + |
| Alprenolol* (Aptin, Betapin; Betacard) Dose: 200–800 mg MDD: 800 mg TPC: 50–200 ng/ml | Lipid (10) | 3.1 | Hepatic | 1–3 | 85 | 3.4 | − |
| Atenolol (Tenormin) Dose: 50–100 mg MDD: 100 mg TPC: 200–500 ng/ml | Water (46–62) | 6–9 | Renal, 95% | 2–4 | 3–10 | 0.7 | + |
| Betaxolol (Betoptic) Dose: 1 drop in eye twice daily MDD: not available | Water (70–90) | 12–22 | Hepatic, 3–12% | — | 50–60 | 4.9–13 | + |
| Esmolol (Brevibloc) Dose: IV 50–500 μg/kg/min (loading dose) MDD: 300 μg/kg/min | Water | 9 min | Hepatic, plasma esterases | — | 55 | 3.4 | + |
| Labetalol (Normodyne, Trandate) Dose: 400–800 mg MDD: 1–2 grams | Water (50) | 6–8 | Hepatic, 95% Blocks alpha (weakly) and beta activity | — | 50 | 11 | − |
| Levobunolol (Betagan) Dose: Ophthalmologic: 1 drop twice daily, 0.5%, 1% | Water (100) | 6.1 | Hepatic | — | — | — | − |
| Metoprolol (Lopressor) Dose: 50–100 mg MDD: 450 mg TPC: 50–100 ng/ml | Lipid (>95) | 3–4 | Hepatic | 1–2 | 10 | 5.6 | + |
| Nadolol (Corgard) Dose: 40–320 mg MDD: 320 mg TPC: 20–400 ng/ml | Water (15–25) | 14–23 | Renal, 70% | 3–4 | 25 | 2.1 | − |
| Oxyprenolol (Trasicor) Dose: 80–320 mg MDD: 480 mg TPC: 80–100 ng/ml | Lipid (70–95) | 1.5–3 | Hepatic | 1–2 | 80 | 1.5 | − |
| Pindolol* (Visken) Dose: 20–60 mg MDD: 60 mg TPC: 50–150 ng/ml | Lipid (>90) | 3–4 | Hepatic, 60%; renal, 40% | 1.25 | 57 | 2.0 | − |
| Practolol* (Eraldin) Dose: 25–600 mg MDD: 800 mg TPC: 1500–5000 ng/ml | Water (100) | 6–8 | Renal No longer available in United States because of adverse reactions | 3 | 40 | — | + |

*Table continued on following page*

TABLE 25. **Pharmacokinetic Properties of Beta Blockers** Continued

| Drug Name | Solubility and Absorption (%) | Plasma t½ (hr) | Elimination Route | Peak Concentration (hr) | Protein Bound (%) | Vd (Liters/kg) | Beta₁ Cardiac Selective |
|---|---|---|---|---|---|---|---|
| Propranolol (Inderal)<br>Dose: 40–160 mg<br>MDD: 480 mg<br>TPC: 50–100 ng/ml | Lipid (100) (70% first pass) | 2–3 | Hepatic; renal (<1%), active hydroxy metabolite | 1.5 | 90–95 | 3.6 | – |
| Sotalol (Beta-cardone, Sotacor)<br>Dose: 80–320 mg<br>MDD: 480 mg<br>TPC: 500–4000 ng/ml | Water (70) | 5–13 | Renal<br>Prolongs QT and may produce torsades de pointes | 2–3 | 54 | 0.7 | – |
| Timolol†‡ (Blocadren)<br>Dose: 20 mg; ophthalmologic (Timoptic, 0.25%, 0.5%), 1 drop twice daily<br>MDD: 60 mg<br>TPC: 5–10 ng/ml | Lipid (>90) | 3–5 | Hepatic, 80%; renal, 20% | 4–5 | <10 | 5.5 | – |

*Partial agonists.
†Substantial first pass.
‡Mitochondrial calcium protection during ischemia.
Abbreviations: MDD = maximum daily dose; TPC = therapeutic plasma concentration.

with peak action in 2 to 4 hours. Half-life is 3 to 4 hours (quinidine gluconate, 8 to 12 hours). Large Vd. Metabolized predominantly by the liver. *Manifestations*: Cinchonism (headache, nausea, vomiting, tinnitus, deafness, diplopia, dilated pupils). Myocardial depression, dysrhythmias, ECG changes—prolongation of PR, QRS, and QT intervals. Rashes and flushing. Hemolysis in glucose-6-phosphate dehydrogenase deficiency. Dementia reported. *Management*: (1) Gastrointestinal decontamination. (2) Monitor ECG and liver function. (3) May need antidysrhythmic drugs and pacemaker and alkalinization.

**Salicylates.** *Toxic dose:* See Table 26. Methyl salicylate (oil of wintergreen): 1 ml equals 1.4 grams of salicylate. One teaspoonful equals 21 adult aspirins. *Toxicokinetics*: Plasma concentration is significant in

30 minutes and peaks in 1 to 2 hours. Half-life is 3 to 6 hours (therapeutic) to 12 to 36 hours (toxic). Urine pH influences urine salicylate elimination. *Manifestations of acute ingestion* (see Table 26): The metabolic disturbance in adults and older children is usually respiratory alkalosis; in children under 5 years of age, the initial respiratory alkalosis will usually change to metabolic or mixed metabolic acidosis and respiratory alkalosis, with acidosis predominating within a few hours.

*Management*: (1) Gastrointestinal decontamination is useful up to 12 hours postingestion, as some factors delay absorption (food, enteric-coated tablets, other drugs); pylorospasm may delay emptying; and concretions may form. Activated charcoal should be administered every 4 hours until stools are black. Concretions

TABLE 26. **Quantities of Aspirin Ingested: Deposition and Manifestations***

| Category | Amount Ingested (mg/kg) | Toxicity Expected | Gastrointestinal Decontamination | Manifestations Anticipated |
|---|---|---|---|---|
| Nontoxic | <150 | No | No | None |
| Usually nontoxic | >150 | No | Yes (home) | None |
| Mild intoxication | 150–200 | Yes | Yes (ECF) | Vomiting, tinnitus, mild hyperventilation |
| Moderate intoxication | 200–300 | Yes | Yes (ECF) | Hyperpnea, lethargy or excitability |
| Severe intoxication | 300–500 | Yes | Yes (ECF) | Coma, convulsions, severe hyperpnea |
| Very severe intoxication | >500 | Yes | Yes (ECF) | Potentially fatal |

*See toxic dose indications for gastrointestinal decontamination.
*Abbreviation:* ECF = emergency care facility.

TABLE 27. **Recommendations for Fluid Management for Moderate or Severe Salicylism***

| Purpose | Rate (ml/kg/hr) | Duration (hr) | mEq/Liter | | | | Glucose (%) |
|---|---|---|---|---|---|---|---|
| | | | Na | K | Cl | HCO₃ | |
| Volume expansion | 20 | 0.5–1.0 | 100 | 0 | 77 | 23 | 5–10 |

Administered as 0.45% saline with 23 mEq/liter NaHCO₃

| | | | Na | K | Cl | HCO₃ | Glucose (%) |
|---|---|---|---|---|---|---|---|
| Hydration Ongoing losses Alkalinization | 4–8 | Until therapeutic blood serum concentration 30 mg/dl | 56 | 40 | 56 | 1–2 mEq/kg child; 50–100 mEq adult | 5–10 |

Administered as 0.33% saline and NaHCO₃ to obtain urine pH 7.5–8.0, blood pH 7.5

| | | | mEq/kg/day | | | |
|---|---|---|---|---|---|---|
| Maintenance | 2–6 | — | 3 | 2 | 4 | |

*For severe acidosis pH < 7.15, may require 1–2 mEq/kg of sodium bicarbonate every 1–2 hr. Usual fluid loss is 200–300 ml/kg, but carefully monitor for fluid overload. Potassium may be needed in excess of 40 mEq/liter when alkalinizing.

may be removed by lavage, whole-body irrigation, endoscopy, or gastrostomy. (2) Intravenous fluid should be given as recommended in Table 27. Alkalinization enhances salicylate excretion. Potassium is essential to produce adequate alkalinization. Monitor *both* the urine *and* blood pH. Do not use the urine pH alone to assess the need for alkalinization (Antidote 35, Table 4). (3) Fluid retention can be treated with mannitol (20%), 0.5 gram per kg over 30 minutes, or furosemide, 1 mg per kg intravenously. (4) Hyperpyrexia should be treated with external cooling. (5) Abnormal bleeding or hypoprothrombinemia will need vitamin K, 10 to 50 mg intravenously, and, if bleeding continues, fresh blood or platelet transfusion (Antidote 38, Table 4). (6) Dialysis (hemodialysis) or hemoperfusion is indicated if there is persistent acidosis (pH < 7.1) and lack of response to fluid or alkali in 6 hours; if serum salicylate levels are initially greater than 160 mg per dl or greater than 130 mg per dl at 6 hours postingestion (do *not* use the salicylate level as the sole criterion for dialysis); or if there are coma and uncontrollable seizures, congestive heart failure, acute renal failure, and progressive deterioration despite good management. (7) Chronic toxicity is usually a more severe intoxication because of the cumulative pharmocokinetics of salicylates. Management needs are outlined in Table 28.

*Laboratory aids*: The metabolic acidosis of salicylism has a moderately elevated anion gap. Hyper- or hypo-glycemia may exist. Serum salicylate levels used in conjunction with the Done nomogram (Figure 3) are useful predictors of expected severity following *acute single ingestions*. The Done nomogram is *not* useful in chronic intoxications, methyl salicylate, phenyl salicylate, or homomethyl salicylate ingestions. The salicylate level for use in the Done nomogram should be obtained 6 hours postingestion. Before 6 hours, levels in the toxic range should be treated, and patients with levels below the toxic range should be retested if a potentially toxic dose is ingested. Monitor urine output, urine pH, electrolytes, arterial blood gases, blood glucose, prothrombin time, renal function, serum salicylate level, and urine salicylate with the ferric chloride test. Arterial blood pH should be kept at 7.5. *Prognosis*: Persistent vigorous treatment of salicylate ingestion is essential, as recovery has occurred despite decerebrate rigidity.

**Sedative Hypnotics, Nonbarbiturate.** See Table 29. *Management* is primarily supportive (especially intubation and ventilator therapy with continuous positive airway pressure for adult respiratory distress syndrome) and with the use of hemoperfusion or hemodialysis in patients who are severely intoxicated and fail to respond to good supportive care and whose intoxication is life-threatening. Avoid emesis because of rapid onset of convulsions, apnea, and coma. (1) *Chloral hydrate* management includes cautious gastrointestinal decontamination. Avoid the use of epinephrine

TABLE 28. **Management of Chronic Salicylate Intoxication**

| Classification | Urine pH | Blood pH | Hydration | NaHCO₃ (mEq/liter) | Potassium (mEq/liter) |
|---|---|---|---|---|---|
| Mild | Alkaline | Alkaline | Yes | No† | 20 |
| Moderate | Acid* | Alkaline | Yes | pH 7.5† | 40 |
| Severe | Acid | Acid | Yes | pH 7.5 | 40‡ 80§ |

*Paradoxical acid urine and alkaline blood indicate potassium depletion.
†Bicarbonate administered to keep blood pH 7.5 and urine pH 7.5–8.0.
‡Normal serum potassium and ECG.
§Low serum potassium and/or abnormal ECG indicating potassium deficiency.

TABLE 29. **Nonbarbiturate Sedative Hypnotic Drugs**

| Drug | Absorption and Toxic Dose | Peak (hr) | Vd (Liter/kg) | Protein Bound (%) | Elimination Route | Serum Half-life (hr) | Toxic Level (μg/ml) | Manifestations and Comment* |
|---|---|---|---|---|---|---|---|---|
| Chloral hydrate (Noctec) | Rapid TD, 2 grams FD, 4–10 grams | 1–2 | 0.75–0.9 | 40 | Hepatic 90% to active metabolite trichloroethanol (TCE) | 4–8 | 100 (80 TCE—very toxic) | Pear-like odor; dysrhythmias (especially ventricular), hepatotoxicity, irritant to mucosa of GI tract; ARDS; radiopaque capsules |
| Ethchlorvynol (Placidyl) | Rapid TD, 2.5 grams FD, 5 grams | 1–2 | 3–4 | 35–50 | Hepatic 90% | 10–25 in OD over 100 | 20–80 | Prolonged coma up to 200 hr, apnea, hypothermia, pulmonary edema, pink gastric aspirate, pungent odor |
| Glutethimide (Doriden) (highest mortality of all sedative hypnotics, 14%) | Slow, erratic TD, 5 grams FD, 10 grams | 6 | Large, 2–2.7 | 50 | Hepatic 98% to toxic metabolite 4-hydroxyglutarimide | 10 in OD over 100 | 20–80 | Prolonged, cyclic coma up to 120 hr, anticholinergic signs, convulsions, recurrent apnea, hyperthermia |
| Meprobamate (Equanil, Miltown) | Rapid TD, 10 grams | 4–8 | 10 | 20 | Hepatic 90% | 6–16 | 30–100 | Coma, convulsions, pulmonary edema, apnea, concretions in stomach |
| Methaqualone (Quaaludes, "love drugs") | Rapid TD, 800 mg FD, 125 mg/kg | 1–3 | 2–6 | 80 | Hepatic 90% | 10–40 | 8–10 | Hypertonia, hyper-reflexia, convulsions, apnea, acts "drunk," bleeding tendencies |
| Methyprylon (Noludar) | Rapid TD, 3 grams | 2–4 | 1–2 | — | Hepatic 97% | 3–6; over 8 in OD over 50 | 30 | Hyperactive coma lasts 30 hr, miosis, persistent hypotension, pulmonary edema; mortality rare |

*Comment includes other features besides the typical manifestations of all these agents—coma, respiratory depression, psychologic and physiologic withdrawal, hypotension, hypothermia (except glutethimide hyperthermia).

*Abbreviations:* TD = toxic dose; FD = fatal dose; OD = overdose; ARDS = adult respiratory distress syndrome; GI = gastrointestinal.

and catecholamines that may produce dysrhythmias. Propranolol, 0.1 mg per kg in 1-mg increments, appears to be more effective than lidocaine for ventricular dysrhythmias. (2) *Ethchlorvynol* management includes gastrointestinal decontamination up to 12 hours postingestion. Resin hemoperfusion (Amberlite XAD-4) is the best method of extracorporeal removal when other measures fail in a life-threatening situation (ingestion of over 10 grams or 100 mg per kg, with serum levels of over 100 μg per ml in the first 12 hours or 70 μg per ml after 12 hours in patients with prolonged life-threatening coma). External rewarming if temperature is below 32° C. (3) *Glutethimide* management includes gastrointestinal decontamination up to 24 hours postingestion. Concretions may form. Resin hemoperfusion appears to be the best method of extracorporeal removal in life-threatening protracted coma when the patient has ingested over 10 grams and has a serum level of over 30 micrograms per ml. Treat hyperthermia with external cooling. (4) *Meprobamate* management includes gastrointestinal decontamination up to 12 hours postingestion, with charcoal hemoperfusion in prolonged coma with life-threatening complications. Concretions may form in the stomach and may require breaking up or surgical removal. (5) *Methaqualone* management includes gastrointestinal decontamination. Forced diuresis, dialysis, and hemoperfusion are not indicated. Fatalities are rare. (6) *Methyprylon* management includes gastrointestinal decontamination and may require treatment of the hypotension with vasopressors of the alpha adrenergic variety—levarterenol (Levophed). The hypotension usually does not respond to position or fluids alone. This is a dialyzable drug, but dialysis usually is not necessary. Fatalities are rare.

**Strychnine.** Primarily available as a rodenticide and

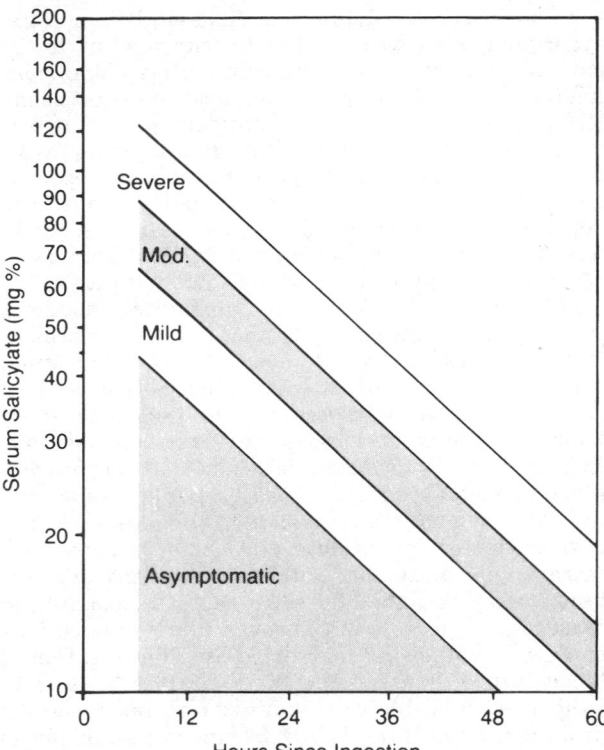

**Figure 3.** The Done nomogram for salicylate intoxication. For limitations of use, see *Laboratory aids*. (Redrawn from Done A: Salicylate intoxication: significance of measurements of salicylate in blood in cases of acute ingestion. Reproduced by permission of Pediatrics 26:800, 1960.)

component of cathartics and "tonics." Adulterant of "street drugs," particularly marijuana and cocaine. *Toxic dose*: 5 to 10 mg; fatal in doses of 15 to 30 mg. *Toxicokinetics*: Rapid absorption. Manifestations may occur within 15 to 30 minutes. Low protein binding. Hepatic metabolism, which appears to be saturable. Twenty per cent is excreted in urine. Has been found in the urine up to 48 hours after a 700-mg dose. *Manifestations*: Interferes with postsynaptic neurotransmitter inhibition by glycine. Hyperacusis is often the first sign. Mild cases—face stiffness (trismus and risus sardonicus). Moderate cases—extensor muscle thrusts. Severe cases—tetanic convulsions with opisthotonos. Death occurs within 1 to 3 hours after ingestion. The prognosis for survival improves if the patient survives beyond 5 hours. The complications of intoxication are lactic acidosis, hyperthermia, rhabdomyolysis and renal damage from precipitation of myoglobin in the renal tubules, and death from hypoxia. *Management*: (1) Emesis is contraindicated because of rapid absorption and the early onset of seizures. Gastric aspiration and lavage may be used after the seizures are controlled. Activated charcoal should be given and repeated. (2) Control convulsions with diazepam or phenobarbital. (3) Supportive care for respiratory depression. (4) Acid diuresis and dialysis do not appear to be justified on the basis of available studies. (5) Paralysis with assisted ventilation is useful.

**Tear Gas** (Lacrimators). CS (chlorobenzylidine), "riot control"; CN powder (chloroacetophenone, 1 per cent); Mace (chloroacetophenone). *Management*: Dermal and ocular decontamination. Protect attendants from contamination. Ophthalmologic evaluation. Oxygen therapy may be needed for dyspnea and respiratory distress.

**Theophylline.** *Toxic dose*: Acute, single dose greater than 10 mg per kg yields mild toxicity. Greater than 20 mg per kg, moderate manifestations. *Toxicokinetics*: Absorption is complete. Peak levels occur within 60 to 90 minutes after ingestion of liquid preparations; 1 to 3 hours after regular tablets; and 3 to 10 hours after slow-release preparations. Vd, 0.3 to 0.7 liter per kg. Protein binding, 15 to 40%. Half-life varies: 3.5 hours average in a child and 4.5 hours in an adult (range from 3 to 9 hours). In neonates and young infants the drug's half-life is much longer. Overdose increases the half-life. *Elimination*: Hepatic metabolism, 90% (demethylation and oxidation); 8 to 10% is excreted unchanged in the urine. *Manifestations*: Acute toxicity generally correlates with blood levels; chronic toxicity does not. Ten to 20 μg per ml is the therapeutic range, but some mild gastrointestinal toxicity may occur. Twenty to 40 μg per ml is moderate toxicity, with gastrointestinal and CNS stimulation. Over 50 μg per ml—seizures and dysrhythmias may occur, but they may also occur at lower levels and without gastrointestinal symptoms. Children tolerate higher serum levels. Chronic intoxication is more serious and difficult to treat. Many factors increase theophylline concentration.

*Management*: (1) Gastrointestinal decontamination in acute overdose, up to 4 hours with regular preparations and up to 8 to 12 hours with slow-release preparations. Test aspirate or vomitus for blood. Give activated charcoal every 4 hours. Do not induce emesis if hematemesis exists. (2) Monitor ECG, obtain theophylline levels every 4 hours until in the therapeutic range of 10 to 20 μg per ml. (3) Control seizures with diazepam. If coma, convulsions, or vomiting exists, intubate immediately. (4) Hypotension is treated with fluid challenge and if this fails, vasopressors. (5) Hematemesis is managed with iced saline lavage and blood replacement if needed. (6) Charcoal hemoperfusion is the management of choice in life-threatening convulsions, dysrhythmias, hematemesis, or intractable vomiting refractory to conventional measures. Differences in slow-release preparations from regular preparations: few or no gastrointestinal symptoms with high levels; peak concentration times may be 10 to 24 hours postingestion; and onset of seizures may occur 10 to 12 hours postingestion. *Laboratory aids*: Monitor theophylline levels, check for occult blood in vomitus and stools, monitor vital signs and hemoglobin and hematocrit (for hemorrhage). Monitor cardiac, renal, and hepatic function, electrolytes, blood glucose, arterial blood gases, and acid-base balance.

**Toluene.** See Hydrocarbons.

**Tranquilizers.** See Sedative Hypnotics.

**Trichloroethylene.** See Hydrocarbons.

**Tricyclic Antidepressants** (TCAD). These agents are generally rapidly absorbed from the gastrointestinal tract, but absorption may be prolonged in overdose owing to anticholinergic action. Their bioavailability has considerable variation among patients, and they are highly bound to plasma and tissue proteins. Protein binding decreases with decreasing pH. The Vd is large, usually 10 to 20 liters per kg. The TCAD are metabolized primarily in the liver. $N$-Demethylation of the tertiary amines yields the active secondary amine metabolites; hydroxylation gives rise to inactive metabolites. Forty per cent is excreted in the feces and only 3% in the urine unchanged. The t½ varies from 9 to 198 hours. In an overdose, the half-life may be much longer. Tricyclic tertiary amines (metabolized to active metabolites) are amitriptyline (Elavil), imipramine (Tofranil), and doxepin (Sinequan). Tricyclic secondary amines (metabolized to nonactive metabolites) are desipramine (Norpramin, Pertofrane), protriptyline (Vivactil), and nortriptyline (Aventyl). Tricyclic dibenzoxazepine (metabolized to a major metabolite) is amoxapine (Asendin).

*Manifestations*: The onset of action varies from less than 1 hour to 12 hours after ingestion. The phases of intoxication are (1) consciousness with dry mouth, mydriasis, ataxia, increased deep tendon reflexes, and changes in the ST segment; (2) Stages I and II coma with hypertension, tachycardia above 160, mydriasis, and supraventricular tachycardia; and (3) Stages III and IV coma with hypotension, heart rate under 120, respiratory depression, tonic-clonic seizures, and ventricular dysrhythmias. The CNS effects occur early, and seizures are common. *Cardiovascular toxicity* is frequent in the serious poisonings and results from anticholinergic effects, sympathomimetic activity (by blocking reuptake of catecholamines), quinidine activity, catecholamine depletion, and alpha-adrenergic blockage. Cardiotoxic effects include cardiac dysrhythmias, hypertension, hypotension, and pulmonary edema.

*Toxic dose*: The TCAD have a narrow margin of safety. In a child, a 375-mg dose and in adults, as little as 500 to 750 mg has been fatal. The following dosages may serve as a guide to the degree of toxicity: Less than 10 mg per kg produces light coma, mydriasis, and tachycardia and has a good prognosis. At 20 mg per kg, Stage III manifestations are produced. At 30 mg per kg, fatalities may result. At 50 mg per kg, the mortality rate is increased. Over 70 mg per kg is rarely survived. Therapeutic blood levels are in the range of 50 to 170 ng per ml. If the QRS interval is less than 0.10 second for 6 hours, the prognosis is good. If it is greater than 0.10 second, seizures may occur, and if it is over 0.16 second, serious dysrhythmia may occur.

NEWER ANTIDEPRESSANTS. Amoxapine (Asendin) allegedly has less cardiotoxicity. Patients with amoxapine overdose may develop the syndrome of seizures, rhabdomyolysis, and acute renal tubular necrosis. Recent reports indicate more fatalities with amoxapine

than with TCAD. Maprotiline (Ludiomil) is a tetracyclic compound with cardiac toxicity similar to the existing tricyclic antidepressant drugs. Trazodone hydrochloric acid (Desyrel) is an antidepressant chemically unrelated to the other antidepressants. It produces less serious toxicity, although orthostatic hypotension, vertigo, and priapism have been reported. Bupropion (Wellbutrin) is a phenylaminoketone antidepressant that produces dose-related seizures. Nomifensine (Merital) was withdrawn in 1986 because of reports of hemolytic anemia associated with it.

*Management*: (1) Maintenance of vital functions. Intensive care unit care until there are no abnormalities in the ECG for 24 to 48 hours. (2) Gastrointestinal decontamination (omit emesis) if the patient is alert. Intact pills have been recovered by lavage up to 18 hours after ingestion. Suspected cases should have ECG monitoring. (3) Activated charcoal cathartic every 4 to 6 hours and continuous nasogastric suction for the first 48 hours may interrupt enterohepatic recycling of tricyclic antidepressants. (4) Control seizures with intravenous diazepam. Intravenous phenytoin (Dilantin) may be added for seizures not responding to diazepam alone. (5) All cardiovascular complications of TCAD should *first* be treated by alkalinization of blood with sodium bicarbonate to a pH of 7.5 to 7.55 (Antidote 35, Table 4). Alkalinization increases the protein binding of the TCAD. Serum potassium levels should be followed, as a sudden increase in blood pH can aggravate or precipitate hypokalemia. Specific cardiovascular complications should be treated as follows: *Hypotension*—norepinephrine (Levophed), a predominantly alpha-adrenergic drug, is preferred over dopamine. (Hypertension that occurs early rarely requires treatment.) *Serious conduction defects* are best managed with phenytoin, and patients may need a temporary transvenous pacemaker. *Sinus tachycardia* usually does not require treatment. *Supraventricular tachycardia* that does not respond to alkalinization alone may be treated with phenytoin, physostigmine, or synchronized cardioversion. *Ventricular tachycardia*—after alkalinization and phenytoin, intravenous lidocaine (for one dose only) may be required for persistent ventricular tachycardia. Synchronized cardioversion may be needed if lidocaine fails. *Ventricular fibrillation* should be treated with direct current countershock. *Torsades de pointes* is treated with isoproterenol, lidocaine, phenytoin, and atrial or ventricular overdrive pacing to shorten the QT interval. *Laboratory aids*: Arterial blood gases with blood pH, ECG, serum electrolytes, blood urea nitrogen and creatinine, serum phenytoin level, urine output, and, in severe cases, central venous pressure and/or PAWP should be monitored.

**Turpentine.** See Hydrocarbons.

**Xylene.** See Hydrocarbons.

# Section 18

# Appendices and Index

## LABORATORY VALUES OF CLINICAL IMPORTANCE

method of
REX B. CONN, M.D.
*Thomas Jefferson University*
*Philadelphia, Pennsylvania*

Reference values for laboratory tests serve as indispensible benchmarks when evaluating laboratory data on an individual patient. However, reference values should not be considered equivalent to normal values, because in medicine it is a logical impossibility to define normality. There can be no sharp dividing line between normal and abnormal values, and there is a gradual transition during any pathologic process from what is clearly normal to a value that is clearly abnormal.

Reference values are derived from statistical studies on subjects believed to have no condition that might affect the measurement being evaluated. An important consideration is that the reference ranges derived by these statistical methods encompass only 95% of the reference population. Thus, a value slightly outside the range might be due to a chance distribution or to an underlying pathologic process.

A single reference range for all individuals may be inadequate for some measurements. Values obtained on presumably normal persons may vary because of age, sex, body build, race, environment, and state of gastrointestinal absorption. Another consideration is that values for some constituents found in a "normal" population may reflect a general disorder in the population rather than normality. Thus, reference values for serum cholesterol level now indicate the "desirable" range rather than that actually found in the reference population.

Tables of reference values must be revised and updated frequently to reflect the addition of new tests, the deletion of obsolete tests, and changes in techniques used in the clinical laboratory. As with many other aspects of medicine, widespread use of computers has both simplified and complicated application of reference ranges. Most laboratory computer systems permit use of as many as one or two dozen age- and sex-corrected ranges for each constituent, and the appropriate range is indicated on each patient's report. Serum alkaline phosphatase determination is an example of a test in which the values change dramatically with age and differ between sexes. The computer handles this well, but one can imagine how the following tables would appear if up to a dozen ranges were included for each test listed.

### THE INTERNATIONAL SYSTEM OF UNITS FOR LABORATORY MEASUREMENTS (LE SYSTÈME INTERNATIONAL D'UNITÉS)

The United States is the only major industrialized country that has not adopted the International System of Units (abbreviated S.I. units) for expressing measurements in all areas of science and industry. The medical profession in the United States has been remarkably firm in its opposition to introduction of S.I. units, even though many American medical journals express laboratory data only in S.I. units. A much more significant change occurred some 35 years ago when the apothecaries' system was abandoned in favor of the metric system for expressing drug dosages, and it appears to be only a matter of time until the International System is adopted. Because of this, the following information on S.I. units is being reprinted from *Current Therapy 1990.*

The International System is a coherent approach to all types of measurement that utilizes seven dimensionally independent basic quantities: mass, length, time, thermodynamic temperature, electrical current, luminous intensity, and amount of substance. Each of these quan-

TABLE 1. **Base Units**

| Property | Base Unit | Symbol |
|---|---|---|
| Length | meter | m |
| Mass | kilogram | kg |
| Amount of substance | mole | mol |
| Time | second | s |
| Thermodynamic temperature | kelvin | K |
| Electrical current | ampere | A |
| Luminous intensity | candela | cd |

TABLE 2. **Derived Units**

| Derived Property | Derived Unit | Symbol |
|---|---|---|
| Area | square meter | $m^2$ |
| Volume | cubic meter | $m^3$ |
| | liter | L |
| Mass concentration | kilogram/cubic meter | $kg/m^3$ |
| | gram/liter | g/L |
| Substance concentration | mole/cubic meter | $mol/m^3$ |
| | mole/liter | mol/L |
| Temperature | degree Celsius | C = K − 273.15 |

tities is expressed in a clearly defined *base unit* (Table 1).

Two or more base units may be combined to provide *derived units* (Table 2) for expressing other measurements such as mass concentration (kilograms per cubic meter) and velocity (meters per second). Standardized prefixes (Table 3) for base and derived units are used to express fractions or multiples of the base units so that any measurement can be expressed in a value between 0.001 and 1000.

### Medical Applications

The most profound change in laboratory reports will result from expressing concentration as amount per volume (moles per liter) rather than mass per volume (milligrams per 100 milliliters). The advantages of the former expression can be seen in the following:

*Conventional Units*

1.0 gram of hemoglobin
Combines with 1.37 ml of oxygen
Contains 3.4 mg of iron
Forms 34.9 mg of bilirubin

TABLE 3. **Standard Prefixes**

| Prefix | Multiplication Factor | Symbol |
|---|---|---|
| atto | $10^{-18}$ | a |
| femto | $10^{-15}$ | f |
| pico | $10^{-12}$ | p |
| nano | $10^{-9}$ | n |
| micro | $10^{-6}$ | μ |
| milli | $10^{-3}$ | m |
| centi | $10^{-2}$ | c |
| deci | $10^{-1}$ | d |
| deca | $10^1$ | da |
| hecto | $10^2$ | h |
| kilo | $10^3$ | k |
| mega | $10^6$ | M |
| giga | $10^9$ | G |
| tera | $10^{12}$ | T |

*S.I. Units*

1.0 mmol of hemoglobin
Combines with 4.0 mmol of oxygen
Contains 4.0 mmol of iron
Forms 4.0 mmol of bilirubin

Chemical relationships between lactic acid and pyruvic acid and the glucose from which both are derived, as well as the relationship between bilirubin and the binding capacity of albumin, are other examples of chemical relationships that will be clarified by using the new system.

There are a number of laboratory and other medical measurements for which the S.I. units appear to offer little advantage, and some that are disadvantageous because the change would require replacement or revision of instruments such as the sphygmomanometer. The cubic meter is the derived unit for volume; however, it is inappropriately large for medical measurements, and the liter has been retained. Thermodynamic temperature expressed in kelvins is not more informative for medical measurements. Since the Celsius degree is the same as the Kelvin degree, the Celsius scale is used. Celsius rather than centigrade is the preferred term.

Selection of units for expressing enzyme activity presents certain difficulties. Literally dozens of different units have been used in expressing enzyme activity, and interlaboratory comparison of enzyme results is impossible unless the assay system is precisely defined. In 1964, the International Union of Biochemistry attempted to remedy the situation by proposing the International Unit for enzymes. This unit was defined as the amount of enzyme that will catalyze the conversion of 1 μmol of substrate per minute under standard conditions. Difficulties remain, however, as enzyme activity is affected by temperature, pH, the type and amount of substrate, the presence of inhibitors, and other factors. Enzyme activity can be expressed in S.I. units, and the katal has been proposed to express activities of all catalysts, including enzymes. The katal is that amount of enzyme that catalyzes a reaction rate of 1 mol per second. Thus, adoption of the katal as the unit of enzyme activity would provide no more information than is obtained when results are expressed in International Units.

Hydrogen ion concentration in blood is customarily expressed as pH, but in S.I. units it would be expressed in nanomoles per liter. It appears unlikely that the very useful pH scale will be discarded.

Pressure measures, such as blood pressure and partial pressures of blood gases, would be expressed in S.I. units using the pascal, a unit that can be derived from the base units for mass, length, and time. This change probably will not be adopted in the early phases of the conversion to S.I. units. Similarly, a proposed change in expressing osmolality in terms of the depression of freezing point is inappropriate, because osmolality may be calculated from vapor pressure as well as freezing point measurement.

In the following tables, reference ranges for the most commonly used diagnostic tests are given in conventional units and in S.I. units. The conversion of weight per volume (conventional units) to amount per volume (S.I. units) is based on the molecular weight of the analyte. For heterogeneous analytes, for example, gamma globulins, weight per volume must be retained as the unit; however, volume is expressed as the liter rather than as the deciliter as in conventional units. Weight per volume is retained for albumin, to be consistent with the other serum proteins. Hemoglobin is expressed here in S.I. units as the tetramer; in some countries it is expressed as the monomer, in which case the numerical values in S.I. units are four times as great as those shown. Plasma drug concentrations for therapeutic monitoring are not given in S.I. units, since it is unlikely that pharmaceutical manufacturers will change to molar quantities for expressing drug dosages.

## Reference Values in Hematology

| | | Conventional Units | S.I. Units |
|---|---|---|---|
| Acid hemolysis test (Ham) | | No hemolysis | No hemolysis |
| Alkaline phosphatase, leukocyte | | Total score 14–100 | Total score 14–100 |
| Cell counts | | | |
|   Erythrocytes | | | |
|     Males | | $4.6$–$6.2$ million/mm$^3$ | $4.6$–$6.2 \times 10^{12}$/L |
|     Females | | $4.2$–$5.4$ million/mm$^3$ | $4.2$–$5.4 \times 10^{12}$/L |
|     Children (varies with age) | | $4.5$–$5.1$ million/mm$^3$ | $4.5$–$5.1 \times 10^{12}$/L |
|   Leukocytes | | | |
|     Total | | $4500$–$11,000$ mm$^3$ | $4.5$–$11.0 \times 10^9$/L |
|     Differential | *Percentage* | *Absolute* | *Absolute* |
|       Myelocytes | 0 | 0/mm$^3$ | 0/L |
|       Band neutrophils | 3–5 | $150$–$400$/mm$^3$ | $150$–$400 \times 10^6$/L |
|       Segmented neutrophils | 54–62 | $3000$–$5800$/mm$^3$ | $3000$–$5800 \times 10^6$/L |
|       Lymphocytes | 25–33 | $1500$–$3000$/mm$^3$ | $1500$–$3000 \times 10^6$/L |
|       Monocytes | 3–7 | $300$–$500$/mm$^3$ | $300$–$500 \times 10^6$/L |
|       Eosinophils | 1–3 | $50$–$250$/mm$^3$ | $50$–$250 \times 10^6$/L |
|       Basophils | 0–0.75 | $15$–$50$/mm$^3$ | $15$–$50 \times 10^6$/L |
|   Platelets | | $150,000$–$350,000$/mm$^3$ | $150$–$350 \times 10^9$/L |
|   Reticulocytes | | $25,000$–$75,000$/mm$^3$ | $25$–$75 \times 10^9$/L |
| | | 0.5–1.5% of erythrocytes | |
| Coagulation tests | | | |
|   Bleeding time (template) | | 2.75–8.0 min | 2.75–8.0 min |
|   Coagulation time (glass tubes) | | 5–15 min | 5–15 min |
|   Factor VIII and other coagulation factors | | 50–150% of normal | 0.5–1.5% of normal |
|   Fibrin split products (Thrombo-Welco test) | | <10 µg/ml | <10 mg/L |
|   Fibrinogen | | 200–400 mg/dl | 2.0–4.0 g/L |
|   Partial thromboplastin time (PTT) | | 20–35 sec | 20–35 sec |
|   Prothrombin time (PT) | | 12.0–14.0 sec | 12.0–14.0 sec |
| Coombs' test | | | |
|   Direct | | Negative | Negative |
|   Indirect | | Negative | Negative |
| Corpuscular values of erythrocytes | | | |
|   Mean corpuscular hemoglobin (MCH) | | 26–34 pg | 0.40–0.53 fL fmol |
|   Mean corpuscular volume (MCV) | | 80–96 µm$^3$ | 80–96 fL |
|   Mean corpuscular hemoglobin concentration (MCHC) | | 32–36% | 0.32–0.36 |
| Haptoglobin | | 26–185 mg/dl | 260–1850 mg/L |
| Hematocrit | | | |
|   Males | | 40–54 ml/dl | 0.40–0.54 |
|   Females | | 37–47 ml/dl | 0.37–0.47 |
|   Newborns | | 49–54 ml/dl | 0.49–0.54 |
|   Children (varies with age) | | 35–49 ml/dl | 0.35–0.49 |
| Hemoglobin | | | |
|   Males | | 14.0–18.0 grams/dl | 2.17–2.79 mmol/L |
|   Females | | 12.0–16.0 grams/dl | 1.86–2.48 mmol/L |
|   Newborns | | 16.5–19.5 grams/dl | 2.56–3.02 mmol/L |
|   Children (varies with age) | | 11.2–16.5 grams/dl | 1.74–2.56 mmol/L |

*Table continued on following page*

## Reference Values in Hematology *Continued*

| | Conventional Units | S.I. Units |
|---|---|---|
| Hemoglobin, fetal | <1.0% of total | <0.01 of total |
| Hemoglobin $A_{1C}$ | 3–5% of total | 0.03–0.05 of total |
| Hemoglobin $A_2$ | 1.5–3.0% of total | 0.015–0.03 of total |
| Hemoglobin, plasma | 0–5.0 mg/dl | 0–0.8 μmol/L |
| Methemoglobin | 30–130 mg/dl | 4.7–20 μmol/L |
| Sedimentation rate (ESR) | | |
| Wintrobe: Males | 0–5 mm/hr | 0–5 mm/h |
| Females | 0–15 mm/hr | 0–15 mm/h |
| Westergren: Males | 0–15 mm/hr | 0–15 mm/h |
| Females | 0–20 mm/hr | 0–20 mm/h |

## Reference Values for Blood, Plasma, and Serum
### (For some procedures the reference values may vary depending on the method used)

| | Conventional Units | S.I. Units |
|---|---|---|
| Acetoacetate plus acetone, serum | | |
| Qualitative | Negative | Negative |
| Quantitative | 0.3–2.0 mg/dl | 3–20 mg/L |
| Acid phosphatase (thymolphthalein monophosphate substrate), serum | 0.11–0.60 U/L | 0.11–0.60 U/L |
| Adrenocorticotropin (ACTH), plasma | | |
| 6 a.m. | 10–80 pg/ml | 10–80 ng/L |
| 6 p.m. | <50 pg/ml | <50 ng/L |
| Alanine aminotransferase (AST, SGOT), serum | 7–40 U/L | 7–40 U/L |
| Albumin, serum | 3.5–5.5 grams/dl | 33–55 g/L |
| Aldolase, serum | 1.5–12.0 U/L | 1.5–12.0 U/L |
| Aldosterone, plasma | | |
| Supine | 3–10 ng/dl | 0.08–0.30 nmol/L |
| Standing | | |
| Males | 6–22 ng/dl | 0.17–0.61 nmol/L |
| Females | 5–30 ng/dl | 0.14–0.80 nmol/L |
| Alkaline phosphatase (ALP), serum | 20–90 U/L (30° C) | 20–90 U/L (30 C) |
| Ammonia nitrogen, plasma | 15–49 μg/dl | 11–35 μmol/L |
| Amylase, serum | 25–125 U/L | 25–125 U/L |
| Anion gap | 8–16 mEq/L | 8–16 mmol/L |
| Ascorbic acid, blood | 0.4–1.5 mg/dl | 23–85 μmol/L |
| Aspartate aminotransferase (AST, SGPT), serum | 7–40 U/L | 7–40 U/L |
| Base excess, blood | 0 ± 2 mEq/L | 0 ± 2 mmol/L |
| Bicarbonate | | |
| Venous plasma | 23–29 mEq/L | 23–29 mmol/L |
| Arterial blood | 18–23 mEq/L | 18–23 mmol/L |
| Bile acids, serum | 0.3–3.0 mg/dl | 3–30 mg/L |
| Bilirubin, serum | | |
| Conjugated | 0.1–0.4 mg/dl | 1.7–6.8 μmol/L |
| Unconjugated | 0.2–0.7 mg/dl | 3.4–12 μmol/L |
| Total | 0.3–1.1 mg/dl | 5.1–19 μmol/L |
| Calcium, serum | 9.0–11.0 mg/dl | 2.25–2.75 mmol/L |
| Calcium, ionized, serum | 4.25–5.25 mg/dl | 1.05–1.30 mmol/L |
| Carbon dioxide, total, serum or plasma | 24–30 mEq/L | 24–30 mmol/L |
| Carbon dioxide tension ($P_{CO_2}$), blood | 35–45 mmHg | 35–45 mmHg |
| β-Carotene, serum | 40–200 μg/dl | 0.74–3.72 μmol/L |
| Ceruloplasmin, serum | 23–44 mg/dl | 230–440 mg/L |
| Chloride, serum or plasma | 96–106 mEq/L | 96–106 mmol/L |
| Cholesterol, serum or EDTA plasma | | |
| Desirable range | <200 mg/dl | <5.18 mmol/L |
| LDL cholesterol | 60–180 mg/dl | 600–1800 mg/L |
| HDL cholesterol | 30–80 mg/dl | 300–800 mg/L |
| Copper | | |
| Males | 70–140 μg/dl | 11–22 μmol/L |
| Females | 85–155 μg/dl | 13–24 μmol/L |

### Reference Values for Blood, Plasma, and Serum *Continued*
### (For some procedures the reference values may vary depending on the method used)

| | Conventional Units | S.I. Units |
|---|---|---|
| Cortisol, plasma | | |
| 8 a.m. | 6–23 µg/dl | 170–635 nmol/L |
| 4 p.m. | 3–15 µg/dl | 82–413 nmol/L |
| 10 p.m. | <50% of 8 a.m. value | <50% of 8 a.m. value |
| Creatine, serum | 0.2–0.8 mg/dl | 15–61 µmol/L |
| Creatine kinase (CK, CPK), serum | | |
| Males | 55–170 U/L | 55–170 U/L |
| Females | 30–135 U/L | 30–135 U/L |
| Creatine kinase MB isozyme, serum | 0.0–4.7 ng/ml | 0.04–4.7 µg/L |
| Creatinine, serum | 0.6–1.2 mg/dl | 53–106 µmol/L |
| Ferritin, serum | 20–200 ng/ml | 20–200 µg/L |
| Fibrinogen, plasma | 200–400 mg/dl | 2.0–4.0 g/L |
| Folate, serum | 1.8–9.0 ng/ml | 4.1–20.4 nmol/L |
| Erythrocytes | 150–450 ng/ml | 340–1020 nmol/L |
| Follicle-stimulating hormone (FSH), plasma | | |
| Males | 4–25 mU/ml | 4–25 U/L |
| Females | 4–30 mU/ml | 4–30 U/L |
| Postmenopausal | 40–250 mU/ml | 40–250 U/L |
| γ-Glutamyltransferase, serum | | |
| Males | 5–38 U/L | 5–38 U/L |
| Females | 5–29 U/L | 5–29 U/L |
| Gastrin, serum | 0–200 pg/ml | 0–200 ng/L |
| Glucose (fasting), plasma or serum | 70–115 mg/dl | 3.89–6.38 mmol/L |
| Growth hormone (hGH), plasma | 0–10 ng/ml | 0–10 µg/L |
| Haptoglobin, serum | 26–185 mg/dl | 260–1850 mg/L |
| Immunoglobulins, serum | | |
| IgG | 550–1900 mg/dl | 5.5–19.0 g/L |
| IgA | 60–333 mg/dl | 0.60–3.3 g/L |
| IgM | 45–145 mg/dl | 0.45–1.5 g/L |
| IgD | 0.5–3.0 mg/dl | 5–30 mg/L |
| IgE | <500 ng/ml | <500 µg/L |
| Insulin (fasting), plasma | 5–25 µU/ml | 36–179 pmol/L |
| Iron, serum | 75–175 µg/dl | 13–31 µmol/L |
| Iron binding capacity, serum | | |
| Total | 250–410 µg/dl | 45–73 µmol/L |
| Saturation | 20–55% | 0.20–0.55 |
| Lactate | | |
| Venous blood | 4.5–19.8 mg/dl | 0.50–2.2 mmol/L |
| Arterial blood | 4.5–14.4 mg/dl | 0.50–1.6 mmol/L |
| Lactate dehydrogenase (LD, LDH), serum | 100–190 U/L | 100–190 U/L |
| Lipase, serum | 10–140 U/L | 10–140 U/L |
| Lipids, total, serum | 450–850 mg/dl | 4.5–8.5 g/L |
| Luteinizing (LH), serum | | |
| Males | 6–18 IU/L | 6–18 U/L |
| Females | 5–22 IU/L | 5–22 U/L |
| Premenopausal | | |
| Mid-cycle | 3 times baseline | 3 times baseline |
| Postmenopausal | >30 IU/L | >30 U/L |
| Magnesium, serum | 1.8–3.0 mg/dl | 0.75–1.25 mmol/L |
| Osmolality | 286–295 mOsm/kg water | 285–295 mOsm/kg water |
| Oxygen, blood | | |
| Capacity (varies with hemoglobin) | 16–24 vol % | 7.14–10.7 mmol/L |
| Content, arterial | 15–23 vol % | 6.69–10.3 mmol/L |
| Saturation, arterial | 94–100 % | 0.94–1.00 |
| Oxygen tension ($P_{O_2}$), blood | 75–100 mmHg | 75–100 mmHg |
| $P_{50}$ | 26–27 mmHg | 26–27 mmHg |
| pH, arterial blood | 7.35–7.45 | 7.35–7.45 |
| Phenylalanine, serum | <3 mg/dl | <0.18 mmol/L |
| Phosphate, inorganic, serum | 3.0–4.5 mg/dl | 1.0–1.5 mmol/L |
| Potassium, serum or plasma | 3.5–5.0 mEq/L | 3.5–5.0 mmol/L |
| Prolactin, serum | | |
| Males | 1–20 ng/ml | 1–20 µg/L |
| Females | 1–25 ng/ml | 1–25 µg/L |

*Table continued on following page*

## Reference Values for Blood, Plasma, and Serum *Continued*
### (For some procedures the reference values may vary depending on the method used)

|  | Conventional Units | S.I. Units |
|---|---|---|
| Protein, serum | | |
| Total | 6.0–8.0 grams/dl | 60–80 g/L |
| Albumin | 3.5–5.5 grams/dl | 35–55 g/L |
| Alpha$_1$ globulin | 0.2–0.4 grams/dl | 2–4 g/L |
| Alpha$_2$ globulin | 0.5–0.9 grams/dl | 5–9 g/L |
| Beta globulin | 0.6–1.1 grams/dl | 6–11 g/L |
| Gamma globulin | 0.7–1.7 grams/dl | 7–17 g/L |
| Pyruvate, blood | 0.3–0.9 mg/dl | 0.03–0.10 mmol/L |
| Sodium, serum or plasma | 136–145 mEq/L | 136–145 mmol/L |
| Testosterone, plasma | | |
| Males | 275–875 ng/dl | 9.5–30 nmol/L |
| Females | 23–75 ng/dl | 0.8–2.6 nmol/L |
| Pregnant | 38–190 ng/dl | 1.3–6.6 nmol/L |
| Thyroid-stimulating hormone (TSH), serum | 0–7 μU/ml | 0–7 mU/L |
| Thyroxine, free (FT), serum | 1.0–2.1 ng/dl | 13–27 pmol/L |
| Thyroxine (T$_4$), serum | 4.4–9.9 μg/dl | 57–128 nmol/L |
| Triglycerides, serum | 40–150 mg/dl | 0.4–1.5 g/L |
| Triiodothyronine (T$_3$), serum | 150–250 ng/dl | 2.3–3.9 nmol/L |
| Triiodothyronine uptake, resin (T$_3$RU) | 25–38% uptake | 0.25–0.38 uptake |
| Urate, serum | | |
| Males | 2.5–8.0 mg/dl | 0.15–0.48 mmol/L |
| Females | 1.5–7.0 mg/dl | 0.09–0.42 mmol/L |
| Urea, serum or plasma | 24–49 mg/dl | 4.0–8.3 mmol/L |
| Urea nitrogen, serum or plasma | 11–23 mg/dl | 7.9–16.4 mmol/L |
| Viscosity, serum | 1.4–1.8 times water | 1.4–1.8 times water |
| Vitamin A, serum | 20–80 μg/dl | 0.70–2.80 μmol/L |
| Vitamin B$_{12}$, serum | 180–900 pg/ml | 133–664 pmol/L |

## Reference Values for Urine
### (For some procedures the reference values may vary depending on the method used)

|  | Conventional Units | S.I. Units |
|---|---|---|
| Acetone and acetoacetate, qualitative | Negative | Negative |
| Albumin | | |
| Qualitative | Negative | Negative |
| Quantitive | 10–100 mg/24 hr | 0.15–1.5 μmol/24 h |
| Aldosterone | 3–20 μg/24 hr | 8.3–55 nmol/24 h |
| δ-Aminolevulinic acid | 1.3–7.0 mg/24 hr | 10–53 μmol/24 h |
| Amylase | 3–20 U/hr | 3–20 U/h |
| Amylase/creatinine clearance ratio | 1–4% | 0.01–0.04 |
| Bilirubin, qualitative | Negative | Negative |
| Calcium (usual diet) | <250 mg/24 hr | <6.3 mmol/24 h |
| Catecholamines | | |
| Epinephrine | <10 μg/24 hr | <55 nmol/24 h |
| Norepinephrine | <100 μg/24 hr | <590 nmol/24 h |
| Total free catecholamines | 4–126 μg/24 hr | 24–745 nmol/24 h |
| Total metanephrines | 0.1–1.6 mg/24 hr | 0.5–8.1 μmol/24 h |
| Chloride (varies with intake) | 110–250 mEq/24 hr | 110–250 mmol/24 h |
| Copper | 0–50 μg/24 hr | 0–0.80 μmol/24 h |
| Cortisol, free | 10–100 μg/24 hr | 27.6–276 nmol/24 h |
| Creatinine | 15–25 mg/kg body weight/24 hr | 0.13–0.22 mmol/kg body weight/24 h |
| Creatinine clearance (corrected to 1.73 m² body surface area) | | |
| Males | 110–150 ml/min | 110–150 ml/min |
| Females | 105–132 ml/min | 105–150 ml/min |
| Dehydroepiandrosterone | | |
| Males | 0.2–2.0 mg/24 hr | 0.7–6.9 μmol/24 h |
| Females | 0.2–1.8 mg/24 hr | 0.7–6.2 μmol/24 h |

## Reference Values for Urine *Continued*
### (For some procedures the reference values may vary depending on the method used)

| | Conventional Units | S.I. Units |
|---|---|---|
| Estrogens, total | | |
|   Males | 4–25 μg/24 hr | 14–90 nmol/24 h |
|   Females | 5–100 μg/24 hr | 18–360 nmol/24 h |
| Glucose (as reducing substance) | <250 mg/24 hr | <250 mg/24 h |
| Hemoglobin and myoglobin, qualitative | Negative | Negative |
| 17-Hydroxycorticosteroids | | |
|   Males | 3–9 mg/24 hr | 8.3–25 μmol/24 h |
|   Females | 2–8 mg//24 hr | 5.5–22 μmol/24 h |
| 5-Hydroxyindoleacetic acid | | |
|   Qualitative | Negative | Negative |
|   Quantitative | <9 mg/24 hr | <47 μmol/24 h |
| 17-Ketosteroids | | |
|   Males | 6–18 mg/24 hr | 21–62 μmol/24 h |
|   Females | 4–13 mg/24 hr | 14–45 μmol/24 h |
| Magnesium | 6.0–8.5 mEq/24 hr | 3.0–4.2 mmol/24 h |
| Metanephrines (see Catecholamines) | | |
| Osmolality | 38–1400 mOsm/kg water | 38–1400 mmol/kg water |
| pH | 4.6–8.0 | 4.6–8.0 |
| Phenylpyruvic acid, qualitative | Negative | Negative |
| Phosphate | 0.9–1.3 grams/24 hr | 29–42 mmol/24 h |
| Porphobilinogen | | |
|   Qualitative | Negative | Negative |
|   Quantitative | <2.0 mg/24 hr | <9 μmol/24 h |
| Porphyrins | | |
|   Coproporphyrin | 50–250 μg/24 hr | 77–380 nmol/24 h |
|   Uroporphyrin | 10–30 μg/24 hr | 12–36 nmol/24 h |
| Potassium | 25–100 mEq/24 hr | 25–100 mmol/24 h |
| Pregnanediol | | |
|   Males | 0.4–1.4 mg/24 hr | 1.2–4.4 μmol/24 h |
|   Females | | |
|     Proliferative phase | 0.5–1.5 mg/24 hr | 1.6–4.7 μmol/24 h |
|     Luteal phase | 2.0–7.0 mg/24 hr | 6.2–22 μmol/24 h |
|     Postmenopausal | 0.2–1.0 mg/24 hr | 0.6–3.1 μmol/24 h |
| Pregnanetriol | <2.5 mg/24 hr | <7.4 μmol/24 h |
| Protein | | |
|   Qualitative | Negative | Negative |
|   Quantitative | 10–150 mg/24 hr | 10–150 mg/24 h |
| Sodium | 130–260 mEq/24 hr | 130–260 mmol/24 h |
| Specific gravity | 1.003–1.030 | 1.003–1.030 |
| Urate | 200–500 mg/24 hr | 1.2–3.0 mmol/24 h |
| Urobilinogen | <4.0 mg/24 hr | <6.8 μmol/24 h |
| Vanillylmandelic acid (VMA, 4-hydroxy-3-methoxymandelic acid) | 1–8 mg/24 hr | 5–40 μmol/24 h |

## Reference Values for Therapeutic Drug Monitoring

| | Therapeutic Range | Toxic Levels | Proprietary Names |
|---|---|---|---|
| **Antibiotics** | | | |
|   Amikacin, serum | 25–30 μg/ml | Peak: >35 μg/ml<br>Trough: >5–7 μg/ml | Amikin |
|   Chloramphenicol, serum | 10–20 μg/ml | >25 μg/ml | Chloromycetin |
|   Gentamicin, serum | 5–10 μg/ml | Peak: >12 μg/ml<br>Trough: >2 μg/ml | Garamycin |
|   Tobramycin, serum | 5–10 μg/ml | Peak: >12 μg/ml<br>Trough: >2 μg/ml | Nebcin |
| **Anticonvulsants** | | | |
|   Carbamazepine, serum | 5–12 μg/ml | >12 μg/ml | Tegretol |
|   Ethosuximide, serum | 40–100 μg/ml | >100 μg/ml | Zarontin |

*Table continued on following page*

## Reference Values for Therapeutic Drug Monitoring *Continued*

| | Therapeutic Range | Toxic Levels | Proprietary Names |
|---|---|---|---|
| **Anticonvulsants** (*Continued*) | | | |
| Phenobarbital, serum | 10–30 µg/ml | Vary widely because of developed tolerance | |
| Phenytoin, serum | 10–20 µg/ml | >20 µg/ml | Dilantin |
| Primidone, serum | 5–12 µg/ml | >15 µg/ml | Mysoline |
| Valproic acid, serum | 50–100 µg/ml | >100 µg/ml | Depakene |
| **Analgesics** | | | |
| Acetaminophen, serum | 10–20 µg/ml | >250 µg/ml | Tylenol |
| Salicylate, serum | 100–250 µg/ml | >300 µg/ml | Disalcid |
| **Bronchodilator** | | | |
| Theophylline (aminophylline), serum | 10–20 µg/ml | >20 µg/ml | |
| **Cardiovascular Drugs** | | | |
| Digitoxin, serum (specimen must be obtained 12–24 hr after last dose) | 15–25 ng/ml | >25 ng/ml | Crystodigin |
| Digoxin, serum (specimen must be obtained 12–24 hr after last dose) | 0.8–2.0 ng/ml | >2.4 ng/ml | Lanoxin |
| Disopyramide, serum | 2–5 µg/ml | >5 µg/ml | Norpace |
| Lidocaine, serum | 1.5–5.0 µg/ml | >6–8 µg/mL | Xylocaine |
| Procainamide, serum (measured as procainamide + *N*-acetylprocainamide) | 4–10 µg/ml | >16 µg/ml | Pronestyl |
| Propranolol, serum | 50–100 ng/ml | Variable | Inderal |
| Quinidine, serum | 2–5 µg/ml | >10 µg/ml | Cardioquin Quinaglute Quinidex Quinora |
| **Psychopharmacologic Drugs** | | | |
| Amitriptyline, serum (measured as amitriptyline + nortriptyline) | 120–150 ng/ml | >500 ng/ml | Amitril Elavil Endep Limbitrol Triavil |
| Desipramine, serum (measured as desipramine + imipramine) | 150–300 ng/ml | >500 ng/ml | Norpramin Pertofrane |
| Imipramine, serum (measured as imipramine + desipramine) | 150–300 ng/ml | >500 ng/ml | Antipress Imavate Janimine Presamine Tofranil |
| Lithium, serum (obtain specimen 12 hr after last dose) | 0.8–1.2 mEq/L | >2.0 mEq/L | Lithobid |
| Nortriptyline, serum | 50–150 ng/ml | >500 ng/ml | Aventyl Pamelor |

## Reference Values in Toxicology

| | Conventional Units | S.I. Units |
|---|---|---|
| Arsenic | | |
| Blood | 3.5–7.2 µg/dl | 0.47–0.96 µmol/L |
| Urine | >100 µg/24 hr | <1.3 µmol/24 h |
| Bromides, serum | 0 | 0 |
| | Toxic: >17 mEq/L | Toxic: >17 mmol/L |
| Carboxyhemoglobin, blood | <5% saturation | <0.05 saturation |
| Symptoms occur | >20% saturation | >0.20 saturation |
| Ethanol, blood | <0.05 mg/dl (<0.005%) | <1.0 mmol/L |
| Marked intoxication | 300–400 mg/dl (0.3–0.4%) | 65–87 mmol/L |
| Alcoholic stupor | 400–500 mg/dl (0.4–0.5%) | 87–109 mmol/L |
| Coma | >500 mg/dl (>0.5%) | >109 mmol/L |
| Lead | | |
| Blood | 0–40 µg/dl | 0–2 µmol/L |
| Urine | <100 µg/24 hr | <0.48 µmol/24 h |
| Mercury, urine | <100 µg/24 hr | <50 nmol/24 h |

## Reference Values for Cerebrospinal Fluid

|  | Conventional Units | S.I. Units |
|---|---|---|
| Cells | <5/mm³; all mononuclear | <5 × 10⁶/L, all mononuclear |
| Electrophoresis | Predominantly albumin | Predominantly albumin |
| Glucose | 50–75 mg/dl | 2.8–4.2 mmol/L |
|  | (20 mg/dl less than serum) | (1.1 mmol less than serum) |
| IgG |  |  |
|   Children under 14 | <8% of total protein | <0.08 of total protein |
|   Adults | <14% of total protein | <0.14 of total protein |
| IgG index $\left( \dfrac{\text{CSF/serum IgG ratio}}{\text{CSF/serum albumin ratio}} \right)$ | 0.3–0.6 | 0.3–0.6 |
| Oligoclonal banding on electrophoresis | Absent | Absent |
| Pressure | 70–180 mm water | 70–180 mm water |
| Protein, total | 15–45 mg/dl | 150–450 g/L |

## Reference Values for Semen

|  | Conventional Units | S.I. Units |
|---|---|---|
| Volume | 2–5 ml | 2–5 ml |
| Liquefaction | Complete in 15 min | Complete in 15 min |
| Leukocytes | Occasional or absent | Occasional or absent |
| Count | 60–150 million/ml | 60–150 × 10⁶/ml |
| Motility | >80% motile | >0.80 motile |
| Morphology | 80–90% normal forms | 0.80–0.90 normal forms |
| Fructose | >150 mg/dl | >8.33 mmol/L |

## Reference Values for Feces

|  | Conventional Units | S.I. Units |
|---|---|---|
| Bulk | 100–200 grams/24 hr | 100–200 g/24 h |
| Dry matter | 23–32 grams/24 hr | 23–32 g/24 h |
| Fat, total | <6.0 grams/24 hr | <6.0 g/24 h |
| Nitrogen, total | <2.0 grams/24 hr | <2.0 g/24 h |
| Water | Approximately 65% | Approximately 0.65 |

## REFERENCES

1. Brown SS, Mitchell FL, and Young DS (eds): Chemical Diagnosis of Disease. Amsterdam, Elsevier/North-Holland Biomedical Press, 1979.
2. Conn RB (ed): Current Diagnosis, 8th ed. Philadelphia, WB Saunders Co, 1991.
3. Goodman AG, Gilman LS, Rall TW, and Murad F: Goodman and Gilman's The Pharmacological Basis of Therapeutics, 7th ed. New York, Macmillan Co, 1985.
4. Henry JB (ed): Clinical Diagnosis and Management by Laboratory Methods, 18th ed. Philadelphia, WB Saunders Co, 1991.
5. Lundberg GD, Iverson C, and Radulescu G: JAMA 255:2247, 1986
6. Miale JB: Laboratory Medicine-Hematology, 6th ed. St Louis, CV Mosby, 1982.
7. Physicians' Desk Reference, 45th ed. Oradell, NJ, Medical Economics Co, 1991.
8. Tietz NW: Clinical Guide to Laboratory Tests, 2nd ed. Philadelphia, WB Saunders Co, 1990.
9. Tietz NW: Textbook of Clinical Chemistry. Philadelphia, WB Saunders Co, 1986.
10. Williams WJ, Beutler E, Erslev AJ, and Lichtman MA: Hematology, 3rd ed. New York, McGraw-Hill Book Co, 1983.

Some of these values have been established by the Clinical Laboratories at Thomas Jefferson University Hospital and have not been published elsewhere.

## NOMOGRAM FOR THE DETERMINATION OF BODY SURFACE AREA OF CHILDREN AND ADULTS*

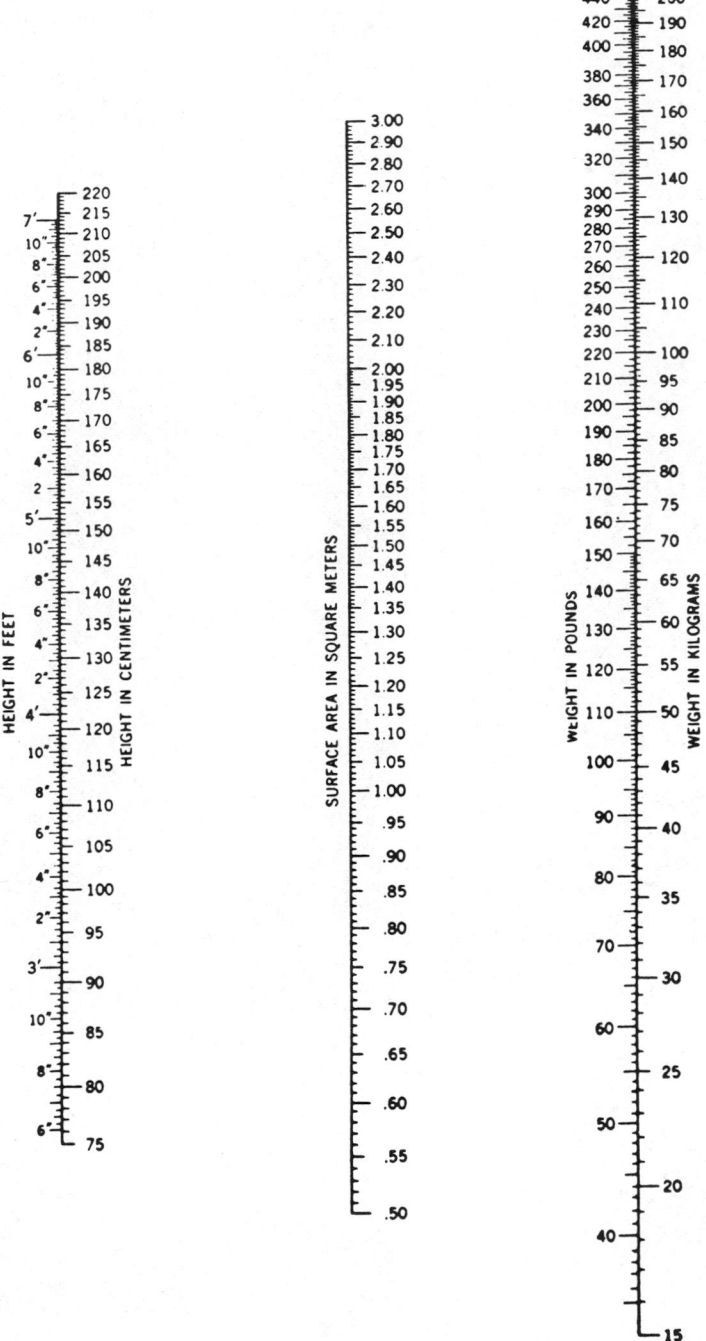

*From Boothby, W. M., and Sandiford, R. B.: Boston Med. Surg. J. *185*:337, 1921.

# Index

Note: Page numbers followed by (t) refer to tables; page numbers in *italics* refer to illustrations.

Effusive pericarditis, 290

Ehrlichiosis, 105

Ejaculation, retrograde, after prostatectomy, 653

Elastic stockings, in management of venous insufficiency, 777

Elbow pain, 929

Elderly patient, endocarditis in, 232(t)
  gout in, 514
  hypertension in, 254–255
  treatment of insomnia in, 31

Elective abortion, 942–943

Electrical burns, 1074

Electroconvulsive therapy, for mania (bipolar disorder), 1059

Electrodesiccation, for leukoplakia, 751
  for skin cancer, 724–725

Electrohydraulic lithotripsy, 678

Electrolyte(s), in body fluids, 558(t)
  in fluid replacement solutions, 12, 54(t), 55(t), 559(t). See also *Fluid replacement therapy.*
  in stool of cholera patients, 54(t), 558(t)
  in total parenteral nutrition, 554, 554(t)

Electrolyte losses, in diarrhea, 558(t)

Electrolyte requirements, in infants and children, 557

Electromechanical dissociation, and cardiac arrest, 196
  management of, *199*

Electron beam therapy, for cutaneous T cell lymphoma, 372, 381

Embolism. See also *Thromboembolism.*
  air, 406–407
  pulmonary, 167–173, 1031
    diagnosis of, 167, *168*
    prophylaxis against, 167–168, 169(t)
    risk factors for, 167, 169(t)
    treatment of, 168–173, 172(t)

Emergency medical service, and management of cardiac arrest, 197

Emergency treatment, of burns, 1072–1074
  of leukemia, 354, 360(t)
  of snake bite, 1086–1087

Emesis. See *Vomiting.*

Emollient(s), for contact dermatitis, 789
  for pruritus, 33

Emollient laxatives, 16

Emotional response, to chronic pain, 3

Emphysema, 135

Empyema, 152–154, *153*

Enalapril, for heart failure, 230, 230(t), 276(t)
  for hypertension, 244(t)
  in glomerular disease, 642

Enalaprilat, for hypertensive emergency, 254(t)

Encainide, for arrhythmias, 217(t)
  effectiveness of, 208(t)
  side effects of, 208(t), 217(t)

Encephalitis, 849
  measles and, 110
  toxoplasmosis and, in AIDS, 38(t), 39, 116, 116(t), 117
  varicella and, 51
  viral, 51, 110, 849–850

Encephalopathy, hepatic, 412, 420–421

Encephalopathy *(Continued)*
  branched-chain amino acids in management of, 554
  fulminant hepatitis and, 455
  lead-induced, 1115
    treatment of, in children, 1116(t)
  Reye's syndrome and, 851

Endarterectomy, carotid, 292, 814

Endemic relapsing fever, 98–100, 99(t)

Endocarditis, infectious, 231–239
  antimicrobials for, 46(t), 233, 234(t)–235(t)
    resistance to, 236
  brucellosis and, 49
  clinical manifestations of, 232(t)
  gonorrhea and, 681(t)
  mitral valve prolapse and, 227
  prophylaxis against, 223(t), 238, 238(t), 239(t)
  prosthetic valve and, 232(t), 238
  Q fever and, 93
  surgery for, 235, 236(t)

Endocrine disorders, and constipation, 15(t)

Endolymphatic hydrops, 847–849

Endometriosis, 989–992, 990(t), 991(t)

Endometrium, cancer of, 1017–1020, 1018(t), 1019(t)

Endotracheal intubation, in child with head injury, 895
  in newborn, 965
  in patient undergoing cesarean section, 958

Endourologic stone extraction, 678

Enflurane, use of, in cesarean section, 958

Enoxacin, for chancroid, 679(t)

*Entamoeba histolytica* infection, 42–43
  treatment of, 13(t), 42–43, 43(t)

Enteral nutrition, 551
  for newborn, 973
  in management of Crohn's disease, 443
  in management of malabsorption, 466

Enteric (typhoid) fever, 121–124

Enterobacteriaceae genera, treatment of bone infection by, 927(t)

*Enterobius vermicularis* infestation, 488(t), 490
  vaginitis due to, 1009

Enterocolitis, necrotizing, in newborn, 978
  salmonellosis and, 120–121

Enterohepatically recirculated drugs, 1090(t)

Enteropathy, eosinophilic, 465
  gluten-sensitive, 462–463
    diet for, 462–463

Enthesitis, 913

Enuresis, 633–635
  after prostatectomy, 652
  after stroke, 817
  diurnal, 632
  in children, 632–633
  mixed, 632
  nocturnal, 632, 633

Environmental control, in management of asthma, 701–702

Eosinophilic enteropathy, 465

Ephedrine, for myasthenia gravis, 862

Ephedrine *(Continued)*
  for neuropathic edema, 884

Epidemic influenza, 67–70

Epidemic relapsing fever, 98–100, 99(t)

Epidermal dehydration, and contact dermatitis, 801

Epididymitis, 635–636, 681

Epidural analgesia/anesthesia, for cesarean section, 956–957, 957(t)
  for vaginal delivery, 953–955

Epiglottitis, 24, 162

Epilepsy, 819–820
  causes of, 820(t), 825
  in adolescents and adults, 819–825
  in infants and children, 825–830
  treatment of, 821–825, 826–830, 827(t)
    in child with head injury, 897
    in patient with brain tumor, 899
    in patient with encephalitis, 850
    therapeutic vs. toxic levels of drugs used in, 1105(t), 1135(t)–1136(t)
  vestibular, 845

Epinephrine, for anaphylactic reaction, 691(t), 692, 713, 714, 715, 793
  in transfusion recipient, 406, 407(t)
  for asthma, 698, 700, 703(t), 707
  for asystole, in cases of myocardial infarction, 268
  for chronic obstructive pulmonary disease, 136(t)
  for croup, 162
  for laryngotracheobronchitis, 24
  in neonatal resuscitation, 964, 964(t)

Epiphrenic diverticula, 426–427, 429

Episodic vertigo, 841–847

Epistaxis, von Willebrand's disease and, 336

Epithelioma cuniculatum, 754

Epstein-Barr virus infection, 87–89

Ergocalciferol, for rickets, 534(t)

Ergonovine, for migraine, 837

Ergot preparations, for Alzheimer's disease, 809
  for headache, 832, 833(t), 839

Erosive lichen planus, 772

Erosive osteoarthritis, cystic, 922–923

Eructation, 9

Eruption(s), creeping, 763
  drug, fixed, 797
  eczematous, id reaction and, 775, 777
  light, polymorphous, 803
  papulosquamous, 727–730

Erysipelas, 757

Erythema, figurate, 783
  fixed, 782–783

Erythema annulare centrifugum, 783

Erythema chronicum migrans, 783
  in Lyme disease, 101

Erythema gyratum repens, 755, 783

Erythema marginatum, 783

Erythema multiforme, 772, 782–783

Erythema nodosum, 783
  in sarcoidosis, 174

Erythema nodosum leprosum, 75–76

Erythrasma, 768

Erythrocyte(s), transfusion of, 397(t), 397–398

Erythrocyte antibodies, hemolytic reaction to, 403, 404

*Process Immediately for 30-day Trial*

# BUSINESS REPLY MAIL

FIRST CLASS MAIL      PERMIT NO. 7135      ORLANDO, FL

POSTAGE WILL BE PAID BY ADDRESSEE

ORDER FULFILLMENT DEPARTMENT

**WB SAUNDERS COMPANY**

Harcourt Brace Jovanovich, Inc.

**6277 SEA HARBOR DR**

**ORLANDO FL 32821-9989**